Dictionary of

Medical Syndromes

Sergio I. Magalini, M.D.

Professor of Clinical Toxicology
Department of Anesthesia and Resuscitation
School of Medicine
Universita Cattolica del Sacro Cuore, Rome

Sabina C. Magalini, M.D.

Department of Surgery
School of Medicine
Universita Cattolica del Sacro Cuore, Rome

Dictionary of

Medical Syndromes

Fourth Edition

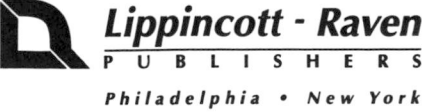

Lippincott - Raven
PUBLISHERS
Philadelphia • New York

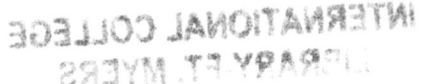

Acquisitions Editor: Stuart Freeman
Developmental Editor: Karen Frame
Senior Production Editor: Molly E. Connors
Production Service: Berliner, Inc.

Fourth Edition

Library of Congress Cataloging-in-Publication Data

Dictionary of medical syndromes / edited by Sergio I. Magalini, Sabina C. Magalini. —
4th ed.
     p.   cm.
  Rev. ed. of: Dictionary of medical syndromes / Sergio I. Magalini, Sabina C.
Magalini, Giovanni de Francisci. 3rd ed. c1990.
  Includes bibliographical references and index.
  ISBN 0-397-58418-0
  1. Syndromes—Dictionaries.   I. Magalini, Sabina I.
II. Magalini, Sergio C.   III. Magalini, Sabina I.   Dictionary of medical syndromes.
  [DNLM: 1. Dictionaries, Medical.   2. Syndrome—dictionaries.
3. Eponyms—dictionaries.   WB 15 D554 1990]
RC69.M33   1997
616'.003—DC20
DNLM/DLC
for Library of Congress   96-41119
                           CIP

9   8   7   6   5   4   3

Preface

In 1970, when this book was first published, I felt a strong urge to write a strenuous defense in the Introduction of the use of eponyms in medicine. At that time it appeared that the prognosis for their survival was extremely poor, and that they required urgent resuscitation (a new discipline only just born at that time). Many colleagues proposed some measure of euthanasia for eponyms as a form of terminology, because they no longer responded to modern, rigid scientific criteria on which to base an unequivocal nomenclature and a definitive taxonomic system.

My attempt at that time was to design a standard grid to give a uniform structure to all the information on each single syndrome, with the aim of making them more scientific as part of an effort to simplify and crystallize these units of knowledge according to the reductionistic spirit of the 1970s (see the Preface to the first edition). Since that time, however, there has been a change of stagelight on "syndrome plays." I avoided structuring them in the monistic system of reference represented by current medical knowledge that is still mainly (if not entirely) directed toward establishing conceptual superunits—diseases—where a definite and absolute rule of cause and effect is imperative. Instead, I attempted to define each one of them independently according to a strict reference to routine medical practice.

From an epistemological analysis of the history of syndromes it can be deduced that they do not represent dead historical documents of past knowledge. Although a few clearly have become obsolete and others have remained in a lethargic state, most of them are strong and show a tenacious grip on life; indeed, some are still being born.

Now, after 25 years, we can see that syndromes not only are surviving, but also are proliferating and reproducing, and that we may, at full tilt, consider them as living entities that cannot be crystallized within rigid, permanent structures, but must be left free to grow and change; finally, we must accept them for the simple fact that they exist and are endowed with a strong power of survival.

Let us try to summarize some of the roles that syndromes play in medical practice. They represent a useful parascientific metalanguage as mnemonics to stabilize our knowledge of particular pathological events. They function as boats or small islands of firm ground to support temporarily our uncertain steps when we move in the fluid realm of pathology; thus providing a sort of resting place where we can stop whenever we try to evaluate the possible relationship between the observed cluster of symptoms and signs and the fragments of memories of established medical knowledge, logical deductions, sensations, and feelings generated by the patient for an observer. They maintain the hermetic message hidden in all pathological manifestations, preserving a certain margin of elasticity; an elasticity not provided by other types of more rigidly codified definitive knowledge of diseases, for which the taxonomy, classification, and defined causes have established what appears to be a definite location. In other words, in a syndrome a symptom or a combination of symptoms may be directly or indirectly generated by different initial events, or be the final or temporary manifestation of a flowing cascade of variable intervening phenomena, whereas the same agent or event may generate different combinations of symptoms.

On balance, syndromes should be considered neither literary realities nor empty nomina of a professional convention; instead they should be considered metaphorical expressions of real practical needs, sources of reflection, doors to mnemonic systems with their roots in the complex medical psyche.

A warning, however, must also be issued concerning the disadvantages and the possible abuses of any nominalistic system where a name, acquiring a final value, loses its transparency and becomes opaque. It thus loses its use as an instrument and becomes instead a final object endowed with attributed reality.

In the physician–patient relationship it is easy to see a situation where the physician knows the name of the disease or of a syndrome and consequently ought to know how to cure it.

How many times in our practice have we used or abused this method! How many patients have we seen leaving our office smiling just for having received the precious gift (usually well paid for) of a mere name, happy to have reached a secure state where something could and would be done to relieve their sickness, and happy to have bought something real, scientific, and concrete! How often do we forget that by selling names easily we create patients and the consequent need for medical treatment, and that, in addition to having pacified the patient's mind, we also have deeply satisfied ourselves for having reached the name of the pathological condition! And, unconsciously, we forget that, as doctors, we usually become strongly bound to that name, especially if we have written it down, and that from then on we must proceed according to established patterns of reasoning and action (the famous accepted standards), possibly losing contact with the real sequence of events, accepting what fits our diagnosis and discharging, ignoring, and no longer even seeing what does not.

Finally, allow me a few last thoughts after 4 years spent in preparing this new edition. It could be said that whoever proposes a new syndrome performs an act of intelligence, since he or she recognizes and inoculates a fragment of truth from the world of events in pathology; whoever uses the syndromes performs an act of acceptable and useful conformity; although whoever has been collecting them for the past 25 years perhaps has been merely acting out his or her own form of paranoia. In writing this book the authors have behaved, not as crusaders aiming at the conquest of a determined objective, but as knights errant, collecting medical syndromes, large or small, pregnant with meaning or bereft of apparent significance, as they encountered them along the path of practice in the wide world of medicine. They did not act according to the rules of standard science, where every piece of evidence or fact, simple or complex, has to be placed and made to fit, like a strangely shaped piece, in an enormous predesigned puzzle, since everything in this world must have its place according to the scientific monistic structure. Instead, they preferred to store them in a neutral, artificial container known as alphabetical order, thus providing the syndrome entities with the benefit of an independent space, where the fantasy needed to rectify the potential errors intrinsic in any scientific dogmatic classification could be easily brought into play; and the freedom to continue to act as freelance, transparent instruments, capable of providing some continuously scanning light to the anima of the dark realm of clinical medicine.

Sergio I. Magalini, M.D.

Acknowledgments

I wish to acknowledge, once more, the contribution of my secretaries, Stefania Croce and Nadia Bruschelli, for typing and retyping the new syndromes and the revised pieces of the updated ones. A particular thanks also goes to Dr. Fabrizio La Mura, M.D., who introduced me to the secrets of navigating the Internet.

Dictionary of

Medical Syndromes

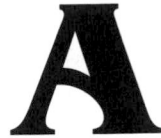

AAGENAES

Synonyms. Cholestasis intrahepatic, recurrent; stasis-lymphedema; cholestasis hereditary Norwegian type.

Symptoms and Signs. Both sexes. From and after birth. In Norwegian kindreds. Jaundice in recurrent episodes. Progressive edema of legs from school age on.

Etiology. Recessive inheritance.

Pathology. Hypoplasia of lymphatic vessels causing lymphedema; obstructive cholestasis with bouts of icterus. Liver shows giant cell transformation in infancy and later fibrosis and eventually cirrhosis.

Therapy. Liver transplantation in end-stage liver failure.

BIBLIOGRAPHY. Aagenaes O, Sigstad H, Bjorn-Hausen R: Lymphedema in hereditary recurrent cholestasis from birth. Arch Dis Child 45:690–699, 1970
Aagenaes O: Hereditary recurrent cholestasis with lymphedema—two new families. Acta Ped Scand 63:465–471, 1974
Desmet VJ: Congenital diseases of intrahepatic bile ducts: variations on the theme "ductal plate malformation." Hepatology 16:1069–1083, 1992

A AND V

Synonyms. A-esotropia; A-exotropia; horizontal—vertical—noncomitant strabismus; V-esotropia; V-exotropia. See Pretectal.

Arbitrary Standards for the Syndromes to Qualify. 1. A-esotropia. Esodeviation greater by 10 diopters in upward gaze than in direct forward gaze. 2. V-esotropia. Esodeviation greater by 15 diopters in downward gaze than in direct forward gaze. 3. A-exotropia. Exodeviation greater by 10 diopters in lower gaze than in direct forward gaze. 4. V-exotropia. Exodeviation greater by 15 diopters in upward gaze than in direct forward gaze.

Etiology. Unknown. Three schools: (1) horizontal tecti school; (2) vertical muscles school; (3) combined school.

Therapy. Value of surgical correction still not assessed. Good and poor results claimed by each of the three schools using procedures based on the etiologic hypothesis.

BIBLIOGRAPHY. Urist MJ: Horizontal squint with secondary vertical deviations. AMA Arch Ophthalmol 46:245–267, 1951
Dunlap EA: Present status of the A and V syndromes. Am J Ophthalmol 52:396–401, 1961
Abrahamsson M, Fabian G, Sjostrand J: Refraction changes in children developing convergent or divergent strabism. Br J Ophthalmol 76:723–727, 1992
Quick MW, Bothe RG: Photographic technique for measuring horizontal and vertical eye alignment throughout the field of gaze. Invest Ophthalmol Vis Sci 33:234–246, 1992

AARSKOG-SCOTT

Synonyms. Facial—digital—genital. FDG; facial dysplasia—short stature—penoscrotal anomalies. AAS; hypertelorism—brachydactyly—shawl scrotum (including Teebi syndrome). See Noonan; Leopard; Robinow and pseudohypoparathyroidism.

Symptoms. Males fully affected; females exhibit partial features. Normal weight and length at birth. Good health. Developmental landmarks within normal limits. In some cases, moderately impaired intelligence or early delay in motor performance, or both. Slow maturation from 3 years on.

Signs. Short stature (100%). *Craniofacial.* Hypertelorism (100%); anomalous superior helices (100%); "widow's peak" (triangular point of scalp hair) (60%); ptosis (30%); hypoplastic maxilla (100%). *Acral.* Small, broad hands and feet (90%); short fingers with single crease (57%); simian crease (28%); mild webbing between fingers (43%); joint laxity (29%); joint restriction (35%). *Abdominal.* Inguinal hernia (57%); protruding umbilicus (100%); cryptorchidism (64%). *Other.* Abnormal cervical vertebrae (90%); pectus excavatum (21%). Shawl scrotum. A new associated anomaly recently described is cystic porencephaly with generalized seizures.

Etiology. X-linked recessive; possible X-linked semidominant mode of inheritance. Autosomal inheritance also reported.

Pathology. See Signs.

Diagnostic Procedures. X-Rays. See Signs. Bone age normal. Growth hormone assay: normal. Karyotype: normal.

Therapy. Trials with growth hormone have failed.

Prognosis. Shortness of stature; no serious mental deficiencies.

BIBLIOGRAPHY. Aarskog D: A familial syndrome of short stature associated with facial dysplasia and genital anomalies. J Pediatr 77:856–861, 1970
Scott CJ Jr: Unusual facies, joint hypermobility, congenital anomaly, and short stature: A new dysmorphic syndrome. In Bergsma D, McKusick VA, Konigsmark BW (eds): The Clinical Delineation of Birth Defects, vol 10, The Endocrine System, pp 240–246. Baltimore, Williams & Wilkins, 1971
Teebi AS, Naguib KK, Al-Awadi S, et al: New autosomal recessive faciodigitogenital syndrome. J Med Genet 25:32–36, 1988

AASE-SMITH

Synonyms. Anemia congenital—triphalangeal thumb; triphalangeal thumb.

Symptoms. Very rare. Occurs in males; present from birth. Delayed closure of fontanels. Pallor. Mild growth deficiency (third percentile). Triphalangeal thumbs; mild radial hypoplasia; narrow shoulders. Ventricular septal defect and others. Hepatosplenomegaly of variable degree. Cleft lip and palate reported.

Etiology. Autosomal recessive and X-linked inheritance have been suggested.

Pathology. Bone marrow. Hypoplasia.

Diagnostic Procedures. *Blood.* Anemia; variable leukopenia. X-ray of skeleton and chest. *Bone marrow cultures.* Fail to stimulate production of erythropoietic precursors. *Dermatoglyphics.* Help to distinguish whether a triphalangeal thumb is indeed a thumb or a duplicated index finger with absence of the thumb.

Therapy. The preferred treatment is frequent blood transfusions for the first 12 months of life. Iron overload is prevented by chelation therapy. The benefit of prednisone is not clear; its use should be avoided if possible during the first year of life because of the serious implications for growth and the developing brain. Bone marrow transplantation may be the ultimate treatment when other therapies fail.

Prognosis. Anemia tends to recede spontaneously with age.

BIBLIOGRAPHY. Aase JN, Smith DW: Congenital anemia and triphalangeal thumbs. J Pediatr 74:471–474, 1969

Pfeiffer RA, Ambs E: Das Aase-Syndrome: autosomal rezessive vertete konnatal insuffiziente Erythropoese und Triphalangie der Daumen. Monatsschr Kinderheilk 131:235–237, 1983

Muis N, Beemer FA, Van Dijken P, Klep-de-Pater JM: The Aase syndrome: case report and review of the literature. Eur J Pediatr 145:153–157, 1986

ABDOMINAL ANGINA

Synonyms. Abdominal intermittent claudication; angina abdominalis; intestinal angina; visceral angina; chronic midgut ischemia; claudicatio intermittens abdominalis; intermittent anemic dysperistalsis; intermittent ischemia of mesenteric arteries; ischemic abdominal; mesenteric vascular insufficiency; vascular abdominal insufficiency; mesenteric arterial insufficiency.

Symptoms. Appear in middle and old age; prevalent in males. Cramping abdominal pain usually developing 15 to 30 minutes after a meal, and lasting 1 to 3 hours (direct correlation between amount of food and intensity and duration of pain). Nausea, vomiting, diarrhea may occur. Weight loss. Clinical manifestation may be chronic and unremitting, recurrent with long remission, or transient.

Signs. Moderate abdominal distension during attacks. Occasionally, systolic bruit in upper part of abdomen.

Etiology and Pathology. Arteriosclerotic narrowing and obliteration of ostia of gastrointestinal branches of the abdominal aorta, usually superior mesenteric artery involved. In intestine, there may be villose atrophy, ulcerations, or small infarctions.

Diagnostic Procedures. *Blood.* Anemia (malnutrition type); leukocytosis (occasional). *Stool.* Occult blood. *X-ray of abdomen.* Negative. *Angiography.* Exposure with patient in lateral position so that the obstruction is not obscured by the aorta.

Therapy. Elective surgical revascularization of superior mesenteric artery, celiac axis, or both. Endoarterectomy, excision, and graft replacement or bypass graft (preferable).

Prognosis. Eventual development of acute intestinal ischemia.

BIBLIOGRAPHY. Schnitzler J: Zur Symptomatologie des Darmarterienverschulussen. Wien Med Wochenschr 51:505–509; 568–572, 1901

Jaxheimer EC, Jewell ER, Persson AU: Chronic intestinal ischemia: The Lahey Clinic approach to management. Surg Clin N Am 64:123–130, 1985

Bergan JJ: Visceral ischemic syndromes: Obstruction of superior mesenteric artery, celiac axis, and inferior mesenteric artery in Sabiston. Textbook of Surgery, 14th ed. Philadelphia, WB Saunders, 1991

Lindsey JL, DeBakey ME, Beall AC: Diagnosis and treatment of diseases of the aorta. In Schlant RC, Alexander RW: Hurst's The Heart, 8th ed, p 2176. New York, McGraw-Hill, 1994

ABDOMINAL APOPLEXY

Synonyms. Massive intraperitoneal hemorrhage; intra-abdominal apoplexy; mesenteric or subperitoneal hemorrhage.

Symptoms. Prevalent in arteriosclerotic hypertensive males. Sudden severe abdominal pain, restlessness, shock.

Signs. Peritoneal irritation.

Etiology and Pathology. Spontaneous rupture of intra-abdominal vessel. Arteriosclerosis and hypertension in young patient; rupture of small localized aneurysm has been suggested. Rupture of superior mesenteric aneurysm mycotic (60% of cases), atherosclerotic (40%).

Diagnostic Procedures. *Blood.* Anemia; leukocytosis. *X-ray.* Flat abdominal plate to evaluate fluid level.

Therapy. Early surgery with suture of bleeding point; endoaneurysmorrhaphy; for branch aneurysms, bowel resection.

Prognosis. Excellent if suture of bleeding point performed in time.

BIBLIOGRAPHY. Cushman GF, Kilgore AR: The syndrome of mesenteric or subperitoneal hemorrhage (abdominal apoplexy). Ann Surg 114:672–681, 1941

Srinivasan V, Turner AG, Blackford HN: Massive intraperitoneal hemorrhage associated with renal pathology. J Urol 151:980–981, 1994

ABDOMINAL COCOON

Symptoms and Signs. Intestinal obstruction, mass of palpable bowel loops in the abdomen, in patients treated by Le Veen shunt.

Etiology. Unknown. Hypotheses include: subacute peritoneal infections, fibrin deposit from increased ascitic fluid turnover. Increased potential for intraperitoneal clotting of ascites caused by chronic disease.

Pathology. Large fibrotic sac wrapping the small bowel in the manner of a cocoon. The examination shows a fibrosing, nonspecific, chronic inflammatory process.

Diagnostic Procedure. Plain X-ray of the abdomen.

Therapy. Surgical lysis of the fibrous cocoon.

Prognosis. Depends on the hepatic disease.

BIBLIOGRAPHY. Cambria RP, Shamberger RC: Small bowel obstruction caused by the abdominal cocoon syndrome: possible association with the LeVeen shunt. Surgery 95:501–503, 1984

ABDOMINAL THORACIC

Synonyms. Thoracoabdominal. Includes all pathologic conditions in which thoracic pathology is manifested by abdominal symptoms and vice versa; for instance, symptoms of gastrointestinal type owing to coronary artery sclerosis or pneumonia, and anginal type of pain owing to gallbladder pathology; pleural effusion secondary to disease below diaphragm (pancreatitis; sequela of abdominal surgery; subphrenic abscess; Meig (see); dialysis; hydronephrosis and urinothorax; cirrhosis; nephrosis uremic pleuritis; glomerulonephritis).

Etiology. Interrelationship of nervous (spinal and autonomous system) reflexes between abdomen and chest.

Pathology. Varies according to lesions determining the reflex mechanism.

Diagnostic Procedures. *Blood.* Leukocytosis in pneumonia with abdominal pathologic changes. *X-rays of chest and abdomen.* Detection of pneumonia or abdominal pathology. *ECG.* Diagnosis of coronary artery diseases.

Therapy. Of the underlying disorder.

Prognosis. According to etiology.

BIBLIOGRAPHY. Long WB, Cohen S: The digestive tract as a cause of chest pain. Am Heart J 100:567–572, 1980

Mellow MH: A gastroenterologist's view of chest pain. Curr Prob Cardiol 7:7–9, 1983

Fraser RS, Paré JAP, Fraser RG, Paré PD: Synopsis of Disease of the Chest, 2nd ed. Philadelphia, WB Saunders, 1994

ABESHOUSE TRIAD

Synonyms. Adrenal cysts.

Symptoms. Flank discomfort; occasionally, gastrointestinal and renal symptoms.

Signs. Palpable mass in homolateral side; radiologically evident downward displacement of kidney.

Etiology. Congenital malformation, endothelial cysts and pseudocysts in the adrenal gland. In differential diagnosis, consider also parasites (Echinococcus) and neoplasia.

Pathology. Majority (39%) are endothelial (angiomatous) cysts and pseudocysts.

Diagnostic Procedures. *Ultrasonography. CT scan. MRI.*

Therapy. Surgical excision.

Prognosis. Lesions benign.

BIBLIOGRAPHY. Doran AG: Cystic tumour of the suprarenal body successfully removed by operation. Br Med J 1:1558–1563, 1908
Abeshouse GA, Goldenstein RB, Abeshouse BS: Adrenal cysts: review of the literature and report of three cases. J Urol 81:711–719, 1959
Sroujeh AS, Farah GR, Haddad MJ: Adrenal cysts: Diagnosis and management. BR J Urol 65:570–575, 1990
Kafagi FA, Gross MD, Shamiro B: Clinical significance of the large adrenal mass. BR J Surg 78:828–833, 1991

ABLEPHARON-MACROSTOMIA

Synonyms. McCarthy-West; AMS.

Symptoms and Signs. In male children. *Face:* triangular, hypertelorism, absence of zygomatic arches. Thin hair, absence of eyelids, internal strabism. *Nose:* small, triangular nostrils. *Macrostomia:* from inadequate fusion of commisures. Ears rudimentary. *Skin:* dry, coarse, skin folds. Webbing between proximal phalanges of fingers. Absence or hypoplasia of nipples. *Genitals:* ambiguous, micropenis. Occasionally cryptorchidism, umbilical hernia. *Intelligence:* retarded development.

Etiology. Unknown. Possibly autosomal recessive inheritance.

Therapy. Plastic and reconstructive surgery.

Prognosis. Poor.

BIBLIOGRAPHY. McCarthy GT, West CM: Ablepheron macrostomia syndrome. Dev Med Child Neurol 19:659–672, 1978
David A, Gordeeff A, Badoual J, et al: Macrostomia, ectropion athrophic skin hypertricosis: another observation. AM J Med Genet 39:112–115, 1991

ABRIKOSSOFF MYOBLASTOMA

Synonyms. Abrikossov tumor; Abrikossoff M and T; granular cell myoblastoma.

Symptoms. Both sexes equal incidence. Onset between 30 and 50 years of age. Seldom in childhood. Asymptomatic or paucisymptomatic.

Signs. Firm, round nodule, sessile or pedunculated, on skin or beneath tongue. Color varies from pink to grayish. Rarely, skin over the tumor ulcerates. Frequently affected are oral tissue (lips, palate, uvula, tongue) and genital tract (vulva).

Etiology. Unknown. Possibly reactive rather than neoplastic in nature.

Pathology. Pseudoepitheliomatous hyperplasia; large cells with acidophilic cytoplasm, small nucleus, large nucleolus, arranged in syncytium. Cells possibly of neural or nerve sheath origin or lipid containing histicytes. Fibers of striated muscle in layers; dyskeratosis.

Therapy. Excision.

Prognosis. Benign tumor of slow growth. Possible recurrence if no wide excision. A malignant, metastasing type reported.

BIBLIOGRAPHY. Abrikossoff A: Ueber Myome, Ausgehend von der quergestreiften willkurlichen Musckulatur. Virchows Arch (Pathol Anat) 260:215–233, 1926
MacKie RM: Soft tissue tumors. In Champion RH, Burton JL, Ebling FJG (eds): Rook/Wilkinson/Ebling Textbook of Dermatology, 5th ed, p 2094. Oxford, Blackwell Scientific, 1992

ACANTHOSIS NIGRICANS, MALIGNANT

Synonyms. Keratosis nigricans, malignant; acanthosis nigricans, paraneoplastic.

Symptoms and Signs. Both sexes equally affected. Lesions may appear at any age, preceding, accompanying, or following other symptoms of presence of malignancies, such as adenocarcinoma or reticulosis. Frequently, pruritus (40%); pigmentation, dryness, roughness of skin, which assumes a gray-brown to black color; hyperkeratosis; papillomatous elevation. Mucosae involved in 50% of cases. Compared to benign form lesions are more copious, extended, and severe, and involve the extremities. It may precede other malignancy by as much as 5 years (usually less). Symptoms and signs of associated malignancy: stomach (60%), uterus, pancreas, intestines, and less frequently: bladder, lung, breast, lymphomas.

Etiology. Unknown; paraneoplastic syndrome. No genetic factor demonstrated.

Pathology. Hyperkeratosis; papillomatosis; acanthosis and pigmentation of variable degree even within single section. Occasionally, horny inclusion cysts.

Diagnostic Procedures. *Blood.* Glycemia (frequent association with lipodystophic diabetes). *Biopsy of skin.* Deposits of glycosaminoglycan in affected skin.

Therapy. Medical or surgical treatment of associated malignancy.

Prognosis. Occasionally, total or partial regression with removal of underlying tumor. Frequently, recurrence.

BIBLIOGRAPHY. Janovsky V. In Unna PG et al (eds): International Atlas Seltener Hautkrankheiten. Leipzig, Leopold Voss, 1890 (plate II)
Pollitzer S. In Unna PG et al (eds), International Atlas Seltener Hautkrankheiten. Leipzig, Leopold Voss, 1890 (plate 10)
Riegel DS, Jacobs MI: Malignant acanthosis nigricans: a review. Dermatol Surg Oncol 6:923–927, 1980
Griffiths WD, Leigh IM, Marks R: Disorders of keratinization. In Champion RH, Burton JL, Ebling FJG (eds): Rook/Wilkinson/Ebling Textbook of Dermatology, 5th ed, p 1386. Oxford, Blackwell Scientific, 1992

ACANTHOSIS NIGRICANS SYNDROMES

1. Acanthosis nigricans, malignant (see).
2. Acanthosis nigricans, familial (benign); benign familial form, nonprogressive (see Acanthosis nigricans, malignant).
3. A. Acanthosis nigricans–insulin resistant (see Miescher I).
   B. Acanthosis nigricans, insulin resistance, acral hypertrophy, muscle cramps (Flier). Two cases described.
   C. Acanthosis nigricans, leprechaunism, insulin resistance (see Donohue).

D. Acanthosis nigricans, pineal hyperplasia, insulin resistant diabetes, somatic abnormalities (see Rabson-Mendenhall).

E. Acanthosis nigricans, lipodystrophy, hyperlipemia, hepatosplenomegaly, insulin resistance (see Lawrence-Seip).

4. Pseudoacanthosis nigricans (see).
5. Gourgerot-Carteaud (see).
6. Rud (see).
7. Leprechaunism.
8. Wilson (see).
9. Obesity.
10. Bloom (see).
11. Crouzon (see).
12. Beare-Stevenson (see).
13. Louis-Bar (see).
14. Stein-Leventhal (see).
15. Observed also in drug induction (nicotine, corticosteroids, pituitary extract, insulin, diethylstilbestrol) hyperphosphatasemia; several endocrinopathies (acromegaly, adrenogenital, Cushing, Addison, Alstrom, Diabetes mellitus: Type A, B, C, hypothyroidism, ovarian hyperthecosis, pinealoma, Prader-Willi, etc.).

BIBLIOGRAPHY. Janovski V. In Unna PG et al (eds): International Atlas Seltener Hautkrankheiten. Leipzig, Leopold Voss, 1890 (plate II)

Pollitzer S. In Unna PG et al (eds): International Atlas Seltener Hautkrankheiten. Leipzig, Leopold Voss, 1890 (plate 10)

Pollitzer S: Acanthosis nigricans: A symptom of a disorder of the abdominal sympathetic. JAMA 53:1369–1373, 1909

Griffiths WD, Leigh IM, Marks R: Disorders of keratinization. In Champion RH, Burton JL, Ebling FJG (eds): Rook/Wilkinson/Ebling Textbook of Dermatology, 5th ed, p 1385. Oxford, Blackwell Scientific, 1992

ACCIDENT-PRONE

Symptoms and Signs. Most common patients are males under age 21. Variable physical, mental, or emotional symptoms result in occurrence of accident. Occasionally, recurrent at same time (hours, weeks, months). More frequent in summer.

Etiology. The child impulsivity and self-harm may be related to problems of parental marital discord or to the withdrawal or depression of a parent.

Therapy. Complete assessment of physical, psychological, and developmental status, careful evaluation of family and especially of parental interactions.

Prognosis. Accidents usually decrease after age 21, but some people remain accident prone for life.

BIBLIOGRAPHY. Nicoli AM Jr: The adolescent. In The Harvard Guide to Modern Psychiatry. Cambridge, Belknap Press of Harvard Univ Press, 1978

ACCOMMODATIVE EFFORT

Symptoms. Blurring of images (asthenopia) with near vision appearing within few minutes after reading, sewing, or observing a near object.

Signs. Measurable abnormality of accommodative functions. Increased amplitude of accommodative adduction. Abnormal relaxation of accommodation induced by relative divergence at close distances. Latent convergence insufficiency.

Etiology. Accommodative fatigue; presbyopia; hyperopia; accommodative paralysis.

Pathology. Depends on etiology.

Diagnostic Procedures. Keep patient under observation until blurring of images appears. Then it is easy to observe typical findings.

Therapy. Correction of latent convergence insufficiency in addition to accommodative effort.

BIBLIOGRAPHY. Hill RV: Accommodative-effort syndrome: pathologic physiology. Am J Ophthalmol 34:423–431, 1951

Carpenter RHS (ed): Eye movements. In Vision and Visual Dysfunction, vol 8. Hondmills/Basingstone/Hampshire, Macmillan, 1991

ACh–AChR INTERACTION ABNORMALITY

Synonyms. See myasthenic syndromes.

Symptoms and Signs. Only one case described. Onset from birth severe generalized symptoms of myasthenia gravis.

Etiology. Autosomal recessive inheritance suspected. Anomalous interaction between ACh and ACh receptor.

BIBLIOGRAPHY. Engel AG, Walls TJ, Nagel A, et al: Newly recognized congenital myasthenic syndromes. I congenital paucity of synaptic vesicles and reduced quantal release. II High conductance fast channel syndrome. III Abnormal acetylcholine receptor (AChR) interaction with acetylcholine. IV AChR deficiency and short channel open time. Prog Brain Res 84:125–137, 1990

ACHARD

Synonyms. Marfan variant.

Symptoms and Signs. Same as in Marfan (see), plus mandibulofacialis dysostosis. Joint laxity limited to hands and feet.

Etiology. Autosomal dominant with incomplete expression (see Marfan). Not recognized as an autonomous clinical entity by many authors.

Diagnostic Procedures. *X-rays:* Brachycephaly, short mandibular rami, and increased gonial angle; various other radiological abnormalities (see Marfan).

BIBLIOGRAPHY. Achard C: Arachnodactylie. Bull Mem Soc Med Hôp Paris 19:834–840, 1902

Duncan PA: The Achard syndrome. Birth Defects 11:69–73, 1975

McKusick VA: Mendelian Inheritance in Man, 7th ed, p 7. Baltimore, Johns Hopkins Univ Press, 1986

ACHARD-THIERS

Synonym. Diabetic bearded woman.

Symptoms. Voice changes; absent or sparse menstruation.

Signs. Hypertrichosis and acne of face; hypertrophy of clitoris; atrophy of breast; obesity; abdominal striae; increased blood pressure.

Etiology. Hyperplasia of adrenal cortex with increased production of androgens and 11-oxysteroids.

Pathology. Hyperplasia or adenoma of adrenal glands; atrophic or sclerotic ovaries; pancreatic changes consisting of increase of islet cells and pericanalicular sclerosis; liver cirrhosis; colloid changes of thyroid.

Diagnostic Procedures. *Blood.* Hyperglycemia; insulin resistance; decreased sugar tolerance. *Urine.* Increased excretion of steroids in urine following adrenocorticotropic hormone (ACTH) stimulation.

Therapy. Surgery of adrenal may be useful.

BIBLIOGRAPHY. Achard C, Thiers J: Le virilisme pilaire et son association a l'insuffisance glycolytique (diabete des femmes avec barbe). Bull Acad Nat Med (Paris) 86:51–66, 1921

Dawber RPR, Ebling FJG, Wojnarowska FT: Disorders of hair. In Champion RH, Burton JL, Ebling FJG (eds): Rook/Wilkinson/Ebling

Textbook of Dermatology, 5th ed, p 2568. Oxford, Blackwell Scientific, 1992

ACHENBACH

Synonyms. Finger apoplexy; paroxysmal hand hematoma.

Symptoms. Appear in both sexes; more frequent in females. Spontaneous severe pain in the hands after strain or temperature changing (e.g., cooling).

Signs. Small, round hematoma with or without edema of affected hand.

Etiology. Unknown; postulated allergic-hyperergic mechanism, neurosympathetic reaction.

Pathology. Blood effusion without rupture of venous walls.

Diagnostic Procedures. *Coagulation test.* Negative. *Pinching test.* Positive (occasionally).

Prognosis. Spontaneous regression in days. Recurrence in the same or opposite hand. In some cases development of phlebectasia.

BIBLIOGRAPHY. Achenbach W: Ematomi parossistici della mano. Athena (Rome) 23:187–189, 1957
Achenbach W: Das Paroxysmale Handhaematom Medizinische 52:2138–2140, 1958
Stieler W, Heinze-Werlitz C: Paroxysmales Fingerhaematom (Achenbach syndrom) Hautartz 41:270–271, 1990

ACHONDROGENESIS Type IV

Radiologically identified as subgroups of the Langer-Saldino (see).

BIBLIOGRAPHY. Whitley CB, Gorlin RJ: Achondrogenesis: nosology with evidence of genetic heterogenecity. Radiology 148:693–698, 1983

ACHONDROPLASIA

Synonyms. Parrot; chondrodystrophia fetalis; hypoplastic chondrodystrophy; achondroplastic dwarfism; rickets fetal; ACH.

Symptoms and Signs. Occurs in both sexes. Dwarfed from birth. *Head.* Bulging; marked saddling of nose; "bulldog-face" appearance. *Extremities.* Absolute diminution in length; disproportionate proximal parts. Fingers pudgy; characteristic "trident hands." *Spine.* kyphosis (seldom); paraplegia may develop in 2nd or 3rd decades. Mild hypotonia; delayed motor progress. Intelligence usually normal. Forme fruste exists where only X-ray findings demonstrate condition.

Etiology. Unknown; autosomal dominant inheritance (10%) or spontaneous mutation (90%).

Pathology. Tubular bones short and proportionally thick. Foramen magnum compressed and small internal hydrocephalus frequent. *Histology.* Epiphyseal line discloses shorter cartilage columns without usual linear arrangement; some cartilage cells show mucinoid derangement.

Diagnostic Procedures. *X-ray.* In infants, excessive separation in ossification centers of vertebrae; caudal narrowing; short iliac wings and changes in sacroiliac curve: ossification centers set into metaphyseal ends. *Blood.* Relative glucose intolerance.

Therapy. Orthopedic-neurologic follow up. Relative intervention, if possible, deferred until full growth. Surgical therapy of some complications, such as hydrocephalus (which results from obstruction at the foramen magnum), dental malocclusion, strabismus (resulting from craniofacial dysmorphism), and spine deformities such as kyphosis. Medical therapy for recurrent otitis media. *Physiotherapy.* Psychological counseling during childhood. Genetic counseling.

Prognosis. Dwarfism in majority of cases; serious neurologic complication in early adulthood in some cases. In the majority of cases, the lifespan is normal; the mean adult height 131.5 cm in men and 125 cm in women.

BIBLIOGRAPHY. von Soemmering JT: Abbildungen und Beschreibungen einiger Misgerburden die sich ecemals auf den anatomischen. Theater zu Cassel befanden, p 30. Mainz, Kurfustlen privilegirten Universituats Buchhandlung, 1791
Parrot JMJ: Sur la malformation achondroplasique et le Dieu Phtah. Bull Soc Anthrop Paris I (3rd sers):296–308, 1878
Fitzsimmons JS: Familial recurrence of achondroplasia. Am J Med Genet 22:609–613, 1985
Nicoletti B et al (eds): Human achondroplasia: A multidisciplinary approach. First Int Symp on Human Achondroplasia, 1986, Rome, Italy. New York, Plenum, 1988
Rimoin DL: Genetic disorders of the osseous system. In Beithon P: McKusick's Heritable Disorders of Connective Tissue, pp 568–578. St Louis, Mosby, 1993

ACHONDROPLASIA REGIONAL–DYSPLASIA ABDOMINAL MUSCLE

Insufficient evidence to substantiate diagnosis. This condition may represent other dwarfisms.

Symptoms and Signs. Regional achondroplasia of ribs and ilium associated with abdominal muscle weakness.

BIBLIOGRAPHY. Caffey J: Achondroplasia of pelvis and lumbosacral spine. Am J Roentgen 80:449–457, 1958
Shapira E, Fischel E, Moses S, et al: Syndrome of incomplete regional achondroplasia (ilium and ribs) with abdominal muscle dysplasia. Arch Dis Child 40:694–697, 1965
Rimoin DL: Genetic disorders of the osseous system. In Beithon P: McKusick's Heritable Disorders of Connective Tissue, 5th ed, pp 568–578. St Louis, Mosby, 1993

ACHOO

Synonyms. Peroutka sneeze; helio-ophthalmic outburst; photic sneeze.

Symptoms. Very common phenomenon (circa 25% of population) in both sexes. Uncontrollable sneezing when passing from dark to bright light (usually sun); from 2 or 3 sneezes to 40 or more.

Etiology. Dominant inheritance. Poorly understood phenomenon. Photic reflex.

BIBLIOGRAPHY. Everett HC: Sneezing in response to light. Neurology 14:483–490, 1964
Peroutka SJ, Peroutka LA: Autosomal dominant transmission of the photic sneeze reflex. New Engl J Med 310:599–600, 1984

AChR DEFICIENCY AND SHORT CHANNEL OPEN TIME

Symptoms and Signs. One case, girl. From birth: respiratory insufficiency; facial dysplasia, ophthalmoplegia.

Etiology. Autosomal recessive (?). Maybe mutation of one of the subunits of ACh receptor.

Diagnostic Procedures. EMG: decremental response at 2 Hz stimulation. Mean single channel conductance: normal, but mean channel open time, short.

Therapy. Anticholinesterase drugs.

BIBLIOGRAPHY. Engel AG, Walls TJ, Nagel A, et al: Newly recognized congenital myasthenic syndromes. I Congenital paucity of synaptic vesicles and reduced quantal release. II High conductance fast channel syndrome. III Abnormal acetylcholine receptor (AChR) interaction with acetylcholine. IV AChR deficiency and short channel open time. Prog Brain Res 84:125–137, 1990

ACHROMATOPSIA

Synonyms. Total color blindness; congenital cone dysfunction; monochromatism; color blindness total; day blindness.

Symptoms. Both sexes affected; rare. Four types recognized:

1. Complete rod monochromatism, evidence since childhood, with subnormal visual acuity 20/50 to 20/200 or less. All objects perceived as gray. Scotopic vision.
2. Atypical rod monochromatism (nonfunctional cone pigment) with pendular nystagmus and photophobia.
3. Blue cone monochromatism with no ophthalmic findings blue cone function preserved.
4. Group of various rare cone and cone-rod dystrophies with onset in adolescence or later, usually macular retinal pigment epithelium atrophy; abnormal green-red color vision.

Signs. Head posture against strong light. Undulatory nystagmus; absence of photopic flicker.

Etiology. Autosomal recessive inheritance types 1, 2, and some subtypes of group 4; sex-linked recessive type 2 and some subtypes of group 4; and autosomal dominant and some subtypes of group 4.

Pathology. No or very few cones; alterations of cone morphology in external area; depigmentation, degeneration, and normal number of cones in macular area.

Diagnostic Procedures. *Test pseudoisochromatic plates. Electroretinography.* Reduction of critical fusion frequencies; reduction of *b* wave and absence of *a* wave.

Therapy. None.

Prognosis. Nonprogressive permanent condition. Visual defects according to degree of involvement from total color blindness to ability to read when holding the book close and shaded from glare. Nystagmus diminishing in adult life.

BIBLIOGRAPHY. Larsen H: Demonstration mikrocopischer Präparate von einem monochromatischen. Augen Klin Monatsbl Augenheilk 72:1, 1924
Voke-Fletcher J: Congenital rod monochromatism in a brother and sister. Mod Probl Ophthal 19:236–237, 1978
Bird AC, Jay B, Hussain AA, et al: Retinal photoreceptor disorders. In Garner A, Klintworth GK (eds): Pathobiology of Ocular Disease: A Dynamic Approach, 2nd ed, p 1224. New York, Marcel Dekker, 1994
Motuisky AG, Deeb SS: Color vision and genetic defects. In Scriver CR, Beaudet AL, Sly WS, et al: The Metabolic and Molecular Bases of Inherited disease, 7th ed, pp 4280–4281. New York, McGraw-Hill, 1995

ACHROMIC NEVI

Synonym. Amelanotic nevus, nevus anemicus.

Symptoms and Signs. Occurs in both sexes; present since birth, or onset early in life. Unilateral or bilateral lack of pigment in a systematized distribution present usually on the trunk; no change in distribution throughout life; no alteration of texture or changes in sensation in affected areas; no pigmented border around achromic area: Under diascopic pressure nevus becomes indistinguishable from branched surrounding skin; rubbing fails to produce vasodilatation.

Etiology. Congenital mesenchymal alteration that inhibits migration of melanoblast precursor cell. Autosomal dominant familial form described. Nevus anemicus may reflect locally increased vascular reactivity to cathecholamines.

Diagnostic Procedures. *Biopsy of skin.* Absence of melanophores. Injection of bradykinin, acetylcholine, 5-hydroxytryptamine nicotine, histamine does not produce vasodilatation; axillary sympathetic block followed by erythema.

Therapy. None or cosmetic.

Prognosis. Permanent condition.

BIBLIOGRAPHY. Lesser E. In Ziemssen HV: Handbook der Hautkrankheiten, Bd 2, p 183. Leipzig, Vogel, 1884
Coupe RL: Unilateral systematized achromic naevus. Dermatologica 134:19–35, 1967
Atherton DJ: Naevi and other developmental defects. In Champion RH, Burton JL, Ebling FJG (eds): Rook/Wilkinson/Ebling Textbook of Dermatology, 5th ed, pp 494–496. Oxford, Blackwell Scientific, 1992

ACID PHOSPHATASE DEFICIENCIES

Synonyms. Rathbun; hypophosphatasia.

Symptoms. Six clinical syndromes have been identified, although there is high variability within each one with some overlapping. See 1) Hypophosphatasia perinatal; 2) Hypophosphatasia infantile; 3) Hypophosphatasia childhood; 4) Hypophosphatasia adulthood; 5) Odontohypophosphatasia; 6) Pseudohypophosphatasia.

Etiology. Deficiency of acid phosphatase in all cell lines. Autosomal recessive inheritance. Mild forms may be transmitted as autosomal dominant trait.

Therapy. No medical treatment. Avoid traditional therapies for rickets or osteomalacia. Enzyme replacement, ALP infusion offer no significant benefits. Cortisone occasionally useful. Nonsteroid anti-inflammatory agents used for periarticular calcium deposition. Antibiotic in case of infections. Supportive treatments: dental care, orthopedic measures for fractures, craniotomy in premature synostosis.

BIBLIOGRAPHY. Rathbun J: Hypophosphatasia Am J Dis Child 75:822–831, 1948
Whyte MP: Hypophosphatasia. In Scriver CR, Beaudet AL, Sly WS, et al: The Metabolic and Molecular Bases of Inherited Disease, 7th ed, pp 4095–4111. New York, McGraw-Hill, 1995

PERINATAL HYPOPHOSPHATASIA

Synonyms. Nadler-Egan; hypophosphatasia perinatal (lethal).

Symptoms and Signs. It is expressed in utero, frequent stillbirth. Caput membranaceum, short limbs ostheochondral spurs may protrude from midportion of forearms and legs. If surviving to delivery: vomiting; hypotonia; lethargy; opisthotonus; seizures; bleeding; recurrent respiratory infections.

Diagnostic Procedures. Assay of lysosomal acid phosphatase in cultured fibroblast and multiple tissues. No activity. Prenatal diagnosis possible. *X-ray.* Skeleton almost completeley demineralized, fractures often present.

Prognosis. Death a few days after birth.

INFANTILE HYPOPHOSPHATASIA

Synonyms. Fraser (D), hypophosphatemic, non rachitic bone disease.

Symptoms and Signs. Both sexes. Onset before sixth month of age. Postnatal development apparently normal, then failure to thrive and features of rickets. Bulging of anterior fontanella, papipilledema, proptosis, mild hypertelorism, brachiocephaly, blue sclerae (occasionally). Predisposition to pneumonia.

Diagnostic Procedures. *Blood and Urine.* Hypercalcemia and hypercalciuria and, evidence of kidney functional impairment. *X-ray.* Characteristic, less marked than those of perinatal form. *Skeletal scintigraphy.*

Prognosis. Variable course after a period of deterioration improvement. Fifty percent of patients die from respiratory infections.

CHILDHOOD HYPOPHOSPHATASIA

Symptoms and Signs. Earlier than 5 years loss of deciduous teeth (aplasia, hypoplasia, and dysplasia of cementum); pain, stiffness, and weakness of muscles, short stature, waddling gait, rachitic deformities.

Diagnostic Procedures. *X-ray.* Characterizing sign: in metaphyseal areas of long bones "tongues of radiolucency." Premature closure of cranial sutures, skull "beaten-copper" appearance. *Dental radiography.* Enlarged pulp chambers and root canals "shell teeth."

Prognosis. May spontaneously improve in adolescence

ADULT HYPOPHOSPHATASIA

Symptoms and Signs. Onset in middle age. Anamnestic memory of premature loss of deciduous teeth and good health in adolescence and younger age. Pain in the feet and discomfort in the lower limbs from stress fractures and pseudofractures. Attacks of pseudogout (see); calcific periarthritis.

Diagnostic Procedures. *X-ray.* Osteopenia; pseudofractures (Looser zone, see); periarticular calcium deposition and ligament ossification; spinal hyperostosis (resembling Forestier-Rotes-Querol, see).

ODONTOHYPOPHOSPHATASIA

Symptoms and Signs. Dental disease without other features of hypophosphasia.

PSEUDOHYPOPHOSPHATASIA

Synonyms. Scriver.

Symptoms and Signs. Extremely rare form with all the feature of infantile form (see) with normal or increased serum alkaline phosphatase.

BIBLIOGRAPHY. Fraser D, Salter RB: The diagnosis and management of the various type of rickets. Ped Clin North Amer 5:417–441, 1958

Scriver CR: Vitamin D dependency (editorial). Pediatrics 45:361–363, 1970

Nadler HL, Egan TJ: Deficiency of lysosomal acid phosphatase: a new familial metabolic disorder. New Engl J Med 282:303–307, 1970

Whyte MP, Teitelbaum SL, Murphy WA, et al: Adult hypophosphatasia: clinical, laboratory, and genetic investigation of a large kindred with review of the literature. Medicine (Baltimore) 58:329, 1979

Moore CA, Wappner RS, Coburn SP, et al: Pseudohypophosphatasia: clinical, radiographic, and biochemical characterization of a second case. Am J Hum Genet 47:A-68, 1990

Whyte MP: Hypophosphatasia. In Scriver CR, Beaudet AL, Sly WS, et al: The Metabolic and Molecular Bases of Inherited Disease, 7th ed, pp 4095–4111. New York, McGraw-Hill, 1995

ACKERMAN (J.L.)

Synonyms. Molar root (pyramidal)—juvenile glaucoma-upper lip deformity; Glaucoma—juvenile—upper lip deformity—dental roots; taurodontism.

Symptoms and Signs. Present from birth. Fused molar roots; single root canal (taurodontism); juvenile glaucoma; sparse body hair; full upper lip (absence of "cupid bow"); thick filtrum. Occasionally, syndactyly and hyperpigmentation of interphalangeal joints of fingers and clinodactyly of fifth finger.

Etiology. Unknown; has appeared in two generations of a family.

BIBLIOGRAPHY. Ackerman JL, Ackerman AL, Ackerman AB: Taurodont, pyramidal and fused molar roots associated with other anomalies in a kindred. Am J Phys Anthrop 38:681–694, 1973

ACRAL FIBROKERATOMA

Synonyms. Digital fibrokeratoma (acquired).

Symptoms. Males more commonly affected than females; onset at any age from 17, but predominant in patients over 60 years of age.

Signs. Growth usually on fingers, with a slight or major resemblance to a rudimentary supernumerary digit. Occasionally, similar growth may appear also on palms or on soles of feet.

Etiology. Possibly reaction to trauma.

Pathology. Core of lesion formed by modified dermis, both reticular and papillary layer features included. Presence of elastic fibers (differential elements with true fibroma). Epithelial covering: acanthosis and hyperkeratosis.

Therapy. Excision.

Prognosis. After rather abrupt appearance, a rapid growth follows until the final size is reached. Lesion remains at maximum size for months or years.

BIBLIOGRAPHY. Hare PJ: Rudimentary polydactyly. Br J Dermatol 66:402–408, 1954

Bart RS, Andrade R, Kopf AW, et al: Acquired digital fibrokeratomas. Arch Dermatol 97:120–129, 1968

MacKie RM: Soft tissue tumors. In Champion RH, Burton JL, Ebling FJG (eds): Rook/Wilkinson/Ebling Textbook of Dermatology, 5th ed, pp 2076–2077. Oxford, Blackwell Scientific, 1992

ACROCALLOSAL

Synonyms. Schinzel; corpus callosum absence—hallux duplication—postaxial polydactyly.

Symptoms and Signs. From birth. Both sexes. Mental retardation; seizures. Macrocephaly; hypertelorism; cleft lip and palate (15%), hallux duplication, postaxial polydactyly; hypospadias, cryptorchidism, inguinal hernias, bipartite right clavicle.

Etiology. Autosomal recessive inheritance (possible). Inverted tandem duplication chromosome 12p13.3-p11.2.

Pathology. Absence of corpus callosum. Congenital cysts of brain and diffuse cortical atrophy.

Diagnostic Procedures. *CT brain scan. MRI.*

BIBLIOGRAPHY. Schinzel A: Post-axial polydactyly hallux duplication, absence of corpus callosum, macroencephaly and severe mental retardation: a new syndrome. Helv Pediatr Acta 34:141–146, 1979

Moechler JB, Pober BR, Holmes, et al: Acrocallosal syndrome: new findings. Am J Med Genet 32:306–310, 1989

Yuksel M, Calishan M, Ogur G, et al: The acrocallosal syndrome in a Turkish boy. J Med Gen 27:48–49, 1990

ACROCEPHALOSYNDACTYLY II

Synonyms. ACS II; Apert-Crouzon; Apert atypical; cephalosyndactyly; Vogt cephalodactyly. Possibly equal to Apert syndrome with unusually marked facial features.

Symptoms and Signs. Present from birth. Head and facial characteristic of Crouzon syndrome (see); extremely hypoplastic maxilla associated with syndactyly (typical of Apert, see; however, less severe).

Etiology. Autosomal inheritance, dominant or recessive type.

BIBLIOGRAPHY. Vogt A: Dyskephalie (Dysostosis craniofacialis, Maladie de Crouzon 1921) und eine neuartige Kombination dieser Krankheit mit Syndaktylie der 4 Extremitaeten (Dyskephalodaktylie). Klin Monatsbl Augenheilkd 90:441–454, 1933
Temtamy SA, McKusick VA: The Genetics of Hand Malformation. New York, National Foundation March of Dimes, 1978
Cohen MM, Kreiborg S: The central nervous system in the Apert syndrome. Am J Med Genet 35:36–45, 1990

ACRODERMATITIS, PERSISTENT

Synonyms. Andrew; Hallopeau; pustular recalcitrant acrodermatitis; acropustulosis acrodermatitis perstans; "Dermatite continue" dermatitis repens pustular acrodermatitis; acrodermatitis continua.

Symptoms and Signs. More common in females; may be seen in children; onset usually in middle age. Starts on fingers or thumbs, frequently following minor trauma or infection with burning and itching. Skin surrounding nail usually first affected by vesicles, pustules, or erosions with hemorrhagic periphery. Then lesions burst, leaving exuding areas that evolve in crusts or eczematous scaling. New lesions appear on other fingers or palms and soles. Seldom, lesions extend to forearm or elbow or evolve into a generalized pustular psoriasis, especially in the elderly.

Etiology. Unknown. Bacterial or infective origin excluded by negative cultures.

Pathology. Early lesions. Wide range of histologic features resembling eczema, intraepithelial vesicles, or pustules. Later lesions. Resemble psoriasis, but without its typical features.

Diagnostic Procedures. *Biopsy.* Repeated in well-chosen sites.

Therapy. Corticosteroids, coal tar, and salicylic acid of limited benefit. X-rays of marginal value. Prolonged courses of tetracycline, in low doses, beneficial in 30% of cases. Removal of foci. Etretinate of relative value because of relapse in course of treatment and local aftereffects (palmo or plantar skin painful). Cyclosporin or radiotherapy (with due precautions) may be beneficial.

Prognosis. Chronic, recurrent condition. May evolve into generalized pustular psoriasis.

BIBLIOGRAPHY. Hallopeau H: Sur les acrodermatites (Polydactylites continues recidivantes). Ann Dermatol Syph 35:473–475, 1897
Andrew GC, Birkman FW, Kelly RJ, et al: Recalcitrant pustular eruptions of the palms and soles. Arch Dermatol Syph 29:548–563, 1934
Camp RDR: Psoriasis. In Champion RH, Burton JL, Ebling FJG (eds): Rook/Wilkinson/Ebling Textbook of Dermatology, 5th ed, pp 1448–1450. Oxford, Blackwell Scientific, 1992

ACRODYSOSTOSIS

Synonyms. Arkless-Graham; Maroteaux-Malamut; acrodysplasia I; see Martin Albright (also indicated with the name acrodysostosis).

Symptoms and Signs. Both sexes affected; onset prenatal. Growth deficiency. Middle ear infections. Brachycephaly; flat nasal bridge; hypoplastic maxilla; prognathism. Shortness of extremities more pronounced in distal parts: hands short, broad; radius, ulna, and distal humerus deformed; cone-shaped epiphyses. Mental deficiency (90% of cases). Hypogonadism. Occasionally, several additional malformations are present: teeth, skin (hypopigmented ulcer), genital, skeletal.

Etiology. Unknown. Sporadic. Older parental age (suggesting autosomal dominant inheritance).

Prognosis. Deformities slowly progressing during growth period with restriction of joint mobility.

BIBLIOGRAPHY. Arkless R, Graham GB: An unusual case of brachydactyly. Am J Roentgen 99:724–739, 1967
Maroteaux P, Malamut G: L'acrodystose. Presse Med 76:2189–2192, 1968
Hernandez RM, Miranda A, Kofman-Alfaro S: Acrodysostosis in two generations: an autosomal dominant syndrome. Clin Genet 39:376–382, 1991

ACROKERATOELASTOIDOSIS

Synonyms. AKE; Costa (OG); focal acral hyperkeratosis.

Symptoms and Signs. Appearance of yellow, nodular, hyperkeratotic lesions on the palms and soles, possibly extending to dorsum of hands and feet. Absence of systemic manifestations.

Etiology. Possible autosomal dominant inheritance.

Pathology. Hyperkeratosis and disorganization of elastic fibers.

Therapy. Vitamin A, and derivatives topical and systemic.

BIBLIOGRAPHY. Costa OG: Acrokeratoelastoidosis: a hitherto undescribed skin disease. Dermatologica 107:164–167, 1953
Greiner J, Kruger J, Palden L, et al: A linkage study of acrokeratoelastoidosis: possible mapping to chromosome 2. Hum Genet 63:222–227, 1983
Griffiths WD, Leigh IM, Marks R: Disorders of keratinization. In Champion RH, Burton JL, Ebling FJG (eds): Rook/Wilkinson/Ebling Textbook of Dermatology, 5th ed, pp 1381–1382. Oxford, Blackwell Scientific, 1992

ACROMEGALOID FACIAL APPEARANCE

Synonyms. AFA; thick lips—oral mucosa.

Symptoms and Signs. From birth. Thickened lips, prominent rugae and phrenula of the intraoral mucosa. Blepharophimosis; highly arched eyebrows. Bulbous nose. Large hands.

Etiology. Proposed autosomal dominant inheritance.

BIBLIOGRAPHY. Hughes HE, McAlpine PJ, Cox DW, et al: An autosomal dominant syndrome with acromegaloid features and thickened oral mucosa. J Med Gen 22:119–125, 1985

ACRO-OSTEOLYSIS

Synonyms. Schinz. See Nélaton.

Symptoms and Signs. Both sexes. Onset at puberty. Recurrent ulcers of fingers and toes. Elimination of bone sequestra. Normal sensitivity.

Etiology. Acquired in workers with vinylchloride. Congenital; autosomal dominant inheritance.

Prognosis. Healing with loss of digits.

BIBLIOGRAPHY. Harms I: Ueber die familiaere Ackro-osteolyse. Fortschr Roentgenstr 80:727–733, 1954
Ross JA: An unusual occupational bone change. In Jeliffe AM, Strickland B (eds): Symposium Ossium. London, Livingstone, 1970
Schinz HR, Baensch WE, Friedl E, et al: Roentgen-diagnostic, vol 1, 969, p 734. New York, Grune & Stratton, 1981
Todd G, Saxe N: Idiopathic phalangeal osteolysis. Arch Dermatol 130:759–769, 1994
Klippel JH, Dieppe PA: Rheumatology, pp 2.10.4, 6.8.7–6.8.8. St Louis, Mosby, 1995

ACROPARESTHESIA

Synonyms. Nothnagel; Putnam; Schultze; nocturnal arm dysesthesias; sciatic arm neuralgia; sleep tetany; tired arm. See also Wartenberg.

Symptoms. Prevalent in women of middle age. Paresthesias, anesthesias, pain in the arm occurring exclusively while patient is lying down. Numbness develops also when sustained grip is used. It always affects the dominant arm. In the morning hand is stiff and can be used freely only after it is massaged.

Signs. Absence of objective signs, even after long duration of the symptoms.

Etiology. Idiopathic form is extremely rare, and direct causes such as compression and irritation, or indirect ones such as heart diseases must always be carefully sought, so that this will not become a diagnosis of escape. The syndrome is observed in rheumatoid arthritis, myxedema, acromegaly, amyloidosis, mucopolysaccharidosis, multiple myeloma.

Pathology. See Etiology. Common finding: thickening of transverse carpal ligaments or synovia of flexor tendons and median nerve compression.

Diagnostic Procedures. *X-ray* of cervical column and shoulder in different projections. *ECG. EMG.* See Etiology.

Therapy. Hydrocortisone beneath carpal ligaments and chlorothiazide or other diuretics. Section of transverse carpal ligaments final treatment.

Prognosis. If true form (extremely rare), recurrent pain without complication and self-limited.

BIBLIOGRAPHY. Nothnagel H: Zur Lehre von den vasomotorischen Neurosen. Dsch Arch Klin Med 2:173–191, 1867
Putnam JJ: A series of cases of paresthesia, mainly of the hands, of periodical recurrence, and possibly of vaso-motor origin. Arch Med NY 4:147–162, 1880
Schultze F: Neber Akroparaesthesie Dsch Z Nervenh 3:300–318, 1893
Ford FR: The tired arm syndrome: a common condition manifest by nocturnal pain in the arm and numbness of the hand. Bull Johns Hopkins Hosp 98:464–466, 1956
Adams RD, Victor M: Principles of Neurology, 5th ed, p 348. New York, McGraw-Hill, 1993

ACROPECTOROVERTEBRAL

Synonyms. F* syndrome.

Symptoms and Signs. Broad, short thumbs with partial duplication of distal phalanx and webbing with index that shows radial deviation; webbing of toes; sternal deformity, spina bifida occulta (L5-S1).

Etiology. Autosomal dominant inheritance.

Diagnostic Procedures. *X-ray of hand.* Fusion of capitate and hammate and, occasionally, other carpal bones.

BIBLIOGRAPHY. Grosse FR, Hermann J, Opitz JM: The F-form of acropectorovertebral dysplasia: the F syndrome. Birth Defects Orig Art Ser V (3):48–63, 1969

ACROPHOBIA

Synonyms. Height vertigo. See also Visual vertigo.

Symptoms and Signs. Frequent in alcoholics. Eccessive fear of heights. Vertigo, panic attacks.

Etiology. Conditioned phobic reaction. Sign of neurosis.

_____
*Initial of family name.

Diagnostic Procedures. Vestibular functions. Psychiatric evaluation.

Therapy. Systematic desensitization, in vivo desensitization on psychotherapy.

Prognosis. Good with therapy.

BIBLIOGRAPHY. Brandt T: Vertigo. Its Multisensory Syndromes, p 296. London, Springer-Verlag, 1991

ACRO-RENAL

Synonyms. Dicker-Opitz.

Symptoms and Signs. Male. Malformations of limbs and kidneys.

Etiology. Dominant inheritance. Not a casual entity but a nonspecific development field defect (?).

BIBLIOGRAPHY. Dicker H, Opitz JM: Associated acral and renal malformation. Birth Defects Orig Art Ser V (3):68–77, 1969
Curran AS, Curran JP: Associated acral and renal malformations: a new syndrome? Pediatrics 49:716–725, 1972

ACRO-RENAL-MANDIBULAR

Synonyms. Halal; split hands and feet—mandibular hypoplasia.

Symptoms and Signs. In two female sibs. Split hands and feet, renal and genital malformations, severe mandibular hypoplasia.

Etiology. Recessive inheritance.

BIBLIOGRAPHY. Halal F, Desgranges MF, Leduc B, et al: Acro-renal-mandibular syndrome. Clin Genet 5:277–284, 1980

ACTINIC KERATOPATHY, CHRONIC

Synonyms. Bietti nodular keratopathy; climatic droplet keratopathy; CAK; Labrador keratopathy; gelatinous dystrophy; spheroidal degeneration of cornea see also photophthalmia

Symptoms and Signs. Male preponderance in most series. Incidence increase with age and type of activity (sun and extreme environmental factor exposure). In absence of evidence of other diseases or inflammation, opacities (oil-like droplets) appear in the periphery of cornea in the horizontal media line. Droplets grow in time in size and number to form a band across cornea. Severity of condition is indicated in grades from trace to grade 4 according to severity of vision reduction (grade 3 on). Droplets may develop also in the conjunctiva.

Etiology. Ultraviolet light is an important cause.

Pathology. Proteinaceous bodies of unidentified type strongly autofluorescent.

Diagnostic Procedures. *Slit lamp biomacroscopy: autofluorescence.*

Therapy. Excision.

Prognosis. Progressing condition if persisting exposure: recurrence after 18 months from excision.

BIBLIOGRAPHY. Forsius H: Climatic changes in the eyes of Eskimos, Lapps and Cheremisses. Acta Ophthalmol (Copenhagen) 50:532–538, 1972
Gray RH, Johnson GJ, Freedman A: Climatic droplet keratopathy. Surv Ophthalmol 36:241–253, 1992
Klintworth GK: Degenerations, depositions and miscellaneous reactions of the ocular anterior segment. In Garner A, Klintworth GK (eds): Pathobiology of Ocular Disease: A Dynamic Approach, 2nd ed, pp 748–752. New York, Marcel Dekker, 1994

ACUTE ACALCULOUS CHOLECYSTITIS

Synonyms. Cholecystitis acute, acalculous.

Symptoms and Signs. Between 6 to 17% of cases of acute cholecystitis occur in the absence of stones; in pediatric population in 50% of cases. Often in patients without a previous history of biliary colics and with various concomitant medical problems (prolonged fasting, total parental nutrition, ventilatory support with positive pressure ventilation, general anesthesia, narcotic analgesic use, intra-abdominal and extra-abdominal surgery, ileus, burns, shock, sepsis, transfusions, postpartum, etc.). Abdominal pains, only in 70% localized to upper quadrant. In the early stage absence of fever, tenderness, and mass.

Etiology. Obstructive (hypomobility, hypovolemia, increased pigment load or nonobstructive vascular infections, etc.) or combination have been reported.

Pathology. Nonspecific and variable, according to etiology.

Diagnostic Procedures. *Echography, CT scan. Blood.* Leukocytosis.

Therapy. Antibiotics; percutaneous cholecystomy particularly indicated (attention not to miss perforation and gangrene).

Prognosis. Overall mortality between 9 to 66% (for acute calculous cholecystatis, 2%), explained by usually severe underlying or associated illness and complications.

BIBLIOGRAPHY. Strasberg SM, Clavien PA: Acute acalculous cholecystitis. In Haubrich WS, Schaffner F, Berk JE (eds): Bockus Gastroenterology, 5th ed, pp 2665–2673. Philadelphia, WB Saunders, 1995

ACYL-CoA DEHYDROGENASE, LONG CHAIN, DEFICIENCY OF

Synonyms. Hale; LCAD; nonketotic hypoglycemia, dicarboxylic aciduria deficit in oxidation of fatty acids; pseudo-Zellweger; pseudoneonatal adrenoleukodystrophy; Acyl coenzyme A oxidase deficiency; peroxisomal 3-oxo-acyl-coenzyme A thiolase deficiency; bifunctional protein deficiency.

Symptoms. In neonatal period, those of adrenoleukodystrophy (see), and in early childhood those of Zellweger (see). Hypoglycemia and respiratory arrest with fasting.

Signs. Cardiomegaly; hepatomegaly; hypotonia.

Etiology. Autosomal recessive inheritance. Deficiency of acyl-CoA dehydrogenase, which oxidizes long-chain fatty acids.

Pathology. Liver: panlobular steatosis, portal fibrosis; no necrosis or cholestasis enlargement.

Diagnostic Procedures. *Blood, tissue, and body fluid.* Low plasma carnitine and high elevation of very long chain fatty acids. *Urine.* No ketones at fasting; dicarboxylic acids; low hydroxy butyrate levels. *Assay for enzyme.* Activity reduced at less than 10%.

Therapy. No specific treatment available. Trial with dietary restriction of fat and supplementation with glycerol-trioleate and glycerol-trierucate (possibility of toxic effects), avoid prolonged fasting. Carnitine administration.

Prognosis. In some cases, death. In survivers, hypotonia and developmental defects.

BIBLIOGRAPHY. Naylor EW, Mosovich LL, Guthrie R, et al: Intermittent nonketotic dicarboxylic aciduria in two siblings with hypoglycemia: an apparent defect in beta-oxidation of fatty acids. J Inherit Metab Dis 3:19–24, 1980
Treem WR, Stanley CA, Hale DE, et al: Hypoglycemia, hypotonia and cardiomyopathy: the evolving clinical picture of long-chain acyl-CoA dehydrogenase deficiency. Pediatrics 87:328–333, 1991

Darmaun D, Haymond MW, Bier DM: Metabolic aspects of fuel homeostasis in the fetus and the neonate. In De Groot LJ (ed): Endocrinology, 3rd ed, p 2779. Philadelphia, WB Saunders, 1995
Weatherall DJ, Ledingham JGG, Warrell DA (eds): Oxford Textbook of Medicine, 3rd ed, p 1441. Oxford, Oxford Med Pub, 1996

ACYL-CoA DEHYDROGENASE, MEDIUM CHAIN, DEFICIENCY OF

Synonyms. Nonketotic hypoglycemia; carnitine deficiency owing to medium-chain acyl-CoA dehydrogenase deficiency; MCADH deficiency, dicarboxylic aciduria defect in beta oxidation of fatty acids.

Symptoms. In adolescence, hypoglycemia, lethargy, coma. Symptoms similar to Reye (see).

Signs. Hepatomegaly.

Etiology. Autosomal recessive inheritance. Deficiency of MCADH that does not permit oxidation of medium-chain fatty acids.

Pathology. *Liver.* Peripheral lobular fatty changes; steatosis.

Diagnostic Procedures. *Blood.* Low serum carnitine. *Urine.* Dicarboxylic aciduria (C6–C14), no ketosis with fasting.

Therapy. Carnitine administration.

Prognosis. If identified and treated: benign condition.

BIBLIOGRAPHY. Naylor EW, Mosovich LL, Guthrie, et al: Intermittent dicarboxylic aciduria and hypoglycemia in two siblings: apparent defect in beta oxidation of fatty acids. (Abst.) Am J Hum Genet 30:35A, 1978
Amendt BA, Rhead WJ: Catalytic defect of medium-chain acyl-coenzyme A dehydrogenase deficiency: lack of both cofactor responsiveness and biochemical heterogeneity in eight patients. Clin Invest 76:963–969, 1985
Darmaun D, Haymond MW, Bier DM: Metabolic aspects of fuel homeostasis in the fetus and the neonate. In De Groot LJ (ed): Endocrinology, 3rd ed, p 2779. Philadelphia, WB Saunders, 1995

ACYL CoA DEHYDROGENASE, SHORT-CHAIN DEFICIENCY

Synonyms. ACADS deficiency; lipid storage myopathy owing to short-chain acyl-CoA dehydrogenase deficiency; SCADH deficiency; SCAD deficiency.

Symptoms and Signs. In infants, failure to thrive, development delay, vomiting, nonketotic hypoglycemia. In adults, weakness on exertion.

Etiology. Defect of SCAD systemic (infantile form) or muscular (adult form). Adult form may be a riboflavin-responsive multiple acyl-CoA dehydrogenase (MAD) deficiency. (See glutaric aciduria type II.)

Pathology. Muscle: lipid storage.

Diagnostic Procedures. *Serum.* Acidosis. *Muscle.* Low concentration of carnitine. *Enzyme studies.* Defect of SCAD.

Therapy. Carnitine supplementation.

Prognosis. In infantile form, death in months or years. In adult form, stable condition.

BIBLIOGRAPHY. Turnbull DM, Bartlett K, Steven DL, et al: Short-chain acyl-CoA dehydrogenase deficiency associated with a lipid storage myopathy and secondary carnitine deficiency. New Engl J Med 311:1232–1236, 1984
Di Donato S, Garavaglia B, Rinaldi M, et al: Clinical and biochemical phenotypes of carnitine deficiency. In Ferrari R, Di Mauro S, Sherwood G (eds): L-Carnitine and Its Roles in Medicine: From Function to Therapy. London, Academy Press, 1992

Darmaun D, Haymond MW, Bier DM: Metabolic aspects of fuel homeostasis in the fetus and the neonate. In De Groot LJ (ed): Endocrinology, 3rd ed, p 2779. Philadelphia, WB Saunders, 1995

ADAMANTIADES-BEHÇET

Synonyms. Behçet; Gilbert (W.); Halushi-Behçet; Touraine; aphthosis; oculobuccogenital; triple symptom complex of Behçet.

Symptoms. Prevalent in young males; more frequent in Mediterranean area. Recurrent every 2 to 3 months and lasting from 1 week to 1 month. Pain and irritation of eyes; disturbed vision (initially unilateral); pain in the mouth (98%) and dysphagia; considerable pain on walking because of painful lesions on scrotum or labia. Other manifestations include fever, arthralgia, malaise; gastrointestinal, lung, and neurologic manifestations (the latter appear between second and fifth year of disease); acute meningomyelitis; meningoencephalitis; dementia; erythema nodosum (80%); arthritis (30% to 60%); parkinsonism.

Signs. Iritis (first manifestation); hypopyon; conjunctivitis; keratitis; retinal hemorrhages. In mouth, aphthae appearing in crops extending to pharynx. On genitals, small papules that ulcerate.

Etiology. Unknown: virus (?); related to collagen diseases (?); possible autosomal dominant inheritance of autoimmune disorder.

Pathology. Nonspecific inflammation; perivascular lymphocytic infiltration of meninges, brain, spinal cord; cerebral edema; destruction of ganglion cells; thrombophlebitis (25%); arterial aneurysm reported in some cases.

Diagnostic Procedures. *Blood.* Anemia; hypergammaglobulinemia; high sedimentation rate; high antiplasmin level lymphocytes, endothelial cells and neutrophil function evaluation. Complement and immunoglobulin studies. *MRI.*

Therapy. Adrenal steroids and antibiotics have doubtful benefits. Chlorambucil reported beneficial; levamisole helps for oral and genital ulcerations; corticosteroids and azathioprine used in relapses. Pulse cyclophosphamide and cyclosporine. IV IgG and low-dose aspirin have been tried with promising results.

Prognosis. Poor; condition recurrent and progressive; vision impaired by recurrent attacks. Oral and genital lesions regress, leaving scarring. Case history of 17 years' duration reported. Central nervous system involvement is cause of death.

BIBLIOGRAPHY. Bluthe L: Zur Kenntnis des recidivirenden Hypopyons (thesis). Heidelberg, 1908
Adamantiades, B: Sur un cas d'iritis a hypopyon recidivant. Ann Ocul 168:271, 1931
Behçet H: Uber rezidivierende Aphthöse, durch ein Virus verursachte Geschwure am Mund, am Auge und an den Genitalien. Derm Wochenschr 105:1152–1157, 1937
Feigenbaum A: Description of Behçet's syndrome in Hippocratic third book of endemic diseases. Br J Ophthalmol 40:355–357, 1956
Rewald E, Jaksic JC: Behçet's syndrome treated with high dose intravenous IgG and low dose aspirin. J Roy Soc Med 83:652–653, 1990
O'Duffy DJ, Kokmen E (eds): Behçet's Disease: Basic and Clinical Aspects. New York, Marcel Dekker, 1991

ADAMS-KERSHNER

Obsolete.

Synonyms. Kershner-Adams. Used to indicate chronic interstitial suppurative pneumonia of unknown origin.

BIBLIOGRAPHY. Kershner RD, Adams WE: Chronic nonspecific suppurative pneumonitis. J Thor Surg 17:495–511, 1948
Desaive P, Leroux G: La pneumonic suppuree non specifique chronique (syndrome der Kershner et Adams). Acta Chir Belgica 52:38–49, 1953

ADAMS-OLIVER

Synonyms. Absence defect of limbs, scalp, skull. Scalp defect—ectrodactyly.

Symptoms and Signs. Both sexes. From birth. Absence of lower extremities and fingers of hands (in some patients, lack of hands or lower legs). Ulcerated area on vertex of scalp, bone defect underneath. Skin and skull lesions similar to those of aplasia cutis congenita (see).

Etiology. Dominant inheritance, variable expressivity. Cases suggesting autosomal recessive inheritance identical to the dominant form also reported.

BIBLIOGRAPHY. Adams FH, Oliver CP: Hereditary deformities in man due to arrested development. J Hered 36:3–7, 1945
Kuster W, Lenz W, Kaariainen H, et al: Congenital scalp defects with distal limb anomalies (Adams-Oliver syndrome) report of ten cases and review of literature. Am J Med Gen 31:99–115, 1988
Atherton DJ: Naevi and other developmental defects. In Champion RH, Burton JL, Ebling FJG (eds): Rook/Wilkinson/Ebling Textbook of Dermatology, 5th ed, pp 519–520. Oxford, Blackwell Scientific, 1992

ADAMS-VICTOR-MANCALL

Synonym. Alcohol myelinolysis pontine; central pontine myelolysis; myelinolysis, central pontine.

Symptoms and Signs. Both sexes affected; onset usually in adulthood, in alcoholic or nutritionally deprived patients. Progressive facial and tongue weakness, speech and deglutition impairment. Occasionally, pseudobulbar phenomena: emotional lability. In some cases, quadriparesis at onset that results in flaccid and areflexic quadriplegia. Positive Babinski. Sensorial alteration frequently observed. Locked-in syndrome. Sphyncters seldom affected. In majority of cases no symptoms or signs of pontine lesion because of small size of lesion or because obscured by coma.

Etiology. Alcoholism or nutritional deficiency. May be associated with various conditions such as Wilson, Wernicke, diabetes, amyloidosis, leukemia, infections, and kidney transplantation.

Pathology. Central pontine myelinolysis of variable extension involving center or basal portion of middle and upper pons. Nerve cells and blood vessels relatively unaffected.

Diagnostic Procedures. *Spinal fluid.* Normal. *Blood.* Anemia and other findings associated with nutritional deficiency; severe electrolyte changes. Reduced serum osmolality, Pco_2 increased. *CT brain scan and MRI.*

Therapy. Thiamine and other vitamins; dietary treatment. Electrolyte deficit correction.

Prognosis. Poor; rapid evolution in 2 to 3 weeks; coma and death. Some patients have survived with intensive treatment.

BIBLIOGRAPHY. Victor M, Adams RD: Effect of alcohol on nervous system. Res Publ Assoc Res Nerv Ment Dis 32:526–573, 1953
Adams RD, Victor M, Mancall EL: Central pontine myelinolysis. Arch Neurol Psychiatr 81:154–161, 1959
Wiederholt WC, Kobayashi RM, Stockard JJ, et al: Central pontine myelinolysis: A clinical reappraisal. Arch Neurol 34:220–227, 1977
Adams RD, Victor M: Principles of Neurology, 5th ed, pp 891–893. New York, McGraw-Hill, 1993

ADDISONIAN SYNDROMES

Synonyms. Addison disease; adrenal cortical insufficiency; melasma suprarenal. Adrenal cortical insufficiency clinically results in two types of syndromes: acute adrenal insufficiency and chronic adrenal insufficiency.

ACUTE ADRENAL INSUFFICIENCY

Synonyms. Addisonian crisis; adrenal crisis; Bernard-Sergent.

Symptoms. Dramatic appearance. Anorexia; nausea; vomiting; back pain; cyanosis; mental torpor.

Signs. Weak pulse; orthostatic hypotension; heart sound weak and soft; supraventricular tachycardia; dehydration; hypothermia; weight loss. Scarce responsiveness to volume expansion and pressor agents. Fever appears when treatment is started.

Etiology. Secretory failure of adrenals; idiopathic (65%), tuberculosis (20%), other causes (15%) including: hemorrhage into adrenals, infections, especially from fungi and less frequently bacterial (see also Waterhouse-Friderichsen); trauma; metastasis; vascular thrombosis; sarcoidosis; amyloidosis; immunodeficiency syndromes; etc. Bilateral adrenalectomy (occurrence not justifiable since must be prevented by proper medications); adrenal cortical atrophy and abrupt discontinuation of cortisone; cortisone-like therapy; tumors and other destructive processes in the region of sella turcica; isolated ACTH deficiency (autoimmune lymphocytic hypophysitis).

Pathology. See etiology. Bilateral adrenal hemorrhage; atrophy (induced by prolonged treatment with adrenal steroids); decreased weight; loss of lipid content of cells of both glomerular and fascicular zones.

Diagnostic Procedures. In such emergency, treat first, refine diagnosis later. *Blood.* Preliminary tests: RBC count; WBC formula (relative lymphocytosis and eosinophilia) blood sugar; sodium (hypo); potassium (hyper); blood urea nitrogen; plasma cortisol level. *X-ray. CT scan. MRI* according to etiologies.

Therapy. Start immediately intravenous (IV) infusion 5% dextrose while waiting for other medications. Hydrocortisone (100–400 mg) added to dextrose and given in 2-hour period (repeated every 6 hours). After 24–36 hours, hydrocortisone (100 mg/day). Penicillin or other antibiotic (even if no sign of infection), plasma, or albumin to counteract shock. Catecholamine only with precaution (after some dextrose and hydrocortisone have been given).

Prognosis. Without treatment, rapidly fatal. With treatment, dramatic improvements. Continue treatment as long as necessary. Do not exceed 3000 ml of fluid a day, especially if sodium-containing solutions are used. Once out of shock, the patient may be maintained on oral medication (prednisone 5 mg in the morning and 2.5 mg in the early evening).

CHRONIC ADRENAL INSUFFICIENCY

Synonym. Addison disease.

Symptoms. Early emotional lability; irritability. The following symptoms appear: asthenia; weakness; easy fatigability (improving with rest and sleep); anorexia; nausea; vomiting; weight loss; abdominal pain; constipation or diarrhea; increase of emotional lability; salt craving; amenorrhea; loss of libido; impotence; muscle cramps; contractures.

Signs. Weight loss (100%); hypotension (90%); hyperpigmentation of skin patches of dark grayish pigmentation in mucosa of mouth, vagina, rectum (90%); asymmetric areas of vitiligo (5%); decrease of body hair; dehydration.

Etiology. Several mechanisms may induce adrenal insufficiency. They are subdivided as primary type and secondary type.

Primary type.

1. Primary atrophy (related to the development of autoantibodies). In this type, the frequent association with extraadrenal endocrine deficiencies (pancreatic, gonadal) has been interpreted as owing to a generalized tendency toward endocrine organ failure with adrenal insufficiency as the most prominent component. (See Multiple endocrine deficiency syndrome.)
2. Infections: tuberculosis; viral, bacterial, and mycotic diseases.
3. Infiltration by leukemia, reticuloendotheliosis, Hodgkin disease, metastatic tumors, amyloidosis.
4. Hemorrhages: trauma; infections; anticoagulant treatment; thrombocytopenia; thrombosis.
5. Congenital familial form. Autosomal dominant, recessive and X-linked.
6. Induced by drugs that alter adrenal cortisol metabolism (triparanol, amphenone 33bis 4-amino-phenyl-2-butanone 1,1-dichloro-2-(o-chlorophenyl)-2-(p-chlorophenyl) ethane).

Secondary type. Pituitary failure owing to tumor; necrosis; iatrogenic (medicamental, surgical, radiologic); suppression of activity; hypothalamic failure to produce corticotropin-releasing factor (CRF).

Pathology. Lesions of adrenal or pituitary (or both) depending on etiology. Over 50% of patients show lymphocyte infiltration of adrenal cortex.

Diagnostic Procedures. Evidence of adrenal insufficiency may be gathered by direct and indirect tests of adrenal functions. Adrenocorticotropic hormone (ACTH) stimulation. The most reliable test for measuring adrenal function directly. Preferable is the IV 8-hour technique (administration of dexamethasone orally to protect from reactions), determination of urinary 17-hydroxysteroid, and 17-ketosteroid or plasma cortisol level or both, used as indexes of adrenal response.

Lack of increase is present in both primary and secondary (pituitary) insufficiencies. To differentiate the two forms, continue injection of ACTH for several days, and repeat determination. If levels increase, secondary type is indicated.

Determination of level of urinary 17-ketosteroid and 17-hydroxycorticosteroid and of plasma cortisol of relative value. *Other diagnostic procedures.* Indirect indications of adrenal insufficiency are given by a group of tests more economical and less complicated, although not very specific, than the previous ones: water load test; salt deprivation test; serum and salivary sodium:potassium ratio; absolute number of circulating eosinophils; glucose tolerance test. Other findings in Addison syndrome are normocytic, normochromic anemia, lymphocytosis presence of antiadrenal antibodies (in about 50% of cases). *X-ray, CT scan, MRI* of skull; of chest (for heart size); of abdomen (adrenal calcification [10%]). *ECG-EEG.* Generalized theta activity; alpha rhythm suppressed; occasionally, delta activity.

For diagnosis of pituitary type, the frequent association of other endocrine defects is important: insulin tolerance test; high cholesterol; low basal metabolic rate; urinary gonadotropins; oligospermia. *Determination of ACTH.* Metyrapone test after prolonged ACTH administration (now a test of only historic interest).

Therapy. A combination of glucocorticoid, mineralocorticoid, and androgenic-anabolic agents. The combination cortisolfluohydrocortisone-fluor-oxymesterone is one of the more recommended.

Prognosis. With adequate treatment normal health may be maintained.

BIBLIOGRAPHY. Addison T: Diseases of suprarenal capsules. London Med Gaz O S 43 (NS 8):517–518, 1849

Chuandi L, Junquing C, Ruohua S, et al: Addison's disease of autosomal dominant inheritance: a report of 11 cases in one family. Kexue Tongbao 30:981–984, 1985

Loriaux DL, McDonald WJ: Adrenal insufficiency. In De Groot LJ (ed): Endocrinology, 3rd ed, pp 1731–1740. Philadelphia, WB Saunders, 1995

ADDISON-BIERMER

Synonyms. Biermer. Addison anemia; Hunter-Addison; Lebert; Biermer-Ehrlich; pernicious anemia

Symptoms and Signs. Presenting complaints: symptoms of anemia (58% of cases); paresthesia (13%); gastrointestinal symptoms (11%); sore tongue or mouth (7%); weight loss (5%); difficulty in walking (3%). Long-term complication: carcinoma of the stomach.

Etiology. The disease occurs in two forms: an adult type (common) and a congenital variety (rare). In the first type, the lack of intrinsic factor (necessary for absorption of vitamin B_{12}) is associated with gastric atrophy and deficiency of many other gastric secretions (achylia gastrica). In the congenital form, only intrinsic factor is lacking, other components of gastric juice remaining normal. An autoimmune mechanism has been postulated.

Pathology. Skin pallor; yellowish hue. Heart dilated, flabby. Fatty changes in parenchymatous viscera, with generalized iron deposition. Extramedullary myeloid metaplasia. Tongue and gastric mucosa atrophic. Neurologic features (see Lichtheim).

Diagnostic Procedures. *Blood.* Macrocytic anemia, poikilocytosis; mean corpuscular volume increased; hemoglobin content of red cell increased. Platelets slightly decreased. Slight to marked hyperbilirubinemia. High serum iron; low folic acid and vitamin B_{12} levels; low serum alkaline phosphatase; high lactic acid dehydrogenase. Antibodies against parietal cells of stomach. Leukocytes. Macropolycytes; some immature cells may be found. *Bone marrow.* Erythroid series; megaloblastosis; hyperplasia. Abnormal myelopoiesis; enlargement of elements, especially metamyelocytes; nuclear changes. *Gastric analysis and gastroscopy.* Achlorhydria and typical changes. Biopsy of stomach mucosa. Typical changes. *Schilling test:* Positive.

Therapy. Vitamin B_{12} lifelong administration.

Prognosis. Good with treatment.

BIBLIOGRAPHY. Addison T: On the Constitutional and Local Effects of Disease of the Suprarenal Capsules. London, S Highly, 1855
Biermer A: Versamml. dtsch. Naturforsch u. Dresden, Aerzte, 1868
Biermer A: Form von progressiver pernicioser Anamie. Korresp Bl Schweiz Arzt 2:15–18, 1872
Lebertt: Handbuch der allgemeinen Pathologie und Therapie. Tubingen, 1876
Hunter W: Pernicious anemia. Its pathology, septic origin, symptoms, diagnosis and treatment. Based upon original investigation. London, 1901
Lee GR: Megaloblastic and nonmegaloblastic macrocytic anemias. In Lee GR, Bithel TC, Foerster J, et al (eds): Wintrobe's Clinical Hematology, 9th ed, pp 750–763. Philadelphia, Lea & Febiger, 1993

ADENINE PHOSPHORIBOSYLTRANSFERASE DEFICIENCY

Synonyms. 2, 8-dihydroxyadenine lithiasis (2, 8-DHA); APRT deficiency.

Symptoms and Signs. From birth, three mutant forms identified: (1) partial deficiency; asymptomatic; (2) complete deficiency (Type I defect in caucasian) urolythiasis with from mild to severe symptoms: colics; hematuria; urinary tract infection, dysuria, passage of gravel or stones. In some cases renal failure; (3) partial deficiency (Type II in Japanese) urolythiasis with related variable symptoms.

Etiology. Autosomal dominant inheritance. Deficiency of adenine phosphoribosyltransferase (chromosome 16).

Pathology. Stones composed of 2, 8-DHA. Because of their radiolucency they often are confused with uric acid.

Diagnostic Procedures. *Blood.* Uric acid normal levels. No immunodeficiency. *Urine.* Normal uric acid, excretion of abnormal adenine derivatives.

Therapy. Diet (purine restriction). Allopurinol. Avoid alkali. Chronic renal failure kidney transplantation.

Prognosis. Depends on degree of renal deficit at moment of discovery.

BIBLIOGRAPHY. Cartier P, Hamet M: Une nouvelle maladie métabolique: le deficit complet en adénine-phosphorybosiltransférase avec lithiase de 2, 8-dihydroxyadénine. CR Acad Sci (Paris) 279:883–886, 1974

Kamatani N, Terai C, Kuroshima S, et al: Genetic and clinical studies on 19 families with adenine phosphoribosyltranferase deficiencies. Human Genet 75:163–168, 1987
Simmonds HA, Sahota AS, Van Acker KJ: Adenine phosphoribosyltransferase deficiency and 2, 8-dihydroxyadenine lithiasis. In Scriver CR, Beaudet AL, Sly WS, et al: The Metabolic and Molecular Bases of Inherited Disease, 7th ed, pp 1707–1719. New York, McGraw-Hill, 1995

ADH-RESISTANT DIABETES INSIPIDUS

Includes all conditions where renal tubular inability to respond to antidiuretic hormone (ADH) predominates over other renal pathologic manifestations that may be present.

Synonyms. Nephrogenic diabetes insipidus; diabetes insipidus nephrogenic type II; vasopressin-resistant diabetes insipidus; water baby.

Etiology. Congenital conditions. (1) Hereditary nephrogenic diabetes insipidus syndrome, or water baby, is due to X-linked inheritance with variable degrees of manifestation in females. The defect resides (improbably) in the mobility of ADH to stimulate renal tubular cAMP (2) Associated with Fanconi or Lightwood syndromes (see).

Acquired Conditions. (1) Hypokalemia; (2) hypercalcemia; (3) Conn syndrome; (4) drug-induced (demethylchlortetracycline, metoxyflurane, lithium); (5) in systemic diseases amiloidosis; in Sjogren.

Pathology. According to etiology.

Diagnostic Procedures. If diabetes insipidus, administration of ADH does not modify symptomatology. Adults often have hyperuricemia.

Therapy. Proper fluid intake, hydrochlorothiazide 0.5–1.5 mg/kg/24 hr in combination with a sodium intake of less than 1 mEq/kg/24 hr; potassium supplements if required. Indomethacin has been effective in some patients.

Prognosis. With early diagnosis and proper therapy: good.

BIBLIOGRAPHY. La Combe Lu: De la polydipsie. L'experiance. J Med Chir 7:305, 1841
Weil A: Ueber die hereditare form des diabetes insipidus. Dtsch Arch Klin Med 93:180–290, 1908
Bichet DG, Razi M, Lonergan M, et al: Hemodynamic and coagulation responses to 1-desamino(8-D-arginine) vasopressin in patients with congenital nephrogenic diabetes insipidus. New Engl J Med 318:881–887, 1988
Baylis PH: Vasopressin and its neurophysin. In De Groot LJ (ed): Endocrinology, 3rd ed, pp 412–415. Philadelphia, WB Saunders, 1995

ADIE

Synonyms. Holmes-Adie; Holmes G. III; Markus; Weill-Reys. When not associated with disturbed deep tendon reflexes: Adie partial; Argyll-Robertson nonluetic; Argyll-Robertson pupil with mydriasis.

This syndrome was fully described before Adie publications (1931): Piltz J 1899; Strasburger J 1902; Saeger J 1902; Markus C 1905; Holmes D 1931.

See pupillotonic pseudotabes.

BIBLIOGRAPHY. Piltz J: Ueber neue Papillenphaenome. Neurol Zentralbl. 18:248–254, 1899
Strasburger J: Pupillentraegheit bei Accommodation und Convergenz. Neurol Zentralbl 21:738–740, 1902
Saeger J: Ueber die sogenänte Myotonische Pupillenbenegung. Neurol Zentralbl 21:1000–1004, 1902
Markus C: Notes on a peculiar pupil phenomenon in two cases of partial iridoplegia. Lancet 2:1257, 1905

Holmes G: Partial iridoplegia with symptoms of other diseases of nervous system. Trans Ophthalmol Soc UK 51:209–228, 1931
Adie WJ: Pseudo-Argyll-Robertson pupils with absent tendon reflexes, a benign disorder simulating tabes dorsalis. Br Med J 1:928–930, 1931

ADIE-CRITCHLEY

Synonyms.   Fulton; forced grasping and groping; premotor cortex.

Symptoms and Signs.   Grasping. When an object is placed in one hand of patient, he grasps it, and it cannot be withdrawn because he involuntarily does not release it. Patient may also be unable to release object voluntarily and if he tries to throw it away, it remains firm in his hand. Groping. The affected hand goes after and attempts to grasp objects that touch it, or grasps other hand when it moves.

Etiology.   Tumor of contralateral frontal lobe superior part of area 6. When syndrome affects both hands, localizing value is lost.

BIBLIOGRAPHY. Adie WJ, Critchley M: Forced grasping and groping. Brain 50:142–170, 1927
Walshe FMR: On the "Syndrome of the premotor cortex" (Fulton) and the definition of the terms "premotor" and "motor": With a consideration of Jackson's views on the cortical representation of movements. Brain 58:49–80, 1935
Grinker RR, Sahs AL: Neurology, 6th ed. Springfield, IN, CC Thomas, 1966

ADRENAL HEMORRHAGE, NEONATAL

Synonyms.   Neonatal adrenal.

Symptoms.   Incidence over 1% of postmortem findings in newborn; onset between 2nd and 7th postnatal days. Occasionally, asymptomatic (and discovered as calcification and adrenal insufficiency in later life). High fever; tachypnea; convulsions; vomiting; collapse.

Signs.   There may be a mass in the flank with overlying skin discoloration; jaundice may also develop. Pallor; cyanosis; skin rash; purpura.

Etiology.   Stress and trauma at birth (leading cause). Physiologic involution of adrenals. Systemic diseases such as thrombocytopenia, syphilis.

Pathology.   In 70% of cases, right adrenal involved; in 5–10% bilateral. From small hemorrhage to destruction of entire gland.

Diagnostic Procedures.   *Blood.* Catecholamines, methoxyamines, and vanillylmandelic acid determination to rule out neuroblastoma. *X-ray.* Lateral abdominal. Retroperitoneal mass. Urography. Kidney displacement. Calcification of adrenal sometimes as early as 12th day of life. *Ultrasonography of abdomen.* Diagnostically may be very helpful.

Therapy.   According to symptomatology. Exploration frequently indicated to differentiate from neuroblastoma. Transfusions; antibiotics; hormone replacement; fluid and electrolyte balance.

Prognosis.   Depends on extension of lesion.

BIBLIOGRAPHY. Goldzieher MA, Gordon MD: Syndrome of adrenal hemorrhage in a newborn. Endocrinology 15:165–181, 1932
Di George Levine LS: Disorders of the adrenal glands. Behrman RE, Kliegman Arvin Nelson: Textbook of Pediatrics, 15th ed, pp 613–614. Philadelphia, WB Saunders, 1995

ADRENOGENITAL SYNDROMES

Synonyms.   Corticosexual; adrenal virilizing; adrenal feminizing; congenital adrenal hyperplasia; adrenal hyperplasia III.

Clinical findings and treatment vary according to etiology, which includes congenital adrenal hyperplasia, feminizing adrenal tumors, viril-

izing adrenal tumors, ill-defined group with hirsutism with or without menstrual disorders. (For last group see Hirsutism.)

A.   CONGENITAL ADRENAL HYPERPLASIA

According with enzymatic defects of adrenal steroidogenesis it may be subdivided into major subtypes: (1) Deficiency of 21-hydroxylase (simple virilizing, salt losing, and nonclassic forms); (2) 11-hydroxylase deficiency (hypertensive classic and nonclassic forms and salt losing variants with additional corticosterone methyl oxidase type I (?) and type II deficiency); (3) 17-hydroxylase deficiency with or without 17,20-lyase deficiency; (4) 3-hydroxysteroid dehydrogenase deficiency (classic and possibly nonclassic forms); (5) cholesterol desmolase deficiency (congenital lipoid hyperplasia).

SIMPLE VIRILIZING FORM

MALE

Symptoms.   Frequency 1/14,000; nonclassic form 0.1–1% (3% in European Jews). Infants a few months old exhibit frequent erections; from 1 to 5 years of age deepening of voice and marked muscular development occur.

Signs.   Macrogenitosomia precox: at a few months of age, penis enlargement with normal small testis, pubic and axillary hair, increased pigmentation (Addison-like), seborrhea; between 1 and 5 years of age, acne; at 8 to 10 years, fusion of epiphysis.

Etiology.   Autosomal recessive mutant gene. Chromosomal location 6p. Enzyme P450 c21. Excessive secretion of adrenal androgens beginning during fetal life. Deficiency of 21-hydroxylase. Increased production of 17-OHP, 4-A. Decreased production of cortisol, increase of ACTH.

Pathology.   *Testis.* Biopsy shows small seminiferous tubules, no Leydig cells; occasionally, hyperplastic adrenal tissue; seldom, testicular maturity and spermatogenesis. *Adrenals.* Markedly enlarged. Not many studies done on this form of adrenal hyperplasia. In young children, glands brownish in color, irregular, cerebriform surface: In older patients, adenomas have been observed (see sodium-losing form for description of microscopic changes).

Diagnostic Procedures.   *Urine.* Increase in excretion of 11-oxysteroids and 17-ketosteroids and pregnanetriol; regression of size of testis with cortisone therapy. Cortisone and glucocorticoids decrease the excretion of 17-ketosteroids and pregnanetriol (last test differentiates this form from virilizing adrenal tumors). Adrenocorticotropic hormone (ACTH) administration. Markedly increases excretion of pregnanetriol and related steroids and causes a moderate rise of androgens and estrogens. Cortisol metabolites show absence of or insufficient response to ACTH (pathognomonic response).

Therapy.   Cortisone or hydrocortisone intramuscularly (IM) at high dose (from 25 to 100 mg, according to age) regulated according to excretion of 17-ketosteroids. After 7–10 days of treatment, maintenance treatment: cortisone IM every third day, or per os daily, adjusting doses to requirement of individual patient.

Prognosis.   Treatment started before age 2 years, normal development; if at later age, no changes in physical appearance or height, but fertility is restored.

FEMALE

Synonyms.   De Crecchio; Apert-Gallais, pseudohermaphroditism, female.

Symptoms.   Rapid and progressive virilization starting from birth; hypertrophic clitoris will have frequent erection. Voice deep; somatic growth accelerated. Pubic and then axillary hair appears between 6 months and 3 years of age. Acne develops early. Somatic growth accelerated. Thick muscles, heavy beard and body hair; no breast development; amenorrhea.

Signs.   Diagnosis easier than in males since at birth various degrees of external genitalia abnormalities are present, resulting in pseudohermaphroditism. Changes may be minimal especially in nonclassic form (simple enlargement of clitoris) to maximal (child is mistaken for a cryptorchid male).

Etiology. See Male.

Pathology. Pseudohermaphroditism with various degrees of abnormal evolution of external genitalia. Five types of abnormality differentiated by the degree of fusion of labial-scrotal folds, development of clitoris, closure of the urogenital sulcus. Ovaries polycystic with thick albuginea, similar to Stein-Leventhal (see). With time, disappearance of follicle and progressive follicular inactivity; cortex entirely stromatous. In rare cases, abnormal adrenal tissue found in the broad ligament. For adrenal changes, see Male.

Diagnostic Procedures. See male plus: nuclear chromatin and chromosomal studies for sex determination. *Urethroscopic examination. X-ray vaginogram* (with injection of radiopaque material).

Therapy. See Male. If condition discovered in early infancy, raise as a female and treat with cortisone. If mistake has been made and child raised as a male, after 3 years of age psychologic evaluation and advice. Hormonal therapy and surgery ideal between 1 and 3 years age. Correction of sex may be considered even in early adult life.

Prognosis. Excellent response. Correction dependent upon degree of abnormalities. Properly treated female may become pregnant. Marked tendency to abortion; in normal offspring normal adrenals function.

BIBLIOGRAPHY. DeCrecchio L: Sopra un caso di apparenza virile in una donna. II. Morgagni 7:151, 1865
Apert M: Dystrophies en relation avec les lésions des capsules surrénales. Bull Soc Pediatr Paris 12:501–518, 1910
Gallais A: Le Syndrome génito-surrénal: Etude anatomo clinique (thesis). Paris, 1912
New MI: Congenital adrenal hyperplasia. In De Groot LJ (ed): Endocrinology, 3rd ed, pp 1813–1835. Philadelphia, WB Saunders, 1995

SODIUM-LOSING FORM

Synonyms. Debré-Fibiger; Fibiger-Debré-von Gierke; Pirie; interrenal androgenic intoxication; salt-wasting CAH.

Symptoms and Signs. Frequency 1/14,000. Appear at 5 to 10 days of age, or later in life if precipitated by infections. Acute adrenal crisis: apathy; anorexia; vomiting; diarrhea; abdominal pain; convulsion; circulatory collapse. In other cases, sudden death without dehydration and circulatory collapse. Severe dehydration; changes in skin color (dusky).

Etiology. See simple virilizing form. Low cortisol secretion contributes to loss of salt.

Pathology. Marked enlargement of zona reticularis and zona fasciculata; atrophy of zona glomerulosa. The adrenal cells are hyperplastic, with eosinophilic cytoplasm, vesicular nuclei, and large nucleoli. Among enlarged hyperpigmented cells, cells with granular cytoplasm, and lipidic vacuoles, often in cordlike arrangements.

Diagnostic Procedures. See simple virilizing form. *Blood.* Hematocrit. Electrolyte studies. High serum potassium appearing before low serum sodium; low bicarbonate. *Electrocardiogram.* Hyperkalemia. *Weight determination. Blood pressure. Nuclear sex chromatin or chromosome studies:* in ambiguous sex.

Therapy. In acute adrenal crisis. (1) Sodium chloride IV (NaCl 0.9% solution) immediately (3 to 6 g NaCl in first 24 hours). (2) Desoxycorticosterone acetate 2 mg IM, if no response. (3) Hydrocortisone 25 mg added to NaCl infusion. After crisis is over (24 to 36 hours). (1) Resumption of oral feeding and 3 to 5 g NaCl a day. (2) Cortisone IM daily; high dose to reach maintenance dose. (3) Then deoxycorticosterone acetate 1 to 2 mg daily. When patient is in good condition. (1) Implantation of 125 mg deoxycorticosterone acetate pellets (effective for 8 to 12 months). Further maintenance. (1) Reimplantation of deoxycorticosterone acetate pellets, or 9-fluorocortisol 5 to 100 μg per day. Mild case. Salt addition to diet only.

BIBLIOGRAPHY. Debré R, Semelaigne G: Hypertrophie considérable des capsules surrénales chez un nourrison mort a 10 mois sans avoir augmente de poid depuis sa naissance. Bull Soc Pediatr Paris 23:270, 1925
New MI: Congenital adrenal hyperplasia. In De Groot LJ (ed): Endocrinology, 3rd ed, pp 1813–1835. Philadelphia, WB Saunders, 1995

HYPERTENSIVE FORM

Synonym. 11-hydroxylase deficiency; adrenal hyperplasia IV.

Symptoms and Signs. Frequency 1/100,000. Moderate to severe hypertension in patient exhibiting symptoms and signs of simple virilizing form (see, respectively, male and female form). Some patients have only minor signs of virilization (nonclassic form).

Etiology. Autosomal recessive inheritance. Chromosomal location 8q Enzyme P450 c11. Deficiency of 11-hydroxylase, which causes absent production of cortisol, increase in ACTH, excessive production of desoxycorticosterone and other cortisol precursors that may cause hypertension.

Pathology. Markedly enlarged adrenals with hyperplastic zona glomerulosa.

Diagnostic Procedures. *Hypertension measurement.* Moderate to severe. *Blood and urine.* Steroid increased DOC, 11-deoxy-cortisol (S); steroid decreased: cortisol, and more or less aldo.

Therapy. Cortisone, as outlined in treatment of simple adrenal hyperplasia of male. Blood pressure responds to treatment.

Prognosis. Good with adequate treatment.

BIBLIOGRAPHY. Birke G, Diczfalusy E, Plantin LO, et al: Familial congenital hyperplasia of the adrenal cortex. Acta Endocrinol (Copenh) 29:55–69, 1958
Hochberg Z, Schechter J, Benderly A, et al: Growth and puberal development in patients with congenital adrenal hyperplasia due to 11-B-hydroxylase deficiency. Am J Dis Child 139:771–776, 1985
New MI: Congenital adrenal hyperplasia. In De Groot LJ (ed) Endocrinology, 3rd ed, pp 1813–1835. Philadelphia, WB Saunders, 1995

17-HYDROXYLASE DEFICIENCY

See Biglieri.

ISOLATED 17,20-LYASE DEFICIENCY

Symptoms and Signs. Both sexes. In males, ambiguous genitalia. Absence of postnatal virilization. At puberal age primary amenorrhea and absence of development of secondary sex characteristics. No hypertension.

Etiology. Autosomal recessive inheritance. Chromosomal location 10. Enzyme 450 c17. Deficient production of 17,20-lyase that impedes synthesis of C 19 sex steroids in adrenals and gonads, and spare cortisol production.

Diagnostic Procedures. *Blood and urine.* Steroid decreased DHEA, testosterone, 4-androstenedione salt metabolism: normal. ACTH or hCG stimulation testing.

BIBLIOGRAPHY. Zachmann M, Prader A: 17–20 Desmolase deficiency. In New MI, Levine LS (eds): Adrenal Diseases in Childhood (Pediatric and Adolescent Endocrinology, vol 13), p 95. Basel, Karger, 1984
Zachmann MM, Kempken B, Manella B, et al: Conversion from pure 17,20-desmolase to combined 17,20-desmolase/17-hydroxylase deficiency with age. Acta Endocr 127:97–99, 1992

FORM WITH 3-HYDROXYSTEROID DEHYDROGENASE DEFICIENCY

Synonyms. Bongiovanni; 3-OH-steroid dehydrogenase deficiency; adrenal hyperplasia II.

Symptoms and Signs. *Female.* Fewer virilization signs than in other form (hypertrophy of clitoris; labial fusion; no displacement of urethral orifice). *Male.* Normal differentiation of external genitals incomplete (perineal hypospadias).

Etiology. Autosomal recessive inheritance. Chromosomal location 1q. Enzyme 3-OH-steroid-dehydrogenase II. 3-Hydroxysteroid dehydrogenase deficiency results in impaired production of testosterone and reduced androgenic activity. Small partial peripheral transformation of dehydroepiandrosterone (DHEA) to testosterone accounts for minor virilization in males and females.

Diagnostic Procedures. *Blood.* Steroid increased. DHEA, 17-OH-pregnenolone; steroid decreased: aldo, testosterone, cortisol. For electrolytes, see sodium-losing form.

Prognosis. Death in early infancy despite medical treatment. In nonclassic form survival possible.

BIBLIOGRAPHY. Bongiovanni AM: Adrenogenital syndrome with deficiency of 3-hydroxysteroid dehydrogenase. J Clin Invest 41:2086–2092, 1962

Zachmann M, Forest MG, De Peretti E: 3–hydroxysteroid dehydrogenase deficiency: follow up study in a girl with pubertal bone age. Hormone Res 11:292–302, 1979

New MI: Congenital adrenal hyperplasia. In De Groot LJ (ed) Endocrinology, 3rd ed, pp 1813–1835. Philadelphia, WB Saunders, 1995

B. CONGENITAL LIPOID HYPERPLASIA OF ADRENAL GLANDS

Synonyms. Praeder-Gunter; cholesterol desmolase deficiency; 20–22 desmolase deficiency; P450 side chain cleavage enzyme; adrenal hyperplasia.

Symptoms and Signs. Weight loss; apathy; anorexia; vomiting; diarrhea. Skin pigmentation. *Male.* Testis in the abdomen or inguinal canal. *Female.* Complete or almost complete female appearance.

Etiology. Autosomal recessive inheritance. Chromosomal location 15 Enzyme 450 scc defect of 3-hydroxysteroid (Bongiovanni syndrome) or altered transformation of cholesterol to pregnenolone. Defect of 20–22 desmolase converting cholesterol to pregnenolone. Mild cases might be confused with 3-hydroxysteroid dehydrogenase deficiency.

Pathology. Enlarged, yellowish, nodular surface caused by focal hyperplasia; cells distended by large deposit of lipoids, rich in cholesterol.

Diagnostic Procedures. Steroid increased: none; steroid decreased: all. Electrolyte changes, see sodium-losing.

Therapy. Cortisone and desoxycorticosterone acetate (temporary response).

Prognosis. Death before 8 months for adrenal insufficiency.

BIBLIOGRAPHY. Praeder A, Gunter HP: Das Syndrom des Pseudohermaphroditismus masculinus bei kongenitaler Nebennierenrindenhyperplasie ohne Androgenüberproduktion (adrenaler Pseudohermaphroditismus masculinus). Helvet Paediatr Acta 10:397–412, 1955

Praeder A, Anders GJ, Habich H: Zur Genetik des kongenitalen adrenogenitalen Syndroms (virilisierende nebennierenhyperplasia). Helvet Paediatr Acta 17:271–284, 1962

New MI: Congenital adrenal hyperplasia. In De Groot LJ (ed) Endocrinology, 3rd ed, pp 1813–1835. Philadelphia, WB Saunders, 1995

C. FEMINIZING ADRENAL TUMORS

Symptoms and Signs. *Young boy.* (Rare). Gynecomastia; accelerated development of bones and musculature. *Young girl.* (Rare, two patients reported). Precocious puberty (3 and 4 years old); breast, pubic, and axillary hair; vaginal bleeding; accelerated development of bones and musculature. *Adult male.* (25 to 66 years old).

Symptoms. Decreased libido and potency; pain at site of tumor.

Signs. Gynecomastia with or without tenderness, and atrophy of testis, areolar pigmentation and seldom secretion; prostate and penis seldom atrophic, generally normal; feminizing hair changes.

Etiology. Carcinomas or adenomas of adrenals.

Pathology. Difficult differentiation between benign and malignant tumors in the adrenal; most or all feminizing tumors believed malignant. Metastasis to lung, liver, local lymph nodes, brain, bones. Contralateral adrenal atrophy or normal atrophic changes in testis.

Diagnostic Procedures. *CT scan, MRI:* evidence of lesion. *Urine.* Estrogens usually highly elevated; 17-ketosteroids increased in most cases; pregnanetriol and pregnanediol usually highly increased; 17-hydroxycorticosteroids in 50% of patients increased. *ACTH stimulation* negative; *cortisone suppression* negative.

Therapy. Surgical removal and X-ray after surgery. Cortisone therapy before and during operation.

Prognosis. Poor. Regression of symptoms and return of spermatogenesis after operation. After surgery frequent appearance of metastasis and death in one year, except in adenomas. In children, more favorable because of earlier diagnosis.

BIBLIOGRAPHY. Bittorf A: Nebennierentumor und Geschelchtsdrüsenausfall beim Manne. Klin Wochenschr 56:776, 1919

Wilkins L: Feminizing adrenal tumor causing gynecomastia in a boy of five years contrasted with virilizing tumor in five-year-old girl; classification of seventy cases of adrenal tumor in children according to their hormonal manifestations and review of eleven cases of feminizing adrenal tumor in adults. J Clin Endocrinol 8:111–132, 1948

Gabrilove JL, Shaima DC, Wotiz HH, et al: Feminizing adrenocortical tumors in the male. Medicine 44:37–53, 1965

Santen RJ: Gynecomastia. In De Groot LJ (ed) Endocrinology, 3rd ed, p 2476. Philadelphia, WB Saunders, 1995

D. VIRILIZING ADRENAL TUMORS

Symptoms and Signs. *Prepubertal female.* From few months to pubertal age. Hirsutism; clitoral hypertrophy; rapid bone and musculature development; no breast development; short stature; no menses at pubertal age. Prepubertal male. Macrogenitosomia Precox. (For other symptoms and signs, see Adrenogenital syndromes: congenital adrenal hyperplasia.) *Adult female.* Usually 30 to 40 years or later; also after menopause. Hirsutism (first sign) beard and mustache and head hair loss: acne; voice change; oligomenorrhea progressing to amenorrhea; clitoral hypertrophy; muscular hypertrophy; loss of fat deposit; breast atrophy; increased libido. *Adult male.* Chance discovery.

Etiology. Carcinomas and adenomas.

Pathology. *Carcinoma.* Usually round, large, localized in one pole of adrenal. Tumor often commixed with some normal tissue; left side more frequent; well vascularized on surface; cellular polymorphism and atypia. *Adenoma.* Normal cells; no mitosis; intact capsule. Difficult differential diagnosis between malignant and benign tumor; frequent metastasis from apparently benign tumor.

Diagnostic Procedures. *CT scan, MRI:* may show tumor. *Urine.* Increase of 17-ketosteroids (with DHEA more than 50% of 17-ketosteroids). *ACTH stimulation* negative. *Cortisone suppression* negative.

Therapy. Surgical removal.

Prognosis. Rapid regression of symptoms after surgery. Virilizing tumor grows slowly. Prognosis, however, depends on degree of malignancy, time of surgery, and presence of metastasis. In malignant type, 3-year survival, 30%. In adenoma, much better.

BIBLIOGRAPHY. Baulieu EE, Peillon F, Migeon CJ: Adrenogenital syndrome. In Eisenstein AB (ed): The Adrenal Cortex. Boston, Little, Brown, 1967

Gabrilove TJ, Seman AT, Sabet R, et al: Virilizing adrenal adenoma with studies on the steroid content of the adrenal venous effluent and a review of the literature. Endocrine Rev 2:462–483, 1981

Kasa-Vubu JZ, Kelch RP: Precocious and delayed puberty: diagnosis and treatment. In De Groot LJ (ed) Endocrinology, 3rd ed, p 1969. Philadelphia, WB Saunders, 1995

ADRENOGENITAL SYNDROMES WITH HIRSUTISM, NONTUMOR FORM

Affects mostly females. Rare cases reported in men.

FEMALE

Synonyms. 21-hydroxylase deficiency mild form; 21-hydroxylase deficiency nonclassical form; cryptic adrenal hyperplasia; simple virilizing adrenal hyperplasia.

Symptoms. Usually patients have normal puberty, menstruation may be normal or abnormal, and some patients become pregnant with normal offspring. Growth accelerated during childhood; premature closure of epiphyses leads to shortened adult stature.

Signs. Important to know date of onset of signs. Hirsutism of various degrees alone or combined with various degrees of masculine habitus and acne.

Etiology. Unknown. Suggested for some cases: partial deficiency of 21-hydroxylase or defect of 11-B-hydroxylase or both. Both forms with and without demonstrated hormonal abnormalities are familial.

A subgroup may be recognized on the basis of the biochemical findings of increased urinary excretion of dehydroepiandrosterone (DHEA), and other androgenic steroids. An increased DHEA excretion combined with hirsutism and menstrual disorders may also be found in mild form of congenital adrenal hyperplasia, simple obesity, Cushing, acromegaly, and mental disorders.

Pathology. In many cases mild form of congenital adrenal hyperplasia. In some cases polycystic ovaries have been found.

Diagnostic Procedures. *Urine.* Increased excretion of pregnanetriol (in 2–3% of total cases); moderate increase of 17-ketosteroids. *Adrenocorticotropic hormone (ACTH) stimulation.* Increase of excretion of pregnanetriol and corticosteroids. *Cortisone suppression.* Decrease of pregnanetriol.

Therapy. Cortisone or synthetic glucocorticoid, prolonged treatment.

Prognosis. With prolonged treatment, decrease of virilization signs. Minor response of hirsutism in some cases; always improvement of menstrual cycles and often correction of sterility.

BIBLIOGRAPHY. Jayle MF, Malassis D, Pinaud H: Excretion de la dehydroepiandrosterone avant et après administration d'ACTH en pathologie surrenalienne. Acta Endocrinol (Copenh) 31:1–32, 1959
Decurt J, Jayle MF, Mauvais-Jarvis P: Virilisme surrenalien para ou postpubertaire avec pregnanetriolurie. Rev Eur Endocrinol 1:17, 1964
Kutten F, Coulin P, Girard F, et al: Late onset adrenal hyperplasia in hirsutism. New Engl J Med 313:224–231, 1985

MALE

Symptoms. Asthenia; sterility.

Signs. Associated with increased hirsutism, gynecomastia.

Etiology. Moderate adrenal hyperplasia. May be partial defect of 21-hydroxylase (?).

Pathology. Adrenal hyperplasia; arrested spermatogenesis.

Diagnostic Procedures. *Sperm count.* Low. *Urine.* Increased 17-ketosteroid (DHEA++) and in some cases, estrogens. *Biopsy of testis.*

Therapy. Cortisone.

Prognosis. Spermatogenesis is resumed following cortisone administration.

BIBLIOGRAPHY. Perloff WW, Hadd HE: The adrenogenital syndrome "Virilizing Type" in an adult male: a case report. Am J Med Sci 234:441–443, 1957

Bigozzi U, Borghi A, Giusti C, et al: An unusual case of adrenal dysfunction in male. J Clin Endocrinol 19:1506–1510, 1959
New MI, White PC, Pang S, et al: The adrenal hyperplasias. In Scriver CR, Beaudet AL, Sly WS, et al: The Metabolic and Molecular Bases of Inherited Disease, 6th ed, pp 1881–1917. New York, McGraw-Hill, 1989

ADRENOLEUKODYSTROPHY

Synonym. ALD; Simerling-Creutzfeld; Addison-Scholz; Addison-Schilder; adrenomyeloneuropathy; AMN; bronze; melanodermic leukodystrophy; sudanophilic leukodystrophy-bronzing of skin-adrenal atrophy; in the past confused with Schilder (see).

Symptoms and Signs. Only males affected. Symptoms and signs of adrenal insufficiency (see Addison) precede neurologic ones (see Schilder) that become evident between 5 and 14 years of age. Onset reported also at various ages, even advanced. Mental development normal to 4–8 year then dementia and progressive neurologic defects. The following subtypes have been identified: Familial form of Addison disease in males without neurologic signs, in females Addison disease with associated mild spastic paraparesis; in young males progressive degeneration of cerebral white matter, often with cortical blindness; in adolescent or young adult males associated cerebral and spinal involvement; in adult males progressive spinal cord degeneration; in heterozygous females chronic nonprogressive spinal cord disorder; in male infants possibly a "connatal" form.

Etiology. Sex-linked recessive inheritance. Gene has been mapped to Xq28. Sporadic forms also described and autosomal recessive inheritance (see Zellweger).

Pathology. *Brain.* Extensive demyelinization or myeloclastic diffuse sclerosis or both; cytoplasmatic inclusion bodies in the macrophages. *Adrenal cortex.* Nests of large eosinophilic cortical cells with hypochromatic nuclei.

Diagnostic Procedures. See Addison. *Cerebrospinal fluid.* Protein elevated; IgG elevated. *CT brain scan and MRI. Tissues* (especially white matter and adrenals) *and body fluids* contain high levels of unbranched fatty acids, ULCFA pentacosamide, tetracosamide.

Therapy. Adrenal hormone replacement is effective for adrenal insufficiency. Diets to normalize ULCFA are in study. Bone marrow transplantation and immunosuppression have been attempted.

Prognosis. Death from 6 months to 4 years from onset of neurologic signs.

BIBLIOGRAPHY. Siemerling E, Creutzfeldt HG: Bronzekrankheit und sklerorisende Encephalomyelitis (diffuse sclerose). Arch Psychiatr Nervenkr 68:217, 1923
Scholz W: Klinische, pathologisch-anatomische underbiologische Undersuchungen bei familiarer, diffuser Hirnsklerose im Kindesalter: Ein Bertrag zur Lehr von den Heredodegenerationem. Z Ges Neurol Psychiatr 99:651–717, 1925
Fanconi A, Prader A, Isler W, et al: Morbus Addison mit Hirnsklerose im Kindesalter. Ein hereditaeres Syndrom mit X-chromosomaler Vererbung? Helv Pediat Acta 18:480–501, 1964
Moser HW, Smith KD, Moser AB: X-linked adrenoleukodystrophy. In Scriver CR, Beaudet AL, Sly WS, et al: The Metabolic and Molecular Bases of Inherited Disease, 7th ed, pp 2325–2349. New York, McGraw-Hill, 1995

ADRENOMYODYSTROPHY

Synonyms. Von Petrykowski.

Symptoms and Signs. Two brothers. Symptoms and signs of Addison (see) plus dystrophic myopathy; chronic constipation, severe psychomotor retardation, terminal massive bladder, megacolon.

Symptoms. Unknown. X-linked recessive phenotype.

Pathology. Liver fatty degeneration. Pituitary: ACTH-producing microadenomas.

Prognosis. Death in early infancy.

BIBLIOGRAPHY. Von Petrykowski W, Beckmann R, Bohm N, et al: Adrenal insufficiency, myopathic hypotonia, severe psychomotor retardation, failure to thrive, constipation and bladder ectasia in two brothers: adrenomyodystrophy. Pediat Res 13:1195, 1979; Helv Pediat Acta 37:387–400, 1982

ADVANCED-SLEEP-PHASE

Synonyms. Insomnia advanced-phase-pattern.

Symptoms and Signs. Usually in healthy elderly persons. Early evening sleep onset (8–9 PM) and early awakening. Forced delaying of onset of sleep does not prevent early awakening.

Etiology. Alteration of normal circadian rhythm of sleep–wake cycle, possibly owing to metabolic alterations.

BIBLIOGRAPHY. Monk TH: Disorders of chronobiology. In Kruger MH, Roth T, Dement WC (eds): Principles and Practice of Sleep Medicine, pp 324–337. Philadelphia, WB Saunders, 1989

ADVERSIVE

Synonym. Compulsory turning.

Symptoms and Signs. Homolateral miosis and turning of head in opposite direction; compulsive turning when patient attempts to progress forward; nystagmus.

Etiology. Following neurosurgery, after ablation of Brodmann area of one frontal lobe; stimulation of red nucleus; nitrogen mustard treatment; neoplastic, inflammatory, or vascular frontal lobe lesions.

Pathology. Ablation of Brodmann area; posterior longitudinal fascicle destruction.

Therapy. Phenylhydantoin.

Prognosis. No recovery.

BIBLIOGRAPHY. Adams RD, Victor M: Principles of Neurology, 5th ed, p 534. New York, McGraw-Hill, 1993

ADYNAMIC BONE DISEASE

Synonyms. Renal adynamic bone.

Symptoms and Signs. Most common in patients with end-stage renal disease (with normal parathyroid function), overtreated with calcium and vitamin D, or with diabetes mellitus or aluminum intoxication. May be asymptomatic or increased fracture rate, and in some cases manifestation of hypogonadism.

Etiology. Decreased ability of bone to take up calcium owing to presence of inhibitors of bone remodeling and deficiency of a factor involved in bone growth and formation. See also symptoms.

Diagnostic Procedures. *Bone biopsy* normal or reduced bone density, absence of bone aluminum. *Blood.* Mild elevation of serum alkaline phosphatase, relatively normal serum parathyroid hormones, hypercalcemia.

Therapy. Control of serum phosphate and calcium; vitamin D analogues.

Prognosis. Increased mortality rate compared with other form of osteodystrophy.

BIBLIOGRAPHY. Moriniere P, Cohen-Solal A, Belbrik S, et al: Disappearance of aluminic bone disease in along term asymptomatic dialysis population restricting Al(OH) intake: emergence of an idiopathic adynamic bone disease not related to aluminum. Nephron 53:93–101, 1989
Hruska KA, Teitelbaum SL: Renal osteodystrophy. New Engl J Med 333:166–174, 1995

AFFERENT LIMB, ACUTE

Synonyms. Blowout of duodenal stump; acute afferent limb.

Symptoms and Signs. After Billroth II gastrectomy and gastroduodenostomy. On fifth to seventh p.o. day acute exacerbation of abdominal pain or fever and discomfort.

Etiology. Obstruction of afferent loop owing to kinking, retroanostomic hernia, or technical misadventure that determines leak of duodenal stump with possible abscess formation.

Diagnostic Procedures. *CT scan; ultrasonography; reintervention:* for second look.

Therapy. Surgery with repair.

Prognosis. Fifty percent mortality.

BIBLIOGRAPHY. Matsusue S, Kashihara S, Takeda H, et al: Three cases of afferent loop obstruction: the role of ultrasonography in the diagnosis. Jpn J Surg 18:709–713, 1988
Donahue PE: Early postoperative and postgastrectomy syndromes in postsurgical syndromes. Gastoenterol Clin N Am 23:215–226, 1994

AFZELIUS (A.)

Synonyms. Lipschutz; erythema chronicum migrans.

Symptoms and Signs. Both sexes affected; onset all ages. More common in Scandinavia; in the USA associated with Lyme arthritis (see). Eruption of single or multiple lesions of erythema annulare centrifugum, expanding to reach massive extension. Meningitic symptoms and signs in a number of cases.

Etiology. Tick (Ixodes) bite. Borrelia spirochete.

Therapy. Penicillin; tetracyclins; and other antibiotics.

Prognosis. Prompt response to treatment.

BIBLIOGRAPHY. Afzelius A: Erythema chronicum migrans. Acta Derm Venereol (Stockh) 2:120–125, 1921
Hellerström S: Erythema chronicum migrans Afzelli. Acta Derm Venereol (Stockh) 11:315–321, 1930
Champion RH: Disorders of blood vessels. In Champion RH, Burton JL, Ebling FJG (eds): Rook/Wilkinson/Ebling Textbook of Dermatology, 5th ed, pp 1014–1015. Oxford, Blackwell Scientific, 1992

AGAMMAGLOBULINEMIA

Synonym. Antibody deficiency.

CONGENITAL

See individual syndromes.

Symptoms and Signs. Normal at birth; onset at about ninth month of life. Increased susceptibility to infections caused by pyogenic bacteria, controlled by antimicrobial chemotherapy. Manifestation of atopy. Failure to thrive as consequence of repeated infections. If surviving, chronic bronchiectasis, a condition similar to rheumatoid arthritis (may precede infection manifestation), and other collagen-like conditions may develop.

Etiology. See immunologic deficiency syndromes.

ACQUIRED

Symptoms. Both sexes affected; onset in adulthood. Susceptibility to recurrent sinusitis, pneumonia, chronic progressive bronchiectasis. Sprue-like syndrome. Protein-losing enteropathy. Arthritic manifestation (rare in this form). Exfoliative dermatitis; nephrotic syndrome (occasionally).

Signs. Hepatosplenomegaly (frequent); evidence of noncaseating granulomas in lungs, skin, liver, spleen (without particular microorganism involved).

Etiology. Associated, through unknown mechanism, with lymphatic system malignancies, or other dysglobulinemic conditions (e.g., myoclonia). Possibility of a congenital type suggested by occurrence in relatives. See Immunologic deficiency syndromes (secondary).

BIBLIOGRAPHY. Butler JL, Cooper MD: Antibody deficiency diseases. In Scriver CR, Beaudet AL, Sly WS, et al: The Metabolic and Molecular Bases of Inherited Disease, 6th ed, pp 2689–2693. New York, McGraw-Hill, 1989
Lukens JN: Immune deficiency diseases: inherited and acquired: In Lee GR, Bithel TC, Foerster J, et al (eds): Wintrobe's Clinical Hematology, 9th ed. Philadelphia, Lea & Febiger, 1993

AGE-RELATED MACULOPATHY

Synonyms. Documented under a variety of eponyms: senile macular degeneration; retina posterior pole colloidal degeneration. Haab; Junius-Khunt; Hutchinson-Tay guttate choroiditis; Doyne honeycomb choroiditis; Holthouse-Batten superficial choroiditis; Malattia levantinese. The different syndromes present several common features but with some clinical differences and different types of inheritance or are sporadic. The most important have been individually reported.

BIBLIOGRAPHY. Haab O: Erkrankungen der Macula Lutea Zentralbl Augenheilkd 9:384–391, 1885
Garner A, Sarks S, Sarks JP: Degenerative and related disorders of the retina and choroid. In Garner A, Klintworth GK (eds): Pathobiology of Ocular Disease: A Dynamic Approach, 2nd ed, p 631. New York, Marcel Dekker, 1994

AGLOSSIA-ADACTYLIA

Synonyms. De Jussieu; Meyer; Hanhart II; hypoglossia-hypodactyly.

Symptoms and Signs. Total or partial absence of tongue; underdeveloped mandible; enlargement of sublingual muscular ridges; hypertrophy of sublingual and submaxillary glands; cleft and high arched palate; lower lip defects; missing lower incisors; bony fusion of dental arches; intraoral bands. Hypoplasia of extremities: from complete peromelia to absence of distal digits; syndactylia; anonychia. Dextrocardia; transposed viscera.

Etiology. Unknown. Intrauterine environmental factors; expression of lack of genes responsible for growth of distal structures(?).

Pathology. See Symptoms and Signs.

Diagnostic Procedures. Chromosome studies. Normal.

Therapy. Depending on manifestation, surgical or orthopedic corrections or both.

Prognosis. If intelligence not impaired and tongue not totally absent, speech not severely affected.

BIBLIOGRAPHY. De Jussieu M: Observation sur la manière dont une fille sans langue s'acquitte des fonctions qui dépendent de cet organe. Hist Acad Roy Soc (Paris) Mem:6–14; 1718–1719

Meyer MW: Über die angeborenen Fehlen der Zunge und die dadurch bedingte Hinderung des Saugens. Jahrb Kinderhulkd 13:328–354, 1849
Hanhart E: Über die Kombination von Peromelie mit Mickrognathie, ein neues Syndrom beim Menschen, entsprechend der Akroteriasis congenita von Wriedt und Mohr beim Rind. Arch Hlaus Stift Vererbungsforsch 25:531–543, 1950
Schuhl JF: L'aglossie-adactylie. A propos d'une observation. Revue de la littérature. Ann Pediatr (Paris) 33:137–140, 1986

AICARDI

Synonyms. Chorioretinal anomalies—corpus callosum agenesis—infantile spasms; corpus callosum (agenesis)—chorioretinal abnormality.

Symptoms. In females only (males, intrauterine death). Infantile spasms, which may become manifest between 1 day and 4 months of age; epileptic attacks; mental abnormalities; hypotonia; delayed postural acquisition.

Signs. Microcephaly and head deformities: biparietal bossing; occipital flattening; plagiocephaly; facial asymmetry; low-set ears; microphthalmia. Cyanosis. Telangiectasia. Vertebral anomalies: hemivertebra; fusion; spina bifida. Rib anomalies. Absence of pupillary reflexes. Specific diagnostic chorioretinopathy. Cleft-lip-palate and holoprosencephaly (seldom).

Etiology. Possibly, single dominant gene of X-chromosome is determinant. Unknown. The current theories include congenital infection, an X-linked genetic defect, and an intrauterine environmental agent.

Pathology. See Signs. Agenesis of corpus callosum.

Diagnostic Procedures. *X-ray, CT brain scan, MR imaging.* Bat-wing deformity of third and lateral ventricles. Typical image of total agenesis of corpus callosum (in most cases) or, less evident, electroencephalography. Hypsarrhythmia asynchronous burst suppression discharges and sleep spindles. *Spinal fluid.* Normal. *Blood and urine.* Normal. *Dermatoglyphics.* High number of digital arches. *Chromosome studies.* Normal. *Ophthalmologic findings.* Microphtalmia, nystagmus, optic nerve colobomas, and pathognomonic chorioretinal lesions: multiple lacunae with the aspect of atrophic white-yellowish, round holes crossed over by vessels. Funnel-shaped disk.

Therapy. Hydrocortisone; adrenocorticotropic hormone (ACTH); antiepileptic compounds.

Prognosis. Manifestations progress with age. Temporary improvement with treatment. High mortality for different causes. If onset of symptoms in adolescent period, greater life expectancy.

BIBLIOGRAPHY. Aicardi J, Chevrie JJ, Rousselie F: Le syndrome spasmes en flexion, agénesie calleuse, anomalies chorio-rétiniennes. Arch Fr Pediatr 26:1103–1120, 1969
Baierl P, Markl A, Thelen M, et al: MR imaging in Aicardi syndrome. AJNR 9:805–806, 1988
Donnenfeld AE, Packer RJ, Zackay EH, et al: Clinical, cytogenic and pedigree findings in 18 cases of Aicardi syndrome. AMJ Med Genet 32:461–467, 1989
Adams RD, Victor M: Principles of Neurology, 5th ed, p 1017. New York, McGraw-Hill, 1993

AICARDI-GOUTIERES

Synonyms. Encephalopathy infantile—calcification basal ganglia—chronic CSF lymphocytosis. See Fahr.

Symptoms and Signs. Normal at birth. Onset at approximately 3 months. Manifestation of encephalopathy, spastic quadraplegia, mental retardation, in some cases microcephaly.

Etiology. Unknown. Possibly autosomal recessive inheritance.

Pathology. Brain: No evidence of infection lymphocytes infiltration. Calcification of basal ganglia.

Diagnostic Procedures. *Blood.* No evidence of infections. *Spinal fluid.* Pleiocytosis. Lymphocytes. *X-rays, CT scan.* Frontal atrophy; hypodensity of white matter, basal ganglia calcification.

Therapy. Symptomatic.

Prognosis. Leads to a progressive vegetative status and early death.

BIBLIOGRAPHY. Aicardi J, Goutieres F: A progressive familial encephalopathy in infancy with calcification of the basal ganglia and chronic cerebrospinal fluid lymphocytosis. Ann Neurol 15:49–54, 1984

Mehta L, Trounce JQ, Moore RJ, et al: Familial calcification of the basal ganglia with cerebrospinal fluid pleocytosis. J Med Gen 23:157–160, 1986

AIDS

Synonyms. Acquired immunodeficiency syndrome; HIV infection.

Symptoms and Signs. In homosexuals, drug addicts, patients treated with blood or derivates, or through vertical transmission from infected mothers to fetus or neonate. Demonstrated in residents of all five continents. Following infection, usually period asymptomatic of variable length, then generalized lymphoadenopathy with or without a constellation of signs and symptoms: termed "the AIDS-related complex" or "ARC": fever, weight loss, diarrhea, fatigue, night sweats. Patients can die from ARC, or develop full-blown AIDS, that is: pneumocystic carinii pneumonia; cytomegalovirus infections; persistent diarrhea; acute or chronic meningitis; progressive dementia; hypercatabolic wasting syndrome; Kaposi sarcoma, and other malignancies.

Etiology. Infection with the human retrovirus HTLV III/LAV (renamed HIV). That selectively attacks cells that express the CD4 membrane glycoprotein in particular T lymphocytes, monocytomacrophages, and neuronal cells.

Diagnostic Procedures and Pathology. Immunologic profile: lymphopenia with a selective deficiency of the T4 subset of lymphocytes (a CD4 cell count of fewer than 200–250 in an HIV-positive subject is diagnostic); presence of antibodies to the retrovirus (enzyme-linked immunoabsorbent assay ELISA and Western blot testing with HIV-antigen is highly specific); isolation of the virus from peripheral blood lymphocytes or other body materials (blood, saliva, bronchoalveolar lavage). Abnormalities associated with progression to symptomatic disease: lowered CD4–positive lymphocytes; raised CD8-positive lymphocytes; anemia; cytopenia; high VES; high microglobulin; high IgA; reduced cellular immune function; reduced HIV-specific cytotoxicity; reduced anti-p24; raised p24; raised viral load; raised syncytium-inducing viral phenotype.

Therapy. Radiation therapy for the transient palliation of Kaposi sarcoma; chemotherapy against the malignant diseases; antimicrobial agents for the various infections; management of fever, of breathlessness, of acute brain syndrome, of wasting syndrome, etc. Specific drugs against the virus have been tried, with variable success: zidovudine; didanosine; zalcitabine; combination therapy. Immune reconstitution: bone marrow transplantation; infusion of histocompatible lymphocytes; IL-2; interferons.

Prognosis. Poor. Mortality once form fully expressed is very likely to approach 100% at the present stage.

BIBLIOGRAPHY. Fauci AS, Masur H, Gellmann EP, et al: The acquired immunodeficiency syndrome: an update. Ann Intern Med 102:800–813, 1985

Fauci A: AIDS: immunopathogenic mechanism and research strategies. Clin Res 35:503–510, 1987

Edelman AS, Zolla-Pazner S: AIDS: A syndrome of immune dysregulation, dysfunction and deficiency. FASEB J 3:22–30, 1989

Weller IVD, Conlon CP, Peto TEA: HIV infection and AIDS. In Weatherall DJ, Ledingham JGG, Warrell DA (eds): Oxford Text- book of Medicine, 3rd ed, pp 467–483. Oxford, Oxford Med Pub, 1996

AIDS EMBRYOPATHY

Symptoms and Signs. Growth failure; microcephaly; hypertelorism; marked prominence and boxlike appearance of the forehead; a flat nasal bridge that, because of the prominent forehead, appears "scooped out" in profile; mild upward or downward obliquity of the eyes; long palpable fissures with blue sclerae; a short nose with flattening of the columella; a well-formed, triangular philtrum; markedly patulous lips.

Etiology. Dysmorphic syndrome associated with intrauterine HTLV-III infection.

Diagnostic Procedures. *Blood.* Antibodies to HTVL-III measured by ELISA or Western blot techniques; after the first 6 months of life immunologic aberrations: reverse T4 to T8 ratios, depressed lymphocyte mitogenic responses, hypergammaglobulinemia.

Therapy. Symptomatic.

Prognosis. Unknown (recently described). Probably poor.

BIBLIOGRAPHY. Marion RW, Wiznia AA, Hutcheon G, Rubinstein A: Human T-cell lymphotropic virus type III (HTLV III) embryopathy. Am J Dis Child 140:638–640, 1986

Barbour SD: Acquired immunodeficiency syndrome of childhood. Pediatr Clin North Amer 34247–268, 1987

Lyman WD, Rubinstein A: Pediatric AIDS: Clinical, pathologic and basic sciences perspective. Proc New York Acad Sci Conf v 693, 1993

Scott GB: Special consideration in children. In Broder S, Merigan TC, Bolognesi D: Textbook of AIDS Medicine, pp 169–181. Baltimore, Williams & Wilkins, 1994

AINHUM

Synonym. Dactylolysis spontanea; Ombanja (Bantu); constricting bands of extremities; including pseudo-ainhum and factitial-ainhum.

Symptoms and Signs. Found mostly in black races in Africa, America, and the Panama Canal Zone. Cases in whites have been reported. Onset between 30 and 40 years of age. True ainhum affects the fifth toe exclusively. In the pseudo-ainhum other fingers and toes encircled by tight constricting bands 0.5 to 1.0 cm wide. Frequently, there is associated hyperkeratosis of palms and soles, and thickening of skin with wart-like formation over joints (usually knee). Absence of systemic manifestations.

Etiology. Abnormal blood supply to the foot in true ainhum. In pseudo-ainhum, associated with various neurologic and ectodermal dysplasias (see Vohwinkel syndrome), erythropoietic protoporphyria, or infections. Dominant inheritance also reported. Factitial owing to self-application of a rubber tourniquet.

Pathology. Connective tissue constricting bands. Epidermal hypertrophy; thickened; bone resorption and skin ulceration of involved digits.

Diagnostic Procedures. *X-ray.* Absorption of the bones. Arteriography: in true ainhum: posterior tibial artery attenuated at the ankle, and absence of plantar arch and its branches.

Therapy. Protection from trauma; control of secondary infections; transverse incision of constricting bands or amputation. In pseudo-ainhum staged Z-plasty also indicated.

Prognosis. Unsatisfactory results from surgery except in pseudo-ainhum, where benefits have been reported with the indicated technique.

BIBLIOGRAPHY. Da Silva JF: On Ainhum. Arch Derm Syph 6:367–376, 1880

Horwitz MT, Tunick I: Ainhum: report of six cases in New York. Arch Derm Syph 36:1058–1063, 1937

Christopher AP, Grattan CEH, Cowan MA: Pseudoainhum and erythropoietic protoporphyria. Br J Dermat 118:113–116, 1988

Burton JL: Disorders of connective tissue. In Champion RH, Burton JL, Ebling FJG (eds): Rook/Wilkinson/Ebling Textbook of Dermatology, 5th ed, pp 1823–1824. Oxford, Blackwell Scientific, 1992

AKINETIC

Synonym. Hypokinetic.

Symptoms. Muscular rigidity associated with slight slowing of voluntary movement. Speech is slow and monotonous. Tremor may be present, mostly in upper extremity and usually hands and forearms; little movement. Disorder of station and gait. Facial expression fixed, with infrequent blinking.

Signs. Cogwheel phenomenon; tendon reflexes normal; Babinski negative.

Etiology. Part of the paralysis agitans (Parkinson) syndrome (see).

Pathology. Multiple lesions, now well defined, affecting the globus pallidus, substantia nigra, and other parts of extrapyramidal system.

Diagnostic Procedures. Neurologic examination. *CT scan. MRI.*

Therapy. Belladonna and derivatives; synthetic substance such as trihexyphenidyl hydrochloride (Artane); cyrimine hydrochloride (Pagitane); procyclidine hydrochloride (Kemadrine), levamphetamine, levodopa; amantadine hydrochloride, imipramine; amieziptyline. Neurosurgical procedures available.

Prognosis. Progressive condition, partially relieved by medical and surgical procedures.

BIBLIOGRAPHY. Adams RD, Victor M: Principles of Neurology, 5th ed, pp 84, 977. New York, McGraw-Hill, 1993

AKINETIC MUTISM

Synonyms. Cairns. Eponym used also as a rather arbitrary designation to indicate various states of impaired cosciousness such as the persistent vegetative state, the locked-in syndrome, the coma vigile, or the abulia.

Symptoms. Silent, brief immobility that characterizes certain subacute or chronic states of altered consciousness in which sleep–wake cycles have returned, but external evidence for mental activity remains almost entirely absent and spontaneous motor activity is lacking.

Etiology. Large bilateral frontal lobe lesions; bilateral diffuse destruction of the cerebral cortical mouth; bilateral hemispheric demyelinizations, hydrocephalus; large bilateral lesions of ganglia; paramedial lesions of the reticular formation of the midbrain.

Diagnostic Procedures. *CAT. MRI. ECG. Sensory evoked potentials. Electroencephalographic brain mapping.*

Therapy. As in persistent vegetative state.

Prognosis. Variable.

BIBLIOGRAPHY. Cairns H, Oldfield RC, Pennybacker JB, et al: Akinetic mutism with an epidermoid cyst of the third ventricle. Braim 64:273, 1941

Adams RD, Victor M: Principles of Neurology, 5th ed, pp 302–303. New York, McGraw-Hill, 1993

ALA DEHYDRATASE DEFICIENCY PORPHYRIA

Synonyms. ALADP, Doss.

Symptoms and Signs. Only six cases reported. Two adolescents: vomiting, pain in arms and legs, mixed motor/sensor, neuropathy, abdominal pain; clinical exacerbation following stress, alcohol. One patient had onset at 2 years of age with general muscle hypotonia, paralysis of legs, and respiratory insufficiency. One adult (63 years old) exhibited polyneuropathy. This patient had also myeloproliferative disease. Two siblings (26 and 28 years of age) exhibited similar porphyric symptoms.

Etiology. Autosomal recessive inheritance. Homozygosity for defective ALA dehydratase.

Diagnostic Procedures. *Urine.* Massive elevation of ALA, elevations of porphyrins. *Blood.* Elevation of porphyrin. *Erythrocytes.* Zn-protoporphirin. *Feces.* Elevation of porphyrins.

Therapy. Supportive. Intravenous glucose.

Prognosis. Good for survival.

BIBLIOGRAPHY. Doss M, Von Tieppermann R, Schneider J, et al: New types of hepatic porphyria with porphobilinogen synthase defeat and intermittent acute clinical manifestation. Klin Wochenschr 57:1123, 1127, 1979

Kappas A, Sassa S, Galbranth RA, et al: The porphyrias. In Scriver CR, Beaudet AL, Sly WS, et al: The Metabolic and Molecular Bases of Inherited Disease, 7th ed, pp 2113–2116. New York, McGraw-Hill, 1995

ALACRIMA, CONGENITAL

Synonyms. Dry eye, including: agenesis of lacrimary glands.

Symptoms and Signs. Congenital form present in children; unilateral form very rare. unilateral form very rare. Deficient lacrimal secretion. Duct orifices may be present or absent, lacrimal points absent or atretic.

Etiology. Sporadic; dominant inheritance reported in some cases. It may be classified into five categories: persistence of normal lack of tears in newborn; neurogenic hyposecretion; absence or hypoplasia of lacrimal gland; associated Riley-Day syndrome; associated anhydrotic ectodermal dysplasia; or in association with other nervous system anomalies, such as aplasia of cranial nerve nuclei or associated with agenesis of salivary glands.

Pathology. According to the above categories. Aplasia of gland, injury or aplasia of trigeminal (V), facial (VII) nerve, or respective nuclei, greater superficial petrosal nerve, sphenopalatine ganglion, geniculate ganglion.

Diagnostic Procedures. See associated syndromes.

Therapy. Protective ointment. In some cases occlusion of the lacrimal puncta is helpful. In severe cases tarsorraphy may be necessary to protect the cornea.

Prognosis. See associated syndromes.

BIBLIOGRAPHY. Thurnam J: Two cases in which the skin, hair, and teeth were very imperfectly developed. Med Chir Trans 31:71–82, 1848

Smith RS, Maddox SF, Collins BE: Congenital alacrima. Arch Ophthalmol 79:45–48, 1968

Milunsky J M, Lee VW, Siegel BS, et al: Agenesis or hypoplasia of major salivary and lacrimal glands. Am J Med Genet 37:371–374, 1990

Uleckas JK, Garel L, Milot J, et al: Orbital scan in congenital alacrima. J Pediat Ophthalmol Strabismus 31:114–117, 1994

Moore BD: Lacrimal system abnormalities. Optom Vis Sci 71:182–183, 1994

ALACTASIA

Synonyms. Lactase deficiency in infancy; lactase isolated intolerance; disaccharide intolerance III, primary adult type hypolactasia.

Symptoms and Signs. Both sexes affected; variable age of onset. Usually intolerance to milk, and other symptoms that appear in adolescence or young adult life, although the symptomatology may begin at 3 to 4 years of age. Quite rare in infants and young children (inherited or of transitory type). In infants, diarrhea, failure to thrive, dehydration. At later age, ill-defined complaint of milk intolerance; irritable bowel syndrome (see).

Etiology. This is actually not a disease because 1/3–1/2 of the population presents lactase intolerance after 5–6 years of age, but on low milk diet does not manifest symptoms. Two phenotypes of lactase absorptions exist: lactase persistence (LACP) and lactase resistance (LACR). To have low lactase digestion capacity (LDC) one has to be homozygous for LACR. Variable: hereditary form autosomal recessive with onset of manifestation at various age; temporary deficiency related to various pathologic conditions; deficiency secondary to reduced mucosal contact time after surgery of gastrointestinal tract.

Pathology. No constant features. Possibly, blunting of duodenal and jejunal villi.

Diagnostic Procedures. *Intestinal biopsy.* Histologic and enzyme assays. *Oral lactose tolerance test.* Development of the syndrome. C-lactose breath test. *Hydrogen breath test. Urine.* Lactosuria.

Therapy. Elimination of lactose from diet.

Prognosis. Except in rare cases in infancy, usually a tolerable condition, which does not produce any severe complication.

BIBLIOGRAPHY. Auricchio S, Rubino A, Semenza G, et al: Isolated intestinal lactase deficiency in the adult. Lancet 2:324, 1963
Dahlqvist A, Hammond B, Crane RK, et al: Intestinal lactase deficiency and lactose intolerance in adults: preliminary report. Gastroenterology 45:488, 1963
Flatz G: The genetic polymorphism of intestinal lactase activity in adult humans. In Scriver CR, Beaudet AL, Sly WS, et al: The Metabolic and Molecular Bases of Inherited Disease, 7th ed, pp 4441–4450. New York, McGraw-Hill, 1995

ALAJOUANINE

Symptoms and Signs. Both sexes affected. In newborn, bilateral facial (VII) and external oculomotor (VI) paralysis; convergent strabismus. Talipes equinovarus.

Etiology. Unknown.

BIBLIOGRAPHY. Alajouanine T, Huc G, Gopcevitch M, et al: Quatre cas d'une affection congénitale caractérisée par une double pied bot, une double paralysie faciale et une double paralysie de la sixième paire. Rev Neurol (Paris) 2:501–511, 1930

ALBATROSS

Synonyms. Postgastrectomy–personality defect. See also Bile reflux.

Symptoms. In patients with (1) history of antisocial behavior, (2) addiction to salicylates or other analgesics, (3) psychiatric illness or personality derangements, who have had any type of surgical treatment for peptic ulcer disease. Abdominal pain without demonstrable cause; intermittent nausea; vomiting; continuing dependency on analgesic drugs; severe nutritional deficiency.

Signs. Lack of correlation between objective signs and symptomatology. Weight loss and other signs of malnutrition.

Etiology. Psychologic derangement focusing its expression in an actual (iatrogenic) anatomic and physiologic defect. Syndrome named after the poem by Coleridge in which the sailor shot the albatross. When calamity followed, his shipmates hung the dead bird around his neck.

Pathology. Some patients have true ulcer; generally no ulcer found at surgery.

Diagnostic Procedures. *X-rays* of gastrointestinal tract.

Therapy. Prophylaxis very important; careful screening of patients with this type of psychologic derangement before surgery. Psychotherapy; correction of malnutrition.

Prognosis. Poor; recurrence of symptoms with request for continuous medical care.

BIBLIOGRAPHY. Johnstone FR, Holubitsky IB, Debas HT: Post-gastrectomy problems in patients with personality defects: the "albatross" syndrome. Can Med Assoc J 96:1559–1564, 1967
Richie WP: Alkaline reflux gastritis in postsurgical syndromes. Gastroent Clin North Am 23:281–294, 1994

ALBERS-SCHÖNBERG I

Synonyms. Henck-Assman; marble bones; ivory bones; osteosclerosis fragilis generalisata; osteopetrosis generalisata. See Carbonic anhydrase II deficiency.

ADULT BENIGN DOMINANT FORM

Synonym. Henck-Assman.

Symptoms. Asymptomatic (50%); fractures (40%); osteomyelitis of mandible (10%); cranial nerve palsy (16%); optic (II), oculomotor (III), facial (VII) nerves optic atrophy. Bone pains most frequently in lumbar areas.

Signs. Nonspecific; frontal bossing (18%); exophthalmos (6%); no hepatosplenomegaly.

Etiology. Unknown; dominant inheritance with variable expression. Suggested abnormality of thyrocalcitonin.

Pathology. Absence or reduction of medullary cavity areas of hematopoiesis in enlarged haversian canals. Noncalcified hyaline cartilage remnants diffuse in the bones. Few fibrils in bone matrix and seldom cross between osteons. Remodeling of bone prominent.

Diagnostic Procedures. *Blood.* Normal, except for increase of acid phosphatase. *X-rays.* Required for diagnosis. Bones symmetrically involved by diffuse sclerotic process is early sign; increased density of diaphyseal region of growing bones.

Therapy. Symptomatic.

Prognosis. Good; normal longevity may be expected with this form. Cranial nerve palsy may be incapacitating, but does not affect longevity.

MALIGNANT RECESSIVE FORM

Symptoms and Signs. Manifestation in childhood. Optic atrophy (78%); poor growth (36%); repeated fractures (28%); deafness (22%); mental retardation (22%); osteomyelitis (18%); facial palsy (10%); splenomegaly (62%); hepatomegaly (48%); frontal bossing (34%); large head (22%); lymphoadenopathy (18%); genu valgum (16%); pectus deformities (8%).

Etiology. Recessive inheritance. Failure of bone resorption.

Pathology. See Benign form. Myeloid metaplasia in spleen and liver.

Diagnostic Procedures. *Blood.* Anemia; thrombocytopenia. Nucleated red cells and immature myeloid elements. Increased acid phosphatases. *X-rays.* Required for diagnosis. Bones symmetrically involved by diffuse sclerotic process is early sign; increased density of diaphyseal region of growing bones.

Therapy. No specific treatment, treat metabolic acidosis till late adolescence. Orthopedic management.

Prognosis. Poor. No patient has lived past 20 years of age. Usually death in infancy because of anemia or infections.

CLINICALLY INTERMEDIATE FORMS

BIBLIOGRAPHY. Albers-Schönberg H: Roentgenbilder einer seltenen Knochenerkrankung. München Med Wochenschr 51:365, 1904

Sly WS, Hu PY: The carbonic anhydrase II deficiency syndrome: osteopetrosis with renal tubular acidosis and cerebral calcification. In Scriver CR, Beaudet AL, Sly WS, et al: The Metabolic and Molecular Bases of Inherited Disease, 7th ed, pp 4113–4124. New York, McGraw-Hill, 1995

ALBERT

Synonyms. Schanz I; Achilles tendon bursitis; achillodynia; hindfoot bursitis; calcaneal bursitis.

Symptoms. Pain and difficulty in walking.

Signs. Swelling of different consistencies (from tense to bony) over posterior part of foot; frequently, hyperkeratosis of overlying skin; associated occasionally with infections.

Etiology. Chronic irritation from shoes; overprominent border of calcaneus; trauma.

Pathology. Bursitis in region of attachment of Achilles tendon. In some cases calcification in the bursae.

Diagnostic Procedures. *X-ray.*

Therapy. Reduction of pressure on inflamed area. Topical cortisone injection. Surgery seldom efficient.

Prognosis. Tendency to relapse.

BIBLIOGRAPHY. Albert E: Achillodynie. Wien Med Presse 34:41–43, 1893

Schanz A: Eine typische Erkrankung der Achilles. Schne Zbl Chir 32:1289–1291, 1905

Klippel JH, Dieppe PA: Rheumatology, pp 5.13.7–5.13.8. St Louis, Mosby, 1995

ALBINISM-MICROCEPHALY-DIGITAL ANOMALIES

Synonyms. Microcephaly—albinism—digital anomalies.

Symptoms and Signs. Both sexes. Microcephaly, oculocutaneous albinism, hypoplasia of fingers and agenesis of the phalanx of toe.

Etiology. Autosomal recessive.

Therapy. Symptomatic. See Albinism, minimal pigment type.

Prognosis. Poor.

BIBLIOGRAPHY. Castro-Gago M, Pombo M, Novo I, et al: Syndrome familiar de microcefalia con albinism oculocutaneo y anomalias digitales. Ann Esp Pediatr 19:128–131, 1983

ALBINISM, OCULAR, AUTOSOMAL RECESSIVE

Synonyms. Autosomal recessive ocular albinism, AROA; OAAR.

Symptoms and Signs. Both sexes equally affected; onset from birth. Skin and hair color normal, with presence of pigmented nevi or freckles (or both) and without increased tendency to skin neoplasia. Eye color presents normal range. Nystagmus and photophobia are present in variable intensities; visual acuity shows moderate to severe decrease.

Etiology. Autosomal recessive inheritance.

Pathology. Melanosomes are normal.

Diagnostic Procedures. *Ophthalmoscopy. Transillumination of iris* shows cartwheel to diaphanus pattern; in males red reflex present; in both sexes there is some retinal pigment in the posterior. *Blood.* Serum

tyrosine and the beta melanocyte-stimulating hormone level are unknown. *Incubation of hair bulb in tyrosine:* pigmentation.

Therapy. None.

Prognosis. Good.

BIBLIOGRAPHY. King RA, Hearing VJ, Creel DJ, et al: Albinism. In Scriver CR, Beaudet AL, Sly WS, et al: The Metabolic and Molecular Bases of Inherited Disease, 7th ed, p 4378. New York, McGraw-Hill, 1995

ALBINISM, OCULAR-LATE ONSET

SENSINEURAL DEAFNESS

Synonyms. Ocular albinism—sensineural deafness, OASD; deafness—ocular albinism. See Margolis-Ziprkowski and Nettleship-Falls.

Symptoms and Signs. In male (Afrikaner). From birth. Typical ocular albinism. In middle age, develop moderate deafness.

Etiology. X-linked recessive inheritance.

Pathology. Typical of this albinism is presence of numerous macromelanosomes on skin biopsy.

BIBLIOGRAPHY. Winship I, Gericke G, Beighton P: X linked inheritance of ocular albinism with late-onset sensorineural deafness. Am J Med Genet 19:797–803, 1984

King RA, Hearing VJ, Creel DJ, et al: Albinism. In Scriver CR, Beaudet AL, Sly WS, et al: The Metabolic and Molecular Bases of Inherited Disease, 7th ed, pp 123, 225. New York, McGraw-Hill, 1995

ALBINISM, OCULAR MINIMAL PIGMENT TYPE

Synonyms. OCA1MP; albinism platinum form.

Symptoms and Signs. From birth. No pigment in skin and eyes. Irides blue to gray. Minimal amount of pigment develops in first decade of life. Iris translucency from + to ++++. Nystagmus present for life. Visual acuity 20/50 to 20/400. Pigmented nevi or freckles possible. Hair: white, turning light yellow with time.

Etiology. Autosomal recessive. Gene involved Tyrosinase, location 11q.

Diagnostic Procedures. *Hairbulb tyrosinase activity.* Nonmeasurable.

Therapy. Protection with a broad-spectrum sunscreen preparation during exposure to sunlight.

Prognosis. Depends on the occurrence of skin cancer.

BIBLIOGRAPHY. King RA, Wirtsehafter JD, Olds DL, et al: Minimal pigment: a new type of oculocutaneous albinism. Clin Genet 29:42–50, 1986

King RA, Hearing VJ, Creel DJ, et al: Albinism. In Scriver CR, Beaudet AL, Sly WS, et al: The Metabolic and Molecular Bases of Inherited Disease, 7th ed, pp 4371–4372. New York, McGraw-Hill, 1995

ALBINISM, OCULAR-TEMPERATURE SENSITIVE

Synonyms. OCA1TS.

Symptoms and Signs. Both sexes. Skin color white, pigmented nevir freckles possible, hair white at birth, after puberty changes on limbs, not on scalp and axilla. Iris blue to gray, translucency ++++, retinal pigment absent, nystagmus, visual acuity strongly reduced.

Etiology. Autosomal recessive inheritance gene involved tyrosinase, location 11q.

Diagnostic Procedures. *Tyrosinase analysis of hairbulb* show that the enzyme is temperature-sensitive losing activity at about 35°C (so that melanin of hairs on cooler areas of body are synthesized).

BIBLIOGRAPHY. King RA, Towsend D, Oetting WS, et al: Temperature sensitive tyrosinase associated with periferal pigmentation in oculocutaneous albinism. J Clin Invest 87:1046–1053, 1991

King RA, Hearing VJ, Creel DJ, et al: Albinism. In Scriver CR, Beaudet AL, Sly WS, et al: The Metabolic and Molecular Bases of Inherited Disease, 7th ed, p 4372. New York, McGraw-Hill, 1995

ALBINISM, OCULAR-TY-NEG

Synonyms. ATN; Garrod albinism; albinism I; oculocutaneous–Ty-neg albinism; OCA1A; tyrosine negative albinism; albinism (complete, perfect).

Symptoms and Signs. Both sexes affected; present from birth. Skin color pink to red; hair color white (for all of life); absence of pigmented nevi and freckles; high incidence of skin neoplasia. Eye color gray to blue, red reflex prominent; iris translucency ++++; retinal pigment absent; visual acuity progressively worsening (practically and legally blind). Marked nystagmus and photophobia.

Etiology. Autosomal recessive inheritance. Mutation of the tyrosinase locus; gene location 11q.

Pathology. Melanosomes in hair bulb show only stage I and II.

Diagnostic Procedures. *Ophthalmoscopy.* Transillumination of iris shows no visible pigment; the red reflex is present; the fundal pigment absent. *Blood.* Serum tyrosinase and the beta melanocyte-stimulating hormone levels are normal. *Incubation of hair bulb in tyrosine:* no pigment formation.

Therapy. None.

Prognosis. Blindness. High incidence of skin neoplasia.

BIBLIOGRAPHY. Wafer L: A new voyage and description of the isthmus of America, giving an account of the author's above, there. Collection of Voyages, 3rd ed, vol 3, pp 261–463. London, 1729

Garrod AE: Inborn errors of metabolism. (Croonian lectures. Lecture I.) Lancet 2:1–7, 1908

King RA, Hearing VJ, Creel DJ, et al: Albinism. In Scriver CR, Beaudet AL, Sly WS, et al: The Metabolic and Molecular Bases of Inherited Disease, 7th ed, p 4369. New York, McGraw-Hill, 1995

ALBINISM, OCULAR-TY-POS

Synonyms. Albinism II; albinoidism; OCA2; Oculocutaneous–Ty-pos albinism; albinism imperfect, albinism incomplete; albinism partial.

Symptoms and Signs. Identified particularly in Africa. In Caucasian minimal in northern Europe moderate increase in southern Europe. Both sexes affected; present from birth. Skin from pink-white to cream color; pigmented nevi may be present, particularly in sun-exposed areas; hair color white-yellow-reddish, darkening with age. Eye color blue, yellow, or brown. Visual acuity defect severe in childhood; vision improving with age; nystagmus and photophobia not as severe as in Albinism, Ty-neg (see).

Etiology. Autosomal recessive inheritance. Gene involved P (pink-eyed dilution) location 15q. Possible association with Prader-Willi (see) and Angelman (see).

Pathology. Melanosomes in hair bulb to early stage III; polyphagosomes.

Diagnostic Procedures. *Ophthalmoscopy.* Transillumination of iris shows pigmented cartwheel at pupil and limbus; red reflex may be absent; fundal pigment in adult absent to reduced. *Blood.* Serum tyrosine level normal to reduced; beta melanocyto-stimulating hormone normal. *Incubation of hair bulb.* In Ty-positive albinism: pigmentation.

Therapy. None.

Prognosis. High incidence of skin neoplasia. Prognosis for vision better than for albinism I.

BIBLIOGRAPHY. Kugelman TP, Van Scott EJ: Tyrosinase activity in melanocytes of human albinos. J Invest Dermatol 37:73, 1961

Witkop CR Jr, Van Scott EJ, Jacoby GA: Evidence for two forms of autosomal recessive albinism in man. Proc II Int Congr Hum Genet, Institute G. Mendel, Rome:1064–1069, 1961

King RA, Hearing VJ, Creel DJ, et al: Albinism. In Scriver CR, Beaudet AL, Sly WS, et al: The Metabolic and Molecular Bases of Inherited Disease, 7th ed, pp 4374–4376. New York, McGraw-Hill, 1995

ALBINISM, OCULAR-YELLOW MUTANT

Synonyms. Amish albinism; oculocutaneous—albinism yellow mutant; OCA1B yellow mutant; xanthous albinism.

Symptoms and Signs. Both sexes affected; present from birth. Skin color pink-white to cream; pigmented nevi and freckles may be present and abundant; hair white at birth, by 6 months yellow reddish. Eyes blue in infancy, tendency to darken with age. Nystagmus of variable intensity (for life); photophobia not extremely severe (+ to ++); reduced vision in infancy tends to improve with age.

Etiology. Autosomal recessive inheritance, gene involved Tyrosinase location 11q.

Pathology. Melanosomes in hair bulb to stage III; polyphagosomes.

Diagnostic Procedures. *Ophthalmoscopy.* Transillumination of iris shows, in adult, cartwheel effect; red reflex present; fundal pigment from absent to ++. *Blood.* Serum tyrosinase level normal. *Incubation of hair bulb in tyrosine:* pigmentation.

Therapy. None.

Prognosis. Fair. Improvement of vision; susceptibility to skin neoplasia unknown.

BIBLIOGRAPHY. King RA, Hearing VJ, Creel DJ, et al: Albinism. In Scriver CR, Beaudet AL, Sly WS, et al: The Metabolic and Molecular Bases of Inherited Disease, 7th ed, pp 4370–4371. New York, McGraw-Hill, 1995

ALBINOIDISM, DOMINANT

The term albinoidism is used to indicate the absence of photophobia and nystagmus.

Symptoms and Signs. Both sexes affected; present from birth. Skin color pink; presence of pigmented nevi or freckles unknown. Eye color blue. Absence of nystagmus and photophobia; vision normal to slightly reduced.

Etiology. Autosomal dominant inheritance.

Diagnostic Procedures. *Blood.* Serum tyrosine level and beta melanocyte-stimulating hormone levels unknown. *Ophthalmoscopy.* Transillumination of iris shows punctate pigmentation; red reflex present; fundus punctate pigmentation.

BIBLIOGRAPHY. Waardenberg PJ: Remarkable Fact in Human Albinism and Leukism. Neederlands, Van Gorkum Assen, 1970

King RA, Hearing VJ, Creel DJ, et al: Albinism. In Scriver CR, Beaudet AL, Sly WS, et al: The Metabolic and Molecular Bases of Inherited Disease, 7th ed, p 4376. New York, McGraw-Hill, 1995

ALBRIGHT-HADORN

Eponym obsolete; used to indicate the occurrence of the hypokalemic periodic paralysis (see) in patients with renal tubular acidosis (see).

BIBLIOGRAPHY. Albright F: Osteomalacia and late rickets, the various etiologies met in the U.S. with emphasis on that resulting from aspecific form of renal acidosis, the therapeutical indications for each etiological subgroup, and the relationship between osteomalacia and Milkman's syndrome. Medicine 25:399–479, 1946

Hadorn W: Osteomalacie mit paroxysmaler hypokaliämisher. Muskellähmung; ein neues Syndrome. Schweiz Med Wochenschr 78:1238–1242, 1948

ALCOHOLIC CARDIOMEGALY-EMPHYSEMA

Symptoms and Signs. Exclusive in chronic alcoholic males. Chronic bronchitis; slow progressive cardiopulmonary insufficiency.

Etiology. Alcohol ingestion; secondary pulmonary infections as complicating factor.

Pathology. Cardiomegaly; chronic bronchitis; lung emphysema.

Diagnostic Procedures. *Blood.* Anemia; pyruvic acid level, liver function test. Pulmonary function tests. *Electrocardiography. X-ray of chest.*

Therapy. Discontinuation of alcohol intake. Thiamine and correction of diet. Antibiotics. Symptomatic for cardiac insufficiency.

Prognosis. Poor; high mortality between 55 to 70 years of age for cardiopulmonary insufficiency.

BIBLIOGRAPHY. Josserand A: Le syndrome gros coeur et emphyseme importante complications viscerale de l'alcoolisme et facteur de surmortalité masculine. Lyon Medical 189:42–44, 1953

Segel LD, Klausner SC, Gnadt JTH, et al: Alcohol and the heart. Med Clin North Am 68:147–161, 1984

Regan TJ: Alcohol and nutritional disease. In Schlant RC, Alexander RW: Hurst's The Heart, 8th ed, pp 1943–1948. New York, McGraw-Hill, 1994

ALCOHOLIC KETOACIDOSIS

Synonyms. Dillon.

Symptoms and Signs. Occurs in chronic alcoholics; onset after a binge of several days. Cessation of food intake and continuous alcohol consumption; persistent vomiting that causes patient to stop alcohol intake. After 12–96 hours; severe dehydration, mental obtundation, and specific metabolic changes. (See Diagnostic Procedures.)

Etiology. Not clearly established. Consequence of alcohol withdrawal (see).

Diagnostic Procedures. *Blood.* Marked metabolic acidosis; hyperketonemia; moderate (and variable) elevation of plasma lactate; glucose normal or slightly elevated.

Therapy. Fluid and electrolyte balance as in diabetic ketoacidosis, prevention of shock and hypokalemia; acid-base derangement correction. Thiamine 50–100 mg; chlordiazepoxide.

Prognosis. Recurrent condition. Possibility of fatality.

BIBLIOGRAPHY. Dillon ES, Dyer WW, Smells LS: Ketone acidosis of nondiabetic adults. Med Clin North Am 24:1813–1822, 1940

Goldstein DB: Pharmacology of Alcohol. New York, Oxford Univ Press, 1983

Regan TJ: Alcohol and nutritional disease. In Schlant RC, Alexander RW: Hurst's The Heart, 8th ed, pp 1943–1948. New York, McGraw-Hill, 1994

ALCOHOLIC NEUROPATHY

Synonym. Alcoholic pseudotabes; neuropathic beri-beri.

Symptoms and Signs. Onset subacute. Burning pain in the legs and feet; muscle tenderness; superficial hyperesthesia; paresthesia in the lower and upper extremities, predominant in the distal parts, progressing to decreased tactile and deep sensibility and paradoxical hyperalgesia, loss of sense of position at passive motion. Weakness of legs; ataxia; muscle weakening and atrophy with fasciculation. Temporary tendon hyperreflexia followed by areflexia. Ulcer and trophic changes of skin.

Etiology. Chronic alcohol intoxication plus nutritional deficiency.

Diagnostic Procedures. *Blood.* Anemia; liver function test. Serology for syphilis. *Gastric juice. Achlorhydria.* Frequent. *Spinal fluid.* Normal.

Therapy. Withdrawal of alcohol; restoration of adequate diet, high caloric, high carbohydrates, vitamin B complex. Prevention of contraction.

Prognosis. Long period to recover. Because of alcohol addiction, possible relapses.

BIBLIOGRAPHY. Kalivas PW, Samson HH (eds): The neurobiology of drug and alcohol addition. Ann New York Ac Sci 1:654, 1992

ALCOHOLIC PARANOIA

See also Othello.

Symptoms and Signs. Usually occurs in males. Delusion of jealousy.

Etiology. Impairment of personality development that leads to alcoholism and to suspicion and distrust; brutality to sexual partners. Alcohol-induced impotence; recurrent panic-like state; paranoid state.

Therapy. Psychotherapy.

Prognosis. Poor. Patient feels better when hospitalized. Return to normal environment produces recurrences.

BIBLIOGRAPHY. Kalivas PW, Samson HH (eds): The neurobiology of drug and alcohol addition. Ann NY Acad Sci 654, 1992

Kaplan HI, Sadock BJ: Comprehensive Textbook of Psychiatry, 6th ed, p 1145. Baltimore, Williams & Wilkins, 1995

ALCOHOLIC, REVERSIBLE ACUTE MUSCULAR

Synonym. Alcoholic muscular cramps.

Symptoms and Signs. Appear in chronic alcoholic patients; spontaneous onset or precipitated by exercise. Muscle aching or cramps; tenderness; weakness; myoglobinuria. Other symptoms and signs of chronic alcoholism. Red conjunctivae, flushing of skin, "whiskey nose"; edema of mucous membranes; characteristic hoarseness; vomiting, diarrhea; coarse tremor.

Etiology. Unknown; possible depression of glycolytic enzymes by ethanol or its metabolites. Secondary defects (e.g., thiamine, magnesium) may also be responsible. Intrinsic muscle defect; alcohol sensitivity(?).

Pathology. Muscles show histologic evidence of necrotic changes.

Diagnostic Procedures. *Blood.* Anemia; hyperkalemia, increased serum glumatic-oxaloacetic transaminase (SGOT); liver function test. *Special studies.* Basal serum creatine phosphokinase activity elevated; ischemic exercise tests, lactic acid-marked rise with exercise. Immunodiffusion studies. Demonstration of antimyoglobin antibody. *Biopsy of muscle. Electromyography. Electrocardiography. Urine.* Myoglobin may be present. *X-ray of chest.* Frequently, cardiomegaly.

Therapy. Discontinuation of alcohol intake; thiamine and correction of diet.

Prognosis. Lesions reversible upon discontinuation of alcohol intake.

BIBLIOGRAPHY. Hed R, Larrson H, Wahlgren F: Acute myoglobinuria: report of a case with fatal outcome. Acta Med (Scand) 152:459–463, 1955

Perkoff GT, Hardy P, Valez-Garcia E: Reversible acute muscular syndrome in chronic alcoholism. New Engl J Med 274:1277–1285, 1966

Regan TJ: Alcohol and nutritional disease. In Schlant RC, Alexander RW: Hurst's The Heart, 8th ed, pp 1943–1948. New York, McGraw-Hill, 1994

ALCOHOL WITHDRAWAL

Synonym. Rum fits; whiskey fits.

Symptoms. In chronic alcoholics when they attempt to stop drinking (most severe symptoms in those who have been drinking the longest). Usually 7 to 48 h after cessation of drinking. Aggravation of tremulousness or "shakes"; severe anxiety; insomnia; inability to concentrate; feeling of unreality. In most severe cases truncal ataxia, nausea, vomiting, diarrhea, abdominal cramps. Hallucination within 24 to 25 days after alcohol withdrawal (25%). Patients remain able to describe hallucinations and communicate coherently. "Rum fits" or grand mal seizures in burst of two to six or more may be first symptoms. Delirium tremens is a combination of severe tremulousness and hallucination in severe form.

Signs. Evidence of dehydration, tachycardia, dilation of pupils, profuse sweating. Increased temperature may be observed. Increased blood pressure.

Etiology. Alcohol withdrawal alone may precipitate syndrome; thiamine deficiency and other nutritional deficiencies concur in determining this syndrome.

Diagnostic Procedures. *Blood.* Liver function test, pyruvate serum level; pyruvate tolerance curve. *EEG* temporary abnormalities that revert to normal in days. Stroboscopic stimulation causes generalized myoclonus or seizures.

Therapy. Benzodiazepines; IV fluids with glucose, electrolytes, and vitamin B complex; complete diet re-evaluation. Antiemetics; antacids; ataractics; anticonvulsants. Lofexidine, atenolol.

Prognosis. Often limited to 3 to 7 days. Delirium tremens mortality estimated between 2% and 12%. Repeated attacks following resumption and discontinuation or increasing or decreasing intake of alcohol. A delayed type of syndrome with milder symptoms is reported that may occur years after discontinuation of alcohol intake.

BIBLIOGRAPHY. Sutton T: Tracts on Delirium Tremens, on Peritonitis, on Some Other Internal Inflammatory Affections and on the Gout. London, Thomas Underwood, 1813

Blake A: A Practical Essay on the Disease Generally Known under the Denomination of Delirium Tremens. London, Burgess Hill, 1825

Lerner WD, Fallon HJ: The alcohol withdrawal syndrome. New Engl J Med 313:951–952, 1985

Adams RD, Victor M: Principles of Neurology, 5th ed, p 912. New York, McGraw-Hill, 1993

ALDER

Synonyms. Alder-Reilly anomaly.

Symptoms and Signs. No particular clinical feature attributable to the presence of anomaly (see Diagnostic Procedures). However, found in association with many syndromes: Hurler; Hunter; Maroteaux-Lamy; and other types of bone and cartilage abnormalities.

Etiology. Dominant inheritance. Incomplete degradation of protein-bound carbohydrate complexes because of enzymatic deficiencies.

Pathology. See Diagnostic Procedures.

Diagnostic Procedures. *Blood.* In leukocytes, presence of azurophil and basophil granulations, larger than normal; similar bodies may be present in lymphocytes and monocytes. Function of leukocytes normal.

Bone marrow. Granulation presence more evident than in peripheral blood.

Therapy. That of associated syndrome.

Prognosis. Permanent characteristic.

BIBLIOGRAPHY. Alder A: Ueber konstitutionell bedingte Granulationveraenderungen der Leukocyten. Dtsch Arch Klin Med 183:372–378, 1939

Reilly WA: Granules in leukocytes in gargoylism. Am J Dis Child 62:489–491, 1941

Athens JW: Qualitative disorders of leukocytes. In Lee GR, Bithel TC, Foerster J, et al (eds): Wintrobe's Clinical Hematology, 9th ed, p 1615. Philadelphia, Lea & Febiger, 1993

ALDOSTERONE SYNTHETASE DEFICIENCY

Synonyms. Ulick; adrenal hyperplasia IV; corticosterone methyloxidase Type II deficiency; CMO II deficiency.

Symptoms and Signs. High incidence in Iranian Jews. From I week to three months of age. Absence of ambiguous genitalia and postnatal virilization. Hypotension that leads to death (from potentially fatal electrolytes abnormalities, salt wasting). Symptoms become less severe as patient ages; in adulthood asymptomatic except for short stature and possible postural hypotension.

Etiology. Autosomal recessive inheritance. Chromosomal location 8q. Deficiency of 18-dehydrogenase or 18-hydroxycorticosterone with impaired production of aldosterone. Sex hormones and glucocorticoids are unaffected.

Diagnostic Procedures. *Blood.* Variable levels of aldosterone (low); plasma renin activity (elevated); 18-hydroxycorticosreone marked elevation; ratio of 18-OH-THA to aldosterone exceeds 5. Severe electrolyte derangements. *Urine.* Ratio of 18-hydroxycorticosterone metabolites to aldosterone greater than 5 (n.v. less than 3.0).

Therapy. 9-fluorocortisone during infancy and early childhood.

Prognosis. From death in infancy to normal lifespan.

BIBLIOGRAPHY. Royer P, Lestradet H, de Menibus CH, et al: Hyperaldosteronisme familial chronique à debut neo-natal. Ann Paediat 8:133–138, 1961

Ulick S, Gautier E, Vetter KK, et al: An aldosterone biosynthetic defect in a salt-losing disorder. J Clin Endocrl Met 24:669–672, 1964

Lee PDK, Patterson BD, Hintz RL, et al: Biochemical diagnosis and management of corticosterone methyl oxidase type II deficiency. J Clin Endocr Met 61:225–229, 1986

New MI: Congenital adrenal hyperplasia. In De Groot LJ (ed): Endocrinology, 3rd ed, pp 1822–1823. Philadelphia, WB Saunders, 1995

ALEXANDER

Synonyms. Factor VII deficiency. Proconvertin deficiency. SPCA deficiency.

Symptoms and Signs. Frequency 1/500,000. From childhood or in adulthood life. Like hemophilia but less severe. Postoperative blood losses are not great. Thromboembolism is possible.

Etiology. Autosomal recessive. Heterozygotes sometimes have hemorrhagic manifestations. Occasionally associated in bronchogenic carcinoma.

Diagnostic Procedures. *Blood.* Quick time lengthened, prothrombin time normal, cephaline and Stypven time normal (different from factor X deficiency; see Christmas).

Therapy. Plasma, purified: protrombin complex. Contraceptives to prevent menorrhagia.

Prognosis. Good.

BIBLIOGRAPHY. Alexander B, Goldstein R, Landwehr G, et al: Congenital SPCA deficiency: a hitherto unrecognised coagulation defect with hemorrhage rectified by serum and serum fractions. J Clin Invest 30:596, 1951

Bithel TC: Hereditary coagulation disorders. In Lee GR, Bithel TC, Foerster J, et al (eds): Wintrobe's Clinical Hematology, 9th ed, pp 1443–1444. Philadelphia, Lea & Febiger, 1993

ALEXANDER (W.S.)

Synonyms. Fibrinoid degeneration of astrocytes; dysmyelogenic leuko-dystrophy-megalobarencephaly; leukodystrophy-megalobarencephaly.

Symptoms and Signs. Prevalent in males, onset in infancy. Retardation of physical and mental development and slow progressive enlargement of head. Frequently, seizures.

Etiology. Metabolic disorder of unknown nature that interferes with myelinization of white matter. Autosomal recessive inheritance reported.

Pathology. Megalencephaly; hydrocephalus. Rosenthal fibers and homogeneous eosinophilic masses scattered in the cortex and white matter in the astrocytes related to blood vessels; prominent demyelinization deposit spreads along all interfaces of central nervous system, including pial-glial and perivascular tissue. Leukodystrophy prevalent in frontal lobe.

Diagnostic Procedures. *Blood and urine.* Normal. *Spinal tap.* Increased pressure. *Electroencephalography. CAT. Ultrasonography.*

Therapy. Symptomatic.

Prognosis. Poor. Progressive condition; death within one to two years from onset. In exceptional cases, a few years of survival from onset.

BIBLIOGRAPHY. Alexander WS: Progressive fibrinoid degeneration of fibrillary astrocytes associated with mental retardation in a hydrocephalic infant. Brain 72:373–381, 1949

Herndon RN, Rubinstein LJ, Freeman JN, et al: Light and electron microscopic observations on Rosenthal fibers in Alexander's disease and in multiple sclerosis. Neuropath Exp Neurol 29:524–551, 1970

Riggs JE, Schochet SS, Nelson J: Asymptomatic adult Alexander's disease: entity or nosological misconception? Neurology 38:152–154, 1988

Iwaki T, Kume-Iwaki, Leim RKH, et al: Alpha-B-crystallin is expressed in nonlenticular tissues and accumulates in Alexander's disease brain. Cell 57:71–78, 1989

Adams RD, Victor M: Principles of Neurology, 5th ed, pp 811–812. New York, McGraw-Hill, 1993

ALEZZANDRINI

Symptoms and Signs. Occurs in adolescence and early adulthood. Unilateral impairment of vision and, after months or years, facial vitiligo and poliosis appear on the same side. Bilateral perceptive deafness occasionally develops.

Etiology. Unknown.

Pathology. Degenerative retinitis.

BIBLIOGRAPHY. Alezzandrini AA: Manifestation unilaterale de degenerescence tapeto-retinienne, de vitiligo, de poliose, de cheveux blancs et d'hypoacousie. Ophthalmologica 147:409–419, 1964

Bleehen SS, Ebling FJG, Champion RH: Disorders of skin colour. In Champion RH, Burton JL, Ebling FJG (eds): Rook/Wilkinson/Ebling Textbook of Dermatology, 5th ed, pp 1612, 2226. Oxford, Blackwell Scientific, 1992

ALIBERT-BAZIN

Synonyms. Auspitz; Vidal-Brocq; Hallopeau-Besnier; mycosis fungoides; cutaneous T cell lymphoma, CTCL. See Sézary.

Symptoms. Rare, more frequent in males (2:1). Onset at any age after seventh year, median age 50–60 years. Pruritus, pain, insomnia.

Signs. Isolated nonspecific eczematous lesions. In some cases at onset, they assume the aspect of generalized erythroderma (Hallopeau-Besnier syndrome). (See also Sézary.) The lesions consist in extending patches of varying hues, which may present bizarre shapes; dry and moderate scaling; no spontaneous vesiculation. This stage lasts many years (4 to 10) and lesions may simulate psoriasis, parapsoriasis, lichen, exfoliative dermatitis, and other conditions. In a second stage they ulcerate (fungate). Typical "leonine facies" with prominent folds in some cases. Lymphadenopathy may be present from onset or develop later.

Etiology. Unknown. Genetic (autosomal recessive), environmental (occupational hazard: petrochemicals, textile, metal, farming never confirmed), infective agents (human retroviruses) have been implicated.

Pathology. Skin lesions show histologic alterations that vary during course of disease. At onset, lesions may be nonspecific. With progression, superficial dermal infiltrates develop, especially perivascularly, formed by lymphocytes, histiocytes, reticular cells, neutrophils, eosinophils, and plasma cells, and frequently also by fragmented nuclei. Mixed with these elements are a variable number of "mycosis cells" (characterized by a large, round, deeply stained nucleus, crenated at its margin). These cells, however, must not be considered specific for this condition. With progression, infiltration of the lower corium and subcutaneous layers. Tumor transformation implies a more monoformic pattern with or without predominance of mycosis or reticular cells, followed by thinning and ulceration of epidermis.

Diagnostic Procedures. *Skin biopsy.* See Pathology. *Lymph node biopsy.* Seldom, pattern of lymphoma; frequently, signs of chronic inflammation. *Bone marrow.* Seldom, mycosis cells; increase of plasma cells. *Blood.* Anemic neutrophilic leukocytosis and eosinophilia (if lymphocytosis, consider Sézary syndrome, see).

Therapy. At onset weak steroid cream, photochemotherapy (PUVA). Total lymphoid irradiation (TLI) electrobeam radiotherapy (EBRT) total body irradiation (TBI) (remission for months), corticosteroids, mechlorethamine, etretinate. Trials with cyclosporin and interferon and combined EBRT and chemotherapy; monoclonal antibody; autologous marrow transplantation also attempted (good results to be confirmed).

Prognosis. Possible evolution into Sézary (see). Median survival approximately five years.

BIBLIOGRAPHY. Alibert JL: Description des maladies de la peau observées à l'Hôpital Saint Louis et exposition des meilleures methodes survies pour leur traitment. Paris, Barrois L'Ainé, 1806

Bazin APE: Leçons théorique et cliniques sur les affections cutanée de nature arthritique et dartreuse, consideerées en ellememes et dans leurs rapports avec les éruptions, scrofuleuses, parasitaires et syphilitiques. Paris, A Delahaye, 1860

Auspitz H: Ein Fall von Granuloma Fungoides. Urtljschr Dermatol 12:123–143, 1885

Auspitz H, Shelley WB: Familial mycosis fungoides revisited. Arch Derm 116:1177–1178, 1980

Greer JP, Salhany KE, King LE Jr: Cutaneous T cell lymphoma: mycosis fungoides and Sézary syndrome. In Lee GR, Bithel TC, Foerster J, et al (eds): Wintrobe's Clinical Hematology, 9th ed, pp 2143–2169. Philadelphia, Lea & Febiger, 1993

ALIBERT I

Synonyms. Hawkin, false keloid; cicatricial keloid; post-traumatic keloid; scar hypertrophy; hypertrophic scars.

Symptoms. Black race particularly susceptible. Females more susceptible. May appear during pregnancy. Rare in infancy and old age. Maximum between puberty and age 30. Local pain; tenderness.

Signs. Three to 4 weeks after trauma, scar begins to thicken and form a reddish plaque, which may continue to grow forming a cord-like excrescence of a more or less bizarre configuration.

Etiology. To be differentiated from true keloid. Local factor or systemic factors (or both) have been called responsible. Both autosomal recessive and dominant inheritance reported.

Pathology. In early stages, impossible to differentiate between false and true keloids: both have perivascular cellular nodules of collagen fibers. Later, in false keloids, the bundles of fibers aggregate and shrink, while elastic fibers appear.

Diagnostic Procedures. Skin biopsy.

Therapy. Early treatment produces best results, radiotherapy; intralesion injection (preceded by liquid nitrogen spray application) or systemic administration of corticosteroids. Retinoic acid application (good results). Surgery as last resort, since spontaneous regression is frequent.

Prognosis. Good response to treatment; spontaneous regression in many cases.

BIBLIOGRAPHY. Alibert JL: Note sur la kéloide. J Univ Sci Med 2:207–216. 1816
Hawkins CH: On warty tumours in cicatrices. London Med Gaz 13:481–482, 1833
MacKie RM: Soft tissue tumors. In Champion RH, Burton JL, Ebling FJG (eds): Rook/Wilkinson/Ebling Textbook of Dermatology, 5th ed, pp 2073–2076. Oxford, Blackwell Scientific, 1992

ALIBERT II

Synonyms. Borovskii; Aleppo boil; Bagdad boil; Biskra button; Chiclero ulcer; Delhi sore; Kandahar sore; Lahore sore; leishmaniasis old world; oriental boil.

Symptoms. Endemic on the Mediterranean coasts and warm countries from Asia to South America. Both sexes and all ages can be affected. Incubation period 1 to 6 months. Malaise; pruritus.

Signs. First stage. Wet or early ulcerative form. Red nodules at site of inoculation, which ulcerate in the center and extend ulcerating edges. Occasionally, small secondary nodules around the main lesion. Second stage. Dry or late ulcerative form. Brown nodules extend into a plaque; after 6 months, ulcerate and, then, crust. Satellite nodules more frequent. Third stage. Leishmaniasis recidivans. Brown papules re-form around area of previous lesion, and slowly coalesce to form lupus-like plaques.

Etiology. Leishmania tropica parasite transmitted by sand fly.

Pathology. Preulceration, dermal infiltrate of histiocytes with Leishman-Donovan (L-D) bodies, surrounded by lymphocytes and plasma cells. After ulceration, large number of neutrophils and reduction of number of L-D bodies.

Diagnostic Procedures. *Biopsy.* From ulcer floor. *Culture in NNM* (Nicolle-Novy-MacNeal) medium and antibiotics. *Montenegro test.*

Therapy. Topical treatment for simple sores. Heating (technically difficult), freezing with CO_2 snow; curatage in local anesthesia; or stibogluconate or meglumine antimoniale infiltrations. Systemic treatment for severe forms. Pentostam intramuscularly or intravenously; steriods may be also useful.

Prognosis. Wet form: After 2 to 6 months, spontaneous healing with residual scar. Dry form: After 8 to 12 months, regression with residual scar. L. recidivans: Exceedingly chronic course.

BIBLIOGRAPHY. Alibert JL: Note sur la pyrophlyctide endémique ou pustule d'Alep. Rev Med Franc et Etrang (Paris) 3:62–68, 1829
Karagezian LA, Kozhniilevshmanioz-Armenii. Vestn Dermatol Venerol 40:61–64, 1966
Bryceson DM, Hay RJ: Parasitic worms and protozoa. In Champion RH, Burton JL, Ebling FJG (eds): Rook/Wilkinson/Ebling Textbook of Dermatology, 5th ed, pp 1252–1258. Oxford, Blackwell Scientific, 1992

ALIBERT III

Synonyms. Barber itch; sycosis vulgaris; coccogenic sycosis; ficosis; mentagra; sycosis simplex; tinea barbae.

Symptoms. Only adult males affected. Pruritus on the face.

Signs. Small annular, moderately scaly lesions on the beard area. Peripheral growth with central healing. May assume features of chronic bacterial folliculitis.

Etiology. Trichophyton mentagrophytes; T. verrucosum; T. violaceum; T. schoenleini.

Pathology. Chronic inflammatory lesions, pustules, or abscess with hyphae in follicles.

Diagnostic Procedures. *Mycologic examination of infected hairs. Cultures.*

Therapy. Scrubbing with soap and water. Fungistatic preparations for topical use. Systemic administration of antimycotic.

Prognosis. Inflammatory lesions may clear spontaneously or persist for months.

BIBLIOGRAPHY. Alibert JL: Déscription Des Maladies de la Peau, vol 2, p 214. Bruxelles, Wahlew, 1825
Highet AS, Hay RJ, Roberts SOB: Bacterial infections. In Champion RH, Burton JL, Ebling FJG (eds): Rook/Wilkinson/Ebling Textbook of Dermatology, 5th ed, pp 976–977. Oxford, Blackwell Scientific, 1992

ALICE IN WONDERLAND

Synonym. Todd.

Symptoms. Bizarre disturbance of body image; macropsia, micropsia feeling of levitation; alteration of sense of passage of time; depersonalization; doubling of personality.

Etiology. Migraine attack; epilepsy; hypnagogic states; schizophrenia; hallucinogenic drugs; various diseases of parietal lobe.

Therapy. Depending upon etiology.

BIBLIOGRAPHY. Todd J: Syndrome of Alice in Wonderland. Can Med Assoc J 73:701–704, 1955
Linn L: Clinical manifestations in psychiatric disorders. In Kaplan HI, Sadock BJ: Comprehensive Textbook of Psychiatry, 6th ed, p 656. Baltimore, Williams & Wilkins, 1995

ALIQUORRHEA

Synonyms. Cerebral ventricular collapse; spontaneous hypoliquorrhea.

Symptoms. Severe headache, increasing when the patient attempts to sit up or stand up; stiff neck; nausea; dizziness; buzzing of ears.

Signs. Bradycardia; Kernig sign; optic disc normal; normal reflexes; no paresis or sensibility disturbance.

Etiology. Unknown. Spontaneous decrease of secretion of spinal fluid, establishing a negative pressure in the cerebrospinal cavity. In addition to rare condition, frequently observed after lumbar puncture, injury and operation of brain, chronic subdural hematomas, and dehydration in general.

Diagnostic Procedures. *Lumbar puncture.* Absent or low cerebrospinal pressure; very little or no fluid obtained; typical air suction through the needle with noise when the patient passes from a sitting position to lying down. Queckenstedt increase in pressure. *Cerebrospinal fluid.* When obtained is blood-tinged or yellowish; protein increased; normal cells. *Blood.* Normal; in some cases, moderate increase of sedimentation rate.

Therapy. Injection of warm Ringer solution into the spinal canal until normal pressure is reached; relieves all symptoms for a day or two.

Prognosis. All patients recovered.

BIBLIOGRAPHY. Ingvar S: Danger of leakage of cerebrospinal fluid after lumbar puncture. Acta Med Scand 58:67–101, 1923

Lindqvist T, Moberg E: Spontaneous hypoliquorrhea; report of a case. Acta Med Scand 132:556–561, 1949

Adams RD, Victor M: Principles of Neurology, 5th ed, pp 549–561. New York, McGraw-Hill, 1993

ALLAN-HERNDON-DUDLEY

Synonyms. Mental retardation (X-linked); hypotonia.

Symptoms and Signs. *Male.* Normal at birth but for hypotonia. At 6 months inability to hold up the head. Dysarthria, ataxia, athetoid movements. Retarded motor development, muscular atrophy. At more advanced age, joint contractures and hyporeflexia. Facies elongated, bitemporal narrowing, large ears.

Etiology. X-linked inheritance suggested. Gene located in Xq21.

Prognosis. Reach adult life; normal stature.

Diagnostic Procedures. *Blood.* Serum cretine kinase, aminoacids: normal.

BIBLIOGRAPHY. Allan W, Herndon CN, Dudley FC: Some examples of the inheritance of mental deficiency; apparently sex-linked idiocy and microcephaly. Am J Ment Defic 48:325–334, 1943–1944

Opitz JM, Sutherland GR: International workshop on the fragile X and X-linked mental retardation. Am J Med Genet 17:5–94, 1984

Stevenson RE, Goodman HO, Schwartz CE, et al: Allan-Herndon syndrome I: clinical studies. Am J Hum Genet 47:446–453, 1990

ALLEMANN

Symptoms and Signs. Club fingers (one element of syndrome). In some cases facial asymmetry and signs relative to degeneration of various motor branches of nerves present as well.

Etiology. Unknown.

Diagnostic Procedures. *Urography.* Duplication of the renal images (second element of syndrome).

BIBLIOGRAPHY. Allemann R: Die klinische Bedeutung familiarer Heredopatie und Mutation für die Urologie. Z Urol 80:641–649, 1936

ALLEN-HINES

Synonym. Lipedema legs.

Symptoms. Frequently, family history of big legs. Almost exclusively in women. Distress (emotional and physical because of the appearance of the leg). Increase of symptoms and signs with warm weather. Emotional

reaction is precipitated by the fact that "fat legs" are considered unattractive in modern societies. Older civilizations and Hottentots, for instance, consider them a sign of beauty.

Signs. Gradual onset; bilateral enlargement of buttocks and legs. Fat and fluid accumulation; sensitivity to pressure; swelling soft; pitting edema minimal. Usually the fat accumulation limited to legs and the rest of body appears normal; occasionally accompanied by generalized obesity. Feet normal in size and configuration.

Etiology. Unknown; possibly constitutional hereditary character.

Therapy. Nonspecific; bed rest induces moderate degree of decrease in size of legs.

Prognosis. Course progressive.

BIBLIOGRAPHY. Allen EV, Hines EA Jr: Lipedema of the legs: a syndrome characterized by fat legs and orthostatic edema. Proc Staff Meet Mayo Clinic 15:184–187, 1940

Wold LE, Hines EA, Allen EV: Lipedema of legs: a syndrome characterized by fat legs and edema. Ann Int Med 34:1243–1250. 1951

ALLEN-MASTERS

Synonyms. Masters-Allen; broad ligament laceration; laceration of uterine support; ligamentum latum laceration.

Symptoms. Occurs mainly in multiparas. Pain in the pelvic region; dyspareunia; dysmenorrhea; backache; urinary frequency; rectal tenesmus.

Signs. Laceration of the posterior aspect of the broad ligament; angiomatous aspect of the blood vessels in broad ligament. Cervix may be moved in any direction with minimal or no movement of the uterus.

Etiology. Unknown. Surgical, traumatic, or precipitated delivery; criminal abortion, excessive packing.

Pathology. Nonspecific inflammatory infiltration; angiomatous aspect of the vessels; cellular necrosis. Endometriosis can often be demonstrated macroscopically and microscopically with the same frequency. Hyperplasia of the venous tissue and neuroma can be found.

Therapy. Suturing the rupture is not enough. It is recommended that after laparotomy the pelvic peritoneum be resected, with the exception of pouch of Douglas.

Prognosis. Good with treatment.

BIBLIOGRAPHY. Allen WM, Masters WH: Traumatic laceration of uterine support: The clinical syndrome and the operative treatment. Am J Obstet Gynecol 70:500–513, 1955

Bret AJ, Bardiaux M, de Brux J: Algies pelviennes d'origine genitale; La pelviperitonite chronique scleroinflammatoire. Etude clinique et histopathologique de 25 cas. A propos du syndrome d'Allen et Masters. Sem Hôp Paris 43:173–182, 1967

Philipp EE, Barnes J, Newton M: Obstetrics and Gynecology, 3rd ed, pp 93–94. London, Heinemann, 1986

ALLERGIC ALVEOLITIS, EXTRINSIC

Clinical features depend on immunologic response of the patient, antigenicity of dust, and intensity and frequency of exposure. Manifestations are similar regardless of the organic dust inhaled.

Symptoms. Develop within 4 to 6 hours of exposure. Cough; dyspnea; chills, fever, malaise, myalgia.

Signs. Bibasilar moist rales; patient appears acutely ill and exhausted.

Etiology. Immunoreactions: type I (allergic reactions); type III (precipitin mediated); type IV (delayed hypersensitivity) involved. Very often serum precipitins against the offending antigen can be detected. Types of dusts responsible give the name to the syndromes.

1. Bagassosis. Dust from moldy sugar cane.
2. Baker asthma. Probably owing to inhalation of molds present in bread.
3. Bible printer. Moldy paper; solutions used for printing.
4. Bird breeder lung. Avian excreta (Avian proteins).
5. Cheese-washer lung. Dust from cheese particles.
6. Christmas tree allergy (Variant of "wood-pulp worker"). Dust from the bark of Christmas tree.
7. Coffee-roaster lung. Dust from green coffee.
8. Coptic (Mummy disease). Dust from mummy bandage.
9. Dog house. Dust from moldy straw mattresses used for dogs.
10. Farmer lung. Dust from grains and hay.
11. Fertilizer induced lung. Fertilizer contamination by streptomyces albus.
12. Fishmeal-worker lung. Fish protein.
13. Humidistat (Humidifier lung; air conditioner pneumonitis; heating system disease). Aerosol of microorganisms or dusts from contaminated heating or cooling system.
14. Malt worker lung. (Brewer lung). Malt dust.
15. Maple bark. Dust from moldy maple bark (see also wood-pulp).
16. Mushroom worker lung (Mushroom picker lung). Dust from cultivated mushrooms in mushroom-growing farms.
17. New Guinea lung thatched roof worker (Streptomyces viridis?).
18. Paprika splitter lung. Paprika dust.
19. Pigeon breeder (bird breeder lung; bird fancier lung). Dust from bird excreta and plumage.
20. Pituitary snuff taker lung. Pituitary powder.
21. Prawn-worker lung. Forced air used to blow meat out of shell. Shell fish proteins.
22. Red cedar asthma. Due to isocynates and plicatic acid present in Western red cedar (thuja plicata).
23. Research-assistant lung. Dust from rat excreta; rat serum proteins.
24. Sequoiosis. Sauna taker lung. Redwood dust (see also wood-pulp).
25. Sewage. Induced hypersensitivity pneumonitis. Contaminated sewage (Cephalosporium sp).
26. Sisal-worker disease. Dust from Agave sisalana fibers.
27. Smallpox handler lung. Aerosol from smallpox lesions (affects medical and nursing staff dealing with smallpox patients).
28. Suberosis. Dust from moldy cork.
29. Tea-grower lung. Dust from moldy tea.
30. Thatched roof disease (Papuan lung; New Guinea lung). Dust from the thatched roof common in New Guinea houses.
31. Tobacco grower lung. Dust from moldy tobacco.
32. Wood-pulp worker lung (Papermill worker disease). Dust from wood-pulp.
33. Woolsorter lung. Dust from wool.

Pathology. Infiltration of alveolar walls by lymphocytes, plasma cells, and histiocytes with foamy cytoplasm; infiltration of the interstitium with mononuclear cells; sometimes, giant cell granulomas.

Diagnostic Procedures. *Blood.* Leukocytosis. Increased IgE and serum precipitins against suspected agent. *Pulmonary function tests.* Decreased vital capacity; decreased pulmonary compliance. *X-ray of chest.* Fine nodular densities. *Bronchoalveolar lavage (BAL).* Increased number of T lymphocytes predominantely of suppressor type. *Lung biopsy.* Bronchiolitis and granulomas.

Therapy. Avoidance of offending antigen; appropriate ventilation of working areas. Corticosteroids; bronchodilators. Oxygen.

Prognosis. Good with prevention. Repeated episodes produce chronic pulmonary and cardiac damage.

BIBLIOGRAPHY. De Francisci G, Magalini SI, Scrascia E: Etiopatogenesi e problemi rianimativi nelle polmoniti da ipersensibilità. Rec Progr Med 66:541–552, 1979

De Francisci G, Magalini SI: Le pneumopatie interstiziali da farmaci. Rec Progr Med 68:65–76, 1980

Chan-Yeung M: Occupational asthma. In Lynch JP, Deremee RA: Immunologically Mediated Pulmonary Diseases, p 306. Philadelphia, Lippincott, 1991

Fink JN: Hypersensitivity pneumonitis. In Lynch JP, Deremee RA: Immunologically Mediated Pulmonary Diseases, p 399. Philadelphia, Lippincott, 1991

ALLERGIC CYSTITIS

Synonyms. Cystitis allergy; food allergy; enuresis allergic.

Symptoms. Strangury; pollakiuria. Enuresis in young children.

Signs. Pain on palpation of suprapubic area.

Etiology. Allergy to specific foods or drugs. In case of enuresis, chocolate, dairy products, and food containing red dyes have been implicated.

Pathology. Bladder wall. Edema and infiltration with eosinophils and monocytic cells.

Diagnostic Procedures. *Urine.* Usually, absence of signs of infection (possibly secondary); occasionally, presence of eosinophils and red cells in sediment. *Cystoscopy.* (To be performed only after acute situation has subsided.) Edema and congestion of bladder wall. *Allergy tests.*

Therapy. Identification of and abstention from ingestion of allergic food or drug. Epinephrine; ephedrine; antihistamines; corticosteroids (usually temporarily useful). Attempts at desensitization.

Prognosis. Tendency to become a chronic condition. Complication of infection frequent. May be cured by avoidance of offending agents or successful desensitization.

BIBLIOGRAPHY. Esperanca M, Gerrard JW: Nocturnal enuresis. Comparison of the effect of imipramine and dietary restriction on bladder capacity. Can Med Assoc J 101:721, 1969

Zaleski A, Shokeri MK, Gerrard JW: Enuresis: Familial incidence and relationship to allergic disorders. Can Med Assoc J 106:30, 1972

Stites DP, Terr AI (eds): Basic and Clinical Immunology. London, Prentice-Hall, 1991

ALLERGIC GASTROENTERITIS

Synonyms. Quincke edema (confusing misused eponym see Quincke I); allergic jejunitis; angioneurotic edema of gastrointestinal tract; eosinophilic gastroenteritis; gastrointestinal idiopathic eosinophilic infiltrations; granuloma eosinophilic stomach. (See also Loeffler.)

Symptoms and Signs. Nearly equal sex distribution; seen in all ages, but most common in the sixth decade. Symptomatology may vary in kind with the organ involved. However, common pattern may be observed: recurrent gastrointestinal disorders lasting many years; vomiting; flatulence; diarrhea; epigastric pain; cramps; heartburn (in class II pain and cramping more prolonged and not intermittent, see Pathology). In some cases also history of melena or hematemesis; pyloric obstruction; cholecystitis and cholelithiasis; history of allergy (in 50% of cases).

Etiology. Unknown. Allergic mechanism (hypersensitivity reaction) postulated for the diffused type (class I); local inciting agents for the circumscribed types (class II).

Pathology. Two classes appear unrelated. Class I (diffused type). (1) Polyenteric: more than one portion of intestine involved; antrum of the stomach characteristically affected with extension to jejunum and ileum. Areas affected are firm, with edematous appearance; omentum and mesentery may appear inflamed or fibrotic; pylorus usually narrowed. Diffuse inflammatory infiltration from submucosa (occasionally also serosa) by mature eosinophils, with rare macrophages and giant cells; occasionally, hyalinization or necrosis of muscles. Mucosa free of involvement. (2) Monoenteric: similar pattern of lesions limited to the stomach. (3) Regional: similar pattern involving only a limited region: prepyloric and pyloric with borders not well defined. Class II (circumscribed type). (1) Regional: pseudotumors located at any site of the gastrointestinal tract; mucosa may be ulcerated; granuloma type of lesion, with rich reticular fibrillar and fibroblastic elements; varying numbers of blood vessels, and inflammatory cells. Scarce eosinophilic infiltration; histiocytes rare. (2) Polypoid pedunculated polyps; microscopically same pattern as regional type.

Diagnostic Procedures. *X-ray.* Varying findings according to location and extension of lesions. In class I, usually smooth concentric narrowing of the antrum; absence of peristalsis in involved area; signs of pyloric obstruction; with bowel involvement, tubular segmental narrowings, alternating with dilated loops. *Blood.* Eosinophilia (up to 60%). *Bone marrow.* High percentage of eosinophils may be found. *Biopsy of lesion.* See Pathology.

Therapy. Conservative treatment with adrenocorticotropic hormone (ACTH) and corticosteroids usually brings prompt control of symptoms and of eosinophilia. When indicated, exploratory laparotomy and biopsy. According to location and extension of lesions, surgical intervention may be decided upon. Usually gastroenterostomy is adequate; in some cases subtotal gastrectomy and total gastrectomy have been performed. According to recent findings, surgery seems necessary only for control of bleeding.

Prognosis. Lesions do not recur after resection. If they recur after conservative treatment, response to successive steroid administrations is prompt.

BIBLIOGRAPHY. Konjetzny GE: Ueber Magenfibrome. Beitr Klin Chir 119:53, 1920

Barrie HJ, Anderson JC: Hypertrophy of pylorus in an adult with massive eosinophil infiltration and giant cell reaction. Lancet II:1007–1009, 1948

Kohler PF, Brown WR: Immunologic aspects of hepatic and gastrointestinal tract disease. JAMA 248:2704–2709, 1982

Stites DP, Terr AI (eds): Basic and clinical immunology. London, Prentice-Hall, 1991

ALLERGIC RHINITIS

Synonyms. Bostocks; Engels atopic hypersensitivity autumnal catarrh; hay fever; immune reaction type 1; pollinosis; see Angelucci and Besnier prurigo.

Symptoms and Signs. Both sexes affected; first manifestation seldom observed before 2 months of age. Atopic infantile eczema frequently is early manifestation (see Unna); allergic rhinitis develops in 30 to 50% of cases of infantile eczema. Accurate family anamnesis reveals history of typical skin or systemic disorders of allergic type. All year around or in particular seasons or special environments (indoor, open air, country, gardens, humid places) attacks of rhinitis, conjuntivitis occasionally followed by asthmatic attack.

Etiology. Interplay of genetic factors (of complex nature, both dominant and recessive reported) and precipitating factors (immunological contact of mucosae with allergens; psychological). Most frequent airborne allergens responsible: pollens, molds, types of dust, dermatophagoides (dust mites).

Pathology. Hypertrophy of nasal and first airway mucosae with eosinophilic infiltration. Frequent development of poliposis.

Diagnostic Procedures. *Blood.* IgE level increased (in 80% of cases); IgG, IgA, IgM usually normal. Eosinophilia; search for specific antibodies (RAST). *Skin tests and provocative tests* (inhalation).

Therapy. General allergic management. Avoid exposure to allergens. Specific treatment for desensibilization: antihistaminics; corticosteroids; Cromolyn sodium.

Prognosis. With age, intensity of symptoms may decrease.

BIBLIOGRAPHY. Bias WB, Marshal DG, Platt-Mills TAE: Genetic control of factor involved in bronchial asthma, hay fever and other allergic states. In Litwin SD (ed): Genetic Determinants of Pulmonary Disease, pp 127–148. New York, Marcel Dekker, 1978

Charpin J, Dry J, Michel FB: Desensibilization des maladies allergiques: allergenes nouveaux, vigilance accrue. La Presse Med 33:1754, 1985

Stites DP, Terr AI (eds): Basic and Clinical Immunology. London, Prentice-Hall, 1991

ALLERGIC SEMINAL

Synonyms. Allergic vulvovaginitis.

Symptoms and Signs. *Vaginal.* Burning and pain during coitus or after ejaculation lasting from 2 to 70 hours. Erythema and edema, bullae on the labia.

Etiology. Family described (mother and four daughters) suggests autosomal dominant inheritance.

Diagnostic Procedures. *Skin test.* Reactivity to seminal fluid. *Blood.* No sperm agglutinating antibody detectable.

Therapy. Antihistaminics per os and/or topical.

BIBLIOGRAPHY. Chang T-W: Familial allergic seminal vulvovaginitis. Am J Obstet Gynecol 126:442–444, 1976

ALLGROVE

Synonyms. Achalasia-Addisonian; glucocorticoid deficiency-achalasia; addisonian-achalasia; alacrima-achalasia-addisonianism; adrenal insufficiency-alacrima-achalasia; triple A; 3A.

Symptoms. Both sexes. Defective tear formation at birth. Addisonian symptoms (onset 2–10 years of age) and achalasia (onset 7.7–17.0 year of age). Recently described associated motor and sensory neuropathy, ataxia, optic atrophy, impaired intelligence and impaired autonomic functions and skin changes in addition to hyperpigmentation, in a few cases hyperkeratosis of palms and cutis anserina.

Etiology. Recessive inheritance, possibly as a result of deletion of autosomal DNA with closely linked genes necessary for normal adrenal and neural function and dermal keratinization, or secondary to metabolic error, or related to degeneration of autonomic nerve supply of adrenals.

Pathology. Absence of the zona fasciculata and almost normal zona glomerulosa.

Diagnostic Procedures. *Blood.* Cortisol deficiency in all cases, and increase of ACTH in some cases, lack of response to ACTH stimulation; recurrent hypoglycemia. Occasionally aldosterone deficiency with evidence of salt loss. *Nerve conduction studies.*

Therapy. See Addisonian syndromes (chronic adrenal insufficiency).

Prognosis. Death may be caused by adrenal crisis.

BIBLIOGRAPHY. Allgrove J, Clayden GS, Grant DB, et al: Familial glucocorticoid deficiency with achalasia of the cardias and deficient tear production. Lancet I:1284–1286, 1978

Dugardeyn C, Anooshiravani M, Christophe C, et al: Achalasia-alacrima-ACTH insensitivity syndrome. J Belg Radiol 76:167–168, 1993

Grant DB, Barnes ND, Dumic M, et al: Neurological and adrenal dysfunction in the adrenal insufficiency-alacrima-achalasia (3A) syndrome. Arch Dis Child 68:779–782, 1993

ALPERS

Synonyms. Christensen-Krabbe; cerebral gray matter diffuse progressive degeneration-hepatic cyrrhosis; gray matter, poliodystrophia cerebri; glioneural juvenalis dystrophy.

Symptoms and Signs. Both sexes. Begins in early life with convulsions followed by progressive spasticity, myoclonus, ataxia, visual disturbance, and finally dementia. Growth retardation and increasing microcephaly: In some cases late onset jaundice and liver cirrhosis (see Alpers-hepatic cirrhosis).

Etiology. Anoxia; postepileptic, sequelae of trauma mentioned among other etiologic factors. Possible cases of autosomal recessive inheritance.

Pathology. Diffuse encephalopathy: degenerative changes in the middle layers of cerebral and cerebellar gray matter, with loss of cells and gliosis (walnut brain). Cerebral white matter and basal ganglia relatively spared.

Diagnostic Procedures. *EEG.* Typical patterns. *CT scan; MRI.* Progessive atrophy. *Brain biopsy.* See pathology.

Therapy. Anticonvulsivant therapy.

Prognosis. Very poor. Status epilepticus often terminating event.

BIBLIOGRAPHY. Alpers BJ: Diffuse progressive degeneration of the gray matter of the cerebrum. Arch Neurol Psychiatr 25:469–505, 1931

Boyd SG, Hardem A, Egger J, et al: Progressive neural degeneration of child with liver disease (Alpers disease). Characteristic neurophysiological feature. Neuropediatrics 17:75–80, 1986

Adams RD, Victor M: Principles of Neurology, 5th ed, p 812. New York, McGraw-Hill, 1993

ALPERS-HUTTENLOCHER

Synonym. Alpers progressive infantile poliodystrophy; liver cirrhosis—Alpers; poliodystrophia cerebri progressiva.

Symptoms and Signs. Both sexes. In early life (15 months), hypotonia, anemia hemorrhagic tendency, trichorrheis; seizures, spasticity, myoclonus, and dementia; later, jaundice, ascites.

Etiology. Recessive inheritance. Unidentified biochemical defect assumed.

Pathology. Diffuse anoxic encephalopathy. Liver cirrhosis.

Diagnostic Procedures. *Electroencephalography:* Typical patterns. *CT scan.* Progessive atrophy. *Brain biopsy.* See pathology. *Liver biopsy.* Fatty degeneration or cirrhosis. *Blood.* Glutathione oxidase deficiency in some cases.

Therapy. Symptomatic.

Prognosis. Death in early infancy for status epilepticus.

BIBLIOGRAPHY. Ford FR, Livingston S, Pryles CV: Familial degeneration of the cerebral gray matter in childhood with convulsions, myoclonus, spasticity, cerebral ataxia, choreoathetosis, dementia, and death in status epilepticus: Differentiation of infantile and juvenile type. J Pediat 39:33–43, 1951

Wefring KW, Lamvik JD: Familial progressive polydystrophy with cirrhosis of liver. Acta Paediatr Scand 56:295–300, 1967

Martin JB: Genetics in neurology. Ann Neurol 34:757–773, 1993

ALPHA-ANTITRYPSIN DEFICIENCY

Synonyms. Antitrypsin; 1AT, protease inhibitor; PI.

Symptoms and Signs. Present from birth or early infancy. No good evidence that modest reduction of concentration of 1AT in plasma per se is associated with disease symptoms and signs reported seem to be a result of the association with other diseases (mainly pulmonary emphysema and liver diseases, less frequently, disorders with immune response and inflammatory components: kidney disease, panniculitis, rheumatoid arthritis, uveitis malignancies and others). Recurrent chest infections and wheezing, related to passive smoking. Cholestatic jaundice eventually remitting (leaving mild liver abnormalities) or progressing to ascites and hepatic failure or, later (in first decade of adolescence), to cirrhosis. Usually onset of clinical manifestations in early adulthood.

Etiology. Deficiency of alpha1–antitrypsin (A-1–AT). Thirty-five different codominant alleles, each contributing to the measured antitryptic activity. Affected individual is (PiZZ) phenotype; heterozygous MZ (PiMZ) relatives are identified by typing (see Diagnostic Procedures). Autosomal recessive inheritance.

Pathology. *Liver.* Severe form micronodular portal cirrhosis; in PiZZ homozygous, presence of cytoplasmic granules in hepatocytes remain PAS positive after diastasis exposure. *Lung.* Panacinar form of emphysema.

Diagnostic Procedures. Electrophoresis typing of Pi (protease inhibitor). Polymorphic variants identified by letters (first alphabetical letters assigned to faster moving forms; slower designated PiZZ; PiMM = homozygous normal). Presence of slower form (PiZZ) responsible for low-serum antitrypsin level.

Therapy. Symptomatic. Alpha 1 antitrypsin intravenous administration once a week. No response (release of A-1–AT) to phenobarbital, estrogen, steroid. Successful portacaval shunt or liver transplantation are followed by good life expectancy.

Prognosis. Variable, from no harmful effects to death in infancy or adult life. Pulmonary emphysema; danazole, stop smoking (concomitant aggravating factor); parenteral administration of synthetic analogs.

BIBLIOGRAPHY. Laurel CB, Erikson S: The electrophoretic alpha 1 globulin pattern of serum in alpha 1 antitrypsin deficiency. Scand J Clin Lab Invest 15:132–140, 1963

Crystal RG: Alpha 1 trypsin deficiency, emphysema and liver disease: genetic basis and strategies for therapy. J Clin Invest 85:1343–1352, 1990

Cox DW: 1–Antitrypsin deficiency. In Scriver CR, Beaudet AL, Sly WS, et al: The Metabolic and Molecular Bases of Inherited Disease, 7th ed, pp 4125–4158. New York, McGraw-Hill, 1995

ALPHA 2–ANTIPLASMIN DEFICIENCY

Synonyms. Miyasato*; alpha 2–AP deficiency; plasmin inhibitor deficiency.

Symptoms and Signs. Rare. From birth, severe hemorrhages from umbilical cord and all other sites; in adult life spontaneous joint hemorrhages; hemothorax.

Etiology. Autosomal recessive.

Diagnostic Procedures. *Blood.* Shortening of time of lysis of clot and euglobulin lysis time. Radioimmunoassay of alpha2–antiplasmin: reduced or absent.

Therapy. Antifibrinolytic agents: tranexamic acid.

Prognosis. Bleeding episodes reduced in frequency and severity by treatment.

BIBLIOGRAPHY. Kluft C, Vellenga E, Brommer EJP: Homozygous alpha-2–antiplasmin deficiency. Lancet II:206, 1979

Kluft C, Nieuwenhuis HK, Rijken DC, et al: Alpha 2 Antiplasmin Enschede: Disfunctional alpha 2 antiplasmin molecule associated with an autosomal recessive hemorrhagic disorder. J Clin Invest 80:1391–1400, 1987

Bithell TC: Hereditary coagulation disorders. In Lee GR, Bithell TC, Foerster J, et al (eds): Wintrobe's Clinical Hematology, 9th ed, p 1447. Philadelphia, Lea & Febiger, 1993

---

*Probands surname.

ALPORT

Synonyms. Dickinson; deafness—nephropathy; hematuria-nephropathy—deafness; hemorrhagic familial nephritis. See Fechtner.

Symptoms. Both sexes affected. Initially asymptomatic. Later progressive renal insufficiency; loss of hearing; reduced vision (in males).

Signs. In the female, hematuria often only manifestation; occasionally nerve deafness complication of renal insufficiency in pregnancy (hypertension edema). In the male, hematuria; albuminuria; cylindruria; recurrent pyelonephritis; usually deafness, auditory nerve or Corti organ; occasionally congenital anomalies of the eyes (cataracts; spherophakia), including Alport-like hereditary nephritis (NALD). Other possible anomalies: inguinal hernia; anomalies of fingers; cryptorchidism; myasthenia; memory of recent event impaired; tumors of central nervous system.

Etiology. Unknown; autosomal dominant inheritance (possibly modified by a sex-linked suppressor gene). An X-linked inheritance is also proposed in some families.

Pathology. Chronic glomerulonephritis with interstitial renal foam cells.

Diagnostic Procedures. *Urine.* Hematuria; albuminuria; cylindruria; hyperaminoaciduria. *Blood.* Increased blood urea nitrogen and creatinine; anemia; megathrombocytopenia (nonconstant). *Ophthalmoscopy.* Fundus albipunctatus; lens alterations. *Audiometry.* Nerve deafness. *X-rays.* Changes related to kidney and cardiac failure and anomalies of urinary system. In some cases, spina bifida; pectus excavatum; renal calcification. *Renal arteriography.*

Therapy. Treatment of pyelonephritis. Kidney transplantation when indicated.

Prognosis. In the female, normal life span except for complications. In male renal failure by the fifth decade.

BIBLIOGRAPHY. Dickinson WH: Diseases of the kidney and urinary derangements, part 2:379. London, Longman, 1875
Alport AC: Hereditary familial congenital hemorrhagic nephritis. Br Med J 1:504–506, 1927
Crawfurd MA: Alport's syndrome. J Med Genet 25:623–627, 1988
Byers PH: Disorders of collagen biosynthesis and structure. In Scriver CR, Beaudet AL, Sly WS, et al: The Metabolic and Molecular Bases of Inherited Disease, 7th ed, pp 4062–4063. New York, McGraw-Hill, 1995

ALSTROEM

Synonyms. Retinitis pigmentosa—deafness—obesity—diabetes mellitus. See Laurence-Moon; Leber II and Bardet-Biedl.

Symptoms and Signs. High incidence in Sweden and Holland. Both sexes. At birth, blindness or marked reduction of vision; nystagmus; neuropathic deafness; acanthosis nigricans; obesity; manifestations of nephropathy and hypogonadism. Absence of polydactyly and mental retardation.

Etiology. Autosomal recessive inheritance.

Pathology. Defect of cones.

Diagnostic Procedures. *Fundus oculi.* In childhood normal; in later life pigmentation or depigmentation; occasionally, narrowing vessels. *Blood.* Hyperuricemia; hypertriglyceridemia. Hyperglycemia (as result of resistance to insulin) hyperprebetalipoproteinemia. *Electroretinography.* Absence or reduction of electrical activity.

Therapy. Symptomatic.

Prognosis. Poor. Possible development of or association with, cataract, keratoconus, or progression of optic atrophy or both.

BIBLIOGRAPHY. Alstroem CH, Hallgren B, Nielson LB, et al: Retinal degeneration combined with obesity, diabetes mellitus and neurogenous deafness. A specific syndrome (not hitherto described) distinct from the Laurence-Moon-Biedl syndrome. A clinical endocrinological and genetic examination based on a large pedigree. Acta Psychiatr Neurol Scand 34 (suppl 129):1–35, 1959
Connolly MB, Jan JE, Couch RM, et al: Hepatic dysfunction in Alstrom disease. Am J Med Genet 40:421–424, 1991

ALTAMIRA

Synonyms. Altamira hemorrhagic.

Symptoms and Signs. Low-grade fever precedes hemorrhages of skin, followed by bleeding of the mucous membranes; asthenia. Hemorrhagic skin lesions caused by insect bites; traumatic hematomas; petecchiae and ecchymoses on the whole surface of the body, or restricted to face and extremities. Small and painless lymph nodes in groin and axillae; seldom, moderate hepatosplenomegaly.

Etiology. The disease is owing to the bite of the black fly Simulium. Affected are immigrants living in an area called Altamira in a forest region of Brazil. No specific etiologic agent has been isolated. This hemorrhagic syndrome may be owing to a hypersensitivity phenomenon or response to a toxin associated with intense black fly bites. Either a direct toxic effect or a hypersensitivity reaction could lead to an arrest of megakaryocyte maturation.

Pathology. Bone marrow biopsy shows increased number of megakaryocytes.

Diagnostic Procedures. *Blood.* Platelets below 100,000; anemia; white blood cells normal; plasma clotting factors normal.

Therapy. Intravenous glucose; prednisone (20 to 40 mg day until symptoms relieved). In severe cases, blood transfusions.

BIBLIOGRAPHY. Pinheiro FP, Bensabath G, Costa D Jr, et al: Haemorrhagic syndrome of Altamira. Lancet I:639–642, 1974
Simpson DHI: Viral hemorrhagic fevers of man. Bull WHO 56:819, 838, 1978

ALUMINUM INTOXICATION

Synonyms. Antacid intoxication; dialysis encephalopathy; pseudohyperparathyroidism; dialysis dementia; phosphate deficiency rickets. See hard water.

Symptoms and Signs. Usually in patients on chronic treatment with aluminum hydroxide for duodenal ulcer, uremia, or in hemodialysis. Muscle weakness; bone pain; in some cases dementia (dialysis dementia).

Etiology. Excessive intake of aluminum (for chronic therapeutic treatment or poisoning).

Pathology. Bone and joints tissue: deposition of aluminum; osteomalacia (without osteitis fibrosa); mineralization defects.

Diagnostic Procedures. *X-rays.* See Pathology. *Blood.* Microcytic anemia; increased Ca level: normal or decreased parathyroid hormone and alkaline phosphatase levels.

Therapy. Desferoxamine. Chelation. Discontinue administration of aluminum preparations.

Prognosis. Good response to treatment.

BIBLIOGRAPHY. Wills MR, Savory F: Aluminium poisoning: dialysis encephalopathy, osteomalacia and anemia. Lancet 22:29–34, 1983
Andress DL, Maloney NA, Cobum FW, et al: Osteomalacia and aplastic bone disease in aluminium related osteodystrophy. J Clin Endocr Met 65:I.11–16, 1987

Stanbury SW, Mawer EB: Metabolic disturbances in acquired osteomalacia. In Cohen RD, Lewis B, Alberti KGMM, et al: The Metabolic Basis of Acquired Disease, pp 1717–1782. London, Ballire Tindall, 1990

ALVEOLAR CAPILLARY BLOCK

Synonyms. Alveolar hypoventilation; interstitial diffuse pulmonary fibrosis. See Hamman-Rich.

Symptoms. Dyspnea on effort; pleuritic pain.

Signs. Digital clubbing (may follow or precede dyspnea). Cyanosis; diffuse fine rales. Frequently, subcutaneous rheumatoid nodules.

Etiology. All conditions that reduce the total oxygen diffusing capacity of the lungs because of alteration of the pulmonary surface (alveolar-capillary block). Diseases of pulmonary interstitium: granulomatosis; scleroderma; rheumatoid arthritis.
Now it is known that the importance of alveolar-capillary block has been greatly exaggerated in the past, because arterial hypoxia in patients at rest with decreased diffusing capacities has been shown to be caused mainly by ventilation-perfusion inequalities and changes in pulmonary capillary blood volume and not by a simple reduction in the oxygen diffusing capacity.

Pathology. Initially, nonspecific interstitial pneumonia; then formation of mature fibrous tissue that evolves into "honeycomb lung"; bronchiectasis.

Diagnostic Procedures. *Blood.* Polycythemia. *X-rays of lung.* Early subacute stage, punctate nodular miliary-like pattern; later, medium to coarse reticulation. Occasionally, pleural effusion. *Pulmonary function test.* Restrictive; ventilatory defect; reduction of diffusing capacity.

Therapy. According to etiology. Adrenal steroid useful in collagen forms. Intensive care; ECG and pulse oxymetry monitoring; oxygen; in severe cases consider mechanical ventilation.

Prognosis. Evolving into congestive heart failure.

BIBLIOGRAPHY. Ellman P, Ball RE: "Rheumatoid disease" with joint and pulmonary manifestations. Br Med J 2:816–820, 1948
Fishman AP, Turino GM, Bergofsky EH: The syndrome of alveolar hypoventilation. Am J Med 23:333–339, 1957
Fraser RS, Paré JAP, Fraser RG, Paré PD: Synopsis of Disease of the Chest, 2nd ed. Philadelphia, WB Saunders, 1994

ALZHEIMER

Synonyms. A D; Presenile dementia. See Pick (A.) arteriopathic dementia; senile dementia (conditon identical but for the age of onset).

Symptoms. Predominant in female; onset usually in fifth or sixth decades. Gradual loss of immediate memory; patient conscious of defect and initially worried about it. Slovenly in dress; speech dysarthric; change in behavior; short temper or euphoria; disorientation in time and space; more need for sleep. Occasionally, hemiparesis; tremor; convulsions.

Signs. Focal signs of central nervous system defects. Hyperreflexia or hyporeflexia.

Etiology. Unknown; autosomal dominant inheritance reported and suggested for most cases. The possible role of virus-like scrapie agents, other viruses and interaction between genetic and environmental agents have been discussed.

Pathology. Shrinking of brain; thickening of pia; diffuse rarefaction of cortex, moderate glial reaction; large number of senile plaques. Neurofibrillar degeneration (dust-like argentophilic bodies or curled ends).

Diagnostic Procedures. *EEG.* Loss of frequencies; slow high-voltage activity. *CT scan, MRI.* Dilatation of ventricles and increased subarachnoid space. *Spinal fluid.* Normal or moderately increased protein.

Therapy. Hydergine-LC has been tried, without success. Acetyl-L-carnetine awaits corroboration. Chlorpromazine and related drugs as symptomatic for aberrant behavior when needed.

Prognosis. Death in 5 to 10 years.

BIBLIOGRAPHY. Alzheimer A: Ueber Einen Eigengartigen Schweren Krankheits: Prozess der Hirnrinde. Zentralbl Nerverkh 25:1134, 1906; 30:177–179, 1907
Thompson TL, Filley CM, Mitchell WD, et al: Lack of efficacy of hydergine in patient with Alzheimer's disease. N Engl J Med 323:445–448, 1990
Berg L: Alzheimer's disease. In Morris JC: Handbook of Dementing Illnesses. New York, Marcel Dekker, 1993

AMAUROSIS FUGAX

Symptoms. Transient visual loss; continuous recurrence may result in complete blindness.

Signs. Depends on etiology. Blood hypertension; polycythemia.

Etiology. Tabagism; hypertension; polycythemia; reduction of cerebral flow, as part of carotid system ischemia syndrome (see), indicating insufficiency of the ophthalmic artery. Microemboli of cholesterol arising from ulcerating arteriosclerotic plaques that temporarily obstruct the retinal artery; as part of syncope, migraine, or insufficiency of the vertebral-basilar system.

Pathology. Depending on etiology. Vascular spasm, if recurrent, results in ischemic retinal necrosis.

Therapy. Application of cold or hot water is beneficial within minutes in recurrent attacks. Elimination or treatment of pathogenetic factors: tobacco; polycythemia; hypertension. Sympathectomy.

Prognosis. Varies according to etiology.

BIBLIOGRAPHY. Moore RF: Medical Ophthalmology. London, Churchill, 1922
Adams RD, Victor M: Principles of Neurology, 5th ed, pp 207, 215, 703. New York, McGraw-Hill, 1993

AMBLYOPIC SCHOOLGIRL

Synonyms. Hysterical amblyopia.

Symptoms and Signs. Amblyopia. Alterations of visual fields: variable abnormal dark adaptation curve. Ring scotomas; hemianopsias.

Etiology. Related directly or indirectly to psychological disturbances.

Therapy. Psychotherapy.

BIBLIOGRAPHY. Schlaegel TF Jr, Quilala FV: Hysterical amblyopia. Arch Ophth 54:875–884, 1955
Manty Jarvi MI: The amblyopic school girl syndrome. J Ped Ophthal Strabys 18:30–33, 1981
Mamelok AE: Psychiatry and ophthalmology. In Kaplan HI, Sadock BJ: Comprehensive Textbook of Psychiatry, 6th ed, p 1255. Baltimore, Williams & Wilkins, 1995

AMELOGENESIS IMPERFECTA

Synonyms. Steinberg; Witkop teeth; microdontia.

Symptoms and Signs. Clusters of enamel defects: smooth, rough, pitted; failure to erupt of many teeth.

Etiology. Six forms recognized: 4 autosomal dominant: A. I. Hypocalcification type (A I H2); A.I. Hypomaturation hypoplasia type—Taurodontism; A.I. Hypoplastic type (including microdontia); Tricho-dento-osseous (see); 3 autosomal recessive: Kohlschutter (see); A.I. Local hypoplastic type; Enamel-renal (see); A.I. Pigmented hypomaturation type; 2 X-linked: A.I. Hypomaturation type (includes snow capped teeth); A.I. Hypoplastic type (AI H1).

BIBLIOGRAPHY. Witkop CJ Jr, Sauk JJ Jr: Heritable defects of enamel. In Stewart RE, Prescott GH: Oral Facial Genetics. St Louis, Mosby, 1976

Crawford PJM, Aldred MJ: Amelogenesis imperfecta with taurodontism and the tricho-dento-osseous syndrome: separate conditions or a spectrum of disease? Clin Med Genet 38:44–50, 1990

AMENORRHEA-GALACTORRHEA-HYPOTHYROIDISM

Symptoms and Signs. Postpartum galactorrhea and amenorrhea, accompanied by all symptoms and signs of hypothyroidism.

Etiology. Unknown. See: Multiple endocrine deficiency (acquired?).

Pathology. Unknown.

Diagnostic Procedures. *Thyroid function.* Hypothyroidism. *X-ray of skull.* Normal sella turcica. *Blood.* Increase in prolactin.

Therapy. Thyroid.

Prognosis. Amenorrhea and galactorrhea as well as hypothyroidism corrected by treatment.

BIBLIOGRAPHY. Ross F, Nusynowitz ML: A syndrome of primary hypothyroidism, amenorrhea, and galactorrhea. J Clin Endocrinol 28:591–595, 1968

Leite V, Cowden EA, Friesen H: Endocrinology pf lactation and nursing: disorders of lactation. In De Groot LJ (eds): Endocrinology, 3rd ed, pp 2235–2236. Philadelphia, WB Saunders, 1995

AMENORRHEA-GALACTORRHEA SYNDROME

Synonyms. Including: Ahumada-del Castillo (Argonz-del Castillo, galactorrhea-amenorrhea in nullipara); Chiari-Frommel (Chiari I, Frommel-Chiari; lactation uterus atrophy; galactorrhea-amenorrhea postpartum); Forbes-Albright (galactorrhea-amenorrhea pituitary enlargement); hyperprolactinemia.

Symptoms and Signs. Association of galactorrhea and amenorrhea concomitant or not with postpartum. Associated with neurological symptoms of pituitary tumor.

Etiology. Increase of prolactin secretion. Adenoma (prolactin secreting) of pituitary.

Diagnostic Procedures. *Blood.* Prolactin values raised; prolactin release test altered (TRH test particularly useful). *CT scan, MRI.* Pituitary enlargement.

Therapy. If tumor, hypophysectomy or radiation. Bromocriptine, lergotrile mesylate.

Prognosis. Avoid pregnancy if pituitary tumor. Depends on stage of disease and treatment.

BIBLIOGRAPHY. Frommel R: Ueber puerperale Atrophie des Uterus. Z Geburtshilfe Gynak 7:305–313, 1882

Chiari JB, Braun C, Spaeth J: Report of diseases of women observed during the years 1848 to 1855, inclusive, in the Department of Gynecology (Municipal Clinic), Vienna Klin. Geburtsh V Gynak:371, 1855

Ahumada JC, del Castillo EB: Sobre un caso de galactorrea y amenorrea. Bol Soc Obst Gin (Buenos Aires) 11:64–72, 1932

Krestin D: Spontaneous lactation associated with enlargement of pituitary, with report of 2 cases. Lancet I:928–930, 1932

Argonz J, del Castillo EB: A syndrome characterized by estrogenic insufficiency, galactorrhea and decreased urinary gonadotropin. J Clin Endocrinol 13:79–87, 1953

Forbes AP, Heunemann PH, Griswald GC, et al: Syndrome characterized by galactorrhea, amenorrhea and low urinary FSH: comparison with acromegaly and normal lactation. J Clin Endocrinol 14:265–271, 1954

Koppelman MCS: Hyperprolactinemia amenorrhea and galactorrhea. Ann Int Med 10:115–121, 1984

Baird DT: Amenorrhea, anovulation, and dysfunctional uterine bleeding. In De Groot LJ (ed): Endocrinology, 3rd ed, p 2065. Philadelphia, WB Saunders, 1995

AMINOPTERIN-LIKE

Synonyms. Pseudoaminopterine.

Symptoms and Signs. No evidence of maternal exposure to the drug. Signs remind of folate angonist syndrome (see). Brachyoturricephaly with cranio synostosis, malar hypoplasia, ogival palate, michrognathia, abnormal ears; mental and physical development retardation.

Etiology. It is an autosomal recessive syndrome, associated with translocation involving chromosome 5 and 10.

BIBLIOGRAPHY. Fraser FC, Anderson RA, Mulvihill SI, et al: An aminopterin-like syndrome without aminopterin. Clin Genet 32:28–34, 1987

Verloes A, Bricteux G, Koulisher L: Pseudoaminopterine syndrome. Am J Med Genet 46:394–397, 1993

AMNESIA, GLOBAL TRANSIENT

Synonyms. Fisher-Adams; transient global amnesia.

Symptoms. Occasionally, abrupt onset of profound memory loss and disorientation without consciousness change; in some cases after sexual intercourse, pain, emotion, or fatigue. No evidence of aphasia or memory alterations.

Signs. Most patients have a history of arterial hypertension. Physical examination otherwise normal.

Etiology. Unknown. Suspected vascular basis, cerebral ischemia in distribution of posterior cerebral arteries supplying inferomedial parts of both temporal areas. Interpreted as a form of temporal lobe epilepsy (?) or of migraine.

Diagnostic Procedures. *EEG.* Negative possible presence of spike discharges that disappear in few months. *MRI and CT brain scan.* Negative.

Therapy. None. Treatment of blood hypertension (if present).

Prognosis. Return of mental state to normality, usually, within 12 to 24 hours. Occurrence of single (usual) or seldom with long intervals repeated episode; successive sexual relations could be asymptomatic.

BIBLIOGRAPHY. Fisher CM, Adams RD: Transient global amnesia. Acta Neurol Scand (suppl) 9:7–83, 1964

Matthew NT, Meyer JS: Pathogenesis and natural history of transient global amnesia. Stroke 5:303–311, 1974

Mayeux R: Sexual intercourse and transient global amnesia. Lancet 1:864, 1979

Adams RD, Victor M: Principles of Neurology, 5th ed, pp 373–374. New York, McGraw-Hill, 1993

AMNIOTIC BAND

Synonyms. Streeter bands; amnion adhesion fetus; ADAM complex; amputation (congenital); constricting bands; terminal transverse defect of arms. Included Ballantyne-Smith

Symptoms and Signs. Uncommon anomalies (disruption, deformation, malformations) that involve the head and, more frequently, the fetal limbs, producing peromelia. Possibly associated: chest deformities; omphalocele; gastroschisis; genital malformations; imperforate anus; hypoplastic lungs; scoliosis; meningomyelocele; ectopia cordis.

Etiology. Unknown (controversial). Sporadic occurrence possible; genetic origin has been considered. (1) Primary lesion within developing limbs mesenchyme, external band or band only secondary (Streeter). (2) Primary abnormality of the amnion and amniotic bands encircling distal part of limbs (Ballantyne-Smith).

Pathology. Rupture of amnion, chorion intact; amniotic bands producing, on vascular basis, necrosis of fetal limbs.

Diagnostic Procedures. *X-rays. Ultrasonography. Amniotic fluid* (elevated alpha fetoprotein), for prenatal diagnosis.

Therapy. In some cases, surgical procedures to remove constricting band.

Prognosis. Permanent alteration, from simple single ring constriction to severe involvement. Fatal.

BIBLIOGRAPHY. Ballantyne JW: Manual of Antenatal Pathology and Hygiene. The Foetus. Edinburgh, W Greene, 1902
Streeter GL: Focal deficiencies in fetal tissues and their relation to intra-uterine amputation. Contrib Embryol Carnegie Inst Washington 22 (126):1–144, 1930
Fiedler JM, Phelan JP: The amniotic band syndrome in monozygotic twins. Am J Obstet Gynecol 146:864–865, 1983
Askins G, Errol G: Congenital constriction band syndrome. J Ped Orthoped 8:461–466, 1988

AMNIOTIC FLUID

Synonym. Amniotic fluid embolism.

Symptoms. Sudden dyspnea; shock. Common in multiparas over 30, with history of hard labor or pitocin administration or both.

Signs. Tachypnea; percussion of lung areas obtuse; cyanosis; hypotension. Uterine relaxation followed by profuse vaginal bleeding.

Etiology. Embolism of amniotic fluid (including squames, lanugo, hairs from the skin, fat, mucin, and bile) into the cardiovascular system causes pulmonary edema, embolic phenomena, depression of fibrinogen in circulation with resulting rise in pulmonary artery pressure and right ventricular failure, followed then by systemic blood fall and shock, and owing to anticoagulant property of amniotic fluid by uncontrollable bleeding.

Pathology. Massive intravascular clotting. Emboli in pulmonary vessels of mucus, amniotic cells, and debris; pulmonary edema.

Diagnostic Procedures. *Blood.* Hypofibrinogenemia; prolonged clotting time. Monitoring of vital parameters.

Therapy. Treatment of shock, importance of monitoring central venous pressure; care to prevent right heart insufficiency. Fibrinogen administration. Heparin and EACA. Real utility vs. risks has to be evaluated further.

Prognosis. Usually fatal. Maternal mortality rate of 1 in 20,000–30,000 deliveries, perhaps even higher. Ten percent of maternal death.

BIBLIOGRAPHY. Weiner AE, Reid DE, Roby CC: The hemostatic activity of amniotic fluid. Science 110:190, 1949
Aguillon A, Andjus A, Grayson A, et al: Amniotic fluid embolism: A review. Obstet Gynecol Surv 17:619–636, 1962
Fraser RS, Paré JAP, Fraser RG, Paré PD: Synopsis of Diseases of the Chest, 2nd ed, pp 562–563. Philadelphia, WB Saunders, 1994

AMOK

Synonyms. Whitman; AMUK.

Symptoms. Reported primarily in Malayan and African people. Occasionally seen in Western countries. Homicidal attack, preceded by period of depression; preoccupation. In an unprovoked outburst of rage patient runs about armed, usually with a knife, and attacks indiscriminately any person or animal that he encounters before he is overpowered or kills himself.

Etiology. Unknown; toxic or chronic psychotic condition; brain syndromes (see). A small pineal tumor was found on autopsy in Whitman (young Texan who shot passersby from a tower).

Therapy. Overpowering and physical restraint of patient. Then specific antitoxic and psychiatric assistance, removing underlying cause. Prevention through education.

BIBLIOGRAPHY. Westermeyer J: A comparison of amok and other homicides in Laos. Am J Psych 129:708–709, 1972
Murphy HBM: History and evolution of syndromes: The striking case of latah and amok. In Hammer M, Salzinger K, Sutton S (eds): Psychopathology: Contribution from the Social, Behavioral and Biological Sciences. New York, Wiley & Sons, 1973
Kaplan HI, Sadock BJ: Comprehensive Textbook of Psychiatry, 6th ed, pp 1055–1056. Baltimore, Williams & Wilkins, 1995

AMORPHOSYNTHESIS

Symptoms. Both sexes affected; onset at all ages. Neglected extrapersonal or personal space. Usually, unawareness or neglect of left side of the body; inability to orientate to same side space. Patient does not integrate perceptions (hearing, visual tactile, kinesthetic) of the affected side in his or her total consciousness.

Etiology. Damage (neoplastic, hemorrhagic) of controlateral parietal lobe.

BIBLIOGRAPHY. Denny-Brown D, Meyer JS, Horenstein S: The significance of perceptual rivalry resulting from parietal lesion. Brain 75:433–471, 1952
Dimond SJ, Blizard DA: Evolution and lateralization of the brain. Ann NY Acad Sci 299:1–501, 1977
Adams RD, Victor M: Principles of Neurology, 5th ed, p 397. New York, McGraw-Hill, 1993

AMOTIVATIONAL

Synonyms. Marijuana toxicity.

Symptoms and Signs. In adolescent marijuana smokers. Energy loss, diminished attentiveness, harmed parental relationship, behavioral disruptions.

Etiology. Marijuana smoking. Many authors contest this syndrome.

BIBLIOGRAPHY. Beaubrun MH, Knight F: Psychiatric assessments of 30 chronic users of cannabis and 30 matched controls. Am J Psychiatr 130:309–311, 1983
Maxwell D: Medical complications of substance abuse. In Ghodse AH, Maxwell D: Substance Abuse and Dependence, pp 176–203. London, Macmillan Press, 1990

AMYLOIDOSIS SYNDROMES

Synonyms. Fibrilloses. At present there is a trend to classify the amyloidosis on the chemical composition of the amyloid fibrils. This is not yet entirely possible since in many forms of systemic amyloidosis, amyloid subunits have not yet been identified. An attempt of general classification recognizes systemic and localized forms, and the systemic forms have been further subdivided into the subtypes (1) Immunoglobulin (AL) (former primary or myeloma (see Kahler-Bozzolo) and other plasma cell dyscrasias (see Waldenstroem and heavy chain) characterized by the presence of Ig light chains (kappa and lambda) and monoclonal immunoglobulin; (2) Reactive (AA) (former secondary) characterized by the presence of amyloid A and chronic inflammatory diseases; (3) Hereditary autosomal dominant inheritance (formerly: familial, heredofamilial), characterized by the presence of subunit proteins (transthyretin, gelsolin, fibrinogen, lysozyme, apolipoprotein A-I;4) 2–microglobulin (see dialysis) characterized by the presence of 2–microglobulin in patients submitted to chronic renal dialysis. The number of mutations in plasma transthyretin associated with amyloidosis are at present over 40, especially in hereditary amyloidosis, and are also multiple for the other subunit proteins, thus chemical classification is impractical from a clinical point of view. Although some overlappings have been identified, the historical old, clinical classification still retains a certain practical value. (See individual syndromes.)

BIBLIOGRAPHY. Benson MD: Amyloidosis. In Scriver CR, Beaudet AL, Sly WS, et al: The Metabolic and Molecular Bases of Inherited Disease, 7th ed, pp 4159–4191. New York, McGraw-Hill, 1995

AMYLOIDOSIS–ATRIAL STANDSTILL, FAMILIAL

Synonyms. Harrison; Maeda; atrial standstill-amyloidosis.

Symptoms and Signs. Onset in the 2nd to 4th decade: bradycardia and cardiomegaly; abdominal pains; absence of peripheral neuropathy, rapid progressive cardiac failure, gastrointestinal disorder, or renal dysfunction.

Etiology. Unknown.

Pathology. Amyloid deposits limited to atrium; and loss of muscle with replacement fibrosis.

Diagnostic Procedures. *ECG.* Bradycardia. Absence of P waves. *X-ray.* Cardiomegaly. *Echocardiogram.* Dilatation of right atrium. *Cardiac catherization.* Absence of waves on right atrial pressure curve. *Biopsy.* See pathology. Atropine and exercise increase frequency but P wave remain absent. *Blood.* Temporary increase of transaminases during abdominal pain episode.

Therapy. Pacemaker; oral anticoagulants.

Prognosis. With treatment condition appears to stabilize.

BIBLIOGRAPHY. Harrison WH, Derric JR: Atrial standstill: a review and presentation of two new cases of familial and unusual nature with reference to epicardial pacing in one Angiology 20:610–617, 1969
Maeda S: Tanaka T, Hayashi T: Familial standstill caused by amyloidosis. Br Heart J 59:498–500, 1988

AMYLOIDOSIS III

Synonyms. Fredriksen; amyloid cardiomyopathy I; Denmark amyloid cardiomyopathy; amyloidosis methionine 111.

Symptoms and Signs. Both sexes affected; onset between 37 and 46 years of age. From dyspnea and rather rapidly progressing right heart failure to cachexia and anasarca. Marked splitting of second sound; extrasystoles.

Etiology. Unknown. Autosomal dominant.

Pathology. Thick-walled heart; amyloid infiltration in pericardium. Infiltration of gastrointestinal tract, including tongue, peripheral nerves, and fat deposits; lack of infiltration of liver, brain, and skeletal muscles. Chemical analysis of post mortem tissues (in the Danish patients) shows amyloid contains transthyretin (former prealbumin) with methionine for leucine substitutionat position 111.

Diagnostic Procedures. *X-ray of chest.* Moderate cardiomegaly. *Electrocardiography.* Two categories: (1) right bundle block, left axis devia-

tion, P-R prolonged; (2) left ventricular hypertrophy with left axis deviation or low voltage in peripheral leads. *Heart catheterization.* Low cardiac output; elevation of pulmonary wedge, right atrial, and pulmonary artery pressures.

Therapy. Diuretics give temporary benefit.

Prognosis. Duration of condition for 2 to 6 years from onset. In some cases sudden death or death from congestive heart failure.

BIBLIOGRAPHY. Fredriksen T, Gotzsche H, Harboe N, et al: Familial primary amyloidosis with severe amyloid heart disease. Am J Med 33:328–348, 1962
Husby G, Ranlov PJ, Sletter K, et al: The amyloid in familial amyloidotic cardiomyopathy of Danish origin is related to prealbumin. In Glenner GG: Proceedings of the IV International Symposium on Amyloidosis. Amsterdam, Excerpta Medica, 1985
Benson MD: Amyloidosis. In Scriver CR, Beaudet AL, Sly WS, et al: The Metabolic and Molecular Bases of Inherited Disease, 7th ed, pp 4159–4191. New York, McGraw-Hill, 1995

AMYLOIDOSIS VII

Synonyms. Oculoleptomeningeal amyloidosis; Ohio amyloidosis.

Symptoms and Signs. Dementia, seizures, strokes, visual deterioration, coma; neurological dysfunctions are episodic.

Etiology. Possibly autosomal dominant. Possible relation with hereditary cerebral hemorrhage not yet clarified.

Pathology. Severe diffuse amyloidosis of leptomeninges and subarachnoid vessels; patchy fibrosis and obliteration of subarachnoid space. Diffuse neuronal loss in brain and cerebellum. Occasional superficial brain infarction. Minimal amyloid deposits in other organs, except vitreous, and retinal membranes and vessels.

BIBLIOGRAPHY. Goten H, Steinberg MC, Farboody GH: Familial oculoleptomeningeal amyloidosis. Brain 103:473–495, 1980
Benson MD, Wallace MR: Amyloidosis. In Scriver CR, Beaudet AL, Sly WS, et al: The Metabolic and Molecular Bases of Inherited Disease, 6th ed, p 2454. New York, McGraw-Hill, 1989

AMYLOIDOSIS IX

Synonyms. Amyloidosis primary cutaneous, familial lichen amyloidosis, Lichen amyloidosis.

Symptoms and Signs. More frequent in South America and Asia. Onset at puberty. Intense pruritis, moderate lichenoid lesions. Absence of other signs. Scratching relieves pruritus by removing core of papules.

Etiology. Autosomal dominant inheritance. Reported also X-linked inheritance.

BIBLIOGRAPHY. Issak L: Localized amyloid cutis associated with psoriasis in siblings. Arch Dermatol Syph 61:859–862, 1950
Sagher F, Shanon J: Amyloidosis cutis: familial occurrence in three generations. Arch Derm 87:171–175, 1963
Newton JA, Jagjvan A, Bhogal B, et al: Familial primary cutaneous amyloidosis. Br J Derm 112:201–208, 1985

AMYLOIDOSIS SYSTEMIC SENILE

Synonyms. Senile systemic amyloidosis; senile cardiac amyloidosis.

Symptoms and Signs. In individual dying over age 80 at post mortem studies. Deposit of amyloid often in heart, and less frequently varying degree of systemic involvement.

Etiology. Unknown.

Pathology. See symptoms and Signs.

BIBLIOGRAPHY. Buerger L, Braunstein H: Senile cardiac amyloidosis. Am J Med 28:357, 1960

Westermark P, Sletten K, Johansson B, et al: Fibril in senile systemic amyloidosis is derived from normal trathyretin. Proc Natl Acad Sci USA 87:2843, 1990

AMYOPLASIA

Synonyms. Constitute a subgroup in the category of arthrogryposis (see).

Symptoms and Signs. Syndrome characterized by an almost absence of muscles, a characteristic medial rotation of the arms, multiple joint contractures and ankylosis. Frequently presence of midfacial capillary hemangioma.

Etiology. Most of cases sporadic.

BIBLIOGRAPHY. Hall JG, Reed SD, Dricoll EP: Amyoplasia: a common, sporadic condition with congenital contractures. Am J Med Genet 15:571–590, 1983

Walton J, Karpati G, Hilton-Jones D: Disorders of Voluntary Muscle, p 810. Edinburgh, Churchill Livingstone, 1994

AMYOTROPHIC LATERAL SCLEROSIS

Synonyms. Charcot amyotrophic lateral sclerosis; ALS; Aran-Duchenne; motor neuron system; progressive spinal muscular atrophy; amyotrophic lateral sclerosis; progressive bulbar palsy.

Symptoms. Predominant in males; onset in the 4th to 6th decades of life. Symmetric weakness in small hand muscles, particularly interossei, thenar, and hypothenar. Fibrillation and atrophy that rapidly appear. Atrophy gradually and progressively extends, involving muscles of arms, shoulders, and trunk.

Signs. Fasciculation and atrophy of affected muscles.

Etiology. Unknown; possibly inherited; toxic (?); nutritional and viruses (?) growth factors (?); pancreatic adenoma; viruses (?), growth factors (?) autoimmunity; free radicals; a theory has been proposed that the accumulation of glutamate in the brain causing eccitotoxicity may lead to damage and death of neurons.

Pathology. Anterior cell of spinal tract affected by degenerative changes; muscle shows typical changes from damaged innervation; connective tissue replacement of muscle fibers.

Diagnostic Procedures. *Blood and urine.* Negative. *Cerebrospinal fluid.* Normal. Evoked Potential. *Chromosomal studies.*

Therapy. Symptomatic; avoidance of contractures; 2-amino-6-trifluoromethosybenzothiazol may produce some benefit, at its maximum, after 9 months of administration (delay of need for tracheostomy).

Prognosis. Progressive without remissions; death in few years.

BIBLIOGRAPHY. Aran FA: Recherches sur une maladie non encour décrit du systéme musculaire (atrophie musculaire progressive). Arch Gen Med (Paris) 24:172–214, 1850

Duchenne, GB: Etude comparée des lésions anatomique dans l'atrophie musculaire progressive et dans la paralysie générale. Union Med Prat Fr 7:202, 1853

Smith RA (ed): Handbook of Amyotrophic lateral sclerosis. New York, Marcel Dekker, 1992

Lipton SA, Rosenberg PA: Excitatory aminoacids as a final pathway for neurologic disorders. New Engl J Med 330:613–622, 1994

Bensimon G, Lacomblez L, Maininger V, et al: A controlled trial of riluzole in amyotrophic lateral sclerosis. New Engl J Med 330:585–591, 1994

ANALBUMINEMIA

Symptoms. Both sexes affected; present at birth. Asymptomatic or asthenia.

Signs. Mild persistent edema; occasionally, arterial hypotension and mild diarrhea.

Etiology. Defective synthesis of albumin. Likely autosomal recessive inheritance.

Pathology. Reported in some cases, but not likely related to the condition: aortic valve insufficiency; skin changes (angiomas; eczema; lipodystrophy); gynecomastia; rheumatoid arthritis. Related to the condition: high concentration of albumin in the tissue and early arteriosclerotic changes. Liver biopsy shows normal pattern and moderate increase of reticuloendothelial system.

Diagnostic Procedures. *Blood.* Protein electrophoresis shows absence of albumin band, increase of most globulin fractions; immunochemical quantitation confirms lack of or extremely low levels of albumin. IgG and IgM, fibrinogen, alpha 1-acidglycoprotein, alpha 1-antitrypsin, haptoglobulin, C-reactive protein, and prealbumin increased. Beta-lipoproteins, cholesterol, and esterified fatty acids are increased. Free fatty acids are normal. Erythrocyte sedimentation, rarely, increased. Serum osmolality reduced 50%. *Test with injection of albumin.* Marked by (55 days) prolonged survival (normal: 13–21 days).

Therapy. None, or repeated injection of albumin advisable in certain physiopathologic conditions (e.g., pregnancy, infections).

Prognosis. Excellent. No known impairment except for lack of albumin. Increased tendency to arteriosclerotic changes.

BISALBUMINEMIA

Symptoms and Signs. None.

Etiology. Unknown; codominant hereditary characterstic with normal and abnormal genes fully expressed.

Diagnostic Procedures. *Protein electrophoresis.* Shows the presence of an abnormal albumin in addition to the normal one.

Therapy. None.

ANOMALOUS ALBUMINEMIA

Congenital abnormality; possibly nonspecifically associated with syndrome of goiter and deafness.

BIBLIOGRAPHY. Bennhold H, Peters H, Roth E: Über einen Fall bon kompletter Analbuminaemie ohne wesentliche klinische Krankheitszeichen. Verh Dsch Ges Inn Med Kong 60:630–634, 1954

Scheurlen PG: Ueber Serumeiweissveranderungen beim Diabetes mellitus. Klin Wochenschr 33:198–205, 1955

Fraser GR, Harris H, Robson EB: A new genetically determined plasmaprotein in man. Lancet I:1023–1024, 1959

Gitlin D, Schmid K, Earle DP, et al: Observations on double albumin. II. A peptide difference between two genetically determined human serum albumins. J Clin Invest 40:820–827, 1961

Dammacco F, Miglietta A, D'Addabbo A, et al: Analbuminemia: report of a case and review of the literature. Vox Sang 39:153–161, 1980

Galliano M, Minchyitti L, Iadarola P, et al: Genetic variants of human serum albumin. Prog Med Lab 2:475–477, 1988

ANCELL

Synonyms. Ancell-Spiegler; Brooke-Fordyce trichoepitheliomas; Spiegler; turban tumors; cylindromatosis.

Symptoms and Signs. Prevalent in females (not definitely established); onset during late childhood or early adolescence. Presence of small scalp lesions (Ancell-Spiegler turban tumors) or facial skin lesions affecting especially nasolabial area (Brooke-Fordyce trichoepitheliomas) or both in the members of affected families. No systemic manifestations.

Etiology. Unknown; autosomal dominant inheritance. Some isolated cases reported (phenocopies).

Pathology. Scalp tumors with appearance of typical cylindromas. Epithelial cell islands surrounded by hyaline membrane. Face tumors, appearance of tricoepitheliomas, cyst-like spaces, and horn cells.

Diagnostic Procedures. *Biopsy.*

Therapy. Surgical excision and skin graft. X-ray therapy (may cause chronic ulceration and risk of neoplastic changes).

Prognosis. Benign lesions; occasionally malignant changes (basal cell epithelioma) have been noted. In one case lung cylindroma.

BIBLIOGRAPHY. Ancell H: History of a remarkable case of tumors, developed on the head and face. Med Chir Trans 25:227–246, 1842

Brooke HG: Epithelioma adenoides cysticum. Br J Dermatol 4:269–286, 1892

Fordyce JA: Multiple benign cystic epitheliomas of the skin. J Cut Dis 10:459–472, 1892

Spiegler E: Ueber Endothelioma der Haut. Arch Dermatol Syph 50:163, 1899

Vernon HJ, Olsen EA, Vollmer RT: Autosomal dominant multiple cylindromas associated whit solitary lung cylindroma J Am Acad Derm 19:397–400, 1988

MacKie RM: Tumors of the skin appendages. In Champion RH, Burton JL, Ebling FJG (eds): Rook/Wilkinson/Ebling Textbook of Dermatology, 5th ed, p 1508. Oxford, Blackwell Scientific, 1992

ANDERMANN

Synonyms. Charlevoix*; corpus callosum agenesis—neuropathy.

Symptoms and Signs. Both sexes. Mental and physical retardation, areflexia, paraparesis. Microcephaly, optic atrophy, seizures. Progressive motor neuropathy.

Etiology. Autosomal recessive inheritance. An X-linked form described with additional brain abnormalities.

Diagnostic Procedures. *CT scan; MRI.*

Therapy. Orthopedic surgery when needed.

Prognosis. Motor neuropathy leads to loss of ambulation by adolescence and progressive scoliosis.

BIBLIOGRAPHY. Andermann F, Andermann E, Goubert M, et al: Familial agenesis of corpus callosum with anterior horn cell disease. Trans Am Neur Ass 97:242–244, 1972

Larbrisseau A, Vanasse M, Brochu P, et al: The Andermann syndrome. Can J Neurol Sci 11:257–261, 1984

ANDERSEN II

Synonyms. Alpha 1,4 glucan: alpha 1,4 glucan 6-gluconyl transferase deficiency; brancher deficiency; amylopectinosis; cirrhosis liver-abnormal glycogen; Cori's type IV glycogenosis; glycogenosis storage disease type IV.

Symptoms. Very rare or difficult to identify. Onset in early infancy, full manifestation between 7th and 12th months. Poor development; repeated respiratory infections; hypotonia.

Signs. Marked hepatosplenomegaly with enlargement of abdomen; ascites; esophageal varices.

*County of Quebec where reporting family resided.

Etiology. Autosomal recessive inheritance (suggested). Alpha 1,4 glucan: alpha 1,4-glucan 6-gluconyl transferase (brancher) deficiency.

Pathology. Liver cirrhosis; complete disruption of architecture; vacuolated cells containing described type of glycogen. Same material (in granular form) has been found in spleen, lymph nodes, lung macrophages, heart, and muscle fibers.

Diagnostic Procedures. *Blood.* Moderate anemia; seldom hypoglycemia, diminished hyperglycemic response to epinephrine and glucagon. Initially, liver function test slightly impaired; then progressive deterioration and hyperbilirubinemia. *EEG.* Nonspecific abnormalities.

Therapy. Treatment for liver failure and ascites. Liver transplantation.

Prognosis. Very poor; invariably fatal. Terminal diarrhea; melena; hyperpyrexia. Older case died before the age of 5. With liver transplant good immediate results, long-term success not known.

BIBLIOGRAPHY. Andersen DH: Studies on glycogen disease with report of a case in which the glycogen was abnormal. In Najjar VA: Carbohydrate Metabolism, pp 28–42. Baltimore, Johns Hopkins Univ Press, 1952

Andersen DH: Familial cirrhosis of the liver with storage of abnormal glycogen. Lab Inv 5:11–20, 1956

Howell RR: Continuing lesson from glycogen storage disease (editorial). New Engl J Med 324:55–56, 1991

Selby R, Starzl TE, Yunis E, et al: Liver transplantation for type IV Glycogen storage disease. New Engl J Med 324:39–42, 1991

Chen YT, Burchell A: Glucogen storage diseases. In Scriver CR, Beaudet AL, Sly WS, et al: The Metabolic and Molecular Bases of Inherited Disease, 7th ed, pp 935–936. New York, McGraw-Hill, 1995

ANDERSON (C.M.)

Synonyms. Hypobetalipoproteinemia—intestinal accumulation of apolipoprotein-like; chylomicron retention.

Symptoms and Signs. Prevalence in males (6:2). Severe diarrhea in infancy and variable degree of growth retardation. As a general rule absence of neuro-ocular symptoms, however, there are reports with neurologic manifestations (decreased tendon reflexes and vibratory sense) and slight mental retardation.

Etiology. Unknown. Genetic relationship to Bassen-Kornzweig (allelic genes?). Autosomal recessive inheritance.

Pathology. Intestinal wall: fat-laden enterocytes with high level of apo-B-48.

Diagnostic Procedures. *Blood.* Hypobetolipoproteins, low HDL, total LDL are about half of normal, Apo B-100 is found in LDL, plus several additional abnormalities of lipid pattern. Acanthocytosis usually absent (few reports of mild manifestation). Hypoalbuminemia. Extremely low tocopherol level. *Eye.* In some cases minor defect in color vision and retinal function. *Intestinal biopsy.* See pathology.

Therapy. Restriction of dietary fats, supply adequate amount of fatty acids supplemented by vitamins A and E

Prognosis. Benign.

BIBLIOGRAPHY. Anderson CM, Towley RRW, Freeman M, et al: Unusual causes of steatorrhea in infancy and chilhood. Med J Austr 2:617–622, 1961

Pessah M, Benlian P, Beucler I, et al: Anderson's disease: genetic exclusion of the apolipoprotein-B gene in two families. J Clin Invest 87:367–370, 1991

Kane JP, Havel RJ: Disorders of the biogenesis and secretion of lipoproteins containing the B apolipoproteins. In Scriver CR, Beaudet AL, Sly WS, et al: The Metabolic and Molecular Bases of Inherited Disease, 7th ed, pp 1870–1871. New York, McGraw-Hill, 1995

ANDERSON (L.G.)

Synonyms. Osteodysplasia familial. (The Melnick-Needles and an autosomal dominant condition, both apparently unrelated, are indicated under the same synonym.)

Symptoms and Signs. Present from birth. Midfacial hypoplasia; mandibular prognathism; pointed chin; mandible with wide angle, increased length, reduced height, and reduced bigonial width. Large ears. Kyphoscoliosis. Hypertension.

Etiology. Unknown; Autosomal recessive inheritance.

Diagnostic Procedures. *X-rays.* Calvaria thinned; mastoid pointed; abnormal ribs; spinous process of cervical vertebra anomalies; superior pubic ramus thin. *Blood.* Hyperuricemia.

BIBLIOGRAPHY. Anderson LG, Cook AJ, Coccaro PJ, et al: Familial osteodysplasia. JAMA 220:1687–1693, 1972
Buchignani JS, Cook AJ, Anderson LG: Roentgenographic findings in familial osteodysplasia. Am J Roentgen 116:602–608, 1972
Schendel S, Delaire J Familial osteodysplasia. Head Neck Surg 4:335–343, 1982

ANDOGSKY

Synonyms. Atopic cataract; cataracta dermatogenes; dermatitis lichenoides pruriens; dermatogenous cataract; nummular eczema; eczema plaques; lichen circumscriptus chronicus (Vidal); pruritus diathesique (Besnier).

Symptoms and Signs. Chronic eczematous skin lesions from childhood, and in 3rd decade of life development of bilateral cataracts. Skin lesions produce lichenification of the skin in the neck, flexor surfaces of extremities, especially elbows and knees. Leonine facies may result from the skin lesions. Atopic keratoconjunctivitis; keratoconus; uveitis; asthma occasionally associated.

Etiology. Unknown; heredity reported in only one case. See mesoectodermal dysplasia syndromes.

Diagnostic Procedures. *Blood.* Occasionally, eosinophilia.

Therapy. Symptomatic; cataract extraction.

Prognosis. Variable.

BIBLIOGRAPHY. Andogsky N: Cataracta dermatogenes. Klin Monatbl Augenheilk 52:824–831, 1914
Thannhauser SJ: Werner's syndrome (progeria of adult) and Tothmund's syndrome: Two types of closely related heredofamilial atrophic dermatosis with juvenile cataracts and endocrine features; a critical study with five new cases. Ann Intern Med 23:559–626, 1945
Reed CE, Friedlaender M: Immunologic aspects of disease of the eye. JAMA 248:2692–2699, 1982
Garner A, Klintworth GK (eds): Pathobiology of Ocular Disease: A Dynamic Approach, 2nd ed. New York, Marcel Dekker, 1994

ANDRADE

Synonyms. Transthyretin abnormality; TTR abnormality; methinine 30-prealbumin defect; amyloidosis I, amyloidosis neuropathic; Portuguese type amyloidosis (including Japanese, British, and Swedish types). FAP type I. See amyloidosis.

Symptoms. Both sexes affected; onset in 2nd to 4th decades. Orthostatic hypotension precedes other symptoms. Insidious slow progression of initial peripheral symmetric paresthesias of lower extremities, to motor weakness (difficulty in walking), and eventually spreading into upper extremities and trunk. Cyclic diarrhea and constipation; impotence. Heat intolerance; hoarseness (rare); occasional blurring of vision.

Signs. Pupils irregular and unequal; sluggish reaction to light. Dissociation of sensory impairment: pain and temperature affected, although vibration and position spared. Tendon reflexes gradually lost. Trophic ulcers on the legs. Muscle wasting not prominent. Occasionally, cardiomegaly. In some families vitreous opacity and exophthalmos may be associated.

Etiology. Unknown. Autosomal dominant inheritance. Substitution of methionine for valine at position 30 of prealbumin molecule.

Pathology. Amyloid material infiltrating autonomic ganglia, spinal nerve roots, and peripheral nerves between fibers and vessel walls. Brain and spinal cord not involved.

Diagnostic Procedures. *Blood.* Normal (occasionally, anemia). *Electrocardiography.* S-T and T wave changes. *Spinal fluid.* Moderate increase of protein. *Biopsy of nerve. X-ray.* Occasionally, osteoporosis of metatarsal and phalanges or circumscribed translucent areas.

Therapy. Symptomatic.

Prognosis. Death occurs in approximately 10 years from cachexia, intercurrent infections, and other complications.

BIBLIOGRAPHY. De Bruyer RS, Stern RO: A case of progressive hypertrophic polyneuritis of Dejerine and Sottas with pathological examination. Brain 52:84–107, 1929
Andrade C: A peculiar form of peripheral neuronopathy: Familial typical generalized amyloidosis with special involvement of the peripheral nerves. Brain 75:408–427, 1952
Benson MD, Dwulet FE: Identification of carriers of variant plasma prealbumin (transthyretin) associated with familial amyloidotic polyneuropathy type I. J Clin Invest 75:71–75, 1985
Benson MD. Amyloidosis. In Scriver CR, Beaudet AL, Sly WS, et al: The Metabolic and Molecular Bases of Inherited Disease, 7th ed, pp 4169–4170. New York, McGraw-Hill, 1995

ANEMIC-HEMATURIC

Synonyms. Hematuria—anemia.

Symptoms and Signs. Vary with season in which they occur. Constant asthenia; fever; tachycardia; anemia; vesiculoerythematous dermatitis may occur in either season. *Summer.* Anorexia; vomiting; gastralgia; diarrhea; jaundice; dehydration; nervousness. *Winter.* Edema; oliguria; hematuria; albuminuria; cylindruria; increase of anemia.

Etiology. Unknown. Epidemic in Argentina, in relation with a regional cattle disease.

Therapy. Symptomatic.

Prognosis. Long convalescence without complication.

BIBLIOGRAPHY. Villar JB: Epidemic anemic-hematuric syndrome. Rev Asoc Med Argent 62:649, 1948 (abst); JAMA 140:364, 1949

ANETODERMA, PERIFOLLICULAR

Synonyms. Macular atrophy; dermatitis atrophicans maculosa. See Jodasson-Pellizari and Schweninger-Buzzi.

Symptoms. Appear in women of advanced age.

Signs. Crops of round-oval, pink, small maculae usually on internal aspects of the thighs, seldom on trunk or face, neck. Larger erythema plaques may be present.

Etiology. Unknown. Endocrine factors (?); fat accumulation (?). Elastase-producing strains of Staphylococcus considered as responsible.

Pathology. Thinning of epidermis; thickening of horny layer; widening of follicles; and formation of keratinized masses. In some cases, prolapse of fatty tissue toward epidermis.

Diagnostic Procedures. None, or biopsy.

Therapy. None. Penicillin topical and general in early stage.

Prognosis. Once developed persistent asymptomatic condition.

BIBLIOGRAPHY. Burton JL: Disorders of connective tissue. In Champion RH, Burton JL, Ebling FJG (eds): Rook/Wilkinson/Ebling Textbook of Dermatology, 5th ed, p 1773. Oxford, Blackwell Scientific, 1992

ANETODERMA PRIMARY

Synonyms. In the past subdivided in Jodassohn-Pellizari (see) and Schweninger-Buzzi (see).

Symptoms and Signs. Rare condition. Both sexes all ages but prevalent in females aged 20–40. Crops of round, pink macules of 0.5–1 cm, enlarging up to 2–3 cm (within 7–14 days) on trunk, thighs, arms, seldom neck and face or elsewhere. Slow fading and flattening centrifugally leaving gray, white, or blue spots of athropic skin, where a finger can be admitted through a ring of normal skin. New lesion may continue to appear and develop as described and sometime coalesce and form large atrophic areas.

Etiology. Unknown. In some cases possible infective origin. Specific lesion (focal elastosis) possibly secondary to release of elastase from inflammatory cells.

Pathology. Early stage: edema and lymphocytic infiltration perivascular and appendicial; later reduction and fragmentation of elastic fibers, reduction of dermal collagen.

Diagnostic Procedures. *Skin biopsy.*

Therapy. Penicillin, antifibrinolytic agents suggested, but found not effective once lesions have progressed to atrophy.

Prognosis. Lesions persist for life; new lesions may continue to develop for years.

BIBLIOGRAPHY. Burton JL: Disorders of connective tissue. In Champion RH, Burton JL, Ebling FJG (eds): Rook/Wilkinson/Ebling Textbook of Dermatology, 5th ed, pp 1773–1775. Oxford, Blackwell Scientific, 1992

ANETODERMA SECONDARY

Same type of lesions of anetoderma primary (see) secondary to several pathologic conditions as syphilis, lupus erythematosus, leprosy, pityriasis drug reaction (penicillin), etc. It includes also anetoderma, perifollicular (see).

ANEURYSM OF AORTA

Synonyms. Dissecting aortic hematoma; dissecting aortic aneurysm; abdominal aortic aneurysm, AAA; aortic aneurysm.

Symptoms. Appears mostly in young men; followed by equal incidence between two sexes; onset from 40 to 70 years of age. Severe anterior chest pain not responding to morphine or responding only to high doses. Strongest at onset (and not progressing as in myocardial infarction) radiating mostly to the back, to the abdomen, legs, neck, and head. Pain in some cases may be missing. Shock; coma; hemiplegia; confusion; weakness of legs.

Signs. Absent or unequal pulsations of carotid, brachial, femoral arteries occurring immediately or within a few hours of onset of pain. Pulsation of sternoclavicular joint. Distension of neck veins, heart systolic, and diastolic murmur (10–15% of cases). Blood pressure high (contrasting with signs of shock, pallor, tachypnea).

Etiology. Dissecting aneurysm of the aorta usually found in association with cystic medial necrosis; in some cases, associated with pregnancy, coarctation of aorta, aortic stenosis, myxedema, atheromatous aortic lesion, aortic abscess. Reported familial autosomal inheritance of condition.

Pathology. Transverse tear of the intima a few cm from aortic valve. Intramural hematoma (sometimes blood re-enters aorta through another intimal lesion). Following De Bakey nomenclature proximal dissection is type I and distal dissection is type III; in type II dissection is limited to the ascending aorta.

Diagnostic Procedures. *ECG.* Left ventricular hypertrophy; no specific changes; pericarditis. *X-ray.* Enlargement of aorta. *Echocardiography, aortography, CT scan, digital subtraction angiography. Blood.* Anemia; leukocytosis; increase of bilirubin. *Urine.* Red blood cell; albumin; casts.

Therapy. Medical treatment only palliative effect and symptomatic. Surgery to create a re-entry into the aorta, and suturing of the false lumen; when possible aortic replacement.

Prognosis. Usually fatal in hours or days; spontaneous re-entry of blood into the aorta improves symptomatology and chance of survival. Surgical treatment mortality about 25%.

Subdivision of the clinical pattern of aneurysm of the aorta on the basis of the dominant clinical symptoms and signs gives five syndromes:

1. Cardiovascular. Hypertension, chest pain, cardiac failure dominate, making the differential diagnosis from that of myocardial infarction very difficult.
2. Cerebral. Neurologic findings with confusion and coma confuse the diagnosis with that of a vascular cerebral accident.
3. Pulmonary. Dyspnea, parenchymal changes, left hemothorax suggest the diagnosis of pneumonia.
4. Abdominal. Pain in the epigastrium is present in 60% of the cases in which pain is a symptom of dissecting aneurysm; hematemesis and melena and in some cases an abdominal mass may simulate intestinal bleeding from peptic ulcer or suggest the diagnosis of a tumor.
5. Renal. Involvement of the renal artery gives pain and hematuria as main symptoms, focusing the attention on the kidney rather than the aorta.

BIBLIOGRAPHY. Baer S, Goldburgh H: The varied clinical syndromes produced by dissecting aneurysm. Am Heart J 35:198–211, 1948
Hirst AE, Hohns VJ Jr, Kime SW Jr: Dissecting aneurysm of aorta: a review of 505 cases. Medicine 37:217–279, 1950
De Bakey ME, Henley WS, Cooley DA: Surgical management of dissecting aneurysms of aorta. J Thorac Cardiovasc Surg 49:130–149, 1965
Johnson G Jr, Avery A, McDougal EG, et al: Aneurysm of the abdominal aorta: incidence in blacks and whites in North Carolina. Arch Surg 120:1138–1140, 1985
Lindsey JL, DeBakey ME, Beall AC: Diagnosis and treatment of diseases of the aorta. In Schlant RC, Alexander RW: Hurst's The Heart, 8th ed, pp 2166–2170. New York, McGraw-Hill, 1994

ANGELMAN

Synonyms. Puppet children; happy puppet. Williams and Frias suggested the use of eponym Angelman syndrome because the term happy puppet may appear derisive and even derogatory to the patient family.

Symptoms. Major fits and frequent infantile spasms; easily provoked and prolonged paroxysms of laughs; jerky puppetlike movements; continuous tongue protrusion; mental deficiency.

Signs. Skull alterations: brachycephaly; microcephaly; occipital depression or flattening; prognathism; incomplete development of choroid.

Etiology. Unknown; very rare form of infantile epilepsy. Sporadic. Considered autosomal recessive inheritance in some cases.

Pathology. Not reported.

Diagnostic Procedures. *X-ray of skull.* Vertical inclination of base. *EEG.* Typical pattern with consistent absence of hypsarrhythmia and presence of symmetric synchronous 2/sec wave and spike activity. The persistence of such patterns represents one of the characteristic elements that differentiate it from the transitional EEG pattern of infantile spasm syndrome. *CT scan.* Unilateral cerebellar atrophy demonstrated in one patient.

Therapy. Prednisone; ethosuximide.

Prognosis. Temporary improvement with therapy.

BIBLIOGRAPHY. Angelman H: "Puppet" children: a report on three cases. Dev Med Child Neurol 7:681–688, 1965

Boyd SG, Harden A, Patton MA: The EEG in early diagnosis of the Angelman (Happy Puppet) syndrome. Eur J Pediatr 147:508–513, 1988

Dorries A Spohr H-L Kunze J Angelman (happy puppet) syndrome: seven new cases documented by cerebral computerized tomography: review of literature Europ J Pediatr 148:270–273, 1988

Fryburg JS, Breg WR, Lindgren V: Diagnosis of Angelman syndrome in infants. Am J Med Genet 38:58–64, 1991

ANGELUCCI

Synonyms. Critical allergic conjunctivitis; spring catarrah; periodic allergic conjunctivitis; vernal conjunctivitis.

Symptoms. Both sexes affected; onset at any age, but mainly in young adults: in patients with allergic condition in the family. Recurrence usually in the spring. Cutaneous or mucous itching with sudden onset and sudden termination. Reaction may always affect the same site or alternate. Lacrimation; photophobia; excitability.

Signs. Conjunctival congestion; generally watery discharge, which may become stringy secretion; granulations on upper tarsus or gelatinous perilimbic areas. Vasomotor lability; tachycardia.

Etiology. Unknown. In the group of allergic diseases.

Pathology. Large cobblestone-like tissue changes, known as giant papillae, most prominent on the upper palpebral conjunctiva. Local synthesis of IgE occurs in them. Histologically, high number of basophils, eosinophils, and mast cells. White opacities (Trantas dots), containing eosinophils, may be seen at the corneoscleral limbus. Their presence parallels the activity of the disease.

Diagnostic Procedures. *Blood.* Occasionally, eosinophilia. Elevated serum IgE levels. *Conjunctival smear.* Negative for bacteria; eosinophilic cells usually present. *Skin test.* Positive for several antigens, especially pollens. *Tears.* Elevated levels of IgE.

Therapy. Topical vasoconstrictors; cold compresses; moving to a cool climate or air conditioning the patient's room can be useful. Topical corticosteroids may relieve symptoms but are not recommended for long-term use because of their ocular side effects (glaucoma, cataract formation, opportunistic infections). Specific treatment for desensitization. Bisodic chromoglycate eye drops and chlorphenamine maleate.

Prognosis. The disease usually subsides with aging of the patient.

BIBLIOGRAPHY. Angelucci A: Di una sindrome sconosciuta negli infermi di catarro primaverile. Arch Ottol (Palermo) 5:270–276, 1897–98

Foeter CS: Ocular manifestation of immune disease. In Garner A, Klintworth GK (eds): Pathobiology of Ocular Disease: A Dynamic Approach, 2nd ed, pp 155–156. New York, Marcel Dekker, 1994

ANGIECTASIS PREGNANCY

Synonym. Hemangiomas in pregnancy.

Symptoms. Occurs in less than 5% of pregnancies. Appearance of well-defined small painful areas, with increased temperature on posterior side of legs during third month of pregnancy.

Signs. Intradermal, raised cluster of blood vessels in the back of legs.

Etiology. Relationship between lesion and female sex hormones has been postulated. More painful lesions observed with lower level of estrogen or pregnanediol.

Therapy. Estrogen administration.

Prognosis. May disappear spontaneously in a few weeks or persist during entire pregnancy. Pain disappears with estrogen administration.

BIBLIOGRAPHY. Rook A, Wilkinson DS, Ebling FJG, et al: Textbook of Dermatology, 4th ed, p 275. Oxford, Blackwell Scientific, 1986

ANGIOIMMUNOBLASTIC LYMPHADENOPATHY

Synonyms. Immunoblastic lymphadenopathy; A.I.L.D., immunoblastic-lymphadenopathy, I.B.L.

Symptoms. Fever; sweating; pruritus; rash; anorexia. Dypsnea.

Signs. Weight loss; generalized lymphadenopathy.

Etiology. Unknown. Abnormal immune state. Aggressive lymphoma or non-neoplastic hyperimmune proliferation of B lymphocytes.

Pathology. Lymph nodes. Loss of architecture; lymphocyte depletion; pleomorphic infiltrate (histiocytes, plasma cells, etc.); vascular proliferation and infiltration by amorphous eosinophilic material. Immunophenotypic studies show that large immunoblasts are actived T cells. Like other angiocentricimmunoproliferative diseases typical involvement of respiratory tract.

Diagnostic Procedures. *Biopsy of lymph node.* See Pathology. *X-rays.* Lung initially has coarse, reticulonodular pattern, then consolidation; mediastinal lymph node enlargement. *Blood.* Hypergammaglobulinemia; polyclonal hypergammaglobulinemia; hemolytic anemia, positive Coombs test.

Therapy. Corticosteroids and immunosuppressive agents.

Prognosis. Poor. Survival time function of degree of stage and chemotherapy sensitivity. If visceral involvement, fulminating course.

BIBLIOGRAPHY. Frizzera G, Moran EM, Rappaport H: Angio-immunoblastic lymphoadenopathy with dysproteinemia. Lancet 1:1070–1073, 1974

Azevedo SJ, Yunis AA: Angioblastic lymphoadenopathy. Am J Hematol 20:301–312, 1985

Frizzera G, Kaneko Y, Sakurai M: Angioimmunoblastic lymphadenopathy and related disorders: a retrospective look in search of definitions. Leukemia 3:1–5, 1989

Isaacson PG, Norton AJ: Extranodal Lymphomas. Edinburgh, Churchill Livingstone, 1994

ANGIOMA, MULTIPLE PROGRESSIVE

Symptoms. Appear in both sexes; onset in infancy or adolescence.

Signs. Bluish, compressible nodules, scattered along the course of a vein appear on face or extremities or both, in the subcutaneous tissue.

Etiology. Possibly congenital malformation.

Pathology. Cavernous angioma.

Therapy. Local destructive measures.

Prognosis. After months or years, spontaneous disappearance.

BIBLIOGRAPHY. Darier J, Auken G: Progressive multiple angioma. Acta Derm Venerol 31:304–307, 1951

MacKie RM: Soft tissue tumors. In Champion RH, Burton JL, Ebling FJG (eds): Rook/Wilkinson/Ebling Textbook of Dermatology, 5th ed, p 2087. Oxford, Blackwell Scientific, 1992

ANGIOMA NEUROCUTANEOUS, HEREDITARY

Synonyms. Hemangiomatosis disseminata.

Symptoms and Signs. Both sexes. Presence of angiomas at various sites with wide distribution on the skin. Sudden hemorrhages, hemiparesis, or strokes. Absence of retinal angiomas or telangiectases.

Etiology. Autosomal dominant.

Pathology. Typical cavernous angiomas.

Therapy. Surgery.

Prognosis. Death at different ages caused by strokes.

BIBLIOGRAPHY. Burke EC, Winkelman RK, Stickland MK: Disseminated hemangiomatosis: the new born with central nervous system involvement. Am J Dis Child 108:418–424, 1964

Zaremba J, Stapien M, Jellowicka M, et al: Hereditary neurocutaneous angioma: a new genetic entity? J Med Genet 16:443–447, 1979

Hurst J, Baraitser M: Hereditary neurocutaneous angiomatous malformations: autosomal dominant inheritance in two families. Clin Genet 33:44–48, 1988

ANGIONEUROTIC EDEMA, HEREDITARY

Synonym. Osler (W)I; angioedema hereditary; HANE; C1 esterase inhibitor deficiency; C1-INH.

Symptoms and Signs. Rare condition. Five percent of cases of angioedema without urticaria and approximately 1% of all cases of angiedema. Both sexes affected; onset in early childhood. Episodes may be elicited by traumas (especially dental). Nausea; vomiting; colic; painless swellings of skin and mucosae; itching. Circumscribed edema in various areas of skin and mucosae; in some cases, signs simulating acute abdomen; in other cases only edema of glottis. In some patients systemic lupus erythematosus and glomerulonephitis.

Etiology. Unknown; autosomal dominant. Different types of C1 esterase inhibitors have been described with different activity levels. Hereditary absence of functional C1 inhibitor causes excessive production and slow catabolism of activated C1, which increases permeability of vessels and starts complement cascade. Angioedema owing to acquired C1-inhibitor deficiency can occur, as a consequence of B-cell lymphoproliferative disorders such as chronic lymphatic leukemia, multiple myeloma, or essential cryoglobulinemia. In this case the defect is caused not by defective synthesis but by markedly increased catabolism of the C1-inhibitor protein.

Diagnostic Procedures. *Blood.* Decreased C2 and C4 component of complement. Measurements of C1-INH, reduction of serum levels of C1, C4, and C2; increased thyroglobulin microsomal antibodies. X-rays during attacks; transient edema of intestinal wall.

Therapy. Prophylaxis of attacks by administration of inhibitors of the conversion of plasminogen to plasmin: anabolic steroids. During attacks; infusion of fresh plasma; or of the preparation of the deficient inhibitor: Danazol and stanozolol (nonvirilizing androgen) with good results. Also epsilon-aminocaproic acid and tranexamic acid.

Prognosis. Response to treatment generally poor; over 20% die of laryngeal obstruction before early middle age.

BIBLIOGRAPHY. Osler W: Hereditary angio-neurotic edema. Am J Med Sci 95:362–367, 1888

Hartmann L: L'oedemic angioneurotique hereditaire a propos de 185 malades et 40 families. Bull Acad Nat Med 167:343–351, 1983

Chappatte O, De Swiet M: Hereditary angioneurotic edema and pregnancy: Case reports and review of literature. Brit J Obstet Gynaec 95:938–942, 1988

Frigas E: Angioedema with acquired deficiency of the C1 inhibitor: a constellation of syndromes. Mayo Clinic Proc 64:1269–1275, 1989

Champion RH: Uricaria. In Champion RH, Burton JL, Ebling FJG (eds): Rook/Wilkinson/Ebling Textbook of Dermatology, 5th ed, pp 1877–1879. Oxford, Blackwell Scientific, 1992

ANGIOTROPIC LARGE CELL LYMPHOMA

Synonyms. Pfleger-Tappeiner; angioendotheliomatosis prolifeans systemisata (misnomer); neoplastic angioendotheliomatosis (misnomer).

Symptoms and Signs. At all ages, predilecting the 7th decade. Both sexes. "De novo" condition or concurrency with non-Hodgkin lymphoma. Varied and not specific skin manifestations: nodules or plaques partly hemorrhagic or ulcerated with or without overlying teleangiectasia. Variable neurologic manifestations: aphasia, mental confusion, progressive muscular weakness, variable focal signs. Occasionally signs of adrenal insufficiency and/or nephrotic syndrome; rarely diffuse intravascular coagulation.

Etiology. Unknown.

Pathology. All organs may be infiltrated (liver, spleen, bone marrow usually initially spared). Capillaries, venules, and small arterioles distended by masses of lymphoid blasts, rarely spilling out of vessels, seldom infarctions except in the brain.

Diagnostic Procedures. *Biopsy. X-ray. CT scan. MRI.*

Therapy. Chemotherapy.

Prognosis. Very poor, median survival 5 months.

BIBLIOGRAPHY. Pfleger L: Tappeiner J Zur Kenntnis der systemisierten Endotheliomatose der cutanen Blutgefaesse (Reticuloendotheliose?) Hautarzt 10:359–363, 1959

Isaacson PG, Norton AJ: Extranodal Lymphomas, pp 323–326. Edinburgh, Churchill Livingstone, 1994

ANHIDROSIS

Synonyms. Hypohidrosis; thermogenic anhidrosis; sweat retention.

Symptoms. Occurs when patients are exposed to high temperature and high humidity. Malaise; weakness; flushing; pruritus; headache; nausea.

Signs. Tachycardia; tachypnea; fever.

Etiology. All causes that prevent sweating (inability to produce or to deliver to skin surface). Congenitally absent or deficient sweat glands; dermatitis; ectodermal dysplasia scars; neurogenic factors; miliaria; endocrine and metabolic conditions; drugs (ganglion-blocking, anticholinergic). It may be inherited as an X-linked trait (see Christ-Siemens-Tourine); autosomal recessive inheritance reported as well. Recently reported a case with generalized anhidrosis with morphologically intact sweat glands, and with the mother showing a similar but milder condition (autosomal dominant inheritance?). Three types of anhidrosis postulated ectodermal dysplasia with generalized anhidrosis and: (1) hair, sweat glands, dental anomaly with or without other congenital defects; (2) simple morphological or functional defect of sweat glands; and (3) no other defects or morphologic sweat gland anomalies.

Diagnostic Procedures. *Colorimetric test.* Absence of sweating. *Muscarinic stimulation.* Reduction of normal response to variable degree.

Therapy. Removal to cooler, dryer place with breeze. Treatment, when feasible, of determining causes.

Prognosis. Severe hyperthermia may develop, sometimes with fatal consequences.

BIBLIOGRAPHY. Wolkin J, Goodman JI, Kelley WE: Failure of sweat mechanism in desert. JAMA 124:478–482, 1944

Mahloudji M, Livingston KE: Familial and congenital simple anhidrosis. Am J Dis Child 113:477–479, 1967

Crump IA, Danks DM: Hypohidrotic ectodermal dysplasia: A study of sweatpore in the X-linked forms and in a family with probable autosomal recessive inheritance. J Pediatr 78:466–473, 1971

Ingberg A: Familial generalized anhidrosis. Isr J Med Sci 26:457–458, 1990

Champion RH: In Champion RH, Burton JL, Ebling FJG (eds): Rook/Wilkinson/Ebling Textbook of Dermatology, 5th ed, p 1575. Oxford, Blackwell Scientific, 1992

ANIRIDIA

Synonyms. Iridemia.

Symptoms and Signs. Frequency in general population 1:50,000 to 1:100,000. Present from birth; usually bilateral (hereditary); or later in any period of life (traumatic). Impaired vision. Vestigial iris; various deformities of anterior eye.

Etiology. (1) Dominant type: mutation of 11p13. (2) Recessive (two-thirds of cases): sporadic, frequently associated with various conditions (cerebellar ataxia; mental retardation with microcephaly; Wilms tumor; Marinesco; Sjögren syndromes). (3) Trauma.

Pathology. Various aspects (see Diagnostic Procedures).

Diagnostic Procedures. *Ophthalmoscopy.* (1) Hereditary dominant: thin iris margin associated or not associated with cataract or glaucoma. (2) Hereditary recessive: macula normal aspect. (3) Traumatic: iridodialysis; iris contracted or sinking (or both); partial inversion; hyphemia; partial dislocation of lens. Sporadic aniridia is associated with an increased incidence of Wilms tumor. *Periodic abdominal examination.* Supplemented by ultrasound examination or intravenous pyelography advised in all children with sporadic aniridia.

Therapy. Hereditary form: none. Traumatic form: cold applications; silk anchoring suture of periphery of iris.

Prognosis. Hereditary: poor. Traumatic: variable according to lesions and time of repair.

BIBLIOGRAPHY. Mollenbach CJ: Congenital defects in internal membrane of the eye. Clinical and genetic aspects. In Opera ex Domo Biologiae Heriditariae Humanae Universitatis Hafniensis, vol 15, p 152. Copenhagen, Munksgaard (ed), 1947

Shaw MW, Falls HF, Neel JV: Congenital aniridia. Am J Hum Gen 12:389–415, 1960

Klintworth GK: Genetically determined disorders affecting the eye. In Garner A, Klintworth GK (eds): Pathobiology of Ocular Disease: A Dynamic Approach, 2nd ed. New York, Marcel Dekker, 1994

ANISMUS

Synonyms. Spastic pelvic floor; rectal outlet obstruction. See also colonic inertia.

Symptoms and Signs. Chronic constipation. Frequently associated bladder dysfunction.

Etiology. Unknown. Paradoxical contraction of pelvic floor muscles and alteration of the anorectal inhibitory reflex involving intrinsic nonadrenergic, noncholinergic inhibitory nerves.

Pathology. Dilatation and evidence of chronic inflammation in anorectal area.

Diagnostic Procedures. *Marker studies.* Prolonged retention of markers in the rectum. *Manometric recording and radionucleide imaging.*

Therapy. That of chronic constipation. Diet, mild laxative, cisapride suppository.

BIBLIOGRAPHY. Martelli H, Devroede G, Arhan P, et al: Mechanisms of idiopathic constipation. Outlet obstruction. Gastroenterology 75:623–631, 1978

Kohh TR: Constipation. In Haubrich WS, Schaffner F, Berk JE (eds): Bockus Gastroenterology, 5th ed, pp 105–106. Philadelphia, WB Saunders, 1995

ANKYLOSED TEETH-CLINODACTYLY

Symptoms and Signs. Abnormal teeth eruption and migration. Mandibular prognatism (mild). Head and face abnormalities. Bilateral clinodactyly (fifth fingers).

Etiology. Autosomal dominant inheritance.

BIBLIOGRAPHY. Pelias MZ, Kinnebrew MC: Autosomal dominant transmission of ankylosed teeth, abnormalities of the jaws and clinodactyly. A four-generation study. Clin Genet 27:496–500, 1985

ANKYLOSING SPONDYLITIS–AORTIC INSUFFICIENCY

Symptoms and Signs. Two percent present aortic regurgitation at 10 years, 30 years later up to 10%. Aortic insufficiency initially silent course, then becomes manifest.

Etiology and Pathology. Inflammatory process extended immediately above and below aortic valve causing aortic insufficiency.

Therapy. That of ankylosing spondylitis. When aortic insufficiency becomes manifest, valve replacement may be considered.

Prognosis. Not particularly severe.

BIBLIOGRAPHY. Graham DC, Smythe HA: The carditis and aortitis of ankylosing spondylitis. Bull Rheumat Dis 9:171–174, 1958

Roberts WC, Hollingsworth JF, Bulkley BH: Combined mitral and aortic regurgitation in ankylosing spondylitis. Am J Med 56:237–243, 1974

Bergfeldt L, Edhag O, Rajs J: HLA-B2-associated heart disease. Am J Med 77:961–967, 1984

Schlant RC, Alexander RW: Hurst's The Heart, 8th ed, pp 1466, 1467, 1928. New York, McGraw-Hill, 1994

ANORECTAL

Synonyms. Antibiotic-associated diarrhea, benign. See Janbon and pseudomembranous enterocolitis.

Symptoms. Burning, anal pruritis, sometimes diarrhea, appearing after administration of large spectrum antibiotic.

Signs. Redness around the anus.

Etiology. Antibiotic modification of intestinal flora. Most frequent causative agent. Clostridium difficile.

Therapy. Discontinuation of antibiotic. Symptomatic: cortisone ointment or suppository.

Prognosis. Recovery in a few days except for possible further development and evolution into Pseudomembranous Enterocolitis (see).

BIBLIOGRAPHY. Finney JMT: Gastroenterostomy for cicatrizing ulcer of the pylorus. Johns Hopkins Hosp Bull 4:53–55, 1893

Borriello SP (ed): Antibiotic-Associated Diarrhea and Colitis. Amsterdam, Martinus Nijhoff, 1984

La Hatte, Tedesco FJ, Shuman BM: Antibiotic-associated injury to the gut. In Haubrich WS, Schaffner F, Berk JE (eds): Bockus Gastro-enterology, 5th ed, pp 1657–1671. Philadelphia, WB Saunders, 1995

ANOREXIA NERVOSA

Synonym. Apepsia hysterica; Magersucht.

Symptoms. Occurs in young girls from adolescence to early adulthood (seldom after 30 years of age) from upper or middle classes. Not eating and other disturbances of eating function because of morbid aversion to food. Amenorrhea may precede weight loss. Occasionally, vomiting, ab-dominal symptoms (belching; sensation of fullness; dull pain; nausea); usually, constipation, occasionally diarrhea. Depression and other neu-rotic symptoms. Continuing vigorous activity despite rapidly increasing cachexia. Closely bound with parents, but with underlying hostility against one or both of them. Lack of sexual adjustment. Weight loss; menstrual disturbance. Seldom observed in adolescent boys.

Signs. Severe cachexia, hypotrichosis.

Etiology. Unknown. Compulsive neurosis with a pattern fixed on re-fusal to eat, frequently following emotional, chronic, or acute emotional trauma.

Pathology. Loss of fat deposits; severe generalized cachexia; osteo-porosis.

Diagnostic Procedures. *Urine.* Determination of follicle-stimulating hormone (FSH), 17–ketosteroids. *X-ray of skull and chest. Blood.* Normal serum protein; anemia, leukopenia; bone marrow hypoplasia.

Therapy. Psychiatric care; if no response, hospitalization and tube feeding. Imipramine (150 mg/day) possibly useful.

Prognosis. Symptomatic recovery or chronic course with fluctuations of symptoms for many years. Mortality 4–30% (inanition or infections). In the male antidepressant medication alone frequently is adequate.

BIBLIOGRAPHY. Morton R: Physiologia or a Treatise of Consumptions. London, 1689
Gull WW: Address in medicine. Lancet II:171–176, 1868
Browning CH, Miller SI: Anorexia nervosa: a study in prognosis and management. Am J Psychiatr 124:1128–1132, 1968
Bhanji S, Jolles FEF, Jolles RAS: Goethe's Ottilie: an early 19th century description of anorexia nervosa. J Royal Soc Med 83:581–585, 1990
Giannini AJ, Slaby AE: The Eating Disorders. Ijmuiden, Netherlands, 1993

ANOSOGNOSIA

Synonyms. Asomatognosia. See Anton-Babinski and Gerstmann.

Symptoms. Inability of the patient to recognize a body or functional defect such as the existence of hemiparesis; blindness (see Anton); postoperative states; vomiting; sphincter incontinence. Denies the ex-istence of the condition and attempts to disprove it by going through psychic process that lets him convince himself that what is said by the physician is false.

Etiology. Organic brain diseases; increased intracranial pressure; bleeding; tumor.

Therapy. Depending upon etiology.

Prognosis. Some cases may respond to treatment.

BIBLIOGRAPHY. Adams RD, Victor M: Principles of Neurology, 5th ed, p 400. New York, McGraw-Hill, 1993

ANOXIC OVERWEAR

Synonyms. Contact lens reaction; pupillary conjunctivitis.

Symptoms and Signs. Refractive error, corneal neovascularization, papillary conjunctivitis.

Etiology. Hydrogel lens reaction owing to reduction in oxygen supply. Allergic or toxic reaction to cleaning and preservative liquids.

Pathology. Endothelial cell changes.

Prognosis. Good with substitution to eyeglasses.

BIBLIOGRAPHY. Binder PS: The physiologic effects of extended wear of soft contact lenses. Ophthalmology 87:745–749, 1980
Morris DA: Ocular trauma. In Garner A, Klintworth GK (eds): Patho-biology of Ocular Disease: A Dynamic Approach, 2nd ed, pp 408–409. New York, Marcel Dekker, 1994

ANTERIOR ABDOMINAL WALL

Synonyms. Abdominal wall anterior.

Symptoms. Two subtypes according to localization of pain: (1) Lower quadrant area right or left; (2) superior margins of upper quadrant. Pain: continuous; sometimes in relation with motion; no relation with food ingestion or evacuation.

Signs. With patient lying on his back, firmly compress with single finger or thumb the painful area and ask the patient to raise both legs a few inches. If pain increases because of the contraction of muscles, it is of abdominal wall origin; if decreased, it is of visceral origin.

Etiology. Unknown. It may be associated with, but independent from, gastrointestinal disorders.

Pathology. No specific changes of muscles.

Diagnostic Procedures. Tests for differential diagnosis of gastro-intestinal diseases.

Therapy. Infiltration of various abdominal layers with hydrocortisone.

BIBLIOGRAPHY. Long C: Myofascial pain syndromes. Henry Ford Hosp Med Bull 4:102–106, 1956
Steinheber FV: Medical conditions mimicking the acute surgical ab-domen. Med Clin N Am 57:1559–1567, 1973
Haubrich WS: Abdominal pain. In Kohh TR: Constipation. In Haubrich WS, Schaffner F, Berk JE (eds): Bockus Gastroenterology, 5th ed, pp 11–29. Philadelphia, WB Saunders, 1995

ANTERIOR CHEST WALL SYNDROMES

Synonyms. Costal margin; costochondral junction; inframammary; pectoralis major; xiphoid process; chest wall pain. See also SAPHO.

Symptoms and Signs. Pain of somatic structures of anterior chest wall associated with marked tenderness on fingertip pressure; not relieved by rest, food, or nitroglycerine. According to localization, five subtypes have been recognized.

1. Pectoralis major syndrome. More frequent on left side. Pain present in the upper half of chest, second and third costal region; on occa-sion pain may radiate to arm. It may exist in association with cardiac disease. Responds to specific treatment (see).
2. Inframammary syndrome. More frequent in women on the left side. Pain present under the breast in the midclavicular line sixth-seventh costal region. It may coexist with gastrointestinal pathology. Re-sponds to specific treatment and when associated with an antispastic and antacids.

3. Costal margin syndrome. Both sides of chest. Pain localized on the margins of the eighth, ninth, and tenth ribs at their conjunction. Responds to specific treatment.
4. Costochondral junction syndrome. Tietze's syndrome (see). Pain in the upper chest at the costochondral junctions. Responds to specific treatment.
5. Xiphoid process syndrome (see).
6. Herpes zoster.
7. Mondor syndrome (see).
8. Thoracic outlet syndromes (see).

Etiology.   Variable, in some cases even psychogenic.

Pathology.   Finding inconsistent; occasionally, lymphocytic infiltration of connective tissue; muscle degeneration. In Tietze syndrome, osteochondritis.

Therapy.   Injections of corticosteroid on the trigger points rapidly relieve the symptoms. If area of pain too extensive, adrenal steroids or derivatives orally, or local ethyl chloride spray.

Prognosis.   Good or depending on possible coexisting associations.

BIBLIOGRAPHY. Prinzmetal M, Massumi R: The anterior chest wall syndrome: Chest pain resembling pain of cardiac origin. JAMA 159:177–184, 1955

Long C: Myofascial pain syndromes. Henry Ford Hosp Med Bull 4:102–106, 1956

O'Rourke R: Chest pain. In Schlant RC, Alexander RW: Hurst's The Heart, 8th ed, pp 464–466. New York, McGraw-Hill, 1994

ANTIPHOSPHOLIPID THROMBOSIS

Synonyms.   APL-T. Includes (A) lupus anticoagulant thrombosis; (B) anticardiolipin antibody thrombosis; and (C) antiphospholipin-fetal wastage.

Symptoms and Signs.   Ratio A/B 1/5. Both syndromes characterized by thombosis, fetal wastage, thrombocytopenia. In antiocardiolipin, frequently thombosis of both arteries and veins, pulmonary embolization and premature coronary artery, cerebrovascular and retinal vascular diseases. In lupus anticoagulant, common association with venous and seldom with artery thrombosis. The clinical pattern in anticardiolipin antibodies may be subdivided in four subtypes (according with areas and organs involved and occurrence of embolization) and the antiphospholin-fetal wastage syndrome. In addition, the anticardiolipins may be associated with cardiac disease (myocardial infarction, cardiac valvular abnormalities, etc.), skin diseases (Sneddon, Degos, livedo vasculitis, etc.); neurologic syndromes (migraine, chorea, Guillen-Barré seizures, optic neuritis), obstetric syndromes (abortion in first trimester; recurrent fetal wastage in second-third trimesters, placental vasculitis, maternal trombocythemia).

Etiology.   All syndromes may be primary or secondary: associated with systemic lupus erythematosus, other connective and autoimmune disorders, and other conditions such lymphomas, virus infections (especially HIV), malignancies (see historical Trusseau), or the administration of a number of drugs (phenitoin, fansidar, quinine, quinidine, hydralazine, procainamide, phenothiazines, alpha-interferon, cocaine, etc.).

Pathology.   Intravascular thrombosis see symptoms and signs.

Diagnostic Procedures.   *Blood coagulation studies* (aPTT unreliable) and search for anticoagulant presence. All idiotypes of anticardiolipin antibodies also must be assessed (IgG, IgM, IgA). *Doppler.*

Therapy.   According to subtypes includes "baby" aspirin heparin, and the addition of corticosteroid only in presence of lupus. Plasmapheresis, plasma exchange, immunoabsorption column, intravenous immunoglobulin.

Prognosis.   Guarded. Early stroke, myocardial infarction, retinal thrombosis, etc. According to clinical patterns and response to preventive measures and treatment.

BIBLIOGRAPHY. Conley CL, Hartmann RC: A hemorrhagic disorder caused by circulating anticoagulant in patients with disseminated lupus erythematosus. J Clin Inves 31:621, 1952

Bick RL, Baker WF: The antiphospholipid and thrombosis syndromes: Common bleeding and clotting disorders. Med Clin N Am 78:667–684, 1994

ANTITHROMBIN III DEFICIENCY

Synonyms.   Hereditary antithrombin III deficiency; ATIII; thrombophilia hereditary—ATIII deficiency.

Symptoms and Signs.   Both sexes. From teenage: thromboembolic disease, phlebitis, and ulcers of lower part of legs.

Etiology.   Autosomal dominant. Thirty-four variants have been described. Some conditions may predispose to acquire this type of deficiency, especially following the use of oral contraceptives: vascular, rheologic, platelet abnormalities, other clotting or fibrinolytic defects, pregnancy collagen disorders, etc.

Diagnostic Procedures.   *Blood.* Antithrombin III assay. Antithrombin III may be greatly reduced or normal (inactive protein).

Therapy.   Coumarin anticoagulants. Attempted alpha 2 macroglobulin.

Prognosis.   Depends on severity of thrombosis.

BIBLIOGRAPHY. Egeberg O: Inherited antithrombin deficiency causing thrombophilia. Thromb Hemost 13:516, 1965

Marcinia KE, Farley CH, De Simone PA: Familial thrombosis due to antithrombin III deficiency. Blood 43:219, 1974

De Stefano V, Leone G: Antithrombin III congenital defects revising classification system. Thromb Haemost 62:820–821, 1989

Mitchell L, Piovella F, Ofosu F, et al: Alpha 2 macroglobulin may provide protection from thromboembolic events in antithrombin III-deficient children. Blood 78:2299–2304, 1991

Bithel TC: Thrombosis and antithrombin therapy. In Lee GR, Bithel TC, Foerster J, et al (eds): Wintrobe's Clinical Hematology, 9th ed, pp 1520–1522. Philadelphia, Lea & Febiger, 1993

ANTLEY-BLIXER

Synonyms.   Acrocephalosynankia; trapezoidocephaly—synostosis; multisynostotic osteodysgenesis—long-bone fractures; osteodysgenesis–multisynostosis—fractures of long bones; acrocephalosynankia; camptomelic dysplasia; short limbed craniosynostotis.

Symptoms and Signs.   From birth. Both sexes. Midface hypoplasia, dysplastic ears, trapezoidocephaly; arachnodactyly; humeroradialsynostosis; femoral bowing; easy bone fractures (frequently connatal).

Etiology.   Sporadic and autosomal recessive inheritance.

Pathology.   Associated possible heart and kidney malformations.

Diagnostic Procedures.   *X-rays.* Craniosynostosis (lamboid and coronal sutures); humeroradial synostosis, bowed femur; sclerosis of vertebral bodies; associated features: clubfoot; arachnodactyly; long bone fractures. *Ultrasound.* Prenatal diagnosis.

Prognosis.   Poor. Respiratory failure as possible cause of death within first 8 months of life.

BIBLIOGRAPHY. Antley RM, Blixen D: Trapezoidocephaly, midface hypoplasia and cartilage abnormalities with multiple synostosis and skeletal fractures. Birth Def Orig Art Ser XI (2):397–401, 1975

Antley RM, Bixler D: Development in trapezoidocephaly–multiple synostosis syndrome. Am J Med Genet 14:149–150, 1983

Herva R, Seppanen U: Multisynostotic osteodysgenesis. Pediatr Radiol 15:63–64, 1985

DeLozier-Blanchet CD: Antley-Bixler syndrome from a prognostic perspective. Am J Med Genet 32:262–263, 1989

ANTON

Synonyms. Denial–visual hallucination; visual anosognosia.

Symptoms. Denial of blindness (the objects described as seen must be regarded as hallucinations); confabulation; allocheiria (reference of sensation to opposite site from stimulus application).

Signs. Blindness.

Etiology. Not well established. Tumor; neurosurgery; arteriosclerosis; bilateral obstruction of occipital region arteries; lesion of calcar or thalamic connections.

Pathology. See Etiology.

Therapy. Symptomatic.

Prognosis. Poor quoad vitam.

BIBLIOGRAPHY. Anton G: Ueber die Selbstwahrnehmung der Herderkrankungen des Gehirns durch den Kranken bie Rindenblindheit und Rindentaubheit. Arch Psychiatr Nervenkr 32:86, 1899

Adam RD, Victor M: Principles of Neurology, 5th ed, p 400. New York, McGraw-Hill, 1993

ANTON-BABINSKI

Synonyms. Asomatoagnosia unilateral.

Symptoms and Signs. In patient with dense left hemiplegia. Conceptual negation of paralysis anosognosia: unawareness or indifference toward the condition expressed by denial of it, admission of weakness, justification by pain that prevents movement, denial of the left part of body as if not belonging and relative neglect of it (dressing apraxia).

Frequently associated: mental derangements, blunted emotivity, illusions, hallucinations of movements, allocheiria, disturbed perception of space.

Etiology and Pathology. Lesion of the cortex, and white matter of the superior parietal lobule. Its variable extension into post-central gyrus, frontal motor areas, and temporal and occipital lobes explains the possible associated anomalies. In right hemiplegia symptoms obscured by concurrent aphasia.

BIBLIOGRAPHY. Anton G: Ueber die Selbstwahrnehmung der Herderkrankungen des Gehinrs durch den Krauken bei Rindenblindheit and Rindentaubheit. Arch Psychiatr Nervenkr 32:86, 1899

Adams RD, Victor M: Principles of Neurology, 5th ed, pp 398, 421. New York, McGraw-Hill, 1993

ANTON-VOGT

Synonyms. Vogt and Vogt; double athetosis; congenital chorea; Hammond athetoid; infantile partial striatal sclerosis; status marmoratus. Including Pincus-Chutorian; Mount-Reback. See Little (W.J.).

Symptoms. Premature infants frequently affected; onset months after birth when complex motor activity develops, such as sitting, standing, and walking. Purposeless, involuntary, slow, sinuous movements of face, neck, trunk, and extremities, exaggerated by activity and excitement. Dysarthria; association with mental and emotional disturbances; con-vulsions. In Pincus-Chutorian cerebellar signs are associated and intellect is spared.

Etiology. Not clear; related to asphyxial disturbances or fetal encephalitis. Autosomal inheritance reported of both dominant and recessive type.

Pathology. Striatum shrunken; ganglion cells absent; structure invaded by thin myelinated fibers (status marmoratus). Findings observed only in some patients.

Diagnostic Procedures. *Electroencephalography. Spinal tap. CT scan. MRI.*

Therapy. In severe cases, section of central portion of cerebral peduncle. Sedative and antispasmodic agents.

Prognosis. Disease static. Manifestations depending on cerebral defects. Mental deficiency of variable degree. Long survival possible (60-year-old reported).

BIBLIOGRAPHY. Athetosis. Medical Times Gaz London 2:747–748, 1871

Anton G: Ueber die Beteiligung der grossen basalen Gehirnganglien bei Bewegungstörungen and Inshesondere. Chorea Jahrh J Psychiatr Neur 14:141–147, 1896

Oppenheim H, Vogt C: Wesen und Localisation der kongennitalen und infantilen Pseudobulbärparalyse. J Psychal Neurol 18:293–308, 1911

Vogt C: Quelques considerations générales á propos du syndrome due Corps strié. J Psychiatr Neurol 18:479–492, 1911

Vogt C, Vogt O: Zur Lehre der Ezkrankungen des Striäten Systems. J Psychol Neurol 25:627–846, 1920

Adams RD, Victor M: Principles of Neurology, 5th ed, pp 839, 1040, 1041. New York, McGraw-Hill, 1993

ANUS, IMPERFORATE

Synonyms. Includes anorectal agenesis, anal agenesis and rectal atresia.

Symptoms and Signs. Present from birth. Anorectal agenesis occurs prevalently in males; anal membranes intact; in both sexes a fistula is almost always present. Absence of communication between rectal sections (anal agenesis or anorectal agenesis without fistula). Absence of emission of meconium, or passage of meconium in the urine, in presence of fistula. After two to three days, abdominal distension. If the point of obstruction is low, digital exploration may reveal defect. In rectal atresia (rare, 2%) both sexes equally affected: rectum ending blindly above pelvic floor with early obstructive symptoms.

Etiology. Hereditary malformation of sex-linked recessive type. Autosomal dominant in association with other malformations see Townes-Brocks and V.A.T.E.R.

Pathology. Anal membrane preventing communication of intestinal lumen. Frequently associated with other malformations of lower intestinal tract (e.g., rectoperineal, rectovescical, rectourethral).

Diagnostic Procedures. *X-ray.* With infant head down, an opaque object inserted in anus: gas level separated from object by a membrane; on plain radiographs gas shadow is above the I point and also shows air in the bladder.

Therapy. Excision of membrane. If underweight (in case of associated anomalies), temporary colostomy to precede more complex intervention.

Prognosis. Good with intervention. In some cases rupture of cecum in labor; fecal impaction and megacolon; residual constipation.

BIBLIOGRAPHY. Weinstein ED: Sex-linked imperforate anus. Pediatrics 35:715–717, 1965

Winkler JM, Weinstein ED: Imperforate anus and heredity. J Ped Surg 5:555–558, 1970

Cywes S Millar AJW: Embriology and anomalies of the intestine. In Haubrich WS, Schaffner F, Berk JE (eds): Bockus Gastroenterology, 5th ed, pp 925–927. Philadelphia, WB Saunders, 1995

ANXIETY-TENSION

Synonym. Anxiety neurosis.

Symptoms. Anxiety manifested by tension in the voice, anxious look; patient characteristically sits on the edge of chair, wipes wet palms. Concern often oriented not to mental reactions, but to the somatic manifestations consisting of muscular hypertension, headache, tight throat, dizziness, blurred vision, precordial distress, rapid heart, spastic colon, diarrhea or constipation, flushing, and all symptoms that are found in the psychologic "alarm reaction." Fatigue-blueness may appear in advanced stages of the condition. Persons physically well-endowed, intelligent, perfectionists, hard-driving, economically and socially successful, not complacent about their situation and symptoms, as opposed to "neurotics," who instead appears complacent, inadequate socially and economically, not equally intelligent.

Signs. Objective changes; gastrointestinal; cardiovascular, and others, corresponding to somatic symptoms.

Etiology and Pathology. Chronic "alarm reaction" with shifting of attention from tangible obstacle to feelings and person himself.

Therapy. Mild sedative. Psychiatric explanation of mechanism of symptoms and training in relaxation. Rhythmic exercises. Vitamins and a combination of betaine hydrochloride and glycocyamine useful in advance states with fatigue symptoms.

Prognosis. Excellent with adequate treatment.

BIBLIOGRAPHY. Dixon HH, et al: Therapy in anxiety states and anxiety complicated by depression. West J Surg 62:338–341, 1954
Freud S: Mourning and melancholia. In The Complete Psychological Works of Sigmund Freud, vol 14, pp 237–258. London, Hogarth, 1957
Barlow DH: Anxiety and Its Disorders: The Nature and Treatment of Anxiety and Panic. New York, Guilford, 1988

AORTA COARCTATION

Synonyms. Coarctation of aorta.

Symptoms. Predominant in males (isthmus) or equal sex distribution (abdominal); onset in two periods: early infancy (dyspnea) and between 20 and 30 years of age. Usually, initially asymptomatic. Constant onset of symptoms in second period. *Minor.* Headache, spontaneous epistaxes; leg fatigue; claudication of leg (abdominal coarctation); dysphagia; ache in the shoulders, tinnitus. *Major.* Symptoms related to congestive heart failure; rupture of anterior aneurysm; endocarditis; and cerebral hemorrhage.

Signs. Physical appearance usually normal; at times athletic (broad chest and shoulders, thin hips and legs). Typical signs: hypertension (systolic) in arms (if proximal to obstruction); hypotension (systolic) in the legs or absence of pulse. Search for collateral vessels (seldom obvious). Forceful pulses in the neck and supraclavicular regions. Systolic murmur (posterior chest interscapular auscultation) over constricted zone.

Etiology. Abnormality of development in embryonal life. Sometimes hereditary.

Pathology. Deformity composed of medial tissue and shown by localized thickening, infolding of aortic wall, which reduces the lumen at arch-descending aorta junction. Bulging above and below constricted segment. Frequent association with other cardiac malformation. *Infantile type.* Aortic isthmus, or proximal involvement. *Adult type.* At or below obliterated ductus insertion distal to isthmus.

Diagnostic Procedures. *Electrocardiography.* Ventricular hypertrophy; left bundle branch block. *X-rays.* Normal to pathognomonic. Signs usually present after 2 years of age: ribs notching posterior at inferior margin (at 6 years of age); left subclavian and descending aortic shadows classic features in isthmus coarctation; deformity of barium-filled esophagus. *Echocardiogram.* Two-dimensional with Doppler interrogation and color flow imaging. *Cardiac catheterization.*

Therapy. *Medical.* According to heart failure (digitalis or diuretics, IV sedation), prostaglandin E, to give relief and allow further assessment and surgery. *Surgical.* Prompt correction in infants who do not respond to medical management, or with other associated defects. Elective correction between 4 and 6 years of age to prevent relatively high occurrence of recoarctation.

Prognosis. Those who survive hazard of infancy reach early adulthood; 25% die before age 20; 50% before 30; 75% before 50. Good results with surgery.

BIBLIOGRAPHY. Meckel JF quoted by Jarcho S: Coarctation of the aorta. Am J Cardiol 7:844–851, 1961
Smallborn JF, Huhta JC, Adams PA, et al: Cross-sectional echocardiographic assessment of coarctation in the sick neonate and infant. Br Heart J 50:349–361, 1984
Perloff JK: The Clinical Recognition of Congenital Heart Disease, 4th ed, pp 132–155. Philadelphia, WB Saunders, 1994

AORTIC ARCH

This syndrome includes: (1) Carotid artery occlusion; (2) vertebral-basilar artery occlusive; (3) subclavian artery occlusive; and (4) subclavian steal.

Symptoms and Signs. Although each of the syndromes shows a particular pattern of symptoms and signs, there is a variable degree of overlapping; lesions of more than one artery, and congenital anatomic variation will further confuse differentiation. In the tables that follow, Jones and colleagues have attempted differentiation of symptoms and signs.

Etiology. Atherosclerosis (in majority of cases); nonspecific arthritis (16%, this last group forms the Takayasu syndrome, see also; trauma; embolization).

Pathology. Atherosclerotic changes of the arterial walls, thrombosis, and neurologic alterations according to artery affected.

Diagnostic Procedures. *Four-vessel arteriography.* Noninvasive techniques: *Echocardiogram.* Two-dimensional with Doppler interrogation and color flow imaging. *Ocular pneumoplethysmography.*

Therapy. Surgical reconstruction procedures.

Prognosis. According to degree and time of occlusion and variations in surgical possibilities and skill, death due to cerebral vascular insufficiency.

Symptoms Associated with Artery Involved

Symptoms	Artery		
	Innominate	Vertebral	Subclavian
Motor-sensory impairment	×		
Seizures	×		
Visual Impairment	×		
Diplopia	×		
Aphasia-dysphasia	×		
Syncope	×	×	
Memory change	×	×	
Lightheadedness	×	×	×
Vertigo		×	×
Arm			×
None			×

Physical Findings Associated with Artery Involved

Findings	Innominate	Vertebral	Subclavian
Blood pressure			
Reduction (arm) 160–30 mmHg	×		×
Pulse change			
Arm	×		×
Neck	×		
Bruit neck	×		×
Neurologic deficits	×		
Ischemic changes			
Hand			×
Subclavian steal			×
			(66.7%)

Jones TW, Thomas GI, Edmark KW: Thoracocervical occlusive disease. Am Surg 33:535–541, 1967

BIBLIOGRAPHY. Broadbent WH: On ingravescent apoplexy. Med Chir Soc London 8:103–108, 1876

Ross RR, McKusick VA: Aortic arch syndromes, diminished or absent pulses in arteries arising from arch of aorta. Arch Intern Med 92:701–740, 1953

Bustamante RA, Milanes B, Casas R, et al: Chronic subclavian-carotid obstruction syndrome (pulseless disease). Angiology 5:479–485, 1954

Davis JB, Grove WJ, Julian OC: Thrombotic occlusion of the branches of the aortic arch, Martorell's syndrome: Report of a case treated surgically. Ann Surg 144:124–126, 1956

Van Mierop LHS, Kutsche LM: Embryology of Heart. In Schlant RC, Alexander RW: Hurst's The Heart, 8th ed, pp 1721–1723. New York, McGraw-Hill, 1994

AORTIC ARCH HYPOPLASIA

Symptoms. Both sexes affected; normal at birth. Onset before 6 weeks of age. Intensity of symptoms according to degree of lesion. Dyspnea; feeding difficulty; failure to thrive. Possibly, development of progressive cardiac failure.

Signs. Cyanosis: mild and involving primarily lower extremities. Acyanosis if associated with large ventricular septal defect. Murmurs absent or minor; seldom, left parasternal systolic murmurs (of associated ventricular septal defect), or midsystolic.

Etiology. Congenital defect. Described also in offspring of mothers with rubella.

Pathology. Uniform tubular narrowing of ascending part and arch of aorta. Seldom present as isolated defect; frequently associated with ventricular septal defect, patent ductus arteriosus, or other malformations.

Diagnostic Procedures. *ECG.* Right atrium and ventricle hypertrophy. *X-ray.* Normal pattern to marked cardiac enlargement and pulmonary venous congestion. *Cardiac catheterization. Echocardiogram.* Two-dimensional with Doppler interrogation and color flow imaging.

Therapy. Corrective plastic surgery.

Prognosis. Variable according to degree of lesion. Amenable to surgical repair. Recoarctation is common and often necessitates a second operation.

BIBLIOGRAPHY. Lev M: Pathologic anatomy and interrelationship of hypoplasia of the aortic arch complex. Lab Invest 1:61–70, 1952

Braunwald E: Heart Disease, vol 2, pp 1003–1004. Philadelphia, WB Saunders, 1980

Van Mierop LHS: Embryology of the heart. In Schlant RC, Alexander RW: Hurst's The Heart, 8th ed, pp 1722–1723, 2166. New York, McGraw-Hill, 1994

AORTIC ATRESIA

Synonyms. Aortic valve atresia.

Symptoms. Predominant in males; at birth may appear normal, but symptoms develop within first few days of life. Critical illness; listlessness; tachypnea.

Signs. Severe pallor; mild to intense cyanosis; edema; absent or diminished arterial pulses; signs of severe pulmonary hypertension; absent heart murmurs; sternal lift. Later, hepatomegaly.

Etiology. Congenital malformation.

Pathology. Complete closure of aortic orifice by fibrous membrane. Hypoplasia of ascending aorta. Mitral valve hypoplasic or atresic. Patent ductus arteriosus.

Diagnostic Procedures. *ECG.* Right ventricular hypertrophy; right atrial P waves. *X-ray.* Cardiomegaly; absence of aortic shadow; pulmonary venous congestion. *M-mode and two-dimensional echocardiography. Cardiac catheterization.*

Therapy. Intravenous prostaglandin E infusion (to maintain ductal patency prior to catheterization and surgery). Palliative surgery; emotional support, genetic counseling for parents.

Prognosis. Fatal within first week. A few children survive a few months (optimal interatrial communication).

BIBLIOGRAPHY. Norwood WJ, Lange P, Hansen DD: Physiologic repair of aortic atresia–hypoplastic: Left heart syndrome. New Engl J Med 308:23–26, 1983

Perloff JK: The Clinical Recognition of Congenital Heart Disease, 4th ed, p 738. Philadelphia, WB Saunders, 1994

AORTIC-LEFT VENTRICULAR TUNNEL

A rare congenital malformation where a tunnel begins in the ascending aorta, lies on the anterior wall, proceeds into the epicardium, penetrates the ventricular septum and empties in subaortic zone of left ventricle.

Symptoms. Early birth or early infancy. Mild symptoms. Few present congestive heart failure, others dyspnea, fatigue, growth failure in weeks or months.

Signs. Bounding arterial pulses, wide pulse pressure, hyperdynamic left ventricular lift. To and from murmur, diastolic sound louder.

Etiology. Unknown.

Diagnostic Procedures. *Cardiac catheterization. Two-dimensional echocardiography with color flow imaging and spectral Doppler interrogation. X-ray.*

Therapy. Medical and early surgical management. Progressive also when mild initial symptoms.

Prognosis. Rapid onset of congestive failure and death if surgery is not performed (80.9% survive surgery).

BIBLIOGRAPHY. Roberts WC, Morrow AG: Aortico-left venticular tunnel. A cause of massive aortic regurgitation and of intracardiac aneurysm. Am J Med 39:662, 1965

Levy MJ, Schachner A, Blieden LC: Aortic–left ventricular tunnel: collective review. J Thorac Cardiovasc Surg 84:102–109, 1982

Perloff JK: The Clinical Recognition of Congenital Heart Disease, 4th ed, pp 117–118. Philadelphia, WB Saunders, 1994

AORTICOPULMONARY WINDOW

Synonyms. Elliotson; aorticopulmonary septal defect; aortopulmonary fistula.

Symptoms and Signs. Both sexes affected; present from birth. Acyanosis; physical underdevelopment. Clinical signs suggest patent ductus arteriosus (see); systolic murmur maximum in third intercostal space. Wide and bounding pulse.

Etiology. Embryological fault resulting in persistence of a round or oval window communication between ascending aorta and pulmonary trunk.

Diagnostic Procedures. *Electrocardiography.* Ventricular hypertrophy with diastolic overload of left heart. *X-rays.* Pattern similar to large patent ductus (left-to-right shunt) and pulmonary hypertension. *Two-dimensional echocardiography with color flowing and Doppler interrogation.*

Therapy. Cardiosurgery.

Prognosis. Early death.

BIBLIOGRAPHY. Elliotson J: Case of malformation of the pulmonary artery and aorta. Lancet I:247–248, 1830

Doty DB, Richardson JV, Falkovsky GE, et al: Aortopulmonary septal defect: hemodynamic angiography and operation. Ann Thorac Surg 32:244–250, 1981

Perloff JK: The Clinical Recognition of Congenital Heart Disease, 4th ed, pp 535–540. Philadelphia, WB Saunders, 1994

AORTOCAVAL FISTULA

A. SPONTANEOUS

Symptoms. Predominant in males (no cases reported in females); onset between 40 and 78 years of age. Pain in the back or abdomen, or both; occasionally, radiation to legs. Dyspnea; anorexia; nausea; vomiting; restlessness; confusion; lethargy; stupor; oliguria; shock.

Signs. Palpable aneurysm; abdominal bruit usually systolic and diastolic, seldom only systolic; cardiomegaly; edema of legs; pulsating vein; ascites; hepatomegaly. Blood pressure: low diastolic; wide pulse pressure.

Etiology. Rupture of aortic aneurysm (usually arteriosclerotic; seldom syphilis; Marfan; mycosis).

Pathology. Fistula of aorta into vena cava; fluid retention (10–15 kg) in legs, abdomen.

Diagnostic Procedures. *Venous pressure.* In legs markedly increased. *Urine.* Hematuria. *Stool.* Presence of blood. *Blood.* Hyperazotemia. *Aortography. CT scan. MRI.*

Therapy. Treatment of shock. Surgical interruption of fistula.

Prognosis. Without operation, survival from 1 hour to 47 days. Cause of death congestive heart failure, shock, rectal hemorrhage, cerebral insufficiency, anuria.

B. TRAUMATIC

Symptoms. Pain in the back or abdomen, occasionally, radiation to legs. Dyspnea; oliguria; anorexia; nausea; vomiting.

Signs. Palpable aneurysm; systolic and diastolic bruit; pulmonary rales; cardiomegaly; edema; ascites; hepatomegaly.

Etiology. Trauma.

Pathology. Formation of fistula between aorta and vena cava.

Diagnostic Procedures. *X-ray. Aortography.*

Therapy. Surgery.

Prognosis. Traumatic form is relatively benign since systemic arterial insufficiency and regional venous hypertension are, if at all, exceptional complications. Without surgery, survival may be for years (mean 5.3 years).

BIBLIOGRAPHY. Syme J: Case XV-Case of spontaneous varicose aneurysm. Edinb Med Surg J 36:105, 1931

Nennhaus HP, Javid H: The distinct syndrome of spontaneous abdominal aortocaval fistula. Am J Med 44:464–473, 1968

Fowler NO: High-cardiac-output states. In Schlant RC, Alexander RW: Hurst's The Heart, 8th ed, p 508. New York, McGraw-Hill, 1994

APERT-GALLAIS

Synonyms. Cooke-Apert; Gallais; genito-suprarenal; suprarenal genital; suprarenal pseudohermaphroditism—virilism—hirsutism.

French designation of the congenital adrenal hyperplasia syndrome in females (see Adrenogenital syndromes). See also Achard-Thiers, Pellizzi, Cushing, and hirsutism.

BIBLIOGRAPHY. Apert M: Dystrophies en relation avec les lésions de capsules surrénales, hirsutisme et progeria. Bull Soc Pediat 12:501–518, 1910

Gallais A: La Syndrome Génito-Surrénale: Étude Anatomo-Clinique (thesis). Paris, 1912

APERT

Synonyms. Acrocephalosyndactyly I; syndactyly-oxycephaly; ACS I.

Symptoms. Headache; visual loss, conductive hearing loss.

Signs. Acrocephaly (head pointed in region of anterior fontanelle); beak-shaped nose; hypoplastic maxilla; occasionally associated with exophthalmos and visual loss. Mental retardation. Cases with normal intelligence reported. Syndactylism of various types, partial or total fusion or webbing of fingers and toes. Other skeletal deformities. Acne vulgaris. Possible visceral (heart, lung, kidney) malformations.

Etiology. Most cases sporadic. Autosomal dominant and recessive cases (?) reported. Old paternal age.

Pathology. Premature fusion of cranial bone; synostosis and synarthrosis; agenesis of bones.

Diagnostic Procedures. *X-ray. MRI. CT scan.* Turrybrachycephaly, premature closure of sutures; dilated cerebral ventricles; syndactyly (mitten hand and sock foot). *Prenatal ultrasonography.*

Therapy. Orthopedic or surgical correction when feasible. Craniectomy early in life.

Prognosis. High mortality rate in early infancy.

BIBLIOGRAPHY. Wheaton SW: Two specimens of congenital cranial deformity in infants associated with fusion of the fingers and toes. Trans Path Soc London 45:238–241, 1894

Apert E: De l'acrocephalosyndactyly. Bull Soc Med Hôp Paris 23:1310–1330, 1906

Cohen MM Jr: Craniosynostosis: Diagnosis, Evaluation and Management. New York, Raven, 1986

Patton MA, Goodship J, Hayward R, et al: Intellectual development in Apert's syndrome. A long term follow up of 29 patients. J Med Gen 25(3):164–167, 1988

APLASIA CUTIS CONGENITA

Synonyms. Catlin marks; skull-scalp defect; congenital absence of skin, including: parietal foramina.

Symptoms and Signs. Lesion(s) present at birth; one (more frequently) or multiple sharply marginated lesions with red glistening base of variable shape. Usually on the scalp (2/3) (may be taken as forceps injuries), frequently close to the midline, less frequently on limbs (1/4), seldom on trunks. Infection possible; meningitis in case of deep lesions reported. Possible associated lesions: limbs ring constriction or anomalies; congenital heart defects; thracheoesophageal fistula; cleft lip-palate; uterus and cervix duplication; cerebral malformations; mental retardation.

Etiology. Most cases sporadic. Autosomal dominant and recessive forms reported (in form involving the scalp). Several types classified.

1. A. C. C. on the scalp without multiple anomalies
2. Adams-Olivier (see)
3. A.C.C. with epidermal nevi
4. A.C.C. overlying developmental malformations
5. A.C.C. associated with fetus papiraceus
6. A.C.C. in epidermolysis bullosa
7. A.C.C. from teratogens (Methimazole) or infection in pregnancy
8. A.C.C. in malformation syndromes (trisomy 13; chromosome 4p deletion; Dellerman-Orthuys; Johanson-Blizzard, Setleis; focal dermal hypoplasia; EEC; etc.)

Pathology. Absence of epidermis and occasionally of dermis and subcutaneous fat; if reepithelization, absence of epidermal appendices and possible hypertrophic scar.

Diagnostic Procedures. *Biopsy of skin.*

Therapy. Prevention of infection; larger lesion: early grafting.

Prognosis. Excellent in absence of complication and for shallow lesions. Spontaneous healing. Occasionally hypertrophic scarring.

BIBLIOGRAPHY. Cordon M: Extrait d'une lettre au sujet de trois enfants de la meme mère nés avec une partie des extremitès deniees de peau. J Med Chir Pharmacie 26:556–557, 1767
Hoffman E: Wien Med Presse 18:552, 1885
Frieden IJ: Aplasia cutis congenita. A clinical review and proposal for classification. J Am Acad Dermatol 14:646–660, 1986
Atherton DJ: Naevi and other developmental defects. In Champion RH, Burton JL, Ebling FJG (eds): Rook/Wilkinson/Ebling Textbook of Dermatology, 5th ed, pp 518–525. Oxford, Blackwell Scientific, 1992

APOLIPOPROTEIN C-II DEFICIENCY, FAMILIAL

Synonyms. Apo C-II deficiency.

Symptoms and Signs. Detection in adulthood. Recurrent abdominal pain resulting from pancreatitis, which may lead to diabetes and its symptoms and signs. No xantomas or hepatomegaly (see LPL deficiency). Anemia.

Etiology. Autosomal recessive inheritance. Absence of apolipoprotein C-II, which is essential for lipoprotein lipase clearance of chylomicron and VLDL from plasma.

Pathology. Pancreas. Acute pancreatitis typical signs.

Diagnostic Procedures. *Blood.* Anemia probably hemolytic. Milky fasting plasma. *Lipids.* Elevated fasting plasma triglycerides mostly of chylomicrons but also (nonconstant) of VLDL; cholesterol high, in VLDL low in LDL and HDL; plasma apolipoprotein A-1 reduced. The lipid pattern may be classified as type 1 or type 5; assay of lipoprotein lipase activity in postheparin plasma.

Therapy. Moderate restriction of fats in diet. Plasma transfusions (containing Apo C-II) cause immediate decrease of plasma triglycerides.

BIBLIOGRAPHY. Breckenridge WC, Little JA, Steiner G, et al: Hypertriglyceridemia associated with deficiency of apolipoprotein C-II. New Engl J Med 298:1265, 1978
Schettler G, Habenicht AJR: Principles and Treatment of Lipoprotein Disorders. Ijmuiden, Netherlands, Springer, 1994
Brunzell JD: Familial lipoprotein lipase deficiency and other causes of the chylomicronemia syndrome. In Scriver CR, Beaudet AL, Sly WS, et al: The Metabolic and Molecular Bases of Inherited Disease, 7th ed, pp 1922–1924. New York, McGraw-Hill, 1995

APOPLEXIA UTERI

Synonyms. Hemorrhagic necrosis senile endometrium.

Symptoms. Vaginal bleeding; symptoms of cardiac decompensation such as cough, dyspnea, chest pain, edema of lower extremities. Symptoms of bleeding in gastrointestinal tract: vomiting of blood; passage of dark stool.

Signs. Signs of cardiac failure; tachycardia; enlargement of heart; enlarged, tender liver; edema of lower extremities. Postmenopausal bleeding with normal pelvic findings.

Etiology. Necrosis of the endometrium.

Pathology. Findings at autopsy: severe generalized and uterine arteriosclerosis. Some form of cardiovascular disease associated with a variable degree of circulatory decompensation.

Therapy. Curettage to rule out endometrial carcinoma. Treatment of the symptoms and of the arteriosclerosis.

Prognosis. Postmenopausal bleeding of this kind has some prognostic significance. Thus, if vaginal bleeding develops in a postmenopausal female with cardiovascular decompensation, it should prompt the consideration of endometrial ischemia as a likely cause. Although of relatively little consequence in itself, this occurrence should alert the physician to the possibility of coincidental or subsequent development of the far more important and severe hemorrhagic necrosis of the bowel.

BIBLIOGRAPHY. Novak ER, Woodruff JD: Gynecologic and Obstetric Pathology with Clinical and Endocrine Relations, 6th ed. Philadelphia, WB Saunders, 1967
Daly JJ, Balogh K Jr: Hemorrhagic necrosis of the senile endometrium ("apoplexia uteri"): relation to superficial hemorrhagic necrosis of the bowel. New Engl J Med 278:709–711, 1968
Gompel C, Silverberg SG: Pathology, Gynecology and Obstetrics, 3rd ed, pp 194–197. Philadelphia, JB Lippincott, 1985

APPARENT MINERALOCORTICOID EXCESS

Synonyms. Mineralocorticod excess, apparent; includes licorice excess.

Symptoms and Signs. In children. Hypertension.

Etiology. Lack of effective 11-hydroxysteroid dehydrogenase in target tissues (mimicking licorice excess that acts as an exogenous inhibitor of 11–OHSD) that prevents cortisol conversion to cortisone by the kidney and thus causes excessive cortisol binding to and activation of renal mineralocorticoid receptor.

Therapy. Inhibit endogenous cortisol secretion with replacement synthetic glucocorticoid.

BIBLIOGRAPHY. Stewart P, Valentino R, Wallace A, et al: Mineralocorticoid activity of licorice: 11-hydroxysteroid dehydrogenase deficiency comes of age. Lancet 2:821–824, 1987

APPLE PEEL

Synonyms. Jejunal atresia; Christmas tree; intestinal atresias.

Symptoms. At birth. Vomiting of bile, abdominal distension, failure to pass meconium.

Signs. At surgery, the distal small bowel comes straight off the cecum and twists around the marginal artery like an apple peel. Other possible anomalies: imperforate anus; biliary atresia; spina bifida; microcephaly; microphthalmos; heart defects; uretero pelvic junction obstruction.

Etiology. Suggested. Autosomal recessive inheritance.

Pathology. Jejunal atresia. Obliteration of superior mesenteric artery may underlie the malformation.

Diagnostic Procedures. *X-ray.* Plain abdominal. *Barium enema. CT scan. Ultrasonography.*

Therapy. Surgery.

Prognosis. Good with surgery.

BIBLIOGRAPHY. Mishalany HG, Najjar FB: Familial jejunal atresia: three cases in one family. J Pediat 73:753–755, 1968

Blyth HM, Dikson JAS: Apple peel syndrome (congenital intestinal atresia): a family study of seven index patients. J Med Genet 6:275–277, 1969

Seashore JH, Collins FS, Markowitz RI, et al: Familial apple peel jejeunal atresia: surgical, genetic and radiographic aspects. Pediatrics 80:540–544, 1987

Haubrich WS, Schaffner F, Berk JE (eds): Bockus Gastroenterology, 5th ed, pp 904–906. Philadelphia, WB Saunders, 1995

APRACTOGNOSIA

Synonyms. Minor parietal, right parieto-occipital.

Symptoms and Signs. Body scheme disturbances: denial of left hemiplegia hemiagnosia; motor hemispontaneity. Apraxia for dressing: difficulty in recognizing the relationship between clothes and body, especially the right-left relation (particularly in difficult maneuver that requires left-right manual performance, such as tightening shoelace and necktie). Vasoconstrictive disabilities: inability to draw a three-dimensional pattern or a complex figure (attempt to reproduce a bicycle or a man is a good test.) Disorders of "spatial thought": unilateral spatial agnosia; disturbed orientation resulting in the inability of the patient to find his way, since he turns constantly to the right. Disturbance of calculation and counting. Opticovestibular disturbances: sensation of vertigo; distortion of subjective horizontal and vertical lines.

Etiology and Pathology. Lesions of the minor (nondominant) cerebral hemisphere, which includes the supramarginal gyrus and part of the angular gyrus, and the posterior part of the first temporal convolution. Surgical excision of the area; vascular, traumatic, neoplastic lesions.

Prognosis. In past surgical cases, improvements of various symptoms.

BIBLIOGRAPHY. Hecaen H, Penfield W, Bertrand C, et al: The syndrome of apractognosia due to lesions of the minor cerebral hemisphere. AMA Arch Neurol Psychiatr 75:400–434, 1956

Adams RD, Victor M: Principles of Neurology, 5th ed, p 398. New York, McGraw-Hill, 1993

ARCHER

Synonym. Uncomplicated supraclavicular aortic stenosis. See hypercalcemia, infantile and Williams-Beuren; supravalvular aortic stenosis, SVAS.

Symptoms and Signs. More frequent in males. History of cyanosis in infancy; inequality between right and left arm and neck pulses; high basal systolic murmur; no systolic click or aortic diastolic murmur. Normal facies and intelligence. Congestive failure may develop.

Etiology. Congenital malformation: (1) Nonfamilial sporadic occurrence; (2) autosomal dominant; (3) incomplete form of infantile hypercalcemia (see).

Pathology. Most frequent lesion, shelf-like thickening or ridge at upper border of Valsalva sinuses; circular narrowing of aorta or long stenotic segment of aorta; fibrous bands from aortic cusps to ridge.

Diagnostic Procedures. *X-ray of chest. Angiocardiography. EEG. Two-dimensional echocardiography with color flow imaging and spectral Doppler interrogation.*

Therapy. Surgical correction; complete correction impossible in some cases.

Prognosis. Reduced longevity.

BIBLIOGRAPHY. Archer RS: Note on a congenital band stretching across the origin of the aorta. Dublin J Med Sci 65:405–406, 1878

Johnson LW, Fishman RA, Schneider B, et al: Familial supravalvular aortic stenosis: report of a large family and review of literature. Chest 70:494–500, 1976

Nugent EW, Plauth WH, Edwards JE, et al: The pathology, pathophysiology recognition and treatment of congenital heart disease. In Schlant RC, Alexander RW: Hurst's The Heart, 8th ed, pp 1794–1795. New York, McGraw-Hill, 1994

A.R.D.S.: ADULT RESPIRATORY DISTRESS

Synonyms. Congestive atelectasis; noncardiogenic pulmonary edema; push-pull pump; septic lung; shock lung; wet lung; white lung; capillary leak-lung edema.

Symptoms and Signs. Onset of respiratory symptoms occurs after 24–48 hours from the initial insult. Tachypnea; labored breathing followed by cyanosis.

Etiology. Tissue damage caused by vasoactive substances released by neutrophils, platelets, and complement activation. Associated with a variety of conditions that may directly or indirectly damage the pulmonary capillary endothelium. Direct damage includes trauma, infections, aspiration, fat embolism. Indirect damage mediated by humoral factors includes sepsis, pancreatitis, shock, DIC, drugs.

Pathology. Pulmonary capillary damage with interstitial damage followed by alveolar edema. Later extensive pulmonary fibrosis.

Diagnostic Procedures. *Blood.* Findings of hypoxemia at gas analysis. *X-ray.* Diffuse pulmonary infiltrates. Reduced lung compliance. Increased shunt fraction and dead space ventilation.

Therapy. Increased inspired oxygen tension. Mechanical ventilation and positive end expiratory pressure (PEEP). Extracorporeal CO_2 elimination. Prostaglandins (PGE_1) under investigation. Cardiovascular support with dopamine.

Prognosis. About 50% mortality. Good recovery for people who survive.

BIBLIOGRAPHY. Ashbaug MDG, Bigelow DB, Petty TL, Levine BE: Acute respiratory distress syndrome in adults. Lancet II:319–323, 1967

Robin ED, Carey LC, Grenvik A, et al: Capillary leak syndrome with pulmonary edema. Arch Int Med 130:66–71, 1972

Editorial: Current opinion. Crit Care 1:1, 1995

A.R.E.D.Y.L.D.

Synonyms. Pinheiro, acrorenal field defect, ectodermal dysplasia, lipoatrophic diabetes.

Symptoms and Signs. Both sexes. Low birth weight; hypotrichosis; mandibular prognatism; peculiar nose; deciduous teeth dysplasia; permanent dentition absent; aplasia or hypoplasia of breast; and features of lipoatrophic diabetes (see) and minor renal disease.

Etiology. Possibly pleitropic recessive gene.

Prognosis. One case death at 1½ years; other alive at time of report in the second decade.

BIBLIOGRAPHY. Pinheiro Freire-Maia N, Chautard Freire-Maia EA, et al: AREDYLD: a syndrome combining an acrorenal field defect, ectodermal dysplasia, lipoatrophic diabetes and other manifestations. Am J Med Genet 16:29–33, 1983

ARGINASE DEFICIENCY

Synonyms. Terheggen; argininemia; hyperargininemia.

Symptoms and Signs. Rare. Onset in neonatal period. Spastic tetraplegia; mental retardation; seizures; hyperactivity; growth failure.

Etiology. Autosomal recessive trait (?). Arginase deficiency. Autosomal recessive.

Diagnostic Procedures. *Blood, urine, cerebrospinal fluid.* Hyperargininemia; chromatographic amino acid screening. Confirmation by determination of arginase activity in red cells or liver tissue. Hyperammoniemia progressivelly rising to three–four times normal level.

Therapy. Low-protein diet. Benzoate and phenylacetate use supported by preliminary results.

Prognosis. Early death or mental and physical retardation.

BIBLIOGRAPHY. Peralta Serrano A: Argininuria, convulsiones y oligofrenia: Un nuevo error innato del metabolismo? Rev Clin Esp 97:176–183, 1965

Brusilow SW, Horwich AL: Urea cycle enzymes. In Scriver CR, Beaudet AL, Sly WS, et al: The Metabolic and Molecular Bases of Inherited Disease, 7th ed, pp 1205–1206. New York, McGraw-Hill, 1995

ARGININOSUCCINASE LYASE DEFICIENCY

Synonyms. Allan; argininosuccinase aciduria; ASase aciduria; ASAL (argininosuccinate lyase) deficiency.

Symptoms and Signs. Both sexes affected; prevalent in females (2:1). Three types according to time of onset.

1. Neonatal (soon after birth). Poor feeding; lethargy; hypothermia; tachypnea; seizures and coma.
2. Subacute. Early infancy feeding difficulties; failure to thrive; seizures; delayed mental milestones; hepatomegaly; friable tufted hair (trichorrhexis nodosa).
3. Late onset. Mental retardation becomes evident in second year of life; history of feeding troubles, vomiting, irritability; intelligence quotient between 30 and 60; seizures; hair changes (see preceding) in 50% of cases.

Etiology. Autosomal recessive inheritance. Deficiency of ASAL activity (chromosome 7).

Pathology. *Nonspecific.* Multiple necrotic foci. *Kidney.* Degenerative alterations; tubular casts. *Myocardium.* Extensive necrosis. *Brain.* Edema; spongy alteration of gray and white matter; swollen astrocytes; demyelinization.

Diagnostic Procedures. *Urine.* Arginosuccinic acid (ASA) in great quantity. *Blood.* Increase of ASA, increase of transaminases and alkaline phosphatases. *Cerebrospinal fluid.* Increase in ASA (compared with blood).

Therapy. Symptomatic. Selective diet (low-protein diet and in small feedings) and activation of other pathways of waste nitogen synthesis and excretion.

Prognosis. *Neonatal type.* Death in the first days. *Subacute type.* Unknown. Late onset type. From severe mental disorder to asymptomatic evolution.

BIBLIOGRAPHY. Brusilow SW, Horwich AL: Urea cycle enzymes. In Scriver CR, Beaudet AL, Sly WS, et al: The Metabolic and Molecular Bases of Inherited Disease, 7th ed, pp 1187–1188. New York, McGraw-Hill, 1995

Rezvani I: Urea cycle and hyperammoninemia. In Behrman RE, Kliegman Arvin Nelson: Textbook of Pediatrics, 15th ed, p 352. Philadelphia, WB Saunders, 1995

ARGYLL ROBERTSON

Synonyms. Robertson spinal miosis; reflex iridoplegia; iridoplegia reflex.

Symptoms and Signs. Vision not significantly affected; associated with various symptoms of syphilis of central nervous system: general paresis, tabes dorsalis. Unilateral or bilateral small pupils that do not react to light but react to accommodation and convergence; dilate poorly or not at all with mydriatic. Usually, unequal and irregular.

Etiology. Syphilis (tabes; meningovascular); alcoholic midbrain changes; diabetes; general paresis; Wernicke syndrome; arteriosclerosis; posttraumatic.

Pathology. Not exactly determined. Lesions of pretectal region to oculomotor nucleus (?), iris (more likely), ciliary ganglion (?). Lesions of axons of ciliary ganglion have been demonstrated.

Diagnostic Procedures. Test for light and convergence accommodation. *Blood and spinal fluid.* Syphilis.

Therapy. None.

Prognosis. Depends upon etiology.

BIBLIOGRAPHY. Robertson DA: On an interesting series of eye-symptoms in a case of spinal disease: with remarks on the action of Belladonna on the iris, etc. Edinb Med J 14:696–708, 1869; Med Classics 1:851–868, 1937

Lebensohn JE: Centenary of the Horner and Argyll Robertson pupillar syndromes. Proc Inst Med Chicago 28:65, 1970

Adams RD, Victor M: Principles of Neurology, 3rd ed, p 209. New York, McGraw-Hill, 1985

ARHINENCEPHALIA

Synonyms. Holoprosencephaly; alobar familial.

Symptoms and Signs. Different types of facial anomalies are included in this type of malformation: cyclopia (see); ethmocephaly (see); cebocephaly (see); median cleft lip; and less severe facial dysmorphisms.

Etiology. Variable; most cases undetermined. Varying degrees of deficit of midline facies development and incomplete morphogenesis of brain, depending on prochordal mesoderm defect. In some cases, chromosomal defects.

Pathology. According to mentioned varieties.

Therapy. Limited to medical assistance to survival measures.

Prognosis. From fair to very poor for survival.

BIBLIOGRAPHY. Ahlfeld F: Die Missbildungen des Menschen. Leipzig, FW Grunow, 1880–1882

Kundrat H: Arhinencephalie als Typische Art von Missbildung. Gratz, Von Leuschner and Lubensky, 1882

Gorlin RJ, Cohen MM, Levin LS: Syndromes of Head and Neck, pp 573–582. Oxford, New York, 1990

ARIAS

Synonyms. Crigler-Najjar type 2; hyperbilirubinemia, intermediate degree; bilirubin defect; partial defect conjugation; hyperbilirubinemia congenital type II. See Gilbert.

Symptoms. Onset from first year of life or later (at 4–30 years of age). Asymptomatic; only occasionally instances of neurologic manifestations.

Signs. Generalized jaundice. Gallstones sometimes present (coincidental?).

Etiology. Autosomal recessive inheritance. Genetic lesion found in the variable region exon for bilirubin-UGT1 resulting in the substitution of a single aminoacid in the N-terminal region of the isoform.

Pathology. Extrahepatic ducts patent; no histologic abnormalities, except for hypertrophy-hyperplasia of smooth endoplasmic reticulum and Golgi apparatus. In limited cases, brain abnormalities.

Diagnostic Procedures. *Blood.* Serum bilirubin (unconjugated type) increased (6–20 mg/100 ml); fasting (24 hours); elevation of bilirubin. *Duodenal aspiration.* Bile pigment: hourly output of bilirubin below calculated production rate. Most pigment in form of monoglucuronide. *Menthol and salicylamide tests.* Abnormal.

Therapy. Phenobarbital (60–180 mg daily); dichlorodiphenyl trichloroethane (chlorophenothane).

Prognosis. Benign disorder; good response to treatment.

BIBLIOGRAPHY. Arias IM: Chronic unconjugated hyperbilirubinemia without overt signs of hemolysis in adolescents and adults. J Clin Invest 41:2233–2245, 1962

Chowdhury JR, Wolkoff AW, Chowdhury NR, Arias IM: Hereditary jaundice and disorders of bilirubin metabolism. In Scriver CR, Beaudet AL, Sly WS, et al: The Metabolic and Molecular Bases of Inherited Disease, 7th ed, pp 2182–2184. New York, McGraw-Hill, 1995

ARIETI-GRAY

Obsolete.

Synonyms. Angiosis, progessive, multiform. See Sturge-Weber.

Symptoms and Signs. Feeblemindness, seizures.

Etiology. See Sturge-Weber.

Pathology. Multiform angiosis with aneurysm of Willis circle and abdominal aorta; subarachnoidal proliferation of capillaries; intracranial calcification.

Diagnostic Procedures. *CT scan. MRI. EEG. Arteriography.*

Therapy. Symptomatic.

Prognosis. Guarded.

BIBLIOGRAPHY. Arieti S, Gray EW: Progessive multiform angiosis. Arch Neurol Psychiatr (Chic) 51:182–191, 1944

ARLT

Synonyms. Egyptian ophthalmia; chronic follicular keratoconjunctivitis; granular conjunctivitis; trachoma; chlamydial keratoconjunctivitis.

Symptoms. Both sexes affected; onset variable, insidious or acute. Initially, photophobia, tears, blepharospasm.

Signs. Swollen eyelids; mucopurulent discharge; preauricular lymph nodes; conjunctival blebs. Later, scarring, lacrimal dysfunction, and corneal opacities.

Etiology. Infection owing to a Bartonella (psittacosis), Lymphogranuloma venereum, transmitted by contact. Infection owing to Chlamydia trachomatis transmitted by contact.

Pathology. Papillary hypertrophy of conjunctiva; corneal invasion by dense fibrous tissue, lymphocyte infiltration. Necrosis of conjunctival follicles followed by scarring (Herbert pits).

Diagnostic Procedures. Agent isolation. Inclusion bodies in epithelial cells.

Therapy. Local and systemic antibiotics (tetracycline per os).

Prognosis. According to treatment. Possible complications: entropion; ectropion; symblepharon; xerosis; blindness. Corneal transplantation if severe scarring.

BIBLIOGRAPHY. Arlt CF, von: Die Kranheiten des Auges. Praga, Credner & Kleinbub, 1851

Persson K, Rönnesiam R, Svanberg L, et al: Neonatal chlamydial eye infection: an epidemiological and clinical study. Br J Ophthalmol 67:700–704, 1983

Feducowiez HB, Stetson S: External Infections of the Eye: Bacterial, Viral, and Mycotic, with Noninfectious and Immunologic Diseases, 3rd ed. Norwalk, CT, Appleton-Century-Crofts, 1985

ARLT-DAVIDSEN

Eponym (obsolete) used to indicate the association: lamellar cataract, brown hypoplasia of the teeth, and epilepsy.

BIBLIOGRAPHY. Moortgat P: Syndromes á Noms Propres. Paris, J Prélat, 1966

ARMENDARES

Synonyms. Craniosynostosis—dwarfism—retinitis pigmentosa.

Symptoms and Signs. Present from birth. Microcephaly; craniosynostosis; cranial asymmetry; small face; short nose; micrognathia; high palate; scanty eyebrows; ptosis eyelids; epicanthal fold; retinitis pigmentosa; ear malformation; intelligence normal; bone age delayed; short fingers with clinodactyly, single palmar crease.

Etiology. Unestablished inheritance; X-linked or autosomal recessive.

Diagnostic Procedure. *Electroretinogram*; diminution b-wave.

BIBLIOGRAPHY. Armendares S, Antillon F, Del Castillo V: A newly recognized inherited syndrome of dwarfism, craniosynostosis, retinitis pigmentosa, and multiple congenital malformation. J Pediatr 85:872–873, 1974

Armendares S, Antillon F, Del Castillo V, et al: A newly recognized inherited syndrome of dwarfism, craniosynostosis retinitis pigmentosa and multiple congenital malformations. Birth Defects 11:49–53, 1975

ARNASON

Synonyms. Gudmundsson, amyloid cerebral deposits; hereditary cerebral hemorrhage; Iceland hereditary cerebral hemorrhage; amyloidosis VI: HCHWA (hereditary cerebral hemorrhage with amyloidosis); gammatrace, defect of; cerebral amyloid angiopathy.

Symptoms and Signs. In Icelandic families. Both sexes affected; onset of cerebral hemorrhages at young age (in one family, at 44 years in first generation; at 30 years in second generation; at 22.5 years in third generation). Variable neurologic symptoms according to site of hemorrhages.

Etiology. Autosomal dominant inheritance.

Pathology. Amyloid deposits in the walls of cerebral vessels. Absence of senile plaques. Minor amyloid infiltration in brain or other visceral parenchyma.

Prognosis. Death on first episode or survival of variable duration; up to 13 years.

BIBLIOGRAPHY. Arnason A: Apoplexie und ihre Vererbung. Acta Psychiatr Neurol (suppl) 7:1–180, 1935

Cosgrove GR, Leblanc R, Meagher-Villemure K, et al: Cerebral amyloid angiopathy. Neurology 35:625–639, 1985

Jensson O, Palsdottir A, Thorsteinsson L, et al : The saga of cystatin C gene mutation causing amyloid angiopathy and brain hemorrhage: clinical genetic studies in Iceland. Clin Genet 36:368–377, 1989

Benson MD: Amyloidosis. In Scriver CR, Beaudet AL, Sly WS, et al: The Metabolic and Molecular Bases of Inherited Disease, 7th ed, p 4179. New York, McGraw-Hill, 1995

ARNDT-GOTTRON

Synonyms. Lichen myxedematous variant papular mucinosis; papular myxedema; scleromyxedema; lichen fibromucinodosis.

Symptoms and Signs. Appear in 3rd to 5th decades. Diffuse thickening of skin underlying lichenoid papular eruption, often in linear patterns, approximately of uniform size. Infiltrations involve the greater part of the body. Distortion of facial features and limitation of finger movements. Lassitude and muscular weakness may be present.

Etiology. Unknown.

Pathology. Proliferation of fibroblasts and deposition of acid mucopolysaccharides in upper section of dermis. Muscles may be infiltrated with lymphocytes.

Diagnostic Procedures. *Biopsy of skin. Blood.* Presence of a paraprotein of the IgG class. *Bone marrow.* Mild plasma cell infiltration.

Therapy. None. Melphalan or cyclophosphamide (attention to toxicity). Corticosteroids useless; dermabrasion of some help.

Prognosis. Poor; no spontaneous resolution; with melphalan, gradual resolution of skin lesions within 3 months.

BIBLIOGRAPHY. Gottron HA: Skleromyxeodem (eine eigenartige Erscheinungsform von Myxothesaurodermie). Arch Derm Syph 199:71–91, 1954

Black MM, Gawkrodger DJ, Seymour CH, et al: Metabolic and nutritional disorders. In Champion RH, Burton JL, Ebling FJG (eds): Rook/Wilkinson/Ebling Textbook of Dermatology, 5th ed, pp 2326–2328. Oxford, Blackwell Scientific, 1992

ARNETH

Not a syndrome but the combination of auscultory sounds modification induced by lung hepatization: bronchial murmur; bronchophony; whispering pectoriloqui.

BIBLIOGRAPHY. Minerbi C: La "sindrome polmonitica di Arneth." La vera natura fisica del fremito vocale tattile. Atti Accad Sc Med Ferrara 3–4:47–49, 1928

ARNOLD-CHIARI

Synonyms. Celand-Arnold-Chiari; Chiari; basilar impression; cerebellomedullary malformation; platybasia.

Symptoms. Both sexes affected. Divided in two major subgroups. Type I onset usually in adolescence or in 3rd or 4th decade, usually not associated with hydrocephalus and presenting recurrent headache, neck pain, paresthesias (transient), urinary frequency, and progressive lower limbs spasticity. Type II (associated with hydrocephalus and or myelomeningocele) symptoms may appear in infancy and presents stridor, wick cry, or respiratory complications with abnormal control of breathing, upper-airway dysfunction, aspiration pneumonia, and cor pulmonale. Particularly, abnormalities in control of ventilation are manifested by hypoventilation, sleep apnea, and prolonged breath-holding spells, or milder manifestations as abnormalities of gait spasticity and progressive incoordination; headache; vomiting; visual disturbances; diplopia; mental dullness.

Signs. Hydrocephalus; papilledema; nystagmus; glossopharyngeal (IX), vagus (X), spinal accessory (XI), and hypoglossal (XII) nerve palsies; posterior and lateral column nerve palsies; signs of cerebellar ataxia.

Etiology and Pathology. Unknown. In type I, congenital malformation of occipital bone and proximal end of cervical spine, determining displacement of cerebellar tonsils through foramen magnum into cervical canal. In type II, anomaly of the hindbrain, failure of pontine flexure and consequent elongation of fourth ventricle and kinking of brain stem with displacement of inferior vermis, pons and medulla into cervical canal.

Diagnostic Procedures. *X-ray. CT brain scan. MRI.* Platybasia; narrowing of foramen magnum. Herniation of cerebral tonsils. *Spinal fluid.* Increased pressure and proteins. Volume of ventricular system and rate of disappearance of radioiodinated serum albumin.

Therapy. Condition may be corrected by neurosurgical procedures. Ventriculoatrial shunting. Early and prolonged ventilatory support can result in favorable outcome.

Prognosis. Differs according to the degree of alterations. In children with extensive deformity, death during first year of life.

BIBLIOGRAPHY. Arnold J: Myelocyste, Transposition von Gewebskeimen und Sympodie. Beitr Path Anat Allg Path 16:1–28, 1894

Chiari H: Ueber Veränderungen des Kleinhirns infolge von Hydrocephalie des Grosshirns. Dtsche Med Wochenschr 17:1172–1175, 1891

Dong ML: Arnold-Chiari malformation type I appearing after tonsillectomy. Anesthesiology 67:120–122, 1987

Haslam RHA: The nervous system. In Behrman Kliegman Arvin: Nelson Textbook of Pediatrics, 15th ed, p 1684. Philadelphia, WB Saunders, 1995

ARNOLD NERVE COUGH

Synonyms. Arnold neuralgia; vagus auricular branch neuralgia.

Symptoms. Reflex cough, caused by friction from clotting, temperature changes; associated with attack of suboccipital stabbing or burning pain, shifting to neck occasionally and to shoulder. Auricular neuralgia may be present. During remission of pain, tenderness and paresthesias of area.

Signs. Pain on pressure on the area posterior to ear.

Etiology. Irritation of auricular branch of vagus (X) nerve.

Pathology. Neuritis or compression of nervous branch by different pathologic process.

Therapy. Removal of cause of irritation when identified. Trial with phenytoin or carbamazepine, analgesics, anti-inflammatories, local anesthetics. In refractory cases: surgical interruption of nerve seldom successful and may cause "anesthesia dolorosa."

Prognosis. Depends upon etiology.

BIBLIOGRAPHY. Alayza Escardo F: Arnold's neuralgia. JAMA 161:391, 1956

Vick NA: Grinker's Neurology, 7th ed. Springfield, IL, Charles C Thomas, 1976

Adams RD, Victor M: Principles of Neurology, 5th ed, p 163. New York, McGraw-Hill, 1993

ARRHYTHMOGENIC RIGHT VENTRICULAR DYSPLASIA

Synonyms. ARVD. See dilated myocardiopathy.

Symptoms and Signs. Recurrent sustained ventricular tachycardia with left branch block dilated myocardiopathy (see).

Etiology. Autosomal dominant inheritance.

Prognosis. Death in the 30–40-year range.

BIBLIOGRAPHY. Pietras RJ, Lam W, Bauernfiend R, et al: Chronic recurrent right ventricular tachycardia in a patient without ischemic heart disease: clinical hemodynamic and angiographic findings. Am Heart J 105:357–366, 1983

Laurent M, Descaves C, Biron Y, et al: Familial form of arrhythmogenic right ventricular dysplasia. Am Heart J 113:827–829, 1987

Myerburg RJ, Kessler KM, Castellanos A: Recognition clinical assessment and management of conduction disturbances. In Schlant RC, Alexander RW: Hurst's The Heart, 8th ed, p 743. New York, McGraw-Hill, 1994

ARTERIAL VARICES

Synonyms. Arteriovenous aneurysm; arteriovenous anastomosis; arteriovenous fistula.

Symptoms. Onset usually at puberty or after straining activities; usually occurs in young persons. Enlargement of the vessels of the lateral side of legs noted; increase in skin temperature may be experienced.

Signs. Enlarged vessels with pulsation synchronous with cardiac pulsation; bruit and thrill may be detected. Arterial-type bleeding.

Etiology. Congenital; arteriovenous connections; familial occurrence.

Diagnostic Procedures. Elevation. Veins remain filled; after pressure rapid refilling. Introduction of needle shows pulsation of syringe barrel. Oxygen saturation higher than recorded in blood from other veins of patient. *Angiography.* Useful on confirming the diagnosis.

Therapy. Surgical excision.

Prognosis. Recurrence after surgery. Repeated interventions.

BIBLIOGRAPHY. Pratt FH: Arterial varices syndrome. Am J Surg 77:456–460, 1949

Szilagyi DE, Smith RF, Elliot JP, Hageman JH: Congenital arteriovenous anomalies of the limbs. Arch Surg 111:423–429, 1976

Braundwald E: Heart Disease, vol 2, p 286. Philadelphia, WB Saunders, 1980

ARTERIOSCLEROSIS OF SPINAL VESSELS

Symptoms. Appear in middle to late age; onset insidious. Weakness starting in one leg, and extending then to the other; intermittent claudication. Urinary urgency, retention, incontinence.

Signs. Hyperreflexion of lower extremities; positive Babinski sign.

Etiology. Arteriosclerotic degeneration of spinal arteries (atherosclerotic process very seldom affects spinal vessels). Arteritis of spinal vessel (syphilis).

Pathology. Nonspecific occlusive arteritis and secondary ischemic atrophy of dorsolumbar cord.

Diagnostic Procedures. *Spinal fluid. Arteriography. Blood serology.*

Therapy. Nonspecific.

Prognosis. Slow or rapid evolution to spastic paraplegia.

BIBLIOGRAPHY. Keschner M, Davison C: Myelytic and myelopathic lesions: arteriosclerotic and arteritic myelopathy. Arch Neurol Psychiatr 29:702–725, 1933

Adams RD, Victor M: Principles of Neurology, 5th ed, p 1093. New York, McGraw-Hill, 1993

ARTERIOVENOUS FISTULA OF CORONARY ARTERY

Synonym. Coronary arteriosystemic fistula.

Symptoms. Both sexes equally affected. Usually, asymptomatic. Growth and development not compromised.

Signs. Continuous, relatively soft murmur that does not peak on second heart sound and that usually becomes evident only after neonatal fall in pulmonary vascular resistance. Increased frequency of respiratory infections. Heart failure may develop after fourth decade.

Etiology. Defective embryogenesis of coronary artery entering right heart chambers, pulmonary artery, or left chambers (coronary arteriosystemic fistula) owing to persistence of primitive intramyocardial sinusoids or faulty development of distal branches.

Pathology. Usually solitary, rarely multiple. A saccular aneurysm may develop especially in adult and shows calcification.

Diagnostic Procedures. *ECG.* Usually normal. *X-ray.* Normal to variable, according to volume of fistula. *Arterial pulse.* Normal; pulse pressure increased. *Two-dimensional echography with color flow imaging and Doppler interrogation. Selective cardiac catheterization or aortography.*

Therapy. *Medical.* Prevention of complication (thrombosis, myocardial ischemia, infective endocarditis, rupture). *Surgical.* Recommended because it is simple, safe, effective.

Prognosis. Good with surgery. Heart failure may develop after age 40.

BIBLIOGRAPHY. Krause W: Ueber den Ursprung einer accessorishen A coronaria cordis aus der A pulmonalis. Medicine 24:225–227, 1865

Perloff JK: The Clinical Recognition of Congenital Heart Disease, 4th ed, pp 562–580. Philadelphia, WB Saunders, 1994

ARTHROGRYPOSIS

Synonyms. Guérin-Stern; Otto; Rocher-Sheldon; Rossi; myodystrophy fetal deformans; amyoplasia congenita, AMC; arthrogryposis multiplex congenita; arthromyodysplasia; see Gordon (H.).

Symptoms. Both sexes equally affected. Limited motion of all joints with the exception of mandibular and spinal. Occasional paralysis of different muscles. Reduced facial gesticulation confers a melancholic aspect.

Signs. Osteoarticular deformity with enlargement of joints, hypoplasia of attached muscles, and zones of thickening of the overlying skin (cardboard aspect), alternated with atrophic tracts. *Arms.* Rotated inward; cylindrical elbows; flexed wrists and fingers. *Legs.* Thighs rotated outward; dislocated hip; extended knees; clubfoot; absence of the fibula (occasional). *Skull.* Premature synostosis; palate defect. *Spine.* Absence of sacrum (occasional). No specific dermatoglyphic alterations.

Etiology. Unknown. Congenital neuromuscular disorder; osteoarticular deformities seem to be secondary to muscular atrophy. Lower motor neuron deficiency present in high proportion of cases. Viral hypotesis, familial form autosomal recessive inheritance (rare).

Pathology. Degeneration of some muscle fibers dispersed among normal ones, with fibrotic changes, and fatty infiltration. Inelastic articular capsules; atrophy of the bone. Degeneration of motor neurons of spinal cord.

Diagnostic Procedures. *Muscle biopsy. X-ray. CT scan. MRI. Bone atrophy. Electromyography.*

Therapy. Surgical mobilization partly successful.

Prognosis. Situation not progressive. Mortality 10% at early age; infections and visceral malformations are the leading causes.

BIBLIOGRAPHY. Paré A: Monstre et prodiges. In Malgaigue JF: Oevres Completes Revues et Collationnees, 3rd ed, p 25. Paris, JB Baillieres, 1573

Otto AW: Monstrorum sexcentorum descriptio anatomica. Bratislava, 1841

Guérin JR: Recherches sur les deformités congénitales chez les monstres. Paris, 1880

Rocher HL: Les raideurs articulaires congénitales multiples. J Med Bordeaux 4:772–780, 1913

Stern WG: Arthrogryposis multiplex congenita. JAMA 81:1507–1510, 1923

Scheldon W: Amyoplasia congenita (multiple congenital articular rigidity, arthrogryposis multiplex congenita). Arch Dis Child (London) 7:117–136, 1932

Rossi E: Le syndrome arthromyodysplasique congénital. Helv Paediatr Acta 2:82–97, 1947

Hall JG, Reed SD, Driscoll EP: Part I Amyoplasia: a common sporadic condition with congenital contractures. Am J Med Gent 15:571–590, 1983

Herring JA: Instructional case: Arthrogryposis. J Pediatr Orthoped 8:353–355, 1988

ARTHROGRYPOSIS, DISTAL TYPE

TYPE I

Symptoms and Signs. From birth. Involvement of hands and feet. See arthrogryposis; variable contraction of other joints.

Etiology. Autosomal dominant inheritance.

Prognosis. Good response to physiotherapy.

TYPE II

Symptoms and Signs. Major involvement of hands and feet associated with other defects: fused cervical vertebrae; cervical pterygia; scoliosis; congenital hip dislocation; contractures of other joints.

Etiology. Autosomal dominant.

Prognosis. Moderate response to physiotherapy.

TYPE II WITH CRANIOFACIAL ABNORMALITIES DOMINANT

Symptoms and Signs. Associated craniofacial abnormalities including asymmetry, hypertelorism, high nasal bridge, malar hypoplasia, arched palate.

Etiology. Autosomal dominant inheritance.

BIBLIOGRAPHY. Lin P, Hall J, Grever R, et al: A new familial arthrogryposis with autosomal dominant type of inheritance. West Pediatr Clin Res Meeting, Carmel, CA, 1977

Kawira EL, Bender HA: An unusual distal arthrogryposis. Am J Med Genet 20:425–429, 1985

Moore CA, Weaver DD: Famial distal arthrogryposis with cranio facial abnormalities: a new subtype of type II? Am J Med Genet 33:231–237, 1989

TYPE II WITH CRANIOFACIAL ABNORMALITIES RECESSIVE WITH HYPOPITUITARISM–MENTAL RETARDATION I

BIBLIOGRAPHY. Chitayat D, Hall JC, Couch RM, et al: Syndrome of mental retardation, facial anomalies, hypopituitarisim and distal arthrogryposis in sibs. Am J Med Genet 37:65–70, 1990

TYPE II WITH CRANIOFACIAL ABNORMALITIES RECESSIVE WITH MENTAL RETARDATION I

BIBLIOGRAPHY. Chitayat D, Hodgkinson KA, Blaichman, et al: Syndrome of mental retardation and distal arthrogryposis in sibs. Am J Med Genet 41:49–51, 1991

ARTHROGRYPOSIS MULTIPLEX CONGENITA, DISTAL, X-LINKED

Three distinctive types of X-linked AMC have been reported with variable manifestations, ranging from mild and moderate to lethal forms.

BIBLIOGRAPHY. Hall JG, Reed SD, Scott CI, et al: Three distinct types of X-linked arthrogryposis seen in six families. Clin Genet 21:81–97, 1982

Hennekam RCM, Barth PG, Van Lookeren Campagne W, et al: A family with severe X-linked arthrogryposis. Europ J Pediat 50:656–660, 1991

ARTHROGRYPOSIS MULTIPLEX CONGENITAL–RENAL HEPATIC ABNORMALITIES

Symptoms and Signs. Males. See Arthrogryposis multiplex congenita, distal, X-linked. Jaundice. Renal impairment.

Etiology. X-linked inheritance.

Pathology. *Kidney.* Tubular cell degeneration and nephrocalcinosis. *Liver.* Black color due to pigmentary deposits.

Prognosis. Death at birth or within first months.

BIBLIOGRAPHY. Nezelof C, Dupart MC, Joubert F, et al: A lethal familial syndrome associating arthrogryposis multiplex congenita, renal dysfunction and a cholestatic and pigmentary liver disease. J Pediat 94:258–260, 1979

Di Rocco M, Reboa E, Barabino A, et al: Arthrogryposis, cholestatic pigmentary liver disease and renal dysfunction: report of a second family. Am J Med Genet 37:237–240, 1990

ARTHROGRYPOSIS, NEUROGENIC

Synonyms. Arthrogryposis multiplex neurogenic.

Symptoms and Signs. Arthrogryposis-like lesions with primary neurologic lesions.

Etiology. Possibly autosomal recessive inheritance. Virus infections considered.

BIBLIOGRAPHY. Ek JI: Cerebral lesions in arthrogryposis multiplex congenita. Acta Pediatr 47:302–316, 1958

Frischknecht W, Branchi L, Pilleri G: Familiaere Arthrogryposis multiplex congenita. Helv Paediat Acta 15:259–279, 1960

Krugliak L, Gadoth N, Bear AJ: Neuropathic form of arthrogryposis multiplex congenita: Report of 3 cases with complete necropsy, including the first reported case of agenesis of muscle spindles. J Neurol Sci 37:179–185, 1978

ARTICHOKE, MODIFICATION OF TASTE BY

Symptoms. Eating an artichoke (Cymara scolymus) makes water taste sweet in some subjects.

Etiology. Temporary alteration in the tongue. Genetic basis unknown.

Pathology. None.

Therapy. None.

BIBLIOGRAPHY. Blakeslee AF: A dinner demonstration of threshold differences in taste and smell. Science 81:504–507, 1935

Bartoshuk LM, Lee CH, Scarpellino R: Sweet taste induced by artichoke. Science 178:988–989, 1972

A.S.A. TRIAD

Synonym. Asthma—nasal polyps—aspirin intolerance.

Symptoms and Signs. Both sexes. Early or late onset in life of asthmatic attacks, nasal polyposis, and aspirin intolerance. Cases with incomplete triad.

Etiology. Recessive inheritance, also dominant reported; possible importance of environmental factors. Probably owing to aspirin inhibition of cyclooxygenase pathway.

BIBLIOGRAPHY. Miller FF: Aspirin-induced bronchial asthma in sisters. Am Allergy 29:263–265, 1971
Von Maur K, Adkinson NF Jr, Van Metre TE Jr, et al: Aspirin intolerance in a family. J Allergy Clin Immun 54:380–395, 1974
Weatherall DJ, Ledingham JGG, Warrell DA (eds): Oxford Textbook of Medicine, 3rd ed, pp 2735, 2849. Oxford, Oxford Med Pub, 1996

ASBOE-HANSEN

See Bloch-Sulzberger. Considered by the authors as the initial phase of the Bloch-Sulzberger syndrome. There is no reason for considering it an autonomous entity.

BIBLIOGRAPHY. Asboe-Hansen G: Bullous keratogenous and pigmentary dermatitis with blood eosinophilia in newborn girls: report of four cases. Arch Dermatol Syph 67:152–157, 1953

ASCHER

Synonyms. Laffer-Ascher; blepharochalasis—thyroid; struma—double lips; blepharochalasis—double lips.

Symptoms and Signs. In several cases swelling of lid onset during first 8 years, in others at puberty. *Eyes.* Blepharochalasis fundamental sign (see Fuchs syndrome for description). Two phases as in Fuchs: (1) Recurrent edemas; (2) atrophy of skin and subcutaneous tissue of eyelids, and prolapse of orbital cavity contents. *Mouth.* Thickening of lips and gums; mucosa gives the aspect of double lips. *Thyroid.* Enlargement (occasional; it usually appears during II decade).

Etiology. Unknown. Localized cutaneous atrophy. This syndrome needs a modern evaluation with new techniques of endocrine studies. Autosomal dominant inheritance.

Pathology. Early localized edema of eyelids and lips. Later, atrophy of skin; subcutaneous with progressive degeneration; disappearance of elastic fibers. In early stages, perivascular lymphocytic infiltration that tends to disappear with progress of the disease has also been noticed. Thyroid alteration not described.

Diagnostic Procedures. *Blood and urine.* Normal. Basal metabolism rate. Usually normal; occasionally slightly elevated. Thyroid scanning radioactive iodine.

Therapy. Some improvements in cases have been obtained with the use of thyroid extract. Plastic surgery for correction of skin defect.

Prognosis. Good result obtainable by plastic correction of defect. Otherwise, progressive condition.

BIBLIOGRAPHY. Neurstaetter O: Über den Lippensaum beim Menschen: seinen Bau seine Entwicklung und seine Bedeotung Jena. Z Med Natur 29:345–390, 1895
Laffer WB: Blepharochalasis report of a case of this trophoneurosis involving also the upper lip. Cleveland Med J 8:131–135, 1909
Ascher KW: Blepharochalasis mit Struma und Doppellippe. Klin Monatsbl Augenheilkd 65:86, 1920
Goldberg R: Floppy eyelid syndrome and blepharochalasis. Am J Ophthalmol 102:376–381, 1986
Pitanguy I: Ascher's syndrome. Head Neck Surg 10:309, 1988

ASEPTIC MENINGITIS

Synonyms. Choriomeningitis, acute benign.

Symptoms. Headache; mild stiffness of neck and back; anorexia; nausea; vomiting.

Signs. Fever; convulsions; papilledema occasionally; absence of normal reflexes; positive Kerning and Brudzinsky signs. Sensory disturbances.

Etiology. Polio, echo, mumps, measles, rubella, coxsackie virus. Leptospirosis; spirochetosis; toxoplasmosis; tuberculosis; trichinosis; cysticercosis cerebri. Serum sickness; vaccines; toxic substances; pyogenic infections contiguous to meninges not adequately treated.

Pathology. Lymphocytic leptomeningeal choroid plexus; ependyma infiltrations; inclusion body in viral etiology.

Diagnostic Procedures. *Cerebrospinal fluid.* Increased in pressure; clear becoming turbid with progression of disease. Sugar, proteins normal or slightly increased, presence of mononuclear cells, usually negative cultures, titer of viral antibodies rising (when virus infection causative). *Blood.* White blood cells; lymphocytosis (virus); polymorphs (bacteria); eosinophils (parasites). *Urine cultures. X-rays of skull.*

Therapy. Depends on etiology.

Prognosis. In aseptic viral meningitis, usually, symptoms and signs subsiding in 7 days; residual fatigue. If other agents responsible, may be extremely severe and fatal if not promptly diagnosed and treated.

BIBLIOGRAPHY. Wallgren A: Une nouvelle maladie infectieuse du systeme nerveux central. Acta Paediatr (Belge) 4:158–182, 1925
Rosenthal MS: Viral infections of the central nervous system. Med Clin N Am 58:593–603, 1974
Melnick Jl: Enteroviruses: polioviruses, coxsackieviruses, echoviruses, and newer enteroviruses. In Fields BN, Knipe DM (eds): Virology, 2nd ed. New York, Raven, 1990

ASHERMAN

Synonyms. Traumatic uterine adhesions; traumatic amenorrhea, endometrial adhesion—uterine synechia.

Symptoms. Amenorrhea (traumatic amenorrhea); repeated abortions; amenorrhea or hypomenorrhea; impaired fertility.

Signs. Cervix uteri occluded; uterine probe cannot be passed into the cervical canal.

Etiology. Dilatation and vigorous curettage of the (especially puerperal) uterus and postabortal infections. According to Asherman: "Most prone to damage, however, are the succulent and hyperemic walls of the puerperal uterus."

Pathology. Two varieties are known: (1) cervical adhesions giving rise to the amenorrhea; and (2) corporeal adhesions, repeated abortions, impaired fertility, and hypomenorrhea. Adhesions in the corpus uteri are either endometrial or, most often, consist of fibromuscular bands.

Diagnostic Procedures. *Hysterography.* Stable filling defects.

Differential Diagnosis. Other causes of amenorrhea; intrauterine polyps.

Therapy. For the cervical type, adequate dilatation of the cervical canal. For the corporeal type, therapy only indicated if symptomatic. It consists of instrumental separation of the adhesions. Prophylaxis, though, is the best way to treat the condition. Postpartum curettage should be avoided.

Prognosis. Good, once condition is recognized and treated.

BIBLIOGRAPHY. Asherman JG: Amenorrhea traumatica (atretica). J Obstet Gynaecol Br Emp 55:25–30, 1948; Traumatic intrauterine adhesions. J Obstet Gynaecol Br Emp 57:892–896, 1950

Dalsace J, Musset R, Netter A, et al: Les synechies uterines. Proceedings XVII Congres Fed Soc Gyn et Obst Langue Francoise, pp 196–252. Marseille, 9–12. Paris, Masson, 1957

Chapman K, Chapman R: Asherman's syndrome: a review of the literature, and a husband and wife's 20-year world-wide experience. J Roy Soc Med 83:576–580, 1990

ASHERSON

Synonyms. Cricopharyngeal achalasia sphincter; upper esophageal sphincter dysfunction.

Symptoms and Signs. Dysphagia (of all degrees of severity), followed immediately by episodes of coughing (mild or severe paroxysms). There is a holdup of swallowed contents in the hypopharynx detectable on a pharyngoscopic mirror, or demonstrable on X-ray, after a radiopaque material is swallowed. In cricopharyngeal achalasia the dysphagia is most noticeable when liquids are swallowed; when there is a "spillover" into the air passage, producing paroxysms of coughing; and when, in extreme cases, the inhaled contents produce pneumonia.

Etiology. The causes are many, but the syndrome is seen at its most extreme in certain cases of sudden bilateral recurrent laryngeal paralysis, and in poliomyelitis with pharyngeal paralysis. It is caused by a neuromuscular incoordination, with failure of relaxation of the cricopharyngeal muscle.

Diagnostic Procedures. *X-ray.* Diagnosis confirmed after a radiopaque swallow: prominent crycopharingeal bar. *Manometric studies.* Hypertensive upper esophageal sphincter.

Therapy. In mild cases, dilatation of the cricopharyngeal sphincter; in severe cases, myotomy of the cricopharyngeal muscle.

BIBLIOGRAPHY. Asherson N: Achalasia of the cricopharyngeal sphincter. J Laryngol Otol 64:747–758, 1950

Bonavina L, Khan MA, De Meester TR: Pharyngoesophageal dysfunction: the role of crycopharyngeal myotomy. Arch Surg 120:541–549, 1985

Richter JE: Motility disorders of the esophagus. In Sleisenger MH, Fordtran JS (eds): Gastrointestinal Disease, Pathophysiology, Diagnosis and Treatment, 5th ed, pp 1083–1122. Philadelphia, WB Saunders, 1992

ASK-UPMARK

Synonyms. Segmental hypoplasia of kidney.

Symptoms and Signs. In young age. Prevalent in female. Blood hypertension.

Etiology. Unknown.

Pathology. Kidney. Outer border showing hypoplastic areas as notches and cavities clearly demarcated from normal tissue. In hypoplastic areas glomeruli small and poorly developed, tubuli fibrotic, dilated, colloid casts or atrophic. Arteries fibroelastic. Endoarteritis.

Diagnostic Procedures. *Intravenous arteriography. CT scan. MRI. Blood.* Evidence of renal insufficiency.

Therapy. If monolateral, surgical removal in toto of affected area. If bilateral and partial removal excluded, medical treatment of hypertension, finally dialysis or transplantation.

Prognosis. Related to early treatment.

BIBLIOGRAPHY. Lyundquist A, Lagergren C: The Ask-Upmark kidney Acta Pathol. Microbiol Scand 56:277–282, 1962

Vaamonde CA, Oster JR: Renal involvement in heredofamilial and congenital disease. In Massry SG, Glassock RJ: Textbook of Nephrology, 3rd ed, p 886. Baltimore, Williams & Wilkins, 1995

ASPARAGUS, URINARY EXCRETION OF ODORIFEROUS COMPONENT OF

Symptoms and Signs. After eating asparagus, urinary excretion of an odoriferous substance, called methanethiol. A subject who is a nonexcretor may become an excretor during pregnancy; the child born probably will be an excretor.

Therapy. None. The syndrome does not have any pathological significance.

BIBLIOGRAPHY. Allison AC, McWhinter KG: Two unifactorial characters for which man is polymorphic. Nature 178:748–749, 1956

ASPARTYLGLYCOSAMINURIA

Synonyms. Fountain.

Symptoms and Signs. More frequent in Finns. Predominant in females. Normal at birth, then after a few months recurrent infections, diarrhea, hernias. Failure to thrive and hepatomegaly. By first decade coarsening of facies, increased acne and photophobia, joint laxity, macroglossia, brachycephaly. Mental deterioration between age 6 and 15. Latter hypotonia or spasticity. Crystal-like lens opacities (33% of cases). Seldom hepatosplenomegaly.

Etiology. Autosomal recessive inheritance. Enzyme defect on chromosome 4 (4q21 qter).

Pathology. In all tissues presence of vacuolated cytoplasm with variable PAS staining.

Diagnostic Procedures. *Blood.* Neutropenia (13/25). Vacuolated lymphocytes (9/25). *Fibroblast cultures.* Defect of metabolism of aspartylglycosamine. Prenatal diagnosis is possible. *X-rays. CT scan. MRI.* Thick calvaria, microcephaly, small sella turcica; vertebral alterations; cortical tinning of tubular bones; pathological fractures. *EEG.* Abnormalities. *Urine.* Aspartylglycosamine.

Therapy. Symptomatic.

Prognosis. Mental deterioration. Death 3th to 5th decade usually caused by pneumonia or pulmonary abscess.

BIBLIOGRAPHY. Jenner FA, Pollitt RJ: Large quantities of 2–acetoamido-1(–1–aspartamido)-1–2–dideoxyglucose in the urine of mentally retarded siblings. Biochem J 103:48, 1967

Antio S: Aspartylglycosaminuria: analysis of thirty-four patients. J Ment Defic Res Monogr Ser 1:1, 1972

Fountain RB: Familial bone anormalities deaf mutism, mental retardation and skin granuloma. Proc Roy Soc Med 67:878–879, 1974

Fryus JP, Dereymaeker A, Hefnagels M, et al: Mental retardation, deafness skeletal abnormalities and coarse face with full lips. Confirmation of the Fountain syndrome. Am J Med Genet 26:551–555, 1987

Thomas GH, Beaudet AL: Disorders of glycoprotein degratation and structure: mannosidosis, mannosidosis, fucosidosis, sialosidosis aspartylglycosaminuria and carbohydrate-deficient glycoprotein syndrome. In Scriver CR, Beaudet AL, Sly WS, et al: The Metabolic and Molecular Bases of Inherited Disease, 7th ed, pp 2532, 2545, 2548. New York, McGraw-Hill, 1995

ASPERGER

Synonyms. Autism variant: See Kanner.

Symptoms and Signs. Usually in boys. Milder degree of autism that in Kanner. Difficult diagnosis. Lack of empathy and deviant styles of verbal and nonverbal communication; idiosyncratic attachment to inanimate objects. Patients develop as eccentric, socially unadapted personalities, usually flat, mirthless but frequently with some particular aptitude (arithmetic, memory of numbers or facts, etc.).

Etiology. Debates as to whether a mild form of Kanner or some other type of disorder as an early manifestation of schizoid personality. It appears to be a form of brain dysfunction, probably with a genetic basis.

Prognosis. Poor. The majority will, as adults, have major psychosociological difficulties.

BIBLIOGRAPHY. Asperger H: Die autistischen psychopathie in kindersalter. Arch Psychiatr Nervenkr 177:76–137, 1944
Weatherall DJ, Ledingham JGG, Warrell DA (eds): Oxford Textbook of Medicine, 3rd ed, p 4108. Oxford, Oxford Med Pub, 1996

ASTERIXIS

Synonyms. Adams-Foley; flapping tremor (misnomer); negative tremor (misnomer).

Symptoms and Signs. Bilateral or unilateral spontaneous or evoked tremor (asking the patient to hold his arms outstretched with hands dorsiflexed or dorsiflex hands and extend fingers while resting forearms on the arms of a chair). Involuntary movements owing to sudden interruption of sustained posture that allows inherent elasticity and gravity to cause movement that patient corrects, frequently overshooting.

Etiology. Observed in normal person during drowsiness. Hepatic encephalopathy, hypercapnia, metabolic and toxic encephalopathy. May be due to phenytoin or other anticonvulsants administration. Unilateral type caused by controlateral anterior cerebral artery infarction or sterotaxic thalamotomy and upper midbrain lesions.

Diagnostic Procedures. *EMG.* Attacks accompanied by silence for a period of 35–200 minutes.

Therapy. That of basic pathology.

Prognosis. Variable, from no pathologic meaning to rather negative sign for the evolution of basic pathology.

BIBLIOGRAPHY. Adams RD, Foley JM: The neurological disorder associated with liver disease. Res Publ Assoc Nerv Ment Dis 32:198, 1953
Adams RD, Victor M: Principles of Neurology, 5th ed, p 88. New York, McGraw-Hill, 1993

ÅSTRÖM-MANCALL-RICHARDSON

Synonym. Multifocal progressive leukoencephalopathy, PML.

Symptoms. Both sexes affected; onset insidious, usually after 40 years of age. Unilateral weakness; dysphagia; visual impairment up to blindness; aphasia; alteration of consciousness up to dementia.

Signs. Hemiparesis; homonymous hemianopia; and other signs associated with myeloproliferative or lymphoproliferative syndromes (see); Besnier-Boeck-Shaumann (see); tuberculosis; primary hypersplenism; Whipple syndrome (see) carcinomatosis; blue sea histiocyte.

Etiology. Viral infection (papovavirus SV 40 and more frequently JC type) in patients with impaired immunologic response, frequently owing to myeloproliferative, neoplastic, infective, chronic granulomatosis conditions.

Pathology. Wide demyelinization (central and peripheral) in perivascular foci, with sparing of axis cylinders; variable cytologic reactions; occasionally, presence of inclusion bodies formed by crystalline arrays of particles similar to papovaviruses.

Diagnostic Procedures. Diagnosis of associated condition. *Spinal fluid.* Pressure normal or slightly elevated; pleocytosis, protein elevated; search for serological evidence of presence of papovaviruses. *Electroencephalography.* Slow wave, diffuse activity; alteration according to localization and extension of lesions.

Therapy. That of associated conditions. Trials with cytosine arabinoside and vidarabine usually without success.

Prognosis. Poor. Remission or improvement may follow the treatment of associated condition. Progressive deterioration. Death usually within 3–20 months of onset.

BIBLIOGRAPHY. Åström K, Mancall EL, Richardson EP Jr: Progressive multifocal leukoencephalopathy: A hitherto unrecognized complication of chronic lymphatic leukemia and Hodgkin's disease. Brain 81:93–111, 1958
Richardson EP Jr: Our evolving understanding of progressive multifocal leukoencephalopathy. Ann NY Acad Sci 230:358–364, 1974
Adams RD, Victor M: Principles of Neurology, 5th ed, p 658. New York, McGraw-Hill, 1993

ASTRONAUT-BONE DEMINERALIZATION

Synonyms. Allison; bone-demineralization; nonuse bone atrophy.

Symptoms and Signs. Appear after periods of prolonged immobilization. From asymptomatic to generalized weakness and articular pain on motion.

Etiology. It has been observed that immobilization (in bed, casting, on orbital flights) produces significant bone demineralization. In astronauts the change has been related to the diet and the immobilization produced by the confinement in the capsule.

Therapy. Gradual exercise and diet rich in calcium may reduce the extent of calcium loss.

Prognosis. Usually good with treatment and return to normal life.

BIBLIOGRAPHY. Allison N, Brooks B: Bone atrophy: A clinical study of the changes in bone which result from non-use. Arch Surg 5:499–526, 1922
Mack PB, La Chance PA, Vose GP, et al: Bone demineralization of foot and hand of Gemini-Titan IV, V, and VII astronauts during orbital flight. Am J Roentg 100:503–511, 1967
Coe FL, Favus MJ: Disorders of Bone and Mineral Metabolism. New York, Raven, 1993
Smith R: Metabolic effects of accidental injury and surgery. In Weatherall DJ, Ledingham JGG, Warrell DA (eds): Oxford Textbook of Medicine, 3rd ed, p 1550. Oxford, Oxford Med Pub, 1996

ASTRONAUT HEMOLYTIC ANEMIA

Synonyms. Hemolytic anemia—hyperbaric oxygen.

Symptoms and Signs. Hemolytic crisis in astronauts exposed to 100% oxygen or patients undergoing hyperbaric oxygen treatment.

Etiology. Unknown.

BIBLIOGRAPHY. Gordon-Smith EG, Contreras M: Acquired haemolytic anemia. In Weatherall DJ, Ledingham JGG, Warrell DA (eds): Oxford Textbook of Medicine, 3rd ed. Oxford, Oxford Med Pub, 1996

ATELOSTEOGENESIS

Synonym. Giant cell chondrodysplasia; spondylo–humero–femoral hypoplasia; AO1; AO2; AO3. See de la Chapelle (possibly equal to AO II); boomerang dysplasia (possibly part of a common spectrum).

Symptoms and Signs. *Facies.* Flat nasal bridge; mild face hypoplasia; micrognathia; cleft palate. *Limbs.* Short, rhizomelic, fingers; deviated joints dislocation; occasionally lack of ossification of single hand bones. *Chest.* Narrow.

Etiology. AO1: sporadic; AO2: autosomal recessive; AO2: sporadic (dominant mutation?).

Pathology. AO1: acellularity with or without giant cells; AO2: cystic areas; AO3: normal or mild hypocellularity. In cartilage of resting zone degenerated chondrocytes, encapsulated in fibrous tissue.

Diagnostic Procedures. *X-rays. Ultrasonography. CT scan.* See signs.

Prognosis. AO1: neonatally lethal; AO2: neonathally lethal; AO3: lethal in infancy.

BIBLIOGRAPHY. Marateaux P, Stanescu V, Stanescu R: Four recently described osteochondrodysplasias. In Papadatos CJ, Bartsocas CS (eds): Skeletal Dysplasias, pp 345–350. New York, Liss, 1982

Rimoin DL, Sillence DO, Lachman RS, et al: Giant cell chondrodysplasia: a second case of a rare lethal newborn skeletal dysplasia. Am J Hum Genet 32:125, 1980

Hunter AGW, Carpenter BF: Atelosteogenesis I and boomerang dysplasia: a question of nosology. Clin Genet 39:471–480, 1991

ATHEROSCLEROSIS OBLITERANS

Synonyms. Arteriosclerosis obliterans; arterial insufficiency of common iliac artery; arterial insufficiency; atherosclerotic occlusive; occlusive arterial chronic; obliterative arteriosclerosis; peripheral arterial. See also Moenckeberg.

Symptoms. Occurs in patients over 40 years of age; 75% are male. Resulting from sudden arterial occlusion or more frequently of slow, insidious progression. Most important symptoms: pain; tightness; cramps that develop while walking and subside with rest, most frequently in the calf, but may occur as well in the foot, thigh, and buttocks (intermittent claudication). With progression of the disease, rest pain (pretrophic) may be present, mostly in the foot and occurring at night; sensory symptoms also may be experienced; hyperesthesia.

Signs. Pallor; cyanosis; trophic changes of the skin; ulcer and gangrene in advanced stage precipitated by trauma; decrease of skin temperature; decrease or absence of arterial pulsations; atrophy of muscle. Elevation pallor and dependent rubor. Later sign: hyporeflexia.

Etiology. Unknown. Risk factors for arteriosclerosis: smoking, diabetes mellitus, hyperlipemia hypertension, obesity.

Pathology. Arteries thrombosed by occluding masses; atheromatous changes of arterial wall; calcareous deposits.

Diagnostic Procedures. *Blood.* Hyperlipemia. *Arterial pulse. Angiography.* Shows site and nature of lesion (calcifications). *Noninvasive diagnostic techniques.* Doppler ultrasonic velocity detector; segmental plethysmography.

Therapy. Conservative; some cases benefit from thromboarteriectomy, vascular graft, and sympathectomy. Protect leg and foot from injuries. Control associated pathologies; diet; walking; refrain from smoking; pain treatment; thromboembolytic therapy. Surgery sometimes feasible.

Prognosis. Progressive.

BIBLIOGRAPHY. Imparato AM, Kim G, Davidson T, et al: Intermittent claudication: its natural course. Surgery 78:795, 1975

Joyce JW: The diagnosis and management of the peripheral arteries and veins. In Schlant RC, Alexander RW: Hurst's The Heart, 8th ed, pp 2185–2188. New York, McGraw-Hill, 1994

ATHROMBIA

Synonyms. Factor 3 platelet deficiency; PF3; platelet factor 3 deficiency (possibly the same syndrome); thrombopathia.

Symptoms. Bleeding tendency.

Etiology. Unknown. Deficient platelet adhesion to collagen fibers. Autosomal recessive or X-linked inheritance discussed.

Diagnostic Procedures. *Coagulation tests.* Platelets do not spread or agglutinate normally on slide. In presence of added adenosine diphosphate (ADP) platelet adhesiveness, aggregation, and factor 3 release becomes normal (differentiates this form from Glanzmann). Type I. Prolonged bleeding time, normal clot retraction, defective Salzman test in presence of PF3. Type II. Altered interaction between platelets and collagen with normal ADP, adrenalin induced aggregation and normal Salzman test.

BIBLIOGRAPHY. Inceman S, Ucar S, Ulutin ON: Athrombia thrombocytopathica. Thromb Diath Haemorrh 4:234–243, 1960

Weiss HJ: Platelet aggregation, adhesion and adenosine diphosphate release in thrombopathia (platelet factor 3 deficiency): a comparison with Glanzmann's thrombasthenia and von Willebrand's disease. Am J Med 43:570–578, 1967

Goldman BA, Aledort LA: Essential athrombia: a family study. Ann Intern Med 76:269–273, 1981

ATHYROTIC HYPOTHYROIDISM

Synonym. Agoitrous hypothyroidism; cretinism, athyrotic; thyroid dysgenesis.

Symptoms. Present at birth. Feeding problems; decreased activity. Severe damage on morphogenesis and function of brain.

Signs. At birth only minor signs of hypothyroidism (see), which become in time progressively more evident. Constipation; jaundice; cold and dry skin; mottling, large tongue; umbilical hernia.

Etiology. Unknown. Simple development defect of sporadic occurrence.

Pathology. Absence of small nonfunctional residue of thyroid gland.

Diagnostic Procedures. See Gull.

Therapy. Thyroid hormone given as soon as possible.

Prognosis. According to time of onset of thyroid hormone administration. Variable grades of brain function impairment.

BIBLIOGRAPHY. Ainger LE, Kelly VC: Familial athyrotic cretinism: report of 3 cases. J Clin Endocr 15:469–475, 1955

Kaplan EL, Shukla M, Hara H, et al: Developmental abnormalities of the thyroid. In De Groot LJ (ed): Endocrinology, 3rd ed, p 893. Philadelphia, WB Saunders, 1995

ATKIN

Synonyms. Oculo—cerebro—acral, (Roberts-like)-ectrodactyly.

Symptoms and Signs. Males. From birth. Microphthalmia, cloudy cornae, cleft lip, malformed ears, webbed neck, split hands and foot, cerebral (cysts), heart, and urogenital malformations.

Etiology. Probably X-linked inheritance.

BIBLIOGRAPHY. Atkin JF, Patil S: Apparently new oculo-cerebro-acral syndrome. Am J Med Genet 19:585–587, 1984

ATLANTOAXIAL SPINE DISLOCATION

Synonyms. Cervical spine dislocation; odontoid dysplasia; atlantoaxial spine subluxation.

Symptoms and Signs. One of the most important clinical manifestations in short stature syndromes. Progressive neuromuscular disturbances ranging from a decrease of physical endurance to paraplegia or sudden death (particularly under anesthesia).

Etiology. Two factors necessary to cause atlanto-axial instability and secondary myelopathy: odontoid hypoplasia or aplasia and ligamentous laxity. It may also occur on rheumatoid arthritis (greater in males).

Pathology. Variable degree of odontoid dysgenesis and ligamentous laxity, plus thick wad of soft tissue posterior to the dysplastic odontoid process; spinal cord compression and displacement to one side of the canal.

Diagnostic Procedures. *X-ray. CT scan. MRI.*

Therapy. Surgical stabilization of involved area; posterior cervical fusion.

Prognosis. After successful stabilization, improvement of neurologic symptoms (increase in strength and physical endurance) within 2 years. If not treated, possibility of sudden death.

BIBLIOGRAPHY. Bailey JA: Disproportionate Short Stature: Diagnosis and Management. Philadelphia, WB Saunders, 1973
Williams JP, Somerville G, Miner ME, Reilly D: Atlanto-axial subluxation and trisomy 21: another perioperative complication. Anesthesiology 67:253–254, 1987
Wordsworth BP: Rheumatoid arthritis. In Weatherall DJ, Ledingham JGG, Warrell DA (eds): Oxford Textbook of Medicine, 3rd ed, p 2959. Oxford, Oxford Med Pub, 1996

ATLAS

Synonyms. Occipital neuralgia.

Symptoms and Signs. In subjects involved in stressful mental work. Nuchal algia with muscle contraction; anxiety, restlessness, depression, and hypochondria. In case of muscular origin also very painful palpation of nucal muscles.

Etiology. Usually psychic background. In other cases muscular inflammation.

Therapy. Rest, massage, antinflammatory agents.

Prognosis. Good, possibility of conversion symptoms, if psychogenic origin.

BIBLIOGRAPHY. Sigwald J, Jamet F: Occipital neuralgias. In Vinken PJ, Bruyn GW: Handbook of Clinical Neurology, vol 5, p 373. Amsterdam, North-Holland, 1968

ATR16

Synonyms. Thalassemia; mental retardation. See also Weatherall.

Symptoms and Signs. Anemia, mental retardation, variable dysmorphic features.

Etiology. Long deletions at the end of chromosome 16, which remove the alpha-globin genes and 1–2 million bases of DNA or more complex rearrangements, such as balanced translocations.

BIBLIOGRAPHY. Weatherall DJ: Disorders of the synthesis or function of haemoglobin. In Weatherall DJ, Ledingham JGG, Warrell DA (eds): Oxford Textbook of Medicine, 3rd ed, p 3511. Oxford, Oxford Med Pub, 1996

ATRIAL SEPTAL DEFECT–ATRIOVENTRICULAR CONDUCTION, PROLONGED

Symptoms and Signs. Complete form in addition to symptoms of atrial septal defect–persistent ostium secundum (see); prolongation of PR interval. Incomplete forms in members of same family (atrial septal defect only or PR prolongation).

Etiology. Autosomal dominant inheritance.

Diagnostic Procedures. See Atrial septal defect–persistent ostium secundum. *Electrocardiography.* PR interval ranging from 0.22–0.56 sec; left axis deviation. Clinical examination of family members of suspected cases. Biochemical marker for the mutant gene.

Therapy. Symptomatic.

Prognosis. Possibility of sudden death.

BIBLIOGRAPHY. Weil MH, Allenstein BJ: A report of congenital heart disease in five members of one family. N Engl J Med 265:661–667, 1961
Pease WE, Mordenberg A, Ladda RL: Familial atrial septal defect with prolonged atrioventricular conduction. Circulation 53:759–762, 1976
Perloff JK: The Clinical Recognition of Congenital Heart Disease, 4th ed, pp 313–316. Philadelphia, WB Saunders, 1994

ATRIAL SEPTAL DEFECT–PERSISTENT OSTIUM PRIMUM

Symptoms and Signs. Pure form is not different from atrial septal defect–persistent ostium secundum (see). For complicated form see endocardial cushion defect. Mitral stenosis and mitral valve prolapse are unusual but important associated defects.

ATRIAL SEPTAL DEFECT–PERSISTENT OSTIUM SECUNDUM

Synonym. Sinus venous defect.

Symptoms and Signs. Ostium secundum: female to male ratio is 1.5:3.5. Usually not detected for years. Children delicate, frail, underweight, normal height. Growth retardation if large left-to-right shunts. Possible recurrent respiratory infections. First sound may be split at left sternal margin and tip; second component is loud. Soft midsystolic murmur after first sound. Conspicuous thrust of right ventricle on left sternal edge.

Etiology. Autosomal dominant or recessive inheritance. Most common congenital condition in adults.

Pathology. Atrial septal defect. In the region of the fossa ovalis; inferior to the fossa or in the upper part of atrium septum (sinus venous variety).

Diagnostic Procedures. *Arterial pulse.* Within normal limit. Jugular venous pulse. Usually normal. *Echocardiography.* Findings characteristic of right ventricular volume overload: (1) increased right ventricular end-diastolic dimension; (2) abnormal motion of the ventricular septum; (3) real-time two-dimensional scans from the apical position to identify the location and size of the atrial defect. *Phonocardiography. ECG.* P-wave normal or peaked; small q-waves in II, III, and aVF leads. *X-ray.* Pulmonary arterial plethora; small aorta; conspicuous pulmonary artery; dilatation of right heart. *Cardiac catheterization.* The oxygen content of blood from the right atrium is much higher than that from the superior vena cava.

Therapy. Surgical treatment according to pulmonary systemic blood flow ratio. For asymptomatic infants and children, surgery is recommended prior to entry into school.

Prognosis. Pulmonary hypertension begins to appear in the early 20s. Passage of time, after adolescence, is associated with an increase in the frequency and severity of symptoms; congestive failure is the most common cause of death in unoperated atrial septal defects.

BIBLIOGRAPHY. Rokitansky CF: Die Defecte der Scheidewände des Herzens Braumüller. Wien, 1875
Haworth SG: Pulmonary vascular disease in secundum atrial septal defect in childhood. Am J Cardiol 51:265–278, 1983

Van Mierop LHS, Kutsche LM: Embryology of Heart. In Schlant RC, Alexander RW: Hurst's The Heart, 8th ed, p 1721. New York, McGraw-Hill, 1994

Perloff JK: The Clinical Recognition of Congenital Heart Disease, 4th ed, pp 349–380. Philadelphia, WB Saunders, 1994

ATRIOVENTRICULAR CONGENITAL HEART BLOCK

Synonyms. Morquio I.

Symptoms. Incidence 1:10,000 to 1:20,000. Appears in children. Both sexes affected; onset from fetal life to adult life. (The later discovered, the less probability of congenital origin.) In many cases no symptoms with exercise tolerance normal or slightly reduced with or without mild dizziness. In a low percentage poor tolerance to stress or continuous febrile illnesses. In some patients recurrent frank syncope with or without convulsions.

Signs. Normal growth, development, and physical aspect. Seldom, cyanosis. Arterial pulse slow; resting rate above 40 beats/min (inappropriate to patient age). Acceleration of 10 to 20 beats/min after exercise. Waterhammer pulse. Heart area palpation: left ventricular impulse prominent. Auscultation: slow rate and regular variation of rhythm; variation in intensity of first sound; grade 2 to 3 midsystolic murmur; normal respiratory splitting of second sound; third heart sound common. Systolic hypertension. Irregular jugular pulsation.

Etiology. Congenital defect in the main stem of the bundle of His.

Pathology. Seventy percent of cases have no other evidence of heart disease; the most frequently associated cardiac malformations are "corrected" transposition of the great arteries (ventricular inversion), single ventricle, and patent ductus arteriosus.

Diagnostic Procedures. *Arterial pulse.* Low rate; pulse pressure; wide arterial upstroke brisk; arterial waves abnormalities. *Venous pulse.* Intermittent common waves; abnormalities of a wave. *ECG.* Inconstant ratio between P-waves. *X-ray.* Normal heart size to moderate increase.

Therapy. Implantation of a permanent pacemaker.

Prognosis. Generally good. In some cases heart may be unable to respond to increased circulation demands, and congestive heart failure and death, especially in neonatal period, may occur.

BIBLIOGRAPHY. Morquio L: Sur une maladie infantile et familiale caractérisée par des modifications permanentes du pouls, des attaques syncopales et epileptiforme et la mort subite. Arch Med Enf 4:467–475, 1901

Myerburg RJ, Kessler KM, Castellanos A: Recognition clinical assessment and management of conduction disturbances. In Schlant RC, Alexander RW, Hurst's The Heart, 8th ed. New York, McGraw-Hill, 1994

Perloff JK: The Clinical Recognition of Congenital Heart Disease, 4th ed, pp 53–66. Philadelphia, WB Saunders, 1994

ATRIOVENTRICULAR SEPTAL DEFECTS

Synonyms. Atrioventricular defect—persistent A-V ostium; ostium atrioventricularis communis; persistent common A-V canal; atrioventricular canal defects; endocardial septal defects.

Symptoms and Signs. Female slightly predominant in incomplete form; equal sex ratio in complete form. Complete form. High incidence in Down syndrome (see). Onset in early infancy. Recurrent respiratory infections; failure to thrive; dyspnea; orthopnea; signs of congestive heart failure. Absent or slight cyanosis accompanying crying or strains. First heart sound single; soft prominent systolic murmur with first sound. At site of left ventricular impulse, murmur of mitral regurgitation radiating toward sternum, becoming evident after a few weeks. At lower left sternal margin, murmur of ventricular septal defect. Second sound shows constant splitting with loud second component. Incomplete form. Onset in childhood according to extent and combination of malformations. Relatively asymptomatic or several symptoms. Murmur of mitral regurgitation or ventricular septal defect. Arrhythmias increasing with age.

Etiology. Defects (singly or in association) of atrial septum, ventricular septum, atrioventricular (A-V) valves, and A-V conduction system.

Diagnostic Procedures. *Electrocardiography.* Sinus rhythm; prolonged P-R; P-wave direction normal peaked and of increased amplitude; QRS left axis deviation and distinctive vectocardiographic patterns. *X-ray.* Pulmonary plethora; cardiomegaly. M-mode and two-dimensional echocardiography with color flow imaging and Doppler interrogation. *Cardiac catheterization. Aortography.*

Therapy. Symptomatic. Cardiac surgery.

Prognosis. Complete form: Death usually in early infancy; some patients may reach childhood. Incomplete form: If surviving childhood, symptoms will be delayed to first or second decades; arrhythmias to complete heart block; susceptibility to infective endocarditis.

BIBLIOGRAPHY. Becker AE, Anderson RH: Atrioventricular septal defects: What's in a name? J Thorac Cardiovasc Surg 83:461–469, 1982

Towbin JA, Roberts R: Cardiovascular diseases due to genetic abnormalies. In Schlant RC, Alexander RW: Hurst's The Heart, 8th ed, p 1728. New York, McGraw-Hill, 1994

Perloff JK: The Clinical Recognition of Congenital Heart Disease, 4th ed, pp 349–380. Philadelphia, WB Saunders, 1994

ATROPHY-DEAFNESS NEUROGENIC-AMYOTHROPHY

Synonyms. Iwashita; Rosenberg-Chutorian. See Treft.

Symptoms and Signs. Both sexes. From birth. Progressive polyneuropathy (similar to Charcot-Marie-Tooth, see); deafness and visual loss.

Etiology. Not established if autosomal dominant, recessive, or X-linked disorder (possible cluster of syndromes).

Pathology. Degeneration of acoustic and optic peripheral nerves.

Prognosis. Progressive disorder. Visual loss in 4th decade.

BIBLIOGRAPHY. Iwashita H, Inone N, Araki S, et al: Optic atrophy, neural deafness and distal neurogenic amyothrophy: report of a family with two affected siblings. Arch Neurol 22:357–364, 1970

Rosenberg RN, Chutorian A: Familial opticoacoustic nerve degeneration and polyneuropathy. Neurology 17:827–832, 1967

Treft RL: Unique hereditary syndrome found involves vision and hearing loss. Ophthal Times, July:12–13, 1983

AUSTIN

Synonyms. Mucosulfatidosis; Multiple sulfatase deficiency; MSD.

Symptoms and Signs. Both sexes. Onset usually before 2 years of age. (Clinical variants include neonatal form with rapid progressive course and late-onset variant with slower course.) Hepatosplenomegaly and dysostosis multiplex (as in Maroteaux-Lamy see) neurodegenerative signs with demyelinization (as in metachromatic leukodystrophy) and ichthyosis; visual deterioration; loss of retinal pigment; grey macula; optic atrophy. Mental deterioration up to vegetative status.

Etiology. Autosomal recessive or X-linked inheritance; genetic locus are dispersed throughout the genome. Enzymes deficient in one of the following: Heparan sulfamidase, iduronate-2-sulfatase, steroid sulfatase, arylsulfatase A, arylsulfatase B, and galactosamine-6-sulfatase.

Pathology. Alder-Reilly granulation of leukocytes; lysosomal inclusions in different tissues.

Diagnostic Procedures. *Urine.* Excessive excretion of glycosaminoglycans and deficiencies of several sulfatase enzymes.

Therapy. Symptomatic. Ichthyosis by Lac-Hydrin (12% ammonium lactate), bone marrow transplantation partial benefits.

Prognosis. Death during first decade.

BIBLIOGRAPHY. Austin JH: Studies in metachromatic leukodystrophy XII. Multiple sulfatase deficiency. Arch Neurol 28:258–264, 1973

Ballabio A, Shapiro LJ: Steroid sulfatase deficiency and X-linked ichthyosis. In Scriver CR, Beaudet AL, Sly WS, et al: The Metabolic and Molecular Bases of Inherited Disease, 7th ed, pp 3015–3017. New York, McGraw-Hill, 1995

AUSTRIAN

Eponym to indicate the triad; alcoholic debilitation, pneumococcal pneumonia, and pneumococcal meningitis.

Prognosis. Poor.

BIBLIOGRAPHY. Strauss AL, Hamburger M: Pneumococcal endocarditis in the penicillin era. Arch Intern Med 118:190–198, 1966

AUTOIMMUNO HEMOLYTIC ANEMIAS

Synonyms. Dreyfus-Dausset-Vidal; Dyke-Young (chronic macrocytic type); Hayem-Widal-Loutit; Lederer-Brill; Lederer anemia (acute transient type);acquired hemolytic anemia; hemolytic anemia; antiglobulin positive hemolytic anemia; immune hemolytic anemia, AIHA; see Dressler; Hemolytic anemia, newborn; and Marchiafava-Micheli.

WARM ANTIBODY TYPE

Symptoms. Slightly more prevalent in females; onset at all ages. Extremely variable clinical features. Onset acute or insidious; occasionally, history of previous infection. From acute hemolytic crisis with pyrexia, shock-like prostration up to coma, to chronic mild anemia with moderate tiredness and exertional dyspnea. Hemoglobinuria frequent feature. Dark stool. Occasional features: superficial thrombophlebitis; gallstones (usually asymptomatic); precordial pain headache; complex neurologic syndrome (Dreyfus-Dausset-Vidal) accompanying hemolytic crisis. Bleeding features (see Evans).

Signs. Pallor; jaundice; splenomegaly; occasionally, liver enlargement.

Etiology. Primary and idiopathic; usually sporadic cases; familial occurrence reported. Occurrence in member of family with other types of autoimmune syndromes (e.g., lupus erythematosus, rheumatoid arthritis, pernicious anemia) suggests the possibility of an hereditary fundamental aberration of immune apparatus. Other associations: virus infections; drug-dependent antibodies; lymphomas; lymphatic leukemia; other nonlymphoreticular tumors.

Pathology. Spleen enlarged; congestion of pulp; histiocytic proliferation; giant cell formation; erythrophagocytosis; myeloid metaplasia. Areas of thrombosis and infarction. Hemosiderosis of spleen and liver. Liver enlarged, congested; occasionally, areas of focal necrosis. Renal lesion may be (seldom) observed. Normoblastic hyperplasia of bone marrow.

Diagnostic Procedures. *Blood.* Variable degree of anemia; usually, macrocytosis; considerable anisopoikilocytosis; spherocytosis; autohemoagglutination; reticulocytosis; small number of siderocytes; normoblastemia; erythrophagocytosis. In acute episode, leukocytosis; in chronic, usually neutropenia. Platelets normal or low (see Evans). Hyperbilirubinemia; haptoglobulin absent in acute stage. Osmotic fragility moderately or markedly increased; autohemolysis markedly increased. Positive Coombs test, direct and indirect. Special techniques to demonstrate special antibodies. Red cell survival time shortened. Normal complement concentration.

Therapy. Corticosteroids; splenectomy. In chronic cases, immunosuppressant agents.

Prognosis. Unpredictable; potentially dangerous. Quick recovery; several relapses; may become chronic. Overall mortality for this condition 50%.

COLD AGGLUTINATION SYNDROME

Synonym. Cryoglobulinemia.

Symptoms. Slightly more prevalent in females; onset usually in older age than warm antibody type; 30–80 years of age. Variable features: anemia and associated symptoms, usually severe and usually more severe in winter, occasionally, main sensory neuropathy may develop; Raynaud phenomenon (see); hemoglobinuria with cold exposure.

Signs. Pallor; jaundice; spleen and liver only occasionally enlarged. Purpuric eruptions followed by hyperpigmentation. Ulceration about ankles.

Etiology. Primary disease or in many cases, secondary to infections such as primary atypical pneumonia (mycoplasma pneumoniae) virus, collagen disorders, lymphoma.

Pathology. See warm antibody type. The possibility, although rare, of acute renal failure reported. Occasionally, tissue gangrene of finger or toes.

Diagnostic Procedures. *Blood.* Anemia; erythrocytes show minor abnormalities when compared with warm agglutination type; seldom erythrophagocytosis; moderate reticulocytosis; autohemoagglutination markedly increased. Osmotic fragility normal or slightly increased. Leukocytes and platelets decreased, normal, or increased. Hyperbilirubinemia variable. Coombs direct positive, cold agglutination test with temperature ranging between 2°C and 28°C. Patient serum may lyse normal erythrocytes in vitro at low temperature (20°C; pH 6.5–7.5). Decreased serum complement. Wasserman and Kahn negative. *Urine.* Increased urobilin all the time; hemoglobinuria associated with cold exposure. *Stool.* Increased stercobilin.

Therapy. Corticosteroid. Avoid exposure to cold.

Prognosis. Relatively benign; usually no recovery (except in the secondary cases), but patients may live many years with the condition.

"MIXED" WARM- AND COLD-REACTIVE ANTIBODIES SYNDROME

Symptoms and Signs. Approximately 8% of all patients with autoimmune hemolytic anemias. Those of a severe hemolysis with chronic and intermittent course.

Etiology. Unknown or secondary: collagen, non-Hodgkin lymphoma, Hodgkin disease, other malignancies. Mediated by two families of antibody: IgG reacting at normal temperature and IgM reacting optimally in the cold.

Therapy. Corticosteroid (dramatic response reported). Avoid exposure to cold.

DRUG-INDUCED IMMUNE HEMOLYTIC ANEMIA

Synonym. Penicillin type hemolytic anemia (1); alpha-methyldopa type hemolytic anemia (2); innocent bystander (stibophen) type hemolytic anemia.

Symptoms and Signs. (1) Patients who have received or being exposed to the drug for a long time. Those of a brisk hemolytic process, without evidence of intravascular hemolysis. (2) Methyldopa is the most common cause of drug-induced immune hemolytic anemia. It occurs in 15% of patients receiving the drug, for longer than 3 months. Those of an insidious and slowly progressive hemolysis, no specific symptoms. (3) Innocent bystander type. In patients with schistosomiasis receiving stibophen, a small amount of drug may cause symptoms and signs of acute intravascular hemolysis and hemoglobinuria; frequent renal failure and possible disseminated intravascular coagulation.

Etiology. (1) Development of antibodies reacting specifically with the drug itself causes hemolysis from the binding of penicillin to the red cell membranes. (2) Mechanism of antierythrocyte antibodies unknown. (3) Circulating antigen-antibody complexes settle on red cells and lead to complement-dependent lysis.

Therapy. (1) Discontinuation of drug and if needed corticosteroid. (2) Discontinuation of drug and if needed corticosteriods, blood transfusion. (3) Discontinuation of drug and if needed blood transfusions, treatment of renal failure, steroids not useful.

BIBLIOGRAPHY. Hayem G: Sur une variété particuliére d'ictére chronique; ictére infectieux chronique splénomégalique. Presse Méd 1:121–125, 1898
Widal F, Abrami P: Types divers d'ictéres hémolytiques non congénitaux, avec anémie; la recherche de la résistance globulaire par le procédé des hématies déplasmatisées. Bull Mem Soc Méd Hôp Paris 24:1127–1169, 1907
Dreyfus B, Dausset J, Vidal G: Étude clinique et hématologique de douze cas d'anémie hémolytique acquise avec anti corps. Rev Hématol 6:349, 1951
Dacie JV: The Haemolytic Anaemias. New York, Grune & Stratton, 1963
Foerster J: Autoimmune hemolytic anemias. In Lee GR, Bithel TC, Foerster J, et al (eds): Wintrobe's Clinical Hematology, 9th ed, pp 1170–1196. Philadelphia, Lea & Febiger, 1993

AUTONOMIC SPINAL

Lesions of the autonomic fibers connected with the spinal cord result in different syndromes according to the level of the lesions.

1. C8–T1 (ciliospinal reflex center): pupillary miosis; enophthalmos; ptosis (Horner syndrome).
2. T1 segment: dilatation of pupil; exophthalmos; upper eyelid elevation; cervical sympathetic chain (Claude Bernard syndrome); perspiration; and vasoconstriction.
3. T1–T6 spinal cord; T1–T4 sympathetic ganglia: tachycardia.
4. T4–T7 (?) spinal cord: inhibition of bronchiolar constriction; upper thoracic sympathetic chain.
5. T2–T9: perspiration and vasoconstriction; upper extremity piloerection; cervical sympathetic chain.
6. T10–L4: perspiration; vasoconstriction, lower extremity piloerection.
7. T5–L4: perspiration; vasoconstriction; thoracic wall and abdomen piloerection.
8. T5–T9: inhibition of gastric muscles and contraction of sphincter.
9. Thoracolumbar ganglionated chain; celiac ganglion, superior mesenteric ganglia; splanchnic nerve: visceral vasoconstriction; inhibition of intestinal wall; contraction of ileocecal sphincter.
10. L1–L2 inferior mesenteric ganglion: vasoconstriction in kidney; constriction of rectal sphincter.
11. L1–L3 inferior mesenteric ganglion: inhibition of detrusor (?) plus constriction of internal sphincter (?) of bladder.
12. S1–S3 and pelvic nerves: contraction of detrusor; relaxation of rectal and vesical sphincters; muscles; erection.

BIBLIOGRAPHY. Vick NA: Grinker's Neurology, 7th ed. Springfield, IL, Charles C Thomas, 1976

AUTOSCOPIC

Synonyms. Lukianowicz; mirror image. See also Capgras and lilliputian.

Symptoms and Signs. Occurs in patients suffering from depression, migraine, epilepsy, schizophrenia: delusion of suddenly experiencing of seeing double (not in color, but as a white or grayish image).

Etiology. Delusional dislocation of body image in the visual sphere. Well-known psychic phenomenon cited in history and literature.

Therapy. That of the basic neurologic psychotic condition.

BIBLIOGRAPHY. Critchley M: Neurological aspects of visual and auditory hallucinations. Br Med J 2:634–639, 1939
Lukianowicz N: Autoscopic phenomena. AMA Arch Neurol Psychiatr 80:199–220, 1958
Kaplan HI, Sadock BJ: Comprehensive Textbook of Psychiatry, 6th ed, p 1040. Baltimore, Williams & Wilkins, 1995

AVELLIS

Synonyms. Ambiguospinothalamic paralysis; Avellis-Longhi; Avellis hemiplegia; palatopharyngeal paralysis; spinothalamic tract-nucleus ambiguous.

Symptoms. Dysphagia; dysphoria; unilateral loss of pain and temperature to trunk and limbs; Horner's syndrome may be associated.

Signs. Paralysis of soft palate and larynx controlateral to the pain and temperature loss.

Etiology. Vascular or inflammatory or neoplastic lesions involving the nucleus ambiguous and the vagus (X) and accessory nerves, and spinothalamic tract.

Pathology. See Etiology. Lesion localized in the medulla or near the jugular foramen.

Therapy. Depends upon etiology.

Prognosis. As in preceding.

BIBLIOGRAPHY. Avellis G: Klinicshe Beitrage zur halbseitigen Kehlkopflähmung. Berl Klin 40:1–26, 1891
Fox SL, West GB Jr: Syndrome of Avellis; review of literature and report of one case. Arch Otolaryngol 46:773–778, 1947
Adams RD, Victor M: Principles of Neurology, 5th ed, p 1173. New York, McGraw-Hill, 1993

AXENFELD

Synonyms. Arcus juvenilis; posterior embryotoxon; Hagedoom syndromes. See Rieger and Reese-Ellsworth.

Signs. Posterior corneal embryotoxon; increased visibility of the Schwalbe line. When associated with other anterior segment disturbances and juvenile glaucoma, the complex is called Reiger. The eponym Axenfeld also is used as synonym for Reiger and Hagedoom mesostromal dysgenesis. This syndrome often is a component of the more complex syndromes that involve oculodentodigital systems, or associated with other diseases and developmental anomalies (Marfan syndrome; dystrophia myotonica; facial deformities).

Etiology. Autosomal dominant inheritance. Developmental arrest with persistence of deficient absorption and atrophy of mesodermal uveal tissue in the angle of anterior chamber (Reiger). Developmental arrest of anterior vitreous body (mesostrom anterior; Hagedoom).

BIBLIOGRAPHY. Axenfeld T: Embryotoxon corneae posterius. Ber Dtsch Ophthalmol Ges 42:301, 1920
Rieger HV: Über Subconjunctivitis epibulbous metastatica bei Parotitis epidemica. Arch Ophthalmol 133:505–507, 1935
Hagedoom A: Congenital anomalies of the anterior segment of the eye. Arch Ophthalmol 17:223–227, 1937
Chitty LS, McCrimmon R, Temple IK, et al: Dominantly inherited syndrome comprising partially absent eye muscles, hydrocephaly, skeletal abnormalities and distinctive facial phenotype. Am J Med Genet 40:417–420 1991

AXENFELD-SCHÜRENBERG

Synonyms. Congenital cyclic oculomotor paralysis.

Symptoms and Signs. Congenital or appear during first year of life. Unilateral oculomotor (III) nerve paralysis, upper lid ptosis, eye abduction, and midriasis (relaxed phase), alternating with the paralysis of automatic contraction (lasting 30 seconds to 1 minute) of the muscle innervated by the oculomotor (III) nerve, with resulting lifting of upper lid, myosis, and deviation of the eye (spastic phase).

Etiology and Pathology. Unknown; possibly congenital. One case reported after trauma.

BIBLIOGRAPHY. Axenfeld T, Schürenberg E: Zur Kenntniss der angeborenen Beweglichkeitdefekete der Augen. Klin Monatsb Augenhleilkd 39:64;844, 1901
Latorre-Morasso S, Agular J: Enfermedad de Axenfeld-Schürenberg. Arch Soc Oftal Hispano Am 1:625–632, 1942
Susac JO, Smith JL: Cyclic oculomotor paralysis. Neurology 24:24–27, 1974
Leigh RJ, Zee DS: The Neurology of Eye Movements. Philadelphia, FA Davis, 1983
Klintworth GK: Ocular involvement in disorders of the nervous system. In Garner A, Klintworth GK (eds): Pathobiology of Ocular Disease: A Dynamic Approach, 2nd ed. New York, Marcel Dekker, 1994

AYERZA-ARRILAGA

Eponym obsolete. Used to indicate a variety of Ayerza syndrome (see), when owing to chronic bronchopulmonary syphilis and to a syphilitic obliterans sclerosis of the pulmonary artery.

BIBLIOGRAPHY. Arrilaga RC: Esclerosis secundaria de la arteria pulmonary y su quadro clinico (cardiacos negros). Buenos Aires, 1912
Garnier M, Delamare V: Dizionario Dei Termini Tecnici e Medicina, 19th ed. Rome, DEMI, 1974

AYERZA

Synonyms. Cardiac block; cardiopathy nigra; pulmonary arteriosclerosis; pulmonary arteritis.

Symptoms and Signs. Gradual onset in 5th decade of life in patients with preceding bronchopulmonary symptomatology. Respiratory insufficiency with severe dyspnea; marked cyanosis of face, hands, and feet. Signs of pulmonary emphysema and right ventricular hypertrophy. Digital clubbing. Occasionally, splenomegaly. Passive congestion of liver.

Etiology. Unknown; associated with diseases of pulmonary artery such as atherosclerosis, syphilis.

Pathology. Hypertrophy of right ventricle; sclerosis with intimal thickening; atheroma formation; loss of elastic fibers with resulting generalized (arterial and arteriolar) narrowing of vascular bed; pulmonary emphysema.

Diagnostic Procedures. *Blood.* Polycythemia. *Pulmonary function tests. X-ray of chest.*

Therapy. Control of secondary polycythemia, congestive failure, and other symptomatic treatments.

Prognosis. Poor.

BIBLIOGRAPHY. Ayerza L: Unpublished clinical lecture at National University of Buenos Aires, 1901
Arrillaga FC: Esclerosis secundaria de la arteria pulmonary su cuadro clinico (Cardiacos negros). Buenos Aires, 1912
Athens JW, Lee GR: Polycythemia: erythrocytosis. In Lee GR, Bithel TC, Foerster J, et al (eds): Wintrobe's Clinical Hematology, 9th ed, p 1252. Philadelphia, Lea & Febiger, 1993

AZOREAN NEUROLOGIC

Synonyms. Machado-Joseph; Joseph; spinopontine atrophy; includes Woods-Schaumburg.

Symptoms and Signs. Both sexes. Onset in fourth decade. In family prevalently descendant from Azores inhabitants, also reported in Japan, the United States, Europe. Variable clinical features. Four phenotypic variations tentatively identified (variations even occur in the same family): (1) cerebellar ataxia, external ophthalmoplegia, pyramidal signs; extrapyramidal signs; (2) same as variation 1 without extrapyramidal signs; (3) same as 1 plus distal muscular atrophy; (4) same as 1 plus neuropathy and parkinsonism.

Etiology. Unknown. Autosomal dominant inheritance.

Pathology. Loss of neurons and gliosis in substantia nigra, nuclei pontis, vestibular nuclei, cranial nerves, Clarke columns and anterior horns.

Diagnostic Procedures. *CT brain scan. MR imaging.* Presence of air in the posterior fossa. *EEG. Electromyography. Cerebrospinal fluid. Blood.* Frequent hyperglycemia.

Prognosis. Progressive condition of ataxia, parkinsonism; limited eye movements, muscle fasciculation, reflex loss in lower limbs, nystagmus, cerebellar tumor, and Babinski sign.

BIBLIOGRAPHY. Boyer SH, Christholm AW, McKusick VA: Cardiac aspect of Friedreich's ataxia. Circulation 25:493–505, 1962
Nakano KK, Dawson DM, Spence A: Machado disease: a hereditary ataxia in Portuguese immigrants to Massachusetts. Neurology 22:49–55, 1972
Woods BT, Schaumburg HH: Nigro-spino-dental degeneration with nuclear ophthalmoplegia. A unique and partially tractable clinicopathological entity. J Neurol Sci 17:149–166, 1972
Barbeau A, Roy M, Cunha L, et al: The natural history of Machado-Joseph disease: an analysis of 138 personally examined cases. Can J Neurol Sci 11:510–525, 1984
Eto K, Sumi SM, Bird TD, et al: Family with dominantly inherited ataxia amyotrophy and periferal sensory loss: spinopontine atrophy or Machado-Joseph Azorean disease in another non-Portuguese family? Arch Neurol 47:968–974, 1990

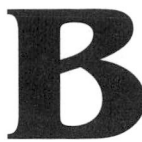

BAASTRUP

Synonyms. Michotte; kissing osteophytes.

Signs. Radiologic syndrome: formation of bridges between closely approximated adjacent osteophytes observed in degenerative joint disease: to be differentiated from other types of senescent vertebral ankylosis (see Forestier-Rotes-Querol and von Bekhterer-Strümpell). Contact of spinus process has to be considered among the many mechanisms determining nerve root compression. Cervical, thoracic, or lumbar vertebrae may be involved.

Diagnostic Procedure. *Roentgenogram.* Necessary to differentiate pathogenic mechanism responsible for the syndromes deriving from compression.

BIBLIOGRAPHY. Baastrup CJ: Proc. spin. vert. lumb. unter einige zwischen diesen liegenden Gelenkbildungen mit pathologischen Prozessen in dieser Region. Rortsch Röntger 48:430–435, 1933
Michotte LJ: Le syndrome des épineuses. Rev Rheum 16:249–258, 1949
Klippel JH, Dieppe PA: Rheumatology, pp 3, 273. St Louis, Mosby Yearbook, 1995

BABINSKI-NAGEOTTE

Obsolete.

Synonyms. Dorsolateral oblongata; hemibulbar; medullary tegmental paralysis. See also Céstan-Chenais and Wallenberg.

Symptoms and Signs. On one side; hemiparesis; sensibility alteration. On the other; cerebellar hemiataxia. Ocular findings: enophthalmus; ptosis; nystagmus; miosis (see Bernard-Horner). Occasionally, analgesia of hemiface, vocal cord, and soft palate and adiadochokinesia, lateral pulsion; dysmetria.

Etiology. Neoplasia; vascular.

Pathology. Lesion of pontobulbar or medullobulbar regions.

Therapy. According to lesion.

Prognosis. Poor.

BIBLIOGRAPHY. Babinski J, Nageotte J: Hémisynergie, latéropulsion et miosis bulbaire. Nouv Icon Salpétrière, p 492. Paris, 1902
Bogorodinski DK, Pojarisski KM, Rasorenova RA, et al: The Babinski-Nageotte syndrome (pathogenesis and correlation with other alternate syndromes). Rev Neurol (Paris) 119:505–512, 1968
Adams RD, Victor M: Principles of Neurology, 5th ed, p 690. New York, McGraw-Hill, 1993

BABINSKI-VAQUEZ

Symptoms and Signs. In syphilitic patients. Argyll Roberts pupilla (see) aortis, altered reflex of quadriceps and triceps surae and signs of chronic meningoencephalities.

Etiology. Syphilis.

BIBLIOGRAPHY. Babinsky JFF: Les troubles pupillaires sans les anéurismes de l'aorte. Bull Soc Méd Hop Paris 18:1121–1124, 1901

BABOON

Synonyms. Allergic contact dermatitis, systematically induced; mercury exanthema.

Symptoms and Signs. In patients with a previous concact sensitivity. Diffuse erythema of the buttocks and erythema of upper inner surface of thighs, occasionally accompanied by erythema of axillae (similar to textile dermatitis from underwear).

Etiology. Reaction provoked (inhalation, ingestion, injection) by several allergens: ampicillin, nickel, mercury, Antabuse, hair dyes in patients with previous sensitization.

Pathology. Biopsy. Leucocytoclastic vasculitis.

Diagnostic Procedures. Closed path tests. Oral challenge with suspected allergen.

Therapy. Symptomatic: cortisone ointments, antihistaminics.

Prognosis. Good.

BIBLIOGRAPHY. Andersen KE, Hjorth N, Menn T: The baboon syndrome: systematically induced allergic contact dermatitis. Contact Derm 10:97–100, 1984

BACILLARY ANGIOMATOSIS

Synonyms. Cat-scratch—HIV; epithelioid angiomatosis; see Petzetakis.

Symptoms and Signs. In HIV-positive or in immunodeficient patients following cat-scratch. Symptoms related to cutaneous, lymphatic, and/or visceral lesions.

Etiology. Caused by a bacillus closely related to rickettsiae.

Pathology. Lesions show vascular proliferation.

Diagnostic Procedures. Culture of microrganisms from lesions. AIDS (see evaluation).

Therapy. Respond to erythromycin and tetracyclines (treatments that are not effective in cat scratch disease).

BIBLIOGRAPHY. Stoler MH, Bonfiglio TA, Steigbigel RT, et al: An atypical subcutaneous infection associated with acquired immune deficiency syndrome. Am J Clin Pathol 80:714–718, 1983
Relman DA, Loutit JS, Schmidt TM, et al: The agent of bacillary angiomatosis: an approach to the identification of uncultured pathogens. N Engl J Med 323:1573, 1990

BACTERIAL OVERGROWTH

Synonyms. Afferent loop; gastrojejunal loop obstruction; stagnant loop; bacterial overgrowth; stasis; blind loop.

Symptoms. Frequently observed in patients who underwent partial gastrectomy and present achlorhydria and stagnant afferent loop; or in patients with Crohn. From asymptomatic to anorexia; nausea; diarrhea; postprandial fullness, and pain in upper abdomen, followed by vomiting of bile, no food (only violent retching induces food vomiting). Fatty foods usually precipitate vomiting.

Signs. Pallor. Lichtheim syndrome signs (see); abdominal distention; palpable mass.

Etiology. Several disorders may be associated with the syndrome. Alteration of gastric acid secretion, presence of normal motor activity of small intestine unimpeded by localized blind loops, inflammation or strictures (postoperative) or abnormal connections between loops with recirculation of bowel content; normally functioning ileo-cecal valve preventing reflux of material from colon in small intestine. Other possible causes, all conditions causing stagnation. Diabetic neuropathy, scleroderma, strictures, diverticula, pseudo-obstruction, chronic pancreatitis, cirrhosis immunodeficiency syndromes, age, etc.

Pathology. Afferent loop of anastomosis may present partial volvulus, herniation, adhesion or simply be too short or too long, signs of inflammation, necrosis, perforation with leakage may be present and variable findings according with basic pathology.

Diagnostic Procedures. *X-ray digestive tract. Blood.* Megaloblastic type of anemia. *Bone marrow.* Schilling test. Small intestine aspirate for bacteriological studies. *Carbon isotope and hydrogen breath tests.*

Therapy. Surgery to remove obstruction. *Medical.* Broad spectrum antibiotic may correct the anemia. If surgery not feasible, administration of antibiotics for 2 weeks every month (risk of allergy or adverse reactions) to be reserved only for clinically severe manifestations. *Nutritional.* To correct and prevent malnutrition.

Prognosis. Chronic or recurrent condition, until when indicated, surgically corrected.

BIBLIOGRAPHY. White WH: On the pathology and prognosis of pernicious anemia. Guy's Hosp Rep 32:149, 1890
Tabaqchali S, Hatzioannou J, Booth CC: Bile salt deconjugation and steatorrhea in patients with the stagnant-loop syndrome. Lancet II:12–16, 1968
Toskes PP: Bacterial overgrowth syndromes. In Haubrich WS, Schaffner F, Berk JE (eds): Bockus Gastroenterology, 5th ed, vol 2, pp 1174–1182. Philadelphia, WB Saunders, 1995

BAELZ

Synonyms. Puente disease; Volkmann cheilitis; Von Baelz; glandular chelitis; cheilitis glandularis apostematosa; myxodermatitis labialis.

Symptoms. Onset from childhood or early adolescence. Suppurative form (Volkmann): pain and tenderness of lower lip.

Signs. Lower lip slightly enlarged; on the internal aspect small orifices from which saliva can be squeezed easily. In the Volkmann variety, crusts and scales cover the orifices.

Etiology. Unknown; developmental defect (?). Frequent association with Ascher.

Pathology. *Simple form.* Sclerosis around hyperplastic salivary glands. *Suppurative form.* Inflammatory infiltration.

Diagnostic Procedures. *Biopsy.*

Therapy. Plastic excision of tissue presenting hyperplastic glands from shaving vermilionectomy to excision of an elongated ellipse of tissue. If other underlying cause such as actinic or atopia treat accordingly.

Prognosis. Both forms may persist for life; in some cases complicated by squamous cell carcinoma (in some series 20–30%).

BIBLIOGRAPHY. von Baelz E Ueber Erkrankungen der Schleimdruesen des Mundes M-hefte prakt Derm 11, 1890
Unna PG: Ueber Erkrankungen der Schleimdruesen der Mundes. M-hefte prackt Derm 11:317–321, 1890
Puente JJ, Acevedo A: Quelitis glandularis. Rev Med Lat Am 22:671–679, 1927

Burton JL: The lips. In Champion RH, Burton JL, Ebling FJG (eds): Rook/Wilkinson/Ebling Textbook of Dermatology, 5th ed, p 2766. Oxford, Blackwell Scientific, 1992

BAGASSE WORKER

Synonyms. Bagassosis. See also allergic alveolitis, extrinsic.

Symptoms. In person working with bagasse, a residue of sugar cane. May be acute, subacute, or chronic. Onset insidious or sudden after exposure to dust from bagasse. Fever, chills, sweat, malaise; dry cough; anorexia, weight loss; aches in the chest, backache; occasionally, hemoptysis (?).

Signs. Tachypnea; tachycardia; hypoxemic signs; fine inspiratory rales in the chest.

Etiology. Hypersensitivity to moldy bagasse.

Pathology. Interstitial pneumonitis.

Diagnostic Procedures. *X-ray.* Of chest. Fine reticular or nodular opacities. *Blood.* Moderate anemia; no eosinophilia; monocytes may be increased. *Skin test.* Positive reaction against specific antigen.

Therapy. Corticosteroids; removal from exposure.

Prognosis. Good if further exposure is prevented; otherwise, chronic pulmonary condition.

BIBLIOGRAPHY. Jamison SC, Hopkins J: Bagassosis, a fungus disease of the lung: Case report. New Orleans Med Surg J 93:580–582, 1941
Nicholson DP: Bagasse worker's lung. Am Rev Respir Dis 97:546–560, 1968
Fraser RS, Paré JAP, Fraser RG, Paré PD: Synopsis of Diseases of the Chest, 2nd ed. Philadelphia, WB Saunders, 1994

BAILEY-CUSHING

Synonyms. Cerebellar midline; archicerebellum; flocculonodular lobe; vermis; vestibulocerebellum; medulloblastoma (misnomer). See Fourth ventricle.

Symptoms. Both sexes affected; male-to-female ratio 3:2 or 3:1; most common in childhood. Unsteadiness in balance, disturbed coordination of the body in space, without appreciable ataxia; walking very poor; good coordination when lying or with body well braced. Headache and vomiting; marked anorexia and weight loss frequent findings.

Etiology. Midline cerebellar tumor, medulloblastoma, other tumors; vascular lesions; chronic alcoholism; idiopathic atrophies seldom affect this part of cerebellum.

Pathology. Medulloblastoma most frequent type of neoplastic lesion.

Diagnostic Procedures. *CT brain scan. MRI. Arteriography. Spinal tap.*

Therapy. Surgery; radiotherapy.

Prognosis. Very poor; survival from months to 2–3 years; 5 years survival with therapy in 60% of cases.

BIBLIOGRAPHY. Bailey P, Cushing H: Medulloblastoma cerebelli: a common type of midcerebellar glioma of childhood. Arch Neurol Psychiatr 14:192–224, 1925
Adams RD, Victor M: Principles of Neurology, 5th ed, p 101. New York, McGraw-Hill, 1993

BAKER CYSTS

Synonyms. Popliteal bursitis; popliteal hernia; popliteal cysts.

Symptoms. Occurs at any age; more frequent in males (15–30 years of age). Mild aching and stiffness of knee, usually unilateral.

Signs. Fluctuating in size; swelling in popliteal space, 10 by 5 cm approximate size; enlargement extends toward Achilles tendon. Limited extension of knee. Transillumination reveals cystic nature of lesion.

Etiology. Unknown; trauma (?). All causes increasing synovial fluid tension. Autosomal dominant inheritance reported in a family.

Pathology. Posterior herniation of capsule of knee or herniation of superior tibiofibular articulation; enlarged semimembranous bursa. Escape of synovial fluid from knee into one of posterior bursae. Moderate inflammatory changes.

Diagnostic Procedures. *Transillumination.* Pneumography contraindicated.

Therapy. Surgical dissection and binding of peduncle. Conservative treatment only temporary effect.

Prognosis. Good if dissection complete; otherwise recurrences.

BIBLIOGRAPHY. Baker WM: Baker's cyst: formation of abnormal synovial cysts in connection with joints. Med Classics 5:805–820, 1941

Toyama WM: Familial popliteal cysts in children. Am J Dis Child 124:486–587, 1972

Insall JN, Windsor RE, Scott WN, et al (ed): Surgery of the Knee. New York, Churchill Livingstone, 1993

Klippel JH, Dieppe PA: Rheumatology, pp 3, 4, 10. St Louis, Mosby Yearbook, 1995

BALINT

Synonym. Psychic paralysis of visual fixation. Few observations of complete form (major syndrome); the minor form presents the same symptoms, but they are inconspicuous and transitory. See amorphosynthesis.

Symptoms and Signs. Inability of the patient to look toward a point that is in his peripheral visual field; inability to move eyes to command and follow objects in motion; inability to estimate distance between two objects standing in different relationships to patient (can see only one at a time). "Optic ataxia": inability to execute voluntary movement in response to visual stimuli. The patient tries to grasp an object, extending his hand in the wrong direction, and reaches the object by chance after repeated attempts. "Disturbed attention": normal attention for all nonvisual stimuli; patient does not turn his head to a sudden light on the side. When walking, bumps against obstacles; cannot find his way although he knows and can describe the route. The symptoms are lateralized and more noticeable on one side. Concomitant symptomatology is represented by some language difficulty, agraphia, and ideomotor apraxia. Tonic and motor phenomena of arms and loss of coordination of two parts of the body. Stereoscopic vision, gnosis, visual memory are preserved.

Etiology and Pathology. Bilateral parieto-occipital lesions. In major syndrome very large lesion involving both occipital and frontal areas. Frontal lesion anatomic or functional (?). Neoplastic; vascular.

Diagnostic Procedures. *CT brain scan. MRI.* Diffuse cortical atrophy. *Electroencephalography. Brain mapping. Spinal fluid. Ophthalmologic examination. Evoked visual potentials.*

Therapy. Depends upon etiology.

Prognosis. Depends upon etiology.

BIBLIOGRAPHY. Balint R: Seelenlähmung des "Schauens," optische Ataxie, räumliche Störung der Aufmerksamkeit. Mschr Psych Neurol 25:51–81, 1909

Hecaen H, DeAjuriaguerra J: Balint's syndrome (psychic paralysis of visual fixation and its minor forms). Brain 77:373–400, 1954

Stieglmayr FS: Balint's syndrome. New Engl J Med 277:660, 1967

Adams RD, Victor M: Principles of Neurology, 5th ed, pp 403–404. New York, McGraw-Hill, 1993

BALCAN MYOCLONUS

Synonyms. Eldridge. See Myoclonic epilepsy.

Symptoms and Signs. Onset 10 years of age. Light sensitive myoclonus, worse attacks at waking.

Etiology. Autosomal recessive inheritance.

Pathology. Loss of Purkinje cells, absence of inclusion bodies.

Diagnostic Procedures. *EEG.* Synchronous, spike-and-wave discharges that may precede attacks.

Therapy. Seizures respond to valproic acid and condition is negatively affected by phenytoin (even death).

Prognosis. Favorable with valproic acid treatment.

BIBLIOGRAPHY. Eldridge R, Iivanainen M, Stern R, et al: "Baltic" myoclonus epilepsy: hereditary disorders of childhood made worse by phenytoin. Lancet 2:838–842, 1983

Adams RD, Victor M: Principles of Neurology, 5th ed, pp 90–91. New York, McGraw-Hill, 1993

BALCAN NEPHRITIS

Synonyms. Yugoslavian chronic endemic nephropathy; southeastern Europe endemic nephropathy; Danubian endemic familial nephropathy, DEFN.

Symptoms. None; negative history of edema; hematuria; upper respiratory infection.

Signs. Usually normal blood pressure; occasionally, hypertension.

Etiology. Unknown. Condition affects one-third of population in endemic areas (small villages along rivers in Yugoslavia, Bulgaria, Romania). People who move out do not develop the disease; people who move in develop the disease in approximately 10 years.

Pathology. With advanced form; small kidney of about 50 g, atrophy of surface of cortex, deeper portion spared; interstitial fibrosis affecting tubules that are hyperplastic with mitotic figures; glomerular lesions seem secondary to tubular lesions. Histology of kidney consistent with primary amyloidosis.

Diagnostic Procedures. *Urine.* Proteinuria, not over 1 g/day; few leukocytes; occasionally, casts. *Blood.* Hyperazotemia (occurring in patients older than 30–40 years); hyperchloremic acidosis.

Therapy. Symptomatic and kidney transplantation.

Prognosis. Slow progression of renal insufficiency over 5–10 years to death. Kidney transplantation possible.

BIBLIOGRAPHY. Hall PW, Dammin GJ, Griggs RC, et al: Investigation of chronic endemic nephropathy in Yugoslavia. Am J Med 39:210–217, 1965

Eknoyan G, Tubulointerstitial nephropathies. In Massry SG, Glassock RJ: Textbook of Nephrology, 3rd ed. Baltimore, 1995

Haubrich WS, Schaffner F, Berk JE (eds): Bockus Gastroenterology, 5th ed, p 1045. Philadelphia, WB Saunders, 1995

BALLANTYNE

Synonyms. Clifford; Runge; gestation prolonged I; placental dysfunction I; postmaturity; prolonged gestation; yellow vernix. See Placental insufficiency.

Symptoms and Signs. Gestation exceeding the date of delivery by 3 weeks. Arrest of increase in weight of fetus. At birth, low weight and alertness of newborn; absence of vernix; skin: dry, colloid-like, and desquamating; umbilical cord, nails, and occasionally all skin stained yellow or greenish. Frequently, respiratory distress.

Etiology. Unknown; attributed to placental insufficiency.

Pathology. Placenta shows avascular chorionic villi. Newborn may exhibit amniotic fluid inhalation.

Diagnostic Procedures. Umbilical vein blood. Low PO_2; high: hemoglobin, blood urea nitrogen, and bilirubin.

BIBLIOGRAPHY. Ballantyne JW: The problem of the postmature infant. J Obstet Gynaecol Br Emp 2:512–554, 1902

Runge H: Ueber einige besondere Merkmale der weber fragener Frucht. Zentralbl Gynaekol 66:1202–1206, 1942

Liggins GC Endocrinology of parturition. In De Groot LJ (ed): Endocrinology, 3rd ed, p 2214. Philadelphia, WB Saunders, 1995

BALLARD

Synonyms. Mu chain; heavy chain (μ); μ HCD.

Symptoms and Signs. Both sexes affected. Less frequent then alpha- or gamma-HCD; hepatomegaly; splenomegaly; pathologic fractures.

Etiology. Unknown. See Pathology. Possibly autoimmune disorder.

Pathology. Infiltration of visceral organs (liver, spleen, lymph nodes) by lymphocytes, vacuolated plasma cells, reticular cells. Most patients exhibit associated chronic lymphocytic leukemia or CCL-like lymphoproliferative disorder, non-Hodgkin lymphoma, and seldom amyloidosis.

Diagnostic Procedures. *Blood.* Hypogammaglobulinemia; presence of a rapidly migrating protein (μ). *Bone marrow.* Presence of vacuolated plasma cells. *Urine.* Frequent presence of protein of Bence-Jones.

Therapy. That of the associated condition. Cyclophosphamide and chlorambucil.

Prognosis. That of the associated condition.

BIBLIOGRAPHY. Ballard HS, Hamilton LM, Mazcus AJ: A new variant of heavy chain disease (μ chain disease). New Engl J Med 282:1060–1062, 1970

Foestert J: Heavy chain diseases. In Lee GR, Bithel TC, Foerster J, et al (eds): Wintrobe's Clinical Hematology, 9th ed, pp 2267–2268. Philadelphia, Lea & Febiger, 1993

BALLER-GEROLD

Synonym. Craniosynostosis—radial aplasia.

Symptoms and Signs. *Head and facies.* Turribrachycephaly; steep forehead; ocular hypertelorism; high nasal bridge; low philtrum; occasionally, epicanthic folds, dysplastic ears. *Extremities.* Radius hypoplastic or absent; ulna short and bowed; carpal bones missing or fused; thumb hypoplastic or missing; knee ankylosis; hip dislocation; varus feet; hypoplasia of third and fourth toe. *Cryptorchidism.* Normal intelligence, occasionally mental retardation.

Etiology. Autosomal recessive inheritance.

Diagnostic Procedures. *X-ray.* Symptoms and signs; craniosynostosis involving coronal suture.

BIBLIOGRAPHY. Baller F: Radiusaplasie und Inzucht. Z Menschl Vererb Konstitutionsl 29:782–790, 1950

Gerold M: Frankturheilung bei einen seltenenen Fall kongenitaler Anomalie der oberen Gliedmassen. Zbl Chir 84:831–843, 1959

Huson SM, Rodger CS, Hall CM, et al: The Baller-Gerold syndrome-phenotypic and cytogenetic overlap with Roberts syndrome J Med Genet 27:371–375, 1990

Dellapiccola B, Zelante L, Mingarelli R, et al: Baller-Gerold syndrome: case report and clinical radiological review. Am Med Genet 42:356–368, 1992

BALÓ

Synonyms. Concentric sclerosis; encephalitis periaxialis concentrica.

Symptoms and Signs. Both sexes affected; onset in childhood. Progressive, spastic paralysis, and symptoms and signs of neurologic disorders according to areas of brain affected.

Etiology. Unknown. Possibly a variety of Schilder (see).

Pathology. Central nervous system: diffuse areas of demyelinization arranged concentrically.

Diagnostic Procedures. *EEG. CT scan. MRI. Spinal tap. Serology.*

Therapy. Symptomatic.

Prognosis. Death in weeks or in 2–3 years.

BIBLIOGRAPHY. Marburg O: Die sogenannte akute multiple Sklerose (Encephalomyelitis periaxialis sceroticans). J Psychiat 27:213–312, 1906

Barré, Moren, Draganesco, et al Encéphalite périaxale diffuse (type Schilder). Syndrom tétraplégique avec stase papillaire. Rev Neurol 2:541–557, 1926

Baló J: Leukoencephalits periaxialis concentrica. Magy norvosi Arch 28:108–264, 1927

Baló J: Encephalitis periaxialis concentrica. Arch Neurol Psychiatr 19:242–264, 1928

Adams RD, Victor M: Principles of Neurology, 5th ed, pp 791–792. New York, McGraw-Hill, 1993

BALSER-FITZ

Synonyms. Fitz; hemorrhagic pancreatitis; pancreatitis acute.

Symptoms. Occurs at any age; slightly higher incidence in female (see Etiology). Unbearably epigastric pain, radiating over large areas, especially on the back, many times may not even be alleviated by opiates; sitting and bending forward partially relieves the intensity of pain, which is usually steady, occasionally colicky. Nausea, vomiting, constipation; shock.

Signs. Fever; tachycardia; weak pulse; hypotension. Skin. Cold, clammy and jaundiced. Abdomen. Seldom, skin discoloration 7 days after onset of pain due to ecchymosis; Grey-Turner signs (on the loin); Cullen's sign (around the umbilicus); tenderness; muscle guarding; auscultatory peristalsis usually normal. Chest: Presence of fluid or atelectasis or pneumonia, especially left lower side (30% of patients).

Etiology. In children, mumps infection or idiopathic. In adults (usually in fifth decade), chronic alcoholism. In adults in sixth decade, biliary tract diseases. Other causes of pancreatitis: parasitic infestation; adrenal steroid administration; hyperparathyroidism; metabolic disorders; trauma; heredity; allergy.

Pathology. Pancreas edematous, friable, hemorrhagic (in some cases this feature may be completely absent); fatty necrosis. Microscopically, acinar necrosis, edema, polymorphonuclear infiltration. In cases of some duration, abscess may develop. Fat necrosis is also observed in mesentery, omentum, and peritoneum. Associated pathology may be found in hepatobiliary tract, spleen, thrombosis, thrombophlebitic legs.

Diagnostic Procedures. *Blood.* Leukocytosis; anemia (not constant); bilirubin elevated; alkaline serum phosphatase elevated; hypocalcemia (confirmatory of diagnosis second day from onset); hyperglycemia (occasionally); plasma antithrombin titer elevated (?); serum amylase high values (immediate rise); serum lipase high values (later rise but longer-lasting). *Urine.* Amylase and lipase high values. Abdominal and thoracic paracentesis. Fluids show high values of amylase and lipase. *Echosonography.* Low readability for gas presence. *X-ray* (plain radiograph of the abdomen). *CT scan. MRI.*

Therapy. Immediate medical management of: fluid loss (to mantain intravascular volume and caloric and plastic apport); shock, pain, prevention of infection, neutralization of the enzymes, calcium if hypocalcemia. Gastric suction; anticholinergic drugs; antibiotics (according to infection). Surgery only in case when diagnosis in doubt, or if present biliary tract infection (cholangitis) but only when pancreatitis has subsided. Peritoneal washout.

Prognosis. Much improved with modern medical treatment, but still very severe. Mortality about 30% with hemorrhagic type and 5% with acute edematous type.

BIBLIOGRAPHY. Balser W: Ueber Fattenneckrose eine zuwellen toedliche Krankheit des Menschen. Arch Pathol Anat 90:520–535, 1882
Fitz R: Acute pancreatitis: A consideration of pancreatic haemorrhage, hemorrhagic, suppurative and gangrenous pancreatitis and disseminated fat-necrosis. Boston Med Surg J 120:181–187; 205–207, 1889
Zoepffel H: Das akute Pancreasoedem, eine Vorstufe der akuten Pancreasnekrose. Deut Zschr Chir 75:301–312, 1922
De Francisci G, Magalini SI, Sollazzi L, et al: Le pancreatiti da farmaci. Etiopatogenesi e problemi rianimativi. Rec Progr Med 72:201–212, 1982
Marshall JB: Acute pancreatitis. A review with an emphasis on new developments. Arch Int Med 153:1185–1198, 1993
Steinberg W, Tenner S: Acute pancreatitis. N Engl J Med 330:1198–1210, 1994

BAMATTER

Synonyms. Walt Disney dwarfism. Geroderma osteoplastic hereditary; osteoplastic geroderma.

Symptoms and Signs. Rare. Full syndrome from early childhood: stunted growth; senile changes in skin; normal scalp hair; microcornea; corneal opacities; articular hyperthrophy; multiple fractures and bone malformations. Forme fruste: partial forms presenting geroderma, osteodysplasia, microphthalmia, glaucoma without dwarfism.

Etiology. Unknown; hereditary X-linked or autosomal recessive. Less severe in female heterozygotes.

Pathology. Osteoporosis. Senile changes in skin.

Diagnostic Procedures. *Hormonal studies. X-ray of skeleton. Biopsy of skin.*

Therapy. None.

Prognosis. Variable according to degree. Generally resulting in dwarfism.

BIBLIOGRAPHY. Bamatter F: Gérodermie osthéodysplastique heréditaire (Un noveau biotype de la progeria). Ann Paediatr 174:126–127, 1950
Lisker R, Hernandez A, Martin-Lavin M, et al: Gerodermia osteodysplastica hereditaria: report of three affected brothers and literature review. Am J Med Genet 3:389–395, 1978
Hunter AGW: Is geroderma osteodysplastica underdiagnosed? J Med Genet 25:843–846, 1988

BAMBERG I

Synonyms. Palmus; saltatory spasm.

Symptoms and Signs. Ambulation jumpy or springy owing to clonic spasms of muscles.

Etiology. Irritation of motor cells of spinal cord.

BIBLIOGRAPHY. Bamberg H: Saltatorischer Reflekskampf, eine merkwürdige Form von Spinal-Irritation. Wein Med Wochenschr 9:49–53, 1859
Adams RD, Victor M: Principles of Neurology, 5th ed, pp 1194–1195. New York, McGraw-Hill, 1993

BAMBERG II

Synonyms. Concato; chronic polyserositis.

Symptoms and Signs. Those relative to the formation and progression of effusion in the pleural and peritoneal cavities.

Etiology. In majority of cases, tubercular disease; in remaining cases, idiopathic.

BIBLIOGRAPHY. Bamberg H: Ueber zwei selrene Herzaffktionen usw. Wien Med Wochenschr 14–25, 1872
Concato L: Sulla poliomenorrea scrofolosa o tisi delle sierose. Gior Intern Sc Med 3:1037–1053, 1881
Davis PDO: Clinical Tubercolosis. London, Chapman and Hall, 1994

BANKER-VICTOR-ADAMS

Synonym. Muscular dystrophy; congenital.

Symptoms and Signs. Onset at birth or early infancy. Variable severity of muscle weakness. Contractures of proximal muscles and trunk. Evidence of cerebral and retinal malformations; mental retardation. Poor sucking and swallowing. May walk when surviving at later age.

Etiology. Autosomal dominant or recessive inheritance. Status of this syndrome difficult to evaluate. Scarce pathologic reports.

Diagnostic Procedures. *Blood.* Slight to moderate elevation of CK. *EMG.* Myopathic pattern.

Prognosis. Variable from benign evolution and reaching second decade to early death.

BIBLIOGRAPHY. Banker BQ, Victor M, Adams RD: Arthogryposis multiplex due to congenital muscolar dystrophy. Brain 80:319, 1957
Adams RD, Victor M: Principles of Neurology, 5th ed, pp 1224–1225. New York, McGraw-Hill, 1993

BANKI

Symptoms and Signs. Hungarian family (three generations). Fusion of lunate and cuneiform bones, clinodactyly, brachymetacarpy, and thin diaphysis.

Etiology. Autosomal dominant inheritance.

BIBLIOGRAPHY. Banki Z: Kombination erblicher Gelenk und Knochenanomalien an der Hand. Fortschr Roentgenstr 103:588–604, 1965

BANNAYAN-RILEY-SMITH

Synonym. Bannayan-Riley-Ruvalcaba; Ruvalcaba-Myhre-Smith; Riley-Smith; Bannayan-Zonana; macrocephaly—multiple lipomas—hemangimata.

Symptoms and Signs. Predominant in male. Subcutaneous hemangiomata (40%) on the trunk and at proximal limbs multiple cutaneous lipomata (75%); pigmented spots of the penis; macrocephaly; pseudopapilledema, large intra-abdominal masses, hamartomatous polyps limited to distal ileum and colon (45%) and abdominal swelling. Fifty percent of cases hypotonia, motor delay, mild to severe mental deficiency.

Sixty percent of patients myopathic process in proximal muscles; 25% seizures.

Etiology. Autosomal dominant inheritance.

Pathology. Mesodermal hamartomas and discrete lipomas, hemangiomas, and seldom lymphoangiomas (10%) or mixed type (20%). In addition to subcutaneous localization, they may be found in intracranial (20%), intrabony (10%), and intestinal (45%) localizazion.

Diagnostic Procedures. *Electromyography. Muscle biopsy. CT scan. X-ray. Sonography of abdomen.*

Prognosis. Tendency to spontaneous improvement.

BIBLIOGRAPHY. Riley HD, Smith WR: Macrocephaly, pseudopapilledema, and multiple hemangiomata. Pediatrics 26:293–300, 1960

Burke EC, Winkelmann RK, Strickland MK: Disseminated hemangiomatosis. Am J Dis Child 108:418–424, 1964

Bannayan GA: Lipomatosis, angiomatosis and macrocephalia: a previously undescribed congenital syndrome. Arch Path 92:1–5, 1971

Zonana J, Davis D, Rimoin DL: Multiple lipomas, hemangiomas and macrocephaly—an autosomal dominant hamartomatous syndrome. Am J Hum Genet 27:97A, 1975

Ruvalcaba RHA, Myhre S, Smith DW: Sotos syndrome with intestinal polyposis and pigmentary changes of the genitalia. Clin Genet 18:413–416, 1980

Cohen MM Jr: Bannayan-Riley-Ruvalcaba syndrome: renaming three formerly recognized syndromes as one etiologic entity. Am J Med Genet 35:291, 1990

Gorlin RJ, Cohen MM, Levin LS: Syndromes of Head and Neck, 3rd ed, pp 336–338. New York, Oxford Press, 1990

BANNWARTH

Synonyms. Garin-Bujadoux-Bannwarth; facial palsy in lymphocytic choriomeningitis; meningoradiculitis Bannwarth. See Lyme (which is a partial manifestation).

Symptoms. Facial palsy (see Bell) occurring during subacute or chronic lymphocytic choriomeningitis.

Etiology. Borrelia burgdorferi producing meningo (poli-) neuritis or radiculitis.

Pathology. Epi or peri or endoneural vasculitis with neuronal degeneration and lympho-plasmacellular infiltration; lynphoplasmocellular meningitis.

Diagnostic Procedures. *Blood and spinal fluid.* Identification of specific antibodies.

Therapy. Penicillin.

BIBLIOGRAPHY. Garin C, Bujadoux A: Paralysie par les tiques. J Méd Lyon 71:765–767, 1922

Bannwarth A: Chronische lymphocytaere Meningitis, entzuendliche Polyneuritis und "Rheumatismus." Ein Beitrag zum Problem "Allergie und Nervensystem." Arch Psychiatr 113:284–376, 1941

Burgdorfer W, Barbour AG, Hayes SC, et al: A tick-borne spirochetosis? Science 216:1317–1319, 1982

Rahn DW, Malawista SE: Lyme disease: Recommendations for diagnosis and treatment. Ann Int Med 114:472–481, 1991

BANTLER

Synonym. Intestinal hemoangiomatosis—mucocutaneous pigmentation; hemoangiomatosis small intestine—mucocutaneous pigmentation.

Symptoms and Signs. Early infancy. Diffuse pigmentary lesions (ephelides, cafe au lait spots) in mucocutaneous zones.

Etiology. Possibly autosomal dominant inheritance. Maybe included in Rendu-Osler (?).

Pathology. Hemoangiomas in the small intestine.

Diagnostic Procedures. *Blood.* Anemia. *X-ray intestine.* Presence of hemoangiomas. *Stools.* Blood.

Therapy. Surgery.

BIBLIOGRAPHY. Bantler M: Hemangiomas of the small intestine associated with mucocutaneous pigmentation. Gastroenterology 38:641–645, 1960

BANTI

Synonyms. Nonfamilial splenic anemia; chronic congestive splenomegaly; fibrocongestive splenomegaly; hepatolienal fibrosis; splenic anemia.

Symptoms. Most frequently occurs in patients under 35 years of age; it may occur even in children. Female to male ratio 2:1. Insidious or sudden onset. Hematemesis; melena; weakness; flatulence; diarrhea, vague indigestion; abdominal pain or distress; epistaxis (30% of cases).

Signs. Pallor and occasionally mild jaundice, or sallow brown pigmentation of skin; liver slightly enlarged; remarkable splenomegaly that occasionally may precede anemia.

Etiology. Portal hypertension, intrahepatic (e.g., cirrhosis, schistosoma) extrahepatic (e.g., portal vein thrombosis compression; aneurysm) that leads to hypersplenism and successive anemization.

Pathology. Spleen weight up to 600–1200 g or more. Capsule thickened and occasionally adherent to adjacent organs. Pulp firm, grayish red; histologically, fibrosis, dilatation of the sinuses, hyaline degenerative changes of the malpighian bodies. Periarterial hemorrhages; periarteriolar siderotic nodules. Liver cirrhosis may not be grossly evident but is found on microscopic examination. Esophageal varices.

Diagnostic Procedures. *Blood.* Normocytic anemia; leukopenia; thrombocytopenia. *Bone marrow.* Myeloid hyperplasia; maturation arrest of myeloid and megakaryocytic series; later erythroid series arrest. *X-rays.* Upper gastrointestinal tract. *Esophageal varices; sodium sulfobromophthalein excretion. Portal venography and pressure. Spleen scan.* After administration of chromium-tagged red cells.

Therapy. Splenectomy (to relieve leukopenia and thrombocytopenia) not useful, however, for reduction in portal hypertension. Splenectomy plus venovenous anastomosis provides a better shunt. Portacaval shunt and side-to-side portacaval anastomosis have reduced operative mortality and prolonged survival. Liver transplantation when indicated.

Prognosis. Slowly evolving course. Hemorrhage may precipitate the situation.

BIBLIOGRAPHY. Banti G: Dell' Anemia splenica. Arch Scuola Anat Patol (Firenze) 2:53–122, 1883

Athens JW Disorders primarily involving the spleen. In Lee GR, Bithel TC, Foerster J, et al (eds): Wintrobe's Clinical Hematology, 9th ed, pp 1711–1713. Philadelphia, Lea & Febiger, 1993

Schwartz ME, Miller CM: Diseases of hepatic blood vessels. In Haubrich WS, Schaffner F, Berk JE (eds): Bockus Gastroenterology, 5th ed, p 2381. Philadelphia, WB Saunders, 1995

BAR

Synonym. Colibacillosis in pregnancy. Eponym used to indicate the manifestations of abdominal pain (gallbladder; ureters; appendix), hyperthermia, and presence of bacteria in the urine during pregnancy.

BIBLIOGRAPHY. Editorial: Bar syndrome or colibacillosis gravidique. JAMA 128:244, 1948

BARAITSER-BURN

Synonyms. Oral—facial—digital IV; OFD IV.

Symptoms and Signs. Difficulty to differenciate from other OFD. Characterized by severe tibial dysphasia.

Etiology. Autosomal recessive inheritance.

BIBLIOGRAPHY. Baratseir M, Burn J, Fixen J: A female infant with feature of Mohr-Majewski syndromes: variable expression, a genetic compound or a distinct entity? J Med Genet 20:65–67, 1983

Burn J, Desateux C, Hall CM, et al: Orofacialdigital syndrome with mesomelic limb shortening. J Med Genet 21:189–192, 1984

Baraitser M: The orofaciodigital (OFD) syndromes. J Med Genet 23:116–119, 1986

Meinecke P, Hayeck H: Orofaciodigital syndrome type IV (Mohr-Mejewski syndrome) with severe expression expanding the know spectrum of anomalies. J Med Genet 27:200–202, 1990

BARAKAT

Synonyms. Nephrosis—deafness—hypoparathyroidism. Deafness—nephrosis—hypoparathyroidism.

Symptoms and Signs. Deafness, hypoparathyroidism manifestations. Nephrosis, steroid resistant. Renal failure.

Etiology. Autosomal recessive inheritance.

Prognosis. Death within a few months.

BIBLIOGRAPHY. Barakat AY, D'Albora JB, Martin MM, et al: Familial nephrosis, nerve deafness and hypoparathyroidism. J Pediatr 91:61–64, 1977

BARANY

Synonyms. Positional vertigo; vertigo, paroxysmal, positional, benign; BPPV.

Symptoms and Signs. More frequently in elderly subjects; male to female ratio 2:1. In young subjects after viral neurolabyrinthitis and in case of post-traumatic forms, male to female ratio 1:1. In first stages only in the morning at awakening then constantly during described maneuver. When the patient is moved from sitting position to recumbency with the head straight or tilted backward and laterally, after a few seconds paroxysm of vertigo, pallor, hypotension, and fright occur that cause him to attempt to sit up and induce nystagmus (vertical-torsional) lasting for 10–15 seconds. From recumbency to sitting same phenomenon reversed. Complaining of a sensation of walking on pillow. Maintenance of head in position stops the attacks or repeating the maneuver several times brings reduction then disappearance of phenomenon. It returns after a protracted period of rest. Absence of abnormalities in hearing or of vestibular paresis.

Etiology. Cupololithiasis of posterior semicircular canal owing to detachment of otoconia from the otoconial layer by spontaneous degeneration or head trauma and settlement in this location. The "heavy cupola" creates an oversensitivity of the posterior canal to angular acceleration thus BPPV is practically an enhanced postrotatory position response, but not a positional response. Also may be owing to postviral labyrinthitis.

Diagnostic Procedures. *Hallpike maneuver* (rapid positions changes from the sitting to the head hanging right or left position): vertigo attach. *Examination with Frenzel's glasses:* nystagmus beating on the undermost ear or upward when gaze directed toward the uppermost ear; fatiguability with repetition. *Otoneurologic examination:* absence of hearing defects.

Therapy. Physical therapy by positioning maneuvers on serial basis. In intractable cases surgical transection of ampullary nerve.

Prognosis. Benign condition with spontaneous recovery in weeks or months (70%), in 20–30%, when untreated, persists, or shows relapses for years.

BIBLIOGRAPHY. Barany R: Vestibularapparat und Centralnerven System. Med Klin 7:1818–1821, 1911

Barany R: Diagnose von Krankheitser scheinumgen im bereiche des otolithenapparates. Acta Otolaryngol (Stock) 2:434–437, 1921

Brandt T: Vertigo. Its multisensory syndromes, p 139. London, Springer-Verlag, 1991

Herdman SJ, Tusa RJ, Zee DS, et al: Single treatment approaches to benign paroxismal vertigo. Arch Otolaryngol Head Neck Surg 119:450–454, 1993

BARBER (H.W.)

Synonyms. Abortive acrodermatitis; palmoplantar pustolosis; pustular bacterid; pustolosis palmoplantaris. Palmoplantar pustolar psoriasiasis. See acrodermatitis, persistent.

Symptoms. Rare. Moderate prevalence in females; onset at any age; more frequent between 40 and 60 years of age. Itching (occasionally, severe at night). Bilateral lesions start and remain on thenar eminences and on the heels: areas glazed and reddish, with scaling and numerous pustules in various stages of evolution.

Etiology. Unknown. Psoriatic or eczematoid origin debated. Considered by some authors to result from a secondary (vasculitic) reaction to foci.

Pathology. Early lesions show hyperkeratosis, parakeratosis, and scarce or absent spongiosis. On pustule area and periphery, granular layer intact, among invading leukocytes lymphocytes predominate. Later, scaling of the pustules with return of the underlying epidermis to normal.

Therapy. Removal of foci occasionally effective. Corticosteroids, coal tar, salicylic acid, roentgen treatment, and prolonged courses of tetracycline of partial benefit.

Prognosis. Protracted course. Remission and relapses.

BIBLIOGRAPHY. Audry C: Les phlycténose récidivantes des extremités (acrodermatites continues de Hallopeau). Ann Dermatol Syph 2:913–928, 1901

Barber HW: Pustular psoriasis of the extremities. Guy's Hosp Rep 86:108–119, 1936

Camp RDR: Psoriasis. In Champion RH, Burton JL, Ebling FJG (eds): Rook/Wilkinson/Ebling Textbook of Dermatology, 5th ed, p 1448. Oxford, Blackwell Scientific, 1992

BARDET-BIEDL

Synonyms. Biedl-Bardet; Laurence-Moon-Bardet-Biedl (incorrect name); see Laurence-Moon. See also Biemond II and Alstroem.

Symptoms. Both sexes. From birth. Mental retardation. Vision loss progressing to blindness. Absence of paraplegia (to distinguish it from Laurence-Moon).

Signs. Obesity; polydactyly; hypogenitalism.

Etiology. Unknown. Autosomal recessive inheritance.

Pathology. *Eyes.* Retinitis pigmentosa. *Kidney.* Renal abnormalities (chronic glomerulonephritis or hydronephrosis). *Liver.* Frequently fibrosis. *Pituitary and gonads.* Abnormalities or features of secondary hypogenitalism.

Diagnostic Procedures. *Electroretinography. Hormonal studies. Chromosomal studies.*

Therapy. Symptomatic.

Prognosis. Usually fatal at early age from infections renal and/or liver insufficiency. If adulthood reached, blindness at 20 years of age (27%); other features stationary.

BIBLIOGRAPHY. Bardet G: Sur une syndrome d'obesité infantile avec polydactylie et retinité pigmentaire (contribution à l'etude des formes cliniques de l'obesité hypophysaire). Thesis Paris, n 479, 1920
Biedl A: Ein Geschwisterpaar mit adiposo-genitaler Distrophie. Dtsch Med Wschr 48:1630, 1922
Schachat AP, Mannence IH: The Bardet-Biedl syndrome and related disorders. Arch Ophthalmol 100:285–288, 1982
Klintworth GK: Genetically determined disorders affecting the eye. In Garner A, Klintworth GK (eds): Pathobiology of Ocular Disease: A Dynamic Approach, 2nd ed, p 762. New York, Marcel Dekker, 1994

BARD

Eponym to indicate pulmonary metastasis from stomach carcinoma.

BIBLIOGRAPHY. Samson M, et al: Syndrom de Bard. Carcinomatose miliaire polmonaire sécondaire à une neoplasie gastrique. Laval Med 33:106–110, 1962

BARE LYMPHOCYTE

Symptoms and Signs. Both sexes. First symptoms at 3–4 months of age. Persistent diarrhea, malabsorption, mucocutaneous candidiasis, bacterial infections of upper and lower respiratory tract.

Etiology. Autosomal recessive inheritance. Part of the class of combined immunodeficiency clinically and immunologically heterogeneous. T-cells are reduced in number because of selective deficit in CDA+ helper T-cells; B-cells normally are present but functionally immature.

Diagnostic Procedures. *Blood.* Lymphocytes lack HLA-A-, B-, C-antigens and beta-2 microglobulin. Low immunoglobulins; Delayed skin sensitivity tests: negative or slight positivity.

Pathology. Normal thymus, lymph nodes: normal in size, absence of germinal centers in reduced follicles.

Therapy. Bone marrow transplantation.

Prognosis. Most cases die in infancy. Good hope comes from bone marrow transplantation.

BIBLIOGRAPHY. Touraine JL, Betuel H, Souillet G, et al: Combined immunodeficiency disease associated with absence of cell-surface HLA-A and B antigens. Lancet I:319–320, 1978
Mercadet A, Cohen D, Dausset J, et al: Genotyping with DNA probes in combined immunodeficiency syndrome with defective expression of HLA. New Engl J Med 312:1287–1292, 1985
Casper JT, Ash AR, Kirchner P, et al: Successful treatment with an unrelated-donor bone marrow transplant in a HLA-deficient patient with severe combined immune deficiency ("Bare lymphocyte syndrome"). J Pediatr 116:262–265, 1990

BARLOW

Barlow originally described a case exhibiting a combination of scurvy and rickets. Today Barlow is used as eponym for infantile scurvy.

Synonyms. Ascorbic acid deficiency; Cheadle-Moeller-Barlow; Moeller-Barlow; sea scurvy; scorbutus; scurvy; subperiosteal hematoma.

Symptoms. Tenderness of legs and pseudoparalysis; irritability; anorexia; diarrhea; hemorrhagic gums.

Signs. Hemorrhagic skin changes (4%); fever (19%); swelling over long bone (14%). Costochondral beading.

Etiology. Vitamin C deficiency.

Pathology. Ecchymotic lesions on gums, skin, mucosae caused by capillary fragility and traumas. Heart enlarged. Lack of osteoid formation, thickening of calcification zones. Cartilage shows spiculae of calcified matrix disarrayed and fractures at the chondro-osteal conjunction. Only some degree of healing at the fracture site. Bone cortex thinned and subperiosteal dissecting hemorrhages present along the shaft of long bones up to the epiphysis.

Diagnostic Procedures. *Blood.* Anemia microcytic, occasionally, macrocytic; low vitamin C level. *Urine.* No excretion of vitamin C after intravenous injection of 200 mg. *X-rays.* Bone cortex appears as "ground glass" dense line at the end of shaft; proximal zone of rarefaction at corners of tibia, radius.

Therapy. Vitamin C.

Prognosis. Very good with specific treatment; some bone changes remain radiologically evident after cure.

BIBLIOGRAPHY. Barlow T: On cases described as "acute rickets" which are probably a combination of scurvy and rickets, the scurvy being an essential, and the rickets a variable element. Med Chir Trans 66:159–220, 1883
Woodruff C: Infantile scurvy, the increasing incidence of scurvy in the Nashville area. JAMA 161:448–456, 1956
Reuler JB, Broudy VC, Cooney TG: Adult scurvy. JAMA 253:805–807, 1985
Smith R: Disorders of the skeleton. In Weatherall DJ, Ledingham JGG, Warrell DA (eds): Oxford Textbook of Medicine, 3rd ed, p 3094. Oxford, Oxford Med Pub, 1996

BARNARD-SCHOLZ

Synonyms. Ophthalmoplegia—retinal degeneration; oculopharyngeal muscular dystrophy. See also Kearns-Sayre and OXPHOS syndromes.

Symptoms and Signs. Both sexes affected; onset at all ages. Unilateral or bilateral progressive weakness of muscles of eyelids, up to severe ptosis; progressive ocular myopathy up to complete ophthalmoplegia. Retinitis pigmentosa. Occasionally present, weakness of facies, neck, and shoulder muscles; hearing defects and heart block.

Etiology. Variable; considered nuclear ophthalmoplegia; ocular myopathy. Autosomal dominant inheritance; recessive also reported.

Therapy. Symptomatic.

Prognosis. Progressive condition.

BIBLIOGRAPHY. Barnard RI, Scholz RO: Ophthalmoplegia and retinal degeneration. Am J Ophthalmol 27:621–624, 1944
Kiloh LG, Nevin S: Progressive dystrophy of the external ocular muscles (ocular myopathy). Brain 74:115–143, 1951
Knoblauch A, Koppel M: Die okulopharingeale Muskeldystrophie. Schweiz Med Wschr 114:557–561, 1984

BARNES (N.D.)

Synonyms. Thoracolaryngopelvic dysplasia; thoracopelvic dysostosis; see Jeune.

Symptoms. Two families reported. Respiratory distress.

Signs. Thorax: "bell-shaped" small, rigid. Larynx: stenotic. Low stature and asthenic build. Absence of renal problems (see Jeune).

Etiology. Autosomal dominant.

Prognosis. Benign course of respiratory problem.

BIBLIOGRAPHY. Barnes ND, Hull D, Symons JS: "Thoracic dystroph." Arch Dis Child 44:11–17, 1969
Bankier A, Danks DM: Thoracic-pelvic dysostosis: a new autosomal form. J Med Genet 20:276–279, 1983

Burn J, Hall C, Marsden D, et al: Autosomal dominant thoracolaryngopelvic dysplasia: Barnes syndrome. J Med Genet 23:45–49, 1986

BARNES (S.)

Obsolete.

Synonyms. Muscular dystrophy; Barnes.

Symptoms and Signs. Protean myopathy: predominantly hypertrophic, pseudohypertrophic, peroneal atrophy; myotonia of some thigh muscles; affecting six generations of same family.

Etiology. Autosomal dominant inheritance.

BIBLIOGRAPHY. Barnes S: Myopathic family, with hypertrophic, pseudohypertrophic, atrophic, and terminal (distal in upper extremities) stages. Brain 55:1–46, 1932

BARRAQUER-SIMONS

Synonyms. Mitchell II; Holländer; Simond; Smith; Weir Mitchell II; lipodystrophy progressiva; see Laignel-Lavastine or Viard (when is accompanied by real hypertrophy of lower part of body).

Symptoms and Signs. Most frequently, onset at 5–15 years of age; prevalent in females (4:1). Symmetric loss of facial fat occurring over some months, with or without disappearance of fat from arms, chest, abdomen, atrophy stops at umbilical line, and lower limbs appear incongruously fat. Mental retardation in some cases. Glomerulonephritis in 50% of cases.

Etiology. Unknown; congenital derangement of mesenchyma. May follow damage of midbrain or diencephalon. Immunologic derangement considered.

Pathology. Absence of fat in indicated locations; kidney frequently affected: enlarged; nephritis in 50% of cases; pyelonephritis; nephrotic changes. Liver occasionally enlarged; mild fibrosis; fat vacuolization.

Diagnostic Procedures. *Blood.* In some cases, disturbed glucose metabolism and hyperlipemia. Blood urea nitrogen and creatinine elevated. Complement components different variations. Occasionally increased thyroid antibodies. *Urine.* Albuminuria; hematuria. *X-ray.* Pyelograms normal or caliceal dilatation with or without ureter dilatations. *Brain CT scan. MRI.* In some cases, abnormal.

Therapy. Symptomatic treatment of kidney condition.

Prognosis. The presence of pathologic kidney findings (mesangiocapillary glomerulo nephritis in 90% of cases) makes the prognosis guarded. Diabetes mellitus develops in 30% of cases. Death reported 10–25 years after onset in a series.

BIBLIOGRAPHY. Mitchell SW: Singular case of absence of adipose matter in upper half of the body. Am J Med Sci 90:105, 1885
Senior B, Gellis SS: The syndromes of total lipodystrophy and of partial lipodystrophy. Pediatrics 33:593–612, 1964
Burton JL, Cunlife WJ: Subcutaneous fat. In Champion RH, Burton JL, Ebling FJG (eds): Rook/Wilkinson/Ebling Textbook of Dermatology, 5th ed, pp 2158–2160. Oxford, Blackwell Scientific, 1992

BARRÉ

Obsolete.

Synonyms. Deiter nucleus; deuterospinal.

Symptoms and Signs. Vertigo, disequilibrium, lateropulsion, "little steps march" sudden falling.

Etiology. It does not clearly fall into the category of vascular syndromes of medulla.

Pathology. No actual study reported. Suggested, on clinical basis, involvement in the initial segments of the two lateral vestibulospinal pathways and sparing of superior connections of Deiter nucleus.

BIBLIOGRAPHY. Barré JA: Essai sur un syndrome des voies vestibulospinales. Soc oto-neuro-ocul. Stasburg 283–288, 1925
Barré JA: La syndrome vestibulaire Taité Méd 15:125, 1949
Currier RD: Syndromes of the medulla oblungata. In Vinken PJ, Bruyn GW: Handbook of Clinical Neurology, vol 2, pp 219–220. Amsterdam, North-Holland, 1969

BARRÉ-LIÉOU

Synonyms. Bartschi-Rochain; Schuetzenberger; Kuhelendahl; cervical arthritis—vertigo; sympathetic posterior cervical; sympathetic cervical; vertigo cervicalis.

Symptoms. Both sexes affected; onset usually after middle life. Headache; pain in eyes; recurrent disturbed vision; pain in the ears; tinnitus and vertigo; vasomotor disturbance of face; occasionally swallowing and phonation may be affected. Pain in cervical region with neck movements; impaired memory and thinking; anxiety and depression.

Signs. Hypoesthesia of cornea; recurrent small ulcers on palpebral fissure (in chronic cervical arthritis).

Etiology and Pathology. Arthritis of third and fourth cervical vertebra; trauma; cervical disk causing irritation of trigeminal (V) and vestibulocochlear (VIII) nerves. There is, however, no evidence that cervical mechanisms may cause vertigo, so the etiopathogenesis of this syndrome still remains obscure.

Diagnostic Procedures. *Audiologic evaluation. Caloric stimulation. Electronystagmography. CT brain scan. MRI. Brainstem auditory evoked potentials. X-ray of cervical spine.*

Therapy. Traction; ultrasound; deep X-rays; thermal; anti-inflammatory therapy. Meclizine, cyclizine, diazepam, scopolamine.

Prognosis. Chronic condition responding to treatment.

BIBLIOGRAPHY. Barré JA: Sur un syndrome sympathique cervical postérieur et sa cause frequente, l'artrite cervicale. Rev Neurol (Paris) 1:1246–1248, 1926
Liéou YC: Syndrome sympathique cervical postérieur et arthrite cervicale chronique. Étude clinique et radiologique (thesis). Strasbourg, 1928
Brandt T: Vertigo: Its Multisensorial Syndromes, pp 277–288. London, Springer-Verlag, 1991

BARRÉ-MASSON

Synonyms. Angiomyoneuroma; glomangioma; glomus tumor; multiple.

Symptoms. Intense pain at sites of lesion (smaller lesion mainly cellular) or painless (angiomatous nature).

Signs. Round, firm, red blue neoformation on skin of distal parts of limbs. Hemorrhagic foci under fingers and toenails. Tumors are present at birth or appear within 20 years. Isolated tumors may appear also later (33 years average age).

Etiology. Unknown. Usually sporadic. Familial occurrence (autosomal dominant) reported.

Pathology. Well-defined masses of vascular channels in association with aggregates of glomus cells.

Therapy. Excision.

Pathogenesis. Responding to treatment; no recurrences after whole tumor removal.

BIBLIOGRAPHY. Masson P: Le glomus neuromyoartériel des régions tactiles et ses tumeurs. Lyon Chir 21:247–280, 1924

Barré JA, Masson P: Étude anatomo-clinique de certaines tumeurs sous-unguéales douloureuses (tumeurs du glomus neuro-myo-artériel des extrémitiés). Bull Soc Fr Dermatol Syph RS 31:148–159, 1924

Rycroft RJG, Meuter MA, Sharvill DE, et al: Hereditary multiple glomus tumors: report of four families and review of literature. Trans St John Hosp Derm Soc 61:70–81, 1975

MacKie RM: Soft tissue tumors. In Champion RH, Burton JL, Ebling FJG (eds): Rook/Wilkinson/Ebling Textbook of Dermatology, 5th ed, p 2086. Oxford, Blackwell Scientific, 1992

BARRETT

Synonyms. Esophagitis—peptic ulcer; gastroesophageal reflux, GER; columnar lined, Barrett metaplasia.

Symptoms. Occurs in middle-aged or elderly people. Male to female ratio 3:1. Recurrent low retrosternal pain and heartburn; pain may radiate to the neck, scapular region, or both arms, especially after eating acidic, hot, or cold food, or while lying down; in later cases, dysphagia; vomiting; melena; hematemesis.

Etiology. Chronic peptic ulcer of the esophagus. Autosomal dominant inheritance also reported.

Pathology. Peptic ulcer in association with esophagitis. When ulcer penetrates through walls of esophagus mediastinal tissue shows fibrosis and inflammatory adenitis; if blood vessel perforates; hemorrhage, mediastinal and pleural suppuration. Microscopically. Developmental, anomalous lining of mucosa with atypical columnar epithelium.

Diagnostic Procedures. *X-ray.* Discrete crater or niche on the esophagus wall, with absence of atypical rugae distal to the crater; spasm above the lesion; stricture because of edema. *Esophagoscopy.* Crater; poorly developed rugae, edema; inflammation; hemorrhage; leukoplakia. *Exfoliative cytology.* Negative for malignancy.

Therapy. Life style modifications, antacids, H2–receptor antagonists omeprazole, metoclopramide; bethanecol; frequently, surgery is required.

Prognosis. Ulcer penetrates, perforates, or bleeds. Possible neoplastic transformation.

BIBLIOGRAPHY. Barrett NR: Chronic peptic ulcer of the oesophagus and oesophagitis. Br J Surg 38:175–182, 1950

Crabb DW, Berk MA, Hall TR, et al: Familial gastroesophageal reflux and development of Barrett's esophagus. Am Int Med 103:52–54, 1985

Heading RC: Barrett's oesophagus. Br Med J 294:461–462, 1987

Spechler SJ: Comparison of medical and surgical therapy for complicated gastroesophageal reflux disease in veterans. New Engl J Med 326:786–792, 1992

Katzka DA: Columnar-lined (Barrett's) esophagus. In Haubrich WS, Schaffner F, Berk JE (eds): Bockus Gastroenterology, 5th ed, vol 2, pp 468–482. Philadelphia, WB Saunders, 1995

BARROW

Synonyms. Short limb dwarfism; congenital heart defect.

Symptoms and Signs. Male. Sloping forehead, prominent nose bridge, narrow palpebral fissures, epicanthic folds, midline capillary hemangioma, and micrognathia. Rhizomelic short limbs. Congenital heart defect.

Etiology. Unknown.

BIBLIOGRAPHY. Barrow M, Fitzsimmons JS: A new syndrome. Short limbs, abnormal facial appearance and congenital heart defect. Am J Med Genet 18:431–433, 1984

BARTH

Synonyms. Cardioskeletal myopathy X-linked; myopathy cardioskeletal X-linked. See OXPHOS syndromes.

Symptoms and Signs. Only in males. Dilated cardiomyopathy, skeletal myopathy. Growth retardation.

Etiology. X-linked inheritance. Mapping of locus: linkage to Xq 28.

Pathology. May be associated with endocardial fibroelastosis. Ultrastructural abnormalities, in mitochondria, in heart muscle and neutrophils, with abnormally shaped cristae, but no paracrystalline inclusions; skeletal muscle. Increased lipid.

Diagnostic Procedures. *Blood.* Decreased plasma free carnitine; prolonged fasting does not cause lactic acidydracrylic acid.

Therapy. See OXPHOS syndromes. Neutropenia. Urine: Increased 3–metylglutaconic acid, and 2-ethyl-hydracrilic acid.

Prognosis. Death from cardiac failure in infancy or early childhood.

BIBLIOGRAPHY. Barth PG, Scholte HR, Berden JA, et al: An X-linked mitochondiral disease affecting cardiac muscle, skeletal muscle and neutrophils leukocytes. J Neurol Sci 62:327–325, 1983

Towbin JA, Roberts R: Cardiovascular diseases due to genetic abnormalities. In Schlant RC, Alexander RW: Hurst's The Heart, 8th ed, p 1740. New York, McGraw-Hill, 1994

BARTON

See Colles and Smith fractures, distinct in dorsal Barton, which has a dorsal marginal fracture, and volar Barton, which has a volar one.

Etiology. Trauma.

Therapy. These fractures may be reduced by closed reduction and cast. If unstable, open reduction is needed.

BIBLIOGRAPHY. Barton JR: Views and treatment of an important injury of the wrist. Med Exam Philadelphia 1:365–368, 1838

Saito H, Takahashi Y, Zenzai K: Intra-articular fractures of the distal radius. Treatment and results. In Vastamaeki M: Current Trends in Hand Surgery. Amsterdam, Excerpta Medica, 1995

BART

Synonyms. Epidermolysis bullosa—skin absence; dysonychia; epidermolysis bullosa dystrophica (Bart type).

Symptoms and Signs. Congenital absence of skin over lower extremities and of nails (or their deformities); blistering of skin and mucosae. It may be considered as a manifestation of epidermolysis bullosa and not as a separate specific entity.

Etiology. Sporadic or autosomal dominant inheritance. Congenital absence of skin may represent "intrauterine" blistering.

Therapy. Protection from trauma. Antibiotics, corticosteroids.

BIBLIOGRAPHY. Bart BJ, Gorlin RJ, Anderson VE, et al: Congenital localized absence of skin and associated abnormalities resembling epidermolysis bullosa: a new syndrome. Arch Derm 93:296–304, 1966

Bowwes-Bavinck JN, van Haeringen A, Ruiter D: Autosomal dominant epidermolysis bullosa dystrophica: are the Cockayne-Touraine, the Pasini and the Bart-types different expressions of the same mutant gene? Clin Genet 31:416–424, 1987

Pye RJ: Bullous eruptions. In Champion RH, Burton JL, Ebling FJG (eds): Rook/Wilkinson/Ebling Textbook of Dermatology, 5th ed, p 1635. Oxford, Blackwell Scientific, 1992

BARTSOCAS-PAPAS

Synonym. Popliteal pterygium, lethal type.

Symptoms and Signs. At birth. Both sexes. Those of popliteal pterygium (see), plus synostosis of hand and foot bone, digital hypoplasia, and syndactyly. Low birthweight, microcephaly, corneal ulcerations, microstomia, cleft lip-palate, aplastic labia majora, bicornuate uterus; mental retardation. Occasionally midfacial port wine stains.

Etiology. Autosomal recessive inheritance.

BIBLIOGRAPHY. Bartsocas CS, Papas CV: Popliteal pterygium syndrome: evidence for a severe autosomal recessive form. J Med Genet 9:222–226, 1972

Hall JG: The lethal multiple pterygium syndromes. Am J Med Genet 17:803–807, 1984

BARTTER CLASSIC

Synonyms. Aldosteronism—normal blood pressure; hyperaldosteronism without hypertension; juxtaglomerular complex hyperplasia—hypoaldosteronism—hypokalemic alkalosis. See Gitelman and hyperprostaglandin E.

Symptoms. Both sexes equal incidence. In patients often born from pregnancy complicated by polyhydramnios (8:18) or premature delivery (7:18). Mental retardation; slow growth (8:18), weakness; polydipsia, polyuria; tendency to dehydration (16:18) Very seldom (see Gitelman) during infancy or before school age episodes of cramps in legs and arms; convulsive seizures (disappearing after potassium administration).

Signs. Dwarfism. Physical and neurologic examination otherwise noncontributory. Normal blood pressure or hypertension.

Etiology. Hyperplasia and hypertrophy of juxtaglomerular apparatus and primary hyperaldosteronism with hypokalemic alkalosis and normal blood pressure. Defect in the loop of Henle. Possibly, aldosteronism and juxtaglomerular abnormalities stem from unknown cause. Prostaglandins appear to be mediators of renin release in this syndrome (see Hyperprostaglandin E syndrome). Suggestion that renal lesion responsible for the adrenal one. Recessive cases of inheritance reported.

Pathology. Adrenal tissue. Hypertrophy of zona glomerulosa. Kidney tissue. Hypertrophy and hyperplasia of juxtaglomerular apparatus; basement membrane continuous throughout length of afferent arteriole, obstructing space normally present between juxtaglomerular wall and macula densa; atrophy of glomeruli.

Diagnostic Procedures. *Blood.* Hypokalemic alkalosis; serum angiotensin II increased. *Urine.* High normal level of calcium. Loss of potassium is in excess of intake. Potassium loss prevented by infusion of albumin and by treatment with aldosterone antagonists, but not prevented by restriction of dietary sodium or treatment with alkalis. Increased aldosterone excretion. Resistance to pressor effect of angiotensin. ADH-resistant renal concentrating defect. *Electrocardiography.* Pattern of hypokalemia. *Electroencephalography.* Diffuse dysrhythmia.

Therapy. Partial adrenalectomy; aldosterone antagonists. Acetylsalicylic acid; indomethacin plus spironolactone, or dyrenium.

Prognosis. Good response and fast improvement with treatment.

BIBLIOGRAPHY. Pronove P, MacCardle RC, Bartter FC: Aldosteronism, hypokalemia, and a unique renal lesion in a five year old boy. Acta Endocrinol (suppl 6) (Copenh) 51:167, 1960

Bartter FC, Pronove P, Gill JR: Hyperplasia of the juxtaglomerular complex with hyperaldosteronism and hypokalemic alkalosis. Am J Med 33:811–828, 1962

Bettinelli A, Bianchetti MG, Girardin E, et al: Use of calcium excretion values to distinguish two forms of primary renal tubular hypokalemic alkalosis: Bartter and Gitelman syndromes J Pediatr 120:38–43, 1992

Editorial correspondence. Gitelman versus Bartter syndrome. J Pediatr 123:671–673, 1993

Crowe P, Ahmad A, O'Byrne K, et al: Bartter's syndrome in two generations of an Irish family. Postgrad Med J 69:791–796, 1993

BASAN

Synonym. Ectodermal dysplasia absent dermatoglyphic—dysonychia.

Symptoms and Signs. Both sexes. Congenital milia on the chin, ruptured bullae on hands and feet, tapering of fingertips, bilateral simian creases, absence of dermatoglyphic patterns.

Etiology. Autosomal dominant inheritance.

BIBLIOGRAPHY. Basan M: Ektodermale Dysplasie, fehlendes Papillarmuster. Nagelveraenderungen und Vierfingerfurche. Arch Klin Exp Derm 222:546–557, 1963

Harper J: Genetics and genodermatoses. In Champion RH, Burton JL, Ebling FJG (eds): Rook/Wilkinson/Ebling Textbook of Dermatology, 5th ed, p 338. Oxford, Blackwell Scientific, 1992

BASILAR ARTERY MIGRAINE

Synonym. Bickerstaff; premenstrual tension headache; vertebrobasilar migraine. See also Migraine.

Symptoms. In all ages. Occurs in both sexes with equal frequency; in girls and young women; associated with menstrual periods. Prodromal visual loss and scintillation in both halves of visual field, followed by dysarthria, ataxia, vertigo, tinnitus, paresthesia of fingers and toes. Consciousness disturbances and or fainting (persisting even for hours) occasionally associated. Attack of severe throbbing, occipital headache, and vomiting occurs within few (up to 45) minutes. No symptoms during intervals between attacks.

Etiology. Circulatory disorder of basilar artery; transitory constriction of main trunk or branches.

Diagnostic Procedures. *Angiography.* Negative. *Electroencephalography. CT brain scan. MRI. Cochlear and vestibular functional studies.* Normal.

Therapy. Symptomatic; diuretics of some benefit.

Prognosis. As patient grows older this syndrome is replaced by "classic" or "common" migraine syndrome (see).

BIBLIOGRAPHY. Bickerstaff ER: Basilar artery migraine. Lancet I:15–17, 1961

Friedman AP: The migraine syndrome. Bull NY Acad Med 44:45–62, 1968

Adams RD, Victor M: Principles of Neurology, 5th ed, pp 153, 268. New York, McGraw-Hill, 1993

BASS

Synonym. Brachymesodactyly—nail dysplasia; brachydactyly type A5—nail dysplasia.

Symptoms and Signs. Both sexes affected; present at birth. Brachydactyly; hypoplastic fingers and toenails; absent middle phalanges in the fingers and lateral four toes; duplicated distal phalanges of thumbs. Hypoplasia of aricular cartilage.

Etiology. Autosomal dominant inheritance.

BIBLIOGRAPHY. Bass HN: Familial absence of middle phalanges with nail dyplasia: a new syndrome. Pediatrics 42:318–323, 1968

BASSEN-KORNZWEIG

Synonyms. Abetalipoproteinemia; acanthocytosis; betalipoprotein deficiency; lipoprotein deficiency, low-density.

Symptoms. Predominant in males (71%); appears in infancy. The patients are normal at birth but usually fail to thrive during the first year; fatty diarrhea; intellectual development slightly retarded; eye trouble (retinitis) that progresses eventually to blindness; ataxia; intentional tremor; slurred speech; muscular weakness; athetoid movements (occasionally); kyphosis; lordosis.

Signs. Height and weight of kyphotic, lordotic infant and child in the lowest percentile. Retinitis pigmentosa; muscular atrophy; signs of malabsorption. Neuropathy involvement signs; ataxia; absence of deep reflexes.

Etiology. Autosomal recessive inheritance. Altered synthesis of ApoB or altered intracellular conjunction of ApoB with lipid.

Pathology. Intestinal mucosa normal length and shape; many lipid droplets in the cells; no lipid in submucosa and lamina propria. Liver fatty infiltration without hepatomegaly; loss of myelin in the nerves. (All data obtained from biopsies.)

Diagnostic Procedures. *Blood.* Appearance and composition of red cells are part of the characteristic of this syndrome. Red cells thorny (acanthocyte); look like crenated cells. Increased susceptibility to mechanical trauma, increased rate of destruction in lysolecithin test. Normal serum does not modify their shape and normal cells are not affected by patient's serum. With Twin solution 80% of the cells revert to normal aspect. Abnormal biochemical composition of their membrane. Blood lipids. Beta-lipoprotein absent; cholesterol low; triglycerides low, total phospholipids low; lecithin and sphingomyelin increased. No chylomicrons, VLDL and LDL. *Stool.* High content of fat; [131]I Triolein study shows decreased absorption; normal xylose, and B_{12} absorption tests. *X-ray.* Usually not diagnostic; from normal to gross alterations. *Biopsy of jejunum.* See Pathology (pathognomonic).

Therapy. Specific therapy is not available; large supplements of vitamins A, D, E, and K are advised. Massive doses of vitamin E (100 mg/kg/24 hr) may arrest neurological and retinal degeneration. Long-chain fat intake must be eliminated; medium-chain triglycerides can be used in the diet. Treatment of hemolysis not required.

Prognosis. Progression of neurologic and ophthalmic symptoms.

BIBLIOGRAPHY. Bassen FA, Kornzweig AL: Malformation of erythrocytes in a case of atypical retinitis pigmentosa. Blood 5:381–387, 1950
Hardman DA, Pullinger CR, Hamilton RL, et al: Molecular and metabolic basis for the metabolic disorder normotriglyceridemic abetalipoproteinrmia. J Clin Invest 88:1722–1729, 1991
Schettler G, Habenicht AJR (eds): Principles and treatment of lipoprotein disorders. New York, Springer, 1994

BATEMAN

Synonyms. Corticosteroid purpura; cushingoid purpura; death blossoms; cachectic purpura; purpura senilis; steroid purpura.

Symptoms and Signs. In old (Bateman) or debilitated (cachectica) people, after prolonged corticosteroid administration, or in person with Cushing syndrome (steroid). Small petechiae and hematomas, especially on forearm and back of hands (1–4 cm in diameter).

Etiology. Shearing injury of dermal vessels from hypermobility, due to lack of fixation by tissues, especially in areas of prolonged actinic exposure.

Pathology. Atrophy of skin; lack of subcutaneous fat; petecchieae and hematomas.

Diagnostic Procedures. *Blood.* Clotting normal; platelets normal.

Therapy. None of proven value.

Prognosis. Hematomas persist for weeks and leave brown pigmentation.

BIBLIOGRAPHY. Bateman T: Delineations of Cutaneous Disease Exhibiting the Characteristic Appearances of the Principle Genera and Species Comprised in the Classification of the Late Dr. Willan, and Completing the Series of Engravings Begun by that Author. London, Longman, 1817
Bithell TC: Bleeding disorders caused by vascular abnormalities. In Lee GR, Bithel TC, Foerster J, et al (eds): Wintrobe's Clinical Hematology, 9th ed, p 1384. Philadelphia, Lea & Febiger, 1993

BATTEN

Synonyms. Batten-Mayou.

Symptoms. Used to indicate the Jansky-Bielchowsky (see) and the Spielmeyer-Vogt (type 2 and 3 of ceroid lipofuscidosis).

BIBLIOGRAPHY. Batten FE: Cerebral degeneration with symmetrical changes in the maculae in two members of a family. Trans Opthalmol Soc UK 23:386–390, 1903
Mayou MS: Cerebral degeneration, with symmetrical changes in the maculae, in three members of a family. Tr Ophth Soc UK 24:142–145, 1904
Adams RD, Victor M: Principles of Neurology, 5th ed, p 832. New York, McGraw-Hill, 1993

BATTEN-TURNER

Synonyms. BTMD; benign congenital muscular dystrophy; muscular dystrophy, congenital benign.

Symptoms. Onset in both sexes in early childhood. Floppiness and frequent falling and stumbling. Slight delay on reaching milestones or early motor development; normal walking; somewhat handicapped in physical exercises.

Signs. Mild weakness of muscles more pronounced on pelvic girdle, neck flexors, and shoulder girdle; absence of contractures and pseudo-hypertrophy.

Etiology. Unknown; hereditary transmission compatible with autosomal recessive pattern; no definite conclusion has been reached, however. Possibly belongs in the group of intermediate and late onset forms of spinal muscular atrophy in childhood.

Pathology. Muscle biopsy shows dystrophic changes that differ from more common type of muscular dystrophy with respect to endomysial fibrosis, degeneration, and regeneration.

Diagnostic Procedures. *Electromyography. Blood.* Serum glutamic-oxaloacetic transaminase (SGOT); creatine kinase; lactic dehydrogenase; aldolase markedly increased. *Biopsy of muscle.*

Therapy. Symptomatic.

Prognosis. Very good; muscular deficiency minimal; stationary and frequently well compensated.

BIBLIOGRAPHY. Batten FE: Three cases of myopathy, infantile type. Brain 26:147–148, 1903
Turner JWA: On amyotonia congenita. Brain 72:25–34, 1949
Zellweger H, Afifi A, McCormick WF, et al: Benign congenital muscular dystrophy: a special form of congenital hypotonia. Clin Pediatr (Phila) 6:655–663, 1967
Adams RD, Victor M: Principles of Neurology, 5th ed, p 1248. New York, McGraw-Hill, 1993

BATTERED BUTTOCK

Synonyms. Fat fracture; traumatic lipoma. See Cluneal nerve.

Symptoms and Signs. Rare. Reported only in females. Aching and tenderness occurring early or late in areas of the buttocks after blunt trauma. Local deformity with a swelling or retraction.

Etiology. Trauma of the buttocks, following different types of accidents.

Pathology. The fat compartments are burst open, with rupture of the septa and shearing off of the anchorage between the skin and deep fascia. Local vascular damage; varying amount of bruising and different sizes of hematoma. Traumatic lipoma formation, after retraction, of detached subcutaneous tissue into the buttock or thigh. Tissue defect above reabsorbed hematoma, and fat swelling below.

Diagnostic Procedures. *Biopsy.*

Therapy. Surgical repair or excision.

Prognosis. In children, swelling may recede with general body growth. In adults, deformity is permanent. Correction of deformity by wide excision gives good results with complete relief of tenderness and pain.

BIBLIOGRAPHY. Meggitt BF, Wilson JN: The battered buttock syndrome-fat fractures. Br J Surg 59:165–169, 1972

BATTERED CHILD

Synonyms. Child abuse; maltreatment of children.

Symptoms and Signs. Bruises confined to the buttocks and lower back; lash marks; traumatic alopecia; bruises and scars, at various stages of healing, over the foreminences; petechiae; burns; subdural hematoma leading to coma, convulsions, and increased intracranial pressure; intra-abdominal injuries, most commonly ruptured liver or spleen. Mental retardation.

Etiology. Maltreatment of children by their parents, guardians, or other caretakers.

Pathology. Hematomas, scars, burns, welts.

Diagnostic Procedures. *X-rays.* Fractures, cortical thickening; sub-periosteal ossification.

Therapy. Institutionalization of the child; proper therapy of the various lesions; psychological help for the family.

Prognosis. The family can be rehabilitated to adequate care of the child only with intensive and comprehensive treatment.

BIBLIOGRAPHY. Green AH: Child maltreatment: recent studies and future directions. J Child. Psychiatr 23:675–678, 1984
Speight N: ABC of child abuse: nonaccidental injury. Br Med J 298:879–881, 1989
Kennedy CTC: Reactions to mechanical and thermal injury. In Champion RH, Burton JL, Ebling FJG (eds): Rook/Wilkinson/Ebling Textbook of Dermatology, 5th ed, pp 818–820. Oxford, Blackwell Scientific, 1992

BAUER

Synonyms. Brachydactyly type A3; brachydactyly—clinodactyly; brachymesophalangy V.

Symptoms and Signs. More frequent in females. Shortening of the middle phalanx of fifth finger with clinodactyly.

Etiology. Autosomal dominant inheritance.

BIBLIOGRAPHY. Bauer B: Eine bischer nicht beobachtete kongenitale, hereditaere Anomalie des Fingerskelettes. Dtsch Z kir 86:252–259, 1907
Herzog KP: Shortened fifth medial phalanges. Am J Phys Anthrop 27:113–118, 1967

BAYFORD-AUTENRIETH

Synonyms. Arkin; dysphagia lusoria.

Symptoms and Signs. Appears in newborn or in infants. Difficulty in swallowing.

Etiology. Abnormal right subclavian artery (especially if originating distal to aorta coarctation) pressing on the esophagus.

Therapy. Surgery.

Prognosis. Good.

BIBLIOGRAPHY. Bayford D: An account on a singular case of obstructed deglutition. Mem Med Soc London 2:271–282, 1789
Autenrieth, Pfleiderer: De Dysphagia lusoria. Arch Physiol Halle 7:145–188, 1807
Mok CK, Cheung KL, Kong SM, et al: Translocating the aberrant right subclavian artery in dysphagia lusoria. Br J Surg 66:113–116, 1979
Perloff JK: The Clinical Recognition of Congenital Heart Disease, 4th ed, p 138. Philadelphia, WB Saunders, 1994

BAZELON

Synonyms. Lesch-Nyhan variant.

Symptoms and Signs. Females affected. Mental retardation; mutilation of lips and hands; absence of choreoathetosis; spasticity or severe growth retardation.

Etiology. Unknown.

Diagnostic Procedures. *Blood.* Hyperuricemia. Erythrocytes: hypoxanthine-guanine-phosphoribosyl transferase (HGPRT) normal. *Urine.* Normal uric acid excretion.

Prognosis. Unknown.

BIBLIOGRAPHY. Bazelon M, Stevens H, Davis M, et al: Mental retardation, self mutilation and hyperuricemia in female. Trans Am Neurol Assoc 93:187–188, 1968

BAZEX I

Synonyms. Follicular atrophoderma; basal cell carcinoma.

Symptoms and Signs. Present from birth. Both sexes. Occasionally facial eczema shortly after birth. Follicular atrophoderma affecting dorsa of hands and feet ("multiple ice pick marks"), occasionally affecting also the exterior surfaces of the lower back. From adolescence multiple basal cell carcinoma of the face. Occasionally associated hypohidrosis (facial or generalized); sparse hair.

Etiology. Unknown. Autosomal dominant inheritance. Possibility of X-linked inheritance reported in one family.

Pathology. Skin biopsy. No true atrophy, but deep and lax follicular hostia of follicles. Basal cells carcinoma resembles melanocitic nevi.

BIBLIOGRAPHY. Bazex A, Dupe A, Chirstol B: Genodermatose complexe de type indetermine associant une hypothricose un etat atrophodermique generalisé et des degenerescences cutanées multiples (epitheliomas-basocellulaires). Bull Soc Fr Derm Syph 71:206, 1964
Gould DJ, Barker DJ: Follicular atrophoderma with multiple basal cell carcinomas (Bazex). Brit J Dermatol 99:431–435, 1986

Harper J: Genetics and genodermatoses. In Champion RH, Burton JL, Ebling FJG (eds): Rook/Wilkinson/Ebling Textbook of Dermatology, 5th ed, pp 333–334. Oxford, Blackwell Scientific, 1992

BAZEX-GRIFFITH

Synonyms. Bazex II; acrokeratosis paraneoplastica.

Symptoms and Signs. Strong prevalence in men. Skin changes develop slowly, often in phases. Hyperkeratotic psoriasisform plaques on hand, feet, nose, ears. Nail thick and fragile, lesions may spread to proximal upper respiratory limbs and trunk. Neoplasia of upper respiratory tract or adenocarcinoma of various other organs. Enlargement of nodes in cervical and submaxillary areas.

Etiology. In the spectra of paraneoplastic syndromes.

Pathology. Not diagnostic dermatitis with inflammatory changes, hyper and parakeratosis.

Therapy. That of primary malignancy.

Prognosis. That of primary malignancy.

BIBLIOGRAPHY. Barriere H: Les dermatoses para-neoplastiques. Ann Med Interne (Paris) 126:177–181, 1979
Bazex A, Griffith WA: Acrokeratosis paraneoplastica: new cutaneous marker of malignancy. Br J Dermatol. 103:301–306, 1980
Pecora AL, Landsman L, Imgrund SP, et al: Acrokeratosis paraneoplastica (Bazex's syndrome): report of a case and review of literature. Arch Dermatol 119:820–826, 1983
Weismann K, Graham RM: Systemic disease and the skin. In Champion RH, Burton JL, Ebling FJG (eds): Rook/Wilkinson/Ebling Textbook of Dermatology, 5th ed, pp 2418–2419. Oxford, Blackwell Scientific, 1992

BAZIN

Synonyms. Erythema induratum; nodular vasculitis; see Whitfield.

Symptoms and Signs. Predominant in women. Chronic and persistent nodular and indurative lesions evolving with the formation of deep ulcers. Affects calves of legs (rather than lower parts, as in Pernio syndrome) during winter months. Lesion may also be observed on arms and breasts. Usually lesions improve, but do not clear completely, during the summer.

Etiology. Tuberculid that affects the backs of legs with perniotic circulation.

Pathology. Nonspecific granuloma, as well as tubercular granuloma with caseation and varying degree of vasculitis and foreign body giant cells reaction. Fibrosis at later stage. Vascular changes may dominate with the exclusion of granulomatous lesions.

Diagnostic Procedures. *Biopsy. Tuberculin skin test. X-ray of thorax.*

Therapy. If tuberculosis or other etiology proved, specific treatment.

Prognosis. Chronic persistent condition. Spontaneous remissions and relapses frequent.

BIBLIOGRAPHY. Bazin APE: Leçons théoriques et cliniques sur la scrofule, considérée en ellemême et dans ses rapports avec la syphilis. La Dartre et L'arthritis, 2nd ed, p 668. Paris, A Delahaye, 1861
Savin R: Mycobacterial infections. In Champion RH, Burton JL, Ebling FJG (eds): Rook/Wilkinson/Ebling Textbook of Dermatology, 5th ed, p 1053. Oxford, Blackwell Scientific, 1992

BAZZANA

Synonyms. Ophthalmoauricular angiospastic; deafness—ophthalmic.

Symptoms. Otosclerosis with progressive deafness. In early stage, attacks of visual field defect; then permanent concentric contraction.

Signs. Trophic alteration of auditory meatus; vasospasm of retina vessels (during attacks).

Etiology. Unknown.

Prognosis. Progressive deafness and visual field contraction.

BIBLIOGRAPHY. Bazzana EC, Lombardo LE, Montanelli M: Otosclerosi e campo visivo. Arch Ital Otol Rinol Lar 61:620–628, 1950
Roy FH: Ocular Syndromes and Systemic Diseases. Orlando, FL, Grune & Stratton, 1985

BEALS I

Synonym. Auriculo-osteodysplasia.

Symptoms. Both sexes affected. Slight limitation of elbow motion. In some patients, limping.

Signs. Elbow dysplasia (characteristic): from mild dysplasia to dislocation, either anterior or posterior. Bilateral, often asymmetric. Hip dysplasia (occasional): bilateral only in female members of affected family. Other skeletal features: torso of masculine appearance; broad shoulders; wide muscular base of the neck; horizontal clavicles; scapular prominence; short metacarpals in some patients. Nails, teeth, and hair normal. Auricular dysplasia; elongation of lobe accompanied by a small posterior lobule. Short stature (consistently) below 50th percentile in height.

Etiology. Unknown; autosomal dominant inheritance.

Pathology. Chrondroectodermal dysplasia.

Therapy. Intermittent bracing in extension and supination to prevent posterior dislocation.

Prognosis. Good; posterior dislocation results in major disability; anterior dislocation in a minor degree of disability.

BIBLIOGRAPHY. Beals RK: Auriculo-osteodysplasia, a syndrome of multiple osseous dysplasia, ear anomaly, and short stature. J Bone Joint Surg (AM) 49:1541–1550, 1967
McKusick VA: Mendelian Inheritance in Man, 10th ed. Baltimore, Johns Hopkins Univ Press, 1992

BEALS-HECHT

Synonyms. Beals II; arachnodactyly Beals; contractural arachnodactyly. See Marfan syndrome.

Symptoms and Signs. Both sexes affected, present from birth. Facies. Micrognathia. Ears: "crumpled," poor conchae; prominent crura. Short neck. Long extremities. Multiple joint contractures most obvious in the hands (tending to improve with age) arachnodactily, dolichostenomelia, kyphoscoliosis, abnormalities external ears. Usually absence of cardiovascular or ocular manifestations.

Etiology. Autosomal dominant inheritance. Considered in the recent past as a mild phenotype of Marfan now genetically distinct since linked to a different fibrillin locus.

Diagnostic Procedures. *X-Rays. CT Scan, MRI.* Bones slight ostopenia; gracile bones; bowing of long bones; elongation of proximal phalanges hands and feet. Occasionally: vertebral malformations; kyphoscoliosis and consequent thoracic constriction and restrictive disease of lungs; esophageal and duodenal atresia; miltral valve prolapse.

Therapy. Orthopedic.

Prognosis. Spontaneous gradual improvement of articular limitation. Kyphoscoliosis usually progressive.

BIBLIOGRAPHY. Epstein CJ, et al: Hereditary dysplasia of bone with kypho-scoliosis, contractures, and abnormally shaped ears. J Ped 73:379–386, 1968

Beals RK, Hecht F: Delineation of another heritable disorder of connective tissue. J Bone Joint Surg 53:987–993, 1971

Hecht F, Beals RK: "New" syndrome of congenital contractural arachnodactyly originally described by Marfan in 1896. Pediatrics 49:574–579, 1972

Ramos Arroyo MA, Weaver DD, Beals RK: Congenital contractural arachnodactyly: report of four additional families and review of literature. Clin Genet 27:570–581, 1985

Bawle E, Quigg MH: Ectopia lentis and aortic root dilatation in congenital contractural arachnodactyly. Am J Med Genet 42:19–21, 1992

BEAN

Synonym. Blue rubber—bleb nevus.

Symptoms and Signs. Both sexes affected; onset in early childhood. Appearance of one or many (hundreds) blue, small, rubbery subcutaneous nodules. Easily compressible and promptly refilling after compression. They vary in color, size, shape, and number and may be tender. Recurrent melena; pallor. Nocturnal pain and regional hyperhidrosis. Subconjunctival hemangioma with overlying fibrosis; hemorrhagic lesion near macula. Variable neurological manifestations.

Etiology. Unknown; autosomal dominant inheritance.

Pathology. Cavernous type hemangioma in the skin (legs and trunk most affected areas) and intestinal wall (small intestine more affected than distal; then colon). Occasionally present in spleen, liver, and central nervous system.

Diagnostic Procedures. *X-ray.* Bowel: single or multiple polypoid filling defects; phlebolith. *Angiography.* Visceral hemoangiomas. *MRI. CT scan.* Head hemangioma, calcification, thrombosis, brain atrophy. *Blood.* Anemia when bleeding occurs.

Therapy. Symptomatic; correction of anemia. Surgery with resection of intestine in repeated or uncontrollable bleeding. Some severe cases required amputation of limbs affected by angiomatous gigantism.

BIBLIOGRAPHY. Gaskoyen: Case of naevus involving the parotid gland, and causing death from suffocation: naevi of the viscere. Trans Path Soc London 11:267, 1860

Bean WW: Vascular Spiders and Related Lesions of the Skin. Springfield, IL, Charles C Thomas, 1958

Oranje AP: Blue rubber bleb nevus syndrome. Pediatr Dermatol 3:304–310, 1986

Atherton DJ: Naevi and other developmental defects. In Champion RH, Burton JL, Ebling FJG (eds): Rook/Wilkinson/Ebling Textbook of Dermatology, 5th ed, pp 500–501. Oxford, Blackwell Scientific, 1992

BEARD

Synonym. Neuroasthenic neurosis.

Symptoms. Both sexes affected, predominant in women especially, in the fourth or fifth decade (information to be reconsidered with modern change in life and modern version of this neurosis). Onset gradual or sudden. Precipitating factors frequently reported by the patient as overwork, emotional strain, progressive infection, or other pathologic conditions. Beard reports 50 symptoms and signs that have been grouped in the following categories: variable muscular spasms and body aches; autonomic nervous system involvement (discharge); heavy limbs and tiredness; phobic neurosis; hopelessness; insomnia; group of miscellaneous complaints, which may represent the temporary or permanent focus of distress (i.e., dyspepsia; impotence). Patients appear tired, apathetic; accomplish all movements with great effort and keep seeking relief from symptoms.

Etiology. Unknown. Various hypotheses according to schools of psychiatry.

Therapy. Psychological evaluation to establish the need for mental manipulation or pharmacological treatment.

Prognosis. Episodic recurrence or unremitting long period or chronic status.

BIBLIOGRAPHY. Beard GM: Neuroasthenia or nervous exhaustion. Boston Med Surg J 80:217–221, 1869

Kaplan HI, Sadock BJ: Comprehensive Textbook of Psychiatry, 6th ed, p 1206. Baltimore, Williams & Wilkins, 1995

BEARE-STEVENSON CUTIS GYRATUM

Synonyms. Beare-Dodge-Nevin; cutis gyratum Beare-Stevenson.

Symptoms and Signs. Both sexes. From birth:clover leaf skull, hypertelorism, cleft palate; palms and soles and/or facial skin and/or axilla and/or perineum; cutis gyratrum; acanthosis nigricans; scrotum bifidum, large umbilical stump. Occasionally craniosynostosis.

Etiology. Unknown. Sporadic.

BIBLIOGRAPHY. Beare JM, Dodge JA, Nevin NC: Cutis gyratum, acanthosis nigricans and other congenital anomalies. A new syndrome. Br J Derm 81:241–247, 1969

Stevenson RE, Ferlanto GJ, Taylor HA: Cutis gyratum and acanthosis nigricans associated with other anomalies: a distinct syndrome. J Pediat 92:950–952, 1978

Pachinger W, Hong D: Zum Krankheitsbild der Cutis verticis gyrata. Z Hantkr 56:275–280, 1981

Gorlin RJ, Cohen MM Jr, Levin LS: Syndromes of Head and Neck, pp 542–544. New York, Oxford Univ Press, 1990

BEARN-KÜNKEL-SLATER

Synonyms. CALH; Künkel; hepatitis lupoid, lupoid hepatitis; hypergammaglobulinemic hepatitis; plasma cell hepatitis; hepatitis chronic active; autoimmune chronic active heparititis; juvenile active cirrhosis.

Symptoms. Prevalent in females, insidious onset usually at puberty; however, may affect anyone from childhood to old age. Asthenia; amenorrhea or menstrual irregularities; epistaxis and gingivorrhagia; hepatalgia; arthralgia; recurrent idiopathic fever episodes; respiratory distress. Later, hematemesis.

Signs. Hirsutism; acne; striae; spider telangiectases; moon facies; obesity; hepatosplenomegaly; jaundice. Later, ascites.

Etiology. Unknown; autoimmmunity (?); variant of lupus erythematosis (?). Immune complex formation and deposition in tissues.

Pathology. Hepatomegaly; from portal fibrosis, to extensive fibrosis (nodular fibro-cirrhosis); marked plasma cells infiltration.

Diagnostic Procedures. *Blood.* Aminotransferase: over five times upper normal limit; Hypergammaglobulinemia (s-IgG 15. 0 g/l); biologic fixative reaction for rheumatoid arthritis (25%); presence of antinuclear antibodies (75%); positive latex reaction for smooth muscle IgG antibodies (90%). Markers for hepatitis. *Biopsy of liver.* See Pathology. Sodium sulfobromophthalein retention.

Therapy. Steroids and immunosuppressants. If indicated, liver transplantation.

Prognosis. Within 10 years of onset, liver insufficiency, bleeding esophageal varices, coma, death. With treatment survival rate improves dramatically. Liver fibrosis may subside, nodular fibrosis/cirrhosis may resolve, especially if treatment is started early.

BIBLIOGRAPHY. Bearn AG, Künkel HG, Slater RJ: The problem of chronic liver disease in young women. Am J Med 21:3–15, 1956

Schvarcz R, Glaumann H, Weiland O: Survival and histological resolution of fibrosis in patients with autoimmune chronic active hepatitis. J Hepatol 18:15–23, 1993

BEAT KNEE

Synonyms. Prepatellar bursitis; carpet layer, coal miner. See also Housemaid knee.

Symptoms and Signs. (1) *Acute.* Local pain, swelling, tenderness. (2) *Chronic.* Chronic distention of one of the prepatellar bursae, usually the one over tibial tubercle. (3) *Infective.* Local wound, abrasion, or swelling (secondary infection of pre-existing bursitis) with all signs of infection.

Etiology. (1)Unaccustomed work involving kneeling or trauma. (2) Long period of kneeling. (3) Direct or indirect infection of bursa.

Pathology. (1) Effusion of serous fluid. (2) Chronic effusion; hemorrhages; loose bodies; adhesions; calcifications. (3) Formation of pus.

Diagnostic Procedures. *X-ray of knee. Prepatellar tap.*

Therapy. (1) Elastic compression; if great pain, aspirate. (2) Use of protecting knee pads; in some cases surgery. (3) Bed rest, systemic antibiotics, or injection into bursa. If suppuration, establish drainage. Fibrosis and synovial thickening with painful nodules do not respond to treatment. Excision of the bursae.

Prognosis. Varies according to extent of lesion and prevention of further damage.

BIBLIOGRAPHY. Smillie LS: Injuries of the Knee Joint, 4th ed. Baltimore, Williams & Wilkins, 1962

Insall JN, Windsor RE, Scott WN, et al (ed): Surgery of the Knee. New York, Churchill Livingstone, 1993

BECKER-REUTER

Synonyms. Becker (SW) I.

Symptoms. Reported in females; appears in early infancy. Asymptomatic.

Signs. On the neck and forearms, presence of discrete or confluent brown macules. Absence of telangiectasias and atrophic changes.

Etiology. Unknown.

BIBLIOGRAPHY. Becker S, Reuter MJ: Familial pigmentary anomaly. Arch Dermatol Syph 40:987–998, 1939

Bleehen SS, Ebling FJG, Champion RH: In Champion RH, Burton JL, Ebling FJG (eds): Rook/Wilkinson/Ebling Textbook of Dermatology, 5th ed, p 1585. Oxford, Blackwell Scientific, 1992

BECKER (P.E.)

Synonyms. Duchenne late type; benign Duchenne muscular dystrophy, BMD; pseudohypertrophic muscular hypertrophy; muscular dystrophy, progressive, tardive.

Symptoms and Signs. Duchenne muscular dystrophy syndrome with later onset (from childhood to early adulthood), and slower rate of progression; pelvic femor involvement (tendency to toe walking) and later pectoral girdle; greater enlargement of calves during adolescence or young adulthood. Muscle pain with exercise is a marked feature. Frequently associated with color blindness. Slight cardiac involvement; normal mental development.

Etiology. Sex-linked recessive inheritance.

Pathology. Muscle biopsy show some differences from Duchenne. More numerous internal nuclei and distinction between type I and type II fibers is quite clear.

Diagnostic Procedures. See Duchenne. Moderate elevation of CK level.

Therapy. Less requirement of orthopedic surgery than in Duchenne.

Prognosis. Longer survival (over fourth decade) and less impairment than Duchenne. Same cause of death; cardiac failure and skeletal disease.

BIBLIOGRAPHY. Becker PE: Eine neue X-chromosomale muskeldystrophie. Acta Psychiat Nervenkr Scand 193:427–448, 1955

Becker PE: Neue ergebnisse der genetik der muskeldystrophien. Acta Genet 7:303–310, 1957

Worton RG, Brooke MH: The X-linked muscular dystrophies. In Scriver CR, Beaudet AL, Sly WS, et al: The Metabolic and Molecular Bases of Inherited Disease, 7th ed, p 4198. New York, McGraw-Hill, 1995

BECKER (S.W.) II

Synonym. Pigmented hairy epidermal nevus; melanosis Becker.

Symptoms. Common condition. All races, both sexes affected; prevalent in young men. May become evident or conspicuous on exposure to sunlight.

Signs. Appearance of irregular pigmentation on shoulder, chest, less frequently in other areas, which spreads to the size of about 20 cm in diameter by confluence of irregular spots, assuming a geographic map aspect. Dark heavy hairs may grow in and around the pigmentated area 1 or 2 years later.

Etiology. Unknown.

Pathology. Minimal changes from normal skin pattern. Central area of lesion may show thickening and elongation of ridges and dermal papillae.

Therapy. None. Cosmetic masking.

Prognosis. Benign lesion.

BIBLIOGRAPHY. Becker SW: Diagnosis and treatment of pigmented nevi. Arch Dermatol Syph 60:44–65, 1949

Atherton DJ: Naevi and other developmental defects. In Champion RH, Burton JL, Ebling FJG (eds): Rook/Wilkinson/Ebling Textbook of Dermatology, 5th ed, p 462. Oxford, Blackwell Scientific, 1992

BECK-IBRAHIM

Synonyms. Candidiasis; moniliasis; cutaneous anergy. Mucocutaneous dysplasia; including familial, chronic, mucocutaneous candidiasis, dominant and recessive type. See also Multiple Endocrine Deficiency.

Symptoms. Cutaneous anergy. Symmetric crusted lesions of skin about the mouth, nose, neck, ears, perineum, buttocks, groin.

Signs. Paronychia with redness and swelling at the base of fingernails and toes. Arrested growth; change of color of hair to white, then alopecia; thrush of mouth. Normal appetite; no diarrhea. Chronic cutaneous fungal infection.

Etiology. Unknown. (1) Late onset form nongenetic type. (2) Early infancy (a) recessive inheritance: relationship to ferritin and/or myeloperoxidase alteration; (b) autosomal dominant: immunodeficiencies (see Diagnostic Procedures).

Diagnostic Procedures. *Cultures from mouth and stool.* For fungi. Monilia, Candida intradermal skin tests; markedly decreased. Contact sensitization. 2,4–dinitro-1–chlorobenzene (DNCB); 2,4–dinitro-1–

fluorobenzene (DNFB) markedly decreased; sensitization by transfer of lymphocytes: absent. *Lymphocytic stimulation with phytohemagglutinin.* Positive; normal lymphocyte count. *Rejection of skin homografts.* Decreased. *Circulating antibody level.* Normal. *Resistance to systemic infection.* Normal. In autosomal dominant form: candida skin test positive and lymphocyte transformation normal under 2 years of age; negative at older age.

Therapy. Systemic and topical Amphotericin, Nystatin, Natamycin, Flucytosine, Ketoconazole. Topical application of alkaline and gentian violet solutions.

Prognosis. Recurrence of skin lesions and alopecia with intermittent regrowth of hair. Dwarfism.

BIBLIOGRAPHY. Beck SC: Ueber das Erythema mycoticum infantile. Derm Stud Unna Ftschr 1:494, 1910

Ibrahim J: Ueber eine Soormykose der Haut im fruhen Saeugligsalter. Arch Kinderheilkcl 55:91–101, 1911

Schultz FW: Two cases of thrush with unusual symptoms and skin manifestations. Am J Dis Child 29:283, 1925

Sams WM Jr, Jorisso JL, Snyderman R, et al: Chronic mucocutaneous candidiasis: immunologic studies of three generations of a single family. Am J Med 67:948–959, 1979

Hay RJ, Roberts SOB, Mackenzie DWR: Mycology. In Champion RH, Burton JL, Ebling FJG (eds): Rook/Wilkinson/Ebling Textbook of Dermatology, 5th ed, pp 1191–1195. Oxford, Blackwell Scientific, 1992

BECK

Synonyms. Davison; anterior spinal artery occlusion; hemianesthetic hemiplegia; medullary; myelomalacia.

Symptoms. Syndrome may follow trauma. Onset sudden, apoplectiform; sometimes symptoms preceded by pain and paresthesias. Vary according to site of lesion.

1. Occlusion of anterior spinal artery of medulla oblongata (Davison): flaccid quadriplegia, loss of discriminative sensation below level of lesion.
2. Occlusion of branches that supply paramedian area of medulla: homolateral paralysis of tongue and contralateral paralysis of arm and leg with altered tactile sensation.
3. Occlusion at thoracolumbar level: muscular atrophy (segmental) and spastic paralysis of legs; occasionally unilateral with contralateral sensory loss; dissociated sensory loss below the lesion.
4. Occlusion of vessels of lower spinal cord: flaccid paralysis of legs with dissociated sensory changes.

Signs. Abolished reflexes of part involved; sensory changes; vibratory and position sense conserved; coldness of skin.

Etiology. Thrombosis (most frequent); neoplastic or other cause occluding vessel; infection; syphilis; atherosclerosis; coarctation of aorta; trauma.

Pathology. Occlusion of artery; softening of spinal cord in zones on anterior horns, anterior half of cord, pyramidal tract, and spinothalamic tracts; myelomalacia and little glial reaction of zone involved.

Diagnostic Procedures. *Cerebrospinal fluid.* Normal or slightly xanthochromic; proteins may be increased. *CT scan. MRI.*

Therapy. Anticoagulants or as indicated by etiology. Control of infections and rehabilitation of bladder.

Prognosis. Variable.

BIBLIOGRAPHY. Spiller WG: Thrombosis of the cervical anterior median spinal artery; syphilitic acute anterior polymyelitis. J Nerv Ment Dis 36:601–613, 1909

Beck K: Das Syndrom des Verschusses der verderen Spinalarterie. Dtsch Z Nervenh 167:164–186, 1951–1952

Johnson JR, Leatherman KD, Holt RT: Anterior decompression of the spinal cord for neurologic deficit. Spine 8:396–405, 1983

Adams RD, Victor M: Principles of Neurology, 5th ed, p 1096. New York, McGraw-Hill, 1993

BECKWITH-WIEDEMANN

Synonyms. BWS; Wiedemann-Beckwith; exomphalos—macroglossia—gigantism, EMG; neonatal hypoglycemia—visceromegaly—macroglossia—microcephaly.

Symptoms. Occurs in newborn; 60% females. Lethargy and poor feeding developing within the first 2 or 3 days after birth; clonic seizures (controlled by intravenous injection of glucose). Elements of congestive heart failure.

Signs. Somatic gigantism at birth, hemihypertrophy or developing postnatally; macroglossia; transverse linear creases of ear lobule; mild microcephaly; hepatomegaly (not essential feature); omphalocele or umbilical hernia; bilateral noncystic renal hyperplasia; cryptorchidism.

Etiology. Unknown. Sporadic; autosomal dominant inheritance reported. Alteration chromosome 11p15 locus.

Pathology. *Kidney.* Immaturity of renal tubules; glomeruli closely packed and normal maturity for infant age. *Liver and muscle.* Biopsy normal. *Pancreas.* Hypertrophy. *Bone marrow.* Normal. *Gonads.* Interstitial cell hyperplasia. *Pituitary.* Amphophilic hyperplasia. *Adrenal glands.* Fetal adrenocortical cytomegaly. Occasionally (20% risk) development of Wilms tumor, adrenal cortical carcinomas, hepatoblastomas, rabdomyosarcomas.

Diagnostic Procedures. *Blood.* Hypoglycemia; normal galactose tolerance test; polycythemia (nonspecific, perhaps secondary to hypoglycemia). *X-ray.* Accelerated bone maturation; metaphysical flaring and overconstriction of diaphyses.

Therapy. Zinc glucagon; cortisone; diazoxide useful to relieve hypoglycemia. Surgical repair of omphalocele, partial resection of tongue to diminish respiratory tract occlusion.

Prognosis. Infant death rate approximately 21%, resulting from congestive heart failure or caused by severe malformation; association (7.5%) with various neoplasias (especially Wilms tumor). Otherwise normal growth.

BIBLIOGRAPHY. Beckwith JB, Wang CI, Donnell GN, et al: Hyperplastic fetal visceromegaly with macroglossia, omphalocele, cytomegaly of adrenal fetal cortex, postnatal somatic gigantism and other abnormalities: Newly recognized syndrome (Abst no 41). Proc Am Pediatr Soc, Seattle, June 16–18, 1964

Wiedemann, HR: Complexe malformatif familial avec hernie ombelicale et macroglossiè–un syndrome nouveau. J Genet Hum 13:223–363, 1964

Pettenati MJ, Haines JL, Higgins RR, et al: Wiedemann-Beckwith syndrome: Presentation of clinical and cytogenetic data on 22 new cases and review of the literature. Hum Genet 74:143–154, 1986

Carlin ME, Escobar LF, Ward RE, et al: A reassessment of Beckwith-Wiedemann syndrome (BWS). Am J Hum Genet 47:(Suppl)A50, 1990

Haber DA, Housman DE: Wilms tumor. In Scriver CR, Beaudet AL, Sly WS, et al: The Metabolic and Molecular Bases of Inherited Disease, 7th ed, pp 666–670. New York, McGraw-Hill, 1995

BEDNAR TUMORS

Synonyms. See Darier-Ferrand.

Symptoms and Signs. Lesions of dermatofibrosarcoma protuberans (see Darier-Ferrand) containing melanin.

BIBLIOGRAPHY. Bednar B: Storiform neurofibromas of the skin, pigmented and non pigmented. Cancer 10:368–375, 1957

BEEMER II

Synonyms. Hydrocephalus; cardiac malformation; dense bone.

Symptoms and Signs. From birth. Hydrocephalus, unusual facies: bulbous nose, broad nasal bridge; ambiguous genitalia. Heart signs related to double-outlet right ventricle.

Etiology. Unknown. Autosomic recessive inheritance.

Diagnostic Procedures. *Blood.* Thrombocytopenia. *X-ray.* Dense bone.

Prognosis. Lethal condition.

BIBLIOGRAPHY. Beemer FA, Ertbruggen I: Peculiar facial appearance, hydrocephalus, double-outlet right ventricle, genital anomalies and dense bones with lethal outcome. Am J Med Genet 19:391–394, 1984

BEEMER-LANGER

Synonyms. Short rib syndrome—Beemer; see Majewski (possibly same condition).

Symptoms and Signs. From birth. Both sexes. Hydrops, ascites. Face: median cleft of upper lips. Chest: narrow and short. Limbs: bowed. No polydactyly. Occasional: visceral malformation.

Etiology. Autosomal recessive inheritance. It may represent a clinical variability in SRP type II (see Majewski) rather than a separate disorder.

Diagnostic Procedures. *Ultrasound.* Prenatal diagnosis. *X-rays.* Same as in Majewski with tibia more developed.

Prognosis. Lethal in perinatal stage.

BIBLIOGRAPHY. Beemer FA, Langer LO Jr, Klep-de Pater JM, et al: A new short rib syndrome: Report of two cases. Am J Med Genet 14:115–123, 1983
Winter RM: A lethal short rib syndrome without polydactyly. J Med Genet 25:349–357, 1988
Hennekam R: Short rib syndrome—Beemer type in sibs. AM J Med Genet 40:230–233, 1991

BEER AND COBALT

Synonym. Beer drinker.

Symptoms. Occurs usually in person with no history of heart disease. Severe dyspnea; abdominal pain; edema.

Signs. Cyanosis; enlargement of heart; venous distension; tachycardia; gallop rhythm; hepatomegaly; edema (in some cases massive); hypotension.

Etiology. Occurs in beer drinkers (average 6–12 bottles a day for years). Possibly beer containing cobalt (added to enrich flavor by manufacturers). No new cases after removing beer containing cobalt from the market.

Pathology. *Heart.* Pale; soft; increase in weight; interstitial edema; enlargement of myofibrils and necrosis. *Liver.* Centrilobular necrosis.

Diagnostic Procedures. *Electrocardiography.* Low voltage; enlargement of P waves; flattened T-waves; right axis deviation. *Blood.* Electrolyte study, metabolic acidosis; enzyme studies, lactic dehydrogenase (LDH) and serum glutamic-oxaloacetic transaminase (SGOT) very high level; hematocrit high (58–60%).

Therapy. Treatment of heart failure; thiamine.

Prognosis. Death 50%.

BIBLIOGRAPHY. McDermott PH: Nutritional deficiency in myocardiopathy. Am J Clin Nutr 18:313, 1966
McDermott PH, Delaney RL, Egan JD, et al: Myocardosis and cardiac failure in men. JAMA 198:253–256, 1966
Sullivan J, Parker M, Carson SB: Tissue cobalt content in "beer drinkers' myocardiopathy." J Lab Clin Med 71:893–911, 1968
Regan TJ: Alcohol and nutritional disease. In Schlant RC, Alexander RW: Hurst's The Heart, 8th ed, pp 1943–1948. New York, McGraw-Hill, 1994

BEHR I

Synonym. Optic atrophy—ataxia.

Symptoms. Both sexes affected, optical atrophy prevalent in males. In infants, disturbed vision, disturbed coordination with ataxia; urinary sphincter weakness, mental deficiency. Forme fruste described with only slight optical atrophies developing later in life in members of affected families.

Signs. Temporal atrophy of optic nerve. Nystagmus; tendon hyperreflexia; positive Babinski. Clubfoot.

Etiology. Autosomal recessive inheritance.

Pathology. Bilateral optic atrophy (mainly papillomacular bundles); slight affection of pyramidal bundles, posterior cords, and spinocerebellar pathways.

Therapy. None.

Prognosis. In full syndrome, death may occur in first or second decade. In forme fruste, normal life with only minor visual impairment.

BIBLIOGRAPHY. Behr C: Die komplizierte, hereditärfamiliäre Optikusatrophie des Kindesalters; ein bisher nicht beschriebener Symptomenkomplex. Klin Monatsbl Augenheilkd 47:138–160, 1909
van Leeuwen A, Babel J, Van Bogaert L, et al: Heredoataxies par degenereescence spino-ponto-cerebelleuse; Leurs manifestations retiniennes, optiques et cochleaires. Rev Otoneuroophtalmol 20:1–226, 1948
Thomas PK, Workman JM, Thage O: Behr's syndrome: a family exhibiting pseudodominant inheritance. J Neural Sci 64:137–148, 1984
Klintworth GK: Genetically determined disorders affecting the eye. In Garner A, Klintworth GK (eds): Pathobiology of Ocular Disease: A Dynamic Approach, 2nd ed, p 828. New York, Marcel Dekker, 1994

BEHR II

Synonyms. Macula lutea retinae adult degeneration: (1) macula lutea retinae presenile degeneration; (2) macular senile degeneration. See age-related maculopathy.

Symptoms. (1) Onset about 20 years of age. (2) Onset from 40–90 years of age. Impairment of central vision.

Signs. Central atrophic degeneration with pigmentary changes in and around macula.

Etiology. Unknown; Autosomal dominant or recessive inheritance.

Therapy. Symptomatic.

Prognosis. Progressive condition.

BIBLIOGRAPHY. Behr C: Die Heredodegeneration der Makula. Klin Monatsbl Augenheilkd 69:469–505, 1920
Bradley AE: Dystrophy of the macula. Am J Ophthalmol 61:1–24, 1966
Garner A, Sarks S, Sarks JP: Degenerative and related disorders of the retina and choroid. In Garner A, Klintworth GK (eds): Pathobiology of Ocular Disease: A Dynamic Approach, 2nd ed, p 631. New York, Marcel Dekker, 1994

BEIGHTON

Synonyms. Osteogenesis imperfecta; opalescent teeth—blue sclerae—Wormian bones—absent fractures. See Osteogenesis imperfecta.

Symptoms and Signs. Those of osteogenesis with moderate osteoporosis. Absence of joint hyperextensibility.

Etiology. Autosomal dominant. Possibly the same as osteogenesis imperfecta type I.

Diagnostic Procedures. *X-ray.* In older patients, mild flattening and biconcavity of vertebrae. Wormian bones.

Prognosis. Good.

BIBLIOGRAPHY. Beighton P: Familial dentinogenesis imperfecta, blue sclerae and Wormian bones without fractures: another type of osteogenesis imperfecta? J Med Genet 18:124–128, 1981

BELL

Synonyms. Bell-Lachmung; facial nerve palsy; refrigeration palsy.

Symptoms. Both sexes (equal distribution) all ages and all times of year, higher incidence in diabetic patients. Sometimes following exposure to cold or draft; most cases begin without apparent reason. Onset (usually) slight fever; pain behind ear; stiffness of neck followed by stiffness of one side of face. Acme of paralysis attained in 48 h or slower up to 5 days. Homolateral lacrimation; difficulty with speech; occasionally, peculiar taste in the mouth or loss of taste in ipsilateral side of tongue. Hyperacousis may occur. Bilateral palsy occasionally occurs.

Signs. Forehead cannot be wrinkled; upper eyelids close slowly or partially and eyeballs roll upward and outward when attempting to close the eyes. Change of voice; inability to whistle.

Etiology. Unknown; familial cases reported. Virus suspected but not proved.

Pathology. (Presumed) swelling and hyperemia of nerve sheath or periostium with compression of facial nerve in the facial canal.

Therapy. Thiamine; adrenal corticoids (prednisone 40–60 mg/day during first week); protection of eyes; massage. In permanent paralysis; anastomosis of end of peripheral nerve with spinal accessory (X) or hypoglossal (XII) nerve to restore tone of facial muscles and allow closure of eyes.

Prognosis. Usually, recovery in 1 or 2 months in 80% of cases. Recovery of taste precedes recovery of motor function. In some cases, residual incomplete or permanent paralysis.

BIBLIOGRAPHY. Bell C: On the nerves; giving an account of some experiments on the structure and functions, which lead to a new arrangement of the system. Phil Trans 111:398–424, 1821
Bell C: On the nerves of the face; being a second paper on that subject (reprint). Med Classics 1:155–169, 1936
Malin JP: Nervus facialis. In Schemidt D, Malin JP (eds): Erkrankungen der Hirnnerven 2 Aufl Thieme. Stuttgart, New York, 1991
Adams RD, Victor M: Principles of Neurology, 5th ed, pp 1175–1176. New York, McGraw-Hill, 1993

BENCZE

Synonyms. Hemifacial hyperplasia—strabismus; facial asymmetry; dental articulation derangement. See Plagiocephaly.

Symptoms and Signs. Both sexes. Facial asymmetry; amblyopia; strabismus; submucous cleft palate. Rest of body normal.

Etiology. Autosomal dominant inheritance.

BIBLIOGRAPHY. Bencze J, Schnitzler A, Walawska J: Dominant inheritance of hemifacial hyperplasia associated with strabismus. Oral Surg 35:489–500, 1973
Kurnit D, Hall JG, Schurtleff DB, et al: An autosomal dominant inherited syndrome of facial asymmetry, esotropia, amblyopia and submucous cleft palate (Bencze syndrome). Clin Genet 16:301–304, 1979

BENEDIKT

Synonyms. Mesencephalic tegmental paralysis; tegmentum; red nucleus (complete).

Symptoms. Disturbed vision owing to complete oculomotor paralysis of the affected side; involuntary movements; coarse tremor at rest, increasing amplitude under emotion and motion, so that the latter may not be controlled. The tremor paresis, and hypoesthesia, as well as hemichorea, are contralateral to ocular paralysis, arm alone, or both arm and leg.

Signs. Complete (upward, downward, inward) oculomotor paralysis; ptosis; external strabismus; loss of reflex to light and accommodation. Tremor and hemichorea.

Etiology. Arteriosclerosis, syphilis, or neoplasm occluding vessels and resulting in softening of side of tegmentum with involvement of afferent fibers of cerebellum pedunculus cerebellaris superior as they pass through the red nucleus on the way to the thalamus.

Diagnostic Procedures. *Neurologic, opthalmologic examinations. Serology. EEG. CT scan. MRI.*

Therapy. Symptomatic and etiologic.

Prognosis. Reserved.

BIBLIOGRAPHY. Benedikt M: Tremblement avec paralysie croisée du moteur oculaire commun. Bull Méd (Paris) 3:547–548, 1889
Adams RD, Victor M: Principle of Neurology, p 1173. New York, McGraw-Hill, 1993

BENNETT

Synonyms. Boxer fracture; carpometacarpal thumb ray fracture; thumb fracture—dislocation; stave of thumb.

Symptom. Extreme pain at base of thumb.

Signs. Tenderness, swelling at base of thumb.

Etiology. Forced metacarpal flexion with fracture of anterior lip over carpal bone and backward dislocation of metacarpal.

Therapy. Prompt reduction; if dislocation persists, application of traction, surgical fixation, and protective strapping.

Prognosis. Possible correction of deformity by prompt fixation. If orthopedic intervention, healing in 6 weeks. Residual pain, subluxation, arthropathic degeneration possible.

BIBLIOGRAPHY. Bennett EH: Fractures of the metacarpal bones of the thumb. Dublin J Med Sci 73:72, 1882
Canale ST: Fractures and dislocations in children. In Crenshaw AH (ed): Campbell's Operative Orthopedics, 7th ed, p 1844. St Louis, CV Mosby, 1987
Sabiston DC: Textbook of Surgery, 16th ed, p 1323. Philadelphia, WB Saunders, 1991

BENSON

Synonyms. Asteroid hyalitis; scintillatio albescens; synchysis scintillans.

Symptoms. Occurs in people of advanced age. Asymptomatic or slight impairment of vision.

Signs. On simple inspection, vitreous appears normal. Slit-lamp examination shows presence of small, variously shaped bodies irregularly distributed. On ophthalmoscopy, bodies appear shiny and cream colored.

Etiology. Unknown.

Pathology. Crystal of calcium polynitrate or stearate (or both) deposited in the vitreous.

Therapy. None.

BIBLIOGRAPHY. Benson AH: A case of "monocular asteroid hyalitis." Trans Ophthalmol Soc UK 14:101–104, 1894
Gartner J: Whipple disease of the central nervous system associated with ophthalmoplegia externa and severe asteroid hyalitis: a clinico-pathological study. Doc Ophthal 49:155–187, 1980
Wiard Streeten BA, Wilson DJ: Disorders of vitreous. In Garner A, Klintworth GK (eds): Pathobiology of Ocular Disease: A Dynamic Approach, 2nd ed, p 731. New York, Marcel Dekker, 1994

BERANT-BERANT

Synonyms. Craniosynostosis—radio ulnar synostosis.

Symptoms and Signs. Dolichocephaly (sagittal synostosis). Monolateral or bilateral radioulnar synostosis.

Etiology. Possibly autosomal dominant with variable expressivity.

BIBLIOGRAPHY. Berant M, Berant N: Radioulnar synostosis and cranio synostosis in one family. J Pediatr 83:88–90, 1973

BERDON

Synonyms. Megacystis—microcolon—intestinal hypoperistalsis, MM1H. See Megaduodenum and/or megacystis.

Symptoms and Signs. Prevalent in females. Onset from early age or later. Intestinal hypoperistalsis symptoms (achalasia), constipation and urinary retention.

Etiology. Unknown. Familial cases reported.

Pathology. Degeneration of smooth intestinal muscles and neuronal abnormalities.

Diagnostic Procedures. *Sonography. X-ray. Biopsy.*

Prognosis. Fatal.

BIBLIOGRAPHY. Berdon WE, Baker DH, Blan WA, et al: Megacystis-microcolon-intestinal hypoperistalsis syndrome: a new case of intestinal obstruction in a newborn: report of radiologic findings in five newborn girls. Am J Roentgen 126:957–964, 1976
Redeman JF, Jemenez JF, Golladay ES, et al: Megacystis-microcolon-intestinal hypoperistalsis syndrome: case report and review of literature. J Urol 131:981–983, 1984
Penman DG, Lilford RJ: The megacystis—microcolon—intestinal hypoperistalsis syndrome: a fatal autosomal recessive condition. J Med Gen 26:66–67, 1989

BERENDES-BRIDGE-GOOD

Synonyms. Chronic granulomatous disease, CGD; dysphagocytosis congenital; granulomatosis familial; septic progressive granulomatosis. See Job.

Symptoms and Signs. In males. (Female heterozygotes only presence of intermediate defective leucocyte bacterial capacity.) From birth, sus-

ceptibility to infection. Development of inflammatory masses of characteristic pathology that compress vital organs. Failure to thrive, reticulo-endothelial hyperplasia, hypergammaglobulinemia, anemia. Infections more frequent from Staphylococcus aureus and enteric bacteria, Candida albicans, aspergillus on skin, mucosae, intestinal tract, Candida esophagitis (with stenosis), chronic enteritis and colics, diarrhea, intestinal obstruction from inflammatory masses (especially gastric antrum) hepatosplenomegaly, suppurative lymphadenitis, hepatic and perihepatic abscesses, osteomyelitis of metacarpals and metatarsals common (Serratia marcescens), pneumonia, granulomatous cystitis, pyelonephritis, renal abscesses, meningitis, salmonella septicemia.

Etiology. Failure of respiratory burst of phagocytes. Two inheritance patterns: (1) X-linked (majority of cases) and (2) autosomal recessive. The defect consists in the incapacity of neutrophils to be activated to respiratory burst by normal stimuli.

Pathology. Masses: Hyperplastic, with chronic inflammation with granulocytes. Histiocytes containing pigmented lipid material. Masses consist of granulomatous tissue. Lymph nodes. Macrophages containing bacteria.

Diagnostic Procedures. *Blood.* Mild anemia, neutrophils increased or normal. Normal B- and T-lymphocyte functions. Serum Ig elevated. Neutrophil chemotaxis, degranulation, and phagocytosis are normal. Abnormalities of bacterial killing action.

Therapy. Supportive. Antibiotics and corticoids of some symptomatic value. Surgical intervention for complications. Gamma-interferon, effective for 5 weeks. Bone marrow transplantation occasionally effective.

Prognosis. From rapidly fatal to compatible with life until middle age. Average life expectancy 5 to 7 years.

BIBLIOGRAPHY. Berendes H, Bridge Good RA: A fatal granulomatosis of childhood: the clinical, pathological, and laboratory features of a new syndrome. Minn Med 40:20–55, 1957
Johnston RB Jr, Newman SL: Chronic granulomatous disease. Pediatr Clin N Am 24:365–376, 1977
Athens JW: Qualitative disorders of leukocytes. In Lee GR, Bithel TC, Foerster J, et al (eds): Wintrobe's Clinical Hematology, 9th ed, pp 1619–1621. Philadelphia, Lea & Febiger, 1993

BERGER

Obsolete.

Symptoms. Weakness and paresthesia of lower limbs without any objective evidence of pathology or associated condition.

Etiology. Unknown.

BIBLIOGRAPHY. Berger O: Ueber eine eigenthümliche Form von Paraesthesie. Bresl Arztl 1:60–61, 1879

BERGER-GOLDBERG

Synonyms. Hardero Porphynuria. See Dobriner.

Symptoms and Signs. Both sexes. At birth. Jaundice, hepatosplenomegaly. From adolescence photosensitivity.

Etiology. Autosomal dominant inheritance.

Diagnostic Procedures. *Blood.* Hemolytic anemia. *Urine. Feces.* High level of coproporphyrin.

Prognosis. Not affecting life span.

BIBLIOGRAPHY. Berger H, Goldberg A: Hereditary coproporphyria. Brit Med J 2:85–88, 1955
Andrews J, Erdjument H, Nicholson DD: Hereditary coproporphyria: incidence in a large English family. J Med Genet 21:341–349, 1984

BERGER-HINGLAIS

Synonyms. IgA nephropathy; mesangial IgA/IgG nephropathy. See hematuria, essential.

Symptoms and Signs. Prevalent in male; mean age of onset 28 years. Recurrent episodes of gross hematuria, following respiratory infections or associated with diarrhea or strenuous exercises. Mild hypertension.

Etiology. Unknown. Entrapment of IgA in glomerular mesangium and activation of complement (spontaneous or consequent to systemic infection?). Autosomal dominant inheritance reported in some families.

Pathology. Focal segmental proliferative glomerulonephritis; glomerular deposits of IgA in mesangial areas, associated with IgG and C3 and fibrin-related antigens. IgA may also be found around skin capillaries.

Diagnostic Procedures. *Urine.* Hematuria with minimal proteinuria. *Renal function.* Normal. *Blood.* Serum IgA levels elevated (not constant) serum complement components normal. *Biopsy of kidney.* Immunofluorescent stain. (See Pathology.)

Therapy. No specific therapy has been shown to influence the natural history of the disease. Ace inhibitors for hypertension and dietary measures. Intermittent steroid and antibiotic therapy has been used. When indicated, kidney transplantation.

Prognosis. Slow progression. Fifty percent of patients develop end-stage renal failure within 25 years of the time of diagnosis. Recurrence of disease rare on transplanted kidney.

BIBLIOGRAPHY. Berger J, Hinglais N: Les dépôts intercapillaires d'IgA-IgG. J Urol Nephrol (Paris) 74:694–695, 1968

Berger J: IgA glomerular deposits in renal disease. Transplant Proc 1:939–944, 1969

Julian B, Warmond A, Van der Wall Bake: IgA nephropathy. In Massry SG, Glassock RJ: Textbook of Nephrology, 3rd ed, pp 752–760. Baltimore, Williams & Wilkins, 1995

BERGSTRAND

Synonym. Osteoid osteoma.

Symptoms. Both sexes affected, onset at 10–25 years of age. Localized pain, exacerbated at night, corresponding to bone location of lesion. Pain worse at night and relieved by aspirin.

Signs. May affect all bones; most frequently involved are tibia and femur, usually in the metaphyseal-epiphyseal region. Tenderness. Localized swelling seldom evident.

Etiology. Neoplastic theory (Jaffe et al) supported by the almost constant sterility of lesion and type of histologic changes; inflammatory theory (Brailsford, Ottolenghi, and others) supported by the occasional presence of hyperthermia. Familial (autosomal recessive) form reported.

Pathology. When process terminates its evolution, lesion appears as round bone nodule more or less vascularized, isolated from adjacent tissue. Histology. Nidus formed by highly vascular cellular connective tissue without any inflammatory feature and surrounded by osteoid or partially calcified trabeculae, which project toward periphery.

Diagnostic Procedures. *Blood and urine.* Normal. *X-ray.* Image of round intracortical or extracortical rarefied nucleus of variable dimension (2–3 mm to 1–2 cm) with one or more zones of increased density. *CT scan.*

Therapy. Excision.

Prognosis. If entire lesion removed, relapses do not occur and symptoms disappear completely.

BIBLIOGRAPHY. Bergstrand H: Ueber eine eigenartige, wahrseheinlich bisher nicht beschriebene osteoblastiehe Krankheit in den dangen Knochen der Hand in des Fusses. Acta Radiol (Stockh) 11:596–613, 1930

Kaye JJ, Arnold WD: Osteoid osteoma in siblings. Clin Orthoped 126:273–275, 1977

Kricun ME: Imaging of bone tumors. Philadelphia, WB Saunders, 1995

BERK-TABATZNIK

Symptoms. From birth. Optic atrophy; spastic quadriparesis.

Signs. Linear growth deficiency; cervical kyphosis; small distal phalanges.

Etiology. Unknown.

Diagnostic Procedures. *X-ray.* Hemivertebral and vertebral wedging (see Signs).

BIBLIOGRAPHY. Berk ME, Tabatznik B: Cervical Kyphosis from posterior hemivertebrae with brachyphalangy and congenital optical atrophy. J Bone Joint Surg (Br) 43:77, 1961

Hartwell EA, Robinson LK, Robinson LH: Congenital optical athrophy and tele-phalangy. The Berk-Tabatznik syndrome. Am J Med Genet 29:383–389, 1988

BERLIN (C.I.)

Synonym. Leukomelanoderma—infantilism—mental retardation—hypodontia—hypotrichosis. See Christ-Siemens-Touraine and Naegeli.

Symptoms and Signs. Both sexes (two males and two females). Physical and mental development retarded. Eruption of teeth delayed. Facies similar to anhydrotic ectodermal dysplasia, with generalized mottled pigmentation of the skin, thickening of palms and soles; body hair sparse or absent; reduced sweating.

Etiology. Unknown; autosomal recessive inheritance.

BIBLIOGRAPHY. Berlin CI: Congenital generalized melanoleucoderma associated with hypodontia, hypotrichosis, stunted growth, and mental retardation occurring in two brothers and two sisters. Dermatologica 123:227–243, 1961

Harper J: Genetics and genodermatoses. In Champion RH, Burton JL, Ebling FJG (eds): Rook/Wilkinson/Ebling Textbook of Dermatology, 5th ed, p 345. Oxford, Blackwell Scientific, 1992

BERLIN I (R.)

Synonyms. Commotio retinae; traumatic retinal edema.

Symptoms. In some cases, gradual loss of central vision and, usually, successive return of it.

Signs. None.

Etiology. Trauma to eye.

Pathology. Retinal edema; cones in fovea destroyed.

Diagnostic Procedures. *Ophthalmoscopy.* Cloudiness of retina; macula appears bright reddish in contrast.

Therapy. Antiedema treatment: corticosteroids; diuretics. Vitamin A.

Prognosis. Usually good recovery.

BIBLIOGRAPHY. Berlin R: Zur sagenarnten Commotio Retinae. Klin Monatsbl Augenheilkd 11:42–78, 1873

Morris DA: Ocular trauma. In Garner A, Klintworth GK (eds): Pathobiology of Ocular Disease: A Dynamic Approach, 2nd ed, pp 394–396. New York, Marcel Dekker, 1994

BERLIN II (R.)

Synonym. Canalis opticus.

Symptoms. After head trauma without direct involvement of eye. Unilateral or bilateral amaurosis.

Signs. In case of complete blindness, absence of pupillary reflexes.

Etiology. Trauma directly or indirectly producing necrosis of ocular nerve fibers.

Pathology. Necrosis of nerve fibers on border of intracanalicular or intracranial segment (or both) of optic (II) nerve. Fractures of optic canal; dislocation or compression of optic nerves are not necessary components of the syndrome.

Therapy. Attempt to relieve pressure useless.

Prognosis. Variable from reversible to irreversible blindness.

BIBLIOGRAPHY. Berlin R: Ueber Sehstörungen nach Verletzung durch stumpfe Gewalt. Klin Monatsbl Augenheilkd 17:1878
Seitz R: Canalis-opticus-syndrome. Ophthalmologica Ann 158:318–324, 1969
Morris DA: Ocular trauma. In Garner A, Klintworth GK (eds): Pathobiology of Ocular Disease: A Dynamic Approach, 2nd ed, p 396. New York, Marcel Dekker, 1994

BERLOQUE

Synonyms. Berlock; berloque dermatitis; contact photosensitization. See Civatte, light eruption, polymorphous and Richl.

Symptoms and Signs. Occurs only in susceptible individuals. Exposure to the light after application of perfumes. Deep brown pigmentation in wide stripes and in pattern formed by trickle of droplets on face, neck, or other areas.

Etiology. Stimulated melanogenesis by light (wavelength above 320 nm) and by furocoumarins (5–methoxypsoralen) of bergamot, lemon oils, and orange peels, usually contained in eau de cologne.

Diagnostic Procedure. Patch tests. Open (light exposed) and closed dressing with suspected perfume.

Therapy. Cosmetic.

Prognosis. Fading of discoloration after weeks or months.

BIBLIOGRAPHY. Freund E: Ueber bisher noch nicht beschriebene künstliche Hautverfarbungen. Derm Wschr 63:931–936, 1916
Harber LC: Berloque dermatitis. Arch Dermatol 90:572–576, 1964
Bleehen SS, Ebling FJG, Champion RH. In Champion RH, Burton JL, Ebling FJG (eds): Rook/Wilkinson/Ebling Textbook of Dermatology, 5th ed, pp 1594–1595. Oxford, Blackwell Scientific, 1992

BERNARD

Synonyms. Claude Bernard; cervical sympathetic irritation. See also Horner.

Symptoms and Signs. Midriasis; eyelid lag; diminished blinking; retraction of upper and, occasionally, of lower, lids; relative enophthalmos. Ipsilateral side of face: vasoconstriction; decreased local temperature; increased sweating; increased lacrimation.

Etiology and Pathology. Irritative lesions of cervical sympathetic system; tumors; aneurysm; infection or any cause of mechanical compression in any location of path of this system mediastinal; cervical; medullar; midbrain.

Diagnostic Procedures. *X-rays of chest, neck, skull. Angiography. CT brain scan. MRI.*

Therapy. Depends upon etiology.

Prognosis. Depends upon etiology.

BIBLIOGRAPHY. Bernard C: Recherches expérimentales sur le grand sympathique et spécialement sur l'influence que le section de ce nerf exerce sur la chaleur animal. CR Soc Biol (Paris) 5:77, 1853
Shafar J: The syndromes of the third neuron of the cervical sympathetic system. Am J Med 40:97–109, 1966
Adams RD, Victor M: Principles of Neurology, 5th ed, pp 470. New York, McGraw-Hill, 1993

BERNARD-SOULIER

Synonyms. Hemorrhagic dystrophic thrombocytopenia; thromboasthenia—thrombocytopenia (autosomal recessive); giant platelet.

Symptoms and Signs. Both sexes affected; present from infancy. Moderate to severe purpura; epistaxis; menorrhagia.

Etiology. Autosomal recessive or codominant inheritance. Decrease or absence in platelet membrane of all four members of the glycoprotein Ib complex. Also lacking the 1s (glycocalcin–receptor for plasma Von Willebrand factor).

Diagnostic Procedures. *Blood.* Giant platelets (up to 8 μm diameter); mild thrombocytopenia; variable abnormalities in PF-3 activity: platelet aggregation by bovine fibrinogen deficient. *Clotting test.* Bleeding time prolonged; clot retraction and platelet aggregation by adenosine triphosphate (ATP) normal. *Bone marrow.* Megakaryocytes normal or increased in number.

Therapy. Supportive. Splenectomy and corticosteroids ineffective. Massive platelet transfusions are of temporary usefulness.

Prognosis. Variable according to intensity of hemorrhagic manifestations.

BIBLIOGRAPHY. Bernard J, Soulier JP: Sur une nouvelle variété de dystrophie thrombocytaire hémorrhagipare congénitale. Bull Mem Soc Med Hôp 64:969–974, 1948
Bithell TC: Qualitative disorders of platelets function. In Lee GR, Bithel TC, Foerster J, et al (eds): Wintrobe's Clinical Hematology, 9th ed, p 1403. Philadelphia, Lea & Febiger, 1993

BERNHARDT-ROTH

Synonyms. Bernhards; Roth; Rot; cutaneous neuritis; meralgia paresthetica; lateral femoral paresthesia.

Symptoms. Paresthesia and numbing in affected leg; burning pain after a long period of standing or walking.

Signs. Decreased objective sensation to touch; pain; temperature (not constant) in the anterolateral surface of thigh.

Etiology. Compression and irritation of lateral femoral cutaneous nerve by clothing or infectious process. Frequent in obesity and diabetes. Postsurgical etiology in several cases, secondary to retroperitoneal tumor. Familial occurrence autosomal dominant has also been reported.

Pathology. Compression neuritis; proliferation of interstitial tissue.

Therapy. Relief of pressure; if symptoms persist, surgical decompression or nerve resection.

Prognosis. Spontaneous remission in few months, occasionally longer (years); good response to treatment.

BIBLIOGRAPHY. Hager W: Neuralgia femoris. Resection des Nerv. Cutan. Femoria Anterior externus Heilung. Dtsch Med Wchnschr 11:218, 1885
Bernhardt M: Ueber isoliert im Gebiete des N. cutaneus femoris externus vorkommende. Parästhesien Neurol Centralbl 14:242–244, 1895

Massey EW: Familial occurrence of meralgia paresthetica. Arch Neurol 35:182, 1987

Adams RD, Victor M: Principles of Neurology, 5th ed, p 1163. New York, McGraw-Hill, 1993

BERNHEIM

Synonyms. Right ventricle failure; right ventricle obstruction-failure.

Symptoms. Two stages: (1) Few or no clinical symptoms; (2a) dyspnea may be absent; (2b) total heart failure, dyspnea, orthopnea, and other symptoms.

Signs. Two stages: (1) Enlargement of right atrium; distension of cervical veins; increased venous pressure; normal circulation time. (2a) Systemic venous enlargement; lungs clear to percussion and ausculation; hepatic enlargement; dependent edema; possibly ascites. Circulation time normal or slightly increased. (2b) Total heart failure.

Etiology. Left ventricular hypertrophy and enlargement, bulging of septum into the right ventricle and obstruction of the blood flow from right atrium. Existence of syndrome denied by some cardiologists (White, Evans), accepted by others (Russek, Zohman, Drago).

Pathology. *First stage.* Left ventricle hypertrophy. *Second stage.* Heart enlargement; left atrium normal size; right atrium dilated; left ventricle enlarged and bulging on the right. Liver markedly congested, enlarged; cardiac cirrhosis. Lung congestion, infarction, and atelectasis from compression of the enlarged heart.

Diagnostic Procedures. *Electrocardiography. Circulation time. X-ray of chest. Fluoroscopy. Cardiac catheterization.*

Therapy. Treatment of hypertension and heart failure.

Prognosis. That of heart failure, modified by treatment.

BIBLIOGRAPHY. Bernheim P: De l' Asistolie Veineuse dans l'hypertrophie du coeur gauche par stenose concomitante du ventricule droit. Rev Med (Paris) 30:785–800, 1910

Drago EE, Aquilina JT: Bernheim's syndrome. Am J Cardiol 14:568–572, 1964

Schlant RC, Sonnenblick EH: Pathophysiology of heart failure. In Schlant RC, Alexander RW: Hurst's The Heart, 8th ed, p 535. New York, McGraw-Hill, 1994

BERNUTH

Obsolete.

Synonyms. von Bernuth; hemophilia sporadica; Eponym used to indicate sporadic hemophilia. See Hemophilia.

BIBLIOGRAPHY. von Bernuth F: Ueber Kapillarbeobachtungen bei Hämophilie und anderen hämorrhagischen Diathesen. Dtsch Arch Klin Med 152:321–330, 1926

BERTOLOTTI

Synonym. Sacralization-scoliosis-sciatica. See also Cotugno.

Symptoms. Numbness; hypersensitivity or pain along the course of sciatic nerve; low back pain; morning stiffness.

Signs. Scoliosis.

Etiology. Sacralization of lumbar vertebrae.

Diagnostic Procedures. *X-ray of spine.* Sacralization of fifth lumbar vertebra. *CT scan. MRI.*

Therapy. Special postural exercises. Salicylates or other analgesic and anti-inflammatory agents. Deep radiation; thermotherapy.

Prognosis. Insidious progression.

BIBLIOGRAPHY. Bertolotti M: Contributo alla conoscenza dei vizi di differenzazione regionale del rachide con speciale riguardo all' assimilazione sacrale della V lombare. Radiol Med (Torino) 4:113–144, 1917

Bertolotti M: Les syndromes lombo-ischialgiques d'origine vertébrale. Rev Neurol (Paris) 29:1112–1125, 1922

BESNIER-BOECK-SCHAUMANN

Synonyms. Boeck sarcoid; Hutchinson-Boeck; Jungling; Mortimer; Schaumann; lupus pernio; benign lymphogranulomatosis; sarcoidosis.

Symptoms. More frequent in females 20–30 years of age. Early stages. Often asymptomatic; fatigue; moderate cough; mild weight loss; vague chest pains. (In Scandinavian countries and Great Britain, acute symptoms of fever, arthralgia, erythema nodosum more frequently observed.) Later stages: expectoration; hemoptysis; cyanosis; dyspnea; difficulty in vision; blindness; Bell palsy. See Loffgren.

Signs. Early stage. Physical examination negative; minor pulmonary changes; rales. Later stage. Adenopathy; cutaneous polymorphic lesions; hepatosplenomegaly (20–25%); iridocyclitis; scleral nodules; chorioretinitis; acute migratory monoarthritis or polyarthritis; fever.

Etiology. Unknown.

Pathology. Granulomatous lesions formed by concentric arrangement of elongated epithelioid cells, giant cells of Langerhans or foreign body type, inclusion body, fibroblasts surrounding lesions; absence of caseation; later, necrosis and fibrosis with formation of scar. Nodules may be found in all involved organs: liver; lung; kidney; heart; central nervous system; skin; lymph nodes; eyes.

Diagnostic Procedures. *Biopsy.* Kveim test positive (obsolete); Mantoux test negative. *Blood.* High sedimentation rate, high alpha and gamma globulins; high alkaline phosphatases; high calcium (10%); anemia (rarely); moderate leukopenia; eosinophilia; thrombocytopenia (when splenic involvement). *Urine.* Hypercalciuria. *Liver biopsy.* See Pathology. *X-ray.* Hilar or paratracheal lymphoadenopathy; later stage, pulmonary parenchymal nodular involvement, then fibrosis. Bone involvement 10%, affecting mostly bones of the hands. Pulmonary function tests: reduction of vital capacity total lung capacity and diffusing capacity of CO (DLCO) in 40–70%. Bronchoalveolar lavage (BAL): allows staging of the disease; gallium-67 scanning; measurement of serum angiotensin converting enzyme (SACE) to assess activity of the disease.

Therapy. Patients with hypercalcemia can be managed with a low calcium diet. Local steroid therapy for ocular sarcoidosis; intradermal steroids for cutaneous lesions. Indications for systemic corticosteroid therapy include progressive pulmonary impairment or respiratory symptoms, ocular involvement, myocardial and central nervous system involvement, disfiguring cutaneous lesions, persistent hypercalcemia or hypercalciuria with renal involvement. The disease is characterized by frequent spontaneous remissions. Alternative agents to corticosteroids include: chloroquine, phenylbutazone, chlorambucil, azathioprine cyclosporine A, etc. In rare cases of endstage pulmonary disease lung or heart lung transplantation have successfully been performed.

Prognosis. Remissions and relapses frequent, with gradual progression. Average survival 10 years. Fatal outcome in about 20% at earlier phases. In North American patients more benign prognosis; symptoms subside and disappear in 2 years in 9 out of 10 patients.

BIBLIOGRAPHY. Besnier E: Lupus pernio de la face; synovites fongueuses (scrofulo-tuberculeuses) symétriques des extrémités superieures. Ann Dermat Syph 10:333–336, 1889

Boeck C: Multiple benign sarcoid of the skin. J Cutan Genito Urin Dis 17:543–550, 1889

Schaumann, J: Sur une forme érythrodermique du lymphogranulome bénin. Ann Dermatol Syph 1:561–574, 1920

Lynch JP, Strieter RM: Sarcoidosis. In Lynch JP, De Remee RA: Immunologically mediated pulmonary diseases, p 189. Philadelphia, JB Lippincott, 1991

BESNIER PRURIGO

Synonyms. Atopic dermatitis (chronic lichenified flexural form); neurodermatitis disseminated; exudative eczema; diathesic prurigo.

Symptoms. Usually follows (also years later) infantile atopic dermatitis. Pruritus on localized lesion (see Signs) often associated with asthma; exacerbations of asthmatic attack and prurigo alternate.

Signs. Patches of lichenized papules most frequently on bend of knees, elbows, face, and wrists.

Etiology. Unknown. Interplay of genetic factors (of complex nature, dominant inheritance or recessive reported) and precipitating factors (immunological, climatic, and psychological). Inherent itchiness of the skin (?).

Pathology. Scratching lesions and lichenification (not constant).

Diagnostic Procedures. *Blood.* IgE increased (80% of cases). IgG, IgA, and IgM usually normal except severe eczema; presence of specific antibodies (RAST). *Skin reactivity.* To allergens, physical (cold, pressure) and pharmacological agents (histamine, nicotine acid esters, acetylcholine).

Therapy. General allergic management (avoid contact or injection of suspected antigens). Specific desensitizations (effective only in few cases); antipruritic agents (antihistamines), hydroxyzine hydrochloride, cortisone (for acute phase), antibiotic (if infection); topical treatment: ointment, with or diluted corticosteroids, zinc, coal tar, ultraviolet light. (Caution: may have opposite effect). In the author's experience, lactic acid-producing organisms and S-adenosyl L-methionine (200 mg daily) have been useful.

Prognosis. Recurrences, sometimes throughout life.

BIBLIOGRAPHY. Besnier E: Première note et observation preliminaire pour servir d'introduction à l'étude des prurigos diasthesiques. Ann Dermatol Syph 3:634–648, 1892
Burton JL: Eczema, lichenification, prurigo and erythroderma. In Champion RH, Burton JL, Ebling FJG (eds): Rook/Wilkinson/Ebling Textbook of Dermatology, 5th ed, p 582. Oxford, Blackwell Scientific, 1992

BETA BLOCKER EMBRYOPATHY

Synonyms. Propanolol embryopathy; including Minoxidil embryopathy.

Symptoms and Signs. In new born from mothers receiving a single beta-blocker or combination of this type of drugs. Variable malformations. Propanolol and/or captopryl: intrauterine growth retardation, transient hypotension, bradycardia, renal failure, hypoglycemia, hyperbilirubinemia. Variable somatic and visceral defects: skull deformities, limb defects, pyloric stenosis, tracheoesophageal fistula, etc. Propanolol + captopril + minoxidil: hypertrichosis, omphalocele, cardiac defect, genitourinary malformations, facial dysmorfism.

Etiology. Fetal toxicity of above mentioned drugs.

Prognosis. Variable according to lesions.

BIBLIOGRAPHY. O'Connor PC, Jick H, Hunter JR, et al: Propanolol and pregnancy outcome Lancet II:1168, 1981
Kaller SG, Patrinos ME, Lambert GH, et al: Hypertrichosis and congenital anomalies associated with maternal use of Minoxidil. Pediatrics 79:434–436, 1987
Schardein JL: Chemically induced birth defects. New York, Marcel Dekker, 1993
Koren G: Maternal-Fetal Toxicity: A Clinicians' Guide, 2nd ed. New York, Marcel Dekker, 1994

BETA-KETOTHIOLASE DEFICIENCY

Synonym. Ketotic hyperglycinemia; alpha-methylacetoaceticaciduria; 3–oxothiolase deficiency.

Symptoms and Signs. In children, episodic ketoacidosis with seizures and hyperammoniemia or psychomotor retardation.

Etiology. Autosomal recessive inheritance. Deficiency of beta-keto-thiolase.

Diagnostic Procedures. *Blood.* Hypoglycinemia, hyperammonemia. *Urine.* Hyperglycinuria, 2–methyl-3–hydroxybutyrate, 2–methylaceto-acetate and butanone (gas chromatographic analysis).

Therapy. Control of ketoacidosis.

Prognosis. Ranging from early death to normal development.

BIBLIOGRAPHY. Daum RS, Lamm PH, Mamer OA, et al: A new disorder of isoleucine catabolism. Lancet II:1289–1290, 1971
Hillman RE, Keating JP: Beta-ketothiolase deficiency as a cause of the ketotic hyperglycinemia syndrome. Pediatrics 53:221–225, 1974
Fukao T, Yamaguchi S, Tomatsu S, et al: Evidence for a structural mutation (ala347-to-thr) in a German family with 3–ketothiolase deficiency. Biochem Biophys Res Commun 179:124–129, 1991

BETA-MANNOSIDOSIS

Synonym. Wenger-Cooper; mannosidosis beta; MNB.

Symptoms and Signs. Only 10 patients in seven families described, all males. Difficult to define the phenotype of this condition. Normal first few monthts of life. Frequent respiratory infections. Coarse facies, mild bone disease, all patients presented mental retardation; behavior aggressive or unstable. Angiokeratoma of scrotum (in two cases). No hepatosplenomegaly.

Etiology. Autosomal recessive inheritance.

Diagnostic Procedures. *Fibroblast and leukocyte culture.* Absence of beta-mannosidase activity. *Urine.* Large amounts of disaccharides, that yield mannose and glucosamine. *CT scan brain.* Normal in the majority of cases, atrophy in most severe cases.

Prognosis. Relatively mild form of storage disease.

BIBLIOGRAPHY. Wenger DA, Sujansky E, Fennessey PV, et al: Human beta-mannosidase deficiency. N Engl J Med 315:1201–1205, 1986
Cooper A, Hatton C, Thornley M, et al: Human beta-mannosidase deficiency. J Inherit Met Dis 11:17–29, 1988
Thomas GH, Beaudet AL: Disorders of glycoprotein degradation and structure, -mannosidosis, -mannosidosis, fucosidosis, sialidosis, aspartylglucosamlnuria, and carbohydrate-deficient glycoprotein syndrome. In Scriver CR, Beaudet AL, Sly WS, et al: The Metabolic and Molecular Bases of Inherited Disease, 7th ed, pp 2537–2539. New York, McGraw-Hill, 1995

BETA-METHYLCROTONYL CoA CARBOXYLASE DEFICIENCY

Synonym. 3–methyl-crotonic aciduria isolated.

Symptoms and Signs. Normal growth and development until an acute episode presentation between 14 and 33 months of age, following a minor infection similar to Reye syndrome (see): feeding difficulty, vomiting, lethargy, apnea, hypotonia, or hyperreflexia, with or without seizures. Peculiar "tomcat odor" of urine.

Etiology. Autosomal recessive inheritance. Deficiency of 3–methyl-crotonyl CoA carboxylase.

Diagnostic Procedures. *Urine.* Increased 3–hydroxyisovaleric acid and 3–methylcrotonylglycine. *Blood.* Hypoglycemia, hyperammonemia, increased hepatic transaminases, mild metabolic acidosis and modest ketonuria, low free carnetine, occasionally neutrophilia.

Therapy. Symptomatic. Diet low in leucine (no clinical improvement). Identified a form responsive to biotin usually ineffective in other cases.

Prognosis. Death at an early age.

BIBLIOGRAPHY. Eldjarn L, Jellum E, Stokke O, et al: Beta hydroxyisovaleric aciduria and beta-methylcrotonylglycinuria: a new error of metabolism. Lancet II:521–522, 1970
Wolf B, Feldman GL: The biotin dependent carboxylase deficiencies. Am J Hum Genet 34:699–716, 1982
Sweetman L, Williams JC: Branched chain organic acidurias. In Scriver CR, Beaudet AL, Sly WS, et al: The Metabolic and Molecular Bases of Inherited Disease, 7th ed, pp 1397–1398. New York, McGraw-Hill, 1995

BETA-THALASSEMIA INTERMEDIA

Symptoms. Intermediate between thalassemia minor and Cooley syndrome.

Etiology. Owing to different genetic interactions.

1. Homozygosity for two mild beta thalassemia genes or double heterozygosity for one mild and one unusually severe gene
2. Homozygosity or double heterozygosity for beta thalassemia genes of unusual severity, but with coinheritance of a modifying factor
3. Heterozygous beta thalassemia of unusual severity

BIBLIOGRAPHY. Bunn HF, Forget BG: Hemoglobin: Molecular Genetic and Clinical Aspects, p 340. Philadelphia, WB Saunders, 1986
Lukens JN: The thalassemias and related disorders: quantitative disorders of hemoglobin synthesis. In Lee GR, Bithel TC, Foerster J, et al (eds): Wintrobe's Clinical Hematology, 9th ed, p 1122. Philadelphia, Lea & Febiger, 1993

BETA-THALASSEMIA MINIMA

Synonyms. Microcythemia minima; heterozygous beta thalassemia.

Symptoms. Asymptomatic. See Silvestroni-Bianco.

Therapy. Physiotherapy.

Prognosis. Mild weakness with ability to work until old age. Normal life expectancy.

BIBLIOGRAPHY. Bunn HF, Forget BG: Hemoglobin: Molecular Genetic and Clinical Aspects, p 340. Philadelphia, WB Saunders, 1986
Lukens JN: The thalassemias and related disorders: quantitative disorders of hemoglobin synthesis. In Lee GR, Bithel TC, Foerster J, et al (eds): Wintrobe's Clinical Hematology, 9th ed, p 1122. Philadelphia, Lea & Febiger, 1993

BETHLEM MYOPATHY

Synonyms. Bethlem-Van Wijngaarden; myopathy with contractures, autosomal dominant early onset type; muscular dystrophy benign congenital.

Symptoms and Signs. From infancy limb girdle weakness (more proximal than distal muscles) that progresses slowly with periods of arrest, contractions of fingers, elbows, and ankles.

Etiology. Autosomal dominant.

Diagnostic Procedures. *Electromygraphy.* Muscle pattern. *Blood.* Serum creatinine kinase normal or slightly raised.

Prognosis. Death from perforation of intestinal ulcers.

BIBLIOGRAPHY. Bethlem J, Van Wijngaarden GK: Benign myopathy, with autosomal dominant inheritance—a report three pedigrees. Brain 99:91–100, 1976
Ballestrazzi A, Granata C, Trentin V, et al: Bethlem myopathy: clinical data of 14 patients in two families. J Neurol Sci 98:(Suppl)461, 1990

BETTLEY

Synonyms. Fetal cutaneointestinal; cutaneous—intestinal—oropharyngeal ulceration. See also Koehlmeir-Degos.

Symptoms and Signs. Macular, blistering and crusting lesions of skin; oroparingeal ulceration, intestinal ulcers.

Etiology. Unknown. Vasculitis? Relevant to Degos syndrome (see) from which, however, it differs clinically and histologically.

Pathology. Cutis and subcutis inflammatory reaction; fibrinoid necrosis of arteriole found in intestinal lesion.

Etiology. Variable patterns of inheritance.

BIBLIOGRAPHY. Bettley FR: A fetal cutaneointestinal syndrome. Br J Derm 72:423–426, 1960
Ryan TJ: Cutaneous vasculitis. In Champion RH, Burton JL, Ebling FJG (eds): Rook/Wilkinson/Ebling Textbook of Dermatology, 5th ed, p 1953. Oxford, Blackwell Scientific, 1992

BEUKES TYPE, HIP DISLASIA

Synonyms. Hip displasia, Beukes type.

Symptoms and Signs. Both sexes in an Afrikaaner family (47 patients). In childhood pain in the hip and progressive crippling in early adulthood. Good general health, absence of extraskeletal manifestations.

Etiology. Autosomal dominant inheritance, with many instances of male-to-male transmission. Could be a type of multiple epiphyseal dysplasia.

Diagnostic Procedures. *X-ray. Skeletal survey.* Major change. Severely flattened and irregular femoral capital epiphyses.

Prognosis. Development of secondary osteoarthrosis at early age.

BIBLIOGRAPHY. Cilliers HJ, Beighton P: Beukes familial hip dysplasia: An autosomal dominant entity. Am J Med Genet 36:386–390, 1990

BEZOLD

Synonyms. Bezold abscess; temporal bone subperiosteal abscess.

Symptoms. Severe pain in perimastoidal region; difficulty in swallowing; sore throat; difficulty in breathing; nuchal rigidity; fever.

Signs. Swelling in the area between the tip of mastoid process and mandible; otorrhea.

Etiology. Otitis media with rupture of tympanic membrane; infiltration of pus into neck musculature.

Pathology. Perforation of inner surface of mastoid into digastric fossa; abscess extending behind sternocleidomastoid muscle, less frequently reaching perivertebral region or thoracic cavity.

Diagnostic Procedures. *Culture of pus. Blood and urine. X-ray of head and neck.*

Therapy. Sinus opening from mastoid process to neck and drainage. Antibiotics.

Prognosis. Recovery following surgery.

BIBLIOGRAPHY. Bezold F: Ein neuer Weg fur Ausbreitung eitriger Entzündung aus den Räumen des Mittelohrs auf die Nachbarschaft und die in diesem Falle einzuschlagende Therapie. Dtsch Med Wochenschr 7:381–385, 1885

BHATTACHARYYA-CONNOR

Synonyms. Sitosterolemia—xanthomatosis; phytosterolemia.

Symptoms and Signs. Rare defect. From childhood, tendon xanthomas, xanthelasma: atherosclerosis of coronaries and large vessels, signs of hemolytic anemia, recurrent arthralgia and arthritis. Splenomegaly (in some cases).

Etiology. Autosomal recessive inheritance. Increased absorption of sitosterol and defective turnover with accumulation in tissues.

Pathology. Xanthomas similar to those of hypercholesterolemia and cerebrotendinous xanthomatosis, coronary vessels aorta are also are affected.

Diagnostic Procedures. *Blood.* High concentrations of sitosterol and compesterol; normal or increased cholesterol concentration. Hemolytic anemia. Platelets: functional defects.

Therapy. Diet low in plant sterols. Cholestyramine. Suggested also neomycin in the supposition that sterol balance is made negative by this drug. Coronary bypass for cardiac complications

Prognosis. Fair. Death by coronary heart disease possible at early age (second to third decade).

BIBLIOGRAPHY. Bhattacharyya AK, Connor WE: Sitosterolemia and xanthamatosis: a newly described lipid storage disease in two sisters. J Clin Invest 53:1033–1043, 1974
Björkhem I, Boberg KM: Inborn errors in bile acid biosynthesis and storage of sterols other than cholesterol. In Scriver CR, Beaudet AL, Sly WS, et al: The Metabolic and Molecular Bases of Inherited Disease, 7th ed, pp 2088–2093. New York, McGraw-Hill, 1995

BIANCHI

Synonym. Alexia—aphasia—apraxia; parietal. See Head-Holmes; Anton-Babinski; Gerstmann; Pick (A).

Symptoms and Signs. Expressive alexia; contralateral to lesion, hemianesthesia with tactile agnosia of corresponding hand and foot. Transient hemiplegia.

Etiology and Pathology. Usually, lesion of left parietal lobe.

BIBLIOGRAPHY. Bianchi L: La sindrome parietale. Med Ital (Napoli) 9:187, 243, 333, 1911
Adams RD, Victor M: Principles of Neurology, 5th ed, pp 396–399. New York, McGraw-Hill, 1993

BIBER-HAAB-DIMMER

Synonyms. Buckler III; Haab-Dimmer; corneal lattice dystrophy; lattice corneal dystrophy I; LCD

Symptoms. Both sexes affected; onset early in life (20–30 years of age). Progressive vision reduction.

Signs. Corneal grayish lines, translucent cotton-like threads, mostly limited to a zone between center of cornea and periphery, not reaching limbus. Dots with distinct borders scattered all over. Cornea clear between opacities.

Etiology. Unknown; autosomal dominant inheritance.

Pathology. Hyaline degeneration involving stromal lamellae without mucopolysaccharide accumulation.

Diagnostic Procedures. Biopsy of cornea.

Therapy. Corneal transplantation.

Prognosis. Good with transplantation.

BIBLIOGRAPHY. Biber H: Ueber einige seltenere Hornhauterkrankungen. Inaugural Dissertation, Zurich, 1890 (cited by Haab O: Die gittrige Keratitis. Z Augenheilkd 2:235–246, 1899)
Kivlin JD, Lovrien EW, Maumenee IH, et al: Linkage analysis in lattice corneal dystrophy. Am J Med Genet 19:387–390, 1984
Rodrigues MM, Rajagopalan S, Jones KA: Anterior and posterior corneal dystrophy. In Garner A, Klintworth GK (eds): Pathobiology of Ocular Disease: A Dynamic Approach, 2nd ed, pp 1000–1003. New York, Marcel Dekker, 1994

BICARBONATE DEFICIT

Symptoms and Signs. Weakness; malaise; headache; nausea; vomiting; abdominal pain; Kussmaul breathing. If condition progresses, respiratory depression develops. Associated clinical manifestation of basic disease: diabetes; uremia; congestive heart failure; distal renal tubular acidosis.

Etiology. Excess of organic or inorganic acid in the body. Excessive production of acids. (1) Diabetic acidosis; (2) starvation; (3) high fever; (4) thyrotoxicosis; (5) violent exercise; (6) shock. Excessive intake of acid. Administration of sodium, calcium, or ammonium chlorides, or of carbonic anhydrase inhibitors; or cation exchange resins, salicylate poisoning (see); methyl alcohol intoxication. Acid retention. In renal diseases. Loss of bases. Diarrhea; fistulas; Lightwood (see); in ureteroenterostomy patients.

Pathology. Depends upon etiology.

Diagnostic Procedures. *Blood.* Leukocytosis (occasional). (1) Uncompensated metabolic acidosis: blood pH low; Pco_2 normal, CO_2 capacity low; bicarbonate low; chloride increased; sodium low; normal or high according to etiology. (2) Compensated metabolic acidosis: pH low or normal; Pco_2 low; CO_2 capacity normal; bicarbonate low; chloride low, normal, or high; sodium low or normal; potassium high. *Urine.* Acid; very high ammonia (in renal disease normal pH).

Therapy. Correct causes (see Etiology); correct electrolyte balance.

Prognosis. Depends upon etiology. In chronic cases, defect persists for years. In acute, may result in death if treatment not adequate.

BIBLIOGRAPHY. Goldberger E: A Primer of Water, Electrolyte, and Acid-base Syndromes, 3rd ed. Philadelphia, Lea & Febiger, 1965
Du Bose TD, Alpern RJ: Renal tubular acidosis. In Scriver CR, Beaudet AL, Sly WS, et al: The Metabolic and Molecular Bases of Inherited Disease, 7th ed, p 3663. New York, McGraw-Hill, 1995

BICIPITAL TENOSYNOVITIS

Synonym. Shoulder tendonitis.

Symptoms. Prevalent in females; onset gradual or abrupt. Especially disturbing during night when resting on affected shoulder. Pain of various degrees; disability (abduction and internal rotation limited).

Signs. Tenderness on anterior area of humeral head over bicipital groove, Yergason sign positive in 50% of cases.

Etiology. Trauma; strain; temperature change; humidity; idiopathic.

Pathology. Inflammatory changes of synovia of bicipital tendon; serofibrinous exudate. According to stage, various degrees of adhesion and involvement of surrounding tissues.

Therapy. *X-ray treatment.* Systemic corticosteroid; local injection of procaine or hydrocortisone; physical therapy. *Exploratory surgery.* Transplantation of tendon to coracoid process or to floor of bicipital groove.

Prognosis. Acute, subacute, chronic types are known to evolve from one stage to another, or start directly as subacute or chronic. Chronic stage lasts weeks or months. Atrophy of biceps and shoulder muscles may develop.

BIBLIOGRAPHY. Pasteur F: Les algies de l'épaule et la physiothérapie la téno-bursite bicipitale. J Radiol Electrol 16:419–426, 1932
Justis EJ Jr: New traumatic disorders. In Crenshaw AH (ed): Campbell's Operative Orthopedics, 7th ed, pp 2259–2260. St Louis, CV Mosby, 1987

BICKEL-FANCONI

Symptoms and Signs. Onset first year of life: failure to thrive, hepatomegaly; abdominal blotting, features of rickets (unresponsive to vitamine D) and severe tubolopathy.

Etiology. Unknown, unclassified glycogen storage disease. It could be involved in mitochondrial respiratory chain.

Diagnostic Procedures. *Blood.* Moderate hyperlatacidemia.

Therapy. Symptomatic.

BIBLIOGRAPHY. Odièvre M Glycogéenose hépatorénale avec tubulopathie complexe. Rev Inter Hepatol 16:1, 1966
Chesney RW, Kaplan BS, Teitel D, et al: Metabolic abnormalities in the idiopathic Fanconi syndrome: studies of carbohydrate metabolism in two patients. Pediatrics 67:113–118, 1981
Scriver CR, Beaudet AL, Sly WS, et al (eds): The Metabolic and Molecular Bases of Inherited Disease, 7th ed, p 394. New York, McGraw-Hill, 1995

BICKERS-ADAMS

Synonyms. X-linked hydrocephalus; hydrocephalus X-linked; aqueductal stenosis.

Symptoms and Signs. Males affected; females carriers (dull intelligence); present from birth. Spasticity, especially lower extremities. Mental deficiency (IQ in the range of 30); hydrocephalus or narrow scaphocephalic cranium. Flexed thumb over palm; short first metacarpal. Occasionally asymmetric and course facies; seizures.

Etiology. X-linked recessive inheritance.

Pathology. Aqueductal stenosis and hydrocephalus. Occasionally, various brain defects.

Diagnostic Procedures. *EEG.* Diffuse abnormalities. *CT brain scan. MRI. X-ray.*

Therapy. Neurosurgical.

Prognosis. Poor.

BIBLIOGRAPHY. Bickers DS, Adams RD: Hereditary stenosis of the aqueduct of Sylvius as a cause of congenital hydrocephalus. Brain 72:246–262, 1949
Fryns JP, Spaepen A, Cassiman JJ, et al: X-linked complicated spastic paraplegia, MASA syndrome and X-linked hydrocephalus owing to congenital stenosis of the aqueductus of Sylvius: variable expression of the same mutation at X q28. J Med Genet 28:429–431, 1991

BIELSCHOWSKY-LUTZ-COGAN

Synonyms. Lhermitte; medial longitudinal fasciculus, MLF; internuclear ophthalmoplegia.

Symptoms. Unilateral or bilateral palsy on conjugate lateral gaze; recognized various possibilities (1) paresis of convergence and paresis of homolateral internal rectus muscle on lateral gaze; (2) homolateral internal rectus muscle paralysis on lateral gaze without alteration of convergence. With maximal abduction elicited a dissociated nystagmus of contralateral eye. Bilateral internuclear ophthalmoplegia is pathognomonic of multiple sclerosis.

Etiology. Any lesion (hemorrhagic, neoplastic, multiple sclerosis traumatic) that affects the medial longitudinal fasciculus, interconnecting third and fourth and sixth nuclei. (1) Anterior internuclear ophthalmoplegia. (2) Posterior internuclear ophthalmoplegia.

Therapy. According to etiology.

Prognosis. According to etiology.

BIBLIOGRAPHY. Bielschowsky A: Die Innervation der musculi recti interni als Seitenwaender. Ber Zusammenkunft Dtsch Ophthalmol Ges 30:164–171, 1902
Lutz, A: Ueber einseitige Ophthalmoplegia. Internuclearis anterior. Graefes Arch Ophthalmol 115:692–717, 1924
Cogan DG, Kubik CS, Smith L: Unilateral internuclear ophthalmoplegia: report of eight clinical cases with one postmortem study. Arch Ophthalmol 44:783–796, 1950
Stroud MH, Newman NM, Keltner JL, Gay AJ: Abducting nystagmus in the medial longitudinal fasciculus (MLF) Syndrome-internuclear ophthalmoplegia (INO). Arch Ophthalmol 92:2–5, 1974
Klintworth GK: Ocular involvement in disorders of the nervous system. In Garner A, Klintworth GK (eds): Pathobiology of Ocular Disease: A Dynamic Approach, 2nd ed, pp 1712–1713. New York, Marcel Dekker, 1994

BIEMOND I

Synonyms. Brachydactyly—nystagmus; cerebellar ataxia; cerebellar ataxia—nystagmus—brachydactyly.

Symptoms and Signs. Mental deficiency; cerebellar ataxia; strabismus, nystagmus; and one short metacarpal and one short metatarsal. Not all members of family present the full syndrome.

Etiology. Possibly autosomal dominant inheritance.

BIBLIOGRAPHY. Biemond A: Brachydactylie, Nystagmus en cerebellaire Ataxie als familiair Syndroom. Nederl T Geneesk 78:1423–1431, 1934

BIEMOND II

Synonym. See Laurence-Moon-Biedl.

Symptoms and Signs. Pituitary dwarfism; mental retardation; iris coloboma; obesity; secondary hypogenitalism; postaxial polydactyly; hydrocephalus; hypospadias.

Etiology. Irregular autosomal dominant inheritance.

BIBLIOGRAPHY. Biemond A: Het syndroom van Laurence-Biedl en een aarverwant nieuw syndroom. Nederl T Geneesk 78:1801–1814, 1934
Schachat AP, Maumence JH: Bardet-Biedl syndrome and related disorders. Arch Ophthalmol 100:285–288, 1982

BIEMOND III

Synonyms. Dearborn; spinothalamic ataxia; congenital pain indifference; analgia congenital; familial analgia; spinothalamic ataxia; pain indifference congenital. See Swanson.

Symptoms. Both sexes affected; normal at birth. Failure to register pain. Usually, normal physical and mental development; occasionally associated with oligophrenia, convulsions; aphasia (auditory); anhidrosis.

Signs. Evidence of repeated injuries both to soft and hard tissues: scars; fractures; joints with Charchot jointlike (see) lesions. Nail is thickened and deformed. Irregular dentition with vertical grooves on teeth. Deep tendon reflexes diminished or absent. Corneal reflexes diminished. Absence of sympathetic reaction to pain. Frequent oral mutilation.

Etiology. Unknown; autosomal recessive inheritance.

Pathology. Cholinesterase-positive nerves present only around eccrine sweat gland. Spinothalamic tract and/or posterior ascending tract occasionally absent. Hypoplasia of pyramidal tracts. Cutaneous nerves reveal only nonmyelinated fibers. Reduction of neurons in autonomic and sensory ganglia.

Therapy. Symptomatic.

Prognosis. Severe, up to total incapacitation.

BIBLIOGRAPHY. Dearborn G: A case of congenital pure analgesia. J Nerv Ment Dis 75:612–615, 1932

Biemond A: Investigation of the brain in a case of congenital and familial analgia. Proc XI Intern Cong Neuropath, London, 1955

Freytag E, Lindenberg R: Neuropathologic findings in patients of a hospital for the mentally deficient: a survey of 359 cases. Johns Hopkins Med J 121:379–392, 1967

Adams RD, Victor M: Principles of Neurology, 5th ed, p 1148. New York, McGraw-Hill, 1993

BIETTI I

Synonyms. Marginal corneal dystrophy; dystrophia marginalis cristallinea cornae; crystalline retinopathy; tapetoretinal degeneration.

Symptoms. Relatively common in China. Both sexes equal incidence. Onset in middle to advanced age (average 30 years). Asymptomatic.

Signs. Recurrent irritation; inflammation. Progressive night blindness, reduction of visual fields. In some families chronic changes may be absent.

Etiology. Unknown. Autosomal recessive trait.

Pathology. Marginal corneal dystrophy with loose connective tissue replacing stroma; limbal area thinned; Descemet's membrane bulging; Bowman's capsule degenerated. Retinal degeneration, sclerosis of choroidal.

Diagnostic Procedures. *Ophthalmoscopy.* Numerous glistening intraretinal dots over the fundus.

Therapy. Symptomatic.

Prognosis. Slow progression. Seldom, eyeball rupture.

BIBLIOGRAPHY. Bietti G: Ueber familiäres Vorkommen von "Retinitis punctata albescens" (verbunden mit "Dystrophia marginalis cristallinea corneae"). Glitzern des Glaskörpers und anderen degenerativen Augenver-änderungen. Klin Monatsbl Augenheilkd 99:937–956, 1937

Hayasake S, Okuyama S: Crystalline retinopathy. Retina 4:177–181, 1984

Wilson DJ, Weleberg RG, Klein ML: Bietti's crystalline dystrophy: a clinicopathologic correlative study. Arch Ophthalmol 107:213–221, 1989

Bird AC, Jay B, Hussain AA, et al: Retinal photoreceptor disorders. In Garner A, Klintworth GK (eds): Pathobiology of Ocular Disease: A Dynamic Approach, 2nd ed, p 1212. New York, Marcel Dekker, 1994

BIGLIERI

Synonyms. Adrenal and gonadal-17–hydroxylase deficiency; hypogonadism–mineral corticoid excess; 17–hydroxylase deficiency, adrenal hyperplasia V. See Adrenogenital syndromes.

Symptoms. Genotype female adults. In male subjects ambiguous genitalia and succesive possible development of breast. In females primary amenorrhea; lack of secondary sexual development; fatigue; episodes of marked muscle weakness; numbness and tingling in extremities; episodes of partial hair loss. Hypertension.

Signs. Undeveloped breasts; scanty body hair; infantile uterus; small ovaries (on palpation). Wrinkling and premature aging of facial skin. Hypertension (only in 17–hydroxylase pure deficiency). A nonclassic form (identified by molecular genetic methods), without all clinical features

Etiology. Congenital defect of either the 17–hydroxylase or the 17–hydroxylase and 17, 20–lyase activities combined; resulting in decreased synthesis of cortisol, estrogens, and androgens; and increased DOC and corticosterone. Chromosomal location 10. Enzyme P450c17.

Pathology. Unknown.

Diagnostic Procedures. *Blood.* Hypokalemia; alkalosis; low secretion rate of cortisol. Injection of adenocorticotropic hormone (ACTH) fails to increase secretion of cortisol. Androsterone and testosterone essentially undetectable. Plasma ACTH markedly increased. *Urine.* Increased 11–oxycorticosteroids; pregnanetriol markedly decreased, 17–ketosteroid apparently normal (no detectable dehydroisoandrosterone and very low conjugated androsterone and etiocholanolone). Excretion of estrone and estradiol low; increase of urinary gonadotropin, increased production of desoxycorticosterone, corticosterone, progesterone, and aldosterone. *Electrocardiography.* Signs of hypokalemia.

Therapy. Dexamethasone 0.5 mg three times a day.

Prognosis. Good response to treatment.

BIBLIOGRAPHY. Biglieri EG, Herron MA, Brust N: 17–hydroxylation deficiency in man. J Clin Invest 45:1946–1954, 1966

Goldsmith O, Solomon DH, Horton R: Hypogonadism and mineralocorticoid excess: the 17–hydroxylase deficiency syndrome. New Engl J Med 277:673–677, 1967

Yanase T, Simpson ER, Waterman MR: 17–alpha-hydroxylase /17, 20–lyase deficiency from clinical investigation to molecular definition. Endocr Rev 12:91–108, 1991

New MI: Congenital adrenal hyperplasia. In De Groot LJ (ed): Endocrinology, 3rd ed, p 1825. Philadelphia, WB Saunders, 1995

BILE REFLUX

Synonym. Alkaline refux gastritis; postgastrectomy; postcholecistectomy. See also Albatross.

Symptoms and Signs. Especially in elderly patients. Usually after gastric surgery or cholecystectomy, occasionally only with no prior surgery. Substernal distress, anorexia, nausea, and vomiting of bile-stained fluid. Many patients, submitted to the Minnesota multiphasic personality inventory profile (MMPP) show abnormal scores for hysteria and hypochondriasis.

Etiology. Reflux of bile into stomach.

Diagnostic Procedures. *Endoscopy.* Of esophagus, stomach, anastomosis, afferent and efferent limbs. *Biopsy.* Of mucosa. *Upper gastrointestinal barium study. Ultrasonography of abdominal organs. Scintigraphy.*

Therapy. *Medical.* Usually disappointing; trials with ursodesoxycholic acid promising. *Surgical.* Roux-en-Y anastomosis (possible development of Roux syndrome, see). Other surgical options: interposition of isopezistaltic jejunal loop between residual stomach and intestine.

Prognosis. Good with surgery. Possible recurrences.

BIBLIOGRAPHY. Buxbaum KL: Bile gastritis occurring after cholecystectomy. Am J Gastroenterol 77:305–311, 1982
Richie WP: Alkaline reflux gastritis in postsurgical syndromes. Gastroent Clin N Am 23:281–294, 1994

BILGINTURAN

Synonym. Brachydactyly-hypertension.

Symptoms and Signs. Short phalanges and metacarpals. Arterial hypertension.

Etiology. Autosomal dominant inheritance.

BIBLIOGRAPHY. Bilginturan N, Zileli S, Karacadag S, et al: Hereditary brachydactyly associated with hypertension. J Med Genet 10:253–259, 1973

BILIARY CAST

Synonyms. Biliary sludge—cast.

Symptoms and Signs. After liver transplantation; long-term parenteral nutrition. Accumulation and concretion of sludge in the biliary tree without anastomotic strictures.

Therapy. Choleretic drugs; surgical revision of biliary reconstruction.

Prognosis. With proper treatment retransplantation can be avoided.

BIBLIOGRAPHY. Chen CL, Wang KL, Chuang JH, et al: Biliary sludge-cast formation following liver transplantation. Hepatogastroenterology 35:22–24, 1988

BILLROTH

Synonyms. Schistosoma haematobium bladder cancer; Bilharziasis bladder cancer.

Symptoms and Signs. In regions endemic for S. haematobium, early onset (40–50 years), especially males. Nicturia, pain, hematuria.

Etiology. Cocarcinogenetic effect of long-term S. haematobium infection.

Pathology. 60–90% squamous cell carcinoma 5–15% adenocarcinomas. Verrocous exophitic grade 1 tumors (70%). Ulcerative endophytic tumors (25%).

Diagnostic Procedures. *Cystoscopy. Urine cytology urography. CT scan.*

Therapy. Surgical. Usually radical anterior pelvic exentration.

Prognosis. Poor.

BIBLIOGRAPHY. Smith JH, Von Lichtenberg F, Stauffer Lehman J: Parasitic diseases of the genito-urinary system. In Campbell's Urology, 6th ed, p 902. Philadelphia, WB Saunders, 1992
Monroe LS: Gastrointestinal parasites. In Haubrich WS, Schaffner F, Berk JE (eds): Bockus Gastroenterology, 5th ed, vol 2, pp 3177–3181. Philadelphia, WB Saunders, 1995

BILLROTH

Synonyms. Traumatic cephalohydrocele; spurious meningocele.

Symptoms and Signs. Appears in children with history of head trauma. Fluid accumulation under scalp.

Etiology. Trauma, with skull fracture and tear of arachnoid.

Diagnostic Procedures. *X-rays. Cerebral CT scan.* Differentiation from hematoma, abscess, meningocele.

Therapy. Usually conservative.

Prognosis. Good, if infection prevented and according to other consequence of trauma.

BIBLIOGRAPHY. Billroth T: Ein Fall von Meningocele spuria cum Fistula ventriculi cerebri. Arch Klin Chir 3:398–412, 1862
Adams RD, Victor M: Principles of Neurology, 5th ed, pp 763–764. New York, McGraw-Hill, 1993

BINDER

Synonym. Maxillonasal dysplasia. See Villaret-Desoilles.

Signs. Present from birth. Flat vertical nose; absence of nasofrontal angle; nasal hypoplasia and flat alae and tip; nostrils crescent-shaped; normal sense of smell. Upper lip convex and poorly developed philtrum; hypoplasia of premaxillary area, flattening of maxillary base and short dental arch; increased gonial angle and flat chin; relative mandibular prognathism.

Etiology. Unknown. Sporadic; possibly, inherited cases. It is considered a surgical entity more than a syndromic entity.

Diagnostic Procedures. *X-rays.* Hypoplasia of anterior nasal spine and of frontal sinuses. Thickness reduction of labial plate of alveolar bone over upper incisors.

BIBLIOGRAPHY. Zuckerland E: Fossae praenasales. Normales und pathologische. Anatomie der nasenhoele und ihrer pneumatische Anhaenge. Wien, W Braunmueller, 1882
Noyes FB: Case report. Angle Orthodon 9:160–165, 1939
Binder KH: Dysostosis maxillo-nasalis: ein arhinencephaler Missbildunskomplex. Dtsch Zahnalzztl Z 17:438–444, 1962
Olow-Nordenzam MAK, Thilander B: The craniofacial morphology in persons with maxillonasal dysplasia (Binder syndrome). Am J Orthodont 95:148–158, 1989
Sheffield LJ, Hallidey JL, Jensen F: Maxillonasal dysplasia (Binder's syndrome) and chondrodysplasia punctata. J Med Genet 28:503–504, 1991

BING-NEEL

Synonym. Macroglobulinemic neuropsychiatric. See Waldenström.

Symptoms. Anorexia; pronounced weight loss; slight elevation of temperature. After variable length of time with these symptoms. In one case, sudden paralysis of arms, legs, whole body, vomiting, headache, no pains, no paresthesia. In a second case, vomiting, dizziness, loss of feeling at end of fingers. In a third case, psychic changes, pain in arm and legs, deep asthenia of arms without paralysis; deep asthenia of legs with probable paresis. In all cases, symptomatology cannot be attributed to any localized process and appears to be caused by disseminated lesions resulting in irregular generalized neurologic patterns.

Signs. Pallor; generalized mild muscular asthenia, decreased fat; patient looks older than chronologic age; lymphadenopathy. Neurologic examination reveals irregular reflexes, alteration paralysis caused by disseminated spinal lesions.

Etiology. See Waldenström.

Pathology. Widespread alteration of nervous system, especially cauda equina, spinal cord, pons, optic nerves, representing the picture of a toxicoinfectious radiculomeningomyeloencephalopathy. Irregular alteration of other organs, no evidence of multiple myeloma.

Diagnostic Procedures. *Blood.* Anemia; marked increase of sedimentation rate; normal white blood cells with prevalence of lymphocytic elements; hyperproteinemia, with hyperglobulinemia; positive test for colloidal lability (Formal gel, SIA test). Bone marrow hyperplastic in only one case; no evidence of myeloma or leukosis. *Urine.* Albuminuria; casts.

Therapy. No therapeutic attempt is reported in the presentation of the original cases. Since this condition seems to be a complication of macroglobulinemic syndromes, for treatment, see Waldenström.

Prognosis. Death follows within 6–12 months from start of neurologic symptomatology.

BIBLIOGRAPHY. Bing J, Neel AV: Two cases of hyperglobulinemia with affection of central nervous system on a toxi-infectious basis. Acta Med Scand 88:492–506, 1936

Bing J, Fog M, Neel AV: Reports of a third case of hyperglobulinemia with affection of central nervous system on toxi-infectious basis. Acta Med Scand 41:409–426, 1937

Edgar R, Dutcher TF: Histopathology of the Bing-Neel syndrome. Neurology 11:239–245, 1961

Foerster J: Waldenstrom's macroglobulinemia. In Lee GR, Bithel TC, Foerster J, et al (eds): Wintrobe's Clinical Hematology, 9th ed, p 2252. Philadelphia, Lea & Febiger, 1993

BINSWANGER

Synonym. Subcortical arteriosclerotic encephalopathy, SAE. See also Senile dementia; Encephalopathy subcortical, vascular.

Symptoms and Signs. Onset at 50–60 years of age. Progressive dementia associated with variable signs of focal cerebral diseases.

Etiology. Arteriosclerosis. Considered as form with no essential difference from the lacunar syndrome (see).

Pathology. Subcortical demyelinization associated with arteriopathy of small arteries of white matter.

Diagnostic Procedures. *Electroencephalography. Angiography. CT brain scan. MRI. Cerebrospinal fluid.* Normal pressure, protein slight increase.

Therapy. Symptomatic.

Prognosis. Slowly progressing condition alternating with periods of stabilization lasting months or years.

BIBLIOGRAPHY. Binswanger O: Die angrenzung der allgemeinen, progressiven Paralyse. Berl Klin Wochenschr 31:1103–1105, 1894

De Reuck J, Crevits L, De Coster W, et al: Pathogenesis of Binswanger chronic progressive subcortical encephalopathy. Neurology 30:920, 1980

Ross GW, Cummings JL: Vascular dementias. In Thal LJ, Moos WH, Gamzu ER (eds): Cognitive Disorders: Pathophysiology and Treatment. New York, Marcel Dekker, 1992

Morris JC: Handbook of Dementing Illnesses. New York, Marcel Dekker, 1993

BIOTINIDASE DEFICIENCY

Synonym. Multiple carboxylase deficiency (late onset).

Symptoms and Signs. Both sexes. Onset of manifestations usually from 1 week to 2 years. Clinical expression highly variable: myoclonic seizures; hypotonia, skin rash and bacterial or fungal infections; alopecia, developmental delay. Less frequently (25–50%) ataxia, lethargy, conjunctivitis, visual abnormalities, deafness. Seldom (10%) hepatosplenomegaly, speech difficulties.

Etiology. Autosomal recessive inheritance. Disorder of biotin recycling.

Pathology. Chronic cerebellar and cerebral degeneration and atrophy; glyosis of white matter and nuclei; subacute necrotizing myelopathy; acute meningoencephalitis.

Diagnostic Procedures. *Biological fluids.* Reduced or absent biotinidase; ketolactic acidosis, organic aciduria. *Urine.* Presence of hydroxyisovaleric acid and other metabolites, including methylcrotonylglycine–hydroxypropionate, methylcitrate, lactate, and triglylglycine. *Immunological studies.* Abnormalities of cellular immunity.

Therapy. Free biotin (5–20 mg/day).

Prognosis. Pronounced and rapid improvement with treatment. Residual damage according to time of onset of treatment.

BIBLIOGRAPHY. Mumich A, Saudubray JM, Carre G et al: Defective biotin absorption in multiple carboxylase deficiency. Lancet 2:263, 1981

Dunkel G, Scriver CR, Clow CL, et al: Prospective ascertainment of complete and partial serum biotinidase deficiency in a newborn. J Inherit Metab Dis 12:131–138, 1989

Wolf B: Disorders of biotin synthesis. In Scriver CR, Beaudet AL, Sly WS, et al: The Metabolic and Molecular Bases of Inherited Disease, 7th ed, pp 3151–3177. New York, McGraw-Hill, 1995

BIRD-HEADED DWARFISM, MONTREAL TYPE

Synonym. See Seckel.

Symptoms. Both sexes. Normal weight at birth. Mental retardation.

Signs. Ptosis. Premature graying and baldness; redundant, wrinkled skin of palms; cryptorchidism.

Etiology. Autosomal recessive inheritance postulated.

BIBLIOGRAPHY. Fitch N, Pinsky L, Lachance RC: A rare form of bird-headed dwarfism with features of premature senility. Am J Dis Child 120:260–264, 1970

McKusick VA: Mendelian Inheritance in Man, 10th ed. Baltimore, Johns Hopkins Univ Press, 1992

BIRNBAUM

Eponym used to indicate a combination of Huntington (see) with cerebellar atrophy.

Synonyms. Progressive chorea-cerebellar atrophy.

BIBLIOGRAPHY. Birnbaum G: Chronisch-progressive Chorea mit Kleinhirnatrophie. Arch Psychiat 114:160–182, 1941

BIRSCH-HIRSCHFIELD

Symptoms and Signs. Onset in old age. Idiopathic hypertrophic parotitis.

BIBLIOGRAPHY. Moortgat P: Syndromes à noms propres. Paris, J Prélat, 1966

BIRT-HOGG-DUBE

Synonyms. Fibrofolliculomas multiple.

Symptoms and Signs. On the face multiple small, white or yellow, papules. Achrocordons and hidradenomas may be present.

Etiology. Autosomal dominant inheritance.

Pathology. Pilosebaceous follicles poorly formed included in a fibrous stroma.

BIBLIOGRAPHY. Birt AR, Hogg GR, Dubé J: Hereditary multiple fibro-folliculomas with trichodiscomas and acrochordons. Arch Dermatol 113:1674–1677, 1977

Scully K, Bargman H, Assaad D: Solitary fibrofolliculoma. J Am Acad Dermatol 11:361–363, 1984

MacKie RM: Tumors of the skin appendages. In Champion RH, Burton JL, Ebling FJG (eds): Rook/Wilkinson/Ebling Textbook of Dermatology, 5th ed, p 2086. Oxford, Blackwell Scientific, 1992

BITTER

Symptoms and Signs. From birth pseudohemihypertrophy of face; sebaceous nevus in the trigeminal and upper cervical region unilaterally or bilaterally in the skin and mucosae. Dwarfism (occasional). Variable malformation of eyes, brain, mouth, and teeth.

Etiology. Observed in newborn with mothers who had received thalidomide.

BIBLIOGRAPHY. Bitter K: Dtsch Zahn-Mund-u. Kieferheilk 56:17–24, 1971

Liebaldt GP, Leiber B: Cutaneous dysplasias associated with neurological disorders. In Vinken PJ, Bruyn GW (eds): Handbook of Clinical Neurology, vol 14, pp 101, 107. Amsterdam, North-Holland, 1975

BIVENTRICULAR TRANSPOSED AORTA AND LEFT VENTRICULAR STENOTIC PULMONARY ARTERY

Symptoms and Signs. Early deep cyanosis with physical endurance not markedly decreased; apical systolic murmur (grade 1); accentuation of second pulmonary sound; left-sided enlargement of the heart; clubbing of fingers and toes.

Etiology. Unknown; congenital malformation.

Pathology. Biventricular transposed aorta and left stenotic pulmonary artery.

Diagnostic Procedures. *X-rays of chest.* Frontal view, concave middle segment; oblique view, concavity disappears and is replaced by prominence of a vessel whose anterior contour is tangent to anterior border of underlying ventricle. Left-sided enlargement of heart chambers. *Simultaneous catheterization and angiocardiography. Electrocardiography.*

Therapy. Symptomatic.

Prognosis. In these cases, in contrast with cases with transposition of great vessels with or without pulmonary stenosis, life is prolonged for unusual length of time (second decade).

BIBLIOGRAPHY. De la Cruz MV, da Rocha JP: An ontogenetic theory for the explanation of congenital malformations involving the truncus and conus. Am Heart J 51:782–805, 1956

De la Cruz MV, Espino-Vela J, Anselmi G: Biventricular transposed aorta and left ventricular stenotic pulmonary artery: an embryologic and pathologic account of a new syndrome whose existence was previously theoretically predicted. Am Heart J 59:902–912, 1960

Van Mierop LHS, Kutsche LM: Embryology of Heart. In Schlant RC, Alexander RW: Hurst's The Heart, 8th ed. New York, McGraw-Hill, 1994

BIXLER

Synonym. Harper dwarf; hypertelorism—microtia—clefting; HMC; deafness—hypertelorism clefting.

Symptoms. In females. From birth: psychomotor retardation, conductive deafness.

Signs. Head: hypertelorism, microtia, microstomia clefting of lip, palate and nose, hypoplastic pinnae or broad nasal tip, short stature.

Heart murmurs. Occasionally: thenar hypoplasia, syndactyly of toes; shortening of fifth fingers.

Etiology. Possibly autosomal recessive inheritance.

Pathology. Heart ASD; endocardial cushion defect; ectopic kidneys; atretic auditory canals.

BIBLIOGRAPHY. Bixler D, Christian JC, Gorlin RJ: Hypertelorism, microtia and facial clefting: a new inherited syndrome. Birth Defects 5:77–81, 1969

Bixler D, Antley RM: Microcephaly dwarfism in sisters. Birth Defects. Orig Art Ser. 10:161–165. Miami, Symposia Specialists, 1974

Baraitser M: The hypertelorism microtia clefting syndrome. J Med Genet 19:387–388, 1982

Gorlin RJ, Cohen MM, Levin LS: Syndromes of Head and Neck, 3rd ed, p 663. New York, Oxford Univ Press, 1990

BIXLER-ANTLEY

Symptoms and Signs. Those of Erdheim I (see) associated with ectopia of the pigment layer of the iris into anterior surface of iris.

BIBLIOGRAPHY. Bixler D, Antley RM: Familial aortic dissection with iris anomalies: a new connective tissue disease syndrome? Birth Defects Orig Art XII (5):229–234, 1976

BJORKMAN-DACIE

Synonyms. Anemia refractaria sideroblastica; ineffective idiopathic erythropoiesis; IRSA; sideroblastic refractory anemia, primary, acquired; refractory normoblastic anemia; refractory anemia-ringed sideroblasts; RARS (FAB classification see Pathology).

Symptoms. Occurs in older adults (average age 66); very seldom in people younger than 50. Onset insidious. Asthenia.

Signs. Mild pallor; modest hepatosplenomegaly (40%).

Etiology. Unknown, acquired condition. Impairment of heme synthetase reaction. Possibly, neoplasia, drug or toxic hypersensitivity reactions, somatic mutation. X-linked inheritance reported (see Pagon). Some investigators opt for leukemic nature of this group of conditions.

Pathology. *Liver.* Marked deposition of iron. *Blood.* Moderate anemia, normocytic or macrocytic type; occasionally, hypochromic; heavily stippled cells, moderate leukothrombocytopenia; leukocyte alkaline phosphatase reduced in 90% of cases; transferrin increased, modest hyperbilirubinemia. *Bone marrow.* Erythroid hyperplasia; lack of PAS positivity in normoblast; megaloblastic changes (20%); increased hemosiderin; ringed sideroblasts. (According to FAB classification: if less than 5% classified as RA if more than 15% as RARS if myeloblasts over 5–20% as RAEB; and if myeloblasts over 20–30% as RAEB-t regardless of number of sideroblasts.)

Therapy. Pyridoxine 50–200 mg/day (usually ineffective). Some patients who did not respond to pyridoxine were able to respond to pyridoxal phosphate, the coenzyme form of the vitamin. Transfusion of packed cells (minimal benefit). Androgens.

Prognosis. About half of the patients are not severely incapacitated by their anemia, which does not progress for many years. In these cases no treatment is required. In cases with significant cardiovascular symptoms: transfuse with packed red cells. Number of transfusions should be kept to a minimum because of iron overload. Some patients respond to large doses of androgens (50–100 mg of oxymetholone per day). Some patients develop leukemia and acute myelofibrosis.

BIBLIOGRAPHY. Bjorkman S: Chronic refractory anemia with sideroblastic bone marrow. Blood 11:250–259, 1956

Dacie JV: Refractory normoblastic anemia. Br J Haematol 5:245–256, 1959

Holmes J, May A, Geddes D, et al: A family study of congenital X-linked sideroblastic anemia. J Med Genet 27:26–28, 1990

Bottomley SS: Sideroblastic anemias. In Lee GR, Bithell TC, Foerster J, et al (eds): Wintrobe's Clinical Hematology, 9th ed, pp 859–861. Philadelphia, Lea & Febiger, 1993

BJORNSTAD-CRANDALL

Synonym. Crandall; deafness—pili torti; pili torti—deafness. See Ronchese.

Symptoms. Both sexes affected; manifested since early infancy. Sensory neuronal hearing loss occurring as a significant association with pili torti (see). Normal psychic development after reaching puberty evidence of secondary hypogonadism.

Etiology. Unknown; autosomal recessive inheritance.

Pathology. Hair shafts. Longitudinal ridging, irregular twisting.

Diagnostic Procedures. *Blood.* Growth hormone and follicular stimulating hormone deficiency.

BIBLIOGRAPHY. Bjornstad R: Pili torti and sensory loss of hearing. Proc XVII Meeting Northen Dermatological Society. Copenhagen, 1965

Crandall BF, Samec L, Sparkes RS, et al: A familial syndrome of deafness, alopecia and hypogonadism. J Pediatr 82:461–465, 1973

Cremers CWJ, Geerts SJ: Sensorineuronal hearing loss and pili torti. Am Otol Rhinol Laryng 88:100–104, 1979

BK MOLE

Synonyms. Clark; Lynch; MLM; dysplastic nevus, hereditary; sporadic familial atypical mole malignant melanoma; F.A.M.M.M.

Symptoms and Signs. Large number of nevi (some very large) with irregular borders and sometime inflammatory flare.

Etiology. Autosomal inheritance with high variability of expressivity. Sporadic cases reported.

Pathology. Nevi with signs of dysplasia.

Diagnostic Procedures. Biopsy (with great precaution).

Therapy. Wide excision and eventually chemotherapy.

Prognosis. High risk of complete malignant transformation and possibility of cancer at other site.

BIBLIOGRAPHY. Norris W: A case of fungoid disease. Edinburg Med Sur J 16:562–565, 1820

Lynch HT, Krush AJ: Heredity and malignant melanoma implication for early cancer detection. Can Med Assoc J 99:17–21, 1968

Clark WH Jr, Reimer RR, Greene M, et al: Origin of familial malignant melanoma from heritable melanocytic lesions "the b-k mole syndrome." Arch Dermatol 114:732–738, 1978

Lynch HT, Fusaro RM, Albano WA, et al: Phenotypic variation in the familial atypical multiple mole-melanoma syndrome (FAMMM). J Med Genet 20:25–29, 1983

Nancarrow DJ, Palmer JM, Walters MK, et al: Exclusion of the familial melanoma locus (MLM) from the PND/D1S47 and MYCL1 regions of chromosome arm 1p in 7 Australian pedigrees. Genomics 12:18–25, 1992

BLACKFAN-DIAMOND

Synonyms. Hypoplastic congenital anemia; red cell, primary asplasia; congenital aregenerative anemia; idiopathic erythroblastopenia; erythrogenesis imperfecta; erythrophthisis; Diamond-Blackfan; Josephs-Diamond-Blackfan; Kaznelson I. See pure red cell aplasia.

Symptoms. Noted at birth or recognized within first 6 months. Male patients appear to be less affected than female. Growth retardation; failure of sexual maturation; seldom, dyspnea; decrease of activity. Few adults with the syndrome have been described.

Signs. Weight at birth lower than normal; pallor; no jaundice. Presence of minor congenital anomalies (occasionally, hepatomegaly; rare, splenomegaly), which initially regress after blood transfusion.

Etiology. Unknown. Familial incidence in some cases (dominant transmission and expression in the heterozygotes). Abnormalities of tryptophan metabolism in some cases. In one case, association with chromosome abnormality. Spectrum of various conditions characterized by pure erythroid deficiency.

Pathology. Pallor; underdevelopment; failure of sexual maturation. Hemosiderosis (secondary to blood transfusion); cirrhosis. Portal hypertension. Osteoporosis.

Diagnostic Procedures. *Blood.* Normocytic, normochromic anemia; reticulocytes (less than 1%): normoblasts; leukocytes and platelets normal. Hypocalcemia. *Bone marrow.* Erythroid deficiency. *Other series.* Normal. *X-rays.* Variable skeletal and visceral anomalies; growth retardation.

Therapy. Blood transfusion. Adrenal cortical steroids induce remission. Splenectomy is of doubtful utility. Bone marrow transplantation good results.

Prognosis. Course insidious and progressive; severe complications from chronic blood transfusions: hemosiderosis, liver damage, spontaneous remissions (permanent or temporary) reported (20% of one series after 8 months to 13 years failed to respond to any treatment).

BIBLIOGRAPHY. Josephs HW: Anemia of infancy and early childhood. Medicine 15:307–451, 1936

Diamond LK, Blackfan KD: Hypoplastic anemia. Am J Dis Child 56:464–467, 1938

Scimeca PG, Weinblatt ME, Slepowitz G, et al: Diamond Blackfan syndrome: an unusual case of hydrops fetalis. Am J Ped Hematol Oncol 10:241–243, 1988

Williams P: Ancytopenia, aplastic anemia, and pure red cell aplasia. In Lee GR, Bithel TC, Foerster J, et al (eds): Wintrobe's Clinical Hematology, 9th ed, pp 935–936. Philadelphia, Lea & Febiger, 1993

BLACK HEEL

Synonyms. Talon noir; calcaneal petecchiae; purpura traumatica pedis.

Symptoms and Signs. Boys predominantly affected, especially if athletically active; usually epidemic occurrence, seldom sporadic. Blackish discoloration in isolated or aggregated specks in horny layer of back or side of heels; seldom in the forefoot (metatarsal area).

Etiology. Unknown; blood extravasion. Reason for epidemic outbreak unknown.

Therapy. Not needed. Felt pad in the shoes may help.

Prognosis. Spontaneous regression at the end of athletic season.

BIBLIOGRAPHY. Bazex A, Salvador R, Dupre A: Plantar chromhidrosis. Bull Soc Fr Dermatol Syph 69:489–490, 1962

Kennedy CTC: Reactions to mechanical and thermal injury. In Champion RH, Burton JL, Ebling FJG (eds): Rook/Wilkinson/Ebling Textbook of Dermatology, 5th ed, pp 787–788. Oxford, Blackwell Scientific, 1992

BLACKOUT

Synonyms. Hydrostatic pressure; negative acceleration.

Symptoms. In passengers in vehicles (especially airplanes) subjected to rapid acceleration or deceleration. Rise of visual threshold; altered perception of intensity of lights and colors, up to complete loss of consciousness.

Signs. Moderate mydriasis; periorbital edema; subconjunctival hemorrhages.

Etiology. Reduction of retinal arterial pressure.

Pathology. Retinal hemorrhages.

Diagnostic Procedures. *Ophthalmoscopy.* Retinal arterial collapse.

Prognosis. Good. Vision restored after cessation of cause.

BIBLIOGRAPHY. Stokes WH: Unusual retinal vascular changes in traumatic injury to the chest. Arch Ophthalmol 7:101–108, 1932
Lyle DJ, Stapp JP, Button RR: Ophthalmological hydrostatic pressure syndrome. Trans Am Ophthalmol Soc 54:121–128, 1956
Hopkirk JAC, Denison DM: Aerospace medicine. In Weatherall DJ, Ledingham JGG, Warrell DA (eds): Oxford Textbook of Medicine, 3rd ed, pp 1193–1204. New York, Oxford Med Pub, 1966

BLACK WIDOW SPIDER BITE

Synonyms. Arachnidism; araneism; Latrodectus mactans bite; latrodectism.

Symptoms. Local. Unnoticed or pain. Systemic. In the regional lymphatic nodes spreading to the lumbar region, the abdomen, the waist, the thighs, and the whole lower extremities. Muscular pain, cramps, tremors, athralgias, fever (maximum intensity for 20 hours). Photophobia. Exocrine secretion (eye, nose, mouth, and skin).

Signs. *Local.* A red, gooseflesh area of 0.5 cm in diameter, increasing in size and intensity. Then a pallid area up to 5 cm in diameter delimited by a reddish, blush circular border; anesthesia dolorosa. *Cardiovascular.* First tachycardia then bradycardia, cardiac failure; extrasystole, first hypotension then hypertension. *Respiratory.* Tachypnea followed by bradypnea, increased bronchial secretion, bronchoconstriction. *Abdomen.* Rigidity of the abdominal wall; liver enlargement or subicterus. *Urogenital.* Oliguria or anuria during the first 12 hours.

Etiology and Pathology. Bite by female black widow spider (13 mm long, completely black with clepsydra-like red marking on the ventral side).

Diagnostic Procedures. Observation of lesion and progression of muscle involvement to differentiate from acute abdomen. *Blood.* Leukocytosis, neutrophilia, lymphopenia, increased erythrocyte sedimentation rate, decrease of sodium and chlorides, increased blood urea nitrogen. *Urine.* Albuminuria; sediment RBC, WBC, and casts.

Therapy. Calcium gluconate (10%) 10 ml intravenously, specific antivenom when available. Hot bath and analgesic (careful with respiratory depression), neostigmine for muscle spasm. Corticosteroid for fast relief.

Prognosis. Rapid recovery, but in children may be fatal.

BIBLIOGRAPHY. Brown HW: Venenating arthropods (centipedes, scorpions, spiders, ticks, wasps, ants, blister beetles, caterpillars). In Beeson PB, McDermott W (eds): Cecil-Loeb Textbook of Medicine, 12th ed, pp 418–419. Philadelphia, WB Saunders, 1967
Burns DA: Diseases caused by arthropods and other noxious animals. In Champion RH, Burton JL, Ebling FJG (eds): Rook/Wilkinson/Ebling Textbook of Dermatology, 5th ed, pp 1265–1269. Oxford, Blackwell Scientific, 1992

BLADDER NECK

Synonym. Urethral; see Female prostatic obstruction and Hunner.

Symptoms. More frequent in females seldom in males and children of both sexes. Initial urinary hesitancy, weak stream; terminal dribbling.

and occasionally suprapubic and lumbar pain, in absence of objective urologic findings. An acute and a chronic form are recognized.

Signs. Increasing volume of residual urine and large decompensated bladder with cellules and diverticula.

Etiology. Narrowing of bladder outlet (congenital); dysfunction of vesical sphincter muscles (spasm of external uretral sphincter); acquired: bladder neck operation or chronic infections and fibrosis of bladder neck. Psychogenic factors considered in some cases. To be differentiated from pseudobladder neck syndrome where the compression is extrinsic (pelvic tumors; pregnancy).

Pathology. See Etiology.

Diagnostic Procedures. *Urine.* Absolute negativity of all analysis for infections of any type (diagnostic criteria). Determination of residual urine volumes. *Cystograms. Cystourethrography. Cystoscopy. Neurologic examination.* To exclude neurogenic bladder. *Calibration of bladder neck.*

Therapy. *Medical.* Electrostimulation, surgical or psychological according to etiology and degree of involvement. High fluid intake may temporarily improve situation.

Prognosis. Good with adequate treatment.

BIBLIOGRAPHY. Davis DM: Vesical orifice obstruction in women and its treatment by transuretral resection. J Urol 73:112, 1955
Ward JN, Lavengood RWJ, Draper JW: Pseudo bladder neck syndrome in women. J Urol 99:65–68, 1968
Wien AJ: Neuromuscular disorders of the lower urinary tract. In Walsh PC, Reik AB, Stamey TA, et al: Campbell's Urology, pp 626–635. Philadelphia, WB Saunders, 1992
Messing EM: Interstitial cystitis and related syndromes. In Walsh PC, Gittes RF, Perlmutter AD, et al: Campbell's Urology, 5th ed, pp 1031–1040. Philadelphia, WB Saunders, 1992
Bailey: Urinary tract infection. In Weatherall DJ, Ledingham JGG, Warrell DA (eds): Oxford Textbook of Medicine, 3rd ed, p 3210. Oxford, Oxford Med Pub, 1996

BLAND-GARLAND-WHITE

Synonyms. Bland-White Garland; coronary left artery of anomalous origin; left coronary artery from pulmonary artery.

Symptoms. Phase 1. Neonatal. Infant appears normal at birth and for a short time afterward. Phase 2. Transitory. Death or survival according to development of adequate intercoronary anastomosis. Distress; myocardial ischemia symptoms and signs. Phase 3. Progressive improvement of symptoms and signs of ischemia. Frequently, dilatation of left side of heart and secondary mitral insufficiency. Arrythmias in later period. Phase 4. Coronary artery steal syndrome (see).

Signs. Enlarged heart, mostly left ventricle; usually, no murmur or apical holosystolic murmur.

Etiology. Congenital anomaly with origin of left coronary artery from pulmonary artery.

Pathology. Necrosis and fibrosis of left ventricle, especially subendocardial and of papillary muscles. Thrombosis of small arteries and arterioles. If patient survives second phase, abundant collateral circulation.

Diagnostic Procedures. *ECG.* Inversion T1 T2, deep Q1. *Retrograde aortography. Cardiac catheterization.* Diagnostic. *Two-dimensional echocardiography with color flow imaging and spectral Doppler interrogation.*

Therapy. If adequate collateral circulation is demonstrated, ligature of anomalous artery at its origin. If collateral circulation inadequate, vascular graft from aorta to the left coronary artery.

Prognosis. Second phase is most dangerous period; death from acute myocardial ischemia. In third phase, death from fatal arrhythmia. Occasionally, asymptomatic or paucisymptomatic cases may reach adolescence or adulthood.

BIBLIOGRAPHY. Brooks H St J: Two cases of an abnormal coronary artery of the heart arising from the pulmonary artery: with some remarks upon the effects of this anomaly in producing cirsoid dilatation of vessels. Trans Acad Med Ireland (Dubl) 3:447–449, 1885

Brooks HS Jr: Two cases of an abnormal coronary artery arising from the pulmonary artery. J Anat Physiol 20:26, 1886

Abrikossoff A: Anaeurysma des linken Harzventrikels mit abnormer abgangstelle der linken Koronaraterie von der Pulmonalis bei einem funsononatlichen Kinde. Virchow's Arch [Pathol Anat] 203:413–420, 1911

Bland EF, et al: Congenital anomalies of the coronary arteries, report of an unusual case associated with cardiac hypertrophy. Am Heart J 8:787–80l, 1932–33

Perloff JK: The Clinical Recognition of Congenital Heart Disease, 4th ed, pp 561–580. Philadelphia, WB Saunders, 1994

BLAST

Synonym. Blast injury.

Symptoms. Dyspnea; pain in ears; partial or complete deafness; pain in the chest or other regions (see Blast scrotum).

Signs. Shock, loss of consciousness; bradycardia; signs of injury in lung, heart, abdominal organs; abdominal distention; petecchiae in eardrum.

Etiology. Phase of overpressure and underpressure after detonation, especially when occurring underwater with subject in immersion.

Pathology. Hemorrhages in lung parenchyma; arterial embolizations; pneumothorax; gut and sinuses. Gas-free tissues such as liver and spleen are undamaged.

Diagnostic Procedures. *Electrocardiography.* Atrial flutter; fibrillation. *Blood.* Hematocrit, electrolytes. *X-ray of chest.* Increased or decreased transparency.

Therapy. According to type and degree of lesions. Tracheal intubation and mechanical ventilation frequently required.

Prognosis. Variable.

BIBLIOGRAPHY. De Candole CA: Blast injury. Can Med Assoc J 96:207–214, 1967

Fishman AP, Pietra GG: Stretched pores, blast injury and neurohemo-dynamic pulmonary edema. Physiologist 23:53–56, 1980

Denison DM: Diving medicine. In Weatherall DJ, Ledingham JGG, Warrell DA (eds): Oxford Textbook of Medicine, 3rd ed, p 11205. Oxford, Oxford Med Pub, 1996

BLAST SCROTUM

Symptoms. See Blast. Pain in the scrotum.

Signs. See Blast; unilateral swelling of testis and epididymis.

Etiology and Pathology. Pressure from blast increases tension on the external inguinal ring preventing circulatory return.

Therapy. Cold packs.

Prognosis. Recovery.

BIBLIOGRAPHY. Swersie AK: Unilateral scrotal swelling following blast injury: a syndrome. Urology 55:292–294, 1946

Cass AS: Testicular trauma. J Urol 129:299–300, 1983

BLATIN

Synonym. Hydatid fremitis. Eponym used to indicate the sign yielded by a hydatis cyst under tension; the hydatid thrill or vibratory sensation is felt on the palm of the hand when this lies flat over the tumor and a finger is percussed. This sign may be elicited, however, with other types of cyst as well.

BIBLIOGRAPHY. MacLaurin C: The symptoms of liver hydatid. Aust Med Gaz 28:295–300, 1909

Barnett LE: Hydatid thrill: its rarity, physical explanation and diagnostic value. N Z Med J 20:277–285, 1921

BLATT

Synonyms. Cranio-oculo-orbital dysrhaphia—meningocele; oculocranio-orbital dysraphia—meningocele; orbitocranioocular dysraphia—meningocele.

Symptoms and Signs. Both sexes affected; present from birth. Anisometropia; meningocele or meningoencephalocele; cranial deformities; facial bone malformation; hypertelorism; microphthalmus; distichiasis; meibonian glands absent.

Etiology. Unknown, autosomal dominant inheritance.

BIBLIOGRAPHY. Blatt N: Cranio-orbito-ocular dysraphia and meningocele. Rev Otoneurophthalmol 33:185–232, 1961

Tessier P: Surgical treatment of genetically caused eyelid and orbito-facial deformities. Buech Augenarzt 50:82–121, 1968

BLEGVAD-HAXTHAUSEN

Obsolete.

Synonyms. Anetoderma—osteogenesis imperfecta; see Osteogenesis imperfecta.

Symptoms and Signs. Both sexes affected. Skin appears thin, translucent, slackening, and shows well-defined round or oval areas of variable size (from milia to coin) of grayish color. Grosser anomalies of skin usually absent, but described in some cases. Eye: blue sclerae: zonal cataract. Partial or total deafness. Multiple bone fractures from minor traumas. Wounds heal slowly, with ample scars. Vascular fragility with easily forming hematomas. Reported associated defects include those of Ehler-Danlos syndrome.

Etiology. Generalized defect in collagen maturation; autosomal dominant heredity. Identical to Ekman's. The macular atrophy of the skin described represents one of the nonconstant signs of the osteogenesis imperfecta.

Pathology. *Dermis.* Thin, increase of argentophil and elastic fibers; immaturity and swelling of collagenous fiber. *Bones.* Osteogenesis imperfecta (see).

Diagnostic Procedures. *Biopsy of skin. X-ray. Skeletal survey.*

Therapy. Symptomatic.

Prognosis. Osteogenesis imperfecta (see).

BIBLIOGRAPHY. Blegvad O, Haxthausen H: Blaa sclerae og tendens til knoglebrud med pletformet hudatrofi og zonulaer catarat. Hospitalstidende 64:609–616, 1921

BLENCKE

Synonym. Calcaneus metaepiphyseal osteodystrophy.

Symptoms and Signs. Pain on the calcaneal region; increased by walking.

Etiology. See Epiphyseal ischemic necrosis.

BLEPHARONASOFACIAL

Synonym. Pashayan-Putterman.

Symptoms and Signs. Both sexes affected; present from birth. *Facies.* Mask-like; telecanthus; lateral displacement and stenosis of lacrimal puncta; nose bulky; broad bridge, midfacial hypoplasia; horizontal cheek furrows; trapezoidal upper lip. *Extremities.* Soft tissue syndactyly. *Joints.* Hyperextensibility. Nervous system. Poor coordination; torsion distonia; positive Babinski sign.

Etiology. Autosomal dominant inheritance.

BIBLIOGRAPHY. Pashayan H, Pruzansky S, Putterman A: A family with bleopharo-naso-facial malformation. Am J Dis Child 125:389–393, 1973
Putterman AM, Pashayan H, Pruzansky S: Eye findings in the blepharo-naso-facial malformation syndrome. Am J Ophthalmol 76:825–831, 1973

BLEPHAROPHIMOSIS-PTOSIS-EPICANTHUS INVERSUS-LACRIMAL STENOSIS

Synonyms. BPES; Komoto triad; Kohn-Romano; Vignes; conjuctival eyelid tetra (CET).

Symptoms. Male predominance, onset from birth. Visual impairment; occasional amblyopia. Normal mental development. Female infertility.

Signs. Telecanthus; microphthalmus; ptosis; epicanthus inversus; blepharophimosis; elongated lid margin. Divergent strabismus; nystagmus; esotropia. Ductus lacrimalis anomalies. Fundus oculi normal. Low-set ears; deformed pinnae. High-arched palate.

Etiology. Unknown, autosomal dominant inheritance. Possibly two types: (1) with infertility of affected females; (2) transmission from both males and females.

Etiology. Plastic surgery; canthoplasty for aesthetics and ocular functional reasons.

BIBLIOGRAPHY. Gazelowski X: Traite des Maladies des Yeux, 2nd ed. Paris, Balliere,1875
Vignes L: Epicanthus héréditaire. Rev Gen Ophthalmol 8:438, 1889
Komoto J: Ptosis operation. Klin Monatsbl Augenheilkd 66:952, 1921
Kohn R, Romano PE: Blepharoptosis, blepharophimosis, epicanthus inversus, and telecanthus: a syndrome with no name. Am J Ophthalmol 72:625–632, 1971
Baraitser M: Blepharophimosis, ptosis, epicanthus inversus syndrome (BPES syndrome). J Med Genet 25:47–51, 1988

BLESSIG-IWANOFF

Synonyms. Iwanoff; retinal cystoid degeneration; retinoschisis.

Symptoms and Signs. Both sexes affected; onset after 50 years of age. Exceptionally noted in infancy. Asymptomatic or sudden impairment of vision.

Etiology. Not entirely clear. Accumulation of a hyaluronidase-sensitive glycosaminoglycan (GAG) in the outer plexiform layer; neural loss is a secondary event.

Pathology. Retinal cyst located primarily in nuclear layers; all layers involved; cystic areas coalescence with adjacent areas; splitting of retina in two layers with eventual detachment.

Diagnostic Procedures. *Ophthalmoscopy.* In retinal periphery small translucent areas or branching channels.

Therapy. Symptomatic.

Prognosis. Variable according to evolution. Usually favorable, but detachment of retina may follow.

BIBLIOGRAPHY. Garner A, Sarks S, Sarks JP: Degenerative and related disorders of the retina and choroid. In Garner A, Klintworth GK (eds): Pathobiology of Ocular Disease: A dynamic Approach, 2nd ed, pp 666–667. New York, Marcel Dekker, 1994

BLINDNESS, TRANSIENT POST-TRAUMATIC

Synonym. Transient postictal hemianopsia; visual loss, temporary post-traumatic. See blackout.

Symptoms. Usually, bilateral total or partial blindness of few minutes or many hours duration; occasionally, only whitish, foggy aspect of visual field; headache; drowsiness; restlessness; agitation.

Signs. Normal pupillary reaction to light or fixed pupils. Fundus oculi normal.

Etiology. Head trauma, especially of parietooccipital regions causing vasospasm, edema.

Diagnostic Procedures. *Electroencephalography.* In early period, slowing of occipital pattern. *CT scan. MRI. Visual evoked potentials.*

Therapy. None; diuretics.

Prognosis. Good. Complete recovery usually within 24 hours. Recurrences possible.

BIBLIOGRAPHY. Walsh FB: Clinical Neurophthalmology, 2nd ed, Baltimore, Williams & Wilkins, 1957
Adams V: Principles of Neurology, p 757. New York, McGraw-Hill, 1993

BLIND POUCH

Symptoms. Usually appears years after surgery with side-to-side intestinal anastomosis. Weakness; failure to gain weight; intermittent diarrhea; cramping abdominal pain. Symptoms in combination or alone. Complication or hemorrhage and perforation possible.

Signs. Pallor; abdominal scar. Tenderness on abdominal palpation. Sometimes soft tissue mass is palpable.

Etiology. Dilated blind ends of small intestine after side-to-side intestinal anastomosis; not to be confused with "blind loop syndrome," which has different clinical, laboratory, and anatomic abnormalities. Today included in Bacterial overgrowth (see).

Pathology. Dilation of afferent and efferent blind pouches; hypertrophy; edema; ulceration of mucosa.

Diagnostic Procedures. *Blood.* Macrocytic or microcytic anemia (in blind loop usually macrocytic anemia). *X-rays.* Demonstration of blind ileal pouch.

Therapy. Surgical correction. End-to-end anastomosis of normal intestine.

Prognosis. Excellent after surgical correction.

BIBLIOGRAPHY. Brief DK, Botsford TW: Primary bleeding from the small intestine in adults: the surgical management. JAMA 184:18–22, 1963
Botsford TW, Gazzaniga AB: Blind pouch syndrome: a complication of side to side intestinal anastomosis. Am J Surg 113:486–490, 1967

BLOCH-SULZBERGER

Synonyms. Block-Siemens; incontinentia pigmenti, cutaneous lineal melanoblastosis. See also Asboe-Hansen. Siemens-Bloch.

Symptoms and Signs. Appears at birth or within one or two years; female to male ratio 10:1. Recurrent inflammatory lesions (papules, vesicle, bullae) initially localized, then spreading in configurate bizarre patterns. Lesions subside after weeks or months and either pass through papillary or warty stages or directly develop into pigmentary macules. Distribution of lesions highly irregular, not corresponding to blood vessels and nerve dermatomes. Resulting macules chocolate, grayish in color, persisting or fading or disappearing or leaving atrophic areas. Localized atrophic alopecia of scalp; dystrophic nails; keratotic areas. Occasionally linear, macular telangiectases. Associated abnormalities present in two-thirds of patients: dental anomalies; strabismus; cataracts; optic atrophy; retinal abnormalities; nervous system disorders (35%); spastic paralysis; epilepsy; microcephaly, mental retardation; deafness; osseous changes with retarded growth; and abnormal development; heart malformation.

Etiology. Congenital familial condition (15%); pedigree patterns in a family suggest X-linked dominance of autosome X translocation with lethality in the male. Other proposed causes: anomalies of ectomesodermal development; viruses, Herpes simplex (?).

Pathology. Deposit of melanin inside and outside melanophores in pigmented area. Other abnormalities described in symptoms.

Diagnostic Procedures. Vesicle fluid contains eosinophils (95%). *Blood.* Eosinophilia (30–50%). *X-rays. CT scan.* Tooth abnormalities and other lesions according to occurrence (see Symptoms). Skeletal abnormality (20%); microcephaly, brain atrophy and/or edema, hydrocephalus.

Therapy. No treatment needed. Corticosteroid perhaps beneficial on vesicular stage. Control of secondary infections.

Prognosis. According to severity of form and organ involvement. Cutaneous involvement without other abnormalities, resolution usually spontaneous, seldom may be recurrent during childhood. Normal life.

BIBLIOGRAPHY. Garrod AE: Peculiar pigmentation of the skin in an infant. Trans Clin Soc London 39:216, 1906

Bardach M: Systematisierte Naevusbildungen bei einem eineiigen Zwillingspaar. Ein Beitrag zur Naevusaetiologie. Z Kinderheilkd 39:542,550, 1925

Bloch B: Eigentümliche bisher nicht beschriebene Pigmentaffektion (Incontinentia pigmenti). Schweiz Med Wochensch 56:404–405, 1926

Sulzberger MB: Ueber eine bisher nicht beschriebene congenitale Pigmentanomalie (Incontinentia pigmenti). Arch Dermatol Syph 154:19–32, 1928

Ciolla JA: Incontinentia pigmenti and X-autosomal translocations. Human Genet 81:269–272, 1989

Bleehen SS, Ebling FJG, Champion RH: Disorders of skin color. In Champion RH, Burton JL, Ebling FJG (eds): Rook/Wilkinson/Ebling Textbook of Dermatology, 5th ed, pp 1580–1582. Oxford, Blackwell Scientific, 1992

BLOODGOOD

Synonyms. Cheatle; Cooper I; Reclus I; Schimmelbusch; Tillaux-Phocas; blue dome; cystic breast; fibrocystic; chronic cystic mastitis; mastopathia chronica cystica.

Symptoms. Occurs in women; onset at 45–55 years of age. Usually, asymptomatic or pain in the breast, especially premenstrually; receding after onset.

Signs. Bilateral masses in the breasts; round, smooth, tense, mobile, not adherent to skin.

Etiology. Unknown; possible hormonal imbalance.

Pathology. Mammary ducts: dilatation; blue brownish cysts filled by turbid fluid; papillary formation inside the cysts.

Diagnostic Procedures. *Mammography. Xerography. Thermography. Biopsy. Hormonal study. Echography.*

Therapy. Vitamin A. Surgery. Danazol for severe pain. Stop coffee, tea, and chocolate (reported improvement). Bromocryptine.

Prognosis. Malignancy transformation (1–6%).

BIBLIOGRAPHY. Cooper A: Illustrations of the Diseases of the Breast. London, Longmans, 1829

Reclus P: La maladie kystique de mamelles. Bull Soc Anat Paris 8:428–433, 1883

Bloodgood JC: The pathology of chronic cystic mastitis of the female breast, with special consideration of the blue-dome cyst. Arch Surg 3:442–445, 1921

Hutter RUP: Goodbye to "fibrocystic disease." N Engl J Med 312:179–181, 1985

Vorherr H: Fibrocystic breast disease: pathophysiology, pathomorphology, clinical picture and management. Am J Obstet Gynecol 154:161–179, 1986

Hindle WH: Breast Disease for Gynecologists. Appleton Lange, 1990

BLOOM I

Synonyms. Lymphedema-ptosis. See Nonne-Milroy-Meige, Falls-Kertesz, and Noonan.

Symptoms and Signs. Lymphedema of legs and ptosis. May be associated with photosensitive reactions.

Etiology. Autosomal dominant inheritance.

BIBLIOGRAPHY. Bloom D: Hereditary lymphedema (Nonne-Milroy-Meige): Report of a family with hereditary lymphedema associated with ptosis of the eyelids in several generations. NY J Med 41:856–863, 1941

Bligard CA, Storer JS: Photosensitivity in infants and children. Dermatol Clin 4:311–319, 1986

Gorlin RJ, Cohen MM Jr, Levin LS: Syndromes of Head and Neck, pp 297–299. New York, Oxford Univ Press, 1992

BLOOM II

Synonyms. Bloom-German; Bloom-Torre-MacKacek; Levi type dwarfism; telangiectasis facial dwarfism.

Symptoms and Signs. Males preponderant. Usually, low birth weight following full-term gestation; facial rash, discoid lupus erythematosus-like hypersensitivity to sun, skin manifestations in other parts of body, erythematous type, areas of increased and decreased pigmentation, hypersensitivity to light; failure to grow. Microcephaly variable; dolichocephaly, with zygomatic hypoplasia, with or without small nose; protruding ears. Occasionally associated, various abnormalities of eyes, ears, extremities, digits. High-pitched voice.

Etiology. Autosomal recessive inheritance.

Pathology. *Skin lesions.* Moderate parakeratosis; absence of granular layer; thin rete of Malpighi; moderate intercellular edema; corium with capillary and perivascular telengiectasis; lymphocytic infiltrates; hyalinized material in superficial corium; eosinophilic stain.

Diagnostic Procedures. *Blood.* Occasionally, immunoglobulin deficiency (IgA, IgM). *Urine.* Normal porphyrin excretion. *X-ray.* Retarded bone growth. *Chromosome study.* Tendency to chromosomal breakage in vitro.

Prognosis. Except for failure to grow, early development appears normal. Increased possibility of malignancies during second and third decade (leukemia, gastrointestinal).

BIBLIOGRAPHY. Bloom D: Congenital telangiectatic erythema resembling lupus erythematosus in dwarfs. Am J Dis Child 88:754–758, 1954

Gretzula JC, Hevia O, Weber PJ: Bloom's syndrome. J Am Acad Dermatol 17:479–488, 1987

German J, Passarge E: Bloom's syndrome, XII. Report for the register for 1987. Clin Genet 35:57–69, 1989

Harper J: Genetics and genodermatoses. In Champion RH, Burton JL,

Ebling FJG (eds): Rook/Wilkinson/Ebling Textbook of Dermatology, 5th ed, pp 352–353. Oxford, Blackwell Scientific, 1992

BLOUNT-BARBER

Synonyms. Erlacher-Blount; tibia Blount; bowlegs; osteochondrosis deformans tibiae; tibia vara. See also Fairbank and Conradi.

Symptoms. *Infantile type.* Appears at 1 or 2 years of age; usually in overweight children. Gradual increasing of leg bowing without apparent cause. Usually bilateral; occasionally unilateral. (Limp in unilateral; waddle in bilateral.) Pain from strain in the knee or foot observed sometimes. *Adolescent type.* Same symptoms appear at 6–12 years of age; usually unilaterally. Higher frequency in blacks.

Signs. Shortening (1–2 cm) of the leg(s) affected. Abrupt angulation with the apex laterally below the knee joint; bulbous enlargement of medial condyle; internal rotation of tibia; abnormal mobility of knee. All other general physical findings are normal.

Etiology. Unknown. Rickets, tuberculosis, syphilis excluded. Faulty growth of epiphyseal cartilage and delayed ossification of the medial or lateral (?) portion of proximal tibial epiphysis. Multifactorial inheritance proposed.

Pathology. In the beak-like prominence, under the epiphysis are islands of hyaline cartilage, with cells in irregular disposition instead of columnar. In adolescent type, arrest of epiphyseal growth rather than dysplasia.

Diagnostic Procedures. *X-ray.* Irregularity of contour of the proximal tibial epiphyseal line. Areas of rarefaction observed in enlarged metaphysis.

Therapy. In infantile type, progressive correction with conservative measures; if severe deformity, osteotomy required. In adolescent type, osteotomy usually required.

Prognosis. Good with adequate correction.

BIBLIOGRAPHY. Blount WP: Tibia vara, osteochondrosis deformans tibiae. Am J Bone Joint Surg 19:1–29, 1937
Enklaar JE: Osteochondrosis deformans (Blount) bij kinderen. Monatschr Kindergeneesk 23:235–238, 1955
Duncan PA, Shapiro LR, Brust MB, et al: Heterogeneity of the Blount's disease. Proc Greenwood Genet Canter 2:109–107, 1983
Ikegawa S, Nakamura K, Kawai S, et al: Blount's disease in a pair of identical twins. Acta Orthop Scand 61:582, 1990
Klippel JH, Dieppe PA: Rheumatology, pp 7.2.5, 7.4.5, 7.35.8. St Louis, Mosby Yearbook, 1995

BLUE COLOR BLINDNESS

Synonyms. Tritanopia; color blindness tritanopia.

Symptoms and Signs. Much rarer than deuteran or protean abnormalities (frequency 1/500 individuals). Retain red or green, lack blue, and yellow color vision. Visual acuity not affected, no clinical or ophthalmic consequences are associated.

Etiology. Autosomal dominant inheritance. Blue pigment gene on chromosome 7.

Prognosis. Defect remains constant for life

BIBLIOGRAPHY. Young T: The Bakerian lecture: on the theory of light and colors. Phil Trans Roy Soc London 92:12–48, 1802
Weitz CJ, Miyake Y, Schizato K, et al: Human tritanopia associated with two amino acid substitution in the blue-sensitive opsin. Am J Med Genet 50:498–507, 1992
Motulski AG, Deeb SS: Color vision and its genetic defects. In Scriver CR, Beaudet AL, Sly WS, et al: The Metabolic and Molecular Bases of Inherited Disease, 7th ed, p 4281. New York, McGraw-Hill, 1995

BLUE DIAPER

Synonyms. Drummond; hypercalcemia-nephrocalcinosis-indicanuria.

Symptoms. Both sexes affected; onset during first year of life. Anorexia; vomiting; constipation; irritability; failure to thrive; fever and recurrent infections; renal failure; reduced visual acuity; tryptophan malabsorption.

Signs. Pallor; dwarfism; depressed nose bridge; prominent epicanthal folds; nystagmus; strabismus; papilledema; optic atrophy. Bluish discoloration of diaper.

Etiology. Metabolic defect (expressed only in the intestine, not in the kidney) that affects only tryptophan (converted by intestinal bacteria to indacan) that through processes of hydrolysis and oxidation is converted to indigotin (indigo blue) in the urine. Thus the name blue diaper. Reported cases from vitamin D intoxication.

Pathology. See Signs. Occasionally, sclerosis of optic foramina. Peripheral retinal atrophy and optic atrophy. Osteosclerosis. Nephrocalcinosis in the cortex; granuloma formation in medulla; periglomerular fibrosis.

Diagnostic Procedures. *Urine.* Indicanuria and other indole derivatives. Reduced inulin and para-aminohippuric acid (PAH) clearances; increased phosphorus excretion. *Stool.* Increase of tryptophan and derivatives. *Blood.* Hypercalciuria; hyperazotemia; hypercreatinemia.

Therapy. Reduction of calcium intake. Corticosteroids.

Prognosis. Poor for function and quoad vitam.

BIBLIOGRAPHY. Drummond KN, Michael AF, Ulstrom RA, et al: The blue diaper syndrome: Familial hypercalcemia with nephrocalcinosis and indicanuria. A new familial disease, with definition of the metabolic abnormality. Am J Med 37:928–948, 1964
Libit SA, Ulstrom RA, Doeden D: Fecal Pseudomonas aeruginosa as a cause of the blue diaper syndrome. J Pediat 81, I:546–547, 1972
Levy HL: Hartnup disorder. In Scriver CR, Beaudet AL, Sly WS, et al: The Metabolic and Molecular Bases of Inherited Disease, 7th ed, p 3634. New York, McGraw-Hill, 1995

BLUE EDEMA

Synonym. Charcot edema syndromes. Eponym used to indicate the whitish blue hue, usually associated with the edema, that occurs in the limbs in hysterical palsy.

BIBLIOGRAPHY. Guinon G: L'oedème bleu de l'hystériques. Prog Med. 12:259–264, 1890

BLUE VELVET

Symptoms. Follow repeated intravenous injections of strong analgesics with talcum filler. Euphoria, excitement, or depression.

Signs. Apical thrust; tachycardia; systolic murmur; pulmonary rales; hepatomegaly; ankle edema.

Etiology. Intravenous injection of paregoric-triphenamine hydrochloride plus talcum filler.

Pathology. Hypertrophy of muscle cells of heart ventricles; pulmonary subedema; centrilobular hepatic necrosis with hemosiderin deposits and talc crystal in lungs and other tissues.

Diagnostic Procedures. *Blood.* Leukocytosis; hypoalbuminemia.

Therapy. Symptomatic.

Prognosis. Poor. Sudden death may follow the injection.

BIBLIOGRAPHY. Gordon BL, Barclay WR, Rogers HC (eds): Current Medical Information and Terminology, 4th ed. Chicago, American Medical Association, 1971

BOBBLE-HEAD DOLL

Symptoms. Appears in childhood. Continuous bobbing of head (3-sec periods); rhythmical extension and flexion of head and arms. The bobbing may be stopped voluntarily, and ceases during sleep and intentional movements. Generalized fine tremor; hypersensitivity to cutaneous stimuli. Mental retardation; impaired vision.

Signs. Moderate hydrocephalus; obesity.

Etiology. Cyst in region of third ventricle.

Pathology. Large cyst in region of third ventricle with thin wall of fibrous tissue; astroglia of blood vessels; no epithelial lining.

Diagnostic Procedures. *Echoencephalography. CT brain scan. MRI. Spinal tap. Aspiration of fluid from cyst.*

Therapy. Aspiration of fluid in the cyst and possible removal. Ventriculo-peritoneal shunt.

Prognosis. After surgery, bobbing stops. Hydrocephalus, diabetes insipidus, and other diencephalic disturbances may persist or stop.

BIBLIOGRAPHY. Benton JW, Nellhaus G, Huttenlocher PR, et al: The bobble-head doll syndrome: report of a unique truncal tremor associated with third ventricular cyst and hydrocephalus in children. Neurology 16:725–729, 1966

Robergue A, Beauvais P, Richardet JM: Syndrome de la poupée à tete ballottante. Bobble-head doll syndrome. Arch Fr Pédiatr 42:377–378, 1985

BOCHDALEK

Synonyms. Hernia Bochdalek; Diaphragmatic hernia, congenital.

Symptoms and Signs. Occurrence 1/2200 live births. Prevalent in males. May be detected *in utero* from the 10th week of life. At birth or soon thereafter infants present respiratory distress, dyspnea, tachypnea, cyanosis, severe retraction, increased chest diameter, bowel sounds are heard on chest auscultation.

Etiology. Defect in the development of pleuroperitoneal fold through which vicera enter the chest, preventing normal lung development.

Pathology. Defect in the left in 88% of cases; in the right 10%; bilateral 2%.

Diagnostic Procedures. *Prenatal echography. Blood* Respiratory acidosis, metabolic acidosis may also be present.

Therapy. Surgery and intensive assistance. ECMO.

Prognosis. Mortality related to degree of pulmonary hypoplasia and associated congenital anomalies.

BIBLIOGRAPHY. Bochdalek VA: Einige Bemerkungen ueber die Entstehung des angeborenen Zerchfellbruches: Alsd Beitrag zur pathologiscen. Anatomie der Hernien Virschr Prakt Heilk Prag 3:89–97, 1848

Sabiston DC: Textbook of Surgery, 14th ed, pp 1163–1165. Philadelphia, WB Saunders, 1991

BODY OF LUYS

Synonyms. Ballism; corpus Luysii; hemiballism subthalamic nucleus.

Symptoms and Signs. Appears in early or adult life. Violent involuntary movements of one or both body sides; movements greater in the proximal portions; more pronounced on arm than leg; intensity so strong as to bruise tissue or break bones. Movements subside during sleep.

Etiology. Lesion of contralateral body of Luys (hemorrhage; softening; tumor; granulomas; trauma; hereditary degenerative disorders). In cases in which the body of Luys has been found intact, lesions of afferent and efferent fibers are suspected to be involved.

Therapy. Nursing; sedatives; chlorpromazine. Neurosurgery; section of cerebral peduncle, incision of precentral gyrus, section of anterior or posterolateral columns of spinal cord.

Prognosis. If progressive, patient dies from exhaustive cardiac insufficiency in a few weeks. If patient survives acute stage, disease may go into remission or symptoms disappear altogether.

BIBLIOGRAPHY. Fisher O: Zur Frage der anatomischen Grundlage der Athetose double und der posthemiplegischen Bewegungsstörung überhaupt. Z Ges Neurol Psychiar 7:463, 1911

Denny-Brown D: The Basal Ganglia. London, Oxford Univ Press, 1962

Adams RD, Victor M: Principles of Neurology, 5th ed, pp 67, 71. New York, McGraw-Hill, 1993

BOERHAAVE

Synonym. Esophagus laceration spontaneous. See Mallory-Weiss syndrome.

Symptoms. Prevalent in males (5:1), more common in fifth and sixth decades. While straining violently to vomit and retch, excruciating pain in the chest, dyspnea, small amount of blood appears in the vomitus, significant hematemesis rare, shock.

Signs. Subcutaneous emphysema, tachycardia.

Etiology. Laceration of esophagus.

Pathology. Laceration linear and longitudinal (usually posterior) of lower part of esophagus, hydrothorax, and pneumothorax.

Diagnostic Procedures. *X-rays of chest. Blood and electrolyte workup.*

Therapy. Emergency blood replacement. Treatment of shock. Surgical repair of rupture. Antibiotics.

Prognosis. If untreated, death within 24 hours (50% of cases) or 48 hours (90%), or in a few days (100%). Treated, the mortality is 35%.

BIBLIOGRAPHY. Boerhaave H: Atrocis, nec descripti prius, morbi historia. Secundum medicae artis leges conscripta. Lugduni Batavorum, Boutesteniana, 1724

Bruno MS, Grier WR, Ober WB: Spontaneous laceration and rupture of esophagus and stomach; Mallory-Weiss syndrome, Boerhaave syndrome, and their variants. Arch Int Med 112:574–583, 1963

Walker WS, Cameron EW, Walbaum PR: Diagnosis and management of spontaneous transmural rupture of esophagus (Boerhaave's syndrome). Br J Surg 72:204–207, 1985

Praga Pilary S, Ward S, Cowen A, et al: Oesophageal ruptures and perforations—a review. Med J Aust 150:246–252, 1989

Achord JL: Nausea and vomiting. In Haubrich WS, Schaffner F, Berk JE (eds): Bockus Gastroenterology, 5th ed, vol 2, p 46. Philadelphia, WB Saunders, 1995

BOERJESON-FORSSMAN-LEHMANN

Synonyms. Mental deficiency—epilepsy—endocrine disorders. See Coffin-Lowry, Bardet-Biedl, Prader-Willi.

Symptoms. Appears in males in complete form, in females variable expression onset in childhood. Epilepsy; mental retardation, nystagmus, seizures (50%), hypotonia.

Signs. Obesity; genital infantilism; short stature (80%) myxedema. *Head-face.* Microcephaly, prominent supraorbital ridge, ptosis, large ears, coarse facies. *Hands.* Small, tappering flexible fingers.

Etiology. Autosomal recessive inheritance. X-linked inheritance.

Diagnostic Procedures. *X-rays. CT scan. MR imaging.* Brain atrophy; skeletal abnormalities. *EEG.* Paucity of alpha rhythms.

BIBLIOGRAPHY. Börjeson M, Forssman H, Lehmann O: Zusammentreffen von'Idiotie, Epilepsie, Zwergwuchs, Keimdruesen Unterfunktion, Myxoedem and morphologischen Besonderheiten als rezessiverbliches Syndrom. II. Inter Kong Psych Entwichg Kind Wien, 1961

Boerjeson M, Forssman H, Lehmann O: An X-linked, recessively inherited syndrome characterized by grave mental deficiency, epilepsy and endocrine disorders. Acta Med Scand 171:13–21, 1962

Turner G, Gedeon A, Mulley J, et al: Borjeson-Forssman-Lehmann syndrome: clinical manifestations and gene localization to Xq26–27. Am J Med Genet 34:463–469, 1989

BOGART-BACALL

Synonyms. See functional voice syndromes.

Symptoms and Signs. Male to female ratio 3:4. In patient subject to vocal abuse (actors, singers, teachers, etc.). Long-lasting fluctuant or intermittent vocal dysfunction with vocal fatigue and breaks, pitch and resonance abnormalities, variable, dysphonia. Dynamic range usually nonaffected, associated with poor breath support for speaking and without muscoloskeletal tension.

Etiology. Voice abuse.

Pathology. None.

Diagnostic Procedures. Transnasal fiberoptic laryngoscopy: most common MTD types 1 and 3; frequency (pitch) analysis; waveform analysis, spectrography, laryngeal airway resistance measurement.

Therapy. Voice rest and voice therapist intervention.

Prognosis. Success of treatment 80%.

BIBLIOGRAPHY. Koufman JA, Blalock PD: Vocal fatigue and dysphonia in the professional voice user. Bogart-Bacall syndrome. Laryngoscope 98:493–498, 1988

BOGORAD

Synonyms. Crocodile tears; gustatory lacrimation.

Symptoms. Unilateral lacrimation on chewing or introduction of strongly flavored food into the mouth.

Signs. Mechanical simulation and chewing without food do not produce lacrimation.

Etiology and Pathology. Sequela of facial paralysis, faulty regeneration of facial nerve fibers where the salivary fibers are directed along the path of lacrimal nerve.

BIBLIOGRAPHY. Bogorad FA: Symptom of crocodile tears. Vrach Delo 11:1328–1330, 1928

Chorobski J: The syndrome of crocodile tears. Arch Neurol Psychiatry 65:299–318, 1951

Gorlin RJ, Cohen MM, Levin LS: Syndromes of the Head and Neck, 3rd ed, pp 615–616. New York, Oxford Univ Press, 1990

BONHOEFFER I

Synonyms. Souquez-Bertrand; Bonhoeffer chorea; Claude; midbrain tremor; nucleus ruber inferior; rubral tremor; rubrospinal cerebellar peduncle.

Symptoms and Signs. Hemianesthesia and, occasionally hemiataxia with paralysis of contralateral eye muscles innervated by oculomotor and trochlear nerves.

Etiology and Pathology. Occlusion (thrombosis, neoplasia) of terminal branches of paramedian artery of inferior part of red nucleus.

Diagnostic Procedures. *Angiography. CT brain scan. MR imaging.*

Therapy. Anticoagulant: surgery if indicated.

Prognosis. Poor.

BIBLIOGRAPHY. Bonhoeffer K: Ein Beitrag zur Lokalisation der choreatischen Bewegungen. Mschr Psychiatr Neurol 1:6–41, 1887

Claude H: Syndrome péducolaire de la région du noyau rouge. Rev Neurol 23:311–313, 1912

Woo E, Haung CY, Chan FL, et al: Claude's syndrome: clinical and computed tomography correlations. J Comp Tomogr 11:208–211, 1987

Adams RD, Victor M: Principles of Neurology, 5th ed, pp 66–67. New York, McGraw-Hill, 1993

BONHOEFFER II

Synonyms. Delirium; toxic psychosis; brain acute cerebral acute exogenous.

Symptoms. Disordered thoughts and behavior; restlessness; stimuli reach mind, but there is lack of recognition and integration; hallucination.

Signs. Confusion; disorientation; rapidly changing behavioral pattern and reactions to stimuli and surroundings; deterioration of conscious motor activity (e.g., dressing, eating). Incontinence of sphincters. Findings depending on specific etiology.

Etiology. Diffuse brain tissue impairment from many causes: toxemia from general infections, exogenous poisons, and drugs; endogenous intoxication; sudden cessation of drugs; infection of nervous system; noninfective cerebral diseases, cerebral anemia; heat stroke; trauma; hypertension.

Pathology. Depends on etiology.

Diagnostic Procedures. *EEG.* Slowing of activity.

Therapy. Correction of medical or surgical (hypertension) conditions; sedatives (phenothyazine; chlordiazepoxide); hypnotic (chloral hydrate).

Prognosis. Good response with proper treatment. Depending on etiology, permanent impairment of cerebral functions in some cases.

BIBLIOGRAPHY. Bonhoeffer K: Die symptomatischen Psychosen im Gefolge von akuten Infektionen und inneren Erkrankungen. Deuticke, Leipzig, Wien, 1910

Bonhoeffer K: Die exogenen Reaktionstypen, Arch Psychiat Nervenkr 58:58, 1917

Hirsch CJ, Caulfield PA: The acute brain syndrome: early recognition and management. G P 35:87–94, 1967

Peter UH: Das exogene paranoid-halluzinatorische Syndrom. Bibl Psychiat Neurol (Basel) 131, 1967

Adams RD, Victor M: Principles of Neurology, 5th ed, pp 359–361. New York, McGraw-Hill, 1993

BONNET-DECHAUME-BLANC

Synonyms. Neuroretinal angiomatosis; cerebroretinal arteriovenous aneurysm. See Wyburn-Mason.

Symptoms. Hemiplegia appearing in early childhood; mental deterioration.

Signs. Babinski positive; abdominal reflexes absent. Auscultation of skull: systolic murmur synchronous with heartbeat. Ophthalmologic examination: unilateral exophthalmia not pulsating, with dilatation of conjunctival vessels; strabimus; nystagmus; absent reflex to light and accommodation. Fundus oculi examination shows diffuse aneurysm, which makes it impossible to differentiate arteries from veins. Heart. Left hypertrophy.

Etiology and Pathology. Congenital nonmalignant aneurysms of retina, thalamus, and mesencephalus.

Diagnostic Procedures. *X-rays.* Cervical column, skull. *Angiography.* Carotid or vertebral. *Phlebography.* Orbit. *CT brain scan. MRI.* See Signs.

Prognosis. According to entity of lesions; blindness of one eye; mental deterioration.

BIBLIOGRAPHY. Bonnet P, Dechaume J, Blanc E: L'anéurysme cirsoúde de la rétine (anéurysme racemeux). Ses relations avec l'anéurysme cirsoúde de la face et avec l'anéurysme cirsoúde du cerveau. J Med Lyon 18:163–178, 1937
Fischgold H, Bregeat P, Le Besnerais Y, et al: Iconographie de l'angiomatose neuroretinene (syndrome de Bonnet, Dechaume et Blanc). Presse Med 60:1790–1792, 1952
Atherton DJ: Naevi and Other Developmental Defects. In Champion RH, Burton JL, Ebling FJG (eds): Rook/Wilkinson/Ebling Textbook of Dermatology, 5th ed, p 493. Oxford, Blackwell Scientific, 1992

BONNET (C.)

Synonym. Charles Bonnet. See Lilliputian.

Symptoms. Appears in aged blind or partially blind persons not exhibiting other mental disorders, frequently at the close of day. Vivid polychromic, microscopic, macroscopic, or normal sized, visual hallucinations, which the patient generally recognizes as such, and discusses as a curiosity, without emotional involvement. Similarity with lilliputian and hypnagogic imagery.

Etiology. See Cerebral, chronic. If lesion can be identified, usually it is situated in occipital lobe or posterior part of temporal lobe.

BIBLIOGRAPHY. Bonnet C: Essai Analytique sur les Facultés de l'Ame, vol 2, pp 176–178. Copenhagen, 1769
de Morsier G: Le syndrome de Charles Bonnet: Hallucinations visuelles des Veillards, sans déficience mentale. Ann Med Psychol (Paris) 2:678–702, 1967
Adams RD, Victor M: Principles of Neurology, 5th ed, pp 401–402. New York, McGraw-Hill, 1993

BONNET (P.)

Synonyms. Trigeminosympathetic; trigemino sympaneuralgia. See Orbital apex.

Symptoms and Signs. Those of Fothergill (see), associated with those of Bernard (see).

BIBLIOGRAPHY. Bonnet P: Les syndromes trigéminosympathiques. Arch Ophthalmol 16:361–379, 1956
Adams RD, Victor M: Principles of Neurology, 5th ed, pp 1170–1174. New York, McGraw-Hill, 1993

BONNIER

Synonym. Deiters nucleus.

Symptoms. Apprehension; somnolence; weakness of limbs; trigeminal neuralgia; oculomotor manifestations. Vertigo and deafness may be associated.

Etiology. Neoplastic; vascular lesion of lateral nucleus of vestibular nerve (Deiters) or vestibular tract.

Pathology. See Etiology.

Diagnostic Procedures. *Audiography. EEG. Angiography. CT scan. MRI.*

Therapy. Surgery if feasible.

Prognosis. Possible improvement.

BIBLIOGRAPHY. Bonnier P: Syndrome du noyau de Deiters. C R Soc Biol Paris 4:1525–1528, 1902
Courrier RD: Syndromes of medulla oblungata. In Vinken PJ, Bruyn GW: Handbook of Clinical Neurology, vol 2, p 220. Amsterdam, North-Holland, 1969
Brandt T: Vertigo Its Multisensorial Syndromes. London, Springer-Verlag, 1991

BONNEAU

Synonyms. Polysyndactyly-cardiac defects.

Symptoms and Signs. In three brothers. Polysyndactyly of toes and syndactyly of fingers; various cardiac congenital defects: single ventricle, atrial or ventricular defects.

Etiology. Possible autosomal recessive inheritance.

BIBLIOGRAPHY. Bonneau JC, Moirot H, Bastard C, et al: Polysyndactylie avec cardiopathie complexeàpropos de trois cas dans une meme fratrie. J Genet Hum 31:93–105, 1983

BÖÖK

Synonyms. Premature hereditary canities; hereditary premature graying hair. PHC.

Symptoms and Signs. Premature cavities; palmoplantar hyperhidrosis; hypodontia of premolars with bicuspid partially or completely lacking.

Etiology. Unknown; autosomal dominant inheritance.

BIBLIOGRAPHY. Böök JA: Clinical and genetical studies of hypodontia; premolar aplasia, hyperhidrosis, and canities prematuria; new hereditary syndrome in man. Am J Hum Genet 2:240–263, 1950
Harper J: Genetics and Genodermatoses. In Champion RH, Burton JL, Ebling FJG (eds): Rook/Wilkinson/Ebling Textbook of Dermatology, 5th ed, p 347. Oxford, Blackwell Scientific, 1992

BOOMERANG DYSPLASIA

Synonyms. See Atelosteogenesis (AO1) (possibly part of same spectrum).

Symptoms and Signs. In Males. Boomerang shaping of long bones of legs. Dwarfism; characteristic facies.

Etiology. Sporadic condition.

Diagnostic Procedures. *X-rays.* Absence of radii and fibulae; boomerang configuration of other bones.

Prognosis. Death in neonatal period.

BIBLIOGRAPHY. Kozolowski T, Tseruta T, Kameda Y, et al: New forms of neonatal death dwarfism: report of three cases. Pediatr Radiol 10:155–160, 1981
Winship I, Creenin B, Beighton T: Boomerang dysplasia. Am J Med Genet 36:440–443, 1990

BORDERLINE

Symptoms. Chief complaint: attention provoking histrionic episodes. No delusion or paranoid symptoms. Five subgroups may be delineated: (1) Expresses anger as main emotion; has no capacity for affection;

depressive loneliness. (2) Attempts to relate but reacts with anger (psychotic borderline). (3) Attempts and persists in seeking relation, but reacts with "repulsion." (4) Reacts with anger to most people, but seeks a mother figure and, failing, becomes depressed (neurotic borderline). (5) Reacts to anger and loneliness; takes a passive attitude awaiting signs as to how to react.

Etiology. Disturbance of ego function.

Therapy. Propanolol, lithium, carbamazepine, and phenytoin reported as beneficial. Persistent psychotherapeutic attempts.

Prognosis. Only some patients may respond to treatment.

BIBLIOGRAPHY. Grinker RR, Werble B, Drye C: The Borderline Syndrome: A Behavioral Study of Ego Functions. New York, Basic Books, 1968
Adams RD, Victor M: Principles of Neurology, 5th ed, p 1308. New York, McGraw-Hill, 1993
Kaplan HI, Sadock BJ: Comprehensive Textbook of Psychiatry, 6th ed. Baltimore, Williams & Wilkins, 1995

BORNHOLM

Synonyms. Dabney grip; Sylvest; devil grip; myalgia endemic; myalgia epidemic; pleurodynia epidemic.

Symptoms. Epidemic occurrence in summer and early autumn; person-to-person contact; incubation 3–5 days. Affects both sexes in all age groups; prevalent in children and young adults. Recurrent episodes of sudden excruciating pain in abdominal or thoracic regions, increased by movement and respiration. Headache, malaise, sore throat, vomiting (especially in early phase of disease) may be present. In infants, convulsions during attacks.

Signs. During attacks, shallow tachypulse and fever. During remissions of attacks, mild tenderness in affected areas, with minor muscle swelling, hyperestesia, and altered reflexes. Pleural rubs may be present.

Etiology. Coxsackie viruses B3 and B5. Other viruses that can be associated with epidemic disease are Coxsackie virus B1 and B2 and echoviruses 1 and 6.

Pathology. No specific changes.

Diagnostic Procedures. *Throat swabs and stool swabs.* Coxsackie B virus. *X-ray of chest.* Negative. *Blood.* Normal findings; increase of neutralizing antibodies against Coxsackie B type.

Therapy. Nonspecific. Analgesic and antipyretics. Bed rest.

Prognosis. Attacks persist for a few days. Patient afraid and usually remains in bed for several days. After apparent recovery, relapses may occur for about 1 month. Complications include orchitis (common, lasting 3–7 days); fibrinous pleurisy (common); aseptic meningitis (rare); pericarditis (in adults); myocarditis (in newborn). Long-lasting immunity.

BIBLIOGRAPHY. Dabney WC: Account of an epidemic resembling dengue which occurred in and around Charlottesville and the University of Virginia in June 1888. Am J Med Sci 96:488–495, 1888
Sylvest E: En Bornholmsk epidemi-Myositis epidemica. Ugeskr Laeger 92:798–801, 1930
Grist NR, Bell EJ: Enteroviruses. In Weatherall DJ, Ledingham JGG, Warrell DA (eds): Oxford Textbook of Medicine, 3rd ed, p 387. Oxford, Oxford Med Pub, 1996

BORNHOLM EYE

Synonyms. Myopia-X linked.

Symptoms and Signs. In person with family origin from Bornholm island (Denmark). Myopia, astigmatism, impared vision. In male also deuteranopia.

Etiology. X-linked inheritance.

Pathology. Moderate hypoplasia of optic nerve heads.

BIBLIOGRAPHY. Haim M, Fledelius HC, Starsholm D: X-linked myopia in a Danish family. Acta Ophthal 66:450–456, 1988
Schwartz M, Haim M, Skarsholm D: X-linked myopia: Bornholm eye disease-linkage to DNA markers on the distal part of Xq. Clin Genet 38:281–286, 1990

BOUCHER-NEUHAUSER

Synonyms. Spinocerebellar ataxia–hypogonadotrophic; hypogonadism—choroidal dystrophy.

Symptoms and Signs. Both sexes. See cerebellar ataxia–hypogonadism. Neurologic signs develop in adolescence and early adulthood (up to forth decade) they may be progressive or non. Ophthalmic manifestations: onset from first to sixth decade and are variably progressing.

Etiology. Autosomal inheritance indicated.

BIBLIOGRAPHY. Boucher BJ, Gibbert FB: "Familial ataxia, hypogonadism and retinal degeneration." Acta Neurol Scand 45:507–510, 1969
Neuhauser G, Opitz JM: Autosomal recessive syndrome of cerebellar ataxia, hypogonatrophic hypogonadism. Clin Genet 7:426–434, 1975
Baroncini A, Franco N, Forabosco A: A new family with chorioretinal dystrophy, spinocerebellar ataxia, and hypogonadotropic hypogonadism (Boucher-Neuhauser syndrome). Clin Genet 39:274–277, 1991

BOUILLAUD

Synonyms. Sokolskii-Bouillaud; rheumatic fever. First report of the triad: endocarditis, pericarditis, and acute inflammation of joints.

BIBLIOGRAPHY. Bouillaud JB: Traité Clinique des Maladies due Coeur, précédé de recherches nouvelles sur l'anatomie et la physiologie de cet organe, vol 2, pp 170–192, 1835
Sokolskii GI: O reumatizme myshechnai tkani serdtsa (rheumatismus cordis). Uchen Zap Imp Mosk Univ 12:568, 1838

BOURNEVILLE

Synonyms. Bourneville-Brissaud; Bourneville-Pringle; Bourneville phakomatosis; adenoma sebaceum (misnomer); epiloia; tuberous sclerosis. See Pringle-Bourneville.

Symptoms and Signs. Clinically characterized triad: (1) mental and physical retardation; (2) epileptic seizures; (3) sebaceous adenomas of skin and warts, polyps, nevi, usually butterfly distribution on the nose bridge and cheeks. Retinal and other tumors in different organs may coexist. Involuntary movements; local paresis.

Etiology. Congenital hereditary autosomal dominant malformations of neuroectodermal system. About 50% of cases appear to be new mutations.

Pathology. *Skin.* Hyperplastic connective or muscular tissue; neurofibromata type (sebaceous adenoma a misnomer). *Retina.* Small, round growths (phakomas). *Brain.* Many nodules on surface of cortex and ventricular surfaces (pearly white); microgyri or macrogyria. Disturbed cytoarchitecture of brain and localized neoplastic formation (various types of gliomas). Pathologic changes may be found in heart, lung, and kidney as well.

Diagnostic Procedures. *X-ray.* Multiple intracranial calcification; osteoporosis of skull and other bones. *CT brain scan. MRI.* Characteristic calcifications. *EEG.* Abnormal in 87% of cases; grossly disorganized hypsarrhythmic pattern.

Therapy. Treatment of seizures; assessment of intellectual function; control of hyperactivity in children can be achieved with methylphenidate or dextroamphetamine. Surgical excision of tumors only if they are symptomatic. Genetic counseling.

Prognosis. Extremely variable. Patients with mild involvement may have a good prognosis. Death may be caused by status epilepticus, brain tumor, renal failure; or rhabdomyoma of the heart.

BIBLIOGRAPHY. Bourneville DM, Brissaud E: Encéphalite ou sclérose tubéreuse des circonvolutions cérébrales. Arch Neurol (Paris) 1:397–412, 1880–1881

Gomez MR: Tuberous Sclerosis. New York, Raven Press, 1979

Jansen LAJ, Sandkuyl LA, Merkens EC, et al: Genetic heterogeneity in tuberous sclerosis. Genomics 8:237–242, 1990

Fahsold R, Rott H-D, Clausen U, et al: Tuberous sclerosis in a child with de novo translocation t (3; 12) (p26. 3; q23. 3). Clin Genet 40:326–328, 1991

Atherton DJ: Naevi and other developmental defects. In Champion RH, Burton JL, Ebling FJG (eds): Rook/Wilkinson/Ebling Textbook of Dermatology, 5th ed, pp 327–331. Oxford, Blackwell Scientific, 1992

BOUVERET

Synonyms. Cotton; Bouveret-Hoffmann; auricular paroxysmal tachycardia idiopathic; paroxysmal atrial tachycardia.

Symptoms. Onset in any age; more frequent in second to fourth decades. In childhood, affects boys almost exclusively. Onset sudden, without warning, occasionally precipitated by emotion or rapid change in position. Sudden thump in the chest; apparent stopping of the heart; precordial discomfort, then palpitation. Occasionally, (1) pain sensation on throat, pulsation in the neck; (2) anxiety, generalized weakness, cold, or sweating may accompany attack; (3) gastrointestinal symptoms, epigastric discomfort, abdominal distention, burping, nausea, vomiting; (4) polyuria during or at termination of attack.

Signs. Tachycardia. Only with prolonged attack or in presence of underlying disease, signs of congestive failure may appear. Pulse rapid and small. Blood pressure may drop (especially systolic with resultant decrease of pulse pressure).

Etiology. Obscure; occasionally associated with biliary tract diseases; in patient with Wolf-Parkinson-White syndrome; a congenital type is known.

Pathology. None; except of associated diseases.

Diagnostic Procedures. *Electrocardiography*. Rapid regular ventricular complex T-waves that are frequently difficult to identify and slightly modified by fusion with P-waves.

Therapy. Reassurance; Valsalva maneuver; Müller maneuver; inducing vomiting; carotid sinus stimulation (unilateral). Sedatives; intravenous digitalis, phenylephrine ajmalinum; levarterenol. Prevention: avoid precipitating causes, if known: mild sedatives, quinidine.

Prognosis. Attacks usually terminate spontaneously, or with maneuvers or medication. Occasionally, prolonged attacks may induce cardiac failure.

BIBLIOGRAPHY. Cotton P: Notes and observation of unusually rapid action of the heart. Br Med J 1:629, 1867

Bouveret L: De la tachycardie essentielle paroxystique. Rev Mid 9:753–793; 837–855, 1889

O'Rourke RA, Silverman ME, Schlant RC: General examination of the patient. In Schlant RC, Alexander RW: Hurst's The Heart, 8th ed, p 237. New York, McGraw-Hill, 1994

BOWEL BYPASS

Synonyms. Intestinal bypass-arthritis-dermatitis; arthritis-dermatitis; bypass disease.

Symptoms and Signs. In 7–10% of patients submitted to surgery of intestinal bypass usually for weight reduction (substituted today by other surgical procedures). In acute form massive abdominal distention similar to intestinal obstruction; milder or chronic forms with persistent diarrhea, hepatic failure, kidney stones, intermittent polyarthritis involving knees and upper extremity joints. Skin in more than 80% of patients urticarial or papulovesiculopustular rash or (seldom) erythema nodosum, ecchymoses, nodular panniculitis or necrobiotic lipomas; emotional troubles.

Etiology. Intestinal bypass causing water and electrolytes imbalance, vitamin deficiency and bacterial overgrowth. Hypothesis: After jejunal bypass intestinal fragments are digested and bind Igs, forming circulating immune complexes that then are deposited in the skin.

Pathology. Arthritis. Findings similar to those of ulcerative colitis or regional colitis (see Chron). Skin sterile, pustular lesions with accumulation of polymorphs and dermal edema up to dermo-epithelial separation.

Diagnostic Procedures. According to manifestations.

Therapy. Usually resolves with antibiotic therapy and metronidazole, vitamin supplementation. Recostruction of bowel may be indicated. Do not use steroideal anti-inflammatory agents.

Prognosis. Good with therapy. Often correction of bypass is necessary.

BIBLIOGRAPHY. Simon S, Sikka JV, Lynfield YL: Bowel bypass syndrome. Cutis 28:545–547, 1981

Stein MB, Schlappner OLA, Boyko W, et al: The interstinal bypass arthritis-dermatitis syndrome. Arth Rheum 24:684–690, 1981

Clarke J, Weiner SR, Bassett LW, et al: Bypass disease. Clin Exp Rheumatol 5:275–287, 1987

Grant JT, Husby G: Joint manifestations in gastrointestinal diseases. Dig Dis 10:295–312, 1992

Roubenoff R: The musculoskeletal system. In Haubrich WS, Schaffner F, Berk JE (eds): Bockus Gastroenterology, 5th ed, vol 2, p 3497. Philadelphia, WB Saunders, 1995

BOWEN (D.A.L.)

Synonym. Tracheobronchopathia osteochondroplastica.

Symptoms and Signs. Predominantly in men over 50 years of age. Dyspnea; hoarseness; cough; expectoration; wheezing; hemoptysis.

Etiology. Unknown. In several cases established relation with amyloidosis.

Pathology. In majority of cases, diagnosis at autopsy. Subcutaneous nodules, usually confined to portion of the trachea and bronchial wall containing cartilage that produce sessile and polypoid growth; seldom, ulcerating.

Diagnostic Procedures. *Bronchoscopy*. Beaded appearance. Pulmonary function tests. Variable degree of alterations. *X-rays*. Variable findings. Bronchial obstruction; evidence of bone formations on lateral and anterior walls of trachea.

Therapy. Symptomatic.

Prognosis. Poor.

BIBLIOGRAPHY. Bowen DAL: Thacheopathia osteoplastica. J Clin Pathol 12:435–439, 1959

Whitehouse G: Tracheopathia osteoplastica: case report. Br J Radiol 41:701–703, 1968

Fraser RG, Paré JAP, Fraser RG, Paré PD: Synopsis of Diseases of the Chest, pp 218, 613. Philadelphia, WB Saunders, 1994

BOWEN (J.F.)

Synonyms. Intradermal carcinoma epidermoid; precancerous dermatosis.

Symptoms. Severe local pruritus (not constant).

Signs. Appears anywhere on skin or mucosal surfaces. Formation of a limited, reddish, scaly area, which progressively enlarges. The whitish scales are removed with difficulty and leave red, granular surface without bleeding. Lesions are slightly raised. Crusting and hyperkeratosis follow and after years, ulceration. Other lesions may form and frequently become confluent.

Etiology. Various theories: considered associated to exposure to trivalent arsenic compounds or to light, or as manifestation of systemic carcinomatosis; frequently observed in transplant patients.

Pathology. Atypical squamous cell proliferation through the entire epidermis. Acanthosis to variable degree. Cells have large hyperchromatic nuclei; frequently, mitosis. Disorganized epidermal structure. Various degrees of inflammatory changes.

Diagnostic Procedures. Biopsy.

Therapy. Destruction by freezing, cauterization, or diathermy. Local 5–fluorouracil application. Surgical excision preferred.

Prognosis. Recurrences not infrequent. It represents a precancerous lesion; 42.6% develop premalignant or malignant lesion of skin within 6–7 years; 25% show primary systemic cancer within 5 years.

BIBLIOGRAPHY. Bowen JF: Precancerous dermatoses: a study of two cases of chronic atypical epithelial proliferation. J Cutan Dis 30:241–255, 1912

MacKie RM: Epidermal skin tumors. In Champion RH, Burton JL, Ebling FJG (eds): Rook/Wilkinson/Ebling Textbook of Dermatology, 5th ed, pp 1481–1483. Oxford, Blackwell Scientific, 1992

BOWEN (P.)

Synonym. Pulmonary faciocamptodactyly ankyloses. See Fraser. Maybe not to be considered a syndrome. Probably the one family described had cerebrohepatorenal syndrome.

Symptoms and Signs. Appears in both sexes during intrauterine life. Small birth weight and reduced length. Respiratory insufficiency. *Facies.* Ear malformation; hypertelorism; depressed nose tip; micrognathia. *Extremities.* Camptodactyly of fingers; talipes equinovarus; ankylosis of knees, fixed in extension, and of hips in semiflexion.

Etiology. Autosomal recessive inheritance.

Pathology. See Signs; plus pulmonary hypoplasia; cardiac defects; in males, cryptorchidism; in females, clitoral hypertrophy. Occasionally, agenesis of corpus callosum, arhinencephalia, cerebellar hypoplasia.

Prognosis. Death in perinatal period.

BIBLIOGRAPHY. Bowen P, Lee C, Zeliweger N, et al: A familial syndrome of multiple congenital defects. Johns Hopkins Hosp Bull 114:402–414, 1964

BOWLER THUMB

Symptoms and Signs. In bowler players. Thick tender area on ulnar side of base of thumb. Tinel sign may be positive, sensibility of thumb usually normal.

Etiology. Repeated friction or pressure on ulnar digital nerve of thumb.

Pathology. Perineural fibrosis and neuroma of the ulnar nerve.

Therapy. Conservative. Rest, splinting, change of type of grip on the ball or change in the thumb hole in the ball. If failure, stop bowling or surgery: removal of perineural fibrosis, mobilization and transposition of the nerve to a more dorsal position.

Prognosis. Good with treatment.

BIBLIOGRAPHY. Dunham W, Haines G, Speinger J: Bowler's thumb (ulnar neuroma of the thumb). Clin Orthop 83:99–101, 1972

Zemel N: Neurovascular disorders. In Jobe FW: Operative Techniques in Upper Extremity Sport Injuries. St Louis, CV Mosby, 1996

BOYD-STEARNS

Obsolete eponym to indicate a Fanconi-like syndrome: dwarfism; rickets; hypophosphatemia; vitamin D resistant; glycosuria; acidosis and hypochloremia. See Prader.

BIBLIOGRAPHY. Boyd JD, Stearns G: Late rickets resembling the Fanconi syndrome. Am J Dis Child 61:1012–1022, 1941

McKusick VA: Heritable Disorders of Connective Tissue, 4th ed, p 749. St Louis, CV Mosby, 1972

BRACHYDACTYLY TYPE C

Symptoms and Signs. Frequent in Mormon families. Various and variable anomalies of digits: brachymetapody, hyperphalangy, symphalangy, brachydactyly of middle phalanx of index and middle finger; triangulation of fifth middle phalanx.

Etiology. Autosomal dominant inheritance (?).

BIBLIOGRAPHY. Pol D: Brachydactylie "Klinodaktylie" hyperphalangie und ihre Grundlagen. Vichow Arch Pat Anat 229:388–530, 1921

Baraitser M, Burn J: Recessively inherited brachydactyly type C. J Med Genet 20:128–129, 1983

BRACHYDACTYLY TYPE E

Synonym. Dwarfism—brachydactyly, type E. See Biemond I, Gorlin-Sedano and pseudopseudohypoparathyroidism.

Symptoms and Signs. Prevalent in females; present from birth. Dwarfism; short limbs, metacarpals, metatarsals, and some phalanges; cone epiphyses. Considered by same authors are distinguishing features. Cases have been described with associated multiple impacted teeth (cryptodontic metacarpalia–Gorlin-Sedano).

Etiology. Autosomal dominant inheritance.

Prognosis. Benign condition.

BIBLIOGRAPHY. Bell J: On brachydactyly and symphalangism. In Treasury of Human Inheritance, vol 5, pp 1–31. London, Cambridge Univ Press, 1951

Riccardi WM, Holmes LB: Brachydactyly, type E. J Pediatr 84:251–254, 1974

Bale AE, Ludwig IH, Heffron LA, et al: Linkage between the genes for Wolfram syndrome and brachydactyly E. Am J Med Genet 20:733–734, 1985

BRACHYRACHIA

Synonyms. Short-spine dysplasia; brachyolmia; includes Hobaeck; Maroteaux brachyolmia.

Symptoms and Signs. Both sexes: normal birth length. In early childhood short-trunk dwarfism becames apparent; frequent scoliosis, limbs normal or slightly shortened. The types identified Type I or Hobaeck type: squared-off platyspondyly, reduced intervertebral spaces, significant end plate irregularity. Type II or Maroteaux type: rounded vertebral edges, minor end plate irregularity, normal intervertebral spaces. occasionally precocious falx cerebri calcification. Type III: similar to type II plus severe cervical platyspondyly.

Etiology. Autosomal dominant inheritance.

Diagnostic Procedures. *X-rays.* Major changes in the spine; vertebral bodies; small, irregular and radiolucent.

BIBLIOGRAPHY. Hobaeck A: Problems of hereditary chondrodysplasia. Oslo (Norway) 1961, Oslo University

Brown DO, McDonald C: Three cases of familial osseous dystrophy. Austr N Z J Surg 3:78–88, 1983

Shohat M, Lachman R, Gruber HE, et al: "Brachyolmia: radiographic and genetic evidence of heterogeneity." Am J Med Genet 33:209–219, 1989

Rimoin DL, Lachman: Genetic disorders of the osseous skeleton. In Beithon PMC: Kusick's Heritable Disorders of Connective Tissue, 5th ed, p 634. St Louis, Mosby, 1993

BRADBURY-EGGLESTON

Synonyms. Idiopathic orthostatic hypotension, IOH, Bradbury-Eggleston triad. See Orthostatic hypotension and Shy-Dragger.

Symptoms and Signs. In middle age. Prevalent in male. Gradual onset postural hypotension with fixed heart rate; heat intolerance; anhidrosis; nocturnal polyuria; deterioration of abdominal, urinary, and anal sphincter functions; impotency.

Etiology. Unknown. Chronic autonomic failure.

Pathology. Degeneration of efferent sympathetic pathway.

Diagnostic Procedures. *Blood.* Low level of epinephrine, that is not modified by change in position or exercise. Low level of plasma dopamine hydrolase. *Metabolic studies.* Absence of vasoconstriction to intra-arterial administration of tyramine; exaggerated response to norepinephrine. *Urine.* Decreased excretion of metabolites of norepinephrine. *Histochemical studies.* In perivascular nerve fibers absence of catecholamine-specific flourescence.

Therapy. Mechanical measures. Volume expanders; pharmacological agents (sympathomimetics, vasoconstrictors, beta receptor blockers, alpha-2 receptor agonists); prostaglandin synthesis inhibitors, antiserotoninergics, MAO inhibitors, vasopressin. Atrial tachypacing (100 rate).

Prognosis. Less severe than in Shy-Dragger. General debilitation and complications.

BIBLIOGRAPHY. Bradbury S, Eggleston C: Postural hypotension: report of three cases. Am Heart J 1:73–86, 1925

Kopin IJ, Polinsky RJ, Oliver JA, et al: Urinary catecholamine metabolites distinguish different types of sympathetic neuronal dysfunction in patients with orthostatic hypotension. J Clin Endocrinol Metab 57:632–637, 1983

Lewis RP, Budoulas H, Schaal SF, et al: Diagnosis and management of syncope. In Schlant RC, Alexander RW: Hurst's The Heart, 8th ed, pp 930–931. New York, McGraw-Hill, 1994

Adams RD, Victor M: Principles of Neurology, 5th ed, p 322. New York, McGraw-Hill, 1993

BRADLEY

Synonyms. Goodall; Spencer; epidemic collapse; epidemic vomiting; hyperemesis hiemis; intestinal grippe; nausea epidemica; nonbacterial gastroenteritis; winter vomiting; viral gastroenteritis.

Symptoms. Both sexes affected; onset at all ages. Onset usually in winter months and early spring. Sudden and explosive epidemic of profuse vomiting, usually beginning in early morning, associated with severe headache, muscular pains, sweating. Fever may be absent (probably in previously exposed subjects) or very high (first episode) but usually is short-lasting (24–48 hours). Diarrhea in some epidemics, or only in some subjects.

Etiology. Viral condition: Rotavirus; most of cases other viruses: Norwalk-like viruses, enteric adenoviruses, astroviruses, and caliciviruses. Rule out epidemic food poisoning and mass hysteria.

Diagnostic Procedures. Usually none necessary. Virus identification.

Therapy. Symptomatic.

Prognosis. Short-lasting condition (2–3 days), occasionally up to 10 days. Within 3 weeks relapses may occur and bronchopulmonar manifestations complicate the relapsing episode.

BIBLIOGRAPHY. Bradley WH: Epidemic nausea and vomiting. Br Med J 1:309–312, 1943

Goodall JF: The winter vomiting disease: a report from general practice. Br Med J 1:197–198, 1954. Epidemic vomiting. Br Med J 2:327–328, 1969

Kapikian AZ, Kim HW, Wyatt RG, et al: Human reoviruslike agent as the major pathogen associated with "winter" gastroenteritis in hospitalized infants and young children. N Engl J Med 294:969–972, 1976

Cleary TJ, Pauley RJ: Viruses. In Haubrich WS, Schaffner F, Berk JE (eds): Bockus Gastroenterology, 5th ed, p 1140. Philadelphia, WB Saunders, 1995

BRAILSFORD

Synonyms. Acrodysplasia II; peripheral dysostosis; PNM.

Symptoms and Signs. Present from birth. Reduced height and weight; short tubular bones of hands and feet; loose skin around fingers. Slow in learning to walk and talk. Frequent respiratory, cutaneous, and ear infections.

Etiology. Autosomal dominant inheritance. Autosomal recessive form reported also by Goodman.

Diagnostic Procedures. *X-rays.* Shortening of metacarpals and metatarsals; all peripheral bones underdeveloped; absent or minor skeletal changes.

Therapy. Treatment of infection.

Prognosis. Infections frequently cause of death. Final height variable from short to normal; normal mental development.

BIBLIOGRAPHY. Brailsford JF: The Radiology of Bones and Joints, 4th ed, p 33. Baltimore, Williams & Wilkins, 1948

Singleton EB, Siggers DC: Peripheral dysostosis. In Bergsma D (ed): Skeletal dysplasias. Amsterdam Excerpta Medica, pp 510–517, 1974

Goodman RM, Weinberg U, Hertz M, et al: Peripheral dysostosis: an autosomal recessive form. Birth Defects Org Art Ser 10(12):137–146, 1974

McNicol, Makris D: L'acrodystosis and protrusio acetabuli. J Bone Joint Surg (Br) 70B:38–39, 1988

BRAIN-BONE-FAT

Synonyms. Hakola; Nasu-Hakola; dementia progressive-lipomembranous, polycystic osteodysplasia; PDLPO; lipomembranous polycystic osteodysplasia LMPO; see Alzheimer.

Symptoms. Most cases in Finland and Japan. Onset in third decade. Following minor accidents or strain: pain and swelling of wrist or ankle. In fourth decade loss of inhibitions; impotency or frigidity. Intestinal motility disorders.

Signs. Tendon reflexes accentuated, pathologic reflexes; myoclonias, seizures. Bone fractures. Development of cysts on hand and foot bones and ends of long bones.

Etiology. Unknown. Autosomal dominant (or recessive?) inheritance. Defective development of vascular bed considered as primary.

Pathology. *Cysts.* Contain jelly-like material; membranous-lamellar structure interposed between fat and collagen tissue. *Brain.* Narrowing of small vessels; calcification of basal ganglia, glyosis and demyelinization of white matter, senile plaques and neurofibrillar nests.

Diagnostic Procedures. *X-ray of skeleton.* Typical cysts, particular in the distal but sometimes also in the proximal ends of bones. *CT or MRI brain.* Dilated ventricles and cortical atrophy. *EEG.* Typical changes. *Biopsy. Blood.* Occasionally leukemia.

Therapy. Symptomatic.

Prognosis. Progressive condition leading to death.

BIBLIOGRAPHY. Hakola HPA: Neuropsychiatric and genetic aspects a new hereditary disease characterized by progressive dementia and lipomembranous polycystic osteodysplasia. Acta Psychiatr Neurol Scand 232(Suppl):1–173, 1972
Nasu T, Tsukahara Y, Tarayame L: A lipid metabolic disease "membranous lipodistrophic" an autopsy case demonstrating numerous peculiar membrane-structures composed of compound lipid in bone and bone marrow and various adipose tissues. Acta Path Jpn 23:539–558, 1973
Bird TD, Koerker RM, Leaird BJ, et al: Lipomembranous polycystic osteodysplasia (brain, bone and fat disease): a genetic cause of presenile dementia. Neurology 33:81–86, 1983

BRAIN, CHRONIC

Synonyms. Dementia; feeblemindedness; mental retardation; cerebral chronic. (Generic definition that includes several specific syndromes with confusional state as common element.)

Symptoms and Signs. Failure of memory, particularly for recent events, is presenting symptom. Decline in work efficiency, with or without anxiety and depression; loss of emotional balance; irritability; sometimes rush of sexual feeling. Hygiene and appearance deteriorated; dysarthria; aphasia.

Etiology and Pathogenesis. Idiopathic degenerative diseases; endocrine-metabolic conditions; vascular insufficiency; nutritional deficiency; intoxication; encephalitis-meningitis; tumor.

Pathology. Related to etiology; destruction of nerve cells and fiber of cortex and diencephalon.

Diagnostic Procedures. Search for etiology.

Therapy. According to etiology; general care; in depression or anxiety, specific agents.

Prognosis. Depends on etiology; usually progressive.

BIBLIOGRAPHY. Busse EW: Geriatrics today—an overview. Am J Psychiatr 123:1226–1233, 1967
Adams RD, Victor M: Principles of Neurology, 5th ed, pp 353–376. New York, McGraw-Hill, 1993
Kaplan HI, Sadock BJ: Comprehensive Textbook of Psychiatry, 6th ed. Baltimore, Williams & Wilkins, 1995

BRAIN PURPURA

Synonym. Pericapillary encephalorrhagia.

Symptoms and Signs. Suddenly the patient (of various ages) becomes stuporous or comatose without focal neurological signs.

Etiology. Unknown. It may complicate viral pneumonia and some intoxication (arsenic) or be sporadic.

Pathology. Small hemorrhagic pericapillary lesions (1–2 mm) in the white matter, corpus callosum, centrum ovale, or cerebellar peduncles. Destruction of adjacent myelin and axis cylinders. Absence of inflammatory changes.

Diagnostic Procedures. *Cerebral spinal fluid.* Normal or moderate increase of proteins. *EEG. CT brain scan.*

Therapy. None specific.

Prognosis. Variable.

BIBLIOGRAPHY. Adams RD, Victor M: Principles of Neurology, 5th ed, pp 733–734. New York, McGraw-Hill, 1993

BRAIN (W.R.)

Synonyms. Exophthalmic ophthalmoplegia; orbit pseudo-tumor; superior orbital fissure.

Symptoms. Prevalent in males: later age of onset compared to exophthalmic goiter. Onset gradual. Both eyes may be involved or one eye's exophthalmos may precede that in the other by months. Pain; ophthalmoplegia; vision not affected (usually); no sensory disturbances of first branch of trigeminal (V) nerve.

Signs. Exophthalmos; edema of eyelid; chemosis.

Etiology. It may develop in patient with or without hyperthyroidism. Unknown; possibly low-grade infection.

Pathology. Inflammatory mass in ocular muscles.

Diagnostic Procedures. *X-ray. CT scan. MRI of skull. Angiography.*

Therapy. Steroids; antibiotics. Partial suture of the lids to protect eyes. Seldom needed, removal of roof or orbit and canal of optic nerve through anterior craniotomy.

Prognosis. Good response to treatment with improvement of vision. Usually progression spontaneously stops.

BIBLIOGRAPHY. Brain WR: Exophthalmic ophthalmoplegie. Q J Med 7:293, 1938
Ingalls RG: Tumor of the Orbit and Allied Pseudotumors. Springfield, IL, Charles C Thomas, 1953
Lakke JPWF: Superior orbital fissure syndrome. Arch Neurol 7:289–300, 1962
Adams RD, Victor M: Principles of Neurology, 5th ed, p 1234. New York, McGraw-Hill, 1993

BRAIN TUMOR–NEUROASTHENIA

Synonym. Pseudoneurotic brain tumor. See also Amorphosynthesis; organic brain.

Symptoms. Fatigue; weight loss; vague headache; slow speech; depression and emotional instability (irritability, fits of anger or depression, insomnia, decrease or loss of libido and potency).

Etiology. Initial stage precedes objective signs of brain tumor.

Pathology. Brain tumors (neoplastic aneurysm).

Diagnostic Procedures. *CT scan. MRI. X-ray of skull. Angiography. EEG. Spinal fluid.*

Therapy. Surgery when feasible.

Prognosis. Early diagnosis important because psychotic symptoms may mask organic disease and make the prognosis unfavorable because of the delayed treatment.

BIBLIOGRAPHY. Horenstein S: Effects of cerebrovascular disease on personality and emotionality. In Benton AL (ed): Behavioral Changes in Cerebrovascular Disease, p 171. New York, Harper & Row, 1970
Kaplan HI, Sadock BJ: Comprehensive Textbook of Psychiatry, 6th ed, pp 196, 1574. Baltimore, Williams & Wilkins, 1995

BRANCHIO-OTO-URETERAL

Synonyms. BOU.

Symptoms and Signs. Sensorineural hearing loss: preauricular pit or tags.

Etiology. Suggested autosomal dominant inheritance.

Pathology. Duplication of ureters or bifid renal pelvices.

BIBLIOGRAPHY. Fraser FC, Ayme S, Hala F, et al: "Autosomal dominant duplication of the renal collecting system, hearing loss and external ear anomalies: a new syndrome?" AM J Med Genet 14:473–478, 1983

BRANDT

Synonyms. Danbolt-Closs; acrodermatitis enteropathica.

Symptoms. Appears in both sexes; onset in early infancy. Gastrointestinal troubles with intermittent diarrhea. In acute phase, psychic disturbances of schizoid type. Retarded growth rate; photophobia.

Signs. Symmetric rash involving face, ears, back of scalp, buttocks, elbows, and knees, and hands and feet, starting as vesiculobullous, then drying to erythematosquamous type. Paronychia and dysonychia; alopecia; loss of eyebrows and eyelashes; conjunctivitis; blepharitis; scattered superficial opacities of cornea.

Etiology. Autosomal recessive inheritance (?). Possibly a defect of zinc absorption at jejunal level. Reported cases of AIDS manifesting as Brandt syndrome.

Pathology. Histopathologic changes in the skin and gastrointestinal tract are nonspecific; a cytoplasmic inclusion body has been noted in the Paneth cells.

Diagnostic Procedures. *Biopsy of skin. Study of digestive enzymes. Blood.* Low serum zinc.

Therapy. Oral therapy with zinc compounds: 50 mg of zinc sulfate, acetate, or gluconate daily for infants and up to 150 mg daily for children. Plasma zinc levels should be monitored.

Prognosis. Without treatment, fatal within 10 years of onset. With treatment, disease kept under control until puberty. Long remission occurs often, including remission of corneal opacities and of cerebral atrophy.

BIBLIOGRAPHY. Brandt T: Dermatitis in children with disturbances of the general condition and the absorption of food elements. Acta Dermatol Venereol 17:513–546, 1936
Danbolt N, Closs K: Akrodermatitis enteropathica. Acta Dermatol Vernereol 23:127–169, 1942
Koletzko B, Bretschneider A, Bremer HJ: Fatty acid composition of plasma lipids in acrodermatitis enteropathica before and after zinc supplementation. Eur J Pediatr 143:310–314, 1985
Tong TK, Andrew LR, Albert A, et al: Childhood acquired immune deficiency syndrome manifesting as acrodermatitis enteropathica. J Pediatr 108:426–428, 1986
Ammon HV: Diarrhea and constipation. In Haubrich WS, Schaffner F, Berk JE (eds): Bockus Gastroenterology, 5th ed, p 94. Philadelphia, WB Saunders, 1995

BRANDYWINE* DENTINOGENESIS IMPERFECTION

Synonyms. Shields III; dentinogenesis imperfecta.

Symptoms and Signs. Found in southern Maryland. Crown of both deciduous and permanent teeth eroded and pulp exposed. Dentin color amber and smooth. No stigmata or osteogenesis imperfecta.

Etiology. Autosomal dominant inheritance. May be same entity or separate mutation of Capdepont (see).

---

*Isolate in southern Maryland.

Diagnostic Procedures. *X-ray of teeth.* Large pulp chambers and root canals, which become reduced with age.

BIBLIOGRAPHY. Schimmelpfennig CB, McDonald RE: Enamel and dentine aplasia. Oral Surg 6:1444–1449, 1953
Shields ED, Bixler D, El-Kaqfrawy AM: A proposed classification for heritable human dentin defect with a descriptin of a new entity. Arch Oral Biol 18:543–553, 1973
Boughman JA, Halloran SL, Roulston D, et al: An autosomal dominant form of juvenile periodontitis: its localization to chromosome 4 and linkage to dentinogenesis imperfecta and Gc. J Craniofac Genet Dev Biol 6:341–350, 1986

BRAUER

Synonyms. Focal facial dermal dysplasia; forceps marks. See Hidrotic ectodermal dysplasia, and Tylosis and Setleis.

Symptoms and Signs. Both sexes affected; present from birth. Scar-like defects at the temporal regions (similar to forceps lesions). Median furrow on the chin; scar-like lesion. Eyebrows slanted up and outward; eyelashes absent or multiple in upper and absent in lower lids. Protuberant nose.

Etiology. Unknown; autosomal dominant inheritance.

Pathology. *Skin.* Mesodermal dysplasia with absence of subcutaneous fat and contiguity of muscles and skin.

Prognosis. High incidence of abdominal neoplasia in one affected family.

BIBLIOGRAPHY. Brauer A: Heréditarer symmetrischer systematisierter Naevus aplasticus bei 38 Personen. Derm Wochschr 89:1163–1168, 1929
McGeoch AH, Reed WB: Familial focal facial dermal dysplasia. Arch Derm 107:591–596, 1973
Magid ML, Prendiville JS, Esterly NB: Focal facial dermal dysplasia: bitemporal lesions resembling aplasia cutis congenita. J Am Acad Derm 18:1203–1207, 1988
Harper J: Genetics and genodermatoses. In Champion RH, Burton JL, Ebling FJG (eds): Rook/Wilkinson/Ebling Textbook of Dermatology, 5th ed, p 358. Oxford, Blackwell Scientific, 1992

BRAUN-FALCO

Synonym. Circumscribed cutis laxa; localized abdominal wall atrophy.

Symptoms and Signs. Present from birth. Presence of cutis laxa lesions on thorax and anterior abdominal muscles; thorax deformity; mediastinal hernia.

Etiology. Unknown. See Cutis laxa syndromes.

Pathology. See Cutis laxa syndromes.

BIBLIOGRAPHY. Braun-Falco O: Angeborene Dermatochalasis als Leitsymptom eines Symptomkomplexes. Arch Klin Exp Dermatol 220:166–182, 1964
Burton JL: Disorders of connective tissue. In Champion RH, Burton JL, Ebling FJG (eds): Rook/Wilkinson/Ebling Textbook of Dermatology, 5th ed, p 1782. Oxford, Blackwell Scientific, 1992

BRAZILIAN PEMPHIGUS FOLIACEUS

Synonyms. Amendola; Vieira; fogo selvagem; wildfire pemphigus.

Symptoms. Endemic in Brazil (state of Sao Paulo in particular). All ethnic groups and ages affected (benign course if onset before 30 years of age). Fever; chills; localized pain (enhanced by movements).

Signs. Bullae initiate on face, frequently affecting eyes (anterior pole cloudiness 5%) and chest; then become generalized and evolve into pustules, crusts, and exfoliate (pemphigus-like); Nikolsky sign; mucosa not involved.

Etiology. Unknown; possibly an infectious condition associated with endocrine disorders. Simulium pruinosum suspected vector.

Pathology. In upper epidermis, acanthosis, derma infiltration. In older lesions, acanthosis, papillomatosis, hyperkeratosis.

Diagnostic Procedures. Biopsy. Indirect immunofluorescence specific antibodies.

Therapy. Symptomatic. Local and oral corticosteroids.

Prognosis. Evolution in 2 weeks to 1 year. Complications: ocular lesions; gonadal lesions; impotence. Possibly fatal.

BIBLIOGRAPHY. Vieira JP: Pemphigus foliaceus (fogo salvagem). Arch Dermatol Syphilol 41:858–863, 1940

Amendola F: Cataracte no pemfigo foliáceo (nota previa). Rev Paul Med 26:286, 1945

Sevadjian C: Nosology of Brazilian pemphigus foliaceus. Int J Dermatol 18:781–786, 1979

Pye RJ: Bullous eruptions. In Champion RH, Burton JL, Ebling FJG (eds): Rook/Wilkinson/Ebling Textbook of Dermatology, 5th ed, pp 1646–1647. Oxford, Blackwell Scientific, 1992

BRAZILIAN PURPURIC FEVER

Symptoms and Signs. Occurs in children 3 months to 8 years old. Fever, vomiting, and abdominal pain, followed by purpura and death. The initial symptom is often a purulent conjunctivitis. The illness often is complicated by disseminated intravascular coagulation (DIC).

Etiology. Infection with Haemophilus influenzae type B. Cases have been described in Brazil town of Promissao (Sao Paulo state) and in Central Australia.

Pathology. Ischemia of upper and lower limbs in cases of DIC.

Diagnostic Procedures. *Blood cultures.*

Therapy. Symptomatic treatment of shock: antibiotics as suggested by blood cultures. Usually the Haemophilus is susceptible to ampicillin, cefotaxime, chloramphenicol, and cotrimoxaxole.

Prognosis. Poor.

BIBLIOGRAPHY. Centers for Disease Control. CDC preliminary report: epidemic purpuric fever among children–Brazil. MMWR 34:217–219, 1985

McIntyre P, Wheaton G, Erlich J, Hansman D: Brasilian purpuric fever in central Australia. Lancet II:112, 1987

BREAST-FEEDING-HYPERBILIRUBINEMIA

Synonyms. Transient nonhemolytic unconjugated hyperbilirubinemia associated with breast feeding; Hyperbilirubinemia breast feeding; maternal milk hyperbilirubinemia; breast milk jaundice.

Symptoms and Signs. Both sexes. From birth, only in breast-fed children. Progressive jaundice. Ameliorated only by discontinuation of breast feeding. No kernicterus.

Etiology. Presence of inhibitor of UDP-glucuronyl transferase in maternal milk: 3 alpha, 20 beta-pregnanediol.

Diagnostic Procedures. *Blood.* Unconjugated hyperbilirubinemia. Maternal milk. 3 alpha-20 betapregnanediol.

Prognosis. Recession of jaundice with onset of artificial feeding.

BIBLIOGRAPHY. Arthur LJH, Bevan BR, Holton JB: Neonatal hyperbilirubinemia and breast feeding. Dev Med Child Neurol 8:279, 1966

Chowdhury JR, Wolkoff Chowdhury NRAW, Arias IM: Hereditary jaundice and disorders of bilirubin metabolism. In Scriver CR, Beaudet AL, Sly WS, et al: The Metabolic and Molecular Bases of Inherited Disease, 7th ed, p 2178. New York, McGraw-Hill, 1995

BREGEAT

Synonym. Oculo-orbital-thalamo-encephalic angiomatosis.

Symptoms and Signs. From birth. Angiomatosis of eye and orbit, controlateral forehead. Variable neurological signs according to extension of thalamoencephalic angioma.

Etiology. Unknown. Sporadic.

Pathology. Angioma in thalamus extending to choroidal plexus.

Diagnostic Procedures. *CT brain scan. MRI. Angiography.*

Therapy. Evaluation for possible neurosurgery.

Prognosis. Variable.

BIBLIOGRAPHY. Brégeat P, Juge P, Pouliquen Y, et al: A propos d'une angiomatose orbitothalancéphalique. Bull Mem Soc Franc Ophthal 71:581–594, 1958

Chonnette G, Auriel M: Classification de angiodysplasies et tumeurs vasculaires. Rev Stom Clin Maxillo Fac 87:1–5, 1986

BREMER

Synonyms. Passow; status dysraphicus; dysraphism; myelodyplasia. Clinically includes Arnold-Chiari (see); Dandy Walker (see); Klippel-Feil (see); Ostrum-Furst and Nielsen (see). See also Curtius I (possibly same syndrome) hemihypertrophy; Goldenhar.

Symptoms and Signs. Spina bifida (open or closed) constant feature; muscular weakness; mental deficiencies, trophic changes; facial hemiatrophy; abducens (VI) and facial (VII) nerve paralysis; anesthesia first branch of trigeminal (V) nerve; myosis; heterochromia iridis; cervical rib symptoms; kyphoscoliosis; sacral hypertrichosis; enuresis or other symptoms of sphincter weakness; anisomastia; extremities malformations.

Etiology. Irregular dominant inheritance, in some families recessive form described. Disorders of the anlage of spinal cord owing to abnormalities appearing during tubulation and closure of primary medullary plate.

BIBLIOGRAPHY. Fuchs A: Ueber den klinischen Nachweis Kongenitaler Defectbildungen in den Unteren Rueckenmarksabschnitten. Wien Med Wschr 59:2142, 1909

Bremer FW: Klinische Untersuchung zur Aetiologie der Syringomyelie Dtsch. Z Nervenheilk 95, 1926

Curtis F: Lorenz Ueber den Status dysraphicus. Z Neurol 149:1, 1933

Passow A: Analogie und Koordination von Symptomen der Arachnodactylie und des Status dysraphicus (zur Frage der Wesensgleichheit beider Komplexe). Klin Monatsbl Augenheilkd 94:102–103, 1935

Bremer FW: Status dysraphicus und Syringomyelie. Fortschr Neurol Psychiatr 14:109–122, 1942

Liebaldt GP, Leiber B: Cutaneous dysplasias associated with neurologic disorders: Synopsis and differential diagnosis. In Vinken PJ, Bruyn GW (eds): Handbook of Clinical Neurology, vol 14, p 111. Amsterdam, North-Holland, 1972

BRENNEMANN

Synonyms. Mesenteric lymphangitis; idiopathic; lymphadenitis; pseudotuberculous mesenteric; retroperitoneal Brennemann.

Symptoms. Usually in children under 15 years of age. Abdominal pain; nausea; vomiting; fever; following upper respiratory tract infection.

Signs. Pain in lower abdominal quadrant; rebound tenderness; not as severe as in appendicitis. Upper tract respiratory inflammation.

Etiology. Viral infections (adenovirus and others).

Pathology. Mesenteric and retroperitoneal adenitis.

Diagnostic Procedures. Leukocytosis; occasionally, increase of lymphomonocytic elements (virocytes).

Therapy. It is good to operate because of the almost impossible differential diagnosis with acute appendicitis. If diagnosed, treatment is supportive. Specific vaccines are being tested.

Prognosis. Spontaneous recovery. In some young children the occurrence of intussusception has been reported.

BIBLIOGRAPHY. Brennemann J: The abdominal pain of throat infection. Am J Dis Child 22:493–499, 1921
Fox JP, Hall CE, Cooney MK: The Seattle virus. Watch VII. Observations of adenovirus infections. Am J Epidemiol 10:362–386, 1977
Nance FC: Diseases of the peritoneum, retroperitoneum, mesentery and omentum. In Haubrich WS, Schaffner F, Berk JE (eds): Bockus Gastroenterology, 5th ed, vol 2, p 3093. Philadelphia, WB Saunders, 1995

BRENNER

Synonym. Ovarian; fibroepithelioma ovary.

Symptoms. Appears in elderly women. Asymptomatic or postmenopausal recurrent bleeding.

Signs. Possibly, adnexal mass on palpation.

Etiology. Unknown (obsolete entity).

Pathology. Benign ovarian tumor: small, well-capsulated, usually unilateral, seldom estrogenic.

Diagnostic Procedure. *Ultrasonography or CT scan. Surgical exploration.*

Therapy. Removal.

Prognosis. Good.

BIBLIOGRAPHY. Brenner F: Das Ophoroma folliculare. Frankf Zschr Pathol 1:150–171, 1907
Scully RE: Tumors of the ovary and maldeveloped gonads. Armed Forces Inst Path Fasc 16, 1979
Scully RE: Ovarian tumors with endocrine manifestations. In De Groot LJ (ed): Endocrinology, 3rd ed, p 2117. Philadelphia, WB Saunders, 1995

BRETT

Synonym. Janus. Eponym used to indicate an occasional radiologic finding: clear lung on one side and opaque shadow on the other side. This aspect is observed in Fallot's tetralogy (see) with atresia of a branch of pulmonary artery or in case of truncus ateriosus with solitary pulmonary artery.

BIBLIOGRAPHY. Bret J: Le syndrome de Janus. Arch Mal Coeur 49:468–472, 1956
Perloff JK: The Clinical Recognition of Congenital Heart Disease. Philadelphia, WB Saunders, 1978

BRETONNEAU

Synonyms. Diphtheric croup; Diphtheritis, Malignant angina.

BIBLIOGRAPHY. Bretonneau PF: Des inflammations spéciales du tissue muqueux, et in particulier de la diphthtérite, ou inflammation pelliculaire. Paris, Crevot, 1926

BREUS MOLE

Synonyms. Hematomole.

Pathology. Tuberous subchorional hematoma of decidua.

Diagnostic Procedures. *Echography.*

Therapy. Surgery.

BIBLIOGRAPHY. Breus C: Das Tuberoese subchoriale Haematom der Decidua; eine typische Form der Molenschwangershaft. Leipzig, Deuticke, 1892

BRIDGE JUMPING

Symptoms. Prevalent in white males, age 25–34. Repeated episodes common; exacerbated by media publicity, which leads to clusters; usually, occurrence affected by season, holiday, and weather; predilection for particular bridges.

Etiology. Variable, but common psychological characteristics. Exhibitionist personality; depression associated with stress. Frequently also association with alcohol or drug ingestion.

Therapy. Prevention at different level when "on site" and have identified the intention: establish communication; stabilize environment; coordinate harbor patrol; if possible, physically prevent jump or fall in water.

Prognosis. Variable. Often unsuccessful in suicide attempts.

BIBLIOGRAPHY. Pascarelli EF, Katz IB, Nolte C: The epidemiology of bridge jumping. Presented at the 32nd Conference Internationale Médicine Catastrophe, Monte Carlo, April 6–9, 1979
Kaplan HI, Sadock BJ: Comprehensive Textbook of Psychiatry, 6th ed. Baltimore, Williams & Wilkins, 1995

BRIESKY

Synonyms. Leukokraurosis vulvae; kraurosis vulvae; senile genital atrophy; vulvae senile atrophy.

Symptoms. Pruritus (mild and inconstant); dyspareunia; easy traumatism.

Signs. Gradual shrinkage of labia, clitoris, and frenulum. Dryness of mucosa. Leukoplakia may be associated. Vaginitis frequent (responsible for symptoms).

Etiology. Postmenopausal or postovariectomy hormonal deficiencies; or loss of response to hormone (Seabright-Bantam type, see). Obsolete since the older classification of senile atrophy and primary vulvar atrophy relate both to physiological effects of aging and "do not indicate to a specific form of disease." The syndrome today has been subdivided in the following conditions: benign dermatoses of the vulva (lichenification, psoriasis, lichen planus, seborrheic dermatitis, eczematous dermatitis); vulvar epithelial hyperplasia (with and without atypia); lichen sclerosus; leucoderma; infections; Bowen (see) and Paget (see).

Pathology. Thinning of epithelium; hyperkeratinization; elastic tissue altered; collagenous tissue increased. Associated inflammatory feature. See Etiology.

Therapy. Estrogens (particularly useful for vaginitis, less for atrophy). Local estrogen cream. For benign dermatoses antibiotics and antimycotic topical therapy.

Prognosis. Frequent exacerbation. Irreversible condition.

BIBLIOGRAPHY. Briesky A: Die Krankheiten der Vagina Hand. Allerg Spec Chir 4:1–256, 1879

Ive FA: The umbilical perianal and genital regions. In Champion RH, Burton JL, Ebling FJG (eds): Rook/Wilkinson/Ebling Textbook of Dermatology, 5th ed, pp 2849–2854. Oxford, Blackwell Scientific, 1992

BRIGHT

Synonyms. Acute bacterial nephritis; acute glomerulonephritis; acute nephritis; postinfective glomerulonephritis; poststreptococcal glomerulonephritis; PSGN.

Symptoms. Prevalent in males; onset at any age; highest incidence 3–7 years of age. Ten days after airway infection: fatigue; anorexia; cephalalgia; backache; abdominal pain; vomiting; somnolence; dyspnea; oliguria; hematuria.

Signs. Edema of face, less frequently of legs; tachycardia; hypertension; basal rales; moderate temperature elevation.

Etiology. Streptococcal infection by nephrogenic strains (type 4–12 in respiratory infection and a type 49 in impetigo) or other infection (staphylococcal; pneumococcal; viral) causing glomerular damage through the following pathogenetic mechanisms: immunologic reactions; vascular diseases; abnormalities of coagulation; and metabolic defects. In some cases mechanism remains unknown (type 1–12, 18, 25, 49, 55, 57, 60), or suspected (31, 52, 56, 59, 61). Group C streptococcus pathogenetic mechanisms: immune complex (IgG and C3).

Pathology. Kidney. Enlarged, edematous, pale, with punctate hemorrhages or gray spots on surface. Capsule tense; cortex smooth; medulla congested. Glomeruli swollen, filled with cells covering the tuft network. Immunoflourescence reveals granular pattern.

Diagnostic Procedures. *Blood.* Elevated blood urea nitrogen; occasionally, anemia; leukocytosis. Antistreptolysin, antistaphylolysin (and others) titers increased. Increased red cell sedimentation rate. *Urine.* Red blood cells; casts of various type (RBC, epithelial, granular); proteinuria (lower than 2 g/day); decreased sodium excretion. *Renal function tests.* Abnormal in 50% of cases. Renal biopsy: See Pathology. *Light microscopy.* Enlarged glomeruli capillary lumen occluded by mesangial and endothelial cells and infiltrated by leukocytes. Few crescents. *Electron microscopy.* Electron-dense deposits (lumps) on the endothelial side of basement membrane. *Immunofluorescence.* Three patterns: starry sky, mesangeal, and garland, which are deposits of IgG and C3.

Therapy. Bed rest; low protein and low sodium diet; antihypertensive agents; antibiotics.

Prognosis. More intense and severe onset implies a more guarded prognosis. A few deaths from pulmonary edema, hypertensive encephalopathy, or infection; 1% fatality for renal failure. Some patients exhibit proteinuria and hematuria for weeks or months and finally recover; some may develop a chronic condition; 90% of children are finally completely cured; 50% of adults develop chronic glomerular disease.

BIBLIOGRAPHY. Bright R: Cases and observations illustrative of renal disease accompanied with the secretion of albuminous urine. Guy's Hosp Rep London 1:338–400, 1836

Rinberg Y, Fraley EE: The renal mass. In Massry SG, Glassock RJ: Textbook of Nephrology, 3rd ed, p 573. Baltimore, Williams & Wilkins, 1995

BRILL-SYMMERS

Obsolete.

Synonyms. Brill-Boehr-Rosenthal; Symmers; macrofollicular lymphoblastoma; giant follicular lymphoma; giant cell lymphosarcoma; nodular lymphosarcoma. Eponym used to indicate a "clinicohistologic" entity, which is no longer considered distinct, but is classified into the broader category of non-Hodgkins lymphomas. The clinical element was a distinctly superior survival and the histologic feature of a well-differentiated lymphocytic-follicular pattern as compared with other follicular varieties of lymphomas. In later stages 50% lose the follicular pattern and present unstructured cellular infiltration, modifications that usually precede the fatal outcome.

BIBLIOGRAPHY. Brill NE, Boehr G, Rosenthal N: Generalized giant follicle hyperplasia of lymph nodes and spleen: a hitherto undescribed type. JAMA 84:668–671, 1925

Symmers D: Follicular lymphadenopathy with splenomegaly: A newly recognized disease of the lymphatic system. Arch Pathol 3:816–820, 1927

Dumont J: La maladie de Brill-Symmers. Concours Med 103:2437–2453, 1981

Greer JP, Macon WR, List AF, et al: Non-Hodgkin lymphomas. In Lee GR, Bithel TC, Foerster J, et al (eds): Wintrobe's Clinical Hematology, 9th ed, p 2092. Philadelphia, Lea & Febiger, 1993

BRILL-ZINSSER

Synonyms. Eponym used to indicate recrudescence of typhoid fever even years after intial episode.

BIBLIOGRAPHY. Brill NE: An acute infectionus disease of unknown origin. A clinical study based on 221 cases. Am J Med Sci 139:484–502, 1910

Zinsser H: Rats, Lice and History, p 111. Boston, Atlantic Monthly Press, 1935

BRIQUET

Synonyms. Conversion reaction; hysteria conversion; hysterical neurosis.

Symptoms. Prevalent in females; caution for diagnosis in men (rare). Onset in adolescence or later. Prodromal manifestation at earlier age frequent; lack of energy; laziness; somatic symptoms recorded in 30% of cases; flirtatiousness of female; juvenile sexual offense. In women, high incidence of polysurgery. In men, history of criminal acts and drinking. Anxious impulse converted to functional symptoms: motor and sensory disturbances not related to neural pathway but to anatomic distribution (e.g., glove, stocking areas); hemiplegia, paraplegia, disorders of phonation, hearing, sight. Frequently, symptoms arise when patient tries to evade an unpleasant situation.

Etiology. Psychiatric disorder related (not invariably, however) to sexual dysfunction. Use of sexual signals to convey nonsexual messages (placate aggression?). Association with antisocial personality.

Therapy. Psychotherapy.

Prognosis. Tendency to convert to new symptoms; better prognosis for monosymptomatic hysteria in adult life.

BIBLIOGRAPHY. Briquet P: Traité clinique et thérapeutique de l'hysterie. Paris, Bailliere, 1859

Kaplan HI, Sadock BJ: Comprehensive Textbook of Psychiatry, 6th ed, pp 1258–1259. Baltimore, Williams & Wilkins, 1995

BRISSAUD-MARIE

Synonyms. Conversion reaction; conversion hysteria; hysterical neurosis. See also Briquet.

Symptoms. Glossolabial hemispasm.

Etiology. Conversion reaction.

BIBLIOGRAPHY. Brissaud E, Marie P: De la déviation faciale dans l'hémiplégie hystérique. Pro Med, 5:84, 1887

Freedman AM, Kaplan HI, Sadock BJ: Comprehensive Textbook of Psychiatry, 4th ed. Baltimore, Williams & Wilkins, 1985

BRISSAUD-SICARD

Synonym. Brissaud IV; Brissaud I; Brissaud-Lereboullet; pons inferior-anterolateral; hemicraniosis. See Millard-Grubler; and Raymond-Foville.

Symptoms and Signs. Unilateral facial spasm with contralateral paralysis of limbs.

Etiology and Pathology. Irritative lesion of the anterolateral and inferior pons. Pyramidal tract before it crosses VII nucleus.

BIBLIOGRAPHY. Brissaud E: Reserches anatomo-pathologiques et physiologiques sur la contracture permanente des hémiplégiques. Versailles 206, 1880
Brissaud EA, Sicard J: Type special de syndrome alterne. Rev Neurol (Paris) 16:86, 1908
Kaplan HI, Sadock BJ: Comprehensive Textbook of psychiatry, 6th ed, pp 1258–1259. Baltimore, Williams & Wilkins, 1995

BRISTOWE

Synonym. Corpus callosum tumor. See Marchiafava-Bignami.

Symptoms. Not distinctive; more marked form of mental changes seen from involvement of one of frontal lobes; difficulty in concentration; personality changes; memory disturbances; psychoses; negativism and disregard of requests and commands. Apraxia of left hand (in tumor affecting anterior portion of corpus collosum).

Diagnostic Procedures. *Cerebrospinal fluid.* Xanthochromia; pleocytosis. *CT brain scan. MRI.* Distortion of one or both lateral ventricles and third ventricle.

Prognosis. Progressive: stupor; coma; death.

BIBLIOGRAPHY. Plater F: Observationum Bale 1:13–16, 1614
Bristowe JS: Cases of tumour of the corpus callosum. Brain 7:315–333, 1884
Ironside R, Guttmacher M: The corpus callosum and its tumors. Brain 52:442–483, 1929
Alpers BJ, Grant FC: The clinical syndrome of corpus callosum. Arch Neurol Psychiatr 25:67–86, 1931
Elliot FA: The corpus callosum, cingolate gyrus, septum pellucidum, septal area and fornix. In Vinken PJ, Bruyn GW: Handbook of Clinical Neurology, vol 2, p 760. Amsterdam, North-Holland, 1969
Slooff ACJ, Slooff JL: Supratentorial tumor in children. In Vinken PJ, Bruyn GW: Handbook of Clinical Neurology, vol 17, p 507. Amsterdam, North-Holland, 1975

BROADBENT

Synonyms. Ingravescent apoplexy; intraventricular brain hemorrhage.

Symptoms and Signs. Sudden loss of consciousness (from stupor to deep coma) preceded, usually, by severe headache or vomiting or both; Cheyne-Stokes respiration or other breathing abnormalities; generalized flaccidity or focal signs; cerebral shock or diaschisis (loss of functional continuity among various centers of neural pathways). Blood hypertension.

Etiology. Primary subarachnoid hemorrhage with sudden and imposing invasion of blood into ventricular system. Hypertension; trauma.

Pathology. Subarachnoid hemorrhage.

Diagnostic Procedures. *Spinal fluid. Blood. EEG. Angiography. CT brain scan. MRI.*

Therapy. Intensive care; antiedema treatment (with caution).

Prognosis. Severe.

BIBLIOGRAPHY. Broadbent WH: On ingravescent apoplexy. Med Chir Soc London 8:103–108, 1876
Adams RD, Victor M: Principles of Neurology, 5th ed, pp 542–543. New York, McGraw-Hill, 1993

BROCA APHASIA

Synonyms. Expressive aphasia; aphasia expressive; motor aphasia; verbal aphasia.

Symptoms. Predominant impairment of expressive speech; resulting in inability to find words that express thoughts. In Broca's aphasia, the patient may say a few words (i.e., habitual expressions, words of well-known songs) but cannot write. This differs from other forms of aphasia. The patient shows a preserved ability to think in abstraction; and the recognition of his ineptitude and mistakes even if accompanied by some minor difficulty in understanding. Repeated failure causes despair and irritation manifests.

Etiology. Lesions of the posterior part of third frontal convolution and lower part of precentral convolution of dominant hemisphere.

Prognosis. A certain degree of recovery sometimes occurs as other hemisphere asserts itself.

BIBLIOGRAPHY. Broca P: Sur le siège de la faculté du language articulé, avec deux observations d'aphémie. Bull Soc Anat (Paris) 36:330–357, 1861
Adams RD, Victor M: Principles of Neurology, 5th ed, pp 413–414, 416–418. New York, McGraw-Hill, 1993

BROCK

Synonyms. Graham-Burford-Mayer; lung, middle lobe; middle lobe.

Symptoms. Can be observed at any age; onset acute febrile episode. Recurrent hemoptysis and pneumonitis. In interval between episodes, chronic cough and fatigability.

Signs. During acute episodes, signs of pneumonia; in interval, signs of bronchiectasis or chronic suppuration.

Etiology. No single factor responsible; any inflammatory process that results in hilar lymphadenopathy and compression of middle lobe (right) or lingula (left) bronchus, with consequent atelectasis and pneumonitis.

Pathology. Enlargement of peribronchial lymph nodes that encircle the bronchus of middle lobe; obstructive pneumonitis of the middle lobe; bronchiectasis and destruction of lung parenchyma.

Diagnostic Procedures. *X-ray of chest. Bronchoscopy. Bronchography.*

Therapy. Surgical extirpation of affected lobe. Antibiotics only induce remission. Responds well to antibiotics. Surgery rarely required.

Prognosis. Good after surgery.

BIBLIOGRAPHY. Brock RC, Cann RJ, Dickinson JR: Tuberculosis mediastinal lymphadenitis in childhood: secondary effects on lungs. Guy's Hosp Rep London 97:295–317, 1937
Graham EA, Burford TH, Mayer JH: Middle lobe syndrome. Postgrad Med 4:29–34, 1948
Saterfield JL, Virapony C, Clare FC: Computed tomography of combined right upper and middle lobe collapse. J Comp Assist Tomogr 12:383–387, 1988

BROCQ-PAUTRIER

Synonyms. Median rhomboid glossitis, glossite losangique médiane.

Symptoms and Signs. Present in 0.3% of population. Syndrome becomes clinically manifest in third or fourth decade or later. Asymptomatic or burning while eating spicy foods and dryness of mouth. Accidental notice of area on the midline of base of tongue, smooth and devoid of papillae, or elevated and nodular. Sometimes associated candidiasis of palate.

Etiology. Considered in the past as a developmental defect; persistency of tuberculum impar. Today considered associated with candidosis (immune defect may predispose to lesion).

Pathology. Epithelial thickening; acanthosis; slight hyperkeratosis; fibrosis extending into muscular layer.

Diagnostic Procedures. In case of doubt, biopsy (seldom required).

Therapy. Refrain from smoking and antifungal treatment.

Prognosis. Good results with treatment.

BIBLIOGRAPHY. Brocq L, Pautrier LM: Glossite losangique médiane de la face dorsale de la langue. Ann Dermatol Syph 5:1–18, 1914
Touyz LZG, Peters E: Candidal infection of the tongue with non specific inflammation of the palate. Oral Surg 63:304–308, 1987
Kabani S, Cataldo E: Oral manifestations of gasrointestinal disease. In Haubrich WS, Schaffner F, Berk JE (eds): Bockus Gastroenterology, 5th ed, pp 3313–3314. Philadelphia, WB Saunders, 1995

BRODIE I

Synonyms. Brodie abscess; suppurative focal osteomyelitis.

Symptoms. Initially asymptomatic (for years). Intermittent pain at end of a long bone (e.g., tibia); possible fever.

Signs. Initially none, then edema and erythema of skin of painful zone; fusiform swelling of affected bone; localized bone tenderness.

Etiology. Chronic bone abscess where necrotic debris and infective agents have usually been walled off; 50% Staphylococcus aureus, 20% culture negative. Some surgeons call any bone abscess "Brodie abscess."

Pathology. Ulceration of head of bone; encapsulated abscess included in sclerosed bone.

Diagnostic Procedures. *Blood.* Occasionally, leucocytosis. *X-rays.* Bone area rarefacted in metaphysis, well demarcated. *Biopsy.*

Therapy. Drilling and evacuation (Brodie), or excision (preferred).

Prognosis. Excellent with excision. Otherwise, spontaneous remission and possible relapses.

BIBLIOGRAPHY. Brodie BC: An account of some cases of chronic abscess of the tibia. Med Chir Tr London 17:239–249, 1832
Klippel JH, Dieppe PA: Rheumatology. St Louis, Mosby, 1994 pp 4.3.4, 7.43.2, 7.43.3

BRODIE II

Synonyms. Breast adenofibroma; breast cystosarcoma phylloides.

Symptoms. Pain in the breast.

Signs. Usually absent; or distortion of breast contour; nipple flattened; no retraction.

Etiology. Unknown.

Pathology. Benign tumor; nodular, gray-white color. Fibroblastic proliferation, stroma rich cellularity; epithelial growth not prominent; intracanalicular invasion.

Diagnostic Procedures. *Mammography. Ultrasonography. Thermography.*

Therapy. Surgical excision.

Prognosis. Benign; seldom metastasis.

BIBLIOGRAPHY. Brodie BC: Lectures on serocystic tumors of the breast. Lond Med Gaz 25:808–814, 1939
Briggs RM, Walter M, Rosenthal D: Cystosarcoma phylloides in adolescent female patients. Am J Surg 146:712–714, 1983
Hindle WH: Breast Disease for Gynecologists. Appleton Lange, 1990

BRODIN

Synonym. Appendicitis–duodenal stenosis.

Symptoms. Double symptomatology related to duodenal stenosis and appendicitis-like condition.

Etiology. Mesenteric lymphadenitis.

BIBLIOGRAPHY. Brodin M: L'appendice cronique. Son diagnostic par la palpation abdominale en position verticale et son retentissement duodénal avec arrêt en "genu inferius" mis en évidence par l'étude radiologique de la traversée digestive. Presse Med 49:619–621, 1941

BROMHIDROSIS

Synonym. Osmidrosis.

Symptoms. Malodorous sweating. (Marked individual and racial variations in social acceptability.)

Signs. Generalized and, frequently, associated with hyperhidrosis. Localized forms (axillae, feet, genitalia).

Etiology. Eccrine secretion per se is odorless; however, various substances may be excreted with it (garlic; onions; arsenic; sulfinylidric compounds). Bacterial decomposition liberates fatty acids with characteristic odor in gout, diabetes, scurvy, and typhoid.

Therapy. Omission of particular foods from diet. Washing of involved areas and application of antibacterial agents. Agents to control hyperhidrosis, such as aluminum salts and anticholinergic drugs, of little benefit.

Prognosis. Good response to treatment.

BIBLIOGRAPHY. Hurley HJ, Shelley WB: The Human Apocrine Sweat Gland in Health and Disease. Springfield, IL, Charles C Thomas, 1960
Smith M, Smith LG, Levinson B: The use of smell in differential diagnosis. Lancet II:1452, 1982

BRONCHIOLITIS OBLITERANS

Synonym. BOOP, bronchiolitis obliterans organizing pneumonia; panbronchiolitis diffuse, respiratory bronchiolitis; marrow and heart–lung transplant bronchiolitis; cocaine bronchiolitis.

Symptoms and Signs. Are generally the same for all forms (see Etiology): cough, flu-like illness, progressively leading to dyspnea that may resolve or not.

Etiology. Various types of etiology determine all the same clinical patterns but there are different diseases.

Acute and chronic bronchiolitis. Respiratory syncytial virus in infants, viral bronchiolitis (may be adeno) in adults.

Diffuse panbronchiolitis in Japanese, Chinese, and Koreans. Age 30–70 years, prevalent in males. Associated with chronic parasinusitis. Pseudomonas in sputum indicates terminal disease. Survival at 10 years is 30%.

Respiratory bronchiolitis-interstitial lung disease. In smokers 30 to 60 years. Regresses with cortisone and suspension of smoke. Similar to desquamative interstitial pneumonia (see).

Idiopathic bronchiolitis obliterans. Sporadic cases with no obvious inciting cause or associated connective tissue disorder. After corticosteroids stabilization and progression to end-stage lung disease.

Toxic fume exposure. To nitrogen dioxide, sulfur dioxide. Eye, nose, and throat irritation and after weeks bronchiolitis obliterans.

Postinfectious bronchiolitis obliterans. After viral or mycoplasma infection.

In connective tissue disease. Rheumatoid arthritis, scleroderma, LES, eosinophilic fascitis, polymyalgia rheumatica.

Drug-related penicillamine, gold.

Bone marrow transplantation associated. In 10% of bone marrow patients who develop graft versus host disease.

Heart–lung transplantion associated. In males 20–40 years. Probably owing to repeated infections.

Aspiration of activated charcoal (charcoal lung).

Aspiration of cocaine.

Bronchiolitis obliterans organizing pneumoniae (BOOP).

Symptoms and Signs. In both sexes, second–seventh decade, not related to smoking. After flu-like illness, cough and dyspnea.

Etiology. Unknown.

Diagnostic Procedures. *Chest radiogram.* Bilateral patchy infiltrates. *Pulmonary function studies.* Low vital capacity abnormal capacity.

Pathology. Open lung biopsy. Epithelial damage of peribronchiolar alveolar septa. Bronchoalveolar lavage: increased number of cells, lymphocytes, and eosinophils.

Therapy. Prednisone 1 mg/kg for at least 3 months tapering down for one year. Relapses may occur.

Prognosis. In 65% complete resolution; in 20% chronic symptoms and pulmonary dysfunction; in 5% death.

BIBLIOGRAPHY. Ramazzini B: De morbis artificum diatriba Modena A. Capponi Ed, 1770 Utrecht G. Van de Water Ed (IIrd) 1703 Padova, GB Conzetto Ed (III ed), 1713
Lange W: Uber eine eigenthumliche Erktankung der kleinen Bronchien und Bronchilen. Dtsch Arch Klin Med 70:342–364, 1901
Liebow AA: Pulmonary angiitis and granulomatosis. Ann Rev Respir Dis 108:1–18, 1973
Elper GR: Bronchiolitis obliterans; and Lynch JP, Fantone JC: Other pulmonary granulomatous vasculitic syndromes. In Lynch JP, De Remee RA: Immunologically Mediated Pulmonary Diseases, pp 156, 307. Philadelphia, JB Lippincott, 1991

BRONCHOCENTRIC GRANULOMATOSIS

Synonym. BCG, see allergic bronchopulmonary aspergillosis.

Symptoms and Signs. In adults, fever, cough, malaise, dyspnea, wheezing. In 75% history of asthma from birth. In some cases sinusitis, skin rash, glomerulonephritis.

Etiology. Probably an histologic expression of allergic bronchopulmonary aspergillosis or hypersensitivity response to infectious granulomatous processes such as TB, echinococcus, histoplasmosis, coccidioidomycosis, rheumathoid arthritis.

Pathology. *Biopsy.* Infiltration of bronchiolar walls by inflammatory cells, bronchial lumen filled with necrotic exudate. Granulomatoid inflammation of bronchiolar mucosa. Extensive necrosis. Aspergillus hyphae sometimes visible.

Diagnostic Procedures. *Chest X-ray.* Patchy pulmonary infiltrates, segmental or lobar atelectasia. *Blood.* Eosinophilia. Culture for aspergillus and other fungi.

Therapy. That of underlying condition. Corticosteroids.

Prognosis. Good; tied to resolution of underlying disease.

BIBLIOGRAPHY. Liebow AA: Pulmonary angiitis and granulomatosis. Ann Rev Respir Dis 108:1–18, 1973
Lynch JP, Fantone JC: Other pulmonary granulomatous vasculitic syndromes. In Lynch JP, De Remee RA: Immunologically Mediated Pulmonary Diseases, p 307. Philadelphia, JB Lippincott, 1991

BRONZE BABY

Symptoms and Signs. In infants. Brown-gray coloration of the skin following phototherapy.

Etiology. Phototherapy inducing bilirubin changes: formation of photoproduct and copper products.

Diagnostic Procedures. *Blood.* Hyperbilirubinemia. Liver echography. *Urine.* Typical brown-gray color. Hyperbilirubinuria.

Therapy. Discontinuation of phototherapy.

Prognosis. Discoloration reversible unless presence of liver disease.

BIBLIOGRAPHY. Kopelman AE, Brown RS, Odell GB: The bronze baby syndrome: a complication of phototherapy. J Pediatr 81:466–472, 1972
Rubaltelli FF, Jori G, Reddi E: Bronze baby syndrome: a new porphyrine-related disorder. Pediatr Res 17:327–330, 1983
Purcell SM, Wians FH, Ackerman NB, et al: Hyperbilirubinemia in bronze baby syndrome. J Am Acad Dermatol 16:172–177, 1987

BROOKS

Synonyms. Immunodeficiency-6; IMD6; severe combined immunodeficiency disease, X-linked 2; SCIDX2.

Symptoms and Signs. In males. Age of patients ranges from 2.5–34 years. Recurrent infections: sinusitis, otitis, respiratory disorders; varicella (severe), papilloma virus infections.

Etiology. X-linked inheritance.

Pathology. Scarceness of lymphoid tissues.

Diagnostic Procedures. *Blood.* Normal concentration of immunoglobulins, restricted formation of IgG antibodies to immunogens; normal number of B- and NK-cells, decreased number of CD4 (+), CD8 (+) T-lymphocytes, decreased proliferative response of blood B-cells to allogenic cells, mitogens, and antigens.

Therapy. If needed specific gammaglobulins.

Prognosis. Fair span of survival time. Some cases have reproduced unaffected males and carrier females.

BIBLIOGRAPHY. Brooks EG, Schmaltieg FC, Wirt DP, et al: A novel X-linked combined immunodeficiency disease. J Clin Invest 86:1623–1631, 1990

BROSSARD

Obsolete.

Synonyms. Scapulo, distal.

Symptoms and Signs. Onset after first decade. Atrophy and weakness of small foot and calf muscles, and of adductors and recti abdominis, and then of shoulder muscles. Fasciculation, but no signs of reaction or degeneration.

Etiology. Unknown.

BIBLIOGRAPHY. Brossard J: Etude clinique sur un forme héréditaire d'atrophie musculaire progressive débutant par les membres inférieur (type fémoral avec griffe des orteils), p 174. Paris, Steiheil, 1886
Kaeser HE: Scapulo-peroneal syndromes. In Vinken PJ, Bruyn GW: Handbook of Clinical Neurology, vol 22, p 63. Amsterdam, North-Holland, 1975

BROWN

Synonyms. Superior oblique tendon sheath; tendon sheath adherence.

Symptoms. Both sexes affected; present from birth. Congenital strabismus; bilateral ptosis; backward head tilt. Palpebral fissure may widen when attempting upward gaze. Adduction and abduction restricted or abolished. Associated choroidal coloboma.

Etiology. Drug and toxins. Retrobulbar injection of anesthetics.

Pathology. Shortening of sheath of superior oblique muscle and attachment to the troclea. Decreased elasticity of conjunctiva.

Therapy. Surgery.

BIBLIOGRAPHY. Brown HW: Congenital structural motor anomalies. In Allen JH (ed): Strabismus. Ophthalmic Symposium. St Louis, CV Mosby, 1950
Goldhammer J, Smith JL: Acquired intermittent Brown's syndrome. Neurology 24:666–668, 1974
Crawford JS: Surgical treatment of true Brown's syndrome. Am J Ophthal 81:289–295, 1976
Sprague Eustis H, O'Reilly C, Crawford JS: Management of superior oblique palsy after surgery for true Brown's syndrome. J Pediatr Ophthalmol Strabismus 24:10–16, 1987
Erie JC: Acquired Brown's syndrome after peribulbar anesthesia. Am J Ophthalmol 109:349–330, 1990

BROWN BOWEL

Synonyms. Vitamin E deficiency; malabsorption vitamin E; BBS; tocoferol deficiency.

Symptoms and Signs. In patients with malabsorption syndromes and steathorrhea; intestinal pseudobstruction; diverticolosis; GI bleeding; impairment of smooth muscle function at surgical intervention; obstruction of brown intestinal wall.

Etiology. Vitamin E deficiency owing to malabsorption syndromes as causing deposition of lipofuscin in the tunica muscolaris. Possible smooth muscle mithocondrial myopathy.

Pathology. Brown pigmentation of intestinal wall. Lipofuscin accumulation.

Diagnostic Procedures. Evaluation of presence of celiac sprue chronic pancreatitis and degree of malabsorption. *Blood.* Decreased vitamin E.

Therapy. Vitamin E partially useful in early stage of disease. Possible prevention of gastrointestinal carcinoma.

Prognosis. High frequency of gastrointestinal adenocarcinomas (colon), pseudobstruction, GI bleeding.

BIBLIOGRAPHY. Foster CS: The brown bowel syndrome. A possible smooth muscle mitochondrial myopathy. Histopathology 3:1–17, 1979
Horn T, Svendsen LB, Nielsen R: Brown bowel syndrome: review of the literature and presentation of cases. Scand J Gastroenterol 25:66–72, 1990
Reynaert H, Debeuckelaerte S, DeWaele B, et al: The brown bowel syndrome and gastrointestinal adenocarconoma. J Clin Gastroenterol 16:48–51, 1993

BROWN OCULOCUTANEOUS ALBINISM

Synonym. Albinism ocolocutaneous, Brown type.

Symptoms and Signs. In Africans and New Guineans. Recently descibed in Caucasians. Medium brown hair, light brown skin, hazel eyes; iris translucency ++ to ++++; moderate, persistent for life nystagmus, photophobia; visual acuity 20/60 to 20/200; pigmented nevi or freckles absent; pachidermia and keratoses.

Etiology. Autosomal recessive. Defect of pigment accumulation. Gene location chromosome 9p (?).

Pathology. Hair bulbs. Melanosomes in all stages but slight pigment accumulation.

Diagnostic Procedures. *Ophthalmoscopy.* Light retinal pigmentation. Incubation of hair bulb. Low tyrosine incorporation.

Therapy. None.

Prognosis. Low accumulation of pigment with age.

BIBLIOGRAPHY. King RA, Creel D, Cervanka J, et al: Albinism in Nigeria with delineation of new recessive oculocutaneous type. Clin Genet 17:259–262, 1980
King RA, Hearing VJ, Creel DJ, et al: Albinism. In Scriver CR, Beaudet AL, Sly WS, et al: The Metabolic and Molecular Bases of Inherited Disease, 7th ed, p 4376. New York, McGraw-Hill, 1995

BROWN RECLUSE SPIDER BITE

Synonyms. Arachnidism; araneism; Loxosceles reclusa.

Symptoms. Stinging sensation, not too painful; pain follows within 2–8 hours accompanied by nausea, arthralgia, abdominal cramps, and fever, vomiting, delirium.

Signs. Blister on the skin with surrounding area of hemorrhage, which subsequently ulcerates and may become gangrenous. Occasionally, morbilliform, petechial rash appearing within 24–48 hours of bite.

Etiology. Venom from bite by a spider (brown recluse; fiddler spider; Loxosceles reclusa) native to the central and southern states of the United States.

Pathology. Ischemic hemorrhagic necrosis from one to several centimeters in diameter. Dermoepidermal separation, clots occluding small arterioles; moderate inflammatory infiltrate.

Diagnostic Procedures. *Blood.* May show hemolytic anemia and thrombocytopenia, especially in children; leukocytosis. *Urine.* Proteinuria; hemoglobinuria.

Therapy. Corticosteroids (prompt administration) good to prevent necrosis and systemic effect of venom. Skin graft for large lesion, poor take.

Prognosis. In children (if not treated), severe. Death may follow. Healing time of lesion proportional to size.

BIBLIOGRAPHY. Atkins JA, Wingo CW, Sodeman WA: Probable cause of necrotic spider bite in midwest. Science 126:73, 1957
Dillaha CJ, Jansen GT, Honeycutt WM, et al: North American loxoscelism: necrotic bite of the brown recluse spider. JAMA 188:33–36, 1964
Burns DA: Diseases caused by arthropods and other noxious animals. In Champion RH, Burton JL, Ebling FJG (eds): Rook/Wilkinson/Ebling Textbook of Dermatology, 5th ed, pp 2849–2854. Oxford, Blackwell Scientific, 1992

BROWN-SEQUARD

Synonyms. Hemiparaplegic; spastic spinal monoplegia.

Symptoms. Unilateral paralysis of voluntary motion below the level of lesion; segmental atrophy and sensory loss at the level of lesion; contralateral analgesia and thermanesthesia few segments below the lesion; sphincteral disturbances.

Signs. At the side of lesion, increase in muscle tone; increase in deep reflexes; clonus and Babinski sign.

Etiology. Lesion of one lateral half of spinal cord. Hemisection from wound; localized pressure from vertebral, meningeal, neoplastic, degenerative, infectious diseases. Pure forms are rare; lesions can spare part of the one half or extend to other side.

Pathology. Depends upon etiology.

Diagnostic Procedures. *Cerebrospinal fluid.* Increase in protein. *X-ray. CT scan. MRI.*

Therapy. In case of trauma, avoid manipulation and use care in transporting of patient. Avoid overdistension of bladder and prevent infection. General hygienic care of patient, avoiding soiling and decubitus ulcers; fluid intake and metabolic status care. Early activity to avoid osteoporosis and hypercalcemia. Surgery if indicated.

Prognosis. Quoad vitam good with proper care. In case of compression or partial lesion, good degree of functional recovery.

BIBLIOGRAPHY. Dundas R: Case of concussion of the spine, tending to confirm the opinion that nerves of sensation and of motion are distinct. Edinburgh Med Surg J 23:304, 1825
Brown-Sequard CE: De la transmission croisée del impression sentitives par la moelle épinière. C R Soc Biol (Paris) 2:33–34, 1851
Koehler PJ, Endtz LJ: The Brown Sequard syndrome. True or false? Arch Neurol 43:921–924, 1986
Adams RD, Victor M: Principles of Neurology, 5th ed, p 143. New York, McGraw-Hill, 1993

BROWN-VIALETTO-VAN LAERE

Synonyms. Bulbar palsy—perceptive deafness; pontobulbar palsy—deafness.

Symptoms and Signs. Most cases female. Onset in childhood. Irregularly progressive. Multiple cranial nerves (usually VII, IX, X, XI, XII; seldom III, V, VI) and spinal nerve palsies. Producing clumsiness and weakness of arms, shaking, sleepiness, shortness of breath, speech and swallowing difficulties.

Etiology. Genetically heterogeneous with autosomal recessive or dominant inheritance or alternatively caused by a mutant gene on chromosome X.

Therapy. Treatment with steroid produces temporary improvement.

Prognosis. Progessive condition with respiratory function deterioration as cause of death.

BIBLIOGRAPHY. Brown CH: Infantile amyotrophic lateral sclerosis of the family type. J Nerve Ment Dis 21:707–716, 1894
Vialetto E: Contributo alla forma ereditaria della paralisi bulbare progressiva. Riv Sper Freniatr 40:1–24, 1936
Van Laere J: Paralysie bulbo-pontine chronique progressive familial avec surdité: un cas de syndrome de Klippel-Trenaunay de la même fatric (problems diagnostiques et genetiques). Rev Neurol 115:289–295, 1966
Hawkins SA, Nevin NC, Harding AE: Pontobulbar palsy and neurosensory deafnass (Brown-Vialetto-Van Laere syndrome) with possible autosomal dominant inheritance. J Med Genet 27:176–179, 1990

BRUCK

Synonyms. Osteogenesis imperfecta-joint contractures.

Symptoms and Signs. Both sexes. Onset during embriologic development (seventh week on). At birth features of arthrigryposis multiplex aggravated in early infancy by minor traumas; sclerae and teeth normal.

Etiology. Autosomal recessive inheritance.

Diagnostic Procedures. *Echography. X-ray.* Wormian bones.

Therapy. Symptomatic.

Prognosis. Severe physical impairment.

BIBLIOGRAPHY. Bruck A: Ueber eine seltene Form von Erkrankung der Knochen und Gelenke. Dtsch Med Wchnschr 23:152–155, 1897
Viljoen D, Versfeld G, Beighton P: Osteogenesis imperfecta with congenital joint contractures (Bruck syndrome). Clin Genet 36:122–126, 1989

BRUCK-DE LANGE

Synonyms. Cornelia De Lange II; De Lange II; extrapyramidal-muscular hypertrophy; Lange II; mental deficiency–muscular hypertrophy; muscular hypertrophy, cerebral.

Symptoms and Signs. Present from birth. All muscles, or only selected muscle groups, larger and firmer than normal (athletic look). Head may be small and deformed. Muscle rigidity (extrapyramidal type); tendon reflexes normal. Mental deficiency.

Etiology. Possibly autosomal recessive inheritance.

Pathology. *Brain.* Numerous cavities in white matter, thalami, microgyria, and polygyria.

Diagnostic Procedures. *X-rays of skull. Electroencephalography. CT brain scan. MRI. Serum enzymes. Electromyography.*

Therapy. None.

Prognosis. Poor; all patients died within a few months.

BIBLIOGRAPHY. Bruck F: Ueber einen Fall von congenitaler Makroglossie, combiniert mit allgemeiner wahrer Muskelhypertrophie und Idiotie. Dtsch Med Wochenschr 15:229–232, 1889
De Lange C: Congenital hypertrophy of muscles, extrapyramidal motor disturbances and mental deficiency. Am J Dis Child 48:243–268, 1934
Wharton BA: An unusual variety of muscular dystrophy. Lancet I, 248–249, 1965
Adams RD, Victor M: Principles of Neurology, 5th ed, pp 1194, 1278. New York, McGraw-Hill, 1993

BRUEGHEL

Synonyms. Meige; Lingual-facial-oromandibular spasms. See Buccolingual masticatory.

Symptoms and Signs. More frequent in women. Onset usually in the sixth decade. Forceful opening of mouth, lip retraction, spasm of platisma, and tongue protrusion; or clamped jaw and pursed lips. Spastic or spasmodic. Dysphonia and blepharospasm, torticollis, trunk, and/or limbs dystonia variably associated.

Etiology and Pathology. Not clearly assessed. Neuroleptics may induce similar manifestations (see Buccolingul masticatory). In one instance reported foci of neuron loss in the stratum.

Therapy. Many drugs used with constantly poor results. Some success with injections of botulin toxin in affected muscles.

BIBLIOGRAPHY. Jankovic J, Ford J: Blepharospasm and orofacial-cervical dystonia: Clinical and pharmacological findings in 100 patients. Ann Neurol 13:402–411, 1983
Denislic M, Pirtosek Z, Vodusek DB, et al: Botulinum toxin in the treatment of neurological disorders. In Soput D, Zorec R: Toxin and exocytosis. Ann NY Acad Sci 710:76–87, 1994

BRUNAUER

Synonyms. Brauer-Brunauer-Fuhs; Fuhs; keratoderma palmoplantaris dissipatum; palmoplatar keratoderma punctate; included Buschke-Fischer (keratoderma palmoplantaris maculosa disseminata).

Symptoms and Signs. Various patterns. Both sexes. Onset second or third decade. Diffuse punctate thickening of palms and soles and islands of keratoderma at pressure points. Occasionally associated corneal opacities, pili torti, sensorineural hearing loss, hypohidrosis, dental abnormalities.

Etiology. Autosomal dominant inheritance and sporadic.

Therapy. Trials with retinoic acid.

Prognosis. Benign condition.

BIBLIOGRAPHY. Brunauer SR: Zur Symptomatologie und Histologie der kongenitalen Dyskeratosen. Dermatol Z 42:6–26, 1925
Fuhs H: Uber das seltene Syndrom von kongenitalen Keratosen an Haut und Kornea. Dermatol Z 53:538–542, 1928
Griffiths WAD, Leigh IM, Marks R: Disorders of Keratinization. In Champion RH, Burton JL, Ebling FJG (eds): Rook/Wilkinson/Ebling Textbook of Dermatology, 5th ed, p 1371. Oxford, Blackwell Scientific, 1992

BRUNS

Synonym. Postural change; vertigo Bruns.

Symptoms. Sudden development of attacks of vertigo, headache, and vomiting on change of posture of head (extension more than flexion). Freedom from symptoms between attacks. Amaurosis; flashes of light; irregular breathing; occasionally, syncope with apnea.

Signs. Constant anterior flexion of head at midline or with lateral flexion. Neck muscles firmly contracted. Tachycardia.

Etiology. Organic lesion of fourth ventricle or adjacent structures. Tumor, cysticercosis, colloid cyst. Obstruction of flow of cerebrospinal fluid or disturbance of vestibular mechanism or both.

Pathology. See Etiology.

Diagnostic Procedures. *X-ray. CT scan. MRI of skull. Angiography. EEG. Spinal tap* (with caution).

Therapy. Neurosurgery if feasible.

Prognosis. Depends on etiology.

BIBLIOGRAPHY. Bruns O: Neuropathologische Demonstrationen. Neurol Centrabl 21:561–567, 1902
Brandt T: Vertigo: Its Multisensory Syndromes. London, Springer-Verlag, 1991

BRUSA-TORRICELLI

Synonyms. Miller; aniridia—Wilms tumor; AGR triad; del 11p; chromosome 11p deletion; including Wilms tumor—aniridia—gonadoblastoma—mental retardation; WAGR. See also Beckwith-Wiedemann; Klippel-Trénaunay.

Symptoms and Signs. Advanced maternal age. Both sexes affected; more frequent in males. Congenital sporadic aniridia (see). Nephroblastoma, which develops before the age of 3 years. Associated frequently: cataract and glaucoma; mental retardation; microcephaly; growth retardation, genitourinary anomalies (hypospadias, cryptorchidism); external ear malformation; Seldom; facial dysmorphism; umbilical and inguinal hernias.

Etiology. Unknown. Aniridia generically sporadic (with rare exception). Wilms tumor (40% congenital; 60% sporadic). The association is probably genetic, of autosomal dominant type or dependent from chromosomal deletion (11, p 13). Environmental factors cannot be excluded in initiating germinal and the postzygotic mutations.

Pathology. See Aniridia. Nephroblastoma. Cells and tissue suggesting abortive renal elements of mesodermal origin.

Diagnostic Procedures. See Aniridia. *X-rays of abdomen. Retrograde pyelogram. Kidney scan. Ultrasonography. CT scan. MRI.*

Therapy. Surgery. Chemotherapy.

Prognosis. Poor. Ninety percent survival rate with surgery. Chemotherapy and roentgentherapy.

BIBLIOGRAPHY. Brusa P, Torricelli C: Nefroblastoma di Wilms ed affezioni renali congenite nelle casistiche dell' IIPAI di Milano. Minerva Pediatr 5:457–463, 1953
Miller RW, Fraumeni JF, Manning MD: Association of Wilm's tumor with aniridia, hemihypertrophy and other congenital malformation. New Engl J Med 270:922–927, 1964
François J, Concke D, Coppieters R: Aniridia-Wilm's tumor syndrome. Ophthalmologica 174:35–39, 1977
Nelson LB, Spaeth GL, Nowinski TS, et al: Aniridia: A Review. Sur Ophthalmol 28:621–642, 1984
Mannens M, Bleeker-Wagemaker EM, Bliek J, et al: Autosomal dominant aniridia linked to the chromosome 11 pm13 markers catalase and 11S 151 in a large Dutch family. Cytogenet Cell Genet 52:32–36, 1989
Haber DA, Housman DE: Wilms tumor. In Scriver CR, Beaudet AL, Sly WS, et al: The Metabolic and Molecular Bases of Inherited Disease, 7th ed, pp 668–670. New York, McGraw-Hill, 1995

BRUSHFIELD-WYATT

Symptoms and Signs. Trigeminal port wine lesion with calcified angioma in cerebral hemisphere. See Wyburn-Mason.

BIBLIOGRAPHY. Brushfield T, Wyatt W: Hemiplegie associated with extensive naevus and mental defect. Br J Child Dis 24:98–106, 1927
Brinton BD: Brushfield-Wyatt syndrome. Proc R Soc Med 26:846–847, 1933

BRUTON

Synonyms. Immunodeficiency I; sex-linked agammaglobulinemia; XLA; X-linked agammaglobulinemia; hypogammaglobulinemia X-linked.

Symptoms and Signs. Appears only in males; healthy up to 5–12 months of age, then onset of severe infections. In about 50% rheumatoid arthritis-like manifestation (large joints) scleroderma diffuse vasculituis. High frequency of atopic eczema; poisoning; allergic rhinitis; asthenia; in few cases chronic diarrhea and malabsorption. Paucity of palpable lymph nodes, digital clubbing; growth retardation.

Etiology. Unknown; sex-linked recessive inheritance. Gene for XLA mapped to the long arm of X chromosome (q21.3–22).

Pathology. Thymus normal; plasma cells absent; lack of germinal centers and poorly developed crypts of tonsils and of appendix, absence of Peyer's patches. Lymph node architecture: absence of germinal centers and poorly developed follicles.

Diagnostic Procedures. *Blood.* Complete absence of all types of immunoglobulin; normal cellular immunity. Absence of antibody responses even to the strongest antigens.

Therapy. Antibiotic and gammaglobulin (monthly intervals).

Prognosis. Death delayed by treatment, but inevitable in late infancy, early childhood usually by pulmonary infection.

BIBLIOGRAPHY. Bruton OC: Agammaglobulinemia. Pediatrics 9:722–728, 1952

Lederman HM, Winkelstein JA: X-linked agammaglobulinemia: an analysis of 96 patients. Medicine 64:145–156, 1985

Schuurman RKB, Mensinnk EJBM, Sandkuyl LA, et al: Early diagnosis in X-linked agammaglobulinaemia. Europ J Pediat 147:93–95, 1988

Lukens JN: Immune deficiency diseases: Inherited and acquired. In Lee GR, Bithel TC, Foerster J, et al (eds): Wintrobe's Clinical Hematology, 9th ed, pp 1677–1678. Philadelphia, Lea & Febiger, 1993

BRUYN-WENT

Synonyms. Leber-spastic paraplegia; spastic paraplegia-Leber.

Symptoms and Signs. In infancy spastic paraplegia first in the legs then in the arms; athetosis, dysarthria, dystonic position of hands. In adolescence progressive loss of vision (optic atrophy appears to conform to all diagnostic criteria of Leber-see).

Etiology. Unknown. Sex-linked inheritance.

Prognosis. Progression of various symptoms leads the patient to walk on hands and knees, athetosis on every movement.

BIBLIOGRAPHY. Bruyn GW, Went LN: A sex-linked heterodegenerative neurological disorder associated with Lebers's optic atrophy. Part I. Clinical studies. J Neurol Sci 1:59–80, 1964

Gilman S, Romanul FCA: Hereditary dystonic paraplegia with amyotrophy and mental deficiency clinical and neuropathological characteristics. In Vinken PJ, Bruyn GW (eds): Handbook of Clinical Neurology, vol 22, p 454. Amsterdam, North-Holland, 1975

BUCCOLINGUAL MASTICATORY

Synonyms. Tardive dyskinesia; orofacial dyskinesia, including Rabbit syndrome. See also Brueghel.

Symptoms and Signs. In patients (0.5–40%) assuming neuroleptics from youth. Stereotyped involuntary tongue protrusion, lip smacking, puckering, and chewing. Can be associated with chorea, athetosis, dystonia, myoclonus, tics, and facial grimacing, or perioral tremor (Rabbit Syndrome). Movements are accentuated in stress and disappear during sleep.

Etiology. Extrapyramidal effects of neuroleptics. Dopamine receptor hypersensitivity.

Therapy. Withdrawal of neuroleptic.

Prognosis. Variable. Slow remission of signs or permanent tardive dyskinesia.

BIBLIOGRAPHY. Jeste D, Plotking SG, Sinha S, et al: Tardive dyskinesia: reversible and persistent. Arch Gen Psychiatr 36:585–590, 1979

Burke RE: Tardive dyskinesia: current clinical issue. Neurology 34:1348–1353, 1984

Adams RD, Victor M: Principles of Neurology, 5th ed, p 935. New York, McGraw-Hill, 1993

BUCHANAN

Synonym. Truncus arteriosus.

Symptoms. Slight male predominance; onset in first week of life or early infancy. Dyspnea; recurrent respiratory infections; failure to thrive.

Signs. Normal birth weight. Cyanosis or dusky hue on crying or during efforts (nonconstant). Murmur (becomes evident with onset of symptomatology) harsh, systolic, at the base and left sternal edge; over upper sternum continuous bruit; clear and loud second sound; thrill maximal over base.

Etiology. Congential heart malformation, possibly viral etiology; some familial cases reported.

Pathology. Unique great artery originating from the base of the heart and providing the systemic, pulmonary, and coronary circulation. Three varieties distinguished: (1) undivided aorta and pulmonary trunk with a single valve; (2) aortic trunk without pulmonary valve, main pulmonary artery, or branches; (3) undivided aorta and pulmonary trunk with two normal semilunar valves.

Diagnostic Procedures. *Blood.* Polycythemia. *Electrocardiography.* Right axis deviation. *X-rays.* Cardiomegaly; concave shadow at left of sternum; absence of pulmonary conus; increase in pulmonary vascularization. *Angiography.* See Pathology. *Catheterization.* Shunt at aortic, pulmonary areas. Two-dimensional echocardiography with color flow and Doppler interrogation.

Therapy. Surgical correction.

Prognosis. Mortality 25%. Average survival poor when large pulmonary arterial branches originate from short main pulmonary artery. Longevity if pulmonary arteries are small. If pulmonary circulation regulated, occasionally, survival into third or fourth decade.

BIBLIOGRAPHY. Buchanan G: Malformation of the heart; undivided truncus arteriosus; heart otherwise troubled. Trans Pathol Soc Lond 15:89–91, 1864

Ebert PA: Truncus arteriosus. In Glenn WL, Banc AE, Geha AS, et al: Thoracic and Cariovascular Surgery, p 785. Norwalk, CT, Appleton-Century-Crofts, 1983

Perloff JK: The Clinical Recognition of Congenital Heart Disease, 4th ed, pp 686–702. Philadelphia, WB Saunders, 1994

BUCKEY

Synonym. Hyperimmunoglobulinemia E. See Job.

Symptoms. From birth. Initially vesicular eczema then non specific excoriated, papular, and pustular eruption with prevalent staphylococcal infections and skin abscesses that favors scalp and proximal flexures. Respiratory distress. Bronchopneumopathies, lung abscesses, and empiemas. Suppurating lymphoadenopathies. Growth failure. Occasionally osteoporosis and fractures. Seldom asthma and allergic rhinitis.

Etiology. Unknown.

Pathology. Pulmonary abscesses. Mycotic or staphyloccocal.

Diagnostic Procedures. *Blood.* IgE over 5000 Ul/ml. Eosinophilia. Neutrophils increased. Polynucleates: defect of chemotaxis.

Therapy. Antibiotics. Antimycotics. Cimetidine.

Prognosis. Poor. Repeated infections.

BIBLIOGRAPHY. Buckley RH, Wrag BB, Belmaker EZ: Extreme hyperimmunoglobulinemia E and undue susceptibility to infections. Pediatrics 49:59–70, 1972

Buckey RH, Sampsom HA: The hyperimmunoglobulinemia E syndrome. In Franklin EC (ed): Clinical Immunology Update, pp 147–162. Edinburgh, Churchill Livingston, 1981

Anderson DC, Kishimoto TK, Smith CW: Leukocyte adhesion deficiency and other disorders of leukocyte adherence and motility. In Scriver CR, Beaudet AL, Sly WS, et al: The Metabolic and Molecular Bases of Inherited Disease, 7th ed, pp 3981–3982. New York, McGraw-Hill, 1995

BUCKLED INNOMINATE ARTERY

Synonyms. Innominate artery kinking; kinked innominate artery; innominate artery buckling.

Symptoms. Occurs usually in middle-aged, obese women with hypertension. Painless; occasionally intermittent swelling on left side of neck. Swelling and gurgling sensation in the left side of neck occasionally also are observed.

Etiology. Buckling of innominate artery that compresses the left innominate vein against sternum.

Pathology. Loss of elasticity of artery, and buckling of innominate artery.

Diagnostic Procedures. *Angiography.* To differentiate from arteriovenous fistula, cervical pseudoaneurysm, superior vena cava syndrome, subclavian, and axillary vein thrombosis. *Ultrasound techniques and arteriography employing digital subtraction imaging.*

Therapy. Surgery not necessary.

Prognosis. Good.

BIBLIOGRAPHY. Smith KS: The kinked innominate vein. Br Heart J 22:110–116, 1960

Coppola ED, Seller R: Isolated distention of the left external jugular vein: a clinical sign of the syndrome of the buckled innominate artery. Ann Surg 167:586–589, 1968

BUDD-CHIARI

Synonyms. Chiari II: Rokitansky; von Rokitansky I; hepatic vein thrombosis; liver veins occlusion; hepatic veins thrombosis.

Symptoms. More common in males. *Acute.* Sudden abdominal epigastric pain with nausea and vomiting. *Chronic.* Gradual and intermittent symptomatology and signs.

Signs. Progessive tender hepatomegaly; ascites; edema of legs; abdominal collateral vein distention; mild splenomegaly. Occasionally jaundice and hemorrhages from esophageal varices.

Etiology. Acute or chronic obstruction of major hepatic veins by thrombus or tumor or myeloproliferative disorders. Reported also after taking oral contraceptives, aflatoxin, azathioprine, carmustine, doxorubicin, 6-mercaptopurine, 6-thioguanine, vincristine, pyrrolizidine alkaloid, and after liver transplantation. Role of congenital malformation discussed. In two-thirds of patients, etiology unknown.

Pathology. Hepatomegaly; smooth, cirrhotic liver; with irregular fatty degeneration; centrilobular atrophy, hepatic veins closed; ascites; congestive splenomegaly.

Diagnostic Procedures. *Liver function tests.* Moderate increase of bilirubin; alkaline phosphates high. *Biopsy of liver. Portal pressure measurement. Isotope liver scan. Arteriography and venography.* Selective. *Ultrasonography.* Thickened walls of hepatic veins stenosis. Proximal dilatation. Thrombosis. Doppler slow flow and identification of obstruction. *CT scan. MR imaging.*

Therapy. Surgery when indicated. Fibrinolytic agents, anticoagulants, diuretics. Peritoneovenous shunt. Liver transplantation when indicated.

Prognosis. Acute. Death possibly in few days. Chronic. Survivial for months, possibly years.

BIBLIOGRAPHY. Budd G: On Disease of the Liver, p 143. London, JA Churchill, 1845

Chiari H: Ueber die selbstandige Phlebitis obliterans der Haupstaemme der Venae hepaticae als Todesurache. Beitr Pathol Anat (Jeune) 26:1–17, 1899

Selzer G, Parker RGF: Senecio poisoning exhibiting as Chiari's syndrome: a report of 12 cases. Am J Pathol 27:885–907, 1951

Murphy FB, Steinberg HV, Shires GT III, et al: The Budd-Chiari syndrome: a review. AJR 147:9–25, 1986

Schwartz ME, Miller CM: Diseases of the hepatic blood vessels. In Schaffner F: Nonalcoholic fatty liver. In Haubrich WS, Schaffner F,

Berk JE (eds): Bockus Gastroenterology, 5th ed, pp 2387–2390. Philadelphia, WB Saunders, 1995

BUERGER

Synonyms. Winiwarter-Manteuffel-Buerger; Von Winiwarter-Buerger; Billroth-Von Winiwarter; endarteritis obliterans; presenile gangrene; thromboangiitis obliterans.

Symptoms. Occurs almost exclusively in males; larger incidence at 28–50 years of age. Severe pain of extremities at rest (first symptom in four-fifths of cases), resembling that of intermittent claudication, which usually causes insomnia. Vasomotor manifestations frequent: cold sensation at extremities; cold hypersensibility; sudden sweating; dyshidrosis, occasionally, Raynaud phenomenon (see).

Signs. At onset, discrepancy between intensity of symptoms and scarce physical signs; occasionally, however, these signs may represent the first manifestation: trophic changes, ulcerations, and gangrene. It is interesting that the course is represented by progression and regression of signs. Frequent migratory phlebitis, preceding or accompanying arterial disease. Absence or decreased dorsal pedal or posterior dorsal pulse or both; normal proximal pulse.

Etiology. Unknown. Several hypothesis considered: (1) Tobacco intoxication; (2) cold; (3) malnutrition; (4) traumas (to be considered aggravating or favoring agents); (5) infections; (6) collagen disorder; (7) atherosclerosis.

Pathology. Nonsuppurative segmental perivascular reaction, which joins artery, vein, and nerve bundle and makes their separation difficult. High frequency of involvement of superficial veins; scarce involvement of deep veins. Segmental red thrombi; frequently, integrity of inner elastic wall; moderate interstitial fibrosis of the media; constantly present, adventitous sclerosis.

Diagnostic Procedures. *Blood.* Usually, normal value of glycemia and of lipidic pattern; frequently increased viscosity and platelet number. *X-rays.* Occasionally, osteoporosis and osteomyelitis of phalanges. *Angiography.* Site of lesion always distal, bilateral, but not symmetric; great arterial trunks normal; absence of image of arteriovenous shunts; reduction of arterial caliber. *Vasodilation tests. Vasospasm. Doppler.*

Therapy. Antibiotics (in case of positive direct or indirect demonstration of infections); fibrinolytic and anticlotting agents; cortisone or antiinflammatory agents or both; local treatment of infections and gangrene; analgesics. Surgery: sympathectomy; arterial reconstructive surgery may be attempted with uncertain results.

Prognosis. Little response to any kinds of treatment except occasionally to the tobacco abstinence, which may induce remission. Increased incidence of myocardial infarction.

BIBLIOGRAPHY. Von Winiwarter F: Ueber eine eigentumliche Form Endocarditis und Endophlebitis mit Gangran des Fusses. Arch Klin Berlin 23:202–226, 1879

Buerger L: Thromboangitis obliterans: A study of the vascular lesions leading to presenile spontaneous gangrene. Ann J Med Soc 136:567–580, 1908

Joyce JW: The diagnosis and management of diseases of the peripheral arteries and veins. In Schlant RC, Alexander RW: Hurst's The Heart, 8th ed, p 2186. New York, McGraw-Hill, 1994

BUERGER-GRUETZ

Synonyms. Familial lipoprotein lipase deficiency; lipoprotein lipase deficiency, lipoid hepatosplenomegalia; hyperlipemia essential; fat-induced hyperlipemia; hyperchylomicronemia familial; hyperlipoproteinemia type I; LPL.

Symptoms. Rare. Both sexes equally affected; age of detection usually early childhood; onset as soon as child begins intake of fat. Attacks of colicky abdominal pain (it may simulate acute abdomen); pain is avoided by eliminating ingestion of fatty foods; failure to thrive; malaise and anorexia; no nausea or vomiting. Fever may occur with attacks.

Signs. Appearance of xanthomas (50%) of eruptive type at any site including mucous membranes–yellow nodules on erythematous base. Fading and completely disappearing in a few weeks. Signs of peritoneal irritation. Hepatosplenomegaly, tenderness in splenic region. Lipemia retinalis. Heterozygotes only have recurrent acute pancreatitis episodes.

Etiology. Autosomal recessive inheritance. Structural defects in LPL gene. Absence (homozygotes) or decreased activity (heterozygotes) of lipoprotein lipase that clears chylomicrons from plasma.

Pathology. Skin xanthomas; foam cells found in all tissues rich in reticulum cells (e.g., bone marrow; spleen; liver). Evidence of repeated pancreatitis.

Diagnostic Procedures. *Blood.* Characteristic aspect (white-cap top; clear below) of plasma when blood left at 4°C. Type I hyperlipoproteinemia. Very low-density lipoproteins (VLDL), low-density lipoproteins (LDL) (?), high-density lipoproteins (HDL) normal or decreased; cholesterol increased; tryglycerides increased. Attacks reproduced by ingestion of fat. Drop of triglycerides and clearing of plasma after 7 days of low-fat diet. Leukocytosis during attacks. Liver function test and glucose tolerance tests. Normal. Assay of LPI activity in plasma or adipose tissue.

Therapy. Decrease fat (animal and vegetable) intake to 20–25% of caloric intake. Glycerides of medium-chain fatty acids available to substitute for regular fat. Restriction of alcohol and some drugs as estrogens, diuretics, isotretinoin, and beta-adrenergic blocking agents.

Prognosis. This group of patients seems to be remarkably immune to atheromatous complications when compared with other types of hyperlipemia groups. Particular danger owing to repeated pancreatitis.

BIBLIOGRAPHY. Bürger M, Grütz O: Ueber hepatosplenomegale Lipoidose mit xanthomatoesen Veränderungen in Haut und Schleimhaeuten. Arch Dermatol Syph 166:542–575, 1932
Gaqne C, Brun LD, Julien P, et al: Primary lipoprotein lipase activity deficiency: clinical investigation of a French Canadian population. Can Med Assoc J 140:405–411, 1989
Schettler G, Habenicht AJR (eds): Principles and Treatment of Lipoprotein Disorders. New York, Springer, 1994
Brunzell JD: Familial lipoprotein lipase deficiency and other causes of chilomicronemia syndrome. In Scriver CR, Beaudet AL, Sly WS, et al: The Metabolic and Molecular Bases of Inherited Disease, 7th ed, pp 1919–1922. New York, McGraw-Hill, 1995

BULLDOG

Synonym. Simpson dysmorphia; Golabi-Rosen; Simpson-Golabi-Behmel; dysplasia gigantism, X-linked.

Symptoms. In males. *Facies.* Large protruding jaw, wide nasal bridge, upturned nose tip, macroglossia. *Limbs.* Broad, short hands and fingers. Broad stocky body. Cardiac arrhythmias major component (?) of the syndrome. Normal intelligence, or occasionally, mild mental retardation.

Etiology. Unknown. X-linked inheritance.

Prognosis. When patients reach adulthood (usual height above average), they lose some of the clumsiness and general distinguishing features become less apparent. Cardiac arrhythmias may be a cause of death.

BIBLIOGRAPHY. Simpson JL, New M, Laudey S, et al: A previously unrecognized X-linked syndrome of dysmorphia. Birth Defect Org Art Ser XI (2):18–24, 1973
Golabi M, Rosen L: A new X-linked mental retardation-overgrowth syndrome. Am J Med Genet 17:345–358, 1984

Behmel A, Plochl E, Rosenkranz W: A new X-linked dysplasia gigantism syndrome: identical with the Simpson dysplasia syndrome? Hum Genet 67:409–413, 1984
Konig R, Fuchs S, Kern C, et al: Simpson-Golabi-Behmel syndrome with severe cardiac arrhythmias. Am J Med Genet 38:244–247, 1991

BULL EYE RETINOPATHY

Synonyms. Phenothiazine retinopathy.

Symptoms and Signs. In patients receiving phenothiazine derivatives: blurred vision, difficulty in night vision and of colors and variable field defect. In these patients may be present as well corneal conjunctival lenticular and periocular abnormalities.

Etiology. Phenothiazine conjugates with melanin of pigment of retina causing its degeneration and the characteristic aspect of bull's eye.

Pathology. Individual RPE cells are larger than normal and contain increased amounts of lipofuscin, melanolysosomes, and curvilinear bodies.

Diagnostic Procedures. Fluorescine angiography. Electroretinogram.

Therapy. Modulate use of drug according to frequent ophthalmologic controls.

Prognosis. Damage is dose-related, but there is a return to normal when drug is discontinued.

BIBLIOGRAPHY. Potts AM: Uveal pigment and phenothiazine compounds. Trans Am Ophthal Soc 60:517–552, 1962
Scoggs MW, Klintworth GK: Drugs and toxins. In Garner A, Klintworth GK (eds): Pathobiology of Ocular Disease: A Dynamic Approach, 2nd ed, p 1173. New York, Marcel Dekker, 1994

BULLOSIS DIABETICORUM

Synonyms. Cope.

Symptoms and Signs. Rare complication in diabetes mellitus (50 cases reported). Bulbus lesions (clear or hemorrhagic fluid) localized on the legs (no trauma or exposure to sun). Absence of peripheral inflammatory changes. Nikolski's sign negative.

Etiology. Unknown. Not clear nosographic definition. Metabolic.

Pathology. Bulla with clear or hemorrhagic fluid intra- or subepidermic. Scarce dermic inflammatory infiltration (lymphomonocytes). Restitutio ad integrum or atrophic evolution.

Diagnostic Procedures. *Blood.* Diabetes mellitus. All other tests negative, including anti-nuclear and anti-DNA antibodies.

Therapy. Suction of fluid by aspiration.

Prognosis. Usually complete healing without scar or residual atrophic changes.

BIBLIOGRAPHY. Cope RL: Spontaneous bulla formation in the skin of diabetes mellitus. Ann Int Med 32:964–967, 1950
Alinovi A, Iorini M: La bullosis diabeticorum. Segnalazione di un caso clinico. Rec Prog Med 83:143–144, 1992

BUREAU-BARRIERE

Synonyms. Perforating foot ulcer acquired; sensory radicular neuropathy acquired. See Nelaton, Morvan, Trophic ulcer foot. Acropathy ulcero-mutilans nonfamilial.

Symptoms and Signs. Prevalent in males (almost exclusively); onset in adulthood. Usually in people with chronic malnutrition; frequently in alcoholics. Physical trauma to feet frequently contributory factor. Transient bullous lesion resulting in single or multiple perforating indolent ulcer of soles. Floor of ulcer granulating and crusting. Progressive deformity of foot with shortening and broadening to assume a cuboid shape. Cyanosis and hyperhidrosis of affected foot. Sensory changes: sock-like distribution, loss of temperature sensibility; touch and pain usually only partly affected. Deep sense preserved. Tendon and plantar reflexes normal.

Etiology. Peripheral trophic changes of nervous origin; protein deficiency; alcoholism.

Pathology. *Spinal cord.* Absence of syringomyelia. *Peripheral nerves.* Posterior roots and sciatic trunk degenerative changes.

Diagnostic Procedures. *X-ray of foot.* Early arthritis of interphalangeal or metatarsal phalangeal joint; later absorption of bone; partial dislocation. *Oscillometry. Arteriography. Blood.* Possible positivity of liver function test. *Spinal fluid.* Normal. *Nonpictorial tracer techniques, Doppler, thermography.*

Therapy. Protection from shearing forces: plaster cast or "Scotchcast Boot" (3M UK Ltd., Lughborough, Leicestershire, UK). Surgical intervention (increases deformity); sympathectomy; diet; vitamins.

Prognosis. Chronic course; increasing deformity, bouts of inflammation; elimination of bone sequestra. Good response to sympathectomy.

BIBLIOGRAPHY. Bureau Y, Barrière H: Aeropathies pseudo-syringo myélignes des membres inférieurs. Essai d'interprétation nosographique. Sem Hop Paris 31:1419–1429, 1955

Burden AC, Jones GR, Jones R, Blandford RL: Use of the "Scotchcast Boot" in treating diabetic foot ulcers. Br Med J 286:1555–1557, 1983

Savin JA: Skin and nervous system. In Eady RAJ: Prenatal diagnosis of skin disease. In Champion RH, Burton JL, Ebling FJG (eds): Rook/Wilkinson/Ebling Textbook of Dermatology, 5th ed, pp 2469–2470. Oxford, Blackwell Scientific, 1992

BURKA

Variant of Dubin-Johnson (see).

BIBLIOGRAPHY. Burka ER, Brick JB, Wolfe HR: "Lipochrome" hepatosis without jaundice. A variant of Dubin-Johnson syndrome. Am J Med Sci 242:746–749, 1961

BURKE (R.M.)

Synonyms. De Martini-Balestra; lobar lung atrophy; progressive pulmonary dystrophy. See also Vanishing lung syndromes.

Symptoms. Onset slow or rapid, and symptoms related to rapidity of progression. Cough; dyspnea; pain in the chest (if rapid evolution).

Signs. Reduction or absence of breath sound over involved areas. Wheezing; diaphragmatic depression.

Etiology. Formation or expansion of blebs or bullae in lungs. Various degree of obstruction causing pulmonary emphysema.

Pathology. Pulmonary emphysema; presence of blebs or bullae or both.

Diagnostic Procedures. *X-rays.* Considered a radiologic syndrome and represented by progressive decrease of pulmonary density, compression or fanning out of bronchi.

Therapy. If localized bullae, consider resection.

Prognosis. Generally poor.

BIBLIOGRAPHY. Burke RM: Vanishing lungs: a case reported of bullous emphysema. Radiology 28:367–371, 1937

Martini A de, Balestra G: Sindromi di rarefazione polmonare con particolare riguardo alla atrofia polmonare idiopatica. Minerva Med 2:917–926, 1951

Fraser RS, Parè JAP, Fraser RG Paré PD: Synopsis of Diseases of the Chest. Philadelphia, WB Saunders, 1994

BURKITT

Synonyms. African lymphoma; maxillary lymphosarcoma; nonleukemic lymphoma.

Symptoms and Signs. Slightly prevalent in males. Present in central equatorial Africa, cases reported from other non-African areas (United States, Colombia, India). Onset in infancy to adolescence. Tumor mass of jaw (approximately 50%), salivary glands, cervical lymph nodes, or abdomen. In Africa, facial bone involvement prevalent. (In other countries, abdominal tumors predominate.)

Etiology. It is not established if this syndrome represents a different pathologic entity from conventional lymphosarcoma. Causally related to Epstein-Barr virus (mechanism still unknown). Chromosomal alterations reported (8, 2, 14, 22).

Pathology. Jaw; liver; mostly visceral lymph nodes. Microscopically, lymphoblastic neoplastic cells and actively phagocyting histiocytes. Absence of leukemia. Criteria for classification of this form are: (1) histology as described; (2) clinical presentation and tumor localization similar to that reported for African cases.

Diagnostic Procedures. *Biopsy of tumor.* Bone marrow. *Blood.* Negative for leukemia. In Africans, levels of IgG increased and IgM decreased. In Americans, IgG normal or decreased and IgM normal.

Therapy. X-rays and antiblastic chemotherapeutic agents. Particularly responsive to cyclophosphamide alone or in combination (vincristine, methotrexate, and cytosine arabinoside).

Prognosis. More than 50% complete remission after first dose of cyclophosphamide. Dissemination does not exclude a good prognosis. Spontaneous remission also reported.

BIBLIOGRAPHY. Burkitt D: A sarcoma involving the jaws in African children. Br J Surg 46:218–223, 1958

Burkitt DP: The discovery of Burkitt's lymphoma. Cancer 51:1777–1786, 1983

Greer JP, Macon WR, List AF, et al: Non-Hodgkin's lymphomas. In Lee GR, Bithel TC, Foerster J, et al (eds): Wintrobe's Clinical Hematology, 9th ed, p 2084. Philadelphia, Lea & Febiger, 1993

BURNETT

Synonyms. Milk-alkali; milk drinker; milk poisoning.

Symptoms. Weakness; headache; dizziness; depression; nausea; vomiting; anorexia.

Signs. Conjunctivitis; ocular band keratitis; mental confusion or psychosis.

Etiology. Excessive intake of milk or soluble alkali as in therapy for peptic ulcer.

Pathology. Nephrocalcinosis; deposit of calcium in different tissues.

Diagnostic Procedures. *Blood.* Hypercalcemia; hyperazotemia; milk alkalosis; alkaline phosphatases normal or slightly elevated. *Urine.* Calcium and phosphates within normal ranges. *X-ray.* Nephrocalcinosis; calcification periarticular and in other tissues.

Therapy. Discontinuation of milk and alkali; intravenous administration of sodium chloride.

Prognosis. Recovery with treatment.

BIBLIOGRAPHY. Burnett C, Commons RR, Albright F, et al: Hypercalcemia without hypercalcuria or hypophosphatemia, calcinosis and renal in-

sufficiency: a syndrome following prolonged intake of milk and alkali. New Engl J Med 240:787–794, 1949
Cameron AJ, Spence MP: Chronic milk-alkali syndrome after prolonged excessive intake of antacid tablets. Br Med J 3:656–657, 1967
Pounder RE, Fraser AG: Diagnosis, medical management and complications. In Haubrich WS, Schaffner F, Berk JE (eds): Bockus Gastroenterology, 5th ed, p 764. Philadelphia, WB Saunders, 1995

BURNING HANDS

Symptoms. Burning dysesthesia and paresthesia in the hands.

Etiology. Attributed to concussion of spinal cord.

Diagnostic Procedures. *X-rays. CT scan. MRI of spine.* Evidence of trauma. Somatosensory evoked potentials: decrease of positive waves.

BIBLIOGRAPHY. Maroon JC: Burning hands in football spinal cord injuries. JAMA 238:2049–2051, 1977
Wilberger JE, Abla A, Maroon JC: Burning hands syndrome revisited. Neurosurgery 19:1038–1040, 1986

BURNING TONGUE

Synonym. Glossodynia; oral dysesthesia.

Symptoms. Prevalent in middle-aged or elderly women. Especially when tired or promoted by eating hot or spicy foods. Occasionally relieved by eating or drinking. Patients complain of spontaneous intense burning pain of tongue. Occasionally also report unpleasant taste. Cancerphobia or venerealphobia.

Signs. None.

Etiology. Psychological origin. Neurologic disorder (?).

Pathology. None.

Diagnostic Procedures. *Blood test.* To rule out anemia, deficiency states. *X-ray.* Gastrointestinal. To rule out reflux from hiatus hernia.

Therapy. Medical measures useless. If severe symptoms, antidepressants and psychiatric help.

Prognosis. Persistence of symptoms in spite of reassurance and treatment.

BIBLIOGRAPHY. Ziskin DE, Moulton R: Glossodynia: study of idiopathic orolingual pain. J Am Dent Assoc 33:1422–1432, 1946
Karshan M: Studies in etiology of idiopathic orolingual paresthesias. Am J Dig Dis 19:341–344, 1952
Van der Waal I: The Burning Mouth Syndrome. Copenhagen, Munksgaard, 1990

BURNOUT

Synonym. Chronic stress syndrome.

Symptoms and Signs. Impairment of short-term memory, decreased memory storage, decreased attention span, tendency to view minor problems as major, racing thoughts, negative thoughts that stick in the mind, rigid and stubborn positions, feelings of being victimized, loss of sense of humor, demanding behavior; increased muscular tension, tremulousness, palpitations, a feeling of pulsation in the body, epigastric gnawing, retrosternal oppression; self-medication, sometimes drug addiction.

Etiology. Chronic stress that stems from various factors such as low pay, long hours, dead-end career, too much paperwork, inadequate training, no appreciation by clients or by supervisors, powerlessness.

Therapy. Psychiatric counseling; taking the person out of the environment (forced vacation); restructuring the life style to reduce stress to

tolerable levels; marital, family, recreational, economic, and work adjustments.

Prognosis. Good.

BIBLIOGRAPHY. Freundenberger HJ: The staff burnout syndrome in alternative institutions. Psychother Res Pract 12:73–82, 1975
Wilson WP: Burnout and other stress syndromes. South Med J 79:1327–1330, 1986

BURTON

Symptoms and Signs. Both sexes. From birth. Microstomia, pursed lips, dislocated lenses (at about 2 years of age). Kniest-like skeletal dysplasia (see). Growth retardation. Limbs short and bowed. Joints stiff and enlarged.

Etiology. Unknown.

Pathology. Cartilage scattered, dense patches with altered column formations and large collagen bundles. Large and mature chondrocytes.

Diagnostic Procedures. *X-ray.* Long bones, dumbbell-shaped; vertebrae flattened; lumbosacral angle increased. Chest bell-shaped.

BIBLIOGRAPHY. Burton BK, Sumner T, Langer LO: A new skeletal dysplasia: Clinical, radiologic and pathologic findings. J Pediatr 109:642–648, 1986

BURY

Synonyms. Crocker-Williams; erythema elevatum diutinum; erythema multiform variant; cutaneous vasculitis.

Symptoms and Signs. Prevalent in males; onset in middle age. Slow, usually symmetric eruption of papulae or nodules on back of hands aggravated by cold. Occasionally, extensor area of kness, elbows, wrists, ankles, or buttocks may be involved. Plaques of irregular shape initially soft, then harden. Polyarthritis may be associated.

Etiology. Unknown; belongs to the group of cutaneous vasculitis.

Pathology. Pericapillary hyaline degeneration; endothelial swelling; inflammatory infiltrate with leukocytoclasis; lymphocytes; histiocytes; few eosinophils; and plasma cells. Fibrosis supervenes at later stage.

Diagnostic Procedures. *Biopsy.*

Therapy. Nonspecific; moderate reduction of lesion by topical injection with steroids. Dapsone may produce very good remission.

Prognosis. After years, lesions may clear spontaneously.

BIBLIOGRAPHY. Bury SJ: A case of erythema with remarkable nodular thickening and induration of the skin associated with intermittent albuminuria. Illus Med Neur (London) 2:145–148, 1889
Crocker HR, William C: Erythema elevatum diutinum. Br J Dermatol 6:33, 1894
Ryan TJ: Cutaneous vasculitis. In Champion RH, Burton JL, Ebling FJG (eds): Rook/Wilkinson/Ebling Textbook of Dermatology, 5th ed, pp 1929–1930. Oxford, Blackwell Scientific, 1992

BUSCHKE I

Synonym. Scleredema adultorum.

Symptoms and Signs. Prevalent in females, onset at all ages (29% before 10 years, 22% 10–20 years). History of preceding infection (days or weeks before). Moderate fever, malaise, myalgia, and arthralgia. Appearance of symmetric skin induration, nonpitting with sharp outline that separates it from normal skin on neck or face, difficulty in opening mouth; occasionally difficulty in swallowing. Skin induration later involves shoulders, arms, trunk, seldom other areas. Occasionally, pleuropericardial effusion; eyes and parotid involvement.

Etiology. Unknown; possibly lymphatic channel obstruction or hormone (estrogen) derangement.

Pathology. Epidermis normal. Dermal swelling and degenerative changes of collagen, spaces, and fenestration; metachromatic stain; increase in mast cells.

Diagnostic Procedures. *Biopsy. Blood.* Normal, except moderate increase of sedimentation rate. Lupus erythematosis (LE) IgA, IgG paraprotein reported; antistreptolysin O titer increased. *Electrocardiography.* Negative. Reversible changes.

Therapy. Trial with cortical steroids, thyroid hormone. Local injections of hyaluronidase and fybrinolytic.

Prognosis. Usually, spontaneous remission in a few months, occasionally persistence for years.

BIBLIOGRAPHY. Piffard HG: An Elementary Treatise on Diseases of the Skin, for the Use of Students and Practitioners. London, Macmillan, 1876
Buschke A: Ueber Scleroedem. Berl Klin Wockensckr 39:955–957, 1902
Rowell NR, Goodfield MJ: The connective tissue diseases. In Champion RH, Burton JL, Ebling FJG (eds): Rook/Wilkinson/Ebling Textbook of Dermatology, 5th ed, pp 2275–2276. Oxford, Blackwell Scientific, 1992

BUSCHKE-FISHER-BRAUER

Synonym. Keratosis palmoplantaris papulosa. See Brunauer and Greither (same conditions).

Symptoms and Signs. Both sexes. Onset 15–30 years of age. Female less severe manifestations. Keratosis on palms and plants with papular aspect.

Etiology. Autosomal dominant inheritance or sporadic.

Prognosis. Possible development of internal malignancy.

BIBLIOGRAPHY. Schirren V, Dinger R: Untersuchungen ber keratosis palmoplantaris papulosa. Arch Klin Exp Derm 221:481–495, 1965
Salomon T, Stalic V, Lazovic-Tepavac O, et al: Peculiar findings in a family with keratoderma palmo-plantaris papulosa, Buschke-Fisher-Brauer. Hum Genet 60:314–319, 1982
Griffiths WAD, Leigh IM, Marks R: Disorders of keratinization. In Champion RH, Burton JL, Ebling FJG (eds): Rook/Wilkinson/Ebling Textbook of Dermatology, 5th ed, p 1381. Oxford, Blackwell Scientific, 1992

BUSCHKE-OLLENDORFF

Synonyms. Curth; Albers-Schönberg II; dermatofibrosis lenticularis disseminata (Schreus); osteopoikilosis; dermo-osteopoikilosis; osteopathia condensans disseminata

Symptoms. Both sexes affected. Asymptomatic. Cutaneous signs may appear from the second decade, but, usually, become incidentally evident in adult life.

Signs. Firm, small, skin-colored or yellowish nodules (less than 1 cm in diameter) located on posterior aspect of thighs and buttocks, occasionally on arms and trunk, never on the face. They are usually arranged in streaks, not in constant relation with distribution of bone lesions. (See Osteodermopoikilosis.) Keloids occur with high intensity.

Etiology. Autosomal dominant heredity. This syndrome represents one manifestation of osteodermopoikilosis where both the components, skin lesions (Schreus') and bone lesions (Albers-Schönberg's I, see), are evident.

Pathology. Skin patterns varying from disordered arrangement of fibroblasts and collagen fibers to histocytoma characteristics. Hyperplasia of collagen in the corium.

Diagnostic Procedures. *Biopsy of skin.* Greater amount of elastic fibers in dermis; clumps of elastin coated with free fibrils. *X-rays of skeleton.* Small foci of sclerosis (differential diagnosis with osteoblastic metastasis). *Bone imaging.* Normal uptake of 99mTc pyrophosphate.

Therapy. Symptomatic.

Prognosis. Benign; once complete development reached no further changes.

BIBLIOGRAPHY. Buschke A, Ollendorff H: Ein Fall von Dermatosfibrosis lenticularis disseminata und Osteopathia condensans disseminata. Dermatol Wochenschr 86:257–262, 1928
Albers-Schönberg H: Eine seltene, bisher nicht bekannte Strukturanomalie des Skelettes. Fortsch Geb Roentgenstrahlen 23:174, 1915
Stieda A: Ueber umschriebene Knochenverdichtungen im Bereich der substantia spongiosa im Röntgenbilde Beitr Z Klin Chir 45:700–703, 1905
Ayling RM, Evans PEL: Giant cell tumor in a patient with osteopoikilosis. Acta Orthop Scand 59:74–76, 1988
Rimoin DL, Lachman RS: Genetic disorders of the osseous skeleton. In Beighton P: McKusick's Heritable Disorders of Connective Tissue, 5th ed, p 657. St Louis, CV Mosby, 1993

BUSQUET

Synonyms. Metatarsal periostitis; osteoperiostitis ossificans metatarsal. See Epiphyseal syndromes.

Symptoms and Signs. Pain in foot enhanced by walking.

Etiology. Unknown.

Pathology. Osteoperiostitis of metatarsal bones and exostosis.

BIBLIOGRAPHY. Busquet B: L'Ostéo-périostite ossifiante des metatarsiens. Rev Chir 17:1065–1099, 1897

BUSSIERE-ESCOBAR

Obsolete.

Synonyms. Escobar; multiple pterygium; see also Arthrogryposis.

Symptoms and Signs. Small stature; ptosis of eyelids, canthal folds, micrognathia; pterygia of neck, axillae, elbows, and knees; camptodactyly, syndactyly. *Feet.* Equinovarus or rocker bottom. Cryptorchidism; absence of labia major. Anomalies of vertebra or limbs.

Etiology. Autosomal recessive.

Therapy. Surgical.

Prognosis. Good quoad vitam.

BIBLIOGRAPHY. Escobar V, Bixler D, Gleiser S, et al: Multiple pterygium syndrome. Am J Dis Child 132:609–611, 1978

BYAR-JURKIEWICZ

Synonyms. See Cowden.

Symptoms and Signs. Congenital. Macrogengivae and hypertrichosis followed latter in life by giant fibroadenoma of the breast; secondary kyphosis.

Etiology. Unknown.

BIBLIOGRAPHY. Byars LT, Jurkiewicz M: Congenital macrogingiviae and hypertrichosis with subsequent giant fibroadenoma of the breast. Plast Reconstr Surg 27:608–612, 1961

Gorlin RJ, Cohen MM, Levin LS: Syndromes of Head and Neck, p 360. New York, Oxford Univ Press, 1990

BYERS

Synonyms. Spondyloepiphyseal dysplasia—punctate corneal dystrophy.

Symptoms and Signs. Both sexes; from infancy. Those of spondiloepiphyseal dystrophy, congenital (see) and punctuate corneal dystrophy that do not interfere with vision.

Etiology. Autosomal dominant inheritance. Suggested defect of a noncollagenous component of connective tissue.

Diagnostic Procedures. *X-rays.* Pattern differing from classic SED.

BIBLIOGRAPHY. Byers PH, Holbrook KA, Hall JG, et al: A new variety of spondiloepiphyseal dysplasa characterized by punctate corneal dystrophy and abnormal collagen fibrils. Hum Genet 40:157–169, 1978

BYLER

Synonyms. Fatal familial, intrahepatic cholestasis; intrahepatic familial jaundice cholestasis; cholestasis intrahepatic fatal, familial.

Symptoms. Both sexes affected in members of an Amish family (named Byler; other ethnic origins reported); present from early infancy. Recurrent bouts of jaundice often associated with infection episodes. Epistaxis; pruritus, foul-smelling stools. Stunted growth.

Signs. Icterus; protuberant abdomen; appearance of chronic illness. Hepatosplenomegaly.

Etiology. Congenital biochemical abnormality with recurrent cholestasis owing to defect of excretion of conjugated bile salts. Autosomal recessive inheritance.

Pathology. Liver cirrhosis.

Diagnostic Procedures. *Blood.* Hyperbilirubinemia; high serum alkaline phosphatase; normal or low serum cholesterol; hypoprothrombinemia. *Stool.* Light color; steatorrhea. *Urine.* Dark; hyperbilirubinuria.

Therapy. Symptomatic phenobarbital, cholestyramine, and medium triglyceride formula. Vitamin E. Liver transplantation when indicated.

Prognosis. Symptomatic improvement with treatment, but no effect on progressive nature of disease. Death at ages varying between 17 months and 8 years.

BIBLIOGRAPHY. Clayton RJ, Iber FL, Buebner BH: Byler's disease: fatal familial intrahepatic cholestasis in an Amish kindred (abst). J Pediatr 67:1025–1028, 1965

Sokol RJ, Guggenheim MA, Iannaccone ST, et al: Improved neurologic function after long-term correction of vitamin E deficiency in children with chronic familial intrahepatic cholestasis. Acta Neuropath 58:187–192, 1985

Saudubray J-M, Charpentier C: Clinical phenotypes: diagnosis/algorithms. In Scriver CR, Beaudet AL, Sly WS, et al: The Metabolic and Molecular Bases of Inherited Disease, 7th ed, p 389. New York, McGraw-Hill, 1995

BYWATERS

Synonyms. Paxson; muscular necrosis compression; ischemic muscular necrosis; crush; myorenal; see Young-Paxson.

Symptoms. Pain where trauma has occurred; thirst; nausea; oliguria; anuria; shock.

Signs. Signs of injury; hypertension; signs of moderate or severe shock.

Etiology. Extensive trauma of soft tissue; prolonged tissue ischemia (as from use of parachute harness).

Pathology. Injured muscles; loss of pigments. Kidney pigmentary casts occluding tubules with degeneration of tubular epithelium.

Diagnostic Procedures. *Blood.* Hyperkalemia; hyponatremia; hyperazotemia (maximum between sixth and ninth day following injury). *Urine.* Myoglobinuria; hematuria; proteinuria; glucosuria; pigmentary and granular casts. *Electrocardiography.* Signs of hyperkalemia.

Therapy. Fluid balance and liquid diet, with minimum protein and potassium. If hyperkalemia present, intravenous calcium indicated (better to use cation exchange enemas). If transfusion indicated, drain plasma to remove potassium. If acidosis symptoms are present; small amount of sodium bicarbonate. Hemodialysis with artificial kidney often indicated. When the patient resumes diuresis, liberal amounts of fluid and control of electrolyte balance.

Prognosis. Less severe than in the past because of medical management and prevention of complication; infection; lung edema; cardiac insufficiency.

BIBLIOGRAPHY. Bywaters EGL, Beall D: Crush injuries with impairment of renal function. Br Med J 1:427–432, 1941

Paxson NF, Golub LJ, Hunter RM: The crush syndrome in obstetrics and gynecology. JAMA 131:500–504, 1946

Glassock RJ: Hematuria and pigmenturia. In Massry SG, Glassock RJ: Textbook of Nephrology, 3rd ed, pp 563–564. Baltimore, Williams & Wilkins, 1995

BYWATERS LESIONS

Symptoms and Signs. Small, painless reddish-brown infarcts on nail folds or maculopapular, hemorrhagic, painful lesions on digital pads.

Etiology. Necrotizing angiitis observed primarily in rheumatoid disease and in many other vasculites.

Therapy. That of the basic disorders. Role of penicillamine to be evaluated.

Prognosis. Lesions first darken, then are extruded. Pitted scarring may result.

BIBLIOGRAPHY. Bywaters ECL: Peripheral vascular obstruction in rheumatoid arthritis and its relationship to other vascular lesions. Ann Rheumat Dis 16:84–103, 1957

Ryan TJ: Cutaneous vasculitis. In Champion RH, Burton JL, Ebling FJG (eds): Rook/Wilkinson/Ebling Textbook of Dermatology, 5th ed, p 1921. Oxford, Blackwell Scientific, 1992

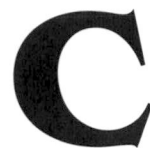

C-TRIGONOCEPHALY

Synonyms. Opitz (J. M.); C syndrome; MCA/MR syndrome.

Symptoms and Signs. Anomaly of the anterior cranium and frontal cortex (trigonocephaly), the root of the nose (broad nasal bridge, epicanthus, and short nose), and palate (thick anterior alveolar ridges); abnormalities of the limbs (polysyndactyly, bridged palmar creases, short limbs, and joint dislocations and/or contractures); visceral defects (congenital heart defects, cryptorchidism, and abnormal lobulations of the lungs and kidneys). Auricular, mandibular, skin, and genital abnormalities can occur, as well as hypotonia, strabismus, and psychomotor retardation.

Etiology. Autosomal recessive inheritance.

Pathology. In autopsied cases, there has been a suggestion of defective nervous system myelination.

Diagnostic Procedures. *Chromosome study.* Normal. *X-ray. MRI. CT scan.* Anomalies of the skull and face.

Therapy. Neurosurgery; other type of surgery when indicated.

Prognosis. About one-half of the cases have died within the first year. All survivors have mental retardation.

BIBLIOGRAPHY. Opitz JM, Johnson RC, McCreadie SR, Smith DW: The C syndrome of multiple congenital anomalies. Birth Defects V (2):161–166, 1969

Opitz JM: C syndrome. In: Birth Defects Compendium, 2nd ed, pp 160–161. New York, Alan R. Liss, 1979

Antley RM, Sung Hwang D, Theopold W, et al: Further delineation of the C (trigonocephaly) syndrome. Am J Med Genet 9:147–163, 1981

Flatz SD, Schinzel A, Doehring E, et al: Opitz trigonocephaly syndrome: report of two cases. Eur J Pediatr 141:183–185, 1984

CACCHI-RICCI

Synonyms. Medullary sponge kidney; MSK; nephrospongiosis (inaccurate term); precaliceal diffuse canalicular ectasia;. tubuloectasia; sponge kidney (inaccurate term); see Polycystic disease.

Symptoms. Both sexes equally affected; onset of detection from 3 weeks of age to 71 years. Uncomplicated form usually asymptomatic. Pain in loin (38%); colic (28%); nocturnal polyuria (28%); occasional polydipsia.

Signs. Seldom, enlargement of kidneys (observed mostly in children).

Etiology. Unknown; usually sporadic occasionally congenital and familial. Dysembryoplastic origin, comparable to that responsible for polycystic disease (see), or secondary to neonatal obstruction; progressive dystrophy in the collective tubules, analogous to cystic degeneration of mucous membranes. Families reported with autosomal dominant inheritance.

Pathology. Few reports. Precaliceal canalicular ectasia; enlarged medulla and integrity and normal dimension of cortex. Histologic findings in the medulla: cystic tubular dilatation alternated with areas of normal tissue; cysts communicating with excretory tract; basement membrane of ectasic area is thinned.

Diagnostic Procedures. *Blood.* Protein level occasionally elevated; uric acid level increased (in 50% of cases); serum alkaline phosphatase often moderately increased; calcium normal. *Urine.* Proteinuria (50%); blood usually absent, leukocyturia (50%). *Renal function tests.* Usually normal, except for presence of manifest defect in concentrating ability. *Urography.* "Bunches of flowers prolonging the calices." The precaliceal canalicular ectasia defines the condition.

Therapy. Symptomatic. Prevention of urinary infection and dehydration. Thiazide diuretics reduce stone forming in cases of hypercalciuria.

Prognosis. Benign clinical course.

BIBLIOGRAPHY. Lenarduzzi G: Reperto pielografico poco comune (dilatazione della vie urinarie intrarenali). Radiol Med (Torino) 26:346, 1939

Cacchi R, Ricci V: Sopra una rara et forse ancora non descritta affezione cistica della piramidi renali (rene a spugna). Atti Soc Ital Urol 21:59–63, 1948

Chamberlin BC, Hagge WW, Stickler GB: Juvenile nephronophthysis and medullary cystic disease. Mayo Clin Proc 52:485–491, 1977

Chapman AB, Gabow PA: Hereditary and congenital renal cystic diseases. In Massry SG, Glassock RJ: Textbook of Nephrology, 3rd ed, pp 922–923. Baltimore, Williams & Wilkins, 1995

C.A.D.A.S.I.L.

Synonyms. Cerebral autosomal dominant arteriopathy-subcortical infarct-leucoencephalopathy; Fisher lipohyalinosis; lipohyalinosis, vascular encephalopathy, chronic familial; encephalopathy, vascular, chronic, familial. See Lacunar (same condition).

Symptoms and Signs. Age of onset mean 45 (s.d. 10.6) years of age. Earlier may precede symptomatology attacks of migraine, ischemic attacks, mood cyclical alterations. Recurrent subcortical ischemic events (84%)with deterioration of gait and mobility and good initial recovery, becoming less complete with successive episodes; progressive or stepwise subcortical dementia with eventual pseudobulbar palsy (31%); migraine with aura (22%); mood disorders with severe depression episodes (20%). Blood hypertension.

Etiology. Autosomal dominant inheritance. Recently mapped to chromosome 19.

Pathology. Involves both cerebral white matter and deep nuclei. Small discrete infarctions (lacunes) and larger areas of diffuse infarction. With extensive demyelination, gliosis, and perivascular dilatation (leucoencephalopathy); thickening and hyalinization of media of small penetrating or perforating end-arteries and arterioles from peripheral and internal circulation.

Diagnostic Procedures. *Four-vessel angiography.* Normal or narrowing of small branches of cerebral arteries. *CSF.* Usually normal. *MRI.* Prominent signal abnormalities.

Therapy. Symptomatic; usually poor response to drugs.

Prognosis. Mean age of death 64.5 (s.d. 10.6).

BIBLIOGRAPHY. Sourander P, Walinder J: Hereditary multi-infarct dementia: Morphological and clinical studies of a new disease. Acta Neuropathol (Berlin) 39:247–254, 1977

Chabriat H, Vahedi K, Iba-Zizen MT, et al: Clinical specrum of CASADIL: A study of 7 families. Lancet 346:934–939, 1995

Broe GA, Bennett HP: Multiple subcortical infarction CASADIL in context. Lancet 346:919–920, 1995

CAFFEY-SILVERMAN

Synonyms. Caffey-Smith; DeToni-Silverman-Caffey; Roske-DeToni-Caffey; Smith-Caffey; infantile cortical hyperostoses, hyperplastic hyperostosis; hyperplastic periostosis.

Symptoms. Prevalent in females. Onset in early infancy (less than 5 months); occasionally, lesion of bone observed radiographically prenatally. Sudden onset; irritability; fever; conjunctivitis; swelling of bones; tenderness and movement limitation of affected parts.

Signs. Sudden swelling of jaw and face (occasionally, swelling starts in extremities and only after a few days involves the face) and other parts of the body. No discoloration, edema, or increase of temperature of skin overlying bone swellings; no lymphadenopathy.

Etiology. Unknown; autosomal dominant inheritance. Collagen disease (?); virus infection (?).

Pathology. Cortical thickening caused by normal but immature lamellar bone. No inflammatory changes. In acute stage, periosteum is loose. A gelatinous alteration is present with mitotic figures and mucinous changes extending to neighboring tendons and fascias. Later, muscular necrosis and fibrous change.

Diagnostic Procedures. *Blood.* Moderate anemia; moderate increase of neutrophils; increase in sedimentation rate and of serum phosphatase. *Urine and cerebrospinal fluid.* Normal. *X-ray.* Thickening of cortex of bones involved; thickening or patchy sclerosis remains after remission of acute stage.

Therapy. Symptomatic.

Prognosis. Variable course from complete disappearance of swelling in a few weeks, with or without local relapse or involvement of other bones for months or years, to fatality (rare).

BIBLIOGRAPHY. Roske G: Eine eigenartige Knochener Krankung im Sauglingsalter. Mschr Kinderheilk 47:385–393, 1930
Caffey J, Silverman WA: Infantile cortical hyperostoses: Preliminary report on a new syndrome. Am J Roentgen 54:1–16, 1945
Caffey J: Infantile cortical hyperostoses: A review of the clinical and radiographic features. Proc R Soc Med 50:347–354, 1956
Borochowitz Z, Gozal D, Misselevitch I, et al: Familial Caffey's disease and late recurrence in a child. Clin Genet 40:329–335, 1991

CAIRNS

Synonym. Tubercular arachnoiditis-hydrocephalus.

Symptoms and Signs. Occurs in children who have survived meningitis. Symptomatology similar to that caused by a posterior fossa neoplasm; communicating or noncommunicating hydrocephalus; occasionally, impaired vision and presence of visual field defects (chiasma lesions); focal symptoms (cerebral cortex lesions).

Etiology. Chronic arachnoiditis following tubercular meningitis (may occur also after other types of meningitis or spontaneous subarachnoid hemorrhage) caused by intracranial adhesions of leptomeninges.

Pathology. Adhesive leptomeningitis over posterior fossa and chiasma or less frequently involving the cortex. Thick arachnoid with chronic inflammatory cell reaction.

Diagnostic Procedures. *CT brain scan. MRI.*

Therapy. Antibiotics and chemoterapy. Surgery when lesion localized.

Prognosis. Fair with modern medical and surgical methods.

BIBLIOGRAPHY. Cairns H: Surgical aspects of meningitis. Br Med J 1:969–976, 1949

Adams RD, Victor M: Principles of Neurology, 5th ed, pp 1099–1100. New York, McGraw-Hill, 1993

CAISSON

Synonyms. Aerobullosis; aeroembolism; bends; chokes; decompression sickness; diver.

Symptoms. Occurs in SCUBA divers (and workers in caissons and tunnels) working under high pressures, when brought back without slow decompression to atmospheric pressure; onset possibly hours after decompression. Headache; weakness; nausea; vomiting; vertigo with tinnitus; dyspnea; chokes; nonproductive cough; occasionally paraplegia with paralysis of bladder and bowel; hemiplegia; shock; convulsions; back and articular pains (bends); abdominal pain; pruritus.

Signs. Tachypnea with shallow respiration; shock, hypotension; bradycardia.

Etiology. Bubbles of nitrogen released in the blood and migrating into different tissues.

Pathology. Infarctions of the brain, spinal cord, and other tissues.

Therapy. Prevention by slow decompression in hyperbaric chamber. When symptoms occur, rapid recompression followed by slow decompression. Administration of antiaggregating drugs (e.g., acetylsalicylic acid) and corticosteroids.

BIBLIOGRAPHY. Bassoe P: The late manifestations of compressed air disease. Am J Med Sci 165:526–542, 1913
Cockett AT, Pauley SM, Zehl DM, et al: Pathophysiology of bends and decompression sickness: An overview with emphasis on treatment. Arch Surg 114:296–301, 1979
Margulies ADC: A short course in diving medicine. Ann Emerg Med 16:689–701, 1987
Weatherall DJ, Ledingham JGG, Warrell DA (eds): Oxford Textbook of Medicine, 3rd ed, pp 1199, 1208–1209, 4128–4129. Oxford, Oxford Med Pub, 1996

CALCAREOUS TENDONITIS

Symptoms. Occurs in sedentary workers; prevalent in males; age of onset 35–60 years, right shoulder affected twice as frequently as left shoulder. Pain, tenderness, and limited mobility of shoulder, of different intensities and degrees. Fever only occasionally (in acute attacks).

Signs. Arm voluntarily fixed, adducted to side; forearm flexed, impaired movement of abduction and external rotation in particular. Tenderness on lateral area of humeral head, above insertion of deltoid.

Etiology. Trauma; idiopathic.

Pathology. Inflammation of one or more of rotator tendons with deposition of calcium around the tendon. Supraspinatus most frequently involved.

Diagnostic Procedures. *X-ray.* Calcific deposit in area of tendon involved. *Blood.* Leukocytosis and elevated erythrosedimentation rate only in acute attacks.

Therapy. Rest; analgesics; physical therapy; X-ray therapy; injection of procain or steroids; washing out bursa with saline injection. Treatment has to be conducted according to symptomatology, stressing the simple, conservative measures whenever possible.

Prognosis. Acute symptoms may persist for days. Spontaneous remission (abrupt or gradual) frequent. Subacute and chronic forms may persist longer.

BIBLIOGRAPHY. Weatherall DJ, Ledingham JGG, Warrell DA (eds): Oxford Textbook of Medicine, 3rd ed, p 2991. Oxford, Oxford Med Pub, 1996

CALCARINA

Symptoms and Signs. Hemi- or quadrant anopsia of eye of controlateral site.

Etiology. Thrombosis secondary to atherosclerosis or embolia of the calcarina artery.

BIBLIOGRAPHY. Hoff H, Tschabitscher H: Die Gefasssyndrome des Grosshir. Munch Med Wscher 101:589, 1959

CALCINOSIS UNIVERSALIS

Synonyms. Teutschlaender; interstitial calcinosis; metabolic calcinosis; myositis ossificans, progressive; see Patin.

Symptoms. Both sexes affected (mostly girls); onset during first two decades of life. Varies according to extent of abnormal calcium deposition in the skin, subcutaneous tissues, fascia, muscles, nerve sheaths, tendons, and visceral organs (seldom). Vague history of nonspecific fever; weakness; painful, stiff joints.

Signs. Irregularly shaped plaques palpable beneath the skin and in deeper tissues. Most frequently in periarticular locations; seldom involving the joints directly. At first, painless, and overlying skin freely movable and normal; then pain and tenderness develop; finally, necrosis and ulceration of skin with discharge of chalk-like material. Sinus tract difficult to heal. Superimposed infections.

Etiology. Unknown; possibly mucopolysaccharides disorder. Reported associated with numerous collagen disorders: scleroderma, dermatomyositis; lupus erythematosus; rheumatoid arthritis; myositis ossificans.

Pathology. Granular deposits of mineral material (apatite crystals) with fibrous reaction of connective tissue; occasional giant cells.

Diagnostic Procedures. *X-ray.* Calcific deposits of various size and shape, mostly as dense lines along course of muscles, tendons, and nerves. *Blood.* Normal. *Urine.* Normal. Differential diagnosis includes studies for parasitic infestations, renal insufficiency, vitamin D intoxication, hyperparathyroidism, hypoparathyroidism, pseudohypoparathyroidism, Burnett (see).

Therapy. No specific treatment. Various trials, including adrenal steroids, edetate (EDTA), cellulose phosphate, and low calcium diet. Results vary, but usually poor.

Prognosis. Calcium deposits may disappear spontaneously and return in years. Chronic course. Septicemia frequently develops when ulcerations occur.

BIBLIOGRAPHY. Teissier LL: Du diabete phosphatique; recherches et variations des phosphates dans les urines (thesis), p 439. Paris, 1876
Teutschlaender O: Ueber progressive Lipogranulomatose der Muskulatur. Klin Wchschr 14:451–453, 1935
Leistyna JA, Hassan AH: Interstitial calcinosis: Report of a case and a review of the literature. Am J Dis Child 107:96–101, 1964
Klippel JH, Dieppe PA: Rheumatology, pp 6.8.8, 6.10.4, 6.12.5. St Louis, CV Mosby, 1994
Weatherall DJ, Ledingham JGG, Warrell DA (eds): Oxford Textbook of Medicine, 3rd ed, p 3093. Oxford, Oxford Med Pub, 1996

CALCIPHYLAXIS

Synonyms. Ischemic necrosis skin-muscles.

Symptoms and Signs. In patients with advanced renal failure, or after long dialysis or after well functioning kidney transplant. Calcification of arteries, ischemic lesions of skin muscles and subcutaneous fat without gangrene or ulcerations.

Etiology. Unknown. Frequently present secondary hyperparathyroidism. Steroids (in transplanted patients) may play a role.

Pathology. Extensive medial calcification of arteries.

Therapy. Parathyroidectomy (significant improvement).

Prognosis. May die from secondary infections.

BIBLIOGRAPHY. Gipstein RM, Coburn JW, Adams JA, et al: Calciphylaxis in man: A syndrome of tissue necrosis and vascular calcification in 11 patients with chronic renal failure. Arch Intern Med 136:1273–1280, 1976
Salusky IB, Ramirez JA, Coburn JW: The renal osteodystrophies. In De Groot LJ: Endocrinology, 3rd ed, p 1158. Philadelphia, WB Saunders, 1995

CALVARIAL DOUGHNUT–OSTEOPOROSIS–DENTINOGENESIS IMPERFECTA

Synonyms. Doughnut lesions of skull.

Symptoms and Signs. Very rare. Both sexes. Multiple fractures; lumpy head; dental caries; underdeveloped teeth.

Etiology. Autosomal dominant inheritance.

Diagnostic Procedures. *Blood.* Serum alkaline phosphatase increased. *X-rays.* Osteoporosis; specific calvarial doughnut lesions. Dentinogenesis imperfecta; deformities from multiple fractures.

BIBLIOGRAPHY. Bartlett JE, Kishore PRS: Familial "doughnut" lesions of the skull. Radiology 119:385–387, 1976
Aube' L, Vallieres M, Lemay M: Lesions en beignet de la voute cranienne: une dysplasie osseuse hereditaire. J Can Ass Radiol 39:204–208, 1988

CALVARIAL HYPEROSTOSIS

Synonyms. See Gardner.

Symptoms and Signs. From infancy, in males. Fronto-parietal bones prominence, without premature cranial suture closure. Not other bones affected.

Etiology. X-linked recessive inheritance.

Pathology. Biopsy of bone lesion: presence of vacuolated histiocytes.

BIBLIOGRAPHY. Pagon RA, Beckwith JB, Ward BH: Calvarial hyperostosis: a benign X-linked recessive disorder. Clin Genet 29:73–78, 1986

CAMERA

Synonyms. Osteopathic lumbosciatalgia; neuralgic osteopathy.

Symptoms. Occurs in middle-aged patients. Pain that may affect practically any bone; intermittent and progressively increasing, sudden onset without apparent cause or following trauma. Difficulty of precise localization because of the diffuse character of pain or of its occasional radiation. Typical exacerbation during night. Contraction of neighboring muscles. Loss of weight. Lack of response to any medical, orthopedic, or physical treatment.

Signs. Absence of bone swelling and change in temperature of overlying skin. Presence of trigger point not larger than 1 cm over affected bone that can be found with the fingertip and better localized with a needle.

Etiology. Localized bone fibrosis and hyperemia.

Pathology. Partial marrow fibrosis; increased number of osteocytes; bone hyperemia.

Diagnostic Procedures. *X-ray. CT scan. MRI.* Negative. Localization of trigger point.

Therapy. Removal of trigger zone of the bone.

Prognosis. Good results with treatment in about 80% of cases.

BIBLIOGRAPHY. Bertola L, Pedrocca A: Osteopatie nevralgiformi lombos-ciatalgiche a localizzazioni vertebrali e paravertebrali (Sindrome del Camera). Minerva Ortop 4:215–218, 1953
Weatherall DJ, Ledingham JGG, Warrell DA (eds): Oxford Textbook of Medicine, 3rd ed, pp 240–241. Oxford, Oxford Med Pub, 1996

CAMPAILLA-MARTINELLI

Synonym. Maroteaux-Campailla-Martinelli; Hunter-Thompson type (variant of); Zwerwuchs; acromesomelic dwarfism. Achromesomeler nanisme acromésolique.

Symptoms and Signs. Normal at birth. Growth deficiences during first year. Frontal prominence, short nose, short distal limbs, coned epiphyses, limited elbow extension. Lower thoracic kyphosis. Large great toe, corneal clouding. Intelligence normal.

Etiology. Autosomal recessive.

Diagnostic Procedures. *X-rays.* Diagnosis at 2 years of age (see Signs).

BIBLIOGRAPHY. Maroteaux P, Martinelli B, Campailla E: Le nanisme acromesomelique. Presse Med 79:1839–1842, 1971
Campailla E, Martinelli B: Deficit staturale con micromesomelia. Minerva Ortop 22:180–184, 1971
Langer LO, et al: Acromesomelic dwarfism manifestations in childhood. Am J Med Genet 1:87–100, 1977
Langer LO Jr, Cervenka J, Camargo M: A severe autosomal recessive acromesomelic dysplasia, the Hunter-Thompson type, and comparison with the Grebe type. Hum Genet 81:323–328, 1989

CAMPTOCORMIA

Synonym. Hysterical back pain. See Briquet.

Symptom. Pain in lumbar area.

Signs. Extreme flexion of spine; normal orthopedic and neurologic findings. Correction of posture on recumbency or by suggestion.

Etiology. Conversion reaction.

BIBLIOGRAPHY. Rockwood CA, Eilert RE: Camptocormia. J Bone Joint Surg 51:553–556, 1969
Weatherall DJ, Ledingham JGG, Warrell DA (eds): Oxford Textbook of Medicine, 3rd ed, p 4209. Oxford, Oxford Med Pub, 1996

CAMPTODACTYLY–CLEFT PALATE–CLUB FOOT

Synonyms. Gordon (H.); Moldenhauer; Nielson; arthrogryposis multiplex congenita, distal, type IIa.

Symptoms and Signs. Both sexes. Camptodactyly, cleft palate, and club foot or minor anomalies of foot. Usually all three anomalies present or one of them can be missing in some members of the families (cleft palate most frequently missing).

Etiology. Unknown. Autosomal dominant inheritance. Penetrance reduced more in females than in males.

BIBLIOGRAPHY. Moldenhauer E: Zur Klinik des Nielsen-syndromes. Derm Wschir 150:594–611, 1964
Gordon H, Davies D, Berman MM: Camptodactyly, cleft palate and club foot syndrome showing the autosomal dominant pattern of inheritance. J Med Genet 6:266–279, 1969
Hall JC, Reed SD, Greene G: The distal arthrogryphosis: Delineation of new entities: Review and nosologic discussion. Ann J Med Genet 11:185–239, 1982

CAMPTODACTYLY–ICHTHIOSIS

Synonyms. Ichthiosis—camptodactyly.

Symptoms and Signs. Generalized muscular hypoplasia; motor development delay; flexures ichthiosis, reduced facial mobility; distal arthrogryposis; windmill-vane camptodactyly; vertical talus.

Etiology. Autosomal recessive.

BIBLIOGRAPHY. Baraitser M, Burn J, Fixsen J: A recessively inherited wind-mill-vane camptodactyly ichthiosis syndrome. J Med Genet 20:125–127, 1983

CAMPTOMELIC DYSPLASIA I

Synonyms. CMD I; Camptomelic dwarfism.

Symptoms. Both sexes affected; present from birth. Frequent respiratory insufficiency; feeding problems; failure to thrive; severe cerebral deficiency.

Signs. At birth, length reduced; subcutaneous fat scarce. Micromelia; bowed tibiae and femora; cutaneous dimple over tibial bend; fibular hypoplasia; foot deformities. Flat facies; hypertelorism; micrognathia; cleft palate. Thorax narrow; scoliosis. Sex reversal may occur in XY individuals.

Etiology. Unknown; most cases sporadic; autosomal recessive inheritance. In two cases observed translocation including long arm of chromosome 17.

Pathology. Tracheomalacia; various degrees of cerebral malformations.

Diagnostic Procedures. *X-rays.* Skeletal survey. Numerous skeletal malformations of long and flat bones.

Therapy. Generally medical.

Prognosis. Extremely poor. Most patients die from respiratory conditions within the first few weeks of life.

BIBLIOGRAPHY. Bound JP, Finaly HVL, Rose FC: Congenital anterior angulation of the tibia. Arch Dis Child 27:179–184, 1952
Môroteaux P, Spranger JW, Opitz JM, et al: Le syndrome campto-melique. Presse Med 22:1157–1162, 1971
Pazzaglia VE, Beluffi G: Radiology and histopathology of the bent limbs in camptomelic dysplasia. Implications in the aetiology of the disease and review of theories. Pediatr Radiol 17:50–55, 1987
Ferguson-Smith MA, Goodfellow PN: SRY and primary sex reversal syndromes. In Scriver CR, Beaudet AL, Sly WS, et al: The Metabolic and Molecular Bases of Inherited Disease, 7th ed, p 744. New York, McGraw-Hill, 1995

CAMPTOMELIC DYSPLASIA II

Synonyms. CMD II, camptomelic—long-limb type.

Symptoms and Signs. See Camptomelic Dysplasia I except for long limbs.

Etiology. May be autosomal recessive. Effect of drugs on embryo. Questioned: the difference from CMD I.

BIBLIOGRAPHY. Khajavi A, Lachman R, Rimoin D, et al: Heterogeneity in the camptomelic syndromes: Long and short varieties. Radiology 120:641–647, 1976

Spranger J: Advances in bone dysplasia. Sixth Int Congr Hum Genet, Jerusalem, 1981

CAMURATI-ENGELMANN

Synonyms. Engelmann; Ribbing; Lehman-Ribbing-Mueller; Mueller-Ribbing-Clémant; progressive diaphyseal dysplasia; osteopathia hyperostotica multiplex infantilis; multiple epiphyseal dysplasia tarda (type Ic); MEDT (Ic).

Symptoms. Both sexes affected. Manifestation onset before age 30, often before age 10. Severe bone pain in the legs. Delayed walking; failure to gain weight; anorexia; headaches; deafness; diplopia; pain; weakness of legs; wide-based gait.

Signs. Underdevelopment; elongation of legs; atrophy of muscles; bilateral symmetric fusiform enlargement of diaphyses of long bones; genu varum; genu valgum; coxa valga; scoliosis. Hypogonadism; hepatosplenomegaly; various ocular findings (exophthalmos; hypertelorism; cataract; papilledema). Less frequently, changes also in flat bones, ribs, and pelvis. Face bones unaffected. (See Craniodiaphyseal dysostosis.)

Etiology. Unknown; autosomal dominant inheritance with wide variance in expression.

Pathology. Subcortical hyperostosis; simple thickening of lamellae of compact bones. Muscular atrophy.

Diagnostic Procedures. *Blood.* Anemia, leukopenia, increased erythrocyte sedimetation rate. Normal calcium, potassium, and alkaline phosphatase. *X-ray.* Cortical thickening; fusiform osteosclerotic enlargement of diaphyses of tubular bones; normal epiphyses and metaphyses.

Therapy. Cortisone treatment beneficial for pain and reduction of bone changes; if optic nerve compression neurosurgical intervention.

Prognosis. Progressive condition, but not affecting life expectancy, and not too disabling.

BIBLIOGRAPHY. Cockayne EA: Case for diagnosis. Proc R Soc Med 13:132–136, 1920

Camurati M: Di un raro caso di osteite simmetrica ereditaria degli arti inferiori. Chir Organi Mov 6:662–665, 1922

Engelmann G: Ein Fall von Osteopathia hyperostotica (scleroticans), multiplex infantilis. Fortschr Geb Röntgehstr 39:1101–1106, 1928

Ribbing S: Studien ueber heriditaere multiple Epiphysenstoerungen. Acta Radiol (Suppl) (Stockh) 34:1–105, 1937

Mueller W: Das Bildung der multiplen erblichen Stoerungen der epiphysenverknoecherung. Z Orthop 69:257, 1939

Ribbing S: Hereditary multiple diaphyseal sclerosis. Acta Radiol 31:522–536, 1949

Bye AME: Progressive diaphyseal dysplasia and a low muscle carnetine. Pediatr Radiol 18:340, 1988

Weatherall DJ, Ledingham JGG, Warrell DA (eds): Oxford Textbook of Medicine, 3rd ed, p 3089. Oxford, Oxford Med Pub, 1996

CANAVAN

Synonyms. Van Bogaert-Bertrand; aspartoacyclase deficiency; spongy degeneration of white matter; encephalopathia spongiotica; cerebral white matter, spongy degeneration, infantile.

Symptoms. Relatively more frequent in Jews. Both sexes affected; onset in infancy (2nd–9th month). Poor head control and hypotonia followed by seizures and spastic paralysis, regression of psychomotor functions, lethargy blindness; occasionally, deafness. Loss of very early milestones. Late decerebrate or decorticated posturing.

Signs. Enlargement of head; separation of sutures. Neurologic signs of spastic paralysis; pathologic reflexes. Patients present blond hair and light complexion in contrast with darker complexion of unaffected members of family.

Etiology. Unknown; autosomal recessive inheritance. Deficiency of aspartoacylase.

Pathology. Increased weight and volume of brain. Small cystic spaces (spongy degeneration) in white matter, basal ganglia, and cerebellum; diffuse demyelinization. Optic atrophy.

Diagnostic Procedures. *CSF.* Occasionally increased protein; derivated metabolites of n-acetyl-L-aspartic acid. *Urine.* Increased n-acetylaspartic acid. *Enzyme analysis of cultured fibroblast.* Activity of aspartoacylase decreased. *CT scan. MR imaging.* Brain enlarged, ventricle relatively normal, decreased attenuation of white matter.

Therapy. Symptomatic.

Prognosis. Death in weeks or usually within first three years; prolonged survival in some cases, especially in cases with later onset.

BIBLIOGRAPHY. Globus JH, Strauss I: Progressive degenerative subcortical encephalopathy (Schilder's disease). Arch Neurol Psychiatr 20:1190, 1928

Canavan MM: Schilder's encephalitis periaxialis diffusa, report of a case in a child aged sixteen and one-half months. Arch Neurol Psychiatr 25:299–308, 1931

Van Bogaert L, Bertrard I: Sur une idiotie familiale avec dégénerescence spongieuse du névraxe. Acta Neurol Belg 49:672–687, 1949

Beaudet AL: Aspartoacylase deficiency (Canavan disease). In Scriver CR, Beaudet AL, Sly WS, et al: The Metabolic and Molecular Bases of Inherited Disease, 7th ed, pp 4599–4605. New York, McGraw-Hill, 1995

CANINE TOOTH

Synonym. Superior oblique palsy class VII.

Symptoms and Signs. Brown syndrome (see). Restriction of the upward gaze.

Etiology. Trauma to the trochlear area. Strengthening (with or without residual palsy) of the superior oblique, and underaction of the inferior oblique of the same side; or combination of trauma to the trochlea and closed head trauma producing a fourth nerve palsy.

BIBLIOGRAPHY. Ellis FH, Helveston EM: Superior oblique palsy: Diagnosis and classification. Int Ophthal Clin 16:127–135, 1976

Fraunfelder FT, Roy FH: Current Ocular Therapy, 2nd ed. Philadelphia, WB Saunders, 1984

CANNON-DE LA PAZ

Synonyms. Cannon reflex; Cannon (W.B.).

Symptoms. Flushing, hot skin; tachycardia; increased sweating.

Etiology. Emotional stress. Increase of epinephrine secretion.

BIBLIOGRAPHY. Cannon WB, De la Paz D: Emotional stimulation of adrenal secretion. Am J Physiol 28:64–70, 1911

CANNON (A.B.)

Synonyms. White folded gingivostomatitis; pachydermia oralis; nevus spongiosus albus mucosae; white sponge nevus mucosae.

Symptoms. Both sexes affected; onset at any age. Asymptomatic.

Signs. Oral and labial mucosae exhibit white, thickened, folded, spongy lesions. Occasionally, same lesions in anal and vaginal mucosae.

Etiology. Unknown; autosomal dominant inheritance.

Pathology. Acanthosis; parakeratosis; hyperkeratosis; vacuolated cells.

Diagnostic Procedures. *Biopsy.*

Therapy. Reassurance on innocuousness of lesion.

Prognosis. Chronic condition, excellent prognosis.

BIBLIOGRAPHY. Cannon AB: White sponge nevus of mucosa (naevus spongiosus albus mucosae). Arch Dermatol Syph 31:365–370, 1935

Witkop CJ, Shankle CH, Graham JB, et al: Hereditary benign intra-epithelial dyskeratosis; II. Oral manifestations and hereditary transmission. Arch Pathol 70:696–711, 1960

Scully C: The oral cavity. In Champion RH, Burton JL, Ebling FJG (eds): Rook/Wilkinson/Ebling Textbook of Dermatology, 5th ed, p 2702. Oxford, Blackwell Scientific, 1992

CANTRELL PENTALOGY

Synonyms. Septum transversum; thoracoabdominal wall defect; pentalogy Cantrell.

Symptoms and Signs. Midline supraumbilical abdominal wall defect; defect of lower sternum; deficiency of anterior diaphragmatic pericardium; congenital intracardiac malformation (80% ventricular septal defect). Two-thirds of patients also have muscular diverticulum of the apical portion of left ventricle.

BIBLIOGRAPHY. Cantrell JR, Haller JA, Ravitch MM: A syndrome of congenital defects involving the abdominal wall, sternum, diaphragm, pericardium and heart. Surg Gynecol Obstet 107:602–614, 1958

Lubinski M, Angle C, Marsh PW, et al: Syndrome of amelogenesis imperfecta, nephrocalcinosis impeared renal concentration and possible abnormality of calcium metabolism. Am J Med Genet 20:233–243, 1985

Zacharion Z, Daums R, Roth H, et al: Das Cantrellsche Syndrom. Z Kinderchir 42:255–259, 1987

Fox JE, Gloster ES, Mirchandami R: Trisomy 18 with Cantrell pentalogy in a stillborn infant. Am J Med Genet 31:391–394, 1988

CANTU I

Symptoms and Signs. In adolescence brown macules develop on the face, forearms and feet: palms and soles are hyperkeratotic.

Etiology. Autosomal dominant mutation.

Therapy. Symptomatic.

BIBLIOGRAPHY. Cantu JM, Sanchez-Corona J, Fragoso R, et al: A "new" autosomal dominant genodermatosis characterized by hyperpigmented spots and palmoplantar hyperkeratisis. Clin Genet 14:165–168, 1978

CANTU II

Symptoms and Signs. Mild mental retardation; short stature; macrocranium; prominent forehead; hypertelorism; exophthalmos; cardiac anomalies; cutis laxa; wrinkled palms and soles; joint hyperextensibility; wide ribs; small vertebral bodies.

Etiology. Probable autosomal dominant mutation. The father's age in each case was advanced (45–55).

Therapy. Symptomatic.

Prognosis. Good if successful treatment of cardiac anomalies. Mental retardation.

BIBLIOGRAPHY. Cantu JM, Sanchez-Corona J, Hernandes A, Mazara Z, Garcia-Cruz D: Individualization of a syndrome with mental defi-

ciency, macrocranium, peculiar facies, and cardiac and skeletal anomalies. Clin Genet 22:172–179, 1982

"CAP"

Synonyms. Subsarcollemal—segmental myofibrillolysis; myopathy congenital with Caps.

Symptoms and Signs. Few cases reported. Myopathy from birth.

Etiology. Unknown. Congenital condition.

Pathology. *Muscle.* Large subsarcolemmal areas of sarcoma-like structures without ATPase activity and myosin filaments (caps).

Therapy. None.

Prognosis. Mild progressive condition.

BIBLIOGRAPHY. Fidzianska A, Badurska B, Runiewicz B, et al: "Cap disease": A new congenital myopathy. Neurology 31:1113–1120, 1981

Goebel HH, Lenard HG: Congenital myopathies. In Rowland LP, Di Mauro S (eds): Handbook of Clinical Neurology, vol 18, p 331 (62). Myopathies. Amsterdam, Elsevier, 1992

CAPDEPONT

Synonyms. Schields II; Stainton; brown teeth; dentinogenesis II imperfecta; opalescent dentin; hypoplastic tooth enamel; pitted teeth; DGI1.

Signs. Both sexes affected. Teeth smaller than normal; color orange, slightly translucent; all or most of teeth become progressively worn down to gum level. Same appearance and wearing occur in deciduous and permanent teeth.

Etiology. Unknown. Autosomal dominant inheritance. If coexistence with osteogenesis imperfecta, is called Schields II.

Pathology. Tooth roots slender; pulp chambers small, cavities uncommon. Dentinal structure disrupted with typical histologic features. Decreased hardness with nontubular character of dentin.

Diagnostic Procedures. *Blood.* Normal; serum phosphate high in some cases. *X-ray.* Of teeth and skeletal survey.

Therapy. Removal of teeth; prosthesis.

Prognosis. Edentia.

BIBLIOGRAPHY. Stainton CW: Crownless teeth. Dental Cosmos 24:972, 1892

Capdepont C: Dystrophic dentaire non encore décrite type héréditaire et familial. Rev Stomat 12:550–561, 1905

Schields ED, Bixler D, El-Kafrawy AM: A proposed classification for hereditable human dentine defect with a description of a new entity. Arch Oral Biol 18:543–553, 1973

Corney G, Ball S, Noades JE: Linkage studies on dentinogenesis imperfecta DGI1. Cytogenet Cell Genet 37:439, 1984

CAPGRAS

Synonyms. Illusion of doubles; phantom double.

Symptoms. Prevalent in women. Patient with otherwise clear consciousness believes that a double has replaced another person, who, as a rule, is a key figure for the patient at time of onset of symptoms (if married, always the husband or wife accordingly). Patient continues to be firmly convinced of this, despite all evidence presented to the contrary. Admits a strong resemblance, but denies the person identity.

Etiology. Unknown. Complex psychopathologic characteristic clinical pattern, associated with paranoid psychosis of schizophrenic or affective type and other psychiatric conditions. No organic basis to the condition, but rather functional condition.

Therapy. No treatment for the syndrome. Treatment of associated psychotic symptoms.

Prognosis. Psychosis may respond to treatment and the illusion of double persist, or vice versa. Changing the attitude of object of delusion toward the patient may improve response.

BIBLIOGRAPHY. Capgras J, Reboul-Lachaux J: Illusion des sosies dans un délire systématisé chronique. Bull Soc Clin Méd Ment 11:6–16, 1923
Enoch MO, Trethowan WH, Barker JC: Some Uncommon Psychiatric Syndromes. Baltimore, Williams & Wilkins, 1967
Kimura A: Review of 106 cases with the syndrome of Capgras. Bibl Psychiat 164:121–130, 1986
Kaplan HI, Sadock BJ: Comprehensive Textbook of Psychiatry, 6th ed, p 1040. Baltimore, Williams & Wilkins, 1995

CAPLAN

Synonyms. Colinet-Caplan; rheumatoid lung silicosis; rheumatoid arthritis–pneumoconiosis; silicoarthritis.

Symptoms and Signs. Usually in patient exposed to fibrogenic dust. Migratory painful joint swelling and other symptoms of rheumatoid arthritis preceding or following pulmonary pathology (cough; mild dyspnea; hemoptysis) with typical chest radiologic pattern.

Etiology. Rheumatoid arthritis or rheumatoid state, plus exposure to fibrogenic dust (as in miner, quarry worker, grinder, wheel worker). Whether exposure to dust plays a role in enhancing or determining the rheumatoid conditions is under discussion.

Pathology. Thickened alveolar septa, and patches of fibrosis. Granulomas with central necrosis with epithelioid cells and giant cells; coalescence of several nodules with necrotic center and formation of cavitations. Rheumatoid endoarteritis.

Diagnostic Procedures. *Blood.* Elevated sedimentation rate; positive latex and Waaler-Rose tests. *X-ray.* Typical alteration of joints and of chest showing multiple and bilateral lung nodules (0.5–5.0 cm in size), frequently peripheral. Negative search for tubercle, bacillus fungi, and negative skin tests for those diseases. *Pulmonary function tests.*

Therapy. Steroid affecting the lung lesions; chloroquine.

Prognosis. The same as rheumatoid arthritis; spontaneous remission of pulmonary lesions make the evaluation of treatment difficult.

BIBLIOGRAPHY. Caplan A: Certain unusual radiological appearances in chest of coal miners suffering from rheumatoid arthritis. Thorax 8:29–37, 1953
Colinet E: Polyarthite chronique evolutive et silicose pulmonaire. Acta Physiother Rheum Belg 8:37–41, 1953
Caplan A, Payne RB, Withey JL: A broader concept of Caplan's syndrome related to rheumatoid factors. Thorax 17:205–212, 1962
Ezenwa AO: Prevalence of rheumatoid pneumoconiosis (Caplan's syndrome) in metal miners. CMA J 120:1492–1494, 1979
Klippel JH, Dieppe PA: Rheumatology, pp 2.4.5, 3.4.2, 3.5.3. St Louis, CV Mosby, 1995

CAPSULAR THROMBOSIS

Symptoms. Complete paralysis involving face, arms, and legs; contractures; occasionally hemianopsia; aphasia (if lesion on dominant side).

Signs. Exaggerated deep reflexes; positive Babinski.

Etiology. Thrombosis or other cause of occlusion of perforating branches alone.

Pathology. Thrombosis of perforating arteries; edema of perfused zone including lenticular nucleus and extrapyramidal pathway (spastic component of syndrome).

Diagnostic Procedures. *Neurologic examination. Arteriography. Electroencephalography. Cerebrospinal fluid. CT scan. MRI brain scan.*

Therapy. Anticoagulant.

Prognosis. Hemiplegia recedes as innervation from ipsilateral hemisphere asserts itself; recovery more marked on leg than arm.

BIBLIOGRAPHY. Fisher CM: Capsular infarct: The underlying vascular lesions. Arch Neurol 36:65–73, 1979
Adams RD, Victor M: Principles of Neurology, 5th ed, p 698. New York, McGraw-Hill, 1993

CAPSULOTHALAMIC (OBSOLETE)

See Capsular thrombosis syndrome.

Symptoms and Signs. Homolateral hemiplegia and hemianesthesia; emotional lability.

Etiology. Lesion (tumor) of internal capsule and thalamus or thalamic sensory fibers.

CAPUTE-RIMOIN-KONIGSMARK

Symptoms and Signs. From birth. Deafness (inner ear); from the end of first year generalized disseminated lentigines light or dark brown color (0.5–2.0 cm) concentrated mostly on the face. Vestibular function not affected. Occasionally syndactyly, and systolic murmur over pulmonary artery.

Etiology. Autosomal dominant inheritance.

BIBLIOGRAPHY. Capute AJ, Rimoin DL, Konigsmark NB, et al: Congenital deafness and multiple lentigines. Arch Derm 100:207–213, 1969

CARBAMYL PHOSPHATE

Synonyms. CPS I deficiency; hyperammonemia type I caused by carbamyl phosphate synthetase deficiency.

Symptoms. Heterogeneous features reported. Both sexes affected; onset in first days or weeks of life. Symptoms consistent with features of Reye syndrome: vomiting; lethargy; seizures, dehydration after onset of feeding. In some cases death at birth.

Etiology. Deficiency of carbamyl phosphate synthetase; possibility of other underlying enzyme defects has been considered. Autosomal recessive inheritance. (Short arm of chromosome 2.)

Diagnostic Procedures. *Blood.* Hyperammonemia (in absence of specific amino acid abnormalities), metabolic acidosis; leukocytes show deficiency of carbamyl synthetase (CBS). *Enzyme studies.* Two forms of carbamyl phosphate synthetase are recognized: lethal and delayed onset. *Liver biopsy.*

Therapy. Subtraction of protein from diet; correction of acidosis. Sodium phenylbutyrate; citrulline. Dialysis.

Prognosis. Frequently, death in neonatal age. Patients surviving longer are severely retarded and have neuronal deficits.

BIBLIOGRAPHY. Freeman JM, Micholson JF, Masland WS, et al: Ammonia intoxication due to a congenital defect in urea synthesis. J Pediatr 65:1039–1040, 1964
Granot E, Matoth I, Lotan C, et al: Partial carbamylphosphate synthetase deficiency, simulating Reye's syndrome in a nine-year old girl. Isr J Med Sci. 22:463–465, 1986

Haraguchi Y, Uchino T, Takiguchi M, et al: Cloning and sequence of a cDNA encoding human carbamyl phosphate synthetase I: molecular analysis of hyperammoniemia. Gene 107:335–340, 1991

Brusilow SW, Horwich AL: Urea cycle enzymes. In Scriver CR, Beaudet AL, Sly WS, et al: The Metabolic and Molecular Bases of Inherited Disease, 7th ed, pp 1187–1188. New York, McGraw-Hill, 1995

CARBOHYDRATE-DEFICIENT GLYCOPROTEIN

Synonyms. CDG.

Symptoms and Signs. Both sexes. From birth. Growth failure, prominent fat pads in the buttocks, lower limbs atrophy, strabismus and retinal degeneration, mental retardation, ataxia, peripheral neuropathy, skeletal abnormalities (owing to neurologic involvement), liver dysfunction. Occasionally, episodic stupor, or coma, or stroke-like episodes, pericardial or other effusions.

Etiology. Favored autosomal recessive inheritance. Basic biochemical defect not yet identified.

Pathology. *Liver.* Steatosis and fibrosis. *Muscle.* Minimal changes. *Sural nerve.* Attenuation of myelin sheaths and presence of multivacuolar myelinoid Schwann cells. Olivopontocerebellar, and portions of brain stem atrophy or cell loss and gliosis. Loss of Purkinje and granule cells in the cerebellar cortex. *Retina.* Marked degeneration.

Diagnostic Procedures. *Blood.* Presence of carbohydrate-deficient transferrin; low thyroxin-binding globulin; haptoglobin; transcortin; apolipoprotein B, cholesterol; coagulation factors; and various peptide and glycopeptide hormones; increased arylsulfatase, AST and, ALT. Electrophoresis of glycoproteins various abnormaties. *Cerebrospinal fluid.* Increased proteins and fluctuating levels of glycoproteins and peptide hormones, increased. *CT scan. MRI.* See Symptoms and Signs. *EEG.* Usually normal. *Nerve conduction study.* Decreased conduction.

Prognosis. Patients reach adulthood with the development and complications of all the mentioned deficits including hypogonadism.

BIBLIOGRAPHY. Jaeken J, Eggermont E, Stibler H: An apparent homozygous X-linked disorder with carbohydrate-deficient serum glycoproteins. Lancet II:1398, 1987

Jaeken J, Carchon H: The carbohydrate-deficient glycoprotein syndromes. Recent Dev Int Pediatr 860, 1993

CARBON DIOXIDE NARCOSIS

Synonyms. Anoxic encephalopathy; hypoventilation; hypoxic encephalopathy; pulmonary insufficiency. See Ondine curse.

Symptoms. Minor. Headache; nausea; anorexia. Severe. Delirium (see Brain, acute). If patient is anoxic, pallor, cyanosis, or shock. Delirium may persist after hypoxia is no longer present.

Signs. Decreased respiratory rate and depth. Patients with ineffective lungs are tachypnoic, but practically hypoventilating. Papilledema. Insufficient ventilatory drive in patient with normal lungs.

Etiology and Pathology. Respiratory acidosis; metabolic alkalosis; bicarbonate ingestion alkalosis; hypokalemic alkalosis; depressant drug poisoning; head trauma; pickwickian syndrome; heart disease; diuretic therapy; Cushing; Conn; myxedema-coma syndromes.

Diagnostic Procedures. *Blood.* Serum pH; serum bicarbonates; electrolytes determination; arterial blood oxygen tension; hemoglobin; glucose level. *Spinal fluid.* Increased pressure.

Therapy. If patient is delirious and awake, keep in quiet, isolated surroundings with light on; small dose of paraldehyde; avoid other sedatives; oxygen at reduced concentration, intermittent positive-pressure breathing. If anemia present, blood transfusion; electrolyte and fluid balance.

Prognosis. Correction of systemic disorder produces remission of symptoms; encephalopathy, when present, improves more slowly than systemic illness. Severe hypoxia may result in death or leave permanent neurologic sequelae. See posthypoxic syndromes.

BIBLIOGRAPHY. Miller A, Bader RA, Bader M: The neurologic syndrome due to marked hypercapnia with papilledema. Am J Med 33:309–318, 1962

Adams RD, Victor M: Principles of Neurology, 5th ed, p 879. New York, McGraw-Hill, 1993

CARCINOID

Synonyms. Bjoerck; Hedlinger; Scholte; Thorson-Bjoerck; Cassidy; argentaffinoma; carcinoid major; flush

Symptoms. Slight prevalence in males; age of presentation in males 18–80 years, in females 33–80 years. Intermittent diarrhea; abdominal pain; cutaneous flushing; asthmatic attacks; weight loss. Arthralgias.

Signs. Cutaneous rash (resembling pellagra); telangiectasis; precordial murmur. A precordial lift (right ventricular type) and systolic thrill palpable. Distention of jugular veins in upright position; hepatomegaly (occasionally, pulsating liver). Occasionally, peripheral edema and ascites.

Etiology. Tumors derived from the APUD cells (amine precursor uptake and decarboxylation). The syndrome usually is determined by metastatic carcinoid tumor. The symptom complex occurs in less than 10% of patients with this tumor. The pathogenesis of different symptoms and pathologic findings of this syndrome are not yet definitely assessed. Excessive production of either serotonin, bradykinin, histamine, or catecholamines has been considered as responsible for the symptoms. Possibly, different biologically active substances are elaborated and released in different combination, thus explaining also the variability of the clinical symptoms that have been described in patients with carcinoid tumor in different organs (e.g., bronchial, gastric).

Pathology. Primary tumor may originate in any part of the epithelium of gastrointestinal tract from cardias to anus, and in the epithelium of biliary and pancreatic ducts from enterochromoaffin and argentoaffin cells. In addition, it may (although rarely) originate in the bronchial epithelium. Metastasis to liver, lymph nodes, lungs, and bones. Fibrous valve formation on both tricuspid and pulmonary valves of heart. Occasionally, involvement of one gland is more extensive than the other; systemic veins may also be involved. Involvement of left side rare. At microscopy with staining methods argyrophil reaction in those containing serotonin.

Diagnostic Procedures. *Urine.* Excretion of high amount of 5-hydroxy-3-indol-acetic acid (5HIAA). *Plasma.* 5HIAA; serotonin. *X-ray of chest, gastrointestinal tract, and bones. Biopsy. Electrocardiography. Liver ultrasonography. CT scan. MRI. Celiac angiography.*

Therapy. Surgical removal of primary lesions (e.g., bronchi, ovaries) leads to cure. Embolization of hepatic artery. For liver metastasis, removal for cure or treatment with chemotherapeutic agents (usually disappointing). Interferon (good [36%] or partial [52%] response) hepatic artery embolization; radiotherapy. Pharmacologic treatment to inhibit synthesis of 5-HT, parachlorophenylalanine, alphamethyldopa, or kallikrein and bradykinin, aprotinin (Trasylol). To prevent release of active substances: somatostatin, octreotide (especially for diarrhea control) alpha adrenergic blocking agents. To inhibit action of active substances, methysergide.

Prognosis. Ileal tumor (primary and metastasis) growth is very slow; bronchial and pancreatic faster. Extremely variable prognosis; cardiac and metabolic features severe aggravating factors. The mean survival is 36 months after first flushing episode; 25% 6-year survival.

BIBLIOGRAPHY. Lubarsch O: Über den primaren Krebs des Ileum nebst Bernerkungen über das gleichzeitige Vorkom men von Kiebs und tuberkulose. Virchow Arch (A) 3:280–317, 1888

Oberndorfer S: Karcinoide Tumoren des Dünndarms. Frank F. Z Pathol 1:426–29, 1907

Cassidy MA: Abdominal carcinomatosis with probable adrenal involvement. Proc R Soc Med London 24:139, 1930–1931

Thomson A, Biorck CB, Yorkam G, et al: Malignant carcinoid of the small intestine with metastases to the liver, valvular disease of the right side of the heart (pulmonary stenosis and tricuspid regurgitation without septal defects), peripheral vasomotor symptoms, bronchoconstriction, and unusual type of cyanosis: a clinical and pathological syndrome. Am Heart J 47:795–817, 1954

Vinik AIR, Enar IP: Neuroendocrine tumors of carcinoid variety. In De Groot LJ (ed): Endocrinology, 3rd ed, pp 2803–2814. Philadelphia, WB Saunders, 1995

CARDIAC RADIATION

High doses of X-ray radiation damage the heart and pericardium following radiotherapy for thoracic cancer. A spectrum of syndromes is observed that, however, cannot be differentiated clinically, from others, without recognizing different etiologic agents.

1. Acute pericarditis.
   a. During radiation.
   b. Delayed.
2. Chronic pericarditis.
   a. Effusion.
   b. Constrictive, associated with myocardial fibrosis and endocardial fibroelastosis.
3. Coronary artery disease with myocardial infarction.
4. Mitral insufficiency and myocardial disease.

BIBLIOGRAPHY. Stewart JR, Cohn KE, Fajardo LF, et al: Radiation induced heart disease: A study of twenty-five patients. Radiology 89:302–310, 1967

Stewart JR, Fajardo LF: Radiation-induced heart disease: Clinical and experimental aspects. Radiol Clin North Am 511–513, 1971

Crawley IS, Schlant RC: Effect of noncardiac drugs electricity and radiation on the heart. In Schlant RC, Alexander RW: Hurst's The Heart, 8th ed, p 2000. New York, McGraw-Hill, 1994

CARDIOMEGALY, FAMILIAL

Synonyms. Cardiomyopathy, familial idiopathic; see Hypertrophic cardiomyopathy; Evans (W.).

Symptoms and Signs. Various clinical patterns. "Hypertrophic congestive" types with various clinical courses, from extremely severe (death in first day) to survival.

Etiology. Various inherited traits; autosomal dominant and recessive types described.

BIBLIOGRAPHY. Evans W: Familial cardiomegaly. Br Heart J 11:68–82, 1949

Whitfield AGW: Familial cardiomyopathy. Q J Med 30:119–134, 1961

Maron BJ, Roberts WC: Hypertrophic cardiomyopathy. In Schlant RC, Alexander RW: Hurst's The Heart, 8th ed, pp 1627–1628. New York, McGraw-Hill, 1994

CARDIOMEGALY, IDIOPATHIC

Synonyms. Abramo-Fiedler; Fiedler; Becker; Meadow (see); adult fibroelastosis; alcoholic heart; cardiac hypertrophy (unknown etiology); cardiovascular collagenosis; pernicious myocarditis; noncoronary cardiomyopathy; nutrition heart; obscure cardiopathy; South African cardiomyopathy.

Cluster of syndromes today subdivided in three major groups:

1. Dilated myocardiopathy (see).
2. Hypertrophic cardiomegaly (see).
3. Restrictive/obliterative cardiomegaly (see Davies).

BIBLIOGRAPHY. Liouville H: Rètrècissemt cardiaque sous aortique. Gaz Med Paris 24:161–1563, 1869

Hallopeau M: Rètrècissement ventriculo-aortique. Gaz Med Paris 24:683–684, 1869

Uber akute interstitielle Myokarditis in Festschrift zur Feier des funfzigjahrigen Bestehens des Stadkrankenhauses zu Dresden-Friedrichstadt. Dresden, pp 1–20. W. Baensch 1899

Becker BJP, Chatgidakis CB, Van Lingen B: Cardiovascular collagenosis with parietal endocardial thrombosis: A clinical pathologic study of forty cases. Circulation 7:345–356, 1953

Maron BJ, Roberts WC: Hypertrophic cardiomyopathy. In Schlant RC, Alexander RW: Hurst's The Heart, 8th ed, pp 1621–1635. New York, McGraw-Hill, 1994

CARDIOPULMONARY–MENTAL RETARDATION–AUTOPHAGIC VACUOLAR MYOPATHY

Synonyms. Lysosomal glycogen storage disease with normal acid maltase activity; pseudoglycogenosis II; glycogen cardiomyopathy.

Symptoms and Signs. Greater expression in males. In adolescence nonobstructive cardiomyopathy, proximal limb weakness, mental retardation.

Etiology. Autosomal dominant. Lysosomal disorders. Unknown biochemical cause.

Pathology. Muscle: autophagic vacuoles with accumulation of glycogen and other residues.

Therapy. Heart transplant.

Prognosis. Mean age of death: women 35, men 16 years of age. Heart transplant guarantees survival.

BIBLIOGRAPHY. Danon MJ, Oh SJ, Di Mauro S, et al: Lysosomal glycogen storage disease with normal acid maltase. Neurology 31:51–57, 1981

Byrne E, Dennet X, Crotty B, et al: Dominantly inherited cardioskeletal myopathy with lysosomal glycogen storage and normal acid maltase levels. Brain 109:523–536, 1986

Dworzac F, Cosazza F, Morandi L, et al: Heart transplant in a patient with lysosomal glycogen storage disease with normal acid maltase. Neurology 41:421, 1991

CARINI

Synonyms. Seeligman; alligator baby; collodion baby; lamellar exfoliation; newborn desquamation; includes lamellar ichthyosis.

Symptoms and Signs. Infant bright red with generalized or partial shiny collodion-like covering that after a few days dries and peels off in large sheets, but may repeatedly reform. Manifestations of underlying diseases (see Etiology) eventually appear.

Etiology. *Mild.* In normal infant. *Moderate.* Lamellar ichthyosis. (Autosomal recessive inheritance). *Severe.* Ichthyosiform erythroderma. Ichthyosis vulgaris and sex-linked ichthyosis.

Pathology. Parakeratotic horny layer shedding and that of underlying condition.

Therapy. Usually none. In severe forms, that of underlying disease. Emolients and keratolytic; isotretinol and etretinate.

Prognosis. Depends on underlying disease.

BIBLIOGRAPHY. Seeligman E: De Epidermis, Imprimis neonatorum desquamatione (inaugural dissertation). Berlin, 1841

Carini A: Di una forma attenuata della cosidetta "ittiosi sebacea." Gior Ital Mal Venereol 36:82–88, 1895

Griffiths WAD, Leigh IM, Marks R: Disorders of keratinization. In Champion RH, Burton JL, Ebling FJG (eds): Rook/Wilkinson/Ebling Textbook of Dermatology, 5th ed, pp 1338–1340. Oxford, Blackwell Scientific, 1992

CARL SMITH

Synonyms. Lymphocytosis, acute infectious.

Symptoms and Signs. Most frequent in children, occasionally in young adults. Incubation 2–3 weeks. Frequently asymptomatic or seldom nonspecific signs. Fever: moderate; morbilliform eruption, pharyngeal exanthema; diarrhea, abdominal distension; latent meningeal reaction; cervical or generalized adenopathy; moderate splenomegaly.

Etiology. Infective agent suggested by epidemiology, but not clearly assessed; possibly more than one type of enterovirus could be responsible.

Pathology. Lymph nodes: nondiagnostic degeneration of follicles and sinus reticuloendothelial proliferation.

Diagnostic Procedures. *Blood.* Normal except for hyperlymphocytosis (population T-CD4) over 20,000 up to 120,000, early onset and returning to normal value in 3–6 weeks. Occasionally moderate eosinophilia, Paul Bunnuel negative. *Bone marrow.* Normal except for lymphocytosis (30–40%). *Cerebrospinal fluid.* Occasionally lymphocytosis.

Therapy. Symptomatic.

Prognosis. Spontaneous recovery.

BIBLIOGRAPHY. Smith CH: Acute infectious lymphocytosis: A specific infection. JAMA 125:342, 1944

Leborrier M: Lymphocytose infecteuse (Maladie de Carl Smith). Encycl Med Chir (Paris) Sang 13009:B10–2, 1988

Athens JW: Variations of leukocytes in disease. In Lee GR, Bithel TC, Foerster J, et al (eds): Wintrobe's Clinical Hematology, 9th ed, p 1578. Philadelphia, Lea & Febiger, 1993

CARMI

Synonyms. Aplasia cutis-gastrointestinal atresia; skin absence—epidermolysis bullosa.

Symptoms and Signs. Both sexes. From birth. Aplasia cutis usually involving predominantly the scalp. Difficulty in feeding from atresia in variable localization (pyloric, esophageal). Occasionally associated: lid ectropion, axillary pterygia.

Etiology. Unknown. Autosomal recessive inheritance.

Diagnostic Procedures. *In gestational period high alpha protein in amniotic fluid. X-ray of digestive tract. Skin biopsy.*

BIBLIOGRAPHY. Leschot NJ, Treffers PE, Beckel-Bloenkolk MJ, et al: Severe congenital skin defects in a newborn: Case report and relevance of several obstetrical parameters. Eur J Obstet Gynecol Reprod Biol 10:381–388, 1980

Carmi S, Sofer S, Karplus M, et al: Aplasia cutis congenita in two sibs discordant for pyloric atresia. Am J Med Genet 11:319–328, 1982

Vivona G, Frontali M, Di Nunzio ML, et al: Aplasia cutis congenita and/or epidermolysis bullosa. Am J Hum Genet 26:497–502, 1987

Atherton DJ: Naevi and other developmental defects. In Champion RH, Burton JL, Ebling FJG (eds): Rook/Wilkinson/Ebling Textbook of Dermatology, 5th ed, pp 521–522. Oxford, Blackwell Scientific, 1992

CARNEVALE

Symptoms and Signs. Two males sibs. Mental retardation. Downslanting palpebrae, ptosis of upper eyelids, convergent strabism. *Limbs:* Limited extension of forearms, hip dysplasia. Abdominal diastasis; cryptorchidism.

Etiology. Unknown.

BIBLIOGRAPHY. Carnevale F, Krajewska G, Fischetto R: New syndrome: ptosis of eyelids, strabismus, diastasis recti, hip defect, cryptorchidism, and development delay in two sibs. Am J Med Genet 33:186–189, 1989

CARNEY I

Synonyms. Triad Carney.

Symptoms and Signs. Prevalent in young women. Symptoms and signs related to the combination of two or three of the following tumors: Pulmonary chondroma; extra-adrenal paraganglioma and gastric lyomyosarcoma.

Etiology. Unknown.

BIBLIOGRAPHY. Carney JA. Shegs SG, Gordon H: The triad of gastric lyomyosarcoma, functioning extra-adrenal paraganglioma and pulmonary chondroma. N Engl J Med 296:1517–1518, 1977

CARNEY II

Synonyms. Carney complex; Russell-Rees; Cushing disease—atrial myxoma—pigmentation; mixoma—spotty pigmentation—endocrine overactivity; nevi—atrial mixoma; mixoid neurofibroma—ephelides; N.A.M.E.; adrenocortical nodular dysplasia; lentiginal mixoma; mucocutaneous mixoma-blue nevi, LAMB; lentigines-atrial mixoma.

Symptoms and Signs. Both sexes. At birth: red hair, fair skin. Development in first weeks (68%) of pigmented lesions (BLU-NEVI) extended to all regions and becoming more evident in summer; subcutaneous mixoid neurofibromata (57%) and cardiac symptoms owing to atrial mixoma. In the teens diagnosis of Cushing III (see); in some cases endocrine adenomatosis: pituitary, testis, thyroid, etc with relative clinical manifestations (sexual precocity, acromegaly), occasionally hemangiomas syndactily, hypertelorism, low IQ.

Etiology. Autosomal dominant inheritance.

Pathology. Mixoid liposarcoma of skin and in heart cavities(atrial ventricular). Adrenal: typical lesions of microadenomatosis or primary adrenocortical nodular dysplasia, with foci of eosinophilic giant cells. In cases of testicular tumors (9 out of 17 cases) usually bilateral and multicentric lesions (Sertoli cell, Leyding cell, or adrenocortical rest tumor).

Diagnostic Procedures. *Blood.* Evaluation of adrenal function and of endocrine glands. *X-ray. CT scan. Ultrasonography. MR imaging.*

Therapy. Surgery for atrial mixoma excision. Medical for endocrine disorders.

Prognosis. Variable acccording to localization and extension of tumors.

BIBLIOGRAPHY. Frankenfeld RH: Bilateral mixoma of the heart. Ann Int Med 53:827, 1960

Russell Rees J, Ross FGM, Keen G: Lentiginosis and left atrial mixoma. Br Heart J 35:874–876, 1973

Atherton DJ, Pitcher DW, Wells RS, et al: A syndrome of various cutaneous pigmented lesions, mixoid neurofibromata, and atrial mixoma: the NAME syndrome. Br J Dermatol 103:421–429, 1980

Carney JA, Gordon H, Carpenter PC et al: The complex of mixomas spotty pigmentation and endocrine overactivity. Medicine 64:270–283, 1985

Young W Jr, Carney JA, Musa BV, et al: Familial Cushing's syndrome due to primary pigmented adrenocortical disease reinvestigation 50 years later. N Engl J Med 321:1659–1664, 1989

Koopman RJJ, Happle R: Autosomal dominant transmisson of the NAME syndrome. Hum Genet 86:300–304, 1991

Weatherall DJ, Ledingham JGG, Warrell DA (eds): Oxford Textbook of Medicine, 3rd ed, pp 1642, 2472, 3795. Oxford, Oxford Med Pub, 1996

CARNITINE DEFICIENCY PRIMARY SYSTEMIC

Synonyms. Cardiomyopathy familial—carnitine deficiency.

Symptoms and Signs. From childhood, weakness, hypotonia, hypoketotic hypoglycemic encephalopathy, failure to thrive, anemia, cardiomyopathy.

Etiology. Defect of high affinity, low concentration, carrier mediated carnitine uptake mechanism. Autosomal recessive inheritance.

Pathology. Muscle: lipid storage.

Diagnostic Procedures. *Serum.* Very low carnitine concentration (10 micromoles n.v. 35–70). *Urine:* Carnitine leak, no other abnormal organic acids. *ECG.* Enlarged and peaked T-waves, left ventricular hypertrophy. *Muscle biopsy.*

Therapy. Oral carnitine supplementation.

Prognosis. Unexplained sudden death, probably owing to untreated condition. Good with therapy.

BIBLIOGRAPHY. Waber LJ, Valle D, Neill C, Di Mauro S, et al: Carnitine deficiency presenting as familial cardiomyopathy: a treatable defect in carnitine transport. J Pediatr 101:700, 1982

Tein I, Di Mauro S: Primary systemic carnitine deficiency manifested by carnitine-responsive cardiomyopathy. In Ferrari R, Di Mauro S, Sherwood G (eds): L-Carnitine and Its Roles in Medicine: From Function to Therapy, pp 155–184. London, Academic Press, 1992

CARNOSINASE DEFICIENCY

Synonyms. Carnosinemia, hyper-β-carnosinemia.

Symptoms and Signs. Appears in first month of life. Myoclonic and grand mal seizures. Severe psychomotor retardation.

Etiology. Probably autosomal recessive, but X-linked type inheritance cannot be excluded. Lack of degradation of carnosine in serum as a result of deficient carnosinase.

Diagnostic Procedures. *Blood plasma.* Carnosinemia increased at least twice normal range (also when on a protein-free diet). Serum carnosinase activity lacking (usually low in normal infants). *Spinal fluid.* High concentration of homocarnosine. *Urine.* Excretion of carnosine. *Electroencephalography.*

Therapy. Trial with low-protein diet. Intravenous carnosinase replacement.

Prognosis. Poor.

BIBLIOGRAPHY. Perry TL, Hansen S, Tischler B, et al: Carnosinemia: A new metabolic disorder associated with neurologic disease and mental defect. N Engl J Med 277:1219–1227, 1967

Scriver CR, Gibson KM: Disorders of aminoacids in free and peptide-linked forms. In Scriver CR, Beaudet AL, Sly WS, et al: The Metabolic and Molecular Bases of Inherited Disease, 7th ed, pp 1362–1363. New York, McGraw-Hill, 1995

CAROLI

Synonym. Congenital biliary ectasias.

Symptoms. Both sexes affected; onset in first years of life or later (frequently around 35 years of age). Nausea; vomiting; gastralgia; fever. Asymptomatic forms have been described.

Signs. Hepatomegaly. Occasionally, jaundice or subicterus.

Etiology. Unknown; probably autosomal recessive inheritance. Defect of proliferation of some tracts of epithelium, which gives origin to biliary tracts, with resulting intrahepatic cysts. Frequent association with polycystic kidney, infantile type (see).

Pathology. Pure form. Congenital, sectorial, round, oval, or digitate dilatations of intrahepatic biliary tracts (rare). Normal epithelium with tendency to pseudopapillomatosis. Normal hepatic parenchyma. In 66% of cases, associated dilatations of extrahepatic biliary tract; occasionally, association with Cacchi-Ricci syndrome (see). Fibrocholangiomatosis form. Associated with the above features, diffuse hepatic fibrosis, and portal hypertension (form more frequent, especially in children). Fibrocirrhosis. Splenomegaly. Lithiasis frequently associated with both forms.

Diagnostic Procedures. *X-ray. Cholangiography.* Integrated with tomography, and selective angiography. *CT scan. Blood and urine.* Changes secondary to lithiasic obstruction, portal hypertension, and infections.

Therapy. According to localization, surgery or symptomatic medical treatment. Liver transplantation gives good results.

Prognosis. Of variable severity according to extension and forms of the condition.

BIBLIOGRAPHY. Caroli J, Couinaud C: Une affection nouvelle, sans doute congénitale, des voies biliaires: La dilatation kystique unilobulaire des canaux hépatiques. Sem Hop Paris 34:496–502, 1958

Bernstein J, Viranuvatti V, Boyer JL: What is Caroli disease? Gastroenterology 63:417–419, 1975

Paris JC, Quandalle P, et al: Un cas de maladie de Caroli associée à un kyste congénital du cholédoque et compliquée d'une lithiase biliaire intra-hépatique. Lille Med 22:226–228, 1977

Bernstein J, Chandra M, Creswell J, et al: Renal-hepatic-pancreatic dysplasia: a syndrome reconsidered. Am J Med Genet 26:391–403, 1987

Beker S, Beker B: Cysts of the liver. In Haubrich WS, Schaffner F, Berk JE (eds): Bockus Gasroenterology, 5th ed, p 2339. Philadelphia, WB Saunders, 1995

CAROTID ARTERY ANEURYSM

Synonym. Internal carotid artery aneurysm.

Symptoms and Signs. Unilateral oculomotor paralysis; loss of pupillary reflexes of light and accommodation (occasionally, pupillary escape); ptosis; pain in the eye or face, or both (trigeminal ganglion compression). Occasionally, homonymous hemianopia, unilateral blindness, optic atrophy; scotoma, headache, attacks of migraine.

Etiology and Pathology. Aneurysm of internal carotid artery. Congenital defect of tunica media, atherosclerosis, trauma, and inflammations usual contributory factors. Twenty-seven percent of all cerebral aneurysms affect this artery.

Diagnostic Procedures. *Angiography. X-ray of skull. CT brain scan.*

Therapy. Surgical intervention.

Prognosis. Variable.

BIBLIOGRAPHY. Dailey EJ, Holloway JA, Murto RE, et al: Evaluation of ocular signs and symptoms in cerebral aneurysms. Arch Ophthalmol 71:463–474, 1964

Joyce JW: The diagnosis and management of diseases of the peripheral arteries and veins. In Schlant RC, Alexander RW, Hurst's The Heart, 8th ed, p 2184. New York, McGraw-Hill, 1994

CAROTID ARTERY—CAVERNOUS SINUS FISTULA

Symptoms. Prodromata of headache and vertigo prior to rupture (rare). Sudden, sharp pain in the eye and headache; seldom, loss of consciousness. Slowly progressing exophthalmos; bruit or thrill, synchronous with heart beat, heard by the patient and described as "buzzing" or "sawing."

Signs. Edema of soft tissues of orbit; superficial vein of eyelid and forehead dilated; partial or total ophthalmoplegia of affected eye. Compression of homolateral common carotid artery suppresses or decreases bruit.

Etiology. Spontaneous or traumatic formation of arteriovenous fistula between internal carotid artery and cavernous sinus.

Diagnostic Procedures. *Ophthalmoscopy.* Pulsation of retinal veins; elevation of optic disk; retinal edema; occasionally, hemorrhages. *X-ray.* (Later). Erosion of sella and sphenoid orbital walls. *Arteriography.* Shows fistula.

Therapy. Ligation of common or internal carotid (possible hemiplegia). Better result obtained by ligating the carotid intracranially above the cavernous sinus. Direct attack on fistula.

Prognosis. Infrequent remission owing to formation of thrombus; possible recurrence from recanalization. Good results with surgery.

BIBLIOGRAPHY. Travers B: A case of aneurysm by anastomosis in the orbit, cured by ligation of common carotid artery. Med Chir Trans 2:1–16, 1817
Troost TB, Glaser JS: Aneurysms, arteriovenous communications and related vascular malformations. In Duane TD (ed): Clinical Ophthalmology, vol 2, pp 16–18. Philadelphia, Harper & Row, 1982
Garner A: Vascular disease. In Garner A, Klintworth GK (eds): Pathobiology of Ocular Disease: A Dynamic Approach, 2nd ed, p 1693. New York, Marcel Dekker, 1994

CAROTID BODY TUMOR

Synonyms. Chemodectoma; nonchromaffin paraganglioma; paragangliomata; glomus jugulare tumor. See also Carotid sinus.

Symptoms. Equal sex distribution; age at onset ranges from second to seventh decade, average age 45 years. Average duration of symptoms before diagnosis, 2.1 years. Frequently asymptomatic. Hoarseness; tinnitus; vertigo; facial nerve palsy; vocal cord palsy. Occasionally cause of transient ischemic attacks.

Signs. Cervical mass that can be moved laterally but not vertically (bilateral in 5% of cases). Hypopharyngeal mass; majority of cervical masses pulsatile; bruit only occasionally.

Etiology. Sporadic; rare familial occurrence with autosomal dominant inheritance.

Pathology. Circumscribed tumor 3–6 cm in diameter, with partial sort of capsule formed by compressed connective tissue arising at the bifurcation of a carotid artery. Red-brown color; focal hemorrhage; very vascular, cells arranged in nest with vascular fibrous septa. Frequently, extension into adventitia.

Diagnostic Procedures. *Angiography of carotid.*

Therapy. Surgical excision.

Prognosis. Usually cured by surgery. Local recurrences; malignant transformation in 5% of cases.

BIBLIOGRAPHY. Chase WH: Familial and bilateral tumors of carotid body. J Pathol Bact 36:1–12, 1933

Lattes R: Nonchromaffin paraganglioma of ganglion nodosum, carotid body, and aortic arch bodies. Cancer 3:667–694, 1950
Oberman HA, Holtz F, Sheffer LA, et al: Chemodectomas (nonchromaffin paraganglioma) of the head and neck. Cancer 21:838–851, 1968
Van Baars FM, Cremers CNRJ, Van Den Broeck P, et al: Familial nonchromaffinic paragangliomas (glomus tumors): Clinical and genetic aspects. Acta Otolaryngol 91:589–593, 1981
Sabiston DC: Textbook of Surgery, 14th ed, pp 1562–1563. Philadelphia, WB Saunders, 1991
Adams RD, Victor M: Principles of Neurology, 5th ed, p 583. New York, McGraw-Hill, 1993

CAROTID KINKING

Symptoms and Signs. Symptoms of cerebral ischemia except if compensation has developed.

Etiology. Because of arteriosclerosis, situated at a point closer to the carotid bifurcation. Same for coiling or tortuosity that becomes more marked when head and neck are flexed and rotated.

Diagnostic Procedures. *CT scan. MRI. Angiography. Doppler.*

Therapy. Vascular surgery may be useful.

BIBLIOGRAPHY. Lie TA: Congenital malformatios of the carotid and vertebral arterial systems including the persistent anastomosis. InVinken PJ, Bruyn GW: Handbook of Clinical Neurology, vol 12, p 294. Amsterdam, North-Holland, 1972

CAROTID SINUS

Synonyms. Weiss-Baker; Charcot-Weiss-Baker; cardio-inhibitory carotid sinus; tight collar; vagal syncope.

Symptoms. More frequent in males over 45 years of age; sudden onset. Headache; transient attack of dizziness; vertigo; fainting; loss of consciousness; convulsions. Unilateral paresthesia; slurred speech.

Signs. Homonymous hemianopia; hemiplegia; bradycardia; drop of blood pressure during attack. Three types of carotid sinus syndrome may be recognized: (1) Vagal type with bradycardia, heart block, or asystole; (2) Depressor type with extensive peripheral dilatation; (3) Type without heart rate and pressure changes (see Weiss-Baker).

Etiology and Pathology. Hypersensitivity of carotid sinus from pressure, tight collar, turning head, shaving, swallowing, or emotion, or may be spontaneous. Atheromatous narrowing of opposite sinus or basilar artery.

Diagnostic Procedures. *Electroencephalography.* Diffuse slow waves. Moderate pressure over carotid sinus reproduces the attack.

Therapy. Prevention by eliminating pressure on the neck (e.g., loose collar). In the depressive type, amphetamine sulfate. In vagal type, atropine sulfate. Surgical denervation of sinus in cases refractory to medical treatment. Ventricular demand pacemaker application.

Prognosis. In simple sensitivity, attack lasts a few minutes. If associated with atheromatous narrowing, serious prognosis.

BIBLIOGRAPHY. Waller A: Experimental researches on the functions of the vagus and the cervical sympathetic nerves in man. Proc R Soc Med 11:302–315, 1862
Charcot JM: Leçons sur les Maladies du Système Nerveux Faites à la Salpétrière. Paris, 1872–1873
Weiss S, Baker JP: The carotid sinus reflex in health and disease. Its role in the causation of fainting and convulsions. Medicine 12:297–354, 1933

Lewis RP, Budoulas H, Schaal SF, et al: Diagnosis and management of syncope. In: Schlant RC, Alexander RW: Hurst's The Heart, 8th ed, pp 932–933. New York, McGraw-Hill, 1994

Weatherall DJ, Ledingham JGG, Warrell DA (eds): Oxford Textbook of Medicine, 3rd ed, p 3926. Oxford, Oxford Med Pub, 1996

CAROTID SYSTEM ISCHEMIA

Synonyms. Carotid artery insufficiency; carotid artery system ischemia; carotid artery occlusion; transient ischemic carotid insufficiency included. See Determann.

Symptoms. Usually appears in adult males. More frequently on left side. Digital compression of carotid bulb in patient with partial or complete obstructive disease may cause syncope. Onset could be intermittent, gradual, or apoplectiform. Intermittent: repetitive with full recovery between attacks; episodes lasting less than 1 hour (rule out hypotension or heart conditions, vertigo, vertebral-basilar ischemia); pain on affected side (inconstant); episodes of temporary homolateral blindness or controlateral hemiplegia or both.

Signs. Absence of pulsation on affected side; bruits over carotid occasionally present; blood pressure determination on both arms to detect differences.

Etiology. Atherosclerosis (leading cause); complication of angiography; closed trauma; digital compression of artery; congenital kinking; hypoplasia of internal carotid artery (see also Fibromuscular dysplasia).

Pathology. Bifurcation of carotid predisposes site of obstruction; atherosclerotic changes; thrombosis.

Diagnostic Procedures. *Angiography.* In high risk group; absence of total agreement on using this test. *Electroencephalography.* Eleven percent of low-voltage, electroencephalogram fast. *CT scan. MR imaging.*

Therapy. Variable, from sympathectomy to endoarterectomy or transposed graft. Anticoagulants.

Prognosis. Quoad vitam fair; various types of residual incapacity.

BIBLIOGRAPHY. Persson AV, Robichaux WT, Silverman M: The natural history of carotid plaque development. Arch Surg 118:1048–1052, 1983

Whisnant JP, Sandok BA, Sundt TM: Carotid endarterectomy for unilateral carotid system transient cerebral ischemia. Mayo Clin Proc 58:171–175, 1983

Dodson TF, Smith RB III: The surgical treatment of peripheral vascular disease. In Schlant RC, Alexander RW: Hurst's The Heart, 8th ed, pp 2197–2199. New York, McGraw-Hill, 1994

CARPAL TUNNEL

Synonyms. Median neuropathy; median neuritis; tardy median palsy; tenosynovitis stenosans—carpal tunnel; thenar amyotrophy, carpal; constrictive median neuropathy. Included Guayon canal.

Symptoms. Prevalent in women; fairly common complaint during pregnancy and in menopause. Numbness, paresthesia, burning pain on index finger, middle finger, or medial half of ring finger, occurring mostly at night and upon waking the patient. Weakness of thumb.

Signs. Anesthesia of thumb and mentioned fingers. Atrophy of thenar eminence; weakness of abductor pollicis and opponens pollicis; thickening and tenderness of flexor tendons; pain increased by flexing wrist to extreme degree; flexion of wrist (and less frequently extension) aggravates symptoms.

Etiology. Most common cause is nonspecific synovitis involving the flexor synovia in carpal tunnel and compressing the median nerve. Precipitating factor may be traumas or disorders such as acromegaly. May be observed in amyloidosis, mucopolysaccharidoses and mucolipidoses. Autosomal dominant inheritance reported (male-to-male transmission).

Pathology. Fibrous proliferation with chronic inflammation and edema of synovial sheaths; fatty or mixedematous fibrous tissue.

Diagnostic Procedures. *Electromyography.* Slow conduction of median nerve and atrophy of muscles. *X-ray.* Of cervical spine to rule out herniated disk. Syringomyelia and muscular atrophy to be considered in differential diagnosis. *Biopsy.* Flexor synovia.

Therapy. Wrist splint for mild symptoms. Better results obtained with surgery sectioning transverse carpal tunnel. Reported that: pyridoxin corrects B_6 deficiency and ameliorates neurologic symptoms.

Prognosis. When occurring in pregnancy 85% of cases recover spontaneously, 15% require surgery, and all obtain complete relief. In about 10%, recurrence of the syndrome with subsequent pregnancies.

BIBLIOGRAPHY. Marie P, Foix C: Atrophie isolée de l'éminence thénar d'origine névritique, rôle du ligament anulaire antérieur du carpe dans la pathogénie de la lésion. Rev Neurol (Paris) 26:647–649, 1913

Serratrice G, Roger J, Guastalla B, et al: Amyotrophies thenariennes familiales d'origine carpienne. Rev Neurol (Paris) 141:746–749, 1985

McDonnell JM, Makley JT, Horwitz SJ: Familial carpal-tunnel syndrome presenting in childhood: report of two cases. J Bone Joint Surg 69A:928–930, 1987

Kuschner SH, Brien WW, Johnson D, et al: Complications associated with carpal tunnel release Orthop Rev 20:346–352, 1991

Klippel JH, Dieppe PA: Rheumatology, pp 3.15.7, 3.15.9. St Louis, CV Mosby, 1995

CARPENTER

Synonyms. Acrocephalopolysyndactyly; acrocephalopolysyndactyly II; ACPS II. See Goodman and Suminitt syndromes (possibly parts of the same spectrum).

Symptoms and Signs. Mental retardation; acrocephaly; peculiar facies; syndactyly (mainly third and fourth fingers); brachymesophalangia; preaxial polydactyly with syndactyly of toes; coxa valga; pes varus. Mild obesity; congenital heart disease; hypogenitalism.

Etiology. Unknown; rare autosomal recessive disorder. Development related to, but genetically distinct from, Apert and the Laurence-Moon-Biedl.

Pathology. See Signs.

Diagnostic Procedures. *X-rays.* Premature closure of cranial sutures; brachymesophalangia; soft tissue syndactyly of hands; preaxial polydactyly and syndactyly of feet; other bone abnormalities.

Therapy. Surgical correction and orthopedic measures when feasible.

BIBLIOGRAPHY. Carpenter G: Two sisters showing malformation of the skull and other congenital abnormalities. Rep Soc Study Dis Child (London) 1:110–118, 1901

Robinson LK, James HE, Maburak SJ, et al: Carpenter's syndrome: Natural history and clinical spectrum. Am J Med Genet 20:461–469, 1985

Cohen DM, Green JG, Miller J, et al: Acrocephalopolysyndactyly type II Carpenter syndrome: clinical spectrum and an attempt at unification with Goodman and Suminitt syndromes. Am J Med Genet 28:311–324, 1987

Gershoni-Baruch R: Carpenter syndrome: marked variability of expression to include Summitt and Goodman syndromes. Am J Med Genet 35:236–240, 1990

CARRARO

Synonyms. Tibia—deafness; deafness—tibia absence.

Symptoms and Signs. Deafness (in four of six sibs); hypoplasia or absence of tibias.

Etiology. Possible linkage of two rare recessive type of inheritances.

BIBLIOGRAPHY. Carraro A: Assenza congenita della tibia e sordomutismo in quattro fratelli. Clin Organi Mov 16:429–438, 1931

Wendler H, Schwartz R: Carraro-Syndrom. Fortschr Roentgenstr. 133:43–46, 1980

CARR-BARR-PLUNKETT

Synonyms. 48 XXXX; tetra-X; XXXX.

Symptoms and Signs. Variable features. Mental retardation (IQ average 55). Midfacial hypoplasia; hypertelorism; micrognathia. Clinodactyly of 5th finger; radial synostosis. Narrow shoulders; web neck. Irregular menstrual cycles.

Diagnostic Procedures. *Chromosome studies.* In 6–9% of cells, three-X chromatin bodies.

Prognosis. Mental deficiency and behavioral problems.

BIBLIOGRAPHY. Carr DH, Barr ML, Plunkett ER: A XXXX sex chromosome complex in two mentally defective females. Can Med Assoc J 84:133–137, 1961

Jones KL: Smith's recognizable patterns of human malformations, p 72. Philadelphia, WB Saunders, 1988

CARRINGTON-LIEBOW

Obsolete.

Synonym. Wegener limited form. See also Liebow-Carrington (probably obsolete).

Symptoms and Signs. Limited form of Wegener's granulomatosis (see) with prevalent pulmonary (with or without limited extrapulmonary) lesions, but without nephritis.

Etiology. Unknown (see).

Therapy. Effectiveness of prednisone uncertain.

Prognosis. Better than in patients with classic symptom triad of Wegener.

BIBLIOGRAPHY. Carrington CB, Liebow AA: Limited forms of angiitis and granulomatosis of Wegener's type. Am J Med 41:497–527, 1966

De Remee RA: Wegener's granulomatosis. In Kynch JP, De Remee RA: Immunologically Mediated Pulmonary Diseases, p 250. Philadelphia, JB Lippincott, 1991

Fraser RS, Paré JAP, Fraser RG, Paré PD: Synopsis of Diseases of the Chest, 2nd ed. Philadelphia, WB Saunders, 1994

CARSON-NEILL

Synonyms. Homocystinuria; cystathionine β-synthase deficiency; CBS deficiency. See also pyridoxine deficiency syndromes.

Symptoms. Both sexes equally affected. Normal parents. Infant appears entirely normal at birth. At 5–6 months may develop seizures followed by paralysis. At 3–5 years, develops dislocation of lenses, mental deficiency (in 66% of patients), delayed speech development, dyslalia, clumsiness, droolings, and thromboembolic accidents.

Signs. In early childhood development of skeletal abnormalities; genu valgum; pes cavus; pectus excavatum or carinatum; kyphoscoliosis; arachnodactyly. Occasionally, also characterized by fine, fair hair, malar flush, livedo reticularis.

Etiology. Autosomal recessive condition characterized by a deficiency of the enzyme cystathionine β-synthetase, which leads to accumulation of homocystine and methionine in blood and spinal fluid, increasing blood coagulation, vascular degeneration, and brain degeneration. Three other causes of homocystinuria are known defect in vitamin B_{12} metabolism, deficiency in N5–10–methylenetetrahydrafolate reductase, selective malabsorption of vitamin B_{12}.

Pathology. In brain, mild diffuse neuronal rarefaction of cortex, hippocampus, basal ganglia; venous infarction and arterial thrombosis. Vessels, medial degeneration of aorta and other elastic arteries. Thrombus formation. Skeletal deformities.

Diagnostic Procedures. *Urine screening test.* Positive cyanide nitroprusside reaction. Confirmatory amino acid chromatography shows presence of homocystine and increased methionine. *Blood.* Increased coagulability; increased platelet adhesiveness; increased level of homocystine and methionine. *Spinal fluid.* Presence of homocystine. *EEG.* Alteration.

Therapy. Low methionine diet supplemented by L-cystine and pyridoxine, folic acid, anticoagulants, and platelet antiaggregating agents.

Prognosis. Death from thrombosis, cerebral, and other organ infarctions.

BIBLIOGRAPHY. Carson NAJ, Neill DW: Metabolic abnormalities detected in a survey of mentally backward individuals in Northern Ireland. Arch Dis Child 37:505–513, 1962

Skovby F: Homocystinuria: Clinical biochemical and genetic aspects of cystathionine β-synthetase and its deficiency in man. Acta Paediat Scand 321(Suppl):1–21, 1985

Visy JM, LeCoz P, Chadefaux B, et al: Homocystinuria due to 5,10-methylenetetrahydrofolate reductase deficiency revealed by stroke in adult siblings. Neurology 41:1313–1315, 1991

Mudd SH, Levy HL, Skovby F: Disorders of transsulfuration. In Scriver CR, Beaudet AL, Sly WS, et al: The Metabolic and Molecular Bases of Inherited Disease, 7th ed, pp 1292–1296. New York, McGraw-Hill, 1995

CARTER–HORSLEY–HUGHES

Synonyms. See polyposis coli juvenile.

Symptoms and Signs. One family described, possibly one variant in the rich family of intestinal polyposis. Characteristic: the diffusion of polyps in the small and large intestine.

Etiology. Autosomal dominant inheritance.

BIBLIOGRAPHY. Carter BN, Horsley GW, Horsley JJ, Hughes RD: A new form of diffuse familial polyposis. A probable genetic explanation. Ann Surg 167:942, 1968

Sabiston DC: Textbook of Surgery, 14th ed, p 805. Philadelphia, WB Saunders, 1991

CARTER-SUKAVAJANA

Synonyms. Cerebello—olivary, atrophy—late rigidity—dementia.

Symptoms and Signs. In males. Variable age for onset from 7–43 years. Ataxia of gait progressing slowly to rigidity and Parkinson symptoms and after years dementia.

Etiology. Sex-linked inheritance. According to clinical and pathological elements this family is very difficult to classify.

Pathology. Diffuse neocortical atrophy with some neuronal loss; mild cell loss in striatum and thalamus; widespread loss of Purkinje and granule cells.

Prognosis. Death few years after onset of dementia.

BIBLIOGRAPHY. Carter HR, Sukavajana C: Familial cerebello-olivary degeneration with late development of rigidity and dementia. Neurol (Minneapolis) 6:876–884, 1956

Eadie MJ: Cerebello-olivary atrophy (Holmes type). In Vinken PJ, Bruyn GW (eds): Handbook of Clinical Neurology, vol 22, pp 411–412. Amsterdam, North-Holland, 1975

CARTILAGE-HAIR HYPOPLASIA

Synonyms. CHH; McKusick metaphyseal chondrodysplasia; metaphyseal dysplasia type A II.

Symptoms. Both sexes affected; disproportionate number of females; onset at birth. Motor milestones normal; frequent infections (bacterial, viral), malabsorption syndrome. Severe myopia. Normal intelligence.

Signs. At birth, short limbs; final height less than 150 cm. Head normal; hair sparse, silky, fine, brittle, short; in males thin silky beard; eyebrows and eyelashes sparse. Joint hypermobility with inability to fully extend elbow; telescoping of the fingers (by pulling them) fingernails short and wide. Foot may be inverted because of overlong fibula. Chest deformity. Abdomen protuberant with prominent veins. High pitched voice in males; delayed hair development in females.

Etiology. Unknown; autosomal recessive inheritance with reduced penetrance.

Pathology. Biopsy of costochondral junction shows achondroplastic-like changes. Lack of pigmented core in hair. Congenital megacolon. Signs of chronic otitis and pulmonary infections. Occasionally, avascular necrosis of femoral head.

Diagnostic Procedures. *Blood.* Normal; neutropenia and abnormal cellular immunity reported in some cases. *X-ray.* In younger patients metaphyseal changes of long bones (irregular sclerosis and cysts; femoral bowing).

Therapy. Medical (antibiotics and treatment of malabsorption) and orthopedic. Leukocyte interferon.

Prognosis. Life span reduced.

BIBLIOGRAPHY. Maroteaux P, Savart P, Lefebre J, et al: Le formes partielles de la dysostose metaphysaire. Presse Med 71:1523–1526, 1963
Perheentupa MO, Kaitila I: Growth of patients with cartilage-hair hypoplasia. March of Dimes Clin Genet Conf Baltimore July 10–13, 1988
Le Merer M, Maroteaux P: Cartilage-hair hypoplasia in infancy: A misleading chondrodysplasia. Eur J Pediatr 150:847–851, 1991

CASSIRER

Synonyms. Acroasphyxia; acrocyanosis; Crocq; Curtius II.

Symptoms. Prevalent in females; onset in peripuberal age. Asymptomatic, or cold or sweating (or both) of extremities, aggravated or caused by cold exposure, emotions. Occasionally relieved by warmth. Paresthesias frequently accompany other symptoms. In some cases, instead of paresthesias, hypoesthesia (anesthetic form) is present.

Signs. Persistent dusky, mottled blue or reddish discoloration of hands and feet, occasionally of ears and nose. Lifting the extremities reduces the cyanosis; absence of frank edema; presence of tissue succulence.

Etiology. Unknown; family history frequently reported. Venular atonia, accompanied by arteriolar hypertony. Cold, humidity, emotion considered as causes. Neurovegetative disturbance, hormonal imbalance have also been considered but not proved.

Pathology. Functional condition. Increase in interstitial fluid. In prolonged chronic cases, possible muscular atrophy and connective tissue proliferation.

Diagnostic Procedures. *Diaphragmatic irides test.* Pressure on acrocya-

nosis zone causes anemia, which regresses slowly and progressively from the edges as a closing diaphragm, as opposed to normal tissue, where color returns to entire area at the same time.

Therapy. Protection from cold. No curative treatment.

Prognosis. Spontaneous remission around the age of 20–25 years; seldom, persistence to advanced age; first pregnancy frequently causes disappearance or marked improvement.

BIBLIOGRAPHY. Cassirer R: Die Vasomotorischtrophiscen. Neurosen Berlin, Karger, 1901
Curtius F, Kruger KH: Das vegetativendoktrine Syndrom der Frau. München, Urban et Schwarzenberg, 1952
Frankel DH, Larson RA, Lorincz Al: Acrolivedosis: A sign of myeloproliferative diseases. Arch Dermatol 123:921–924, 1987
Champion RH: Reactions to cold. In In Champion RH, Burton JL, Ebling FJG (eds): Rook/Wilkinson/Ebling Textbook of Dermatology, 5th ed, p 836. Oxford, Blackwell Scientific, 1992

CAST

Synonym. Dorph; Willet.

Symptoms and Signs. Occurs in patients wearing body casts for orthopedic reasons. Prolonged nausea; repeated vomiting.

Etiology and Pathology. Mechanical compression of fourth portion of duodenum by superior mesenteric artery, resulting in gastric and duodenal dilatation. Intermittent symptoms owing to the fact that flatus intermittently passes.

Diagnostic Procedures. *Blood.* Hypokalemic alkalosis; hypovolemia. *Electrocardiography. X-ray.* Dilated duodenum; linear obstruction at the level of duodenal crossing of superior mesenteric vessels. Presence of a long air-fluid level.

Therapy. Removal of cast; surgical duodenal decompression. Early nasogastric suction.

Prognosis. If adequate treatment not instituted when condition becomes manifest, death from hypovolemia and hypokalemic alkalosis may result.

BIBLIOGRAPHY. Willet A: Fatal vomiting following applications of plaster of Paris-Bandage in case of spinal curvature. St Bartholomew's Hosp Rep 14:333–335, 1878
Dorph MH: The cast syndrome: Review of literature and report of a case. N Engl J Med 243:440–442, 1950
Edmond AS: Scoliosis. In Crenshaw AH (ed): Campbell's Operative Orthopedics, 7th ed, pp 3212–3215. St Louis, CV Mosby, 1987

CASTELLANI

Synonyms. Dermatosis papulosa nigra.

Symptoms and Signs. In blacks (Jamaica and Central America). At time of puberty, more frequent in black or dark brown females. Papules of the face on both malar regions, sparing lower face and chin.

Etiology. Unknown. Autosomal dominant inheritance considered as a variant of seborrheic keratoses.

Pathology. Nevoid developmental defects of pilosebaceous follicles acanthosis, hyperkeratosis.

Therapy. Not requested or diathermy or cautery.

BIBLIOGRAPHY. Castellani A: Observations on some diseases of Central America. J Trop Med Hyg 28:1–14, 1925
MacKie RM: Epidermal skin tumors. In Champion RH, Burton JL, Ebling FJG (eds): Rook/Wilkinson/Ebling Textbook of Dermatology, 5th ed, p 1467. Oxford, Blackwell Scientific, 1992

CASTLEMAN

Synonyms. Lymphoma Castleman; giant lymph-node hyperplasia; angiofollicular lymph node hyperplasia.

Symptoms. First type asymptomatic or second type with constitutional symptoms suggesting collagen disease or various other conditions. Myasthenia gravis, nephrosis, amyloidosis, peripheral neuropathy, Horton.

Signs. The first type, mediastinal mass. The second type, localized adenopathy.

Etiology. Unknown. Systemic. Reactive proliferation of beta lymphocytes. Possible relationship with diseases of plasmacellular type, resulting from faulty immune regulation.

Pathology. Two histologic subtypes that may overlap: hyaline-vascular type (in 80–90% of cases and a plasma cell type [10–20%]) localized or multicentric, generally good preservation of general architecture.

Diagnostic Procedures. *X-rays.* Evidence of localized mediastinal lymph node hyperplasia or of other stations. *Blood.* Laboratory features reminiscing "collagen disorder": anemia, hyperglobulinemia, etc.

Therapy. Radiotherapy.

Prognosis. Chronic course with exacerbation and remission; median survival associated with multicentric type is approximately 30 months; in 25% of cases presenting either B-cell lymphoma or Kaposi sarcoma.

BIBLIOGRAPHY. Castleman B, Inverson L, Pardo Menendez V: "Localized mediastinal lymphonode hyperplasia resembling thymoma." Cancer 9:822–830, 1956
Frizzera G, Massarelli G, Banks PM, et al: A systemic Lymphoproliferation disorder with morphologic features of Castleman's disease. Am J Surg Pathol 7:211–231, 1983
Greer JP, Macon WR, List AF, et al: Non-Hodgkin lymphomas. In Lee GR, Bithel TC, Foerster J, et al (eds): Wintrobe's Clinical Hematology, 9th ed, pp 2092–2093. Philadelphia, Lea & Febiger, 1993

CATAPLEXY

Synonyms. Henneberg (C); tonelessness.

Symptoms. Both sexes affected; onset all ages. Following strong emotions (laughter, fright, anger), and, usually following sleep attacks (seldom preceding them): sudden brief attacks of severe muscle weakness and tone loss; consciousness retained; light attacks may be limited to leg weakness; dropping of jaw; in severe form, total inability to move and total helplessness. Absence of jerking or twitching. Seldom, especially at onset of condition or after medication discontinuation. Status cataplexicus lasting hours.

Signs. Skin color, eye and tendon reflexes normal (may be absent during attacks).

Etiology. Unknown. Possibly a genetically determined susceptibility to the condition. Cataplexy, Narcolepsy (see Gelineau), hypnagogic paralysis (see Rosenthal), hallucinations constitute a clinical tetrade.

Therapy. Imipramine (25mg four times daily) clomipramine (10 mg daily). Second choice in case of failure: protriptyline (15–60 mg daily) or viloxazine (100–300 mg daily).

Prognosis. Attack spontaneous resolves within one to a few minutes. Recurrences at interval of days or weeks. Once started, usually in two-thirds of patients, the condition lasts for life. May occur occasionally in normal individuals without recurrences.

BIBLIOGRAPHY. Mitchell SW: On some of the disorders of sleep. Virginia Med Monthly 2:769–781, (Feb) 1876
Westphal C: Eigetuemlizhe mit Einschlafen verbundene Anfaelle. Arch Psychiat Nervenkr 7:631–635, 1877

Rosenthal C Ueber das verzoegerte psychomotorische Erwachen, seine Entstehung und seine nosologische. Bedeutung Arch Psychiat Berlin 81:159–171, 1927
Wilson SAK: Neurology, pp 1545–1560. London, Arnold, 1940
Passonant P: The history of narcolepsy. In Guilleminault C, Dement WC, Passonant P (eds): Narcolepsy, pp 3–13. New York, Spectrum, 1976
Adams RD, Victor M: Principles of Neurology, 5th ed, pp 345–347. New York, McGraw-Hill, 1993

CATATONIC SCHIZOPHRENIA

Synonyms. Schizophrenia catatonic.

Symptoms. Onset acute in 60% of cases; in 40% chronic progressive decrease of interest, apathy, lack of concentration, stupor mutism, inactivity, commands resisted, food disinterest, incontinence or urine and feces retention. In spite of apparent absence, patients are aware of environment and happenings. Spontaneous remission and possible recurrent periods of excitement, during which tendency to suicide or homicide may became manifest.

Signs. Vacant expression of face, lip pursed, sitting or assuming supine position for hours without motion; occasionally catalepsy. Painful stimulation does not cause reaction.

Etiology. Classified as a schizophrenic syndrome, however, this set of symptoms is now referred more to the manic-depressive group of diseases.

Therapy. Intravenous sodium amytal may abort symptomatology.

Prognosis. Progressing with alternating phases of remission.

BIBLIOGRAPHY. Kraeplin E: Dementia precox and paraphrenia. Barlrey RM (trans), Roberson GM (ed): Edinburgh, Livingstone 1919
Adams RD, Victor M: Principles of Neurology, 5th ed, p 1333. New York, McGraw-Hill, 1993

CAT CRY

Synonyms. LeJeune; B1 deletion; Cri du chat; chromosome 5 short arm deletion; del (5p); 46XX.

Symptoms. Strange high-pitched plaintive cry by an infant, similar to the cry of a cat. Growth retardation; mental retardation.

Signs. Microcephaly; oblique palpebral fissures; epicanthus; moon facies; low-set ears; abnormal palmar dermatoglyphs. Occasionally, micrognathia and strabismus; laryngeal abnormalities (small larynx, small epiglottis). Variable congenital heart disease.

Etiology. Congenital abnormality; de novo deletion of a portion of short arm of chromosome number 5 in the area of p14 to 15, or unbalanced translocation inherited from a carrier parent (15%).

Diagnostic Procedures. *Chromosome study.* Of patient and parents. *Dermatoglyphics.*

Prognosis. Compatible with life, but reduced life span. Mental retardation is invariably severe; speech development is slow. The IQ is most commonly in the 20–30 range. Most patients remain short and underweight, and almost all are microcephalic.

BIBLIOGRAPHY. LeJeune J, Lafourcade J, Berger R, et al: Trois cas de délétion partielle du bras court d'un chromosome 5. C R Acad Sci (D) Paris 257:3098–3102, 1963
MacIntyre MN, Staples WI, Lapolla J, et al: The "cat cry" syndrome. Am J Dis Child 108:538–542, 1964
Wilkins LE, Brown JA, Wolf B: Psychomotor development in 65 home-reared children with cri-du-chat syndrome. J Pediatr 97:401–405, 1980
Gorlin RJ, Cohen MM, Levin LS: Syndromes of Head and Neck, pp 48–49. New York, Oxford, 1990

CAT-EYE

Synonyms. Schachenmann; Schmid-Fraccaro; anal atresia–coloboma iris; partial G-trisomy; trisomy, or tetrasomy 22pter–q11; ocular coloboma–imperforate anus; CES. Coloboma of iris-anal atresia.

Symptoms and Signs. Present from birth. Variable growth deficiency. Mild mental deficiency. Mild hypertelorism; microphthalmos; antimongoloid slant of palpebrae; inferior strabismus; vertical iris coloboma (cat-eye gives the name to the syndrome); cataract; choroidal coloboma. Bilateral prearicular fistulas; umbilical hernia. Anal atresia; occasionally, retrovestibular fistula. Occasionally, heart and kidney malformations.

Etiology. Autosomal dominant inheritance (?). Duplication of q11 region of chromosome 22.

Prognosis. When associated with major chromosomal abnormalities, stillborn or short survival.

BIBLIOGRAPHY. Schachenmann G, Schmid W, Fraccaro M, et al: Chromosomes in coloboma and anal atresia. Lancet 2:290, 1965

Schmid W, Fraccaro M: The cat eye syndrome. Presented at Fourth Conference of Mammalian Cytology and Somatic Cell Genetics, Williamsburg, VA, 1969

Schinzel A, Schmid W, Fraccaro M, et al: The "Cat-eye syndrome": Dicentric small marker chromosome probably derived from a No 22 (tetrasomy 22pter q 11) associated with a characteristic phenotype. Report of 11 patients and delineation of clinical picture. Hum Genet 57:148–158, 1981

Ward J, Sierra IA, D'Croz E: Cat eye syndrome associated with aganglionosis of the small and large intestine. J Med Genet 26:647–648, 1989

CAT SCRATCH

Synonyms. Petzetakis; Debré; Foshay–Mollaret cat-scratch fever; regional nonbacterial lymphadenitis; benign inoculation lymphoreticulosis.

Symptoms. In temperate climate most cases occur in fall and winter. More frequent in children and young adults, in patients who have been scratched or bitten by cats or exposed to penetrating wounds (thorn, splinters, hooks) 7–14 days, or as long as 2 months, before symptoms appear. Slight fever; headache; chills; backache; anorexia; abdominal pain. Alteration of mental status and convulsions, with favorable final prognosis.

Signs. Small area of ulceration surrounded by erythema; vesicles; pustules; regional lymph nodes greatly enlarged, tender with red, hot skin, later (25%) becoming fluctuant; absence of lymphangitis. Spleen occasionally palpable.

Etiology. Caused by a small gram-negative bacterium, the Afipia felis.

Pathology. Lymph node, reticuloendothelial hyperplasia, necrotic centers; irregular microabscesses surrounded by reticular endothelial cells, fibroblasts, macrophages; evolving colliquation.

Diagnostic Procedures. *Hanger–Rose skin test.* Positive. *Rice–Hyde test.* (Incubation of white blood cells with cat-scratch disease skin test antigen). Positive. *Blood.* Slight elevation of sedimentation rate. Slight elevation of eosinophils. *Biopsy.* See Pathology.

Therapy. Aspiration of pus; no incision if liquefaction of lymph node. Antibiotics ineffective.

Prognosis. Fever lasts 2–3 weeks, lymphadenopathy sometimes several months. If sinus complication, encephalitis of variable severity that passes without sequelae.

BIBLIOGRAPHY. Petzetakis M: Monoadénite subaiguë multiple de nature inconnue. Soc Med Athens 16:229, 1935

Debré R, et al: La maladie des griffes de chat. Bull Med Soc Hôp Paris 66:760–769, 1950

Carithers HA: Cat-scratch disease: An overview based on a study of 1200 patients. Am J Dis Child 139:1124–1133, 1985

Carithers HA, Margileth AM: Cat-scratch disease. Acute encephalopathy and other neurologic manifestations. AJDC 145:98–101, 1991

Weatherall DJ, Ledingham JGG, Warrell DA (eds): Oxford Textbook of Medicine, 3rd ed, pp 745–747. Oxford, Oxford Med Pub, 1996

CATEL-MANZKE

Synonyms. Hyperphalangy-clinodactyly of index. Pierre Robin. Pierre-Robin-hyperphalangy-clinodactyly; index finger anomaly-Pierre Robin.

Symptoms and Signs. Mostly in male. Pierre Robin typical signs (see) with anomaly of both indexes. (Both indexes anomaly: accessory ossicle at the base causing ulnar deviation). Also reported in a case dislocatable knees.

Etiology. X-linked recessive inheritance.

BIBLIOGRAPHY. Catel W: Differentialdiagnose von Krankheitssymptomen bei Kindern und Jugendlichen, vol 1, 3rd ed, pp 218–220. Stuttgart, Thiene, 1961

Manzke H: Symmetrische Hyperphalangie des zweiten Fingers durch ein akzessorisches Metarcapale. Fortschir Roentgenst 105:425–427, 1996

Thompson EM, Wintez RM, Williams MJH: A male infant with Catel-Manzke syndrome and dislocable knees. J Med Genet 23:271–273, 1986

CAUCHOIS–EPPINGER–FRUGONI

Synonyms. Opitz (Z); Frugoni; fibrosplenomegaly (congestive); thrombophlebitic splenomegaly. See Banti and Hypersplenism.

Symptoms and Signs. Both sexes affected; onset at all ages. Low-grade or high temperature; abdominal discomfort; "dragging" feeling on left abdominal quadrant. Splenomegaly.

Etiology. Thrombophlebitis of splenic vein.

Diagnostic Procedures. See Banti and Hypersplenism.

Therapy. Antibiotics; anticoagulants; surgery.

Prognosis. Guarded.

BIBLIOGRAPHY. Opitz Z: Zur Kenntnis der thrombophlebitischen Splenomegalie. Jahr Zinderh 107:211–222, 1925

Frugoni C: La splénomegalie thrombophlébitique. Rev Belg Sci Med 10:227–236, 1938

Coon WW: Splenectomy for splenomegaly and secondary hypersplenism. World J Surg 9:437–443, 1985

Athens JW: Disorders primarily involving the spleen. In Lee GR, Bithel TC, Foerster J, et al (eds): Wintrobe's Clinical Hematology, 9th ed, pp 1711–1713. Philadelphia, Lea & Febiger, 1993

CAUDA EQUINA

Synonyms. Chronic arachnoiditis—cauda equina; claudication of cauda equina; filum terminale—cauda equina; pseudoclaudication; conus medullaris; anogenital-vesicle; sacral, including Verbiest; and tethered cord.

Symptoms and Signs. Intense pain in small of back, sciatic region, or perineum. Pain may be unilateral at first (hemicaudal syndrome), but becomes bilateral soon (bilateral sciatica diagnostic of spinal tumor). Sphincter disorders (see Neurogenic bladder syndromes). Flaccid paralysis of gluteal and leg muscles; eventually atrophy and fibrillation. Achilles tendon reflex absent. Occasionally, vascular malformation or lymphosarcoma may infiltrate the region without giving neurologic symptoms but only spasm and shortening of hamstring muscles. A particular variety of this syndrome is represented by the intermittent claudication of the cauda equina (Verbiest), symptoms appearing after walking and usually owing to protrusion of lumbar disk. An acute and a chonic form are considered.

Etiology.   Tumors or other causes (trauma) compressing or infiltrating cauda equina region.

Pathology.   See Signs and Etiology.

Diagnostic Procedures.   *X-ray. Myelography. Cystometrogram. CT scan.*

Therapy.   Surgical decompression.

Prognosis.   Depends upon etiology.

BIBLIOGRAPHY. Dejerine J: La claudication intermittente de la moelle épinière. Presse Med 2:981–984, 1911

Roussy G, Lhermitte J: Le Blesseurs de la Moelle et de la Queue de Cheval. Paris, 1918

Verbiest H: A radicular syndrome from developmental narrowing of the lumbar vertebral canal. J Bone Joint Surg (Br):36:230–237, 1954

Kavanaugh GJ, Svien HJ, Holman CB, et al: "Pseudoclaudication" syndrome produced by compression of the cauda equina. JAMA 206:2477–2481, 1968

Adams RD, Victor M: Principles of Neurology, 5th ed, p 1022. New York, McGraw-Hill, 1993

Weatherall DJ, Ledingham JGG, Warrell DA (eds): Oxford Textbook of Medicine, 3rd ed, pp 3907–3908. Oxford, Oxford Med Pub, 1996

CAUHEPE-FIEUX

Symptoms.   Functional lateral deviation of the jaw.

Etiology.   Persistence of infantile type of deglutition.

BIBLIOGRAPHY. Moortgat P: Syndromes a Noms Propres. Paris, J Prélat, 1966

CAUSALGIA

Synonym.   Traumatic erythromelalgia; erythromelalgia traumatic. See also Mitchell I syndrome.

Symptoms.   Complication in 3% of cases of major nerve injuries. Paroxysmal severe burning pain may localize and especially affect palm of hand or sole of foot. Aggravated by physical and emotional stimuli, cold and dryness; relieved by warmth and humidity.

Signs.   Skin hyperesthetic, often hypoalgesic when tested, cold, smooth, devoid of hairs, discolored, flossy edematous, hyperhydrotic. Trophic changes on nails, curved at the end, brittle. Stiffness of joints.

Etiology.   Incomplete lesions of nerve, usually median and sciatic (60%). Irritation of unsevered sensory fibers; neuritis of periarterial sympathetic fibers.

Pathology.   Incomplete lesion of nerve; atrophied muscles of affected part; atrophy of small bones.

Diagnostic Procedures.   *X-ray.* Atrophy of small bones. *Electromyography. Nerve conduction studies.* Tinel sign. *Sweat test. Skin resistance test. Electrical stimulation.*

Therapy.   Wet dressing for symptomatic relief. Sympathetic ganglia block with procain for temporary relief. Sympathectomy in cases that respond to block.

BIBLIOGRAPHY. Mitchell SW, Morehouse GR, Keen WW: Gunshot Wounds and Other Injuries of the Nerves. Philadelphia, JB Lippincott, 1864

Schott GD: Mechanism of causalgia and related clinical conditions. Brain 109:717, 1986

Schwartzman RJ, McLellant TL: Reflex sympathetic dystrophy: A review. Arch Neurol 44:555, 1987

Adams RD, Victor M: Principles of Neurology, 5th ed, p 1161. New York, McGraw-Hill, 1993

Klippel JH, Dieppe PA: Rheumatology, pp 7.38.1, 7.38.3. St Louis, CV Mosby, 1995

CAVITARY MESENTERIC LYMPH NODE

Symptoms and Signs.   Variable abdominal complaints according to basic condition.

Etiology.   In 50% celiac disease; 25% nonspecific villous atrophy of small bowel; rest miscellaneous conditions.

Pathology.   Mesenteric or retroperitoneal adenopathy, reactive hyperplasia and cavitation of lipid-rich lymph nodes.

Diagnostic Procedures.   *Abdominal. CT scan.* Enlarged mesenteric and retroperitoneal masses of decreased attenuation with or without fluid levels.

Therapy.   According to basic condition.

Prognosis.   According to basic condition.

BIBLIOGRAPHY. Simmonds JP, Rosenthal FD: Lymphoadenopathy in celiac disease. Gut 22:756–758, 1981

Rubesin SE, Laufer I: Radiographic findings in small bowel diseases causing malabsoption. In Haubrich WS, Schaffner F, Berk JE (eds): Bockus Gastroenterology, 5th ed, vol 2, pp 1017–1018. Philadelphia, WB Saunders, 1995

CAYLER

Synonyms.   Asymmetric crying facies—cardiac defect; cardiofacial defect; crying facies—cardiac defect; depression anguli oris muscle.

Symptoms and Signs.   Appears in both sexes; present at birth. Asymmetric crying facies (especially right side); in 5–10% of cases copresence of symptoms and signs of cardiac defect (especially ventricular septal type) associated more or less with variable other anomalies (vertebral; renal; limb).

Etiology.   Unknown. It seems that right-sided asymmetric crying facies is associated with cardiac defect; in left-sided form the association is much less frequent, although left-sided form is much more frequent. Possibly autosomal dominant inheritance.

Pathology.   Facial asymmetry owing to partial agenesis of depressor anguli oris muscle. Cardiac defects.

BIBLIOGRAPHY. Cayler GG: Cardiofacial syndrome. Congenital heart disease and facial weakness, a hitherto unrecognized association. Arch Dis Child 44:69–75, 1969

Perlman M, Reisner SH: Asymmetric crying facies and congenital anomalies. Arch Dis Child 48:627–629, 1973

Perrin P, Worms AM, Marcon F, et al: Le syndrome cardio-faciale de Cayler. A propos de 19 observations. Arch Fr Pediatr 46:257–261, 1989

CEBOCEPHALY

Term derived from name of Cebus monkey. See Arhinencephalia.

Symptoms and Signs.   Hypotelorism; flat incomplete nose; full cheeks; median nostrils; no palate or cleft lips; upper lip forming semicircle with insufficiently developed philtrum and labial tubercle.

Etiology. See Arhinencephaly.

Pathology. Usually halobaroprosencephaly.

BIBLIOGRAPHY. Klopstock A: Familiaerws Vorkommen von Cyklopie und Arrhinencephalie. Mschr Geburtsh Gynaek 56:59–71, 1921
Cohen MM Jr: Haloprosencephaly revisited. Am J Dis Child 127:597, 1974

CEELEN-GELLERSTEDT

Synonyms. Brown pulmonary induration; pulmonary idiopathic hemosiderosis; IPH; essential brown induration lung, immune/idiopathic alveolar hemorrhage (IAH). This condition may be idiopathic or associated with Churg-Strauss, Wegener, Goodpasture, or drugs and chemicals. Pneumohemorrhagic anemia; anemia pneumohemorrhagica (see all). However, it was defined before clinical introduction of antibasement membrane assays, so many cases were misdiagnosed.

Symptoms. Prevalent in males; occurs mostly in childhood; onset sudden. Recurrent episodes of cough, dyspnea, hemoptysis; occasionally, recurrent fever, and abdominal pain.

Signs. Skin pale; sometimes jaundice, and cyanosis. Occasionally, clubbing of fingers and enlargement of spleen.

Etiology. Unknown; recurrent lung hemorrhages; possibly immune reaction. Considered a variety of Goodpasture syndrome, especially in adult form.

Pathology. Hemorrhages and fibrosiderosis of lungs; no generalized hemosiderosis. Lymphoreticular system: changes compatible with immunodeficiency.

Diagnostic Procedures. Exclude other autoimmune condition. *Blood.* Hypochromic anemia; bilirubin increased; normal clotting tests; late secondary polycythemia, decreased gamma-A globulin. *X-ray of lung.* Ill-defined opacities rapidly changing; later diffuse reticulonodular pattern.

Therapy. Steroids of relative benefit in acute episode. Splenectomy has no significant effect.

Prognosis. Death in 3 years from hemorrhage or right heart failure.

BIBLIOGRAPHY. Ceelen W: Die Kreislaufstoerungen der Lungen. In Henke F, Lubarsch O: Handbuch der Speziellen pathologischen Anatomie und Histologie, vol 3, p 10. Berlin, Springer, 1931
Gellerstedt N: Uber die essentielle anaemisierende Form der braunen Lungeninduration. Acta Pathol Microbiol Scand (A) 16:386–400, 1939
Dewes W, Christ F, Overlack A, et al: Idiopathic Ceelen-Gellerstedt pulmononary hemosiderosis. ROFO Mar 146:360–362, 1987
Leatherman JW: Diffuse alveolar hemorrhage in immune and idiopathic disorders. In Lynch JP, De Remee RA: Immunologically mediated pulmonary diseases, p 473. Philadelphia, JB Lippincott, 1991

CENANI-LENZ

Synonyms. Syndactylysm Cenani. See Apert.

Symptoms and Signs. Both sexes. Syndactyly similar to that of Apert (see) plus short ulna and radius with fusion; disorganized phalangeal development; metacarpal fusion. Feet less affected.

Etiology. Autosomal recessive inheritance.

BIBLIOGRAPHY. Liebnam L: Ueber gleichzeitiges Vorkommen von Gliedmassendefekten und osteosklerotischen Systemerkrukung. Ztsch Meusch Vererbungs-und Kostitutionslehre 21:697–703, 1938
Cenani A, Lenz W: Totale syndactylie und totale radioulnare synostose bei zvei Bruedern. Ein Beitrag zur Genetik der Syndactylien Ztschr. Kinderhk 101:181–190, 1967

Pfeiffer RA, Meisel-Stosiek M: Present nosology of the Cenani-Lenz type of syndactyly. Clin Genet 21:74–79, 1982

CENTRAL CORD

Synonyms. Acute central cervical spinal cord injury; central cervical cord.

Symptoms and Signs. After hyperextension injuries in patients with cervical spondylosis or narrow spinal canals. Headache, neck pain, severe burning sensation of face, neck and arms and hands. Stiff neck, spasms of cervical muscles. Tenderness on percussion of back of neck may be present. Dysesthesia of face, usally sparing the central portion; pain in throat and on swallowing. Decrease of strength of deltoid muscles and muscles of arms; tendon reflexes normal or decreased. Slow and gradual improvement of symptoms and signs with rest.

Etiology and Pathology. Selective gray matter vulnerability to cervical trauma usually owing to hyperflexion injury of the neck with anterior compression of the cord at the craniovertebral junction. According to some authors possibility of vascular involvement.

Diagnostic Procedures. *Neurological examination.* See Symptoms and Signs. *Cervical CT and MRI.* Evidence of compression on cord by bony structures (odontoid process), kinking of craniovertebral junction.

Therapy. Rest. Immobilization of neck.

Prognosis. Good with therapy.

BIBLIOGRAPHY. Schneider RC, Cherry G, Pantek H: The syndrome of acute central cervical spinal cord injury. J. Neurosurg 11:546–576, 1954
McGoldrick JM, Marx JA: Traumatic central cord syndrome in a patient with os odontoideum. Ann Emerg Med 18:1358–1361, 1980
Chang HS: Cervical central cord syndrome involving the spinal trigeminal nucleus: A case report. Surg Neurol 44:236–240, 1995

CEREBELLAR ATAXIA–HYPOGONADISM

Synonyms. Holms (G) I; hypogonadotropic hypogonadism—cerebellar ataxia; LHRH deficiency—ataxia; see Boucher-Neuhauser.

Symptoms and Signs. Association of cerebellar syndrome (Marie ataxia, Friedreich ataxia, or neocerebellar) with primary hypogonadism. Partial or total failure of pituitary to stimulate gonadal development at puberty.

Etiology. Syndrome does not represent a homogeneous group. Not known if nervous and endocrine disorders are genetically determined or only fortuitously linked or if pituitary insufficiency is owing to primary dysgenesis or secondary to failure of gonadotropin excretion. Genetic determination of autosomal recessive type shown in some families.

Pathology. See Etiology.

Diagnostic Procedures. *Urine.* Gonodotropin excretion low; increased steroid excretion of a single fraction of adrenal origin reported in some cases. *CT scan. MRI brain scan.* Cerebellar and brain stem atrophy.

Therapy. Hormonal treatment.

Prognosis. Depends on severity of cerebellar syndrome.

BIBLIOGRAPHY. Holmes G: A form of familial degeneration of the cerebellum. Brain 30:466–488, 1907
Matthews WB, Rundle AT: Familial cerebellar ataxia and hypogonadism. Brain 87:463–468, 1964
Abs R, Van Vleymen E, Parizel PM, et al: Congenital cerebellar hypoplasia and hypogonadotrophic hypogonadism. J Neur Sci 98:259–265, 1990
Weatherall DJ, Ledingham JGG, Warrell DA (eds): Oxford Textbook of Medicine, 3rd ed, p 1683. Oxford, Oxford Med Pub, 1996

CEREBELLAR CATALEPSY

Symptoms. Those of cerebellar lesions.

Signs. With patient lying on his back, flex lower extremities at both hips and knees, lift lower extremities from bed and separate the feet. Initially, oscillation of trunk and legs, which later become abnormally fixed.

Etiology. Lesion of cerebellum.

BIBLIOGRAPHY. Babinski J: De l'equilibre volitionnel statique et de l'equilibre volitionnel cinetique. Rev Neurol (Paris) 10:470–474, 1902

Dow RS, Moruzzi G: Physiology and Pathology of the Cerebellum. Minneapolis, Univ of Minnesota Press, 1958

Adams RD, Victor M: Principles of Neurology, 5th ed, p 79. New York, McGraw-Hill, 1993

CEREBELLAR SUPERIOR PEDUNCLE

Synonym. Anterosuperior cerebellar artery.

Symptoms and Signs. Sudden onset without loss of consciousness. Homolateral hypotonia; asthenia; severe difficulty in walking (after ability is regained, leg placed unsteadily in abduction). Contralateral loss of sensibility to pain and temperature, including in head. Occasionally, contralateral loss of hearing. Hyperkinetic movements; palatal myoclonus may be observed occasionally. Horner syndrome occasionally observed. Normal findings: normal swallowing; no palatal weakness or anesthesia in glossopharyngeal zone of distribution; no aphonia; no pyramidal tract signs.

Etiology. Obstruction of anterosuperior cerebellar artery; thrombosis; less frequently, embolism. Neoplasia; inflammation.

Pathology. Gross softening of cerebellum on side affected or lesion of superior cerebellar peduncle (or both).

Diagnostic Procedures. *Arteriography. CT brain scan. MRI. Spinal tap.*

Therapy. Acute stage not major problem since swallowing is not a problem. Rehabilitation to overcome cerebellar deficiency. Surgery when indicated.

Prognosis. Variable according to extension and nature of lesions. Fair recovery frequent.

BIBLIOGRAPHY. Porot A: Hémorragie limitée du pédoncle cérébelleux superiéur droit; hémisyndrome cérébelleux direct. Lyon Méd 106:1137–1141, 1906

Dow RS, Moruzzi G: The Physiology and Pathology of the Cerebellum. Minneapolis, Univ of Minnesota Press, 1958

Adams RD, Victor M: Principles of Neurology, 5th ed, p 721. New York, McGraw-Hill, 1993

CEREBRAL CONCUSSION

Synonym. Brain concussion; see cerebral contusion and Homen.

Symptoms. Period of unconsciousness or disturbance in consciousness (confusion; dazing; stunning) usually lasting less than 5 minutes; and seldom more than 10, following a cerebral concussion. Complete recovery; amnesia consistent accompaniment.

Signs. None, or ecchymosis or discoloration at place of trauma; pallor; superficial respiration; mydriasis; loss of light reflexes; loss of cutaneous and tendon reflexes; hypotension; muscle flaccidity.

Etiology. Injury to head not associated with cerebral lesions such as hemorrhage, contusion, lacerations, or cerebral edema.

Pathology. No gross or microscopic evidence of injury to nervous tissue; small areas of cell loss in cortical areas; or nuclear masses of brain stem.

Diagnostic Procedures. *X-ray of skull. Spinal fluid. Electroencephalography.* Slow, decreased amplitude; occasionally, spikes. *CT brain scan. MRI.*

Therapy. Observation (2–3 days); respiratory assistance. According to symptoms, antiedema treatment (diuretics; corticosteroids; barbiturates).

Prognosis. Usually, complete recovery. Repeated concussion, however, results in the Homen syndrome (see); or if a subacute type of encephalitis develops, the sequelae is named Friedmann syndrome. In children, after minor head injury, it is possible to have a lucid interval with vomiting and mild shock, followed by stupor and recovery in 24 hours. This condition has to be differentiated from the extradural hematoma.

BIBLIOGRAPHY. Gilbert MM: Etiology and treatment of postconcussion syndrome. Headache 8:57–61, 1968

Walt AJ, Wilson RF: Management of Trauma. Philadelphia, Lea & Febiger, 1975

Gennarem TA: Cerebral concussion and diffuse brain injury. In Cooper PR (ed): Head Injury, pp 108–124. Baltimore, Williams & Wilkins, 1987

CEREBRAL CONTUSION

Synonym. Brain contusion. See also Homen and Brain.

Symptoms and Signs. Mild form. Loss of consciousness followed by drowsiness; headache; vertigo. Severe form. Loss of consciousness; hypotension; hypothermia; shallow breathing; arrhythmias; loss of reflexes; pupils unequal; ocular palsies. Later, delirium. Associated with fracture or laceration or both: paraplegia; focal signs; seizures; respiratory arrest.

Etiology. Direct head trauma or rebound.

Pathology. Brain edema from capillary oozing to intracerebral hemorrhages.

Therapy. Corticosteroids; diuretics (glycerol; mannitol); fluid restriction; if needed, respiratory assistance; if needed, intracranial pressure monitoring and surgery.

Prognosis. Variable according to extent of lesions.

BIBLIOGRAPHY. Graham DI, Adams JH, Gennarem TA: Pathology of brain damage in head injury. In Cooper PR (ed): Head Injury, pp 72–88. Baltimore, Williams & Wilkins, 1987

Adams RD, Victor M: Principles of Neurology, 5th ed, p 732. New York, McGraw-Hill, 1993

Weatherall DJ, Ledingham JGG, Warrell DA (eds): Oxford Textbook of Medicine, 3rd ed, p 4044. Oxford, Oxford Med Pub, 1996

CEREBRAL MALARIA

Many clinical varieties of this syndrome may be recognized; they may simulate many different conditions.

Symptoms and Signs. According to different types:

1. Meningitic
2. Monoplegic and hemiplegic
3. Myelitic
4. Ataxic
5. Disseminated sclerotic
6. Bulbar
7. Cerebellar
8. Polyneuritic
9. Korsakoff
10. Aphasic
11. Acute personality change

Etiology. Plasmodium falciparum.

Pathology. Cerebral edema; perivascular hemorrhages. Thrombosis of intracerebral vessels by pigment and clumped erythrocytes and endothelial proliferation (actual vessel occlusion denied by some authors).

Diagnostic Procedures. *Blood.* Demonstration of parasites. *Spinal tap.* Completely normal or slight increase in pressure. In some cases pleocytosis and protein increase.

Therapy. Quinine sulfate; pyrimethamine; sulfadiazine. If patient is comatose or vomiting, quinine intramuscularly and pyrimethamine and sulfadiazine by nasogastric tube. Diphenylhydantoin and sedative. Fluid balance. Relief of CSF increased pressure (diuretics, glycerol, mannitol, barbiturates, phenylhydantoin).

Prognosis. Severe. With early treatment, good. Usually, recovery without permanent neurologic sequelae.

BIBLIOGRAPHY. Brill NQ, Pellicano VL: Estivoautumnal malaria with frontal lobe syndrome. JAMA 121:1150–1152, 1943

Daroff RB, Deller JJ, Kastl AJ, et al: Cerebral malaria. JAMA 121:1150–1152, 1943

Scrascia E, Magalini SI: Trattamento rianimativo nelle sindromi renali e cerebrali da infestazione malarica. Minerva Anestesiol 38:329–334, 1972

De Francisci G, Magalini SI: Terapia intensiva nella malaria cerebrale. Rec Prog Med 74:873–874, 1983

Weatherall DJ, Ledingham JGG, Warrell DA (eds): Oxford Textbook of Medicine, 3rd ed, pp 846–847, 4124. Oxford, Oxford Med Pub, 1996

CEREBRAL RADIATION

Synonym. Brain radiation necrosis. See also Postirradiation vascular insufficiency.

Symptoms and Signs. Usually in patient with acromegaly resistant to radiation treatment, which is treated with heavy doses or multiple courses of ionizing radiation. Syndrome develops 7–12 months after last treatment. Variable symptomatology: headache; convulsions; paresis; impairment of memory; emotional lability; aphasia; stupor.

Etiology. Degenerative process of nervous cells owing to direct effect of radiation and, at least in part, to ischemic origin from postirradiation vasculopathy.

Pathology. Marked damage to neurons; glial degeneration and delayed reparative glial response. Proliferation of collagen; vascular endothelial proliferation; thrombosis; hyalinization of basement membranes.

Diagnostic Procedures. *Arteriography. CT brain scan. MRI. Spinal fluid.*

Therapy. Anticoagulants; craniotomy; removal of gliomatous tissue when feasible.

Prognosis. Progressive, often fatal condition.

BIBLIOGRAPHY. Fisher AW, Holfelder H: Lakales Amyloid im Gehirn eine Spätfolge von Rontgenbestrahlungen. Dtsch Z Chir 227:475–483, 1930

Peck FC Jr, McGovern ER: Radiation necrosis of the brain in acromegaly. J Neurosurg 25:536–542, 1966

AMA: A guide to the hospital management to injury arising from exposure to or involving ionizing radiation. AMA, 1985

CEREBROCOSTOMANTIBULAR

Synonyms. CCM; McNicholl; rib gap defects–micrognathia.

Symptoms. Both sexes affected; evident from birth. Perinatal asphyxia.

Primary or secondary mental handicap; indistinct speech; severe unusual cough.

Signs. Palatal defect; micrognathia; severe costovertebral defect (rib segmentation–fusion of ribs to vertebrae). In one case, elbow hypoplasia, defect of sacrum and coccyx. In another, webbing of the neck and area of skin redundance.

Etiology. Unknown. Autosomal dominant or recessive inheritance.

Pathology. See Signs. Malformed tracheal cartilages.

Diagnostic Procedures. *X-ray of chest. Ultrasound.* Deficiency of posterior portion of affected ribs (diagnostic).

Therapy. Symptomatic.

Prognosis. In most cases, early fatality.

BIBLIOGRAPHY. Smith DW, Theiler K, Schachenmann G: Rib-gap defect with micrognathia, malformed tracheal cartilages, and redundant skin: A new pattern of defective development. J Pediatr 69:799–803, 1966

McNicholl B, Egan-Mitchell B, Murray JP, et al: Cerebro-costo-mantibular syndrome: A new familial developmental disorder. Arch Dis Child 45:421–424, 1970

Schroer RJ, Meyer LC: Cerebro-costo-mandibular syndrome. Proc Greenwood Genet Center 4:55–59, 1985

Drossou-Agakidou V, Andreou A, et al: Cerebrocostomantibular syndrome in four sibs, two pair of twins. J Med Genet 28:704–707, 1991

CEROID LIPOFUSCINOSIS

Synonyms. Neuronal ceroid-lipofuscinosis juvenile type; juvenile cerebroretinal degeneration; amaurotic family juvenile idiocy. Includes (1) Santavuori-Haltia (see); (2) Jansky-Bielchovsky (see) (3) Spielmeyer-Vogt (see); (4) Kufs (see). Other synonyms: Batten (see); Unverricht-Lundborg. See also Pelizaeus-Merzbacher and Tay-Sachs.

BIBLIOGRAPHY. Batten FE: Cerebral degeneration with symmetrical changes in the maculae in two members of a family. Trans Opthalmol Soc UK 23:386–390, 1902

Vogt H: Ueber familiäre amaurotische Idiotie und verwandte Krankheitsbilder. Mschr Psychiat 18:161–71,310–57, 1905

Spielmeyer W: Klinische und anatomische Untersuchungen über einen besonderen Fall von amaurotischer Idiotie. Nissle Beitr Nerv Geistes Krh, Berlin, 1908

Gardiner M, Sandford A, Deadman M, et al: Batten disease (Spielmeyer-Vogt disease Juvenile onset neuronal ceroid-lipofuscinosis) gene (CLN3) maps to human chromosome 16. Genomics 8:387–390, 1990

CERVICAL AORTA

Symptoms. Vascular ring, dysphagia, dyspnea, stridor, brassy cough, usually occurring at the end of childhood or adolescent period. See Bayford-Autenrieth.

Signs. Pulsatile mass on the right side of neck above the clavicle; murmur and thrill over the mass; compression of pulsatile mass produces marked diminution or obliteration of femoral pulses.

Etiology. Aortic arch anomaly.

Pathology. Right aortic arch retained in cervical region; retroesophageal course; left common carotid artery originates from ascending aorta; right subclavian artery originates directly or through a common duct with right common carotid artery near apex of aorta arch; left subclavian artery originates distally to retroesophageal segments of aorta.

Diagnostic Procedures. *Esophagography.* Two-dimensional. *Echography with color flow imaging and Doppler.* Angiography seldom necessary.

Therapy. Removal of first rib on the right to make room for aortic growth and prevention of vascular symptoms and degenerative phenomena. Consider aortic resection and intrathoracic graft.

Prognosis. If not relieved, early degenerative phenomena of aorta wall, erosion, and possibly rupture.

BIBLIOGRAPHY. Beaven TED, Fatti L: Ligature of aortic arch in the neck. Br J Surg 34:414–416, 1946
Massumi R, Wiener L, Charif P: The syndrome of cervical aorta; report of a case and review of the previous cases. Am J Cardiol 11:678–685, 1963
McCue CM, Mauck HP Jr, Tingelstad JB, et al: Cervical aortic arch. Am J Dis Child 125:738–742, 1973
Van Mierop LHS, Kutsche LM: Embryology of Heart. In: Schlant RC, Alexander RW: Hurst's The Heart, 8th ed, pp 1722–1723. New York, McGraw-Hill, 1994

CERVICAL CORD ANTERIOR

Synonyms. Cervical cord, anterior.

Symptoms and Signs. Complete motor loss of pain and temperature differentiation below level of injury with spared deep touch, position, and vibratory sensation.

Etiology. Direct trauma from spinal hyperextension, hyperflexion extrusion of intervertebral disk, or secondary to lesion of anterior spinal artery system.

Therapy. Trial with corticosteroid immediately after trauma or surgery.

Prognosis. Complete paralysis and absolute loss of pain and temperature sensation lasts usually 48 hours but sensation is never recovered completely below the affected level.

BIBLIOGRAPHY. Schneider RC, Kaln EA: Chronic neurological sequelae of acute trauma to the spine and spinal cord. Part II: The syndrome of chronic anterior spinal cord injury or compression: herniated intervertebral discs. J Bone Joint Surg 41A:449–456, 1959
Adams RD, Victor M: Principles of Neurology, 5th ed, p 471. New York, McGraw-Hill, 1993
Weatherall DJ, Ledingham JGG, Warrell DA (eds): Oxford Textbook of Medicine, 3rd ed, pp 2959, 3906. Oxford, Oxford Med Pub, 1996

CERVICAL RIB

Synonym. First thoracic rib. See Thoracic outlet syndromes.

Symptoms. Usually appears in adult life after trauma to the shoulder, stretching of the arm, pregnancy. Usually unilateral (although supernumerary ribs may be bilateral) and more frequent in female patients. Pain on the ulnar border increased by movement; weakness of hand, arm, shoulder; numbness, tingling, and sensory loss on the same ulnar distribution.

Signs. Cyanosis; edema; coolness; spastic vasomotor; muscular atrophy; pulse weak on affected side; occasionally, bony mass palpable in supraclavicular fossa.

Etiology. Supernumerary cervical rib arising from seventh cervical vertebra, irritating the brachial plexus, restricting it between the rib and the scalenus anticus muscle. Autosomal dominant inheritance reported.

Pathology. Neuritis; atrophy of muscles involved.

Diagnostic Procedures. *Adson test.* Positive (costoclavicular and hyperadduction maneuvers). *X-ray.* Shows the supernumerary cervical rib(s).

Therapy. Proper support of shoulder with pillows may relieve syndrome without surgery. Surgery: section or removal inferior part of scalenus anticus. Differential diagnosis with cervical disk that may produce same syndrome.

Prognosis. Recovery with removal of compression.

BIBLIOGRAPHY. Willshire: Supernumerary first rib. Lancet 2:633, 1860
Murphy T: Brachial neuritis caused by pressure of first rib. Aust Med J 15:582–585, 1910
Weston WJ: Genetically determined cervical ribs: A family study. Br J Radiol 29:455–456, 1956
Holst S: Cervical rib and associated vascular complications. J Oslo City Hosp 13:173–182, 1963
Weatherall DJ, Ledingham JGG, Warrell DA (eds): Oxford Textbook of Medicine, 3rd ed, p 3903. Oxford, Oxford Med Pub, 1996

CERVICAL SPONDYLOTIC MYELOPATHY

Synonyms. Cervical disk degeneration, chronic; cord-compression-radiculopathy, myelopathic; hard disk. See Stookey.

Symptoms and Signs. In middle age (mean 53 years). Male to female ratio 4:1. Insidious onset from 1 week to 20 years (mean 1 year). Usually a wide-spaced gait may be the initial manifestation. Five different neurologic levels may be involved alone or in combination with cord and root symptoms causing spasticity (98%), weakness, spinothalamic deficits, post column deficits, small muscle atrophy, fasciculation, sphincter disturbances, local cervical and radicular pain, paresthesias, dermatosomal or segmental sensory deficits. The variability of symptoms combination brought to various subclassifications. For instance, subclassified as lateral or radicular; medial or spinal, combined medial-lateral; vascular syndromes; or as transverse lesion; motor system; central cord, the Brown Sèguard; and brachialgia syndrome.

Etiology. Chronic canal impingement usually by spondilotic spurs. Compression of anterior spinal artery or radicular supplying arteries may be major responsible factor. To be distinguished from the acute disk herniation often, related to a (sub)traumatic event.

Pathology. Cord and roots degeneration from altered vascular supply.

Diagnostic Procedures. *X-ray. CT scan. MRI. Neurologic evaluation. Electromyography.*

Therapy. Immobilization by a cervical collar.

Prognosis. No patients appear to return to a full normal state; seldom spontaneous regression, frequent slow, steady progression. Improvement obtained by treatment.

BIBLIOGRAPHY. Peet MM. Echols DH: Herniation of nucleus pulposus. Cause of compression of spinal cord. Arch Neurol Psychiatr 32:924–932, 1934
Brain WR: Rupture of the intervertebral disk in the cervical region. Proc R Soc Med 49:509, 1948
Montgomery DM, Brower RS: Cervical spondylotic myelopathy: Clinical syndrome and natural history. Orth Clin N Am 23:487–493, 1992

CERVIX, ANNULAR DETACHMENT OF

Synonym. Traumatic avulsion of cervix uteri.

Symptoms and Signs. Unusual bleeding after delivery of child. Detached cervix may be covering the head of the child: cardinal's sign. On inspection of the cervix, might see the partial circular tearing: bucket-handle detachment. Often on inspection, cervix is hanging by a strand of tissue.

Etiology. Predisposing factors are prolonged labor, cervical dystocia, more prevalent in primiparas, cephalopelvic disproportion, length of cervix (an unusually long cervix prevents the external os from opening in normal manner).

Pathology. The detachment of cervix may result in partial circular tearing, a bucket-handle detachment; the detached portion may be closely applied to child's head like a cardinal's cap, or may be found hanging by a strand of tissue after child's birth. Microscopic picture. Acute congestion; hemorrhage; edema; necrosis.

Therapy. Prevention. Early recognition and treatment of cervical dystocia. Treatment after detachment. If incomplete, pedicle divided between clamps and base transfixed. Culture from the vaginal vault, and prophylactic chemotherapy. In management of future pregnancies, elective cesarean section indicated.

Prognosis. *Mother.* Hemorrhage uncommon; puerperal sepsis responsible for a high maternal mortality. *Fetus.* Fetal mortality 30–40% primarily owing to failure of recognition of the cervical dystocia.

BIBLIOGRAPHY. Ingraham CB, Taylor ES: Spontaneous annular detachment of the cervix during labor. Am J Obstet Gynecol 53:873–877, 1947

Fliegner JR: Spontaneous annular detachment of the cervix. Med J Aust 1:438–441, 1968

Cunningham FG, MacDonald PC, Gant NF, et al (eds): Williams Obstetrics, pp 533–534. Englewood Cliffs, NJ, Prentice-Hall, 1993

CERVÒS-NAVARRO

Synonyms. Inflammatory reticuloendotheliosis; encephalitis Cervòs-Navarro.

Symptoms and Signs. Those of an acute, subacute, or chronic encephalitis.

Etiology. In the past considered as malignant; today considered as host reaction to different stimuli. Difficult to asses differences among a large group of alleged different entities that appear to be in most cases variants of one another.

Pathology. Perivascular infiltration with lymphocytes, reticuloendothelial and plasma cells, histiocytes, and argirophilic elements.

BIBLIOGRAPHY. Cervòs-Navarro J Beitrag zur Zytopathologie der Entzuendung im Zentralnervensystem Proc IIIrd Int Congr Neuropathol, Brussels, 1957

Hubert JWA: Tumors of the reticuloendothelial system. In Vinken PJ, Bruyn GW: Handbook of Clinical Neurology, vol 18 pp 234, 241. Amsterdam, North-Holland, 1975

CESTAN-CHENAIS

Synonym. Cestan II. Chenais; oblongata. Type I and II.

Symptoms and Signs. Pharyngolaryngeal or glossopharyngeal paralysis (Avellis'). Contralateral cerebellar hemiataxia; sensibility alterations; ipsilateral enophthalmos; ptosis, nystagmus; miosis (Babinski-Nageotte).

Etiology. Thrombosis; inflammation; neoplasia producing vertebral artery lesion (medially to posterior inferior cerebellar arteries and anterior spinal branches). Supported the existence of at least two genetic variants of the syndrome CMT I and II, whereas an X-linked form is designated as CMT 2 (numerology very confusing).

Pathology. Infarct lesion of lateral portion of medulla oblongata. See Etiology.

Diagnostic Procedures. *Arteriography. CT brain scan. MRI.*

Therapy. Depends upon etiology.

Prognosis. Depends upon etiology.

BIBLIOGRAPHY. Hoffman J: Ueber progressive neurotiscbe Muskelatrophie. Arch Psychiat Nervenkr 20:660, 1889

Cestan RJ, Chenais J: Du myosis dans certaines lésions bulbaires en foyer (hémiplégie du type Avellis associée au syndrome oculaire sympathique). Gaz d Höp 76:1229–1233, 1903

Berciano J, Combarros O, Figols J, et al: Hereditary motor and sensory neuropathy type II. Brain 109:879–914, 1986

CHANARIN-DORFMAN

Synonyms. Triglyceride storage–impaired long-chain fatty acid oxidation; ichthyotic–neutral lipid storage; ichthyosiform erythroderma–leukocyte vacuolization.

Symptoms and Signs. Both sexes. From infancy. Ichthyosis, hepatosplenomegaly. In some cases delayed development (in middle age) of cataracts, nystagmus, deafness, ataxia, areflexia.

Etiology. Multisystem nonlysosomal triglyceride storage, decreased oxidation of oleate. Possibly autosomal recessive inheritance.

Pathology. Triglyceride intracellular infiltration (not membrane enclosed) in many organs: liver, spleen, muscle, central nervous system, intestinal leukocytes.

Diagnostic Procedures. *Blood.* Hypertriglyceridemia; leukocytes: vacuolated. (Jordan's anomaly). Absence of ketone bodies on fasting. *Cerebrospinal fluid.* After onset of neurologic manifestation: increased protein. *Electromyography.* Mild primary myopathy.

Therapy. Diet with medium-chain triglycerides.

Prognosis. Diet reverses hepatosplenomegaly. Survival into adulthood with development of quoted manifestations.

BIBLIOGRAPHY. Dorfman ML, Hershko C, Eisenberg S, et al: Ichthyosiform dermatosis with systemic lipidosis. Arch Dermatol 110:261–266, 1974

Chanarin I, Patel A, Slavin G, et al: Neutral lipid storage disease: A new disorder with impaired long-chain fatty oxidation. Br Med J I:553–555, 1975

Williams ML, Koch TK, O'Donnell JJ, et al: Ichthyosis and neutral lipid storage disease. Am J Med Genet 20:711–726, 1985

Musumeci S, D'Agata A, Romano C, et al: Ichthyosis and neutral lipid storage disease. Am J Med Genet 29:377–382, 1988

CHANDLER (P.A.)

Synonyms. See also Iridocorneal endothelial and Cogan Reese.

Symptoms. Visual blurring.

Signs. Eccentric pupil. Corneal dystrophy and edema; atrophy of iris.

Etiology. Unknown.

Pathology. Glaucoma from occlusion of angle by anterior peripheral synechiae. Iris stromal atrophy, unilateral corneal edema, iridocorneal adhesions, normal or slightly raised intraocular pressure.

BIBLIOGRAPHY. Chandler PA: Atrophy of the stroma of iris, endothelial dystrophy, corneal edema and glaucoma. Am J Ophthamol 41:607–615, 1956

Yanoff M: Iridocorneal endothelial syndrome: unification of a disease spectrum. Surv Ophthalmol 24:1–2, 1979

Garner A, Klintworth GK (eds): Pathobiology of Ocular Disease: A Dynamic Approach, second ed, pp 459, 762, 777, 778, 1424. New York, Marcel Dekker, 1994

CHANDLER (S.A.)

Synonyms. Femoral head idiopathic necrosis; hip osteochondritis dissecans. See Epiphyseal ischemic necrosis, Koenig (F.), and observation hip.

Symptoms and Signs. Male predominance; onset in middle age. Unilateral or symmetric pain of the hip and occasionally of the knee.

Etiology. See Epiphyseal ischemic necrosis.

BIBLIOGRAPHY. Chandler SA: Aseptic necrosis of the head of the femur. Wisc Med J 35:583–618, 1936

CHANDRA-KHETARPAL

Synonym. Levocardia—bronchiectasis—sinus abnormality. See Kartagener.

Symptoms and Signs. Present from infancy. Repeated fever episodes with symptoms and signs of bronchiectasis. Evidence at physical examination of levocardia.

Etiology. Unknown; congenital malformation.

Pathology. Levocardia; bronchiectasis; paranasal sinus not developed.

Diagnostic Procedures. *X-ray of chest and skull. Bronchoscopy. Bronchography. Electrocardiography. Sputum culture.*

Therapy. Antibiotics. If feasible, surgery to excise part of the lung with bronchiectasis.

Prognosis. Repeated infectious episodes.

BIBLIOGRAPHY. Chandra RK, Khetarpal SK: Levocardia with bronchiectasis and paranasal sinus abnormalities. Indian J Pediar 30:78–80, 1963
Datta P: Chandra's syndrome. Lancet 2:1350–1351, 1968
Nugent EW, Plauth WH, Edwards JE, et al: The pathology, pathophysiology, recognition and treatment of congenital heart disease. In Schlant RC, Alexander RW, Hurst's The Heart, 8th ed, p 1808. New York, McGraw-Hill, 1994

CHARCOT ANGINA CRURIS

Synonyms. Angina cruris; angiosclerotic paroxystic myasthenia; intermittent claudication; claudication intermittens.

Symptoms and Signs. Observed, usually, in elderly persons. Pain, cramps, tension, weakness and temperature reduction of upper and, more frequently, lower extremities, which occurs after exercise and recedes after rest.

Etiology. Reduced vascular bed and blood supply not adequate to metabolic needs of tissues. Atherosclerosis; Moenckberg (see); Buerger (see); Leriche (see); other vasculopathic processes.

Diagnostic Procedures. *Angiography. Doppler.*

Therapy. Thrombolytic, acetylsalicylic acid. Vasodilators of doubtful benefit. According to the etiology; sympathectomy, bypass, arterial grafts.

Prognosis. Improved by treatment.

BIBLIOGRAPHY. Charcot JM: Sur la claudication intermittente observée dans un cas d'oblitération de l'une des artères iliaques primitives. C R Soc Biol (Paris) 5:225–258, 1858
Lindsay J Jr, De Bakey ME, Beall AC: Diagnosis of diseases of the aorta. In Schlant RC, Alexander RW: Hurst's The Heart, 8th ed, p 2177. New York, McGraw-Hill, 1994
Klippel JH, Dieppe PA: Rheumatology, p 2.7.1. St Louis, CV Mosby, 1995

CHARCOT-BOUCHARD ANEURYSM

Obsolete.

Symptoms and Signs. Those of a brain hemorrhage.

Etiology. Atheromatous process and not, as previously thought, an angioitis.

Pathology. Small spherical cortical hemorrhages and small dissecting aneurysm (described as genuine miliary aneurism) that in reality do not indicate a real aneurysmatic distension of defective arteries, but simply the presence of adventitial hematomas developed during an apoplectic crisis; in fact, vascular wall (intima and muscularis) are intact.

BIBLIOGRAPHY. Charcot JM, Bouchard C: Nouvelles reserches sur la pathogénie de l'hémorrhagie cérébrale Arch Physiol Norm. et Pathol (Paris) 1:11, 643, 725, 1868
Schwartz P: Apopletic lesions of brain in adults. In Vinken PJ, Bruyn GW: Handbook of Clinical Neurology, vol 11, pp 578–582, 587. Amsterdam, North-Holland, 1976
Weatherall DJ, Ledingham JGG, Warrell DA (eds): Oxford Textbook of Medicine, 3rd ed, pp 2534, 2956. Oxford, Oxford Med Pub, 1996

CHARCOT INTERMITTENT BILIARY FEVER

Synonyms. Charcot triad (according to gastroenterologists). Intermittent biliary fever; secondary cholangitis. Chronic acalculous cholangitis. See Cholangitis primary, sclerosing and Hanot-Roessle.

Symptoms. More frequent in females; onset in middle age. Recurrent episodes of dull or colicky pains in right hypochondrium radiating to the back, accompanied by chills and hyperthermia; nausea, vomiting, anorexia.

Signs. Weight loss; hepatomegaly, hepatalgia. Occasionally, subicterus.

Etiology. Infection of various extrahepatic ducts, enhanced by mechanical or functional obstruction, lithogenic bile and reduced gallbladder ejection.

Pathology. Purulent (or nonpurulent) inflammation of intrahepatic and extrahepatic ducts; dilatation above obstruction and bile stasis; variable hepatic cell damage.

Diagnostic Procedures. *Blood.* Acute stage leukocytosis; positive culture; hyperbilirubinemia; increased alkaline phosphatase and other enzymes. *Urine.* Bilirubinemia. *Scintigraphy. Cholangiography.* Splenic portography; angiography. *CT liver scan. Ultrasonography.*

Therapy. Antibiotics; antispastics; litholytic; surgery to be considered.

Prognosis. Spontaneous temporary remissions may characterize course according to degree of obstruction. Variability depends on treatment. In some cases, once hepatic damage has developed, it may tend to progress slowly, even after obstruction is removed and the infection cured.

BIBLIOGRAPHY. Slesinger MH, Fordtran JS: Gastrointestinal Disease, p 1314. Philadelphia, WB Saunders, 1978
Zeman RK: Non invasive imaging of the biliary tract. In Haubrich WS, Schaffner F, Berk JE (eds): Bockus Gastroenterology, 5th ed, p 2585. Philadelphia, WB Saunders, 1995

CHARCOT JOINTS

Synonyms. Neurogenic arthropathy; tabetic osteoarthropathy.

Symptoms. Prevalent in males; onset usually after 40 years of age; usually, insidious onset. Painful joint swelling (degree of discomfort disproportionally milder than degree of swelling). Other signs of neurologic abnormalities from basic condition frequently not reported by patient.

Signs. Joint (single or groups) swelling with effusion; initially, hypermobility, warmth, tenderness; followed by deformity, instability, coarse crepitation. On palpation, "bag of nuts."

Etiology. Initially associated with tabes dorsalis of syphilitic origin; other conditions responsible are diabetic neuropathy, syringomyelia, myelomeningocele, and various spontaneous or traumatic central and peripheral nervous system pathologies.

Pathology. Combination of destructive and hypertrophic changes; erosion of cartilage; destruction of menisci; loose body formation and osteophyte growth, which may extend to shaft of bone or into ligaments and muscle. Subluxation. Effusion frequently hemorrhagic; synovial inflammatory reaction.

Diagnostic Procedures. *X-ray.* See Pathology. *Blood. Spinal fluid.* Identification of primary pathology. See Etiology.

Therapy. Immobilization and reduction of patient weight. Surgical and orthopedic measures in accord with nature of basic condition and degree of lesion.

Prognosis. Usually, progressive condition; poorly responsive to specific and general types of treatment.

BIBLIOGRAPHY. Charcot JM: Sur quelques arthropathies qui paraissent dépendre d'une lésion du cerveau ou de la moelle épinère. Arch Physiol 1:161–178; 370–400, 1868
Jaspan JB, Green AJ: The neuropathies of diabetes. In De Groot LJ (ed): Endocrinology, 3rd ed, p 1555. Philadelphia, WB Saunders, 1995
Weatherall DJ, Ledingham JGG, Warrell DA (eds): Oxford Textbook of Medicine, 3rd ed, pp 2979, 3002. Oxford, Oxford Med Pub, 1996

CHARCOT-MARIE-TOOTH

Synonyms. Charcot-Marie-Tooth-Hoffman; Tooth; peroneal muscular atrophy; progressive neural muscular atrophy; motor sensory neuropathy, hereditary; HMSN. Type I and II.

Symptoms. Begins in puberty or early adult life. Abnormalities of gait or clumsiness in running, weakness, paresthesia in legs; absence of tendon deep reflexes; later weakness and atrophy of hands, then arms. Occasionally sensory changes.

Signs. Foot drop or clubfoot; atrophy progressing slowly from peroneal to other muscles of legs (stork legs or inverted champagne bottle). Atrophy progressing from hands (final claw hand appearance) to arms. Shoulders, hips, trunk well developed. Loss of deep sensibility and reflexes of parts affected.

Etiology. Unknown; hereditary (dominant or recessive, sex-linked inheritance). Siblings may show abortive form of the disease.

Pathology. Segmental demyelinization of peripheral nerves (e.g., peroneal, tibial); degenerative changes of anterior horn cells, dorsal columns; myopathic changes may be present.

Diagnostic Procedures. *Electromyography. Nerve conduction.* Two major categories CMT1 decreased motor nerve conduction; CMT2 normal. *Spinal fluid.* Normal; occasionally, slight increase in proteins. *X-rays.* Nerve root enlargement; muscle atrophy. Associated anomalies: scoliosis, vertebral anomalies; hip dysplasia, coxa valga.

Therapy. Orthopedic support.

Prognosis. Very slow progression; seldom totally incapacitating; frequently becomes stationary.

BIBLIOGRAPHY. Charcot JM, Marie P: Sur une forme particulière d'atrophie musculaire progressive, souvent familiare débutant pas les pieds et les jambes et atteignant plus tard les mains. Rev Med 6:97–138, 1886
Tooth HH: The Peroneal Type of Progressive Muscular Atrophy. London, Lewis, 1886
Ballabio A, Zoghbi HY: Charcot-Marie-Tooth disease and hereditary neuropathy with liability to pressure palsy. In Scriver CR, Beaudet AL, Sly WS, et al: The Metabolic and Molecular Bases of Inherited Disease, 7th ed, pp 4569–4574. New York, McGraw-Hill, 1995

CHARCOT TRIAD

According to neurologists. The triad consists of (1) nystagmus; (2) scanning speech; (3) intention tremor. This syndrome was considered pathognomonic for multiple sclerosis; however, it is seen only occasionally and in advanced cases of long duration.

BIBLIOGRAPHY. Charcot JM: Diagnostic des formes frustes de la sclérose en plaques. Prog Med 7:97–99, 1879

CHARCOT TRIAD II

According to gastroenterologists the triad consists of (1) biliary colic; (2) fever and chills; (3) jaundice; present in 50–75% of patients with acute cholangitis. (See Charcot intermittent biliary fever.)

CHARCOT-WILBRAND

Symptoms. Visual agnosia; agraphia; associated occasionally with Gerstmann (see).

Etiology. Lesion of the artery of the angular gyrus of dominant side.

BIBLIOGRAPHY. Charcot JM: Sur un Cas de Ceocite' Verbales. Ouvres Completes de Charcot. Paris, Delahaye Lecrosnier, 1887
Tyler HR: Cerebral disorders of vision. In Smith JL (ed): Neuro-Ophthalmology, vol 4. St Louis, CV Mosby, 1968
Sabiston DC, Textbook of Surgery, 14th ed, p 1066. Philadelphia, WB Saunders, 1991
Adams RD, Victor M: Principles of Neurology, 5th ed, pp 221–222. New York, McGraw-Hill, 1993

C.H.A.R.G.E

Synonyms. Coloboma, heart defects, atresia of the choane, retarded growth and development, genital hypoplasia (and), ear anomalies and/or deafness. See Cat eye.

Symptoms and Signs. Rare. From birth. *Eyes:* coloboma and/or microphthalmia, strabismus, iris defects, lens abnormalities. *Heart:* Tetralogy of Fallot (see), ventriculoseptal defect, endocardial cushion defect, pulmonary stenosis, aortic stenosis, etc. *Nose:* Atresia of choanae. *Genital:* Hypoplasia and/or urinary tract anomalies. *Ears:* Malformations and/or hearing loss. *Peripheral nervous system:* Unilateral VII nerve palsy. *Face:* Facial asymmetry, cleft lip and palate, pharyngeal incoordination and swallowing problems. *Limbs:* Short 5th fingers, syndactyly. *GI tract:* Tracheoesophageal fistula and esophageal atresia.

Etiology. No chromosome abnormalities reported, suggested derangement in migration of neural crest cells and caudal presumptive mesodermal cells between fifth and sixth weeks of gestation. Autosomal dominant, recessive and X-linked cases have been reported. May reflect a common phenotypic pathway for various genetic defects (genetic heterogeneity).

Pathology. See Symptoms and Signs.

Diagnostic Procedures. *Ocular examination. Slit lamp microscopy. ENT examination. Echocardiogram. Radiography. CT scan. MRI of skeleton.*

Therapy. Nutrition if swallowing difficulties. Ophtalmic followup for possible retinal detachment.

Prognosis. Life with mild to profound mental retardation.

BIBLIOGRAPHY. Lang J: Ueber Chanenatresie (Hereditaet derselben). Mschr Oherenheilk 46:970–1001, 1912
Hall BD: Choanal atresia and associated multiple anomalies. J Pediatr 95:395–398, 1979

Koletzko B, Majewski F: Congenital anomalies in patients with choanal atresia: CHARGE association. Eur J Pediatr 142:271–275, 1984

Kushnick T, Wiley JE, Palmer SM: Agonadism in 46 XY patient with CHARGE association. Am J Med Genet 42:96–99, 1992

CHARLES RUPPE

Synonyms. Eponym (obsolete) of French literature to indicate a form of fibrous monostotic dysplasia of mandible (ossifying fibroma).

BIBLIOGRAPHY. Hoboek A: Fibrous dysplasia, fibro-osteoma, osteoma of the facial bones and of the skull. Acta Radiol (Stockh) 36:97–113, 1951

CHARMAT

Obsolete. Eponym used to indicate a clinical African syndrome due to macroglobulinemia with splenomegaly.

BIBLIOGRAPHY. Charmat G, Demarchi J, Reynaud R, et al: Le syndrome splénomégalie avec macroglobulinémie. Un nouvel aspect des splénomégalies en Afrique Noire. Presse Med 67:11–12, 1957

CHARLIN

Synonyms. Charlin-Sluder; Harris; nasal nerve; nasociliaris nerve; ganglion ciliare. See also Sluder.

Symptoms and Signs. Identical to cluster headache (see), with the postulated difference that inflammatory changes of eyes may be more severe (pseudopurulent conjunctivitis; keratitis; corneal ulcers, iritis).

Therapy. Cocaine applications in the anterior part of nasal fossa give rapid relief of ocular symptoms.

Prognosis. Very painful, recurrent episodes may induce suicide.

BIBLIOGRAPHY. Charlin C: Sindrome del nervio nasal. Dia Méd 2:839, 1930

Pan H: Differential Diagnosis of Eye Diseases, p 98. Philadelphia, WB Saunders, 1978

Olen J (chairman): Classification and diagnostic criteria for headhache disorders cranial neuralgia and facial pain. Cephalalgia 8:(Suppl 7), 1988

Cady RK, Fox AW: Treating the Headache Patient. New York, Marcel Dekker, 1994

CHASSAIGNAC

Synonyms. Chassaignac-Laehmung; nursemaid elbow; pulled elbow.

Symptoms and Signs. Appears in infants, especially if they have hypermobile tendency. Pain in the arms preventing movements and thus simulating a paralytic condition.

Etiology. Referred to excessive traumatic muscle stretching producing subluxation.

Diagnostic Procedures. *X-ray.*

Therapy. Reposition tramite supination of forearm.

Prognosis. Tendency to relapse.

BIBLIOGRAPHY. Chassaignac PME: De la paralysie douloureus de jeunes enfants. Arch Gen Med 7:653–669, 1856

Piroth P, Gharib M: Die traumatische Subluxation des Radius Koepfchens (Chassaignac). Dtsch Med Wschz 101:1520–1523, 1976

Chard MD: The elbow. In Klippel JH, Dieppe PA: Rheumatology, p 5.9.3. St Louis, CV Mosby, 1995

CHATTLE

Synonym. Laryngeal nerve duosyndrome.

Symptoms and Signs. Appears in newborn. Weakness or unilateral palsy of facial muscles; weakness or palsy of vocal cords or of muscles (or both) of deglutition on contralateral side.

Etiology. Forced flexed lateral position in utero, which causes compression of laryngeal nerve between the thyroid cartilage and the thyroid or crycoid cartilage.

Therapy. B complex vitamins.

Prognosis. According to degree of nerve lesion and possibility of functional restoration.

BIBLIOGRAPHY. Chattle CC: A duosyndrome of the laryngeal nerve. Am J Dis Child 91:14–18, 1956

CHAVANY-BRUNHES

Synonyms. Fritzsche; falx calcification; see Fahr.

Symptoms and Signs. Variable degree of psychoneurotic manifestations; cephalalgic attacks following stress, fatigue or keeping the head in a fixed position for a prolonged period of time. Oligophrenia in some cases (Fritzsche).

Etiology. Unknown; may be familial (autosomal recessive trait).

Diagnostic Procedures. *X-ray of skull.* Calcification of falx, or other areas of scattered calcification (Fritzsche).

Therapy. Analgesic.

Prognosis. Variable.

BIBLIOGRAPHY. Chavany JA, Brunhes J: Syndromes céphalgique et psycho-névrotique avec calcification de la faux du cerveau. Rev Neurol (Paris) 69:113–131, 1938

Fritzsche R: Eine familiar auftretende Form von Oligophrenia mit röntgenolish machwzisbaren symmetrischen Kalkablagerungen in Gehirn, besonders in den Stammganglien. Schweiz Arch Neurol Neurochir Psychiatr 35:1, 1935

Adams RD, Victor M: Principles of Neurology, 5th ed, pp 838–839. New York, McGraw-Hill, 1993

CHEDIAK-HIGASHI

Synonyms. Bégnez-César; Chediak-Steinbrinck-Higashi; oculocutaneous albinism; leukocytic anomaly—albinism; gigantism peroxidase granules—granulation; anomaly leucocytes: gigantism of cytoplasmic organelles.

Symptoms. Photophobia; shifting nystagmus on exposure to light. Weakness; fever not related to infections; cerebellar tremor; dysmetria may be present as well as paralysis. Progressive peripheral neuropathy.

Signs. Decreased pigmentation of skin, hair, and eyes. Red, tender nodules, pustules and crusted ulcers of the skin may occasionally be found. Underdevelopment; moderate hepatomegaly; occasionally, splenomegaly and lymphadenopathy.

Etiology. Unknown; autosomal recessive inheritance. Hypopigmentation caused by an unknown primary defects that interests many types of cells, including melanocytes.

Pathology. Hepatosplenomegaly; lymphoadenopathy; bone changes. Often associated with lymphomas. Histiocytic infiltration of brain and other tissue.

Diagnostic Procedures. *Blood.* Typical abnormalities in the granulation and nuclear structure of all types of leukocytes: gigantic, monstrous peroxidase-positive granules; cytoplasmic inclusion and Döhle bodies. Anemia; thrombocytopenia. *Bone marrow.* Large eosinophilic inclusion bodies in myeloblasts and promyelocytes.

Therapy. None specific; prevention of infection. Long-term treatment with ascorbic acid.

Prognosis. Poor; high susceptibility to infection (not related to deficient antibody production). Lymphomas and hemorrhage (because of thrombocytopenia) usually are cause of death.

BIBLIOGRAPHY. Steinbrinck W: Ueber eine neue Granulationsanomalie der Leukocyten. Dtsch Archiv Klin Med 193:577–581, 1948
Chédiak M: Nouvelle anomalie leucocytaire de caractère constitutionel et familial. Rev Hématol 7:362–367, 1952
Béguez-Cesar A: Neutropenia crònica maligna familiar con granulaciones atipicas de los leucocitos. Bol Soc Cub Ped 15:900–910, 1953
Higashi O: Congenital gigantism of peroxidase granules; first case ever reported of qualitative abnormality of peroxidase. Tohoku J Exp Med 59:315–332, 1954
Scriver CR, Beaudet AL, Sly WS, et al: The Metabolic and Molecular Bases of Inherited Disease, 7th ed, pp 3348–3350, 4377–4378. New York, McGraw-Hill, 1995

CHERRY RED SPOT MYOCLONUS

Synonym. Sialidosis type I.

Symptoms and Signs. Cherry red spot in the macula present before the patient is 10 years old possibly fading in the chronic stage, myoclonus, which is precipitated by voluntary movement, the thought of movement, light touch, passive joint movement and sound, but not by light. Insidious visual loss. Intellect relatively spared.

Etiology. Storage of sialidated glycopeptides and glycolipids in the brain and liver owing to the deficiency of alpha-neuroaminidase (sialidase). Autosomal recessive inheritance.

Pathology. Morphologic changes reflect a storage process in lysosomes of retinal ganglion cells, cortical neurons, neurons of the myoenteric plexus, hepatocytes, and Kupffer cells.

Diagnostic Procedures. *Electroencephalography. Electromyography. Liver biopsy. Urine.* Excretion of large amount of sialidated oligosaccharides

Therapy. 5-hydroxytryptophan.

Prognosis. Myoclonus and visual loss can be very crippling.

BIBLIOGRAPHY. Rapin I, Goldfischer S, Katzman R, et al: The cherry red spot–myoclonus syndrome. Ann Neurol 3:234–242, 1978
Gascon G, Wallenberg B, Daif et al: Successful treatment of cherry spot-myoclonus syndrome with 5–hydroxytryptophan. Ann Neurol 24:453–4551, 1988
Scriver CR, Beaudet AL, Sly WS, et al: The Metabolic and Molecular Bases of Inherited Disease, 7th ed, pp 2535, 2533, 2542, 2544. New York, McGraw-Hill, 1995

CHESHIRE CAT

Synonym. Lanthanic. Refers to no specific disease complex, but to the two following possible categories embracing all diseases:

1. Patients showing all symptoms and signs of a well-defined entity, which the pathology findings fail to confirm.
2. Patients with a lanthanic condition (presence of the disease but no symptoms or signs, or awareness of them by the patient, so that medical help is not sought), or patients who do not show the entire diagnostic spectrum of the condition (*formes frustes*).

This term, proposed by Bywaters to describe the syndrome, is taken from *Alice in Wonderland* in which Alice saw the grin without the cat, and because of its lack of ears she felt it was useless to attempt to speak to it.

This situation exemplifies the difficulty encountered by the physician in dealing with pathologic entities unexpressed or not fully expressed.

BIBLIOGRAPHY. Feinstein AR: Clinical Judgment. Baltimore, Williams & Wilkins, 1967
Bywaters EGL: The Cheshire cat syndrome. Postgrad Med J 44:19–22, 1968

CHESTER-ERDHEIM

Obsolete.

Synonym. Erdheim-Chester; lipogranulomas of bones; bone lipogranulomatosis.

Symptoms and Signs. Onset fifth–seventh decades. Fever, weight loss, polyuria. Bone pain; Chest pain; cough; sinus discharge; symptoms and signs of cardiac failure; pulmonary and renal disease; hepatosplenomegaly; xanthoma of eyelids.

Etiology. Unknown.

Pathology. Diffuse lipogranulomatosis, lesions of bone and visceral organs.

Diagnostic Procedures. *X-ray, CT scan. MRI. Sonography.* See Pathology. Retroperitoneal and visceral infiltration and signs of pleural effusion. *Bone marrow biopsy:* Hystocytes lipid-laden. *Blood:* Evidence of secondary infections. *Urine:* Diabetes insipidus.

BIBLIOGRAPHY. Chester W: Uber Lipoidgranulomatos. Virchows Arch. 279:561–602, 1930
Miller RL, Sheeler LR, Baller TW, et al: Erdheim-Chester disease: case report and review of literature. Am J Med 80:1230–1236, 1936

CHESTER PORPHYRIA

Synonym. Porphyria Chester (Chester, England).

Symptoms and Signs. Neurovisceral symptoms. Absence of photosensitivity.

Etiology. Variant of porphyria (see).

Diagnostic Procedures. Variable excretion patterns resembling that of other forms of porphyria or intermediate. Enzyme study in peripheral blood cells reveal dual deficiency (reduced activity of protoporphobilinogen oxidase and of PBG deaminase).

Therapy. See other porphyrine derangements.

BIBLIOGRAPHY. McColl KEL, Moore MR, Thompson GG, et al: Chester porphyria—biochemical studies of a new form of acute porphyria. Lancet II:796–799, 1985
Quadiri MR, Church SE, McColl KEL, et al: Chester porphyria—a clinical study of a new form of porphyria. Br Med J 292:455–459, 1986

CHILAIDITI

Synonym. Wanderleber.

Symptoms. In adults, very often asymptomatic; in children, symptomatology is instead well evident. Abdominal pain frequently associated with vomiting, occurring typically at the end of day when maximum distention occurs; pain relieved by lying down. Less frequent symptoms; anorexia; constipation and passage of flatus; air swallowing.

Signs. Abdominal distention; liver dullness absent; liver edge results at palpation significantly lowered.

Etiology and Pathology. Altered relationship of liver, colon, and diaphragm, where the colon interposes itself between liver and diaphragm.

Intestinal distention; paralysis of diaphragm; abnormalities of liver ligaments. In children, aerophagia and abdominal distention seem to be among the main causes.

Diagnostic Procedures. *X-ray.* Colon partially or totally interposed between liver and diaphragm.

Therapy. Lying down relieves most of the symptoms. Avoiding gassy foods and aerophagy, abdominal belt. Surgery has been suggested, but seems a too drastic procedure for a usually rather mild situation.

Prognosis. Improvement of symptoms with age has been reported.

BIBLIOGRAPHY. Chilaiditi D: Zur Frage der Hepatoptose und Ptose im allgemeinen im Anschluss an drei Fälle von temporären, partieller Leberverlagerung. Fortschr Rontgenstr Berl 16:173–208, 1910

Jackson ADM, Hodson CJ: Interposition of the colon between liver and diaphragm (Chilaiditi's syndrome) in children. Arch Dis Child 32:151–158, 1957

Melester T, Burt ME: Chilaiditi's syndrome report of three cases. JAMA 254:944–945, 1985

CHINESE RESTAURANT

Synonyms. Glutamic acid toxicity; post-sino-cibal; sin-cib-sin. Food migraine, hot-dog headache; restaurant.

Symptoms. Onset within 15–25 minutes of an abundant meal in a Chinese restaurant. Burning sensation in the back of the neck. Followed by burning over forearms and anterior chest and substernal discomfort. Followed by infraorbital pressure and tightness.

Signs. None; no erythema or sign of muscular contraction in areas of burning or constriction.

Etiology. In susceptible person, monosodium glutamate (5 g) used in Chinese cooking. Nonsusceptible person will have no reaction with even 25 g. Inborn error of metabolism. Autosomal recessive inheritance.

Therapy. Symptomatic.

Prognosis. As many as eight episodes a day can be survived, as proved by the personal experience of a dedicated physician very fond of Chinese food.

BIBLIOGRAPHY. Kwok RHM: Chinese restaurant syndrome. New Engl J Med 278:1122, 1968

Lehrer L: Possible significance of adverse reaction to glutamate in humans. Fed Proc 35:2205–2212, 1976

De Francisci G, Parisi N, Magalini SI: La sindrome del ristorante Cinese. Rec Prog Med 70:353–357, 1981

Settipane GA: The restaurant syndrome. New Engl Reg Allergy Proc 8:39–46, 1987

Weatherall DJ, Ledingham JGG, Warrell DA (eds): Oxford Textbook of Medicine, 3rd ed, p 1844. Oxford, Oxford Med Pub, 1996

CHIN QUIVERING

Synonyms. Mentalis muscle tremor; trembling chin.

Symptoms and Signs. Both sexes affected; present from birth. Chin quivering (fine, transitory tremor) caused by emotion or activities that require concentration. Tremor stops during sleep. Possible interference with speech and occasional association with nystagmus. Reported also, nocturnal myoclonus and tongue biting.

Etiology. Autosomal dominant inheritance with complete penetrance.

Prognosis. Attacks decreasing in frequency with age.

BIBLIOGRAPHY. Massaro (NI) Vingt-six cas de genio-spasme en cinq generations Rev Neurolog 2:534, 1894

Frey E: Ein Streng dominant aerbiches Kirmmuskelzittern. Dtsch Z Nervenheilk 115:9–26, 1930

Gorlin JK, Pinborg JJ, Cohen MM Jr: Syndromes of the Head and Neck, 2nd ed, pp 208–209. New York, McGraw-Hill, 1976

CHIRAY

Synonyms. Biliary atony; biliary hypotonic; cholecystic atony; lazy gallbladder.

Symptoms. Dyspepsia; anorexia; nausea; intolerance to fatty foods; attack of pain in right hypochondrium frequently radiating to the back; headache; nervous depression.

Signs. Pain on palpation of right hypochondrium.

Etiology. Motor disorder of gallbladder; atonic state that determines full capacity of distention so that any sudden increase in pressure results in pain. Other motor disorders such as spasmodic gallbladder or hypertension produce exactly the same symptomatology; secondary to impaired flow, because of sphincter of Oddi spasm or organic impediment.

Pathology. Gallbladder is flaccid; neck poorly visualized. Secondary inflammation of bile ducts and gallbladder may be present.

Diagnostic Procedures. *Cholecystography. Gallbladder scintigraphy. Timed biliary drainage. Cholecystokinin provocative test.*

Therapy. Stimulation of gallbladder contraction with cholecystokinetic foods plus biliary salts. In hyperkinetic conditions, opposite diet has to be used. Vitamin B complex; exercises. Relief of tension and fatigue; psychotherapy.

Prognosis. Good with adequate treatment.

BIBLIOGRAPHY. Chiray M: Etat actuel de le cholecystoatonic. In Albot e Poilleux: Les Voies Biliares. Paris, Masson, 1953

Toouli J: Motility disorders of the biliary tract. In Haubrich WS, Schaffner F, Berk JE (eds): Bockus Gastroenterology, 5th ed, vol 2, pp 2792–2801. Philadelphia, WB Saunders, 1995

CHLOASMA

Synonyms. Liver spot; melasma.

Symptoms. All racial groups; but more frequent in darker-complexioned individuals (especially Spanish descent, living in areas with strong sun radiation). Frequent in women during the entire reproductive period (with onset frequently in pregnancy) and/or in menopause; or induced by contraceptives, cosmetics, phototoxic, antiepileptic drugs. Rarely occurring in men (10%). Asymptomatic.

Signs. Symmetric brown mask-like patches involving cheeks and forehead with three clinical patterns of hyperpigmentation—centrofacial, malar, and mantibular—sometimes also genitalia and breast.

Etiology. Unknown; attributed to genetic influence, UV exposure, endocrine mechanism (thyroid dysfunction) (in some cases, produced by progestional steroids or hydantoin).

Pathology. Increased deposition of melanin in skin basal, suprabasal and stratum corneum layers.

Diagnostic Procedures. *Pregnancy test. Hormonal studies:* leutinizing hormones increased, serum estradiol decreased. Thyroid antibodies may be increased. *Wood light examination.*

Therapy. Challenging. Consider risk: benefit of each type of treatment, that may include from cosmetics to broad spectrum sunscreens, hydroquinone with or without addition of tretinoin, salicylic acid, or glycolic acid. Used as well: azelaic acid. Alpha-hydroxy acid preparation, including glycolic acid; retinoic acid; chemical peel; laser therapy.

Prognosis. After pregnancy or use of progesteron usually fades; it may, however, persist or recur in many cases.

BIBLIOGRAPHY. The Bible. My skin is black upon me; and my bones are burned with heat! Job 30:30

Newcomber VD, Lindberg HC, Sternberg, TH: A melanosis of the face ("chloasma"). AMA Arch Dermatol 83:284–299, 1961

Grimes PE: Melasma. Arch Dermatol 131:1453–1457, 1995

CHLOROMA

Synonyms. Myeloblastoma; Granulocytic sarcomas.

Symptoms and Signs. Extramedullary solid tumor in periosteal and perineural regions (facial bones, spinal cord); other sites skin, gingiva, uterus, and testis.

Etiology. Unknown.

Pathology. The name chloroma is a result of the greenish hue of the tumor. Collection of AML blasts. See Symptoms and Signs.

Diagnostic Procedures. *Blood:* Evidence of acute leukemia.

Therapy. Chemiotherapy. Consider autologous or allogenic marrow transplantation.

Prognosis. Very poor.

BIBLIOGRAPHY. Abe R, Umezu H, Uchida T, et al: Myeloblastoma with an 8; 21 chromosome translocation in acute myeloblastic leukemia. Cancer 58:1260–1264, 1986

Ruitinga P: Diagnostiek van Inwendige Ziekten. Amsterdam, Scheltema and Holkema, 1951

Greer JP, Kinney MC: Acute non-lymphocytic leukemia. In Lee GR, Bithel TC, Foerster J, et al (eds): Wintrobe's Clinical Hematology, 9th ed, pp 1935–1936. Philadelphia, Lea & Febiger, 1993

CHLOROQUINE RETINOPATHY

Synonyms. Toxic maculopathy. See Bull eye retinopathy.

Symptoms and Signs. After longstanding chloroquine therapy (rheumatoid arthritis, dermatologic disorders), impairment of visual acuity.

Etiology. Peripheral pigmentary retinopathy of toxic nature to optic atrophy.

Diagnostic Procedures. *Fundoscopy:* Diffuse mottling of affected central area, then pale ring corresponding to atrophic retinal pigment epithelium surrounding central focus that remains pigmented (Bull's eye macula).

Therapy. Suspension of chloroquine therapy.

Prognosis. Usually permanent lesion.

BIBLIOGRAPHY. Potts AM: Uveal pigment and phenothiazine compounds. Trans Am Ophthal Soc 60:517–552, 1962

Scoggs MW, Klintworth GK: Drugs and toxins. In Garner A, Klintworth GK (eds): Pathobiology of Ocular Disease: A Dynamic Approach, 2nd ed, p 1173. New York, Marcel Dekker, 1994

CHOLANGIOPATHY, INFANTILE DESTRUCTIVE

Synonyms. Infantile, destructive cholangiopathy.

Symptoms and Signs. From paucisymptomatic to persistent conspicuous cholestasis. In cases paucisymptomatic recurrent or chronic cholestatis in young adulthood possible.

Etiology. Includes the Alagille syndrome (see) and a rapid fatal nonsyndromatic intrahepatic biliary atresia. Chromosomal defect (see Alagille) or intrauterine viral infection have been considered as responsible for the biliary atresia. A rare form of sarcoidosis also is associated with a similar condition.

Pathology. Extrahepatic and paucity or atresia of intrahepatic biliary ducts.

Therapy. Variable according to manifestation from none to liver transplantation.

Prognosis. From asymptomatic to fatal.

BIBLIOGRAPHY. Schaffner F: Cholestasis. In Haubrich WS, Schaffner F, Berk JE (eds): Bockus Gastroenterology, 5th ed, vol 2, pp 1948–1949. Philadelphia, WB Saunders, 1995

CHOLANGITIS, PRIMARY SCLEROSING

Synonyms. Fibrosing cholangitis; chronic obliterative cholangitis; primary sclerosing cholangitis.

Symptoms. More frequent in males (70%); onset middle age (39). Initially, even for years, asymptomatic. Pruritus; jaundice, dragging or pain in right upper abdominal quadrant; anorexia, nausea and vomiting; occasionally chills.

Signs. Jaundice (after 1 week of discomfort or pain); occasionally hepatomegaly, weight loss.

Etiology. Unknown. Stenosing inflammatory process of bile ducts. Frequently associated with ulcerative colitis, less frequently with Crohn, Ormond, mediastinal fibrosis, or retro-orbital tumor. Genetic and immunologic factors may play a part in the etiopathogenesis.

Pathology. Thickening of entire system of extrahepatic bile ducts and occasionally edema of adjacent tissues. Collagen scar with few inflammatory cells. Seldom, involvement of intrahepatic ducts. Lymph nodes enlarged.

Diagnostic Procedures. *Blood:* White blood cells increase; eosinophilia; hyperbilirubinemia. Antimitochondrial antibodies usually absent. An increased level of alkaline phosphatase in young men, particularly if affected by the ulcerative colitis that is strongly suggestive for this syndrome. *Intravenous and oral cholangiography.* Failure of ducts to become opaque. *Retrograde and transhepatic cholangiography:* Good diagnostic results. *Biopsy of liver:* Bile stasis; periportal fibrosis.

Therapy. None can favorably affect the course. Surgery. Ductal dilatation and insertion of T or V tubes (left for 6 months or longer). Systemic corticosteroids, methotrexate, ursodiol, liver transplantation improves prospect for longer survival.

Prognosis. Outcome unpredictable; from complete recovery to secondary biliary cirrhosis or related to associated conditions.

BIBLIOGRAPHY. Hoffman CEE: Verschluss der Gallenwege durch Verdickung der Wardungen. Arch Pathol Anat Physiol 49:206–215, 1867

Schwartz SI: Primary sclerosing cholangitis. Surg Clin North Am 53:1161–1167, 1973

Javitt NB: Hyperbilirubinemic and cholestatic syndromes. Postgrad Med 65:120–130, 1979

Lee YM, Kaplan MM: Primary sclerosing cholangitis. New Engl J Med 332:924–933, 1995

CHOLERRHEIC ENTEROPATHY

Synonym. Interrupted enterohepatic circulation.

Symptoms. Occurs in patients with ileal disease or ileal resection. Diarrhea; steatorrhea; weight loss.

Etiology. Interrupted enterohepatic circulation of bile salts owing to pathology of ileum (site of reabsorption of bile salts); ulcerative colitis with ileal involvement; regional ileitis; or resection of ileum; conceivably virus enteritis. Increase of turnover rate and synthesis rate of bile salts caused by lack of bile return.

Pathology. See Etiology.

Diagnostic Procedures. *Stool.* Determination of cumulative fecal excretion of labeled bile acid. Determination of rate of absorption of fat, cholesterol, carotene, vitamins D, E, and K.

Therapy. Dilemma: Administration of bile salts corrects the malabsorption, but worsens diarrhea. In three patients, however, it increased absorption of lipids and corrected diarrhea. Cholestyramine reduces diarrhea, but increases steatorrhea.

Prognosis. Natural history of this recently established syndrome is unknown. It is thought that with time liver may stop compensatory hyperproduction of bile and upper intestine or large intestine may develop ability to absorb bile, and finally large intestine may become refractory to the cathartic effects of bile salts.

BIBLIOGRAPHY. Hofmann AF: The syndrome of ileal disease and the broken enterohepatic circulation: Cholerrheic enteropathy. Gastroenterology 52:752–757, 1967
Everson GT, Kern F Jr: Bile acid and cholesterol homeostasis. In Haubrich WS, Schaffner J, Berk JE (eds): Bockus Gastroenterology, 5th ed, vol 2, p 992. Philadelphia, WB Saunders, 1995

CHOLESTEROL PERICARDITIS

Synonym. Alexander (JS); pericardial effusion chronic.

Symptoms and Signs. Both sexes. In all ages from adolescence. Symptomatic, recurrent pericardial effusions that eventually lead to constricting calcific pericarditis.

Etiology. Unknown. A familial occurrence also reported (autosomal recessive?).

Diagnostic Procedures. *Chest X-rays. Electrocardiography. Echocardiography. Pericardial tapping:* Fluid with abundant cholesterol crystals (gold-paint aspect).

Therapy. Symptomatic.

Prognosis. Cardiac failure.

BIBLIOGRAPHY. Alexander JS: A pericardial effusion of gold paint appearance due to the presence of cholesterin. Br Med J 2:463, 1919
Stanley RJ, Subramanian R, Lie JT: Cholesterol pericarditis terminating as constrictive calcific pericarditis; follow-up study of patient with 40 years history of disease. Am J Cardiol 46:511–514, 1980
Shabetai R: Diseases of pericardium. In Schlant RC, Alexander RW, et al: Hurst's The Heart, 8th ed, p 1670. New York, McGraw-Hill, 1994

CHOLESTERYL ESTER HYDROLASE DEFICIENCY

Synonyms. CESD; hepatic cholesteryl storage; cholesteryl ester storage disease; polycorie cholestérolique. See also Wolman.

Symptoms. Both sexes affected; prevalent in females; detection between 2 and 23 years of age. Hepatomegaly (constant sign) may be present at birth, or become evident later; splenomegaly is frequently present. Absence of jaundice, signs of malabsorption and of neurologic involvement.

Etiology. Deficiency of acid cholesteryl ester hydrolase. Autosomal recessive inheritance.

Pathology. Three categories of findings respectively related to (1) intralysosomal storage of lipids; (2) portal hypertension; (3) atherosclerosis. *Liver.* Prominent lipid accumulation; enlarged, orange color; septal fibrosis (or cirrhosis); focal periportal accumulation of lymphocytes, plasma cells, and foamy macrocytes. *Spleen.* May be similarly infiltrated. *Intestine.* May show infiltration with extracellular lipids and foamy cells. Lipids stored in cells are cholesteryl esters.

Diagnostic Procedures. *Blood.* Hyperbetalipoproteinemia; cholesterol and cholesteryl ester markedly increased; total lipids normal. Anemia.

Biopsy of liver. See Pathology. *Bone marrow.* Foamy cells or normal. *Fibroblast culture.* Demonstration of cholesteryl ester hydrolase deficiency.

Therapy. None. Lovastatin has proved useful in reducing plasma lipids.

Prognosis. Patients survive into adulthood, reported to live past 40 years of age.

BIBLIOGRAPHY. Fredrickson DS: Newly recognized disorders of cholesterol metabolism. Ann Intern Med 58:718–719, 1963
Desai PK, Astrin KH, Thung SN, et al: Cholesteryl ester storage disease: pathological changes in an affected fetus. Am J Med Genet 26:689–698, 1987
Assman G, Seedorf U: Acid lipase deficiency: Wolman disease and cholesteryl ester storage disease. In Scriver CR, Beaudet AL, Sly WS, et al: The Metabolic and Molecular Bases of Inherited Disease, 7th ed, pp 2567–2570. New York, McGraw-Hill, 1995

CHONDRODYSPLASIA PUNCTATA—X-LINKED

Synonyms. CDPX, CPX.

Symptoms and Signs. Males homozygous usually die; females survive. Similar to Conradi (see) and as distinctive features: pigmentary lesions of the skin (whorled or linear) that evolve toward ichthyosis, follicular atrophoderma, cicatrical alopecia and hypoplasia of distal phalanges. Cerebral involvement, asymmetric cataracts.

Etiology. X-linked dominant.

Prognosis. Fatal or extremely severe in males.

BIBLIOGRAPHY. Spranger JW, Opitz JM, Bibber V: Heterogeneity of chondrodysplasia punctata. Hum Genet 11:190–212, 1971
Apple R: X-linked dominant chondrodysplasia punctata. Review of the literature and report of a case. Hum Genet 53:65–73, 1979
Kalter DC, Atherton DJ, Clayton PT: X-linked dominant Conradi-Hunerman syndrome presenting as congenital erythroderma. J Am Acad Derm 21:248–256, 1989

CHONDROMALACIA PATELLAE

Synonym. Aleman.

Symptoms and Signs. Prevalent in middle-aged women; early onset possibly owing to recurrent patellar subluxation or dislocation. Frequently bilateral; crepitus on knee extension; then pain, snapping, and catching and, finally, extensive effusion.

Etiology. Friction of patellofemoral joint aggravated by excessive mobility (subluxation).

Diagnostic Procedures. *X-rays.*

Therapy. *Preventive.* Medial transfer of patellar tendon insertion; plication of medial capsule and alignment correction. *Curative.* Strain relief or, in severe case, patellectomy.

Prognosis. According to efficiency of treatment. Patellectomy restores function.

BIBLIOGRAPHY. Aleman O: Chondromalacia posttraumatic patellae. Acta Chir Scand 63:149–152, 1928
Bronitsky JB: Chondromalacia patellae. J Bone and Joint Surg 29:931–945, 1947
Klippel JH, Dieppe PA: Rheumatology, p 5.12.9. St Louis, CV Mosby, 1995

CHORDA TYMPANI

Symptoms. After surgery or injury to submandibular gland. After eating: flushing and sweating limited to the skin of the chin and submental region (see Frey).

Etiology. Faulty regeneration of injured nerve fibers.

Therapy. Blockage of lingual nerve proximal to the chorda tympani.

BIBLIOGRAPHY. Urprus V, et al: Localized abnormal flushing and sweating on eating. Brain 57:443–493, 1934

Young AG: Unilateral sweating of the submental region after eating (Chorda tympani syndrome). Br Med J 2:976–979, 1956

Bailey BMW, Pearce DE: Gustatory sweating following submandibular gland removal. Br Dent J 158:17–18, 1985

Gorlin RJ, Cohen MM, Levin LS: Syndromes of the Head and Neck, 3rd ed, p 615. New York, Oxford Press, 1990

Weatherall DJ, Ledingham JGG, Warrell DA (eds): Oxford Textbook of Medicine, 3rd ed, p 3878. Oxford, Oxford Med Pub, 1996

CHOREA, HEREDITARY, BENIGN

Synonyms. Chorea, hereditary, progressive-without dementia.

Symptoms and Signs. Early onset of choreic attacks. No intellectual impairment.

Etiology. Autosomal dominant inheritance with reduced penetrance in females.

Therapy. From cortisone administration reported reduction in frequency and amplitude of chorea attacks.

Prognosis. Benign condition. Situation remains stable or improves.

BIBLIOGRAPHY. Pincus JC, Chutorian A: Familial benign chorea with intention tremor: A clinical entity. J Pediat 70:724–729, 1967

Haerer AF, Currier RD, Jackson JF: Hereditary nonprogressive chorea of early onset. N Engl J Med 276:1220–1224, 1967

Schady W, Meara RJ: Hereditary progressive chorea without dementia. J Neurol Neurosurg Psychiatr 51:295–297 1988

CHOREA GRAVIDARUM

Symptoms. Choreiform movement occurring during pregnancy, usually starting in first trimester. In young primiparas, occasionally recurrent in successive pregnancies.

Therapy. Only if very severe case, termination of pregnancy.

Prognosis. After termination of pregnancy, further attacks may recur years later in about 30% of cases.

BIBLIOGRAPHY. Adams RD, Victor M: Principles of Neurology, 5th ed, pp 66–67. New York, McGraw-Hill, 1993

Weatherall DJ, Ledingham JGG, Warrell DA (eds): Oxford Textbook of Medicine, 3rd ed, p 1769. Oxford, Oxford Med Pub, 1996

CHOREA, SENILE

Synonym. Chronic progressive nonhereditary chorea.

Symptoms. Sudden onset after 50 years of age. The same symptoms as in other forms of chorea; rarely, mental deterioration; only changes in emotion and memory.

Etiology. Brain changes secondary to vascular pathology.

Pathology. Degenerative lesion of large and small cells of putamen and corpus striatum. Atherosclerotic vascular changes. Infection and drug therapy.

Therapy. Haloperidol (2–10 mg/day).

Prognosis. Slowly progressing disability. In cases of infections or drugs may disappear after a few weeks.

BIBLIOGRAPHY. Alcock NS: Note on pathology of senile chorea (nonhereditary). Brain 59:376–387, 1936

Adams RD, Victor M: Principles of Neurology, 5th ed, p 972. New York, McGraw-Hill, 1993

CHOREIFORM

Synonym. Dubini; Henoch I; Bergeron; Morvan; Muratow (see text). Different obsolete pathologic entities that have in common the symptoms of choreiform movements. The symptom chorea is a major feature of many distinct nosographical entities that may be differentiated on the basis of different etiology, response to therapy, and prognosis.

BIBLIOGRAPHY. Dubini A: Primi cenni sulla corea elettrica. Ann Univ Med (Milano), 117:5–50, 1846

Henoch E: Beitrage zur Kinderheilkunde. Berlin, A Hirschwald, 1861

Huntington G: On chorea. Med Surg Reporter 26:317–321, 1872

Berland, R: Traitement par le tartre stibié d'une forme de la chorée dite électrique. Poitiers, 1880

Morvan AM: De la chorée fibrillaire. Gaz Hebd Méd 27:173–176, 1890

Muratow W: Zur Pathogenese der Hemichorea postapoplectica. Monatsschr Psychiatr Neurol 5:180–192, 1899

Bremme H: Ein Beitrag zur Bindearmchorea. Monatsschr Psychiat Neurol Berl 45:107–120, 1919

Tsiminakis Y: Zur Localisation der Hemichorea. Arb Neurol Wien Univ 35:57–75, 1933

Wolff PH, Hurnitz I: The choreiform syndrome. Dev Med Child Neurol 8:160–165, 1966

CHORIOCARCINOMA

Synonyms. Chorioepithelioma; syncytioma malignum.

Symptoms. Choriocarcinoma nearly always follows hydatidiform mole, abortion, or term pregnancy. Bleeding from the uterus during pregnancy in the second trimester of pregnancy. Very often, however, first symptoms and signs are related to metastases to lungs, liver, brain, or other areas.

Etiology. Unknown.

Pathology. Composed of both syncytial and cytotrophoblastic cells that do not form chorionic villi, but grow and destroy the uterine muscle.

Therapy. Hysterectomy and excision of all localized and accessible metastases. In advanced cases chemotherapy (e.g., methotrexate).

Prognosis. After chemotherapy, even if metasteses are present, 5-year arrest expected in 85% of cases.

BIBLIOGRAPHY. Lurain JR, Brewer JI, Torok EE, et al: Natural history of hydatidiform mole after primary evacuation. Am J Obstet Gynecol 145:591–595, 1983

Szulman AE: Syndromes of hydatidiform moles. Partial versus complete. J Reprod Med 29:788–791, 1984

Scully RE: Ovarian tumors with endocrine manifestations. In De Groot LJ: Endocrinology, 3rd ed, p 2121. Philadelphia, WB Saunders, 1995

CHORIOCARCINOMA, INFANTILE

Symptoms. Both sexes affected; onset between 5 weeks and 7 months. Anemia; hemopthysis; hematemesis; hematuria or melena.

Signs. Hepatomegaly; breast enlargement; growth of pubic hair; abdominal mass may be palpated.

Etiology. Choriocarcinoma metastasized from placenta during intrauterine life.

Pathology. Choriocarcinoma in lung, liver, occasionally subcutaneous, adrenals, brain.

Diagnostic Procedures. *X-ray.* Presence of mass in lung. *Urine.* Chorionic gonadotropin marked elevation.

Therapy. Methotrexate.

Prognosis. Death is usually rapid. Early recognition important because it will lead to diagnosis and treatment of mother.

BIBLIOGRAPHY. Emery JL: Chorionepithelioma in a newborn male child with hyperplasia of the interstitial cells of the testis. J Pathol Bacteriol 64:735–739, 1952

Witzleben CL, Bruninga, G: Infantile choriocarcinoma: A characteristic syndrome. J Pediatr 73:374–378, 1968

Voüte PA, Barrett A, Bloom HJC, Lemerle J, Neidhardt NK (eds): Cancer in Children: Clinical Management. Berlin, Springer Verlag, 1986

Schaffer, Avery: Diseases of Newborn, p 1026. Philadelphia, WB Saunders, 1991

CHORIORETINOPATHY, CENTRAL SEROUS

Synonyms. Idiopathic central serous chororetinopathy, choroidopathy; central serous chorioretinopathy; CSC.

Symptoms and Signs. Affects healthy young adults, mostly men. Usually monolateral. If bilateral second eye is affected after few weeks. Premonitory transient blurred vision, then scotoma. Visual acuity moderately decreased, induced hyperopia, micropsia and metamorphopsia, color perception decreased, dark adaptation prolonged, stereopsis sometimes impaired.

Etiology. Idiopathic.

Diagnostic Procedures. *Ophthamoscopy:* Circular raised area in the macular region caused by serous detachment of sensory retina. *Fluorangiography:* Focal spot hyperfluorescence, later smokestack appearance. *Microscopy:* Subretinal proteinaceous fluid pink staining between sensory retina and underlying pigment epithelium, retinal photoreceptors normal.

Therapy. Correction of induced hyperopia with pus.

Prognosis. Lesions persist 2–3 months, leaving minimal residual macular pigmentation but normal vision. May recur. In recurrent cases, irreversible changes occur. Subretinal neovascularization or hemorrhagic detachment is rare.

BIBLIOGRAPHY. Wessing A: Central serous retinopathy and related lesions. Mod Probl Ophthalmol 9:148, 1971

CHOROIDAL ARTERY, ANTERIOR

Synonyms. Von Monakow; Monakow; Foix; choroidal artery anterior. See Dejerinne-Roussy.

Symptoms and Signs. Hemiplegia; hemianesthesia, hemianopia; contralateral to lesion. Cognitive function usually spared. Actual clinical pattern rather variable and the hemianesthesia and hemianopia may be partial.

Etiology. Vascular end degenerative or neoplastic origin, with a more discrete participation of thalamus compared with other thalamic syndromes.

Pathology. Softening and hemorrhage on posterior part of internal capsule; globus pallidus; lateral geniculate body; and area of origin of optic nerve.

Diagnostic Procedures. *Spinal tap. Angiography. CT brain scan.*

Therapy. Symptomatic, or surgery if indicated.

Prognosis. Poor, depending on site of occlusion.

BIBLIOGRAPHY. Kolinsko A: Ueber die Beziehung der Arteria choroidea anterior zum hinteren Schenkel der inneren Kapsul des Genhirnes. Vienna, 1891

Steegmann AT, Roberts DJ: The syndrome of the anterior choroidal artery. JAMA 104:1695–1697, 1935

Masson M, Decroix JP, Henin D, et al: Syndrome de l'artère choroidienne antérieure. Rev Neurol 139:547–552, 1983

Adams RD, Victor M: Principles of Neurology, 5th ed, p 683. New York, McGraw-Hill, 1993

CHOROIDAL DYSTROPHY, CENTRAL AREOLAR

Synonyms. Geographic atrophy of pigment epithelium and choriocapillaries; central areolar choroidal atrophy; central areolar choroidal sclerosis.

Symptoms and Signs. In elderly subjects, bilateral. Difficulty passing from light to dark. Loss of visual acuity, eventually central scotoma.

Etiology. Unknown. Inheritance may be autosomal dominant or recessive.

Diagnostic Procedures. *Fundus:* Early stages, simple pigment mottling; ultimately, pigment epithelial atrophy leads to exposure of large choroidal vessels that become visible as white streaks.

Pathology. Total degeneration and virtual absence of choriocapillaris channels in late stages. Bruch membrane is intact, but atrophy of overlying pigment epithelium and retina occurs.

Therapy. None.

Prognosis. Central scotoma.

BIBLIOGRAPHY. Sorsby A, Crick R: Central areolar choroidal sclerosis. Br J Ophthal 37:129, 1953

Willerson D, Aaberg T: Senile macular degeneration and geographic atrophy of retinal pigment epithelium. Br J Ophthal 62:551–553, 1978

Bird AC, Jay B, Hussain AA, et al: Retinal photoreceptor disorders. In Garner A, Klintworth GK (eds): Pathobiology of Ocular Disease: A Dynamic Approach, 2nd ed, p 1221. New York, Marcel Dekker, 1994

CHOROIDEREMIA

Synonyms. Tapetochoroidal dystrophy progressive, TCD, choroidal sclerosis.

Symptoms. Prevalent in male. Early age: night blindness; constriction of visual fields; reduction of central vision. In some cases mental retardation. Reported mental retardation, deafness, and obesity (in cases of microdeletions Xq21).

Signs. *In males:* complete atrophy of choroid and retina. *In females:* remarkable fundoscopic changes (without visual defects).

Etiology. Abiotrophy (not congenital absence, as the name choroideremia indicates) of choroid, progressing slowly. X-linked inheritance. Choroideremia locus mapped to band q21 on X-chromosome.

Prognosis. Progressive loss of vision.

BIBLIOGRAPHY. Wilmer W: Atlas of Fundus Oculi. New York, MacMillan, 1934

Shapira TM, Sitney JA: Choroideremia. Am J Ophthalmol 26:182–183, 1943

Karua J: Choroideremia: a clinical and genetic study of 84 Finnish patients and 126 female carriers. Acta Ophthal Suppl 176:1–68, 1986

Fodor E, Lee RT, O'Donnell JJ: Analysis of choroideraemia gene. Letter Nature 351:614, 1991

Bird AC, Jay B, Hussain AA, et al: Retinal photoreceptor disorders. In Garner A, Klintworth GK (eds): Pathobiology of Ocular Disease: A Dynamic Approach, 2nd ed, pp 1215–1217. New York, Marcel Dekker, 1994

CHRISTIAN I

Synonyms. Adducted thumb; arthrogryposis—cleft palate—craniosynostosis; Christian-Andrews-Conneally; thumb, congenital clasp.

Symptoms and Signs. Both sexes affected; present from birth. Dysphagia; respiratory problems; Hypotonia; muscular fibrillation and cramps; mental retardation; seizures; craniosynostosis; microcephaly; prominent occiput; hypertelorism; antimongoloid slant; ophthalmoplegia; ear abnormalities; cleft palate. Torticollis. Camptodactyly; abducted thumbs; Hirsutism. Occasionally, reduced extension of elbow and knees.

Etiology. Autosomal recessive inheritance.

Pathology. See Symptoms and Signs. Laryngomalacia. Dysmyelinization and glial proliferation in white matter of brain. Muscle: myopathic changes.

BIBLIOGRAPHY. Christian JC, Andrews PA, Conneally PM, et al: The adducted thumb syndrome: An autosomal recessive disease with arthrogryposis, dysmyelinization, craniostenosis and cleft palate. Clin Genet 2:95–103, 1971
Kunze J, Park W, Hansen KH, et al: Adducted thumb syndrome: report of a new case and a diagnostic approach. Eur J Pediatr 141:122–126, 1983

CHRISTIAN II

Synonyms. Brachydactyly preaxial–allux varus–thumb abduction.

Symptoms and Signs. Both sexes affected to similar degree. Short thumbs and halluxes with varism. Metacarpal, metatarsal, and distal phalanges short, proximal and medial phalanges normal.

Etiology. Autosomal dominant inheritance.

BIBLIOGRAPHY. Christian JC, Chu KS, Franken EA, et al: Dominant preaxial brachydactyly with hallux varus and thumb abduction. Am J Hum Genet 24:694–701, 1972

CHRISTMAS

Synonyms. Factor IX deficiency; hemophilia B; plasma thromboplastin component; PTC deficiency.

Symptoms and Signs. Virtually limited to males. Almost identical with those of hemophilia, classic (see). Usually milder; variation of severity correlated with degree of deficiency of plasma thromboplastin component.

Etiology. Congenital deficiency of factor IX. X-linked recessive type of inheritance. Seldom observed in females. See Hemophilia, classic, for explanation. Several factor IX variants have been recognized.

Diagnostic Procedures. *Blood.* Normal bleeding time; normal or prolonged clotting time; usually abnormal thromboplastin generation test; abnormal absorbed plasma reagent in factor IX deficiency; abnormal serum reagent in factor IX deficiency; normal or abnormal prothombin consumption test; factor IX assay diagnostic; normal one-stage prothrombin time.

Therapy. As in hemophilia, stored plasma may be used, or combination of lyophilized factor IX-X-prothrombin commercially available (Bebulin).

Prognosis. Prognosis depends on severity of defect; grossly like classic hemophilia.

BIBLIOGRAPHY. Biggs R, Douglas AS, MacFarlane RG. Christmas disease: A condition previously mistaken for haemophilia. Br Med J 2:1378–1382, 1952
Schulman I, Smith CH: Hemorrhagic disease in an infant due to deficiency of a previously undescribed clotting factor. Blood 7:794–807, 1952
Bithell TC: Hereditary coagulation disorders. In Lee GR, Bithel TC, Foerster J et al (eds): Wintrobe's Clinical Hematology, 9th ed, pp 1437–1438. Philadelphia, Lea & Febiger, 1993

CHRIST-SIEMENS-TOURAINE

Synonyms. CST; Guilford; Siemens; Thurman; Wedderhorn; Weech; anhidrotic-ectodermal dysplasia; EDA; congenital ectodermal defect; ectodermal dysplasia, anhidrotic; hypohidrotic ectodermal dysplasia; HED; see Jacquet and Rapp-Hodgkin.

Symptoms. Prevalent in males; onset from birth. Temperature disturbances owing to reduced or absent perspiration. Increased respiratory infections; dysphagia; poor physical and mental development. Some cases with signs of adrenal medullary insufficiency (see Addison).

Signs. Hypotrichosis and partial or total anodontia (characteristic features). Various degrees of intensity of manifestations. Complete form: smooth, soft, dry skin; prominent frontal ridges and chin; sunken cheeks; thick lips; large ears; saddle nose; defects of nails; occasionally, congenital cataract.

Etiology. X-linked inheritance (severe) with different penetrance and occasionally some manifestation in female carriers; EDA locus is probably located 10 cm distal to DXS1 on proximal Xq between DXS1 and DXYS1. Autosomal dominant and recessive instances of inheritance also reported.

Pathology. Exocrine sweat glands absent or rudimentary; apocrine glands, hair follicles and sebaceous glands may be normal, hypoplastic, or absent.

Diagnostic Procedures. *Sweat tests. Biopsy of skin. Blood.* In some cases protein-bound serum thyroxine is increased.

Therapy. Avoidance of exposure to hot environment.

Prognosis. Incurable condition.

BIBLIOGRAPHY. Thurnam J: Two cases in which the skin, hair and teeth were very imprerfectly developed. Proc Roy Med Chir Soc 31:71–82, 1848
Darwin CH: The Variation of Animals and Plants under Domestication, 2nd ed, p 319. London, John Murray, 1875
Christ J: Uber die Kongenit ectodermalen Defeckte und ihre Beziehungen zu einanden; vikariirendes Pigment fuer Haarbildung. Arch Dermatol Syph 116:685–703, 1913
Week AA: Hereditary ectodermal dysplasia (congenital ectodermal defect). A report of two cases. Am J Dis Child 7:766–790, 1929
Siemens HW: Studien ueber Veredung von Hautkrankheiten. XII Anhidrosis hipotrichotica Arch Dermatol Syph 175:567–577, 1937
Touraine A: L'Anidrose avec hypotricose et anodontic Polydysplasie ectodérmique héréditaire. Presse Med 44:145–149, 1946
Crawford PJM, Aldred MJ, Clarke A: Clinical and radiographic dental findings in X-linked hypohidrotic ectodermal dysplasia. J Med Genet 28:181–185, 1991
Harper J: Genetics and genodermatoses. In Champion RH, Burton JL, Ebling FJG (eds): Rook/Wilkinson/Ebling Textbook of Dermatology, 5th ed, pp 335–337. Oxford, Blackwell Scientific, 1992

CHROMHIDROSIS

See Pseudochromhydrosis.

Symptoms and Signs. Rare in recognizable form. Slightly colored sweat (yellow, blue, or green) seen in 10% of population. May become manifested continuously or intermittently. Both sexes affected; prevalent in females of any age. Site most frequently involved is face (lower eyelids); less frequently, axillae, groin, breast, and hands. Colors can be black, violet, blue, brown, yellow, green, and seldom, red.

Etiology. Granules of lipofuscin in apocrine glands. Commonest cause is ingested drugs or dyes.

Pathology. Large amount of lipofuscin in apocrine glands.

Diagnostic Procedures. *Sweat tests.* Examination with ultraviolet light and chromatography.

Therapy. Surgical: excision of sweat gland involved.

Prognosis. Persistent condition. Good response to surgery.

BIBLIOGRAPHY. Le Roy de Méricourt H: Chromidrose rose. Arch Gen de Med, Nov 1857. Bull Acad Med 13:425–428, 1884
Hurley HJ, Shelley WB: The Human Apocrine Sweat Gland in Health and Disease. Springfield, IL, Charles C Thomas, 1960
Champion RH: Disorders of sweat glands. In Champion RH, Burton JL, Ebling FJG (eds): Rook/Wilkinson/Ebling Textbook of Dermatology, 5th ed, p 1761. Oxford, Blackwell Scientific, 1992

CHROMOSOME 1p, PARTIAL DELETION

Synonyms. 1p/21p translocation.

Symptoms and Signs. In a short, profoundly mentally retarded, microcephalic, 4-year-old girl. Cleft palate and lip, amaurosis and facial dysmorphism.

Etiology. Deletion of a terminal portion of 1p36.

BIBLIOGRAPHY. Yunis E, Quintero L, Leibovici M: Monosomy 1pter. Hum Genet 56:279–282, 1981
Schinzel A: Catalogue of Unbalanced Chromosome Aberrations in Man, pp 71–72. Berlin, DeGruyter, 1984

CHROMOSOME 1q, PARTIAL TRISOMY

Synonyms. Trisomy 1; dup (1q).

Symptoms and Signs. Low birth weight, neonatal death. Facial dysmorphisms: triangular shape with synophrys, beaked nose, midfacial hypoplasia, long philtrum, thick lips, short mandible, prenatal and postnatal growth retardation; microcephaly; heart defects, gastrointestinal tract stenoses, cleft palate, corneal opacities, and microphthalmia. Thymic hypoplasia or aplasia.

Etiology. Partial trisomy of chromosome 1q (1q2 qter).

Prognosis. Many of the patients described died early after birth. All survivors were severely mentally retarded.

BIBLIOGRAPHY. Norwood TH, Hoehn H: Trisomy for the long arm of human chromosome 1. Hum Genet 25:79–82, 1974
Rehder H, Friedrich U: Partial trisomy 1q syndrome. Clin Genet 15:534–540, 1979
Lungarotti MS, Falorni A, Calabro A, et al: De novo duplication 1q32–q42: Variability of phenotypic features in partial trisomics. J Med Genet 17:398–402, 1980
Chia NL, Bousfield LR, Poon CC, et al: Trisomy 1q (q42–qter) confirmation of a syndrome. Clin Genet 34:224–229, 1988

CHROMOSOME 1q, PROXIMAL DELETION

Synonyms. Del (1q), proximal.

Symptoms and Signs. Severe intrauterine and postnatal growth retardation, microbrachycephaly, profound mental deficiency; round facies

with frontal bossing, sparse eyebrows, small mandible; small and dysplastic earlobes; inguinal hernias; hypoplastic genitalia; short and broad hands and feet.

Etiology. Interstitial deletion of the long arm of chromosome 1 (q21 to 23 q25), q25rq32) (q42 or 43rqter).

Prognosis. Poor.

BIBLIOGRAPHY. Crandall BF, Falk RE: Craniosynostosis, profound growth retardation, unusual facies and multiple minor anomalies associated with intercalary delation. 46, XX, del (1)(q24, q31). Am J Hum Genet 26:23a, 1974
Estévez de Pablo C, Garcia-Sagredo JM, Ferro MT, et al: Interstitial delation in the long arms of chromosome 1. 46, XY, del (1)(pterq22. q25qter). J Med Genet 17:483–486, 1980
Schinzel A, Schmid W: Interstitial deletion of the long arm of chromosome 1, del (1) (q21q25) in a profoundly retarded 8-year-old girl with multiple anomalies. Clin Genet 18:305–313, 1980
Taysi K, Sekhon GS, Hillman RE: A new syndrome of proximal deletion of chromosome 1: 1q, 21–23–q-25. Am J Med Genet 13:423–430, 1982
Schinzel A: Catalogue of Unbalanced Chromosome Aberrations in Man, pp 71–72. Berlin, DeGruyter, 1984

CHROMOSOME 1q, TERMINAL DELETION

Synonyms. Del (1q) terminal.

Symptoms and Signs. Mild intrauterine growth deficiency; severe postnatal growth deficiency; microcephaly; profound mental retardation with muscular hypotonia and seizures; microbrachicephaly; facial dysmorphisms: inner epicanthic folds, upslanting palpebral fissures, bulbous nose with flat bridge; scoliosis; genital ambiguity; minor skeletal anomalies. High pitched cry. Forty percent heart defects.

Etiology. Variable terminal deletions of the long arm of chromosome 1.

BIBLIOGRAPHY. Juberg RC, Haney NR, Stallard R: New deletion syndrome: 1q 42. Am J Hum Genet 33:455–463, 1981
Zabel BU, Baumann WA: 1q deletion syndrome. Clin Genet 19:544–545, 1981
Tolkendorf E, Hinkel GK, Gabriel A: A new case of deletion 1q 42 syndrome. Clin Genet 35:289–292, 1989

CHROMOSOME 2p, PARTIAL DELETION

Symptoms and Signs. It is not possible to define a common clinical pattern from the variable somatic malformations.

Etiology. Del (2) (pterp23).

BIBLIOGRAPHY. Emanuel BS, Zackai EH, van Dike DC, et al: Deletion mapping: further evidence for the location of acid phosphatase (ACP1) within 2p23. Am J Med Genet 4:167–172, 1979

CHROMOSOME 2p, PARTIAL DUPLICATION

Synonyms. Dup (2p) partial.

Symptoms and Signs. Variable type and degrees of malformations according to type of chromosomal defect.

Etiology. Several aberrations of this chromosome have been found single or in association with other chromosomal defects. Dup (2)(pterp24) and del(2)(q34qter); dup (2)(pterp23); dup (2)(pterp21); dup (2)(p24p21); dup (2)(p23p24); dup (2)(p11q14), dup (2)(q24q34); dup (2)(q31 qter); dup (2)(q32to34 qter); etc.

BIBLIOGRAPHY. Bender K, Reinwein H, Gorman LZ, et al: Familiaere 2/C-

Translocation. 46, XYt(2p–; Cp+)und 46, XX, Cp+. Hum Genet 8:94–104, 1969

Cassidy SB, Heller RM, Chazen EM, et al: The chromosome 2 distal short arm trisomy syndrome. J Paediatr 91:934–938, 1977

Rosenfeld W, Verma RS, Jhaveri R, et al: Partial duplication for the short arm of chromosome 2: The 2p23 syndrome. Am Genet (Paris) 25:28–31, 1982

Schinzel A: Catalogue of Unbalanced Chromosome Aberrations in Man, pp 107–112. Berlin, de Gruyter, 1984

CHROMOSOME 2q, PARTIAL DELETION

Synonyms. Del (2q).

Symptoms and Signs. *First form:* Children with somatic and mental retardation. Microcephaly. *Nose:* Small. *Eyes:* Cataracts, microphthalmia, ptosis. *Mouth:* Cleft palate (100%), micrognathia. *Fingers:* Deformities. *Heart:* Congenital defects.

II form: As above except for nose prominency.

Etiology. I form. Deletion q21–q31. II form. Deletion 2q31–q33.

BIBLIOGRAPHY. Fryus JP, van Bosstraete N, Malbrain H: Interstitial deletion of the long arm of chromosome 2 in a polymalformed newborn; kariotype 46 XX, del (2) (q 21 q 24). Hum Genet 39:233–238, 1977

Ramer JC, Ladda RC, Frankel CA: A review of phenotype-kariotype correlations in individuals with interstitial delations of long arm of chromosome 2. Am J Med Genet 32:359–363, 1989

CHROMOSOME 2q, PARTIAL DUPLICATION

Synonyms. Dup 2q.

Symptoms and Signs. Weight and length at birth: normal. *Constant:* Mental retardation. *Frequent:* Frontal bossing, microbrachycephaly, hypertelorism, short beaked nose, abnormal pinnae, elongated filtrum, cleft palate. *Occasional:* Reduced vision, myopia, exotropia, glaucoma, nystagmus, iris defects, fundus lesions. Kyphosis, clinodactyly V finger.

Etiology. Partial trisomy 2q; deletion (q31 qter to q34 qter).

BIBLIOGRAPHY. Shapiro LR, Warburton D: Interstitial translocation in man. Lancet 2:712–713, 1972

Rosenthal IM: Trisomy of the distal portion of chromosome 2: a new familial syndrome associated with mental retardation and characteristic facies. Am J Hum Genet 26:73A, 1974

Kyllerman M, Wahlstrom J, Wesrerbrg B, et al: Delineation of a characteristic phenotype in distal trisomy 2 q. Helv Paediatr Acta 39:499–508, 1984

CHROMOSOME 3/B TRANSLOCATION

Synonym. Chromosome 3/B translocation.

Signs. Affected offspring comprised 41% of the progeny of female carriers. In contrast, only 12% of the progeny of male carriers were affected, and these included miscarriages only and no congenitally malformed children. The newborn presents with the following congenital anomalies: low birth weight; micrognathia; small ears; cleft lip and palate; coloboma; cloudy cornea; proptosis; strabismus; cardiac defects: ventricular septal defect; atrial septal defect; absent ductus arteriosus; pulmonary arterial diverticulum; right aortic arch; absent pulmonic valve.

Etiology. Chromosomal anomaly. It is associated with a translocation between a chromosome 3 and member of the B group (no. 4–5). The anomaly is transmitted by the female carrier but not, for some unknown reason, by the male carrier. This differential transmission is similar to that associated with that for Down syndrome with a familial 13–15/21 (D/G) translocation.

Pathology. See Signs.

Therapy. Symptomatic.

Prognosis. Guarded.

BIBLIOGRAPHY. Walzer S, Favara B, Ming PM, et al: A new translocation syndrome (3/B). N Engl J Med 275:290–298, 1966

CHROMOSOME 3p, PARTIAL DELETION

Synonym. Del (3p).

Symptoms and Signs. Asymmetry of the skull and facies, low frontal and nuchal hairline; hypertelorism; synophrys; upslanting palpebral fissures; epicanthic folds; ptosis; strabismus; narrow nose with prominent bridge; long philtrum; small and protruding ears; scoliosis; small fingers and toes; supernumerary postaxial digits in hands and feet; minor renal and cardiovascular anomalies (40%); pre- and postnatal growth retardation and delayed bone maturation; mental retardation.

Etiology. Partial deletion of the short arm of chromosome 3.

Prognosis. Mental retardation.

BIBLIOGRAPHY. Fineman RM, Hecht F, Ablow RC, et al: Chromosome 3 duplication q/deletion p syndrome. Pediatrics 61:611–618, 1978

Merrild U, Berggreen S, Hansen L, et al: Partial deletion of the short arm of chromosome 3. Eur J Pediatr 136:211–216, 1981

Schwyzer U, Binkert F, Caflisch U, et al: Terminal deletion of the short arm of chromosome 3, del (3 pter-p25): A recognizable syndrome. Helv Paediatr Acta 42:309–315, 1987

Meinecke P: Terminal delation of chromosome 3p in adults: A fourth observation. Am J Med Genet 33:108–112, 1989

CHROMOSOME 3p, PARTIAL DUPLICATION

Synonym. Dup (3p).

Symptoms and Signs. Retardation of growth. Facial clefts; heart malformations (85%); renal anomalies; syndactyly of fingers; choanal atresia; microphthalmia; accessory nipples; esophageal atresia; atresia of colon and rectum; genital anomalies (75% of males); mental deficiency (100%); excessive fingertip whorls (90%).

Etiology. Trisomy for the distal end of the short arm of chromosome 3.

Prognosis. Incidence of death in second year is 40%. Facies became less distinctive with age.

BIBLIOGRAPHY. Yunis JJ: Trisomy for the distal end of the short arm of chromosome 3. A syndrome. Am J Dis Child 132:30–33, 1978

Braga S, Schmidt A: Clinical and cytogenetic spectrum of duplication 3p. Eur J Pediatr 138:195–197, 1982

Reiss JA, Scheffield LJ, Sutherland GR: Partial trisomy 3p syndrome. Clin Genet 30:50–58, 1986

Watson MS, Dowton SB, Rohrbaugh J: Case of direct insertion within a chromosome 3 leading to a chromosome 3p duplication in an offspring. Am J Med Genet 36:172–174, 1990

CHROMOSOME 3q, PARTIAL DUPLICATION

Synonyms. Dup (3q). See De Lange.

Symptoms and Signs. From birth. Mental retardation. Seizures (85%). Constant craniofacial anomalies: craniosynostosis (frequent). Hypertrichosis; synophrys, upslanting of palpebral fissures, broad nose, anteverted nostrils, long upper lip, prominent maxilla, downturned mouth-corners, cleft palate (80%). Short neck. Hand anomalies; omphalocele (25%). Abnormalities of urogenital system (50%).

Etiology. Pericentric inversion of chromosome 3 or balanced translocation.

Pathology. See Signs. Brain anomalies: polymicrogyria, hypoplastic olfactory bulbs.

Prognosis. Death before first year of life in 33%.

BIBLIOGRAPHY. Falek A, Schmidt R, Jervis GA: Familial de Lange syndrome with chromosomal abnormalities. Pediatrics 37:92–101, 1966
Tranebjaerg L, Bdekmark UB, Dyhr-Nielsen M: Partial trisomy 3 q syndrome inherited from familial t(3, 9) (q 26. 1; p 23). Clin Genet 32:137–143, 1987

CHROMOSOME 4p, PARTIAL DUPLICATION

Synonym. Wilson (M.G.). Trisomy for the short arm of chromosome 4; dup (4p).

Symptoms and Signs. Both sexes with no predilection. Prenatal onset growth deficiency. Hypertonia during infancy followed by hypotonia. Seizures. Abnormal EEG. Microcephaly, prominent forehead, bulbous nose with depressed or flat nasal bridge; macroglossia, irregular teeth, small pointed mandible; frequently enlarged ears with abnormal helix and anthelix; short neck. Clinodactyly of fifth fingers, campodactyly, hypoplastic finger and toenails. Micropenis, hypospadias, cryptorchidism. Kyphoscoliosis.

Etiology. Trisomy for part of most of the short arm of chromosome 4.

Pathology. Various malformation findings as outlined above.

Diagnostic Procedures. *Chromosome study.*

Therapy. Symptomatic.

Prognosis. One-third of reported cases died during early infancy. Severe mental deficiency is present in 100% (IQ between 20 and 65) of those who survive (without visceral anomalies, such as cardiac or renal defects occasionally present). Life span does not seem to be impaired. Feeding problems are frequent in the neonatal period, and respiratory difficulties are a common complication.

BIBLIOGRAPHY. Wilson MG, Towner JW, Coffin GS, Forsman I: Inherited pericentric inversion of chromosome no. 4. Am J Hum Genet 22:679–683, 1970
Dallapiccola B, Mastroiacovo PP, Montali E, et al: Trisomy 4p: Five new observations and overview. Clin Genet 12:344–356, 1977
Reynolds JF, Schires MA, Wyandt HE et al: Trisomy 4 p in four relatives: Variability and lack of distinct features in phenotypic expression. Clin Genet 24:365–374, 1983
Rogers RC: Partial trisomy of 4p. Proc Greenwood Genet Center 5:29–38, 1986

CHROMOSOME 5p, PARTIAL DUPLICATION

Synonym. Dup (5p); trisomy 5p.

Symptoms and Signs. Postnatal growth retardation. Hypotonia, seizures. Slender extremities with long fingers. Club feet. Jowly appearance. Macrodolicocephaly; hypertelorism, palpebrae upward slanting, narrowed palpebral fissures; low nasal bridge and bulbous nose; coloboma of iris with or without microphtalmia; full lips and macroglossia; hiatal or other hernias; congenital heart defects; anal atresia; malformations of gut and kidneys.

Etiology. Complete or partial trisomy for chromosome 5.

Prognosis. High frequency of early death caused by fatal infections. Mental retardation in the survivors.

BIBLIOGRAPHY. Briblecombe FSW, Lewis FJ, Vowles M: Complete 5p trisomy: 1 case and 1q translocations in 6 generations. J Med Genet 14:271–274, 1977

Leschot NJ, Lim KS: Complete trisomy 5p; de novo translocation (2; 5) (q36; p11) with isochromosome 5p. Case report and review of the literature. Hum Genet 46:271–278, 1979
Kleczkowska A, Fryns JP, Moerman P, et al: Trisomy of the short arm of chromosome 5. Autopsy data in a malformed newborn with INV DUP (5) (13. 1–p15. 3). Clin Genet 32:49–56, 1987

CHROMOSOME 5q, PARTIAL DELETION

Synonyms. See Cat cry.

CHROMOSOME 5q, PARTIAL DUPLICATION

Synonyms. Dup (5q); trisomy 5q.

Symptoms. Severe mental retardation, failure to thrive.

Signs. Low birth weight. Microcephaly. Forehead; hypertelorism, palpebral fissure: downward slanting, epicanthal folds, strabismus; pinnae: large; long philtrum; upper lip: large; micrognathia. Occasionally heart and muscoloskeletal defects.

Etiology. Trisomy for 5q31–5 qter.

BIBLIOGRAPHY. Zabel B, Baumann W, Gehler J: Partial trisomy for short and long arms of chromosome No 5. J Med Genet 15:143–147, 1978
Elias-Jones A: The Trisomy (5) (q 31–q ter) syndrome. Study of a family with a 5(4; 14) translocation. Arch Dis Childhood 63:427–431, 1988

CHROMOSOME 6p, PARTIAL DUPLICATION

Synonyms. Dup (6p).

Symptoms. Low birth weight. Feeding and respiratory and eventually vision problems.

Signs. Craniosynostosis. High forehead, flat occiputum, wide fontanel, ptosis, strabismus, blepharophimosis, microcornea, cataracts. *Nose:* Short, flat round, long philtrum. *Mouth:* Small, lips thin. *Ears:* Low-set pinnae, poor lobes. Cardiac defects (65%). Less frequently renal and musculoskeletal defects.

Etiology. Partial trisomy 6p from parenteral translocation or inversion duplication.

BIBLIOGRAPHY. Turleau C, Papadakov–Lagoyanni SE, Sbyrakis S: La trisome 6p partielle. Ann Génét 21:88–91, 1978
Cote GB: Partial trisomy 6p with kariotype 46, XY ter (22) t (6; 22) (p22; q13) mat. J Med Genet 15:479–481, 1978
Wauters JG, Bossuyt PJ, Roelen L, et al: Application of fluorescence in situ hybridization for early prenatal diagnosis of partial trisomy 6/p monosomy 2q due to a familial percentric inversion. Clin Genet 44:262–269, 1993

CHROMOSOME 6q, PARTIAL DELETION

Synonyms. Del (6q).

Symptoms and Signs. Mental retardation. *Head:* Microcephaly. *Facies:* Asymmetric. *Eyes:* Palpebral fissure upslanting, hypertelorism, microphthalmia, strabismus; epicantal folds. *Nose:* Prominent, broad bridge, long philtrum. *Ears:* Pinnae low-set, large. *Mouth/upper lip:* Thin, cleft palate. Micrognathia. *Neck:* Short. *Hands:* Anomalies (50%). *Heart:* Occasional abnormalities.

Etiology. Chromosome 6q deletion.

BIBLIOGRAPHY. Milosevic J, Kalicanin P: Long arm deletion of chromosome no. 6 in mentally retarded boy with multiple physical malformations. J Ment Def Res 19:139–144, 1975

Young RS, Fidone GS, Reider-Garcia PA: Deletion of the long arm of chromosome 6. Two new cases and review of literature. Am J Med Genet 20:21–29, 1985

CHROMOSOME 6q, PARTIAL DUPLICATION

Synonyms. Dup (6q); trisomy 6q.

Symptoms and Signs. Severe physical and mental retardation. *Head:* Mycrobrachycephaly or turricephaly. *Forehead:* Prominent flat occiput. *Facies:* Flat; eyes: almond-shape; microphthalmia; hypertelorism, palpebrae downslanted. *Nose:* Short. *Nasal bridge:* Broad and flat. *Ears:* Low set. *Mouth:* Thin lips, lower with middle indentation, micrognathia. *Neck:* Short, webbed. *Joints:* Contracted. *Heart:* Occasional defects.

Etiology. Partial 6q trisomy from balanced parental translocation or inversion.

Prognosis. Normal life in absence of cardiac defects.

BIBLIOGRAPHY. Robertson KP, Thermon TF, Tracy MC: Acrocephalosyndactyly and partial trisomy 6. Birth Defects 11:267–271, 1975
Pierpont MEM, MacCarthy KG, Knoblock WH: Partial trisomy 6 q and bilateral retinal detachment. Ophthalmol Paediatr Genet 7:175–180, 1986

CHROMOSOME 7p, PARTIAL DELETION

Synonyms. Del (7p).

Symptoms and Signs. Mental development from normal to severe retardation. *Head:* Craniosynostosis of variable degree: turricephaly, microcephaly, prominent occiput and/or forehead, trigonocephaly, asymmetry, etc. *Facies:* Nevus flameous (see). *Eyes:* Hypotelorism, palpebral downward slanted, ptosis, epicanthal folds. *Nose:* Saddle-shaped. *Ears:* Pinnae low-set, dysplastic. *Heart and genitals:* Malformations (50%).

Etiology. Chromosome 7 short arm deletion.

BIBLIOGRAPHY. Zackai EG, Breg WR: Ring chromosome 7 with variable phenotype expression. Cytogenet Cell Genet 12:40–48, 1973
Hinkel GK, Tolkendorf E, Bergan J: 7p-deletion-syndrome. Mschr Kinderheilkd 136:824–827, 1988

CHROMOSOME 7p, PARTIAL DUPLICATION

Synonyms. Dup (7p); trisomy 7p.

Symptoms and Signs. Severe mental retardation. Dolichocephaly, wide fontanellae, hypertelorism. *Nose:* Short, beaked, micrognathia. Occasionally craniostenosis, skeletal anomalies and cardiac defects.

Etiology. Partial trisomy 7p chromosome.

Prognosis. Few cases survive infancy.

BIBLIOGRAPHY. Alfi OS, Donnell GN, Kramer SL: Partial trisomy of long arm of chromosome 7. J Md Gen 10:187–189, 1973
Larson LM, Vasdahl WA, Jaolal SM: Partial trisomy 7p associated with familial 7 p; 22 q translocation. J Med Genet 14:258–261, 1977
Moore CM, Pfeiffer RA, Craig-Holmes AP: Partial trisomy 7 p in two families resulting from different balanced translocation. Clin Genet 21:112–121, 1982

CHROMOSOME 7q, PARTIAL DELETION

Synonyms. Del (7q).

Symptoms and Signs. Pre-/postnatal growth and severe mental retardation. Feeding problems, hypotonia. *Head:* Microcephaly, prominent forehead. *Nose:* Broad bridge, bulbous tip. *Eye:* Anomalies. *Ears:* Large pinnae. *Mouth:* Large, micrognathia, cleft lip with or without cleft palate (25%). *Neck:* Short. Occasionally heart, genital, and skeletal defects.

Etiology. Deletion of 7q32–7q ter. Deletion 7q21–7q32 does not produce an identifiable syndrome.

BIBLIOGRAPHY. Harris EL, Wappner RS, Palmer CG: 7 deletion syndrome (7q32–7q ter.) Clin Genet 12:233–238, 1977
Young RS, Weaver DD, Kulolich MF: Terminal and interstitial deletions of long arm of chromosome 7. Am J Med Genet 17:437–480, 1984

CHROMOSOME 7q, PARTIAL DUPLICATION

Synonyms. Dup (7q); trisomy 7p.

Symptoms and Signs. Six groups have been described. All have in common physical and mental retardation, apparent hypertelorism, and low-set ears. The form owing to 7q31–7q ter presents: *Head:* Fontanellae large, forehead prominent. *Eyes:* Palpebral fissures downslanting, eyelashes long. *Nose:* Short, long philtrum. *Mouth:* Downcurved upper lip, cleft palate; micrognathia. Early death. Forms caused by 7q32–7q ter do not have cleft palate and have in addition hypotonia, epicanthal folds strabismus, scoliosis, and congenital hip dislocation. Total trisomy (rare) associated with Potter (see).

BIBLIOGRAPHY. Vogel W, Siebers JW, Reinwein H: Partial trisomy 7q. Ann Génét 16:277–280, 1973
Johnson DD, Michels VV, Aas MA: Duplication of 7q31.2–7q ter and deficiency of 18q ter: Report of 2 patients and literature review. Am J Med Genet 25:477–488, 1986
Park JP, McDermet MK, Moeschler JB, et al: A case of de novo translocation 7; 10 and duplication 7p, deletion 10p phenotype. Ann Genet 36:217–220, 1993

CHROMOSOME 8p, PARTIAL DELETION

Synonym. Del (8p).

Symptoms and Signs. Pre- and postnatal growth retardation; microcephaly and moderate to severe mental retardation; congenital nystagmus, short nose, long upper lip; barrel chest with widely spaced nipples; hypospadias and cryptorchidism; congenital heart defects (65%); genital anomalies; inguinal hernias; vertebral anomalies. With growth lessening of facial changes. Minor hand anomalies in 50%.

Etiology. Deletion of short arm of chromosome 8.

Prognosis. Depends on heart defects; mild mental retardation in the survivors.

BIBLIOGRAPHY. Lubs HA, Lubs ML: New cytogenetic techniques applied to a series of children with mental retardation. Nobel Symp 23:240–250, 1973
Orye E, Craen M: A new chromosome deletion syndrome. Report of a patient with 46 XY, 8p-chromosome constitution. Clin Genet 9:289–301, 1976
Patil SR, Hanson JW: Partial deletion of the short arm of chromosome 8 syndrome. J Genet Hum 28:123–129, 1980
Dobyns WB, Dewald GW, Carlson RO: Deficiency of chromosome 8p 21. 1–8pter: case report and review of the literature. Am J Med Genet 22:125–134, 1985

CHROMOSOME 8

Synonym. Warkany; C-group trisomy; trisomy 8 mosaicism.

Symptoms. Both sexes affected; male to female ratio 5:1. Present from birth. Variable degrees of mental deficiency; poor coordination. Estimated frequency 1:25,000–1:50,000.

Signs. Forehead prominent; scaphocephaly; hypertelorism; eyes deeply set; strabismus; corneal opacities; nasal root broad; nares enlarged; lips full (Maya lip); micrognathia; ears cupped; cleft palate. Camptodactyly of fingers and toes. Other occasional defects of bones and urogenital system (40%). Thirty percent has slender trunk and pelvis. Spinal deformities and scoliosis. Cardiac anomalies in 25%. Cryptorchidism in 50%.

Etiology. Trisomy 8 full or in majority mosaics C/normal.

Pathology. Agenesis of the corpus callosum increased.

Diagnostic Procedures. Chromosome studies. *Blood.* Occasionally anemia or leukopenia or both.

Therapy. Symptomatic.

Prognosis. Variable according to ratio of trisomal-to-normal cells. Survival is less restricted than in most other chromosome aberrations: less than one-tenth of all patients died during the first 2 years of life, and most of these were victims of cardiac failure, hydrocephalus internus or infections. Some cases with normal karyotype from cultured leukocytes but trisomy 8 in skin fibroblasts can have an IQ estimated in the 70s and can lead a nearly normal life.

BIBLIOGRAPHY. Warkany J, Rubenstein JH, Soukup SW, et al: Mental retardation, absence of patellae and other malformations with chromosomal mosaicism. J Pediatr 61:803, 1962
Pfeiffer RA, Schellong G, Koseniw W: Chromosomen-anomalienin den Blutzellen eines Kindesmit multiplen. Abartungen Klin Wochenschr 40:1058, 1962
Caspersson T, Lindsten J, Zeck L, et al: Four patients with trisomy 8 identified by the fluorescence and Giemsa bonding techniques. J Med Genet 9:1–7, 1972
Annerén G, Frodis E, Jorulf H: Trisomy 8 syndrome. The rib anomaly and some new features in two cases. Helv Paediatr Acta 36:465–472, 1981
Gagliardi AR, Tajara EH, Varella-Garcia M, et al: Trisomy 8 mosaicism. J Med Genet 15:70–73, 1978

CHROMOSOME 8p, PARTIAL DUPLICATION

Synonyms. Dup 8p; trisomy partial 8p.

Symptoms. Severe mental retardation.

Signs. *Head:* Forehead high frontal and parietal bossing; temple retraction. *Facies:* Round, full cheeks, low nasal bridge, anteverted nostril, mouth wide, everted lower lip, cleft palate and/or uvula. *Ear lobes:* Large. *Neck:* Short. Heart, genital, and skeletal malformations.

Etiology. Partial trisomy 8p.

Pathology. See Signs and frequent absence of corpus callosum.

BIBLIOGRAPHY. Funderburk SJ, Barret CT, Klisak I: Report of a trisomy 8 p infant with carrier father. Ann Génét 21:219–222, 1978
Walker AP, Bocian M: Partial duplication 8q–q21.2 in two sibs with maternally derived insertional and reciprocal translocations. Am J Med Genet 27:3–22, 1987

CHROMOSOME 8q, PARTIAL DUPLICATION

Synonyms. Dup 8q; trisomy, partial 8q.

Symptoms. Mental retardation (IQ 20–70).

Signs. Variable and inconstant signs. Low birth weight (35%); hypertelorism (35%); prominent forehead; flat occiput (35%); short- and broad-based nosed (40%); beaked nose (25%); thin upper lip and lower lip drooping (40%); low-set pinnae (65%). Skeletal anomalies (40%). Heart defects.

Etiology. Chromosome 8q partial duplication.

BIBLIOGRAPHY. Rethoré MD, Aurias A, Couturier J: Chromosome 8: trisomie complete et trisomies segmentaires. Ann Génét 20:5–11, 1977
Walker AP, Bocian M: Partial duplication 8q–q21.2 in two sibs with maternally derived insertional and reciprocal translocation. Am J Med Genet 27:3–22, 1987

CHROMOSOME 9/MOSAIC

Synonym. Haslam.

Symptoms and Signs. Prenatal onset growth deficiency; severe mental deficiency; craniofacial anomalies: sloping forehead with narrow bifrontal diameter; upslanting, short palpebral fissures, deeply set eyes; prominent nasal bridge with short root, small fleshy tip, and slit-like nostrils; micrognathia, low-set, posteriorly rotated and misshapen ears. Skeletal anomalies. Joint anomalies, including abnormal position or function of hips, knees, feet, elbows, and digits; kyphoscoliosis; narrow chest. Other abnormalities: heart defects in about two-thirds of cases, micropenis, cryptorchidism, renal malformations, cystic dilatation of fourth ventricle with lack of midline fusion of cerebellum.

Etiology. Trisomy for chromosome 9.

Diagnostic Procedures. Chromosome study.

Pathology. The anomalies listed above.

Therapy. Symptomatic.

Prognosis. Poor. Death before fourth month of life.

BIBLIOGRAPHY. Haslam R, Broske SP, Moore CM, et al: Trisomy 9 mosaicism, with multiple congenital anomalies. J Med Genet 10:180–184, 1973
Sanchez JM, Fijtman N, Migliorini AM: Report of a new case and clinical delineation of mosaic trisomy 9 syndrome. J Med Genet 19:384–386, 1982
Levy I, Levy Y, Mammon Z, et al: Gastrointestinal abnormalities in the syndrome of mosaic trisomy 9. J Med Genet 26:280–281, 1989

CHROMOSOME 9p DUPLICATION

Synonym. Rethore; dup (9p); trisomy 9p.

Symptoms and Signs. Growth deficiency, primarily of postnatal onset. Delayed puberty such that some patients continue to grow up to the middle of their third decade; severe mental deficiency; microcephaly, hypertelorism; downslanting palpebral fissures, deep-set eyes, prominent nose, down-turned corners of the mouth, cup-shaped ears; short fingers and toes with dystrophic nails; kyphoscoliosis, usually developing during the second decade; congenital heart defects in 5–10% of cases and cleft lip or palate in 35%.

Etiology. Trisomy for the entire short arm of chromosome 9. If only the distal half of 9p is duplicated, the clinical picture is less severe.

Pathology. Malformation findings as outlined above.

Diagnostic Procedures. Chromosome study.

Therapy. Symptomatic.

Prognosis. Of reported patients 5–10% have died in early childhood. The others survived but with mental deficiency and variable degree of handicaps.

BIBLIOGRAPHY. Rethore MO, Larget-Piet L, Abony D, et al: Sur quatre cas de trisomie pour le bras court du chromosome 9. Individualisation d'une nouvelle entité morbide. Ann Genet (Paris) 13:217–232, 1970
Shih L, Diamond N, Searle B, et al: Pure 9p trisomy resulting from maternal mosaicism. Am J Hum Genet 31:110A, 1979
Ginsberg J, Soukup S, Bendon RW: Further observations of ocular pathology in Trisomy 9. J Pediatr Ophthalmol Strabismus 26:146–149, 1989

CHROMOSOME 9p, PARTIAL DELETION

Synonym. Del (9p).

Symptoms and Signs. Trigonocephaly (90%) with a prominent metopica and depressed temples, synophrys and bushy eyebrows, upslanting palpebral fissures (75%), mild hypertelorism, pseudoexophthalmos, midface hypoplasia with short nose and depressed nasal bridge and anteverted nares; small mandible, irregular teeth, high and narrow palate; small posteriorly rotated ears with hypoplastic, adherent lobules and prominent anthelices, and a short and webbed broad neck; wide-set nipples, inguinal and umbelical hernias, scoliosis, diastasis recti, genital anomalies, foot position anomalies (long fingers and toes); mental retardation is frequent, as well as seizure disorders. Cardiac defects (65%).

Etiology. Deletion of the short arm of chromosome 9.

Prognosis. Many adult patients have been reported. Signs may change with age. Mental disorders are frequent in the survivors. Some patients develop leukemia or lymphomas.

BIBLIOGRAPHY. Alfi O, Donnell GN, Grandall BF, et al: Deletion of the short arm of chromosome 9 (46, 9p-): A new deletion syndrome. Ann Genet (Paris) 16:17–22, 1973
Funderburk SJ, Sparkes RS, Klisak I: The 9p-syndrome. J Med Genet 16:75–79, 1979
Wishiewski L, Szymanska J, Niezabitowska A, et al: Two new cases of 9p-syndrome. Klin Paediatr 192:270–274, 1980
Huret JL, Leonard C, Forestier B, et al: Eleven new cases of del (9p) and features from 80 cases. J Med Genet 25:741–749, 1988

CHROMOSOME 9q, PARTIAL DUPLICATION

Synonyms. Dup (9q); trisomy 9q.

Symptoms and Signs. Mental retardation severe. Microdolichocephaly, deep set eyes, nose prominent and beaked, pinnae large, microretrognathia. Cleft lip/palate (35%). Long digits with limited mobility. Occasionally heart and skeletal defects.

Etiology. Duplication in 9q.

BIBLIOGRAPHY. Schwanitz G, Schamberger U, Rott HD: Partial trisomy 9 in the case of familial translocation 8/9 mat. Ann Génét 17:163–166, 1974
Soltan HC, Jung GH, Pyatt Z: Partial trisomy 9q resulting from familial translocation t(9; 16)(q 32; q 24). Clin Génét 25:449–454, 1984

CHROMOSOME 10p, PARTIAL DELETION

Synonym. Del (10p).

Symptoms and Signs. Majority males. Newborns are moderately underweight with widely open fontanels, square-shaped face with high forehead, microcephaly, down slanting palpebral fissures, ptosis of the upper eyelids, short nose with anteverted nostrils and broad and flat bridge, receding mandible, posteriorly rotated and mishaped ears; genital anomalies. Heart anomalies (40%). Frequently babies present feeding difficulties and infections.

Etiology. Deletion of the short arm of chromosome 10.

Prognosis. Many patients die early in life (50%). The survivors are growth retarded, with moderate to severe mental retardation and seizures.

BIBLIOGRAPHY. Berger R, Laroche JC, Toubas PL: Deletion of the short arm of chromosome 10. Acta Paediatr Scand 66:659–662, 1977
Klep-de-Pater JM, Bijllsma JP, Alkema FMJ: Partial monosomy 10p syndrome. Eur J Pediatr 137:243–246, 1981
Greenberg F, Valdes C, Rosenblatt HM, et al: Hypoparathyroidism and T-cell immune defect in a patient with 10 p deletion syndrome. J Pediatr 109:489–492, 1986
Kiss P, Osztovics M: 10p monosomy, a phenotypic variant. Ann Genet 36:232, 1993

CHROMOSOME 10p, PARTIAL DUPLICATION

Synonym. Dup (10p); trisomy 10p.

Symptoms and Signs. Pre- and postnatal growth and mental retardation; dolichocephaly, defective ossification of the calvarian bones, with wide sutures and fontanelles, craniofacial disproportion, narrow face with high forehead, flat nasal bridge, long philtrum, retroposition of the mandible, low-set, posteriorly rotated prominent and dysplastic ears, low hair line; dislocated lips, clubfeet; fine, dry hair, atrophic skin; male genital hypoplasia. Other malformations frequently associated are: cleft lip and palate, heart defects, hypoplasia of the diaphragm, bile duct atresia, cystic kidneys.

Etiology. Trisomy for the short arm of chromosome 10.

Prognosis. Almost half of the patients described died perinatally or during the early postnatal course of asphyxia, prolonged jaundice, feeding difficulties, seizures. The survivors showed muscular hypotonia and underdevelopment, hyperreflexia, diminished activity, and motor and mental deficiency.

BIBLIOGRAPHY. Grosse KP, Schwanitz H, Singer, et al: Partial trisomy 10p in two generations. Human-Genetik 29:141–144, 1975
Yunis E, Silva R, Giraldo A: Trisomy 10p. Ann Genet (Paris) 19:57–60, 1976
Stall C, Willard D: La trisomie 10p. A propos d'une observation d'une translocation maternelle. Pediatrie 35:251–255, 1980
Gonzalez CH, Billerbeck AE, Takayama LC, et al: Duplication 10p in a girl due to maternal translocation t (10; 14) (p11; p12). Am J Med Genet 14:159–167, 1983

CHROMOSOME 10q, PARTIAL DELETION

Synonyms. Del (10q).

Symptoms and Signs. Prevalent in female. Severe mental and physical retardation and nonconstant or specific signs of malformation of face.

Etiology. Deletion of 10q.

BIBLIOGRAPHY. Turleau C, De Grouchy J, Ponsot G: Monosomy 10q ter. Hum Genet 47:233–237, 1979
Wulfsberg EA, Weaver RP, Cunnif CM: Chromosome 10q ter deletion syndrome. A review and report of three new cases. Am J Med Genet 32:364–367, 1989

CHROMOSOME 10q, PARTIAL DUPLICATION

Synonym. Yunis-Sanchez; dup (10q), including trisomy 10q25 qter.

Symptoms and Signs. Majority males. Prenatal onset growth deficiency; mean birth weight 2.7 kg; microcephaly; flat face with high forehead and high arched eyebrows; ptosis; short palpebral fissures; microphthalmia; broad and depressed nasal bridge, bow-shaped mouth with prominent upper lip; cleft palate; malformed; posteriorly rotated ears; campodactyly, proximally placed thumbs, syndactyly between second and third toes, foot position anomalies; heart and renal malformations; kyphoscoliosis; pectus excavatum; cryptorchidism. Occasional abnormalities: brain malformations, ocular anomalies, malrotation of the gut, hypospadias, vertebral malformations. In 10q25 qter also marked hypotonia, microcephaly.

Etiology. Trisomy 10q24 qter, the distal segment of the long arm of chromosome 10. Trisomy 10q25 qter produces distinct clinical picture.

Pathology. Various malformations as outlined above.

Diagnostic Procedures. Chromosome study.

Therapy. Symptomatic.

Prognosis. Poor. One-half of the reported patients died of heart defects; surviving children showed marked mental deficiency.

BIBLIOGRAPHY. Yunis J, Sanchez O: A new syndrome resulting from partial trisomy for the distal third of the long arm of chromosome 10. J Pediatr 84:567–570, 1974

Klep-de Pater JM, Bijlsma JB, de France HF, et al: Partial trisomy 10q. A recognizable syndrome. Hum Genet 46:29–40, 1979

Taysi K, Yang V, Monaghan N: Partial trisomy 10q in three unrelated patients. Ann Génét 26:79–85, 1983

CHROMOSOME 11p, PARTIAL DUPLICATION

Synonyms. Dup (11p); trisomy 11p.

Symptoms and Signs. Severe developmental retardation, no common consistent findings.

BIBLIOGRAPHY. Palmer CG, Poland C, Reed T, et al: Partial trisomy 11, 46, XX, −3, −20, +der3, +der20, t(3:11:20), resulting from a complex maternal rearrangement of chromosome 3, 11, 20. Human Genet 31:219–225, 1976

Bajolle F, Rullier J, Picard AM, et al: Trisomie partielle pour la partie du bras court d'un chromosome 11 par translocation 11/5 paternelle Ann Génét 21:181–185, 1978

CHROMOSOME 11q, PARTIAL DELETION

Synonym. Monosomy 11q; del (11q).

Symptoms and Signs. Females 80%. Frequent respiratory infections. Trigonocephaly (85%), upslanting palpebral fissures, inner epicanthic folds, ptosis of the upper lids, depressed bridge and short tip of the nose with anteverted nares, cup-shaped upper lip, and receding mandible; heart malformations (65%): single ventricle with hypoplasia of the left ventricle with or without atresia of the mitral valve; coloboma of the iris, optic atrophy; pyloric stenosis; anal stenosis; hydronephrosis, cystic kidneys and duplication of kidneys. Minor digital anomalies and joint contractures (70%).

Etiology. Deletion of the long arm of chromosome 11.

Diagnostic Procedures. *Blood:* Thrombocytopenia 50%.

Prognosis. Twenty-five percent of the patients described died within the first days to months of life, from cardiac and respiratory failure. Survivors were short, microcephalic, and often affected by mental retardation.

BIBLIOGRAPHY. Turleau C, Chavin-Colin F, Robin M, et al: Monosomic partielle 11q et trigonocephalie: Un nouveau syndrome. Ann Genet (Paris) 18:257–260, 1975

Lee ML, Sciorra LJ: Partial monosomy of the long arm of chromosome 11 in a severely affected child. Ann Genet (Paris) 24:51–53, 1981

Helmuth RA: Holoprosencephaly, ear anomalies, congenital heart defect and microphallus in a patient with 11q mosaicism. Am J Med Genet 32:178–181, 1989

CHROMOSOME 11q, PARTIAL DUPLICATION

Synonyms. Dup (11q); trisomy, partial 11q.

Symptoms. Low birth weight and reduced postnatal growth. Mental retardation from minimal to moderate (85%). Hypertonia (25%)

Signs. Variable head. Hypertelorism, epicanthal folds strabismus.

Nose: Large, beaked. *Ears:* Preauricular tags or pits. *Mouth:* Lower lip retracted, mandible small; cleft palate (60%). Occasionally, criptorchydism (35%) anal atresia (15%). Heart (40%) and musculoskeletal (30%) defects.

Etiology. Two main types of translocation 11q/22q (inherited from mother) or 11q 23–11 qter.

BIBLIOGRAPHY. Aurias A, Laurent C: Trisomy 11 q individualization d'un nouveau syndrome. Am Génét 18:189–191, 1975

Greig F: Duplication 11 (q 22 - q ter) in a infant. A case report with review. Am Génét 28:185–188, 1989

CHROMOSOME 12 TRISOMY

Synonym. Duplication of the short arm of chromosome 12; dup (12p).

Symptoms and Signs. Midface hypoplasia, shallow orbits, epicanthal folds, flat, wide bridge and upturned tip of the nose and small ears; turribrachycephaly with high forehead, irregular and bushy eyebrows, a long, poorly modeled philtrum, everted lower lip, large tongue, full cheeks; short, broad hands and fingers, and clinodactyly of little fingers; congenital heart defects; microphthalmia, aniridia; cleft palate; and atresia; mental retardation.

Etiology. Duplication of the short arm of chromosome 12.

BIBLIOGRAPHY. Alfi OS, Lange M: Trisomy 12p, a clinically recognizable syndrome. Birth Defects XIII (3b):231–232, 1977

Qazi QH, Kanachanapoomi R, Cooper R, et al: Duplication (12p) and hypoplastic left heart. Am J Med Genet 9:195–199, 1981

CHROMOSOME 13q, PARTIAL DELETION

Synonyms. Del (13q); Lele.

Symptoms. Variable pattern of features present in about 50% of cases. Prenatal onset. Growth deficiency. At birth; muscle hypotony, reduced vision. *Head:* Microcephaly; tendency to trigonocephaly (50%) and other severe skull-brain defects (holoprosencephaly); hypertelorism; ptosis; lid antimongoloid slant; microphthalmia, coloboma; nasal bridge and maxilla prominence; micrognathia; delayed and abnormal dentition. *Ears:* Low set and large. *Neck:* Short and webbed. *Hands:* Thumbs absent or small; fifth finger brachyphalangia. *Feet:* Short, large toe; pes equinovarus. *Genitalia:* Hypospadias; cryptorchidism (60%). Cardiac defect (35%). Retinoblastoma occasional finding that seems related to the genetic condition.

Etiology. Partial deletion of the long arm of chromosome 13. No hereditary factor.

Pathology. Several malformative findings as outlined above.

Diagnostic Procedures. *Chromosome studies. X-rays.* Dilated cerebral ventricles and cisterna cerebellomedullaris; poroencephalia.

Therapy. Symptomatic.

Prognosis. Quoad vitam, variable survival into adulthood. Severe mental retardation. Osteosarcomas and synovial sarcomas.

BIBLIOGRAPHY. Lele KP, Penrose LS, Stallarf HB: Chromosome deletion in a case of retinoblastoma. Ann Hum Genet 27:171–174, 1963

Parcheta B: Clinical features in a case of ring chromosome 13. Eur J Pediatr 144:409–412, 1985

Wilson WG, Campochiaro PA, Conway BP, et al: Deletion (13) (q14. 1q14. 3) in two generations. Variability of ocular manifestations and definition of the phenotype. Am J Med Genet 28:675–683, 1987

CHROMOSOME 14q, PARTIAL DELETION

Synonyms. Del (14q).

Symptoms. Severe mental retardation, hypotonia seizures. Visual impairment. Recurrent respiratory infections.

Signs. Microcephaly, flat occiput, epicanthal folds, face narrow, elongated; palpebral fissures slanting downward. *Nose:* Flat bridge; pinnae: low-set, micrognathia. *Neck:* Short.

Etiology. Deletion of long arm (14q) of chromosome 14.

Pathology. Lateral ventricles enlarged.

Diagnostic Procedures. Fundus oculi: retinitis with specific hyperpigmentation and yellow-white spots in the macula.

Prognosis. Prolonged survival.

BIBLIOGRAPHY. Jalbert P, Sele B, Jalbert H: Chromosome 14 en anneau chez des jemelles monozygotes. Ann Génét 20:59–62, 1977
Caille B, Rethorte MO, Raul O, et al: Deux nouvelles observations de chromosome 14 en anneau. Ann Pédiatr 32:441–446, 1985

CHROMOSOME 14q, PARTIAL DUPLICATION

Synonyms. Dup (14q).

Symptoms and Signs. Physical pre-post-natal and mental retardation. *Face:* Large and asymmetric, chubby cheeks; hypertelorism. *Nose:* Broad; carp mouth; rotated pinnae prominent antitragus. Micrognathia. Cleft palate (50%). *Male:* Hypogenitalism. Variable brain, heart, and lung defects.

Etiology. Chromosome 14q partial trisomy.

BIBLIOGRAPHY. Raoul O, Rethore MO, Dutriliaux B, et al: Trisomic 14 q partielle. Ann Génét 18:35–39, 1975
Turleau C, DeGrouchy J, Chavin-Colin F, et al: La trisomy 14 q distale. Ann Génét 26:165–170, 1983

CHROMOSOME 15q, PARTIAL DELETION

Synonyms. Del (15q); ring 15 chromosome.

Symptoms and Signs. Prenatal growth retardation (100%). Mental retardation (95%). Microcephaly (85%). Hypertelorism (45%). *Face:* Triangular (40%). *Limbs:* Anomalies. Heart defects (30%). Café-au-lait spots (30%). *Male:* Hypogonadism.

Etiology. Deletion of 15q.

BIBLIOGRAPHY. Turner B: Cytogenetic studies in mental retardation. Proc Austr Assoc Neurol 1:41–54, 1963
Fryus JP, Timmermans J, D'Hondt F: Ring chromosome 15 syndrome. Hum Genet 51:43–48, 1979
Butler MG, Fogo AB, Fuchs DA: Two patients with ring chromosome 15 syndrome. Am J Med Gent 29:149–154, 1988

CHROMOSOME 15q, PARTIAL DUPLICATION

Synonyms. Dup (15q); trisomy, partial 15q.

Symptoms and Signs. Severe mental and growth retardation (100%). Hypotonia (frequent) seizures (30%). In case of unbalanced translocation. *Head:* Microdolichocephaly (occasionally hydrocephalus) palpebral fissures slanting downward. *Nose:* Bulbous, pinnae malformed, palate: cleft, micrognathia. In case of distal q arm. *Head:* Microcephaly, sloping forehead. *Facies:* Asymmetric puffy cheeks, palpebral fissure short and downslanting, ptosis. *Nose:* Prominent, broad bridge, long philtrum. *Mouth:* down-turned, palate arched; micrognathia. *Neck:* Short. Skeletal and heart defects.

Etiology. Various types of dup 15q from partial to complete.

BIBLIOGRAPHY. Pffeiffer RA, Kassel E: Partial trisomy 15 q 1. Hum Genet 33:77–83, 1976
Lacro RV, Jones Kl, Mascarello JT: Duplication of distal 15 q. Am J Med Genet 26:719–728, 1987

CHROMOSOME 16p PARTIAL DUPLICATION

Synonyms. Dup (16p); trisomy 16p.

Symptoms and Signs. Severe mental retardation. Microcephaly, hypertelorism, pinnae low-set, maxilla prominent, micrognathia; aplasia or hypoplasia thumb, ASD. Heart defects.

Etiology. Duplication 16p.

Prognosis. Fifty percent die in infancy.

BIBLIOGRAPHY. Leschot NJ, De Nef JJ, Geraedts JP: Five familial cases with a trisomy 16 p syndrome due to translocation. Clin Genet 16:205–214, 1979

CHROMOSOME 16q, PARTIAL DELETION

Synonyms. Del (16q).

Symptoms and Signs. Prenatal and postnatal growth and development retarded. Hypotonia, weak suction. *Head:* Microcephaly, high forehead, prominent metopic suture, large fontanellae, palpebral fissure narrow. *Nose:* Small upturned. *Ears:* Low-set, micrognathia. *Neck:* Short. Occasionally cleft palate and natal teeth. Muscoloskeletal, heart, and intestinal defects.

Etiology. Interstitial and terminal deletion of chromosome 16q.

BIBLIOGRAPHY. Yunis E, Gonzales JT, Torres de Caballeros OM: Partial monosomy 16q. Human Genet 38:347–350, 1977
Rivera H, Vargas-Moyeda E, Moeller M: Monosomy 16 q: A distinct syndrome. Clin Genet 28:84–86, 1985

CHROMOSOME 16q, PARTIAL DUPLICATION

Synonyms. Dup (16q); trisomy 16q.

Symptoms and Signs. Frequent abortion in first trimester. Few liveborn. Low birth weight, severe physical-motor and mental retardation. *Facies:* Round, frontal bossing; glabella prominent, hypertelorism. *Nose:* Bridge depressed, tip round, nostrils anteverted. *Pinnae:* Low set. Maxilla prominent. Hypertrichosis, cryptorchidism, foot defects, contractures.

Etiology. Trisomy 16q.

Prognosis. Early death.

BIBLIOGRAPHY. Francke V: Quinacrine mustard fluorescence of human chromosomes: characterization of unusual translocations. Am J Med Genet 24:189–213, 1972
Garau A, Crisponi G, Peretti D: Trisomy 16 q 21-q ter. Human Genet 53:165–167, 1980

CHROMOSOME 17p, PARTIAL DELETION

Synonyms. Del (17p); Smith-Magenis.

Symptoms and Signs. No definitive clinical pattern identified. Delayed development, brachycephaly, facial hypoplasia, broad nasal bridge, hearing defect, prognathism, short hands.

Etiology. Del (17p11.2).

BIBLIOGRAPHY. Smith ACM, McGavran L, Waidstein G, et al: Deletion of the 17 short arm in 2 patients with facial clefts. Am J Hum Genet 34:410A, 1982

Bridge J, Sanger W, Mosher G, et al: Partial delation of distal 17 q. Am J Med Genet 21:225–229, 1985

Fan YS, Farrell SA: Prenatal diagnosis of interstitial delation of 17 (p11.2 p11.2) (Smith-Magenis syndrome). Am J Med Genet 49:253–254, 1994

CHROMOSOME 17p, PARTIAL DUPLICATION

Synonyms. Dup (17p); trisomy 17p.

Symptoms and Signs. Somatic and mental retardation. Microcephaly, hypertelorism, palpebral fissures narrow, nasal bridge broad. *Ears:* Low set. *Mouth:* Open, mirognathia. *Neck:* Short and webbed. *Fingers:* Long and tapered, flexed. Hypoplasia of male genitals.

Etiology. Partial trisomy 17p.

BIBLIOGRAPHY. Latta E, Hoo JJ: Trisomy of the short arm of chromosome 17. Human Genet 23:213–217, 1974

Feldmann GM, Baumer JG, Sparkes RS: The dup (17 p) syndrome. Am J Med Genet 11:299–304, 1982

CHROMOSOME 17q, PARTIAL DUPLICATION

Synonyms. Dup (17q); trisomy 17q.

Symptoms and Signs. Central nervous system anomalies. Short stature, psychomotor retardation. *Head:* Microcephaly, plagiocephaly, frontal bossing, temporal retraction, hypertelorism. *Facies:* Asymmetric, widow's peak, palpebral fissure usually slanting downward. *Nasal bridge:* Flat. *Mouth:* Wide with downward corners. Cleft lip and/or palate (50%). Pinnae low-set and malformed. *Neck:* Short. *Joints:* Hyperlaxity. Skeletal, heart (50%,) and renal defects. *Males:* Cryptorchidism.

Etiology. Majority involvement of bands q21, q22, or q23 qter, seldom duplication of distal part of 17q.

BIBLIOGRAPHY. Berberich M, Carey JC, Lawce HJ: Duplication (partial trisomy) of the distal long arm of chromosome 17: a new clinically recognizable chromosome disorder. Birth Defects 14:287–295, 1978

Bridge J, Sanger W, Mosher G: Partial duplication of distal 17 q. Am J Med Genet 22:229–235, 1985

CHROMOSOME 18p, PARTIAL DELETION

Synonyms. Monosomy-18, partial short arm; del (18p); De Grouchy-Lamy-Thieffry.

Symptoms and Signs. Few patients (15%) severely affected, most (80%) only minor malformation and mild mental retardation. Present from birth. Variable pattern of features: dysphagia; mental retardation; delayed speech (until 9 years of age); oliguria; rheumatoid-like manifestations (rare). *Head:* Microcephaly; moon facies; hypertelorism; flat bridge of nose; eye lid ptosis; epicanthal folds; mongolism or antimongolian slant; strabismus; nystagmus (rare); cataract; wide mouth; micrognathia; large ears. *Extremities.* Small hands and feet. *Skin.* Alopecia (rare); depigmentation (rare); holoprosencephaly-arhinencephalia defects (rare).

Etiology. Deletion of short arm of chromosome 18 (clinically similar to Cat cry, see).

Diagnostic Procedures. Chromosome studies.

Prognosis. Quoad vitam good (except for cases with holoprosencephaly). Reproduction possible. Mild to severe mental deficiency.

BIBLIOGRAPHY. DeGrouchy J, Lamy M, Thieffry S, et al: Dysmorphie complexe avec des oligophrenie: deletion des bras courts d'un chromosome 17–18. Ct R Acad Sci 256:1028, 1963

Habedank M, Trost-Brinkhues G: Monosomy 18p– and pure 18p in a family with translocation (7; 18). J Med Genet 20:377–379, 1983

Gardner RJM, Sutherland GR: Chromosome abnormalities and genetic counseling, p 150. New York, Oxford Univ Press, 1989

CHROMOSOME 18q, PARTIAL DELETION

Synonyms. De Grouchy II; del (18q).

Symptoms and Signs. Both sexes affected. Gross mental retardation, growth deficiency, seizures, microcephaly; hypotonia (100%), poor coordination, nystagmus, conductive deafness (50%), microcephaly; talipes equinovarus; midface retruded (85%), deeply set eyes; epicanthic folds (42%) strabysmus, skin nodules in nasal folds; tapering fingers, widely separated nipples. In males, minute penis, cryptorchidism. In females, hypoplastic labia minora. Congenital cardiac defects (35%). Inguinal hernias (30%). Abnormal implantation of second toes (84%). Osteoarticular anomalies (50%).

Etiology. Deletion of the long arm of chromosome 18.

Diagnostic Procedures. *Chromosome studies. Blood.* Occasionally, absence of IgA globulin.

Therapy. Symptomatic.

Prognosis. From severe handicap to fair prognosis; short stature below 50th percentile (68%). Ten percent die in first few months of life.

BIBLIOGRAPHY. De Grouchy J, Royer P, Salmon CH, et al: Deletion partielle des bras longs du chromosome 18. Pathol Biol 12:5–79, 1964

Insley J: Syndrome associated with a deficiency of part of the long arm of chromosome no. 18. Arch Dis Child 42:140–146, 1967

Wilson MG, Towner JW, Forsman I, et al: Syndromes associated with deletion of the long arm of chromosome 18 (del) (18 q). Am J Med Genet 3:155–174, 1979

Gardner RJM, Sutherland GR: Chromosome abnormalities and genetic counseling, p 150. New York, Oxford Univ Press, 1989

CHROMOSOME 19q, PARTIAL DUPLICATION

Synonyms. Dup (19q); trisomy 19q.

Symptoms and Signs. Mental retardation, poor physical pre- and postnatal development. Hypotonia. Microbrachycephaly, wide open sutures, palpebral fissures downward slanting, hypertelorism, ptosis, nose short, mouth downturned, cleft palate, neck short. Thorax: barrel-shaped. Skeletal defects.

Etiology. Trisomy distal part long arm 19 chromosome.

BIBLIOGRAPHY. Lange M, Alfi OS: Trisomy 19 q. Ann Génét 19:17–21, 1976

Chen H, Yu CW, Wood MJ, et al: Mosaic trisomy 19 syndrome. Ann Génét 24:32–33, 1981

CHROMOSOME 20p, PARTIAL DUPLICATION

Synonyms. Dup (20p).

Symptoms and Signs. In most cases, normal growth; mild to moderate mental deficiency, hypotonia, poor coordination, ataxia, tremor. *Craniofacial anomalies:* Brachycephaly, upslanting palpebral fissures, blepharophimosis, hypotelorism or hypertelorism; flat nasal bridge with anteverted nares, large and poorly formed ears. *Limb anomalies:* Cubitus valgus, small and tapering fingers, foot position defects. *Other:* Vertebral defects, kyphoscoliosis, umbilical or inguinal hernias, genital hypoplasia with cryptorchidism. *Occasional abnormalities:* Cardiac defects (Fallot's tetralogy), renal malformations, atretic ear canals, iridal colobomata, myopia, strabismus, cataract, hydrocephalus.

Etiology. Trisomy 20.

Therapy. Symptomatic.

Prognosis. Depends on the presence of major anomalies (cardiac). In some cases, patients with mild mental deficiency and no major malformations were not detected before the birth of a second affected sibling.

BIBLIOGRAPHY. Pan SF, Fatora SR, Haas JE, et al: Trisomy of chromosome 20. Clin Genet 9:449–453, 1975
Nevin NC, Nevin J, Thompson W: Trisomy 20 mosaicism in amniotic fluid cell culture. Clin Genet 15:440–443, 1979
Lurie IW, Rumyantseva NV, Zaletajev DV, et al: Trisomy 20p. J Génét Hum 33:67–75, 1985

CHROMOSOME 21q, PARTIAL DELETION

Synonyms. Antimongolism; G-deletion; long arm 21 deletion; monosomy-21 partial; 21g–; G-deletion syndrome; del 21q.

Symptoms and Signs. Mental and growth retardation; muscle hypertonia. *Head:* Microcephaly occiput prominent. *Facies:* Downward slope of eyes (antimongoloid); blepharochalasis; epicanthal folds; occasional cataracts; large external ear; wide external auditory canal; prominent nasal bridge, dysmorphic large pinnae. *Mouth:* Harp-like, bifid uvula; micrognathia. *Neck:* Short. *Gut:* Pyloric stenosis. *Genitals:* Ambiguous cryptorchidism; hypospadias; skeletal system shows retarded growth and various defects; nails dystrophic; normal palmar folds. Seldom heart defects.

Etiology. Deletion of a part of chromosome 21.

Pathology. See Signs.

Diagnostic Procedures. Chromosome studies. Difficulty to diferentiate defects between 21 and 22 chromosome, from this some difficulties in the characterization of the syndrome in the past. *Blood.* Thrombocytopenia; eosinophilia; normal or elevated leukocyte alkaline phosphatase.

Therapy. Symptomatic.

Prognosis. Usually death within first year of life.

BIBLIOGRAPHY. Lejeune J, Berger R, Rethoré MO, et al: Monosomie partielle pour un petit acrocentrique. CR Acad Sci (Paris) 259:4187–4190, 1964
Greenwood RD, Sommer A: Monosomy G: Case report and review of literature. J Med Genet 8:496–500, 1971
Fryns JP, D'Hondt F, Goddeeris P, et al: Full monosomy 21: A clinically recognizable syndrome? Hum Genet 37:155–159, 1977
Carpenter NJ: Partial deletion 21. Case report with biochemical studies and review. J Med Genet 24:706–708, 1987

CHROMOSOME 22q, PARTIAL DELETION

Synonyms. Del (22q). See Di George.

Symptoms and Signs. Atypical. Mental retardation ingravescent with age. Hypotonic. Poor motor coordination. *Head:* Decreased circumference (65%). *Face:* Round in young age. *Eyes:* Wide horizontal, palpebrae almond-shaped, epicanthal folds. Ptosis (35%). *Nose:* Bulbous tip in infancy. Large pinnae.

Etiology. Loss of distal part of long arm of chromosome 22 often resulting in a ring.

BIBLIOGRAPHY. Rethoré MO, Noel B, Couturier J: Le syndrome 2 (22) A propos de quatre nouvelles observations. Ann Génét 111:117, 1978

CHRONIC FATIGUE

To request written information, including information on CFS support groups, contact Chronic Fatigue Syndrome Society, Inc, PO Box 230108, Portland, OR 97223, 503-684-5261.

Synonyms. Akureyri; Royal Free disease; Lake Tahoe; Epstein-Barr virus reactivation, chronic EBV; Iceland disease; CFS; mononucleosis-like, chronic neuromyasthenia; postinfectious neuromyasthenia; postviral fatigue; epidemic neuromyasthenia; neuromyasthenia, sporadic; asthenia, chronic; yuppie disease; viral chronic hyperfatigability; chronic spasmophilia; low NK cell; myalgic encephalomyelitis; see Beard, Burnout and Sick building.

Symptoms. Affects people of all ages, races, and classes. Prevalence in young Caucasian women. Sometimes symptoms follow EBV infections. Onset sudden, headache, sore throat, low-grade fever, fatigue, weakness, arthralgia, inability to concentrate, paresthesias, paresis, anorexia, nausea, vomiting, diarrhea, depression, crying. Feeling of tiredness enhanced by physical or emotional stress, persisting for at least 6 months to years.

Signs. Onset: Tenderness of lymph nodes and other signs mimicking those of flu. In the second phase, absence of physical findings. Some authors consider for diagnosis major and minor criteria.

Major criteria.

1. New onset of persisting or relapsing severe fatigue (over 50% impairment of activity) lasting 6 months or longer
2. Absence of other illnesses

Minor criteria.

1. Mild fever
2. Sore throat
3. Painful lymph nodes
4. Generalized muscle weakness and myalgia
5. Headache
6. Migratory arthralgia
7. Neuropsychologic complaints: photophobia, transient scotomas, forgetfulness, irritability, confusion, inability to concentrate, depression, sleep disturbances

Etiology. Still debated. Previously considered anemia, hypoglycemia, allergy, candidiasis; more recently considered chronic virus infection (Epstein-Barr virus, human herpes virus). Other possible causes are immune system dysfunctions; alteration of cytokine release (overproduction of IL-1, IL-2, and interferons).

Pathology. Unknown.

Diagnostic Procedures. Nonspecific. *Blood.* High antibody levels against any virus (CMV, HS1, measles); abnormal production of interferon or abnormality of 2,5–oligoadenylate synthetase, lack of antibodies to some protein components of EBV, abnormal NK cell function.

Therapy. No treatment proved effective. Antivirals, antidepressants, immunomodulation tried.

Prognosis. Nonprogressive disease. Symptoms reach stable state early in the course and thereafter wax and wane. Some cases of spontaneous recovery reported.

BIBLIOGRAPHY. Albrecht R, Oliver VL, Poskanzer DC: Epidemic neuroasthenia: Outbreak in a convent in New York State. JAMA 187:904–907, 1964
Holmes GP, Kaplan JE, Gantz NM, et al: Chronic fatigue syndrome: A working case definition. Ann Intern Med 108:387–389, 1988
Straus SE: Chronic Fatigue Syndrome. New York, Marcel Dekker, 1995

CHUDLEY

Synonyms. Mental retardation—distinctive mouth—obesity—hypogonadism.

Symptoms. In males. From infancy. Severe mental retardation.

Signs. Short stature, mild obesity, hypogonadism, low total finger ridge comit, typical facies: bitemporal narrowness, palpebral fissures: almond-shaped; nasal bridge: depressed with anteverted nares; upper lip: short and inverted V; macrostomia.

Etiology. X-linked inheritance.

BIBLIOGRAPHY. Chudley AE, Lowry RB, Hoar DI: Mental retardation, distinct facial changes, short stature, obesity, and hypogonadism: a new X-linked mental retardation syndrome. Am J Med Genet 31:741–751, 1988

CHYLOMICRONEMIA SYNDROMES

Three inherited disorders are responsible for this manifestation:

1. Buerger-Gruetz (see)
2. apolipoprotein C-II deficiency (see)
3. lipoprotein lipase inibitor, familial (see) and may be observed in cases of:
4. combined lipoprotein, familial (see).

BIBLIOGRAPHY. Brunzell JD: Familial lipoprotein lipase deficiency and other causes of the chylomicronemia syndrome. In Scriver CR, Beaudet AL, Sly WS, et al: The Metabolic and Molecular Bases of Inherited Disease, 7th ed, p 1913. New York, McGraw-Hill, 1995

CHYLOMICRON RETENTION

Synonyms. Hypolipoproteinemia—selective deletion of APO B-48.

Symptoms and Signs. Male to female ratio 6:2. In infancy or childhood. Severe diarrhea (fat malabsorption); varying degree of growth retardation. Occasionally signs of rickets, acanthocytosis, and neurologic manifestations.

Etiology. Autosomal (X-linked) recessive inheritance. Complex mechanism of inheritance. Defects in several steps of lipidation. Translocation and secretion of apo B-48.

Pathology. Small bowel biopsy: Fat-laden enterocytes with high level of apo B-48.

Diagnostic Procedures. *Blood:* Absence of chylomicrons in plasma after fat ingestion. LDL, apo B and apo A-I levels about half normal value, low vitamin E levels. Occasionally hypoalbuminemia. Acanthocytosis.

Therapy. Restriction of dietary fats with adequate amount of fatty acids, vitamins E and A.

Prognosis. Variable. According to earliness and maintanence of treatment.

BIBLIOGRAPHY. Anderson CM, Townley RRW, Freeman JP: Unusual causes of steatorrhea in infancy and childhood. Med J Aust 11:617, 1961
Kane JP, Havel RJ: Disorders of the biogenesis and secretion of lipoproteins containing the B apolipoproteons. In Scriver CR, Beaudet AL, Sly WS, et al: The Metabolic and Molecular Bases of Inherited Disease, 7th ed, pp 1870–1871. New York, McGraw-Hill, 1995

CINDERELLA

Synonyms. Ramirez; ashy dermatosis; dermatosis cenicienta; erythema dyschromicum perstans; erythema chromicum—figuratum—melanodermicum.

Symptoms and Signs. Both sexes affected; onset from childhood to adulthood. No systemic symptoms or internal manifestations. Disseminated macular lesions "ash gray" in color appearing in the trunk, arms, and face, in both exposed and unexposed areas, sparing palms, soles,

and scalp. Various lesions enlarge with coalescence and form bizarre patterns. Early lesions slightly elevated; zone of pigmentation and hypopigmentation may be observed on the same lesion.

Etiology. Unknown.

Pathology. Active phase. Malpighian layer vacuolization of cells; edema of dermal papillae; moderate perivasculitis in upper third of cutis; infiltrate consisting of histiocytes; small round cells and macrophages containing melanin granules. Inactive phase. Histologic pattern resembling incontinentia pigmenti.

Diagnostic Procedures. *Biopsy of skin. Serology.* To exclude pinta.

Therapy. Cosmesis.

Prognosis. Good.

BIBLIOGRAPHY. Ramirez CO: Los cenicientos: problema clinico. Proc I Cent Amer Cong Derm San Salvadore, Dec. 5–8:122–130, 1952
Knox JM, Dodge BG, Freeman RG: Erythema dyschromicum perstans. Arch Dermatol 97:262–272, 1968
Novick NL, Phelps R: Erythema dyschromicum persistans. Int J Dermatol 24:630–633, 1985
Bleehen SS, Ebling FJG, Champlon RH: Disorders of skin color. In Champion RH, Burton JL, Ebling FJG (eds): Rook/Wilkinson/Ebling Textbook of Dermatology, 5th ed, pp 1595–1596. Oxford, Blackwell Scientific, 1992

CIRCUMVALLATE PLACENTA

Synonym. Placenta circumvallata.

Symptoms and Signs. From affected mothers pregnancy complicated by polyhydramnios. Infants showing cutaneous and intracranial hemorrhages, central nervous system depression, skeletal abnormalities frequently death from respiratory insufficiency.

Etiology. A gene-determined defect (autosomal recessive inheritance).

BIBLIOGRAPHY. Morgan J: Circumvallate placenta. J Obstet Gynaec Br Comm 62:899–900, 1955
Cunningham FG, MacDonald PC, Gant NF, et al (eds): Williams Obstetrics, p 741. Englewood Cliffs, NJ, Prentice-Hall, 1993

CITELLI

Synonym. Aprosexia; adenoidal facies.

Symptoms and Signs. Occurs in children. Loss of power of concentration; insomnia or drowsiness; mental retardation. Facial changes owing to respiratory obstruction may develop.

Etiology. Large adenoids or chronic severe sinus infection.

Therapy. Medical or surgical.

BIBLIOGRAPHY. Citelli S: Vegetazioni adenoidi e sordomutismo. Boll Mal Orecchio Gola Naso 22:141–150, 1904
Weatherall DJ, Ledingham JGG, Warrell DA (eds): Oxford Textbook of Medicine, 3rd ed, p 2611. Oxford, Oxford Med Pub, 1996

CITRULLINEMIA

Synonyms. Argininosuccinate synthetase deficiency; ASA synthetase deficiency; ASS deficiency; citrullinuria.

Symptoms and Signs. Prevalent in Japanese males. Four types have been identified.

1. *Neonatal.* Normal at birth; onset after first days of life. Vomiting; irritability; lethargy; hypotonia or hypertonia of muscles; tachypnea; convulsions; coma.

2. *Subacute.* Initially, normal physical and mental development; onset insidious. Poor feeding and attacks of vomiting followed by tremor, ataxia, convulsions, and delayed physical and mental development. Occasionally, hepatomegaly.
3. *Asymptomatic or mild.* Asymptomatic.
4. *Atypical.* Recurrent episodes of irritability, insomnia, visual alterations, delirium. Normal physical and mental development. Enuresis is constant in all types.

Etiology. Autosomal recessive inheritance. Argininosuccinic acid synthetase deficiency. Mutations causing human citrullinemia are extremely etereogenous and explain different clinical patterns.

Pathology. *Liver.* Nonspecific signs of fatty degeneration. *Brain.* Edema, degeneration of neurons and myelin; presence of enlarged glial cells with lipoid accumulation.

Diagnostic Procedures. *Blood. Urine. Spinal fluid:* High level of citrulline. Hyperammonemia.

1. *Neonatal.* Hyperammonemia after infections; metabolic acidosis; hypoglycemia, hypocalcemia; serum glutamic-pyruvic transaminase (SGPT) increased.
2. *Subacute.* SGOT increased; deficiency of plasma thromboplastin component; blood urea nitrogen low. *EEG:* abnormal. *CT scan, MRI:* cortical atrophy.

Therapy. Nonspecific. Low-protein diet.

1. *Neonatal.* Death in first weeks or months of life.
2. *Subacute.* Physical and mental development delayed.
3. *Asymptomatic.* Development within normal range.
4. *Atypical.* After long period of normal life, spastic paraparesis.

BIBLIOGRAPHY. McMurray WC, Mohyuddin F, et al: Citrullinuria. A new aminoaciduria with mental retardation. Lancet 1:38, 1962
McMurray WC, Rathbun JC, Mohynddin F, et al: Citrullinemia. Pediatrics 32:347–357, 1963
Kobayashi K, Rosenbloom C, Beaudett AL, et al: Additional mutations in argininosuccinate synthetase causing citrullinemia. Mol Biol Med 8:95–100, 1991
Brusilov SW, Horwich AL: Urea cycle enzymes. In Scriver CR, Beaudet AL, Sly WS, et al: The Metabolic and Molecular Bases of Inherited Disease, 7th ed, pp 1203–1204. New York, McGraw-Hill, 1995

CIUFFO

Synonyms. Pulmonic stenosis; atrial septal defect; ECG abnormality.

Symptoms and Signs. Both sexes. A family reported. Clinical evidence of pulmonic stenosis, second type of atrial septal defect (widely and fixedly split second heart sound).

Etiology. Autosomal dominant inheritance.

Diagnostic Procedures. *Electrocardiogram:* Unique changes: superior axis (-88 degrees in the mother) and absence of anterior forces in the precordial leads.

Therapy. Cardiosurgery.

Prognosis. Good with treatment.

BIBLIOGRAPHY. Ciuffo AA, Cunningham E, Traill TA: Familial pulmonary valve stenosis, atrial septal defect and unique electrocardiogram abnormalities. J Med Genet 22:311–313, 1985

CIVATTE

Synonyms. Civatte poikiloderma. See also Riehl and Berloque.

Symptoms and Signs. Relatively common, especially in the mild form; occurs in middle-aged women. Pruritus; erythema; edema; followed by reticulated reddish brown pigmentation and telangiectasia, forming irregular, generally symmetric patches on the cheeks and sides of neck but sparing areas not exposed to light.

Etiology. Unknown. Attributed to photodynamic substances in cosmetics. Probably identical to Riehl.

Pathology. Atrophic macules on skin, covered by white adherent scales.

Therapy. Avoid use of cosmetics and protection of skin from actinic exposure.

Prognosis. Irregular development with remissions or relapses, in some cases progressing to reticular atrophy.

BIBLIOGRAPHY. Civatte A: Poikilodermie réticulée pigmentaire du visage et du cou. Ann Dermatol Syph 4:605–620, 1923
Bleehen SS, Ebling FJG, Champlon RH: Disorders of skin color. In Champion RH, Burton JL, Ebling FJG (eds): Rook/Wilkinson/Ebling Textbook of Dermatology, 5th ed, p 1997. Oxford, Blackwell Scientific, 1992

CLAM DIGGER ITCH

Synonyms. Dermatitis schistosomiasis; cutaneous schistosomiasis; cercaria dermatitis; swimmer itch; marine dermatitis; sea bather eruption.

Symptoms and Signs. Appears in clam diggers and sea bathers on east and west coasts of United States, after few minutes of penetration of cercariae (see Etiology). Intense itching lasting half an hour and leaving small macules; hours later, macules become papules; some pustules accompanied by local edema and severe itching (scratching lesions). Symptoms reach their peak in 3 days and subside in 7 days.

Etiology. Cercarial dermatitis: Penetration in the skin by cercariae of different types of schistosomes, avian or mammalian. Adult worms carried mostly by migratory birds and transmitted to sea snails who transmit them to bathers. Marine dermatitis: salt water and other agents frequently not identifiable.

Pathology. Cercariae in the skin with inflammatory reaction.

Diagnostic Procedures. Identification of infesting agent.

Therapy. Antipruritic and antihistamine topical application. For prevention, destruction of snails on beaches (copper sulfate), and in the water (copper carbonate 2½ lbs/1000 sq ft of bottom of sea along beaches). Drying skin after swimming reduces the infestation remarkably.

Prognosis. Spontaneous recovery in 7 days; repeated infestation more severe.

BIBLIOGRAPHY. Cort WW: Studies on schistosome dermatitis: Status of knowledge after more than 22 years. Am J Hyg 52:251–307, 1950
Weatherall DJ, Ledingham JGG, Warrell DA (eds): Oxford Textbook of Medicine, 3rd ed, pp 970, 975. Oxford, Oxford Med Pub, 1996

CLARKE-HADEFIELD

Obsolete.

Synonyms. Andersen I; pancreas hypoplasia; pancreatic infantilism. See cystic fibrosis.

Symptoms and Signs. Both sexes affected; onset at early age. Delayed growth and development; poor muscles; lack of subcutaneous fat; digestive troubles comparable with mucoviscidosis (see). Usually, absence of respiratory complication. Occasionally, associated with hematologic alterations (see Shwachman).

Etiology. Unknown; congenital exocrine hypoplasia of pancreas on genetic basis.

Pathology. Atrophic pancreas; hepatomegaly.

Diagnostic Procedures. *Stool.* Bulky, fatty. *Pancreatic enzyme determination.* In duodenal secretion, blood, urine, stools. *Biopsy of pancreas.* (No danger of fistula because of lack of enzymes). *Sweat test.* Normal.

Therapy. Pancreatic enzyme administration.

Prognosis. Better than in mucoviscidosis syndrome.

BIBLIOGRAPHY. Clarke C, Hadefield G: Congenital pancreatic disease with infantilism. J Med 17:358–364, 1924
Andersen DH: Cystic fibrosis of the pancreas and its relation to celiac disease. Am J Dis Child 56:344–399, 1938
Bodian M, Sheldon W, Lightwood R: Congenital hypoplasia of the exocrine pancreas. Acta Paediatr Scand (Stockh) 53:282–293, 1964

CLARKSON

Synonyms. Capillary leak, idiopathic systemic capillary leak; systemic capillary leak; see Cyclical edema.

Symptoms and Signs. Rare condition. Onset at 42.6 years, possibility of onset in early childhood. Episodes of severe shock-like syndrome (that spare the lung vasculature) and angio-edematous manifestations.

Etiology. Triggering factors unknown. Exudation of proteins with weight of up to 900,000 daltons and fluids into organs.

Diagnostic Procedures. *Blood.* Hemoconcentration. Presence of an abnormal pataprotein (monoclonal gammopathy). *Urine.* Absence of Bence-Jones protein.

Therapy. Symptomatic. Fluid and crystalloids replacement.

Prognosis. One year from onset survival 22/23, 5-year survival 8/14.

BIBLIOGRAPHY. Clarkson B, Thompson D, Horwith M, et al: Cyclical edema and shock due to increase capillary permeability. Am J Med 29:193–216, 1960
Ewan PW, Lachmann PJ, Morice A, et al: Treatment of systemic capillary leak syndrome. Lancet II:1496, 1988
Foeldvari I, Waida E, Junker AK: Systemic capillary leak syndrome in a child. J Ped 127:739–741, 1995

CLIVUS EDGE

Synonyms. See Foix-Jefferson and Orbital apex.

Symptoms and Signs. Myosis followed by mydriasis and sluggish pupil reaction; paresis of extraocular muscles.

Etiology. Rise in intracranial pressure on the roots of oculomotor nerve that push against bone at the entrance into cavernous sinus.

Pathology. Subdural hematoma, temporal bone tumor. Supraclinoid aneurysm.

Diagnostic Procedures. *CT scan. MR imaging.*

BIBLIOGRAPHY. Fischer-Brugge E: Anatomische Ursachen functionaler kreislangstoerungen des Gehirns und am N. Oculomotorius. Bruns' Beitrage Klin Chir 181:323–336, 1951
Roy A: Ocular Syndromes and Systemic Disease, Orlando, FL, Grune & Stratton, 1985
Adams RD, Victor M: Principles of Neurology, 5th ed, p 611. New York, McGraw-Hill, 1993

CLOQUET

Synonyms. Femoral hernia; crural hernia; hernia femoralis.

BIBLIOGRAPHY. Cloquet JR: Reserches anatomiques sur les hernies de l'abdomen Paris 1817 (Thesis)

Sabiston DC: Textbook of Surgery, 14th ed, p 1145. Philadelphia, WB Saunders, 1991

CLOUGH-RICHTER

Obsolete.

Synonym. Erythrocyte autoagglutination. Of historical interest; one of the first reports of red cell autoagglutination.

BIBLIOGRAPHY. Clough MC, Richter IM: A study of an autoagglutinin occurring in a human serum. Bull Johns Hopkins Hosp 29:86–93, 1918

CLOUSTON

Synonyms. Hidrotic ectodermal dysplasia; ectodermal dysplasia, hidrotic.

Symptoms and Signs. Both sexes affected; present from infancy. Dystrophy of nails; thickened; striated; discolored or thin; short and brittle (may be the only manifestation). Repeated paronychial infections. Skin on edges of nail, finger joints, knuckles, knees, elbows may occasionally be thickened. Hyperkeratosis of palms and soles. In complete form, hair fine, sparse, or absent; usually hair defect develops at puberty. Normal sweating; normal teeth; physical development normal or slightly impaired. Mental development normal or retarded. Strabismus. In one family bilateral cataracts.

Etiology. Unknown; autosomal dominant inheritance.

Pathology. Hyperkeratosis.

Diagnostic Procedures. Biopsy of skin.

Therapy. None.

Prognosis. Sexual development normal. Life expectancy not affected, except in some homozygous states, where it may be fatal.

BIBLIOGRAPHY. Clouston HR: A hereditary ectodermal dystrophy. Can Med Assoc J 21:18–31, 1929
Escobar V, Goldblatt LI, Bixler D, et al: Clouston syndrome: An ultrastructural study. J Clin Genet 24:140–146, 1983
Harper J: Genetics and genodermatoses. In Champion RH, Burton JL, Ebling FJG (eds): Rook/Wilkinson/Ebling Textbook of Dermatology, 5th ed, p 339. Oxford, Blackwell Scientific, 1992

CLOVERLEAF SKULL

Synonyms. Gruber; hydrocephalus chondrodystrophicus congenitum; Kleeblattschaedel anomaly; trefoil skull.

Symptoms and Signs. Both sexes affected. Almost all affected children are born dead. Reported in two adults. Grotesque trilobed skull; downward displacement of the ears; exophthalmos; beak nose with deeply recessed nasal root; prognathism. In the majority of cases, associated deformities of bones (achondroplasia); seldom, ankylosis of elbows have been observed.

Etiology. Etiologically and pathogenetically heterogeneous. Abnormality of ossification resulting in intrauterine synostosis of coronal and lambdoid sutures with hydrocephalus. May be considered, according to recent view, more a sign than a syndrome. It may be observed as isolated anomaly or associated with various pathologic conditions such as Apert (see), Crouzon (see), thanatophoric dwarfism (see); limb bony ankylosing; Carpenters (see), Pfeiffer (see), and other congenital syndromes.

Pathology. Characteristic skull deformity and musculoskeletal alteration (see Signs). Hydrocephaly is common; small cerebellum; cerebellar herniation; polymicrogyria and other brain anomalies.

Prognosis. According to severity.

BIBLIOGRAPHY. Vrolik W: Tabulae ad illustrandam embriogenesin Hominis et Mammalium GMP. London, 1849

Gruber GB: Veber einen akrocephalen Reliefschaedel. Ein Beitrag zur Frage der partiellen Chondrodystrophie. Beitr Path Anat 97:9–12, 1936

Holtermüeller K, Wiedemann HR: Kleeblattschädel syndrome. Med Wcknschr 14:439–446, 1960

Cohen MM Jr: Cloverleaf syndrome update. Proc Greenwood Genet Center 6:186–187, 1987

Clark RD, Eteson D: Kleeblattschaedel association with Saethre-Chotzen syndrome. Third Manchester Birth Defects Conference Manchester, October 25–28, 1988

CLUNEAL NERVE

Synonyms. Episacroiliac lipoma; gluteal. See also Battered buttock.

Symptoms. Low back pain from mild to extremely severe radiation of pain along the distribution of cluneal nerves (buttock; back of hip) occasionally referred pain in the groin or extremities (burning; aching; rarely, sharp or stabbing). Various postures and actions aggravate pain such as sitting, bending, lying, or walking.

Signs. Localized tender area 2 cm in diameter in low lumbar or episacroiliac areas; injection over the deep fascia in trigger point must relieve the symptomatology for longer than half an hour. Occasionally, fatty nodules are observed at the site of trigger zone; restriction of spinal mobility is observed in 62% of cases.

Etiology. Establishment of trigger zone by a violent or minor trauma that initiates degenerative changes of subcutaneous tissue, increase of fibrous stroma, and hypersensitization of sensory nerves to mechanical stimuli (tension).

Pathology. No definite pathology has been observed.

Diagnostic Procedures. See Signs.

Therapy. Surgical differentation of trigger area of tenderness or cluneal neurectomy.

Prognosis. With surgery, 79% excellent results, 11% good results, the remaining recurrent cluneal nerve syndrome.

BIBLIOGRAPHY. Strong EK, Davila JC: The cluneal nerve syndrome. 26:417–429, 1957

Dawson DM, Hallett M, Millender LH: Entrapment Neuropathies, 2nd ed. Boston, Little, Brown, 1990

CLUSTER HEADACHE

Synonyms. Horton II; Bing-Horton; Charlin. Harris; Vallery-Radot; Symond-ache; histamine cephalalgia; paroxysmal cephalalgia, nocturnal orbital; ciliary neuralgia; erythroprosopalgia; vascular headache; periodic migrainous neuralgia; including Sjaastad-Dale; chronic paroxysmal hemicrania.

Symptoms. Affects men 30–40 years old; rare in females. No prodromes. Severe, unilateral aching pain beginning in the infraorbital area, and spreading, increasing in intensity on homolateral side of head and neck. Symptoms appear usually during the night at the same time, regularly several times a day for days or weeks (cluster) followed by remission of days or years. Precipitated occasionally by alcohol or heat; cold brings relief. Pain reaches peak in 10 minutes, attack lasts 1–3 hours; no sequelae. Nostril of same side usually feels obstructed and may have watery discharge. Repeated sweating same side of face also reported. No nausea or vomiting. Recurrences occasionally seasonal.

Signs. Flushing of affected side of face; conjunctiva congested. Occasionally, Horner's sign and bradycardia.

Etiology. Unknown; allergy excluded by all tests or at least not confirmed. Possibly, basic psychological disturbance.

Diagnostic Procedures. *Thermography.* Unique spotted pattern of hypothermia in 66% of patients, which does not change in presence or absence of attacks or vasoactive drugs. *EEG. CT scan. MRI. PET.*

Therapy. All failed including psychotherapy. Symptomatic treatments: ergotamine tartrate seems to bring some symptomatic relief. Intranasal cocaine or subcutaneous sumatriptan to abort an attack. Predisone for cases refractory to above indicated treatments. Trial with lithium carbonate. Amitriptyline has been tried with some success. Nonsteroid anti-inflamatory agents also employed.

Prognosis. See Symptoms. A particular form "the chronic paroxysmal hemicrania" known also as Sjaastad-Dale is characterized by many attacks in a day lasting for years. (This form seems to respond to indomethacin.)

BIBLIOGRAPHY. Bing R: Lehrbuch der Nervenkrankheiten. Berlin, 1913

Harris BT: Neuritis and Neuralgia. London, 1926

Bing R: Ueber traumatische Erythromelalgie und Erythroprosopalgie. Nervenarzt 3:506–512, 1930

Vallery-Radot P, Blamoutier P: Syndrome de vasodilatation hemicephalique d'origine sympathique (hemicranie, hemihydrorrhea, hemilarmoiement). Bull Mem Soc Med Hop Paris 49:1488–1493, 1925

Charlin C: La sindrome del nervo nasale. Boll Ocul (Firenze) 10:921–936, 1931

Horton BT: The use of histamine in the treatment of specific types of headaches. JAMA 116:377–383, 1941

Saper JR: Ergotamine dependency—a review. Headache 27:435–438, 1987

Cady RK, Fox AW: Treating the Headache Patient. New York, Marcel Dekker, 1994

CLUTTON

Synonym. Syphilitic knee synovitis.

Symptoms and Signs. Usually, an insidious onset at 6–16 years of age. Symmetric, indolent, chronic swelling of joints (knee 85%); occasionally recurrent. In few cases, acute or subacute. Periarticular redness, pain, limitation of motion; fever; systemic manifestations. Seldom, polyarticular involvement.

Etiology. Congenital syphilis. Difficult differential diagnosis when not associated with other manifestations of congenital syphilis.

Pathology. Chronic hydrarthrosis; no damage to joints; involves soft tissues exclusively.

Diagnostic Procedures. *Serology.* Synovial fluid aspiration. Rich in lymphocytes. *Biopsy of joint. X-rays.* Negative except for presence of fluid.

Therapy. No response to antibiotics.

Prognosis. Good response to conservative treatment and complete recovery.

BIBLIOGRAPHY. Clutton HH: Symmetrical synovitis of the knee in hereditary syphilis. Lancet 1:391–393, 1886

Weatherall DJ, Ledingham JGG, Warrell DA (eds): Oxford Textbook of Medicine, 3rd ed, p 3002. Oxford, Oxford Med Pub, 1996

COAL MINER ELBOW

Synonyms. Olecranon bursitis; student elbow.

Symptoms. Pain in the elbow.

Signs. Tenderness; swelling of elbow; limitation of movement.

Etiology. Trauma by repeated jolts (e.g., with pneumatic hammer) or friction; associated with elbow disease, gout, arthritis, or unknown causes.

Pathology. Bursitis; degeneration of lining of bursa; adhesion and thickening of wall, villi with intra-articular calcifications.

Diagnostic Procedures. *X-ray.* Intra-articular calcification.

Therapy. Rest and physical therapy (heat); deep X-ray if not responsive; or infiltration with procain or hydrocortisone for acute pain. When indicated excision of the bursa.

Prognosis. Good if traumatic causes removed. The progression of condition may result in atrophy of the joint.

BIBLIOGRAPHY. Weatherall DJ, Ledingham JGG, Warrell DA (eds): Oxford Textbook of Medicine, 3rd ed, pp 2975–2976, 2981. Oxford, Oxford Med Pub, 1996

COATS

Synonyms. Exudative retinitis. Leber miliary aneurysma; retinal teleangiectasia; retinitis hemorrhagica externa.

Symptoms. Prevalent in male children or adolescents (juvenile form). For adult form see Hyperlipemic retinitis. Development of photophobia with cloudy vision, usually unilateral.

Signs. *Group I.* Presence of deep, yellowish, massive exudate in and under external retina, producing localized solid elevation of the retina. No evidence of hemorrhage or vascular changes. *Group II.* Marked changes of small retinal arterioles, fresh hemorrhages; plus abovementioned retinal findings. *Group III.* Reported association with hearing loss, muscular weakness, and mental retardation.

Etiology. Unknown; in juvenile form, supposed intermediary tissue factor that precipitates cholesterol. In adult form, chronic inflammation and hypercholesterolemia as trigger mechanism. Toxoplasmosis may be responsible in some cases; in group III possible autosomal recessive inheritance.

Pathology. Massive exudate formed primarily by free cholesterol esters in external retina and subretinal space, containing foam cells and hemosiderin pigment. Minor inflammatory changes of nongranulomatous type and adhesion between choroid and subretinal organized mass. Same findings in juvenile and adult forms.

Diagnostic Procedures. *Blood.* In juvenile form, blood lipids are normal; in adult form, blood lipids are elevated (cholesterol in particular). *Sabin-Feldman dye test.* Positive in some patients.

Therapy. Diathermy; corticosteroids have limited efficacy.

Prognosis. Progressive loss of visual acuity.

BIBLIOGRAPHY. Coats G: Forms of retinal disease with massive exudation. R Lond Ophthalmol Hosp Rep 17:440–525, 1908
Chang M, McLean IW, Merritt JC: Coats' disease: A study of 62 histologically confirmed cases. J Pediatr Ophthalmol Strabismus 21:163–168, 1984
Haik BG: Advanced Coats' disease. Trans Am Ophthalmol Soc 89:371–376, 1991
Lee ST, Friedman SM, Rubin ML: Cystoid macular edema secondary to juxtavalvular teleangiectasis in Coats disease. Ophthalic Surg 22:218–221, 1991
Garner A: Vascular diseases. In Garner A, Klintworth GK (eds): Pathobiology of Ocular Disease: A Dynamic Approach, 2nd ed, pp 1689–1690. New York, Marcel Dekker, 1994

COBB

Synonyms. Cushing-Bailey-Cobb; cutomucomeningospinal angiomatosis; angiomatosis, cutaneomeningospinal. See Sturge-Weber.

Symptoms and Signs. From birth: Port wine or angiokeratomatous lesion in dermatomal distribution on trunk or extremities. In childhood or adolescence: Spastic paralysis of one or both extremities and sensory loss below level of spinal lesion.

Etiology. Unknown. Reported possible autosomal dominant inheritance.

Pathology. Angioma of spinal cord.

Diagnostic Procedures. *CT scan. Angiography. MRI.*

Therapy. Neurosurgery.

Prognosis. Good with early treatment.

BIBLIOGRAPHY. Cobb S: Hemangioma of the spinal cord associated with skin naevi of these same metamers. Am Surg 62:641–649, 1915
Cusching H, Bailey P: Hemangiomas of cerebellum and retina. Arch Ophth 57:447–456, 1928
Atherton DJ: Naevi and other developmental defects. In Champion RH, Burton JL, Ebling FJG (eds): Rook/Wilkinson/Ebling Textbook of Dermatology, 5th ed, p 489. Oxford, Blackwell Scientific, 1992

COCAINE EMBRYOPATHY

Symptoms and Signs. Reduced weight at birth, stillborn 0.8%; cardiopathy (4%), transposition of large arteries; right heart hypoplasia; encephalopathy (2%); intraparietal encephalocele.

Etiology. Intranasal or intravenous inhalation in pregnancy (1–5 weeks).

BIBLIOGRAPHY. Bingol N, Fuchs M, Diaz V, et al: Teratogenicity of cocaine in humans. J Pediatr 110:93–96, 1987
Roland EH, Volpe JJ: Effect of maternal cocaine use on the fetus and newborn review of literature. Pediatr Neurosc 15:88–94, 1989

COCHRANE

Obsolete.

Synonym. Leucine-sensitive hypoglycemia. See leucine metabolism defects.

BIBLIOGRAPHY. Cochrane WA, Payne WW, Simpkiss MJ, et al: Familial hypoglycemia precipitated by amino acids. J Clin Invest 35:411–422, 1956
Ebbin AJ, Huntley C, Tranquada RE: Symptomatic leucine sensitivity in mother and daughter. Metabolism 16:926–932, 1967

COCKAYNE

Synonyms. Neill-Dingwall; deafness–dwarfism–retinal atrophy; progeroid nanism. See Blooms and also De Santis-Cacchione and Kaposi II.

Symptoms. Onset in second year of life after normal infancy. Cutaneous photosensitivity with pigmentation and scars; decrease of vision; progressive deafness; mental deficiency; unsteady gait.

Signs. Dwarfism with long extremities and large hands and feet. Musculoskeletal abnormalities: flexion deformities of extremities; kyphosis; thickened skull: loss of subcutaneous fat. Senile face; sunken eyes; thin nose; prognathism. Cataracts, ulceration of cornea, degenerative retinopathy (salt and pepper fundus). Optic atrophy poor pupillary response to mydriatics. Hepatosplenomegaly in some cases; older patients sexually underdeveloped.

Etiology. Unknown; hereditary disorders (autosomal recessive type, at least three allelic types with some clinical variability, i.e., early onset in type II). Trisomy in group 19–20. In other cases, normal karyotype.

Pathology. Microcephaly. Cerebral cortex and cerebrum atrophic. Patchy or tigroid demyelinization greatest in occipital lobe. Pericapillary calcification in the cortex, basal ganglia, and cerebellum; larger artery and arteriole mineralization.

Diagnostic Procedures. *Chromosome study. X-rays of skull and extremities.* Intracranial calcification; marble epiphyses in some digits. The ultraviolet (UV) sensitivity of cultured fibroblast cells derived from patients with this syndrome has been studied. The depression of RNA synthesis after UV irradiation is variable among the individual patients, and the level of UV sensitivity does not parallel the severity of the clinical manifestations.

Therapy. Symptomatic.

Prognosis. Progressive deterioration to blindness, deafness, paralysis, inanition, and death in adolescence or early adulthood. Aspiration pneumonia constitutes a leading cause of death.

BIBLIOGRAPHY. Cockayne EA: Dwarfism with retinal atrophy and deafness. Arch Dis Child 11:1–8, 1936
Nance MA, Berry SA: Cockayne syndrome: review of 140 cases. Am J Med Genet 42:68–84, 1992
Klintworth GK: Ocular involvement in disorders of the nervous system. In Garner A, Klintworth GK (eds): Pathobiology of Ocular Disease: A Dynamic Approach, 2nd ed, p 1729. New York, Marcel Dekker, 1994

COCKAYNE-TOURAINE

Synonyms. Weber-Cockayne; hyperplastic epidermolysis bullosa, epidermolysis bullosa hyperplastic; hyperplastic epidermolysis bullosa. Including Kallin.

Symptoms and Signs. Both sexes affected, onset in early infancy or later (also in adulthood). Appearance of bullae, usually after trauma, also spontaneous. Head and limbs mostly affected; scarring and occasionally mutilation results. Normal mental and physical development. Frequent association with ichthyosis, keratosis pilaris, tylosis with hyperhidrosis, and dystrophic nails; hypertrichosis. Involvement of mucosa 20%.

Etiology. Unknown; autosomal dominant inheritance. It may be also an autosomal recessive trait (Kallin Syndrome, from name of patient).

Therapy. Symptomatic; antibiotics; corticosteroids. Protection from trauma. Prevention of bullae: frictioning with ice water.

Prognosis. According to severity of form and age of onset.

BIBLIOGRAPHY. Touraine A: L'heredite en Medicine. Paris, Mason, 1855
Elliot GT: Two cases of epidermolysis bullosa. J Cutan Genitourin Dis 13:10–18, 1895
Weber FP: Recurrent bullous eruptions of the feet in a child. Proc R Soc Med 19:72, 1938
Cockayne EA: Recurrent bullous eruption of the feet. Br J Dermatol Syph 50:358–362, 1938
Mulley JC, Turner T, Nicholls C, et al: Genetic linkage analysis of epidermolysis bullosa dystrophica Cockayne-Touraine type. Clin Genet 28:31–35, 1985
Pye RJ: Bullous eruptions. In Champion RH, Burton JL, Ebling FJG (eds): Rook/Wilkinson/Ebling Textbook of Dermatology, 5th ed, pp 1626–1627. Oxford, Blackwell Scientific, 1992

COCKTAIL PARTY

Synonyms. Chronic brain–hydrocephalus; chatter-box; hyperactivity. ADHD; pseudointelligence. See Strawpeter.

Symptoms. Occurs in children with arrested hydrocephalus (either spontaneous or therapeutic). Characteristic behavior pattern consisting of high sociability, pseudo brightness, excessive talkativeness without complete understanding what they are talking about. Characteristic scanning speech owing to a combination of moderate dysrhythmia and altered intonation pattern. This syndrome is associated, more or less, with the neurologic symptoms and signs related to chronic infantile hydrocephalus.

Etiology. Infantile hydrocephalus. Consider multigenerational genetic vulnerability.

Therapy. Psychostimulant, antidepressant, other therapy (pharmacological psychiatric) according to symptoms.

Prognosis. Educational ability of these patients is relatively poor compared with their conversational ability.

BIBLIOGRAPHY. Bleuler E: Veraultnisbloedsinn. Allg 2 Psychiat 71:537–586, 1914
Ingram TT, Naughton JA: Paediatric and psychological aspects of cerebral palsy associated with hydrocephalus. Dev Med Child Neurol 4:287–292, 1962
Hagberg B, Sjorgen I: The chronic brain syndrome of infantile hydrocephalus; a follow-up study of 63 spontaneously arrested cases. Am J Dis Child 112:189–196, 1966
Accardo PJ, Blondis TA, Whitman BY: Attention Deficit Disorders and Hyperactivity in Children. New York, Marcel Dekker, 1991

CODMAN

Synonym. Chondroblastoma benign.

Symptoms. Four hundred cases well documented. Prevalent in males; onset usually in adolescence or young adult age. Localized pain and limited motion of contiguous joint.

Signs. Swelling and tenderness at epiphyseal extremities of long bones (femur, tibia, and radius in particular); overlying skin is warmer and local muscles show atrophy.

Etiology. Unknown.

Pathology. Foci of necrosis; inflammatory changes; hemorrhages; fibrous scarring and presence of spindle cells; scattered multinucleated giant and polyhedral cells with large central nuclei.

Diagnostic Procedures. X-ray. Well-defined area of rarefaction with surrounding thin zone of denser bone; periosteal thickening.

Therapy. Excision.

Prognosis. Seldom, malignant transformation. Possibility of pathologic fractures.

BIBLIOGRAPHY. Codman EA: Epiphyseal chondromatous giant cell tumours of the upper end of the humerus. Surg Gynecol Obstet 32:543–548, 1931
Carnesale PG: Sometime malignant tumors of the bone. In Crenshaw AH (ed): Campbell's Operative Orthopedics, 7th ed, p 765. St Louis, CV Mosby, 1987

COENZYME Q10 DEFICIENCY

Synonyms. CoQ10 deficiency. See Oxphos syndrome.

Symptoms and Signs. Two cases reported (sisters). Exercise intolerance, recurrent myoglobinuria, slowly progressive weakness of axial and proximal limb muscles. Seizures, cerebellar syndrome, learning disability.

Etiology. Probably defect of CoQ10.

Pathology. Muscle biopsy: Increased lipid droplets and mitochondrial in type I fibers.

Diagnostic Procedures. *Blood.* Lactic acidosis, increased serum CK.

Therapy. Replacement therapy.

Prognosis. Amelioration with therapy.

BIBLIOGRAPHY. Ogasahara S, Engel AG, Frens D, et al: Muscle coenzyme

Q deficiency in familial mitochondrial encephalomyopathy. Proc Natl Acad Sci 86:2379–2382, 1989

COFFIN-LOWRY

Symptoms. Occurs in males (females carriers): onset in postnatal period. Mild growth deficiency; severe mental deficiency; muscle weakness. No speech capability.

Signs. *In males. Head.* Mild hypertelorism; downslanting palpebrae; prominent brows; maxillar hypoplasia; thick alae and nasal septum. *Extremities.* Hands large and soft; fingers tapering; clubbing of the distal phalanges (Hippocratism); accessory thenar crease; flat feet; lax ligaments. *Trunk.* Pectus carinatum and short bifid sternum; vertebral defects; thoracolumbar scoliosis. *In females.* Milder features. Anomalies of the genitourinary tract have been reported; congenital microureteral junction; vesicoureteral reflux; absence of one kidney; massive hydronephrosis.

Etiology. X-linked semidominant inheritance. Autosomal recessive inheritance has been proposed.

Pathology. Ultrastructural studies of skin and conjunctiva: suggestion of lysosomal storage disease.

Diagnostic Procedures. *X-rays. Intravenous pyelography.*

Therapy. Symptomatic.

Prognosis. In males, severe mental deficiency. Stooped posture; muscular weakness.

BIBLIOGRAPHY. Coffin GS, Siris E, Wegienke LC: Mental retardation with osteocartilagenous anomalies. Am J Dis Child 112:205–213, 1966
Lowry RB, Miller JR, and Fraser FC: A New dominant gene mental retardation syndrome: associated with small stature, tapering fingers, characteristic facies, and possible hydrocephalus. Am J Dis Child 121:496–500, 1971
Young ID: The Coffin-Lowry syndrome. J Med Genet 25:344–348, 1988
Miyazaki K, Yamanaka T, Ishida Y, et al: Calcified ligamenta flava in a patient with Coffin-Lowry syndrome: biochemical analysis of glycosaminoglycans. Jpn J Hum Genet 35:215–221, 1990

COFFIN-SIRIS

Synonym. Dwarfism—onychodysplasia; fifth digit. See also Meadow and Senior.

Symptoms. Both sexes affected (female to male ratio 4:1); present from birth. Feeding problems; recurrent respiratory infections; mental deficiency (100%); hypotonia (100%) (from mild to severe).

Signs. Growth deficiency (85%). Lombosacral hirsutism (100%); sparse scalp hair (80%). Microcephaly (65%); full lips. Fifth fingernail hypoplastic or absent. (100%) Toenails hypoplastic or absent. Lax joints (elbow dislocation); small patellae. Occasionally, variable skin, skeletal, genital cardiac defects and Dandy-Walker (see).

Etiology. Unknown. Sporadic, possibly autosomal dominant inheritance with variable expression.

BIBLIOGRAPHY. Coffin GS, Siris E: Mental retardation with absent fifth fingernail and terminal phalanx. Am J Dis Child 119:433–439, 1970
Haspeslagh M, Fryns JP, van den Berghe H: The Coffin-Siris syndrome: Report of a family and further delineation. Clin Genet 26:374–378, 1984
Levy P, Baraitser M: Coffin-Siris syndrome. J Med Genet 28:338–341, 1991

COGAN I

Symptoms. Sex distribution: equal, usually occurs in young adults.

Acute vestibule auditory symptoms precede ophthalmic manifestations (confused with Menière, see): nausea, vomiting, tinnitus, vertigo, rapid development of deafness. Eye symptoms: Photophobic watering, unilateral or bilateral blurring of vision, pain in the eye. Myalgia and convulsion have also been reported.

Signs. Nystagmus, eye redness, ciliary injection, mild iritis, fluffy opacities in the cornea; corneal ulceration and vascularization (rare today because of early treatment by corticosteroids); orbital pseudo tumor papillitis and edema, uveitis, retinal hemorrhage, and maculopathy. Systemic manifestations in 50% of cases: aortitis, aortic valve insufficiency, gastrointestinal hemorrhages.

Etiology. Initially described in association with deafness, lymphoadenopathy, and musculoskeletal diseases.

Pathology. *Eye:* See Signs. *Histology:* Lympho and plasma cells infiltration in the cornea with neovascularization.

Diagnostic Procedures. *Blood:* Leukocytosis and mild eosinophilia, erythrocytes sedimentation rate increased, complement concentration; protein and immunoglobulins, anti-DNA antibodies; nuclear rheumatoid factor: normal; cryoglobulin: increased in 23% of cases. *Electrocardiography:* Aortic valvular disease. *Kidney function test:* Altered in 50% of cases. *Chest X-ray:* Aortic valve insufficiency.

Therapy. Ciclophosphamide or cyclosporin helpful in severe cases. Cyclopegic (under ophtalmological supervision). Cardiosurgery for specific complication.

Prognosis. In 63% of cases serious outcome. Deafness (43%), blindness (8%), aortic insufficiency (14%), death from the disease (9%).

BIBLIOGRAPHY. Cogan DG: Syndrome of non syphilitic interstitial keratitis and vestibulo auditory symptoms. Arch Ophthalmol 33:144–149, 1945
Vollertsen RS: Vasculitis and Cogan's syndrome. Reumat Dis Clin N Am 16:433–439, 1990
Editorial: Cogan's syndrome. The Lancet 337:1011–1011, 1991

COGAN II

Synonyms. Oculomotor apraxia.

Symptoms and Signs. Observed only in children, prevalent in males. Patient unable to turn eyes quickly when asked to look at an object while he is lying on his side, or when his attention is suddenly attracted. To compensate he turns his head, but in doing so, the eyes deviate to the opposite side because of the vestibular reflex. To focus on the object he has to turn his head farther; in this way, he can fixate on the object. The entire cycle occurs in less than 1 second, with a jerky movement of the head. He may carry out such movement when free from stimulus. The mechanism of oculomotor apraxia is the opposite of what occurs in normal person, who first moves the eyes and then the head.

Etiology. Unknown. Congenital condition (in one case carbon monoxide intoxication of mother in second month of pregnancy, and the condition associated with extrapyramidal disease). May occur in ataxia-telangiectasia. Possibly also autosomal recessive inheritance.

Therapy. None.

Prognosis. Unknown; condition not handicapping except for difficulty in reading and making quick turns.

BIBLIOGRAPHY. Wilson SAK: A contribution to the study of apraxia: With a review of literature. Brain 31:164–216, 1908
Cogan DG: Type of congenital ocular motor apraxia presenting jerky head movements. Jackson Memorial Lecture Trans Am Acad Ophthalmol 56:853–862, 1952
Gross-Tsur V, Har-Even Y, Gutman I, et al: Oculomotor apraxia: the presenting sign of Gaucher disease. Pediatr Neurol 5:128–129, 1989
Adams RD, Victor M: Principles of Neurology, 5th ed, p 1036. New York, McGraw-Hill, 1993

COGAN III

Synonym. Cogan-Guerry; corneal dystrophy, epitelial basement membrane; corneal dystrophy, map-dot-fingerprint type; microcystic corneal dystrophy; MDFP.

Symptoms and Signs. May occur in children, most cases in middle-aged or elderly women. Commonly asymptomatic, or mild visual blurring or foreign body sensation. Pain may be caused by associated recurrent erosions. Eyes (on slit-lamp examination): gray, coarse epithelial lines (geographic pattern map) and whitish refractile lines (fingerprints).

Etiology. Nonspecific reaction to a variety of noxious stimuli. Autosomal dominant inheritance reported.

Pathology. Epithelial microcysts and vesicles; loose epithelium eventually pulls off; apparently abnormal basement membrane; loss of hemidesmosomes.

Therapy. Symptomatic for associated lesions.

Prognosis. Relatively nonprogressing condition. In individual with recurrent epithelial erosions usually follows keropathy.

BIBLIOGRAPHY. Cogan DG, Donaldson DD, Kuwabara I, et al: Microcystic dystrophy of the corneal epithelium. Trans Am Ophthalmol Soc 62:213–225, 1964

Werblin TP, Hirst LW, Stark WJ, et al: Prevalence of map-dot-fingerprint changes in cornea. Br J Ophthalmol 65:401–409, 1981

Rodrigues MM, Rajagopalan S, Jones KA: Anterior and posterior corneal dystrophy. In Garner A, Klintworth GK (eds): Pathobiology of Ocular Disease: A Dynamic Approach, 2nd ed, pp 771–773. New York, Marcel Dekker, 1994

COGAN-REESE

Synonym. Descemet membrane; naevus-iritis; iris naevus; NVDE; nodular, unilateral glaucoma.

Symptoms and Signs. Heterochromia of iris (darker the affected eye); multiple pigmented cells cluster in the iris. Unilateral glaucoma; cornea guttata; ectopia of pupil; ectopic uvea.

Etiology. Unknown.

Pathology. Proliferation of endothelial cells.

Therapy. Conservative management by constant observation and if treatment required local resection. (Because lesion may not be a melanoma, iris melanomas behave benignly and seldom metastasize. The eye is otherwise normal, after iridectomy possible accurate histopathologic studies and further decisions.)

BIBLIOGRAPHY. Cogan DG, Reese AB: A syndrome of iris nodules, ectopic Descemet's membrane and unilateral glaucoma. Doc Ophthalmol 26:424–433, 1969

Daicker B, Sturrock G, Guggenheim R: Clinicopathologische Korrelation bei Cogan-Reese Syndrom. Klin Mbl Augenheilk 180:531–538, 1982

Grossniklaus HE, Green WR: Uveal tumors. In Garner A, Klintworth GK (eds): Pathobiology of Ocular Disease: A Dynamic Approach, 2nd ed, pp 1447–1449. New York, Marcel Dekker, 1994

COHEN

Synonyms. Pepper (family name); cerebral-obesity-ocular-skeletal; hypotonia-obesity-cerebral-skeletal.

Symptoms and Signs. Onset from birth. Craniofacial anomalies. Microcephaly; microphthalmia; antimongoloid slant of lids; strabismus; myopia; micrognathia; narrow, high-arched palate; short filtrum. Skeletal abnormalities. Tapering extremities; simian creases; syndactyly; joint hyperextensibility; cubitus valgus; genus varus; scoliosis; lordosis. Muscle hypotonia. Mental retardation. Obesity (onset in middle childhood). Periureteric obstruction. Seizures (possibly new features).

Etiology. Unknown; possibly, autosomal recessive inheritance with variable expressivity. This syndrome presents characteristics in common with Prader-Willi (see) and Laurence-Moon-Biedl (see).

Diagnostic Procedures. *Chromosome studies.* Normal. *Electroencephalography.* Diffuse, high-voltage spikes and wave discharge.

BIBLIOGRAPHY. Hall BD, Smith DW: Prader-Willi syndrome. J Pediatr 81:286–293, 1972

Cohen MM: A new syndrome with hypotonia, obesity, mental deficiency, and facial, oral, ocular and limb anomalies. J Pediatr 83:280–284, 1973

North C, Patton MA, Baraitser M, et al: The clinical features of the Cohen's syndrome: Further case reports. J Med Genet 22:131–134, 1985

Steinlein O, Tariverdian G, Boll Hu T: Tapetoretinal degeneration in brothers with apparent Cohen syndrome: nosology with Mirhosseini-Holmes-Walton. Am J Med Genet 41:196–200, 1991

COINDET

Synonyms. Job Basedow (misnomer); iodide-induced thyrotoxicosis.

Symptoms and Signs. After administration of pharmacologic doses of iodine the following complications may develop:

1. Iodide-induced thyroiditis
2. Iodide-induced thyrotoxicosis
3. Iodide goiter with or without hypothyroidism (see Iatrogenic hypothyroidism).

Acute painful thyroid enlargement that recedes with discontinuation of treatment. Male to female ratio 1:3; exophthalmos absent; goiter; symptoms and signs of hyperthyroidism (see Flajani).

Etiology. In subject with pre-existing or with absent thyroid disease immediately or even years after following administration of: amiodarone; KJ; benzidiazone; radiographic contrast; iodochlorohydroxyquinoline; seaweed; topical application of iodide preparation.

Pathology. Thyroid gland usually nodular.

Diagnostic Procedures. *Blood.* Hyperthyroxinemia (100%); hypertriiodothyroninemia (79%); antithyroid antibodies absent.

Therapy. Response to antithyroid agents 60%.

Prognosis. Self-limited course in about 40% of cases.

BIBLIOGRAPHY. Coindet JR: Nouvelle recherches sur les effect de l'iode. Am Chim Phys 16:252, 1821

Fradkin JE, Wolff J: Iodide-induced thyrotoxicosis. Medicine 62:1–20, 1983

McKenzie JM, Zakarija M: Hyperthyroidism. In De Groot LJ (ed): Endocrinology, 3rd ed, p 684. Philadelphia, WB Saunders, 1995

COITAL CEPHALALGIA

Symptoms and Signs. Both sexes. Male to female ratio 5:4/1. History of migraine in 47% of cases. During intercourse acute headache, lasting 30 minutes to 24 hours; occasionally severe.

Etiology. Unknown.

Diagnostic Procedures. *EEG. CT scan. MRI. Evoked potentials.*

Therapy. Propanolol (40–80 mg) before intercourse, that may be discontinued after one month symptom-free.

Prognosis. It recurs with each intercouse for several months.

BIBLIOGRAPHY. Pearce JMS: Headache. J of Neurol Neurosurg Psychiatr 57:134–144, 1944

COLCOTT-FOX

Synonyms. Tilbury Fox; cutaneous abscesses infantilis; impetigo contagiosa streptogenes; impetigo simplex; porrigo.

Symptoms and Signs. Occurs in feeble and debilitated infants. Development of multiple abscesses of skin following infection of sweat glands (periporitis).

Etiology. Staphylococcal infection. Two forms recognized. Nonbullous impetigo (Staphylococcus aureus or Streptococcus or both); bullous impetigo (staphylococcal).

Pathology. That of subcutaneous abscess.

Diagnostic Procedures. *Culture of pus. Bacteriologic examination.*

Therapy. Care of environmental factors (temperature and humidity); nutritional and fluid balance. Antibiotics.

Prognosis. Good.

BIBLIOGRAPHY. Fox WT: On impetigo contagiosa or porrigo. Br Med J 1:467–469, 495–496; 607–609, 1864
Atherton DJ: The neonate. In Champion RH, Burton JL, Ebling FJG (eds): Rook/Wilkinson/Ebling Textbook of Dermatology, 5th ed, p 415. Oxford, Blackwell Scientific, 1992

COLD HYPERSENSITIVITY

Symptoms. Disturbing reactions experienced when immersed in water.

Signs. Failure to decrease heart rate when immersed in water below body temperature.

Etiology. Lack of emotional adjustment (fear) or failure to compensate physiologically (hypersensitivity to cold). Body immersion normally produces bradycardia that is enhanced by immersion of head.

Diagnostic Procedures. *Heart rate.* Determination of variation of heart rate according to temperature of water in which immersed. *Ice cube test.* Ice cube held in contact with forearm for 3 minutes. A wheal, slightly raised with erythematous peripheral reaction, appears in persons with hypersensitivity to cold.

BIBLIOGRAPHY. Horton BT, Gabrielson MA: Hypersensitivity to cold: A condition dangerous to swimmers. Res Q 11:119–126, 1940
Tuttle WW, Templin JL: Study of normal cardiac response to water below body temperature with special reference to submersion syndrome. J Lab Clin Med 28:271–276, 1942
Grover RF, Reeves JT, Rowell LB, et al: The influence of environmental factors on the cardiovascular system. In Schlant RC, Alexander RW: Hurst's The Heart, 8th ed, p 2124. New York, McGraw-Hill, 1994
Weatherall DJ, Ledingham JGG, Warrell DA (eds): Oxford Textbook of Medicine, 3rd ed, p 2366. Oxford, Oxford Med Pub, 1996

COLD PANNICULITIS (CHILDREN)

Synonym. Haxthausen II; pseudosclerema; subcutaneous fat necrosis; adiponecrosis subcutanea neonatorum; including "popsicle" panniculitis.

Symptoms and Signs. Occurs in healthy, well-nourished newborns; onset frequently after exposure to cool air. Angle of mouth in case of frequent sucking of ice-pops. Formation of movable indurated subepidermal masses on the cheeks or other body areas (e.g., trunk; extremities).

Etiology. Immaturity of subcutaneous fat (excessive saturated fatty acids with high solidification point) exposed to cold or secondary to traumatic injuries. Maternal pre-eclampsia; diabetes also has been considered.

Pathology. Necrosis of subcutaneous fat with perivascular inflammatory reaction. Giant cells containing needlelike crystals.

Therapy. Prevention: None specific. If hypercalcemia, calcium and vitamin D restriction, furosemide, corticosteroids.

Prognosis. Complete spontaneous resolution in 3–4 months. In rare cases, if visceral fat involved or severe hypercalcemia, may be fatal.

BIBLIOGRAPHY. Hochsinger C: Ueber eine akute kongelative Zellgewebsverhartung in der submental Regionen bei Kinder. Monatsschr Kinderheilk 1:323–327, 1902
Fabyan M: Disseminated fat necrosis occurring in an infant without other lesions. Bull Johns Hopkins Hosp 18:349, 1907
Haxthausen H: Adiponecrosis a frigore. Br J Dermatol 53:83–89, 1941
Lowe LB: Cold panniculitis in children. Am J Dis Child 115:709–713, 1968
Burton JL, Cunlife WJ: Subcutaneous fat. In Champion RH, Burton JL, Ebling FJG (eds): Rook/Wilkinson/Ebling Textbook of Dermatology, 5th ed, p 2148. Oxford, Blackwell Scientific, 1992

COLD URTICARIA (FAMILIAL)

Synonyms. Cold hypersensitivity. See Mucke-Wells.

Symptoms and Signs. In area exposed to cold: skin wheals, pain and swelling of joint; chills and fever.

Etiology. Autosomal dominant inheritance; systemic amyloidosis may be observed in cases with cold urticaria.

Diagnostic Procedures. *Blood.* Leukocytosis during attacks.

Therapy. Avoid unprotected exposure to cold. Antihistamines, cyproheptadine. Desensitization to cold may be attempted if the patient has the patience to carry it out.

Prognosis. Persistent condition.

BIBLIOGRAPHY. Kile RL, Rush HA: A case of cold urticaria with unusual family history. JAMA 114:1067–1068, 1940
Witherspoon FG, White CB, Bazemore JM, et al: Familial urticaria due to cold. Arch Dermatol Syph 58:52–55, 1948
Weatherall DJ, Ledingham JGG, Warrell DA (eds): Oxford Textbook of Medicine, 3rd ed, pp 3770–3771. Oxford, Oxford Med Pub, 1996

COLEMAN-MEREDITH

Symptoms and Signs. Combination of symptoms and signs related to one lesion (or multiple) of the occipital-cervical shoulder girdle associated with those relative to cord injury.

BIBLIOGRAPHY. Coleman CC, Meredith JM: Treatment of fracture dislocation of the spine associated with cord injury. JAMA 11:2168–2172, 1938
Freemann BL III: Fractures dislocation and fracture dislocation of spine. In Crenshaw AH (ed): Campbell's Operative Orthopedics, 7th ed, pp 3109–3142. St Louis, CV Mosby, 1987

COLLAGENOMA, CUTANEOUS FAMILIAL

Synonyms. Cardiomyopathy—hypogonadism—collagenoma.

Symptoms and Signs. Both sexes. In postpubertal period, appearance of multiple cutaneous nodules, movable with the skin, on trunk and proximal arms. Possibly, association with disease of other organs; no common denominator; however, in organ system involvement, including signs related to moderate myocardiopathy, hypogonadism, eye and sensorineural ear trouble, recurrent vasculitis.

Etiology. Autosomal dominant inheritance.

Pathology. Localized thickening of the dermis resulting from increased collagen.

Therapy. Symptomatic.

Prognosis. All patients reached adulthood.

BIBLIOGRAPHY. Henderson RR, Wheeler CE, Abele DC, et al: Familial cutaneous collagenoma. Arch Dermatol 98:23–27, 1968
Sacks HN, Crawley IS, Ward JA, et al: Familial cardiomyopathy, hypogonadism and collagenoma. Ann Intern Med 93:813–817, 1980
Atherton DJ: Naevi and Other Developmental Defects. In Champion RH, Burton JL, Ebling FJG (eds): Rook/Wilkinson/Ebling Textbook of Dermatology, 5th ed, p 463. Oxford, Blackwell Scientific, 1992

COLLAGENOSIS, FAMILIAL REACTIVE PERFORATING

Synonyms. PC; Mehregan.

Symptoms and Signs. Both sexes. Onset in early childhood. Recurrent umbilicated papules on the skin that resolve spontaneously in 2 months.

Etiology. Autosomal recessive inheritance. Trauma and cold are triggering factors.

Pathology. Extrusion of collagen fibers through epidermis.

BIBLIOGRAPHY. Mehregan AH, Schwartz OD, Livingood CS: Reactive perforating collagenosis. Arch Dermatol 96:277–282, 1967
Poliak SC, Lebwhol MC, Parris A, et al: Reactive perforating collagenosis associated with diabetes mellitus. N Engl J Med 306:81–84, 1982
Trattner A, Ingber A, Sandbang M: Mucosal involvement in reactive perforating collagenosis. J Am Acad Dermat 25:1079–1081, 1991

COLLAGENOUS COLITIS

Synonyms. Lindstom; watery diarrhea-colitis; enterocolitis, collagenous.

Symptoms and Signs. More common in females than in males (20:1), usually in the sixth decade, pediatric patients described as well. Chronic diarrhea (30 bowel movements a day) with colicky abdominal pain, mucus in stool, minor weight loss. Increased incidence of autoimmune phenomena and diseases and manifestation of drug allergies.

Etiology. Unknown. Hypothesized inflammatory origin or fibrosis owing to local abnormal collagen synthesis.

Pathology. Colonic biopsy linear fibrous thickening presenting as subepithelial band composed of type I and III collagen.

Diagnostic Procedures. *Stool.* Exclude malabsorption. Usually mild steatorrhea.

Therapy. Symptomatic: diphenoxylate, loperamide, dicyclamine, sulphasalaxazine, 5–aminosalicylic acid and prednisone (effective in 100% of cases).

Prognosis. Spontaneous remission is possible, otherwise good response to treatments.

BIBLIOGRAPHY. Lindsrom CG: "Collagenous colitis" with watery diarrhea—a new entity. Pathol Eur 11:87–89, 1976
Maxson CJ, Klein HD, Rubin W: Atypical forms of inflammatory bowel disease. Med Clin N Amer 78:1259–1273, 1994
Schiller LR: Microscopic and collagenous colitis. In Haubrich WS, Schaffner F, Berk JE (eds): Bockus Gastroenterology, 5th ed, p 1700. Philadelphia, WB Saunders, 1995

COLLES

Synonym. Hyperextension fracture.

Symptoms. Occurs usually in elderly persons. Pain in the wrist; numbness in the fingers; reduced radioulnar motion.

Signs. Tenderness at the lower end of radius; swelling and ecchymosis; distal fragment displaced backward; mass over dorsal aspect of wrist; deformity at "silver fork."

Pathology. Nonarticular fracture of distal radius with volar angulation and dorsal displacement.

Etiology. Extension, compression (indirect) trauma, as in falling on outstretched hand.

Therapy. May be treated successfully nonoperatively. Open reduction and internal fixation are needed when radial shortening in young patients or marked crushing.

BIBLIOGRAPHY. Colles A: On the fractures of the carpal extremity of the radius. Edinburgh Med Surg J 10:182–186, 1814
Saito H, Takahaschi Y, Zenzai K: Intra-articular fracture of distal radius: treatment and results. In Vastamaeki M: Current Trends in Hand Surgery, pp 131–138. Netherland, Excerpta Medica, 1995

COLLET-BONNET

Symptoms and Signs. Villaret retroparotid syndrome combined with facial palsy (primary or secondary).

Etiology. Scirrhous parotid tumor.

BIBLIOGRAPHY. Collet FJ, Bonnet P: Le syndrome paralytique du cancer de la parotide. Lyon chir 435, 1923

COLLET-SICARD

Synonyms. Sicard; Vernet-Sargnon; condyloposterior lacerated foramen; glossolaryngoscapulopharyngeal hemiplegia; pharyngeal paralysis; posterior laterocondylar space; retroparotid space. See Villaret and Vernet-Sargnon.

Symptoms and Signs. Difficulty in swallowing; nasal regurgitation; loss of sensation over posterior third of tongue; hoarseness; paralysis of sternocleidomastoid and trapezius muscles; hemiatrophy of tongue.

Etiology and Pathology. Lesions of the last four cranial nerves (glossopharyngeal; vagus; spinal accessory; hypoglossal) by tumor, adenopathies, aneurysm, penetrating injuries, infections.

BIBLIOGRAPHY. Collet FJ: Sur un nouveau syndrome paralytique pharyngolaryngé par blessure de guerre (hémiplégie glosso-laryngoscapulopharyngée). Lyon Méd 124:121–129, 1916
Sicard JA: Syndrome du carrefour condylo-déchiré postérieur (type pur de paralysie des quatre derniers nerfs craniens). Marseilles Méd 53:385–397, 1916–1917
Svien HJ, Baker HL, Rivers MH: Jugular foramen syndrome and allied syndromes. Neurology 13:797–809, 1963
Adams RD, Victor M: Principles of Neurology, 5th ed, p 1172. New York, McGraw-Hill, 1993

COLONIC INERTIA

Synonyms. Slow transit constipation. See also anismus.

Symptoms and Signs. Chronic constipation.

Etiology. Idiopathic. Disorder of colon motility with delayed transit. Lack of postprandial propagating colon contraction associated with movement of intraluminal content.

Diagnostic Procedures. *Marker studies.* Prolonged retention of markers in the rectum. Manometric recording and radionucleide imaging.

Therapy. That of chronic constipation. Diet, mild laxative cisapride, suppository.

BIBLIOGRAPHY. Preston DM, Lennard-Jones JE: Severe chronic constipation of young women: idiopathic slow transit constipation. Gut 27:41–48, 1986
Kohh TR: Constipation. In Haubrich WS, Schaffner F, Berk JE (eds): Bockus Gastroenterology, 5th ed, vol 2, pp 105–106. Philadelphia, WB Saunders, 1995

COLOR BLINDNESS, BLUE-MONOCONE-MONOCHROMATE TYPE

Synonyms. CBBM, partial color blindness, achromatopsia incomplete.

Symptoms and Signs. Defective vision of blue color that worsens with age.

Etiology. X-linked. Progressive abiotrophy.

Diagnostic Procedures. *Pseudoisochromatic plates.* (Ishihara plates). *Electroretinography.* Fundus: young age normal; at 50–60 years, macular scarring.

Prognosis. Progressive anomaly.

BIBLIOGRAPHY. Huddart J: An account of persons who could not distinguish colors. Philos Trans R Soc 67:260, 1777
Sloan LL: Congenital achromatopsia. J Ophthalmol Soc Am 44:117–128, 1954
Nathans J, Davenport CM, Maumenee IH, et al: Molecular genetics of human blue cone monochromacy. Science 245:831–838, 1989

COLOR BLINDNESS, PARTIAL DEUTAN SERIES

Synonyms. CBD, DCB, deuteranopia, daltonism; green color blindness.

Symptoms and Signs. Predominant in males, but also possible in women. From birth, defective vision of colors blue and green.

Etiology. X-linked.

Diagnostic Procedures. *Holmgren test; Ishihara plates.*

Prognosis. Traffic light problems.

BIBLIOGRAPHY. Dalton J: Extraordinary facts relating to the vision colours, with observation. Mem Literary Philos Soc: Manchester 5:28–45, 1798
Purrello M, Nussbaum R, Rinaldi A, et al: Old and new genetics help ordering loci at the telomere of the human X-chromosome long arm. Hum Genet 65:295–299, 1984
Drummond-Borg M, Deeb SS, Motulsky AG: Molecular patterns of X-chromosome-linked color vision genes among 134 men of European ancestry. Proc Natl Acad Sci 86:983–987, 1989

COLOR BLINDNESS, PARTIAL PROTEAN SERIES

Synonyms. CBP, protanopia; red color blindness.

Symptoms and Signs. From birth. Both sexes. Defective vision of color red.

Etiology. X-linked inheritance. A two-locus hypothesis is supported by some observations.

Diagnostic Procedures. *Holmgren test; Ishihara plates.*

BIBLIOGRAPHY. Waaler GH: Uber die Erblichkeitsvethaeltnisse der verscheidenen Arten von angeborener Rotgruenblindheit. Z Induckt Abstammungs Vererbungse 45:279–333, 1927
Drummond-Borg M, Deeb S, Motulsky AG: Molecular basis of abnormal red-green color vision: a family with three types of color vision defects. Am J Med Genet 43:675–683, 1988

COLOR BLINDNESS, PARTIAL TRITANOMALY

Synonym. Tritanomalous color blindness.

Symptoms and Signs. In males. Patients retain red and green, but lack blue and yellow sensory mechanisms.

Etiology. X-linked.

Diagnostic Procedures. *Holmgren test; Ishihara plates.*

BIBLIOGRAPHY. Kalmus H: Diagnosis and Genetics of Defective Color Vision, p 59. Oxford, Pergamon, 1965
Weitz CJ, Miyake Y, Schizato K, et al: Human tritanopia associated with two amino acid substitution in the blue-sensitive opsin. Am J Hum Genet 50:498–507, 1992

COMBETTE

Obsolete.

Synonyms. Cerebellar aplasia; congenital cerebellar; Nonne; Nonne-Marie. See cerebello-parenchymal atrophies.

BIBLIOGRAPHY. Combette: Absence complete du cervelet, des pedoncules postérieurs et de la protuberance cerebrale chez une jeune fille morte dans sa onzieme annee. Bull Soc Anat Paris 5:148–157, 1831
Crouzon O: Athrophie cerebelleuse idiotique in Etudes sur les maladies familiales nerveuses et dystrophiques, Paris, 1929, pp 90–111
Dow RS, Moruzzi G: The Physiology and Pathology of the Cerebellum. Minneapolis, Univ of Minnesota Press, 1958

COMBINED HYPERLIPEMIA, FAMILIAL

Synonym. FCH; hypelipoproteinemia type IIb; combined hyperlipidemia, combined, familial; hypertriglyceridemia, familial.

Symptoms and Signs. 1–2% of European and North American population. Both sexes affected; age of detection second–sixth decades. Uncertain clinical features. Moderate obesity. Hypertension, increased risk of coronary heart disease. Absence of pancreatic involvement and only rarely xanthomas.

Etiology. Autosomal dominant inheritance. The syndrome encompasses a wide variety of several biochemical defects (see Chylomicronemia syndromes). The phenotype is that of hyperlipoproteinemia IV (see).

Pathology. Nonspecific.

Diagnostic Procedures. *Blood.* Type IV hyperlipoproteinemia (in mild form) type V (in severe form) plasma turbid, no cream layer; elevated level of apo B; very low-density lipoproteins (VLDL) increased; chylomicrons "absent"; low-density lipoproteins (LDL) not increased; cholesterol normal; triglycerides increased. Fasting hyperglycemia; insulin resistance; glucose intolerance, hyperuricemia.

Therapy. No specific treatment. Carbohydrate and caloric restriction. Clorofibrate. Trial with human plasma if associated with apolipoprotein II deficiency (drop of triglycerides lasting 6 days). New antilipemic agents under investigation: Lovastatin; fluvastatin; nicotinic acid combined with bile acid-binding resins.

Prognosis. Associated with myocardial ischemia and early death.

BIBLIOGRAPHY. Goldstein JL, Schrott HG, Hazzard WR, et al: Hyperlipemia in coronary artery disease. II. Genetic analysis of lipid levels in 176 families and delineation of a new inherited disorder, combined hyperlipemia. J Clin Invest 52:1544, 1973

Schettler G, Habenicht AJR (eds): Principles and Treatment of Lipoprotein Disorders. New York, Springer, 1994

Kane JP, Havel RJ: Disorders of the biogenesis and secretion of lipoproteins containing the B apolipoproteins. In Scriver CR, Beaudet AL, Sly WS, et al: The Metabolic and Molecular Bases of Inherited Disease, 7th ed, pp 1872–1874. New York, McGraw-Hill, 1995

COMFORT-STEINBERG

Synonyms. Recidivant pancreatitis; hereditary pancreatitis; pancreatitis, hereditary.

Symptoms and Signs. Onset in childhood or adolescence (4–15 years); no sex prevalence. May begin in an acute or chronic form. Recurrent episodes of abdominal pain with repeated episodes of Balser-Fitz's syndrome. Several years later, development of diabetes mellitus symptoms. In some members of the family, diabetes not preceded by pain. In two of three families reported, episodes of hemorrhagic pleural or ascitic effusions.

Etiology. Unknown; genetic transmission, of autosomal dominant type. Suggestion that hypotrophy of Oddi sphincter could be owing to an inherited factor.

Pathology. Progressive destruction of pancreas; each acute relapse leaves increased damage in the gland. Fibroblastic proliferation and fibrosis; infiltration with lymphocytes, plasma cells; atrophy of acinar cells; frequently, calcium deposit.

Diagnostic Procedures. *X-ray. CT scan. MRI. Sonography.* Calcification in the pancreas. Pancreas scan with isotopes. *Blood.* Glucose. *Stool.* Steatorrhea and determination of pancreatic enzymes. *Urine.* Glucose; no aminoaciduria (except in one family, where this finding was reported, resembling recessive type of cystinuria); urinary amylase increased during episodes of pain. *Duodenal fluid. Determination of enzymes.*

Therapy. Symptomatic: pancreatic enzymes. Trial with steroids. In one family, surgical procedures to drain pancreatic ducts relieved symptoms. In another family, no benefit from surgery.

Prognosis. Chronic relapsing condition with progressive functional and anatomic damage. To be differentiated from acute relapsing pancreatitis where pancreas recovers completely between attacks. Increased incidence of pancreatic carcinoma possible; insufficient data, however, to incriminate genetic relationship for this association.

BIBLIOGRAPHY. Comfort MW, Gambill EE, Baggenstoss AH: Chronic relapsing pancreatitis: A study of 29 cases without associated disease of biliary or gastrointestinal tract. Gastroenterology 6:239–285, 1946

Comfort MW, Steinberg AG: Pedigree of family with hereditary chronic relapsing pancreatitis. Gastroenterology 21:54–63, 1952

Weizman Z, Durie PR: Acute pancreatitis in childhood. J Pediatr 113:24–29, 1988

COMLY

Synonyms. Methemoglobinemia, acquired; well methemoglobinemia. See also Stakis-Talma.

Symptoms and Signs. Usually observed in children living in rural environment or in zone not served by aqueduct. Cyanosis of mucosae and skin (occasionally, misdiagnosis of congenital heart disease). According to the entity of intoxication, metabolic and respiratory symptoms may manifest.

Etiology. Nitrates present in well water inducing formation of methemoglobin.

Pathology. Absence of typical findings, except the cyanotic hue of skin.

Diagnostic Procedures. *Blood.* Presence of methemoglobin; absence of other alteration. *Electrocardiography.* Normal (see Symptoms).

Therapy. Stop ingestion of contaminated water. In severe case methylene blue, 1 mg/kg body weight in a 1 g/dl solution given intravenously over 5 minutes. A second dose of 2 mg/kg can be given if cyanosis has not cleared within 1 hour. Doses exceeding 7 mg/kg can be toxic. Ascorbic acid (300–500 mg daily orally) can be useful but its action is slow. Therapy with methylene blue is very dangerous in patients with G6PD deficiency (may trigger hemolytic episodes). The only way to treat these patients is by exchange transfusion.

Prognosis. Good.

BIBLIOGRAPHY. Comly HH: Cyanosis in infants caused by nitrates in well water. JAMA 129:112–116, 1945

Lukens JN: Methemoglobinemia and other disorders accompanied by cyanosis. In Lee GR, Bithel TC, Foerster J, et al (eds): Wintrobe's Clinical Hematology, 9th ed, pp 1263–1265. Philadelphia, Lea & Febiger, 1993

COMPLEX I DEFICIENCY

Synonyms. Mitochondria NADH dehydrogenase, component of complex I; mitochondrial myopathy with deficiency of respiratory chain NDH-CoQ reductase infantile. Fatal multisystem disorders—myopathy. Complex I (NADH: ubiquinone oxidoreductase, EC 1.6.5.3.) has 25 polypeptide subunits so many defects and clinical patterns are possible. For clinical syndromes caused by their defects see OXPHOS syndromes.

COMPLEX II DEFICIENCY

Synonyms. Mitochondrial respiratory chain, complex deficiency; succinate CoQ reductase deficiency. Complex II (Succinate: ubiquinone oxidoreductase, EC 1.3.5.1.) contains four polypeptide subunits. For the clinical syndromes caused by their defects see OXPHOS syndromes.

COMPLEX III DEFICIENCY

Synonyms. Mitochondrial complex III deficiency.

Etiology. Biochemically heterogenous defects of complex III (Ubiquinone: ferrocytochrome c oxydoreductase or cytochrome bc1 complex, EC1.10.2.2), of isolated muscle mitocondria. For the clinical syndromes caused by these defects see OXPHOS syndromes.

COMPLEX IV DEFICIENCY

Synonyms. Benign infantile myopathy; fatal infantile myopathy. Cytochrome c oxidase, COX deficiency. Complex IV (Ferrocytochrome c:oxygen oxidoreductase or cytochrome c oxidase, EC 1.9.3.1). Defect of subunit VIIa in severe form. In benign form temporary alteration of COX activity. For clinical syndromes caused by their possible defects see OXPHOS syndromes.

COMPLEX V DEFICIENCY

Complex V (ATP synthase, EC 3.6.1. 34) is composed of 12 or 13 units. For clinical syndromes caused by their possible defects see OXPHOS syndromes.

BIBLIOGRAPHY. Morgan-Hughes JA, Darveniza P, Landon DN, et al: A mytochondrial myopathy with a deficiency of respiratory chain NADH-CoQ reductase activity. J Neurol Sci 43:27–46, 1979

Bet L, Bresolin N, Maggio M, et al: A case of mitochondrial myopathy, lactic acidosis and complex I deficiency. J Neurol 237:399–404, 1990

Garavaglia B, Antozzi C, Grotti F, et al: A mitochondrial myopathy with complex II deficiency. Neurology 40:294, 1990

Spiro AJ, Moore CL, Prineas JW, et al: A cytochrome related inherited disorder of nervous system and muscle. Arch Neurol 23:103–112, 1970

Di Mauro S, Zeviani M, Bonilla E, et al: Cytochrome C oxidase deficiency. Trans Biochem Soc 13:651, 1985

Di Mauro S, Lombes A, Nakase H, et al: Cytochrome C oxidase deficiency. Pediatr Res 28:526–541, 1990

Di Mauro S: Mitochondrial encephalomyopahies. In RN Rosenberg (ed): Molecular and Genetic Basis of Neurological Disease, pp 665–694. Stoneham, CT, Butterworth, 1993

Shoffner JM, Wallace DC: Oxidative phosphorylation diseases. In Scriver CR, Beaudet AL, Sly WS, et al: The Metabolic and Molecular Bases of Inherited Disease, 7th ed, pp 1535–1609. New York, McGraw-Hill, 1995

CONDORELLI

Obsolete.

Synonyms. Mediastinal obesity. See also Pickwickian.

Symptoms. Occurs in obese people. Slight cyanosis of the face, which becomes more marked on recumbency; episodes of tonicoclonic muscular contractions; alterations of the sleeping rhythm, and alteration of frequency and rhythm of breathing when lying down.

Signs. Diffuse obesity; lack of edema; cyanosis of face; turgor and lack of pulsation of external jugular veins; spasm of vessels on funduscopic examination.

Etiology. Fat infiltration in the mediastinum and water-salt retention.

Pathology. Generalized obesity and mediastinal fat infiltration that constricts the venous margin of the heart and the vascular stem.

Diagnostic Procedures. *Venous pressure.* Markedly increased (diagnostic). *X-ray. Radiochymography. ECG. Echocardiography. EEG.*

Therapy. Strict diet; nicotinic acid (when vasospasm predominates); digitalis (if cardiovascular failure); thyroid (if hypothyroidism).

Prognosis. Regression of symptoms immediately follows weight loss.

BIBLIOGRAPHY. Condorelli L: Fisiopatologia clinica del mediastino (sistemazione su base anatomo-fisiologiche delle sindromi mediastiniche sensu strictiori). Cong Soc Ital Med Int 48:1–163, 1947

Marrazza P, Zilli E: La sindrome venosa degli adiposi di Condorelli, contributo casistico. Policlinico Sez Part 61:12–22, 1954

CONE-ROD DYSTROPHY

Synonym. CDH; CORD; CRD; retinal cone dystrophy.

Symptoms and Signs. Both sexes, onset from childhood in the first decade. Progressive constriction of peripheral visual fields.

Etiology. Autosomal dominant. Probably defect lies in the region 18q21–q22.

Pathology. Eye: Dystrophy of retinal photoreceptors and pigment epithelium; abiotrophic degeneration of rods and cones; accumulation of lipofucsin granules in retinal pigment epithelium.

Diagnostic Procedures. Fundoscopy.

Prognosis. Inexorable progression to blindness.

BIBLIOGRAPHY. Hittner HM, Murphree AL, Garcia CA, et al: Dominant cone-rod dystrophy. Docum Ophthal 39:29–52, 1975

Rabb MS, Tso MOM, Fishman GA:Cone rod dystrophy: A clinical and histopathologic report. Ophthalmology 93:1443–1451, 1986

Bird AC, Jay B, Hussain AA, et al: Retinal photoreceptor disorders. In Garner A, Klintworth GK (eds): Pathobiology of Ocular Disease: A Dynamic Approach, 2nd ed, p 1223. New York, Marcel Dekker, 1994

CONN

Synonyms. Conn-Louis; aldosterone-producing adenoma; mineral corticoid excess, primary.

Symptoms. More common in women, usually in patients 30–50 years of age. Many cases asymptomatic. Central or frontal headache; nicturia; or return to diurnal urinary excretion when patient lying in bed during the day; polydipsia and polyuria (over 2.5 l in 50% of cases); mild asthenia (early); presthesias. More frequent in females; tetany (more frequent in males) muscle weakness or paralysis (in advanced cases and very frequent in Chinese patients).

Signs. Arterial hypertension; optic fundi may show narrow tortuous arteries (no marked vasospasm or papilledema). Heart normal size; later may enlarge. Loss of deep tendon reflexes (late sign; edema rare).

Etiology. Primary aldosteronism owing to a solitary adrenocortical adenoma (60%) producing inappropriate amount of aldosterone partially under the effect of normal adrenocorticotropic (ACTH) response; idiopathic hyperaldostronism (34%); angiotensin II-responsive adenoma (5%); aldosterone-producing carcinoma; primary adrenal hyperplasia; glucocorticoid-suppressible hyperaldosteronism; familial; ectopic aldosterone-producing adenomas and carcinomas (each form about 1%).

Pathology. Small adrenal adenoma (66% of cases), more frequently on left adrenal. If near surface, evident; if in the gland, enlargement and increased consistency of gland. Bilateral hyperplasia of zona glomerulosa (33% of cases).

Diagnostic Procedures. *Blood.* Increased aldosterone concentration; low or hyporesponsive renin activity; low potassium level; study of potassium balance by administering potassium salt; of sodium balance, reduction of sodium intake results in a rise of serum potassium. Serum sodium concentration and carbon dioxide-combining power increased (in advanced cases). *Urine.* Increased potassium excretion; increased aldosterone excretion. With administration of spironolactone, increased sodium excretion and decreased potassium excretion. *Plasma renin.* Diminished. Adrenal venography and adrenal vein sampling. *Electrocardiography.* Sagging ST segments; inverted T-waves; large U-waves and prolonged ST interval (changes reverting to normal after spironolactone administration or potassium replacement). Administration of thiazide, or other diuretics, reveals in early cases the latent potassium-wasting tendency. Tetany may be elicited by hyperventilation or by compression of artery (Trousseau maneuver). *CT scan. MRI. Adrenal scintigraphy.*

Therapy. Unilateral adrenalectomy after preparation with spironolactone if unilateral adenoma. Diet with less than 80 mEq of sodium/day. If bilateral hyperplasia: long-term high-dose spironolactone (side-effects: malaise, gynecomastia, impotence) and eventually surgery. In patient with adverse effects from spironolactone: amiloride.

Prognosis. With surgery in unilateral cases cure in 90% of cases; in bilateral cases: reversion of electrolyte disorder, but frequently blood pressure does not normalize.

BIBLIOGRAPHY. Conn JW: Primary aldosteronism: A new clinical syndrome. J Lab Clin Med 45:3–17, 1955

Edwards CRW: Primary mineralocorticoid excess syndromes. In De Groot LJ (ed): Endocrinology, 3rd ed, pp 1775–1779. Philadelphia, WB Saunders, 1995

CONRADI

Synonyms. Huenermann; chondrodystrophia calcificans congenita;

dysplasia epiphysialis punctata; stippled epiphyses; koala bear dominant.

Symptoms and Signs. Occurs in infancy. Approximately 25% of patients have a distinctive ichthyosiform eruption at birth; thick, yellow, tightly adherent keratinized plaques are distributed in a whorled pattern over the entire body, which may be intensely erythematous. Slow growth, absent cataracts, muscle contractures. Visual trouble; shortening of proximal long bones; scoliosis. Other skeletal abnormalities including macrocephaly or microcephaly; hypertelorism; syndactyly; club foot. Mild mental deficiency. Congenital vascular defects, like severe pulmonary arterial stenoses, may be present.

Etiology. Unknown; autosomal dominant disorder or fresh gene mutation affecting bones and ectodermal structures. May be considered a form of multiple epiphyseal dysplasia.

Pathology. Calcific areas in epiphyses of hips, knees, shoulder, wrists. Other malformations (see Symptoms and Signs). The histologic changes include hyperkeratosis that penetrates to the depths of the hair follicles.

Diagnostic Procedures. *X-ray.* Characteristic presence of multiple punctate calcific deposits in epiphyses during infancy. Various skeletal abnormalities (see Signs). In patients who survive, epiphysis calcifications disappear between first and third years of life. *Chromosome studies.* Normal. *Urine.* Moderate nonspecific aminoaciduria. *Echocardiography.* Dilatation of the right ventricle; signs of pulmonary hypertension.

Therapy. Symptomatic. Orthopedic.

Prognosis. Infants with full syndrome usually die during the first year of life. Survivors exhibit multiple skeletal, ocular, and mental (more or less) debilitating defects. Abnormal calcification disappears by age 1–4 years.

BIBLIOGRAPHY. Conradi E: Vorzeitges Auftreten von Kochen und eigenartigen Verkalkungskernen bei Chondrodystrophia fötalis hypoplastica, Histologische und Röntgenuntersuchungen. J Kinderheilk 80:86–97, 1914
Huenermann C: Chondrodystrophia calcificans congenita als abortive Form der Chondrodystrophye. Kinderheilk 51:1–19, 1931
Marini JC: Heritable collagen disorders. In Klippel JH, Dieppe PA: Rheumatology, pp 7.45.2, 7.45.3. St Louis, CV Mosby, 1994

CONSCIOUS IMMOBILITY

Synonyms. Night nurse paralysis; writer cramp, loss of lip (in instrumentalists), occupational neurosis, focal dystonia.

Symptoms and Signs. Affects nurses of both sexes (60% according to one author); also reported in people driving cars or engaged in navigation or engaged in other skilled motor acts as piano playing, etc. Occurs at any time of day or night and lasts a few seconds. Brief transient disability of voluntary muscles with full awareness of it and inability to terminate it; speech impossible. Not associated with other symptoms.

Etiology. Some features are in common with cataplexy; psychogenic conversion discussed. Probably an intention spasm, where discrete movements are impaired by spreading innervation of unneeded muscles.

BIBLIOGRAPHY. Rudolf G de M: A Conscious Immobility. Bristol, J Wright, 1969
Adams RD, Victor M: Principles of Neurology, 5th ed, p 96. New York, McGraw-Hill, 1993

CONTRACTED BLADDER

Synonym. Schistosomal contracted bladder.

Symptoms and Signs. In late chronic active stage of S. haemetobium infection. Deep, hard, lower abdominal and pelvic pain; urgency, frequency, and incontinence.

Etiology. Oviposition of S. haematobium eggs in deep detrusor muscle with dense fibrous sandy patches.

Pathology. Late S. haematobium infection. Bladder lumen reduced to 50 ml.

Diagnostic Procedures. *Urine.* S. haematobium eggs.

Diagnostic Procedures. Vesical denervation, urinary shunting cup-patch neocystoplasty, and vesical overdistension plus schistosomicidal chemiotherapy.

Prognosis. Possible evolution toward bladder cancer.

BIBLIOGRAPHY. Smith JH, Von Lichtenberg F, Staugger Lehman J: Parasitic diseases of the genitourinary system. In Campbell's Urology, 6th ed, p 900. Philadelphia, WB Saunders, 1992

CONVISART

Eponym used to indicate Fallot syndrome (see) with dextroposed aorta.

BIBLIOGRAPHY. Convisart JN: Traité des Mal du Coeur, vol 2. Paris, 1814
Perloff JK: The Clinical Recognition of Congenital Heart Disease, 2nd ed, p 445. Philadelphia, WB Saunders, 1978

CONWAY

Synonym. Bowed long bones; prenatal bowing.

Symptoms and Signs. Both sexes. Congenital uncomplicated prenatal symmetrical bowing of long bones with dimpling.

Etiology. Not specific. Various conditions cause the syndrome: osteogenesis imperfecta, hypophosphatasic and camptomelic dysplasia.

Prognosis. Self-corrective course.

BIBLIOGRAPHY. Conway TJ: Prenatal bowing and angulation of long bones: a description of its occurrence in a brother and sister. Am Di. Child 95:305–308, 1958
Kapur S, Van Vloten A: Isolated congenital bowed long bones. Clin Genet 29:165–167, 1986

COOPERMAN-MIURA

Synonym. Uvula tongue malposture.

Symptoms. Respiratory disorders; headache; facial pain, often of an intensity suggesting trifacial neuralgia; temporomandibular disarticulations.

Signs. Various degrees of irritation of the covering tissues of the dorsum of the tongue and uvula. Mandibular retrusion. Narrowing of respiratory and alimentary pathways. Abnormalities of the dental plane of occlusion.

Etiology. Underlying cause of irritative phenomena is postural. Mandibular protrusion as seen in Stone Age skulls was a protective mechanism that functioned to preserve head, neck, and throat physiology.

Pathology. Possible presence of potential lesions in such specialized fields of neuropathy, otitis, sinusitis, allergic hypersensitivity, and asthma.

Diagnostic Procedures. Visual examination of uvula tongue malposture during mandibular opening, noting abnormalities of orthopedic gait of the mandible. Observation of nasal breathing. Interpretation of dental plane of occlusion.

Therapy. Mechanical correction of uvula tongue malposture. Intervention by metal or nonmetal oropharyngeal wedges.

Prognosis. Favorable by oral wedge intervention restoring anatomic and physiologic derangements.

BIBLIOGRAPHY. Cooperman HN: New approaches to establishing the plane of occlusion and freeway space in dentures. Dent Dig 71:202, 1965

Cooperman HN, Miura N, Vanhakendover S, Rich H: Uvula tongue malposture. A new approach to Costen's syndrome. Dent Diamond (Japan) 2:127–129, 1977

Miura N, Ueno K, Karasawa J: Dental technology of myodontics. Quintessence, Tokyo, 1987

COOPER I

Synonyms. Breast fibrosis; irritable breast; mastodynia; mammary neuralgia.

Symptoms. Occurs in women; onset from 30–35 years of age. Mammary pain; menometrorrhagia.

Signs. In mammary tissue (usually unilaterally) in upper external quadrant presence of palpable, indurated, mass; process not well defined.

Etiology. Unknown. Considered excessive internal secretion of estriol.

Pathology. Mass formed by whitish, homogeneous tissue, which includes and compresses epithelial structures; atrophy of the latter.

Diagnostic Procedures. *Mammography.* May show calcification. *Echo. Xerography. Thermography.*

Therapy. Vitamin A. Surgery. Bromocriptine or danazol (in cyclic mastalgia). Excision of wedge of the areola (painful nipple).

BIBLIOGRAPHY. Cooper A: Illustration of the Diseases of the Breast. London, Longman, 1829

COOPER II

Synonyms. Lyon; Zuelzer; genitofemoral causalgia; testis neuralgia; pudendal neuralgia.

Symptoms. Recurrent annoying pain of testis.

Etiology. Unknown. May be considered a form of psychalgias when organic cause cannot be found. May be considered as part of the pudendal neuralgia (Zuelzer) or genitofemoral causalgia (Lyon).

Therapy. Mild analgesic; psychotherapy if indicated.

Prognosis. Possible conversion to other symptoms.

BIBLIOGRAPHY. Cooper A: Observations on the Structures and Diseases of the Testis. London, Longman, 1830

Adams RD, Victor M: Principles of Neurology, 5th ed, p 1161. New York, McGraw-Hill, 1993

COOPER HERNIA

Synonyms. Retroperitoneal hernia; hernia retroperitonealis.

BIBLIOGRAPHY. Cooper A: The anatomy and surgical treatment of abdominal hernia London 1827. In Sabiston DC: Textbook of Surgery, 14th ed, p 1144. Philadelphia, WB Saunders, 1991

CORDS

Synonym. Angiopathia retinae juvenilis.

Symptoms. Occurs in children, more frequent in boys (9–10 years peak of incidence), seldom in adolescents or young adults. Reduction of visual fields. Usually unilateral, predominantly on the temporal side.

Signs. Extensive creamy or yellowish exudates within and in the back of retina, occasionally hemorrhages and glistening spots in the detached retina.

Etiology. Possible underlying vascular defect of the retina, primary inflammatory states. Toxocariasis the most common agent. Exceptional familial tendency.

Pathology. Leakage of plasma into retinal tissue, followed by phagocytes that become engorged with lipids (balloon cells); cholesterol crystallizes and causes multinucleated cell response thrombosis; optic and nerve atrophy; latter sclerotic changes.

Therapy. Specific according to infection. Anticoagulants.

Prognosis. Variable according to degree reached by condition before the treatment. Possible progression to blindness.

BIBLIOGRAPHY. Cords R: Papillitis und Glaukom zugleich ein Beitrang zur juvenilen Phlebitis der zentral Vein. Graefes Arch Ophthalmol 105:916–963, 1931

Garner A: Vascular diseases. In Garner A, Klintworth GK (eds): Pathobiology of Ocular Disease: A Dynamic Approach, 2nd ed, pp 1689–1690. New York, Marcel Dekker, 1994

CORK WORKER

Synonyms. Maple-bark worker suberosis. See Allergic alveolitis, extrinsic.

Symptoms. Occurs in persons working with cork; onset insidious. Cough; malaise; weight loss; or sudden fever, dry cough.

Signs. Diffuse fine rales over both sides of chest.

Etiology. Hypersensitivity to moldy cork dust.

Pathology. Interstitial pneumonitis; eosinophil cell infiltration; fibrosis.

Diagnostic Procedures. *Blood.* Eosinophilia. Presence of specific serum precipitin against moldy cork dust. *X-ray.* Increased bronchovascular maskings; diffuse nodular, reticular infiltration. In acute phase, patchy densities.

Therapy. Corticosteroids.

Prognosis. Acute attacks resolve spontaneously in 24–48 hours after removal from exposure. Recurrences on re-exposure. Chronic pulmonary fibrosis if re-exposure not prevented.

BIBLIOGRAPHY. Emanuel DA, Lawton BR, Wensel FJ: Maple-bark disease, pneumoconiosis due to coniosporum corticale. New Engl J Med 266:333–337, 1962

Avila R, Villar TG: Suberosis-respiratory disease in cork workers. Lancet 1:620–621, 1968

CORNEA GUTTATA—ANTERIOR POLAR CATARACT

Synonyms. Dohlman; cataract, anterior, polar–cornea guttata.

Symptoms and Signs. In patients of Scandinavian origin. Cataracts sometimes evident at birth, more often appear between 3 and 10 years of age that become stationary after puberty. Impairment of vision. Central cornea (cornea guttata) affected more severly than periphery.

Etiology. Autosomal dominant inheritance.

Prognosis. Visual impairment of different degree.

BIBLIOGRAPHY. Dohlman C-H: Familial congenital cornea guttata in association with anterior polar cataract. Acta Ophthalmol. 29:445–473, 1951

Traboulzi EI, Weinberg RJ: Familal congenital cornea guttata with anterior polar cataracts. Am J Ophthalmol 108:123–125, 1989

CORNEAL DERMOIDS—SHORT STATURE

Symptoms and Signs. Corneal opacities, short stature.

Etiology. Autosomal recessive trait and linked phenotypes.

Pathology. Cornea: abnormal mesoblastic tissue covered by epithelium.

Diagnostic Procedures. *Slit-lamp examination.* Corneas with superficial and vascularized tissue. *Corneal biopsy.* See Pathology.

Therapy. In severe cases, corneal transplantation.

Prognosis. It depends on the extent of corneal involvement.

BIBLIOGRAPHY. Guizar-Vazquez J, Luengas-Munoz FS, Antillon F: Brief clinical report: Corneal dermoids and short stature in brother and sister. A new syndrome? Am J Med Genet 8:229–234, 1981

Igbal MA, Citayat D, Hahm SYE, et al: Linkage of gene for corneal dermoids with the DXS 43 (Xp22. 2–p22. 1) locus. Am J Hum Genet 41:A171, 1987

CORNEAL DYSTROPHY, POLYMORPHOUS POSTERIOR

Synonyms. Schlichting; corneal dystrophy, hereditary nonprogressive; PPCD; posterior polymorphous corneal dystrophy.

Symptoms. Both sexes affected. Minor or no decrease of visual acuity. Nonprogressive or extremely slowly progressive; rarely may be associated with glaucoma.

Signs. Faint haze in corneas.

Etiology. Unknown; autosomal dominant inheritance.

Pathology. Lesion limited to Descemet membrane and endothelium. Multiple small nodular and larger vesicle excrescences of Descemet membrane, some protruding into anterior chamber, equally distributed all over the membrane. Descemet membrane shows faint cloudiness between lesions.

Diagnostic Procedures. Slit-lamp examination.

Prognosis. Nonprogressive; seldom associated with rupture of Descemet membrane and glaucoma.

BIBLIOGRAPHY. Koeppe L: Klinische Beobachtungen mit der Nernstspalmlampe und dem Hornhautmikroscop. Graefe Arch Klin Exp Ophthalmol 91:363–379, 1916

Rodriguez MM, Sun TT, Krachmer J, et al: Posterior polymorphous corneal dystrophy recent development. Birth Defect Orig Art Ser 18(6):476–491, 1982

CORNEAL HYPOHESTESIA FAMILIAL

Synonyms. Trigeminal anesthesia familial.

Symptoms. Corneal hypohesthesia, no abnormalities of skin sensation in the area of distribution of V cranial nerve. In another family trigeminal anesthesia.

Signs. Punctate epithelial corneal erosions.

Etiology. Autosomal dominant inheritance.

Diagnostic Procedures. *MR imaging.* Hypoplastic state of trigeminal nerve and Gasser's ganglia.

BIBLIOGRAPHY. Purcell JJ Jr, Kratcner JA: Familial corneal Hypoplasia. Arch Ophthal 97:872–874, 1979

Keys CL, Sugar J, Mafee MF: Familial trigeminal anesthesia. Arch Ophthal 108:1720–1723, 1990

CORNEAL-RETINAL INFLAMMATORY

Synonyms. Anterior segment inflammation-cystoid macular edema. See Irvine Gass.

Symptoms and Signs. In subject with inflammation of anterior segment, also secondary to IOL implantation: photophobia, decrease of visual acuity.

Etiology. Inflammatory products produced by inflammation of anterior chamber (prostaglandins and others) decompensate corneal function and determine cystoid macular edema. See also Irvine-Gass.

Diagnostic Procedures. *Ophthalmoscopy. Fluorescin angiography.*

Therapy. Removal of IOL if necessary.

Prognosis. Fair.

BIBLIOGRAPHY. Ostbaum SA, Galin Ma: Cystoid macular edema and ocular inflammation: the corneo-retinal inflammatory syndrome. Trans Ophthalmol Soc UK 99:187–191, 1979

Miyake K, Asakura M, Kobayashi H: Effect of intraocular lens fixation on the blood-acqueous barrier. AM J Ophthalmol 98:451–455, 1984

Apple DJ, Rabb MF: Ocular Pathology, p 156. St Louis, CV Mosby, 1991

CORONARY ARTERY STEAL

See Intramural coronary artery aneurysm and left coronary artery arising from pulmonary artery (IV phase).

Symptoms. Onset in childhood shortly after adequate collateral circulation has developed or when a communication between coronary arteries and heart chambers or intramural coronary aneurysm steals blood from coronary circulation. Onset in later life, in cases of abnormal origin of left coronary artery from pulmonary artery. Angina; dyspnea; fatigue on exertion.

Signs. Harsh systolic and diastolic murmur along left sternal border and on apex.

Etiology. See Symptoms.

Pathology. See Symptoms.

Diagnostic Procedures. *Electrocardiography.* Two-dimensional echocardiography with color flow imaging and spectral Doppler interrogation. *Cardiac catheterization.* Blood from coronary artery flows in retrograde direction. *X-ray of chest.*

Therapy. If evidence of adequate collateral circulation, ligation of anomalous arteries at their origins. If intramural coronary aneurysm, closure of aneurysmal neck and approximation of walls.

Prognosis. Good when surgery indicated and performed.

BIBLIOGRAPHY. Bane AE, Baum S, Blakemore WS, et al: A later stage of anomalous coronary circulation with origin of the left coronary artery from the pulmonary artery. Circulation 36:878–885, 1967

Factor SM, Bache RJ: Pathophysiology of myocardial ischemia. In Schlant RC, Alexander RW: Hurst's The Heart, 8th ed, pp 1037–1038. New York, McGraw-Hill, 1994

CORPUS CALLOSUM AGENESIS

Synonym. See Andermann.

Symptoms and Signs. Rare condition with variable clinical findings. None, or convulsions and mental deficiencies. Macrocephaly or microcephaly. Lack of neuropathy (see Andermann).

Etiology. Unknown. Many genetic causes. Autosomal recessive. For partial agenesis reported X-linked inheritance.

Pathology. Corpus callosum agenesis with frequent association of other developmental defects: absent septum pellucidum; microgyria; arteriovenous malformations.

Diagnostic Procedures. *CT brain scan. MRI.* Third ventricle extending between lateral ventricles.

Prognosis. According to associated defects; various degrees of mental retardation, but normal mental development and normal life are possible.

BIBLIOGRAPHY. Alpers BJ, Grant FC: The clinical syndrome of the corpus callosum. Arch Neurol Psychiat 25:67–86, 1931

Kaplan P: X-linked recessive inheritance of agenesis of the corpus callosum. J Med Genet 20:122–124, 1983

daSilva EO: Callosal defect microcephaly, severe mental retardation and other anomalies in three sibs. Am J Med Genet 29:4837–4843, 1988

Weatherall DJ, Ledingham JGG, Warrell DA (eds): Oxford Textbook of Medicine, 3rd ed, p 4113. Oxford, Oxford Med Pub, 1996

CORPUS LUTEUM INSUFFICIENCY

Synonym. Luteal phase, inadequate.

Symptoms. History of abortion, particularly habitual abortion.

Etiology. Poor endogenous secretion of progesterone hormone during the luteal phase of menstrual cycle.

Diagnostic Procedures. *Blood.* Low level of pregnanediol excretion during the initial phase of menstrual cycle. *Biopsy of endometrium on 24th day of cycle.* Poor secretory response; lowered cell storage of glucose, alkaline phosphatase, and other enzymes. Documentation in two cycles.

Therapy. Once diagnosis is established by history and endometrial biopsy, a plan should be set to treat this syndrome during (1) preconceptional period; (2) implantation period; (3) postconceptional period.

1. *During the preconceptional period.* Progesterone intramuscular (IM) vaginal suppository daily during luteal phase, or daily injection of progesterone in oil starting at the rise of basic body temperature until onset of menses. Use of clomiphene citrate or human chorionic gonadotropin (hCG) every other day in luteal phase have also been proposed.
2. *If pregnancy occurs.*Long-acting progestational agents (e.g., Delalutin) until week 28. If spotting occurs, dosage increase.

Prognosis. Good for successful pregnancy with adequate treatment.

BIBLIOGRAPHY. Davajan V, Israel R: Infertility causes, evaluation and treatment. In De Groot LJ, Cahill GH Jr, Odell WD (eds): Endocrinology, p 2089. New York, Grune & Stratton, 1995

CORRIGAN (A.B.)

Synonyms. Rheumatoid arthritis, benign of aged.

Symptoms and Signs. In aged patients, often males, abrupt onset. Involvement of shoulders, hips, and knees joints.

Etiology. Unknown.

Diagnostic Procedures. *Blood.* Negative tests for rheumatoid factor.

Prognosis. Spontaneous remission in one year.

BIBLIOGRAPHY. Corrigan AB, Robinson RG, Terenty TR, et al: Benign rheumatoid arthritis of the aged. Br Med J 1:444–446, 1974

Cooney LM Jr: Special problems and presenting in the elderly. In Klippel JH, Dieppe PA: Rheumatology, p 2.11.2. St Louis, CV Mosby, 1995

CORRIGAN (D.J.)

Synonyms. Congenital aortic regurgitation; congenital aortic valve insufficiency; congenital regurgitation.

Symptoms. Great prevalance in males. Usually asymptomatic for long period of life span. Then, weakness; inappropriate diaphoresis; lethargy; awareness of neck pulsations or heart contractions; vascular pain on carotid, subclavian, or thoracic and abdominal aorta; exertional dyspnea. In some cases, sudden intractable cardiac failure.

Signs. Rapid pulse rise and collapse (Corrigan pulse); high blood pressure with high pulse pressure; Quincke pulse; anteroposterior head shaing; chest palpation (apex heart heaving); displaced left and downward; high-pitched diastolic murmur; blowing decrescendo (best heard with patient sitting or standing and leaning forward); Austin-Flint murmur.

Etiology. Congenital malformation; most commonly bicuspid aortic valve.

Pathology. Hypertrophy of left ventricle. Several possible defects and associations: unicuspid, unicommisural aortic valve; bicuspid, tricuspid, quadricuspid valves; associated with subvalvular aortic stenosis (see), supravalvular aortic stenosis (see) or ventricular septal defect.

Diagnostic Procedures. *ECG.* In mild form, normal. In severe form, R-waves tall in left precordium; S-waves deep in right precordium; depression of ST segment; T-wave inversion in DI, aVL, V5, V6 leads. *X-ray.* Enlargement of left ventricle; dilatation of ascending aorta. *Two-dimensional echocardiography, with spectral Doppler interrogation and color flow imaging.*

Therapy. Prevention of bacterial endocarditis. Eventually, consideration for surgery. Ideally surgery should be performed before clinical symptoms of heart failure develop.

Prognosis. Normal life and insidious progression of condition and sudden manifestation in young adults. Acute form may present a much faster evolution and a stormy course. All forms eventually lead to cardiac failure. For valve replacement the early mortality is approximately 2–3%; late results are mostly related to the junctional status of the left ventricle.

BIBLIOGRAPHY. Corrigan DJ: On permanent patency of the mouth of the aorta or inadequacy of the aortic valves. Edinburgh Med Surg J 37:225–245, 1832

Schlant RC, Alexander RW: Hurst's The Heart, 8th ed, pp 1466–1477. New York, McGraw-Hill, 1994

Perloff JK: The Clinical Recognition of Congenital Heart Disease, 4th ed, pp 117–125. Philadelphia, WB Saunders 1994

COR TRIATRIATUM

Synonym. Stenosis of common pulmonary vein.

Symptoms. Both sexes affected; onset in early age (not in newborn; occasionally in adolescence or in adulthood). Seldom completely asymptomatic (mild obstruction). Cyanosis; failure to thrive; exertional dyspnea; tachypnea; orthopnea; cough; irritability. With later onset; exertional dyspnea, then episodes of pulmonary edema. Recurrent hemophthysis.

Signs. Normal or growth retardation and aspects of chronic illness. On auscultation, first sound normal or loud and snapping; second sound loud pulmonic component. Murmurs may be absent or systolic, diastolic, or continuous types may be present.

Etiology. Congenital malformation.

Pathology. Drainage of pulmonary vein into an accessory left atrial chamber proximal to left atrium.

Diagnostic Procedures. *Electrocardiography.* P-waves peaked (right atrial involvement); right axis deviation and variable right ventricle hypertrophy. *X-ray.* Pulmonary venous congestion; ground glass aspect; acute pulmonary edema (on attacks). Heart size normal or marked cardiomegaly. *Two-dimensional echocardiography with Doppler interrogation and color flow imaging.*

Therapy. Medical management. Treatment of intercurrent infections: (Congestive failure and bacterial endocarditis). If symptoms appear, surgical removal of diaphragm is indicated.

Prognosis. Interval between onset of symptoms and death usually short. Extremely variable survival according to degree of lesions, from death in early infancy to survival in the fourth decade without symptoms. Progressive pulmonary venous hypertension and congestion with right-sided heart failure.

BIBLIOGRAPHY. Andral G: Précis d'Anatomie Pathologique, Paris, vol 2, p 313. Gaben, 1829
Borst M: Ein Cor triatriatum. Verh Dtsch Ges Pathol 178–192, 1905
Ostman-Smith I, Silverman NH, Oldershaw P, et al: Cor triatriatum sinistrum. Diagnostic features on cross-sectional echocardiography. Br Heart J 54:211–219, 1984
Perloff JK: The Clinical Recognition of Congenital Heart Disease, 4th ed, pp 178–185. Philadelphia, WB Saunders 1994

COTE-KATSANTONI

Symptoms and Signs. In infancy. Retarded somatic and mental development; ectodermal dysplasia.

Etiology. Unknown.

Diagnostic Procedures. *Blood.* Neutropenia; evidence of malabsorption.

BIBLIOGRAPHY. Coté GB, Katsantoni A: Osteosclerosis and ectodermal dysplasia. Prog Clin Biol Res 104:161–162, 1982
Blau EB: Ectodermal dysplasia, osteosclerosis, atrial, septal defect malabsorption, neutropenia, growth and mental retardation: the Coté-Katsantoni syndrome? Am J Med Genet Mar 26:729–732, 1987

COT-SIDES

Symptoms and Signs. Falling out of a bed with its cot-sides up. Loss of consciousness. It occurs in brain-damaged patients (trauma, cerebral vascular accidents, neoplasms).

Pathology. Those of the original injury or illness, plus signs of recent contusion or generalized brain edema.

Diagnostic Procedures. *CT brain scan.*

Therapy. Surgical intervention when indicated. Prevention: strapping in, or heavy sedation, or both, in brain-damaged person who can climb out of bed and fall.

Prognosis. Poor. In most of the patients described, coma persists until death in a few days.

BIBLIOGRAPHY. Crompton R: Cot-sides syndrome, medico-legal entity. Lancet 1:1278–1279, 1985

COSSIO-BERCONSKY

Eponym used to indicate the association of interatrial communication and Pick (F.) (see).

BIBLIOGRAPHY. Cossio P, Berconsky I: Communication interauricolar y sinfisis pericardica. Rev Argent Cardiol 3:360–366, 1936

COSTELLO-DENT

Synonyms. Hypohyperparathyroidism. Eponym used to indicate a clinical syndrome represented by the combination of mild tetany (attributed to hypothyroidism) and osteitis fibrosa generalisata.

BIBLIOGRAPHY. Costello JM, Dent CE: Hypohyperparathyroidism. Arch Dis Child 38:397–407, 1963

COSTEN

Synonym. Temporomandibular joint.

Symptoms. Headache; facial pain; stuffy sensations in the ears; tinnitus; earache; impaired hearing; dizziness; nystagmus, burning throat, mouth, and tongue.

Signs. Herpes in external auditory canal.

Etiology. Overaction of jaw joint, followed by development of a loose joint produced by absorption of meniscus, condyles, and bone (Costen). Myofascial trigger zone that produces, through an unknown mechanism, all symptoms when the area is stimulated by various stimuli such as heat, cold, pressure, needling (Freese).

Pathology. Erosion of glenoid or mandibular fossa with impaction of the condyles.

Diagnostic Procedures. *X-ray of jaw.*

Therapy. Dental correction of malocclusions; injection of corticosteroids in temporomandibular joint.

BIBLIOGRAPHY. Costen JB: A syndrome of ear and sinus symptoms dependent upon disturbed function of the temporomandibular joint. Ann Otol Rhinol Laryngol 43:1–15, 1934
Costen JB: Classification and treatment of temporomandibular joint problems. J Michigan Med Soc 55:673–677, 1956
Harris TB, Birchenbaugh J, Gier RE: Temporomandibular joint disorders. A basic review. Mo Dent J 66:18–20, 1986
Klippel JH, Dieppe PA: Rheumatology, pp 5.14.1–5. St Louis, CV Mosby, 1995

COTARD

Synonym. Delirium of total negation.

Symptoms. Patient complains of having lost everything: possessions; strength; part of (blood; heart; intestine) or entire body. Also, world does not exist for him anymore, and paradoxically he feels that he has become immortal. Other megalomelancholic ideas may be present.

Etiology. Unknown. Seen especially in manic-depressive patients or in certain brain syndromes.

Therapy. Acute syndrome lasts only a few days or weeks. Responds to treatment of basic disorder.

BIBLIOGRAPHY. Cotard J: Du délire des negations. Arch Neurol 4:152–282, 1882
Kaplan HI: Comprehensive Textbook of Psychiatry, 4th ed, p 1232. Baltimore, Williams & Wilkins, 1985

COTTLE

Synonym. Wide nose.

Symptoms. Occurs at any age; more common in older people, and in females, especially after menopause. Exacerbated in spring and fall and in winter when going into the cold from a warm room. Tearing; sensation of dryness in the eyes and nasal mucosa; nasal mucosal crusting.

Signs. Keratoconjunctivitis sicca and rhinitis sicca. Epiphora; nasal index and tip index disproportion.

Etiology. Failure in the conduction of tears, without organic obstruction of drainage passage. Hypertrophy of inferior turbinate, occluding Hasner valve; insufficiency of buffer system of nasal vestibule on expiration and nasal valve in inspiration.

Diagnostic Procedures. *Schirmer test.* Positive. *Cotton test.*

Therapy. Small cotton ball placed in the vestibule (of such size as not to constitute an obstruction) and determined if less effort needed in breathing. Usually beneficial within 5 minutes: decrease of lacrimation, and conjunctiva and nasal mucosa become moist. Initially, cotton ball worn continuously; then when needed.

Prognosis. Wearing cotton ball permits healing; and size of lobule may be considerably reduced.

BIBLIOGRAPHY. Cottle MH: Structure and function of nasal vestibule. Arch Otolaryngol 62:173–181, 1955
Gunderson HC: The wide nose. Presented at the American Rhinological Society, Chicago, Oct. 11, 1956
Gaynon IE: Lacrimal insufficiency, keratoconjunctivitis sicca and malfunction of the inferior turbinate in the wide nose or open nasal space syndrome (Cottle). Am J Ophthalmol 53:614–618, 1962

COTTON-BERG

Synonyms. Proximal end tibia fracture; fender fracture. Eponym used to indicate a fracture of the external side of tibial head resulting from a violent abduction and the consequent impact against the external condyle of the femur.

BIBLIOGRAPHY. Cotton FJ, Berg R: Fender fracture of the tibia and the knee. N Engl J Med 201:989–995, 1929
Sisk TD: Fractures of lower extremities. In Crenshaw AH (ed): Campbell's Operative Orthopedics, 7th ed, pp 1637–1653. St Louis, CV Mosby, 1987

COTUGNO

Synonyms. Sciatic neuritis; sciatica. See also Facets and Putti-Chavany.

Symptoms. Occurs most often in males, onset usually abrupt. Unilateral pain in posterior portions of thighs and back of leg, worsened by movement, sneezing, coughing.

Signs. Weakness of leg involved, especially below knee; ankle jerk absent; sensory impairment. Tenderness on palpation along course of sciatic nerve; loss of lumbar curve. Gaenslen sign; Patrick sign; straight-leg raising test; Lasègue's sign; Ober test.

Etiology and Pathology. Most frequent. Radicular compression and neuritis of L4–5 interspace by herniation of intervertebral disk. Other causes. Tumor (primary or metastatic); infection; arthritic changes; fractures of spine; pelvic conditions compressing the nerve (e.g., pregnancy; neoplasm; abscess).

Diagnostic Procedures. *X-ray of spine. MRI. CT scan. Spinal tap.* Increase of total protein.

Therapy. Rest; analgesic; anti-inflammatory agent; vitamin B_{12}; physiotherapy. According to etiology, surgery or antibiotics.

Prognosis. Usually subacute or chronic course. Increasing in days to a maximum, then receding gradually.

BIBLIOGRAPHY. Cotugno D: De ischiade nervosa commentarius. Napoli Frates Simonis 1764; Vienna, Gräffer, 1770
Cotugno D: A Treatise of the Nervous Sciatica, or Nervous Hip Gout. London, Wilkie, 1775

COUGH SYNCOPE

Synonyms. Charcot vertigo; laryngeal epilepsy; post-tussive; tussive syncope; laryngeal vertigo.

Symptoms. Occurs most frequently in middle-aged men who excessively indulge in tobacco, alcohol, and food. Following cough attack (dry, unproductive, paroxysmal, with intense muscular effort); burning or tingling of larynx may precede cough. Sudden syncope (occurs within seconds; no sequelae; frequently no memory of consciousness loss).

Signs. Usually pyknic, slightly obese patient. Frequent signs of respiratory tract infections, emphysema, or bronchial asthma. During syncope, complete muscle relaxation, and patient falls or slumps. Face congested, then pale; diaphoresis frequent; convulsion rare (10%).

Etiology. Not clearly defined. Relation to epilepsy, and narcolepsy-cataplexy (Gelineau, see) has been discussed, but elements of differentiation exist to establish this syndrome as an autonomous clinical entity.

Diagnostic Procedures. *Serology.* To differentiate from laryngeal crisis of tabes dorsalis. *Electroencephalography.* To differentiate from epilepsy. *X-ray of chest.*

Therapy. No treatment during attack. Treatment of underlying respiratory condition. Procaine block of superior laryngeal nerve in refractory cases. Change in diet and smoking habits.

Prognosis. Attacks generally benign and of little consequence; death, however, may occur. Cure of respiratory condition prevents recurrences of attacks.

BIBLIOGRAPHY. Charcot JM: Seance du 19 Novembre 1876. Gaz Med Paris 5:588–589, 1876
Lewis RP, Budoulas H, Schaal SF, et al: Diagnosis and management of syncope. In: Schlant RC, Alexander RW: Hurst's The Heart, 8th ed, p 933. New York, McGraw-Hill, 1994

COUNTER-DISASTER

See Disaster.

Symptoms and Signs. Psychological state that drives uninjured or slightly injured people to volunteer after the disaster to participate in extremely vigorous rescue activity. They become physically overexerted and perform with poor efficiency. Danger of becoming careless, especially in applying first aid measures.

Therapy. Education and training.

BIBLIOGRAPHY. Garb S, Eng E: Disaster Handbook. New York, Springer, 1964

COURVOISIER-TERRIER

Synonym. Bard-Pic; ampulla of Vater obstruction.

Signs. Courvoisier law: Palpable distended gallbladder indicates a neoplasm as cause of obstructive jaundice. Important sign, but not invariably present; gallbladder may be distended, but not palpable.

BIBLIOGRAPHY. Bard L, Pic A: Contribution a l'étude clinique et anatomo-pathologique du Cancer primitif du pancreas. Rev Med Par 8:257–282; 363–405, 1888
Courvoisier LG: Casuistischstatistische Beiträge zur Pathologie und Chirurgie der Gallenwege, pp 57–58. Leipzig, Vogel, 1890
Vergese A, Berk SL: Courvoisier's law. Lancet 1:99, 1986

COUVADE

Synonym. Male pseudopregnancy.

Symptoms. Occurs in men whose wives are pregnant; usually symptoms start in third month of wife's pregnancy. Mostly gastrointestinal symptoms: appetite loss; toothache; nausea; vomiting; morning sickness; constipation; diarrhea. Abdominal swelling rare (see Simpson). Tension and anxiety may be present or absent. Different from delusion of pregnancy: patient with couvade syndrome never has the idea of being pregnant.

Etiology. Unknown; this neurotic development appears equivalent to the couvade ritual, which was practiced since antiquity and is still practiced in different parts of the world by many races. It consists of the father retiring at time of wife's labor, mimicking labor pain, receiving the attention due to the parturient woman.

Therapy. None; symptoms disappear with termination of wife's pregnancy.

Prognosis. Self-limited, very benign neurosis. In some cases, recurrence on successive pregnancies of wife.

BIBLIOGRAPHY. Taylor EB: Research into the Early History of Mankind and the Development of Civilization, 2nd ed, p 301. London, Murray, 1865
Bogren LY: The couvade syndrome: Background variables. Acta Psychiatr Scand 70:316–320, 1984
Kaplan HI, Sadock BJ: Comprehensive Textbook of Psychiatry, 4th ed, p 934. Baltimore, Williams & Wilkins, 1985

COUVELAIRE

Synonyms. Uteroplacental apoplexy; premature separation of placenta, abruptio placentae (see Defibrinating).

Symptoms. Vaginal bleeding, and shock out of proportion to external bleeding; local pain and tenderness.

Signs. Tender and firm uterus; rapid enlargement of uterus. Fetal signs: sudden, violent movement of the fetus; changes in rate and quality of heart sounds.

Etiology. By definition, placental detachment after the 24th week. Cause unknown. Predisposing factors: toxemia; hypertension; chronic glomerulonephritis; trauma; chronic vascular disease.

Pathology. Retroplacental hematoma occurring between basal decidua and myometrium; rupture into amniotic sac. In severe cases, extensive hemorrhagic infiltration occurs between muscle bundles producing bluish mottling of uterus, broad ligaments, tubes, and ovaries—Couvelaire uterus. Complication of separation: hypofibrinogenemia (see Defibrinating syndrome); acute renal failure.

Diagnostic Procedures. Ultrasound examination.

Therapy. Depends on stage of labor, efficiency of uterine contractions, period of gestation, and actual or potential infection. (1) Watchful expectancy; (2) rupture of membranes; (3) cesarean section. Cesarean section limited to (1) severe detachment seen early and fetus living; (2) patients in whom cervix is uneffaced, and undilated; (3) those showing no progress in labor after rupture. Replacement of blood; intravenous (IV) infusion of fibrinogen; IV infusion of epsilon-aminocaproic acid. Occasionally a cesarean hysterectomy is necessary if bleeding is uncontrollable.

Prognosis. Fetal mortality around 40%; maternal mortality under 1%.

BIBLIOGRAPHY. Couvelaire A: Traitment chirurgical des hémorrhagies utero-placentaires avec décollement du placenta normalment inséré. Ann Gynecol Obstet (Paris) 8:591–608, 1911
De Lee JB: A case of fatal hemorrhagic diathesis, with premature detachment of the placenta. Am J Obstet 44:785–792, 1901

Monteiro AA, Inocencio AC, Jorge CS: Placental abruption with disseminated intravascular coagulopathy in the second trimester of pregnancy with fetal survival. Br J Obstet Gynecol 94:811–812, 1987
Bithell TC: Acquired coagulation disorders. In Lee GR, Bithel TC, Foerster J, et al (eds): Wintrobe's Clinical Cematology, 9th ed, pp 1481–1482. Philadelphia, Lea & Febiger, 1993

COWDEN*

Synonyms. Lloyd-Dennis; hamartoma, multiple; MHAM; dysplastic gangliocytoma of the cerebellum; included Lhermitte-Duclos (see) (is today considered part of the multiple hamartoma syndrome).

Symptoms and Signs. Both sexes. Onset usually end of second–third decade. Recurrent diarrhea (in some cases). Seizures and cerebellar signs (Lhermitte-Duclos). Virginal hypertrophy of breasts (70% of females); also fibroadenomas fibrocystic disease, adenocarcinoma (25%). Macrocephaly; Bird-like facies; hypoplastic mandible and maxilla, high-arched palate; scrotal tongue; papillomatosis of lips and oral mucosa. Also, frequent multiple thyroid adenomas, scoliosis, and pectus excavatum. Skin: typical lesions lichenoid or papillomatous papules or small nodules mostly localized around eyelids, alae nasi, mouth, pinnas, neck, and dorsa of hands and forearms (76%). Trichilemmomas. Punctate keratoses on palms and soles. Frequent association with various tumor and hamartomas.

Etiology. Autosomal dominant inheritance.

Pathology. Hamartomatous polyps of intestine in some cases (60%).

Diagnostic Procedures. *Skin biopsy.* Hair follicles hamartomas (pattern of trichilemmomas).

Therapy. Surgery.

Prognosis. Fair; one case developed acute myelogenous leukemia; high frequency of breast cancer in females.

BIBLIOGRAPHY. Lhermitte J, Duclos P: Sur un ganglioneurome diffuse du cortex du cervelet. Bull Assoc Franc Cancer 9:99–107, 1920
Costello MJ: A case for diagnosis (keratosis follicularis?) Arch Dermatol Syph 44:109–110, 1941
Lloyd KM, II, Dennis M: Cowden's disease, a possible new symptom complex with multiple system involvement. Ann Intern Med 58:136–142, 1963
Starink TM: The Cowden Syndrome and other familial Multiple Hair Tumors (sic) syndromes. Amsterdam, Free Univ Press, 1986
Padberg GW, Schot JDL, Wielvoye GJ, et al: Lhermitte-Duclos disease and Cowden disease: a single phakomatosis. Ann Neurol 29:517–523, 1991
Albrecht S, Haber RM, Goodman JC et al: Cowden syndome and Lhermitte-Duclos disease. Cancer 70:869–876, 1992

CRAIN

Synonym. Erosive osteoarthritis.

Symptoms and Signs. Predominantly affects women; onset in middle age or postmenopause. Episodes of painful inflammations of distal interphalangeal joints, followed by proximal joint involvement. Recurrent for years, with long intermittent periods of complete remission (up to 10 years). Presence of mucous cysts over affected joints (to be differentiated from Heberden nodes, see).

Etiology. Unknown; hereditary condition or sporadic.

Pathology. Bony ankylosis; juxta-articular bone erosions; proliferative synovitis.

Diagnostic Procedures. *Blood.* Sedimentation rate normal; rheumatoid factor normal. *X-rays.* Cartilage loss; osteophyte formation; sub-

---

*Name of affected family.

chondral sclerosis; juxta-articular bone erosion. Absence of findings of generalized osteoarthritis.

Therapy. Corticosteroids and anti-inflammatory agents during attacks.

Prognosis. Evolution toward severe functional impairment.

BIBLIOGRAPHY. Crain DG: Interphalangeal osteoarthritis. JAMA 175:1049–1053, 1961
Weatherall DJ, Ledingham JGG, Warrell DA (eds): Oxford Textbook of Medicine, 3rd ed, p 2949. Oxford, Oxford Med Pub, 1996

CRANE-HEISE

Synonyms. Cleft lip/palate; clavicle/ribs agenesis; talipes equinovarus.

Symptoms and Signs. Intrauterine delayed development. *Head.* Large, hypertelorism, nasal bridge: depressed. *Facies.* Small, micrognathia, cleft lip/palate. *Neck.* Short. *Limbs.* Soft tissue syndactyly of digits. Talipes equinovarus. *Genitals.* Penis short, cryptorchidisms.

Etiology. Autosomal recessive inheritance.

Diagnostic procedures. *X-rays.* Calvaria poorly mineralized cervical vertebrae; clavicle absent; scapulae small, radial heads dislocated.

Prognosis. Apparently lethal.

BIBLIOGRAPHY. Crane JP, Heise RL: New syndrome in three affected siblings. Pediatrics 68:235–237, 1981

CRANIODIAPHYSEAL DYSOSTOSIS

Synonym. CDD; see Craniometaphyseal dysplasia and Camurati-Engelmann; leontiasis ossea; van Buchem.

Symptoms. Both sexes affected; present from infancy, becoming symptomatic within first few years. Nasal obstruction; anorexia; vomiting; blindness; deafness; mental retardation.

Signs. Marked facial distortion; widened ribs; clavicles thickened in midportions.

Etiology. Unknown; autosomal recessive trait.

Pathology. Sclerosis of skull bones; paranasal sinuses overgrown. In long bones thin-cortex, uniform thickness of shafts; in metacarpals and metatarsals, some degree of ballooning in midportions with thin cortex.

Diagnostic Procedures. *Blood.* Normal calcium, phosphorus, and alkaline phosphatase. *X-rays of bones.* Facial and cranial thickening and distortion. Long bones: diaphyseal endostosis and shaped as "policeman stick."

Therapy. Surgical correction of nerve compression.

Prognosis. Poor; condition more severe than Pyle. Faster progression to blindness and death.

BIBLIOGRAPHY. De Souza O: Leontiasis ossea. Porto Alegre (Brazil) Faculdade de Med Rev Dos Cursos 13:47–54, 1927
Macpherson RI: Craniodiaphyseal dysplasia, a disease or group of diseases? J Can Assoc Radiol 25:22–23, 1974
Levy MH, Kozlowski K: Cranial-dyaphyseal dysplasia report of a case. Australas Radiol 31:431–435, 1987
Brueton LA, Winter RM: Craniodiaphyseal dysplasia. J Med Genet 27:701–706, 1990

CRANIO-FRONTONASAL

Symptoms and Signs. Prevalent in female with more severe manifestations. From birth. *Head.* Brachycephaly, plagiocephaly, dolichocephaly, broad forehead. *Face.* Symmetry, mild face hypoplasia, hypertelorism, broad nose, esotropia or exotropia, telechantus, high arched palate, cleft lip and palate. *Teeth.* Abonormalities. *Limbs.* Clavicle pseudoarthrosis, short fifth finger, broad digits, long fingers, syndactyly, campodactyly. *Trunk.* Short stature, scoliosis, neck and chest anomalies. *Genitals.* Hypospadias, shawl scrotum.

Etiology. Presumed X-linked inheritance with metabolic interference.

BIBLIOGRAPHY. Cohen MM Jr: Craniofrontonasal dysplasia. Birth Defects 15:85–89, 1979
Kwee ML, Zindhout D: Inheritance of cranio-fronto-nasal syndrome. Am J Med Genet 30:841–842, 1988

CRANIOMETAPHYSEAL DYSPLASIA

Synonym. See Craniodiaphyseal dysostosis and Pyle.

Symptoms and Signs. Both sexes affected; onset from infancy. Deafness; blindness; facial paralysis; multiple involvement of cranial nerves. Normal intelligence. Leonine facies; complete nasal obstruction (in recessive form).

Etiology. Both autosomal recessive and dominant inheritance.

Pathology. Hyperostosis of cranial and facial bones with compression of cranial nerves at foramina. Metaphyseal changes of long bones (club-like rather than like Erlenmeyer flask, flask shape is more typical of Pyle, see).

Diagnostic Procedures. *X-rays.* See Pathology.

Therapy. Surgical decompression of nerves.

Prognosis. Recessive form more severe. Without treatment, extremely severe incapacitation.

BIBLIOGRAPHY. Spranger JW, Paulsen K, Lehmann W: Die kraniometaphysare. Dysplasia. Z Kinderheilk 93:64–79, 1965
Carnevale A, Grether P, Castillo V, et al: Autosomal dominant craniometaphyseal dysplasia: Clinical variability. Clin Genet 23:17–22, 1983
Hudgius RJ, Edwards MDB: Craniometaphyseal dysplasia associated with hydrocephalus: case report. Neurosurgery 29:617–618, 1987

CRESCENTIC GLOMERULONEPHRITIS

Synonyms. Rapidly progressive glomerulonephitis; extracapillary proliferative glomerulonephritis. Includes: antiglomerular basement membrane antibody-mediated; crescentic glomerulonephritis; immune complex mediated crescentic glomerulonephritis; ANCA-associated glomerulonephitis.

Symptoms and Signs. Usually young or middle-aged males (in women at any age). Sometimes preceded by exposure to hydrocarbon fumes or respiratory illness (in 30% of cases preceding streptococcal infection). Onset seldom acute, usually insidious. Anorexia; fever; myalgia; or abdominal pain; diarrhea; smoky urine; oliguria (more severe than in acute nephritic syndrome). Blood hypertension (less severe than in acute nephritic).

Etiology. Not a specific disease but a pathological entity caused by inflammation from different etiologies. Three major immunopathologic categories recognized: immune complex-mediated (lupus glomerulonephrites, IgA nephropathy-including Schoenlein-Henoch; acute post infectious, fibrillary glomerulopathy, membranoproliferative glomerulonephritis types I and II); anti-GBM antibody-mediated (Goodpasture; anti-GBM glomerulonephritis without lung hemorrhage); ANCA associated (pauciimmunecrescentic); Wegener, microscopic polyarteritis.

Pathology. Light microscopy. Accumulation of cells (crescents) in Bowman space in a variable percentual (25–80%) of glomeruli; in time, glomerular sclerosis. Electromicroscopy. Widened zones in subendothelial space with detachment gaps in basement membrane. Immunofluorescence. Glomeruli with linear deposits of IgG (rarely IgA); C3 deposits are rare.

Diagnostic Procedures. *Urine.* Dysmorphic RBC, casts. Decreased glomerular filtration rate. *Blood.* Circulating antiglomerular basement membrane antibodies; signs of uremia. HLA-DR2 in 85% of patients. Fibrin degradation products high in urine and serum. *Biopsy of arteries.* Presence of arteritis in different percent according to forms.

Therapy. According to cause, severity and stage: earlier immunosuppression steroids; cyclophosphamide; azathioprine; role of plasmapheresis discussed.

Prognosis. Without therapy, progression to renal insufficiency in 6 months. With therapy, better prognosis. Renal transplantation is followed by a 10–30% recurrence of disease.

BIBLIOGRAPHY. Couser WG: Rapidly progressive glomerulonephitis: classification, pathogenetic mechanisms and therapy. Am J Kidney Dis 11:449–464, 1988

Jennette JC, Falk JR: Crescentic glomerulonephritis. In Massry SG, Glassock RJ: Textbook of Nephrology, 3rd ed, pp 742–746. Baltimore, Williams & Wilkins, 1995

CRETINISM, SPORADIC

Synonyms. Congenital hypothyroidism. Includes endemic cretinism. See Kocher-Debre-Semelaigne.

Symptoms and Signs. Both sexes affected at birth; overweight; lethargy; facies with heavy expression; eyes pig-like; nystagmus; large tongue; mouth open; later, drooling and delayed dentition; yellow tint on cheek; hypothermia; altered tone of voice; persistent neonatal jaundice; protuberant belly; umbilical hernia; skin dry, flabby, and cold; hair coarse. Failure to thrive; poor appetite; constipation. Cardiomegaly (occasionally); slow pulse. In endemic cretinism, frequently deafness. In 50% of cases; ataxia, muscular hypotonia, diplegia. Clumsy gait. Delayed sexual development. Mental development retarded. Final result dwarfism and imbecility. Occasionally goiter.

Etiology. Variable. Usually autosomal recessive in all types of syndromes described. Can be owing to complete lack (athyreosis), to reduced thyroid function because of enzyme defects; impaired thyroid response to thyrotropin, thyroid stimulating hormone (TSH) defective production, failure of iodide transport, failure to form organic iodine, defect of peroxidase, failure of coupling of iodotyrosines. Endemic in particular areas (Crete, Beotia, Alpine Valleys). Failure of iodotyrosine deiodinase activity, altered thyroglobulin synthesis, deficiency of TBG.

Pathology. Many features of delayed development (cerebral, skeletal). Generally, marked hypertrophy of pituitary.

Diagnostic Procedures. *Blood.* Free thyroxine (FT4), total thyroxine (TT4) decreased; TSH increased. *X-ray of knee.* Absent calcification of epiphyses. Numerous other signs of delayed skeletal growth. The different forms described require for the diagnosis complex thyroid stimulating and inhibiting tests that distinguish the various enzymatic defects.

Therapy. Thyroid hormone started as soon as possible and maintained at adequate levels.

Prognosis. Strictly correlated with time of onset and adequacy and maintenance of therapy. Normal physical and mental development possible with correct treatment.

BIBLIOGRAPHY. Saldanha PH, Toledo SPA: Inherited hypothyroidism unresponsive to thyrotropin in man. Rev Bras Genet 11:803–804, 1988

Utiger RD: Hypothyroidism. In De Groot LJ (ed): Endocrinology, 3rd ed, pp 752–757. Philadelphia, WB Saunders, 1995

CREUTZFELDT-JAKOB

Synonyms. In addition to a (possibly) proper Creutzfeld-Jakob syndrome, under the same heading or and under a number of various synonims (in a very confusing fashion), several disorders have been indicated (and with particular frequency, corticostriatal spinal degeneration or Heidenhain syndrome, see); corticostiatospinal degeneration, spastic pseudosclerosis, Jakob-Creutzfeldt; spastic paraplegia, Parkinson dementia–ALS complex of Guam; Davidson corticopallidospinal degeneration; corticostriatospinal presenile degeneration; presenile polyencephalic; Nevin-Jones; atrophia spongiforme cerebrale; Brownell-Oppenheimer; progressive dementia, "Mad Cow," etc.

Symptoms. Both sexes affected; onset between the fifth and sixth decades of life. Some affected patients in their 20s have been reported. Prodromic symptoms: vague psychic disturbances that progress within a few months to dementia. Neurasthenia followed by confusion; disorientation; weakness; stiffness of limbs; choreoathetoid movements; dysarthria; cortical blindness.

Signs. Spastic weakness of extremities; unsteady ataxic gait; nystagmus; rigidity; tremor; athetosis; localized amyotrophies; decreased abdominal and increased tendon reflexes; occasionally, positive Babinski.

Etiology. The syndrome at least in some of the entities included under this heading is transmitted by a virus that withstands usual methods of sterilization. (Equipment that has come in contact with tissue or blood from these patients should be autoclaved for 1 hour.) The natural route of transmission of this disease is unknown. Because it occurs both in a sporadic and familial form, in some families there could be a genetic susceptibility to the infection.

Pathology. Diffuse neuronal degeneration of cerebral cortex (deeper layers), basal ganglia, descending corticospinal tracts; status spongiosus, neuroglial reaction.

Diagnostic Procedures. *Spinal fluid.* Normal. *CT scan. MRI. EEG.*

Therapy. Symptomatic.

Prognosis. Rapid course; death in 12–16 months in infective cases, in 5–10 years in other ones.

BIBLIOGRAPHY. Creutzfeldt HG: Ueber eine eigenartige herdformige Erkrankung des Zentralnervensystems. In Nissl F, Alzheimer A: Histologie und Histopathologie. Jena, Fischer, Arbeit Erganzungband, 1921

Jacob A: Ueber eigenartige Erkrankungen des Zentralnervensystems mit bemerkenswertem anatomischen Befunde (Spatische Pseudosklerose-Encephalomyelopathie mit disseminierten Degenerationsherden). Zschr Ges Neurol Psychiat 64:147–228, 1921

Adams RD, Victor M: Principles of Neurology, 5th ed, pp 973–974. New York, McGraw-Hill, 1993

Bjornsson J, Carp RI, Love A (eds): Slow infections of the central nervous system. Proc New York Acad Sci N9434, 1994

CREYX-LEVY

Synonyms. Sjögren reverse (see); ophthalmorhinostomato hygrosi.

Symptoms and Signs. Generalized hypersecretions (lacrimal; nasal; oral; gastric). Cervical arthritis.

Etiology. Unknown.

Diagnostic Procedures. *Blood.* In some cases, leukopenia, eosinophilia, and thrombocytopenia; increase of erythrocyte sedimentation rate; hypochloremia. *Gastric juice.* Hyperchlorhydria. *X-ray of skeleton.* Calcification of cervical vertebrae, ligaments, and cervical lymph nodes. *Sialography. Schitzmer test.*

Therapy. Hypersecretion is not affected by atropine and derivates. Trials with corticosteroids.

Prognosis. Chronic condition responding poorly to treatment.

BIBLIOGRAPHY. Creyx M, Lévy J: Syndrome d'opthalmo-rhino-stomatoxérose, dit des "Gougerot-Sjoegren," sindrome d'opththalmo-rhino-stomato-hygrose. Bull Soc Med Hop 64:1123–1128, 1948

CRIGLER-NAJJAR TYPE I

Synonyms. Congenital hyperbilirubinemia; congenital familial non-hemolytic jaundice.

Symptoms and Signs. Both sexes affected. Jaundice appears in first few days after birth. Majority of cases develop central nervous system symptomatology resembling kernicterus (see). Recurrent fever; no hepatomegaly or splenomegaly.

Etiology. Congenital absence (or marked reduction?) of glucoronyl transferase activity resulting in the lack of conjugation of bilirubin with gluconuride and high level of indirect bilirubin in blood and brain damage (kernicterus). Autosomal recessive inheritance.

Pathology. *Liver.* Normal parenchymal cells; bilirubin in hepatic canaliculi. *Brain.* Basal nuclei stained with bile.

Diagnostic Procedures. *Blood.* High level of indirect bilirubin with considerable fluctuation; absence of incompatibility of blood group. Failure to respond to phenobarbital treatment. *Liver function test.* Normal. *Urine.* Absence of bilirubin; urobilinogenuria. *Stool.* Reduced fecal urobilinogen. *Cholangiography.* Patency of extrahepatic bile duct. *Biopsy of liver.*

Therapy. Continuous extracorporeal perfusion; plasmapheresis; peritoneal dialysis with albumin; cholestyramine orally; phototherapy.

Prognosis. Fatal in early infancy, amount of brain damage determining prognosis. Patients without brain involvement survive. Patients without early brain involvement survive but may have kernicterus at later age.

BIBLIOGRAPHY. Crigler JF, Najjar V: A congenital familial non-hemolytic jaundice with kernicterus. Pediatrics 10:169–179, 1952
van Es HHG, Goldhoorn BJ, Paul-Abrahamse M, et al: Immuno-chemical analysis of uridine diphosphate-glucuronosyltransferase in four patients with Crigler-Najjar syndrome type I. J Clin Invest 85:1199–1205, 1990

CRISSCROSS HEART

Synonyms. Upstairs-downstairs heart, superoinferior heart; atrioventricular connection discordant.

Symptoms and Signs. Rare. Cyanosis or heart failure or both.

Etiology. Unknown. Congenital condition.

Pathology. Atrioventricular spatial relation that places each ventricle in a contralateral position to its associated atrium.

Diagnostic Procedures. *Cardiac catherization. Angiography. Echography. CT scan. MRI.*

Therapy. Palliative surgery in infancy.

Prognosis. Poor.

BIBLIOGRAPHY. Vaan Praagh S, La Corte M, Falows KE, et al: Superoinferior ventricles: Anatomic and angiographic findings in ten post-mortem cases. In Van Praagh R, Takao A (eds): Etiology and Morphogenesis of Congenital Heart Disease. Mount Kisco, NY, Futura Publishing, 1980
Attie F, Munoz-Castellanos L, Ovseyevitz J, et al: Crossed atrioventricular connections. Am Heart J 99:163–172, 1980
Perloff JK: The Clinical Recognition of Congenital Heart Disease, 4th ed, p 72. Philadelphia, WB Saunders, 1994

CRISWICK-SCHEPENS

Synonyms. Vitroretinopathy (familial exudation). Exudative vitreo-retinopathy familial. FEVR.

Symptoms and Signs. Vitreous detachment with organized membrane. Displacement of macula snowflakes opacities. Recurrent vitreous hemorrhages.

Etiology. Autosomal dominant or X-linked recessive inheritance.

Pathology. Vitreous hemorrhages. Secondary cataract. Phitis bulbi, retinal detachment.

Diagnostic Procedures. Fluorescein angiography.

Prognosis. After 20 years of age stops progression.

BIBLIOGRAPHY. Criswick VG, Schepens CL: Familial exudative vitreo-retinopathy. Am J Ophthalmol 68:578–594, 1969
Heydenreich A: Kongenitale Retinoschisis und weitere vitreo-retinale Degenerationen und ihre Differentialdiagnose. Faha Ophthalmol (Leipzig), 11:3–14, 1986

CRITICAL ILLNESS NEUROPATHY

Synonyms. CIN; polyneuropathy—intensive care.

Symptoms and Signs. Both sexes equal incidence. As part or following the combination of sepsis, respiratory failure, polyneuropathy, and long hospitalization in a intensive care department. It occurs in 70% of these cases. This neuropathy may be easily mistaken for weakness and debility associated with the long immobilization. Greater distal than proximal weakness, areflexia, or hyporeflexia.

Etiology. Unknown.

Pathology. Nerve biopsy: primary axonal degeneration of motor and sensory fibers without inflammation; muscle: scattered atrophic fibers.

Diagnostic Procedures. *Electrodiagnostic studies.* Significant compound muscle action potential amplitude reduction and significant amplitude reduction of sensory nerve action potentials. *Blood.* Creatinine phosphokinase normal or slightly elevated.

Therapy. Early aggressive rehabilitation may lead to favorable outcome.

Prognosis. Most patients who survive septic event will recover from polyneuropathy; however, some patients do not recover and in others recovery may take years.

BIBLIOGRAPHY. Bolton CF, Gilbert JJ, Hahn F, et al: Polyneuropathy in critically ill patients. J Neurol Neurosurg Psychiatr 47:1223–1231, 1984
Jarrett SR, Mogelof JS: Critical illness neuropathy: Diagnosis and management. Arch Phys Med Rehab 76:688–691, 1995

CROHN

Synonyms. Crohn-Lesniowsky; regional enteritis.

Symptoms. Slight prevalence in males; Jewish people most frequently affected; onset at any age; average 25 years. Symptoms variable according to anatomic location and amount of involvement. Onset usually mild, insidious symptoms: borborygmus; bloating; flatulence; mild abdominal cramps and mild diarrhea; occasional temperature elevation. Slow progression to more severe symptoms: (1) Pain (85% of patients), peristaltic type with or without diarrhea; cramps usually do not subside following defecation; with more advanced disease pain becomes constant. Initially pain localized in periumbilical region; may mimic "acute appendicitis"; later corresponds to site of the lesion. (2) Diarrhea (90%), soft or semiliquid, seldom liquid; tenesmus rare, except if perineal lesions have developed. (3) Fever (33%), not accompanied by chills. (4) Perianal-perirectal fistulas (20%). (5) Symptoms of bowel obstruction or perforation in stomach or duodenal localization; nausea, vomiting, ulcerlike pain dominant symptoms. (6) Melena (4%). Systemic manifestation: fever; weight loss; polyarthritis (5%); rarely, erythema nodosum; pyoderma gangrenosum; nervousness; tension; depression.

When condition begins in childhood, growth retardation and delayed maturation are observed.

Signs. Abdominal distention; tenderness on palpation of abdomen in region corresponding to areas of involvement. Mass in right lower quadrant frequently may be palpated.

Etiology. Unknown; possibly included in the autoimmune group of diseases. Familial cases reported (10% of cases).

Pathology. Lesion may occur in any part of intestine, from stomach to rectum. Terminal ileum involved in 75% of cases. Areas of lesions alternated with normal areas. Affected tract appears rigid, thickened. Serosa covered by mesenteric fat and fibrostenotic exudate; chronic subserous inflammation. Mesentery edematous, rubbery, with several enlarged lymph nodes. (When fistulas have developed, matting of intestinal loops.) Marked narrowing of intestinal lumen; mucosal ulcerations and nodularity; frequently, lesions stop abruptly at ileocecal junction; however, in some cases may continue into proximal colon. Histology. Mucosa inflamed, ulcerated, or atrophic. Submucosa thickened, with granulomatous formations, with or without giant cells. Granulomas also are found in subserosa and lymph nodes. Muscular coat normal. Marked fibrotic changes in submucosa and subserosa.

Diagnostic Procedures. *Blood.* Moderate anemia; leukocytosis; hypoproteinemia; hypoprothrombinemia (frequent); electrolyte alterations; hypocalcemia. *X-ray.* Early, blunting, flattening, thickening of plica circulares; lumen and contour irregularities. Later, longitudinal ulcerations; finally; uniform, rigid tube with disappearance of mucosal pattern and various degree of narrowing of the lumen (initially spastic; later stenotic, Kantors sign), alternated with skipped areas of normal intestine are characteristic features.

Therapy. *Medical.* Diet; correction of anemia; rest; psychotherapy; anticholinergic drugs; sedatives; salicylazosulfapyridine (most effective antibacterial); adrenal steroids, nitrogen mustard, Azathioprine (Imuran®). *Surgical.* Resection of affected tracts.

Prognosis. More severe in young people; milder in old-age onset. Frequent remission and relapses. Relapses after surgical procedures frequent. With treatment, patients may have relatively good health most of the time.

BIBLIOGRAPHY. Leśniowski A: Przyczynek Do Chirurgii Kiszek. Medycyna 31:460–464, 483–489, 514–518, 1903
Crohn BB, Ginzburg L, Oppenheimer GD: Regional ileitis. JAMA 99:1323–1329, 1932
Teahon K, Bjanarson I, Pearson M, et al: Ten years' experience with an elemental diet in the management of Crohn's disease. Gut 31:1133–1137, 1990
Weatherall DJ, Ledingham JGG, Warrell DA (eds): Oxford Textbook of Medicine, 3rd ed, pp 1936–1943. Oxford, Oxford Med Pub, 1996

CROME

Symptoms. In females. Epileptic attacks. Mental retardation. Visual impairment.

Signs. Congenital cataracts; small stature.

Etiology. Autosomal recessive inheritance.

Pathology. Encephalopathy. Renal tubular necrosis.

Prognosis. Death (4 and 8 months).

BIBLIOGRAPHY. Crome L, Duckett S, Franklin AW: Congenital cataracts, renal tubular necrosis and encephalopathy in two sisters. Arch Dis Child 38:505–519, 1963

CRONKHITE-CANADA

Synonyms. Alopecia—polyposis—skin pigmentation—onychotrophia.

Symptoms and Signs. Prevalent in females. Diffuse brownish pigmentation of skin (more intense at body folds); alopecia, onychotrophia. These changes may precede or follow gastrointestinal complaints: nausea; vomiting; diarrhea.

Etiology. Unknown; nonfamilial form of generalized gastrointestinal polyposis.

Pathology. Benign adenomatous polyps affecting practically the entire gastrointestinal mucosa.

Diagnostic Procedures. *X-rays of gastrointestinal tract. Biopsy.*

Therapy. In some patients, malabsorption is partly corrected by removal of polyps. Endoscopic resection. Gastrectomy, hemicolectomy according to prevalence of polyps in different regions. Generally bowel resection is to be avoided. Medical regimens have scarce success.

Prognosis. Usually fatal within 18 months from onset of diarrhea. Remission reported after surgery. Some patients may have a long survival time.

BIBLIOGRAPHY. Cronkhite LW, Canada WJ: Generalized gastrointestinal polyposis. New Engl J Med 252:1011–1015, 1955
Nishihi M, Takasugi S, et al: Cronkhite-Canada syndrome: a case report and analytical review of 37 cases reported in Japan Hiroshima. J Med Sci 33:607–614, 1984
Lynch PM: Polyposis syndromes. In Haubrich WS, Schaffner F, Berk JE (eds): Bockus Gastroenterology, 5th ed, vol 2, p 1739. Philadelphia, WB Saunders, 1995

CROSBY

Obsolete. Used to indicate: Non Spherocityc hereditary hemolytic anemia.

BIBLIOGRAPHY. Crosby WH: Hereditary non-spherocytic hemolzytic anemia. Blood 5:233–253, 1950

CROSS

Synonyms. Kramer (family name); gingival fibromatosis—hypopigmentation—microphthalmia—oligophrenia—athetosis. Hypopigmentation—oculocerebral; oculo-cerebral—hypopigmentation.

Symptoms and Signs. Rare. Four cases described; present from birth. Skin pink with presence of pigmented nevi and freckles; hair white to light blond. Eye color, gray blue; microphthalmia, cataracts. Nystagmus very marked; blindness; oligophrenia; athetosis; gingival fibromatosis.

Etiology. Autosomal recessive inheritance.

Pathology. Melanosomes in hair bulb scanty, from stage III to IV.

Diagnostic Procedures. *Blood.* Serum tyrosine levels normal; beta melanocyte-stimulating hormone level unknown. *Incubation of hair with tyrosine. Pigmentation.*

Therapy. Symptomatic.

Prognosis. Poor.

BIBLIOGRAPHY. Cross HE, McKusick VA, Breen W: A new oculocerebral syndrome with hypopigmentation. J Pediatr 70:398–406, 1967
Fryus JP, Dereymaeker AM, Heremans G, et al: Oculocerebral syndrome with hypopigmentation (Cross syndrome): report of two siblings born to consanguineons parents. Clin Genet 34:81–84, 1988
Courtens W, Broeckx W, Ledoux M, et al: Oculocerebral hypopigmentation syndrome (Cross syndrome) in a gypsy child. Acta Pediatr Scand 78:806–810, 1989
Weatherall DJ, Ledingham JGG, Warrell DA (eds): Oxford Textbook of Medicine, 3rd ed, p 3759. Oxford, Oxford Med Pub, 1996

CROSTI

Synonym. Winkelmann; high-grade β-cell lymphoma; large cell lymphoma—follicular center origin; reticulohistiocytoma of dorsum.

Symptoms and Signs. Male to female ratio, 1:6. Age, 22–92, median 58. Usually single, less freqently multiple red or violaceous, nodular masses of variable size, seldom ulcerated. Predilected areas: back, less freqently, neck and trunk. Seldom any other area of body.

Etiology. Unknown.

Pathology. In early stage superficial and deep perivascular distribution, then extension into subcutis. Sparing of Grenz zone and epidermis. Lymphoid follicles may be present, typical or reactive. Cytology: pleomorfic population, medium size to large cells with twisted or multilobulated nuclei and large pale eosinophilic cytoplasm. Other cells are small T-cells at the periphery and eosinophils and histocytes.

Diagnostic Procedures. *Biopsy.* Marker studies: in the majority of β-cell series markers CD20 and CD22, only a few staining for immunoglobulins.

Therapy. Radiotherapy; chemotherapy; cortisone.

Prognosis. Good. If recurrence still sensitive to radiotherapy and chemotherapy Only 2–5% spread beyond the skin. If spreading occurs prognosis of high-grade nodal lymphoma.

BIBLIOGRAPHY. Crosti A: Mycosis fongoide et rèticulo-histiocytome cutanè malin. Minerva Dermatol 26:3–11, 1951
Toonstra J, Van Der Putte SC, Kalsbeek GL: Multilobated cutaneous T cell lymphoma. Report of two cases resembling Crosti's reticulosis. Dermatologica 166(3):128–135, 1983
Isaacson PG, Norton AJ: Extranodal Lymphomas, pp 178–182. Edinburgh, Churchill Livingstone, 1994

CROUZON

Synonyms. Apert-Crouzon; Virchow oxycephaly; Vogt cephalosyndactyly; pseudo-Crouzon (Franceschetti); craniofacial dysostosis; oxycephaly—acrocephaly.

Symptoms. More frequent in males; present at birth. Headache, subnormal mental development; moderate hearing loss; progressive visual loss. In mild cases, vision may not be severely affected.

Signs. Exophthalmos (possible luxation of globe); bluish sclerae; widely separated eyes (hypertelorism); obliquity of palpebral fissure; outer canthus slanting downward; nystagmus; divergent strabismus; papilledema. Beak-shaped nose; hypoplastic maxilla; short upper lip, and protruding lower lip; head pointed in region of anterior fontanelle.

Etiology. Premature closure of cranial bones; transmitted as dominant trait.

Pathology. Premature closure of cranial bones with secondary brain damage owing to intracranial hypertension.

Diagnostic Procedures. *Spinal fluid.* Increased pressure. *X-ray.* Facial-cranial abnormalities.

Therapy. Open affected sutures widely and prevent closure by interposition of polyethylene; if marked exophthalmos, orbital decompression.

Prognosis. Good with surgery.

BIBLIOGRAPHY. Crouzon MO: Dysostose craniofaciale héréditaire. Presse Med 20:737–739, 1912
Vogt A: Dyskephalie (Dysostosis Craniofacialis, Maladie de Crouzon 1921) und neuartige Kombination dieser Krankheit mit Sybdaktylie der 4 Extremitaeten (Dyskephalodaktylie). Klin Monatsbl Augenheilkd 90:441–454, 1933
Rollnick BR: Germinal mosaicism in Crouzon syndrome. Clin Genet 33:145–150, 1988

CROW-FUKASE

Synonyms. Takatsuki, Shinpo; P.E.P., P.O.E.M.S.; polyneuropathy-organomegaly-endocrinopathy-monoclonal protein-skin lesions.

Symptoms and Signs. Usually younger than other patients with myeloma. Chronic progressive peripheral sensorimotor polyneuropathy. Weakness, loss of general reflexes and vibratory and position. Skin changes: diffuse hyperpigmentation, hypertrichosis, and hair thickening. Anasarca-pitting edema on the lower extremities. Ascites and pleural effusion. Gynecomastia and impotence in men and amenorrhea in women. Hepatosplenomegaly and generalized lymphadenopathy; papilledema; fever; hyperhidrosis; finger clubbing.

Etiology. Abnormal proliferation of plasma cells.

Pathology. *Nerve biopsy:* Axonal degeneration and segmental demyelination. *Lymph node biopsy:* Capillary proliferation and sheets of mature plasma cells in the interfollicular tissue. Bony lesions solitary in 50% of cases with strong sclerotic component.

Diagnostic Procedures. *Nerve conduction velocities (motor and sensory).* Slow. *Cerebrospinal fluid.* Elevated protein level. *Blood.* Hyperglobulinemia M-component typically inferior to 30 g/L. IgG (occasionally IgA) characterized by lambda chains; low testosterone level hypercalcemia; hyperprolactinemia. *X-rays.* Skeletal sclerotic and lytic lesions. *Bone marrow.* Plasma cells over 5%.

Therapy. Prednisone; cyclophosphamide; radiation therapy.

Prognosis. Transient improvement with therapy. Death in a few years.

BIBLIOGRAPHY. Crow RS: Periferal neuritis in myelomatosis. Br Med J 2:802–804, 1956
Shinpo S, Nishitani H, Tsunematsu T, et al: Solitary plasmacytoma with polyneuritis and endocrine disturbances (in Japanese). Nippon Rinsho 26:2444–2456, 1968
Takatsuki K, Ucchiyama T, Sagawa K, et al: Plasma cell dyscrasia with polyneuropathy and endocrine disorder: review of 32 patients. In Seno S, Takaku F, Irino S (eds): Topics in Hematology, pp 454–457. Amsterdam, Excerpta Medica, 1977
Takanishi T, Sobue I, Toyokura Y: The Crow-Fukase syndrome: A study of 102 cases in Japan. Neurology (Cleveland) 34:712–720, 1984
Toyokuni S, Ebina Y, Okada S, et al: Report of a patient with POEMS/Takatsuki/Crow-Fukase syndrome associated with focal spinal pachymeningeal amyloidosis. Cancer 70:882–886, 1992
Foerster J: Multiple Myeloma. In Lee GR, Bithel TC, Foerster J, et al (eds): Wintrobe's Clinical Hematology, 9th ed, pp 2223–2224. Philadelphia, Lea & Febiger, 1993

C.R.S.T. SYNDROME

Synonyms. Thibierge-Weissenbach; calcinosis–Raynaud phenomenon–sclerodactyly–telangiectasis; progessive systemic sclerosis; including C.R.E.S.T. (E for esophageal involvement). See Calcinosis universalis; Profichet.

Symptoms. Prevalent in females; condition at an average age of 45 years. Reported only in whites. No family history of telangiectasia. First symptoms referable to hands. Bleeding manifestations rare (epistaxis; melena; or from cutaneous telangiectasis). Raynaud's phenomenon; dysphagia.

Signs. Placques of calcinosis on different subcutaneous locations; hands usually involved. Sclerodactyly, telangiectasia on different cutaneous locations (face and hands involved). Mucosae occasionally involved.

Etiology. Unknown; belongs in the group of collagen disorders. Relation with scleroderma not clearly defined (different prognosis). Possible relation with Rendu-Osler-Weber syndrome; several criteria for differential diagnosis: lack of familial occurrence; prevalence in female.

Pathology. Dilated capillaries and venules; absence of muscular and elastic tissue, covered by thinned epithelium. Skin in sclerodermatoid lesion compatible with but not typical of scleroderma.

Diagnostic Procedures. *X-ray.* Subcutaneous calcinosis. *Esophageal studies.* Abnormal pattern compatible with scleroderma. *Blood.* Normal calcium, phosphorus, and alkaline phosphatases; total protein and electrophoresis. *L.E. test.* Negative. No anemia or white blood cell abnormalities. *Renal and liver tests.* Usually normal. *Urine.* Normal.

Therapy. Sympathectomy for Raynaud phenomenon. Corticosteroids, prostacyclin, dextran dipenicillamine, plasmapheresis, azathioprine.

Prognosis. Slow progressive evolution even in presence of systemic manifestations. Average followup of 15 years. (In scleroderma, 5 yr survival about 50%.)

BIBLIOGRAPHY. Thibierge G, Weissenbach RJ: Concrétions calcaires sous-cutanées at sclérodermie. Ann Dermatol Syph 2:129–155, 1911
Ouyang A, Cohen S: Motility disorders of the esophagus. In Haubrich WS, Schaffner F, Berk JE (eds): Bockus Gastroenterology, 5th ed, vol 2, pp 431–433. Philadelphia, WB Saunders, 1995

CRUVEILHIER-BAUMGARTEN

Synonym. Baumgarten portal hypertension variant.

Symptoms. Digestive troubles; hematemesis.

Signs. Abdominal distention; prominent periumbilical (caput medusae) and thoracoabdominal veins; continuous venus hum and thrill on the periumbilical region; small liver; splenomegaly.

Etiology. Failure of obliteration of umbilical vein; or noncirrhotic portal hypertension.

Pathology. Congestive splenomegaly; development of collateral circulation, including esophageal varices.

Diagnostic Procedures. *Liver function test.* Altered. *Blood.* Anemia; leukopenia; thrombocytopenia (in hypersplenism). *Abdominal phlebography.* Determination of portal hypertension.

Therapy. Portacaval shunt or splenectomy and splenorenal anastomosis.

BIBLIOGRAPHY. Cruveilhier J: Maladies des veines. In Anatomie Pathologique du Corps Humain, vol 1, p 16. Paris, Baillière, 1829–1835
Von Baumgarten P: Ueber vollstandiges Offenbleiben der Vena umbilicalis; zugleich ein Beitrag zur Frage des Morbus Banti, p 6; Baumgartens, Arbeiten, 1908, Arb Geb Path Anat Inst Tubing 6:93, 1907
Schwartz ME, Miller CM: Diseases of the hepatic blood vessels. In Haubrich WS, Schaffner F, Berk JE (eds): Bockus Gastroenterology, 5th ed, vol 2, p 2834. Philadelphia, WB Saunders, 1995

CRYPTORCHIDISM

Synonym. Testicular ectopia.

Symptoms and Signs. Disturbed testicular descent, so that testis remains in the inguinal canal or migrates in suprapubic, femoral, or perineal area. At birth, incidence of this abnormality is 2.7%, figure declining to 1% at age 3 months. Associated renal anomalies possible (in inherited cases).

Etiology. Unclear; anatomic factors (preventing migration) seem predominant, but concurrence of genetic factors seems possible. Autosomal recessive inheritance. Pituitary hypogonadism in mother seems a predisposing factor.

Pathology. Dislocation of testis (see Symptoms). Possible abnormality of germinal epithelium.

Diagnostic Procedures. *Endocrine and cytogenetic studies, testicular biopsy (at time or during surgery).* To rule out possibility of genetic disorders; in unilateral cryptorchidism controlateral scrotal testis in adulthood is normal only in 25% of cases. *Blood.* Testosterone level increase follows administration of human chorionic gonadotropins (hCG).

Therapy. *Medical.* Human chorionic gonadotropin 2000 IU three times a week for 6 weeks; if needed the cycle may be repeated once. *Surgical.* Positioning of testis into scrotum. In case of adult with inguinal retained testis in adulthood yearly evaluation; if adominal, better orchiectomy.

Prognosis. In majority of cases, spontaneous descent of testis in correct position. Increased frequency of development of testicular cancer (occurring beween 20 and 44 years of age, less common afterward); orchidoplexy does not reduce risk.

BIBLIOGRAPHY. Corbus BC, O'Connor VJ: The familial occurrence of undescended testis. Report in six brothers with testicular anomalies. Surg Gynecol Obstet 34:237–240, 1922
Winters SJ: Clinical disorders of the testis. In De Groot LJ (ed): Endocrinology, 3rd ed, pp 2389–2390. Philadelphia, WB Saunders, 1995

CRYPTOTHYROIDISM

Synonym. Lingual thyroid; suprahyoid-infrahyoid thyroid

Symptoms and Signs. From asymptomatic to dysphagia, dysphonia, dyspnea, or choking sensation and various signs of hypothyroidism. Discovery in infancy, childhood, or later of an accidental mass on the back of tongue or supra or infrahyoid zone, that may be mistaken for a thyroglossal duct cyst.

Etiology. Unknown. Could be a hereditary condition.

Diagnostic Procedures. *Radioisotope scanning.*

Therapy. Thyroid hormone to suppress and reduce size of ectopic thyroid. Autotransplantation can be tried. Remove if normal thyroid tissue is also present to prevent, even if rare, neoplastic evolution.

BIBLIOGRAPHY. McGirr EM, Hutchinson JH: Dysgenesis of the thyroid gland as a cause of cretinism and juvenile myxedema. J Clin Endocrinol Metab 15:668–679, 1955
Kaplan EL, Shukla M, Hara H, et al: Developmental abnormalities of the thyroid. In De Groot LJ (ed): Endocrinology, 3rd ed, pp 895–896. Philadelphia, WB Saunders, 1995

CUBITAL CANAL, ELBOW

Symptoms and Signs. Weakness of flexor carpi ulnaris, flexor digitorum profundus, of fourth and fifth fingers, and intrinsic muscles, sensory loss extending to the dorsum of the ulnar aspect of hand.

Etiology and Pathology. Synovitis of elbow extending extra articulary, or large olecranon bursa causing ulnar nerve pain at cubital canal.

Therapy. Anti-inflammatory agents or surgery.

BIBLIOGRAPHY. Nakano KK: The entrapment neuropathies of rheumatoid arthritis. Orthop Clin N Amer 6:873–860, 1975
Dawson DM, Hallett M, Millender LH: Entrapment Neuropathies, 2nd ed. Boston, Little, Brown, 1990

CURLING ULCER

Synonym. Gastrointestinal postburn ulcer. See von-Rokitanski-Cushing.

Symptoms and Signs. Clinical onset at various times after burns; serious bleeding begins usually between the fourth and tenth day. Repeated, severe rectal bleeding, occurring after severe burning. Gastrointestinal perforation with peritonitis may occur. The full-blown episode of severe gastrointestinal bleeding after burning is relatively rare (2–4%). Moderate gastrointestinal bleeding, however, seems to be much more frequent (58%). Hematemesis and melena occur with equal frequency.

Etiology. Unknown. Curling ulcer (active gastrointestinal hemorrhage) represents the end point of common, usually concealed, gastrointestinal ulceration with microscopic hemorrhages.

Pathology. Ulceration may be found in any part of the gastrointestinal tract from esophagus to terminal ileum (posterior duodenum more frequent location).

Diagnostic Procedures. *Stool.* Blood determination.

Therapy. Intense antacid program as soon as burned patient able to take fluid. Cimetidine (800 mg to 2g/day intravenously or orally) and pirenzepine bichloridrate (75–125 mg/day) have been suggested as prophylactic measures. Initial treatment: Gastric lavage with chilled solutions and systemic antibiotics (if sepsis). Infusion of vasopressin into left gastric artery through a placed catheter. Blood replacement. Surgery with same principles of therapy for treatment of gastrointestinal hemorrhages.

Prognosis. Very severe if massive bleeding unless rapid treatment is instituted.

BIBLIOGRAPHY. Curling TB: On acute ulceration of the duodenum in cases of burn. Medico-Chir Trans (London) 25:260–281, 1942
Ivarsson L, Sjodahl R, Haglund U (eds): Proceeding from a symposium: Acute mucosal damage to the stomach. Scand J Gastroenterol (Suppl 105):5 (all issue), 1984
Haubrich WS, Schaffner F, Berk JE (eds): Bockus Gastroenterology, 5th ed, p 754. Philadelphia, WB Saunders, 1995

CURRARINO

Synonyms. Kennedy (RLJ); A.S.P. association; anorectal-sacral-presacral anomalies; anus imperforate complex; imperforate anus complex.

Symptoms. From birth, both sexes. Greater incidence in females. Recurrent meningitis; various grade of intestinal constipation or obstruction. Progressive neurologic manifestations.

Signs. Anorectal anomalies (stenosis, atresia, ectopia, altered function); sacral bone defects; presacral defect (meningocele, lipomas, hamartoma, teratoma, cysts) involving rectum and neurocanal.

Etiology. Autosomal dominant inheritance (50%).

Diagnostic Procedures. *X-rays. CT scan. MRI. Ultrasonography.* See Pathology. Occasionally, lipomeningocele, low conus, dural ectasia, dysplastic conus.

Therapy. Neurosurgery.

Prognosis. Variable. First considered as a stable condition, today considered as progressive but amenable to improvement (spontaneous or therapeutic).

BIBLIOGRAPHY. Kennedy RLJ: An unusual rectal polyp: anterior sacral meningocele. Surg Gynecol Obs 43:803–804, 1926
Currarino G, Coln D, Votteler T: Triad of anorectal, sacral and presacral anomalies. Am J Roentgenol Obs 137:395–398, 1981
Tunell WP, Austin JC, Barnes PD, et al: Neuroradiologic evaluation of sacral abnormalities on imperforate anus complex. J Ped Surg 22:58–61, 1987
Janneck C, Holthusen W: Die Curarino-Trias-Brobachtung von 4 aellen Z. Kindechir 43:112–116, 1988

CURRARINO-SILVERMAN

Synonyms. Silverman II; pigeon breast; pectus carinatum.

Symptoms. Both sexes affected; onset from infancy. Asymptomatic; occasionally, dyspnea.

Signs. Projection of sternum outward. Thoracic anteroposterior diameter increased and lateral decreased.

Etiology. Variable. (1) Hereditary form; autosomal dominant; (2) rickets; (3) secondary; other conditions (see Marfan).

Pathology. Accelerated obliteration of sutures, which causes the pectus carinatum; secondary excessive growth of ribs. Hypertrophy of posterolateral section of diaphragm; hypotrophy of ventral part.

Therapy. Surgery.

Prognosis. Stable condition. Good esthetic and functional results with surgical correction.

BIBLIOGRAPHY. Currarino G, Silverman FN: Premature obliteration of the sternal sutures and pigeon breast deformity. Radiology 70:532–540, 1958
Pickard LR, Tepas JJ, Shermeta DW, et al: Pectus carinatum. Results of surgical therapy. J Pediatr Surg 14:228–230, 1979
Shneerson JM: Disorders of the thoracic cage and diaphragm. In Oxford Textbook of Medicine, 3rd ed, p 2875. Oxford, Oxford Med Pub, 1996

CURTIUS I

Obsolete.

Synonyms. Friedreich; Steiner; ectodermal dysplasia–ocular malformation; hemifacial microsomic–radial defects. See also Hemihypertrophy, Bremer; First arch; Goldenhar.

Symptoms. Males more frequently affected; onset from birth, but may become accentuated at puberty. Asymptomatic or variable according to signs. Frequently, amblyopia, reduced capacity to thermal regulation, mental retardation (15–20%).

Signs. Abnormalities may be segmented, unilateral, or crossed. Frequently, ichthyosis vulgaris (see). Hypertelorism; telangiectasia; absent or sparse eyebrows and eyelashes; decreased tear secretion; congenital cataract; coloboma, hypodontia, and unilateral tooth enlargment; occasionally: dyscephaly; tongue enlarged and thicker on involved side. Associated defects of limbs (unilateral macrodactyly; polydactyly; syndactyly; clubfoot; and long bone enlargement) may be present.

Etiology. Autosomal dominant inheritance, occasionally recessive. Suggested to be a form of Goldenhar (see) and overlaps with Bremer (see).

Pathology. Only a limited number of autopsies. Nonspecific pathologic changes. Frequent enlargement of kidney and adrenal gland.

Diagnostic Procedures. *Dental X-ray.* Abnormalities; greater diameter of canine early diagnostic sign.

Therapy. Symptomatic; plastic reconstruction of structures involved after completion of maturation.

Prognosis. Variable according to degree of involvement of neurologic structures.

BIBLIOGRAPHY. Barwell R: Case of unilateral hypertrophy of the head and face involving bones and soft parts. Trans Pathol Soc Lond 32:282–284, 1881
Meckel JF: Ueber die seitliche Asymmetrie im teirischen Korper, anatomische physiologisches Beobachtungen und Untersuchungen, p 147. Halle, Renger, 1822

Curtius F: Kongenitaler partieller Piesenwuchs mit endocrien Stoerungen. Dtsch Arch Klin Med 147:310–319, 1925

Jongbloet PH: Goldenhar syndrome and overlapping dysplasias. J Med Genet 24:616–620, 1987

CUSHING I

Synonyms. Acoustic neuroma; angle tumor; cerebellopontine angle; pontocerebellar angle tumor.

Symptoms and Signs. Prevalent in females (3:1); onset of acoustic neuroma in majority of cases between third and sixth decades; onset of glioma before age 20. Chronology of onset of symptoms is of utmost importance for differential diagnosis. Headache; vomiting; vertigo; tinnitus; dimness of vision. Cranial nerve involvement, particularly trigeminal (V), abducens (VI), facial (VII), and acoustic (VIII) (more frequent in extracerebral lesions), with relative symptomatology. Cerebellar symptoms include ataxia of extremities; lower extremities more affected than upper ones; adiadochokinesia; spontaneous nystagmus; pyramidal tract signs may be present. Later, with increasing intracranial pressure, other symptoms, such as olfactory loss, may also occur. Bilateral forms also described.

Etiology. Neoplastic or vascular (less frequently) pontine angle lesion. Brain stem may be primary or secondary site of involvement. Extracerebral lesions may also induce the syndrome. Bilateral forms are hereditary with autosomal dominant transmission.

Pathology. Acoustic neuroma originates in peripheral part of vestibular division of acoustic (VIII) nerve. Oval and well circumscribed; adapt to the wall of posterior fossa and stretches and compresses adjacent nerves and brain stem.

Diagnostic Procedures. *Arteriography. CT brain scan. MRI. Spinal tap.*

Therapy. Surgery if feasible.

Prognosis. Poor; average life expectancy of untreated patients is 3.5–5 years after diagnosis. Good results with surgery.

BIBLIOGRAPHY. Wishart JH: Case of tumours in skull dura mater and brain. Edinburgh Med Surg J 18:393, 1822

Cushing HW: Tumors of the nervus acusticus and the Syndrome of the Cerebello Pontine Angle. Philadelphia, WB Saunders, 1917

Keschner M, Grossman M: Cerebellar symptomatology evaluation on the basis of intracerebral and extracerebral lesions. Arch Neurol Psychiatr 19:78–94, 1928

Eldridge R: Central neurofibromatosis with bilateral acoustic neuroma. Adv Neurol 29:57–65, 1981

Weatherall DJ, Ledingham JGG, Warrell DA (eds): Oxford Textbook of Medicine, 3rd ed, pp 3874–3875. Oxford, Oxford Med Pub, 1996

CUSHING II

Synonyms. Chiasmal; suprasellar meningioma; optic tract; upper omonymous quadrantanopia.

Symptoms. Usually occurs in adults. Characterized by three elements. Initial decrease of lateral or central vision: (1) bitemporal field defects, usually progressive; (2) primary optic atrophy, total blindness may result; (3) essentially normal sella turcica (see Diagnostic Procedures).

Etiology. Usually a suprasellar meningioma (Cushing original description), other space-occupying lesions in the region of optic chiasm, such as craniopharyngiomas, pituitary adenoma, giant aneurysm, chiasmal glioma, nasopharyngeal carcinoma, colloid cyst of third ventricle, or remote lesions that produce dilatation of third ventricle and secondary chiasm compression.

Diagnostic Procedures. *X-ray of skull.* Essentially normal sella turcica. With modern techniques it is possible, however, to detect bone reaction in the area of tuberculum sellae. Occasionally, calcification may be present in suprasellar meningioma. *MRI. CT brain scan. Angiography.*

Therapy. Surgery.

Prognosis. Depends on etiology and extent of lesions.

BIBLIOGRAPHY. Cushing H: Chiasmal syndrome of primary optic atrophy and bitemporal field defects in adults with normal sella turcica. Arch Ophthalmol 3:505–551, 1930

Bebin J, Knighton RS: Chiasmatic syndrome. Henry Ford Hosp Med J 16:223–233, 1968

Weatherall DJ, Ledingham JGG, Warrell DA (eds): Oxford Textbook of Medicine, 3rd ed, pp 3867–3869. Oxford, Oxford Med Pub, 1996

CUSHING III

Synonyms. Adrenal cortex adenoma; adrenal cortex carcinoma; pituitary basophilism.

Different clinical forms may be recognized: (1) adrenal neoplasm; (2) Cushing disease; (3) ectopic ACTH syndrome (see).

CUSHING DISEASE

Symptoms and Signs. See Cushing syndrome owing to benign or malignant neoplasm of the adrenal.

Etiology. Inappropriate levels of ACTH produced by pituitary, resulting in adrenal hyperplasia.

Pathology. Pituitary adenoma or hyperfunction; bilateral adrenal hyperplasia; other organs and tissue involved (see Pathology of Cushing syndrome).

Diagnostic Procedures. *Blood.* Increase of plasma ACTH or prolonged secretion during the day. Increased 17–hydroxycorticoids. Hematologic and biochemical changes (see Diagnostic Procedures of Cushing syndrome). *Urine.* Some changes as in Cushing syndrome. ACTH stimulation. Threefold to fivefold increase of urinary 17-hydroxycorticoids. Metyrapone responsiveness. Qualitatively normal. Dexamethasone suppression. Response only to high doses.

Therapy. If pituitary tumor with sellar enlargement, ablation of pituitary; if no enlargement, choice of adrenal ablation or pituitary ablation. Radiation of pituitary gland when partially removed or not neurologically aggressive. Implantation of 90-yttrium rods in the pituitary gland. If adrenal ablation (fastest method to control severe hypercortisonism), substitutive therapy has to be instituted and followed for life. Good results also with pharmacologic treatment: cyproheptadine; bromocriptine; aminoglutethimide or o,p8DDD.

Prognosis. Good result with adequate treatment. If patient is not treated, death in 5 years.

ECTOPIC ACTH SYNDROME

Listed separately under Ectopic ACTH.

CYCLICAL CUSHING

Synonyms. Periodic Cushing; transient Cushing.

Symptoms and Signs. Intermittent, cyclic or intermittent mild symptoms and reduced signs of Cushing syndrome (see).

Etiology. Cushing disease, ectopic ACTH secretion, and primary adrenal derangements most frequent causes. Thymus, lung, stomach, kidney tumors as causes of ectopic ACTH secretion.

Diagnostic Procedures. See preceding with the possible variants. Response to hydrocortisone or hydrocortisone is variable (conflicting patterns of response) during active phase and in quiescent periods. Discrepant urine tests also reported with elevated 17-hydroxysteroids and normal urine free cortisol excretion. Dynamic tests must be carried out for prolonged periods to evidentiate failure to suppress serum cortisol with 1 mg dexametazone, with elevated urine cortisol excretion.

Therapy. Diet; diuretics.

Prognosis. Guarded.

BIBLIOGRAPHY. Cushing H: The basophil adenomas of the pituitary body and their clinical manifestations (pituitary basophilism). Bull Johns Hopkins Hosp 50:137–195, 1932

Zondek H: Die Krankeiten der endokrinen Drusen, p 371. Berlin, Springer, 1923

Zondek H, Leszynsky HE: Transient Cushing syndrome with report of a case. Br Med J 1:197–200, 1956

Wolff SM, Adler RC, Buskirk ER, et al: A syndrome of periodic hypothalamic discharge. Am J Med 36:956–967, 1964

Nieman L, Cutler GB: Cushing's syndrome. In De Groot LJ (ED): Endocrinology, 3rd ed, pp 1741–1769. Philadelphia, WB Saunders, 1995

CUSHING SYNDROME CAUSED BY BENIGN OR MALIGNANT NEOPLASM OF THE ADRENALS

Symptoms. Weakness; fatigability; oligomenorrhea; backache; loss of libido; loss of potency in man; mental aberrations from simple irritability to schizophrenia.

Signs. Obesity of face, neck, trunk, or generalized plethoric face; purple striae of abdomen and legs; ecchymosis; peripheral edema; hirsutism; hypertension; enlarged heart.

Etiology. Neoplasm of adrenal that secretes cortisol autonomously, not dependent on adrenocorticotropic hormone (ACTH) stimulation, with suppression of ACTH production and atrophy of normal adrenal tissue.

Pathology. Carcinoma or benign adenoma of adrenals; atrophy of normal adrenal tissue. Heart enlarged; obesity generalized or with typical distribution; osteoporosis; atrophy of muscles; nephrosclerosis and nephrocalcinosis; hyperplasia of islet of pancreas; atrophy of pituitary.

Diagnostic Procedures. *Urine.* Increased urinary 17–ketosteroids; 17–hydroxy-corticoids; glycosuria. *Blood.* Decreased plasma ACTH level; increased plasma 17–hydroxycorticoid; decreased lymphocytes and eosinophils; increased neutrophils and red cells; increased sugar and cholesterol. ACTH stimulation. Lack of response with malignant tumor; normal response in benign adenoma. Metyrapone responsiveness. Failure to respond; response in benign adenoma. Dexamethasone suppression. Lack of response; response in benign adenoma. *X-ray.* Osteoporosis; pyelogram possibly showing adrenal tumor; nephrocalcinosis. *CT scan. MRI.*

Therapy. Surgical removal of tumor; adequate coverage with cortisol for acute adrenal insufficiency. After surgery, administration of cortisol for 1 year or longer, plus ACTH to stimulate atrophic tissue. If tumor cannot be removed, administration of 2, 28–bis-(2–chlorophenyl, 4–chlorophenyl)-1, 1–dichloroethane (o, p8 DDD) or Metyrapone.

Prognosis. Good in benign adenoma; good if malignant tumor removed in time and no metastasis has occurred.

BIBLIOGRAPHY. See Cushing disease.

CUTIS LAXA SYNDROMES

Synonyms. Chalasodermia; dermatochalasia; dermatolysis; dermatomegaly; cutis pendula; elastosis systemica (with internal manifestation). See De Barsy syndrome.

CONGENITAL

Symptoms and Signs. Present at birth or noticed within first months

of life, frequently after episodes of edema. Loss of elasticity of skin; formation of skin folds, particularly noticeable on face and trunk, progressing during infancy and becoming less evident after puberty. Many infants have a hoarse cry, probably because of laxity of the vocal cords. Adult males exhibit infantile genitalia and impotence. General development is normal. Frequently respiratory insufficiency because of emphysema and resulting in cor pulmonale. Occasionally, symptoms and signs related to presence of esophagus, duodenum, ileum, and bladder diverticula.

Etiology. Autosomal dominant and X-linked inheritance described. Deficiency of lysyloxidase activity, low levels of copper (disorder of copper metabolism?). X-linked inheritance described (see Occipital horn).

Pathology. Skin thickness normal. Elastic fibers reduced, shortened, and degenerated. Increase of mucopolysaccharides. Other tissues may show similar changes. Tortuous artery; pulmonary stenosis; aortic dilatation.

Diagnostic Procedures. *Biopsy of skin.* See Pathology. *Blood and other fluids.* Normal if not affected by respiratory or gastrointestinal complications. *Pulmonary function tests. X-ray of chest and gastrointestinal tract.* Differential diagnosis with Ehlers-Danlos, Grönblad-Stranberg-Touraine; von Recklinghausen II; Donahue, Debré-Fittke.

Therapy. Plastic surgery sometimes useful. Pulmonary treatment when needed.

Prognosis. Patients with forms without emphysema have normal life expectancy; otherwise early death. Recessive inheritance more severe (lethal). Dominant inheritance milder course; frequently only cosmetic problem.

ACQUIRED

Symptoms and Signs. Appears at puberty or later, preceded by episodes of angioedema or inflammatory process. Slow development of skin changes represented by folding, generalized or limited to face, body, or neck. Vascular fragility and purpura. Occasionally respiratory insufficiency owing to emphysema or gastroenteric manifestation.

Etiology. Unknown.

Pathology. See Congenital form.

Therapy. See Congenital form.

Prognosis. Determined by intensity, progression, and pulmonary complications.

BIBLIOGRAPHY. Alibert JL: Histoire d'un berger des environs de Gisores (dermatose Hypermorphe). Monog Dermatol 2:719, 1883

Variot G, Cailliau F: Peau ridée sénile chez un enfant de deaux ans. Agénesie de réseux élastique du derme. Bull Soc Méd Hôp (Paris) 43:989–994, 1919

Vaglio R: Un caso di cutis laxa. Pediatria (Napoli) 31:321–323, 1923

Weber FP: Chalasodermia or "loose skin" and its relationship to subcutaneous fibroids or calcareous nodules, etc. Urol Cutan Rev 27:407–409, 1923

van Maldergem L, Ogur G, Yuksel M: Facial anomalies in congenital cutis laxa with retarded growth and skeletal dysplasia. Am J Med Genet 32:265, 1989

Burton JL: Disorders of connective tissue. In Champion RH, Burton JL, Ebling FJG (eds): Rook/Wilkinson/Ebling Textbook of Dermatology, 5th ed, pp 1770–1772. Oxford, Blackwell Scientific, 1992

CUTIS MARMORATA

Synonyms. Marble skin. See also Livedo reticularis and Van Lohuizen; telangioectasia congenita. CMTC, included cutis marmorata.

Symptoms. None.

Signs. Manifested especially in children (50% of cases); less frequently in adults and young women. With cold exposure bluish red mottling of skin, which subsides in warm environment. Areas more affected are extremities and pectoral region. Frequently associated with Cassirer (see), Pernio (see), and erythrocyanosis. In some cases association with telangiactasis and superficial erosions.

Etiology. Unknown. Considered a physiologic reflex. Could be a mild form of Livedo reticularis (see).

Pathology. Spasmodic narrowing of arterioles with dilatation of capillaries and venules.

Diagnostic Procedures. For severe form see Livedo reticularis.

Therapy. Symptomatic.

Prognosis. Benign (physiologic condition); in majority of cases it may evolve into Livedo reticularis.

BIBLIOGRAPHY. Van Lohuizen CHJ: Uber eine seltene angeborene Hautanomalie. (Cutis marmorata telangectatica congenita). Acta Dermatol Venerol 3:202–211, 1922

Champion RH: Livedo reticularis; A review. Br J Dermatol 77:167–179, 1965

Champion RH: Reactions to Cold. In Champion RH, Burton JL, Ebling FJG (eds): Rook/Wilkinson/Ebling Textbook of Dermatology, 5th ed, pp 838–839. Oxford, Blackwell Scientific, 1992

CUTIS VERTICIS GYRATA

Synonyms. Unna II; Perin-Audry; bulldog scalp; gyrate scalp; washboard scalp; see Rosental-Kloepfer.

Symptoms and Signs. Both sexes affected, onset at all ages. Presence of folds and furrows of scalp and face, imparting to scalp a corrugated or gyrate appearance. Isolated sign or component of other syndromes: (1) Touraine-Salente-Golé; (2) Marie; (3) microcephalic idiocy; (4) myxedema; (5) local inflammatory or traumatic causes; (6) melanocytic nevi. Frequently associated with mental deficiencies; in one family thyroid aplasia reported.

Etiology. Autosomal inheritance.

Pathology. Hypertrophy of cutis; according to etiology.

Therapy. None. In nevoid form, plastic surgery.

BIBLIOGRAPHY. Robert A: Journal de Chirurgie par Malgaigne Paris 1:125–126, 1843

McDowall TW: Case of abnormal development of the scalp. J Ment Sci 39:62–64, 1893

Jadassohn J: Eine eigentuemliche Furchung, Erweiterung und Verdickung der Haut am Hinterkopf. Verh Dtsch Dermatol Ges, IX Kongress, S 451, 1906

Unna PG: Cutis verticis gyrata. Monatsschr Prakt Dermatol 45:227, 1907

Akesson HO: Cutis verticis gyrata and mental deficiencies in Sweden I. Epidemiological and clinical aspects. Acta Med Scand 175:115–127, 1964

Dawber RPR, Ebling FJG, Wojnarowska FT: Disorders of Hair. In Champion RH, Burton JL, Ebling FJG (eds): Rook/Wilkinson/Ebling Textbook of Dermatology, 5th ed, p 2637. Oxford, Blackwell Scientific, 1992

CYCLICAL EDEMA

Synonyms. Edema, cyclic, idiopathic. See also Clarkson; Angioneurotic edema, hereditary, periodic edema, and Leg stasis.

Symptoms. In women edema begins to collect mostly in legs when they assume the standing position. In many cases edema disappears when patient is lying down; in some cases recumbency does not help, and the edema becomes generalized. In the premenstrual period symp-

tom may be aggravated. Many patients appear emotionally disturbed, hysterical, or psychotic.

Signs. Edema that recedes with bed rest.

Etiology. Unknown; possibly aldosterone hypersecretion or increased permeability of capillaries of legs.

Diagnostic Procedures. Useful to exclude other causes of edema; diseases of heart, liver, kidneys, veins, thyroid; and simple water and sodium retention.

Therapy. Bed rest; elastic stockings. Diuretic; low-salt diet; aldosterone antagonists, vasopressor agents. In some cases refractory to above treatment, exploration and excision of adenomas or hyperplastic adrenal tissue if found.

BIBLIOGRAPHY. Mach RS, Fabre J, Muller, AF et al: Idiopathique edeme par retention sodique avec hyperaldosteronurie. Bull Mem Soc Med Hop (Paris) 71:726–732, 1955

Leutscher JA, Dowdy, AJ, Arustein AR, et al: Idiopathic oedema and increased aldosterone excretion. In Balien E (ed): C.I.O.M.S. Symposium on Aldosterone. Oxford, Blackwell, 1964

Luetscher JA: Disorders associated with altered secretion of aldosterone. In Eisenstein AB (ed): The Adrenal Cortex. Boston, Little, Brown, 1967

Champion RH: Urticaria. In Champion RH, Burton JL, Ebling FJG (eds): Rook/Wilkinson/Ebling Textbook of Dermatology, 5th ed, p 1878. Oxford, Blackwell Scientific, 1992

CYCLIC NEUTROPENIA

Synonyms. Cyclic agranulocytosis; myelocytic periodic; cyclic leukopenia; periodic neutropenia; periodemitis mucosa necrotica, recurrent I. neutropenia, cyclic hematopoiesis.

Symptoms. Most cases from infancy present cyclic (21 day) recurrence of fever, malaise, and ulcer in the oral mucous membranes associated with recurrent neutropenia. Occasionally associated are arthralgia, abdominal pain, conjunctivitis, sore throat, headache, lymphadenitis, skin ulcers, ischiorectal and vaginal infections, and mental depression. In few cases onset in the sixth–seventh decades of life.

Signs. Splenomegaly and the recurrent lesions mentioned earlier.

Etiology. Recurrent deficit of myelopoiesis at primitive cell level; autosomal dominant inheritance in some cases, sporadic in the others.

Pathology. Spleen shows different degree of vascular and perivascular hyalinization.

Diagnostic Procedures. *Blood.* During attacks leukopenia; recurrent depression of neutrophils. Occasionally also thrombocytopenia. Return to normal values in intervals. *Bone marrow.* Maturation arrest of myeloid series during cycle.

Therapy. Splenectomy. Has some effect on number of neutrophils; recurrent symptoms persist. Corticosteroid. Have some symptomatic effect on lesions and fever while administered. Bone marrow transplantation tried with some success. Daily injection of rhG-CSF reduces severity and numers of clinical manifestations with minimal side effects.

Prognosis. Persistence of recurrent manifestation despite any known treatment.

BIBLIOGRAPHY. Leale M: Recurrent furunculosis in an infant showing an unusual blood picture. JAMA 54:1854, 1910

Rutledge BH, Hansen-Prüss OC, Thayer WS: Recurrent agranulocytosis. Bull Johns Hopkins Hosp 46:369–389, 1930

Wright DG, Dale DC, Fauci AS, et al: Human cyclic neutropenia: Clinical review and long-term follow-up of patients. Medicine 60:1–13, 1981

Athens JW, Neutropenia. In Lee GR, Bithel TC, Foerster J, et al (eds):

Wintrobe's Clinical Hematology, 9th ed, pp 1603–1605. Philadelphia, Lea & Febiger, 1993

CYCLIC STRABISMUS

Synonyms. Periodic esotrophia, alternate-day squint.

Symptoms and Signs. Both sexes from infancy. Cycles of 24 hours with eyes alternatively straight and crossed. Frequent strabismus in the other members of the family.

Etiology. Unknown. Autosomal dominant trait.

BIBLIOGRAPHY. Richter CP: Clock-mechanism esotrophia in children (alternate-day squint). Johns Hopkins Med J 122:218–223, 1968
Friendly DS, Manson RA, Albert DG: Cyclic strabismus. A case study. Doc Ophthalmol 34:189–202, 1973

CYCLIC THROMBOCYTOPENIA

Synonyms. Thrombocytopenia cyclic; including Garcia. See also Tidal platelet dysgenesis.

Symptoms and Signs. Most common in women. Trombocytopenia during menstrual periods. Increased bleeding tendency of not significant extent. In the inter periods thrombocytosis.

Etiology. Unknown. No correlation with endocrine factors. In some cases reported autosomal dominant inheritance (Garcia).

Diagnostic Procedures. *Blood.* Intermittent periods of thrombocytosis and thrombocytopenia. *Bone marrow.* Contemporaneous change of megakariocytes from hyperplasia to hypoplasia.

Therapy. None.

Prognosis. Benign condition.

BIBLIOGRAPHY. Skoog WA, Lawrence JS, Adams WS: A metabolic study of a patient with idiopathic cyclical thrombocytopenia purpura. Blood 12:844–850, 1957
Lewis ML: Cyclic thrombocytopenia: a thrombopoietin deficiency? J Clin Pathol 27:242–246, 1974
Aranda E, Dorantes S: Garcia's disease: Cyclic thrombocytopenic purpura in a child and abnormal platelet count in his family. Scand J Haematol 18:39–46, 1977
Bithell TC: Miscellaneous forms of thrombocytopenia. In Lee GR, Bithell TC, Foerster J, et al: Wintrobe's Clinical Hematology, p 1366. Philadelphia, Lea & Febiger, 1993

CYCLIC VOMITING, IDIOPATHIC

Symptoms and Signs. In children before the age of six. Repeated cyclic episodes of vomiting.

Pathology. Unknown. Psychosomatic versus neurologic causes discussed.

Diagnostic Procedures. *EEG.* To rule out migraine. *X-ray. Echography.* To rule out anatomic obstructions.

Therapy. Antiemetics (with little effect).

Prognosis. Disappears spontaneously before adolescence.

BIBLIOGRAPHY. Hoyt CS, Strickler GB: A study of 44 children with the syndrome of recurrent (cyclic) vomiting. Pediatrics 25:775–780, 1960
Achord JL: Nausea and vomiting. In Haubrich WS, Schaffner F, Berk JE (eds): Bockus Gastroenterology, 5th ed, vol 2, p 46. Philadelphia, WB Saunders, 1995

CYCLIST PALSY

Synonyms. Ulnar nerve compression; handlebar palsy.

Symptoms and Signs. In bicycle riders. Neuropathy usually involving both motor and sensory components of ulnar nerve. Commonly affects dominant hand.

Etiology. Repeated compressures on the hand and extended position of the wrist that stretch and compress the ulnar nerve.

Pathology. Neuritis of ulnar nerve.

Diagnostic Procedures. *Distal sensory latencies of ulnar nerve.*

Therapy. Proper position of the rider on bicycle, frequent position changes, padded gloves and handlebars, and when needed interruption of difficult ride with short periods of rest.

Prognosis. Spontaneous resolution with reduction or temporary cessation of riding.

BIBLIOGRAPHY. Eckman PB, Perlstein G, Altrocchi PH: Ulnar neuropathy in bicycle riders. Arch Neurol 32:130–131, 1975
Zemel N: Neurovascular disorders. In Jobe FW: Operative Techniques in Upper Extremity Sport Injuries. St Louis, CV Mosby, 1996

CYCLOPIA

Synonyms. Oddi; Fraser; synopsy.

Symptoms and Signs. The most extreme form of holoprosencephaly. Single eye globe with varying degrees of doubling of intrinsic ocular structures, arhinia and a blind-ending proboscis located under the median eye.

Etiology. Inherited condition caused by deletion of a small chromosomal segment.

Diagnostic Procedures. *Karyogram.* Reveals presence of a missing third chromosome and a supplementary chromosome in C group. Same karyogram noted in healthy relatives.

BIBLIOGRAPHY. Ellis R: On a rare form of twin monstrosity. Trans Obstet Soc 7:160–164, 1865
Pfitzer P, Muntefering H: Cyclopism as an hereditary malformation. Nature 217:1071–1072, 1968
Gorlin RJ, Cohen MM Jr, Levin LS: Syndromes of Head and Neck, p 573. New York, Oxford 1990

CYLINDRIC SPIRALS MYOPATHY

Synonyms. Myopathy cylindric spirals; inclusion body myopathy.

Symptoms and Signs. From birth. Cramps, muscle stiffness, post-effort muscle tightness, percussion myotonia.

Etiology. Autosomal dominant inheritance.

Pathology. Muscle inclusion bodies represented by cylindrical spirals in subsarcolemmal region.

Diagnostic Procedures. *EMG. Muscle biopsy.*

Therapy. Symptomatic.

Prognosis. Lifelong condition.

BIBLIOGRAPHY. Bove KE, Iannaccone ST, Hilton PK, et al: Cylindrical spirals in a familial neuromuscolar disorder. Ann Neurol 7:550–556, 1980
Goebel HH, Lenard HG: Congenital myopathies. In Handbook of Clinical Neurology, 18 (62): Rowland LP, Di Mauro S (eds): The Myopathies, p 331. Amsterdam, Elsevier, 1992

CYRIAX

Synonyms. Davies-Colley; slipping rib. See Anterior chest wall.

Symptoms. Pain in the chest, which may be dull and recurrent or very sharp and associated with symptoms of shock. It may be elicited by sneezing, deep inspiration, movement of arm. Occasionally, patient feels a snapping, "slipping of something" just before the onset of pain.

Signs. Compression of cartilage of rib involved always reproduces symptomatology.

Etiology and Pathology. Injury of the interchondral synovial membrane of the first three false ribs (8th, ninth, and tenth) that allows the anterior end of the rib to curl under the cartilage and compress the intercostal nerve and sympathetic fibers. Trauma direct or indirect (false movements) or idiopathic.

Therapy. Surgical or conservative. The three principal methods of treatment are reassurance, injection of the affected area with local anesthetic, and surgical excision of the affected cartilage (in few cases, two or more cartilages).

Prognosis. Complete recovery. Diagnosis of this condition may prevent useless abdominal surgery or wrong treatment for nonexistent heart conditions.

BIBLIOGRAPHY. Cyriax EJ: On various conditions that may simulate referred pain of visceral disease. Practitioner 102:314–322, 1919
Telford KM: The slipping rib syndrome. Can Med Assoc J 62:463–465, 1950
Porter GE: Slipping rib syndrome: An infrequently recognized entity in children: A report of three cases and review of the literature. Pediatrics 76:810–813, 1985
Weatherall DJ, Ledingham JGG, Warrell DA (eds): Oxford Textbook of Medicine, 3rd ed, p 3890. Oxford, Oxford Med Pub, 1996

CYSTATHIONINURIA

Synonyms. Cystathionase deficiency; CTH deficiency.

Symptoms and Signs. Rare condition. No clinical abnormalities are characteristically associated with this enzyme deficiency, but the following have been encountered: congenital defects (e.g., club foot, small ears); acromegaly; motor and mental retardation; cataract; diabetes mellitus and insipidus.

Etiology. Gamma cystathionase deficiency: genetic heterogeneity; autosomal inheritance. Relatives of those patients also had increased cystathionine level; however, they were asymptomatic. The relationship between metabolic defect and malformations may be coincidental.

Pathology. *Brain.* Diffuse atrophy. *Liver.* Smaller than normal; pale; fibrotic. *Heart.* Fatty degeneration (data based only on one autopsy).

Diagnostic Procedures. *Plasma, cerebrospinal fluid, and urine.* Marked increases of cystathionine. Head: *CT scan. MRI.*

Therapy. Pyridoxine reduces concentration of cystathionine. Only in some patients (expression of genetic heterogeneity). Low methionine diet.

Prognosis. Relatives of patients with the metabolic defect remained completely asymptomatic. Both patients reached advanced age despite mental and physical defects.

BIBLIOGRAPHY. Harris H, Penrose LS, Thomas DHH: Cystathioninuria. Ann Hum Genet 23:442, 1959
Scriver CR, Beaudet AL, Sly WS, et al: The Metabolic and Molecular Bases of Inherited Disease, 7th ed, pp 199, 1287, 1310, 1313, 1441. New York, McGraw-Hill, 1995

CYSTIC DUCT

Synonyms. Infundibulocystic; organic gallbladder syphopathy; gallbladder stasis; precholecystectomy.

Symptoms. Prevalent in women with numerous pregnancies. Sharp pain in the area of gallbladder, sometimes radiating to the back following fatty food ingestion.

Signs. Tenderness over gallbladder region; gallbladder may be palpated. Minimal jaundice.

Etiology. Mechanical, noncalculous, partial obstruction of the cystic duct. Forceful contraction of gallbladder to overcome resistance to bile flow.

Pathology. Constrictive bands, adhesions, kinking of cystic duct; adherence of gallbladder with resulting angulation of infundibulocystic junction. Congenital or acquired cystic stenosis. All are possible findings. Gallbladder normal or slightly inflamed.

Diagnostic Procedures. *Cholecystography.* Determination of biliary drainage by serial cholecystography or cholecystokinin cholecystography.

Therapy. Surgical.

Prognosis. Following surgery, complete and lasting recovery.

BIBLIOGRAPHY. Schieden V: Uber die "Stauungsgallenblase." Zentralbl Chir 41:1257, 1920
Camishion RC, Goldstein F: Partial noncalculous cystic duct obstruction (cystic duct syndrome). Surg Clin North Am 47:1107–1114, 1967
Corazziari E, Torsoli A: Dysfunction of the sphincter of Oddi. In Haubrich WS, Schaffner F, Berk JE (eds): Bockus Gastroenterology, 5th ed, vol 2, pp 2802–2811. Philadelphia, WB Saunders, 1995

CYSTIC DUCT STUMP

Synonyms. Oddi; deformed gallbladder; cystic duct remnant.

Symptoms. Appears a few months or years after cholecystectomy. Pain in right epichondrium; radiation to right shoulder. Nausea; vomiting; chills and fever (rare).

Signs. Jaundice in high percentage of cases. Pain on Murphy maneuver.

Etiology. Formation of a pouch or sac on stump of gall bladder or behind the common duct below the junction of left and right hepatic ducts.

Pathology. Cystic formation containing concentrated bile and occasionally calculi; choledochitis.

Diagnostic Procedures. *Intravenous cholangiography.* CPRE.

Therapy. Surgery.

Prognosis. Good.

BIBLIOGRAPHY. Oddi R: Effetti dell' estirpazione della cistifellea. Bull Sci Med di Bologna 21:194–202, 1888
Peterson FR: Re-formed gallbladder review of 27 cases. Tr West SA 51:203–220, 1942
Hopkins SF: The problem of the cystic duct remnant. Surg Gynecol Obstet 148:531–533, 1979
Corazziari E, Torsoli A: Dysfunction of the sphincter of Oddi. In Haubrich WS, Schaffner F, Berk JE (eds): Bockus Gastroenterology, 5th ed, vol 2, pp 2802–2811. Philadelphia, WB Saunders, 1995

CYSTIC FIBROSIS

Synonyms. CF; Clarke-Hadefield (see). Fibrocystic, meconium ileus (see), mucoviscidosis.

Symptoms and Signs. Prevalence of 1:2000 live births. May start from birth with meconium ileus (see). Pulmonary involvement starts in childhood with obstruction of small airways, recurrent infection, bronchiolitis, barrel chest deformity, growth retardation, cyanosis, digital clubbing. More frequent infections with Staphylococcus aureus and Pseudomonas aeruginosa. Cor pulmonale in late phases of disease. Later in life obstruction of pancreatic ducts and loss of pancreatic enzyme activity with progressive absent weight gain, abdominal distention, frequent evacuation with bulky, oily stool, and rectal prolapse. Pancreatitis is not frequent. A meconium ileus equivalent of adulthood may appear in 21% of patients with intestinal obstruction. Focal biliary cirrhosis is present in 25% of patients and can present itself as a persistent neonatal icterus. In later life this can evolve (2–3%) into partial hypertension and splenomegaly. Liver complications are seen only in patients with pancreatic insufficiency. Adult males are infertile in 98% of cases because of mechanical obstruction of vas deferens. In females delayed puberty and various gynecologic malformations; pregnancy is possible. Visual defects, venous engorgement of retinal veins and blurring of the optic nerve head are possible. Salivary glands are enlarged. Sweat is rich in Na+ and Cl– because of decreased transductal reabsorption.

Etiology. Generalized defect of exocrine glands that causes thick mucous secretions in many organs and variable patterns of clinical manifestations. Autosomal recessive, either single mutant allele or genetic heteroegenicity. CF has coincidental occurrence with other congenital diseases (Down, cri-du-chat, agammaglobulinemia, Wiskott-Aldrich).

Diagnostic Procedures. Sweat test method of Gibson-Cooke with quantitative pilocarpine ionophoresis: chloride concentration above 60 mEq/liter is consistent with diagnosis of CF. Anamnesis with characteristic symptoms and signs.

Therapy. Psychosocial support and qualified long-term medical assistance. Surgery for intestinal obstruction often needed. Adequate nutritional support, prevention of pulmonary infections. Transplantation of most affected organ (except lung) useful.

Prognosis. Variable. Prognosis is determined by degree of pulmonary involvement. Prognosis has improved in the last three decades. Mean age 21 years in 1978.

BIBLIOGRAPHY. Fanconi G, Uehlinger E, Knauuer C: Das Coeliakie Syndrom be: angeborener zystischer Pankreasfibrose und Bronkiektasien. Wien Med Wockenschr 86:753–756, 1936

Andersen DH: Cystic fibrosis of pancreas and its relation to celiac disease: Clinical and pathological study. Am J Dis Child 56:344–399, 1938

Di Santa Agnese P, Blanc W: A distinctive type of biliary cirrhosis of the liver associated with cystic fibrosis of the pancreas. Pediatrics 18:387–408, 1956

Tausing LM: Cystic fibrosis. Stuttgart, New York, Thieme, 1984

Weatherall DJ, Ledingham JGG, Warrell DA (eds): Oxford Textbook of Medicine, 3rd ed, pp 2746–2755. Oxford, Oxford Med Pub, 1996

CYSTINOSIS

Synonyms. Abderhalden-Kaufman-Lignac-Fanconi-Debré; cystindiathesis. Metabolic disorder characterized biochemically by an abnormally high intracellular content of free cystine. There are three forms of the disease:

1. Infantile nephropathic (see also Fanconi)
2. Benign
3. Intermediate

INFANTILE NEPHROPATHIC

Synonyms. Fanconi-De Toni, cystinosis, early onset.

Symptoms and Signs. Onset at 6 months. Polyuria, polydipsia, recur-

rent fever, growth retardation, rickets, acidosis, clinical picture of Fanconi-De Toni syndrome (see). Mentally normal, hydrocephalus. Blond hair, fair complexion, severe photophobia.

Etiology. Autosomal recessive. Impaired cystine transport across lysosomal membrane.

Diagnostic Procedures. *Urine.* Glycosuria, organic aciduria, aminoaciduria, proteinuria. *Eye transillumination.* Homogenously dispersed tinsel-like refractile opacities, cornea, and conjunctiva. *Bone marrow.* Presence of cystine crystals.

Pathology. Specific lesion deposition of cystine crystals in all organs (not brain and muscle). Kidney: characteristic "swan neck" deformity of tubule, cystine crystals in cornea and conjunctiva. Peripheral retinopathy.

Therapy. Symptomatic, vitamin D, penicillamine, dithiothreitol (DTT), cysteamine, ascorbic acid, diet, renal transplantation.

Prognosis. Poor quoad vitam. Better with kidney transplantation but death in second decade.

BENIGN

Synonyms. Cystinosis. Adult non-nephropathic type.

Symptoms and Signs. Both sexes affected. Detection at various ages, childhood asymptomatic: normal growth, absence of skin pigmentation, rickets, retinopathy. Incidental discovery during routine ophthalmic examination.

Diagnostic Procedures. Slit-light transillumination.

Pathology. Cystine deposits in cornea.

Prognosis. Good.

INTERMEDIATE

Synonyms. Late-onset cystinosis, adolescent cystinosis, nephropathic.

Symptoms and Signs. Late onset in adolescence. No complete Fanconi syndrome. Same as infantile form but less severe. Photophobia, chronic headaches.

Etiology. Either double heterozygotes with one gene of infantile form and one benign form or genetic compounds.

Pathology. Renal biopsy: glomerular changes.

BIBLIOGRAPHY. Abderhalden F: Familiare cystindiathese. Z Physiol Chem (Strassb) 38:557–561, 1903

Garrod AE: Inborn error of metabolism. Lancet Z Lecture I, p 1; Lecture II, p 73; lecture III, p 142; lecture IV, p 214, 1908

Weatherall DJ, Ledingham JGG, Warrell DA (eds): Oxford Textbook of Medicine, 3rd ed, pp 1355–1356. Oxford, Oxford Med Pub, 1996

CYSTINURIA

Symptoms and Signs. Males affected more seriously than females. Formation of renal stones by the age of 30 in 50% of cases, with typical clinical manifestation (e.g., pain, hematuria). The majority of these patients are of small stature (because of malabsorption and loss of the essential amino acid, lysine). Prevalence 1:7000.

Etiology. Inherited condition. Characterized by altered transepithelial transport mechanism of the amino acid, expressed primarily in kidney and intestine, as excessive urinary excretion of cystine, lysine, arginine, and ornithine. Two forms of inheritance patterns: (1) Autosomal recessive (with heterozygote with normal urine); (2) incomplete recessive (with heterozygote with some amount of mentioned amino acids in the urine). This syndrome is not to be confused with Abderhalden-Kaufman-Lignac and Lignac-Debré-Fanconi (see), and with other syndromes where cystinuria occurs as part of general aminoaciduria (e.g.,

Fanconi-De Toni syndrome, Wilson's syndrome).

Pathology. Renal calculosis with secondary inflammatory and fibrotic changes of kidney parenchyma.

Diagnostic Procedures. *Urine.* Excessive excretion of amino acids mentioned in etiology; passage of cystine stone; hematuria; proteinuria. *X-ray.* Intravenous pyelogram.

Therapy. Diet with reduced methionine (maintains urine alkalinity) and abundant in volume. Kidney transplantation.

Prognosis. Except for formation of stone and small stature, would be a benign disorder. Without kidney transplantation death at end of fourth decade.

BIBLIOGRAPHY. Wollaston WH: On Cystic oxide, a new species of urinary calculus. Phil Trans Roy Soc London 100:223–230, 1810
Garrod AE: The Croonian lectures on inborn errors of metabolism. Lancet 2: Lecture I, p 1; Lecture II, p 73; Lecture III, p 142; Lecture IV, p 214, 1908
Segal S, Thier SO: Cystinuria. In Scriver CR, Beaudet AL, Sly WS, et al: The Metabolic and Molecular Bases of Inherited Disease, 6th ed, pp 2479–2496. New York, McGraw-Hill, 1989
Stephens AD: Cystynuria and its treatment: 25 years experience at St. Bartholomew's Hospital. J Inherit Metab Dis 12:197–209, 1989
Weatherall DJ, Ledingham JGG, Warrell DA (eds): Oxford Textbook of Medicine, 3rd ed, pp 1356–1357. Oxford, Oxford Med Pub, 1996

CYSTITIS, IRRADIATION

Synonym. Radiation cystitis.

Symptoms. Both sexes affected, onset at least 1–10 years after radiation treatment. Pollakiuria; stranguria, incontinence; hematuria.

Signs. Pain at palpation over bladder.

Etiology. X-ray; radium treatment of pelvic condition.

Pathology. *Mild.* Mild mucosal inflammatory edematous changes; dilation of submucosal vessels and increased vascularization. *Severe.* Ulcerative necrotic generalized lesions. *Chronic.* Defined lesions; bulbous edema; ulcerative necrotic lesions.

Diagnostic Procedures. *Urine.* Proteinuria; hematuria; presence of white blood cells and cellular debris.

Therapy. Antinflammatory agents. Antibiotics.

Prognosis. Generally, remission; in severe cases, fibrosis and reduction of bladder capacity and formation of fistulas, and evolution toward bladder cancer.

BIBLIOGRAPHY. Duncan RE, Bennett DW, Evans AT, et al: Radiation induced bladder tumors. J Urol 118:43–48, 1977
Sella A, Dexeus FH, Chong C, et al: Radiation therapy associated with invasive bladder tumors. Urol 33:185–192, 1989

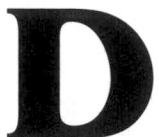

D

DABSKA

Synonyms. Endovascular papillary angioendothelioma; endothelioma endovascular papillary.

Symptoms and Signs. In infants and children. Diffuse swelling on any side of body.

Etiology. Unknown.

Pathology. Anastomosing vessels, some containing papillary projections (renal glomeruli-like) occasionally locally invasive or metastasing to regional lymphnodes.

Diagnostic Procedures. *Biopsy.* Cells positive for factor VIII associated antigen; negative for class II markers.

Therapy. Wide surgical excision.

Prognosis. Good with treatment. Possible metastasis.

BIBLIOGRAPHY. Dabska M: Malignant endovascular angioendothelioma of childhood. Cancer 24:503–509, 1969

Morgan J, Robinson NJ, Rosen LB, et al: Malignant endovascular papillary angioendothelioma. Am J Dermopathol 11:64–68, 1989

D'ACOSTA

Synonyms. Acosta; acute mountain sickness; altitude anoxia; altitude sickness; hypobarism—acute mountain sickness. See Monge syndrome.

Symptoms and Signs. Occurs 4–6 hours after reaching high altitude, or later (96 hours). Variability in intensity of symptoms, according to altitude. Pulsatile headache; nausea; vomiting; anorexia; insomnia; irritability. In some cases, symptoms may progress to confusion, coma, and death. Signs of pulmonary edema may also develop.

Etiology. Hypoxia; inappropriate secretion of antidiuretic and corticoadrenal hormones; fluid retention; hypervolemia. Increase in ventilation stimulated by hypoxia and resulting in hypocapnia and respiratory alkalosis.

Pathology. Cerebral and pulmonary edema.

Therapy. Diuretics. Acetazolamide, 250 mg every 8 hours prior to and during the ascent to altitude. (The drug acts by increasing renal excretion of bicarbonate and reducing the extent of the respiratory alkalosis.) In severe cases, prompt transfer to lower altitude. Oxygen and cardiopulmonary resuscitation in cases of pulmonary edema.

Prognosis. Minor symptoms disappear after 4–8 days of acclimatization. In severe cases, without treatment death can occur. The return at lower altitude immediately improves the clinical manifestations.

BIBLIOGRAPHY. D'Acosta J: Efecto estraño que hace en ciertas terras de Indias el aire, coviento que corre. Nella sua Historia Natural y Moral de las Indias Forms, vol 3. Sevilla, Juan de Leon, 1950

Blume FD, Boyers SJ, Braverman LE, et al: Impaired osmoregulation at high altitudes. Studies on Mt Everest. JAMA 252:524–526, 1984

Grover RF, Reeves JT, Rowell LB, et al: The influence of environmental factors on the cardiovascular system. In Schlant RC, Alexander RW: Hurst's The Heart, 8th ed, pp 2117–2122. New York, McGraw-Hill, 1994

DA COSTA (J.M.)

Synonyms. Neurocirculatory asthenia, cardiac neurosis; effort syndrome (misnomer); nervous heart; soldier heart. See Orthostatic. The designation "effort syndrome" has been dropped, since symptoms and signs of this syndrome closely resemble those of emotion and fear, rather than those of "effort" in normal subject, and depend on central stimulation.

BIBLIOGRAPHY. DaCosta JM: On irritable heart: A clinical study of a form of functional cardiac disorder and its consequences. Am J Med Sci 61:17–52, 1871

Sheehan DV: Panic attacks and the cardiovascular system. In Schlant RC, Alexander RW: Hurst's The Heart, 8th ed, pp 2099–2100. New York, McGraw-Hill, 1994

DAHLBERG

Synonyms. Lymphedema—hypoparathyroidism; hypoparathyroidism—lymphedema.

Symptoms and Signs. Broad nasal bridge, displacement of inner canthi, noted after birth. Described in two brothers. Congenital lymphedema; signs of hypoparathyroidism (see hypoparathyroidism syndromes); nephropathy; mitral valve prolapse; and brachytelephalangy; bilateral cataract (in one case developed at age 19 years).

Etiology. Unknown. Possibly autosomal recessive or X-linked inheritance.

Diagnostic Procedures. *Blood.* See hypoparathyroidism plus evidence of renal failure (slowly developing). *X-ray.* Suspect pulmonary lymphagiectasis. Pleural thickening, chest. *ECG.*

Therapy. Symptomatic; in one case kidney transplant necessary.

Prognosis. Both cases were recognized in adult life.

BIBLIOGRAPHY. Dahlberg PJ, Borer WZ, Newcomer KL, et al: Autosomal or X-linked recessive syndrome of congenital lymphedema, hypoparathyroidism, nephropathy, prolapsing mitral valve and brachytelephalangy. Ann J Med Genet 16:99–104, 1983

DANA I

Synonyms. Essential benign tremor; hereditary benign tremor; presenile tremor; tremor, benign, hereditary.

Symptoms. Both sexes affected; on the average onset at 50 years of age and later in women than men, extending progressively. More or less rhythmic, fine, or coarse tremor (rate 4–12/sec). Present when there is increase in muscle tone (static tremor), and in movement (kinetic or intentional). Enhanced by emotion, fatigue, and cold; relieved by rest, sedation, and sleep. Affects mostly hands, arms, neck, and head; trunk occasionally may be involved.

Signs. Lack of parkinsonian signs (rigidity; postural flexion; mask face). No deficit of reflexes or sensations; no pathologic reflexes; good coordination. Mild extrapyramidal symptoms.

Etiology. Unknown; autosomal dominant inheritance. Earlier appearance in subsequent generation noted.

Pathology. Not contributory to interpret nature of disorder.

Diagnostic Procedures. *Thyroid function studies.* Negative. *Electromyography.* Negative. *Spinal fluid.* Negative.

Therapy. Nonspecific; some benefit from sedatives.

Prognosis. Benign course. After more or less rapid progression, the situation becomes stabilized, and patients are not incapacitated.

BIBLIOGRAPHY. Dana CL: Hereditary tremor; A hitherto undescribed form of motor neurosis. Am J Med Sci 94:386–393, 1887

Critchley M: Observation on essential (heredofamilial) tremor. Brain 72:113–139, 1949

Busenbark KL, Nash J, Hubble JP, et al: Is essential tremor benign? Neurology 41:1982–1983, 1991

DANDY

Synonyms. Infraclinoid. See orbital apex.

Symptoms and Signs. Only alleged minor differences with orbital apex syndrome (see).

Etiology and Pathology. Aneurysm of internal carotid artery in the anterior part of cavernous sinus.

Diagnostic Procedures. *X-ray. CT scan. MRI. Angiography.* Erosion of anterior clinoid process and occasionally thinning of lateral wall of optical canal.

BIBLIOGRAPHY. Dandy WE: Intracranial Arterial Aneurysm. Ithaca, NY, Comstock Pub Com, 1944

Roger J, Bille J, Vigoroux RA: Multiple cranial nerve palsies. In Vinken PJ, Bruyn GW: Handbook of Clinical Neurology, vol 2, p 88. Amsterdam, North-Holland, 1969

DANDY-WALKER

Synonyms. Luschka-Magendie foramina atresia; Sylvius aqueduct obstructed; hydrocephalus internal; noncommunicating hydrocephalus; see also Arnold-Chiari.

Symptoms. Vomiting, hyperirritability, convulsions.

Signs. Progressive enlargement of the head; congested veins in the scalp; bulging of anterior fontanelle; separated cranial sutures; papilledema, bradycardia; bradypnea.

Etiology. Internal hydrocephalus developing in utero and other unidentified primitive factors responsible for the development of following malformations: complete or partial obstruction of foramina of Luschka and Magendie owing to a noninvolution of posterior medullary velum of fourth ventricle, which persists as a thick membrane, and other midline malformations (e.g., agenesis of corpus callosum). In some cases, occurrence of the syndrome in siblings suggests a recessive inheritance.

Pathology. Dolichocephaly; thinning of occipital squama; high insertion of tentorium and lateral sinuses; dilatation of fourth ventricle; cerebellum displaced by the cyst-like dilatation and consequent partial or complete aplasia of the vermis. Additional midline malformations may occasionally be present. Brain and cerebellar cortex affected first; white matter contains fat from distruction of myelin. Proliferation of glia.

Diagnostic Procedures. Fetal hydrocephalus diagnosed by antenatal *ultrasound examination*; postnatally: *CT scan. MRI.*

Therapy. Surgical treatment during the first week of life: simultaneous shunting of both the ventricles and the cyst through the same valve in the peritoneum.

Prognosis. Poor.

BIBLIOGRAPHY. Dandy WE, Blackfan KD: Internal hydrocephalus: An experimental clinical and pathological study. Am J Dis Child 8:406–485, 1914

Dandy WE: The diagnosis and treatment of hydrocephalus due to occlusion of the formina of Magendie and Luschka. Surg Gynecol Obstet 32:112–124, 1921

Walker AE: A case of congenital atresia of the foramina of Luschka and Magendie: Surgical cure. J Neuropathol Exp Neurol 3:368–373, 1944

Stoll C, Huber C, Alembik Y, et al: Dandy-Walker variant malformation, spastic paraplegia, and mental retardation in two sibs. Am J Med Genet 37:124–127, 1990

DANCE MANIA

Synonyms. In the past: France, danse de St Guy. Italy, tarantulism, stellio, astaragazza. Other countries, chorea lasciva, chorea imaginatica; chorea, St Viti; St Viti chorea. In the present: shake; rock 'n roll; Saturday night fever; break dance; house; techno; trance.

Symptoms and Signs. Epidemic dance psychosis, in some cultures with religious implications: Shamanism, Dervish, Macumba, etc.

Etiology. In the past and today a collection of minor or major psychotic derangements, often under the influence of respectively old or modern drugs (however, in the past with this terminology, especially in sporadic cases, many other organic pathologic conditions were included: chorea minor, ballism, spinocerebellar degenerations, paralysis agitans, and chorea hereditaria).

Prognosis. Prolonged state of agitation, exhaustion may lead to very serious consequences, including death from organ failure or traumatic accidents.

BIBLIOGRAPHY. Von Hohenheim PATB (Paracelsus): Opera omnia medico-chimica-chirurgica. Genua Antoni & Turnes, 1658

Sydenham T: Schedulae Monitoria de Novae Febris Ingressae, 1686

Baglivi I: De anatomie, morsu et effectibus. Tarantulae Lugd Bat 35–40, 1699

Bruyn GW: Huntington's chorea: Historical, clinical and laboratory synopsis. In Vinken PJ, Bruyn GW: Handbook of Clinical Neurology, vol 6, p 300. Amsterdam, North-Holland, 1968

DARIER-FERRAND

Synonyms. Dermatofibroma protuberans; dermatofibrosarcoma progressive, recurrent; protuberans dermatofibroma.

Symptoms and Signs. Rare. Equal incidence in both sexes in adult life. Small, hard nodules infiltrating the skin that may enlarge to form freely movable plaques or may become pedunculated. They appear mostly in the trunk and flexural regions. Later they become painful, fixate to the underlying structure, ulcerate, and discharge.

Etiology. Unknown. Nodules may appear in area previously traumatized. Malignant tumor.

Pathology. Well-differentiated fibrosarcoma. Uniform fibroblasts extending up to dermoepithelial junction and down to subcutaneous fat; peripherally, they blend into normal dermis. Occasionally, modest, mitotic activity. The arrangement is that of spokes of a wheel. Blood vessels scarce and difficult to identify. Older lesions show mucoid degeneration.

Diagnostic Procedures. *Biopsy.*

Therapy. Surgical excision providing large margin of healthy tissue to prevent recurrence.

Prognosis. Slow growth over periods of months or years. Metastasis and spread to lymph nodes very rare. Recurrence after excision 20% (owing to inadequate removal of tissue).

BIBLIOGRAPHY. Darier J, Ferrand M: Dermatofibromes progressive et récidivante ou fibro-sarcomes de la peau. Ann Dermatol Syph 5:45–62, 1924

Burkhardt BR, Soule EH, Winkelmann RK, et al: Dermatofibrosarcoma protuberans. Study of fifty-six cases. Am J Surg 111:638–644, 1966

MacKie RM: Soft tissue tumors. In Champion RH, Burton JL, Ebling FJG (eds): Rook/Wilkinson/Ebling Textbook of Dermatology, 5th ed, pp 2078–2979. Oxford, Blackwell Scientific, 1992

DARIER-ROUSSY

Synonym. Subcutaneous sarcoidosis.

Symptoms and Signs. Subcutaneous nodules on the trunk, thighs, shoulders, symmetric distribution, skin-colored or bluish red, slowly evolving without ulceration.

Etiology. Sarcoidosis; possibly other causes. See Besnier-Boeck-Schaumann.

Pathology. See Besnier-Boeck-Schaumann.

BIBLIOGRAPHY. Darier J, Roussy G: Des sarcoides soubcutanees; contribution à l'étude des tuberculides ou tuberculose atténuees de l'hypoderme. Arch Méd Exp Anat 18:1–50, 1906

James DG, Epstein WL: Cutaneous sarcoidosis. In James DG (ed): Sarcoidosis and Other Granulomatous Disorders. New York, Marcel Dekker, 1994

DARIER-WHITE

Synonyms. Darier I; White; dyskeratosis follicularis vegetans; keratosis follicularis; psorospermosis; keratosis follicularis. See Hopf and Gougerot-Hailey-Hailey.

Symptoms and Signs. Both sexes affected; onset in childhood (10–20 years). Many confluent flesh-colored keratotic papules forming greasy crusted areas, vegetating and malodorous, on the seborrheic areas of head, neck, back, abdomen, and groin. Seldom, hair loss. Punctate keratosis on palms and soles. Palmoplantar keratoderma (10%). Seldom, hemorrhagic macules in hands and feet. Normally general health remains unaffected. Occasionally (10%), lesions are in zosteriform pattern and limited to one half of body. Mucosae of mouth, esophagus, genitals, and anus may exhibit white umbilicate papules; hypertrophy of gums may also occur. Onychodystrophy. Seldom associated: small stature; low intelligence; genital hypoplasia. Exacerbations may follow corticosteroid administration or exposure to UV radiation.

Etiology. Unknown; autosomal dominant inheritance. Defect in synthesis, organization, maturation of tonofilament-desmosome complex.

Pathology. Early, fissures above basal layer, later extending through Malpighian layer. Around lacunae small separated groups of cells enlarged with dark nuclei, clear cytoplasm, and glistening ring (partial keratosis). Hyperkeratosis; parakeratosis; acanthosis of different degrees.

Diagnostic Procedures. *Biopsy of skin. Blood.* Low vitamin A level. *X-ray of chest.* Diffuse fibrosis with nodulation mainly affecting lower lobes. Polycystic kidney or kidney agenesis; occasionally, cystic changes in the bones.

Therapy. In mild cases none or simple emolients and avoid exposure to sun. For more severe forms: etretinate or isotretinoin. Dermoabrasion for very severe forms.

Prognosis. Chronic benign condition. Treatment may give excellent, moderate, or no improvement. Relapses when treatment is discontinued. Degree of mental retardation variable, from institutional care required to normal life.

BIBLIOGRAPHY. Darier J: Psorospermose folliculaire vegetante. Etude anatomo-pathologique d'une affection cutanée non décrite ou com-

preise dans le groupe des acnés sébacées, cornées, hypertrophiantes, des kératoses (ichtyoses) folliculaires, etc. Ann Dermatol Syph 10:597–612, 1889

White JC: A case of keratosis (ichthyosis) follicularis. J Cutan Genitourin Dis 7:201–209, 1889

Oxholm A, Oxholm P, Da Cunha Bagn F, et al: Abnormal essential fatty acid metabolism in Darier's disease. Arch Dermatol 126:1308–1311, 1990

Griffiths WAD, Leigh IM, Marks R: Disorders of Keratinization. In Champion RH, Burton JL, Ebling FJG (eds): Rook/Wilkinson/Ebling Textbook of Dermatology, 5th ed, pp 1362–1366. Oxford, Blackwell Scientific, 1992

DARROW-GAMBLE

Synonyms. Gamble-Darrow; hypochloremic congenital alkalosis—diarrhea; chlorurrhea; chloride diarrhea, familial; WDHA; watery diarrhea—hypokalemia—achlorhydria.

Symptoms. Usually prematurity; watery profuse diarrhea; no vomiting; failure to gain weight; good appetite except in period of dehydration.

Signs. Abdominal distention with a marked "ladder" pattern suggesting a (false) intestinal obstruction.

Etiology. Defective jejunal brush-border Na/H exchange. Possibly, autosomal recessive inheritance.

Pathology. Juxtaglomerular hyperplasia.

Diagnostic Procedures. *Blood.* Low plasma chloride; high bicarbonate; low sodium; normal potassium (except when diarrhea is severe); elevated pH (7. 64); normal blood urea nitrogen (BUN), sugar, protein, and calcium. Hyperreninemia, increased aldosterone levels. *Stool.* High chloride; low sodium; acid pH. *Stomach and duodenal secretion.* Normal. *Urine.* Occasionally, pH higher than that of plasma; no chloride; little sodium; variable amount of potassium.

Therapy. Intermittent intravenous administration of sodium chloride and potassium chloride initially and then orally (over 4 g potassium chloride daily).

Prognosis. With treatment, growth almost normal; stools remain loose, causing little inconvenience; danger in period of febrile illness and warm weather.

BIBLIOGRAPHY. Gamble J: Congenital alkalosis with diarrhea. J Pediatr 26:509–518, 1945

Darrow DC: Congenital alkalosis with diarrhea. J Pediatr 26:519–532, 1945

Booth IW, Strange G, Murer H, et al: Defective jejunal brush-border Na+/H+ exchange: A cause of congenital diarrhea. Lancet I:1066–1069, 1985

Perheentupa J: The Finnish disease heritage: a personal look. Acta Paed. 84:1094 –1099, 1995

Weatherall DJ, Ledingham JGG, Warrell DA (eds): Oxford Textbook of Medicine, 3rd ed, p 1706. Oxford, Oxford Med Pub, 1996

DAVID (W.)

Synonym. Purpura feminarum typica.

Symptoms and Signs. Occurs in women during reproductive period. Hemorrhages from gums and other mucosal areas periodically recurring, usually during menstrual periods.

Etiology. David believes that a deficit of ovarian hormones is the cause of the syndrome.

Diagnostic Procedures. *Blood.* Complete clotting studies; evaluation of hormonal activities. *Evaluation of psychic balance.* See Psychogenic purpura.

BIBLIOGRAPHY. Hyde JH: A contribution to the study of bleeding stigmata. J Cutan Dis 15:557, 1897

David W: Ueber Purpura–Erkrankungen bei Frauen. Med Klin 22:1755–1756, 1926

Agle DP, Ratnoff OD: Purpura as a psychosomatic entity. Arch Intern Med 109:685–694, 1962

Bithell TC: Bleeding disorders caused by vascular abnormalities. In Lee GR, Bithel TC, Foerster J, et al (eds): Wintrobe's Clinical Hematology, 9th ed. Philadelphia, Lea & Febiger, 1993

DAVID-STICKLER

Synonyms. Wagner; Wagner-Stickler; Cervenka; Stickler; arthro-opththalmopathy; clefting; hyaloid-retina degeneration—palatoschisis; see Marshall, Weissbacher-Zweymuller; Favre and Nance-Insley.

Symptoms. Both sexes affected; onset at birth. Congenital progressive myopia, astygmatism, vitreocorneal degeneration; blindness. Hypermobility of joints; in childhood, onset of stiffness and articular pain. Progressive deafness (sensorineural type).

Signs. Nasal bridge depressed; maxillar hypoplasia; philtrum prolonged; occasionally: cleft palate. Arthropathy, primarily affected: knees, hips, and spine; less severely, wrists, elbows, and ankles. Articular bony enlargement and hypermobility and then deforming changes (3rd and fourth decades). Phthisical or glaucomatous blind eyes; chronic uveitis; keropathy; chorioretinal degeneration; total retinal detachment (during first decade). Skeletal abnormalities. Mitral valve prolapse (50%).

Etiology. Autosomal dominant inheritance. Included by David in mucopolysaccharidosis group (not confirmed by other authors). Abnormal development of epiphyseal plate. Confused relationship with Marshall and Weissbacher-Zweymuller syndromes; possibly part of a spectrum including Wagner–Stikler, Weissmuller–Zweigberg, Pierre Robin, Kniest, SED congenital.

Pathology. See Signs.

Diagnostic Procedures. *X-rays of skeleton.* Eccentro-orthochondrodysplasia (Morquio). *Ophthalmoscopy. Audiography. Blood and urine.* Normal.

Therapy. Orthopedic.

Prognosis. Blindness during first decade. Severe arthropathy by third or fourth decade.

BIBLIOGRAPHY. David B: Ueber einen dominanten Erbgang beieiner polyopen enchondralen Dysostose typ Pfaundler-Hurler. Z Orthop 84:657–660, 1953

Strickler GB, Pugh DG: Hereditary progressive arthroophthalmopathy: II. Additional observations of vertebral abnormalities, a hearing defect, and a report of a similar case. Mayo Clin Proc 42:495–500, 1967

Temple IK: Stickler's syndrome. J Med Genet 26:119–126, 1989

Heathcote G: Collagen and its disorders. In Garner A, Klintworth GK (eds): Pathobiology of Ocular Disease: A Dynamic Approach, 2nd ed, p 1063. New York, Marcel Dekker, 1994

DAVIES

Synonyms. Endomyocardial tropical fibrosis; EMF; mural tropical endomyocardial fibrosis. Tropical endomyocardial fibrosis; eosinophilic tropical endomyocardial fibrosis; see Loeffer. endomyocardial.

Symptoms. Reported mostly in Uganda; cases in Sri Lanka, South America, and other African countries. No sex or racial predominance; onset before adolescence. Dyspnea; palpitation; cough; occasionally, chest pains. Fever in initial period then usually subsiding, in some cases prolonged.

Signs. Peripheral edemas. Digital clubbing; cyanosis; jaundice. Early

apical systolic murmur, and S3 opening snap (after S2). Diminution of cardiac pulsation (constrictive, pericarditis-like).

Etiology. Unknown. Primary myocardial condition with thrombosis and endocardial disease. Considered as possible causes: excessive serotonin; malnutrition; parasites; viruses; anemia; hypersensitivity. Suggested infective origin.

Pathology. *Early stage.* Endocardial and inner myocardial cells of connective tissue are swollen with mucopolysaccharides and covered by fibrin; thrombus formation followed by fibroblastic proliferation. *Late stage.* Extensive, white, endocardial thickening mostly at left ventricular apex; right ventricle similarly thickened, but less extensively affected.

Diagnostic Procedures. *ECG.* No consistent pattern. *X-rays.* Massive pericardial effusion; right atrial dilatation; dilatation right infundibular vestibulum. Pulmonary hypertension; enlargement of main pulmonary artery. *Blood.* Eosinophilia (occasional). *Biopsy of endocardium by right heart catheterization.* See Pathology. *Angiography. Echography. Radionuclide imaging.*

Therapy. Symptomatic. Corticosteroids. Surgical treatment useful on short term. Heart transplantation.

Prognosis. Survival 1–2 years from onset of symptoms; longer survival (8–12 years) possible. Good with transplantation.

BIBLIOGRAPHY. Davies JPN: Endocardial fibrosis in Africans. East Afr Med J 25:10–14, 1948

Davies JPN, Cales RM: Some considerations regarding obscure diseases affecting the mural endocardium. Am Heart J 59:600–631, 1960

Shabetai R: Restrictive cardiomyopathy. In Schlant RC, Alexander RW: Hurst's The Heart, 8th ed, p 1645. New York, McGraw-Hill, 1994

DAVIS (J.A.)

Synonyms. Achondroplasia—Swiss-type agammaglobulinemia. Dysplasia metaphyseal (type B-III); metaphyseal dysostosis (type B-III); thymolymphopenia—metaphyseal dysostosis. See Swiss type agammaglobulinemia and X-linked hypogammaglobulinemia—isolated growth hormone deficiency.

Symptoms. Both sexes affected; present from birth. High susceptibility to infections.

Signs. Absence of hair and eyebrows; ichthyosiform lesions; erythroderma; cutis laxa; short limb dwarfism.

Etiology. Unknown; autosomal recessive inheritance (suggested) or X-linked.

Diagnostic Procedures. *Blood.* See Swiss-type agammaglobulinemia. *X-rays of long bones.* Short (femora more so than humeri); metaphyseal widening; irregularity of growth plates; pelvic abnormalities; hands, skull, fibula normal.

Therapy. Antibiotics; immunoglobulins; blood transfusion (with caution and preferably after removal of white cells and injection of blood older than 21 days). Bone marrow transplantation.

Prognosis. Poor. Death frequently before reaching first year.

BIBLIOGRAPHY. Davis JA: A case of Swiss type agammaglobulinemia and achondroplasia. Br Med J 2:1371, 1966

Ammann AJ, Sutliff W, Nillinchick E: Antibody-mediated immunodeficiency in short limbed dwarfism. J Pediatr 84:200–203, 1974

DAVIS (M.D.)

Synonym. Rheumatoid arthritis—uveitis.

Symptoms. Most frequent in children, but occurs at all ages. Symptoms of rheumatoid arthritis; trouble with vision; pain; lacrimation; photophobia.

Signs. Those of rheumatoid arthritis. Uveitis; iridocyclitis; less frequently, scleritis; secondary formation of band-shaped keratopathy; choroidal inflammation. Occasionally, hepatosplenomegaly.

Etiology. Unknown; possibly, collagen disorder or autoimmune condition.

Pathology. See Signs.

Diagnostic Procedures. *Blood.* Sedimentation rate. R.A. test.

Therapy. Systemic and topical (eye) corticosteroids.

Prognosis. Often poor.

BIBLIOGRAPHY. Davis MD: Endogenous uveitis in children: Associated band-shaped keratopathy and rheumatoid arthritis. Arch Ophthalmol 50:443–454, 1953
Hakin KN, Lightman S: The eye in systemic immune disorders. In Garner A, Klintworth GK (eds): Pathobiology of Ocular Disease: A Dynamic Approach, 2nd ed, p 188. New York, Marcel Dekker, 1994

DAWIDENKOW

Synonyms. Scapulo-peroneal of Dawidenkow.

Symptoms and Signs. Onset at 14–26 years of age, seldom later, up to 40 years. Symptoms and signs similar, but not identical to scapolo-peroneal muscular atrophy but in addition sensory disturbances in typical glove and stocking distribution, fasciculations, and sometimes degeneration and pes equinus. Pelvic girdle and hands never involved.

Etiology. Sporadic or autosomal dominant inheritance

Prognosis. Benign noninvalidating course.

BIBLIOGRAPHY. Oransky W: Ueber einen hereditaeren Typus progressiver Muskeldystrophie. Dtsch Z Nervenheilk 99:147–155, 1927
Dawidenkow S: Ueber die neurotische Muskel-atrophie Charcot-Marie. Klinisch-genetische Studien Z ges. Neurol Psychiat 107:259, 1927
Kaeser HE: Scapulo-peroneal syndrome. In Vinken PJ, Bruyn GW (eds): Handbook of Clinical Neurology, vol 22, pp 59–60. Amsterdam. North-Holland, 1985
Stevenson WG, Perloff JK, Weiss JN, et al: Facioscapulohumeral muscular dystrophy: Evidence for selective, genetic electrophysiologic cardiac involvement. J Am Coll Cardiol 15:292–299, 1990

DEAD FETUS

Synonyms. Macerated fetus; macerated stillborn.

Symptoms and Signs. Diagnosis may be based on clinical manifestation of hemorrhages, or (better) on fibrinogen determination on patients who are known or suspected to be carrying a dead fetus in uterus. The latter method allows recognition of three grades of the syndrome.

1. Potential. No hemorrhages; fibrinogen declining to or below 150 mg/100 dl with or without evidence of fibrinolysis.
2. Occult. No hemorrhages; fibrinogen below 90 mg/100 dl, or fibrinolytic activity high.
3. Overt. Hemorrhages of unclottable blood because of hypofibrinogenemia and hyperfibrinolysis.

Etiology. Death of fetus after 4–5 weeks of retention. Maternal absorption into the circulation of products of pregnancy (amniotic fluid and products of autolysis of fetus) and activation of fibrinolytic mechanism resulting in slow defibrination of blood.

Pathology. Fetus dead; sign of intravascular coagulation and fibrinolysis of the clots.

Diagnostic Procedures. *Blood.* Serial determination of fibrinogen levels. *X-ray.* To demonstrate death of fetus.

Therapy. Rupture of membranes early in labor. A traumatic delivery, administration of fibrinogen, antifibrinolytic agents, and heparin as indicated.

Prognosis. Enormously improved with recognition and adequate treatment.

BIBLIOGRAPHY. Weiner AE, Reid DE, Roby CC, et al: Coagulation defects with intrauterine death from Rh sensitization. Am J Obstet Gynecol 60:1015–1022, 1950
Hodgkinson CP, Thompson RJ, Hodari AA: Dead fetus syndrome. Clin Obstet Gynecol 7:349–360, 1964
Pilipp EE, Barnes J, Newton M: Obstetrics and Gynecology, 3rd ed, p 360. London, William Heinemann, 1986
Bithell TC: Acquired coagulation disorders. In Lee GR, Bithel TC, Foerster J, et al (eds): Wintrobe's Clinical Hematology, 9th ed. Philadelphia, Lea & Febiger, 1993

DEAFNESS CONDUCTIVE—MALFORMED EXTERNAL EARS

Synonyms. Ear malformations; deafness.

Symptoms and Signs. Both sexes. Congenital conductive deafness; malformed, low-set external ears. Occasionally mental retardation and symptoms and signs of hypogonadism.

Etiology. Autosomal recessive inheritance.

BIBLIOGRAPHY. Mengel MC, Konigsmark BW, Berlin CI, et al: Conductive hearing loss and malformed low-set ears, as a possible recessive syndrome. J Med Genet 6:14–21, 1969
Cantu JM, Ruenes R, Garcia-Cruz D: Autosomal recessive sensory neural-conductive deafness and pinna anomalies. Hum Genet 40:231–234, 1978

DEAFNESS, CONGENITAL—OTITIC MENINGITIS

Synonym. Cerebrospinal otorrhea meningitis—congenital deafness.

Symptoms. Congenital unilateral deafness. Otorrhea without history of trauma. Recurrent episodes of meningitis.

Etiology. Unknown (possibly virus infection or trauma). Congenital malformation of inner ear with communication of middle ear and encephalic cavity through the vestibule of the labyrinth.

Pathology. See Etiology.

Diagnostic Procedures. *X-ray. Basal cisternography. CT. MRI brain scan.*

Therapy. Surgical correction through direct transaural approach.

Prognosis. Good when corrected.

BIBLIOGRAPHY. Neuzelius C: Spontaneous cerebrospinal fluid otorrhea due to congenital malformation. Acta Otolaryngol (Stockh) 39:314, 1951
Barr B, Wersall J: Cerebrospinal otorrhea with meningitis in congenital deafness. Arch Otolaryngol 81:26–28, 1965
Stool S, Leeds NE, Shulman K: The syndrome of congenital deafness and otitic meningitis: Diagnosis and management. J Pediatr 71:547–552, 1967

DEAFNESS-HYPOPITUITARISM, AUTOSOMAL RECESSIVE

Symptoms and Signs. Two sisters neurosensory deafness; hypopituitary dwarfism.

Etiology. Autosomal recessive inheritance.

BIBLIOGRAPHY. Winkelmann W, Behtge H, Pfeiffer RA: Hypothalamo-hypophysaerer Minderwuchs mit innenohrschwerhoerigkeit bei zwei Schwertern. Internist 13:52–56, 1972

DEAFNESS-HYPOGONADISM, X-LINKED, RECESSIVE

Symptoms and Signs. Male. Association of primary hearing loss and primary hypogonadim. Heterochromia of iris (partial).

Etiology. X-linked recessive inheritance.

BIBLIOGRAPHY. Myhre SA, Ruvalcaba RHA, Kelley VC: Congenital deafness and hypogondism. A new X-linked recessive disorder. Clin Genet 22:299–307, 1982

DEAFNESS, OPTIC ATROPHY

Synonym. Gernet.

Symptoms and Signs. Both sexes. Congenital deafness. Late in life progressive optic atrophy leading to mild visual impairment.

Etiology. Unknown. Autosomal dominant inheritance.

BIBLIOGRAPHY. Gernet H: Kombination mit Tanbheit. Dtsch Ophthalmol Ges 65:545–547, 1964
Konigsmark BK, Knox DL, Husserl IE, et al: Dominant congenital deafness and progressive optic nerve atrophy. Arch Ophthalmol 91:99–103, 1974

DEAFNESS SENSORINEURAL, AUTOSOMAL DOMINANT

Synonyms. Includes: Dominant congenital severe sensorineural deafness; deafness progressive hightone; deafness midtone neural; deafness progressive lowtone (see Konigsmark); deafness low frequency, mixed conductive sensorineural; deafness unilateral.

Symptoms and Signs. Deafness for itself is not a syndrome, however, some dominant pedigrees have been described, with different clinical characteristics. Usually all other findings are normal except for an occasional mild retardation of mental development. The time of onset is variable from birth to adult life. Slow progression of hearing loss in a period of decades. For this type of inherited deafness in association with other findings, see individual syndromes.

Etiology. Sporadic pseudodominance and autosomal dominant inheritance.

Pathology. From normal to severe alteration of organ of Corti.

Diagnostic Procedures. *Audiometry, MRI, and CT to exclude malformations.*

Therapy. Sometimes auditory aids may be useful.

Prognosis. By adult life total deafness or only for some tones.

BIBLIOGRAPHY. Fay EA: Marriages of the deaf in America. Washington Volta Bureau, 1898
Konigsmark BW, Salman S, Haskin SH, et al: Dominant midfrequency hearing loss. Ann Otolaryngol 79:1–12, 1970
Parving A: Inherited low frequency hearning loss: a new mixed conductive-sensorineural entity? Scand Audiol 13:47–56, 1984
Higashi K: Heterogeneity of dominant high frequency sensorineural deafness. Clin Genet 33:424–428, 1988
Everberg G: Unilateral anacusis. Clinical, radiological and genetic investigation. Acta Otolaryngol 158:Suppl 366–374, 1990

DEAFNESS SENSORINEURAL, AUTOSOMAL RECESSIVE

Synonyms. Deafmutism (misnomer), congenital deafness I and II, recessive congenital deafness; deafness inner ear. Includes Michel; Mondini; Alexander; Bing-Siebenmann; Scheibe; Pendred; Usher.

Symptoms and Signs. From birth deafness and secondary mutism (correctable by training). According to a first classification three inherited recessive syndromes have been described: Pendred (10%), Uscher (see), and deafness with EKG changes. Another classification (Ormerod) describes them as follows: Michel type (lack development of internal ear), Mondini-Alexander type (see), Bing-Siebenmann (bony labyrinth normal, but membranous parts immature—often associated with retinitis pigmentosa), Scheibe (malformation of cochlea and saccule; this type is present in Waardenburg [see]); Siebenmann type (changes in the middle ear with thyroid hormone deficiency; mixomatous changes in the middle ear; microtia and meatus atassia). The defects are usually isolated, but may be associated also with middle ear bony and fibrous defects or other abnormalities. In addition to the reported forms other recessive forms of congenital deafness have been identified where various associated features may be found. (See individual syndromes.)

Etiology. Genetic studies evidence the existence of at least two allelic recessive, phenotypically nondistinguishable forms of congenital deafness (deafness congenital I and II).

Diagnostic Procedures. *X-rays. CT scan. MRI. Audiology.*

Therapy. Early detection, special education, seldom surgery may play a role.

Prognosis. Variable according to lesions and treatments. With adequate training it is possible to acquire the capacity to speak.

BIBLIOGRAPHY. Meniere P: Reserches sur l'origine de la surdinite. Gaz Med Paris (Ser 3):223, 1846
Ormerod FC: The pathology of congenital deafness. J Laryng 74:919–950, 1960
Fraser GR: Profound childhood deafness. J Med Genet 1:118–151, 1964
Kenigsmark BW, Gorlin RJ: Genetic and Metabolic Deafness. Philadelphia, WB Saunders, 1976
Brownstein Z, Friedlander Y, Peritz E, et al: Estimated number of loci for autosomal recessive severe nerve deafness within the Israeli Jewish population, with implications for genetic counseling. Am J Med Genet 41:306–312, 1991

DEAFNESS SENSORINEURAL AND CONDUCTIVE, X-LINKED

Symptoms and Signs. In males. In all continents. Both types of perceptive and conductive deafness have been reported with this type of inheritance.

BIBLIOGRAPHY. Wilde WR. Practical Observations on Aural Surgery and the Nature and Diagnosis of Diseases of the Ear. London, Churchill, 1853
Reardon W: Sex linked deafness: Wilde revisited. J Med Genet 27:376–379, 1990

DEAN-BARNES

Synonyms. Porphyria cutanea tarda hereditaria; mixed hepatic porphyria, porphyria variegate; Porphyria cutanea tarda type II; uroporphyrinogen decarboxylase deficiency. South African genetic porphyria. Royal malady (because members of British royalty suffered from it), including type I (sporadic).

Symptoms. Both sexes affected. In women milder manifestations; may be more pronounced during pregnancy. In South Africa Afrikaaners

3:1000 incidence. Clinical onset difficult to determine because of variability of intensity and type of skin lesions. Usually noticed in third decade of life. (1) Skin manifestation (in 50% of patients, the only finding): increased sensitivity to light and minor mechanical traumas; erythema; edema; bullae healing with moderate scarring; hyperpigmentation or atrophic depigmented areas. (2) Abdominal and neurologic symptoms and signs identical with those observed in Swedish type of porphyria (see). These are usually precipitated by ingestion of barbiturates and other drugs.

Etiology. Type I: sporadic 50% deficiency of URO limited to liver plus additional environmental factors to elicit manifestations of the syndrome: Type II: autosomal dominant inheritance. Fifty percent deficient activity of uroporphyrinogen (URO) decarboxylase in many tissues.

Pathology. Absence of particular findings with the exception of high concentration of porphyrin precursors in the liver.

Diagnostic Procedures. *Stool.* Increased concentration of protoporphyrin and coproporphyrin in all patients (also in asymptomatic or paucisymptomatic). *Urine.* During attacks, larger amounts of aminolevulinic acid and porphobilinogen and porphyrins. *Blood.* Electrolytes imbalance (excessive vomiting; fluid loss).

Therapy. Eliminate exposure to alcohol; estrogens; phlebotomies (every 2 weeks). Reduce iron overload as in hemochromatosis; oral chloroquine (0.5–1.0 g/day for several days). Sunscreening agents. Erythopoietin possible future useful agent in complicated cases, i.e., renal failure.

Prognosis. During acute attack of abdominal pain, 25% mortality. Overall mortality not significantly increased, however, because many patients never have acute attacks, but only skin manifestations.

BIBLIOGRAPHY. Barnes, HD: Further South African cases of porphyrinuria. S Afr J Clin Sci 2:117–169, 1951
Dean G: Porphyria. Br Med J 2:1291–1294, 1953
Roberts AG, Elder GH, Newcombe RG, et al: Heterogeneity of familial porphyria cutanea tarda. J Med Genet 25:669–676, 1988
Lee GR. Porphyria. In Lee GR, Bithel TC, Foerster J, et al (eds): Wintrobe's Clinical Hematology, 9th ed, pp 1277–1280. Philadelphia, Lea & Febiger, 1993

DE BARSY

Synonyms. Cutis laxa-corneal clouding-mental retardation; progeroid De Barsy.

Symptoms and Signs. Both sexes. From birth. Cutis laxa (see). Cloudy corneas. Delayed psychomotor development and hypotonic dwarfism. Facies progeria-like, normal hair. Thumbs, great toes and hips dislocation, hyperreflexia; occasionally: cataract.

Etiology. Unknown. Cases sporadic. Possibly autosomal recessive inheritance.

Pathology. Skin: elastic fibers frayed, scarce and with low density. Collagen fiber network: normal.

BIBLIOGRAPHY. De Barsy AM, Moens E, Dierckx L: Dwarfism, oligophrenia and degeneration of the elastic tissue in skin and cornea. A new syndrome? Helv Paediatr Acta 23:305–313, 1968
Pontz BF, Zepp F, Stoss H: Biochemical, morphological and immunological findings in a patient with cutis laxa associated inborn disorder (De Barsy's syndrome). Eur J Pediatr 134:428–434, 1986
Karnes PS, Shamban AT, Olsen DR, et al: De Barsy syndrome: report of a case, literature review and elastin gene expression studies of the skin. Am J Med Genet 42:29–34, 1992

DEBRE-FITTKE

Synonym. Cutis laxa»dysostosis; cutis laxa recessive type II.

Symptoms and Signs. Skin and viscera. Those described in cutis laxa congenital form (see). Associated from birth with persistent fontanelles, moderate oxycephaly, hip dislocation. Isolated features of pigeon breast, flat feet, scoliosis. Weak joints may also be present in relatives of patients.

Etiology. Probably autosomal recessive inheritance.

Pathology. See Cutis laxa congenital form.

Therapy. See Cutis laxa congenital form.

Prognosis. Good quoad vitam.

BIBLIOGRAPHY. Debré R, Marie J, Seringe P: "Cutis laxa" avec dystrophies osseuses. Bull Soc Méd Hôp 53:1038–1039, 1937
Fittke H: Ueber eine ungewöhliche Form "multipler Erbubartung" (Chalodermie und Dysostose). Z Kinderheilk 63:510–523, 1942
Fitzsimmonds JS, Fitzsimmonds EM, Guibert PR, et al: Variable clinical presentation of cutis laxa. Clin Genet 28:284–295, 1985
Ogur G, Yuksel-Apak M, Demiryont M: Syndrome of congenital cutis laxa with ligamentous laxity and delayed development: report of a brother and sister from Turkey. Am J Med Genet 37:6–9, 1990

DE CLERAMBAULT

Synonyms. Clerambault I; Kandinski; erotomania pure.

Symptoms. Generally occurs in women. Sudden onset in a state of clear consciousness. Delusional belief that a man is profoundly in love with the patient. Person selected is usually a prominent public figure, older than the patient or her husband, with whom only a brief acquaintance exists. Other features that usually coexist are her interpretations of his reaction to her approaches expressing, not rejection, but a form of love, and belief that presents received from husband or other friends are secretly sent by him. Attempts with sexual intent, or actual assaults on the object of affection frequently occur.

Etiology. Unknown; erotomania may exist as autonomous entity or be premonitory syndrome of other psychosis, or occasionally just a symptom of psychosis of a paranoid type. This psychiatric entity rests upon a basis of unsatisfied affection associated with a rebellious tendency.

Therapy. Some cases respond to pharmacotherapy and some to electroconvulsive treatment. Hospitalization becomes necessary, especially if patient becomes actively aggressive.

Prognosis. Pure form chronic, stable, and persistently vehement. Persists usually for many years. When their approaches have been rejected, patients may become aggressive against victim or relatives.

BIBLIOGRAPHY. De Clérambault GG: Les Psychoses Passionelles; Oevre psychiatrique. Paris, Presses Universitaires, 1942
Jordan HW, Howe G: De Clerambault syndrome (erotomania): A review and case presentation. J Natl Med Assoc 72:979–985, 1980
Remington GJ, Jeffries JJ: Erotomanic delusions and electroconvulsive therapy: A case series. J Clin Psychiatr 55:306–308, 1994
Kaplan HI, Sadock BJ: Comprehensive Textbook of Psychiatry, 6th ed, p 169. Baltimore, Williams & Wilkins, 1995

DEFECATION SYNCOPE

Symptoms and Signs. In elderly. Usually after arising from bed at night or during disimpaction. Frequently associated, AV block, sinus bradycardia.

Etiology. Sudden decompression of rectum.

Diagnostic Procedures. *Electrocardiography. Valsalva maneuver.* May reproduce syncope. *X-ray of chest (to exclude pulmonary embolism).*

Prognosis. Good. Related to basic condition.

BIBLIOGRAPHY. Pathy MS: Defecation syncope. Age Ageing 7:233–238, 1978

Lewis RP, Budoulas H, Schaal SF, et al: Diagnosis and management of syncope. In Schlant RC, Alexander RW: Hurst's The Heart, 8th ed, p 934. New York, McGraw-Hill, 1994

DEFIBRINATING

Synonyms. Consumption coagulopathy; defibrination; disseminated intravascular coagulation. Compared with congenital hypofibrinogenemia or afibrinogenemia, deficiency of fibrinogen may develop in many pathologic conditions. The hemorrhages and bleeding become dramatic features of the following conditions:

1. High hematocrit and inadequate fibrinogen to form good clot
Cyanotic congenital heart disease. Vaquez-Osler
2. Impaired synthesis of fibrinogen
Hepatic diseases (rare). Amyloidosis
3. Excessive utilization and secondary general deficiency
Massive venous thrombosis
De Gimard
Moschcowitz
Waterhouse-Friderichsen
Giant cavernous hemangioma
Incompatible blood administration
Abruptio placenta
Dead fetus
Septic abortion
Amniotic fluid
Neoplastic diseases–hypofibrinogenemia
Extracorporeal circulation
4. Fibrinolysis
Primary form (hyperplasminemia)
Iatrogenic (administration of plasminogen activator). Endogenous release (surgery of lung; prostate; brain, neoplasm)
Deficiency inhibitors (liver disease)
Other proteolytic enzymes (leukemias). Secondary (association of defibrination and fibrinolysis)
Placenta previa
Dead fetus
Amniotic fluid
De Gimard
Lymphomas
Leukemias
Kasabach-Merritt
Waterhouse-Friderichsen
Overwhelming infections

See individual syndromes for symptoms, signs, and therapy.

BIBLIOGRAPHY. Fletcher AP, Alkjaersig N, Sherry S: Pathogenesis of the coagulation defect developing during pathological plasma proteolytic (fibrinolytic) states. I. The significance of fibrinogen proteolysis and circulating fibrinogen breakdown products. J Clin Invest 41:896–916, 1962

Sharp AA: Pathological fibrinolysis. Br Med Bull 20:240–245, 1964

Bithell TC: Acquired coagulation disorders. In Lee GR, Bithel TC, Foerster J, et al (eds): Wintrobe's Clinical Hematology, 9th ed, pp 1480–1483. Philadelphia, Lea & Febiger, 1993

DE GIMARD

Synonyms. Sheldon; purpura gangrenosa hemorrhagica; purpura fulminans.

Symptoms and Signs. Appears most often in children, in association with various infections (viral, streptococcal) or with pregnancy; sudden onset. Fever; prostration; diffuse skin ecchymosis; no involvement of mucosae; gangrene may occur rapidly. In childhood, gangrene and auto amputation of distal extremities, bleeding (gastrointestinal and CNS).

Etiology. Neisseria meningitidis infection in children with immature protein C and S systems that causes dermal microvascular thrombosis.

Pathology. In addition to hemorrhagic manifestation (Schwartzmann-type reaction in the skin), extensive intravascular thrombosis may occur.

Diagnostic Procedures. *Blood.* Usually, no abnormal coagulation; however, in some cases, deficiency of factor V, excess antithrombin, hypofibrinogenemia.

Therapy. Treatment of infection; general supportive treatment; heparin; fibrinogen; hyperbaric oxygenation.

Prognosis. Rapid, fatal course of 1–4 days.

BIBLIOGRAPHY. De Gimard M: Purpura hemorrhagique primitif au purpura infectieux primitif (thesis). Paris, 1844

Sheldon JH: Purpura neonatica. A possible clinical application of the Schwartzman phenomenon. Arch Dis Child 22:7–13, 1947

Marcinia KE, Wilson HD, Marlar RA: Neonatal purpura fulminans: A genetic disorder related to the absence of protein C in blood. Blood 65:15–20, 1985

Bithell TC: Bleeding disorders caused by vascular abnormalities. In Lee GR, Bithel TC, Foerster J, et al (eds): Wintrobe's Clinical Hematology, 9th ed, p 1376. Philadelphia, Lea & Febiger, 1993

DEGOS ACANTHOMA

Synonym. Clear cell acanthoma; acanthoma, clear cell.

Symptoms and Signs. Both sexes equally affected; onset from middle age. Single or multiple lesions formed by brown plaques, marginated, reddish, scaly, occurring mostly on limbs.

Etiology. Unknown.

Pathology. Acanthosis and papillomatosis with cells with clear cytoplasm and infiltration by granulocytes.

Diagnostic Procedures. Biopsy.

Therapy. Excision.

Prognosis. No reports of recurrence after excision or spontaneous disappearing.

BIBLIOGRAPHY. Degos R, Dehort J, Civatte J, et al: Epidermal tumour with an usual appearance: Clear cell acanthoma. Ann Dermatol Syph 9:361–371, 1962

MacKie RM: Epidermal skin tumors. In Champion RH, Burton JL, Ebling FJG (eds): Rook/Wilkinson/Ebling Textbook of Dermatology, 5th ed, p 1469. Oxford, Blackwell Scientific, 1992

DEGOS II

Synonyms. Erythrokeratoderma en cocardes.

Symptoms and Signs. From birth, fixed, erythematous, well demarcated plaques predilecting extensor surfaces, and round plaques with concentrical erythema and scaling that appear and disappear. Absence of palm keratoderma, but palm scaling erythrokeratolysis may be present.

Etiology. Autosomal dominant inheritance.

BIBLIOGRAPHY. Degos R, Delzant O, Morival H: Erytheme desquamatif en plaques congenital et familial (genodermatose nouvelle?) Bull Soc Fr Dem Syph 54:442–444, 1947

Griffiths WAD, Leigh IM, Marks R: Disorders of keratinization. In Champion RH, Burton JL, Ebling FJG (eds): Rook/Wilkinson/Ebling Textbook of Dermatology, 5th ed, p 1350. Oxford, Blackwell Scientific, 1992

DE HASS-HOUTSMULLER

Synonyms. Passow.

Symptoms and Signs. Association of von Recklinghausen (see) and Fuchs heterochromia (see).

BIBLIOGRAPHY. De Hass EBH, Houtsmiller AJ: Een patient met heterochromie van Fuchsen ziekte van Recklinghausen. Ned T Geneesk 106:1853–1857, 1962

DE JEANS

Synonym. Orbital floor.

Symptoms and Signs. Intense pain in superior maxillary region; hypoesthesia and paresthesia in area of first and second branch of trigeminal (V) nerve; exophthalmos; diplopia.

Etiology. Any lesion (e.g., infection; tumor) involving floor of orbit.

Pathology. See Etiology.

Diagnostic Procedures. *X-ray of skull. Cultures.*

Therapy. Depends on etiology.

Prognosis. Extension of lesion to cranial cavity may occur.

BIBLIOGRAPHY. DeJans MC: Le syndrome du plancher de l'orbite. Bull Mem Soc Fr Ophthalmol 48:473–485, 1935
Adams RD, Victor M: Principles of Neurology, 5th ed, p 590. New York, McGraw-Hill, 1993

DEJERINE-KLUMPKE

Synonyms. Klumpke; brachial plexus neuritis; lower radicular; paralysis brachial plexus.

Symptoms. Pain; hyperesthesia or lack of sensation on medial side of arm; weakness and then paralysis of hand. Disturbed vision.

Signs. Atrophy of interosseous, thenar, hypothenar, flexor carpi ulnaris, flexor digitorum muscles; sensory changes ulnar side of arm. Enophthalmos; myosis, narrowed palpebral fissure; hemifacial sweating (Horner).

Etiology. Lesion affecting inner cord of brachial plexus (eighth cervical to first thoracic) and sympathetic fibers. Infection and tumor (50%); trauma (50%).

Therapy. Depends on etiology.

Prognosis. Depends on etiology.

BIBLIOGRAPHY. Klumpke A: Contribution à l'étude des paralysies radiculaires du plexus brachial; paralysies radiculaires totales; paralysies radiculaires inférieures; de la participation des filets sympathiques oculopupillaires dans ces paralysies. Rev Med (Paris) 5:591–616; 739–790, 1885
Bauer J: Letter-Augusta Dejerine-Klumpke (Historical review). Ann Intern Med 81:128, 1974
Adams RD, Victor M: Principles of Neurology, 5th ed, p 1158. New York, McGraw-Hill, 1993

DEJERINE-MOUZON

Synonyms. Parietal lobe; pseudothalamic (Foix) see Foix.

Symptoms and Signs. Impairment of pain, thermal, tactile, and vibratory sense in half of body. In some cases with subcortical parietal lesions hyperpathia similar to that of Dèjerine-Roussy (see). If dominant lobe involved possibly aphasia, tactile agnosia, or Gerstman syndrome (see); in nondominant lesions possibly anagnosia.

Etiology. Lesions of parietal cortex (neoplastic hemorrhagic; degenerative, etc.).

Diagnostic Procedures. *CT scan. MR imaging. Evoked potentials. EEG.*

Therapy. According to nature and extent of lesion.

Prognosis. Variable usually poor.

BIBLIOGRAPHY. Botez MI: Parietal lobe syndromes. In Handbook of Clinical Neurology, vol 45, pp 63–85. Frederiks JAM (ed): Clinical Neuropathology. Amsterdam, Elsevier, 1985

DEJERINE "ONION PEEL SENSORY LOSS"

Symptoms. Sensory loss starting from mouth and nose and extending concentrically outward: "onion peel distribution."

Etiology. Lesions of medulla oblongata affecting the trigeminal (V) nerve centers.

BIBLIOGRAPHY. Déjérine J: Semiologie des Affections du Systeme Nerveux. Paris, Masson, 1914
Schneider RC, McGillicuddy JE: Concomitant craniocerebral and spinal trauma. In Vinken PJ, Bruyn GW: Handbook of Clinical Neurology, vol 24, pp 163–165. Amsterdam, North-Holland, 1976

DEJERINE RADICULAR

Eponym indicating the radicular pain and motor, sensorial, and trophic changes in areas of distribution of nerves compressed or irritated by any cause, mechanical (see Discogenic syndromes) or inflammatory, at nerve root site within dural cavity. To be differentiated from peripheral neuritis.

BIBLIOGRAPHY. Déjérine J: Semiologie des Affections du Systeme Nerveux. Paris, Masson, 1914

DEJERINE-ROUSSY

Synonyms. Thalamic hyperesthetic anesthesia; retrolenticular.

Symptoms and Signs. Complete hemianesthesia (contralateral to site of lesion), involving superficial, deep, and stereognostic sensations (face often spared). Threshold for stimuli raised considerably, but when sensation is elicited, intense and unpleasant reaction. Cold in particular elicits strong reaction, often accompanied by violent motor reaction. Passive movements and position apperception decreased or absent. Thalamic hyperpathia or phenomenon of central pain caused by unappreciated stimuli or central thalamic lesions. Occasionally, temporary flaccid hemiplegia or hemiparesis; hemiataxia with choreoathetoid movements and dysarthria; emotional overreactions.

Etiology. Thrombosis of thalamogeniculate artery, neoplastic lesion affecting nucleus ventralis posterolateralis of thalamus. May occur also with lesion of the white matter of parietal lobe.

Pathology. Edema; hemorrhagic softening of thalamus unilateral.

Therapy. General; symptomatic care. Amitriptyline, imipramine, thioridazine, fluphenazine. Surgery last resort since increases the sensory defect.

Prognosis. Progressive to complete loss of hemibody position. Relieved occasionally by surgery of frontal lobe.

BIBLIOGRAPHY. Déjérine J, Roussy G: Le syndrome thalamique. Rev Neurol (Paris) 14:521–532, 1906
Bogousslavsky J, Regli F, Uske A: Thalamic infarcts: Clinical syndromes etiology, and prognosis. Neurology 38:837–848, 1988

Combier J, Graveleau PH: Thalamic syndromes. In Vinken PJ, Bruyn GW: Handbook of Clinical Neurology, vol 45, pp 87–95. Amsterdam, Elsevier, 1985

Adams RD, Victor M: Principles of Neurology, 5th ed, pp 144–145. New York, McGraw-Hill, 1993

DEJERINE-SOTTAS

Synonyms. Gombault; Dejerine-Thomas; interstitial hypertrophic radiculoneuropathy; hypertrophic interstitial infantile neuritis. See Roussy-Levy; Charcot-Marie-Tooth, Roussy-Cornie.

Symptoms. Onset in infancy or early adolescence. Weakness and atrophy beginning in lower extremities and later spreading to upper ones (resembling Charchot-Marie-Tooth). Marked sensory loss in all four extremities; incoordination of arms.

Signs. Kyphoscoliosis; clubfoot; fasciculation; areflexia; Romberg sign; miosis; nystagmus; increase in size of nerve trunks.

Etiology. Unknown; possibly includes different entities; considerable difference in inheritance reported in various groups. Recessive and dominant types. Autosomal dominant inheritance.

Pathology. Hypertrophic neuropathy (onion bulb formation in histology).

Diagnostic Procedures. *Blood and urine.* Negative. *Spinal fluid.* (In some groups of patients, increase of protein.) *Biopsy of nerve.* See Pathology. *Electromyography. X-rays.* Vertebral anomalies.

Therapy. Symptomatic.

Prognosis. Progressive condition; death from complications in third–fourth decade.

BIBLIOGRAPHY. Déjérine J, Sottas S: Sur la névrite interstitielle, hypertrophique et progressive de l'enfant. CR Soc Biol 2:43–53, 1890

Ouvrier RA, McLeod JC, Conchin TE: The hypertrophic forms of hereditary motor and sensory neuropathy. A study of hypertrophic Charcot-Marie-Tooth disease (HMSN II) and Dejerine-Sottas disease (HMSN III) in childhood. Brain 110:121–148, 1987

Adams RD, Victor M: Principles of Neurology, 5th ed, pp 1149–1150. New York, McGraw-Hill, 1993

DEJERINE-THOMAS

Synonyms. Presenile ataxia; olivopontocerebellar; pontoolivocerebellar. See olivocerebellar degeneration syndromes and Friedreich ataxia and Menzel.

Symptoms. Onset in middle life or later. Progressive ataxia of extremity and trunk. Dysarthria; oscillation of head and body. Mental deterioration. Later sphincters affected.

Signs. Wavering gait; rigidity and extrapyramidal signs; nystagmus; deep reflexes exaggerated; Babinski sign.

Etiology. Unknown.

Pathology. Atrophy of cortex of cerebellum, olivary, pontine, and arcuate nuclei, middle cerebellar peduncle.

Diagnostic Procedures. *CT scan. MRI. Neuroimaging.*

Therapy. Symptomatic.

Prognosis. Progression in 5–10 years to total incapacitation. Death from intercurrent diseases.

BIBLIOGRAPHY. Déjérine J, Thomas A: L'atrophie olivo-ponto-cérébelleuse. Nov Iconog Salpêt 13:330–370, 1900

Geary JR, Earll KM, Rose AS: Olivopontocerebellar atrophy. Neurology 6:218–224, 1956

Jellinger K: Pallidal, pallidonigral and pallidoluysionigral degenerations

including association with thalamic and dentate degenerations. In Vinken PJ, Bruyn GW, Klawans HL (eds): Handbook of Clinical Neurology, vol 49, p 450. Amsterdam, Elsevier, 1986

DEJERINE TOXIC PARAPLEGIA

Obsolete. Paraplegia from peripheral nevritis and ataxia from opioid abuse. Presently paraplegia observed in opioid addiction is referred to as compression from sleeping in malposition (see Saturday night).

BIBLIOGRAPHY. Dejerine J: Sur un cas de paraplegie par nevrites peripheriques chez une ataxique morphinomane (Contribution al'etude de la nevrite peripherique). Comp Rend Soc Biol Paris 4:137–143, 1887

DE LA CHAPELLE

Synonyms. "Ring around the chondrocyte" dysplasia; neonatal osseous dysplasia I.

Symptoms and Signs. Both sexes. Limbs extremely short; fibula and ulna triangular; cleft palate; small thorax, genitourinary system anomalies. Respiratory insufficiency cause of death (laryneal stenosis, tracheobronchomalacia).

Etiology. Autosomal recessive inheritance.

Pathology. Cartilage from respiratory system abnormal: tracheobronchomalacia, pulmonary hypoplasia. Heart: patent foramen ovale and ductus Botalli. Typical: resting cartilage contains "ring" around chondrocytes.

Diagnostic Procedures. *Blood.* Evidence of variable hematologic abnormalities and endocrine dysfunctions. *X-ray.* See signs.

Therapy. Symptomatic.

Prognosis. Neonatal death.

BIBLIOGRAPHY. De la Chapelle A, Maroteaux P, Havu N, et al: Une rare dysplasie osseuse letale de la transmission recessive autosomique. Arch Franch Pediat 29:759–770, 1972

Whytley CB, Burke BA, Granroth G, et al: De la Chapelle dysplasia. Am J Med Genet 25:29–39, 1986

Stern HJ, Graham JM Jr, Lachman RS, et al: Atelosteogenesis type III: A distinct skeletal dysplasia with features overlapping atelosteogenesis and oto-palato-digital syndrome type II. Am J Med Genet 36:183–195, 1990

DE LANGE I

Synonyms. Brachmann-de Lange; Cornelia De Lange I; Amsterdam dwarfism; Amstelodamensis typus degenerativus.

Symptoms and Signs. Prenatal growth retardation. Females prevalence in the lower birth weight group. *Skin.* Hirsutism of face; forehead; back, cutis marmorata; perioral pale cyanosis. *Head.* Brachycephaly or microbrachycephaly. *Eyebrows.* Long, usually meeting on midline. *Eyes.* Exotropia, usually alternating. *Ears.* Low set. *Nose.* Small, upturned. *Mouth.* Widely spaced teeth; upper lip small midline beak; lower lip corresponding notch, angles downward. *Arms.* Limited extension at the elbow. *Hands.* Simian crease; thumb proximally inserted or absent; fingers small, incurved; some rudimentary or absent. Difference between two hands. *Feet.* Syndactyly, partial or total. *Other.* Mental retardation, limited vocabulary or no speech. Walking possible with assistance or alone. Development and weight gain markedly impaired. Epilepsy (20%). Congenital heart defect (17%).

Etiology. Unknown; most cases sporadic; discussed genetic basis probably autosomal dominant inheritance. (In some cases chromosomal abnormalities have been reported: apparent translocation of major portion of one chromosome of G group to chromosome A3 and other group alterations.) Environmental damage during gestation excluded.

Pathology. See Signs. Developmental anomalies of brain; microcephaly and convolutional distortion; abnormality of gastrointestinal system; occasionally, cardiac malformations.

Diagnostic Procedures. *Chromosome study. Blood, urine, and cerebrospinal fluid.*Usually normal. *Nitrogen balance study, basal metabolic rate.* Usually normal; paradoxically with the severe growth failure. *Endocrinologic studies.* For possible associated defects and differential diagnosis. *Prenatal diagnosis.* Plasma protein A suggested as a marker.

Therapy. Symptomatic.

Prognosis. Progressive condition. Intestinal obstruction, infections, complications often cause of death.

BIBLIOGRAPHY. Brachmann E: Ein Fall von symmetrischer. Monodactylie Durch Ulnadefekt Jb Kinderheilk 84:224–235, 1916
De Lange C: Sur un type nouveau de dé-génération (typus Amstelodamensis). Arch Med Enfant 36:713–719, 1933
Hawley PP, Jackson LG, Kurnit DM: Sixty-four patients with Brachmann–De Lange syndrome: A survey. Am J Med Genet 20:453–459, 1985
Filippi G: The de Lange syndrome: report of 15 cases. Clin Genet 35:343–363, 1989
Adams RD, Victor M: Principles of Neurology, 5th ed, pp 1018–1019. New York, McGraw-Hill, 1993

DELAYED-SLEEP-PHASE

Synonyms. Insomnia delayed-phase-pattern.

Symptoms and Signs. Usually in healthy elderly persons. Chronic inability to fall asleep at conventional time (usually not before 3–6 AM) subject may sleep normally until 11 AM–2 PM or awake early in the morning and usually sleep 1 or 2 hours in the afternoon.

Etiology. Alteration of normal circadian rhythm of sleep–wake cycle, possibly owing to metabolic alterations.

Therapy. Melatonine at 10 PM and strong light exposure at time of awakening.

BIBLIOGRAPHY. Monk TH: Disorders of chronobiology. In Kruger MH, Roth T, Dement WC (eds): Principles and Practice of Sleep Medicine, pp 324–337. Philadelphia, WB Saunders, 1989
DeGroot LJ: Endocrinology, 3rd ed. Philadelphia, WB Saunders, 1995

DEL CASTILLO

Synonyms. Germinal aplasia; testicular dysgenesis (Sertoli cell only). See Male pseudohermaphroditism, incomplete hereditary (Type I).

Symptoms. Sterility; normal libido and erection.

Signs. Normally developed man with all secondary sexual characteristics; testis small or normal.

Etiology. Either X-linked inheritance or male limited autosomal dominant or recessive inheritance has been proposed. The same findings observed after exposure to radiation or cancer chemotherapy.

Pathology. Seminiferous tubules with Sertoli cells; little or absent tubular fibrosis; no germinal cells. Leydig cells normal.

Diagnostic Procedures. *Sperm count.* Low. *Urine.* Decreased 17–ketosteroids; normal FSH hormone.

Therapy. None.

Prognosis. When caused by radiation, damage may be reversible.

BIBLIOGRAPHY. Del Castillo E, Trabucco A, de la Balze FA: Syndrome

produced by absence of germinal epithelium without impairment of Sertoli or Leydig cells. J Clin Endocrinol 7:493–502, 1947
Chaganti RSK, Jhanwar SC, Ehrenbard LT, et al: Genetically determined asynapsis, spermatogenic degeneration and infertility in men. Am J Hum Genet 32:833–848, 1980
Winter SJ: Clinical disorders of the testis. In DeGroot LJ (ed): Endocrinology, 3rd ed, p 2391. Philadelphia, WB Saunders, 1995

DELLEMAN-ORTHUYS

Synonyms. Oculo-cerebro-cutaneous.

Symptoms and Signs. Both sexes. From birth. *Skin.* Areas of aplasia and tags (about 1 cm in diameter) predominantly around eyes and nose; rings of denser hair growth around scalp lesions. Orbital cysts, microphthalmia, colobomas, skull defects and neurological pathological manifestations.

Etiology. Unknown. Sporadic mosaicism from a mutant gene (?).

Pathology. Histopathology of skin lesions not reported. Skull defects and cerebral malformations (poroencephalopathy and corpus callosum agenesis).

BIBLIOGRAPHY. Delleman JW, Orthuys JWE: Orbital cyst in addition to congenital cerebral and focal dermal malformations: A new entity? Clin Genet 19:191–198, 1981
Glorgi PL, Gabrielli O, Catassi C, et al: Oculocerebrocutaneous syndrome: A description of a new case. Eur J Pediatr 148:325–326, 1989

DEMARQUAY

Synonyms. Demarquay-Richet; Van der Woude; cleft lip—palate; lip pit—cleft palate.

Symptoms and Signs. No sex predominance or limitation; very rare (1:75,000–1:100,000). Fistulas of lower lip appearing as pits or humps on vermillion part of lip, usually equidistant from midline, or, occasionally, with different degrees of asymmetry. Different depths of depression; usually asymptomatic or secreting small amount of saliva. All types of clefts. Some members of family may have double lower lip only. Association with other malformations found: anomalies of extremities; popliteal pterygia; anomalies of genitourinary tract.

Etiology. Unknown; autosomal dominant inheritance with variable expressivity of the trait; high degree of penetrance (80%). Pits expressed more frequently than clefts.

Pathology. Fistula lined by stratified squamous epithelium; large epithelial cells with small nuclei also found. Serous acini and mucous acini may be present.

Therapy. Surgical excision; correction of cleft.

BIBLIOGRAPHY. Demarquay JN: Quelques considerations sur le bec-delievre. Gaz Med Paris 13:52–54, 1845
Van der Woude A: Fistula labii inferioris congenita and its association with cleft lip and palate. Am J Hum Genet 6:244–256, 1954
Burdick AB, Bixler D, Puckett CL: Genetic analysis in families with Van der Woude syndrome. J Craniofac Genet Dev Biol 5:181–208, 1985

DEMENTIA PARALYTICA

Synonyms. General paralysis of the insane; paretic neurosyphilis; general paresis; syphilitic paresis.

Symptoms. Combination of psychotic and neurologic symptoms. *Psychotic.* Demented; expansive; agitated; depressive, with possible variation and interlacing of manifestations in same individual. First symptoms, usually, impairment of efficiency and disorientation, memory failure, dream-like activity, delusional states, emotional changes, defect in judgment. Patient usually does not worry over his condition. *Neurologic.* Headache; body pains; vague muscle weakness; hyporeactive midriasis or Argyll Robertson (see); variable reflex changes; slurred speech; tremor; Lissauer paralysis (see).

Etiology.   Late form of syphilis.

Pathology.   Leptomeninges cloudy, thickened, arachnoid adherent to pia; atrophy of brain with hydrocephalus ex vacuo; infiltration of leptomeninges greatest at frontal pole, extending into cortex and into adventitial spaces; increased iron content of brain; involvement of ganglion cells (degeneration); glia increased; presence of free spirochetes.

Diagnostic Procedures.   *Spinal fluid.* Positive serologic tests; increased (monocytic) cells and proteins. *Blood.* Serologic tests. *CT scan. MRI.* Brain shrinkage.

Therapy.   Penicillin. Symptomatic and nursing care.

Prognosis.   Progressive course. Death in 3 years; delayed by prompt and full treatment.

BIBLIOGRAPHY. Morris J C (ed): Handbook of Dementing Illnesses. New York, Marcel Dekker, 1993

DE MEYER

Synonym.   Median cleft face; frontonasal dysplasia.

Symptoms and Signs.   Both sexes affected; present from birth. Midline frontal bone. Extremely variable degree of deficits: widow's peak; hypertelorism. Nasal tip: Variable degree of alteration from notched broad to divided nostrils; absence of prolabia with median cleft lip or without cleft palate. Mental deficiency severe in 8% of cases, mild in 12%.

Etiology.   Unknown. Sporadic. Both autosomal dominant and recessive inheritance proposed.

Therapy.   Cosmetic surgery.

Prognosis.   Good quoad vitam; usually, normal mental development.

BIBLIOGRAPHY. Hoppe I: Eine angeborene Spaltung der Nase. Press Med 2:164–165, 1859
De Meyer W: The median cleft face syndrome. Differential diagnosis of cranium bifidum occultum, hypertelorism and median cleft nose, lip and palate. Neurology 17:961–971, 1967
Kwee ML, Lindhout D: Frontonasal dysplasia, coronal craniosynostosis, pre- and postaxial polydactyly and split nails: A new autosomal dominant mutant with reduced penetrance and variable expression? Clin Genet 24:200–205, 1983
Naidich TP, Osborn RE, Bener B, et al: Median cleft face syndrome: MR and CT data from 11 children. J Comput Assist Tomogr 12:57–64, 1988

DE MORGAN

Synonyms.   Capillary angioma; senile angioma; cayenne pepper spots; rub spots; papillary varix; telagiectasias, spider angiomas.

Symptoms and Signs.   Elderly persons affected; occasionally appears in younger people. Predominantly affects face and ears. Small, red masses, not branching, of dilated vascular loops.

Etiology.   Unknown; immunologic reaction considered. Dilatation of venules.

Pathology.   Dilated, thin-walled venules, without vascular tissue proliferation; decrease of elastic tissue in layers of corium.

Therapy.   Cosmetic.

Prognosis.   Persistent and progressive condition.

BIBLIOGRAPHY. De Morgan C: The Origin of Cancer. Considered with Reference to the Treatment of the Disease. London, Churchill, 1872
Bean WB: Vascular Spiders and Related Lesions of the Skin. Springfield, Charles C Thomas, 1958
Bithell TC: Bleeding disorders caused by vascular abnormalities. In Lee GR, Bithel TC, Foerster J, et al (eds): Wintrobe's Clinical Hematology, 9th ed. Philadelphia, Lea & Febiger, 1993

DE MORSIER I

Synonyms.   Morsier I; acromegalo-epileptic; epileptic-endocrine; see Penfield.

Symptoms.   Appears in first decade of life. Seizures or other epileptic manifestations (spasm, myoclonus). Mental deterioration; precocious puberty.

Signs.   Accelerated growth and weight increase; acromegalic aspect in some cases. All signs of precocious sexual development.

Etiology and Pathology.   Possible causes: infundibular, mammilary, or epiphyseal tumors, inflammatory lesions with meningoencephalitis; traumatic lesions.

Diagnostic Procedures.   *Electroencephalography.* Pattern consistent with subcortical deep lesion. *CT brain scan. MR imaging. Pituitary hormonal excretion studies.*

Therapy.   That of the type of epilepsy.

Prognosis.   Poor; mental deterioration constant feature.

BIBLIOGRAPHY. De Morsier G: Pathologie du diencéphale. Les syndromes psicologiques et syndromes sensorio-moteurs. Schweiz Arch Neurol Psychiatr 54:161–226, 1944
Bondin G, Barbizet J: D'association epilepsieendocrinopathie. Rev Neurol (Paris) 91:330–347, 1954
De Morsier G: Contribution à l'étude clinique des altérations de la formation réticulée: Le syndrome sensorio-moteur et psychologique. J Neurol Sci 4:15–49, 1966
Kohler MC: L'association comitialité, croissance excessive et puberté précoce, arrieration mentale, une forme particuliere de séquelles d'encephalopathies ou d'encéphalite infantile. J Med Lyon 48:1437–1530, 1967

DENIAL

Symptoms.   Patient denies objective deficits, such as blindness, paralysis, speech defects (see Anton and Cotard). When confronted with evidence, vigorously denies that affected part (e.g., extremities) belongs to him.

Etiology.   Disturbed psychology related to personality changes, usually caused by structural brain damage.

BIBLIOGRAPHY. Kaplan HI, Sadock BJ: Comprehensive Textbook of Psychiatry, 6th ed. Baltimore, Williams & Wilkins, 1995

DENNIE-MARFAN

Synonyms.   Paralysis, congenital syphilitic; juvenile paresis; syphilitic congenital paralysis. See Hutchinson triad.

Symptoms and Signs.   Both sexes affected; onset insidious or acute in infancy or childhood. Acute vomiting; fever; convulsions; loss of consciousness; spastic or flaccid tetraplegia; development of mental retardation. Insidious, slow progression from weakness to tetraparesis.

Etiology.   Congenital syphilitic infection.

Pathology.   Diffuse syphilitic lesions in brain, cerebellum, and spinal cord.

Diagnostic Procedures. *Blood. Spinal fluid. Serology. EEG.*

Therapy. Penicillin.

Prognosis. Locomotor symptoms recede with treatment. Mental retardation remains.

BIBLIOGRAPHY. Dennie C: Partial paralysis of the lower extremities in children accompanied by backward mental development. Am J Syph 13:157–163, 1929

Adams RD, Victor M: Principles of Neurology, 5th ed, pp 623–625. New York, McGraw-Hill

DENNY-BROWN I

Synonyms. Carcinomatous neuromyopathy; myopathy—sensorial paraneoplastic neuropathy; paraneoplastic neuromyopathy.

Symptoms and Signs. Many neurologic syndromes (seldom in the pure form; usually in variable combinations) occur in patients with neoplastic diseases. Peripheral neuropathies; radiculopathies; posterior root degeneration; myelopathies; cerebellar degeneration; dementia. These syndromes can cause disability that is out of proportion with the neoplastic condition and thus dominates the clinical aspect. In addition, neuromuscular involvement may precede the discovery of tumor.

Etiology. Unknown. Most tumors may be associated with these manifestations.

Therapy. Early surgery of neoplasia.

Prognosis. Early surgery may be extremely rewarding for the control of the paraneoplastic syndromes.

BIBLIOGRAPHY. Denny-Brown N: Primary sensory neuropathy with muscular changes by carcinoma. J Neurol 2:73–87, 1948

Tyler HR: Paraneoplastic syndromes of nerve, muscle and neuromuscular junction. Ann NY Acad Sci 230:348–357, 1974

Adams RD, Victor M: Principles of Neurology, 5th ed, p 1009. New York, McGraw-Hill, 1993

DENYS-DRASH

Synonyms. Drash; Wilms tumor—pseudohermaphroditism; nephropathy; Wilms tumor—genital anomalies, including Frasier.

Symptoms and Signs. Rare. From birth: Severe urogenital malformations causing final renal failure before 2 years of age; pseudohermaphroditism (ambiguous or female external genitalia); and Wilms tumor (see Epstein).

Etiology. Mutation in the zinc finger domains of one WT1 gene, affecting DNA sequence recognition. Autosomal dominant inheritance; in two families mutations shown to arise "de novo." XY kariotype most frequent but also 46,XXY or 46XX.

Pathology. Nephropathy, focal or diffuse mesangial sclerosis: Streak gonads, gonadoblastoma. Wilms tumor.

Diagnostic Procedures. *Chromosomal studies, kidney echography.*

Therapy. Surgery for malformations, kidney transplantation.

Prognosis. Poor.

BIBLIOGRAPHY. Frasier SB, Bashore RA, Mosier HD: Gonadoblastoma associated with pure gonadal dysgenesis in monozygotic twins. J Pediat 64:740–745, 1964

Denys P, Malvaux P, van den Bergh H, et al: Association d'un syndrome anatomo-pathologique de pseudohermaphoditisme masculin, d'une tumor de Wilms, d'une nephropathie parenchymateuse et d'un mosaicisme XX/XY. Arch Fanc Pediat 24:729–739, 1967

Drash A, Sherman F, Hartmann WH, et al: A syndrome of pseudoher-

maphroditism, Wilms' tumor, hypertension, and degenerative renal disease. J Pediatr 76:565–593, 1970

Moorthy AV, Chesney RW, Lubinsky M: Chronic renal failure and XY gonadal dysgenesis: Frasier syndrome—a commentary on reported cases. AM J Med Genet Suppl 3:297–302, 1987

Pelletier J, Bruening W, Kashtan CE, et al: Germline mutations in the Wilm's tumor suppressor gene are associated with abnormal urogenital development in Denys-Drash syndrome. Cell 67:437–447, 1991

DE QUERVAIN I

Synonyms. Quervain I; clasped thumb, congenital; flexor pollicis longus—stenosing tendovaginitis; pollex varus; snapping thumb; trigger thumb.

Symptoms. More frequent in adults (prevalent in females) than in children (equal sex distribution); insidious onset. In adults, in addition to the thumb, other fingers may be involved; in children, limited to the thumb. Adult reports a snapping phenomenon in the distal interphalangeal joint. In children, mother reports that child has the thumb in fixed flexion.

Signs. Small nontender mass palpable at metacarpophalangeal articulation. Frequently, both thumbs present nodule, if snapping phenomenon is present in only one hand.

Etiology. Congenital, traumatic, or both. Snapping caused by the passage of the bulbous tendon through narrowed sheath both in extension and flexion.

Pathology. Local thickening of tendon sheath. Microscopic inflammatory changes according to duration of condition.

Therapy. Surgery.

Prognosis. Complete correction by surgery.

BIBLIOGRAPHY. De Quervain F: Ueber eine Form von chronischer Tendovaginitis. Cor Bl Schweiz Arzte (Basel) 25:389–394, 1895

Hauck G: Ueber eine Tendovaginitis stenosans der Beugeschnenscheide mit dem Phanomen des schnellende Finger. Arch Klin Chir 123:233–258, 1923

Weckesser EC, Reed JR, Heiple KG: Congenital clasped thumb (congenital flexion-adduction deformity of the thumb): A syndrome, not a specific entity. J Bone Joint Surg (Am) 50:1417–1428, 1968

Milford L: Carpal tunnel and ulnar tunnel syndrome. In Crenshaw AH (ed): Campbell's Operative Orthopedics, 7th ed, pp 462–463. St Louis, CV Mosby, 1987

DE QUERVAIN II

Synonyms. Quervain II; giant cell thyroiditis; granulomatous thyroiditis; pseudotuberculous thyroiditis; acute nonsuppurative thyroiditis; subacute thyroiditis.

Symptoms. More common in middle-aged women; onset dramatic, often after infection of respiratory tract. Hyperthermia; sweating; malaise; agitation; diffuse myalgia; cephalalgia; pain in thyroid area radiating to ear or face; dysphagia.

Signs. Moderate enlargement and tenderness of thyroid. Tachycardia.

Etiology. Unknown. Viral infection and autoimmune nature considered possibilities.

Pathology. Thyroid enlarged, firm, pale; capsule not involved. Histology. Inflammatory changes, fibrous scarring. Presence of pseudotubercles (clusters of fibroblasts, lymphocyte macrophages, plasma cells, arranged around giant cells) among normal tissue.

Diagnostic Procedures. *Blood.* Leukocytosis or normal white blood cell count; increased erythrocyte sedimentation rate; moderate increase of protein-bound iodine; thyroid autobodies seldom present. *Basal metabolic rate.* Normal. *Ultrasonography.* Hypoechogenicity of affected areas. *Thyroid scan.* Typical reduction of iodine uptake. *Biopsy.* Fine needle aspiration: see Pathology.

Therapy. Rest. Analgesics and anti-inflammatory agents. For severe symptoms, short trials with corticosteroid (3 weeks). For refractory form roentgen treatment of thyroid area (300–400 r) advised by some authors.

Prognosis. Usually, spontaneous regression with possible relapses of decreasing intensity.

BIBLIOGRAPHY. Mygind H: Thyroiditis akuta simplex. Laryngol 91:181–193, 1985
De Quervain F: Ueber acute, nicht eiterige Thyroiditis. Arch Klin Chir 67:706–714, 1902
Magalini SI, Pericoli F: La tiroidite subacuta: Osservazione su alcuni aspetti ematochimici e coagulativi. Minerva Med 2:2–16, 1955
Hamburger JI: The various presentations of thyroiditis: Diagnostic considerations. Ann Intern Med 104:219–221, 1986
Volpé R: Subacute and sclerosing thyroiditis. In De Groot LJ (ed): Endocrinology, 3rd ed, pp 742–747, 1599. Philadelphia, WB Saunders, 1995

DERCUM

Synonyms. Anders; adiposis dolorosa; fibrolipomatosis dolorosa; lipalgia; lipomatosis dolorosa.

Symptoms. Prevalent in women 40–60 years of age. Pain in part of body where localized accumulation of fat occurs. Asthenia; headache; frequently amenorrhea and ecchymoses; diminution of sweating; terminally, mental depression and deterioration.

Signs. Subcutaneous accumulation of elevated, dry, reddish or bluish fat; anesthesia and diminished cutaneous sensibility.

Etiology. Unknown; autonomous existence of clinical entity is doubted. Considered as part of generalized obesity.

Pathology. Multiple, nodular subcutaneous fat accumulation and degeneration.

Diagnostic Procedures. Nonspecific.

Therapy. Weight reduction, excision of tumors, lidocaine intravenously.

Prognosis. Long progressive course. Cardiac failure often terminal episode.

BIBLIOGRAPHY. Dercum FX: Three cases of an hitherto unclassified affection resembling in its grosser aspects obesity, but associated with special nervous symptoms, adiposis dolorosa. Am J Med Sci 104:521–535, 1892
Joseph HL: Adiposis dolorosa (Dercum's disease). Arch Dermatol 74:332, 1956
Burton JL, Cunlife WJ: Subcutaneous fat. In Champion RH, Burton JL, Ebling FJG (eds): Rook/Wilkinson/Ebling Textbook of Dermatology, 5th ed, pp 2153–2154. Oxford, Blackwell Scientific, 1992

DERMAL ERYTHROPOIESIS

Synonyms. Erythropoiesis, dermic; dermic erythropoiesis.

Symptoms and Signs. Appears in newborn. Generalized hemorrhagic-purpuric rash. Individual lesions 2–7 mm in diameter, raised dark blue magenta, slowly regressing and disappearing in 3–4 weeks. Hepatomegaly; splenomegaly; jaundice (not constant); lymphadenopathy.

Etiology. Associated with intrauterine viral infections; cytomegalo-virus demonstrated in some cases; rubella strongly considered in other cases.

Pathology. *Skin.* Poorly delimited aggregates of large nucleated cells; erythroblasts in different stages of maturation from normoblast to orthochromatic erythroblast, and nonnucleated erythrocytes. Absence of myeloid elements, megakaryocytes, and lymphocytes. Erythroblast plaques present exclusively in extravascular sites. Other pathologic findings consistent with cytomegalic infections or other virus infection (e.g., hepatitis, encephalitis). Various congenital malformations.

Diagnostic Procedures. *Blood.* Anemia; reticulocytosis; thrombocytopenia; hyperbilirubinemia. *Virus cultures. Biopsy of liver by needle.*

Therapy. Symptomatic.

Prognosis. Rash completely disappears in 3–4 weeks. Life expectancy depends on associated pathologic involvement and malformations.

BIBLIOGRAPHY. Dieterich H: Studien uber extramedullare Blutbildung bei chirugichen Erkrankungen. Arch Klin Chir 134:166–175, 1925
Brough AJ, Jones D, Page RH, et al: Dermal erythropoiesis in neonatal infants. Pediatrics 40:627–635, 1967

DERMATITIS ARTEFACTA

Synonyms. Factitial dermatitis; neurotic excoriation. See Purpura, psychogenic.

Symptoms. Prevalent in adolescent women or young adults; rare in children, except if mental retardation is present; connected with malingering for reluctant induction in armed services or for insurance claims. Peculiar patient demeanor. Strong denial of self-infliction of lesions and display of ingenuity and cunning. Complaint of unusual sensation in the skin.

Signs. Cutaneous lesions that widely vary in configuration and distribution, usually localized in areas easily reached by patient's hands. Pattern of lesion does not conform with known pathologic process.

Etiology. Hysterical derangement; calls attention to patient or compensates for psychological disturbance, inferiority complex, lack of sexual satisfaction, or malingering.

Pathology. Acute or chronic inflammation resulting from nail, glass fragments, or knife scratching, caustic application, cigarette burning.

Diagnostic Procedures. Differential diagnosis with polyarteritis nodosa (see) and porphyria tarda (see).

Therapy. Psychiatric treatment. Once nature of lesions is suspected, firm dressing and supervision.

Prognosis. In cases where the simple basic emotional problem is identified the situation can be cured. Generally expression of deep disturbance bodes poor prognosis.

BIBLIOGRAPHY. Bithell TC: Bleeding disorders caused by vascular abnormalities. In Lee GR, Bithel TC, Foerster J, et al (eds): Wintrobe's Clinical Hematology, 9th ed. Philadelphia, Lea & Febiger, 1993
Kaplan HI, Sadock BJ: Comprehensive Textbook of Psychiatry, 6th ed, pp 1530–1531. Baltimore, Williams & Wilkins, 1995

DERMATITIS, RADIATION

Synonyms. Radiodermatitis; roentgen poikiloderma; roentgen atrophy. Two forms are recognized: acute and chronic types.

ACUTE

Symptoms and Signs. The course is divided into four phases:

1. Erythema and edema of exposed areas that progress for 48 hours and then rapidly subside.
2. Absence of symptoms and signs for 1–4 days.
3. Erythema with occasional blood extravasation into involved areas; progressive formation of vesicles and bullae; third week after exposure bullae dessicate and desquamate.
4. Regression of signs; however, areas greatly injured do not heal.

Etiology. Exposure to roentgen rays.

Pathology. In acute stage, hydropic alterations in epidermis. In dermis, inflammatory infiltrates, edema, homogenization of collagen bundles.

Therapy. Corticosteroids for topical and systemic use.

Prognosis. According to intensity of exposure.

CHRONIC

Symptoms and Signs. Slow progressive formation of telangiectasis, pigmentation, atrophy, and finally ulceration of areas exposed.

Etiology. Repeated, small doses of X-rays.

Pathology. Atrophy, hyperplasia, and finally neoplasia, involving all skin components.

Therapy. Small areas can be excised and skin grafts applied.

Prognosis. Malignant incidence 10–28%.

BIBLIOGRAPHY. Spittle MF: Radiotherapy and reactions to ionizing radiation. In Champion RH, Burton JL, Ebling FJG (eds): Rook/Wilkinson/Ebling Textbook of Dermatology, 5th ed, pp 3089–3091. Oxford, Blackwell Scientific, 1992

DERMATOOSTEOLYSIS, KIRGHIZIAN TYPE

Synonyms. Kirghizian type dermato-osteolysis; Kozlova.

Symptoms. Both sexes. From infancy. Recurrent skin ulceration, arthralgia, fever, visual impairment, or blindness. Oligodontia; nail dystrophy, keratitis.

Signs. Fistolous osteolysis around joints.

Etiology. Autosomal recessive.

BIBLIOGRAPHY. Kozlova SI, Altshuler BA, Kravchenko VA: Self limited autosomal recessive syndrome of skin ulceration, arthro-osteolysis with pseudoacromegaly, keratitis and oligodontia in a Kirghizian family. Am J Med Genet 15:205–210, 1983

DERRY

Synonyms. Generalized gangliosidosis type 2; gangliosidosis type 2 GM1; infantile/juvenile GM1 gangliosidosis type 2.

Symptoms. Both sexes affected; onset in early infancy (at 6–20 months). Locomotor ataxia present from 1 year of age. Internal strabismus; loss of coordinated movements and speech; weakness of extremities, then spasticity; mental and motor deterioration up to lethargy; startle response to sound; seizures; late blindness; recurrent respiratory infections.

Signs. Normal facies. Macrocephaly. Occasionally skeletal dysplasia. This type of gangliosidosis usually does not have facial and peripheral edema, hepatosplenomegaly, macular cherry spot, and macroglossia.

Etiology. Autosomal recessive inheritance. Enzyme defect: acid beta galactosidase deficiency; difference in residual enzyme activity could explain the phenotypic difference between types 1 and 2, rate of storage in type 2 being slower. Defect on chromosome 3.

Pathology. Neuronal lipoidosis and renal epithelial ballooning similar to type 1; visceral histiocytosis not as pronounced.

Diagnostic Procedures. *Blood.* Vacuolated lymphocytes. *Bone marrow.* Foamy cells and vacuolated lymphocytes. *Urine.* Moderate amount of mucopolysaccharide; assay of beta-galactosidase. *X-rays.* Mild changes of long bones; vertebral beaking; modeling deformity of pelvis. *Fibroblast culture.* Assay of beta-galactosidase activity.

Therapy. Symptomatic.

Prognosis. Death at 3–10 years of age, usually from overwhelming infection.

BIBLIOGRAPHY. Derry DM: Late infantile systemic lipidosis: Delineation of two types. Neurology 18:340–348, 1968
Suzuki Y, Sakuraba H, Oshima A, O'Brien JS: Galactosidase deficiency. In Scriver CR, Beaudet AL, Sly WS, et al: The Metabolic and Molecular Bases of Inherited Disease, 7th ed, pp 2787–2789. New York, McGraw-Hill, 1995

DE SANCTIS-CACCHIONE

Synonyms. Xerodermic idiocy; xeroderma pigmentosum—idiocy; xeroderma pigmentosum types A, B, D, and G. See Kaposi II.

Symptoms and Signs. Both sexes affected; onset in infancy or early childhood. *Dermatologic.* Lentigines and areas of pigmentation. Manifestations of xeroderma pigmentosum are dependent on age and environment (sun sensitivity). Skin tumor, usually basal and squamous cell carcinoma and, less frequently, malignant melanoma. Alterated dermatoglyphic pattern. *Neurologic.* Microcephaly; speech disorders; mental deficiency; spastic paralysis; convulsions; cerebellar ataxia. *Ocular.* Photophobia; keratitis; ectropion. *Endocrine.* Stunted growth; gonadal hypoplasia; hepatomegaly, pneumonia. *Type A.* Classical form of the syndrome with all the described characteristics. *Type B.* Symptoms of XP and Cockayne syndrome (see). *Type D.* Neurologic symptoms develop in later life than in group A. Sometimes associated with trichotiodystrophy. *Type G.* All signs but no development of tumors. *Type H.* Associated with Cockayne syndrome (see) (may not represent distinct group). Type I neurologic form.

Etiology. Autosomal recessive inheritance. Affected children are unable to repair DNA damaged by ultraviolet light and are sensitive to light in the wavelength range of 280–310 nm (UVB). Defective capacity of performing excision repair of damaged DNA at pyrimidine dimers because of enzyme deficiencies. The various forms all have different enzymatic alterations in that fibroblasts from one group of patients may correct defects of another group of patients when hybridized.

Pathology. Disturbances of pigmentation and maturation of epidermal cells, resulting eventually in malignant transformation, basal and squamous cell, and melanoma. Small brain; gliosis; loss of neurons.

Diagnostic Procedures. *Biopsy of skin. Electroencephalography.* Abnormalities. *X-ray. CT scan. MRI.* Microcephaly, ventricular dilatation, premature closure of sutures. Extremely small sella turcica. *Urine.* Occasionally, porphyrinuria, low excretion of 17–ketosteroid. *Cell culture study. Blood.* Increased serum copper and cholesterol level.

Therapy. Surgical excision of lesions that show neoplastic changes. Grafting of skin from nonlight-exposed areas; topical antimitotic agents (5-fluorouracil); genetic counseling, patient and family education.

Prognosis. When the condition shows the neoplastic tendency, poor. Affected families should have genetic counseling. The defect is detectable in cells cultured from amniotic fluid, so amniocentesis can provide an early diagnosis during pregnancy.

BIBLIOGRAPHY. Pick FJ: Ueber Melanosis lenticularis progressiva. Vschratol Derm Syph 11:3–32, 1884
DeSanctis C, Cacchione A: L'idiozia xerodermica. Riv Sper Freniat 56:269–292, 1932
Jung EG: Xeroderma Pigmentosum. Int J Dermatol 25:629–633, 1986
Cleaver JE, Kraemer KH: Xeroderma pigmentosum and Cockayne syndrome. In Scriver CR, Beaudet AL, Sly WS, et al: The Metabolic and

Molecular Bases of Inherited Disease, 7th ed, p 4407. New York, McGraw-Hill, 1995

DESBUQUOIS

Synonyms. Micromelic dwarfism—vertebral, metaphyseal abnormalities—carpometatarsal ossification.

Symptoms and Signs. Both sexes. Recognized in first year of life. Micromelic dwarfism, narrow chest, vertebral and metaphyseal abnormalities and advanced carpometatarsal ossification. Occasionally glaucoma, mental retardation. Findings in the hand are distinctive: presence of extraossification centres that may cause finger deviation (this sign may not be any longer evident after 1 year of age). Before accomplishment of one year of age: coronal cleft of vertebrae.

Etiology. Autosomal recessive inheritance.

BIBLIOGRAPHY. Desbuquois G, Grenier B, Michel J, et al: Nanisme chondro-dystrophique avec ossification anarchique et polymalformations chez deux soeurs. Arch Franch Pediat 23:573–587, 1966

Le Merrer M, Young ID, Stanescu V, et al: Desbuquois syndrome. Eur J Pediat 150:793–796, 1991

DESMOND

Synonyms. Senter; keratosis—ichthyosis—deafness; KID; ichthyosiform erythroderma—sensorineural deafness.

Symptoms and Signs. Both sexes equal ratio. Those of Ichthyosiform erythroderma (see), plus sensorineural deafness; vascularized corneas (not constant features); cryptorchidism, variable flexion contractures. In some cases in middle age: hepatomegaly, hepatic cirrhosis, evidence of glycogen storage.

Etiology. Glycogen storage disease. Possibly autosomal recessive and dominant inheritance, as well as sporadic form discussed.

Pathology. Glycogen deposit in skin and visceral tissue. Liver cirrhosis.

Therapy. Liver transplantation according to evolution of cirrhosis.

Prognosis. Patients may not reach middle age.

BIBLIOGRAPHY. Desmond F, Bar J, Chevillard Y: Erythrodermia ichthyosiforme congenital seche, surdi-mutite, hepatomegalie de transmission recessive autosomique etude d'une famille. Bull Soc Fran Derm Syph 78:585, 1971

Senter TP, Jones KL, Sakati N, et al: Atypical ichthyosiform erythroderma and congenital sensorineural deafness. A distinct syndrome. J Pediatr 92:68–72, 1978

Wilson GN, Squires RH Jr, Weinberg AG: Keratitis, Hepatitis Ichthyosis and deafness: report and review of KID syndrome. AM J Med Genet 40:255–259, 1991

DE SOUZA

Synonym. Amyloidosis, cutaneous bullous.

Symptoms and Signs. One family reported. One male, three females. Onset 10–13 years of age. Bulbous lesions mainly around the joints.

Etiology. Autosomal recessive.

BIBLIOGRAPHY. De Souza AR: Amyloidoise cutanea bulhosa familial: Observacao de 4 casos. Rev Hosp Clin Fac Med Sao Paulo 18:413–417, 1963

Sohar E, Gafni J: The hereditary amyloidoses: their place in the research of amyloidoses. In Wegelius O, Pasternack A (eds): Amyloidosis, pp 175–182. London, Academic Press, 1976

DESQUAMATIVE INTERSTITIAL PNEUMONIA

Synonyms. DIP. See "Usual" interstitial pneumonia.

Symptoms. Prevalent in adults. In 50% of cases preceded by a nonspecific upper respiratory infection. Gradual onset of dypsnea, dry cough, weight loss, anorexia, and fatigability. Arthralgia and myalgia may be present.

Signs. Cyanosis (in half of adult patients); finger clubbing. Physical examination unrevealing.

Etiology. Unknown. Response to a variety of insults (e.g., infections, drugs, and toxic agents). DIP is probably an early stage in the development of the more commonly observed UIP (usual interstitial pneumonitis).

Pathology. Lungs diffusely nodular and stiff. Diffuse massive proliferation of alveolar lining cells; cell masses well preserved; some mitotic figures. Some containing PAS-positive, iron-negative, golden brown pigment granules. Minimal interstitial inflammation; moderate thickening of alveolar septa; absence of necrosis; bronchioles normal. At the periphery of lung, small lymphoid center.

Diagnostic Procedures. *X-ray of chest.* Ground glass wedge-shaped opacity at the bases, radiating from hilus. Hilar adenopathy may be present. *Electrocardiography.* Right ventricular predominance. *Pulmonary function.* Hyperventilation; decreased arterial oxygen tension; elevated alveolar arterial oxygen gradient. *Biopsy of lung.* See Pathology.

Therapy. Corticosteroids.

Prognosis. Dramatic response to steroid treatment. Relapses follow withdrawal of treatment. Process generally irreversible, but more benign course than other chronic interstitial pneumonias. Over a period of 10 years after diagnosis, 16% mortality. In some cases, cure with complete reversibility and no sequelae.

BIBLIOGRAPHY. Liebow AA, Steer A, Billingsley JG: Desquamative interstitial pneumonia. Am J Med 39:369–404, 1965

Schneider RM, Nevius DB, Brown HZ: Desquamative interstitial pneumonia in a four-year-old child. N Engl J Med 277:1056–1058, 1967

Fraser RS, Paré JAP, Fraser RG, Paré PD: Synopsis of Diseases of the Chest, 2nd ed. Philadelphia, WB Saunders, 1994

DETERMANN

Synonyms. Angiosclerotic intermittent akinesia; angiosclerotic intermittent dyskinesia; angiosclerotic paroxysmal myasthenia. See Carotid system ischemia.

Symptoms. Transitory attacks of hypokinesia or akinesia expressed usually as poverty of movements (disinclination to use an affected part or to engage it freely in all natural actions of the body).

Etiology. Atherosclerosis. See Carotid artery system ischemia.

BIBLIOGRAPHY. Determann H: "Intermittierendes Hinken" eines Armes, der Zunge und der Beine (Dyskinesia intermittens angiosclerotica). Dtsch Z Nervenb 29:152–162, 1905

Vick NA: Grinker's Neurology, 7th ed. Springfield, IL: Charles C Thomas, 1976

DEUTSCHLAENDER

Synonyms. March foot; march fracture.

Symptoms. Slow onset of mild, persistent pain in the foot while walking.

Signs. Tenderness on dorsum of foot; lump palpable in region of second or third metatarsal.

Etiology. Prolonged and repeated marches; inadequate footwear.

Pathology. Fracture of second or third metatarsal; formation of bone callus around fracture.

Diagnostic Procedures. *X-ray.* See Pathology.

Therapy. Rest. Change of footwear.

Prognosis. Good, if adequate treatment and possible avoidance of determining cause.

BIBLIOGRAPHY. Deutschlaender CW: Ueber entzuendliche Mittel-fuss-geschmieleste. Arch Klin Chir 118:530–548, 1921

Fam AG: The ankle and the foot. In Klippel JH, Dieppe PA: Rheumatology, p 5.13.10. St Louis, CV Mosby, 1995

DE VAAL

Synonyms. Congenital aleukia; reticular dysgenesis; panaleukia, hematopoietic hypoplasia.

Symptoms and Signs. Severe intractable infections in first few days of life.

Etiology. Unknown. Lack of development of almost complete degree, at the most primitive level of leukocyte system. Autosomal recessive inheritance proposed.

Pathology. *Thymus.* Represented by few immature lobules and fibrous connective tissue; absence of small lymphocytes; presence of so-called large lymphocytes, reticular cells; no differentiation between cortex and medulla in the lobules; Hassell body absent. *Lymph nodes.* Slightly enlarged; formed by cells similar to the ones seen in the thymus and cells resembling plasma cells; few lymphocytes scattered at the periphery of nodes; no primary follicles and germinal centers. *Spleen.* Normal size; substitution of Malpighi follicles by clear zones of reticular cells and plasma cell-like cells. Groups of cocci; absence of granulocytes. Intestinal mucosa. Accumulation of similar cells; small lymphocytes practically absent; granulocytes absent despite zones of ulcerations and erosion. *Bone marrow.* Complete absence of myeloid series; normal erythroid series and megakaryocytes; rarely, monocytes. *Other tissues.* Focal necrosis; groups of cocci, lack of granulocytes close to bacterial colonies.

Diagnostic Procedures. *Blood.* Complete agranulocytosis; presence of only few large lymphocytes and monocytes.

Therapy. Antibiotics and symptomatic. Bone marrow transplantation.

Prognosis. Death within a few days after birth with therapy.

BIBLIOGRAPHY. De Vaal OM, Seynhaeve V: Reticular dysgenesia. Lancet 2:1123–1125, 1959

Gitlin D, Vawter G, Craig JM: Thymic alymphoplasia and congenital aleukocytosis. Pediatrics 33:184–192, 1964

Roper M, Parmley RT, Crist WM, et al: Severe congenital leukopenia (reticular dysgenesis): Immunologic and morphologic characterization of leukocytes. Am J Dis Child 138:832–835, 1985

Athens JW: Qualitative disorders of leukocytes. In Lee GR, Bithel TC, Foerster J, et al (eds): Wintrobe's Clinical Hematology, 9th ed, p 1603. Philadelphia, Lea & Febiger, 1993

DEVERGIE

Synonyms. Hebra; Kaposi IV; Tarral-Besnier; lichen ruber acuminatus; pityriasis rubra pilaris.

Symptoms. Both sexes affected; onset at any age. At onset, slight pruritus.

Signs. When it begins in early infancy, insidious appearance of signs; scaling of scalp and face; generalized erythema; reddening, thickening, and scaling of palms and soles; follicular papules firm and red, present-ing a horny cap, especially on proximal phalanges, knees, and elbows, rare on limbs, and still less frequently on trunk; lesions may group into plaques. Almost all cases, however, begin after 15 years of age. Same signs as preceding, developing rapidly (in days) into follicular plaques (in weeks). Milder forms are common both in children and adults.

Etiology. *Infantile form.* Autosomal dominant heredity suggested. *Adult form.* No demonstration of genetic factors.

Pathology. The histologic changes are not characteristic: acanthosis; hyperkeratosis; cellular perinuclear vacuolization; mild secondary inflammatory alterations.

Diagnostic Procedures. *Biopsy of cutaneous lesions. Blood.* Decrease of vitamin A level (frequent). *Liver function tests.* Altered (in adult form).

Therapy. In adult form, recommended rest and bland applications, if erythrodermic phase is active, of etretionate or isotretinoin. High doses of vitamin A may be effective, but of limited use because of toxic effects. Addition of corticosteroids is ineffective. Folic acid antagonists and other cytostatic agents may produce a temporary improvement. In congenital forms, all therapeutic trials have little effect.

Prognosis. Course is variable. Hereditary type is less severe and manifestation may last for entire life; the acquired type is more severe; however, in some cases, complete remission may occur within months. Association with neuromuscular diseases has been reported. Severe forms may be associated with very low intelligence, requiring institutional care.

BIBLIOGRAPHY. Devergie MG: Pityriasis pilaris, maladie de la peau non décrite par les dermatologistes. Gaz Hebd Méd 3:197–201, 1856

Kaposi M: Lichen ruber acuminatus und Lichen ruber planus. Arch Dermatol Syph 31:1–32, 1895

Griffiths WAD, Leigh IM, Marks R: Disorders of keratinization. In Champion RH, Burton JL, Ebling FJG (eds): Rook/Wilkinson/Ebling Textbook of Dermatology, 5th ed, pp 1358–1362. Oxford, Blackwell Scientific, 1992

DEVIC

Synonyms. Devic-Gauld; Erb-Devic; optic myelitis neuritis; optic neuromyelitis; optic neuritis; ophthalmoneuromyelitis; ophthalmoencephalomyelitis, neuromyelitis optica.

Symptoms. Occurs at any age; more common 20–50 years of age. Nonspecific upper respiratory infection may precede neurologic manifestations. Acute loss of vision with central scotoma; rapidly progressing ascending myelitis with loss of sphincter control. Headache, consciousness changes, convulsion.

Etiology. Unknown. Sequel of immunological reaction; considered by some authors as manifestation of multiple sclerosis. Familial cases reported. Considered also as a particular clinical variation of Leber I.

Pathology. Areas of softening in both white and gray matter in brain and spinal cord; axis cylinders destroyed; microglial response; mild leptomeningeal reaction. Complete necrosis and cavitation may be observed. Neuritis in optic nerve.

Diagnostic Procedures. *Cerebrospinal fluid.* Normal or protein elevation; increased lymphocytes; occasionally, spinal block. *Ophthalmoscopy.* Bilateral optic neuritis; from mild edema of optic disk to optic atrophy.

Therapy. General care; prevention of infection.

Prognosis. Variable from complete remission to repeated attacks with finally paraplegia and blindness, or vision recovery in about 50%, with variable residual impairment. Mortality 50%.

BIBLIOGRAPHY. Allbutt TC: On the ophthalmoscopic signs of spinal disease. Lancet 1:76–78, 1870

Erb W: Ueber das Zusammenkommen Von Neuritis optica und Myelitis subacuta. Arch Psychiatr Norvenkr 1:146–157, 1880

Seguin EC: On the coincidence of optic neuritis and subacute transverse myelitis. J Nerv Ment Dis 7:177–188, 1880

Devic ME: Myélite subaigue compliquée de nérvite optique. Bull Med Par 8:1033–1034, 1894

Gault F: De la neuromyélite optique aiguë (Thesis). Lyon, 1894

Chusid MJ, Williamson SJ, Murphy JV, et al: Neuromyelitis optica (Devic's disease) following varicella infection. J Pediatr 95:737–738, 1979

Klintworth GK: Ocular involvement in disorders of the nervous system. In Garner A, Klintworth GK (eds): Pathobiology of Ocular Disease: A Dynamic Approach, 2nd ed, p 1717. New York, Marcel Dekker, 1994

DIABETES INSIPIDUS, NEUROHYPOPHYSEAL

Synonym. Neurohypophyseal diabetes insipidus; diabetes insipidus, cranial type.

Symptoms. Prevalent in males; onset usually at young age. Insatiable polydipsia; polyuria; pale urine, occasionally up to 15–30 liters a day. Dehydration; constipation.

Signs. Dryness of skin and mucosae.

Etiology. Lesion damaging structure of hypothalamic neurohypophyseal tract; trauma; surgery; tumor; granulomas. Idiopathic (approximately 30%). In some cases autoimmune process. Two inherited forms known: a sex-linked recessive and an autosomal dominant.

Pathology. Pathologic lesion according to cause (see Etiology). Secondary dilatation and hypertrophy of bladder with megaloureter.

Diagnostic Procedures. *Urine.* Low specific gravity. *X-ray of skull. CT. MRI brain scan. Spinal tap. Secretory function test.* Nicotine; hypertonic saline solution; vasopressin.

Therapy. Correction of determining cause, if possible. Replacement treatment with vasopressin (nasal insufflation, or intramuscular administration). Chlorothiazide or hydrochlorothiazide with vasopressin. Desaminocys-D-arginine-vasopressin (DDAVP).

Prognosis. Usually, condition lasts for life. Transient forms with spontaneous recovery are sometimes observed after trauma or neurosurgery. Development of resistance or allergy to vasopressin complicates treatment.

BIBLIOGRAPHY. Weil A: Veber die hereditaere Form des Diabetes insipidus. Virchows Arch Pathol Anat 95:70–95, 1884

Forssman H: On hereditary diabetes insipidus with special reference to a sex-linked form. Acta Med Scand 159(Suppl):1–196, 1945

Pedersen EB, Lamm LU, Albertsen K, et al: Familial cranial diabetes insipidus: A report of five families: Genetic, diagnostic and therapeutical aspects. QJ Med 57:883–896, 1985

Laing RBS, Dean JCS, Pearson DWM, et al: Facial dysmorphism: a marker of autosomal dominant cranial diabetes insipidus. J Med Genet 28:544–546, 1991

Baylis PH: Vasopressin and its neurophysin. In De Groot LJ (ed): Endocrinology, 3rd ed, pp 412–415. Philadelphia, WB Saunders, 1995

DIABETES MELLITUS

Symptoms. Both sexes affected. *Type I:* onset at all ages. *Type II:* Usually in middle age. Polyuria; thirst; enuresis; increased appetite and loss of weight (in children more than in adults); pruritus (vulvae; generalized); premature loosening of the teeth; asthenia; somnolence; impotence; history of delivering large babies and hydramnios.

Signs. *Ocular.* Premature cataract; retinopathy; microaneurysms; vitreous and retinal hemorrhages. *Dermal.* Mycotic infections (Candida albicans); xanthochromia; xanthomatous tumors. *Cardiovascular.* Atherosclerotic vascular occlusion; nonhealing leg ulcers with gangrene; edema; heart failure. *Renal.* Kimmelstiel-Wilson syndrome; nephrosclerosis; chronic pyelonephritis; papillary necrosis. *Neurologic.* Peripheral neuritis; areflexia; loss of vibration sense; neurogenic bladder; nocturnal diarrhea; coma.

Etiology. *Type I.* (Insulin dependent diabetes mellitus)—10% of all patients—has susceptibility gene in region HLAD of chromosome 6 and is associated with certain HLA antigens B8, BW15, DW3, DW4 and with islet cell antibodies. Likely, type I diabetes results from an infection or toxic environmental insult to pancreatic B-cells of genetically predisposed individuals. In this form, circulating insulin is absent. In this group a subgroup (about 10%), type IB presents associated autoimmune endocrine diseases. *Type II.* (Non-insulin-dependent diabetes mellitus)–90% of all patients–is transmitted as an autosomal dominant trait on chromosome 11. A secretory defect exists in beta cells and insulin resistance depends on failure of tyrosine kinase activation following the binding of insulin to receptor. Other conditions may cause this syndrome, such as malnutrition, pancreatic diseases, other endocrinopathies, certain drugs, or genetic defects. A special category is represented by impaired glucose tolerance (IGT), or paraphysiologic condition such as pregnancy.

Diagnostic Procedures. *Urine.* Glycosuria; ketonuria. *Blood.* Hyperglycemia; ketosis; hypercholesterolemia. Glucose tolerance test. Insulin tolerance test. Ornithene test. For insulin reserve. Good to detect a latent diabetic state. Cortisone test. Decreased glucose tolerance after cortisone therapy. Insulin antibodies demonstration in blood or tissues. *Biopsy of skin and muscles. X-ray of abdomen. Calcification of aorta.*

Differential Diagnosis. To differentiate from pentosuria and fructosuria, use Tes-tape (specific for glucose). DeToni-Fanconi syndrome; renal glycosuria; alimentary hyperglycemia (e.g., dumping syndrome; starvation; liver disease).

Complications. *Acute.* Ketosis; acidosis; coma (see Diabetic ketoacidosis); insulin allergy (local, usually). *Chronic.* Premature arteriosclerosis with leg ulcers; neuropathy; ocular disorders, Kimmelstiel-Wilson (intracapillary glomerulosclerosis; hypertension; proteinuria; edema); pyelonephritis; papillary necrosis; skin lesions; xanthomas; chronic pyogenic infections; increased incidence of tuberculosis; insulin resistance.

Therapy. Correct diet and avoid obesity. Vitamin B complex. Insulin therapy. Indications: (1) diabetes mellitus, especially in older and obese; (2) pancreatectomy; (3) diabetic coma. Crystalline insulin. Short-acting (6–8 hours); used most frequently in (1) diabetic coma; (2) postprandial blood sugar elevation; (3) after surgical operations. Protamine zinc insulin (PZI). Long-acting (up to 40 hours); used in very mild forms of hyperglycemia. Intermediate. Neutral protamine Hagedorn (NPH) globin insulin, zinc insulin (lente, semilente). Mixtures. Most commonly used are 2:1 and 3:1 crystalline: PZI; 2:1 and 3:1 NPH: crystalline. Toxicity. Iatrogenic hypoglycemic syndrome (hypoglycemia, especially if the patient fails to eat or after long exercise, manifested by weakness, hunger, sweating, irritability, faintness, tremors, convulsions.) If patient is conscious, give orange juice and sugar. If the patient is unconscious, administer: (1) 20–30 ml of 50% glucose intravenously (IV) (treatment of choice); (2) epinephrine 0.5 ml subcutaneously; (3) glucagone 1 mg IV. Insulin allergic reactions are rare. Frequent instead is lipoatrophy (atrophy of subcutaneous fat at the site of injection). Oral hypoglycemic agents. Indications: (1) adult type diabetes; (2) mild degree diabetes without complications; (3) good responsiveness (fall of blood sugar to 110 mg in 4 hours after administration of 3.0 mg of these drugs); (4) insulin-resistant diabetes. Contraindicated in juvenile diabetes and in diabetes with complications (ketosis; infections). Sulfonylurea. Tolbutamide (Orinase); chlorpropamide (Diabinese), acetohexamide (Dymelor). Dosage. Chlorpropamide: 0.5 g per os daily initially, then 0.1 g daily. Tolbutamide: 1 g three times a day. Acetohexamide: 250 mg initially. Biguanides. Indications: (1) may replace insulin therapy or sulfonylurea; (2) in combination with insulin in some juvenile diabetes. Dosage: Phenformin (DBI): 25 mg three times a day per os initially, increasing slowly. Long acting (DBI-TD): 50 mg daily. Pancreas transplantation.

Prognosis. The outlook for the juvenile diabetic is not so favorable as compared to the adult diabetic who is adequately treated. Factors affecting the prognosis: pregnancy (increased mortality rate of babies; hydramnios; toxemia; edema; prolonged gestation; atherosclerosis; trauma; infections; emotional stress often precipitate the disease in susceptible persons). Periods of insulin resistance (treated with corticosteroids). Periods of increased sensitivity to insulin with hypoglycemia. Central and peripheral nervous degeneration. Prophylaxis: No marriage between diabetics. Individual with family history of diabetes should not marry with members of similar families. Avoidance of obesity.

BIBLIOGRAPHY. Fajans SS: Diabetes mellitus: Description etiology and pathogenesis natural history and testing procedures. In De Groot L, Cahill GF Jr, Odell WD, et al (eds): Endocrinology, p. 1007. New York, Grune & Stratton, 1979

Various authors: Alberti KGMM, Krall LP (eds): The Diabetes Annual. Amsterdam, Elsevier, 1987

Fajans SS: Diabetes mellitus: definition, classification, tests. In De Groot LJ (ed): Endocrinology, 3rd ed, pp 1411–1422. Philadelphia, WB Saunders, 1995

DIABETES MELLITUS, TRANSIENT NEONATAL

Synonym. Transient neonatal diabetes.

Symptoms and Signs. Babies usually born at term; emaciation and underweight; absence of subcutaneous fat; skin not dry or wrinkled. Poor weight gain; polyuria; polydipsia. Frequent development of infections; abscess; fever.

Etiology. Pancreatic cell unable to produce adequate insulin. Mother with low blood sugar (alimentary; overproduction of insulin) or placental disease that prevents normal transport of sugar from mother to fetus, or primary delayed maturation of islet-cell cells.

Pathology. Dehydration; absence of subcutaneous fat.

Diagnostic Procedures. *Blood.* High fasting blood sugar; diabetic glucose tolerance curve. *Urine.* Glycosuria; absence of ketonuria.

Therapy. Insulin; adequate formula; antibiotic for infections.

Prognosis. Self-correcting condition between 7 days to 18 months. Childs blood sugar and glucose tolerance curve normal. In cases not detected, death may occur from inanition, marasmas. Mental retardation also may be observed in some cases.

BIBLIOGRAPHY. Gerrard JW, Chin W: The syndrome of transient diabetes. J Pediatr 61:89–93, 1962

Lernmark A: Insulin-dependent (type I) diabetes: etiology, pathogenesis and natural history. In De Groot LJ (ed): Endocrinology, 3rd ed, p 1425. Philadelphia, WB Saunders, 1995

DIABETES, TRANSITORY MENINGITIS

Symptoms and Signs. Those of meningitis (see). This syndrome may be observed in about 25% of meningococcal meningitis as well as in tuberculous meningitis.

Etiology. Etiologic agents of meningitis (Mycobacterium tuberculosis; meningococcus) affect endocrine regulation of carbohydrate metabolism through damage of thalamus, hypothalamus, pituitary, adrenals, pancreas, liver.

Pathology. *Central nervous system.* Basilar accumulation of exudate and changes typical of meningitis. Prominent microscopic changes limited to pituitary and adrenals, with various degrees of cellular swelling and degeneration. *Pancreas.* No definite changes.

Diagnostic Procedures. *Blood.* Hyperglycemia and acidosis. *Urine.* Glycosuria and acetone. *Spinal tap.* Findings of meningitis (diagnosis may be impeded if diabetic acidosis only considered).

Therapy. Treat meningitis and do not be misled by the diabetic findings.

Prognosis. That of meningitis. The diabetic findings are transitory and disappear at time of convalescence from meningitis.

BIBLIOGRAPHY. Loeb M: Ein erklarungs Versuch der verschiedenartigen Temperaturverhaltnisse bei der tuberculosen Basilarmeningitis. Dsch Arch Klin Med 34:433, 1883–1884

Fox MJ, Kuzma JF, Washam WT: Transitory diabetic syndrome associated with meningococcic meningitis. Arch Intern Med 79:614–621, 1947

Edwards MS, Baker CJ: Complications and sequelae of meningococcal infections in children. J Pediatr 99:540–545, 1981

DIABETES, TRUE RENAL

Synonyms. Renal glycosuria; glycosuria renal.

Symptoms and Signs. Both sexes affected. Peak of first diagnosis at age of military service. Asymptomatic (in pregnancy or starvation). Constant glycosuria of variable severity, 10 –100 g/25 hour; independent from diet. In Type O glycosuria: dehydration and ketosis during starvation or pregnancy.

Etiology. A group of different genetic abnormalities. One group identified as autosomal dominant inheritance; another, recessive type. Relationship with diabetes mellitus must be established for every case; many patients belong to diabetic families.

Pathology. In some patients, structural defects of proximal convoluted tubules have been shown.

Diagnostic Procedures. *Urine.* Glycosuria. *Blood.* Normal glycemia. Glycosylated hemoglobin fraction normal. Glucose tolerance test: normal or slightly flat; decrease in maximal glucose reabsorptive capacity (Tmg).

Therapy. None.

Prognosis. Excellent. Normal life and survival; usually patients do not develop diabetes mellitus.

BIBLIOGRAPHY. Hjärne UA: Study of orthoglycaemic glycosuria with particular reference to its hereditability. Acta Med Scand 67:422–495, 1927

Desjeix JF, Turk E, Wright E: Congenital selective Na^+ d-glucose cotransport defects leading to renal glycosuria and congenital selective intestinal malabsorption of glucose and galactose. In Scriver CR, Beaudet AL, Sly WS, et al: The Metabolic and Molecular Bases of Inherited Disease, 7th ed, pp 3572–3577. New York, McGraw-Hill, 1995

DIABETIC KETOACIDOSIS

Symptoms. Occurs more frequently in juvenile diabetes. Ketosis. Mild nausea; thirst; malaise. Acidosis. Vomiting; drowsiness; hyperpnea.

Signs. Skin and mucosa dry; eyeball soft; fruity odor to breath; deep breathing (Kussmaul); fever; coma.

Etiology. Precipitating factors: infections; vomiting; diarrhea; circulatory failure; in patient with diabetes (see Diabetes mellitus).

Diagnostic Procedures. *Urine.* Sugar increased; acetone increased. *Blood.* Acetone increased. Test at the bedside and start treatment without waiting for the rest of chemistry. Differential diagnosis with hypoglycemic coma solved by the response to glucose intravenous (IV) injection. Blood sugar increased, blood urea nitrogen (BUN) increased, sodium decreased, potassium increased. *Electrocardiography. X-ray. Cultures. Sensitivity test.* In infections.

Therapy. Simple ketosis. Hospitalization indicated. Start treatment of infection, circulatory or other complications. Diet (three main meals, three light). Short-acting insulin after every meal. Acidosis. Insulin (liberal and repeated use of short-acting insulin): (1) In severe cases, 100–200 IU (half IV, half subcutaneously (s.c.); every 2 hours additional 50 IU until ketonuria disappears. (2) If no change in 6 hours increase insulin (sign of insulin resistance requiring massive dose). Fluid and electrolytes. (1) Initial isotonic or slightly hypotonic fluid, 2–3 l given rapidly; sodium chloride plus sodium lactate or sodium chloride plus sodium bicarbonate. (3) After improvement in blood sugar, start glucose 5% in hypotonic multiple electrolytes (sodium 40 mEq/l; potassium 30–40 mEq/l). Correction of precipitating and complicating factors (infection; circulatory failure; renal disease; pancreatitis; surgical abdomen). If coma results, hospitalization. If differential diagnosis requires, start glucose 5% IV and watch for response. If shock occurs, plasma, vasopressor, insulin as outlined for acidosis; fluid as outlined for acidosis. Follow-up. Electrocardiography; electrolyte studies. As soon as patient is conscious, 200 ml of fruit juice. As soon as ketonuria starts to recede, 200 ml of milk every 3–4 hours and insulin (25–35 IU).

Prognosis. When severe, death if adequate treatment not instituted at once.

BIBLIOGRAPHY. Winegrad AI, Morrison AD: Diabetic ketosis, non ketotic hyperosmolar coma and lactic acidosis. In De Groot LJ, Cahill GF Jr, Odell WD, et al (eds): Endocrinology, p 1025. New York, Grune & Stratton, 1979
Foster DW, Mc Garry JD: Diabetes mellitus acute complications, ketoacidosis, hyperosmolar coma, lactic acidosis. In De Groot LJ (ed): Endocrinology, 3rd ed, pp 1506, 1521–1522. Philadelphia, WB Saunders, 1995

DIABETIC MYELOPATHY

Synonyms. Diabetic amyotrophy; diabetic myelopathy. See Diabetic pseudotabes. Diabetic neuropathy; mononeuropathy multiplex.

Symptoms. Both sexes affected; diabetic patients in the fifth–7th decades. Pain in the leg, severe, asymmetric, occasionally unilateral, maximal in hip and thigh.

Signs. Asymmetric wasting of muscles, and loss of tendon reflexes. Fasciculation. Lack of objective sensory disturbances; tenderness; ulcers. Normal vibration sense at the ankles; Babinski extensor response.

Etiology. Diabetes (doubtful if this condition exists as a separate entity). Part of radicular lesions of diabetes. This syndrome is, according to the authors, mainly motor as contrasted with the diabetic pseudotabes, which is mainly sensory. Actually several clinical syndromes may go under this denomination: acute mononeuropathy; mononeuropathy multiplex; symmetric motor and sensorial loss with subacute or chronic evolution.

Pathology. Not reported, indirect indication of cord lesion.

Diagnostic Procedures. *Spinal fluid.* High protein level. *Electromyography.* Partial denervation of leg muscles; no fibrillation activity. *Blood. Enzymes.*

Therapy. Diet; insulin; vitamin B complex; physical therapy.

Prognosis. Variable form, rapid improvement with treatment. Unremitting course, possibly, spontaneous improvement.

BIBLIOGRAPHY. Bruns L: Ueber neuritische Lähmungen beim Diabetes mellitus. Berl Klin Wochenschr 27:509–515, 1890
Garland H, Taverner D: Diabetic myelopathy. Br Med J 1:1405–1408, 1953
Adams RD, Victor M: Principles of Neurology, 5th ed, pp 1136–1138. New York, McGraw-Hill, 1993
Jaspan JB, Green AJ: The neuropathies of diabetes. In De Groot LJ (ed): Endocrinology, 3rd ed, pp 1536–1568. Philadelphia, WB Saunders, 1995

DIABETIC PSEUDOTABES

See Pseudotabetic and Diabetic myelopathy.

Symptoms and Signs. In diabetic patients, shooting pain, more intense at night; cutaneous hyperesthesia. Charcot joints, impotence, neurogenic bladder may be associated.

Etiology. Diabetes; radicular and peripheral neuropathy rather than myelopathy. Clinically the following syndromes may be distinguished frequently overlapping with those indicated in diabetic myelopathy: (1) symmetric primary sensory polyneuropathy affecting mainly feet and legs slowly progressing; (2) autonomic neuropathy involving bowel, bladder, and circulation; (3) painful thoracoabdominal radiculopathy.

Diagnostic Procedures. *Blood.* Demonstration of diabetes mellitus. *Serology.* Negative for syphilis. *Spinal tap.* Normal or slight increase in protein.

Therapy. That of diabetes, plus vitamin B complex.

Prognosis. Variable, occasionally good response to treatment.

BIBLIOGRAPHY. Gowers WR: Diseases of Nervous System. London, Churchill-Livingston, 1938
Adams RD, Victor M: Principles of Neurology, 5th ed, pp 1136–1138. New York, McGraw-Hill, 1993
Jaspan JB, Green AJ: The neuropathies of diabetes. In De Groot LJ, Endocrinology, 3rd ed, pp 1536–1538. Philadelphia, WB Saunders, 1995

DIALLINAS-AMALRIC

Synonyms. Amalric; deafness—macular dystrophy.

Symptoms. Both sexes affected; onset early infancy (in acquired type, from birth; in inherited type, at 5 years). Partial deafness (50–60%); minor troubles of vision with normal visual fields, dark vision, and color vision.

Signs. Reddish fovea in marked contrast with deep grayish background; occasionally, pigmentation extends in streak to the periphery, usually bilateral. Heterochromic iridis.

Etiology. Unknown; hereditary (autosomal recessive) or embryopathic; postnatal infections.

Pathology. In most cases, labyrinthal changes; in inherited cases, cochlear involvement.

Diagnostic Procedures. *Electroretinography.* Normal.

Therapy. Symptomatic.

Prognosis. No progressive macular degeneration. Deafness progressive in hereditary cases; nonprogressive in acquired type.

BIBLIOGRAPHY. Diallinas NP: Les altérations oculaires chez les sourds-muets. J Genet Hum 8:225–262, 1959
Amalric P: Nouveau type de degénérescence tapetoretinienne au cours de la surdimutité. Bull Soc Ophthalmol Fr 73:196–212, 1960
Remky H, Klier A, Kobor J: Maculadystrophie bei Taubstummheit (syndrom von Amalric). Klin Monatsbl Augenheilkd 114:180–187, 1964
Konigsmark BW, Knox DL, Husserls IE, et al: Dominant congenital deafness and progressive optic nerve atrophy. Arch Ophthalmol 91:99–103, 1974

DIAPHYSEAL MEDULLARY STENOSIS–BONE MALIGNANCY

Synonyms. Hardcastle; bone dysplasia—medullary fibrosarcoma; malignant fibrous hystocytoma.

Symptoms and Signs. Both sexes. Second to fifth decade. Minimal trauma cause bone fracture. Cataract; bone malignancy (9/23) (fibrosarcoma).

Etiology. Autosomal dominant inheritance.

Pathology. Malignant fibrous hystocytoma. Diaphyseal medullary stenosis with cortical thickening; methaphyseal striation and cystic changes.

Prognosis. Highly aggressive tumor.

BIBLIOGRAPHY. Arnold WH: Hereditary bone dysplasia with sarcomatous degeneration. Am Intern Med 78:902–906, 1973
Hardcastle P, Nade S, Arnold W: Hereditary bone dysplasia with malignant change report of three families. J Bone Joint Surg 68:1079–1089, 1986

DIAPHRAGM, CONGENITAL ABSENCE

Synonyms. Lewis-Besant; diaphragm unilateral agenesis.

Symptoms and Signs. Both sexes affected. Respiratory insufficiency and then heart failure and death.

Etiology. Congenital unilateral or bilateral absence of diaphragm (often associated with other muscle defects: pectoralis; abdominal) causing a displacement of abdominal viscera into thoracic cavity and determining lung collapse. Multifactorial factors. Autosomal recessive and X-linked inheritance reported.

Therapy. Plastic surgery. Intensive care; mechanical ventilation. In severe cases, extracorporeal membrane oxygenation (ECMO).

Prognosis. Poor.

BIBLIOGRAPHY. Lewis AJ, Besant DF: Muscular dystrophy in infancy. J Pediatr 60:376–384, 1962
Wolff G: Familial congenital diaphragmatic defect: Review and conclusions. Hum Genet 54:1–5, 1980
Farag TI, Issa MA, Mahfuz ES: Discordant, nonsyndromic congenital diaphragmatic defect in sibs. J Med Genet 26:781–782, 1989
Haubrich WS: Diaphragmatic hernias. In Haubrich WS, Schaffner F, Berk JE (eds): Bockus Gastroenterology, 5th ed, p 437. Philadelphia, WB Saunders, 1995

DIAPHRAGM EVENTRATIO

Symptoms. Asymptomatic or minor symptoms (postprandial fullness; eructation; dyspnea).

Signs. In recumbent position, peristaltic sounds in the chest.

Etiology. Congenital. Atrophy or relaxation (hemilateral or total) of diaphragm, without phrenic nerve deficit.

Pathology. Involved part of diaphragm thinner, with muscle degeneration; atelectasia, or aplasia of part of compressed lung. Displacement of mediastinum.

Diagnostic Procedures. *X-ray of chest and abdomen. Pulmonary function test.*

Therapy. If needed to improve ventilation, surgery to strengthen diaphragm through plication.

Prognosis. Good.

BIBLIOGRAPHY. Norio R, Kaariainen H, Rapala J, et al: Familial congenital diaphragmatic defects: Aspects of etiology, prenatal diagnosis and treatment. Am J Med Genet 17:417–483, 1984
Haubrich WS: Diaphragmatic hernias. In Haubrich WS, Schaffner F, Berk JE (eds): Bockus Gastroenterology, 5th ed, p 438. Philadelphia, WB Saunders, 1995

DIAPHRAGM RUPTURE

Symptoms. Intense dyspnea; sharp pain in abdominal region and shoulder; vomiting.

Signs. Reduced expansion of inferior edge of lung. Distant respiratory sounds; rales.

Etiology. Trauma (e.g., car accident, surgery). Complication of abdominal or thoracic conditions.

Pathology. Diaphragmatic laceration; possibly, herniation of intestinal loop or omentum into thorax.

Diagnostic Procedures. *X-ray of chest and abdomen.*

Therapy. If shock occurs, control of evolution and indicated treatment. Plastic surgery.

Prognosis. Generally good, determined by associated lesions. Possibly development of diaphragmatic hernia.

BIBLIOGRAPHY. Cox EF: Blunt abdominal trauma: A 5–year analysis of 870 patients requiring celiotomy. Ann Surg 199:467–474, 1984
Haubrich WS: Diaphragmatic hernias. In Haubrich WS, Schaffner F, Berk JE (eds): Bockus Gastroenterology, 5th ed, p 438. Philadelphia, WB Saunders, 1995

DIAPHYSEAL ACLASIS

Synonyms. Exostosis external, multiple; chondromatosis multiple hereditary; osteochondromatosis.

Symptoms and Signs. Both sexes. Increased severity in males. From birth to early childhood: diaphyseal-juxtaepiphyseal outgrowths leading to various types of deformity. The growth of the exostosis slows down at adolescence. Areas most frequently affected: knees, pelvis, ribs. Shortness of stature variable.

Etiology. Autosomal dominant.

Pathology. Exostosis capped by hyaline cartilage.

Diagnostic Procedures. *X-rays. CT. MRI.* All bone may be involved; exostosis from metaphyses and apex directed away from epiphyses; shortening of ulna and fibula. *Bone scintigraphy. Ultrasound.* Overlying cystic bursae.

Therapy. Orthopedic procedures when needed.

Prognosis. No new growths occur in adult life; 2–10% incidence of sarcoma only in adulthood.

BIBLIOGRAPHY. Krooth RS, Macklin MT, Hilbish TF: Diaphyseal aclasis (multiple exostoses) in Guam. Am J Hum Genet 13:340–347, 1961
Peterson HA: Multiple hereditary osteochondromata. Clin Orthop 239:222–230, 1989

DIASTROPHIC DWARFISM

Synonyms. Diastrophic dysplasia; DD; cherub dwarf.

Symptoms. Both sexes affected; present from birth. Frequent respiratory infection. Severe functional impairment of hand and foot functions. Delayed motor milestones. Fertility reduced.

Signs. At birth, weight normal, length reduced. Micromelia: forearms and legs more involved than distal parts of limbs. Stiff fingers, "hitchhiker" thumb; club foot. Joint contractures. Scoliosis. Variable webbing at joints. Ear lobe deformities with hypertrophic cartilages (86%); cleft palate (common). Facies normal; however, occasionally, beaking of nose; broad nasal bridge; midface hemangiomas.

Etiology. Autosomal recessive. Wide variability of expression. Metabolic defect of chondrocyte that causes death and/or defect in synthesis of collagen and/or proteoglycan.

Pathology. Cartilaginous deformities and muscle contraction leading to severe joint stiffness. Irregular arrangement of cartilage cells and capillaries in the epiphyses.

Diagnostic Procedures. *X-ray. CT scan. MR imaging. Ultrasound of skeleton.* Multiple joint deformities, especially of hands and feet; long bone deviation; bowing of large metaphyses; scoliosis or kyphoscoliosis (66%).

Therapy. Orthopedic treatment; deformities are prone to early recurrences after correction.

Prognosis. Mortality rate high, especially in neonatal and early infancy periods, generally from respiratory infections. In survivors, good general health; normal mental development; severe orthopedic problems.

BIBLIOGRAPHY. Lamy M, Maroteaux P: Le nanisme diastrophique. Paris, Presse Med 68:1977–1980, 1960

Gustavson K-H, Holmgren G, Jagell S, et al: Lethal and non-lethal diastrophic dysplasia: A study of 14 Swedish cases. Clin Genet 28:321–334, 1985

Gallop TR, Eisier A: Prenatal ultrasound diagnosis of diastrophic dysplasia at 16 weeks. Am J Med Genet 27:321–324, 1987

Perheentupa J: The Finnish disease heritage: A personal look. Acta Paed. 84:1094–1099. 1995

DIBASIC AMINOACIDURIA I

Symptoms and Signs. Generally Finnish population, rare in other populations. Asymptomatic. Possible mild intestinal malabsorption; mental retardation.

Etiology. Autosomal recessive inheritance.

Diagnostic Procedures. *Urine.* High excretion of lysine, ornithine, and arginine. *Blood.* Normal plasma level of said amino acids. Impaired intestinal absorption of L-cystine. Homozygotes, protein intolerance. Heterozygotes, normal or protein intolerance.

BIBLIOGRAPHY. Whilar DT, Scriver CR: Hyperbasicaminoaciduria: An inherited disorder of amino acid transport. Pediatr Res 2:525–534, 1968

Simell O: Lysinuric protein intolerance and other cationic aminoaciduria: as. In Scriver CR, Beaudet AL, Sly WS, et al: The Metabolic and Molecular Bases of Inherited Disease, 7th ed, p 3611. New York, McGraw-Hill, 1995

DIETLEN

Synonym. Pericardial diaphragmatic adhesion.

Symptoms and Signs. During inspiration, tachycardia and feeling of epicardial tension.

Etiology. Complication of pericarditis, pleurisy, or diaphragmatitis, with formation of adhesions between pericardium and diaphragm.

Pathology. See Etiology.

Diagnostic Procedures. *Electrocardiography.* Flutter during inspiration. *X-ray and Kinocardiography of chest to demonstrate adhesions.*

Therapy. If needed, surgery.

Prognosis. Good.

BIBLIOGRAPHY. Dietlen H: Herz und Gefaesse im Roentgenbild. Ein Lehrbuch. Leipzig, Barth, 1923

DIETL

Synonyms. Floating kidney; movable kidney; nephroptosis; ren mobilis.

Symptoms. More frequent in older, thin females. When standing, acute pain in lumbar area, possible radiation to genitals; nausea and vomiting and feeling of general prostration. Oliguria. When lying down, symptoms subside.

Signs. Palpable movable kidney.

Etiology. Often related to an aberrant vessel or loss of perirenal fat and defective renal fascia. Frequently follows a rapid loss of weight. Associated with visceroptosis.

Pathology. Reduction of fat in perirenal tissue.

Diagnostic Procedures. *X-rays. Excretory urography; ultrasonography, renal scan.* Show kidney mobility or presence of abnormality of vessels.

Therapy. Weight gain; proper posture; exercises to strengthen muscle; surgery.

Prognosis. Good with treatment or various complications may arise (e.g., kinking of ureters; hydronephrosis).

BIBLIOGRAPHY. Dietl J: Merki wedrujace i ich uwiezquienie. Przegl Lek 3:225–227, 1864

Dietl J: Wandernde Nieren und deren Einklemmung. Wien Med Wochenschr 14:253–256, 579–581, 593–595, 1864

Homsy TL, Mehta PH, Huot D, et al: Intermittent hydronephrosis. A diagnostic challenge. J Urol 140:1222–1226, 1988

Resnick MI, Kursh ED: Extrinsic obstruction of the ureter. In Walsh PC, Retik AB, Stamey TA, et al: Campbell's Urology, 6th ed, pp 533–569. Baltimore, WB Saunders, 1992

DIETRICH

Synonyms. Dysplasia, epiphyseal-metacarpal type III b; metacarpal epiphyseal necrosis; MEDT type III b; multiple epiphyseal dysplasia type III b. See also Multiple epiphyseal dysplasias.

Symptoms. Both sexes affected; onset in infancy and up to 18 years of age. Pain and limitation of movements in toe joints.

Signs. Fusiform enlargement of proximal interphalangeal joints, especially of second and third metatarsal bones, less frequently of other digits. Later, possible digital shortening.

Etiology. Unknown; in some cases proven autosomal dominant; in other cases, suspected recessive-type inheritance.

Pathology. Avascular osteolysis in epiphyseal-diaphyseal zone of digits.

Diagnostic Procedures. *X-rays of hands and feet.* Destruction of cartilages; lacunae of bone reabsorption; hazy outline; shortening of phalangeal epiphyses.

Therapy. Symptomatic.

Prognosis. Severe deformities. Spontaneous arrest after closure of epiphyses. Eventual regeneration of cartilage.

BIBLIOGRAPHY. Odman P: Hereditary enchondral dysostosis: Twelve cases in three generations mainly with peripheral location. Acta Radiol 52:97–113, 1959

DI GEORGE

Synonyms. Parathyroid-thymic aplasia; pharyngeal (3–4) pouch; third-fourth pouch/arch; immunodeficiency, cellular—hypoparathyroidism. See Shprintzen.

Symptoms and Signs. Both sexes affected (male predominance 2:1);

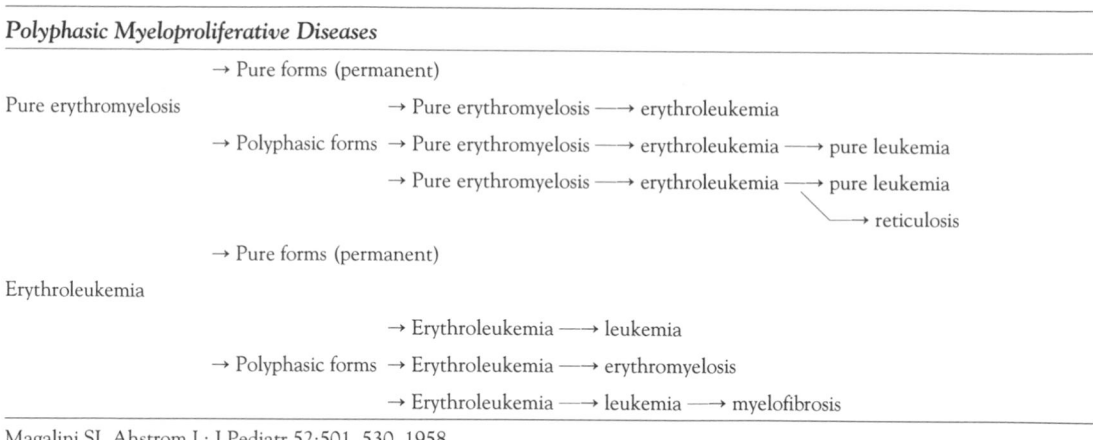

Polyphasic Myeloproliferative Diseases

Magalini SI, Ahstrom L: J Pediatr 52:501–530, 1958

early onset. Severe infection; diarrhea; tetany; Chostek, Trousseau signs. Dehydration; pulmonary and mucosal infections. Several malformations (60%): microcephaly, hypertelorism; down slanting palpebral fissures; ear anomalies. Symptoms from congenital heart defects. Aortic arch anomalies; ventricular septal defects and other congenital cardiac defects (only 5% have normal heart).

Etiology. Unknown. Sporadic; Associated also with deletion of proximal 22q or distal 10p and with fetal alcohol syndrome (see).

Pathology. Congenital absence, hypoplasia, ectopia of parathyroid; absence of thymus.

Diagnostic Procedures. *Blood.* Anemia; progressive lymphopenia; hypocalcemia; high phosphorus; hypoglobulinemia; normal immunoglobulins. Cellular immunity: diminished. *X-rays. CT scan. MR imaging. Sonography.* Evidence of cardiac heart defects.

Therapy. Calcium; parathormone; antibiotics; thymus transplant. Bone marrow transplant should be considered, especially when a fetal thymus is unobtainable and an HLA-matched sibling is available.

Prognosis. Very poor; death from infections, cardiovascular defects, or seizures within the first month or second year of life.

BIBLIOGRAPHY. Boettiger E, Wernstedt W: Toelic verlaufender Fall von Spasmophilic bei einem Brustkinde mit Anomalien des Thymus und der Parathyroidea. Acta Ped Scand 6:373–382, 1922
Lobdell, DH: Congenital absence of parathyroid glands. Arch Pathol 67:412–415, 1959
Di George AM (moderator): New concept of cellular basis of immunity. (Discussion of Cooper MD, Peterson RDA, Good RA). J Pediatr 67:907–908, 1965
Lukens JN: Immune deficiency diseases: Inherited and acquired. In Lee GR, Bithel TC, Foerster J, et al (eds): Wintrobe's Clinical Hematology, 9th ed, p 1688. Philadelphia, Lea & Febiger, 1993

DIGITOTALAR DYSMORPHISM

Synonyms. Ulnar drift. See arthrogryposis multiplex congenita, distal type.

Symptoms and Signs. Ulnar deviation of fingers. Adduction and flexor deformity of thumbs, bilateral vertical talus and rockerbottom feet. Mild reduction of stature.

Etiology. Autosomal dominant inheritance.

BIBLIOGRAPHY. Sallis JG, Beighton P: Dominantly inherited digitotalar dysmorphism. J Bone Joint Surg 54:509–515, 1972

Dhaliwal AS, Myeres TL: Digitotalar dysmorphism. Orthopedic Rev 14:90–94, 1985

DI GUGLIELMO I

Synonyms. Erythremia; erythroblastomatosis; erythroleukemia; erythromyelosis; Helmeyer-Schoener; Guglielmo I.

ACUTE

Three types of disorders may be distinguished: (1) pure form; (2) mixed form; (3) transient (see Table).

Symptoms. Male prevalence over 50 years of age. Tiredness; shortness of breath on exertion; occasionally, early bruising; bleeding from gums; fever. Bone pain may be main initial complaint.

Signs. Pallor; occasionally, petecchiae and ecchymosis; hepatosplenomegaly; moderate irregular lymphadenopathy.

Etiology. Unknown. Familial cases with autosomal dominant inheritance have been reported.

Pathology. Hepatomegaly; splenomegaly; lymphadenopathy. Infiltration with pathologic erythroid elements in spleen, lymph nodes, liver, heart, skin, muscle, esophagus, stomach, adrenal, kidney, and gonads. Focal necrosis of spleen. Frequently, superimposed fungi (Candida; Mucor) growth. Some cases end with total bone marrow aplasia and metaplastic infiltration of different organs.

Diagnostic Procedures. *Blood.* Presence of nucleated red cells in different stages of maturation with numerous pathologic features. Hypergammaglobulinemia, Coombs test positive in many cases. *Bone marrow.* Prevalence of erythroid elements with anaplastic, dysplastic changes. Prominent megaloblastic changes in erythroid precursor (over 50% of nucleated marrow cells and at least 30% of myeloblasts). Ringed sideroblast with specific stain. Decreased number of megakaryocytes.

Therapy. Blood transfusion and symptomatic. Most of these cases are completely refractory to steroids and chemotherapy. Transient forms and mixed form may respond to corticocosteroids and chemotherapy with partial or total remission.

BIBLIOGRAPHY. Copelli M: Di una emopatia sistemizzata rappresentata da una iperplasia eritoblastica. Pathologica 4:460–465, 1912
Di Guglielmo G: Un caso di eritroleucemia. Folia Med 3:319, 1917
Di Guglielmo G: Eritremie acute. Rel 29th Congr di Med Int Roma, 1923
Peterson HR Jr, Bowlds CF, Yam LT: Familial DiGuglielmo syndrome. Cancer 54:932–938, 1984

Greer JP, Kinney MC: Acute nonlymphocytic leukemia. In Lee GR, Bithel TC, Foerster J, et al (eds): Wintrobe's Clinical Hematology, 9th ed, p 1927. Philadelphia, Lea & Febiger, 1993

CHRONIC

Symptoms and Signs. Weakness; chronic refractory anemia; splenomegaly usually treated for years before gradual appearance of nucleated red cells in peripheral blood.

Etiology. Unknown; similar or identical with refractory normoblastic anemia (possibly preleukemic phase).

Pathology. See Acute form.

Diagnostic Procedures. *Blood.* Anemia; anisocytosis; poikilocytosis; siderocytes; scarce reticulocytosis. *Bone marrow.* Hyperplastic erythroid series; frequently, megaloblastic features; increased mitosis; bizarre erythrocyte morphology; erythrophagocytosis.

Therapy. Symptomatic; megaloblastic changes not affected by vitamin B_{12} or folic acid.

Prognosis. Progressive deterioration with increasing number of circulating nucleated red cells. Evolution into aplastic phase; blastic crisis (sudden increase of nucleolar cells in peripheral blood) may precede death that occurs within 2–5 years from first appearance of nucleated cells in circulation.

BIBLIOGRAPHY. Baldini M, Fudenberg HH, Fukutake K, et al: The anemia of the Di Guglielmo syndrome. Blood 14:334–366, 1959
Thurm RH, Casey MJ, Emerson CP: Chronic Di Guglielmo syndrome. Am J Med Sci 44:399–405, 1967

DIHYDROPYRIMIDINE DEHYDROGENASE DEFICIENCY

Synonyms. DPT deficiency; thymine-uraciluria, hereditary; pyridinemia, familial; flouorouracil toxicity, sensitivity to.

Symptoms and Signs. Two forms described: (1) Metabolic early in life; seizures, mental development, hypertonia; hyperreflexia; microcephaly; (2) pharmacokinetic. Onset after exposure to 5–fluorouracil: stomatitis, hair loss, diarrhea, fever; weight loss; ataxia, neurologic symptoms progessing to coma; encephalopathy.

Etiology. Deficiency of dihydropyrymidine dehydrogenase (EC1.3.1.2). Autosomal recessive inheritance.

Pathology. Brain dysmyelination.

Diagnostic Procedures. *Urine.* Excess of uracil, thymine, and 5–hydroxymethyluracil. *Blood.* In metabolic form: elevated level of pyrimidine, pharmacokinetic form. Thrombocytopenia, neutropenia

BIBLIOGRAPHY. Berglund G, Greter J, Lindstedt S, et al: Urinary excretion of thymine and uracil in a two-year-old child with a malignant tumor of the brain. Clin Chem 25:1325–1328, 1979
Scriver CR, Gibson KM: Disorders of and amino acids in free and peptide-linked forms. In Scriver CR, Beaudet AL, Sly WS, et al: The Metabolic and Molecular Bases of Inherited Disease, 7th ed, pp 1351–1353. New York, McGraw-Hill, 1995

DILATED MYOCARDIOPATHY

Synonyms. Abramo-Fiedler; Fiedler; Meadow; Becker; fibroelastosis, adult; alcoholic heart disease; cardiac hypertrophy—unknown etiology; cardiovascular collagenosis; pernicious myocarditis chronic; endocardial fibrosis; noncoronary cardiomyopathy; nutritional heart disease; obscure cardiopathy; subendocardial fibroelastosis; South African cardiomyopathy. Including Keshan. See Cardiomegaly, idiopathic; Loeffler endocardial and Davis.

Symptoms. Prevalent in males (78%); mean age of clinical onset 34 years. Easy fatigability; exertional dyspnea; palpitations; ankle swelling (in late afternoon); progressing to orthopnea, paroxysmal nocturnal dyspnea, effort syncope, right upper abdominal quadrant pain.

Signs. Cardiac enlargement: first sound normal; pulmonic component of second sound accentuated (when other signs of congestion develop); pathologic third sound; occasionally, murmurs of secondary mitral or tricuspid insufficiency. Hepatomegaly; positive liver-jugular sign.

Etiology. Spectrum of conditions includes alcohol abuse, systemic arterial hypertension, pregnancy (see Meadow), genetic factors, microvascular spasm, infectious and immunologic derangements, toxic cobalt (see Beer and cobalt), selenium deficiency (Keshan disease), catecholamine thyroid hormone increase and autonomic function derangements.

Pathology. Massive increase in heart size up to 1000 g. Chronic inflammatory change; fibroplastic proliferation of myocardium, of endocardium, thickened in patchy fashion, and occasionally also of pericardium. Passive congestion of liver.

Diagnostic Procedures. *X-ray of chest.* Cardiomegaly, both ventricles dilated; occasionally also atria, right more than left one; pleural effusion occasionally present. *EEG. Phonocardiogram. Echocardiogram. Radionuclide imaging. Angiocardiogram. Endomyocardial biopsy.*

Therapy. Symptomatic; diuretics.

Prognosis. Unexpected death may occur from myocardial irritability or embolic phenomena, hemoptysis, hemiplegia.

BIBLIOGRAPHY. Fiedler A: Ueber akute interstitielle Myokarditis. In Festschrift zur Feier des fünfzigjährigen Bestehens des Stadtkrankenhauses zu Dresden-Friedrichstadt, pp 1–20. Dresden, W Baensch, 1899
Gilbert EM, Bristow MR: Idiopathic dilated cardiomyopathy. In Schlant RC, Alexander RW: Hurst's The Heart, 8th ed, pp 1609–1619. New York, McGraw-Hill, 1994

DI MAURO-DI MAURO

Synonyms. Carnitine palmitoyil-transferase deficiency; myopathic CPT deficiency.

Symptoms and Signs. Highly prevalent in male. In female very rare and milder manifestations. Between attacks normal muscle function. Sustained muscular exertion causes aching (cramp-like), rapid fatigue. In first or second decade attacks of myoglobinuria after cold exposure, caloric deprivation (low carbohydrate, high fat diet in particular), fever, vomiting.

Etiology. Deficiency of carnitine palmitoyl-transferase, probably autosomal recessive inheritance with low penetrance in females.

Pathology. Lipid accumulation in vacuoles, mainly in type I muscle fibers.

Diagnostic Procedures. *Blood.* Elevation of triglycerides. Normal rise of serum lactate following exercise. *Urine.* Myoglobinuria after ischemic exercise.

Therapy. Low fat diet, and extra carbohydrate before exercise.

Prognosis. Good with treatment.

BIBLIOGRAPHY. Di Mauro S, Di Mauro PMM: Muscle carnitine palmitoyl-transferase deficiency and myoglobinuria. Science 182:924–931, 1973
Ferrari R, Di Mauro S, Sherwood G (eds): L-Carnitine and Its Role in Medicine: From Function to Therapy. London, Academic, 1992

DI MAURO-HARTLAGE

Synonym. Muscle phosphorylase deficiency type I; McArdle, atypical variant of.

Symptoms and Signs. From birth generalized, rapidly progressive muscle weakness.

Etiology. Probably defect of phosphorilase on chromosome 11q13.

Diagnostic Procedures. See McArdle. No detectable phosphorylase activity in muscle.

Pathology. Muscle histology: disorganization of myofibrils by excesses of glycogen in intermyofibrillar space.

Therapy. Symptomatic.

Prognosis. Poor. Death in a few weeks from respiratory failure.

BIBLIOGRAPHY. Di Mauro S, Hartlage PL: Fatal infantile form of muscle phosphorylase deficiency. Neurology 28:1124–1129, 1978
De La Marza M, Patten BM, Williams JC, Chambers JP: Myophosphorylase deficiency: A new cause of infantile hypotonia simulating infantile muscular atrophy. Neurology 30:402, 1980
Abarbanel JM, Bashan N, Potashnik R, et al: Adult muscle phosphorilase b kinase deficiency. Neurology 36:560–562, 1986
Mllstein JM, Herron TM, Haas JE: Fatal infantile muscle phosphorilase deficiency. J Child Neurol 4:186–188, 1989

DIMMER

Synonym. Keratitis nummularis.

Symptoms. Onset after minor ocular trauma. Ocular pain; photophobia; excessive lacrimation.

Signs. Diskoid infiltration of superficial layers of cornea without consensual conjunctivitis.

Etiology. Trauma.

Therapy. Topical application of analgesic and antibiotics.

Prognosis. Slow progression and then healing.

BIBLIOGRAPHY. Dimmer F: Ueber eine der Keratitis nummularis mahestehende Hirnhutentzuendung. Augenheilkd 13:621–635, 1905

DI SAIA

Synonyms. Coumarin; fetal warfarin; anticoagulant fetal.

Symptoms. Both sexes affected; present from birth. Poor feeding; variable degree of mental deficiency; hypotonia; seizures; visual impairment to blindness; respiratory infections.

Signs. Growth deficiency of prenatal onset. Nose hypoplasia, low bridge; mild ocular hypertelorism; short neck; brachydactyly. Cardiovascular anomalies.

Etiology. Warfarin taken by mother during pregnancy. The critical period of exposure is 6–9 weeks gestation. Most of the effects on bones are secondary to the inhibition of gamma-carboxylation of glutamyl residues of osteocalcins in the developing bone. Central nervous system abnormalities are associated with exposure in the second or third trimester and are related to hemorrhage in the nervous tissues of the fetus. Thirty-five percent of infants exposed die prenatally or show serious defects.

Diagnostic Procedures. *X-ray.* Stippled mineralization in vertebrae, epiphyses, cartilage.

Prognosis. For CNS manifestations, poor.

BIBLIOGRAPHY. Di Saia PJ: Pregnancy and delivery of a patient with Stan-Edwards mitral valve prosthesis. Report of a case. Obstet Gynecol 28:469–471, 1966
Shaul WL, Emery H, Hall JC: Chondrodysplasia punctate and maternal warfarin use during pregnancy. Am J Dis Child 129:360–362, 1975
Leonard CO: Vitamin K responsive bleeding disorder. A genocopy the

warfarin embryopathy. In Smith DW: Conference on Malformations and Morphogenesis. Reenville, SC, Aug 1987
Koren G (ed): Maternal-fetal Toxicology, 2nd ed. New York, Marcel Dekker, 1994

DISASTER

Symptoms. Response of person involved in disaster, injured or not. (Does not apply to person who arrives at site of disaster later.) Four stages may be distinguished:

1. Few minutes to hours. Stunned; apathetic; not responding to directions; disorganized behavior regarding injury or priority of activities.
2. Several days. Suggestibility; tries to be helpful with reduced efficiency; minimizes his need of care. Onset of guilty feeling because he survived and could not help others.
3. Few weeks. Mild euphoria; enthusiasm for rebuilding and repairing damages; feeling of identification with community.
4. Eventually fading and disappearing into normality. Hypercriticism; annoyance.

BIBLIOGRAPHY. Garb S, Garb E: Disaster Handbook. New York, Springer-Verlag, 1964
Stutman RK, Bliss EL: Posttraumatic stress disorder, hypnotizability, and imagery. Am J Psychiatr 142:741–743, 1985
Manni C, Magalini SI (eds): Emergency and Disaster Medicine. Heidelberg, Berlin, Springer-Verlag, 1985

DISCOGENIC

Syndromes owing to nerve root or spinal cord compression by herniation of nucleus pulposus or narrowing of intervertebral disks with reduction of space. Local and radicular pain.

BIBLIOGRAPHY. Schmorl G: Die pathogische Anatomie der Wirbelsäule. Verh Dtsh Orthop Ges 21:3–41, 1927
Schmorl G: Ueber die an den Wirbelbandscheiben vorkommenden Ausdehnughs-und Zerresisungsvorgänge und die dadurch an ihnen und der Wirbelspongiosa hervorgerufenen Veränderungen. Verh Dtsch Pathol Ges 22:250–262, 1927
Weatherall DJ, Ledingham JGG, Warrell DA (eds): Oxford Textbook of Medicine, 3rd ed, pp 3906–3907. Oxford, Oxford Med Pub, 1996

DISTAL OSTEOSCLEROSIS

Symptoms and Signs. In a South African family mixed European. Both sexes. From infancy. Asymptomatic. Distal segment of forearms widened.

Etiology. Autosomal dominant inheritance.

Diagnostic Procedures. *X-rays.* Hyperostosis of distal portions of forearms and legs and calvarium, mild sclerosis of base of skull, pelvis, femoral neck and pedicles of vertebrae.

BIBLIOGRAPHY. Beighton P, Macrae M, Korzlowski K: Distal osteosclerosis. Clin Genet 18:298–304, 1980

DISTICHIASIS–HEART AND VASCULATURE ANOMALIES

Symptoms and Signs. Reported combination of distichiasis and variable heart (ventricular septal defect, patent ductus arteriosus, sinus bradycardia, wandering atrial pacemaker) and vasculature (edema, varicosities, arterial disease of legs) in members of both sexes of a family.

Etiology. Autosomal dominant.

BIBLIOGRAPHY. Goldstein S, Qazi QM, Fitzgerald J, et al: Distichiasis, congenital heart defects and mixed peripheral vascular anomalies. Am J Med Genet 20:283–294, 1985

DISTICHIASIS-LYMPHEDEMA

Synonym. Lymphedema—distichiasis.

Symptoms and Signs. Both sexes affected. Extra eyelashes that cause eye irritation. Lymphedema of limbs, especially below knees, that becomes manifest at adolescence. Occasionally, epidural spinal cysts and vertebral anomalies.

Etiology. Autosomal dominant inheritance.

Therapy. Eyelash removal and surgery for lymphedema has little effectiveness; frequent recurrences.

BIBLIOGRAPHY. Kuhnt H: Ueber distichiasis (congenital) vera. Z Augenhk 2:46, 1899
Falls HS, Dertesz ED: A new syndrome combining pterygium colli with developmental anomalies of the eyelids and lymphatics of the lower extremities. Trans Am Ophthalmol Soc 62:248–275, 1964
Dale RF: Primary lymphedema when found with distichiasis is of the type defined as bilateral hyperplasia by lymphography. J Med Genet 24:170–171, 1987

DIVERSION COLITIS

Symptoms and Signs. After colostomy with diversion of fecal stream: mucus or bloody rectal discharge, crampy abdominal pains, tenesmus.

Etiology. Unknown. Overgrowth of normal bacterial flora, pathogens or prolonged contact with luminal toxins. Colonic nutritional deficiency (?).

Pathology. Colon biopsy. Acute and chronic inflammatory infiltrata, patchy lymphoid infiltration areas.

Diagnostic Procedures. *Coloscopy.* Nonspecific colitis.

Therapy. Reanastomosis of excluded segment.

Prognosis. In 2–3 months, resolution of the condition.

BIBLIOGRAPHY. Morson BC, Dawson IMP: Gastrointestinal Pathology. London, Blackwell Scientific, 1972
Glotzer DJ, Glick ME, Goldman H: Proctitis and colitis following diversion of the fecal stream. Gastroenterology 80:438–441, 1981
Maxson CJ, Klein HD, Rubin W: Atypical forms of inflammatory bowel disease. Med Clin N Amer 78:1259–1273, 1994

DIVER SYNCOPE

Symptoms and Signs. Loss of consciousness (even sudden death) during underwater diving.

Etiology. Poorly understood. Several factors in combination may be responsible: age, hypoxia, "diving reflex," cold hypersensitivity (see).

Prognosis. "Per se" fair.

BIBLIOGRAPHY. Lewis RP, Budoulas H, Schaal SF, et al: Diagnosis and management of syncope. In: Schlant RC, Alexander RW: Hurst's The Heart, 8th ed, p 934. New York, McGraw-Hill, 1994
Weatherall DJ, Ledingham JGG, Warrell DA (eds): Oxford Textbook of Medicine, 3rd ed, pp 1204–1211. Oxford, Oxford Med Pub, 1996

DIVRY-VAN BOGAERT

Synonyms. Bogaert-Divry; Van Bogaert-Divry; angiomatosis, cortico-meningeal, diffuse.

Symptoms. Present from infancy. Spastic diplegia; seizures; physical and mental developmental retardation.

Signs. Cutis marmorata; generalized acrocyanosis; trophic changes of nails; occasionally, hypertricosis.

Etiology. Unknown; autosomal recessive inheritance.

Pathology. Angiomatosis of cortex and meninges (not calcific); diffuse sclerosis.

Therapy. Symptomatic.

Prognosis. Poor.

BIBLIOGRAPHY. Divry P, Van Bogaert L: Une maladie familiale caractérisée par une diffuse corticomeningée non calcifiante et une démyélinisation progressive de angiomatose la substance blanche. J Neurol Neurosurg Psychiatr 19:41–54, 1946
Owen LG, Hanno R: Neurocutaneous syndromes. Cutis 21:848–851, 1978
Bussone G, Parati EA, Boiardi A, et al: Divry Van Bogaert syndrome. Clinical and ultrastructural findings. Arch Neurol 41:560–562, 1984

DNA AUTOSENSITIVITY

Synonyms. Autosensitization DNA; purpura, DNA sensitivity.

Symptoms and Signs. All female patients in good health. Painful spot in the extremities preceding appearance of wheal or tender nodules. In 2–48 hours, wheals or red nodules evolve into hematomas that spread circumferentially with a diameter of 10–12 cm, sometimes from mid-thigh to ankle or from elbow to fingertips. Lesions appear in crops at intervals of 2–4 weeks.

Etiology. Unknown; autosensitization to deoxyribonucleic acid (DNA) limited to extremities.

Pathology. *Biopsy of skin.* Feulgen-positive masses resembling hematoxylin bodies in lesions 20–72 hours old. In older lesions, infiltration with mature lymphocytes in the adventitia of small dermal vessels.

Diagnostic Procedures. Injection of DNA preparation in the skin of extremities reproduces the specific lesions. Injection in the skin of trunk gives a negative result. For differential diagnosis: Injection of red cell membranes. Negative result (see Gardener-Diamond). *Injection of histamine.* Negative. *Lupus erythematosus test.* Negative. *Coagulation studies.* Negative.

Therapy. Dramatic result with administration of chloroquine or primaquine, complete cessation of pain and tenderness; immediate recurrence of symptoms when therapy is stopped. Corticosteroids or antihistamines or psychotherapy are ineffective.

Prognosis. Chronic recurrent condition.

BIBLIOGRAPHY. Levin MB, Pinkus H: Autosensitivity to deoxyribonucleic acid (DNA). Report of a case with inflammatory skin lesions controlled by chloroquine. N Engl J Med 264:533–537, 1961
Little AS, Bell HE: Painful subcutaneous hemorrhages of the extremities with unusual reactions to injected deoxyribonucleic acid. Ann Intern Med 60:886–891, 1964
Bithell TC: Bleeding disorders caused by vascular abnormalities. In Lee GR, Bithel TC, Foerster J, et al (eds): Wintrobe's Clinical Hematology, 9th ed, p 1385. Philadelphia, Lea & Febiger, 1993

DOAN-WISEMAN

Synonyms. Wiseman-Doan; neutropenia, primary splenic; splenic neutropenia (primary); splenic panhematopenia; see Neutropenic.

Symptoms. Prevalent in females. Fever; pain in left hypochondrium.

Signs. Various degrees of splenomegaly.

Etiology. Unknown; splenic selective dysfunction with trapping and destruction of granulocytes. Often associated with other features of hypersplenism, anemia, thrombocytopenia (see Doan-Wright).

Pathology. Spleen enlarged; active phagocytosis of granulocytes. In bone marrow, normal cellularity or slight decrease of mature granulocytes.

Diagnostic Procedures. *Blood.* Marked neutropenia. Search for leukocytes antibodies. *Spleen scan. Bone marrow.*

Therapy. Splenectomy.

Prognosis. Normalization of granulocyte count.

BIBLIOGRAPHY. Wiseman BK, Doan CA: Primary splenic neutropenia. A newly recognized syndrome closely related to congenital hemolytic icterus and essential thrombocytopenic purpura. Ann Intern Med 16:1097–1117, 1942
Doan CA, Wright CS: Primary congenital and secondary acquired splenic panhematopenia. Blood 1:10–26, 1946
Athens JW: Disorders primarily involving the spleen. In Lee GR, Bithel TC, Foerster J, et al (eds): Wintrobe's Clinical Hematology, 9th ed, pp 1708–1709. Philadelphia, Lea & Febiger, 1993

DOAN-WRIGHT

Synonyms. Wright-Doan; splenic neutropenia(acquired); splenic panhematopenia.

Symptoms and Signs. Both sexes affected; onset at all ages; acute or gradual onset. All clinical manifestations of anemia, thrombocytopenia, neutropenia. Splenomegaly; no lymphadenopathy.

Etiology. Variable causes of spleen pathologic changes: infiltration, cyst neoplasms.

Pathology. *Spleen.* Congestion; erythrophagocytosis; granulocyte phagocytosis; megakaryocytosis. *Bone marrow.* Hyperplasia of all series of production; erythrocytic; myelocytic; megakaryocytic.

Diagnostic Procedures. *Blood.* Anemia; variable reticulocytosis; neutropenia; thrombocytopenia; variable hyperbilirubinemia. *Coombs and agglutination tests.* Negative. *Hepatosplenoechography.*

Therapy. Splenectomy.

Prognosis. Condition may be present for weeks or years; periodic recurrences with spontaneous return to normal values reported. Splenectomy is followed by return of blood elements to normal values.

BIBLIOGRAPHY. Doan CA, Wright CS: Primary congenital and secondarily acquired splenic panhematopenia. Blood 1:10–26, 1946
Athens JW: Disorders primarily involving the spleen. In Lee GR, Bithel TC, Foerster J, et al (eds): Wintrobe's Clinical Hematology, 9th ed, pp 1710–1711. Philadelphia, Lea & Febiger, 1993

DOBRINER

Synonyms. Berger-Goldberg; Watson; HCP; coproporphyria hereditaria; porphyria hepatica II; coproporphyrinogen oxidase deficiency.

Symptoms and Signs. Both sexes affected; onset at various ages. Usually latent before puberty. From completely asymptomatic form (50%) to intermittent attacks of abdominal pain and neurologic and psychiatric manifestations (usually associated with signs of hepatic insufficiency). Acute attacks may be precipitated by drugs. Photosensitivity is present only during attacks.

Etiology. Autosomal dominant inheritance; 50% deficiency of coproporphyrin oxidase. Primary partial block in conversion of coproporphyrinogen III to protoporphyrinogen IX.

Pathology. Absence of particular findings.

Diagnostic Procedures. *Stool.* Increased excretion of coproporphyrin III (95% isomer III); increase of coproporphyrin, ALA and PBG.

Therapy. Supportive treatment: high carbohydrate intake. Heme arginate should be tried.

Prognosis. From asymptomatic to fatal attacks.

BIBLIOGRAPHY. Dobriner K: Simultaneous excretion of coproporphyrin I and III in a case of chronic porphyria. Proc Soc Exp Biol Med 35:175–176, 1936
Watson CJ, Schwartz S, Schulze W, et al: Studies on coproporphyrin III. Idiopathic coproporphyrinuria a hitherto unrecognized form characterized by lack of symptoms in spite of the excretion of large amounts of coproporphyrin. J Clin Invest 28:465–468, 1949
Lee GR: Porphyria. In Lee GR, Bithel TC, Foerster J, et al (eds): Wintrobe's Clinical Hematology, 9th ed, pp 1289–1290. Philadelphia, Lea & Febiger, 1993

DOCKHORN

Synonyms. Alport syndrome variant; hereditary nephropathy without deafness. Alport syndrome features without associated deafness.

BIBLIOGRAPHY. Dockhorn RJ: Hereditary nephropathy without deafness. Am J Dis Child 114:135–138, 1967

DOEGE-POTTER

Used to indicate hypoglycemia, presumably related to the production of circulating agents capable of insulin-like action, in cases of mesenchymal tumors (see Paraneoplastic syndromes).

BIBLIOGRAPHY. Doege KW: Fibro-sarcoma of the mediastinum. Ann Surg 92:955–969, 1930
Potter RP: Intrathoracic tumors. Case report. Radiology 14:60–61, 1930
Sabiston DC: Textbook of Surgery, 14th ed, p 1777. Philadelphia, WB Saunders, 1991

DOEHLE-HELLER

Synonyms. Syphilitic aorta; cardiovascular syphilis.

Symptoms. Both sexes affected but prevalent in males; average age at onset was 35–55 years (today higher, 60–65 years). In untreated cases of syphilis, present in 75% of cases. Clinically manifested in only 10% of affected individuals. Symptoms related to complications: coronary ostial stenosis; aortic insufficiency; aneurysm.

Signs. Described as a characteristic "loud bell-like or tambor-like second aortic sound"; however, this sign is not specific for this condition. A rough aortic systolic murmur of some significance. (Both signs assume high suggestive value if associated with positive serology for syphilis, in patients over 40 years of age, and in absence of hypertension.)

Etiology. Infection by Treponema pallidum. This syndrome usually develops 10–25 years after onset of primary syphilitic infection. Inadequacy of early antisyphilitic therapy to be considered among etiologic factors.

Pathology. The lesions are those of syphilitic infection, originating in the aorta or myocardium. Distinctive features: intimal bluish gray plaques; wrinkling of inner aspects of aorta, radial or parallel grooves; sharp demarcation between lesions and healthy areas. Most severe lesions usually located in the ascending aorta above sinus aorta. The histologic changes affect adventia, media (productive mesoarteritis), and intima, with specific inflammatory changes and scarring.

Diagnostic Procedures. *Blood. Serology. Electrocardiography. X-ray of chest. Angiocardiography.*

Therapy. Penicillin and other antibiotics. Surgical treatment.

Prognosis. Condition most frequently diagnosed at autopsy. Uncomplicated forms, relatively benign prognosis. Asymptomatic phase lasts an average of 6 years. Symptomatic phase, formerly considered ominous prognostic sign, today ascertained to last an average of 6.5 years. If heart failure occurs, prognosis becomes very doubtful.

BIBLIOGRAPHY. Döhle KG: Ein Fall von eigentümlicher Aortener-Krankung bei einem Syphilitischen. Kiel, Lipsius und Tischer, 1885
Heller AL: Ueber die syphilitische Aortitis und ihre Bedeutung für die Entstehung von Aneurysmen. Verh Dtsch Pathol Ges p. 346, 1900
Stone J: Syphilis and the cardiovascular system. In Schlant RC, Alexander RW: Hurst's The Heart, 8th ed, pp 1949–1952. New York, McGraw-Hill, 1994

DOHI

Synonyms. Acropigmentation, Dohi; dyschromatosis extremitis, symmetric.

Symptoms. Relatively frequent in Japan; described also in Europe. Both sexes affected; onset in infancy or early childhood. Asymptomatic.

Signs. Mottled pigmentation and depigmentation on back of hands and feet, occasionally, on upper and lower limbs. Face not affected, except for few small maculae.

Etiology. Unknown. Autosomal dominant inheritance.

BIBLIOGRAPHY. Komaya G: Symmetrische Pigmentanomalie der Extremitaeten. Arch Dermatol Syph 147:389–393, 1924
Siemens HW: Acromelanosis albo-punctate. Dermatologica 128:86–87, 1964
Bleehen SS, Ebling FJG, Champion RH: Disorders of skin color. In Champion RH, Burton JL, Ebling FJG (eds): Rook/Wilkinson/Ebling Textbook of Dermatology, 5th ed, p 1585. Oxford, Blackwell Scientific, 1992

DONOHUE

Synonym. Leprechaunism.

Symptoms. Born from shorter gestation. Prevalent in females (2:1). Failure to thrive; mental retardation; retarded osseous development; sexual precocity.

Signs. Marasmic broad nose; hypertelorism; large ears. *Body.* Hirsutism; lack of adipose tissue; nipples and external genitals are hypertrophic.

Etiology. Unknown; familial condition; possibly, recessive inheritance; frequently demonstrated in consanguinity of parents; absence of chromosomal defect. Pathogenetic mechanism: defect in a component of the cellular insulin receptor that is common to the receptor and the insulin-like growth factor.

Pathology. Morphologic changes described. *Pituitary.* Prevalence of chromophobe cells. *Ovary.* Premature follicular maturation with no evidence of luteinization. *Pancreas.* Hyperplasia of islet of Langerhans. *Kidney.* Calcium deposit in collecting tubules. *Liver.* Hemosiderosis. Generalized lymphocyte depletion. *Bones.* Delayed growth. *Skin.* Fragmentation of elastic and collagen fibers.

Diagnostic Procedures. *Blood.* Hypoglycemia, elevated plasma insulin, impaired glucose homeostasis, absence of anti-insulin receptor antibodies, altered insulin receptor binding and response to insulin. *Urine.* High level of epidermal growth factor. Low gonadotropin excretion; high 17-ketosteroid excretion.

Prognosis. Frequently, death at early age.

BIBLIOGRAPHY. Donohue, WL: Dysendocrinism. J Pediatr 32:739–748, 1948

Frindik JP, Kemp SF, Fiser RH, Schedewie H, Elders JM: Phenotypic expression in Donohue syndrome (leprechaunism): A role for epidermal growth factor. J Pediatr 107:428–429, 1985
Lindhout D, et al: Leprechaunism: from phenotype to genotype. David W Smith Conference on Malformations and Morphogenesis. Madrid, Spain, 1989

D.O.O.R.

Synonyms. Deafness, onychoosteodystrophy recessive; see Robinson G.C.

Symptoms and Signs. Both sexes. Mental retardation, seizures, sensorineuronal deafness, onycodystrophy, triphalangeal thumbs, abnormal dermatoglyphics.

Etiology. Autosomal recessive and dominant (DOO) inheritance.

Diagnostic Procedures. *Blood and urine.* Increased organic acid 2-oxoglutarate. *X-rays.* Phalangeal anomalies; occasionally spinal anomalies, short femoral neck and metaphysial spur femur distal end.

BIBLIOGRAPHY. Feinmesser M, Zelig S: Congenital deafness associated with onychodystrophy. Arch Otolaryng 74:507–508, 1961
Patton MA, Winter RM, Krywawych S, et al: Raised 2–oxoglutarate in the DOOR syndrome. J Med Genet 22:139, 1985

DORMANDY-PORTER

Obsolete.

Synonyms. Fructose-galactose. See fructose intolerance, hereditary.

BIBLIOGRAPHY. Dormandy TL, Porter RJ: Familial fructose and galactose intolerance. Lancet 1:1189–1194, 1961
Gitzelmann R, Steinman B, Van den Berghe G: Disorders of fructose metabolism. In Scriver CR, Beaudet AL, Sly WS, et al: The Metabolic and Molecular Bases of Inherited Disease, 6th ed, p 407. New York, McGraw-Hill, 1989

DOUBLE

Synonyms. Combination of Alzheimer (see) and Pick (see).

BIBLIOGRAPHY. Moyano BA: Coloracion de la neuroglia por el metodo de Holzer. Semin Med 2:1919, 1930
Berlin L: Presenile sclerosis (Alzheimer's disease) with features resembling Pick's disease. Arch Neurol Pschiatr 61:369, 1949
Adams RD, Victor M: Principles of Neurology, 5th ed, p 966. New York, McGraw-Hill, 1993

DOUBLE CORTEX

Synonyms. Diffuse cortical dysplasia; neuronal migration benign disorder.

Symptoms and Signs. Rare. All female. Age of onset of epilepsy (various forms: drop attacks, generalized clonic or tonic-clonic seizures, infantile spasms) between 2 months and 11 years. Delayed aquisition of developmental milestones. Varible degrees of mental retardation. Occasionally mild dysarthria, mild bilateral pyramidal syndrome.

Etiology. Unknown. Possible action of prenatal factor, maternal drug or X-ray exposure.

Pathology. From biopsy specimen: "Well-preserved isocortical lamination in cortical layers 1–4. Layer 5 and 6 could not be clearly separated. Layer 6 merged with U fibers of white matter. Beneath a further thin band of well myelinated white matter, coalescent clusters of large, unlaminated, well differentiated ganglion cells."

Diagnostic Procedures. *EEG.* Varible epileptic patterns. *MRI (diagnostic).* Band of subcortical gray matter, heteropia underlying the cortical mantle and separated by a thin rim of white matter, most obvious in frontocentroparietal region.

Therapy. Symptomatic; partial results with callosotomy.

Prognosis. Good for survival.

BIBLIOGRAPHY. Jacob H: Genetisch verschiedene Gruppen entwicklungsgestoerter Gehirne Z ges. Neurol Psychiat 160:615–648, 1938
Palmini A, Andermann F, Aicardi J, et al: Diffuse cortical dysplasia or the "double cortex" syndrome: the clinical and epileptic spectrum in ten patients. Neurology 41:1656–1662, 1991

DOUBLE OUTLET–LEFT VENTRICLE

Symptoms. Extremely rare: less than 5% of double outlet ventricles. Major cyanosis of variable degree according to magnitude of pulmonary arterial blood flow; clinical manifestations similar to tricuspid atresia, tetralogy of Fallot, or transposition of great arteries with ventricular septal defect.

Etiology. Unknown.

Pathology. Both great vessels arise above morphologic left ventricle. Ventricular septal defect, pulmonary stenosis. Tricuspid valve abnormalities and right ventricular hypoplasia are frequently associated.

Diagnostic Procedures. *ECG. X-rays.* Two-dimensional echocardiography with color flow imaging and spectral Doppler interrogation. Results according to association with subaortic ventricular defect and pulmonary stenosis or no pulmonary stenosis.

Therapy. Surgical.

Prognosis. Therapy of palliative value.

BIBLIOGRAPHY. Sakakiara S, Takao A, Arai T, et al: Both great vessels arising from left ventricle. Bull Heart Inst J 10:66, 1967
Van Praagh R, Weinberg PM, Srebo JP: Double-outlet left ventricle. In Moss AJ, Adams FH, Emmanoulides C, et al (eds): Heart Disease in Infants, Children and Adolescents, 4th ed. Baltimore, Williams & Wilkins, 1989
Perloff JK: The Clinical Recognition of Congenital Heart Disease, 4th ed, pp 505–506. Philadelphia, WB Saunders, 1994

DOUBLE OUTLET–RIGHT VENTRICLE I

Synonym. Right ventricular origin of both great arteries—subaortic ventricular septal defect—without pulmonic stenosis. Two clinical types classified: (a) with low pulmonary vascular resistance: and (b) with high pulmonary vascular resistance.

Symptoms and Signs. Male to female ratio 1.7:1. Transient cyanosis (temporary high pulmonary vascular resistance). Bulging active precordium with right and left ventricular impulses, left parasternal systolic thrill and murmur of ventricular septal defect, loud pulmonary component of second sound with close splitting and apical mid-diastolic murmur. Early congestive heart failure, poor growth and development.

Etiology. Congenital malformation.

Pathology. Complex anatomy. Aorta usually positioned to the right of and anterior to the pulmonary trunk or side by side with the aorta to the right. Ventricular septal defect, is subaortic. Pulmonary stenosis frequently coexists.

Diagnostic Procedures. *Electrocardiography.* Right ventricular hypertrophy; biatrial P-waves. *X-ray.* Cardiomegaly; pulmonary congestion. *Two-dimensional echocardiography* with color flow imaging and spectral Doppler interrogation.

Therapy. Surgical correction.

Prognosis. According to degree of defects. Chronic heart failure.

BIBLIOGRAPHY. Peacock TB: On Malformations of the Human Heart, 2nd ed, London, J Churchill and Sons, 1866
Perloff JK: The Clinical Recognition of Congenital Heart Disease, 4th ed, pp 488–493. Philadelphia, WB Saunders, 1994

DOUBLE OUTLET–RIGHT VENTRICLE II

Synonyms. Right ventricle origin of both great arteries; infracristae ventricular septal defect; absence of pulmonic stenosis.

Symptoms and Signs. Both sexes equally affected; present from birth. Initially, cyanosis and digital clubbing mild or absent; later both may appear. Retarded growth; frequent respiratory infections; early congestive heart failure; overactive bulging precordium; both right and left systolic impulses; murmur of ventricular septal defect; loud pulmonic component of second sound.

Etiology. Congenital malformation.

Pathology. Right ventricular origin of both great arteries with infracristal ventricular septal defect and no pulmonic stenosis.

Diagnostic Procedures. *Electrocardiography.* Counterclockwise depolarization with left axis deviation. *X-ray.* Cardiomegaly; pulmonary congestion. *Two-dimensional echocardiography* with color flow imaging and spectral Doppler interrogation (diagnostic).

Therapy. Surgical correction.

Prognosis. According to degree of defects. In patients who survive infancy, chronic heart failure from progessive pulmonary vascular obstruction (resembling Eisenmenger complex, see).

BIBLIOGRAPHY. Nugent EW, Plauth WH, Edwards JE, et al: The pathology, pathophysiology, recognition, and treatment of congenital heart disease. In Schlant RC, Alexander RW: Hurst's The Heart, 8th ed, p 1807. New York, McGraw-Hill, 1994
Perloff JK: The Clinical Recognition of Congenital Heart Disease, 4th ed, pp 488–493. Philadelphia, WB Saunders, 1994

DOUBLE OUTLET–RIGHT VENTRICLE IV

Synonyms. Right ventricular origin of both great arteries; subaortic ventricular defect; pulmonic stenosis.

Symptoms and Signs. Both sexes affected. Symptoms present at birth or delayed and progressive. Cyanosis early sign; initially may be intermittent or delayed. Other symptoms and signs similar to Fallot tetralogy (see), including squatting. Symptoms may vary from mild to very severe (complete pulmonary atresia). Signs that differentiate this diagnosis from Fallot are palpable left ventricular impulse with fourth heart sound and a holosystolic murmur at lower sternal left edge.

Etiology. Congenital malformation.

Pathology. Ventricular origin of both great arteries from right ventricle; ventricular septal defect located below crista supraventricularis (rarely above) and variable degree of pulmonic stenosis.

Diagnostic Procedures. *Electrocardiography.* Left axis deviation; counterclockwise depolarization. PR interval is often prolonged. P-waves variable according degree of obstructions. *X-ray.* Rounded cardiac apex (in Fallot tetralogy, boot-shaped). *Selective angiocardiography. Two-dimensional echocardiography* with color flow imaging and spectral Doppler interrogation (diagnostic).

Therapy. Surgical correction.

Prognosis. According to degree of defects and treatment.

BIBLIOGRAPHY. Braun K, De Vries A, Feingold DS, et al: Complete dextroposition of aorta, pulmonary stenosis, interventricular septal defect, and patent foramen ovale. Am Heart J 43:773–780, 1952

Nugent EW, Plauth WH, Edwards JE, et al: The pathology, pathophysiology, recognition, and treatment of congenital heart disease. In Schlant RC, Alexander RW: Hurst's The Heart, 8th ed, p 1807. New York, McGraw-Hill, 1994

Perloff JK: The Clinical Recognition of Congenital Heart Disease, 4th ed, pp 493–498. Philadelphia, WB Saunders, 1994

DOUBLE WHAMMY

Synonym. Voluntary eye propulsion; eye propulsion.

Symptoms. Ability to voluntarily propel and retract one or both eyes.

Etiology. Phenomenon produced by contracting superior and inferior obliques while relaxing all rectus muscles, and successive moderate contraction of orbicularis muscle.

Pathology. After years of propulsion, no apparent damage to eyeballs and optic nerve.

BIBLIOGRAPHY. Friedenwald H: Luxation and avulsion of eyeball during birth. Am J Ophthalmol 1:9–12, 1918

Ferrer H: Voluntary propulsion of both eyeballs. Am J Ophthalmol 11:833–855, 1928

Walsh TJ, Gilman M: Voluntary propulsion of the eyes. Am J Ophthalmol 67:583–585, 1960

DOWAGER HUMP

Symptoms and Signs. Prevalent in elderly females. Marked thoracic kyphosis.

Etiology. Osteoporotic fractures.

BIBLIOGRAPHY. Klippel JH, Dieppe PA: Rheumatology, p 7.32.5. St Louis, CV Mosby, 1995

DOWLING-DEGOS

Synonyms. Reticular pigmented anomaly of flexures, see Haber and Kitamura.

Symptoms and Signs. Present in adult life (fourth decade). Asymptomatic. On axillae and groin (also other areas affected: intergluteal, inframammary, neck, limbs, trunk, etc.), pigmented macules (freckle-like) symmetrical and progressivelly extending. Occasionally comedo-like lesions, pitted acniform scars, near angle of mouth. Mental retardation and trichilemmal cysts.

Etiology. Autosomal dominant inheritance.

Pathology. Acanthosis with elongation of rete ridges and increased melanin at the tips.

Prognosis. Progressive condition.

BIBLIOGRAPHY. Dowling GB, Freudenthal WA: A case of acanthosis nigricans. Br J Dermatol 50:467–471, 1938

Degos R, Ossipowski B: Dermatose pigmentaire réticulée de plis (dicussion de l'acanthosis nigricans). Ann Dermatol Syphilgr 81:147–151, 1954

Harper J: Genetics and genodermatoses. In Champion RH, Burton JL, Ebling FJG (eds): Rook/Wilkinson/Ebling Textbook of Dermatology, 5th ed, p 370. Oxford, Blackwell Scientific, 1992

DOWLING-MEARA

Synonyms. Epidermolysis, herpetiform simple; herpetiform simple epidermolysis bullosa.

Symptoms and Signs. In infancy. Severe and extensive blistering, occasionally involving also mucosae with plaque-like lesions, spontaneous herpetiform serous and hemorrhagic blistering of trunks (distinctive feature). Occasionally loss of nails that regrow normally. Improvement with fever and in the summer.

Etiology. Autosomal dominant inheritance.

Pathology. Initial blister initiating in the basal cells; cytolysis followed by inflammation. Electron microscopy: In cytoplasm large clumps of keratin tonofilaments.

Therapy. Prolonged warm saline soaks. Fever may induce remission.

Prognosis. Condition improving with age. Usually blisters leave no scars.

BIBLIOGRAPHY. Dowling GB, Meara RH: Epidermolysis bullosa resembling juvenile dermatitis herpetiformis. Br J Dermatol 66:139–143, 1954

Hacham-Zadeh S, Rappersberger K, Livschin R, et al: Epidermolysis bullosa herpetiformis Dowling-Meara in a large family. Am J Acad Dermatol 18:702–706, 1988

Pye RJ: Bullous eruptions. In Champion RH, Burton JL, Ebling FJG (eds): Rook/Wilkinson/Ebling Textbook of Dermatology, 5th ed, pp 1627–1628. Oxford, Blackwell Scientific, 1992

DOWN

Synonyms. Trisomy 21; trisomy 22; trisomy G1. Mongolian idiocy; mongolism (are improper eponyms used in the past and that must be deleted from literature in relation to Down syndrome).

Symptoms. Both sexes, all races affected. Incidence related to maternal age. Twenty-five-year-old mother, 1:2000; 35-year-old mother, 1:200; over 40–year-old mother, 1:40 or higher incidence. Two populations: one with high mortality in first year of life or stillborn and another that survives infancy. Mental retardation (IQ 20–60) becoming evident to parent at end of first year of life. Usually, child is happy, affable, and affectionate; walking, speech, and toilet training delayed until 2–3 years of age. Generalized hypotonia. Persistent infection and obstructive symptoms of nose. Delayed puberty. In female, early menopause.

Signs. Newborn small, remaining short of stature; tendency to overweight. *Extremities.* Short limbs, hands square; fingers short and stubby; feet short with poorly developed arch. *Dermatoglyphic.* Changes of dermal ridge pattern allows objective diagnosis. *Pelvis.* Iliac wing wide and flat, small iliac angle. *Head.* Small; occiput flat; neck short and thick. *Eyes.* Hypotelorism; small orbital sockets; upper outward slant of palpebral fissures. Iris usually blue or grey, small whitish speckles (Brusfield spots). Squint common; later in life cataracts frequent. *Nose.* Small; hypoplasia of maxilla; protrusion of tongue; thickened, fissured (scrotal) lower lip may enlarge and hang down in later life. *Teeth.* Malocclusion. Signs of congenital heart defects (in 50% of cases). In neonatal period in some cases, atresia of duodenum. *Genitals.* In male, genitalia undescended and small penis. In female, genitalia show large labia majora and small labia minora. Occasional abnormalities: seizures; strabismus; nystagmus; keratoconus; cataract; low placement of ears; web neck; funnel or pigeon breast; tracheoesophageal fistula; duodenal atresia. The incidence of leukemia is about 1:95, or close to 1%.

Etiology. Chromosomal anomalies that usually cause delay in physical, intellectual, and language development: (1) Nondisjunction trisomy 21 "regular mongol" (most common variety); (2) "de novo" translocation (relatively rare); (3) inherited translocation (very rare); (4) mongol mosaicism. Full trisomy 21, 94%; 21 trisomy/normal mosaicism 2, 4%; translocation cases (equal D/G and G/G) 3, 3%.

Pathology. See Signs. In 50%, congenital heart malformations: large cushion septal defect; atrioventricularis communis (most common); frequently tetralogy of Fallot and other types. Fatty metamorphosis in liver (69%); portal tract abnormalities (96%); amyloidosis (8%). Testis frequently undescended; azospermia; absence of part or all of epididymis.

Diagnostic Procedures. *Dermatoglyphic and chromosome studies.* See Etiology. *Blood.* Acute leukemia three times more common than in comparable age group. Alkaline phosphatase of leukocytes increased. A number of enzymes are also increased.

Therapy. No cure; help family to adjust to situation. Treat repeated respiratory infections and heart conditions when present.

Prognosis. Highest mortality in the first month of life (8%). Survival first year 80%; second year 85%; fifth year 76% and small decrease thereafter. Congenital heart conditions decrease survival as well as low birth weight, maternal age (equal or higher than 35) and status of regional medical care.

BIBLIOGRAPHY. Down JLH: Observations on an ethnic classification of idiots. Clin Lect Rep London Hosp 3:259–262, 1866

Roberts DF, Callow MH: Origin of the additional chromosome in Down's syndrome: A study of 20 families. J Med Genet 17:363–367, 1980

Hartley XY: A summary of recent research into the development of children with Down's syndrome. J Ment Defic Res 30:1–14, 1986

Mastroiacovo P, Bertollini R, Corchia C: Survival of children with Down syndrome in Italy. Am J Med Genet 42:208–212, 1992

DOWNBEAT NYSTAGMUS–VERTIGO

Synonym. Vertigo—downbeat nystagmus; vertigo—downbeat nystagmus. See also Upbeat nystagmus vertigo.

Symptoms and Signs. Both sexes. All ages, rare in children. Downbeat nystagmus in the primary position of gaze that is not suppressed by fixation. Enhanced on lateral gaze of head extension. Associated with oscillopsia and imbalance, tendency to fall backward.

Etiology. Tonic imbalance of vertical semicircular canal reflexes modulated by otoliths. Cerebellar ectopia or degeneration. Alcoholic cerebellar degeneration. Drugs: phenytoin, carbamazepine, lithium, etc. Multiple sclerosis tumor, hematoma, vascular diseases, encephalitis, deficiency of vitamin B_{12}, and magnesium depletion. Congenital hereditary form reported.

Pathology. Lesion either on the floor of the fourth ventricle between vestibular nuclei or vestibulocerebellar flocculus.

Diagnostic Procedures. *EEG. CT scan. MRI. Electronystagmography.*

Therapy. Depends on etiology. Surgery. Congenital form may receed spontaneously. Clonazepam and baclofen suppress downbeat nystagmus. Physical balance training.

Prognosis. Depends on etiology.

BIBLIOGRAPHY. Cogan DG: Downbeat nystagmus. Arch Ophthalmol 80:757–768, 1968

Bixeman WW: Congenital hereditary downbeat nystagmus. Canadian J Ophthalmol 18:344–348, 1983

Brandt T: Vertigo: Its Multisensory Syndromes, pp 99–107. London, Springer-Verlag, 1991

DOW-VAN BOGAERT

Synonym. See Choreiform syndromes.

BIBLIOGRAPHY. Dow RS, Van Bogaert L: On complex involuntary move-

ments appearing late following the resection of a cerebellar hemisphere. J Belge de Neurol Psychiatr 38:803–807, 1938

DOYNE

Synonyms. Honeycomb retinal degeneration presently included in the group of age-related maculopathy (see) and Holthouse-Batten.

Symptoms and Signs. Both sexes affected; onset in third decade. Formation of white spots in peripapillary areas, and usually in the macular area as well. Between fourth and fifth decades lesions multiply; finally, white bodies become confluent to produce a white confluent atrophic area. Visual deterioration progressive in 75% of cases (white bodies on nasal side of optic disk pathognomonic of this form).

Etiology. Unknown; autosomal dominant transmission.

Pathology. Nodular thickening of Bruch membrane; choroid normal; evolution to homogeneous atrophy involving optic disk and macular area.

Diagnostic Procedures. Ophthalmologic examination.

Prognosis. Progressive visual deterioration. Absence of lesion in macular area in a 35-year-old patient can be regarded as a favorable prognostic sign.

BIBLIOGRAPHY. Doyne RW: Peculiar condition of choroiditis occurring in several members of the same family. Trans Ophthamol Soc UK 19:71, 1899

Pearce WG: Doyne's honey-comb retinal degeneration. Br J Ophthalmol 52:73–78, 1968

Garner A, Sarks S, Sarks JP: Degenerative and related disorders of the retina and choroid. In Garner A, Klintworth GK (eds): Pathobiology of Ocular Disease: A Dynamic Approach, 2nd ed, p 631. New York, Marcel Dekker, 1994

DREIFUSS-EMERY

Synonyms. Emery-Dreifuss (X-linked); scapuloperoneal X-linked; humeroperoneal neuromuscular; rigid spine. The classification of this syndrome is still very confused.

Symptoms and Signs. Prevalence in males. Only few females described. Onset 4–5 years of age. Muscle weakness, initially involving the lower extremities (tendency to walk on tip-toes, followed in the early teens by waddling gait), then by marked weakness of shoulder girdle muscles. Increase lumbar lordosis, flexion deformities of elbows. Mild pectus excavatum, cardiac involvement and absence of muscular pseudohypertrophy. Mental retardation. Heart conduction anomalies sometimes observed.

Etiology. Unknown. X-linked inheritance. An autosomal dominant form identified with various clinical differences. See Emery-Dreifuss, autosomal dominant.

Prognosis. Remarkably different among cases: usually no reduction of life span; death from severe cardic arrhythmia possible.

BIBLIOGRAPHY. Cestan R, LeJonne NI: Une myopathy avec retractions familiales. Nous. Iconog. Salpetriere 15:38–52, 1902

Dreiffus FE, Hogan GR: Survival in X-linked chromosomal muscular dystrophy. Neurology 11:734–737, 1961

Emery AEH, Dreifuss FE: Unusual type of benign X-linked muscular dystrophy. J Neurol Neurosurg Psychiatry 29:338–342, 1966

Dubowitz V: Rigid spine syndrome: A muscle syndrome in search of a name. Proc Roy Soc Med 66:219–220, 1973

Thomas PK, Petty RKH: Emery–Dreifuss muscular dystrophy. J Med Genet 22:138–139, 1985

McKusick VA: Mendelian Inheritance in Man, 10th ed, p 1916. Baltimore, Johns Hopkins, 1992

DRESBACH

Synonyms. Hemolytic elliptocytic anemia, hereditary ovalocytosis, hereditary elliptocytosis (HE), hereditary pyropoikilocytosis (HPP) which probably represents a more severe form of the same disease. Five clinical phenotypes have been described.

1. MILD HE

Symptoms and Signs. All races, no anemia or splenomegaly, mild hemolysis. Elliptocytosis is a morphologic curiosity except in cases (5–20%) in which cirrhosis, infectious mononucleosis, or malaria decompensate the disease. Cases of mild HE with abnormal erythropoiesis are described in southern Italians.

Etiology. Autosomal dominant.

Diagnostic Procedures. *Blood smear.* More than 30% of RBC are elliptocytes.

Therapy. When necessary, splenectomy.

Prognosis. Good.

2. MILD HE WITH POIKILOCYTOSIS IN INFANCY

Symptoms and Signs. Neonatal jaundice, hemolytic anemia in childhood. Predominant in blacks. In adult life only mild HE.

Etiology. Autosomal dominant.

Diagnostic Procedures. *Blood smear of parents.* One will have mild HE. *Blood smear.* Poikilocytes or elliptocytes.

Therapy. Splenectomy usually not necessary.

Prognosis. Good.

3. SPHEROCYTIC HE

Symptoms and Signs. Families of European descent. Hemolysis always present. Splenomegaly.

Etiology. Autosomal dominant.

Diagnostic Procedures. *Blood smear.* Elliptocytosis and spherocytosis.

Therapy. Splenectomy often necessary.

Prognosis. Good.

4. STOMATOCYTIC HE

Symptoms and Signs. Only in aborigines of Melanesia. Mild hemolysis.

Etiology. Autosomal recessive.

Diagnostic Procedures. *Blood smear.* Roundish elliptocytes traversed by one or two bars (appearance of double stomatocytes).

Therapy. Symptomatic.

Prognosis. Good.

5. HEREDITARY PYROPOIKILOCYTOSIS (HPP)

Symptoms and Signs. In blacks. In childhood severe hemolytic anemia with complications, growth retardation, frontal bossing.

Etiology. Unknown. Maybe autosomal recessive.

Diagnostic Procedures. *Blood smear.* Extreme poikilocytosis with spherocytes, elliptocytes, triangulocytes. Abnormal thermal sensitivity of blood.

Therapy. Splenectomy.

Prognosis. Severe.

BIBLIOGRAPHY. Dresbach M: Elliptical human red corpuscles. Science 19:469–470, 1904
Bunn HF, Forget BG: Hemoglobin: Molecular, Genetic and Clinical Aspects. Philadelphia, WB Saunders, 1986

DRESSLER (D.)

Synonyms. Donath-Landsteiner; Harley; paroxysmal cold hemoglobinuria. See Hemolytic anemia of newborn.

Symptoms. Both sexes affected; onset at all ages (syphilitic type onset in young group). Paroxysmal attacks of hemoglobinuria; in some patients frequent episodes induced by minor cold exposure; in others, rare attacks induced by exposure to very low temperature. From a few minutes to hours after exposure to cold (also limited to an area of the body) pains in the back and legs, abdominal cramps, headache, shaking chills, hyperpyrexia, and hemoglobinuria lasting a few hours; temporary enlargement of spleen and jaundice with each attack. Abortive attacks may occur with simple hemoglobinuria without systemic manifestations. Vasomotor phenomena. Paresthesias; urticaria; cyanosis; Raynaud phenomena with or without gangrene observed in several cases.

Etiology. Congenital syphilis (chronic type), idiopathic (acute transient type and chronic type), or associated with cold agglutinin.

Pathology. That of congenital syphilis when it is the cause.

Diagnostic Procedures. *Blood.* Anemia after attack; all findings of hemolytic crisis; leukopenia followed by neutrophilic leukocytosis; erythrophagocytosis. Donath-Landsteiner antibody test. Positive, "biphasic test." *Serology.* For syphilis. Coombs test (and other studies). For differential diagnosis of other hemolytic anemias. Rosenbach test (immersion of extremity in cold water induces hemolytic crisis). Erlich test (ligature around finger). Immersion in icy water: demonstration of local hemoglobinemia. *Urine.* Presence of hemoglobin and methemoglobin.

Therapy. Antisyphilitic treatment (when syphilis demonstrated). In idiopathic case, no specific treatment. Adrenocorticotropic hormone (ACTH) and steroid reported beneficial. Avoidance of exposure to cold.

Prognosis. Usually chronic, relatively benign condition; seldom cause of severe anemia or death. Great variability of clinical manifestations, from simple, minimal hemoglobinuria after exposure to intense cold to repeated attacks with minimal temperature variations.

BIBLIOGRAPHY. Elliotson J: Diseases of the heart united with ague. Lancet 1:500–501, 1832
Dressler DR: Ein Fall von intermittirender Albuminurie und Chromaturie. Arch Pathol Anat Physiol 6:264–266, 1853
Donath J, Landsteiner K: Ueber paroxysmale Hämoglobinurie. Münch Med Wochenschr 51:1590–1593, 1904
Foerster J: Autoimmune hemolytic anemias. In Lee GR, Bithell TC, Foerster J, et al (eds): Wintrobe's Clinical Hematology, 9th ed, pp 1184–1186. Philadelphia, Lea & Febiger, 1993

DRESSLER (W.)

Synonym. Postmyocardial infarction; pericarditis, postinfarction.

Symptoms and Signs. Develops after 2–10 weeks in 3–4% of cases of recent myocardial infarction. Fever; chest pain; symptoms and signs of pericarditis, pleurisy, and pneumonitis; tendency to recurrences, although the full picture (including pericarditis and pneumonia) is not always present.

Etiology. Unknown. Some evidence has been found that an antigen produced by myocardial necrosis may induce the formation of autoantibodies.

Pathology. That of myocardial infarction, pleurisy, pneumonia.

Diagnostic Procedures. *Blood.* Increase of sedimentation rate and leukocytosis; demonstration of heart autoantibodies. *Blood cultures. X-ray of chest. Electrocardiography.*

Therapy. Corticosteroids, indomethacin, aspirin.

Prognosis. Good response to corticosteroids. Danger of cardiac tamponade, especially with patients on anticoagulant. Repeated episodes last for 1–2 weeks (exceptionally, 3–6 weeks); recurrences may occur up to 12 months.

BIBLIOGRAPHY. Solof LA, Zatuchini J, Janton DH, et al: Reactivation of rheumatic fever following mitral commisurotomy. Circulation 8:481–493, 1953
Dressler W: A complication of myocardial infarction resembling idiopathic recurrent benign pericarditis. Circulation 12:697, 1955
Dressler W: The post myocardial infarction syndrome: report on forty-four cases. Arch Int Med 103:28–42, 1959
Shabetai R: Diseases of pericardium. In Schlant RC, Alexander RW, et al: Hurst's The Heart, 8th ed, p 1667. New York, McGraw-Hill, 1994

DREUW (M.)

Synonym. Alopecia parvimaculata.

Symptoms and Signs. Both sexes affected; onset at all ages. Usually, epidemic outbreaks. Rapid development of several small, irregular patches of alopecia.

Etiology. Unknown.

Pathology. Lymphocytic infiltration around hair follicle, sparing the bulbs, followed by atrophic, sclerotic changes. Sebaceous glands and hair follicles disappear; sweat glands remain.

Therapy. None.

Prognosis. The hair may regrow or permanent bald scars remain.

BIBLIOGRAPHY. Dreuw M: Ueber epidemische Alopecia; Vorlaufige Mitteilung. Monatsschr Prakt Dermatol 51:18–22, 1910
Hofer W: Sporadisches Auftreten von Alopecia parvimaculata. Dermatol Wochenschr 149:381–386, 1964
Dawber RPR, Ebling FJG, Wojnarowska FT: Disorders of hair. In Champion RH, Burton JL, Ebling FJG (eds): Rook/Wilkinson/Ebling Textbook of Dermatology, 5th ed, p 2601. Oxford, Blackwell Scientific, 1992

DREW

Synonym. Intermittent touch. See also pseudophakic bullous keratopathy.

Symptoms and Signs. After cataract surgery. Decrease of vision.

Etiology. Intermittent touch of inappropriately placed IOL causes corneal decomposition.

Pathology. Ciliary flush, localized corneal changes. Cystoid macular edema.

BIBLIOGRAPHY. Drew RC: Intermittent touch syndrome. Arch Ophthalmol 100:1440, 1982
Apple DJ, Rabb MF: Ocular Pathology, 4th ed, p 154. St Louis, Mosby Yearbook, 1991

DREYFUS

Obsolete.

Synonym. Platyspondylysis.

Symptoms. Short neck; slow development of kyphoscoliosis; joint laxity; muscle weakness; batracian (frog-like) abdomen; short stature.

Etiology. Unknown. Not a clear entity. Individual manifestations and their associations are present in many syndromes.

BIBLIOGRAPHY. Dreyfus JR: Ueber ein neues mit allgemeiner wahrer oder scheinbarer Breitwirbligkeit (Platyspondylia vera aut spuria generalisata) ein hergehends Syndrom. Jahr Kinderheilkd 150:42–54, 1938

DROBIN

Synonym. Renal-ocular.

Symptoms. Fever, myalgias, conjunctival/scleral injection of eyes, enlargement of lymph nodes.

Signs. Ophthalmologic examination: acute iritis. Blood tests: abnormal renal function.

Etiology. Unknown; probably it is a viral-like illness.

Pathology. Renal biopsy: acute interstitial nephritis that can be mononuclear or eosinophilic; bone marrow, lymph nodes: granulomas.

Diagnostic Procedures. *Blood screening for kidney function. Renal biopsy. Lymph node or bone marrow biopsies.*

Differential Diagnosis. Tuberculosis, sarcoidosis, Wegener granulomatosis, collagen vascular disorder, Behçet disease, syphilis, toxoplasmosis, cytomegalovirus infection, leprosy, *Chlamydia psittaci* infection, herpes simplex infection.

Therapy. Steroids, e.g., prednisone, 60 mg/day, tapered after 1 month to 30 mg/day. Topical steroids and atropine on the affected eye.

Prognosis. Good.

BIBLIOGRAPHY. Drobin RS, Vernier RL, Fish AL: Acute eosinophilic interstitial nephritis and renal failure with bone marrow-lymph node granulomas and anterior uveitis. A new syndrome. Am J Med 59:325–333, 1975
Steinman TI, Silva P: Acute interstitial nephritis and iritis. Renal-ocular syndrome. Am J Med 77:189–191, 1984

DUANE

Synonyms. Stilling; Stilling-Türk-Duane; Türk-Stilling; eye retraction; retraction.

Symptoms and Signs. Prevalent in females; onset from birth. Unilateral and in 15–20% bilateral deficiency of convergence and occasionally up or down deviation on adduction. Reduction or loss of abduction of the globe; retraction on adduction with occasional limitation of this movement; narrowing of palpebral fissure in adduction and widening in attempts of abduction. Pupillary changes; heterochromia iridis. Frequently associated, Klippel-Feil (see) and various malformations of face, ears, and teeth. Provided classification, for instance Type I paresis of abduction, retraction of eyeball on adduction; type II paresis of adduction, retaction of eyeball on attempted adduction; type III paresis of vertical motors, increased eyeball retraction and narrowing of palpebral fissure on adduction.

Etiology. Congenital defect; Ascribed to malformation or cicatrization of lateral rectus muscle, of its fascia, or of the fascial sheath from birth trauma (tenon capsule). Today attributed rather to central nervous system (probably supranuclear) lesion determining a paradoxical synergism of the external and internal rectus muscles instead of the usual antagonism. This etiologic hypothesis is based on characteristic electromyographic response; histologic evidence still not provided.

Pathology. Alteration of external rectus muscle occasionally observed. Pathologic changes may be central (supranuclear lesion); aberrant innervation affects oculomotor (III) and facial (VII) nerves. The syndrome has been described in association with cerebral arteriovenous malformation and with other associated malformations that have been simplified into four categories: skeletal, auricular, ocular, and neural.

Diagnostic Procedures. *Electromyography. Pattern of eye muscles. CT brain scan. MRI. Cerebral arteriography.* When indicated.

Therapy. When electromyography shows paradoxical innervation, surgery for correction is contraindicated. Surgical correction of associated anomalies.

BIBLIOGRAPHY. Stilling J: Untersuchungen ueber die ntstehung der Lurzsichtigkeit. Wiesbaden S 13, 1887

Türk S: Ueber Retractions-bwegungen der Augen. Dsch Med Wchschr 22:199, 1896

Duane A: Congenital deficiency of abduction, associated with impairment of adduction, retraction movements, contraction of palpebral fissure and oblique movements of the eye. Arch Ophthalmol 34:133–159, 1905

Parks MM: Ophthalmoplegic syndromes and trauma. In Duane TD, Jaeger EA (eds): Clinical Ophthalmology. Philadelphia, Harper & Row, 1987

DUBIN-JOHNSON

Synonyms. Sprinz-Nelson; Dubin-Sprinz; black liver—jaundice; icterus—hepatic pigmentation; chronic idiopathic jaundice.

Symptoms. Both sexes affected; onset in childhood or adult life. In women, occasionally unmasked by contraceptive pills or pregnancy. Intermittent episodes of jaundice associated with mild pain in right hypochondrium. Absence of pruritus. Occasionally weakness, fatigue. Frequent occurrence in Persian Jews associated with factor VII deficiency.

Signs. Mild enlargement of liver and tenderness.

Etiology. Autosomal recessive inheritance. Primary defect in secretion of conjugated bilirubin and other organic anions.

Pathology. *Liver.* Black color; deposit of melanin-like pigment in parenchymal cells; especially centrilobular areas; normal bile canaliculi, no fibrosis or inflammation; Kupffer cells no pigment.

Diagnostic Procedures. *Blood.* Increased conjugated bilirubin; serum alkaline phosphatases normal; sodium sulfobromophthalein level increased. *Urine.* Bilirubinuria; abnormal distribution of coproporphyrin isomer I and III (pathognomonic). *Cholecystography. Ultrasound.* Often, lack of visualization of biliary system. *Biopsy of liver.* Diagnostic (see Pathology).

Therapy. None; advise the patient about benign and congenital nature of condition and reassure on no need for unnecessary surgery.

Prognosis. Good; no limitation on normal life.

BIBLIOGRAPHY. Dubin IN, Johnson FB: Chronic idiopathic jaundice with unidentified pigment in liver cells: New clinicopathologic entity with report of 12 cases. Medicine 33:155–197, 1954

Sprinz H, Nelson RS: Persistent non-hemolytic hyperbilirubinemia associated with lipochrome-like pigment in liver cells: Report of 4 cases. Ann Intern Med 41:952–962, 1954

Chowdhury JR, Wolkoff AW, Chowdhury NR, et al: Hereditary jaundice and disorders of bilirubin metabolism. In Scriver CR, Beaudet AL, Sly WS, et al: The Metabolic and Molecular Bases of Inherited Disease, 7th ed, p 2188. New York, McGraw-Hill, 1995

DUBOWITZ

Synonyms. Dwarfism, eczema, peculiar facies.

Symptoms. Both sexes affected; present from birth. Mental deficiencies mild to moderate (35%); hyperactivity (60%); speech delayed (60%) stubborness; shyness; high-pitched cry (50%). Feeding difficulties (65%); diarrhea; rhinorrhea; otitis.

Signs. Low birth weight. *Head.* Microcephaly (mild); small facies; shallow supraorbital ridge; hypertelorism, short palpebral fissures; lateral telecanthus; palpebral ptosis; micrognathia; caries. *Face and flexural areas.* Eczema; scarce hair; missing or reduced lateral eyebrows. Occasionally cleft palate (35%), pes planus, cryptorchidism, hypospadia (70%). *Vascular (arterial) abnormalities.* Right internal carotid artery occlusion; aberrant right subclavian artery; coarctation of the aorta.

Etiology. Autosomal recessive inheritance.

Therapy. Surgical correction of vascular abnormalities.

Prognosis. Eczema recedes between second and fourth year of age. Deficient speech development. Proportioned dwarfism. Association with leukemia, lymphoma, aplastic anemia, neuroblastoma.

BIBLIOGRAPHY. Dubowitz V: Familial low birth weight dwarfism with unusual facies and a skin eruption. J Med Genet 2:12–17, 1969

Shuper A, Merlob P, Weitz R, et al: The diagnosis of Dubowitz syndrome in the neonatal period—A case report. Eur J Pediatr 145:151–152, 1986

Ilyina HG, Lurie IW: Dubowitz syndrome: Possible evidence for a subclinical subtype. Am J Med Genet 35:561–565, 1990

DUCHENNE I

Synonyms. Progressive bulbar palsy; labioglossolaryngeal paralysis.

Symptoms. Onset at 50–60 years of age. Progressive speech defect, from minor defect in articulation to the production of incomprehensible sound (laryngeal). Mastication and deglutition defect with occasional nasal regurgitation; drooling; gait and movement affected by spasticity of extremities; occasionally ophthalmoplegia. Loss of emotional control with episodes of sudden laughing and crying.

Signs. Weakness of facial muscles; spasticity of extremity muscles; hyperreflexia.

Etiology. Degeneration of the bulbar nuclei of trigeminal (V), facial (VII), glossopharyngeal (IX), vagus (X), and hypoglossal (XII) nerves, in association with other degenerative disorders, or primary. Considered as a variant of amyotrophic lateral sclerosis (see Aran-Duchenne).

Pathology. Degeneration of mentioned nuclei and corticobulbar tracts. Atrophic changes and glial reaction.

Therapy. Symptomatic.

Prognosis. Poor; involvement of respiratory centers cause of death.

BIBLIOGRAPHY. Duchenne G: Paralysie musculaire progressive de la langue, du voile du palais et des lèvres: Affection non encore décrite comme espéche morbide distincte. Arch Gen Med 16:283–296, 1860

Adams RD, Victor M: Principles of Neurology, 5th ed, p 1181. New York, McGraw-Hill, 1993

DUCHENNE II

Synonyms. Duchenne-Griesinger; Landouzy-Duchenne; pseudohypertrophic muscular dystrophy; muscular dystrophy, pseudohypertrophic, progressive; DMD.

Symptoms. Incidence 1/3500 male births (see also Duchenne dystrophy in females); onset at first–sixth years. Waddling gait; frequent falling; clumsiness. Gower maneuver to arise when lying on the floor. Axial and proximal girdle muscles of lower and then upper extremities involved before distal girdle muscles. Eventually, patient becomes confined to wheelchair and contractures develop. Frequent respiratory infections; frequent gastric dilatation; one third of patients are mentally retarded.

Signs. Pseudohypertrophy of calves and occasionally of deltoid triceps and other muscles. Palpation reveals doughy consistency. Scoliosis, muscular atrophy, and contractures develop when patient can no longer walk. Cardiac enlargement and sinus tachycardia.

Etiology. Two-thirds sex-linked recessive inheritance; one-third sporadic. Defect on Xp 21 that determines deficiency of structural protein dystrophin, normally adherent to muscle plasma membrane. Lack of protein determines muscle cell death, with several episodes of regeneration and final fatty substitution of muscle fibers. Possibility of a group with autosomal recessive type has been discussed.

Pathology. Muscle pale; fish-like. Biopsy shows necrotic and degenerating muscle fibers occurring in clusters, successively falling apart with invasion by macrophages and inflammatory cells.

Diagnostic Procedures. *Blood.* Aldolase; creatine phosphatase, serum glutamic-oxaloacetic transaminase (SGOT), glutamic-pyruvic transaminase (GPT), lactic dehydrogenase, increased during course of disease; in advanced disease revert to normal or remain only slightly elevated. *Electroencephalography. Electromyography:* Abnormalities of conduction. *Biopsy of muscle.*

Therapy. Exercise and activity to limit of tolerance. Bracing, surgery (in young patients, fasciotomy), and orthopedic measures prolong self-sufficiency.

Prognosis. Confinement to wheelchair usually at 9–12 years of age. Velocity of progression of disease grossly inverse proportionate to age of onset; 75% of patients die by the age of 20. Mortality rate drops sharply after that age; 5% remain alive at age 50. Sudden death from myocardial failure, respiratory infections.

BIBLIOGRAPHY. Duchenne GB: Recherches sur la paralysie musculaire pseudohypertrophique, ou paralysie myosclérosique. Arch Gen Med 11:5–25, 179–209; 305–321; 421–443, 552–588, 1868
Adams RD, Victor M: Principles of Neurology, 5th ed, pp 1218–1219. New York, McGraw-Hill, 1993

DUCHENNE DYSTROPHY IN FEMALES

Symptoms and Signs. Only females are carriers of the condition, since it has a recessive sex-linked type of transmission. Carrier without clinical manifestations may be identified in approximately 80% of cases by biochemical studies: increase of creatine kinase. Occasionally, female may present typical clinical symptoms of Duchenne syndrome. The course is usually mild and slowly evolving.

Etiology. Unknown. Occurrence of clinical form of syndrome in female difficult to explain because of inheritance type of pattern. The following possibilities considered: (1) chromosomal mosaicism; (2) possible existence of an autosomal type of transmission; (3) Lyon hypothesis.

BIBLIOGRAPHY. Pearson CM, Fowler WM, Wright SW: X-chromosome mosaicism in females with muscular dystrophy. Proc Natl Acad Sci USA 50:24, 1963
Verellen–Dumolin C, Freund M, De Meyer R, et al: Expression of X-linked muscular dystrophy in a female due to translocation involving X p21 and non-random inactivation of the normal X-chromosome. Hum Genet 67:115–119, 1984
Greggs RC, Fischbeck KH: X-linked muscular dystrophies. In Rowland LP, Di Mauro S (eds): Handbook of Clinical Neurology, vol 18. Myopathies, p 117. Amsterdam, Elsevier, 1992

DUCKERT

Synonyms. Laki-Lorand; factor XIII deficiency; fibrinase deficiency; fibrin stabilizing factor; FSF deficiency; LL factor.

Symptoms and Signs. Prevalent in males. After birth bleeding from umbilicus. Usually after injury episode of serious bleeding. Wounds heal slowly and may break repeatedly. Hematomas; hematuria.

Etiology. Genetic polymorphism autosomal inheritance.

Diagnostic Procedures. *Blood.* Clotting tests normal. Fibrin prepared from patient soluble in 5 molar urea or 1% monoacetic acid.

Therapy. Transfusion of small amount of plasma (also stored) controls bleeding. Fibrin life (3–5 days).

Prognosis. Intracranial bleeding frequent cause of death. Good response to treatment; long survival possible.

BIBLIOGRAPHY. Duckert I, Jung E, Shmerling DH: A hitherto undescribed congenital haemorrhagic diathesis probably due to fibrin stabilizing factor deficiency. Thromb Diath Haemorrh 5:179–186, 1960
Berliner S, Lusky A, Zivelin A, et al: Hereditary factor XIII deficiency: report of four families and definition of the carrier state. Br J Haematol 56:495–505, 1984
Board PG, Chapple R, Coggan M: Haplotypes of the coagulation factor XIII: A subunit locus in normal and deficient subjects. Am J Med Genet 42:712–717, 1988
Saito M, Asukura H, Yoshida T, et al: A familial factor XIII subunit B deficiency. Br J Haematol 74:290–294, 1990

DUCTUS ARTERIOSUS, PATENT

Synonyms. Patent ductus arteriosus. Botallo duct patency (misnomer).

Symptoms. Symptoms usually are restricted to patients with large shunts that produce heart failure. Prevalent in females (3:1). In most cases, asymptomatic, in few cases exertional dyspnea, palpitation, fatigability. Occasionally, physical underdevelopment. Cardiac failure sooner or later. Frequent complication; bacterial endocarditis.

Signs. Pallor; habitus gracilis. *Heart.* Typical Gibson murmur: machinery-like occupying most of systole and diastole, with characteristic crescendo-systolic thrill over site of maximal intensity of sound. Second pulmonic sound accentuated; high pulse pressure; occasionally, a Corrigan pulse; capillary pulsation; pistol-shot femoral pulse and radial pulses may be unequal.

Etiology. Unknown. Reported as inherited recessive characteristic, or autosomal dominant inheritance. Maternal rubella complication.

Pathology. Patency of ductus arteriosus, uncomplicated or associated with other cardiac anomalies. In uncomplicated cases, pulmonary artery and branches become dilated, as well as both ventricles, which also show different degree of hypertrophy.

Diagnostic Procedures. *Two-dimensional echography* with color flow imaging and spectral Doppler interrogation. *X-ray. Angiocardiography.* Prominence of pulmonic arc in left upper portion of heart silhouette. *Electrocardiography.*

Therapy. Surgical (closure of ductus) and medical (Indomethacin).

Prognosis. Excellent; complete recovery with surgery in uncomplicated cases. If not treated, cardiac failure and endocarditis cause death.

BIBLIOGRAPHY. Carcano GB: 1593. In Castiglioni A: A History of Medicine. New York, Knopf, 1947
Wells HG: Persistent patency of the ductus arteriosus. Am J Med Sci 136:381, 1908

Marquis RM: The continuous murmur of persistence of the ductus arteriosus: An historical review. Eur Heart J 1:465–478, 1980
Nugent EW, Plauth WH, Edwards JE, et al: The pathology, pathophysiology, recognition, and treatment of congenital heart disease. In Schlant RC, Alexander RW: Hurst's The Heart, 8th ed, pp 1782–1785. New York, McGraw-Hill, 1994
Perloff JK: The Clinical Recognition of Congenital Heart Disease, 4th ed, pp 510–545. Philadelphia, WB Saunders, 1994

DUCTUS ARTERIOSUS, PATENT REVERSED FLOW

Symptoms. Usually present at birth. Exertional dyspnea; squatting occasionally present. Patent ductus is more common in the premature infant, especially those with birth asphyxia or respiratory distress syndrome.

Signs. Cyanosis (increasing with exercise) more intense in lower half of the body and in left hand rather than right. Clubbing may involve only lower extremities. Only a faint systolic murmur in third left interspace or no murmur. Seldom, diastolic murmur on left sternal border, loud with diastolic thrill.

Etiology. Unknown; patent ductus arteriosus with high pulmonary vascular resistance and reversed flow from pulmonary artery to aorta.

Pathology. Patency of ductus arteriosus. Hypertrophy of right ventricle. Pulmonary arteries normal or with occlusive lesions.

Diagnostic Procedures. *X-ray.* Prominence of pulmonary artery and its branches; sharp cutoff of small peripheral pulmonary artery. *Angiocardiography. Electrocardiography. Cardiac catheterization. Pressure determination. Oximetry. H-mode echocardiography. Pulsed Doppler ultrasonography.*

Therapy. Surgery usually contraindicated when pulmonary pressure very high and with shunt reversal. When transient (exertional) reversal of flow, surgery may be highly beneficial.

Prognosis. Smaller degree of myocardial insufficiency than in simple patent ductus arteriosus. High incidence of bacterial endocarditis. Patient may live for many years.

BIBLIOGRAPHY. Keith JD, Rowe RD, Vland P: Heart Disease in Infancy and Childhood, 3rd ed. New York, Macmillan, 1978
Nugent EW, Plauth WH, Edwards JE, et al: The pathology, pathophysiology, recognition, and treatment of congenital heart disease. In Schlant RC, Alexander RW: Hurst's The Heart, 8th ed, pp 1782–1785. New York, McGraw-Hill, 1994
Perloff JK: The Clinical Recognition of Congenital Heart Disease, 4th ed, p 510. Philadelphia, WB Saunders, 1994

DUDLEY-KLINGENSTEIN

Synonyms. Jejunum neoplasm. See Peutz-Jeghers and Gardner.

Symptoms. Combination of melena and abdominal pain, simulating a gastroduodenal lesion.

Signs. Pallor; tachycardia; abdominal distention.

Etiology. Benign or malignant lesion of jejunum.

Diagnostic Procedures. *X-ray of gastrointestinal tract.* Negative for gastroduodenal ulcer (pyloric spasm may be observed occasionally); jejunum shows filling defect. *Gastric fluid.* Usually, normal or low values of chlorhydric acid. *Blood.* Posthemorrhagic anemia.

Therapy. Surgery.

Prognosis. Depends on nature of lesion.

BIBLIOGRAPHY. Dudley HD: Vascular tumors of the small intestine with symptoms simulating peptic ulcer. Surg Clin North Am 14:1331–1337, 1934
Klingenstein P: Benign neoplasms of the small intestine complicated by severe hemorrhage: Report of two cases operative intervention and recovery. J Mt Sinai Hosp 4:972–979, 1938
Perzin KH, Bridge MF: Adenomas of the small intestine: A clinicopathologic review of 51 cases and a study of their relationship to carcinoma. Cancer 48:799–819, 1981
Bogoch A: Bleeding from the alimentary tract. In Haubrich WS, Schaffner F, Berk JE (eds): Bockus Gastroenterology, 5th ed, vol 2, p 66. Philadelphia, WB Saunders, 1995

DUHRING

Synonyms. Brocq-Duhring; dermatitis herpetiformis; dermatitis multiformis.

Symptoms and Signs. Prevalent in males (2:1); onset usually from 20–55 years of age; occasionally, in child over 5 years of age. Onset acute or gradual. Pruritus; pleomorphic, symmetric skin eruptions: erythematous, urticarial, papular, vesicular, or bullous that excoriate easily (small papules without blistering also seen); eczematous, exudative; or lichenified. Progressive pigmentation at site of lesion (in 50% of cases). Lesion affects extensor aspects of extremities, especially knees, elbows, and buttocks. Also frequently involved, axillary folds, shoulders, trunk, and face. Seldom, mucosal lesions. Occasionally, laryngeal involvement. Majority of patients: asymptomatic or paucisymptomatic gluten enteropathy.

Etiology. Unknown. Role of gluten not yet clearly established.

Pathology. Accumulation of neutrophils and eosinophils within dermal papillae; in vicinity of early blisters, formation of subepidermal vesicles. No advanced acantholysis. Villous atrophy in small bowel.

Diagnostic Procedures. *Biopsy. Blood.* Occasionally, increase of circulating eosinophils. A variety of antibodies in some patients (antithyroid, antireticulin, antigluten, and antigliadin); IgA-containing immune complexes in 25% of patients, more rarely IgG or IgM complexes. HLA B8 present in 85–95%, strong association with DRw3 and HLA-DQw2.

Therapy. Prolonged treatment with maintenance doses of dapsone. Sulfapyridine better tolerated by some patients. Topical application of corticosteroids (symptomatic).

Prognosis. Long course, remissions, and relapses; 20–30% with permanent or prolonged remission.

BIBLIOGRAPHY. Fox WT: A clinical study of hydroa. Arch Derm (Philad) 6:12–52, 1880
Duhring LA: Dermatitis herpetiformis. JAMA 3:225–229, 1884
Brocq L: De la dermatite Herpetiforme de Duhring. Ann Dermatol Syph 9:1–20, 1888
Duhring LA: Selected Monographs on Dermatology. London, New Sydenham Soc, 1893
Hall RP: The pathogenesis of dermatitis herpetiformis: recent advances. J Am Acad Dermat 16:1129–1144, 1987
Pye RJ: Bullous eruptions. In Champion RH, Burton JL, Ebling FJG (eds): Rook/Wilkinson/Ebling Textbook of Dermatology, 5th ed, pp 1658–1663. Oxford, Blackwell Scientific, 1992

DUKES-FILATOW

Obsolete. Eponym used to indicate Rubeola.

BIBLIOGRAPHY. Filatow NF: Vorlesungen ueber akute Infektionkrankheiten in Kindersalter. Uebers. Von L. Polosky Wein 383, 1897
Dukes C: On the confusion of two different diseases under the name of rubeola (rose-rash). Lancet II 89–94, 1900

DUMON-RADERMECKER

Synonyms. Amaurotic idiocy tardive-epilepsy.

Symptoms and Signs. Both sexes. During childhood: severe mental retardation, seizures. Late onset (fifth–sixth decade) ataxia (broad-based gait, intentional tremor, strong emotional component, accompanied by action hypertonia), dysarthria both cerebellar and pseudobulbar. Pyramidal signs absent. Only in one case optic atrophy.

Etiology. Autosomal dominant inheritance.

Pathology. Massive cytoplasmic deposits (probably glycolipid) in the nerve cells of cerebellar and cerebral cortex, thalamus, reticular formation, and some cranial nerve nuclei. Moderate cerebral and cerebellar atrophy.

Diagnostic Procedures. *CT scan. MRI. EEG. Fundus oculi.*

Therapy. Symptomatic.

Prognosis. Does not shorten life span of patients.

BIBLIOGRAPHY. Dumon-Raedermecker M Form très tardives d'idiotie amaurotique dans une souche d'ologophrénie congénitale avec epilepsie Acta Neurol Belg 65:778–807, 1965

DUNCAN

(Name of first patient described.)

Synonyms. Epstein-Barr; immunodeficiency-5; immunodeficiency, X-linked progressive, variable; ineffective immunological response; X-linked lymphoproliferative; XLP; infectious mono, susceptibility to.

Symptoms and Signs. In males. Described also in females. Fulminant hepatic failure and/or aplastic anemia. If they survive first week become hypogammaglobulinemic or develop malignant B-cell lymphomas.

Etiology. Unknown. Patients are clinically and immunologically normal before encountering EBV. After EBV infection antibody and cytotoxic reactions become exaggerated and uncontrolled, destroying hepatocytes, and hematopoietic and immune system cells. X-linked inheritance.

Pathology. *Liver.* Acute liver degeneration. *Blood.* Aplastic anemia, possible multiple rapidly developing lymphomas. *Bone marrow, lymphonodes, liver, and spleen.* Plasmocytoid lymphocytes, mature plasma cells and histiocytes.

Diagnostic Procedures. *Blood.* Antibody response to EBV abnormal, followed by rapid deterioration of B- and T-cell function. *Bone marrow.* See Pathology.

Therapy. In candidates, immunoprophylaxis for EBV (when becomes available). Acyclovir ineffective.

Prognosis. Death in first week in 80%.

BIBLIOGRAPHY. Purtillo DT, Carsel CK, Yaung JPS: Fatal infections mononucleosis in familial lymphohistiocytosis. N Engl J Med 201:736, 1991
Purtillo DT, Grierson HL: Methods of detection of new families with X-linked lymphoproliferative disease. Cancer Genet Cytogenet 51:143–153, 1991

DUNNINGAM

Synonyms. Kobberling-Dunningam, lipoatrophic diabetes; lipodystrophy familial of limbs and lower trunk; reverse partial lipodystrophy. See Berardinelli.

Symptoms and Signs. Only in females, full-blown condition. Only rare instances of male occurrence (?) reported. Fat accumulation on the neck, shoulders, and genitalia, lean muscular limbs phlebectasia. Thickened nails; premature eruption of teeth and macrodontia of upper central incisors with palatal cups from cingulum; open bite; tongue with filiform and fungiform papillae. Two types delineated:

1. Loss of subcutaneous fat limited to limbs saving face and trunk.
2. Involving also trunk, except vulva (pseudolabial hypertrophy).

Etiology. Sporadic and autosomal dominant inheritance (probable).

Pathology. Same as in lipoatrophic diabetes plus pineal hyperplasia.

Diagnostic Procedures. *Blood.* Hyperglycemia insulin resistant; type IV hyperlipoproteinemia, occasionally hypouricemia.

BIBLIOGRAPHY. Dunningam MG, Cochrane M, Kelly A, et al: Familial lipoatrophic diabetes with dominant transmission. Q J Med 43:33–48, 1974
Kobberlin J, Dunningam MG: Familial partial lipodystrophy: two types of an X-linked dominant syndrome. Lethal in the hemizygous state. J Med Genet 23:120–127, 1986
Reardon W, Temple IK, MacKinnon H, et al: Partial lipodystrophy syndromes, a further male case. Clin Genet 38:391–395, 1990

DUPLAY

Synonyms. Subacromial bursitis; scapulohumeral bursitis; subdeltoid bursitis; frozen shoulder; periarticular fibrositis shoulder; scapulohumeral periarthritis; shoulder adhesive capsulitis.

Symptoms. Occurs after 40 years of age; prevalent in women (seldom before menopause); in older men, and in sedentary workers. Gradually increasing pain in the shoulder during abduction and internal rotation, up to severe debilitating pain. Pain radiates to the arm and forearm, occasionally to scapular area.

Signs. Scapulohumeral fixation; arm adducted. Tenderness on palpation in various areas of shoulder.

Etiology. Trauma (15%); idiopathic (85%); frequently observed after periods of inactivity; muscle spasm in anxiety and depression; associated with some visceral diseases.

Pathology. Adhesive capsulitis arising from joint lining and spreading to it from other extrarticular joint structures.

Diagnostic Procedures. *X-ray.* Negative. After 2–3 months, demineralization of upper humerus.

Therapy. Moderate exercise initially; treatment of emotional aspects. In chronic cases; X-ray treatment, systemic corticosteroids, hydrocortisone injections. Surgery: closed or open manipulation.

Prognosis. Chronic course and prolonged disability frequent. Response to treatment not as good as in calcareous tendonitis.

BIBLIOGRAPHY. Duplay ES: De la peri-arthrite scapulo-humerale et des raideurs de l'épaule qui en sont la conséquence. Arch Gen Med 20:513–542, 1872
Haslock I: Back pain and periarticular disease. In Weatherall DJ, Ledingham JGG, Warrell DA (eds): Oxford Textbook of Medicine, 3rd ed, p 2995. Oxford, Oxford Med Pub, 1996

DUPRE

Synonym. Meningism.

Symptoms. Occurs mostly in infancy and childhood. Suddenly during the onset of an acute febrile disease: headache; neck stiffness; occasionally, convulsion and coma.

Signs. Positive Kernig sign.

Etiology. Increase in pressure of spinal fluid during the onset of acute febrile disease owing to relative hemodilution and filtration through choroid plexus.

Diagnostic Procedures. *Cerebrospinal fluid.* Increased pressure; increased proteins; negative bacteriologic studies; negative virus studies.

Therapy. Diuretics and control of pressure.

Prognosis. Spontaneous recovery within a few days.

BIBLIOGRAPHY. Dupré E: Le méningisme. Cong Fr Med 1:411–423, 1895
Adams RD, Victor M: Principles of Neurology, 5th ed, pp 647–650. New York, McGraw-Hill, 1993

DUPUYTREN

Synonym. Palmo-plantar fibromatosis.

Symptoms. Prevalent in males (6:1); high familial incidence; gradual increase of incidence with age, especially after 40 years of age. Unilateral or bilateral involvement. Right hand more frequently affected. Fingers affected in the following order: little, middle, index. Pain on the palm of hands. Progressive loss of function of hand owing to inability to extend fingers.

Signs. Small nodular thickening of palmar connective tissue, especially over fourth and fifth fingers. Puckering of palmar skin. Various degrees of flexion contracture of fingers.

Etiology. Unknown; autosomal dominant inheritance. Associated with many different pathologic conditions: epilepsy; pulmonary tuberculosis; chronic alcoholism; Steinbrocker; Peyronie. Free radical production secondary to ischemia may play some role and so does the increased concentration of hypoxanthine.

Pathology. Small nodules or thickening of palmar connective tissues overlying tendons of fingers; adherence between fascia and skin, successive appearance of fibrous bands from nodules to base of fingers.

Therapy. For pain (in nodular stage) reassurance of benign nature of pain. Ultrasound; heat; exercises; local injection of steroids (in early phase). Allopurinol to reduce free radicals and vitamin C and E as free radical scavengers. Surgery after contracture begins according to degree of involvement; best results after active phase has subsided.

Prognosis. Different degrees and speeds of evolution in different patients. Chronic benign condition that leads, however, to severe incapacitation. In some patients, fibrosis may remain nonprogressive for years.

BIBLIOGRAPHY. Dupuytren G: De la rétraction des doigts par suite d'une affection de l'aponévrose palmaire. Operation chirurgicale, qui couvient dans le cas. J Univ Hebd Med Chir Prat, Paris 5:352–365, 1831
Dupuytren G: Permanent retraction of the fingers, produced by an affection of the palmar fascia. Lancet 2:222, 1833–1834
Ranta H, Knif J, Ranta K: Familial hypodontia associated with Dupuytren's disease. Scand J Dent Res 98:457–460, 1990

DURAL SINUS THROMBOSIS

Symptoms. Often occurs in debilitated children or in postpartum period. Headache; nausea; vomiting; chills; remittent fever; tachycardia; convulsions; stupor and variable symptoms according to localization and eventual embolization.

Signs. Swelling of optic disks; engorgement of scalp veins; palpation of thrombosed vessel when extended to jugular vein.

Etiology. *Noninfective.* Malnutrition; heart conditions; trauma; postpartum; tumor; polycythemia. *Infective.* All kinds of infection spreading from middle ear and mastoid.

Pathology. Occlusion of the vessel by thrombus, bacteria, fibrin leukocytes; secondary thrombosis of almost all cortical veins; some of them rupture and cause hemorrhages, cerebral softening, edema, and abscess.

Diagnostic Procedures. *CT brain scan. MRI. Spinal fluid.* Leukocytosis; pressure and protein increased. *Blood.* Leukocytosis.

Therapy. Antibiotics; thrombolytics; anticoagulants.

Prognosis. Poor.

BIBLIOGRAPHY. Smith JC: Primary cerebral thrombophlebitis. JAMA 148:613–616, 1952
Crawford SC, Digre KB, Palmer CA: Thrombosis of the deep venous drainage of the brain in adults. Arch Neurol 52:1101–1108, 1995

DURAND

Synonyms. Lactose intolerance congenital; hypolactasia neonatal, neonatal lactose intolerance. See lactase deficiency.

Symptoms. Both sexes neonatal. Vomiting, failure to thrive.

Signs. Dehydratation; cataracts.

Etiology. Abnormal permeability of gastric mucosa. Autosomal dominant inheritance.

Pathology. Liver and brain degenerative processes.

Diagnostic Procedures. *Urine.* Lactosuria and disacchariduria, aminoaciduria. *Blood.* Acidosis, evidence of liver and kidney damage. *Jejunal biopsy.* Lactase activity normal.

Therapy. Change to milk-free diet.

Prognosis. Rapid recovery with change in diet; after 6 months patients tolerate normal diet. If not treated may be fatal.

BIBLIOGRAPHY. Durand P: Lattosuria idiopatica in una paziente con diarrea cronica ed acidosi. Minerva Pediatr 1:706–711, 1958
Hoskova A, Sabecky J, Mcskos A, et al: Severe lactose intolerance with lactosuria and vomiting. Arch Dis Child, 55:304–316, 1980
Semenza G, Auricchio S: Small-intestinal disaccharides. In Scriver CR, Beaudet AL, Sly WS, et al: The Metabolic and Molecular Bases of Inherited Disease, 7th ed, p 4467. New York, McGraw-Hill, 1995

DURAND I

Synonyms. Alpha-fucosidase acid deficiency; alpha-fucosidase deficiency; fucosidosis.

Symptoms. A concentration of patients in Calabria region of southern Italy. Two forms today identified: a fatal infantile form (type I) (60%) and milder form with adult survival (type II) (40%). Both sexes affected; normal at birth. Psychomotor retardation becoming evident by 12–15 months of age. Different degrees of severity. Progressive deterioration. Spasticity; tremor; loss of contact with environment; frequent infections.

Signs. Facies becoming coarse; development of spondyloepiphyseal dysplasia; kyphoscoliosis; cornea clear and fundus normal; angiokeratoma corposis diffusum (see Fabry). Vessels of the gums may be dilated and tongue large.

Etiology. Autosomal recessive inheritance; lack of acid alpha-fucosidase. Genetic polymorphism or heterogeneity may explain different clinical patterns (see Prognosis). Enzyme defect on chromosome 1.

Pathology. *Liver.* Abnormal lysosomes; vacuoles resembling those of Hurler syndrome, or containing stocks of circular lamellae. *Brain.* Half-empty vacuoles (without Zebra bodies). *Skin.* Full-blown diffuse angiokeratoma to minor vascular lesions.

Diagnostic Procedures. *Blood.* Vacuolization of lymphocytes. Deficient activity of lysosomal enzyme alpha-fucosidase in all cells and tissues, serum, and urine. *X-ray.* Minor skeletal alterations. *Sweat.* Increased sodium chloride content. Prenatal diagnosis is possible.

Therapy. Symptomatic.

Prognosis. Two types clearly distinguishable: (1) death before sixth year of life; (2) death in early adulthood (with more marked clinical signs).

BIBLIOGRAPHY. Durand P: A new mucopolysaccharide lipid storage disease. Lancet 2:1313–1314, 1966

Thomas GH, Beaudet AL: Disorders of glycoprotein degradation and structure: mannosidosis, fucosidosis, sialidosis, and aspartyl-glycosaminuria and carbohydrate-deficient glycoprotein syndrome. In Scriver CR, Beaudet AL, Sly WS, et al: The Metabolic and Molecular Bases of Inherited Disease, 7th ed, pp 2539–2542. New York, McGraw-Hill, 1995

DURAND-NICOLAS-FAVRE

Synonyms. Lymphogranuloma venereum.

Symptoms and Signs. Both sexes. Incubation 5–21 days. From sexual intercourse or contact with contaminated material. First phase: evanescent external genitalia lesions. After their disappearance lymphnodes enlargement, suppuration, and multiple drainage. According to sexual practice proctitis, tenesmus and eventually rectal strictures.

Etiology. *Chlamydial throchomatis* infection.

Pathology. Inguinal buboes bilateral, lymphnode fusion and breaking to form sinuses with discharges and scarring.

Diagnostic Procedures. *Blood.* Positive complement fixation test. IgM more specific for acute infection.

Therapy. Tetracyclines, Doxycycline, Erythromycin.

Prognosis. Good with early treatment.

BIBLIOGRAPHY. Durand M, Nicolas J, Fevre M: Lymphogranulomatose inguinale subacque d'origine génitale probable, peut etre vénérienne. Bull Soc Med Hop Paris 35:274–288, 1913

Martin DH, Mroczkowski TF, Dalu ZA: A controlled trial of a single dose of azithromycin for the treatment of Chlamydial urethritis and cervicitis. N Engl J Med 327:921–925, 1992

DUVERNOI

Synonyms. Abdominal gas cyst; intestinal emphysema, bullous; cystic lymphopneumatosis; emphysema intestinalis; intestine gas cyst; peritoneal pneumatosis; pneumatosis cystoides intestinalis; PCI.

Symptoms. Present in both sexes; onset at all ages (greatest incidence in males 30–50 years of age and females 60–70 years). Nonspecific. Alternating diarrhea and stypsis; abdominal distention; vague pains; rectal bleeding; partial or complete (rare) intestinal obstruction.

Signs. Crepitant, nontender, abdominal masses, plus signs of various complications, when occurring.

Etiology. Idiopathic (primary) (15%) or as complication, through unknown pathogenic mechanism due to other intestinal conditions (see Pathology). In infants, consequences of bacterial invasion. Particular diet (i.e., unpolished rice) may induce condition in animals.

Pathology. Multiple gas-filled cysts in gastrointestinal tract and occasionally in other organs of abdominal cavity. Size of cysts variable from microscopic to many centimeters in diameter. Cysts (thin-walled) break easily. Small bowel most frequent site. Other pathology of gastrointestinal tract frequently associated: pyloric stenosis; appendicitis; regional enteritis; ulcerative colitis; tubercular enteritis.

Diagnostic Procedures. *X-ray of intestine.* Clusters of radiolucent areas following course of bowel; pneumoperitoneum (occasionally); Chilaiditi (see). *Sigmoidoscopy (when sigmoid involved).* Submucosal cystic lesions.

Therapy. Secondary forms: Treat underlying condition. In both primary and secondary forms: Hyperbaric O_2 treatment, or let the patient breath O_2 by mask for several days. Dietary adjustment, antibiotics to modify intestinal flora. Surgery seldom needed except in secondary forms.

Prognosis. That of underlying condition. Cysts may disappear spontaneously or persist for a long time without serious symptoms.

BIBLIOGRAPHY. Combalusier: Pneumopathologie ou traité de maladies venteuses, vol 1, p 19. Paris, 1745

Duvernoi JC: Anatomische Beobachtungen der Unter der aussern und innern Haut der gedarme Eingeschlossenen Luft Phys Med Abhandl Acad Wissench Petersb 2:182, 1783

Bang, BLF: Luftholdige kyster i väggen af ileum og i nydannet bindeväv pä sammes serosa. Nord Med Ark, 8:1–15, 1876

Brandt LJ, Simon DM: Pneumatosis cystoides intestinalis. In Haubrich WF, Schaffner F, Berk JE (eds): Bockus Gastroenterology, 5th ed, vol 2, pp 1685–1693. Philadelphia, WB Saunders, 1995

DWARFISM, ENVIRONMENTAL

Synonyms. Deprivation dwarfism; emotional dwarfism; environmental failure to thrive; growth failure—maternal deprivation; maternal deprivation; sensory deprivation; psychological dwarfism.

Symptoms. Appears in infants or children. Failure to thrive; height-growth failure with subsequent correction in presence of appropriate nurturing. Mental retardation with subsequent acceleration when environment is changed. Apathy; intense irritability; withdrawal and defense against any kind of approach. May be present: vomiting; diarrhea; acute or chronic respiratory infections; anemia; neuromuscular disorders; signs of traumas (see Battered child syndrome). In some instances, failure to thrive may be observed in presence of a voracious appetite.

Etiology. Neglect or physical abuse or both. In the family, psychosocial factors, financial deprivation, sexual incompatibility or promiscuity in parents, familial illness, physical abuse, inexperience in mothering, unwanted pregnancy.

Pathology. Weight below third percentile; height below normal; signs of physical abuse.

Diagnostic Procedures. *Evaluation of familial psychosocial factors. X-ray. Blood. Urine. Endocrine studies.*

Therapy. Removal from environment or correction of negative environmental factors.

Prognosis. Good if adequate treatment possible.

BIBLIOGRAPHY. Talbot NB, Sobel EH, Burke BS, et al: Dwarfism in healthy children: Its possible relation to emotional, nutritional, and endocrine disturbances. N Engl J Med 236:783–793, 1947

Ruddy RM, Scanlin TF: Abnormal sweat electrolytes in a case of celiac disease and a case of psychological failure to thrive. Review of other reported causes. Clin Pediatr 26:83–89, 1987

Save M, Job JB, Chaussain JL: Les retards de croissance psychogénes. Etude critique des élements de diagnostic. Arch Fr Pediatr 44:331–338, 1987

Weatherall DJ, Ledingham JGG, Warrell DA (eds): Oxford Textbook of Medicine, 3rd ed, pp 1281–1283. Oxford, Oxford Med Pub, 1996

DWARFISM–IMMUNOPATHY–ASTHMA

Synonym. Asthma—dwarfism—high IgA.

Symptoms. Both sexes affected; onset age 4–5 months. Recurrent attacks of asthma; between attacks, no respiratory symptoms. Four to 5 years later, seasonal episodes of nasal congestion, sneezing, nasal itching.

Signs. Shortness of stature.

Etiology. Unknown; genetically related defect of not yet established type.

Diagnostic Procedures. *Blood.* Great elevation of IgA globulin; depressed IgM concentrations.

Therapy. Asthma and atopic allergy respond well to sympatholytics and prednisone.

Prognosis. Persistent condition; mild; usually not requiring hospitalization.

BIBLIOGRAPHY. Huntley CC, Johnson HW, Lyerly AD: Asthma, short stature and elevated gamma IgA globulins. Am J Dis Child 109:353–358, 1965

Sly RM, Heimlich EM: Identical twins with short stature, elevated IgA, and asthma. Ann Allerg 25:578–586, 1967

DYGGVE-MELCHIOR-CLAUSEN

Synonyms. Dyggve-Melchior-Clausen dwarfism; pseudo-Morquio type A; Smith-McCort (included).

Symptoms and Signs. Diagnosed within first year. In autosomal form: mild to moderate mental retardation; microcephaly. In X-linked normal intelligence and minor microcephaly. Short trunk dwarfism. Exaggerated lordosis. Fingers clawed and with limited extension. Waddling gait.

Etiology. Autosomal recessive inheritance and X-linked recessive (Smith-McCort). Erroneously interpreted as a mucopolysaccharidosis; the alleged lysosomal storage has not been demonstrated.

Pathology. Presence of focal nests of few (2–20) necrotic cells scattered into resting cartilage, surrounded by calcified fibrotic rings.

Diagnostic Procedures. *X-ray. Skeletal survey.* Spine with generalized platyspondylosis; irregularity of iliac crest (lace-bordered); flaring of metaphyses. *Urine.* Search for and identification of mucopolysaccharides that will exclude the diagnosis. Reported elevated chondroitin sulfate-N-acetylgalactosamine 6-sulfate sulfatase and reduced aryl sulfatase glycoprotein-AMP-metabolism.

Therapy. Symptomatic.

Prognosis. In autosomal form atlantoaxial instability predisposes to cord compression. By 5–6 years of age dwarfism becomes evident; adult height 115–130 cm (autosomal); 130–150 (X-linked form).

BIBLIOGRAPHY. Dyggve HV, Melchior JC, Clausen J: Morquio-Ulrich's disease; An inborn error of metabolism? Arch Dis Child 37:525–534, 1962

Schlaepfer R, Rampini S, Wiesmann U: Das Dyggve-Melchior-Clausen-Syndrome: Fallbeschreibung und Literaturnebersicht. Helv Paediatr Acta 36:543–559, 1981

Beighton P: Dyggve-Melchior-Clausen syndrome. J Med Genet 27:512–515, 1990

DYKE-DAVIDOFF-MASSON

Synonyms. Cerebral hemiatrophy; DDM.

Symptoms and Signs. Both sexes affected; present from birth. Cerebral hemiatrophy with homolateral skull and sinus hypertrophy. Mental retardation; seizures; difficulty and impairment of speech development.

Etiology. Unknown. Normal chromosomal pattern.

Diagnostic Procedures. *X-rays of skull.* Hemihypotrophy of skull and sinuses. *CT brain scan.* Hemireduction of brain size. *Electroencephalography.* Abnormal. *Dermatoglyphic pattern.* Normal. *Urine.* Amino acid excretion normal or increased.

Therapy. Anticonvulsants.

Prognosis. Not adequately known.

BIBLIOGRAPHY. Dyke CG, Davidoff LM, Masson CB: Cerebral hemiatrophy with homolateral hypertrophy of the skull and sinuses. Surg Gynecol Obstet 57:588–600, 1933

Parker CE, Harris N, Mavalwala J: Dyke-Davidoff-Masson syndrome; five cases: Studies and deductions from dermatoglyphics. Clin Pediatr 11:228–292, 1972

DYKE-YOUNG

Obsolete. Used in the past to indicate macrocytic hemolytic anemia.

BIBLIOGRAPHY. Dyke SC, Young F: Macrocytic hemolytic anemia associated with increased red cell fragility. Lancet II:817–821, 1938

DYSBARISM

Gas nitrogen and fat embolism occurring in fliers who rapidly reach high altitude. Symptomatology, signs, etiology, pathology, see Caisson.

BIBLIOGRAPHY. Niess OK, Stonehill RR: Dysbarism: A jet age problem of all physicians. Dis Chest 44:121–125, 1963

Weatherall DJ, Ledingham JGG, Warrell DA (eds): Oxford Textbook of Medicine, 3rd ed, pp 1202–1203. Oxford, Oxford Med Pub, 1996

DYSCHROMATOSIS UNIVERSALIS HEREDITARIA

Synonym. Includes dyschromatosis symmetrica hereditaria. See Dohi (probably same condition).

Symptoms and Signs. Both sexes. Only in Japanese. Onset first or second year of life. Pigmented flecks and spots over all the body, varying in size, shape, and color; frequently sparing the face and concentrating on the abdomen. No associated defects.

Etiology. Autosomal recessive (quasidominant) difficult to assess because of frequent consanguineous marriages in the family.

BIBLIOGRAPHY. Suenaga M: Genetical studies on skin disease, VII. Dyschromatosis universalis hereditaria in five generations. Tohoku J Exp Med 55:373–376, 1952

Westerhoff W, Beeher FA, Cormane RM, et al: Hereditary congenital hypopigmented and hyperpigmented macules. Arch Dermatol 114:931–936, 1978

DYSFIBRINOGENEMIA, HEREDITARY

Symptoms and Signs. Usually, asymptomatic or minor bleeding problems.

Etiology. Functionally defective fibrinogen. One hundred and sixty different types of abnormal fibrinogen have been identified; they are designated by place of discovery (e.g., Paris I, Baltimore, Detroit). Incomplete dominant or codominant autosomal inheritance.

Diagnostic Procedures. *Blood.* Usually clot forms, but at abnormally slow rate.

Therapy. Symptomatic.

Prognosis. Good.

BIBLIOGRAPHY. Menache D: Dysfibrinogenemie constitutionnelle et familiale Proc IX Cong Eur Soc Hematol 1255–1259, 1963

Bithell TC: Hereditary coagulation disorders. In Lee GR, Bithel TC, Foerster J, et al (eds): Wintrobe's Clinical Hematology, 9th ed, pp 1439–1442. Philadelphia, Lea & Febiger, 1993

DYSKINETIC CILIA

Synonyms. Afzelius; Kartagener incomplete; Polynesian bronchiectasis; immotile cilia. See also Kartagener.

Symptoms and Signs. Prevalence 1:40,000. Symptoms and signs the same as in Kartagener. Half the affected patients have situs viscerum inversus. Males are sterile.

Syndrome is diagnosed in: (1) patients with complete Kartagener; (2) men without situs inversus but typical history (chronic bronchitis and rhinitis) with living but immobile spermatozoa; (3) patients without situs inversus but with typical clinical signs and sibs with complete Kartagener; (4) patients without situs inversus but with clinical signs if biopsy shows classical signs of ciliary immotility.

From birth. Neonatal asphyxia; chronic bronchial disease; chronic rhinitis; nasal polyps; chronic sinusitis; otitis. *In childhood.* Bronchiectases; moderate hearing loss; recurrent headaches. Dextrocardia. Rare associated polydactyly anomalies.

Etiology. Recessive autosomal inheritance owing to abnormal structure and function of body cilia because of defective protein formation.

Pathology. Electron microscopy. Variable alterations of cilia structure.

Diagnostic Procedures. *Sperm.* Examination of cilia is easier in ejaculate when spermatozoa are poorly motile or immotile. *Biopsy or brushing of nasal canti, bronchi, middle ear, nasal polyps, or endometrium* show same alterations. *Radioactive aerosol.* Mucociliary transport absent or reduced. *X-ray.* Bronchial wall thickening, hyperinflation, segmental atelectasis and bronchiectasis.

Therapy. Symptomatic. Surgery for complications. Abstinence from smoking.

Prognosis. Good quoad vitam. Decrease of pulmonary function with age. Sterility in males.

BIBLIOGRAPHY. Afzelius BA: A human syndrome caused by immotile cilia. Science 193:317–319, 1976

Afzelius AB, Mosberg B: The immotile-cilia syndrome including Kartagener's syndrome. In Stanbury JB, Wyngaarden JB, Fredrickson DS, et al: The Metabolic and Molecular Bases of Inherited Disease, 5th ed, p 1986. New York, McGraw-Hill, 1983

Reyes de la Rocha S, Pysher TJ, Leonard JC: Dyskinetic cilia syndrome: clinical, radiography and scintigraphic findings. Pediatr Radiol 17:97–103, 1987

Fraser RS, Paré JAP, Fraser RG, Paré PD: Synopsis of Diseases of the Chest, 2nd ed, pp 680–683. Philadelphia, WB Saunders, 1994

DYSLEXIA

Synonyms. Hinshelwood; word blindness; reading disability. Includes dysgraphia and acaculia. See Gerstmann.

Symptoms and Signs. Specific reading disability (inability to derive meaning from printed words; significant discrepancy between measured intelligence and reading activity); spelling and writing disability in spite of the ability to recognize letters. Ability to recognize symbols, drawings, diagrams usually is stored. Persistent reversal of letters indicative symptoms. Higher incidence of left-handness in subjects and members of the family. Frequently associated acalculia (difficulties with numbers). Associated speech defects seen especially in males.

Etiology. Autosomal dominant inheritance with reduced penetrance in females; sex-linked recessive inheritance also reported.

Pathology. Reported cytoarchitectonic abnormalities in the left cerebral hemisphere and posterior language area on the left.

Diagnostic Procedures. *CT scan.* Increased prevalence of relative symmetry (reversed or atypical symmetry) of the temporal planes of the two hemispheres.

Therapy. Special educational training and drilling.

Prognosis. With treatment and steady drilling the defect may be overcome slowly. Adult may partially compensate for the manifestation that is more evident in childhood.

BIBLIOGRAPHY. Hinshelwood J: A case of dyslexia—a peculiar form of word blindness. Lancet 2:1454, 1896

Hallgreen B: Specific dyslexia (congenital word blindness, a clinical and genetic study). Acta Psychiat Neurol Scand 65(Suppl) 1:287, 1950

Kinsbourne M: Disorders of mental development. In Menkes JH (ed): Textbook of Child Neurology, 3rd ed, pp 764–801. Philadelphia, Lea & Febiger, 1985

De Fries JC, Fulker DW, la Buda MC: Evidence for a genetic aetiology in reading disability of twins. Nature 329:537–539, 1987

Adams RD, Victor M: Principles of Neurology, 5th ed, pp 916–917. New York, McGraw-Hill, 1993

DYSOSTOSCLEROSIS

Synonyms. Osteosclerosis—platyspondily.

Symptoms. Prevalent in male (11/12). In childhood. Tendency to fractures. Progressive motor and mental retardation. Reduced visual acuity to blindness, facial palsy.

Signs. Short stature. Facies: narrow midface, beak-like nose, micrognathia, abnormal teeth with chalky enamel and premature loss; depressed skin plaques; flattened nails.

Etiology. Autosomal recessive inheritance (?).

Pathology. Bone: transition of cartilage to bone abnormalities; defect of resorption of calcified cartilage.

Diagnostic Procedures. *X-rays. CT scan. MR imaging.* Head sclerosis of vault, base, and mastoids; lack of pneumatization of paranasal sinuses; narrowing of cranial nerves foramina. Vertebral: punctate sclerosis; flattening. Ribs, sternum, clavicles, scapulae: sclerotic changes. Tubular bones club-shaped, thin cortex, areas with coarse trabeculae; multiple fractures.

Therapy. Symptomatic.

Prognosis. Poor.

BIBLIOGRAPHY. Ellis RWB: Osteopetrosis (marble bones: Albers-Schonberg disease, osteosclerosis fragilis generalisata, congenital osteosclerosis). Proc Roy Soc Med 27:1563–1571, 1934

Houston GS, Gerrard JW, Ives EJ: Dysosteosclerosis. Am J Roentgen 130:988–991, 1978

Fryns JP: Dysosteosclerosis in a mentally retarded boy. Acta Paediatric Belg 33:53–56, 1980

Rimoin DL: Genetic disorders of the osseous system. In Beithon P: McKusick's Heritable Disorders of Connective Tissue, pp 652–656. St Louis, CV Mosby, 1993

DYSPHASIC DEMENTIA

Synonyms. See Pick and Alzheimer.

Symptoms and Signs. In males: progressive dementia; severe dysphasia; paralysis agitans. In one family, bulemia.

Etiology. Unknown. Autosomal dominant inheritance.

Pathology. Typical findings of Pick (see) Alzheimer (see), Parkinson and nonspecific spongiform degeneration of superficial cortical layers.

Therapy. Symptomatic. Trial with tacrine chloridrate.

Prognosis. Progressive condition.

BIBLIOGRAPHY. Kim RC, Collins GH, Parisi JE, et al: Familial dementia of adult onset with pathological findings of a 'non-specific' nature. Brain 104:61–78, 1981

Morris JC (ed): Handbook of Dementing Illnesses. New York, Marcel Dekker, 1993

DYSTOCIA-DYSTROPHIA

Synonyms. Bradytocia; dyspituitaric dystocia.

Symptoms and Signs. Occurs in females who are of stocky build, somewhat bull-necked with broad shoulders, short thighs, and tendency to obesity. May have male distribution of hair; hands are stubby with middle three fingers of approximately same length. Bony structure of pelvis: android-type giving rise to deep transverse arrest and difficulties of delivery at the outlet. The cervix is small and dimensions of vagina are skimpy. These patients are rather subfertile. Spasmodic dysmenorrhea is very common, have tendency to abortion, incidence of eclampsia is high. Labor starts with fetal head often high and in majority cases occiput posterior; membranes rupture early in labor.

Etiology. Abnormalities of pelvis form.

Pathology. Nothing unusual, except the android-type of pelvis.

Therapy. Close observation during labor, and recourse to cesarean section if necessary.

Prognosis. Good if carefully observed during antepartum period and intrapartum period.

BIBLIOGRAPHY. Horner DA: Bradytocia; a study based on 500 cases in the Chicago Lying-In Hospital. Surg Gynecol Obstet 44:194–201, 1927

Williams B: Dystocia dystrophia syndrome. J Obstet Gynecol Br Emp 49:412–425, 1942

Cunningham FG, MacDonald PC, Gant NF, et al (eds): Williams Obstetrics, pp 475–491. Englewood Cliffs, NJ, Prentice-Hall, 1993

DYSTONIA-DEAFNESS

Synonym. Scribanu; deafness—dystonia.

Symptoms and Signs. In male deafness onset in infancy; in childhood: dysartria, bizarre posture of head and neck, hyperactivity, progressive symptoms that lead to inability to walk and talk.

Etiology. X-linked inheritance.

Pathology. Neuronal loss and gliosis of basal ganglia.

Prognosis. Death in the second decade. Forme fruste (only deafness, 1 case), survival into adulthood.

BIBLIOGRAPHY. Scribanu N, Kennedy C: Familial syndrome with dystonia, neuronal deafness and possibly intellectual impairment: Clinical course and pathologic findings. Neurol 14:235–243, 1976

DYSURIA-PYURIA

Synonyms. Acute urethral; see Honeymoon cystitis.

Symptoms and Signs. Most frequent in young women, acute dysuria and pollakiuria.

Etiology. In 88% lower urinary tract infection with coliforms or staphylococci or *Chlamydia trachomatis*; in other cases unknown.

Diagnostic Procedures. *Urine.* Culture.

Therapy. Antibiotics. Good results with doxycycline.

Prognosis. In cases with infections prompt remission. In the others prolonged condition.

BIBLIOGRAPHY. Komaroff AL, Friedland G: The dysuria-piuria syndrome. N Engl J Med 303:452–454, 1980

Forland M: Dysuria and frequency. In Massry SG, Glassock RJ: Textbook of Nephrology, 3rd ed, p 555. Baltimore, Williams & Wilkins, 1995

DZIERSZYNSKY

Obsolete.

Synonyms. Hyperplastic periosteal dystrophy; see also Van Buchem. Eponym used to indicate a generalized hyperosteosis particularly affecting cranium, clavicles, sternum, and phalanges. Hereditary condition.

BIBLIOGRAPHY. Dzierszynsky W: Dystrophia periostales, hyperplastica familiaris. Zbl Ges Neurol 2:547, 1913

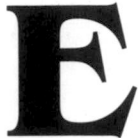

E-FEROL

Symptoms and Signs. In low-birth-weight infants. Progressive clinical deterioration, thrombocytopenia, renal dysfunction, cholestasis, ascites.

Etiology. Total parenteral nutrition, in infants whose birth weight is lower than 1500 g, supplemented with E-ferol, an intravenous vitamin E preparation.

Diagnostic Procedures. Blood chemistry.

Pathology. Progressive hepatic injury characterized initially by Küpffer cell exfoliation, central lobular accumulation of cellular debris, and centrally accentuated panlobular congestion. Late stage: progressive intralobular cholestasis, inflammation of hepatic venules, and extensive sinusoidal veno-occlusion by fibrosis.

Therapy. Symptomatic.

Prognosis. Poor.

BIBLIOGRAPHY. Bove KE, Kosmetatos N, Wedig KE, et al: Vasculopathic hepatotoxicity associated with E-ferol syndrome in low birth weight infants. JAMA 254:2422–2430, 1985
Avery GB, Fletcher MA, McDonald MC: Neonatology, 4th ed. Philadelphia, JB Lippincott, 1994

EAGLES

Synonyms. Styloid process elongated; epihyal bone. See Glomus.

Symptoms. Pain in the throat, referred to the ear; dysphagia, sensation of foreign body in tonsillar area.

Signs. Palpation of styloid process through the tonsillar fossa produces pain.

Etiology. Physical irritation of nerves and vessels passing near tip of styloid process. Not all prolonged styloid process produce pain, and typical pain may be observed in some cases in absence of abnormal process. Same symptoms observed also in case of fracture of the process.

Pathology. From normal to prolonged or fractured styloid process. Usually mineralized.

Diagnostic Procedures. *X-rays. CT scan. MRI.*

Therapy. Surgical intervention debated.

Prognosis. Chronic recurrent manifestations.

BIBLIOGRAPHY. Eagle WW: Elongated styloid process. Report of two cases. Arch Otolaryngol 25:584–587, 1937
Camarda AJ, Deschamps C, Forest D: Styloid chain ossification: a discussion of etiology. Oral Surg 67:508–520, 1989

EALES

Synonyms. Periphlebitis retinae; retinal periphlebitis; retinal vasculitis; vasculitis retinae.

Symptoms and Signs. Prevalent in males; affects primarily young adults. Occurs in stress situation, after trauma, or after awakening. Sudden loss of vision usually in one eye, or vision impairment (scotoma; floating spots); occasionally associated with ataxia; paresthesias; speech disorders.

Etiology. Variable. Autoimmune process triggered by exogenous insult. Infective: tuberculosis; focal infection (dental; tonsillar; sinus); syphilis; multiple sclerosis; hemopathies: hemoglobin anomalies; Bassen-Kornzweig; Buerger.

Pathology. Retina vasculitis. The primary form originates in venules; the secondary, after uveitis process. Retinal hemorrhages; detachment of retina. Common feature, infiltration of retinal veins and peripheral cuffing by lymphocytes, plasma cells, and occasionally granulomatous reaction and multinucleated cells.

Diagnostic Procedures. *Ophthalmoscopy.* See Pathology.

Therapy. Topical atropine, hydrocortisone. Photocoagulation of aneurysms and neovascularization.

Prognosis. Progressive condition with improvements and recurrences; complications owing to thrombosis and necrosis. Tendency to involve both eyes.

BIBLIOGRAPHY. Eales H: Cases of retinal haemorrhage associated with epistaxis and constipation. Birmingham Med Rev 9:262–273, 1880
Elliot AJ: Periphlebitis retinae. In Duane TD (ed): Clinical Ophthalmology, vol 3. Philadelphia, Harper & Row, 1986
Garner A: Vascular disease. In Garner A, Klintworth GK (eds): Pathobiology of Ocular Disease: A Dynamic Approach, 2nd ed, pp 1690–1691. New York, Marcel Dekker, 1994

EAR CHOLESTEATOMA

Synonyms. Aural cholesteroleosis; cholesteatoma.

Symptoms. Onset in childhood or adolescence. Gradual onset of facial paralysis; homolateral deafness; tinnitus.

Signs. Loss of vestibular caloric response.

Etiology. Epidermoid theory; traumatic theory; metaplastic theory; inflammation theory.

Pathology. Cholesteatoma occupying antrum, usually unilateral with or without otic perforation.

Diagnostic Procedures. *X-rays. Otoscopy. Exploration.*

Therapy. Surgery.

Prognosis. Patient with family history followed, and if lesion is discovered, prophylactic treatment before it becomes secondarily infected. Facial paralysis does not show complete recovery after surgery when chronic infection has supervened.

BIBLIOGRAPHY. Cushing H: A large epidermal cholesteatoma. Surg Gynecol Obstet 51:334, 1928
Brosnan ML: Primary cholesteatomas of temporal bone. Arch Otolaryngol 86:363–366, 1967
Weatherall DJ, Ledingham JGG, Warrell DA (eds): Oxford Textbook of Medicine, 3rd ed, p 4033. Oxford, Oxford Med Pub, 1996

EATON-LAMBERT

Synonyms. Lambert-Eaton; LEMS; bronchial carcinoma—myasthenia; see Erb-Goldflam and paraneoplastic.

Symptoms and Signs. Male to female ratio 4.7:1; 70% of males and 25% of females have associated malignancy (80% small cell carcinoma of lung). Nonmalignant LEMS is associated with autoimmune diseases. There may be association with subacute cerebellar degeneration and ataxia. Onset in middle life. Weakness and increased fatigabilty of trunkal and proximal limb muscles; mild transient ocular symptoms; decreased salivation; dry mouth; decrease lacrimation and sweat; orthostatism; impotence; hypoactivity or absence of tendon reflexes with return to normality after muscle exercise.

Etiology. Acquired immune disease in which pathogenic autoantibodies deplete the voltage-sensitive calcium channels (VSCC) of the motor nerve terminal by antigenic modulation. The deficiency of VSCC restarts ingress of calcium in motor nerve terminal during activity and so quantal release. A high proportion of LEMS patients presents small-cell carcinoma of lung that expresses VSCC. Autoantibodies form that crossreact with VSCC of motor neuron terminal.

Pathology. Bronchial carcinoma (oat cell or anaplastic).

Diagnostic Procedures. *Neostigmine.* (Prostigmine and edrophonium chloride [Tensilon]) tests. Negative or feebly positive. *X-ray of chest. Bronchography. Bronchoscopy. EMG (needle).* Reduction of compound muscle action potential that gradually attains normal amplitude after tetanic stimulation or maximal voluntary activity.

Therapy. High voltage radiation, chemotherapy for carcinoma or both; or surgery if feasible. 4-Aminopyridine and 3-4-diaminopyridine can be useful but present problems because side effects. Plasmapheresis can be effective and so high doses of i.v. injection of immunoglobulins. Azathioprine and cyclosporine and corticosteroids are clinically useful.

Prognosis. According to degree of diffusion or metastasis of carcinoma. Non-neoplastic LEMS has better prognosis.

BIBLIOGRAPHY. Anderson JH, Churchill-Davidson HD, Richardson AT: Bronchial neoplasm with myasthenia. Lancet 2:1291–1293, 1953
Lambert EH, Eaton LM, Rooke ED: Defect of neuromuscular conduction associated with malignant neoplasm. Am J Physiol 187:612–613, 1956
O'Neill JH: The Lambert-Eaton myasthenic syndrome. A review of 50 cases. Brain III:577–586, 1988
Penn AS, Richman DP, Ruff RL, et al (eds): Myasthenia gravis and related disorders. Experimental and clinical aspects. Ann NY Acad Sci 681, 1993
Lisak RP: Handbook of Myasthenia Gravis and Myasthenic Syndromes. New York, Marcel Dekker, 1994

EBSTEIN

Synonym. Tricuspid valve anomaly.

Symptoms. Both sexes equally affected. Asymptomatic for years or dyspnea and fatigability; squatting unusual.

Signs. Cyanosis at birth or delayed, or recurrent with increasing severity. Moderate clubbing of fingers and toes. Paroxysmal arrhythmias; heart markedly enlarged; characteristic triple or quadruple rhythm; systolic murmur on left border of sternum, at apex. In many cases apical diastolic murmur as well.

Etiology. Congenital heart defect, with downward displacement of tricuspid valve into right ventricle, and deformation of valve leaflets. Familiar occurrence with autosomal recessive phenotype.

Pathology. As described, with atrialization of right ventricle above the valve. Right ventricle decreased in volume. Patency of foramen ovale in many cases and interatrial septal defect. Association with other cardiac anomalies frequent.

Diagnostic Procedures. *ECG.* Right bundle branch block and prolonged P-R interval; tall P-waves; atrial tachycardia; premature beats and flutter frequent. *Two-dimensional echocardiography with color flow imaging and Doppler interrogation. Fluoroscopy. X-ray.* Enlargement of right atrium; small pulmonary artery; oligemic lung fields. *Angiocardiography.* Enormous right atrium. *Catheterization.* Right atrium increased pressure; evidence of right-to-left left-to-right shunts.

Therapy. Surgery produces variable results. Medical therapy symptomatic: to prevent and treat complications of cyanosis and endocarditis and treat heart failure; extracorporeal membrane oxygenation: successful in critical neonates.

Prognosis. Variable; 50% of patients diagnosed in infancy experience early death; others may survive to middle life. Average life span 22 years. Late survival into the ninth decade. Arhythmias, heart failure, complication of cyanosis, low cardiac output if intact atrial septum are causes of death.

BIBLIOGRAPHY. Ebstein W: Ueber einen sehr seltenen Fall von Insuffiziens der Valvula tricuspidalis, bedingt durch eine angeborene hochgradige Fahlbildung derselben. Arch Anat Physiol 238–254, 1866 (translated by Schiebler GL, Gravenstein JS, Van Mierop LHS). Am J Cardiol 22:867, 1968
Watson H: Natural history of Ebstein's animaly of tricuspid valve in childhood and adolescence. An international co-operative study of 505 cases. Br Heart J 36:417–427, 1974
McIntosh N, Chitayat D, Bardanis M, et al: Ebstein anomaly: report of familiar occurrence and prenatal diagnosis. Am J Med Genet 42:307–309, 1992
Nugent EW, Plauth WH, Edwards JE, et al: The pathology, pathophysiology recognition and treatment of congenital heart disease. In Schlant RC, Alexander RW: Hurst's The Heart, 8th ed, pp 1804–1808. New York, McGraw-Hill, 1994
Perloff JK: The Clinical Recognition of Congenital Heart Disease, 4th ed, pp 247–266. Philadelphia, WB Saunders, 1994

ECTODERMAL HYPOHIDROTIC DYSPLASIA

Symptoms and Signs. Facies: typical: Teeth: missing (most). Hair: thin, sparse, slow growing; Hypohidrosis, Nails: usually normal.

Etiology. X linked; autosomal recessive or dominant inheritance.

BIBLIOGRAPHY. Passarge E, Nuzum CT, Schembert WK. Anhidrotic ectodermal dysplasia an autosomal recessive trait in an inbred kindred. Humangenetik 3:181–185, 1966

ECTOPIA LENTIS-ECTOPIA PUPIL

Symptoms and Signs. Lens and pupil usually displaced in opposite direction. No skeletal, visceral or metabolic disorders associated.

Etiology. Clearly assessed autosomal recessive inheritance.

BIBLIOGRAPHY. Waardenburg PJ: Ueber das Erblichkeitsmoment bei angeborenen Ektopie der Pupille und Linse. Genetica 6:337–382, 1924
Calley A, Lloyd IC, Ridgway A et al: Ectopia lentis et pupillae the genetic aspects and differential diagnosis. J Med Gent 28:791–794, 1991

ECTOPIA LENTIS SIMPLEX

Synonyms. Usher

Symptoms and Signs. Usually in short person. Ectopia lentis may be associated with Marfan, Weill-Marchesani syndrome or isolated symptoms as joint stiffness.

Etiology. Autosomal dominant (also recessive may occur) inheritance.

Therapy. Surgery.

Prognosis. Two forms distinguished a benign stationary and a progressive one.

BIBLIOGRAPHY. Usher CH: A pedigree of congenital dislocation of lenses. Biometrika 16:273–282, 1924

Jaureguy BM, Hall JG: Isolated congenital ectopia lentis with autosomal dominant inheritance. Clin Genet 15:97–109, 1979

Stevenson RE, Schreoer RJ, Taylor HA et al: Dislocated lens dolichostenomelia and joint stiffness. Proc Grennwood Gent Center 1:16–22, 1982

Garner A, Klintworth GK (eds): Pathobiology of Ocular Disease: a Dynamic Approach, 2nd ed, pp 12, 486, 815, 821. New York, Marcel Dekker, 1994

ECTOPIC ACTH

Synonyms. ACTH ectopic secretion. See Cushing.

Symptoms. More frequent in men: weakness; fatigability. In women: oligomenorrhea, polyuria, polydipsia. Symptoms due to the adrenocorticotropic hormone (ACTH) producing tumor (e.g., lung; pancreas).

Signs. Ecchymosis; edema; lymphoadenopathy or evidence of obstruction of superior vena cava (see); hyperpigmentation; carcinomatous neuropathy, and/or myopathy; seldom hirsutism and acne. Most of the signs of classic Cushing do not have time to develop because of the fast course of the disease; typical obesity usually does not appear; hypertension has been observed only in some cases.

Etiology. Tumors of lung: oat-cell carcinoma (60%), bronchial adenoma (carcinoid type 4%), thymus (10%) pancreas (10%), and less frequently: breast, prostate, parathyroid, thyroid, ovary, sympathicoblasts, producing ACTH, which induces adrenal hyperplasia.

Pathology. Lung tumor; oat cell carcinoma. Carcinomas of various endocrine glands mentioned. Early features of Cushing.

Diagnostic Procedures. *Blood.* High level of plasma ACTH; increased cortisol. *Urine.* Increased 17-ketosteroids and 17-hydroxycorticoids; other typical changes due to excessive cortisol production and changes due to primary tumor. *ACTH stimulation.* Varying responses according to level of circulating ACTH. *Metyrapone responsiveness.* Varies according to level of circulating cortisol. *Dexamethasone suppression.* Negative response also with high doses.

Therapy. Usually inoperable at time of discovery; some cases operated in time have been cured. Chemotherapy. Metyrapone alone or in combination with aminoglutethimide; ketoconazole; octreotide.

Prognosis. Poor, death owing to primary tumor and metastasis. Better prognosis for pheochromocytoma, thymoma, bronchial carcinoid, paraganglioma.

BIBLIOGRAPHY. Brown WH: A case of pluriglandular syndrome. Lancet 2:1022–1023, 1928

Strott CA, Nugent CA, Tyler FH: Cushing's syndrome caused by bronchial adenomas. Am J Med 44:97–104, 1968

Sherwood LM: Paraneoplastic endocrine disorders (ectopic hormone syndromes). In De Groot LJ (ed): Endocrinology, 3rd ed, pp 2769–2774. Philadelphia, WB Saunders, 1995

ECTOPIC PREGNANCY

Symptoms. Incidence, 1:300 pregnancies. Precipitating incidents leading to rupture are straining at stool, coitus, or bimanual pelvic examination. Irregular bleeding; usually skipping of one period, then vaginal bleeding coming 1 day or more later. Dull aching pain most common symptom. Referred shoulder pain when free intraperitoneal bleeding. Fainting and shock when massive intraperitoneal bleeding.

Signs. Palpable tender mass at the time of the examination. Sometimes signs of pelvic irritation. Bluish discoloration around the umbilicus (Cullen sign).

Etiology. Chronic pelvic inflammatory disease, secondary to IUD application, gonorrhea or other infections affecting the endosalpinx. Endometriosis; genital tuberculosis; congenital factors.

Pathology. Any fertilized ovum implanting outside the uterine cavity is called ectopic. Varieties: tubal pregnancy (most common); interstitial pregnancy; ampullar pregnancy; cornual pregnancy; cervical pregnancy; ovarian pregnancy; abdominal pregnancy (primary and secondary); intraligamentary pregnancy. Fate of the implanted fertilized ovum: rupture with blood loss into peritoneal cavity; rupture between the two leaves of the broad ligament; abortion via the fimbriated end of the fallopian tube; or abdominal pregnancy, secondary variety.

Diagnostic Procedures. In addition to the history and physical examination: *Culdocentesis* (tapping of cul-de-sac). *Pregnancy test.* The important point is to have a "high index of suspicion" every time a woman in the reproductive period of her life gives a history of amenorrhea or pelvic pain. *Echography. Laparoscopy.*

Therapy. Surgical; exploratory laparotomy and removal of the affected tube. In some rare cases, salpingostomy, removal of the implanted ovum, and preservation of the affected tube. Medical: methetrexate.

Prognosis. Good if treatment is instituted as soon as diagnosis is made.

BIBLIOGRAPHY. Cunningham FG, MacDonald PC, Gant NF, et al (eds): Williams Obstetrics, pp 691–719. Englewood Cliffs, NJ, Prentice-Hall, 1993

ECTRODACTYLY

Synonyms. Birch-Jensen; split hand or foot; finger aborted; brachydactyly type B; lobster claw.

Symptoms and Signs. Both sexes. Congenital. Varieties of malformations that affect one or both hands and occasionally feet. Typical form (lobster claw) with absence of central rays, and atypical form (monodactyly) with deficiency of radial rays and no cleft. Either type may be present in the same family or on different limbs of same person. Isolated type of malformations or in association with other somatic malformations such as:

1. Ectrodactyly; polydactyly.
2. Ectrodactyly; tibia absence.

Synonyms. Tibia absence-split hand or foot; cleft hand-tibia absence.

3. Ectrodactyly; cleft palate (ECP).
4. Ectrodactyly; ectodermal dysplasia; cleft palate.

Synonyms. EEC; Rosselli-Giulienetti.

5. Ectrodactyly; ectodermal dysplasia without cleft palate.
6. Ectrodactyly; mantibulofacial dysostosis.
7. Karsh-Neugebauer (see).
8. Ectrodactyly; uropathy; diaphragmatic defects.
9. Split hand or foot; hypodontia.

Etiology. Term ectrodactyly is not specific. It must be reserved to indicate "transverse terminal aphalangy," "adactyly," or "acheiria"; however, currently it is used to indicate this nosographic condition. Usually sporadic when isolated; and hereditary (autosomal dominant inheritance and possibility of recessive forms discussed) when associated with the other mentioned malformations.

Pathology. Anatomically two types. Typical lobster claw and monodactyly.

Diagnostic Procedures. *X-ray.*

Therapy. Orthopedic reconstruction when feasible, according to type or severity of lesion.

Prognosis. Variable.

BIBLIOGRAPHY. White WH, Baker H: Case of congenital deformity of femora, absence of tibiae and malformation of feet and hands. Trans Clin Soc London 21:295–297, 1888

Birch-Jensen A: Congenital Deformities of the Upper Extremities. Copenhagen Ejnar Munksgaard, 1949

Opitz JM, Frias JL, Cohen MM Jr: The ECP syndrome an other autosomal dominant cause of monodactylous ectrodactyly. Eur J Pediatr 133:217–220, 1980

Rosselli D, Giulenetti R: Ectrodermal dysplasia. Br J Plast Surg 14:190–204, 1961

Tetany SA, McKusick VA: The Genetics of Hand Malformations. New York, Alan R Liss, 1978

Czeizel A, Lesonci A: Split hand, obstructive urinary anomalies, spina bifida or diaphragmatic defect syndrome with autosomal dominant inheritance. Human Genet 77:203–204, 1987

Wallis CE: Ectrodactyly (split hand/split foot) and ectodermal dysplasia with normal lip and palate in a four generation kindred. Clin Genet 34:252–257, 1988

Sharland M, Patton MA, Hill L: Ectrodactyly of hands and feet in a child with a complex translocation including 7q 21. 2. Am J Med Genet 39:413–414, 1991

EDELMANN

Obsolete.

Synonyms. Pancreatohepatic; hepatopancreatic. A rather poorly defined syndrome. This designation has been used to indicate an atrophic or hypotrophic pancreatitis with fatty liver infiltration. The liver infiltration is considered secondary to the pancreatic insufficiency.

BIBLIOGRAPHY. Edelmann A: Ueber eine bisher nicht beachtetes panchreo-hepatisches Syndrome. Wien Klin Wochenschr 49:1336–1339, 1936

Snell AM, Comfort MW: Hepatic lesions presumably secondary to pancreatic lithiasis and atrophy. Am J Dig Dis 4:217, 1937

Cole WH, Howe JS: The pancreaticohepatic syndrome. Surgery 8:19–33, 1940

Kessel L: Acute transient hyperlipemia due to hepatopancreatic damage in chronic alcoholics (Zieve's syndrome). Am J Med 32:747–757, 1962

EDWARDS

Synonyms. Trisomy E; trisomy 16–18; trisomy 18; chromosome 18 trisomy.

Symptoms. Second to trisomy 21 in frequency. Prevalent in females; paternal and maternal age above normal; onset from fetal life. Small for gestational age, frequently born post-term; failure to thrive; difficulty in feeding; generalized hypertonicity with rigidity in flexion of the limbs and seizures. Mental retardation.

Signs. Babies thin, frail; prominent occiput; low-set and malformed ears; receding chin; protruding eyes. Corneal opacity, optic disk coloboma. Congenital heart disease: typically ventricular septal defects and valve anomalies Frequently, umbilical and inguinal hernias. Cryptorchidism. Characteristic: tight flexion of fingers across the palm; index finger overlapping over third digit; occasionally syndactyly; fingers cannot be extended. Convex sole of foot ("rocker-bottom feet"); no hyperreflexia.

Etiology. Trisomy in group E chromosomes (18 possibly the deviant pair). Nondisjunction of maternal gamete or possibly balanced translocation. Carrier either parent or mosaicism.

Pathology. Frequently, abnormalities of cerebral or cerebellar development. Spina bifida; meningomyelocele; high incidence of Meckel diverticulum; esophageal atresia; heterotopic pancreatic tissue; atresia of extrahepatic biliary tree; malrotation of colon; several cardiovascular abnormalities; multiple renal cysts; radial malformation.

Diagnostic Procedures. *Chromosome study.* Trisomy E group. *Dermatoglyphics.* Transversal palmar crease present with greater frequency than in normal. *Blood.* Congenital thrombocytopenia in some cases.

Therapy. Symptomatic.

Prognosis. Mean survival time in male patient, 58.5 days; in females, 282 days. Patients seldom survive to second year.

BIBLIOGRAPHY. Edwards JH, Harnden DG, Cameron AH, et al: A new trisomic syndrome. Lancet 1:787–790, 1960

Rabinowitz JG, Moseley JE, Mitty HA, et al: Trisomy 18, esophageal atresia, anomalies of the radius, and congenital hypoplastic thrombocytopenia. Radiology 89:488–491, 1967

Moerman P, Fryns JP, Goddeeris P, et al: Spectrum of clinical and autopsy findings in trisomy 18 syndrome. J Genet Hum 30:17–38, 1982

Avery GB, Fletcher MA, McDonald MC: Neonatology, 4th ed. Philadelphia, JB Lippincott, 1994

EGGER

Synonyms. Joubert-oro-facio-digital anomalies; Dandy-Walker-postaxial polydactyly; Joubert-Boltshauser.

Symptoms. Both sexes. Features of Joubert (see) or Dandy-Walker (see). Respiratory anomalies: tachypnea (up to 95/mn) and irregular respiratory rate.

Signs. Lobulated tongue, with hamartomata, toe and finger polydactyly.

Etiology. Autosomal recessive inheritance.

Pathology. Posterior fossa cyst continuous with fourth ventricle, partial or total absence of cerebellar vermis, occasionally hydrocephalus.

Diagnostic Procedures. *CT scan. MRI.*

BIBLIOGRAPHY. Egger J, Bellman MH, Ross EM, et al: Joubert-Boltshauser syndrome with polydactyly in siblings. J Neurol Neurosurg Psychiat 45:737–739, 1982

Pierquin G, Deroover J, Levi S, et al: Dandy-Walker malformation with postaxial polydactyly: A new syndrome? Am J Med Genet 33:483–484, 1989

EHLERS-DANLOS

Synonyms. Meekeren-Ehlers-Danlos; Danlos; Sack; Van Meekerent I Chernogubov dermatorrhexia; arthrochalasis—dermatorrhexis—dermatocutis hyperelastica; E-D; fibrodysplasia elastica generalisata; India rubber skin; rubber man; Sack-Barabas; Viljoin; Hernandez; Friedman-Harrod; Beasly-Cohen.

Symptoms. Described primarily in people of European ancestry. Both sexes affected (some authors report male prevalence); recognized from birth. Several clinical forms have been outlined.

ED I (gravis type). Frequently, prematurity; skin hyperextensible, marked bruisability; severe and generalized joint hypermobility. Delayed sitting and walking; unsteadiness with falling and fractures; varicose veins; mitral valve prolapse, dilatation of the aortic root. Face: epicanthal folds (25%), blue sclerae (10%), myopia, strabismus, Gorlin sign (tip of tongue touches nose); alterations of the teeth. Aracnodactyly.

ED II (mitis type). Milder manifestations; joint hypermobility may be limited to hands and feet.

ED III (benign hypermobile type). Joint laxity, skin hyperextensibility, mild connective tissue fragility.

ED IV (ecchymotic; Sack type; Sack-Barabas syndrome). Minimal skin involvement; moderate or minimal joint involvement; marked bruisability; extensive ecchymosis; pigmented scar over bony prominences. Frequently, visceral rupture. It has been divided in three forms according to etiology.

Type A: autosomal dominant.

Type B: autosomal recessive in which the biochemical defect is diminished type III collagen synthesis.

Type C: of unknown etiology in which there is an intracellular accumulation of type III collagen. It has been divided in two forms. In subtype A, lysyl oxidase is deficient, and in subtype B, the biochemical defect is unknown. Frequently, visceral rupture.

ED V (X-linked form). Marked skin hyperextensibility; moderate joint hypermobility; moderate vascular fragility.

ED VI (Hydroxylysine-deficient collagen or ocular type, autosomal recessive type). Predominance of ocular abnormalities over other features. Biochemical diagnosis: low hydroxylysine residue from collagen. Two types have been described: one with autosomal recessive inheritance and procollagen aminoprotease deficiency, and one of sporadic occurrence with a structural mutation of $pro\alpha_2$ (I).

ED VII (procollagen-persistent type; arthrocalasis multiplex congenita). Floppiness in infancy; moderate skin and vascular abnormalities; marked joint hypermobility. Dwarfism.

ED VIII (periodontitis type). Autosomal dominant. Mild skin hyperelasticity, joint hypermobility and bruisability, moderate cutaneous fragility, and severe periodontitis leading to premature loss of teeth and alveolar bone absorption.

ED IX. (See Occipital horn.) There is a defect of copper metabolism.

ED X (fibronectin defect). Joint hyperexsensibility, thin skin, platelets agglutination defect, petecchiae, narrow pelvis.

In addition the following forms have been described:

TYPE VILJOIN. Similar to type III; differs in cause of the severity of joint complications and the presence of wormian bones in the skull.

TYPE HERNANDEZ (Progeriod form). Joints hyperextensibility, easy bruisability, hernias, mental retardation, wrinkled facies, short stature, curly hair, winged scapulae, cryptorchidism, multiple nevi. Defects seem to be based on alteration of proteodermatan sulfate biosynthesis.

TYPE FRIEDMAN-HARROD (ED type unspecified). Scoliosis, hernias, mild joint hypermobility, periodontiasis, aortic rupture, allergies.

TYPE BEASLEY-COHEN. Mental retardation, hyperelasticity of skin of hands, mild scarring, decreased muscle mass, hearing deficit.

Etiology. Various types of inheritance. First three varieties are autosomal dominant. ED IV is autosomal dominant or recessive. Type V is X-linked. Type VI is autosomal recessive. Types VII and VIII are autosomal dominant. Type IX is X-linked. Type X is autosomal recessive.

Pathology. Debated, no consistent findings. Loose fragmented elastic tissue observed in some cases in the skin ligaments and joint capsules (whether result of trauma or primary abnormality not established). Pseudotumors formed by noncapsulated fat, with calcification of connective tissue, vascular proliferation, and cystic formation. Organization of collagen bundles into an intermeshing network. ED I, II, and III: increased collagen fibril diameter. ED IV, C: small collagen fibril diameter with dilatation of rough endoplasmic reticulum. ED V B: increased collagen fibril diameter. ED VI: small fibril diameter.

Diagnostic Procedures. See individual types for biochemical defects.

Therapy. Avoidance of traumas; drainage of large hematomas. Orthopedic measures sometimes necessary. Surgical procedures, with caution because of eventual dehiscence.

Prognosis. Good quoad vitam. According to intensity of manifestations, joint hypermobility is reduced with age. Complication from visceral malformation occasionally is cause of death.

BIBLIOGRAPHY. Van Meekeren JA: De dilatabilitata extraordinaria cutis. In: Observations Medico-Chirurgicales. Amsterdam, 1682
Tschernogobow A: Cutis laxa. Mhft Prokt Derm 14:76, 1892
Ehlers E: Cutis laxa, Neigung zu Haemorrhagien in der Haut lockerung mehrerer Artikulationen. Dermatol Z 8:173–174, 1901
Danlos H: Un cas de cutis laxa avec tumeurs par contusion chronique des coudes et des genoux. Bull Soc Fr Dermatol Syph 19:70–72, 1908
Beasley RP, Cohen MM Jr: A new presumably autosomal recessive form of Ehlers-Danlos syndrome. Clin Genet 16:19–24, 1979
Beighthon P: The Ehlers-Danlos Syndrome. London, Heinemann, 1970
Jessee EF, Oven DS, Sagar KB: The benign hypermobile joint syndrome. Arthritis Rheum 23:1053–1056 1980
Friedman JM, Harrod MJE: An unusual connective tissue disease in mother and son: A new type of Ehlers-Danlos syndrome? Clin Genet 21:168–173, 1982
Hernandez A, Aguirre-Negrete MG, Gonzales-Flores S, et al: Ehlers-Danlos syndrome featured with progeriod facies and mild mental retardation: Further delineation of the syndrome. Clin Genet:30:456–461, 1986
Viljoen D, Goldblatt J, Thompson D, et al: Ehlers-Danlos syndrome: Yet another type? Clin Genet 32:196–201, 1987
Weebury RR: Ehlers-Danlos syndrome: Historical review, report of two cases in one family, and treatment needs. J Dent Child:56:220–224, 1989
Byers PH: Disorders of collagen biosynthesis and structure. In Scriver CR, Beaudet AL, Sly WS, et al: The Metabolic and Molecular Bases of Inherited Disease, 7th ed, pp 4051–4061. New York, McGraw-Hill, 1995

EHRENFRIED

Synonyms. Diaphyseal aclasis; metaphyseal aclasis; hereditary deforming chondrodysplasia; chondromatosis externa; hereditary deforming dyschondroplasia; multiple hereditary exostosis; multiple osteochondromatosis, exostoses multiple.

Symptoms and Signs. Deformity of extremities, including hands (short metacarpal); short stature; excrescence at diaphyseal end of bones; ribs and scapula also involved, never the skull. Neurologic complications from nerve or spinal cord compression.

Etiology. Unknown; autosomal dominant inheritance.

Pathology. Cartilage excrescences. Sarcomatous transformation frequent.

Diagnostic Procedures. *X-ray*. *Blood*. Normal.

Therapy. Decompression if indicated.

Prognosis. Consider possible malignant transformation.

BIBLIOGRAPHY. Ehrenfried A: Multiple cartilaginous exostoses hereditary deforming chondrodysplasia. A brief report on a little known disease. JAMA 64:1642–1646, 1915
Jaffe HL: Hereditary multiple exostosis. Arch Pathol 36:335–337, 1943
Hennekam RCM: Hereditary multiple exostoses. J Med Genet 28:262–266, 1991
Horton WA, Hecth JT: The chondrodysplasias. In Royce PM, Steinmann B (eds): Connective Tissue and Its Heritable Disorders: Molecular, Genetic and Medical Aspects, pp 641–675. New York, Wiley-Liss, 1993

EHRET

Synonyms. Postantalgic posture atrophia; postantalgic atrophy. See astronaut bone reabsorption.

Symptoms. Pain, reduced functional capacities of involved muscle groups.

Signs. Muscle contracture and atrophy.

Etiology. After period of immobilization of muscle groups owing to painful stimuli.

Therapy. Gradual physical therapy.

Prognosis. Good for anatomic and functional recovery.

BIBLIOGRAPHY. Ehret H: Ueber eine functionelle Lähmungsform der peronealmuskel traumatischen Ursprunges. Arch Unfall 2:32–56, 1898
Weatherall DJ, Ledingham JGG, Warrell DA (eds): Oxford Textbook of Medicine. 3rd ed, p 3057. Oxford, Oxford Med Pub, 1996

EHRLICHIOSIS

Synonyms. Human granulocytic ehrlichiosis; HGE.

Symptoms and Signs. Reported in the upper Midwest (mostly Minnesota and Wisconsin). Both sexes, all ages. Usually following outdoor activity. Temperature at least of 37.6°C, headache, myalgias, chills. Seldom rash. More severe manifestations in patients aged, anemic.

Etiology. A Rickettsia-like coccobacillus, obligate intracellular temporarily named *Human granulocitic Ehrlichia*. Very likely transmitted by a tick bite, potential mammalian reservoir still unknown.

Diagnostic Procedures. *Blood.* Anemia, leukopenia, thrombocytopenia, presence of morulae in neutrophils. Polymerase chain reaction positive for HGE in 50% range, serum indirect immunofluorescent antibodies assays (*E. equi* as antigen) of acute or convalescent blood samples: presence of antibodies over 90% of cases. *X-ray.* Pulmonary infiltration in few cases.

Therapy. Doxycycline.

Prognosis. Acute phase range from few to 14 days. Fatality rate calculated in 4.9% in a group studied.

BIBLIOGRAPHY. Maeda K, Markowitz N, Hawley RC, et al: Human infection with Erlichia canis: A leukocytic riskettsia. New Engl J Med 316:853–856, 1987
Bakken JS, Krueth J, Wilson-Noedskog C, et al: Clinical and laboratory characteristics of Human granulocytic ehrlichiosis. JAMA 275:199–205, 1996

EISENLOHR

Synonym. Bulbar paralysis variant.

BIBLIOGRAPHY. Eisenlohr C: Ueber Abscesse in der Medulla oblungata. Dtsch Med Wchsch 19:111–113, 1892

EISENMENGER

Symptoms. Both sexes equally affected. Exertional dyspnea. Delayed physical development; repeated pulmonary infections with occasional hemoptysis. Cough may be the dominant symptom in later life.

Signs. *Infancy.* Moderate cardiomegaly; thrill on left sternal border; systolic murmur; diastolic rumble. *Adolescence, early adult life.* Cyanosis; clubbing of fingers and toes.

Etiology. Congenital heart defect. Left-to-right shunt (ventricular, occasionally also atrial) reverted to right-to-left by pulmonary hypertension.

Pathology. Ventricular septal defect, patent ductus arteriosus, or atrial septal defect. Hypertrophy of both ventricles. Pulmonary artery dilated. Lung fibrosis.

Diagnostic Procedures. *EEG.* Left axis deviation in infants; right axis deviation in older children. Short circulation time. *Two-dimensional echocardiography. Pulmonary function tests.* Oxygen saturation decreased in older children. *X-ray.* Enlargement of right ventricle, prominent main pulmonary artery and central branches with cutoff of peripheral branches. *Catheterization.* Increased pressure in pulmonary artery; increased oxygen in right ventricle. *Blood.* Increased number of red blood cells.

Therapy. Symptomatic. Surgical intervention is generally felt to be contraindicated because elevated pulmonary vascular resistance persists or increases after surgical closure of the defect. Heart transplantation.

Prognosis. Most patients die from heart failure, thrombosis, or endocarditis before reaching 30 years of age if not transplanted.

BIBLIOGRAPHY. Eisenmenger V: Die angeborenen Defekte der Kommerscheidewand des Herzens. Z Klin Med (suppl) 32:1–28, 1897
Abbott ME: Congenital heart disease. In Nelson's Loose Leaf Medicine, vol 5. New York, Thomas Nelson and Sons, 1932
Nugent EW, Plauth WH, Edwards JE, et al: The pathology, pathophysiology recognition and treatment of congenital heart disease. In Schlant RC, Alexander RW: Hurst's The Heart, 8th ed, pp 1767, 1770, 1830–1831. New York, McGraw-Hill, 1994
Perloff JK: The Clinical Recognition of Congenital Heart Disease, 4th ed, pp 402–403, 406–407. Philadelphia, WB Saunders, 1994

EKMAN-LOBSTEIN

Synonyms. OI type IV. See Osteogenesis imperfecta with normal sclerae and absence of deafness.

Etiology. Autosomal dominant.

Diagnostic Procedures. See OI.

Pathology. See OI.

BIBLIOGRAPHY. Ekman OJ: Dissertation Medica. Descriptionem et Casus Aliquot Osteomalaciae Sistems. Uppsala, 1788
Lobstein JG, CFM: Lehrbuch der patologischen Anatomie, vol II, p 179. Stuttgart, 1835
Sillence DO, Jenn A, Danks DM: Genetic hetereogeneity in osteogenesis imperfecta. J Med Genet 16:101–116, 1979
Tsipouras P, Schwartz RC, Goldberg JD, et al: Prenatal prediction of osteogenesis imperfecta (OI type IV): Exclusion of inheritance using a collagen probe. J Med Genet 24:496–409, 1987

ELBOW-KNEE MEDT

Synonyms. Multiple epiphyseal dysplasia; MEDT type III C.

Symptoms and Signs. Limitation of elbow movements; occasionally also of knees, and development of osteochondromas.

Etiology. Unknown. Autosomal dominant inheritance.

BIBLIOGRAPHY. Maroteaux P: Spondyloepiphyseal dysplasias and metatropic dwarfism. Birth Defects 9:35–41, 1969
Maroteaux P, Spranger J: The spondylometaphyseal dysplasias: A tentative classification. Pediatr Radiol 21:293–297, 1991

ELECTROSHOCK-INDUCED PSYCHOTIC

Synonym. Psychosis postelectroshock.

Symptoms. Occurs in some patients who undergo electroconvulsive treatment. Intellectual changes, memory impairment; emotional, organic changes; euphoria or complete affective dullness; hallucination may occur.

Etiology. Intensity of these symptoms depends (not constantly) on number and spacing of the treatments.

Therapy. When in excitement state, barbiturate intravenously.

Prognosis. Acute psychotic symptoms disappear in 1 or 2 weeks; memory defect may persist longer.

BIBLIOGRAPHY. Sackeim HA: The cognitive effects of electroconvulsive therapy. In Thal LJ, Moos WH, Gamzu ER: Cognitive disorders: Pathophysiology and treatment. New York, Marcel Dekker, 1992

ELEJALDE

Synonyms. Acrocephalopolydactylous dysplasia.

Symptoms and Signs. Overweight at birth "pseudohydropic" aspect; acrocephaly; craniostenosis; polydactyly; exophthalmos; cystic kidneys.

Etiology. Autosomal recessive inheritance.

BIBLIOGRAPHY. Elejalde BR. Giraldo C. Jemenez R. et al: Acrocephalopolydactylous dysplasia. BDOAS 13(3B):53–56, 1977

ELIAKIM

Synonym. Hepatic granulomas; granulomatous hepatitis (term to be avoided).

Symptoms. Both sexes affected. Polymyalgialike illness; hyperthermia; hepatomegaly. Those of the underlying disorder.

Etiology. A wide variety of infectious diseases: bacterial, mycobacterial, spirochetal, viral, rickettsial, fungal, parasitic. Hepatobiliary disorders. Systemic disorders: sarcoidosis; Wegener granulomatosis; inflammatory bowel disease; chronic granulomatous disease; granulomatous arteritis; melanoma; Hodgkin disease; drugs and other exogenous agents.

Pathology. Compact collection of mature mononuclear phagocytes. Epithelioid cells. Giant cells and necrosis.

Diagnostic Procedures. *Biopsy of liver.* Granulomas. *Blood.* Mild abnormalities of liver test (particularly of alkaline phosphatase). Hyperbilirubinemia (25% of cases).

Therapy. Moderate doses of corticosteroids. Antibiotics of no use. Treatment of the underlying disorder.

Prognosis. When the underlying disorder can be successfully treated or an offending exogenous agent eliminated, liver dysfunction disappears. Granulomas may persist for a variable length of time.

BIBLIOGRAPHY. Eliakim M, Eisenberg S, Levij I, et al: Granulomatous hepatitis accompanying a self limited febrile illness. Lancet 1:1348–1352, 1968
Lefkowitch JH: Hepatic granulomas. In Haubrich WS, Schaffner F, Berk JE (eds): Bockus Gastroenterology, 5th ed, vol 2, pp 2317–2324. Philadelphia, WB Saunders, 1995

ELLIS-VAN CREVELD

Synonyms. Acrodysplasia III; chondroectodermal dysplasia; mesoectodermal dysplasia; chondrodysplasia ectodermica; chondrodysplasia tridermica.

Symptoms and Signs. Polydactyly, especially hands; dysplasia of nails and teeth; dwarfism; shortening of extremities; mostly proximal (contrast with achondroplasia). Fusion of metacarpal bones; knock-knees owing to defect of proximal tibia. Features of congenital heart defects often associated (mostly atrial septal defect). Small thorax; genital anomalies; mental retardation (30%).

Etiology. Unknown; autosomal recessive inheritance. Occurs in the Amish group in Pennsylvania (5:1000 births).

Pathology. Ectodermal, chondral dysplasia. Failure of epiphysis to produce columnar cartilage. Deformity of proximal metaphyses of the tibia; accelerated maturation of bones and fusion in hands and feet.

Diagnostic Procedures. *X-rays. CT scan.* Bowed femur, humerus et genu valgum; short medial and long lateral slope of metaphysis; shortening of fibula, ribs, and tubular bones in general; small sciatic notch; synmetacarpalism; polydactyly; skull and spine normal. *Ultrasound.* For prenatal diagnosis.

Therapy. Cardiac surgery. Orthopedic and orthodontic procedures.

Prognosis. Thirty percent die in first 2 weeks of life. Dwarfism in those who survive. Heart failure frequent cause of death.

BIBLIOGRAPHY. Thomas: Ueber einen Fall von hereditaeren Polydaktylie mit Anomalien der Zaehne. Dtsc Mschr Zaehnheilkd 6:407–408, 1888
Ellis RWB, Van Creveld S: A syndrome characterized by ectodermal dysplasia, polydactyly; chondrodysplasia, and congenital morbus cordis: Report of three cases. Arch Dis Child 15:65–84, 1940
Harper J: Genetics and genodermatoses. In Champion RH, Burton JL, Ebling FJG (eds): Rook/Wilkinson/Ebling Textbook of Dermatology, 5th ed, p 341. Oxford, Blackwell Scientific, 1992

ELPENOR

Synonyms. Dipsomania; alcoholic hallucinosis; postalcoholic behavior. See Alcoholic syndromes.

Symptoms. After abuse of alcohol, sedative drugs, or hallucinogens, when awakening in unknown surroundings and still partially or totally without contact with consciousness, patient behaves abnormally, antisocially, endangering himself or others.

Etiology and Pathology. *Intoxication.* Complication of alcoholism or drug use. The name of the syndrome is taken from mythologic character, Elpenor, described by Homer in the Odyssey: "The youngest man among us, Elpenor, a lad / Not any too brave or bright, had gone apart / From his friends in the hallowed halls of Circe, seeking / Fresh air. Heavy with wine, he went to sleep. Then hearing the noise and bustle of his comrades. / Stirring about, he sprang up, but forgot the long / Ladder by which he came up and proceeded to fall / Headlong from the roof, breaking his neck / His Soul went down to Hades."

BIBLIOGRAPHY. Carrot E, Velluz J, Rigal: Syndrome d'Elpenor. Press Med 55:573, 1947
Rees Ennis: The Odyssey of Homer (Newly Translated for the Modern Reader), p 171. New York, Random House, 1960
Walin SJ, Mello MK: The effects of alcohol on dreams and hallucinations in alcohol addicts. Ann NY Acad Sci 215:266–302, 1973
Stephens DN, Dahlke F, Duka T: Consequences of drug and ethanol use on cognitive function. In Thal LJ, Moos WH, Gamzu ER: Cognitive disorders: Pathophysiology and treatment. New York, Marcel Dekker, 1992

ELSAHY-WATERS

Synonyms. Branchioskeletogenital; BSG.

Symptoms. Reported in three male siblings. Seizures; mental retardation.

Signs. Pectus excavatum; penoscrotal hypospadias. *Facies.* Brachycephaly; midfacial hypoplasia. *Eyes.* Hypertelorism; strabismus; nystagmus; mild ptosis. *Nose.* Broad bridge; wide tip. *Mouth.* Submucous palatal cleft; multiple jaw cysts; dysplastic dentin.

Etiology. Autosomal recessive (?), X-linked (?) inheritance.

BIBLIOGRAPHY. Elsahy NI, Waters WR: The branchioskeleto-genital syndrome. Plast Reconstr Surg 48:542–550, 1971

ELSBERG

Synonyms. Primary genital herpes; acute urinary retention-genital herpes.

Symptoms and Signs. In women, acute urinary retention.

Etiology. Herpes infection that determines motor and sensitive neuropathy of sacral nervous fibers.

Pathology. That of herpes infection.

Diagnostic Procedures. Urodynamic studies.

Therapy. That of herpes infection; catheterization, and in cases that persist over 5–7 weeks sovrapubic catheter.

Prognosis. Condition usually lasts 4–10 days. Rarely condition persists over 5–7 weeks.

BIBLIOGRAPHY. Hemrika DJ, Schutte MF, Bleker OP: Elsberg syndrome: a neurological basis for acute urinary retention in patients with genital herpes. Obstet Gynecol 68:37S, 1986

ELSCHNIG I

Synonym. Meibonian conjunctivitis. Including Elschnig pearls.

Symptoms and Signs. Smarting of eyes; ocular scratching sensation; photophobia; minimal visual impairment.

Signs. Conjunctivitis. Foamy secretion. Formation of large globules (pearls).

Etiology. Chronic inflammation frequently following removal of a cataract or trauma to the lens.

Pathology. Chronic conjunctivitis with hyperplasia of tarsal glands.

Therapy. Topical anti-inflammatory agents; antibiotics. Epithelial or other nucleated lens fibers proliferate and produce abortive lens fibers.

Prognosis. Benign.

BIBLIOGRAPHY. Elschnig A: Beitrag zur Aetiologie und Therapie der chronischen Conjunctivitis. Dtsch Med Wochenshr 34:1133–1135, 1908
Klintworth GK, Garner A: The causes, types and morphology of cataracts. In Garner A, Klintworth GK (eds): Pathobiology of Ocular Disease: A Dynamic Approach, 2nd ed, p 516. New York, Marcel Dekker, 1994

ELSCHNIG II

Symptoms and Signs. Present from birth. Palpebral fissures extending laterally; lateral canthus displaced out and downward; lower eyelids ectropion; hypertelorism; frequently, cleft palate and lip.

BIBLIOGRAPHY. Elschnig A: Zur Kenntnis der Anomalien der Lidspaltenform. Klin Monatsbl Augenheilkd 50:17–30, 1912

EMBOLISM, PARADOXICAL

Synonym. Cardiac anomaly–cerebral abscess.

Symptoms. May occur at any age. Patients with cardiac anomaly with right-to-left shunt; headache; stiff neck; drowsiness; fever, indicating a possible protective role of the pulmonary capillary bed in removing bacteria from blood.

Signs. Hemiplegia; aphasia; jacksonian convulsion, coma. Other signs of expanding intracranial lesions or meningitis.

Etiology. Acute infective process of central nervous system in patients with congenital cardiac anomaly.

Pathology. Patient with right-to-left cardiac shunt. Usually, single abscess in central nervous system. Occasionally, meningitis.

Diagnostic Procedures. *Blood.* Polycythemia; leukocytosis. *Cerebrospinal fluid.* Increased pressure; increased proteins. (If meningitis, increased leukocytes.) *X-ray of skull. Angiography. CT brain and vertebrae scan.*

Therapy. Antibiotics; surgery if lesions are localized.

Prognosis. Guarded.

BIBLIOGRAPHY. Farre JR: Pathological Researches. Essay I. On malformations of the human heart; illustrated by numerous cases, and preceded by some observations on the method of improving the diagnostic part of medicine. London, Longman, 1814
Gintrac E: Observations et recherches sur la cyanose ou maladie bleue. Paris, Pinard, 1824
Ballet G: Des abscès du cerveau consécutifs à certaines malformations cardiaques. Arch Gen Med 145:659–667, 1880
Chambers WR: Brain abscess associated with pulmonary arteriovenous fistula. Ann Surg 141:276–277, 1955
Ezekowitz MD: Systemic Cardiac Embolism. New York, Marcel Dekker, 1993

EMERY-DREIFUSS

Synonyms. EDMD; muscular dystrophy tardive; scapuloperoneal, X-linked; humero-peroneal neuromuscular. See rigid spine.

Symptoms and Signs. In males. Onset in the first decade of life. European workshop on EDMD (1991) defines this syndrome according to the following criteria:

1. Early contractures of Achilles tendons, elbows, and spine.
2. Slowly progressing muscle wasting and weakness with a predominantly humeral (upper arm) and peroneal (lower leg) distribution, bilateral and approximately symmetrical.
3. Cardiac conduction defect or other evidence of cardiomyopathy.
4. Muscle biopsy showing myopathic features or overdystrophy.
5. Pedigree consistent with unequivocal X-linked inheritance. In some instances the syndrome may present only some of the criteria (i.e., 1, 2, 3, and/or 4).

Toe walking, partial flexion of the elbows, inability to fully flex the neck and spine. Absence of major muscle weakness and of hypertrophy. In early adulthood emerges the final component of the clinical syndrome: atrial conduction abnormalities, with chest pain and recurrent syncope. The cardiac arrhythmia, however, may be seen in childhood, or not appear until the sixth decade, or may be seen without muscle weakness. Some female carriers have developed heart block.

Etiology. X-linked inheritance, with penetrance of 100% in males. Gene defects unknown but locus is close to Xq28.

Pathology. *Muscle biopsies.* Predominance of type II fibers; changes suggesting dystrophy, including fibrosis, necrosis, and marked variation in fiber size.

Diagnostic Procedures. *Blood.* Serum creatine kinase activity elevated (3–10 times; in Duchenne dystrophy it is elevated 50–200 times). EMG pattern is myopathic, with motor unit potentials of short duration and reduced amplitude. *ECG.* Characteristic is atrial paralisis. Early ECG changes include low amplitude, P-waves and first degree heart block, then Luciani-Wenkback (see). Later on complete block and ventricular arrhythmias.

Therapy. Pacemaker, if severe conduction defects are present.

Prognosis. Most children tolerate their undiagnosed disorder through the first 10 years because of the slow insidious progression and resultant mild disability. The rhythm disturbance, if untreated, proves fatal by middle adulthood. Sudden death possible. Frequent TIA for atrial embolism.

BIBLIOGRAPHY. Dreifuss FE, Hogan GR: Survival in X-chromosomal muscular dystrophy. Neurology 11:734–737, 1961

Emery A, Dreifuss F: Unusual type of benign X-linked muscular dystrophy. J Neurol Neurosurg Psychiatr 29:338–342, 1966

Emery AEH: Emery-Dreifuss syndrome. J Med Genet 26:637–641, 1989

Morrison P, Jago RH: Emery-Dreifuss muscular dystrophy. Anaesthesia 46:33–35, 1991

Hopkins LC, Warren ST: Emery-Dreifuss muscular dystrophy. In Vinken PJ, Buyn GW, Klawans HL: Handbook of Clinical Neurology: The Myopathies, vol 62, p 145. Amsterdam, Elsevier, 1992

EMERY-NELSON

Synonym. Hand—foot—flat facies.

Symptoms and Signs. Both sexes affected; present from birth. Unusual facies; long philtrum; flatness, flexion and extension deformities of hands; clawed toes. Retarded physical and mental development.

Etiology. Unknown. Autosomal dominant (?) inheritance with variable expressivity.

BIBLIOGRAPHY. Emery AEH, Nelson MM: A familial syndrome of short stature, deformities of hands and feet and an unusual facies. J Med Genet 7:379–382, 1970

Gorlin RJ, Cohen MM Jr, Levin LS: Syndromes of the Head and Neck, 3rd ed, p 838. New York, McGraw-Hill, 1990

EMPTY SELLA, ACQUIRED

Symptoms. Occurs after treatment of pituitary tumors by surgery, isotopes, X-ray. Reduced visual acuity that in some cases, can evolve into blindness. Hemianopia; top quadrantanopsia; central scotoma (occasionally).

Signs. Irregular visual field defects; pale optic disks. Acromegalia or other manifestations due to the tumor do not belong to the syndrome.

Etiology. X-ray damage and secondary atrophy or scar with mechanical action altering chiasm, optic nerve, or vascular tree.

Pathology. Empty and enlarged sella. See Etiology.

Diagnostic Procedures. Exclude recurrence of tumor (with similar symptomatology). *X-ray.* Enlarged sella. *CT brain scan. MRI.* May reveal air in the sella.

Therapy. Symptomatic.

Prognosis. Poor.

BIBLIOGRAPHY. Busch W: Die Morphologie der Sella turcica und ihre Beziehungen zur Hypophyse. Virchows Atch ath Anat 320:437–458, 1951

Colby MY Jr, Kearns TP: Radiation therapy of pituitary adenomas with associated visual impairment. Proc Staff Meet Mayo Clin 37:15–24, 1962

Lee WM, Adams JE: The empty sella syndrome. J Neurosurg 28:351–356, 1968

Barbarino A, De Marinis L, Mancini A, et al: Prolactin dynamics in normoprolactinemic primary empty sella: Correlation with intracranial pressure. Hormone Res 27:141–151, 1987

Melmed S: Tumor mass effects of lesions in the hypothalamus and pituitary. In De Groot LJ (ed): Endocrinology, 3rd ed, p 458. Philadelphia, WB Saunders, 1995

EMPTY SELLA, PRIMARY

Symptoms and Signs. In absence of surgery or radiotherapy. Familial form. Finding of empty sella turcica (radiologically) associated to osteosclerosis, meningoceles (thoracic or lumbar), wormian bones, moderate dwarfism, facial structure abnormalities. Sporadic cases in obese, middle-aged women with normal pituitary function.

Diagnostic Procedures. See Empty sella, acquired.

BIBLIOGRAPHY. Busch W: Die Morphologie der Sella turcica und ihre Beziehungen zur Hypophyse. Virchows Atch Anat 320:437–458, 1951

Engles EP: Roetnographic demonstration of a hypophysial subaracnoid space. Am J Roent 80:1001–1004, 1958

Melmed S: Tumor mass effects of lesions in the hypothalamus and pituitary. In De Groot LJ (ed): Endocrinology, 3rd ed, p 458. Philadelphia, WB Saunders, 1995

ENAMEL-RENAL

Synonyms. Lubinsky.

Symptoms and Signs. Both sexes. Teeth: absence of enamel in primary and secondary dentition. Dagger-shaped teeth. At age 2-4 onset of life long nocturnal enureris, and polyuria. Later, malignant hypertension and uremia.

Etiology. Autosomal recessive inheritance. Abnormality of vitamin K dependent calcium binging proteins?

Pathology. *Teeth.* Calcification of pulp. *Kidney.* Punctate nephrocalcinosis.

Diagnostic Procedures. *Blood.* Increased osteocolin. *Urine.* Decreased deltacarboxyglutamic acid, calciuria and phosphaturia. *X-ray.* Nephrocalcinosis.

Therapy. Kidney transplantation. Dialysis.

Prognosis. Death in the third decade.

BIBLIOGRAPHY. McGibbon D: Generalized enamel hypoplasia and renal dysfunction. Aust Dent 3 17:61–63, 1972

Lubinsky M, Angle C, Marsh PW, et al: Syndrome of amelogenesis imperfecta, nephrocalcinosis, impaired renal concentration and possible abnormality of calcium metabolism. Am J Med Genet 20:233–243, 1985

ENCEPHALITIC PARKINSONISM

See Parkinson syndrome.

Symptoms and Signs. Gradual onset at any age from childhood. Involvement frequently limited; seldom generalized. Rigidity symptoms and signs prevalent over tremor component. Ptyalism almost constant; pupillary reaction often impaired. Face and scalp covered with greasy secretion. Frequently associated with other sequelae of encephalitis: tics; spasms; behavioral changes; respiratory disorders.

Etiology. Complication of von Economo type of encephalitis. Exposure to certain toxins (manganese dust, carbon disulfide); severe CO poisoning and some drugs: neuroleptic, reserpine, metoclopramide.

Pathology. Lesions of substantia nigra and globus pallidus.

Diagnostic Procedures. See Parkinson.

Therapy. See Parkinson.

Prognosis. See Parkinson.

BIBLIOGRAPHY. Current concepts and controversies in Parkinson's disease (editorial). Can J Neurol Sci 11 (Suppl):1984

Morris JC: Handbook of Dementing Illnesses. New York, Marcel Dekker, 1993.

ENCEPHALOMYELITIS, DISSEMINATED ACUTE

Synonyms. Acute perivascular myelinoclasis; postinfective encephalomyelitis; postexanthematous encephalomyelitis; postvaccinal encephalomyelitis.

Symptoms and Signs. Occurs in both sexes; onset at all ages; associated with virus infection (e.g., measles or after vaccination), basal infection, or without recognizable preceding illness. Onset explosive. Cranial palsies; optic neuritis; vertigo; nausea; vomiting. Then development of paraplegia, hemiplegia, diffuse brain stem signs, and slight fever.

Etiology. Unknown, possibly allergic reaction. Relationship with multiple sclerosis (see) in idiopathic cases not established, but clinically the two conditions are undistinguishable.

Pathology. Similar to multiple sclerosis syndrome (see). In acute cases, marked lymphocytic infiltration.

Diagnostic Procedures. *Blood.* Leukocytosis. *Spinal fluid.* Moderate pleocytosis.

Therapy. In acute form (not postinfective) some benefit from adrenocorticotropic hormone (ACTH) and cortical steroids. Symptomatic.

Prognosis. Variable; from rapid steady progression with groups of symptoms appearing and receding, to sequelae or complete recovery.

BIBLIOGRAPHY. Greenfield JG: Acute disseminated encephalomyelitis as a sequel to influenza. J Pathol Bacteriol 33:453, 1930
Miller HG, Evans MJ: Prognosis in acute disseminated encephalomyelitis, with a note on neuromyelitis optica. J Med 87:347–379, 1953
Adams RD, Victor M: Principles of Neurology, 5th ed, pp 792–794. New York, McGraw-Hill, 1993

ENCEPHALOPATHY, HYPERTENSIVE

See Hypothalamic carrefour and Page.

Symptoms. Intermittent, often transient headache; apathy; anorexia; vomiting; generalized weakness; temporary amaurosis. Convulsion and transient paralysis also frequently seen.

Signs. Marked elevation of blood pressure; hypertensive retinopathy; enlarged heart.

Etiology. Essential hypertension (malignant phase) or secondary hypertension to glomerulonephritis; eclampsia; pheochromocytoma; Cushing; hyperaldosteronism.

Pathology. Vasculocerebral alteration with subintimal hyalinization; hypertrophy of media; cerebral hemorrhage; thrombosis; edema.

Diagnostic Procedures. To determine etiology of blood hypertension. *Blood.* Blood urea nitrogen and protein increased. Increased pressure. *Ophthalmoscopy.* Retinal hemorrhages; bilateral papilledema. *Electrocardiography.* Left ventricular hypertrophy.

Therapy. That for hypertension.

Prognosis. Usually a bad prognostic sign in essential malignant hypertension. In secondary correctable hypertension, good response to treatment.

BIBLIOGRAPHY. Adams RD, Victor M: Principles of Neurology, 5th ed, pp 734–735, 888. New York, McGraw-Hill, 1993
Weatherall DJ, Ledingham JGG, Warrell DA (eds): Oxford Textbook of Medicine, 3rd ed, p 2543. Oxford, Oxford Med Pub, 1996

ENDOCARDIAL FIBROELASTOSIS, SECONDARY

Synonyms. Fibroelastosis, endocardial, secondary. See Weinberg-Himmelfarb.

Symptoms and Signs. Onset at same age as primary form (see Weinberg-Himmelfarb) or later; in adult life after myocardial infarction. Symptoms and signs of Weinberg-Himmelfarb, plus those of associated malformation or pathology: aortic stenosis; coarctation of aorta; anomalous origin of left coronary artery from pulmonary trunk; hypoplastic left heart (see); generalized glycogenosis and others. Respiratory distress, mostly rales in the lung fields, enlarged heart, gallop rhythm, no significant murmur early in the illness.

Diagnostic Procedures. *X-ray.* Heart massively enlarged with left atrial dilatation; left lower lobe atelectasis. *Electrocardiography.* Left ventricular and left atrial hypertrophy. *Two-dimensional echocardiography. Cardiac catheterization.*

Therapy. Medical treatment of heart failure (digitalis and diuretics), L-carnitine if carnitine levels (plasma, muscle) are reduced; restriction of activity. Cardiac transplant attempted.

BIBLIOGRAPHY. Perloff JK: The Clinical Recognition of Congenital Heart Disease, 4th ed, pp 174, 189–197. Philadelphia, WB Saunders, 1994
Shabetai R: Restrictive cardiomyopathy. In Schlant RC, Alexander RW: Hurst's The Heart, 8th ed. New York, McGraw-Hill, 1994

ENDOMETRIOSIS

Symptoms. Found most frequently among women in the higher socioeconomic group; median age 37 years. Characteristics of patient with endometriosis: underweight; overanxious; intelligent and perfectionist; marriage and childbearing are deferred for prolonged periods. Disease occurs only after the female begins to menstruate and regresses after menopause. Rarely seen in women with anovulatory cycles, but common in those who have uninterrupted cyclic menstruation. Endometriosis improves during pregnancy and during artificially induced anovulation. Frequent pregnancies seem to prevent the disease. Endometriosis is associated with infertility. Progressive, severe suprapubic pain during menstruation or just before menstruation; dyspareunia; painful defecation; premenstrual staining; hypermenorrhea; dysuria; hematuria.

Etiology. Unknown, but numerous theories. *Sampson theory.* Viable endometrial fragments are regurgitated with menstrual blood into peritoneal cavity with subsequent implantation. *Meyer theory.* Peritoneal mesothelium possessed totipotency and therefore, may be converted into endometrial tissue. *Hertig theory.* Formation of a fibrinopurulent exudate; organization by endometrial stroma; formation of glandlike spaces. Familial occurrence reported (autosomal dominant).

Diagnostic Procedures. *Pelvic examination. Culdoscopy. Laparotomy.* Differential diagnosis: adenomyosis uteri, pelvic inflammatory disease, nonspecific adhesions; ovarian carcinoma.

Pathology. Commonest site is ovary; other areas include uterosacral ligaments, rectovaginal septum, sigmoid colon, lower genital tract, round ligaments, pelvic peritoneum, small intestine, umbilicus, laparotomy scars, bladder, ureter, breasts, pleura, lung. *Microscopically.* Endometrial epithelium, glands or glandlike structures, stroma, hemorrhage.

Therapy. The aims of therapy: analgesia; resolution of endometriocystic deposits and when wanted, restoration of fertility. Choice of medical and/or surgical approaches is dictated by clinical data and previous response to treatments.

1. Observation and analgesia is beneficial to those patients having only minimal involvement.
2. Ovulation may be suppressed by danazol; progestagens (medroxyprogesterone, dydrogesterone; norethisterone acetate, and lyroestrenol) gestrinone and Gn RH agonists. Pseudopregnancy should be contin-

ued for a minimum of 9 months, and if extensive endometriosis, should be extended to 12–24 months.

3. Conservative surgery includes lysis of adhesions, removal of endometrial implants and endometrial cysts of ovary, presacral neurectomy, uterine suspension.

4. Radical surgery consists of total hysterectomy and bilateral salpingo oophorectomy, and hormone replacement therapy

BIBLIOGRAPHY. Hinson JM Jr, Brigham KL, Danieli J: Catamenial pneumothorax in sisters. Chest 80:633–635, 1981

Shaw RW: Treatment of endometriosis. Lancet 340:1267–1270, 1992

END PLATE AChE DEFICIENCY, CONGENITAL

Symptoms and Signs. In both sexes. From childhood: weakness and abnormal fatigability. Poor suck, cry and episodes of respiratory distress. Motor milestones delayed. Most muscles affected. Ophthalmoparesis (50% of cases); on standing: lordosis and scoliosis after few seconds. Older patients fixed scoliosis and atrophy of some arm muscles.

Etiology. Autosomal recessive inheritance. Absence of acetylcholinesterase from end plate, so ACh remains.

BIBLIOGRAPHY. Engel AG, Lambert EH, Gomez MR: A new myasthenic syndrome with end plate acetylcholinesterase deficiency, small nerve terminals and reduced acetylcholine release. Ann Neurol 1:315–330, 1977

Hutchinson DO, Engel AG, Walls TJ, et al: The spectrum of congenital end-plate acetylcholinesterase deficiency. In Penn AS, Richman DP, Ruff RL (eds): Myasthenia gravis and related disorders: Experimental and clinical aspects. Ann NY Acad Sci 681:469–486, 1993

ENGEL

Synonyms. Cardiomyopathic carnitine deficiency, myopathic carnitine deficiency. Carnitine deficiency I. See Karpati and Di Mauro-Di Mauro.

Symptoms and Signs. Rare condition, affects families of Germanic origin. Early onset (occasionally in adult life) progressive skeletal muscle weakness. Symptoms enhanced by fatigue, and fasting. Occasionally cardiomyopathy evidence.

Etiology. Various causes: biosynthetic defects, defects in transport of carnitine. Autosomal recessive phenotype postulated.

Pathology. Lipid storage myopathy.

Diagnostic Procedures. *ECG.* High theta waves in mid precordial leads. *Blood.* Low level of carnitine and increased level of muscle enzymes in plasma.

Therapy. Carnitine administration (2–4 g/d); prednisone, low-fat high carbohydrate diet.

Prognosis. Good with early therapy.

BIBLIOGRAPHY. Engel AG, Angelini C: Carnetine deficiency of human skeletal muscle with associated lipid storage myopathy: A new syndrome. Science 179:899–901, 1973

Hart ZH, Chang CH, Di Mauro S, et al: Muscle carnitine deficiency and fatal cardiomyopathy. Neurology 28:147, 1978

Waber LJ, Valle D, Neill C, et al: Carnitine deficiency presenting as familial cardiomyopathy: A treatable defect in carnitine transport. J Pediatr 101:700, 1982

Pepine CJ: The therapeutical potential of carnitine in cardiovascular disorders. Clin Ther 13:2–21, 1991

Ferrari R, DiMauro S, Sherwood G (eds): L-carnitine and its role in medicine: from function to therapy. London, Academic Press, 1992

ENGEL-ARING

Synonym. Periodic hypothalamic discharge. See Grahmann and Transient Cushing.

Symptoms. Recurrent at intervals of weeks or 2–3 months, or sporadic episodes lasting 3–5 days. Nausea, vomiting, thirst, fever, mental depression, and withdrawal; weight loss. In intervals; weight regained and normal life. Rapid weight gain precedes attacks.

Signs. Obesity; centripetal distribution; no "buffalo hump"; purple striae on abdomen and buttocks. Blood hypertension and tachycardia during attacks. Neurologic and ophthalmologic examination may be normal or abnormal.

Etiology and Pathology. Unknown; trauma or infection of central nervous system determining alteration of thermoregulatory mechanism and intermittent type of hyperadrenocorticism. Cystic soft degeneration of lateral thalamus and dorsomedial nucleus (in one case hypothalamus not involved).

Diagnostic Procedures. *Blood.* During attacks leukocytosis (up to 20,000); neutrophilia; sedimentation rate slightly increased; fall of potassium, normal sodium and chloride; rise of cholesterol. *Urine.* Normal during interval. During attacks, abrupt increase of 17-ketosteroids and 17-hydroxycorticoid excretion. *ECG.* Normal. *X-ray of chest and skull; of gastrointestinal tract:* stomach dilatation; spasm of pylorus during attacks (normal in interval).

Therapy. Dexamethasone prevents attacks.

Prognosis. Recurrence with temporary remission with treatment.

BIBLIOGRAPHY. Engel GL, Aring CD: Hypothalamic attacks with thalamic lesion. Arch Neurol Psychiatr 54:37–50, 1945

Wolff SM, Adler RC, Buskirk ER, et al: A syndrome of periodic hypothalamic discharge. Am J Med 36:956–967, 1964

Nieman L, Cutler GB Jr: Cushing's syndrome. In De Groot LJ (ed): Endocrinology, 3rd ed, p 1760. Philadelphia, WB Saunders, 1995

ENGEL-VON RECKLINGHAUSEN

Synonyms. Recklinghausen II; von Recklinghausen II; osteitis fibrosa generalisata; parathyroid osteitis; renal osteodystrophy; glomerular rickets.

Symptoms. Manifestations of nephritis or primary or secondary hyperparathyroidism. Arthralgia; fractures.

Signs. Bowing of long bones; spinal and chest deformities.

Etiology. Various conditions may cause this syndrome: (1) chronic nephritis; (2) primary and secondary hyperparathyroidism.

Pathology. That of underlying disease. *Bone.* Increased osteoblastic-osteoclastic activity. Formation of cysts in rarefied bones. Fibrous replacement of bone marrow cavities. *Kidney.* Renal calculi.

Diagnostic Procedures. *X-ray.* Typical findings.

Therapy and Prognosis. According to etiology. It may indicate kidney transplantation.

	Hyperparathryoidism	Acidosis
Blood		
Calcium	Increased	Normal or decreased
Phosphorous	Decreased	Increased
Alkaline phosphatase	Increased	Normal
Urine		
Calcium	Decreased	Decreased
Phosphorous	Increased or normal	Decreased
(NPN)*	Increased (late)	Increased

*nonprotein nitrogen

BIBLIOGRAPHY. von Recklinghausen F: Untersuchungen über Rachitis und Osteomalacie. Jena, G Fisher, 1910

Engel G: Ueber einen Fall cystoider Entartung des gesamten Skeletts. Giessen, 1864

Kanis JA: Renal bone disease. In Weatherall DJ, Ledingham JGG, Warrell DA (eds): Oxford Textbook of Medicine, 3rd ed, pp 3322–3330. Oxford, Oxford Med Pub, 1996

ENTEROPATHIC ARTHRITIS

Synonyms. Acute toxic arthritis; ulcerative colitis; colitic-arthritis. Dermatosis—arthritis—bowel; reactive arthritis. See Reiter.

Symptoms and Signs. Same sex incidence as that of Crohn (see) and ulcerative colitis. Onset at all ages; more common from 25–45 years of age. Bouts of arthritic manifestation associated with enteric symptoms, usually initially involving only a few joints and frequently migrating to others. Prevalence of distal extremity joint involvement and big articulations over hands and feet.

Etiology. Controversial entity. Some authors consider the arthritic condition (sterile arthritis) to be a complication of chronic ulcerative colitis, regional enteritis, and Whipple disease; 15% of patients with jejunal bypass develop symmetric polyarticular inflammation. Enteric infections more frequently associated are shigella species, salmonella species, campylobacter, yersinia species. Many others distinguish this entity as an autonomous association. The form is recognized by the American Rheumatism Association.

Pathology. That of Crohn or ulcerative colitis and arthritis (indistinguishable from that of rheumatoid arthritis).

Diagnostic Procedures. *Blood.* Leukocytosis; high sedimentation rate; hemoglobin reduced. *X-ray.* Nonspecific and minor alterations; usually rheumatoid factor absent. *Synovial fluid.* Total leukocytes 4000–40,000, polymorphs 75–98%; increased viscosity.

Therapy. Nonsteroid antinflammatory agent (variable results). Corticosteroids for treatment of enteritis, possibly secondarily benefiting arthritis. If monoarticular, intra-articular corticosteroids useful.

Prognosis. In 50% of cases, attack lasts less than 1 month; in 10% more than 1 year. One or two attacks for 1 year or less. Final outcome is determined by the evolution of enteric manifestation. Chonicization in 3% circa.

BIBLIOGRAPHY. Hench PS: Nelson's Loose-Leaf Surgery, p 104. New York. Nelson & Son, 1935

Jorizzo JL: Bowel associated dermatosis-arthritis syndrome. Arch Intern Med 144:738–740, 1984

Roubenoff R: The musculoskeletal system. In Haubrich WS, Schaffner F, Berk JE (eds): Bockus Gastroenterology, 5th ed, vol 2, p 3494. Philadelphia, WB Saunders, 1995

ENTEROPATHY-ASSOCIATED T-CELL LYMPHOMA

Synonyms. EATCL.

Symptoms and Signs. In both sexes, 1:1. In patients with malabsorption or celiac disease and/or dermatitis herpetiform, common in the Middle East. Age: fourth–seventh decades, sporadically in younger age. Further deterioration of patient chronic condition, seldom acute abdomen.

Etiology. Unknown.

Pathology. Villous atrophy, crypt hyperplasia, lymphomatous nodules with large T-cell origin in multiple segments of distal small intestine and with early dissemination in mesenteric lymph nodes, liver, speen, bone marrow, lung, and skin.

Diagnostic Procedures. *X-ray. CT scan. MRI. Endoscopy. Biopsy. Stool analysis. Blood.* Normal white cell count and differential, rising IgA titers.

Therapy. Chemotherapy and adjuvant therapies, surgery only for complications.

Prognosis. Very unfavorable except in rare case where resection is followed by long remission.

BIBLIOGRAPHY. Mairly NH, Makie FP: The clinical and biochemical syndrome in lymphoadenoma and allied disease involving the mesenteric lymph glands. Br Med J 1:3972–3980, 1937

Turowski GA, Basson MD: Primary malignant lymphoma of the intestine. Am J Surg 169:433–441, 1995

ENTHESITIS

Synonym. Polyenthesitis; myoenthesitis.* See also fibromyalgia and Overuse syndromes.

Symptoms. Includes all syndromes deriving from degenerative or inflammatory changes, with problems at the joints with slight swelling or without signs. Order of frequency of enthesis involment: sacroiliac, humerus epicondile, calcaneus, coracoid process, and patella.

Etiology. Lesions resulting from microtrauma or macrotrauma (local mechanical disorders); or observed in the pathology of ankylosing spondilytis (systemic disorders) viral infection also prospected. It is used, also, as a diagnostic term when a disease within the category of spondyloarthropathies remains unclassifiable. Possibility of inheritance also considered.

Pathology. From bioptic samples. Thickening and induration, yellow discoloration and edema, granulation with mononuclear infiltration, small vessel proliferation.

Diagnostic Procedures. *X-ray. Scintigraphy. Blood. Biopsy.*

Therapy. Good response to anti-inflammatory agents (phenylbutazone, salazopyrine etc.). Excision of tender and swollen area seldom indicated.

Prognosis. Chronic condition, lasting years.

BIBLIOGRAPHY. La Cava G: Apparato musculo tendineo e sport. Minerva Med 55:461–463, 1964

Schichikawa K, Tanenaka Y, Yokiota M, et al: Polyenthesitis. Rheum Dis N Am 18:203–213, 1992

Weatherall DJ, Ledingham JGG, Warrell DA (eds): Oxford Textbook of Medicine, 3rd ed, pp 2947, 4324. Oxford, Oxford Med Pub, 1996

ENTRAPMENT

Synonym. Compartmental.

Symptoms. Pain of muscle groups, occasionally more severe at rest and during the night; hypoesthesia; paresthesia; muscular weakness.

Signs. Tenderness; muscle atrophy. Pressure on trigger point elicits localized pain in affected areas.

Etiology. Anatomic constriction of peripheral nerve. These are the most frequent sites of entrapment:

Spinoglenoid notch–median.
Carpal tunnel–median.
Bicipital groove–ulnar.
Cubital tunnel–ulnar.
Palmar fascia-pisiform bone–ulnar.
Heads on pronator muscle–anterior interosseous.

---

*The anatomofunctional structural complex that is interposed between muscles and bones or joint structures is named the myoenthesic apparatus.

Inguinal ligament–lateral femoral cutaneous.
Obturator canal–obturator.
Tarsal tunnel–posterior tibial.
Plantar fascia: heads of IV–IV metatarsal–plantar.

See individual syndromes.

BIBLIOGRAPHY. Dawson DM, Hallett M, Millender LH: Entrapment Neuropathies, 2nd ed. Boston, Little, Brown, 1990
Klippel JH, Dieppe PA: Rheumatology, pp 5.19.1, 5.19.12. St Louis, CV Mosby, 1995

ENURESIS

Synonyms. Bed wetting; primary enuresis; secondary enuresis.

Symptoms and Signs. Between 4 and 5 years of age 10–15% of children continue to wet the bed. In adulthood symptoms present in 1–3%. Primary enuresis. No intercurrent episodes of dryness. Secondary enuresis. Periods of dry months and relapses. Episode usually occurs in first third of night.

Etiology. Primary form. Family history; organic conditions (e.g., urologic obstruction, epispadias). Secondary form. Psychologic factors (relapses caused also by organic factors, i.e., intercurring diseases).

Diagnostic Procedures. Rule out organic conditions. Assess psychologic status. Sleep study. Enuresis episodes usually in NREM (rapid eye movement) sleep; follows a burst of K-complex waves and body movements.

Therapy. Correct organic conditions. Parent and child education. Imipramine.

Prognosis. Variable according to nature of condition and treatment. Suspension of imipramine causes relapses. Most children outgrow syndrome.

BIBLIOGRAPHY. Gastant H, Broughton R: A clinical and polygraphic study of episodic phenomena during sleep. Recent Adv Biol Psychiatr 7:197–223, 1969
Starfield B: Enuresis: Its pathogenesis and management. Clin Pediatr 11:343–350, 1972
Adams RD, Victor M: Principles of Neurology, 5th ed, pp 348, 475, 522. New York, McGraw-Hill, 1993

EOSINOPHILIA–MYALGIA

Synonym. L-Tryptophan-associated esosinophilia-myalgia; tryptophan-associated eosinophilia-myalgia; myalgia-eosinophilia.

Symptoms. After ingestion of L-tryptophan for periods lasting from 10 days to several months with doses ranging from 500 mg to 6 g/d onset of the following symptoms: fatigue (90% of cases), xerostomia (47%), fever (40%), weight loss (70%), myalgia; usually proximal disabling episodic muscle spasms (100%), articular symptoms (44%), cough and dyspnea (60%), sensorimotor polyneuropathyy (34%) predominantly axonal.

Signs. Nonspecific diffuse erythematous macules (47%), ecchymosis (9%); massive edema of extremities and trunk (47%); absence of muscle tenderness; articular swelling and/or tenderness; after 3–9 months mucinous papules (resolving in 3–9 months); in 55% of cases late appearance of skin chronic induration resembling scleroderma (see) especially in the extremities (25%) less in the trunk (18%) and breast (7%); alopecia (80%).

Etiology. Unknown cause and pathogenesis. Additional studies needed to assess role of agents identified in the batches of L-tryptophan implicated in the epidemic of 1989.

Pathology. Scleroderma-like skin changes: myositis with eosinophilic infiltration.

Diagnostic Procedures. *Blood.* Variable leukocytosis (median 14,000), eosinophilia (100 cells/micro/l). Moderate trombocytosis. Frequent absence of increased muscle enzymes. Increased serum aldolase (60%). Antinuclear antibodies (38%). *X-ray.* Chest: transient pulmonary infiltrates; joints:synovitis.

Therapy. Corticosteroids.

Prognosis. Evolution toward scleroderma-like changes. Progressive clinical involvement of 1–4 organ system. Corticosteroid therapy does not have significant clinical effect. Extremely low percentage near resolution of symptoms. Death in some cases (not significant difference between treated and untreated cases).

BIBLIOGRAPHY. CDC Eosinophilia-myalgia syndrome. New Mexico MMWR 38:765–767, 1989
Martin RW, Daffy J, Engel AG, et al: The clinical spectrum of the eosinophilia-myalgia syndrome associated with L-tryptophan ingestion: clinical features in 20 patients and aspects of pathophysiology. Ann Intern Med 113:124–134, 1990
Tazelaar HD, Myers JL, Drage CW, et al: Pulmonary disease associated with L-tryptophan-induced eosinophilic myalgia syndrome: Clinical and pathological features. Chest 97:1032–1036, 1990
Leed D, Kaufman LD, Barry L, et al: Clinical follow-up and immunogenetic studies of 32 patients with eosinophilia-myalgia syndrome. Lancet 337:1071–1074, 1991
Coutant G, Blètry O: Pathologie de l'èosinophile: Aspect cliniques, prognostiques et therapeutiques. Edit Tech Encycl Mèd Chir Paris France. Hèmatology 13-009-A10 p3, 1993

EOSINOPHILIC GASTROENTERITIS

Synonyms. Allergic jejunitis; allergic gastroenteritis; angioneurotic edema of gastrointestinal tract; eosinophilic gastroenteritis; gastrointestinal idiopathic eosinophilic infiltrations; granuloma eosinophilic stomach. (See also Loeffler and Quincke I.)

Symptoms and Signs. Nearly equal sex distribution; seen in all ages, but most common in the sixth decade. Symptomatology may vary in kind with the organ involved. However, common pattern may be observed: recurrent gastrointestinal disorders lasting many years; vomiting; flatulence; diarrhea; epigastric pain; cramps; heartburn (in Class II pain and cramping more prolonged and not intermittent; see Pathology). In some cases also history of melena or hematemesis; pyloric obstruction; cholecystitis and cholelithiasis; history of allergy (in 50% of cases).

Etiology. Unknown. Allergic mechanism (hypersensitivity reaction) postulated for the diffused type (Class I); local inciting agents for the circumscribed types (Class II), i.e., parasites.

Pathology. Two classes appear unrelated. Class I (diffuse type). (1) Polyenteric: more than one portion of intestine involved; antrum of the stomach characteristically affected with extension to jejunum and ileum. Areas affected are firm, with edematous appearance; omentum and mesentery may appear inflamed or fibrotic; pylorus usually narrowed. Diffuse inflammatory infiltration from submucosa (occasionally also serosa) by mature eosinophils, with rare macrophages and giant cells; occasionally, hyalinization or necrosis of muscles. Mucosa free of involvement. (2) Monoenteric: similar pattern of lesions limited to the stomach. (3) Regional: similar pattern involving only a limited region; prepyloric and pyloric with borders not well defined. Class II (circumscribed type). (1) Regional: pseudotumors located at any site of the gastrointestinal tract; mucosa may be ulcerated; granuloma type of lesion, with rich reticular fibrillar and fibroblastic elements; varying numbers of blood vessels and inflammatory cells. Scarce eosinophilic infiltration; histiocytes rare. (2) Polypoid pedunculated polyps; microscopically same pattern as regional type.

Diagnostic Procedures. *X-ray.* Varying findings according to location and extension of lesions. In Class I, usually smooth concentric narrowing of the antrum; absence of peristalsis in involved area; signs of pyloric obstruction; with bowel involvement, tubular segmental narrowings, alternating with dilated loops. *Blood.* Eosinophilia (up to 60%) increased Ig E. *Bone marrow.* High percentage of eosinophils. *Biopsy of lesion.* See Pathology.

Therapy. Conservative treatment with adrenocorticotropic hormone (ACTH) and corticosteroids usually brings prompt control of symptoms and of eosinophilia. When indicated, exploratory laparotomy and biopsy. According to location and extension of lesions, surgical intervention may be decided on. Usually gastroenterostomy is adequate; in some cases subtotal gastrectomy and total gastrectomy have been performed. According to recent findings, surgery seems necessary only for control of bleeding.

Prognosis. Lesions do not recur after resection. If they recur after conservative treatment, response to successive steroid administrations is prompt.

BIBLIOGRAPHY. Konjetzny GE: Ueber Magenfibrome. Beitr Klin Chir 119:53, 1920
Barrie HJ, Anderson JC: Hypertrophy of pylorus in an adult with massive eosinophil infiltration and giant cell reaction. Lancet II:1007–1009, 1948
Lane RE: Eosinophilic gastroenteritis. Northwest Med 66:357–359, 1967
Mathelier-Fusade P, Leynardier F: Gastroenterite eosinophila. Presse Méd 11:93, 1994

EOSINOPHIL LUNG, SECONDARY

Synonym. Secondary pulmonary eosinophilic infiltrate.

Symptoms and Signs. Same clinical findings as in Loeffler. Occasionally, recurrent episodes; tropical eosinophilia. (This term includes only infection by Wucheria bancrofti and Brugia malayi.)

Etiology. *Parasites.* Ascaris; trichina; entamoeba; hookworms; filaria; toxocara; schistosomes; lung fluke; strongyloides; trichuris; liver fluke; tapeworms; echinococcus. *Infections.* Tuberculosis; coccidiomycosis; brucellosis; viral and bacterial pneumonia; bronchiectasis. *Neoplastic.* Hodgkin disease; eosinophilic granuloma, eosinophilic leukemia. *Collagen diseases.* Periarteritis; rheumatoid arthritis; rheumatic fever. *Allergies.* Asthma; hay fever; eczema; serum sickness; Dressler syndrome; drugs. *Others.* Fat embolism, aspiration pneumonia; idiopathic familial eosinophilia with pneumonia.

Pathology. Pulmonary eosinophilic infiltrates plus specific findings according to etiology.

Diagnostic Procedures. *Blood.* Eosinophilia. *Sputum.* Eosinophilia. *X-ray of chest.* Pulmonary infiltrates plus specific findings according to etiology. *Specific complement fixation tests for parasites.*

Therapy. Corticosteroids highly effective, except when contraindicated by particular etiology. Specific treatment according to etiology.

Prognosis. Good response to steroids; possible recurrences. Depends on etiology.

BIBLIOGRAPHY. Reeder WH, Goodrich BE: Pulmonary infiltration with eosinophilia (P. I. E. syndrome). Ann Int Med 36:1217–1240, 1952
Hall JW, Kozak M, Spink WW: Pulmonary infiltrates, pericarditis and eosinophilia. Am J Med 36:135–143, 1964
Coutant G, Blètry O: Pathologie de l'èosinophile. Aspect cliniques, prognostiques et therapeutiques. Edit Tech Encycl Mèd Chir Paris France Hèmatology 13-009-A10 p3, 1993

EPIDERMOLYSIS BULLOSA, SIMPLE, OGNA*

Synonyms. Gedde-Dahl; Ogna.

_____
*Name of village in Norway.

Symptoms and Signs. From infancy, both sexes. Traumatic seasonal blistering of palms and soles and seldom other places, distinguished by generalized bruising tendency, onychogryphotic big toenails.

Etiology. Autosomal dominant inheritance. Linkage to erythrocyte glutamic pyruvic transaminase locus.

BIBLIOGRAPHY. Gedde-Dahl T: Epidermolysis bullosa, pp 1–180. Baltimore, Johns Hopkins Press, 1971
Olaisen B, Gedde-Dahl T Jr: GPT-epidermolysis bullosa simplex (EBS Ogna) linkage in man. Human Hered 23:189–196, 1973
Pye RJ: Bullous eruptions. In Champion RH, Burton JL, Ebling FJG (eds): Rook/Wilkinson/Ebling Textbook of Dermatology, 5th ed, pp 1625–1626. Oxford, Blackwell Scientific, 1992

EPILEPTIC AUTOMATISM

After an attack of grand mal or more frequently in psychomotor amnesic epilepsy, patient may wander, avoiding danger; talks and acts without memory of happenings after he comes out of the state and finds himself in unknown surroundings (sometimes in another town).

BIBLIOGRAPHY. Jackson JH: Contribution to the comparative study of convulsions. Brain 9:1–23, 1886
Unvericht H: Die Myoclonie. Berlin, Franz Dentiche, 1918
Temkin O: The Falling Sickness: A History of Epilepsy from the Greeks to the Beginning of Modern Neurology. Baltimore, Johns Hopkins Press, 1945
Ishida Kato: Tonic automation complex: Cases with violent gestural automatism following a brief tonic seizure. Jap J Psychiatr Neurol 47:271–272, 1993
Ebner Dimmer: Automatism with preserved responsivenes: a lateralarizing sign in psychomotor seizures. Neurology 45:61–64, 1995

EPIPHYSEAL ISCHEMIC NECROSIS

Synonyms. Epiphyseal aseptic necrosis; epiphyseal osteochondritis; osteochondritis deformans juvenilis.

Symptoms. Prevalent in males (4:1), except in some forms. See individual syndromes; onset at young age, mostly in childhood, some varieties in adolescence or adult life. Pain corresponding to affected bone, primary epiphyses, or secondary epiphyses. According to bone affected designated by various eponyms:

1. Blencke (see).
2. Chandler S. A. (see).
3. Dietrich (see).
4. Friedrich (see).
5. Kienboeck (see).
6. Köhler I (see).
7. Köhler II (see).
8. Legg-Calvé-Perthes (see).
9. Meyer J (see).
10. Osgood-Slatter (see).
11. Panner (see).
12. Preiser (see).
13. Scheuermann (see).
14. Sever (see).
15. Thiemann (see).

Signs. At site involved, tenderness or palpation, skin changes, swelling, redness, occasionally, thickening.

Etiology. Degeneration and eventual replacement of the osseous nucleus of an epiphysis, due to interference with its blood supply: trauma (?); congenital hereditary factors (?); infection and endocrine disturbances (?).

Pathology. Scanty reports. Osseous nucleus: necrotic; fragmented and compressed; there may be evidence of hemorrhage, cystic degeneration, and fibrosis. Enchondrial plate may be softened and distorted. Histologic changes variable according to the phase in which the analysis is carried out.

Diagnostic Procedures. *X-ray. CT scan. MR imaging.* Similar changes for all types of bones affected. In first stage, scanty modification (bulging of joint capsule; slight displacement of affected bone) followed by osseous manifestations (lucent crescent or other images); later the affected center becomes opaque. Demineralization in surrounding area. In second stage; opacity, fragmentation and flattening of epiphyseal center. In third stage; healing through new bone formation.

Therapy. *Analgesic.* Immobilization, avoidance of weight bearing, and limitation of activity until pain subsides; after: rehabilitation. If a loose body persists in the joint (i.e., in the knee) arthroscopic removal.

Prognosis. Spontaneous recovery in months or years. Complete normal restoration of morphology and function, or, in some cases, persistent malformation owing to irreversible anatomic changes during or following the acute stage.

BIBLIOGRAPHY. Cahill BR, Philips MR, Navarro R: The results of conservative management of juvenile osteochondritis dissecans using joint scintigraphy: A prospective study. Am J Sport Med 17:601, 1989
Twyman RS, Desai K, Aichroth PM: Long term follow-up of osteochondritis dissecans of the knee in children. J Bone Joint Surg (Br) 73:461–464, 1994

EPSTEIN (A.A.)

Synonyms. Idiopathic nephrotic syndrome (INS). Includes various basic pathologic lesions that may represent different diseases. The classification adopted today is based on histopathology, but the clinical entity is approximately the same. Minimal change disease (see). Mesangeal proliferative glomerulonephritis (see). Focal glomerular sclerosis. Diffuse glomerular sclerosis (see). Membranous glomerulonephritis (see). Mesangiocapillary glomerulonephritis types I, II, III (see).

Symptoms and Signs. Insidious onset. Edema (legs and face). Hematuria. Hypertension. Oliguria, anuria possible. Malnutrition. Increased susceptibility to infections. Frequent cardiovascular symptoms and signs. Thromboembolism. Renal vein thrombosis.

Etiology. See individual syndromes.

Diagnostic Procedures. *Urine.* Proteinuria (more than 3.5 g/day), hematuria macroscopic or microscopic. *Blood.* Creatinine and BUN above normal ranges, hypoalbuminemia, electrophoretic alterations (alpha-1 and beta increased). Hyperlipidemia (LDL, VLDL).

Therapy. See individual syndromes.

Prognosis. See individual syndromes.

BIBLIOGRAPHY. Epstein AA: Concerning the causation of edema in chronic parenchymatous nephritis: Methods for its alleviation. Am J Med Sci 154:638–647, 1917
Glassock RJ: Syndromes of glomerular diseases. In Haubrich WS, Schaffner F, Berk JE (eds): Bockus Gastroenterology, 5th ed, vol 2, pp 682–710. Philadelphia, WB Saunders, 1995

EPSTEIN (C.J.)

Synonym. Macrothrombocytopenia—nephritis—deafness.

Symptoms and Signs. Both sexes. Nephropathy. More in females. Hearing loss and nephropathy symptoms identical with those of Alport (see). Hemorrhagic tendency.

Etiology. Unknown. Possibly autosomal dominant trait.

Diagnostic Procedures. *Blood.* Giant thrombocytes, impaired aggrega-

tion with collagen and epinephrine, lack of release of factor III, and adherence to glass. Bleeding time prolonged.

BIBLIOGRAPHY. Epstein CJ, Sahud MA, Piel CF, et al: Hereditary macrothrombocytopenia nephritis and deafness. Ann J Med 52:299–310, 1972
Hansen MS, Behnke O, Pedersen NT, et al: Megathrombocytopenia associated with glomerulonephritis, deafness and aortic cystic media necrosis. Scand J Hemat 21:197–205, 1978

ERB-CHARCOT

Synonyms. Strümpel; Erb IV spastic spinal syphilitic paralysis.

Symptoms. Prevalent in males; onset 2–10 years after infection. Tiredness and stiffness of legs. Dragging feet; urgency and increased frequency of urination; gradual progression to paraplegia; minor sensory changes occur at later stage.

Signs. *Early.* Increase in muscular tone and in deep reflexes; ankle clonus; Babinski positive; abdominal reflexes abolished. *Later.* Minor defects in tactile and proprioceptive spheres.

Etiology. Rare form of spinal syphilis, occurring several years after primary infection.

Pathology. Mild endoarteritis of vessel of spinal cord causing degeneration of lateral column.

Diagnostic Procedures. *Blood and spinal fluid.* Serology to demonstrate syphilitic infections. Differentiate from other numerous causes of spastic paraplegia.

Therapy. Intense antisyphilitic therapy.

Prognosis. Poor; the form does not respond well to treatment.

BIBLIOGRAPHY. Erb, WH: Ueber syphilitische Spinal-paralyse. Neurol Centralbl Leipz 11:161–168, 1892
Adams RD, Victor M: Principles of Neurology, 5th ed, p 626. New York, McGraw-Hill, 1993

ERB-DUCHENNE

Synonyms. Duchenne-Erb; Erb I; brachial plexus paralysis; upper brachial plexus paralysis.

Symptoms and Signs. Arm and forearm adducted and internally rotated and forearm extended and pronated. Flaccid paralysis and wasting of arm and shoulder muscles. No sensation loss, or loss of sensation in a small area on the lower border of deltoid.

Etiology. Lesion occurs during birth when traction of the head or arm is applied, or in twisting arm or shoulder down and backward; or vascular, infective, neoplastic lesion involving the fifth and sixth cervical roots with resulting paralysis of the shoulder and arm muscles.

Therapy. Immobilization of arm to relieve the brachial plexus.

Prognosis. Fair to good in neonatal paralysis; poor in other conditions.

BIBLIOGRAPHY. Duchenne GB: De L'éléctrisation localisée et de son application á la pathologie et á la therapeutique. Paris, Baillière, 1855
Erb W: Ueber eine eigenthümliche Localisation von Lähmungen im Plexus branchialis. Verh Naturh Med 2:130–137, 1874
Adams RD, Victor M: Principles of Neurology, 5th ed, p 1043. New York, McGraw-Hill, 1993

ERB-GOLDFLAM

Synonyms. Erb II; Hoppe-Goldflam; myasthenia gravis pseudoparalytica.

Symptoms and Signs. Annual incidence per milion 2.5–10.4. Prevalence 25–125 per million. Female to male ratio, 6:4. Occurs to any age, but female incidence peaks in third decade and male incidence in sixth seventh decade. Familial cases present before second decade. Abnormal weakness and fatigability of some or all voluntary muscles that increase with repetition or exertion during the day. Improvement with rest and cold, worsened by heat and fever. At onset, transient dyplopia, progressive difficulty in chewing and talking, dyspnea, nasal regurgitation. Proximal limbs muscles and muscles innervated by cranial nerves are more severely affected. No objective sensory deficits, subjective sensory symptoms occasionally described. Spontaneous remissions that last for varying periods.

Signs. Expressionless face; ptosis of upper eyelids; sagging of jaw; manifestation changing during the day, becoming more severe with progression of disease. Reflexes decrease and return to normal after muscle groups rested. Smile resembles a "snarl." Muscle wasting (14% of cases). Classification (Osserman): adult: ocular (group 1) mild generalized (Group 2A), moderately severe generalized (Group 2B), acute fulminating (Group 3), late severe (Group 4). (Thymomas have higher incidence in this group.)

Etiology. Unknown. Anti-Ach R antibodies (IgG1 and IgG2) that bind to a variety of sites on ACh. Receptors on muscle membrane and affect binding of ACh to AChR, affect properties of AChR in channel, cause complement mediated destruction of junctional folds, accelerate degradation of AChR. ACh that cannot bind to AChR remains in the junction and is rapidly destroyed. Possible autosomal recessive inheritance cases described. Thymus hyperplasia and thymoma may play roles in autoimmunization process.

Pathology. No specific alteration in muscle. Presence of lymphorrhages (accumulation of perimysial lymphocytes). Thymus hyperplastic; thymoma occasionally present.

Diagnostic Procedures. *EMG.* (Conventional needle, study of decremental response, single fiber recordings.) *Blood.* Serum anti-AChR antibody titer. In vitro microelectrode studies, ultrastructural studies of neuromuscular function. Anticholinesterase drug test (0.1–0.2 ml of a 10-mg/ml solution of Edrophonium [tensilon] injected IV over 15 seconds): positive. *Provocative tests* (curare; no longer used). *X-ray of chest.* May show thymoma. *Immunocytochemical studies.* IgG and C3, C9 and MAC localized on neuromuscular junction.

Therapy. Pyridostigmine bromide (Mestinon) now generally preferred (60-mg tablets, 180-mg timespan tablets, syrup). From 30 mg every 6 hours to 240 mg every 3–4 hours. Ampules 2 ml (10 mg) for injection. Neostigmine bromide is available in 15-mg tablets (one tablet equivalent to 60 mg tablet of pyridostigmine). Therapy is given to diminish rather than eliminate MG symptoms because side effects of anticholinesterase drugs are fastidious and dangerous.

Cholinergic crisis must be treated with suspension of all therapy, ventilatory support, and intravenous feeding. Refractoriness to drug therapy disappears after a few days of treatment.

Alternate day steroids (prednisone) are safe and indicated for disabling disease not responding to moderate or large dose of anticholinesterase drugs. Various protocols have been adopted.

Azathioprine (2–3 mg/kg/day) and cyclosporin have given good results. Trials with high-dose IV immunoglobulin have given good results. Thymectomy is very effective in all cases, especially in preventing generalization of the disease. Thymoma presents an absolute indication. Plasmapheresis in justified only in life-saving conditions.

Prognosis. Usually progressive; spontaneous remission possible; remission occasionally during pregnancy. Sudden death (myocardial involvement) or death from exhaustion, malnutrition, respiratory insufficiency, and complications. With more aggressive therapy steady fall in mortality. Mortality is now 4% in 5 years. Risk factors age over 40, short history of severe disease, thymoma.

BIBLIOGRAPHY. Willis T: Anima brutorum, pp 404–406. Oxford Theatro Sheldoniano, Oxford, 1672

Erb W: Zur Casuistick der bulbären Lähmungen. Arch Psychiatr Nervenkr 9:325–350, 1879

Goldflam S: Ueber einen scheinbar heilbaren bulbärparalytischen Symptomcomplex mit Betheiligung der Extremitäten. Dsch Z Nerven 4:312–352, 1893

Batocchi AP, Evoli A, Palmisani MT, et al: Early-onset myasthenia gravis: clinical characteristics and response to therapy. Eur J Pediatr 150:66–68, 1990

Engel AG: Myasthenia gravis and myasthenic syndromes. In Roland LP, Di Mauro S: Handbook of Clinical Neurology, vol 18: Myopathies, p 391. Amsterdam, Elsevier, 1992

Penn AS, Richman DP, Ruff RL, et al (eds): Myasthenia Gravis and Related Disorders: Experimental and Clinical Aspects. Ann NY Acad Sci 681, 1993

Lisak RP: Handbook of Myasthenia Gravis and Myasthenic Syndromes. New York, Marcel Dekker, 1994

ERB III

Synonyms. Juvenile muscular dystrophy; superior limb-girdle dystrophy; scapulohumeral muscular dystrophy; scapulohumeral dystrophy; muscular dystrophy I; pelvofemoral muscular dystrophy. Includes: autosomal-recessive muscular dystrophy of infancy, see Leyden-Moebius.

Symptoms. Both sexes equally affected; onset at any age from first to sixth decade, but usually from 20 to 30 years of age. Proximal muscles of arms first involved (Erb type) or more rarely of lumbosacral region (Leyden-Moebius type). Successive involvement of lumbosacral muscles in the first type and of scapulohumeral in the second one, usually occurring within 20 years of the onset. See Duchenne muscular dystrophy (pseudohypertrophy only in few cases) and Landouzy-Déjerine. Involvement of facial muscle as a late event differentiates it from Landouzy-Déjerine (see). Muscle hypertrophy may be present, especially in childhood forms: Inspiratory muscle weakness limits chest expansion and may be considered a form of restrictive lung disease and causes morning headaches, hypersomnia, impaired mental function. In some cases, cardiomyopathy.

Etiology. Unknown. Many cases sporadic; more than one genetic trait may be involved. Family with autosomal recessive type well-demonstrated. Under this and the other various eponyms have been described many conditions, all resulting in similar clustering of symptoms (syndrome).

Pathology. Muscle fiber degeneration. Fibrosis notable feature. Less fat than in Duchenne type.

Diagnostic Procedures. *Serum enzymes.* Aldolase, creatine phosphokinase pyruvate kinase serum glutamic-oxaloacetic transaminase (SGOT), variable elevation, higher value at early stage, normal or slight elevation later. *EEG.* Seldom abnormal. *EMG.* Myopathic findings.

Therapy. Exercise, bracing, surgery.

Prognosis. Contracture develops rapidly only after patient becomes immobilized. Very slow progression. Life span shortened.

BIBLIOGRAPHY. Erb WH: Ueber die "juvenil form" der progressiven Muskelatrophie ihre Beziehungen zur sogneannten Pseudohypertrophie der Muskeln. Isch Arch Klin Med 34:467–519, 1884

Yates JRW, Emery AEH: A population study of adult onset limb-girdle muscular dystrophy. J Med Genet 22:250–257, 1985

Munsat TL, Serratrice G: Facioscapulohumeral and scapuloperoneal syndromes. In Jerusalem F, Sieb JP: The Limb Girdle Syndromes. In Rowland LP, DiMauro S (eds): Handbook of Clinical Neurology, vol 18: Myopathies, pp 161, 179. Amsterdam, Elsevier, 1992

ERDHEIM I

Synonyms. Gsell-Erdheim; Erdheim cystic necrosis of aorta; aorta idiopathic necrosis; annuloaortic ectasia. See Marfan.

Symptoms and Signs. Frequently asymptomatic; or dramatic sequence of aortic rupture. In many cases, associated with various manifestations of Marfan syndrome. Rare. Signs of aortic stenosis (see). In early to late adulthood. Sudden rupture. Aortic aneurysm rupture.

Etiology. Developmental factor or associated with Marfan syndrome (genetic factor); metabolic and toxic factors also considered. Familial occurrence reported (autosomal dominant trait).

Pathology. Wall of aorta separates easily into two layers. Mucoid medial degeneration: loss of muscle and elastic fibers; diffuse ground substance among residual fibers positive for mucopolysaccharide stain.

Therapy. *Cardiosurgery.* Problems related to inconsistency and difficult healing of scar.

Prognosis. Variable.

BIBLIOGRAPHY. Gsell O: Wandnekrosen der Aorta als selbstaendige Erkrankung und ihre Beziehung zur Spontanruptur. Virchows Arch (Pathol) 270:1–36, 1928
Erdheim J: Medionecrosis aortae idiopathica. Virchows Arch (Pathol) 273:454–479, 1929
Rapaport E, Rackley CE, Cohn LH: Aortic valve disease. In Schlant RC, Alexander RW: Hurst's The Heart, 8th ed, pp 1468–1469. New York, McGraw-Hill, 1994

ERDHEIM II

Synonyms. Scaglietti-Dagnini. Acromegalic macrospondylitis. Eponyms used to indicate a particular form of acromegaly, where the bone hypertrophy primarily affects the clavicles, vertebrae, and intervertebral disks causing kyphosis, movement impairment, and pain.

BIBLIOGRAPHY. Erdheim J: Ueber Wirbersaeulenveraen-derungen bei Akromegalie. Virchows Arch (Pathol Anat) 281:197–296, 1931
Scaglietti O, Dagnini G: Sul quadro radiografico delle alterazioni acromegaliche dei corpi vertebrali secondo Erdheim. Radiol Fis Med (Bologna) 2:251–264, 1939

ERNSTER-LUFT

Synonyms. Hypermetabolic mitochondrial; Luft. See OXPHOS syndromes.

Symptoms and Signs. Onset in childhood. Profuse perspiration; polydipsia without polyuria; slenderness despite polyphagia; progressive weakness and hypotonia; tachycardia; elevation of body temperature up to 38.4°C. Tendon reflexes absent.

Etiology. See OXPHOS. Mitochondrial respiration is independent of phosphorylation (loose coupling). Maybe owing to a vicious cycling of calcium uptake and release.

Pathology. Increased number of mitochondria in subsarcolemmic areas with or without inclusions. Thyroid normal.

Diagnostic Procedures. *Basal metabolic rate.* Highly increased (+140 to +210); not changed by antithyroid treatment and by thyroidectomy. *Thyroid function study.* Normal. *Urine.* Creatinuria. *Electromyography.* Myopathic pattern.

Therapy. See OXPHOS syndromes.

Prognosis. Progressive weakness.

BIBLIOGRAPHY. Ernster L, Ikkos D, Luft R: Enzymic activities of human skeletal muscle mitochondria: A tool in clinical metabolic research. Nature 184:1851–1854, 1959
Luft R, Ikkos D, Palmieri G, et al: A case of severe hypermetabolism of nonthyroid origin with a defect in the maintenance of mitochondrial respiratory control. J Clin Invest 41:1776–1804, 1962
Moraes CT, DiMauro S, Zeviani M, et al: Mitochondrial DNA dele-

tions in progressive external ophthalmoplegia and Kearns-Sayre syndrome. N Engl J Med 320:1293–1299, 1989

ERYSIPELOID

Synonyms. Baker-Rosenbach. Klaudes (diffuse septicemic variety); Rosenbach (mild form); seal fingers.

Symptoms. Appears in workers in contact with live infected animals or animal carcasses. High incidence in summer and fall. Three days after inoculation a local dusky erythema develops on upper extremities and extends centrifugally for about 10 cm. Fever (10%). Seldom, severe systemic involvement (form of Klauder) with numerous bullae and plaques; weight loss; arthralgias.

Etiology. Acute (seldom chronic) infection with *Erysipelothrix insidiosa* (formerly *rhusiopathiae*); gram-positive bacillus causative agents of animal (swine) erysipelas and present also in the skin of birds, fish.

Diagnostic Procedures. Culture (in vitro) of biopsy material.

Therapy. Penicillin; tetracyclines; erythromycin.

Prognosis. Resolution in 3–4 days with treatment; in 2 weeks spontaneously; occasionally, protracted with remission and relapses of systemic manifestations.

BIBLIOGRAPHY. Klauder JV: Erysipeloid and swine erysipelas in man. A clinical and bacteriological review: Swine erysipelas in the United States. JAMA 86:536–541, 1926
Highet AS, Hay RJ, Roberts SOB: Bacterial infections. In Champion RH, Burton JL, Ebling FJG (eds): Rook/Wilkinson/Ebling Textbook of Dermatology, 5th ed, pp 992–993. Oxford, Blackwell Scientific, 1992

ERYTHEMA GYRATUM REPENS

See Paraneoplastic syndromes.

Signs. Erythematous lesions spread over the body resembling grain of wood (cypress burl).

Etiology. Associated with visceral malignant tumor. Seldom with tuberculosis.

Diagnostic Procedures. Search for malignancy.

Therapy. That of malignancy.

Prognosis. Poor; skin lesions disappear if tumor cured.

BIBLIOGRAPHY. Rothman S: Ueber Hauterscheinungen bei bosartigen Geschwulsten innerer Organe. Arch Dermatol U. Syph. 149:99–123, 1925
Curth HO: How and why the skin reacts. Ann NY Acad Sci 230:435–442, 1974
Champion RH: Disorder of blood vessels. In Champion RH, Burton JL, Ebling FJG (eds): Rook/Wilkinson/Ebling Textbook of Dermatology, 5th ed, p 1841. Oxford, Blackwell Scientific, 1992

ERYTHEMA MULTIFORME

Synonyms. Dermatostomatitis; ectodermosis erosiva pluriorificialis; erythema papulosum rheumaticum; erythéme polymorphe; herpes iris. See also Stevens-Johnson. At least three major clinical patterns can be recognized: (1) papular or simplex; (2) vesiculobullous; (3) Stevens-Johnson. Atypical cases have also been reported.

PAPULAR OR SIMPLEX

Symptoms. All ages, both sexes affected; male-to-female ratio 3:1.

Moderate malaise; discomfort; myalgia; pruritus; occasionally, mucosal erosions.

Signs. Maculopapules flat, red, increasing in 48 hours to 1–2 cm, assuming (because of change in color in the center) a target pattern. Successive formation at various intervals of crops of new lesions. Limbs generally affected.

VESICULOBULLOUS

Symptoms. More common in children and young adults. Same as above, but of greater intensity and with constant mucosal involvement.

Signs. Erythematous plaque with central bulla and ring of vesicles. Vesicles less abundant than in the papular form.

STEVENS-JOHNSON (see)

Etiology. Unknown. Attacks usually precipitated by a pathologic agent: viral, bacterial, or mycotic infections; neoplasia; collagen diseases; pregnancy; drugs or X-ray exposure. In many cases, however, no correlated condition could be found.

Pathology. *Upper dermis.* Edema; vasodilatation; polymorphs and then lymphohistiocyte infiltration, degenerative changes of small blood vessels and collagen. Absence of acantholysis.

Diagnostic Procedures. Identification of preceding or concomitant pathologic event.

Therapy. Papular. Symptomatic. Vesiculobullous. Corticosteroids for symptomatic relief, plus systemic antibiotics to prevent secondary infections.

Prognosis. Attacks usually of self-limited duration (1–4 weeks). Tendency to recur.

BIBLIOGRAPHY. Ashby DW, Lazar T: Erythema multiforme exudativum major (Stevens-Johnson syndrome). Lancet 1:1091–1095, 1951
Champion RH: Disorder of blood vessels. In Champion RH, Burton JL, Ebling FJG (eds): Rook/Wilkinson/Ebling Textbook of Dermatology, 5th ed, pp 1834–1837. Oxford, Blackwell Scientific, 1992

ERYTHEMA NODOSUM

Synonym. Dermatitis contusiformis. See Loefgren.

Symptoms. Occurs at any age (maximum frequency 20–30 years; rare in children and old people); most common in females (6.7:1). Majority of cases observed from January to June. Painful nodules on pretibial surface, anterior thigh, extensor side of forearms, back of arm, and face. Occasionally, feverishness, malaise, and arthralgia.

Signs. Crops of few or several lesions (2–5 cm in diameter) red, hot; as they involute, changes in color: darker red, greenish, yellow (bruise-like), disappearing in a few days to 3 weeks. Cervical lymphadenopathy frequently associated.

Etiology. Unknown; hypersensitivity reaction. Secondary to numerous viral, bacterial, fungal infections and drugs. Streptococcal infections and sarcoidosis most important in the United States.

Pathology. Perivascular polymorphonuclear infiltration of nodules; dilatation of blood vessels; edema.

Diagnostic Procedures. Search for primary disease. *Blood culture. Skin sensitivity tests. Blood.* Mild anemia, albuminuria; increased sedimentation rate may be present. *X-ray.* Association with hilar lymphadenopathy frequent.

Therapy. That of primary condition. Symptomatic (rest; analgesics). Corticosteroid with caution only when symptoms are severe and when underlying disease does not contraindicate.

Prognosis. Self-resolving in 3–6 weeks. Recurrences possible.

BIBLIOGRAPHY. Willan R: On cutaneous diseases. London, Johnson, 1798
Wilson E: A practical and theoretical treatise on the diagnosis, pathology and treatment of diseases of the skin. London, Churchill, 1842
Ryan TJ: Cutaneous vasculitis. In Champion RH, Burton JL, Ebling FJG (eds): Rook/Wilkinson/Ebling Textbook of Dermatology, 5th ed, pp 1931–1935. Oxford, Blackwell Scientific, 1992

ERYTHROCYANOTIC HEADACHE

Synonyms. Headache erythrocyanotic.

Symptoms and Signs. At awaking from deep sleep: severe, generalized, throbbing headache and flushing of face and erythromelalgia or erythrothermalgia of hands.

Etiology. Mastocytosis; carcinoid; serotonin-producing tumors; pancreatic islets tumor; pheochromocytoma.

Pathology. According to etiology.

Diagnostic Procedures. According to etiology.

Therapy. According to etiology.

Prognosis. According to etiology.

BIBLIOGRAPHY. Adams RD, Victor M: Principles of Neurology, 5th ed, pp 163–164. New York, McGraw-Hill, 1993

ERYTHROCYTIC HYPOPLASIA, ACQUIRED, ACUTE

Synonym. Anemia; acute, acquired, erythrocytic; including Transient erythroblastopenia of childhood.

Symptoms and Signs. Onset at birth or within the first 2 years of life. Acute episodes of acute anemia (aplastic crises) usually following prodromal illness.

Etiology. Possible mechanisms include: a metabolic defect in the handling of tryptophan; action of viruses (in particular, human parvovirus B19); immunologic response to viral infection; toxicity of various drugs against precursor of red cells. When in absence of obvious disorder, the syndrome is defined as transient erythroblastopenia of childhood.

Diagnostic Procedures. *Blood.* Progressive anemia; absence of reticulocytes; return of reticulocytes in about 7 days, anemia may persist longer. With pathogenetic mechanism, evidence of emolysis, virus infections, etc.

Therapy. Symptomatic or according to etiology and evolution, none specific.

Prognosis. Usually spontaneous recovery within 7–10 days with return of reticulocytes.

BIBLIOGRAPHY. Kho LK: Erythroblastopenia (pure red cell aplasia) in childhood in Djakarta. Blood 19:168, 1962
Williams: Pancytopenia, aplastic anemia, and pure red cell aplasia. In Lee GR, Bithel TC, Foerster J, et al (eds): Wintrobe's Clinical Hematology, 9th ed, p 334. Philadelphia, Lea & Febiger, 1993

ERYTHROCYTIC HYPOPLASIA, ACQUIRED, CHRONIC

Synonym. Chronic acquired erythrocytic anemia. See Pure red cell aplasia.

Symptoms and Signs. In adults. Predominant in females. Persistent anemic status.

Etiology. Unknown. Two forms or more have been described as first associated with thymoma (see pure cell aplasia-thymoma) and others not associated with thymoma and presenting immunologic abnormalities or association with various malignant conditions.

Diagnostic Procedures. *Blood.* Normocytic or mildly macrocytic anemia, low reticulocytes; usually normal leukocytes and platelets (with few exceptions). *Serum.* Erythropoietin high. *Bone marrow.* Normal but for scarce number of erythroblasts.

Therapy. Supportive or according to etiology and evolution, none specific. In some cases response to splenectomy, prednisone, cytotoxic agents.

Prognosis. Spontaneous remission rare; relapses common. Mortality related to associated conditions. Hemosiderosis from transfusions frequent.

BIBLIOGRAPHY. Tsai SY, Levin WC: Chronic erythrocytic hypoplasia in adults. Am J Med 22:322–331, 1957
Williams: Pancytopenia, aplastic anemia, and pure red cell aplasia. In Lee GR, Bithel TC, Foerster J, et al (eds): Wintrobe's Clinical Hematology, 9th ed, pp 334–335. Philadelphia, Lea & Febiger, 1993

ERYTHROCYTOSIS, BENIGN FAMILIAL

Synonyms. Benign familial erythrocythemic; familial erythrocytosis; polycythemia, benign familial.

Symptoms. No sex predominance; usually discovered in childhood. Asymptomatic or paucisymptomatic. No thrombotic or hemorrhagic manifestations.

Signs. Splenomegaly of moderate degree in 50% of cases. Congenital disorders may be associated.

Etiology. Autosomal dominant inheritance associated with hemoglobinopathy and other varieties of dominant and recessive type. In some cases (recessive type), consequence of erythopoietin or precursor defect of regulation.

Diagnostic Procedures. *Blood.* Variable degree of erythocytosis; higher in recessive form hematocrit (Hmt greater than 0.1) and lower in dominant (Hmt 0.45–0.60). Studies of hemoglobin type, diphosphoglycerate (DPG) defect. Leukocytes and platelets always within normal limit. Low plasma erythropoietin activity.

Therapy. Usually none.

Prognosis. Good; many years survival without clinical manifestations or according to associated syndrome.

BIBLIOGRAPHY. Bernstein J: Three cases of polycythemia rubra. West London Med J 19:207–208, 1914
Davey MG, Lawrence JR, Lander H, et al: Familial erythrocytosis: A report of two cases and a review. Acta Haematol (Basel) 39:65–74, 1968
Ly B, Meberg A, Kannelonning K, et al: Dominant familial erythrocytosis with low plasma erythropoietin activity: Studies of four cases. Scand J Haemat 30 (Suppl) 39:11–17, 1983
Athens JW, Lee GR: Polycythemia: erythrocytosis. In Lee GR, Bithel TC, Foerster J, et al (eds): Wintrobe's Clinical Hematology, 9th ed, p 1257. Philadelphia, Lea & Febiger, 1993

ERYTHROCYTOSIS NEONATAL

Synonyms. Neonatal polycytemia; plethora neonatal; polycythemia neonatalis.

Symptoms and Signs. By third day after birth, cyanosis, little or no cardiorespiratory distress, occasionally, cardiomegaly (50%). Myoclonic jerks may be present. Moderate hepatosplenomegaly occasionally. Systolic murmur (+), second heart sound normal or slightly increased in intensity, splitting, variable or fixed, narrow or wide. All cardiovascular changes are transient.

Etiology. Different conditions may be responsible for the neonatal polycythemia. (1) Polycythemia with hypervolemia. (a) Twin-to-twin transfusion (see); (b) transfusion maternal–fetal in utero (see); (c) placental transfusion (delay in clamping cord); (d) diabetes in mother; (e) congenital cardiopulmonary defects. (2) Polycythemia without hypervolemia. (a) Placental insufficiency; (b) erythrocytosis, benign familial (see); (c) congenital adrenal hyperplasia with polycythemia; (d) chronic fetal hypoxia.

Pathology. Transitory polycythemia.

Diagnostic Procedures. *Blood.* High hematocrit and hemoglobin level; nucleated erythrocytes; fetal hemoglobin level, beta- alpha-globulin determination; differential red-cell agglutination. *Serial electrocardiography.* Transient and not constant abnormalities. *X-ray of chest.*

Therapy. Continuous oxygen treatment (decreases red cell volume and depresses bone marrow activity); digitalis; phlebotomy when respiratory distress requires.

Prognosis. Excellent: spontaneous or therapeutic remission. Cardiovascular abnormalities disappear after decrease of polycythemia. In some cases, brain damage may result with neurologic sequelae.

BIBLIOGRAPHY. Chaptal J, Jean R, Izarn P, et al: La polyglobulie pathologique néonatale: a propos de cinq observations. Pédiatrie 13:515–525, 1958
Tchernia G, Dreyfus M: Hématologie neo-natale. Encycl Méd Chir (Paris) Sang 13050 a 10 (11, 1979)
Rosenkrantz TS, Oh W: Neonatal polycythemia and hyperviscosity. In Milunsky A, Friedman EA, Gluck L, et al: Advances in Perinatal Medicine, vol 5, p 93. New York, Plenum, 1986
Athens JW, Lee GR: Polycythemia: erythrocytosuis. In Lee GR, Bithel TC, Foerster J, et al (eds): Wintrobe's Clinical Hematology, 9th ed. Philadelphia, Lea & Febiger, 1993

ERYTHROCYTOSIS, SPORADIC

Synonym. Primary erythrocytosis. See Erythocytosis, benign familial. Two subgroups are recognized in this condition, which is characterized by an isolated increase of red cell mass, without any abnormality, known to cause secondary erythrocytosis and lack of familial type of transmission; although possible traits cannot always be excluded. Doubtful autonomy even from a clinical point of view.

1. Cases with pure erythrocytosis without associated abnormalities of growth. Normal leukocytes and platelets; occasionally, slight splenomegaly.
2. Cases with pure erythrocytosis and complex abnormalities of growth and endocrine development. This group may be identical with the cases with diencephalic lesion and erythrocytosis.

BIBLIOGRAPHY. Hottinger A: Beitrage zur Kenntnis der Kindlichen Polycythämie. Klin. Unytersuchungen und hämatolg Studien. Z Kinderheilk 44:61–86, 1927
Nathan M: Erythrémies protopathiques et Diencéphale. Presse Med 39:403–404, 1931
Athens JW, Lee GR: Polycythemia: erythrocytosis. In Lee GR, Bithel TC, Foerster J, et al (eds): Wintrobe's Clinical Hematology, 9th ed, p 1258. Philadelphia, Lea & Febiger, 1993

ERYTHROENZYMOPATHIES OF GLYCOLYTIC PATHWAY

These syndromes are described together because of their similarity and rarity. They represent deficiencies of the ten enzymes of glycolytic pathway and present approximately the same symptoms and signs of pyruvate kinase deficiency (see).

HEXOKINASE

Synonym. HK deficiency.

Symptoms and Signs. Rare. Moderate anemia, does not require regular transfusions. No myopathy or neurologic abnormalities.

Etiology. Autosomal recessive. Four tissue-specific isoenzymes of HK are identifiable; type Ib predominates in reticulocytes. Structural gene for HK I is on chromosome 10 (possible regional assignment 10p11.2).

Therapy. Partial benefit from splenectomy.

GLUCOSEPHOSPHATE ISOMERASE

Synonym. GPI deficiency.

Symptoms and Signs. Frequency second to piruvate deficiency. Hemolytic anemia (from mild to severe) rarely associated with myopathy and/or neurologic abnormalities.

Etiology. Autosomal recessive. Extensive heterogeneity with 34 mutant forms, the dimeric enzyme of 134 kDa is encoded on chromosome 19.

PHOSPHOFRUCTOKINASE

Synonym. PFK deficiency. See Tarui.

Symptoms and Signs. Rare. High male predominance. Onset usually in adolescence or early adulthood. Various clinical phenotypes. Hemolysis (usually well compensated) occasionally associated with myopathy (exercise intolerance or cramps, fatigue, more rapid after high carbohydrate meals), early-onset gout.

Etiology. Autosomal recessive. PFK enzyme is under control of three structural loci, encoded on chromosome 1 cen-q32, 21q22.3 and chromosome 10.

Diagnostic Procedures. *Blood.* Hemolysis usually in absence of anemia. Low 2, 3-DPGlevel. *Hyperuricemia.* After exercise marked increase of ammonia, inosine, and hypoxanthine. *Muscle biopsy.* Absent PFK activity. *MRI of muscle carbohydrate metabolism.*

Prognosis. From death in infancy to minimal manifestation in old age. Patient adjusts well to myopathy.

ALDOLASE DEFICIENCY

Synonym. AL deficiency.

Symptoms and Signs. Very rare. Only three cases reported. Hemolysis and (in one case) mental retardation and dysmorphic features.

Etiology. Autosomal recessive. Aldolase A gene localized to chromosome 16q22-q24.

TRIOSEPHOSPHATE ISOMERASE

Synonym. TPI deficiency.

Symptoms and Signs. Rare. Hemolysis accompanied by progressive neurologic deficit from first month of life.

Etiology. Autosomal recessive. TPI is encoded on the short arm of chromosome 12.

Prognosis. Death in childhood.

PHOSPHOGLYCERATE KINASE

Synonym. PGK deficiency.

Symptoms and Signs. Rare. In males severe hemolytic anemia; variable degree of mental retardation, and movement disorders, hemiplegia, or aphasia, rarely myopathy. In females less evident traits limited to hemolysis.

Etiology. X-linked recessive. PGK has two isoenzymes the PGK-1 (ex-

pressed in all somatic cells) is encoded at Xq13, PGK 2 is an autosomal gene expressed only in spermatozoa.

Therapy. Supportive. Transfusions frequently required. Splenectomy partial benefits.

DIPHOSPHOGLYCERATE MUTASE AND PHOSPHATASE

Synonym. DPGM deficiency.

Symptoms and Signs. Very rare. Ruddy cyanosis, no hemolytic anemia.

Etiology. Autosomal recessive. The SPGM gene assigned to region 7q22-q34.

Diagnostic Procedures. *Blood.* Mild erythrocytosis, near absence of 2, 3-DPG.

Therapy. Requires no therapy.

ENOLASE

Symptoms and Signs. Very rare. Hemolytic anemia. No myopathy or neurologic abnormalities.

Etiology. Autosomal recessive. The enolase gene assigned to chromosome 1p36-pter.

LACTATE DEHYDROGENASE

Synonym. LDH deficiency.

Symptoms and Signs. Very rare. No anemia or overt hemolysis in deficiency of H subunit. Myopathy without hemolysis with lack of M subunit. No neurologic abnormalities.

Etiology. Autosomal recessive. LDH tetrameric enzyme composed of two subunits: H and M. Gene locus for LDH-H assigned to chromosome 12 and LDH-M to chromosome 11.

BIBLIOGRAPHY. Tanaka KR, Paglia DE: Pyruvate kinase and other enzyme deficiency disorders of the erythrocyte. In Scriver CR, Beaudet AL, Sly WS, et al: The Metabolic and Molecular Bases of Inherited Disease, 7th ed, pp 3493–3511. New York, McGraw-Hill, 1995

ESCAMILLA-LISSER

Obsolete.

Synonym. Internal myxedema. This case was reported to draw the attention to visceral manifestations in hypothyroidism with minor external classical manifestations. The so-called internal myxedema, according to these authors, presents ascites, atony of bladder, cardiac atony, intestinal atony, anemia, menorrhagia. All those manifestations respond to specific treatment. Evans first reported the occurrence of ascites and visceral atony in hypothyroidism.

BIBLIOGRAPHY. Evans W: Case of myxedema with ascites and atony of bladder. Endocrinology 26:409–416, 1932
Escamilla RF, Lisser H, Shepardson HC: Internal myxedema: Report of a case showing ascites, cardiac, intestinal and bladder atony, menorrhagia secondary anemia and associated carotinemia. Ann Intern Med 9:297–316, 1935

ESCHELER

Symptoms and Signs. Lateral deviation of moderate amplitude of movements. Difference in muscle tone and bone asymmetry.

Etiology. Congenital asymmetry of tonus and function of propulsive muscles.

BIBLIOGRAPHY. Moortgat P: Syndromes a noms propres. Paris, Prelat, 1966

ESOPHAGEAL, ACHALASIA

Synonyms. Achalasia; cardiospasm; esophageal dystonia; esophageal dyssynergia; functional hiatal stenosis; megaesophagus; krichopharyngeal achalasia, lower esophageal sphincter failure, including Montandon syndrome.

Symptoms. Mostly in whites. Onset at any age; maximal incidence between fourth and sixth decades; equal incidence in both sexes. Onset of acute symptomatology usually abrupt, preceded, however, by minor swallowing abnormalities for years. Feeling of obstruction at the level of xiphoid cartilage. Pain or distress when ingesting food. Intermittent episodes at the beginning; controllable by eating slowly or drinking frequently during meal. Later, symptomatology at any meal plus, occasionally, sensation of fullness behind the sternum. Severe pain substernal may be observed after meal (in Pathology, see type 2). Regurgitation brings relief of symptoms. Regurgitation without nausea of sour or fetid odor, rich in mucous (advanced condition). Weight loss.

Signs. Scanty; determination of swallowing time with stethoscope applied to the xiphoid. In some cases, dilation of veins of neck and face, and cyanosis after meal (relieved by regurgitation); pallor.

Etiology. Not defined. Consequence of neuropathy of myoenteric plexus of esophagus and vagus nerve. Particularly defect of cholinergic innervation; infectious agent? Neurotropic virus? Psychogenic component? Implicated eosinophilic cationic protein (neurotoxic protein of eosinophils). Hereditary and congenital cases reported. Polymyositis may cause a secondary form of achalasia (Montandon syndrome).

Pathology. Dilatation of esophagus; esophagitis. Type 1. Enormous dilatation and thin-walled atrophic vestibule. Type 2. Moderate dilatation; hypertrophic wall vestibule, marked muscular hypertrophy. Esophageal body: decrease of ganglion cells (Lewy bodies) reduction of nerve fibers.

Diagnostic Procedures. *Endoscopy.* Achalasia with dilatation (30%); hiatal hernia (15%); esophagitis (12%); spasm of distal esophagus (10%); normal (24%). *X-ray of esophagus.* Cardiospasm; usually marked or moderate dilatation; diffuse spasm; occasionally, diaphragmatic hernia; strictures; abnormal motor pattern. Marked dilatation evident in latter stages. Hypersensitive response to methacholine during fluoroscopy and manometric studies. Poor or absent relaxation after swallowing; premature contraction of the sphincter; amplitude of contractions greater than 50 cm of water pressure; methacholine test usually positive. Radionuclide studies.

Therapy. Pharmacological: isosorbide dinitrate before meals; calcium channel blockers. Dilatation usually pneumatic. Surgery indicated in about 20% of patients. Modification of Heller myotomy. Correction of malnutrition before surgery.

Prognosis. Good response to treatment (in 95% of cases). Dilation may be repeated several times with good results. Increased incidence of carcinoma.

BIBLIOGRAPHY. Willis T: Pharmaceutice rationalis sive diatribe de medicamentorum operationibus in human corpore. London, Hagae-Comitis A Leers, 1674
Von Mikulicz R: Zur Pathologie und Therapie dem Cardiospasmus. Dtsch Med Wochenschr 30:17–19, 1904
Hurst AF: Some disorders of the esophagus. JAMA 102:582–586, 1943
Montandon A: Pseudo-spasme permanent du bouche de l'aesophage et myoporphiria. Pract oto-rhino-laryng 10:267–281, 1948
Sanderson DR, Ellis FH Jr, Schlegel JF, et al: Syndrome of vigorous achalasia: Clinical and physiologic observations. Dis Chest 52:508–517, 1967
Humeau B, Cloarec D, Simon JP: Doleurs pseudoangineuses d'origine oesophagienne. Resultats de l'esploration fonctionelle et interet du test de distension mecanique par ballonet. Gastroenterol Clin Biol 14:334–1990
Wong RKH, Maydonovitch CL: Achalasia. In Castell DO (ed): The Esophagus, pp 233–260. New York, Little, Brown 1992
Ouyang A, Cohen S: Motility disorders of the esophagus. In Haubrich WS, Schaffner F, Berk JE (eds): Bockus Gastroenterology, 5th ed, pp 423–426. Philadelphia, WB Saunders, 1995

ESOPHAGUS, APOPLEXY

See also Boerhaave and Mallory-Weiss.

Symptoms. Prevalent in later life in females. Severe retrosternal pain that spreads to the lower chest posteriorly.

Signs. Pallor; general distress; shock.

Etiology. Mucosal tear of the lower esophagus; modest blood loss into the lumen. Dissection by blood in the plane of submucosa of the lower esophagus, while the surrounding muscle remains intact. The disorder often is associated with dysfunction of the cardias.

Pathology. See Etiology.

Diagnostic Procedures. *Blood.* Anemia; white blood cells increased. *X-ray.* Of chest with gastrography shows filling defect of the esophagus with the appearance of intramural lesion. *Esophagoscopy.*

Therapy. Nasogastric aspiration; parenteral nutrition; conservative treatment.

Prognosis. Guarded.

BIBLIOGRAPHY. Clark DH, Tankel HT: Pressure rupture and spontaneous perforation of the esophagus. Gut 5:86–89, 1964
Thompson NW, Ernst CB, Fry WJ: The spectrum of emetogenic injury to the esophagus and stomach. Am J Surg 113:13–26, 1967
Smith G, Brunnen PL, Gillanders LA, et al: Oesophageal apoplexy. Lancet 1:390–392, 1974
Ouyang A, Cohen S: Motility disorders of the esophagus. In Haubrich WS, Schaffner F, Berk JE (eds): Bockus Gastroenterology, 5th ed, vol 2, pp 418–436. Philadelphia, WB Saunders, 1995

ESOPHAGUS SPASM, DIFFUSE

Synonyms. Nutcracker esophagus.

Symptoms. Chest pain related to swallowing or not, that mimics angina: oppressive radiation to the neck, jaw, arms, or back. Pain may arise at night. Dysphagia (70%) for solids and liquids. Weight loss from sitophobia (fear of eating).

Etiology. Not defined. Probably neural dysfunction (see esophageal achalasia) or denervation supersensitivity that induces thickening of smooth muscles.

Diagnostic Procedures. *Contrast radiography* (Nutcracker esophagus is a radiologic finding that has given a catchy name to this condition) and endoscopy to exclude neoplastic pathology. *Manometry.* Abnormal contraction in 30% of swallows and hypersensitivity reaction to edrophonium chloride

Therapy. Nifedipine, isosorbide dinitrate, or calcium channel blockers; anticholinergic drugs. Sometimes surgery: large myotomy.

BIBLIOGRAPHY. Sanderson DR, Ellis FH, Schlager JF, et al: Syndrome of vigorous achalasia: Clinical and physiological observations. Dis Chest 52:508–517, 1967
Richter JE, Castell DO: Diffuse esophageal spasm: A reappraisal. Ann Intern Med 100:242–245, 1984
Vantrappen G, Janssen J, Ghillerbert G: The irritable esophagus: A frequent cause of angina-like pain. Lancet I:1232–1234, 1987
Ouyang A, Cohen S: Motility disorders of the esophagus. In Haubrich WS, Schaffner F, Berk JE (eds): Bockus Gastroenterology, 5th ed, pp 423–426. Philadelphia, WB Saunders, 1995

ESPILDORA-LUQUE

Synonyms. Amaurosis-hemiplegia; ophthalmic sylvian. See perisylvian.

Symptoms and Signs. Unilateral blindness; temporary contralateral hemiplegia.

Etiology. Embolus in ophthalmic artery and reflex spasm of middle cerebral artery.

Pathology. See Etiology.

Therapy. None.

Prognosis. Hemiparesis is temporary.

BIBLIOGRAPHY. Espildora-Luque C: Sindrome oftálmico-silviano. Arch Ophthal Hispano-Am 34:616–621, 1934
Geeraets WS: Ocular Syndromes, 3rd ed. Philadelphia, Lea & Febiger, 1976
Adams RD, Victor M: Principles of Neurology, 5th ed, p 227. New York, McGraw-Hill, 1993

ESTREN-DAMESHEK

Synonym. Fanconi I without congenital defect. Constitutional aplastic anemia type II. See Blackfan-Diamond.

Symptoms. Early childhood appearance; weakness; epistaxis; easy bruising; poor development.

Signs. Pallor; ecchymosis; petecchiae. Liver, spleen, and lymph node not palpable.

Etiology. Autosomal recessive inheritance. Familial bone marrow hypoplasia without other congenital defects. See Fanconi I.

Pathology. In bone marrow, quantitative hypoplasia with normal qualitative development of cells. A certain degree of functional hypersplenism postulated.

Diagnostic Procedures. *Blood.* Anemia; leukopenia; thrombocytopenia; high reticulocyte count.

Therapy. Periodic blood transfusions. Testosterone; corticoids. Some cases benefit symptomatically from splenectomy. Bone marrow transplantation attempted with partial results.

Prognosis. Discontinuation of blood transfusions results in death. Possible conversion into leukemia.

BIBLIOGRAPHY. Estren S, Dameshek W: Familial hypoplastic anemia of childhood. Am J Dis Child 73:671–687, 1947
Nowell P, Bergman G, Besa E, et al: Progressive preleukemia with chromosomally abnormal clone in a kindred with Estren-Dameshek variant of Fanconi's anemia. Blood 64:1135–1138, 1984
Deiss A: Non-neoplastic diseases, chemical agents, and hematologic disorders that may precede hematologic neoplasms. In Lee GR, Bithel TC, Foerster J, et al (eds): Wintrobe's Clinical Hematology, 9th ed, p 1947. Philadelphia, Lea & Febiger, 1993

ETHANOLAMINOSIS

Symptoms and Signs. From birth. Cardiomegaly, generalized muscular hypotonia, cerebral dysfunction, failure to thrive.

Etiology. Deficiency of ethanolaminokinase.

Pathology. Deposition of ethanolamine (PAS +) in all tissues.

Diagnostic Procedures. *Urine.* High ethanolamine activity. *X-rays.* Cardiomegaly, hydrocephalus, esophageal ectasia.

Prognosis. Death in childhood.

BIBLIOGRAPHY. Victor KW, Harsteien B, Harms D, Busse H, et al: Ethano-
laminosis: A newly recognized, generalized storage disease with cardiomegaly, cerebral dysfunction and early death. Eur J Pediatr 126:61–75, 1977

ETHMOCEPHALUS

Synonyms. See Arhinencephalia.

Symptoms and Signs. Extreme hypotelorism; absent nose with proboscis; no palate or cleft lips.

Etiology. See Arhinencephalia.

BIBLIOGRAPHY. Aita JA: Congenital Facial Anomalies with Neurologic Defects. Springfield, IL, Charles C Thomas, 1969

ETHMOIDAL NERVE ANTERIOR

Synonyms. Ethmoidal nerve anterior.

Symptoms. Bilateral intense continuous pain over frontal, parietal, occipital, and vertical areas; recurrent aching and stiffness of neck, lasting one or more days.

Signs. Hypersensitive areas around the anterior ethmoidal foramen and over the path of nasal nerves.

Etiology and Pathology. Hypersensitivity reaction owing to surface or intratissue (or both) pressure at the anterior ethmoidal foramen and the foramen of the middle turbinate body causing interference with normal conduction of the action current.

Diagnostic Procedures. Touching the area around the anterior ethmoidal foramen lightly with an applicator causes sharp intense pain. Epinephrine solution 3% applied to the area reduces the symptoms effectively, but temporarily.

Therapy. Epinephrine application; in severe cases resection of the anterior ethmoidal nerves.

Prognosis. Recovery with surgery; improvement with medical treatment.

BIBLIOGRAPHY. Burnham HH: Anterior ethmoidal nerve syndrome: Referred pain and headache from lateral nasal wall. Arch Otolaryngol 50:640–646, 1949

EVANS

The association of idiopathic hemolytic anemia with thrombocytopenia with or without purpuric manifestation, occurring concomitantly or in succession, in absence of any etiologic factors and with demonstrable auto-immune process affecting both red cells and platelets.

BIBLIOGRAPHY. Evans R, Takahashi K, Duane RT et al: Primary thrombocytopenic purpura and acquired hemolytic anemia. Arch Intern Med 87:48–65, 1951
Silverstein MN, Aaro LA, Kempers RD: Evans' syndrome and pregnancy. Am J Med Sci 252:106–111, 1966
Hay EM, Makris M, Winfield J, et al: Evans' syndrome associated with dermatomyositis. Ann Rheum Dis 49:793–794, 1990

EWING

Synonyms. Diffuse bone endothelioma; endothelial myeloma; Ewing sarcoma.

Symptoms. Onset before 30 years of age (80%); prevalent in males. Intermittent pain in any bone, most frequently shafts of long bone and pelvis, increasing with progress of disease. Slight fever.

Signs. Palpation may reveal swelling and increased temperature of overlying skin. Marked pain on pressure.

Etiology. Unknown. Neoplastic proliferation of endothelial cells probably derived by reticular cells of bone marrow.

Pathology. Bone porous, with localized reabsorptions. Tumor found under displaced periostium and within the bone, soft and friable; gray-white areas of necrosis and hemorrhage. New bone formation as a reaction (not by the tumor). Microscopically; small round cells in sheets growing between compartment of well-vascularized connective tissue. Nuclei prominent; little cytoplasm. Mitotic figures.

Diagnostic Procedures. *X-ray.* Periosteal irregularity; areas of different densities of bone marrow; tumor extension parallel to long axis of bone. *Isotope bone scan. Biopsy of bone marrow. Blood.* Leukocytosis; high sedimentation rate. *Electron microscopy.* Helpful in differential diagnosis.

Therapy. X-ray, supervoltage radiation; chemotherapy (cyclophosphamide; methotrexate). Avoid useless surgery.

Prognosis. Five-year survival (10–24%).

BIBLIOGRAPHY. Ewing J: Review and classification of bone sarcomas. Arch Surg 4:485–533, 1922
Burssens AD, Dequeker J: Regional bone diseases. In Klippel JH, Dieppe PA: Rheumatology, pp 7.43.9, 7.43.10. St Louis, CV Mosby, 1994

EXPLODING HEAD

Symptoms and Signs. In both sexes. It occurs with intercourse of several months. Patient in the twilight stage of sleep notices with alarm a sudden, short, very loud noise.

Etiology. Unknown.

Diagnostic Procedures. *EEG. CT scan. MRI. Evoked potential.*

Therapy. None.

Prognosis. Benign condition.

BIBLIOGRAPHY. Pearce JMS: Headache: J Neurol, Neurosurg Psychiatr 57:134–144, 1994

EYELID, CONGENITAL

Synonym. Epicanthus inversus—blepharophimosis—ptosis.

Signs. Bilateral ptosis; epicanthus inversus with telecanthus; palpebral phimosis; or blepharophimosis; deficiency of upper and lower eyelid tissue; elevation of eyebrows; absent supraorbital rims; poorly developed nasal bridge.

Etiology. Unknown. Definite hereditary influence of autosomal dominant type demonstrated in many cases.

Therapy. Canthoplasty and correction of ptosis, implantation of inert materials for reconstruction of supraorbital region and nasoglabellar angle.

Prognosis. Good. Cosmetic and functional results obtained by adequate surgical treatment.

BIBLIOGRAPHY. Blair VP, Brown JB, Hamn WG: Correction of ptosis and epicanthus. Arch Ophthalmol 7:831–846, 1932
Lewis SR, Arons MS, Lynch JB, Blocker TG: The congenital eyelid syndrome. Plast Reconst Surg 39:271–277, 1967
Torczynski E: Developmental anomalies of the eye. In Garner A, Klintworth GK (eds): Pathobiology of Ocular Disease: A Dynamic Approach, 2nd ed, pp 1331–1332. New York, Marcel Dekker, 1994

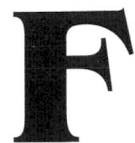

FABER

Synonyms. Hayem-Faber; Knud Faber; Witt; Kaznelson II; achylic chloroanemia; hypochromic chronic anemia; anemia idiopathic hypochromic.

Symptoms. Occurs in women at 30–60 years of age; seldom (4%) in men; frequently in low income class. In convalescence after pregnancy. Menstrual disorders; tiredness; weakness; exertional dyspnea.

Signs. Pallor. In some patients, same constitutional features of pernicious anemia. Light colored eyes; moderate hypertelorism; premature gray hair; nail brittleness.

Etiology. Menstrual disorders; uterine fibroids; hemorrhoids; peptic ulcer; hernia at esophageal hiatus; recurrent epistaxes; hereditary telangiectasia; other causes of chronic blood loss. With present knowledge this syndrome has become obsolete except as a term for the association of hypochromic anemia and achlorhydria and not as a separate entity.

Pathology. According to etiology. In chronic form of anemia, fatty degeneration of myocardium ("tigroid pattern"), cardiac hypertrophy, and dilatation.

Diagnostic Procedures. *Blood.* Hemoglobin determination; red cell indices; serum iron low; iron binding capacity high. *Gastric secretion analysis. Stool.* Occult blood.

Therapy. Iron administration orally, intramuscularly, or intravenously.

Prognosis. Good with treatment and according to etiology.

BIBLIOGRAPHY. Varandaeus: De Morto et Affectione Mulierum Montpellier, 1620
Faber K: Achylia gastrica mit Anaemie. Med Klin 5:1310–1312, 1909
Faber K: Om anaemiske Tilstande ved Achylia gastrica. Berl Klin 50:958–962, 1913
Lange J: Medicinalium Epistolarum Miscellanea Varia et rara. 1554 translation into English by Ruhrach. Am J Dis Child 48:393, 1932
Lee GR: Iron deficiency and iron deficiecy anemia. In Lee GR, Bithel TC, Foerster J, et al (eds): Wintrobe's Clinical Hematology, 9th ed, pp 808–818. Philadelphia, Lea & Febiger, 1993

FABRY

Synonyms. Anderson-Fabry; Ruiter-Pompen; Sweeley-Klionsky; galactosidase A deficiency; GLA; ceramide trihexosidase deficiency; ACD; angiokeratoma corporis diffusum; glycolipid lipidosis; hemorrhagic nodular-glycolipid lipidosis; dystopic lipidosis, hereditary.

Symptoms. Prevalent in males, who present full-blown syndrome; females may present a partial form and female carriers are asymptomatic. Symptoms start in childhood or at puberty. *Family history.* Paresthesia of distal part of extremities with burning pain. Fever precipitated occasionally by variation in temperature or exertion. Frequently, concomitant with the attacks are nausea, vomiting, abdominal pain, dizziness, headache, and generalized weakness.

Signs. Increasing with progression of the disease. Typical cutaneous lesions: telangiectasis of various sizes clustering in areas such as periumbilical, genitals, buttocks, and thighs; bright red or bluish, nonpulsating, partially bleached by pressure. Lack of development of beard and body hair. Edema. Eyes show dilated venules in conjunctiva and retina. Frequent, early corneal and lens opacity. Later, hypertension and signs of cardiovascular disease; lymphedema and renal failure.

Etiology. Sex-linked, incompletely recessive inheritance. Gene encoding. Galactosidase A has been localized to the X-chromosomal region Xq22. Derangement of glycosphingolipid catabolism caused by deficient activity of lysosomal hydrolase-galactosidase A, responsible for an accumulation of globotrial osylceramide and galacto in all tissues.

Pathology. Skin shows telangiectasis or dilated intraepidermal spaces filled with blood; vessel wall in nontelangiectatic zones shows infiltration with glycolipids (ceramide trihexoside) deposited in the endothelial cells and smooth muscles. Identical deposits are observed in the heart, muscles, renal tubules and glomeruli, central nervous system, spleen, liver, bone marrow, lymph nodes, and cornea.

Diagnostic Procedures. *Urine.* Albuminuria (early finding); in sediment increased levels of globotrialosylceramide; vacuolated cells containing glycolipids. Later, casts, hematuria, isosthenuria. *Blood.* Low ceramide-trihexosidase; infusing normal plasma; decline of galactosylglucosylceramide. Later, anemia; hyperazotemia. *Bone marrow.* Typical cells. *Ophthalmologic examination.* Slit-lamp shows characteristic findings.

Therapy. Symptomatic; dexamethasone may help relieve acute symptoms. Low doses of diphenylhydantoin or carbamazepin to relieve discomfort. Plasma exchange. Kidney transplantation.

Prognosis. Recurrent progressive attacks, eventually leading to renal failure and hypertension and cardiovascular disease. Death between 40 and 50 years of age. Females with milder form do not show decreased survival time.

BIBLIOGRAPHY. Fabry J: Ein Beitrag zur Kenntniss der Purpura haemorrhagica nodularis (Purpura papulosa haemorrhagica Hebrae). Arch Dermatol Syph 43:187–200, 1898
Anderson W: A case of angiokeratoma. Br J Dermatol 10:113–117, 1898
Hasholt L, Sorensen SA, Wandal A, et al: Fabry's disease herozygote with a new mutation: Biochemical, ultrastructural and clinical investigations. J Med Genet 27:303–307, 1990
von Scheidt W, Eng CM, Fitzmaurice TF, et al: An atypical variant of Fabry's disease with manifestations confined to the myocardium. New Engl J Med 324:395–399, 1991
Desnick RJ, Ioannou YA, Eng CM: Galactoside A deficiency: Fabry disease. In Scriver CR, Beaudet AL, Sly WS, et al: The Metabolic and Molecular Bases of Inherited Disease, 7th ed, pp 2741–2784. New York, McGraw-Hill, 1995

F.A.C.E.

Synonyms. Facial Afro-Caribbean childhood eruption.

Symptoms and Signs. In Negroid children. Sudden appearance of hypopigmented or monomorphic flesh-colored papules around mouth, eyelids, and ears.

Etiology. Unknown.

Prognosis. The eruption persists for a few months, then spontaneously disappears without residual scarring.

BIBLIOGRAPHY. Marten RH, Presbury DGC, Adamson JE, et al: An unusual papular and acneiform facial eruption in the Negro child. Br J Dermatol 91:435–438, 1976

Williams HC, Ashworth J, Pembroke AC, et al: FACE: Facial Afro-Caribbean childhood eruption. Clin Exper Dermatol 15:163–166, 1990

FACETS

Synonyms. Articular facets; vertebrae; osteoarthritis; spinal osteophytosis.

Symptoms. Vertebral column or radiated pains, usually sciatic; static in type (relieved by certain postures and aggravated by other postures).

Signs. Sciatic scoliosis, homolateral, contralateral, or alternating; muscle spasm. Cardiac enlargement. Flushing of extremities in warm weather.

Etiology. Unknown.

Pathology. Osteoarthritic process with main involvement of vertebral articular facets. Cartilage degeneration, and subluxation of one or both articular processes; muscle spasm; nerve root compression.

Diagnostic Procedures. *X-ray of spine* in different projections. Local injection of the joint as a diagnostic as well as therapeutic procedure.

Therapy. Conservative measures; physical therapy or in rare cases surgical treatment. Lumbosacral ankylosis by bone graft or fusion or removal of the facets.

Prognosis. Recurrent progressive symptomatology responds fairly well to medical treatment or surgical intervention.

BIBLIOGRAPHY. Gormley RK: Low back pain with special reference to the articular facets with presentation of an operative procedure. Coll Papers Mayo Clin 25:813–823, 1933

Maurice-Williams RS: Disorders of spinal nerve roots. In Weatherall DJ, Ledingham JGG, Warrell DA (eds): Oxford Textbook of Medicine, 3rd ed, p 3908. Oxford, Oxford Med Pub, 1996

FACIAL NEURALGIA, ATYPICAL

Synonyms. Atypical facial neuralgia.

Symptoms. Prevalent in young or middle-aged women. Long history of attacks of pain in the face, neck, or head persisting or remitting; not confined to territorial distribution of cranial nerves.

Etiology. Conversion hysteria; hypochondrias; vascular pathology.

Diagnostic Procedures. *X-rays of teeth, sinuses, cervical column.*

Therapy. Antidepressant and antianxiety medication. Only a few cases responded to ergotamine tartrate. Analgesic (addiction frequent); psychotherapy. Refrain from alcohol injection or neurosurgery.

Prognosis. Difficult to cure.

BIBLIOGRAPHY. Harris W: Neuritis and Neuralgia. London, Oxford, 1926

Harris W: An analysis of 1, 433 cases of paroxysmal trigeminal neuralgia (trigeminal-tic) and end-results of gasserian alcohol injection. Brain 63:209–224, 1940

Olen J (Chairman): Classification and diagnostic criteria for headache disorders, cranial neuralgia and facial pain. Cephalalgia 8(Supp7):1988

Adams RD, Victor M: Principles of Neurology, 5th ed, p 168. New York, McGraw-Hill, 1993

FACTITIOUS PURPURA

Synonyms. Devil pinches; bruising simple easy; purpura psychogenic.

Symptoms and Signs. Recurrent painful bruises.

Etiology. Self-inflicted (consciously or unconsciously) bruises.

Pathology. On biopsy; hematoma without evidence of vasculitis.

Diagnostic Procedures. Protection of a designated part with plaster cast (bruises do not appear in protected part). For differential diagnosis see purpura of psychogenic origin and autosensitization purpura.

Therapy. Psychotherapy.

Prognosis. Difficult treatment; occasionally, conversion to other hysterical manifestations.

BIBLIOGRAPHY. Davidson E: Factitious purpura presenting as autoerythrocyte sensitization. Br Med J 1:104, 1964

Bithell TC: Bleeding disorders caused by vascular abnormalities. In Lee GR, Bithel TC, Foerster J, et al (eds): Wintrobe's Clinical Hematology, 9th ed, p 1386. Philadelphia, Lea & Febiger, 1993

FAHR

Synonyms. Cerebral symmetric calcification; striopallidodentate calcinosis; SPD calcinosis; ferrocalcinosis cerebrovascular.

Symptoms. Asymptomatic in many cases. Extrapyramidal disorder of different degree from simple generalized rigidity, athetosis, dystonia to full Parkinson. The extrapyramidal disorder may be progressive and reach full expression in middle life, or occasionally is present from infancy accompanied or not accompanied by mental retardation.

Signs. Small and round head. Optic atrophy.

Etiology. Possibly caused by altered vascular permeability. Associated occasionally with hypoparathyroidism or pseudohypoparathyroidism. Sporadic cases (group 2) from unknown prenatal insult. Familial occurrence reported; autosomal recessive (group 1 with the classic manifestations) and group 3, that appears characterized by progressive encephalopathy with chronic spinal lymphocytosis (see Aicardi-Goutieres); and finally cases with autosomal dominant inheritance (group 4 with mild neurologic symptoms only in the oldest members of the family).

Pathology. Deposit of calcific material in basal ganglia. Usually, initial absence or loss of nerve cell fibers and ground substance. "Mulberry bodies" associated with capillary walls. When there is calcification of capillary walls, extensive rarefaction of cerebral tissue occurs.

Diagnostic Procedures. *X-rays of skull. CT brain scan. MRI.* Demonstration of basal ganglia calcification.

Therapy. Symptomatic; orthopedic procedures if necessary.

Prognosis. Usually, slowly progressive condition in infantile form; poor for mental retardation and spastic features.

BIBLIOGRAPHY. Virchow R: Kalk-Metastasen. Virchows Arch Pathol Anat 8:103–113, 1855

Fahr T: Idiopathische Verkalkung der Hirngefasse. Z Allg Pathol Anat 50:129–133, 1930

Billard C, Dulac O, Boulouche J, et al: Encephalopathy with calcifications of the basal ganglia in children: A reappraisal of Fahr's syndrome with respect to 14 new cases. Neuropediatrics 20:12–19, 1989

Adams RD, Victor M: Principles of Neurology, 5th ed, pp 838–839. New York, McGraw-Hill, 1993

FAHR-VOLHARD

Synonyms. Arteriolar hyperplastic nephrosclerosis; nephrosclerosis, malignant.

Symptoms. Both sexes affected; onset in males 44 years of age, in females 36 years of age. Abrupt onset of intermittent or constant headache; weight loss; followed by dyspnea; impairment of vision (sometimes preceding other symptoms); abdominal pain.

Signs. *Blood.* Hypertension (diastolic greater than 130 mmHg); cardiomegaly; edema; occasionally associated, papilledema, retinopathy (cotton wool exudates and hemorrhages), neurologic abnormalities.

Etiology. Unknown. Associated with malignant hypertension following benign nephrosclerosis or other kidney diseases. Considered as pathogenetic mechanisms: immunologic; derangement in renin, angiotensin, and aldosterone production; disseminated intravascular coagulation.

Pathology. Fibrinoid necrosis of kidney arterioles; endothelial proliferation of afferent arterioles and interlobular arteries.

Diagnostic Procedures. *Urine.* Proteinuria; frequently hematuria (25%); presence of red cell casts. *Blood.* Increased red cell sedimentation rate; in second phase, increased blood urea nitrogen (BUN) and creatinine. *Spinal fluid.* Increased pressure (86%) and protein concentration.

Therapy. Antihypertensive agents; management of renal failure, including dialysis. Kidney transplantation.

Prognosis. Without treatment, death in 15 months. With treatment, mortality at this time reduced to 10–20%; life can be prolonged 5–7 years.

BIBLIOGRAPHY. Fahr G: Hypertension heart, most common form of so-called chronic myocarditis. JAMA 80:981–984, 1924

Fahr G: Hypertension heart. Am J Med Sci 175:453–472, 1928

Campese VM: Clinical aspects and management of essential hypertension. In Massry SG, Glassock RJ: Textbook of Nephrology, 3rd ed, pp 1216–1217. Baltimore, Williams & Wilkins, 1995

FAILED-BACK

Symptoms and Signs. In approximately 25% of patients after disc removal: back and leg pain.

Etiology and Pathology. Possible far lateral disc herniation overlooked or further excretion of more disc material at original site; foramina stenosis; unilateral facet hypertrophy; arachnoiditis or epidural scarring.

Diagnostic Procedures. *CT scan. MR imaging.*

Therapy and Prognosis. Ten percent require surgery (not always successful). Nonsteroidal anti-inflammatory agents, antidepressant, and physiotherapy may be of benefit.

BIBLIOGRAPHY. Long DM: Failed-back syndrome. In Johnson RT (ed): Current Therapy in Neurologic Disease, vol 2, pp 51–53. Toronto, Decker, 1987

Maurice-Williams RS: Disorders of spinal nerve roots. In Weatherall DJ, Ledingham JGG, Warrell DA (eds): Oxford Textbook of Medicine, 3rd ed, p 3908. Oxford, Oxford Med Pub, 1996

FAIRBANK

Synonyms. Epiphyseal dysplasia multiplex tarda; MEDT type Ia; megalia ossium cutis; multiple epiphyseal dysplasia (type Ia); dysplasia epiphysealis hemimelica. See Camurati-Engelmann, Conradi, and Blount-Barber.

Symptoms. Evident at 5–10 years of age. Sometimes pain and difficulty in walking (coxa vara; genu valgum). Patients remain below average height (152 cm). Absence of disability.

Signs. Lesions bilateral and almost symmetric; after puberty some alterations of epiphyseal shape or joint angulation. Hands typically are short and stubby, with narrow, thick nails.

Etiology. Unknown; dominant genetic autosomal inheritance. Rare, autosomal recessive inheritance. Enterogeneity exists within this denomination of epiphyseal dysplasia multiple.

Pathology. Chondrodystrophy affecting only cartilaginous epiphyses.

Cartilage hyaline softer, more mucinous than normal. Multiple centers of ossification may develop at different times in same epiphysis.

Diagnostic Procedures. *X-ray of skeleton.* Multiple ossification centers in epiphyses; epiphyseal union delayed. After puberty, epiphyseal changes. Bone of good structure and well ossified. Occasionally, double patella (seen on lateral views).

Therapy. Physical therapy to provide relief and prevent disability. Surgery to correct deformities delayed.

Prognosis. After puberty, no progression. Possibly, residual deformities may be cured by osteotomy. The patient will be short.

BIBLIOGRAPHY. Barrington-Ward LE: Double coxa vara with other deformities occurring in brother and sister. Lancet 1:157–159, 1913

Fairbank HAT: Generalized disease of skeleton. Proc R Soc Med 28:1611, 1935

Fairbank T: An Atlas of General Affections of the Skeleton. Baltimore, Williams & Wilkins, 1951

Versteylen RJ, et al: Multiple epiphyseal dysplasia complicated by severe osteochondritis dessicans of the knee. Skeletal Radiol 17:407–412, 1988

Klippel JH, Dieppe PA: Rheumatology, pp 7.45.1–7.45.3. St Louis, CV Mosby, 1995

FALCIFORM FOLD, CONGENITAL

Synonym. Persistent hyperplastic primary vitreous; PHPV; posterior hyperplastic primary vitreous.

Symptoms and Signs. Rare, from birth, small eyes. Leukokoria, often bilateral glioma. The anterior chamber is shallow, persistence of posterior part of tunica vasculosa lentis; elongated ciliary processes run centrally to back of lens, break in the posterior capsule, lens coloboma or cataract that may or not develop.

Etiology. Sometimes inherited as autosomic recessive condition. Disembriogenesis. Associated with maternal use of cocaine, deficiency of protein C (inhibitor of the coagulation cascade vitamin K-dependent).

Pathology. Retrolental tissue (undifferenciated neural and fibrous) contains fat, hyaline material, cartilage, and calcifications.

Diagnostic Procedures. *Fundus.* Elongated folding or tenting of retinal tissue from head of optic nerve to retinal periphery or ciliary region.

Prognosis. Progressive disease; eventually massive retinal detachment and phthisis bulbi.

BIBLIOGRAPHY. Pruett R and Schepens C: Posterior hyperplastic primary vitreous. Am J Ophthalmol 69:534–543, 1970

Torczynski E: Developmental anomalies of the eye. In Garner A, Klintworth GK (eds): Pathobiology of Ocular Disease: A Dynamic Approach, 2nd ed, p 1315. New York, Marcel Dekker, 1994

FALLOT

Synonyms. Pulmonic stenosis—ventricular septal defect; Fallot tetralogy.

Symptoms. Both sexes affected; slight male prevalence. Detected weeks or months after birth. Difficulty in feeding; failure to gain weight; poor development. Dyspnea or fatigability on exertion. Orthostatic dyspnea. After a few months of life, paroxysmal attacks of hyperpnea, "hypoxic spell" with increasing cyanosis (alarming manifestation), which disappear before 6 years of age. Characteristic "squatting" when tired or dyspnoic to relieve the symptoms.

Signs. Cyanosis from infancy; at first only when crying or exerting, then persistent. Clubbing of fingers and toes. Heart systolic murmur to the left of sternum (second–third space); systolic thrill. Second sound single for absence of the pulmonic elements. No diastolic murmur. Premedial systolic pulsation may be observed in the second–third interspace.

Etiology. Congenital heart multiple defect. Ventricular septal defect; pulmonic stenosis; dextroposition of aorta and right ventricular hypertrophy. The condition most commonly associated with tetralogy of Fallot is right aortic arch (about 30%).

Diagnostic Procedures. *X-ray.* Heart apex elevated; left lower margin prominent; diminution of pulmonary vessels; lack of pulsation of hilar pulmonary vessels. *Electrocardiography.* Right axis deviation; RS-T depression and inverted T in leads II and III. *Cardiac catheterization.* Right ventricular increased pressure; decrease of pulmonary artery pressure, and oxygen concentration alterations in the various cavities. *Circulation time.* Arm-to-tongue time and right ventricle-to-ear time remarkably shortened. *Blood.* Polycythemia. *Two-dimensional echocardiography* with color flow imaging and spectral Doppler interrogation.

Therapy. Palliative operation: Blalock-Taussig operation and aortic-pulmonary shunt. Open intracardiac repair: valvotomy or infundibular resection. Intracardiac surgical correction in extracorporal circulation. For the severely cyanotic newborn, prostaglandin administration may be of benefit, to open the ductus until surgery can be performed.

Prognosis. Without treatment majority of patients die before 20 years of age from complications. Some patients reach adult life with few symptoms.

BIBLIOGRAPHY. Nicholas Steno (17th century) quoted by Marquis RM: Longevity and the early history of tetralogy of Fallot. Br Med J 1:819, 1956
Fallot A: Contribution à l'anatomie pathologique de la maladie bleue (cyanose cardiaque). Marseille Med 25:77,138;207;210;341;403, 1888
Nugent EW, Plauth WH, Edwards JE, et al: The pathology, pathophysiology, recognition and treatment of congenital heart disease. In Schlant RC, Alexander RW: Hurst's The Heart, 8th ed, pp 1801–1802. New York, McGraw-Hill, 1994
Perloff JK: The Clinical Recognition of Congenital Heart Disease, 4th ed, pp 440–469. Philadelphia, WB Saunders, 1994

FALLOT TETRALOGY—ABSENT PULMONARY ARTERY

Synonym. Pulmonary artery absence; tetralogy of Fallot.

Symptoms and Signs. Both sexes affected; onset in first weeks of life. Cyanosis by 6 months of age that tends to improve with age. For symptoms and signs see Fallot. Left hemithorax (usually) comparatively smaller and the pulmonary stenotic murmur radiates to the upper chest owing to the absence of left pulmonary artery.

Pathology. Fallot tetralogy with associated congenital absence of pulmonary artery (usually the left one)

Diagnostic Procedures. *Electrocardiography. Chest X-ray.* Ipsilateral (usually left) hemitorax comparatively smaller, reduced pulmonary vascularity; aortic root prominent. *Two-dimensional echocardiography with color flow imaging and spectral Doppler interrogation.*

Therapy. Medical or, according to severity, surgical (high risk).

Prognosis. Modified by surgical correction.

BIBLIOGRAPHY. Perloff JK: The Clinical Recognition of Congenital Heart Disease, 4th ed, pp 474–475. Philadelphia, WB Saunders, 1994

FALLOT TETRALOGY—ABSENT PULMONARY VALVE

Synonym. Cheevers; Kurtz-Sprague-White; pulmonary valve absence; Fallot tetralogy.

Symptoms and Signs. Both sexes affected; onset in first weeks of life. Neonatal cyanosis that tends to disappear in a few weeks. Early development of right ventricular failure. Frequent respiratory distress. Emphysema, frequently marked. Right ventricular impulse conspicuous; systolic thrills common; pulmonic ejection sound; absent pulmonic component of pulmonic sound. Gap between aortic component of second sound and onset of diastolic murmur is maximal in second–third intercostal space. Loud midsystolic murmur.

Etiology. Congenital malformation.

Pathology. Absence of pulmonary valve associated with large ventricular septal defect and dilatation of pulmonary trunk and stenotic pulmonary valve ring.

Diagnostic Procedures. *Electrocardiography.* Right axis deviation greater than in classic Fallot. *X-rays.* Marked dilatation of pulmonary trunk and its branches; right ventricle enlarged. Lungs show variable (reduced, normal, or increased) blood flow. *Two-dimensional echocardiography with color flow imaging and spectral Doppler interrogation.*

Therapy. Medical or, according to severity, surgical (high risk).

Prognosis. Modified by surgical correction.

BIBLIOGRAPHY. Cheevers N: Retrecissement congenital de l'orifice pulmonaire. Arch Med Fourth Series 15:488, 1847
Royer BF, Wilson JD: Incomplete heterotaxy with unusual heart malformations. Arch Pediatr 25:881, 1908
Kurtz CM, Sprague HB, White PD: Congenital heart disease: Interventricular septal defects with associated anomalies in series of three cases examined post-mortem and living patient 58 years old with cyanosis and clubbing of fingers. Am Heart J 3:77–90, 1927
Perloff JK: The Clinical Recognition of Congenital Heart Disease, 4th ed, pp 469–473. Philadelphia, WB Saunders, 1994

FALLOT TETRALOGY—BALANCED SHUNT

Symptoms and Signs. Both sexes affected; detected weeks or months after birth. Spells of intermittent cyanosis; hyperpnea and syncope less frequent than in classic form. Physical development normal. Pulmonic murmur longer and louder, frequently with thrill. Soft pulmonic component of second sound.

Etiology. See Fallot, with left-to-right functional shunt.

Diagnostic Procedures. *Electrocardiography.* Well-developed R-waves; small Q in precordial leads. *X-rays.* Normal vascularity of lung; less prominence of the aortic arch; rounded heart apex. *Cardiac catheterization. Two-dimensional echocardiography* with color flow imaging and spectral Doppler interrogation.

Therapy. See Fallot.

Prognosis. Better than that for classic form.

BIBLIOGRAPHY. Perloff JK: The Clinical Recognition of Congenital Heart Disease, 4th ed, p 449. Philadelphia, WB Saunders, 1994
Nugent EW, Plauth WH, Edwards JE, et al: The pathology, pathophysiology, recognition and treatment of congenital heart disease. In Schlant RC, Alexander RW: Hurst's The Heart, 8th ed, pp 1801–1802. New York, McGraw-Hill, 1994

FALLS-KERTESZ

Synonyms. Lymphedema-distichiasis. See Bloom; Noonan and Nonne-Milroy-Meige.

Symptoms and Signs. Photophobia. Late onset lymphedema, and double row of eyelids (distichiasis); cornea irritation up to ulceration: Webbed neck (nonconstant).

Etiology. Autosomal dominant inheritance.

Pathology. Abundant and dilated lymphatic vessels in the legs and thoracic duct absent or congenitally malformed. Congenital heart diseases (16%).

Diagnostic Procedures. *Lymphography.*

Therapy. Symptomatic.

BIBLIOGRAPHY. Neel JV, Schull WJ: Human Heredity, pp 50–51. Univ Chicago Press, 1954

Falls HF, Kertesz ED: A new syndrome combining ptrerygium colli with developmental anomalies of the eyelids and lymphatics of the lower extremities. Trans Am Ophthal Soc 62:248–275, 1964

Dale RF: Primary lymphoedema when found with distichiasis is of the type defined as bilateral hyperplasia by lymphography. J Med Genet 24:170–171, 1987

FALRET

Synonyms. Cyclothymia; folie circulaire; manic-depressive.

Symptoms. In this disorder, there is at least one episode of mania (hypomania; acute delirious mania) and one of depression (simple retardation or acute depression). A brief period of normality may be present between the two states, but in the majority of cases transition is direct.

Etiology. Unknown; considered; hereditary, constitutional, biologic (psychobiologic; metabolic, and from antidepressant drugs), psychologic, and psychodynamic factors.

Therapy. Prevention of suicide attempt (higher risk in moments of transition between the two stages). Assessment of situation and decision to treat at home or to hospitalize. Treatment according to severity of form includes electroconvulsive therapy, drugs, psychotherapy.

Prognosis. States may last days or months. After 45 years of age, shorter periods. Five percent attempt suicide. Long-term prognosis poor.

BIBLIOGRAPHY. Falret JP: Mémoire sur la folie circulaire, forme de la maladie mentale caractérisée par la reproduction successive et régulière de l'état maniaque, de l'état mélancolique, et d'un intervalle lucide plus ou moins prolongé. Bull Acad Imp Med 19:382–400, 1854

Kraepelin E: Maniac-Depressive Insanity and Paranoia. Robertson GM (ed): Edinburgh, Livingstone, 1921

Kaplan HI, Sadock BJ: Comprehensive Textbook of Psychiatry, 6th ed, pp 1070, 2788. Baltimore, Williams & Wilkins, 1995

F.A.M.M.M.

Synonyms. Linch-Clark; BK mole; familial melanoma—dysplastic nevi.

Symptoms and Signs. Numerous large nevi (over 2 cm in diameter) with irregular borders and occasionally inflammatory flare.

Etiology. More than one gene may be involved in the familial form (chromosome 1?). Sporadic form reported.

Pathology. Lesions show dysplastic (architectural, cytological) changes and inflammatory response.

Therapy. Careful followup and surgery.

Prognosis. According to categories A (low incidence of conversion to malignant melanoma), D (multiple lesions and high incidence of malignant evolution).

BIBLIOGRAPHY. Linch HT, Frinchot BC, Lunch JF: Familial atypical multiple mole melanoma syndrome. J Med Genet 15:352–360, 1978

Clark WH, Reimer RR, Greene M, et al: Origins of familial malignant melanomas from heritable melanocytic lesions. Arch Dermatol 114:732–735, 1978

MacKie RM: Melanocytic Nevi and Malignant Melanoma. In Champion RH, Burton JL, Ebling FJG (eds): Rook/Wilkinson/Ebling Text-book of Dermatology, 5th ed, pp 1556–1557. Oxford, Blackwell Scientific, 1992

FANCONI

Synonyms. Fanconi panmyelopathy; aplastic anemia—congenital anomalies; pancytopenia, congenital; infantile familial pernicious-like anemia. Fanconi anemia type 1 and type 2. See Estren-Dameshek.

Symptoms. More common in males (high incidence in siblings); onset in first 8 years of life; tiredness; fatigue; pallor. Recurrent infections; easy bruising; prolonged bleeding, mental retardation; growth retardation.

Signs. Brown, patchy pigmentation of skin; various combinations of congenital abnormalities: microcephaly; microphthalmia; strabismus, deafness; dwarfism; hypogenitalism; hyperreflexia.

Etiology. Defect in the passage of DNA repair-related enzymes from site of synthesis in cytoplasm to the nucleus. Autosomal recessive inheritance. The existence of at least two separate loci has been demonstrated (type 1 and type 2 of the condition).

Pathology. Bone marrow hypoplasia; occasionally, normocellular; rarely, hypercellular. Spleen atrophy (common). Cardiovascular and kidney abnormalities.

Diagnostic Procedures. *Blood.* Pancytopenia; normochromic anemia; macrocytes and target cells observed. Reticulocytes may be slightly increased; white blood cells: usually, neutropenia; immature forms may be noticed. Bilirubin normal; Coombs test negative. Hexokinase lacking in red cells. *Chromosome studies. Bone marrow.* Hyperplasia; inhibition of maturation; definite megaloblastosis, megakaryocytes decreased; increased deposition of hemosiderin; with progress of disease, cellular hypoplasia. *Urine.* Aminoaciduria reported in some patients.

Therapy. *Blood transfusion.* Testosterone and corticosteroids of some use. Surgical or orthopedic correction when indicated. *Splenectomy.* Sometimes moderately beneficial. Bone marrow transplantation with partial results.

Prognosis. High incidence of leukemia in family. Death relatively early after diagnosis (2–4 years) from infections or hemorrhages.

BIBLIOGRAPHY. Fanconi G: Familiare infantile, pernicuoseähnliche Anämie (perniziöses Blutbild und Konstitution). Jahrb Kinderheilk 117:257–280, 1927

Deeg HJ, Storb R, Thomas ED, et al: Fanconi's anemia treated by allogenic marrow transplantation. Blood 61:954–959, 1983

Duckworth-Rysiecki G, Cornish K, et al: Identification of two complementation groups in Fanconi anemia. Somatic Cell Mol Genet 11:35–41, 1985

Auerbach AD, Allen RG: Leukemia and preleukemia in Fanconi anemia patients: a review of the literature and report of the International Fanconi anemia Registry. Cancer Genet Cytogenet 51:1–12, 1991

FANCONI-BICKEL

Synonyms. Bickel-Fanconi; hepatic glycogenosis—renal Fanconi.

Symptoms and Signs. Onset first year of life, failure to thrive; at two years: hepatomegaly and palpable enlarged kidneys; abdominal blotting, features of rickets (unresponsive to vitamin D).

Etiology. Autosomal recessive inheritance. Enzymatic defect not identified. Unclassified glycogen storage disease. The mitochondrial respiratory chain could be involved.

Pathology. Glycogen accumulation in liver and renal cells.

Diagnostic Procedures. *Urine.* Glycosuria, phosphaturia, amino aciduria, bicarbonate wasting. *Blood.* Hypophosphatemia, serum alkaline phosphatase increased. Occasionally: mild hypoglycemia and hyperlactacidemia, hyperlipidemia. *Oral galactose tolerance test.* Impaired. *X-ray.* Pattern of rickets. *Echography.*

Therapy. Symptomatic.

Prognosis. Unknown.

BIBLIOGRAPHY. Fanconi G, Bickel H: Die chronische Aminoacidurie (Aminosaeurediabetes oder nephrotisch-glukosurischer Zwergwuchs bei Glycogenose und der Cystinkrankheit). Helv Paediatr Acta 4:359, 1949
Odièvre M: Glycogéenose hépatorénale avec tubulopathie complexe. Rev Inter Hepatol 16:1, 1966
Chesney RW, Kaplan BS, Teitel D, et al: Metabolic abnormalities in the idiopathic Fanconi syndrome: Studies of carbohydrate metabolism in two patients. Pediatrics 67:113, 1981
Chen YT, Burchell A: Glycogen storage diseases. In Scriver CR, Beaudet AL, Sly WS, et al. The Metabolic and Molecular Bases of Inherited Disease, 7th ed, p 956. New York, McGraw-Hill, 1995

FANCONI-DE TONI

Synonyms. De Toni-Debré-Fanconi; Fanconi renotubular; Fanconi-de Toni-Debré, aminoaciduria—osteomalacia—hyperphosphaturia; nephrotic glycosuric—dwarfism—rickets hypophosphatemic-renal Fanconi. See also cystinosis, benign.

Symptoms. Both sexes affected, normal at birth and during postnatal period; usual onset at 4–6 months of age (Type 1) or at approximately 40 years (Type 2). In the first case failure to thrive; attacks of vomiting; unexplained fever; polyuria; dehydration. In the second loss of height, weakness.

Signs. Rickets.

Etiology. Multiple etiology. Hereditary basis (cystinosis, Lowe, tyrosinemia Type 1; nephrosis familial, galactosemia, glycogen storage disease; hereditary fructose intolerance; Wilson disease) with variable type of inheritance, autosomal dominant or recessive; or acquired as secondary to numerous conditions (myeloma; malignancies; various amino acid metabolism inherited syndromes; expired tetracyclines). Common denominators: proximal renal tubular injury, with functional derangement of excretion of amino acid, glucose, phosphate; urate and bicarbonate; and vitamin D-resistant metabolic bone disease (rickets or osteomalacia). Forms without cystinosis have been described in both adult (see Fanconi renotubular adult type) and children.

Pathology. Cystine deposits in the tissues found only in some cases. Osteomalacia. In kidney (microdissection technique), characteristic lesions affecting nephrons; "swan neck" deformity; shortening of whole proximal convoluted tubule and other aspecific lesions. Pyelonephritis; vacuolization; fibrosis. Frequently, cirrhosis of liver.

Diagnostic Procedures. *Blood.* Chronic acidosis; glucose normal. Phosphate level low initially; with progression of the disease returns to normal level. Calcium normal; phosphorus is low, alkaline phosphatase high, hypokalemia. *Urine.* Glycosuria; phosphaturia; generalized aminoaciduria. *X-ray.* Skeletal rickets.

Therapy. Rickets resistant to vitamin D administration; however, some improvement may be obtained by large doses of this vitamin and supplements of phosphorus. Calcium may also be given with caution (if vitamin D is also given). Shohl solution to control acidosis. Potassium supplement also necessary. Specific drugs (dithiothreitol [DTT], mercaptoethylamine [MEA], ascorbic acid still to be assessed). Dietary measures and renal transplant.

Prognosis. Condition shows a slow progression leading ultimately to death from renal insufficiency and uremia. With treatment, immediate prognosis remarkably improves.

BIBLIOGRAPHY. Fanconi G: Die nicht diabetishen Glykosurien und Hyperglykamien des älteren Kindes. Jahrb Kinderheilk 133:257–300, 1931

de Toni G: Remarks on the relations between renal rickets (renal dwarfism) and renal diabetes. Acta Paediatr Scand 16:479–484, 1933
Debré R, Marie J, Cleret F, et al: Rachitisme tardif coexistent avec une néphrite chronique et une glycosurie. Arch Med Enf 37:597–606, 1934
Bergeron M, Gougoux A, Vinay P: The renal Fanconi syndrome. In Scriver CR, Beaudet AL, Sly WS, et al: The Metabolic and Molecular Bases of Inherited Disease, 7th ed, pp 3691–3704. New York, McGraw-Hill, 1995

FANCONI-HEGGLIN

This eponym has been used to designate a nonspecific positive serology for syphilis in cases of viral pneumonias.

BIBLIOGRAPHY. Fanconi G: Die pseudoluetische, subakute hilifugale Bronchopneumonie des heruntergekommenen Kindes. Schweiz Med Wochenschr 66:821–826, 1936
Hegglin R: Das Wassermann positive Lungeninfiltrat. Hel R Med Acta 7:497–527, 1941

FANCONI-LIKE

Symptoms and Signs. Described in two brothers. Chronic lung infection complicated by repeated bilateral pneumothoraces; osteomyelitis; metastatic lymphadenopathies; multiple cutaneous malignancies; pancytopenia.

Etiology. Unknown. Autosomal recessive phenotype.

Diagnostic Procedures. *Blood.* Pancytopenia, low IgA.

Therapy. One case was responsive to methyltestosterone.

Prognosis. One case died in the mid-twenties.

BIBLIOGRAPHY. Abels D, Reed WB: Fanconi-like syndrome. Immunologic deficiency, pancytopenia and cutaneous malignancies. Arch. Dermatol, 107:419–423, 1973

FANCONI RENOTUBULAR (ADULT FORM)

Synonym. Luder-Sheldon included; renal Fanconi (adult).

Symptoms and Signs. Onset in adulthood. Same features as infantile form (Fanconi-de Toni, see). Osteomalacia; fractures and pseudofractures; pain; deformity.

Etiology. In some cases, may possibly represent a delayed clinical onset of the congenital form (both autosomal dominant or recessive trait). More frequently, secondary to heavy metal intoxication, malignancy, or myeloma.

Pathology. See Fanconi-de Toni; no cystinosis reported in adult form.

Diagnostic Procedures. See Fanconi-de Toni.

Therapy. See Fanconi-de Toni.

Prognosis. Depends on etiology. If etiologic agent is toxin (or other curable cause), complete recovery may be obtained with treatment of primary condition.

BIBLIOGRAPHY. Luder J, Sheldon W: Familial tubular absorption defect of glucose and amino acids. Arch Dis Child 30:160–164, 1955
Patrick A, Cameron JS, Ogg CS: A family with a dominant form of idiopathic Fanconi syndrome leading to renal failure in adult life. Clin Nephrol 16:189–292, 1981
Tieder M, Arie R, Modai D, et al: Elevated serum 1,25-dihydroxy-vitamin D concentration in siblings with primary Fanconi syndrome. New Engl J Med 319:845–849, 1988

Bergeron M, Gougoux A, Vinay P: The renal Fanconi syndrome. In Scriver CR, Beaudet AL, Sly WS, et al: The Metabolic and Molecular Bases of Inherited Disease, 7th ed, pp 3691–3704. New York, McGraw-Hill, 1995

FANCONI-TUERLER

Obsolete.

Synonym. Ataxic diplegia. See Cerebellar syndromes.

Symptoms and Signs. Both sexes equally affected (reported, one family with only boy involved); onset at birth. Cerebellar ataxia; spastic paresis; nystagmus; dysmetria; uncoordinated ocular movements. Mental deficiency.

Etiology. Unknown. Developmental abnormality of oculomotor (III) nerve. Both autosomal dominant and sex-linked inheritances have been reported.

BIBLIOGRAPHY. Fanconi G, Tuerler U: Congenitale Keinhirnatrophie mit supranuclearen Storungen der Motilitat der Augenmusklen. Helv Paediatr Acta 6:479–483, 1951
Pfeiffer RA, Palm D, Junemann G, et al: Nosology of congenital nonprogressive cerebellar ataxia: Report of six cases in three families. Neuropaediatrie 5:91–102, 1974

FARABEE

Synonym. Brachydactyly type A1.

Symptoms and Signs. Proximal phalanges of digits short, middle phalanges rudimentary or fused; short stature. Occasional mental retardation and ankylosis of thumbs.

Etiology. Autosomal dominant inheritance.

BIBLIOGRAPHY. Farabee WC: Hereditary and sexual influence in meristic variation: A study of digital malformations in man. PhD thesis, Harvard Univ, 1903
Pussan C, Lanaerts C, Mathieu M, et al: Dominance reguliere d'une ankylose des pouches avec retard mental se transmettant sur trois generations. J Genet Hum 31:107–114, 1983

FARBER

Synonyms. Farber-Uzman; ceramidase deficiency; N-laurylsphingosine deacilase deficiency; lipogranulomatosis, Farber.

Symptoms and Signs. Onset early months of life. The phenotype has recently been divided in six subtypes with different clinical expression. *Type 1* is the classic syndrome "hoarse cry" (see); laryngeal stridor; swelling of joints of extremities. Skin: infiltrative lesions. Hepatomegaly. Physical and mental development retardation. Diagnostic triad: arthritis, subcutaneous nodules, laryngeal involvement. *Type 2 and 3* present: joints deformities, subcutaneous nodules, and laryngeal involvement, and survive longer. *Type 4* present greater hepatosplenomegaly and die within 6 months, subcutaneous nodules may be absent. *Type 5:* Psychomotor deterioration dominates the picture; viscera are spared. *Type 6* combines Farber and Sandhoff syndromes.

Etiology. Autosomal recessive inheritance. Deficiency of lysosomal acid ceramidase and tissue accumulation of ceramide.

Pathology. *Skin.* Tumefaction, tubular, and nodular (yellowish, firm, 1–2 cm in diameter) in periarticular soft tissues, in other areas of pressure zones in the skin, and in subcutaneous tissues. Oily, yellowish plaques on parietal and visceral serosae. *Histology.* Early: infiltration with sheets of large histiocytes and scattered lymphocytes and plasma cells. Later: histiocyte cytoplasm becomes basophilic, granular, or foamy first, and then vacuolar and necrotic. Fibrosis gradually develops.

Larynx. Lesions similar to the ones described. *Heart.* Valves also similarly involved. Reticular endothelial system. Scarcely involved (bone marrow, spleen, lymph nodes). *Liver.* Enlarged but not involved. Central nervous system. Ballooning of large neurons and glial cells with stored materials, with the characteristics of a nonsulfonated acid mucopolysaccharide: accumulation of ceramide or deficiency of acid ceramidase or both have been demonstrated.

Diagnostic Procedures. *Biopsy of skin.* See Pathology. *Blood.* Moderate leukocytosis (15,000–20,000); anemia; normal cholesterol and total lipids. *X-ray.* Osteoporosis; destructive changes in joints and periarticular calcifications. *Bone marrow.* Occasionally, vacuolated histiocytes. *Biopsy of liver.* Normal. *Urine.* Increased mucopolysaccharide, especially ceramide. Determination of acid ceramidase activity and ceramide. Prenatal diagnosis is possible by monitoring amniocyte ceramidase activity.

Therapy. None specific. Trial with steroids, methotrexate, chlorambucil, and other chemotherapeutic agents with scarce effect.

Prognosis. Progressive course; death within 2 years. Few patients survived into second decade with neurologic problems.

BIBLIOGRAPHY. Farber S: A lipid metabolic disorder—"disseminated lipogranulomatosis." A syndrome with similarity to and important differences from Niemann-Pick and Hand Schüller-Christian disease (abstr). Am J Dis Child 84:499–500, 1952
Moser HW: Ceramidase deficiency: Farber lipogranulomatosis. In Scriver CR, Beaudet AL, Sly WS, et al: The Metabolic and Molecular Bases of Inherited Disease, 7th ed, pp 2589–2599. New York, McGraw-Hill, 1995

FARMER LUNG

Synonyms. Ramazzini; harvester lung; thresher lung. See Allergic alveolitis, extrinsic and silo-filler.

Symptoms. Usually occurs between October and May in farmers exposed to moldy hay or crops. Cough; dyspnea; malaise; fever a few hours after exposure.

Signs. Cyanosis; diffuse rales on both lung fields.

Etiology. Hypersensitivity to a glycopeptide antigen produced by different fungi (thermopolyspora, polyspora, and others) from grains, hay, and other stored vegetable products.

Pathology. Inflammatory granulomatous reaction; frequently, foreign body material in lung parenchyma with secondary bronchopneumonia. In chronic cases, secondary fibrosis and organized endobronchial exudates.

Diagnostic Procedures. *Blood.* Moderate leukocytosis with moderate eosinophilia. *Immunologic studies.* In agar gel; precipitins. *Pulmonary function tests. X-ray of chest.* Fine nodular density measuring 3–5 mm; occasionally, pneumonitis.

Therapy. Excellent results with corticosteriods, removal from exposure.

Prognosis. Attack lasts a few days; occasionally, weeks. Repeated exposure leads to further attacks and development of pulmonary fibrosis, emphysema, chronic bronchitis; may become fatal because of pulmonary insufficiency and cor pulmonale.

BIBLIOGRAPHY. Ramazzini B: De morbis artificum diatriba. Modena A Capponi ed 1700; Utrecht G, Van de Water ed (II ed) 1703 Padova, GB Conzetto ed (IIIed), 1713
Campbell JM: Acute symptoms following work with hay. Br Med J 2:1143–1144, 1932
De Francisci G, Magalini SI, Scrascia E: Etiopatogenesi e problemi rianimativi nelle polmoniti da ipersensibilità. Rec Prog Med 66:541–552, 1979
Elper GR, Silo-filler's disease. A new perspective. Mayo Clin Proc 64:368–370, 1989

FARMER-MUSTIAN

Synonym. Vestibulocerebellar-periodic ataxia; ataxia periodic vestibulocerebellar.

Symptoms and Signs. Both sexes affected; onset in childhood or early adulthood. Episodic attacks of vertigo, diplopia, and ataxia, followed by progressive cerebellar disease.

Etiology. Autosomal dominant inheritance.

Therapy. Attacks of dizziness may be relieved by acetazolamide.

Prognosis. In one family slowly progressive cerebellar ataxia developed, in another one no permanent or progressive cerebellar abnormalities were found.

BIBLIOGRAPHY. Farmer TW, Mustian WM: Vestibulocerebellar ataxia. A newly defined hereditary syndrome with periodic manifestations. Arch Neurol 8:471–480, 1963
Vance JM, Pericak-Vance MA, Payne CS, et al: Linkage and genetic analysis in adult onset periodic vestibulocerebellar ataxia: Report of a new family. Am J Hum Genet 36:785, 1984

FASCIA LATA

Symptoms and Signs. See entrapment.

Etiology. Caused by tightness of fascia lata, compensatory in low back (see), affecting the opening through which the superior peroneal nerve passes.

Therapy. Fasciotomy. In the past, treatment of intervertebral disc protrusion.

BIBLIOGRAPHY. Kopel HP, Thompson WAL: Peripheral entrapment neuropathies. Baltimore, Williams & Willkins, 1963
Dowson DM, Hallett M, Millender LH: Entrapment Neuropathies, 2nd ed. Boston, Little, Brown, 1990

FASCICULATION-WEAKNESS

Synonyms. See stiff man.

Symptoms and Signs. Widespead continous fasciculation lasting for months or years. Mild weakness and chonic easy fatigability. Motor and sensory reflexes are normal.

Etiology. Unknown. Disease of terminal motor nerves.

Pathology. Degeneration and regeneration of motor nerve terminals.

Diagnostic Procedures. *EMG.* Normal (except for fasciculation). *Blood.* Normal enzymes.

Therapy. Fasciculation suppressed by curare and not by nerve block.

Prognosis. Recovery possible.

BIBLIOGRAPHY. Coers C, Telerman-Toppet N, Durda J: Neurogenic benign fasciculation, pseudomyotonia, and pseudotetany. Arch Neurol 38:282, 1981
Adams RD, Victor M: Principles of Neurology, 5th ed, p 1273. New York, McGraw-Hill, 1993

FATAL FAMILIAL INSOMNIA

Synonyms. Insomnia-dysautonomia thalamic, FFI. See prion-related protein syndromes.

Symptoms and Signs. Both sexes. In adults: progressive insomnia, fever, diaphoresis, myosis, sphincter disturbances; subsequently dreamlike status, dysarthria, tremor, and myoclonus, then coma and death.

Etiology. Autosomal dominant caused by mutations in the PrP gene (PRNP) located on short arm of chromosome 20.

Pathology. Limited to anterior and dorsomedial thalamic nuclei neuronal degeneration and reactive astrocytosis; absent spongiosis, vascular or inflammatory changes.

Diagnostic Procedures. *CT scan. MRI. PET. EEG. Brain biopsy.*

Therapy. Symptomatic.

Prognosis. Death at 9 months from onset.

BIBLIOGRAPHY. Little BW, Brown BW, Rodgers-Johnson P, Pearl DP, et al: Familial myoclonic dementia masquerading as Creutzfeld-Jakob disease. Ann Neurol 20:231–239, 1986
Lugaresi E, Medori R, Montagna, et al: Fatal familial insomnia and dysautonomia with selective degeneration of thalamic nuclei. N Engl J Med 315:997–1003, 1986
Medori R, Tritschler H-J, leBlanc A, et al: Fatal familial insomnia, a prion disease with a mutation at codon 178 of the prion protein gene. N Engl J Med 326:444–449, 1992

FAULK-EPSTEIN-JONES

BIBLIOGRAPHY. Faulk WP, Epstein CJ, Jones MD: Cranial nerve anomaly: Familial posterior lumbosacral vertebral fusion and eyelid ptosis. Am Dis Child 119:510–512, 1970

FAVRE

Synonyms. Favre-Chaix; acroangiodermatitis; dermite ochre; stasis purpura; gravitational purpura.

Symptoms and Signs. Prevalent in males. Small macules coalesce to form plaques along venous vessels; usually, in lower legs, extending to feet and upward. Varying shades of yellowish color (ochre).

Etiology. Stasis; venous insufficiency.

Pathology. Skin normal or with mild eczematoid changes. Association with signs of venous stasis, ulceration.

Therapy. Rest; elevation of legs; elastic stockings.

Prognosis. Chronic individual lesions persisting for months or years.

BIBLIOGRAPHY. Favre M: Nouvelle Pratique Dermatologie, vol 5, p 113. Paris, Masson, 1936
Champion RH: Purpura. In Champion RH, Burton JL, Ebling FJG (eds): Rook/Wilkinson/Ebling Textbook of Dermatology, 5th ed, p 1890. Oxford, Blackwell Scientific, 1992

FAVRE-RACOUCHOT

Synonym. Nodular elastoidosis; elastoidosis cutanea nodularis.

Symptoms and Signs. Occurs in people who are chronically exposed to sun. Usually becoming apparent in fourth or fifth decade. Yellowish thickening of skin, with comedones and follicular cysts, especially around the orbits, occasionally in the neck and behind the ears.

Etiology. Reaction to sun.

Pathology. Elastotic degeneration of collagen.

Diagnostic Procedures. *Biopsy.* Of skin.

Therapy. Sunscreens.

Prognosis. Permanent; slowly progressive condition.

BIBLIOGRAPHY. Favre M: Sur une affection kystique des appareils pilosébacés localisee à certaines régions de la face. Bull Soc Fr Dermatol Syph 39:93–96, 1932

Favre M, Racouchot J: L'elastéidose cutanée nodulaire a kystes et á comédons. Ann Dermatol Syph 78:681–702, 1951

Burton JL: Disorders of connective tissue. In Champion RH, Burton JL, Ebling FJG (eds): Rook/Wilkinson/Ebling Textbook of Dermatology, 5th ed, p 1787. Oxford, Blackwell Scientific, 1992

FAZIO-LONDE

Synonyms. Londe; bulbar palsy progressive, infantilis; see Werding-Hoffmann (very likely same syndrome).

Symptoms. Both sexes. From childhood (difference with Werding-Hoffmann where onset is in the first year). Difficult swallowing, absent gag reflex, respiratory difficulty. Facial diplegia, dysarthria; dysphonia. In some cases late development of corticospinal signs.

Signs. Bilateral ptosis, facial weakness, generalized hyporeflexia. Decreased diaphragm motility.

Etiology. Autosomal recessive inheritance.

Pathology. Loss of motor neurons in the hypoglossal, ambiguous, facial, and trigeminal nuclei.

Prognosis. Death within 1–2 years of age.

BIBLIOGRAPHY. Fazio F: Eredità della paralisi bulbare progessiva. Rif Med 4:327, 1892

Londe P: Paralysis bulbaire progressive, infantile et familiale. Rev Med 14:212–254, 1894

Gomez MR, Clearmont V, Bernstein J: Progressive bulbar paralysis in childhood (Fazio-Londe's disease). Report of a case with pathologic evidence of nuclear atrophy. Arch Neurol 6:317–323, 1962

Benjamins D: Progressive bulbar palsy of childhood in siblings. Ann Neurol 8:203, 1980

Adams RD, Victor M: Principles of Neurology, 5th ed, pp 998, 1249. New York, McGraw-Hill, 1993.

FECHTNER*

Synonyms. Acrothrombocytopathy—nephritis—deafness—leukocyte inclusions. Alport syndrome—leukocyte inclusions—macrothrombocytopenia. See Alport.

Symptoms and Signs. Both sexes. Congenital cataracts. Deafness (high tone sensorineural) developing in late infancy. Symptoms and signs of nephritis.

Etiology. Autosomal dominant inheritance.

Diagnostic Procedures. *Blood.* From birth in neutrophils and eosinophils presence of a pale blue cytoplasmic inclusions. Macrothrombocytes. Evidence of renal disease. *Urine.* Moderate proteinuria, from microscopic hematuria to end-stage kidney failure.

Therapy. Symptomatic, up to dialysis or kidney transplantation.

Prognosis. If patient reaches adulthood, that of kidney failure.

BIBLIOGRAPHY. Gershoni-Barunch R, Bamch Y, Viener A, et al: Fechtner syndrome: Clinical and genetic aspects. Am J Med Genet 31:357–367, 1988

Peterson LC, Rao KV, Crosson JT, et al: Fechtner syndrome: A variant of Alport's syndrome with leukocyte inclusions and macrothrombocytemia. Blood 65:397–406, 1985

FEER

Synonyms. Selter; Swift; acrodynia; dermatopolyneuritis; erythredema polyneuropathy; pink disease.

*Family surname of first family described.

Symptoms. Both sexes affected; onset in infancy or early childhood (4 months to 4 years). Restlessness; sleeplessness; hyperhidrosis continua; tremor; muscle flabbiness.

Signs. Cyanosis of fingers, toes, nose; ulcers and gangrene of fingers; ulcer of mucous membranes; loss of healthy teeth; rectal prolapse; exanthemata of palms and soles with exfoliation of large flaps of skin. Muscle hypotonia; tachycardia; blood hypertension; hypertrichosis. Moderate limb hypertrichosis; in some severe cases, may develop on limb, face, or trunk. Fifty percent of cases present ocular findings: proptosis; lacrimation; photophobia; conjunctival itching and injection; midriasis; seldom: keratitis; papilledema; mild optic neuritis.

Etiology. Unknown; possibly toxic or allergic reaction to mercury, infections.

Pathology. *Skin.* In spinous and basal cell layers: acanthosis; papillomatosis; parakeratosis; and necrobiotic changes. *Spinal cord and nerve roots.* Chronic inflammatory changes.

Diagnostic Procedures. *Urine.* Increased excretion of mercury (in some cases).

Therapy. Corticosteroids; dimercaprol in full dosage in severe reaction.

Prognosis. Mortality 10%. Complete recovery in months, occasionally years, with recurrences.

BIBLIOGRAPHY. Feer E: Eine eigenartige Neurose des vegetativen Systems beim Kleinkinde. Ergeb Inn Med 24:100–122, 1923

Spencer PS, Schaumburg HH (eds): Experimental and Clinical Neurotoxicology. Baltimore, Williams & Wilkins, 1980

Dinehart SM, Dillard R, Raimer SS, et al: Cutaneous manifestations of acrodynia (pink disease). Arch Dermatol 124:107–109, 1988

FEGELER

Synonyms. Post-traumatic nevus flammeus; nevus, post-traumatic. See Nevus flammeus.

Symptoms and Signs. Development of nevus flammeus in the area of the trigeminal (V) nerve; homolateral limb weakness and hyperesthesia.

Etiology. Unknown. Ascribed in the past to birth trauma.

Therapy. Nevus can be treated (see Nevus flammeus).

BIBLIOGRAPHY. Fegeler F: Naevus flammeus im Trigeminusgebiet nach Trauma im Rahmen. Eines post-traumatische-vegetativen Syndrome. Arch Dermatol Syph 188:416–422, 1949

FELDAKER

Synonym. Livedo—ulceration. See also Leg stasis. Livedo vasculitis; today grouped with Milian II (see).

Symptoms and Signs. Occurs in middle-aged obese and, frequently, hypertensive women; onset usually during summer. Attacks of edema and aching of legs (occasionally, other sites also), followed by appearance of patches of purplish color or purpura, which ulcerate and produce intense pain, especially at night.

Etiology. Unknown. Combination of various factors: edema; stasis; fibrosis.

Pathology. Mild vasculitis; necrosis of veins and arterioles; vascular walls with cellular infiltrates.

Therapy. Bed rest. Elastic stockings. Treatment of basic conditions: hypertension and obesity.

Prognosis. Protracted course, increasing intensity of manifestations every year. Good quoad vitam.

BIBLIOGRAPHY. Feldaker M, Hines EA Jr, Kierland RR: Livedo reticularis with summer ulcerations. Arch Dermatol 72:31–42, 1955

Ryan TJ: Cutaneous vasculitis. In Champion RH, Burton JL, Ebling FJG (eds): Rook/Wilkinson/Ebling Textbook of Dermatology, 5th ed, p 1945. Oxford, Blackwell Scientific, 1992

FELTY

Synonyms. Rheumatoid arthritis—splenomegaly; neutropenic hypersplenism—arthritis. See Still.

Symptoms. Malaise, fatigability; anorexia; weight loss; joint pains and deformity; recurrent infections, especially oral mucosa; sinusitis; bronchitis; furunculosis; leg ulcers refractory to antibiotic treatment. Occasionally, dragging sensation or pain in left upper quadrant of abdomen.

Signs. Joints with typical alterations of rheumatoid arthritis; spleen enlarged; mild hepatomegaly; generalized lymphadenopathy. Pallor; occasionally, brown pigmentation on exposed surface of extremities.

Etiology. Unknown; variant of rheumatoid arthritis in which there is unusual reticuloendothelial system stimulation with hypersplenism and neutropenia.

Pathology. Joints show typical changes of rheumatoid arthritis in different stages of evolution. Spleen enlarged (240–2400 g). Nonspecific changes, malphighian corpuscles with large germinative center, hyperplasia, reticulum endothelial cells, plasma cells, dilated venus sinuses. Liver within normal limits.

Diagnostic Procedures. *Bone marrow.* Moderate erythroid hyperplasia; marked myeloid hyperplasia with maturation arrest at metamyelocyte level. *Blood.* Moderate hypochromic anemia; moderate thrombocytopenia; marked neutropenia. Latex fixation test often positive; LE test negative; Coombs test negative.

Therapy. Splenectomy beneficial for neutropenia and recurrent infections in most cases. The potential role of recombinant granulocyte colony stimulating factors will be evaluated.

Prognosis. Progression of rheumatoid arthritis disease. The rheumatoid arthritis often precedes the hypersplenism, and neutropenia occasionally appears at the same time, or follows.

BIBLIOGRAPHY. Felty AR: Chronic arthritis in the adult, associated with splenomegaly and leukopenia: A report of five cases of an unusual clinical syndrome. Bull John Hopkins Hosp 35:16–20, 1924

Spivak JL: Felty's syndrome: An analytical review. Johns Hopkins Med J 141:156–162, 1977

Campion G, Maddison PJ, Goulding N, et al: The Felty syndrome: A case-matched study of clinical manifestations and outcome, serological features and immunogenetic associations. Medicine 69:69–80, 1990

FEMALE PROSTATIC OBSTRUCTION

Synonyms. Marion; see bladder neck and Hunner.

Symptoms. Dysuria, from simple difficulty in voiding to complete retention.

Signs. Urinary bladder distension.

Etiology. Inflammation or hypertrophy (or both) of the group of glands surrounding the posterior part of the female urethra.

Diagnostic Procedures. *Urine.* No pathologic findings or varying degree of albuminuria, and variable number of granulocytes in different stages of degeneration (pus). *Cystography.* Filing defect in the region of the internal orifice similar to the defects seen in men in prostatic hypertrophy; in bladder wall, various degree of trabeculation.

Therapy. Transurethral resection.

Prognosis. Good with treatment.

Comment. Not all authors accept hypertrophy of adenomatous tissue equivalent to the male prostate as the pathogenesis of this syndrome. The following have been considered as etiologic factors for the rare obstruction of the neck of bladder observed in women: granulomatous inflammation; neurologic causes; cystocele. (See Bladder neck, clinically identical condition.) Folson and O'Brien, however, presented a good pathologic demonstration of the nature of the tissue in their patients.

BIBLIOGRAPHY. Caulk J: Contracture of the vesical neck in the female. J Urol 6:341–343, 1921

Marion G: De l'hypertrophie congenitale du col vésical. J Urol Méd Chil 23:97–101, 1927

Folson A, O'Brien H: The female obstructing prostrate. JAMA 121:573–580, 1943

Messing EM: Interstitial cystitis and related syndromes. In Walsh PC, Gittes RF, Perlmutter AD, et al: Campbell's Urology, 5th ed, pp 1031–1036. Philadelphia, WB Saunders, 1992

Klahr S: Obstructive nephropathy. In Massry SG, Glassock RJ: Textbook of Nephrology, 3rd ed, pp 530–535. Baltimore, Williams & Wilkins, 1995

FEMORAL-FACIAL

Symptoms and Signs. Both sexes affected, present from birth. Normal intelligence. *Facies.* Palpebral fissures upslanted; short nose; hypoplastic ala nasi; thin upper lip; cleft palate; micrognathia. *Legs.* Short; hypoplasia or absence of femur and fibula; club foot. *Arms.* Hypoplasia of humerus; reduced elbow movements. Lower spine anomalies and variable alteration of pelvis.

Etiology. Unknown. Sporadic. With a single reported exception, father-to-daughter transmission.

Prognosis. Normal intelligence. Ambulatory.

BIBLIOGRAPHY. Franz CH, O'Rahilly R: Congenital skeletal limb deficiencies. J Bone Joint Surg 43:1202–1224, 1961

Daentl DL, Smith DW, Scott CI, et al: Femoral hypoplasia–unusual facies syndrome. J Paediatr 86:107–111, 1975

Burk, U, Riebel T, Held KR, et al: Bilateral femoral dysgenesis with micrognathia, cleft palate, anomalies of the spine and pelvis and foot deformities. Helv Paediatr Acta 36:473–482, 1981

FERGUSON-CRITCHLEY

Synonyms. Spastic paraplegia-ocular-extrapyramidal, hereditary; pseudo-ophthalmoplegia—extrapyramidal.

Symptoms and Signs. Onset in fourth–fifth decades in life. Gait incoordination; mood and affects alteration, tendency to pathological laughter, dysarthria, diplopia, dysesthesia of arms and legs, bladder disorders: hypertonus and hyperreflexia, nystagmus, facial expression becoming immobile and blank, with perioral tremor, twitching of muscles, and resting tremor. Occasionally cerebellar signs. Ocular: limitation or absence of upward and/or lateral deviation of eyes, lid retraction.

Etiology. Regarded as an abiotrophic variant of spinocerebellar ataxia group. Autosomal dominant inheritance.

Pathology. Cerebrum: disarray of cortical architecture, patchy demyelinization of subcortical white matter; cerebellum and brain stem mild neuronal degeneration in dentate nuclei, cerebellar folia thinner and reduction of population of granular layer; thickening of spinal cord leptomeninges; foci of demyelination in dorsal and anterolateral columns.

Diagnostic Procedures. *CT scan. MRI. EEG. CSF.*

Therapy. Symptomatic.

Prognosis. Progression leading to death in 5–16 years.

BIBLIOGRAPHY. Ferguson F, Critchley M: A clinical study of an heredo-familial disease resembling disseminated sclerosis. Brain 52:203–225, 1929

Brown JW: Hereditary spastic paraplegia with ocular and extra-pyramidal symptoms (Ferguson-Critchley syndrome). In Vinken PJ, Bruyn GW (eds): Handbook of Clinical Neurology, vol 22, pp 433–443. Amsterdam, North Holland, 1975

FERGUSON SMITH

Synonyms. Smith keratoacanthoma; epithelioma, self-healing, squamous; multiple keratoacanthomas; multiple molluscum sebaceum; multiple molluscum pseudocarcinomatosum.

Symptoms. Male to female ratio, 3:1; onset in middle life. Asymptomatic or according to location (anus, scrotum, etc.). On the face, less frequently on hands, back of wrists, and forearm, seldom on thighs and chest, rarely on anogenital areas: firm, round, reddish papules that rapidly enlarge and in 1 month reach to 1–2 cm in diameter; the center contains a horny plug, covered more or less by a crust. The lesion evolves or spontaneously resolves in 3 months, but is replaced by others at neighboring sites.

Etiology. Unknown. Autosomal dominant inheritance. Relationship with keratoacanthoma (single) still uncertain.

Pathology. Intradermal tumors of symmetric, globular shape; the epidermis over lesions is thinned. Early lesion formed by multiplying squamous cells; central cells keratinize. Initially similar to a squamous cell carcinoma. In mature form, decrease of peripheral mitosis, enlarging of the core, invasion by inflammatory cells and opening like a flower, finally leaving a scar.

Diagnostic Procedures. *Biopsy.*

Therapy. Curettage or excision. Freezing of lesion at early stage. Radiotherapy. Trial with 13-cis-retinoic acid (teratogenic in pregnant women).

Prognosis. Spontaneous resolution or therapeutic resolution. Depressed scar may remain after healing.

BIBLIOGRAPHY. Fergusson-Smith J: A case of multiple primary squamous celled carcinomata of the skin in a young man, with spontaneous healing. Br J Dermatol 46:267–272, 1934

Hayday RP, Reed ML, Dzubow LM, et al: Treatment of keratoacanthomas with oral 13-cis-retinoic acid. N Engl J Med 303:560–562, 1980

Goudie DR, Yuille MAR, Affara NA, et al: Localization of the gene for multiple self-healing squamous epithelioma (Ferguson-Smith type) to the long arm of chromosome 9. Cytogenet Cell Genet 58:1939, 1991

MacKie RM: Epidermal skin tumors. In Champion RH, Burton JL, Ebling FJG (eds): Rook/Wilkinson/Ebling Textbook of Dermatology, 5th ed, p 1472. Oxford, Blackwell Scientific, 1992

FERRARO

Synonyms. Eponym obsolete; proposed to indicate adult form leukodystrophy.

BIBLIOGRAPHY. Ferraro A: A Familial form of encephalitis periaxialis diffusa. J Nerv Ment Dis 66:329–354; 479–496; 616–620, 1927

Van Bogaert L, Bertrand J: Les leukodystrophies progressives familiales. Rev Neurol II:249–286, 1933

FERTILE EUNUCH

Synonyms. Pasqualini; pseudoeunuchoidism.

Symptoms. No libido or potency; erection rarely occurs.

Signs. Obesity; skin dry; axillary and pubic hair scanty; no beard; penis small, scrotum well formed; testes normal size; prostate small.

Etiology. Not entirely clear; isolated deficiency of luteinizing hormone (LH).

Pathology. Testes normal size; Leydig cells very scarce or absent. Tubules contain normal or reduced number of spermatozoa.

Diagnostic Procedures. *Semen analysis.* Low or normal spermatozoa count. *Blood and urine.* Follicle-stimulating hormone (FSH) normal; LH decreased or undetected; testosterone decreased; 17-ketosteroids markedly decreased. *Biopsy of testes.* See Pathology. *Chromosome studies. X-ray of skull.*

Therapy. Testosterone and human chorionic gonadotropins effective in stimulating spermatogenesis and virilization.

Prognosis. Good response to treatment. More frequent erections and increased spermatozoa count.

BIBLIOGRAPHY. Nathanson I, Towne LE, Aub JC: Normal excretion of sex hormones in childhood. Endocrinology 28:851–865, 1941

Pasqualini RQ, Bur G: Syndrome hipoandrogénica con gametogénesis conservada. Classification de la insuficiencia testicular. Rev Assoc Méd Argent 64:6–10, 1950

Hall JE, Crowley WF Jr: Gonadotropins and the gonad: Normal physiology and their disturbances in clinical endocrine diseases. In De Groot LJ (ed): Endocrinology, 3rd ed, p 255. Philadelphia, WB Saunders, 1995

FETAL ALCOHOL

Synonyms. Ethyl alcohol fetal.

Symptoms. Occurs in 2/1000 children in USA. Both sexes affected; onset from birth. Poor sucking; mild to moderate mental retardation; poor coordination; irritability, apparent hyperacusia; hyperactivity.

Signs. Muscle hypotonia. Growth deficiencies; cerebral nervous system dysfunctions. Microcephaly. Almost pathognomonic are the facial abnormalities: short palpebral fissures; short upturned nose; hypoplastic philtrum; hypoplastic maxilla; thinned upper vermilion. Occasionally; malformations of eyes, ears, and cardiac, urogenital, cutaneous, and skeletal systems.

Etiology. Teratogenic effect of alcohol intake. The evidence to date suggests that chronic consumption of 90 ml of absolute alcohol or more per day (the equivalent of about six "hard" drinks) constitutes a major risk to the fetus. However, no absolutely safe level of ethanol consumption has yet been established.

Pathology. Prenatal insult to cell proliferation leads to diminished fetal cell numbers and limitation of size. In particular, the following effects on the central nervous system are observed: failure or interruption in neuronal and glial migrations; cerebellar dysplasias; heterotopic cell clusters, especially on the brain surface; subsensorial anomalies leading to hydrocephalus.

Diagnostic Procedures. Tests of mental performances; careful clinical examination for detection of characteristic facial anomalies.

Therapy. Symptomatic.

Prognosis. Poor.

BIBLIOGRAPHY. Sullivan WC: A note on the influence of maternal inebriety on the offspring. J Ment Sci 45:489–503, 1899

Lemoine P, et al: Les enfants du parents alcoliques: anomalies observees a propos de 127 cas. Ouest Med 25:477–482, 1968

Malcom MT: Foetal alcohol syndrome. Historical aspects. Alcohol Alcoholism 19:12261–262, 1984

Schardein JL: Chemically Induced Birth Defects, 2nd ed. New York, Marcel Dekker, 1993

Koren G: Maternal-Fetal Toxicology: A Clinician's Guide, 2nd ed. New York, Marcel Dekker, 1994

FETAL DISTRESS

Synonyms. Fetal asphyxia; asphyxia pallida of newborn; intrauterine hypoxia.

Symptoms and Signs. Change in the fetal heart rate and rhythm above 160 or below 100 beats/min, calculated in between uterine contractions. Bradycardia is more significant than fetal tachycardia. Passage of meconium or staining of amniotic fluid with meconium in a cephalic presentation. Changes in acid-base balance of blood detected by using scalp fetal blood.

Etiology. Predisposing factors are prematurity, toxemia of pregnancy, antepartum uterine infection or bleeding, diabetes mellitus, hypertensive disease during pregnancy, Rh isoimmunization and complications during labor and delivery.

Pathology. At autopsy, usually evidence of anoxia.

Diagnostic Procedures. Detection of the cardiac arrhythmia either clinically or through the fetal electrocardiogram. Detection of the acidosis through fetal blood examination. Detection of meconium in cephalic presentation.

Therapy. A pediatrician should be available if possible. In cases of asphyxia (absence of respiration) owing to excessive narcotics, an antidote should be given: nalorphine hydrochloride (5–10 mg intravenously) to mother for 5–15 minutes before delivery or 0.2 mg nalorphine or (better) naloxone hydrochloride (0. 005–0.01 mg/kg) injected into the umbilical vein of the newborn. Respiratory stimulants, such as nikethamide (Coramine) or picrotoxin, have no place in the resuscitation of the newborn. As a general rule, if the newborn at the end of first minute fails to start breathing spontaneously, he is in danger. Without losing any time the trachea must be sucked clear of mucus, endotracheal intubation performed, and artificial respiration started. It can be started with gentle puffs from the mouth at a rate of 16/min, enriched with oxygen. As long as the heart is beating, this should be continued. If the heart stops, external cardiac massage should be started at once, at a rate of 60–80/min. As soon as the newborn starts spontaneous effort for respiration, the endotracheal cannula should be removed. Sodium bicarbonate should not be given unless the infant is being ventilated satisfactorily. Very often the low pH will correct itself with adequate ventilation, restoration of blood volume, and glucose infusion. In any case, the bicarbonate solution should be highly diluted; dilution and slow injection minimize the hazard of acute hyperosmolarity. No time must be wasted on such procedures as slapping of the buttocks of the baby, dilatation of the sphincter ani with finger, immersion of the baby in cold then hot water. Nothing is more harmful to the already handicapped baby.

Prognosis. Depends on the cause of the fetal distress and how rapidly measures for resuscitation are instituted after the diagnosis of the condition.

BIBLIOGRAPHY. Hampton LJ: Resuscitation of the newborn. Clin Obstet Gynecol 3:951–970, 1960
Sunshine P, Benitz WE: Neonatal resuscitation. In Nelson NM (ed): Current Therapy in Neonatal-Perinatal Medicine. Burlington, Ontario, BC Decker, 1986
Dellinger Boehm: Early management of fetal distress in the obstetric patient. Obstet Gynecol Clin N Am 22:215–233, 1995

FETAL FOLATE ANTAGONIST

Synonyms. Aminopterin; methotraxate; folate antagonist, fetal.

Symptoms and Signs. Present at birth. Variable combination of the following: small body; microcephaly; hypoplasia of cranial bones; broad nasal bridge; prominent eyes; micrognathia; cleft palate; low-set ears; short limbs (particularly mesomelic); hypodactyly; talipes equinovarus; hydrocephalus; craniosynostosis.

Etiology. Teratogenic effect of aminopterin and other folate antagonist chemotherapeutic agents.

Diagnostic Procedures. *Skull X-rays.* Lack of normal ossification of the cranial vault at birth, poor ossification of the cranium, and development of multiple wormian bones in follow-up studies, cranium bifidum, aberrant longitudinal suture in the parietal bones, partial craniosynostosis.

Therapy. Neurosurgery (ventriculo-peritoneal shunt, correction of craniosynostosis).

Prognosis. Frequent fetal or early postnatal death; several patients have survived, with handicaps, but normal intelligence.

BIBLIOGRAPHY. Thiersch JB, Philips FS: Effect of 4-amino-pteroglutamic acid (aminopterin) on early pregnancy. Proc Soc Exp Biol Med 74:204–208, 1950
Taybi H, Lachman RS: Radiology of Syndromes, Metabolic Disorders, and Skeletal Dysplasias, 3rd ed. Chicago, Yearbook, 1990
Schardein JL: Chemically Induced Birth Defects, 2nd ed. New York, Marcel Dekker, 1993
Koren G: Maternal-Fetal Toxicology: A Clinician's Guide, 2nd ed. New York, Marcel Dekker, 1994

FETAL HYDANTOIN

Synonyms. Meadows; dilantin fetal.

Symptoms and Signs. Variable; combinations of the following: mild mental deficiency; mild growth deficiency; craniofacial abnormalities (hypertelorism; broad and depressed nasal sella; abnormal ears; gingival hypertrophy; cleft lip and palate); limb abnormalities (hypoplasia of distal phalanges, hypo-onychon) and various others (hirsutism; coarse hair; hernias). Occasionally other malformations may be present; microcephaly; strabismus; congenital heart; pulmonary; gastrointestinal, and genital defects.

Etiology. Teratogenic effect of hydantoin (or combination of hydantoin plus barbiturates) on the fetus. Risk of the complete syndrome 10%; of only some isolated sign 33%.

Therapy. Symptomatic.

Prognosis. Some manifestations regress with growth; gingival hyperplasia, dysonychia. Mild degree of mental deficiency (average IQ of 71).

BIBLIOGRAPHY. Meadow SR: Anticonvulsant drugs and congenital abnormalities. Lancet II:1296, 1968
Hanson JW Teratogen update: Fetal hydantoin effects. Teratology 33:349–353, 1986
Schardein JL: Chemically Induced Birth Defects, 2nd ed. New York, Marcel Dekker, 1993
Koren G: Maternal-Fetal Toxicology: A Clinician's Guide, 2nd ed. New York, Marcel Dekker, 1994

FETAL TOLUENE

Synonyms. Toluene embryopathy.

Symptoms. At birth. Central nervous system dysfunction. Variable alteration of growth.

Signs. Microcephaly. Minor craniofacial and limb anomalies.

Signs. Exposure to aromatic hydrocarbons during pregnancy.

BIBLIOGRAPHY. Hersh JH, Podruch PE, Rogers G, et al: Toluene embriopathy. J Pediatr 106:992–927, 1985
Hersh JH: Toluene embryopathy: Two new cases. J Med Genet 26:333–337, 1989

Schardein JL: Chemically Induced Birth Defects, 2nd ed. New York, Marcel Dekker, 1993

Koren G: Maternal-Fetal Toxicology: A Clinician's Guide, 2nd ed. New York, Marcel Dekker, 1994

FETAL TRIMETHADIONE

Synonyms. German; tridione; oxazolidinediones fetal.

Symptoms. Both sexes affected; prenatal onset. Growth and mental deficiencies. Speech disorders.

Signs. Mild brachycephaly; midfacial hypoplasia and synophrys. Nose short, upturned, with low and broad bridge. Eyebrows upslanted; forehead prominent. Cleft lip and palate. Micrognathia. Ear abnormalities. Signs of cardiac malformations (Fallot tetralogy; septal defects). Genital abnormalities: hypospadias; hypertrophic clitoris. Occasionally, variable abnormalities of skin, gastrointestinal, renal, and skeletal systems.

Etiology. Trimethadione or paramethadione taken in pregnancy. The syndrome becomes manifest in two-thirds of offspring of women who have received the drugs during pregnancy.

Pathology. Cardiac malformations: aortic and/or pulmonic stenosis, hypoplastic left heart, endocardial cushion defect, transposition of great vessels, tetralogy of Fallot.

Therapy. Nonspecific. If these drugs have been used during pregnancy, therapeutic abortion is indicated.

Prognosis. Poor, because of mental deficiency and heart abnormalities.

BIBLIOGRAPHY. German J, Lowal A, Ehlers KH: Trimethadione and human teratogenesis. Teratology 3:349–361, 1970

Zackai E, Mellman MJ, Neider B, et al: The fetal trimethadione syndrome. J Paediatr 87:280–284, 1975

Schardein JL: Chemically Induced Birth Defects, 2nd ed. New York, Marcel Dekker, 1993

Koren G: Maternal-Fetal Toxicology: A Clinician's Guide, 2nd ed. New York, Marcel Dekker, 1994

FETAL VALPROATE

Synonyms. Valproic fetal.

Symptoms and Signs. At birth. Calvaria abnormalities, metopic ridging, trigonocephaly, narrow frontal diameters; midfacial hypoplasia, upturned short nose, broad flat bridge; vermilion border of upper lip. Occasionally respiratory stridor; cleft lip, micrognathia, ear anomalies; tracheomalacia, inguinal hernia, genital, cardiac, and limb anomalies.

Etiology. Valproic acid exposure.

Prognosis. Death in 2–10 years.

BIBLIOGRAPHY. Robert E: Valproate and birth defects. Lancet 2:1142, 1983

Ardinger HH, Atkins F, Blakston RD, et al: Verification of the fetal valproate syndrome phenotype. Am J Med Genet 29:171–185, 1988

Schardein JL: Chemically Induced Birth Defects, 2nd ed. New York, Marcel Dekker, 1993

Koren G: Maternal-Fetal Toxicology: A Clinician's Guide, 2nd ed. New York, Marcel Dekker, 1994

FETAL VITAMIN A

Synonyms. Fetal isotretinoin; etretinate fetal; isotretitoin fetal; retinol fetal.

Symptoms. In newborn from mother treated with "megadoses" of vitamin A or with vitamin A cogeners (isotretinoin, etretinate, etc.). Higher risk between second and fourth week of pregnancy. Cortical blindness, facial nerve palsies; hearing impairment.

Signs. Pattern of defect similar to Di George (see). Microcephaly, hydrocephaly, posterior fossa cysts. *Facies.* Asymmetry, midfacial hypoplasia, metopic synostosis, microphthalmia, oculomotor palsies, cleft lip, palate, microtia. Evidence of (a) cardiovascular anomalies; aorta hypoplasia, VSD, great vessels transposition, left ventricle hypoplasia. (b) Kidney hypoplasia and genitourinary malformation. *Limbs.* Possible various malformations from syndactyly to sirenomelia.

Etiology. Toxic activity of vitamin A or its cogeners.

BIBLIOGRAPHY. Wilson J, Freser FC (eds): Handbook of Teratology. Plenum Press, New York, 1977

Kaiser DL: Retinoid embriopathy: epidemiological perspective. In Koren G (ed): Retinoids in Clinical Practice. New York, Marcel Dekker, 1993

Koren G: Maternal-Fetal Toxicology: A Clinician's Guide, 2nd ed. New York, Marcel Dekker, 1994

FIBRINOID

Symptoms and Signs. In patients with longstanding diabetes. Postvitrectomy (2–14 days) appearance of white gray criss-cross layers of fibrin over retina and behind plane of iris. Visual impairment, rubeosis iris.

Pathology. Retinal detachment. Neovascular glaucoma.

Etiology. Unknown.

BIBLIOGRAPHY. Schepens CL: Clinical and research aspects of subtotal open-sky vitrectomy, 37th ed. Jackson Memorial Lecture. Am J Ophthalmol 92:143–171, 1981

Sebestren JG: Fibrinoid syndrome: A severe complication of vitrectomy surgery in diabetes. Ann Ophthalmol 14:853–856, 1982

FIBROMATOSIS, CONGENITAL-GENERALIZED

Synonyms. Including myofibromatosis juvenile. See Ollier; and fibromuscular dysplasia.

Symptoms and Signs. Onset present at birth or developing during first weeks. Multiple fibroblastic tumors in the skin, muscles, bones, and viscera. Absence of pigmentary skin changes. According to visceral organs involved.

Etiology. Unknown. Familial cases reported (autosomal recessive inheritance).

Pathology. Tumors of fibrous tissue containing also smooth muscle cells and vascular channels (hamartoma type).

Diagnostic Procedures. Biopsy.

Prognosis. From spontaneous remission (rare) to death within 4 months (80%). Internal organ involvement poor prognostic factor.

BIBLIOGRAPHY. Touraine A, Ruel H: La polyfibromatose hereditaire. Am Derm Syph 29:1–5, 1945

Stont AP: Juvenile fibromatoses. Cancer 7:953–978, 1954

Altemani AM, Amstalden EI, Fihlo JM: Congenital generalized fibromatosis causing spinal cord compression. Hum Pathol 16:1063–1065, 1985

Beighton P: Heritable Disorders of Connective Tissue, 5th ed, p 673. St Louis, CV Mosby, 1993

FIBROMATOSIS, GINGIVAL-HANDS, NOSE, AND EARS—ABNORMALITIES—SPLENOMEGALY

Symptoms and Signs. Gingival fibromatosis (see Fibromatosis gingival-hypertrichosis) associated with large soft ears and nose, "whittling" of phalanges, atrophy or dysplasia of nails, hypermobility of joints, hepato- or splenomegaly. Skeletal abnormalities.

Etiology. Autosomal dominant inheritance.

BIBLIOGRAPHY. Laband PF, Habib G, Humphreys GS: Hereditary gingival fibromatosis. Report of an affected family with associated splenomegaly and skeletal and soft tissue abnormalities. Oral Surg 17:339–351, 1964

FIBROMATOSIS, GINGIVAL—PROGRESSIVE DEAFNESS

Synonyms. Gingival fibromatosis—sensorineural deafness.

Symptoms and Signs. Gingival fibromatosis (see fibromatosis gingival; hypertrichosis), progressive sensineural deafness.

Etiology. Autosomal dominant inheritance.

BIBLIOGRAPHY. Jones G, Wilroy RS Jr, McHaney V: Familial fibromatosis associated with progressive deafness in five generations in a family. Birth Defects Org Art Ser XIII (3B):195–201, 1977
Hartfield JK Jr, Bixler D, Hazen RH: Gingival fibromatosis with sensineural hearing loss: An autosomal dominant trait. Am J Med Genet 22:623–627, 1985

FIBROMATOSIS, JUVENILE-HYALINE

Synonyms. Puretic; Murray; juvenile hyaline fibromatosis; hyalinosis systemic.

Symptoms and Signs. Both sexes. Lesions present at birth or appearing in childhood. Face and neck particularly affected. Small pearly papules or nodules and subcutaneous nodules of variable consistency and degree of mobility with possible ulcerations. Frequently associated gengival fibromatosis. Commonly, genus hypertrophy, flexure contraction of joints. Poor muscle development.

Etiology. Altered glycosaminoglycan synthesis. Sporadic or autosomal recessive inheritance.

Pathology. Lesions contain "chondroid cells" in eosinophilic ground substance in the dermis. Dermal collagen and fibrils decreased. In muscle and bone, presence of hyaline materials.

Diagnostic Procedures. *Biopsy. X-ray skeleton.* Osteolytic lesions (possible).

Therapy. Lesions unresponsive to treatment (including radiotherapy); joint contracture may benefit from steroids.

Prognosis. Tumors recur after removal. Persisting in adult life, disabling from joint contractures.

BIBLIOGRAPHY. Murray J: On three peculiar cases of moluscum fibrosum in one family. Med Chir Trans London 56:235–238, 1873
Whitfield A, Robinson AH: A further report on the remarkable series of cases of moluscum fibrosum in children. Communicated to the Society by Dr. John Murray in 1873. Med Chir Trans London 86:293, 1903
Puretic S, Puretic B, Fiser-Herman M, et al: A unique form of mesenchymaldysplasia. Br J Dermatol 74:8–19, 1962
Gorlin RJ, Cohen MM Jr, Levin LS: Syndromes of Head and Neck, pp 849–850. New York, Oxford, 1990
Burton JL: Disorders of connective tissue. In Champion RH, Burton JL, Ebling FJG (eds): Rook/Wilkinson/Ebling Textbook of Dermatology, 5th ed, pp 1805–1809. Oxford, Blackwell Scientific, 1992

FIBROMUSCULAR DYSPLASIA

Synonym. FMD. See Fibromatosis, congenital, generalized.

Symptoms and Signs. Prevalent in females; onset from childhood to middle and later age. Extremely variable manifestations, including blood hypertension, stroke, claudication, myocardial infarction shortly after onset of manifestations.

Etiology. Unknown. Consistent with autosomal dominant inheritance.

Pathology. Small and medium-sized arterial lesions presenting as multiple, small, saccular, dilatations with areas of destruction and fragmentation of the media, alternated with rings of hyperplasia of muscular and fibrous elements of arterial wall. Carotid, cerebral, renal, mesenteric coronary, and iliac arteries may be affected.

Diagnostic Procedures. *Artery biopsy.* See Pathology. According to symptoms. *Angiography.* Lesions of distal two thirds of renal arteries often appearing as a string of beads; alterations may also be found at carotid, coeliac axis, mesenteric, and iliac vessels.

Therapy. Symptomatic. Treatment of hypertension.

Prognosis. Early death.

BIBLIOGRAPHY. Hunt JC, Harrison EG Jr, Kincaid OW, et al: Idiopathic fibrous and fibromuscular stenosis of the renal arteries associated with hypertension. Mayo Clin Proc 37:181–216, 1962
Sandok BA, Houser OW, Baka HL Jr, et al: Fibromuscular dysplasia: Neurologic disorders associated with diseases involving the great vessels of the neck. Arch Neurol 24:462–466, 1971
Rushton AR: The genetics of fibromuscular dysplasia. Arch Intern Med 140:233–236, 1980
Beighton P: Heritable Disorders of Connective Tissue, 5th ed, p 525. St Louis, CV Mosby, 1993

FIBROSIS, MEDIASTINAL IDIOPATHIC

Synonym. Sclerosing mediastinitis; including fibrosclerosis multifocal and retroperitoneal fibrosis familial. See Ormond.

Symptoms. Onset in middle life or later. Dyspnea; cephalalgia; tinnitus; disturbed sensorium; nosebleed; hemophysis. Occasionally, intermittent claudication. In some families associated retoperitoneal fibrosis (see Ormond); sclerosing cholangitis; Riedel thyroiditis (see) and pseudotumor orbitae.

Signs. Facial edema and dusky color; superior vena cava obstruction. Considered a possible manifestation of a collagen disease.

Etiology. Multiple. In most cases, end stage of chronic granulomatous conditions (e.g., histoplasmosis, tuberculosis). Other causes: collagenopathies; methysergide treatment. Autosomal recessive inheritance reported in some families.

Pathology. Mass or plaque of fibrous tissue located in the anterior area of upper mediastinum. Various structures in the area can be compressed: superior vena cava; innominate veins; aorta; pulmonary vessels; esophagus. Dense collagen tissue with variable infiltration of plasma cells, eosinophils.

Diagnostic Procedures. *X-ray.* Widening of upper part of mediastinum. *Biopsy.* See Pathology.

Therapy. For methysergide-induced type, discontinuation of drug. Corticosteroids, surgery.

Prognosis. Progressive condition evolving over years.

BIBLIOGRAPHY. Barrett NR: Idiopathic mediastinal fibrosis. Br J Surg 46:207–218, 1958
Feigin DS, Eggleston JC, Siegelman SS: The multiple roentgen manifestations of sclerosing mediastinitis. Johns Hopkins Med J 144:1–8 1979

Goldbach P, Mohsenifar Z, Salik AI: Familial mediastinal fibrosis associated with seronegative spondylarthropathy. Arthritis Rheum 26:221–225, 1983

Weatherall DJ, Ledingham JGG, Warrell DA (eds): Oxford Textbook of Medicine, 3rd ed, p 3246. Oxford, Oxford Med Pub, 1996

FIBROSITIS

Synonyms. Fibromyositis; rheumatoid myositis; periarticular fibrositis, rheumatism, nonarticular. See S.A.P.H.O.

Symptoms. Pain; stiffness; soreness, especially neck, shoulders, chest, and lower back muscles, with shifting pattern over years, and never uniform over an entire segment. No evidence of associated articular diseases, muscular weakness, atrophy, or neurologic symptoms. Usually accompanied by increased fatigability. All symptoms are worse in morning, relieved by activity, enhanced by cold, dampness, or emotional factors.

Signs. All objective signs are absent except the possible presence of "trigger point," especially painful subcutaneous nodules and spasm of muscles, or segment of muscles.

Etiology. Two types of this syndrome may be recognized: (1) primary type (or true fibrositis) without any underlying systemic disease; (2) secondary type due to rheumatic, infective, bone diseases. For the primary type various hypotheses postulated but not completely satisfactory: (1) local pathology "trigger point"; (2) referred pain from minor and not directly expressed pathologic conditions; (3) psychosomatic. Each of these factors may play a role in this syndrome and often more than one at the same time. (See Polymyalgia.)

Pathology. No pathologic findings have been definitely demonstrated. Some differences have been observed, however, between a control group and fibrositic patients. Fat droplets in muscle fibers; increase of intestinal connective tissue nuclei; lymphocytes and plasma cell infiltrates in painful regions.

Diagnostic Procedures. *Laboratory tests.* All negative. *X-ray.* Negative.

Therapy. Reassurance of the patient on the benign nature of the disease, with explanation of its nature and psychological treatment of tension and other psychic factors (primary or superimposed). Analgesic and antispasmodic treatment; systemic or topical; salicylates and anesthetic; heat; massage.

BIBLIOGRAPHY. Gowers WR: A lecture on lumbago: Its lessons and analogues. Br Med J 1:117–121, 1904

Stockman R: Rheumatism and Arthritis. Edinburgh, Livingstone, 1920

Campbell SM, Clark S, Tindall EA, et al: Clinical characteristics of fibrositis. 1. A "blinded" controlled study of symptoms and tender points. Arthritis Rheum 26:817–824, 1983

Wolfe V, Smithe HA, Yunus MB, et al: The American college of rheumathology. 1990: Criteria for the classification of fibromyalgia. Arthritis Rheumatol 133:160–172, 1990

FICKLER-WINKLER

Synonyms. Olivopontocerebellar II. See Dejerine-Thomas.

Symptoms and Signs. Onset at about 50 years of age. Those of Menzel (see) differing from it in lack of involuntary movements and of sensory changes. In one of the families reported albinism.

Etiology. Autosomal recessive inheritance or pleiotropism.

BIBLIOGRAPHY. Fickler A: Klinische und pathologish-anatomische. Beitraege zu den Erkrankungeer des Kleinhirns. Dtsch Z Nervenheilk 41:306–375, 1911

Winkler C: A case of olivopontine cerebellar atrophy and our concep-

tions of neo- and paleo-cerebellum. Schweiz Arch Neurol Psychiat 13:196–204, 1923

Skre H, Berg K: Cerebellar ataxia and total albinism: A kindred suggesting pleiotropism or linkage. Clin Genet 5:194–204, 1974

FILATOV-DUKES

Synonyms. Dukes; exanthem subitum; fourth disease; pseudorubella; roseola infantum; rose rash.

Symptoms. Onset usually in spring, autumn in children under 2 years of age. Symptoms present in 30% of affected. Mostly sporadic, occasionally limited, epidemic. Incubation period 10–15 days. High temperature (39.5–40°C) lasting 3–4 days without systemic symptoms, except in some cases with convulsions.

Signs. During fever fall or immediately after, rash of pink macular papule arising first on neck and trunk and spreading to face and limbs. Rash lasts 1–2 days. Cervical adenopathy.

Etiology. Human herpes virus 6 (HHV-6).

Diagnostic Procedures. Blood. First 2 days leukocytosis; then leukopenia with relative lymphocytosis.

Therapy. Symptomatic. Soothing bath.

Prognosis. Benign form, completely cured; rare cases of encephalitis.

BIBLIOGRAPHY. Filatov N: Lektsii ob ostrykh infektsionnykh bolezniakh detei. Moskva, 1887 p 113

Dukes C: On the confusion of two different diseases under the name of rubeola (rose-rash) Lancet 2:89–94, 1900

Highet AS, Kurtz J: Viral infections. In Champion RH, Burton JL, Ebling FJG (eds): Rook/Wilkinson/Ebling Textbook of Dermatology, 5th ed, p 895. Oxford, Blackwell Scientific, 1992

FILIPPI

Synonyms. Syndactyly I; microcephaly—mental retardation.

Symptoms and Signs. Both sexes. Severe physical and mental retardation. Syndactyly. Fingers and toes. Microcephaly. Nose broad base.

Etiology. Possibly autosomal recessive inheritance.

BIBLIOGRAPHY. Filippi G: Unusual facial appearance, microcephaly, growth and mental retardation and syndactyly: a new syndrome? Am J Med Genet 22:821–824, 1985

FINCHER

Symptoms and Signs. Rare. Association of sciatica, headache, and presence of blood on lumbar puncture.

Etiology and Pathology. Tumors of the cauda equina, usually ependimoma also; may be caused by extramedullary tumors, causing subarachnoid hemorrhage.

BIBLIOGRAPHY. Fincher EF: Spontaneous subarachnoid hemorrhage in intradual tumors of the lumbar sac: A clinical syndrome. J Neurosurg 8:576–589, 1951

Gil R, Lefevre JP, Les hémorrhagies Méningées des épendimomes encéphaliques et médullaires. Bordeaux Méd 4:325–340, 1971

FINGERPRINT BODY MYOPATHY

Synonyms. Myopathy finger body, benign.

Symptoms and Signs. Those of congenital myopathies (see Goebel). Prominent mental retardation.

Etiology. Possibly sex-linked inheritance.

Diagnostic Procedures. *Muscle biopsy, EMG.*

Therapy. Symptomatic.

Prognosis. Benign condition, not progressive.

BIBLIOGRAPHY. Engel AG, Angelini C, Gomer MR: Fingerprint body myopathy—a newly recognized congenital muscle disease. Mayo Clin Proc 47:377–388, 1972

Fardeau M, Tome FMS, Derambure S: Familial fingerprint body myopathy. Arch Neurol 33:724–725, 1976

Goebel HH, Lenard HG: Congenital myopathies. In Handbook of Clinical Neurology, vol 18: The Myopathies, p 331. Rowland LP, Di Mauro S (eds): Elsevier, Amsterdam, 1992

FINNISH NEPHROSIS

Synonym. Congenital nephrotic; nephrotic, Finnish.

Symptoms. High incidence in Finland (incidence 1/8000) or in people of Finnish extraction. High frequency of maternal toxemia. Onset in first days or weeks of life. Clinical manifestations identical with those of Epstein (nephrosis) that never are evident before the age of 18 months. In 12% of cases pyloric stenosis is the presenting symptom.

Etiology. Autosomal recessive. Absence of heparin sulfate anionic sites in glomerular basement membrane. Disturbed metabolism of type IV collagen.

Pathology. Renal biopsy. Microcystic cortex and renal tubules.

Diagnostic Procedures. Prenatal diagnosis. High α-fetoprotein in *amniotic fluid. Blood and urine* chemical changes identical with Epstein.

Therapy. Steroids and immunosuppressive drugs ineffective.

Prognosis. Death usually before 1 year of age.

BIBLIOGRAPHY. Hallmann N, Hjelt L, Ahvenainen EK: Nephrotic syndrome in newborn and young infants. Ann Paediatr Fenn 2:227–241, 1956

Vernier RL, Klein DJ, Sisson SP, et al: Heparin sulfate-rich anionic sites in human glomerular basement membrane. N Engl J Med 309:1001–1009, 1983

Grahame-Smith HN, Ward PS, Jones RD: Finnish type congenital nephrotic syndrome in twins: Presentation with piloric stenosis. J R Soc Med 81:358, 1988

Perheentupa J: The Finnish disease heritage: A personal look. Acta Paed. 84:1094–1099 1995

FIRST ARCH SYNDROME(S)

This is used as an all-inclusive title to embrace numerous developmental errors of facial bones that have been described under different names. This grouping is justified since all these syndromes are considered as variable manifestations of one basic development error, a faulty vascularization of the first arch during embryonal life (abnormalities of stapedial artery). The different manifestations of the various syndromes depend on the speed with which collateral circulation develops and more or less compensates for this defect.

Etiology. Unknown; a common genetic defect, dominant with variable penetrance will be at the basis of all those syndromes, and the compensatory mechanism (anastomosis) determines its degree of penetrance and consequently the various clinical aspects.

1. Treacher-Collins
2. Pierre Robin
3. Franceschetti-Klein
4. Hypertelorism
5. Goldenhar (?)
6. Cleft lip and cleft palate
7. Some deformities of external and middle ear including deafness

The last two may also occur as a result of environmental agents and various recognized chromosomal disorders, and such cases must not be included in the first arch syndrome.

BIBLIOGRAPHY. McKenzie J: The first arch syndrome. Arch Dis Child 33:477–486, 1958

McKenzie J: The first arch syndrome. Dev Med Child Neurol 8:55–66, 1966

Forfar SC, Arneil GC: Textbook of Pediatrics, 2nd ed. Edinburgh, Churchill-Livingstone, 1978

FISCHER-SARGENT-DRACHMAN

Synonyms. Choreoathetosis, familial inverted; infantile choreoathetosis of Fischer.

Symptoms and Signs. From infancy. Choreic movements predominantly affecting the legs and affecting gait. Normal imtellectual development; no seizures. Occasionally signs of pyramidal tract involvement.

Etiology. Autosomal dominant inheritance.

Prognosis. Progressive course.

BIBLIOGRAPHY. Fischer M, Sargent J, Drachman D: Familial inverted choreoathetosis. Neurology 29:1627–1631, 1979

FISHER (C.M.)

Synonyms. One and a half.

Symptoms and Signs. Both sexes. Onset usually after 20 years of age. Presenting symptoms: vertigo, diplopia, dizziness, difficulty in walking, slurred speech. Development of lateral gaze palsy in one direction with internuclear ophthalmoplegia (INO) in the other direction. In the complete form: one eye fixed at the midline for all lateral movements; the other can only abduct and shows horizontal jerk nystagmus in abduction. Possibly associated other numerous ocular and neurologic signs.

Etiology. Brain stem infarction, multiple sclerosis, pontine glioma-arteriovenous malformation, pontine hemorrhage, basilar artery aneurysm, neoplasia, or metastasis.

Pathology. Unilateral lesion of lower part of dorsal pontine tegmentum affecting ipsilateral paramedian pontine reticular formation, abducens nucleus and internuclear fibers of ipsilateral medial longitudinal fasciculus.

BIBLIOGRAPHY. Bender MG, Weinstein EA: Dissociated monocular nystagmus with paresis of horizontal ocular movements. Arch Ophthamol 21:266–272, 1939

Fisher CM: Some neuro-ophthalmological observations: J Neurol Neurosurg Psychiatr 30:383–392, 1967

Wall M, Vray SH: The one and a half syndrome: A unilateral disorder of the pontine tegmentum. A study of 20 cases and review of the literature. Neurology 33:971, 1983

FISHER (M.)

Synonyms. Guillain-Barré variant; Miller-Fisher; Bickerstaff; ophthalmoplegia-ataxia-areflexia; encephalomyeloradiculopathy disseminated; brain stem areflexia.

Symptoms. Reported in male patients 38–65 years of age. Starting as a respiratory complaint (sore throat; tightness in the chest; pneumonitis; fever; severe headache); after 3–4 days; acute external ophthalmoplegia usually total; diplopia; unilateral or bilateral facial paralysis; cerebellar ataxia; migratory paresthesias of trunk and arms. No mental changes or sensory impairment (or the latter may be minimal); no motor weakness of extremities. Condition may evolve into apneic coma and complete paralysis of motor function of cranial nerves.

Signs. Tendon reflexes abolished; pupillary reflexes sluggish; sensory changes minimal or absent.

Etiology. Viral infection with hypersensitivity (?) of nervous system. May be considered a variant or an atypical form of the Guillain-Barré syndrome.

Pathology. None reported.

Diagnostic Procedures. *Spinal fluid.* Marked albumin-cytologic dissociation. *EEG. CT brain scan* (to rule out hemorrhage). *Acoustic evoked responses.* Preserved. *Motor and sensory nerve conduction studies and EMG.* Electrodiagnostic abnormalities characteristic of an axonal neuropathy or a neuronopathy with predominant sensory nerve changes in the limbs and motor damage in the cranial nerves. The pattern of abnormalities is distinct from the usual features seen in the Guillain-Barré.

Therapy. Cortisone may reduce the acute symptoms.

Prognosis. Self-limited disease of 10–12 weeks, duration with neurologic recovery complete or residual minor paresthesias and horizontal diplopia for some time after recovery.

BIBLIOGRAPHY. Fisher M: An unusual variant of acute idiopathic polyneuritis (syndrome of ophthalmoplegia, ataxia, and areflexia). N Engl J Med 255:57–65, 1956
Bickerstaff ER: Brain stem encephalitis (Bickerstaff's encephalitis). In Vinken PJ, Branyn GN (eds): Handbook of Clinical Neurology, vol 34, pp 605–609. Amsterdam, North Holland, 1978
Al-Din ASN, Jamil A, Shakir R: Coma and brain stem areflexia in brain stem areflexia (Fisher's syndrome). Br Med J 291:535–536, 1985
Fross RD, Daube JR: Neuropathy in the Miller-Fisher syndrome: Clinical and electrophysiologic findings. Neurology 37:1493–1498, 1987

FISHER-VOLAVSEK

Synonyms. Palmo-plantaris keratoma-syringomyelia; onychogryphosis-syringomyelia.

Symptoms. Both sexes affected, present from birth. Congenital malformations (see Signs). Later, developing symptoms of syringomyelia.

Signs. Onychogryphosis; sparse hair of scalp, brows, and lashes. Thickening of terminal digits.

Etiology. Unknown; autosomal dominant inheritance.

BIBLIOGRAPHY. Fisher H: Familiär hereditares Vorkommen von Keratoma Palmare et Plantare. Nagelveranderungen, Haaranomalien und Verdickung der Endglieder der Finger und Zehen in 5 Generationen. Dermatol Z 32:114–142, 1921
Volavsek W: Zur Klinik der Nagelveränderungen und Palmarkeratozen bei Syringomyelie. Arch Dermatol Syph 182:52–57, 1941
Gorlin RJ, Sedano H, Anderson VE: The syndrome of palmar-plantar prekeratosis and premature periodontal destruction of the teeth. J Pediatr 65:895–908, 1964

FISH EYE

Synonyms. Carlson; corneal opacities-dyslipoproteinemia; lipoproteinemia (dys)—corneal opacities. See Tangier and hyperlipoproteinemia.

Symptoms. Described for the first time (man and three daughters) in Finland. Visual impairment (only clinical problem).

Signs. Marked corneal opacities. Corneal appearance resembles those of a boiled fish.

Etiology. Unknown. Probably autosomal dominant inheritance.

Diagnostic Procedures. *Blood.* Cholesterol and percentage of cholesterol esters normal, HDL reduced. Triglycerides elevated: VLDL and LDH triglycerides very high. Lecithincholesterol acyltransferase (LCAT) activity normal or reduced; lipoprotein and hepatic lipases normal; very-low density triglycerides and cholesterol raised.

Therapy. Corneal transplantation.

Prognosis. Unknown. Except for visual impairment general conditions are good.

BIBLIOGRAPHY. Carlson LA, Philipson B: Fish eye disease: A new familial condition with massive corneal opacities and dyslipoproteinaemia. Lancet 2:921–923, 1979
Rees J, Stocks J, Schoulders C, et al: Restriction enzyme analysis of the apolipoprotein A-1 gene in fish eye disease and Tangier disease. Acta Med Scand 215:235–237, 1984
Sketting G, Prydz H: An amino acid exchange in exon I of the human lecithin: Cholesterol acyltransferase (LCAT) gene is associated with fish eye disease. Biochem Biophys Res Commun 182:583–587, 1992
Winder AF: Disorders of lipid and lipoprotein metabolism. In Garner A, Klintworth GK (eds): Pathobiology of Ocular Disease: A Dynamic Approach, 2nd ed, p 1109. New York, Marcel Dekker, 1994

FITCH

Synonyms. Andre; oto-palato-digital type II; cranio-oro-digital; facio-palato-osseus; OPD 2. See Taybi.

Symptoms and Signs. Full syndrome in males. Hypertelorism, frontal bossing, broad nasal bridge, downslanting palpebrae, midface hypoplasia, ears low set, mandibular micrognathia, hearing loss in several cases. From normal mental development to mental retardation. Thorax small, pectus excavatum (occasionally). Short stature, multiple skeletal anomalies. Minor or absent manifestations in female (abnormalities of hands and feet). Separation of form 2 suggested by severity of fibula, clavicle, and rib alterations.

Etiology. X-linked inheritance.

Pathology. Normal chondro-osseus morphology.

Diagnostic Procedures. *Prenatal echography. X-rays.* Multiple skeletal anomalies. Head, thorax, spine (flattened vertebrae) limbs.

Therapy. Symptomatic.

Prognosis. Death usually owing to respiratory infection within first 5 months of life or later (2–3 years).

BIBLIOGRAPHY. Fitch N, Jequier S, Papageorgion A: A familial syndrome of cranial, facial oral and limbs anomalies. Clin Genet 10:226–231, 1976
Andre M, Vigneron J, Didier F: Abnormal facies, cleft palate and generalized dysostosis: a lethal X-linked syndrome. J Pediatr 98:747–752, 1981
Brewster TTG, Lachman RS, Kushner DC, et al: Oto-palato-digital syndrome type 2. Am J Med Genet 20:249–254, 1985
Ogata T, Matsuo N, Nishimura G, et al: Oto-palato-digital syndrome type II: Evidence for intramembranous ossification. Am J Med Genet 36:226–231, 1990
Stratton RF, Bluestone DL: Oto-palato-digital syndrome type II with X-linked cerebellar hypoplasia/hydrocephalus. Am J Med Genet 41:169–172, 1991

FITZGERALD-WILLIAMS-FLAUJEAC TRAIT

Synonym. Kininogen (high molecular weight) deficiency.

Symptoms and Signs. Laboratory curiosity.

Etiology. Autosomal recessive.

Diagnostic Procedures. *Blood.* Prolonged clotting time and partial thromboplastin time. Patient plasma corrects defects in plasma deficient in high molecular weight kininogen.

Therapy. None.

Prognosis. Good.

BIBLIOGRAPHY. Waldman R, Abrahazam J: Fitzgerald Factor: A heretofore unrecognized coagulation factor. Blood 46:761, 1975
Wuepper KD, Miller DR, LaCombe MJ: Flaujeac trait deficiency of human plasma kininogen. J Clin Invest 56:1663, 1975
Cheung PP, Cannizzaro LA, Colman RW: Chromosomal mapping of human kinogen (KNG) to 3q26qter. Cytogen Cell Genet 59:24–26, 1992

FITZ-HUGH AND CURTIS

Synonyms. Stajano; Curtis; gonococcal perihepatitis; subcostal; veneral hepatitis.

Symptoms. Onset in young women 20–30 years of age. Fever may be present. Right upper abdominal pain. Vaginal discharge may be present or absent, as well as pelvic pain.

Signs. Friction rub of hepatic region may be present. Pelvic inflammation and discharge; bartholinitis may be present or minimal. Jaundice (rare).

Etiology. Gonococcal or Chlamydia perihepatitis.

Pathology. Adhesion of the liver and abdominal wall. In one case, necrosis of the liver cells, but few detailed reports of pathologic changes.

Diagnostic Procedures. *Vaginal smear.* For identification of infective agent. *Culture. X-ray. Ultrasonography. Gallbladder studies.* Normal gallbladder, occasionally pericholecystitis.

Therapy. Penicillin.

Prognosis. Excellent with treatment.

BIBLIOGRAPHY. Stajano C: La reaction frenica en ginecologia. Sem Med Buenos Aires 27:243–248, 1920
Curtis AH: Cause of adhesions in right upper quadrant. JAMA 94:1221–1222, 1930
Fitz-Hugh T Jr: Acute gonococcic peritonitis of right upper quadrant in women. JAMA 102:2094–2906, 1934
Vickers FN, Maloney PJ: Gonococcal perihepatitis: Report of three cases with comment on diagnosis and treatment. Arch Intern Med 114:120–123, 1964
Katzman DK, Friedman IM, McDonald CA, et al: Chlamidia trachomatis Fitz Hugh-Curtis syndrome without salpingitis in female adolescents. Am J Dis Child 142:996–998, 1988

FLAJANI

Synonyms. Basedow; von Basedow; Bergie; Graves; March; Parry; thyrotoxicosis; hyperthyroidism; exophthalmic goiter. See Graves ophthalmopathy.

Symptoms. Female predominance, ratio 4:1; onset in third to fifth decade of life. Emotional instability; nervousness; palpitation; intolerance to heat; incessant sweating; occasionally, anorexia; nausea; vomiting; diarrhea; later dyspnea.

Signs. Skin warm and moist; hyperpigmentation. Bilateral (seldom unilateral) exophthalmos; infrequent blinking (Stillwag sign); absence of brow wrinkling when looking up (Joffroy sign); lid lag (Graefe sign); lack of convergence (Moebius sign); thyroid enlarged bilaterally, soft and margins indistinct. Increased cardiac rate; enlargement of heart;

hyperreflexia (recording of Achilles tendon reflex time). Pretibial myxedema (rare). Acropachy (rare).

Etiology. Primary thyroid hyperplasia, occasionally precipitated or initiated by trauma or stress. Metabolic; immunologic, toxic disorders. Sporadic or familial component (40%) autosomal recessive inheritance with relative sex limitation to female.

Pathology. Thyroid enlarged, smooth, elastic, friable; deep fissure in sulci giving nodular aspect. Hyperplasia and hypertrophy of acinar cells; vesicular nuclei; depletion of colloid; enlarged intrafollicular spaces; increased lymph follicles.

Diagnostic Procedures. *Basal metabolic rate.* Increased. *Blood.* TSH (a normal value incompatitible with diagnosis). Increased protein-bound iodine; increased butanol-extracted iodine fraction; serum T4, T3 (T4-binding globulin) levels, and antithyroid antibodies, lymphocytosis, reduced cholesterol level; occasionally macrocytic anemia. *Scan.* Increased uptake of radioactive iodine, and T3; repeat scanning after thyroid-stimulating hormone (TSH). *EKG phonocardiogram. EEG.*

Therapy. Radioactive iodine; iodide; antithyroid drugs; combination of blockade and sedation; lithium carbonate; X-ray treatment; surgery (partial resection of thyroid).

Prognosis. If untreated, progression of symptoms to cardiac failure, through remission and relapses, spontaneous cure possible. Good results with treatments.

BIBLIOGRAPHY. Flajani G: Osservazione LXVII: Sopra un tumor freddo nell'anterior parte del dotto detto broncocele. In Collezione d'Osservazioni e Riflessioni di Chirurgia, G. Flajani, Vol. 3, Rome, p 270. S. Michele A. Ripa Presso Lino Contedini, 1802
Parry CH: Collections from the Unpublished Papers of the Late Caleb Hillier Parry, vol 2, pp 11–28. London, 1825
Graves RJ: Clinical lectures. London Med Surg J 7:516, 1835
von Basedow CA: Exophthalmos durch Hypertrophie des Zellgewebes in der Augenhohle. Wochenschr ges Heilkunde 13:197–204; 220–228, 1840
McKenzie JM, Zakarija M: Hyperthyroidism. In De Groot LJ (ed): Endocrinology, 3rd ed, pp 682–711. Philadelphia, WB Saunders, 1995

FLECK

Synonyms. Hypohidrosis—diabetes insipidus.

Symptoms and Signs. Hypohidrosis, hypotrichosis, anodontia, syndactyly, coloboma; symptoms of diabetes insipidus (see) and of hematopoietic disorders.

Etiology. Unknown.

BIBLIOGRAPHY. Fleck F: Klinische Beobachtungen einer ungewoehnlichen, sporadischen Form von ektodermal-mesodermer Keimblattdysplasie. Dermatol Wochenschr 132:994–1007, 1955

FLECKED RETINA

See also Kandori.

Symptoms and Signs. Normal peripheral visual fields. Slightly abnormal dark adaptation. Abnormal electrooculogram. High incidence of macular abnormalities. Stationary status of minor abnormalities of peripheral retina function. Similar fluorescein staining patterns (fluorescein angiography).

Etiology. Includes three ophthalmoscopically distinct entities: (1) fundus flavimaculatus (suggested autosomal recessive type of inheritance); (2) fundus colloid bodies or drusen (possibly familial congenital condition); (3) fundus albipunctatus (possibly familial congenital condition).

Pathology. Fundus flavimaculatus: distinctive changes in the pigmented epithelium; normal neuroepithelium, Bruch membrane, and choroid. Lesion represented by deposition of acid mucopolysaccharides. Fundus colloid bodies: round or oval lesions of various sizes frequently with calcification and found in far periphery. They may be confluent and form different conglomerate patterns. Fundus albipunctatus: Uniform, dotlike lesion never confluent.

BIBLIOGRAPHY. Krill AE, Klien BA: Flecked retina syndrome. Arch Ophthalmol 74:496–508, 1965
Klien BA, Krill AE: Fundus flavimaculatus. Am J Ophthalmol 64:3–23, 1967
Sabel Aish SF, Dajani B: Benign familiar fleck retina. Br J Ophthalmol 64:652–659, 1980

FLEGEL

Synonym. Hyperkeratosis—lenticularis perstans. See Kyrle.

Symptoms and Signs. Both sexes. Onset after 30 years of age. Starts on dorsa of feet and in some cases successively involves the legs, thighs, arms, and dorsum of hands and seldom the trunk. Pink, reddish brown scaly papules (1–5 mm).

Etiology. Autosomal dominant inheritance.

Pathology. Parakeratotic hyperkeratosis over a flattened epidermis. Lymphocytic infiltration only subpapulae. Lack of Odlan bodies in affected epidermis.

Prognosis. In some families reported high incidence of skin tumors (squamous, basal cell carcinoma) in nonaffected areas.

BIBLIOGRAPHY. Flegel H: Hyperkeratosis lenticularis perstans. Hautarzt 9:362–364, 1958
Beau SF: The genetics of hyperkeratosis lenticularis perstans. Arch Dermatol 106:102, 1982
Griffiths WAD, Leight IM, Marks R: Disorders of cheratinization. In Champion RH, Burton JL, Ebling FJG (eds): Rook/Wilkinson/Ebling Textbook of Dermatology, 5th ed, pp 1367–1369. Oxford, Blackwell Scientific, 1992

FLEISCHNER

Synonyms. Disc-like atelectasis; reflex atelectasis. Eponym used to indicate not a syndrome but the radiologic linear or discoid shadow located in the lower third of one lung or both lungs. Shadow indicates the presence of atelectasis due to hypomobility of diaphragm because of thoracic or abdominal disease.

BIBLIOGRAPHY. Fleischner F: Plattenförmige Atelecthasen in der Unterlappen der Lunge. Fortschr Geb Roentgen 54:315–321, 1936

FLEISHER

Synonyms. Hypogammaglobulinemia-isolated growth hormone deficiency-X linked; growth hormone deficiency—hypogammaglobulinemia; agammaglobulinemia-growth hormone deficiency.

Symptoms. From early age recurrent infections, especially sinopulmonary.

Signs. Delayed puberty. Short stature.

Etiology. X-linked inheritance.

Diagnostic Procedures. *Blood.* Marked deficiency of immunoglobulins. Reduction or lack of circulating B-lymphocytes. Absence of specific

antibodies production. Deficient response of growth hormone to insulin, arginin and levodopa. *X-rays.* Retarded bone age.

Therapy. Globulin administration. Growth hormone.

Prognosis. Fair with treatment.

BIBLIOGRAPHY. Fleisher TA, White RM, Broder S, et al: X-linked hypogammaglobulinemia and isolated growth hormone deficiency. N Engl J Med 302:1429–1434, 1980
Monago V, Mahgnie M, Terrasciano L, et al: X-linked agammaglobulinemia and isolated growth hormone deficiency. Acta Paediatr Scand 80:563–566, 1991
Lukens JN: Immune deficiency diseases, inherited and acquired. In Lee GR, Bithel TC, Foerster J, et al (eds): Wintrobe's Clinical Hematology, 9th ed, p 1687. Philadelphia, Lea & Febiger, 1993

FLETCHER TRAIT

Synonym. Prekallikrein deficiency; PK deficiency.

Symptoms and Signs. Presently a laboratory curiosity. The physiological importance of the kallikrein activities remains to be assesed.

Etiology. Autosomal recessive.

Diagnostic Procedures. *Blood.* Clotting time and partial thromboplastin time prolonged, corrected by preincubation with kaolin and phospholipid.

Prognosis. Good.

BIBLIOGRAPHY. Wuepper KD: Prekallikrein deficiency in man. J Exp Med 138:1345, 1973
Seligsohn U, Griffin JH: Contact activation and factor XI. In Scriver CR, Beaudet AL, Sly WS, et al: The Metabolic and Molecular Bases of Inherited Disease, 7th ed, pp 3293–3295. New York, McGraw-Hill, 1995

FLOATING-HARBOR*

Synonyms. Pelletier-Leisti

Symptoms and Signs. Both sexes. Birthweight and length below fifth percentile, triangular facies, prominent occiput, deep set eyes, large nose; thin lips, short philtrum; wide downturned mouth; short neck; hirsutism; brachydactyly and clinodactyly; loose joints; hypoplastic penis; mental retardation, and speech delay.

Etiology. Autosomal dominant (?).

BIBLIOGRAPHY. Pelletier G, Feingold M: Case report 1: Syndrome Ident 1:8–9, 1973
Leisti et al: The Floating-Harbor syndrome. Birth Defects 11:305–309, 1975
Gorlin RJ, Cohen MM Jr, Levin LS: Syndromes of Head and Neck, p 914. New York, Oxford Univ Press, 1990

FLOPPY EYELID

Symptoms and Signs. Usually in obese individual development of a soft rubbery tarsus that allows eversion of upper eyelid and causes papillary conjunctivitis. Keratoconus.

Etiology. Eyelid eversion during sleep. Unilateral according to prefered side, bilateral in patients who sleep in prone position.

BIBLIOGRAPHY. Parrunovic A, Ilic B: Floppy eyelid syndrome associated with keratoconus. Br J Ophthalmol 72:634–635, 1988
Negris R: Floppy eyelid syndrome associated keratoconus. J Am Ophthal Assoc 63:316–319, 1992

---

*Name derived by the double description from patients from Boston Floating, and Harbor General Hospitals.

FLOPPY INFANT SYNDROMES

Synonyms. Limp child.

1. Myelopathic and neuropathic causes
   Werding-Hoffmann
   Oppenheim
   Walton
   Guillain-Barré
   Poliomyelitis
   Spinal tumors
   Transverse myelopathy, traumatic or of different nature

2. Encephalopathic causes
   Mental deficiency (especially Down)
   Progressive encephalopathy (especially Tay-Sachs)
   Brain tumors
   Riley-Day
   Cerebral palsies

3. Neuromuscular transmission
   Erb-Goldflam
   Abnormal neuromuscular junctions

4. Myopathic causes
   Infantile muscular dystrophies
   Polymyositis syndrome
   Glycogen storage
   Shy-Magee
   Universal muscular hypoplasias

5. Tendon and ligament syndromes
   Ehlers-Danlos syndrome
   Arachnodactyly
   Congenital laxity of ligaments
   Arthrogryposis

6. Osteogenic causes
   Osteogenesis imperfecta syndrome
   Rickets
   Barlow
   Parrot

7. Nonmuscular causes
   Malnutrition
   Vitamin deficiencies
   Chronic diseases
   Acute illness or infections
   Endocrinopathies (especially hypothyroidism and hypopituitarism)
   Metabolic syndromes

BIBLIOGRAPHY. Walton JN: The limp child. J Neurol Neurosurg Psychiatry 20:144–154, 1957
Paine RS: The future of the "Floppy Infant." A follow-up study of 133 patients. Dev Med Child 5:115–124, 1963
Walton J: The floppy infant syndrome. In Weatherall DJ, Ledingham JGG, Warrell DA (eds): Oxford Textbook of Medicine, 3rd ed, pp 4150–4151. Oxford, Oxford Med Pub, 1996

FLOPPY VALVE

Synonyms. Midsystolic click—late systolic murmur; click murmur; billowing mitral valve. See Marfan; mitral valve prolapse; Barlow (JB).

Symptoms. The most common valvular heart disease (3% of the population). Female prevalence. Chest pain, nonexertional and sometimes prolonged; weakness, fatigue, palpitations, light headedness, dyspnea. Sometimes symptoms are vague or absent.

Signs. Many patients may present thoracic or other skeletal malformations. One or more midsystolic clicks, which generally occur 0.1 second or more after the first heart sound; late systolic murmur. Dysrhythmias, low blood pressure. Tall slender body; narrow chest, pectus excavatum; hypomastia, occasionally joint hypermobility; spontaneous pneumotorax.

Etiology/Pathology. Autosomal dominant inheritance. Myxomatous degeneration of the mitral valve. Often the syndrome is associated with Marfan syndrome, osteogenesis imperfecta, and other connective tissue diseases.

Diagnostic Procedures. *ECG.* T-wave inversions in leads II, III, and aVF and occasionally in V5 and V6; ventricular ectopic beats; supraventricular tachycardia. *Echocardiography.* Typical findings. *Cardiac catheterization.* Abnormalities in left ventriculography studies. Evaluation for presence of bacterial endocarditis. *X-rays.* Cardiomegaly; minimal left atrial enlargement. Ballooning of posterior leaflet of mitral valve. *Two-dimensional Doppler, 24-hour ECG monitoring.*

Therapy. Beta-adrenergic blockade; antiarrhythmic therapy; prophylaxis against endocarditis at the time of dental or surgical procedures. Drugs that may cause tachycardia, a reduction in peripheral vascular resistance, or a reduction in venous return can increase the prolapse. Progressive mitral regurgitation requiring valve replacement rarely appears.

Prognosis. In most patients the clinical course is benign. The incidence of complications is around 15%. These include progressive mitral regurgitation, bacterial endocarditis, ventricular arrhythmias. In some cases sudden death.

BIBLIOGRAPHY. Barlow JN et al: The significance of late systolic murmur. Am Heart J 66:443, 1963
Barlow JB, Pocock WA: Billowing, floppy, prolapsed or flail mitral valves. Am J Cardiol 55:501–502, 1985
Levy D, Savage D: Prevalence and clinical features of mitral valve prolapse. Am Heart J 113:1281–1290, 1987
Gaasch WH, O'Rourke RA, Cohn LH, et al: Mitral valve disease. In Nugent EW, Plauth Edwards JE, Schlant RC, Alexander RW: Hurst's The Heart, 8th ed, pp 1502–1510. New York, McGraw-Hill, 1994

FLUCKIGER

Synonym. Cyanosis—digital clubbing; hepatopathy.

Symptoms. Both sexes, all ages affected; most frequent in children. Cyanosis with or without dyspnea; clubbing of fingers develops after initiation of hepatic cirrhosis.

Etiology. The possible development of arteriovenous fistulas in the lungs owing to release of a humoral substance from diseased liver (ferritin?) in susceptible individuals (familial trend?) has been proposed as a mechanism to explain this syndrome. Possibly autosomal recessive inheritance.

Pathology. Liver cirrhosis. Microvenoarteriolar fistulas in lung.

Diagnostic Procedures. *Blood.* Secondary polycythemia; changes found in liver cirrhosis; arterial oxygen desaturation. *Dye dilution studies.* Indirect evidence of lung arteriovenous shunt. *X-rays.* Do not reveal lung alteration.

Therapy. None or portal shunt to decrease hypertension. Liver transplantation when necessary.

Prognosis. Poor; that of liver cirrhosis. Cyanosis and clubbing progressive.

BIBLIOGRAPHY. Fluckiger M: Vorkommen von trommelschlagel-förmigen Fingerendphalangen ohne chronische Veränderungen an den Lungen oder am Herzen. Wein Med 34:1457, 1884
Silverman A, Cooper MD, Moller JH, et al: Syndrome of cyanosis, digital clubbing, and hepatic disease in siblings. J Pediatr 72:70–80, 1968

FLYNN-AIRD

Synonyms. See Werner, Refsum, Cockayne.

Symptoms and Signs. Both sexes. From birth. *Eye.* Blindness. Cataracts, atypical retinitis pigmentosa, myopia. *Teeth.* Marked caries. *Ear.* (At age 7) progressive sensineural deafness. *Skin.* Atrophy, chronic ulcers. *Joints.* Stiffness. *Dementia, ataxia, peripheral neuritis, epilepsy.*

Etiology. Unknown. Autosomal dominant inheritance.

Diagnostic Procedures. *X-ray skeleton.* Cyst changes. *Cerebrospinal fluid.* Increased proteins.

BIBLIOGRAPHY. Flynn P, Aird RB: A neuroectodermal syndrome of dominant inheritance. J Neurol Sci 2:161–182, 1965
Konigsmark BW, Gorlin RJ: Genetic and Metabolic Deafness. Philadelphia, WB Saunders, 1976

FOCAL FIBROCARTILAGINEOUS DYSPLASIA

Synonyms. Tibia vara—focal fibrocartilagineous dysplasia.

Symptoms and Signs. Onset after first year of life. Gross unilateral bowing of proximal tibia.

Etiology. Focal presence of fibrocartilagineous tissue that does not calcify, thus causing various deformations of tibia.

Pathology. *Bone biopsy.* Plaque of dense fibrous tissue in the contest of tibia. Periostal reaction may be present.

Diagnostic Procedures. *X-ray. Bone biopsy.*

Therapy. Conservative management.

Prognosis. Spontaneous resolution of deformity.

BIBLIOGRAPHY. Bell SN, Campbell PE, Cole WG, et al: Tibia vara caused by focal fibrocartilagenous dysplasia: Three case reports. J Bone Joint Surg (Br) 67:780–784, 1985
Olney BW, Cole WG, Menelaus MB: Three additional cases of fibrocartilaginous dysplasia causing tibia vara. J Pediat Orthop 10:405–407, 1990
Kariya Y, Taniguchi K, Yogisawa H, et al: Focal fibrocartilaginous dysplasia consideration of a healing process. J Pediat Orthop 11:545–547, 1991

FOCAL GLOMERULAR SCLEROSIS

Synonyms. Lohlein; Rich.

Symptoms and Signs. Those of idiopathic nephrotic syndrome (see Epstein).

Etiology. Unknown. Probably, immune complex disease. Maybe it is only a superimposed lesion on minimal change disease or on minimal proliferative glomerulonephritis.

Pathology. Light microscopy. Segmental sclerosis of glomeruli owing to increased mesangial matrix and basement membrane. Tubular changes. Electron microscopy. Foot process alterations, mesangial cell hyperplasia. Immunofluorescence. IgM, C1q, C3 irregular granular distribution.

Therapy. Corticosteroids; alkylating agents; cyclosporin A; renal transplantation.

Prognosis. Rapid progression to renal failure. Recurrence of disease in grafts.

BIBLIOGRAPHY. Lohlein MH: Uber die entzundlichen Veranderungen der Glomeruli der menschliehen Nieren und ihre Bedeutung für die Nephritis. Leipzig, Hirzel, 1907
Rich AR: A hitherto unrecognized vulnerability of the juxta medullary glomeruli in lipoid nephrosis. Bull Johns Hopkins Hosp 100:A3, 1957
Meyrier AY: Focal segmental glomerulosclerosis. In Massry SG, Glassock RJ: Textbook of Nephrology, 3rd ed, pp 719–726. Baltimore, Williams & Wilkins, 1995

FOERSTER

Obsolete.

Synonym. Atonic–astatic Foerster; atonic congenital diplegia; atonic–astatic; cerebral diplegia; see "Floppy infant" syndrome.

Symptoms. Present at birth. Marked muscular hypotony; hypermobility of joints; severe mental defect; dysarthria. Absence of paresis; convulsions; sphincter incontinency.

Signs. Normal deep and superficial reflexes; absence of muscular atrophy; occasionally, strabismus. When the child is kept in standing position all body muscles may temporarily become hypertonic.

Etiology. Unknown; only in some cases positive serology for syphilis. Familial cases reported. Clinical features in common with both Creutzfeld-Jakob and dystrophia myotonica. Consanguinity described suggests autosomal recessive inheritance.

Pathology. Sclerotic lesions of frontal lobes involving the motor centers.

Diagnostic Procedures. *Blood. Serology. CSF. EEG. Electromyography. CT scan. MRI.*

Therapy. Nonspecific.

Prognosis. Improvement of muscular hypotonia observed, and in some cases it becomes possible to sit, and also walk with support; mental deterioration does not improve, and language usually does not develop.

BIBLIOGRAPHY. Foerster O: Der atonisch-astatische Typus der infantilen Cerebrallähmung. Arch Klin Med 48:216–244, 1909
Van Rossum A: Foerster's atonic-astatic syndrome. In Recent Neurological Research, Elsevier, 1959
Denny-Brown D: The Basal Ganglia. London, Oxford Univ Press, 1962

FOIX

Synonym. Red nucleus; includes red nucleus superior and red nucleus crossed.

Symptoms and Signs. Superior red nucleus type: cerebellar ataxia; usually associated with hyperkinesia; without oculomotor paralysis and crossed red nucleus type as above plus involvement of third nerve.

Etiology. Lesion limited to the anterior portion of red nucleus or extending to posterior part (the oculomotor roots pass through the posterior part of the nucleus).

BIBLIOGRAPHY. Foix C: Le syndromes de la region thalamique. Presse Med 33:113–117, 1925
Crouzon OJ, Dereux J, Kenzinger J: Paralisies pseudobulbaires d'origine protubérantielle (association d'un syndrome pseudobulbaire et d'un syndrome cérébélleux). Rev Neurol 2:747–753, 1925
Hiller F: The vascular syndromes of the basilar and vertebral arteries and their branches. J Nerv Ment Dis 116:988–1016, 1952
Adams RD, Victor M: Principles of Neurology, 5th ed, p 685. New York, McGraw-Hill, 1993

FOIX-ALAJOUANINE

Synonyms. Spinal cord hemangioma; necrotizing subacute myelitis;

angiodysgenetic radiculomyelomalacia; radiculomyelomalacia angiodysgenetic.

Symptoms. Spastic paraplegia; then flaccid amyotrophia; sensory loss first dissociated then complete. Sphincters involved.

Signs. Tendon reflexes abolished.

Etiology. Foix et al: proliferative endomeso-vasculitis. Moersh et al: vascular lesions. Neubuerger et al: hyperplasia and hyalinosis of vascular walls.

Circulation of spinal cord may also be compromised by aorta operations or aortography.

Pathology. Necrosis of spinal cord without inflammation; amyotrophy. Dysgenesis of spinal vessels with hyperplasia and hyalinosis of walls.

Diagnostic Procedures. *Cerebrospinal fluid.* Protein increased. *X-ray. CT scan; MRI.*

Therapy. Symptomatic.

Prognosis. Subacute course; death in 1 or 2 years.

BIBLIOGRAPHY. Foix C, Alajouanine T: La myelite necrotique subaique. Rev Neurol 2:1, 1926
Neuberger KT, Freed CG, Denst J: Vasal component in syndrome of Foix and Alajouanine: "subacute necrotizing myelitis." Arch Pathol 55:73–83, 1953
Adams RD, Victor M: Principles of Neurology, 5th ed, pp 1091–1092, 1097. New York, McGraw-Hill, 1993

FOIX-CHAVANY-MARIE

Synonyms. Faciopharyngoglossomasticatory diplegia; bilateral anterior opercular; opercular, bilateral, anterior; perisylvian stroke.

Symptoms and Signs. Usually at middle to late age (developmental form reported). Usually previous staged strokes (after second–third infarct). Acute onset; no impairment of consciousness; bilateral paralysis of voluntary movements of nerves V, VII, IX, X, XII; nerves III, IV, VI, XI, spared; preservation of automatic movements. Only occasionally (or left from previous stroke) paralysis of superior limbs, seldom of inferior.

Etiology. Vascular lesion; in congenital cases failure of opercula to form completely.

Pathology. Lesion in the two anterior opercula. In developmental cases bilateral perysylvian cortical dysplasia.

Diagnostic Procedures. *CT scan. MRI. EEG.*

Therapy. Symptomatic.

Prognosis. Survival outlook good; chances of recovery not so; partial improvement (not constant) after 30 days.

BIBLIOGRAPHY. Magnus A: Fall von Aufhebung des Willenseinflusses auf einige Hirnnerven Mullers. Arch Anat Physiol Wissensch Med, pp 258–266, 1837
Foix C, ChavanyJa Marie J: Diplégie facio-linguo-masticatrice d'origene cortico-sous-cortical sans paralysie des membres. Rev Neurol 33:214–219, 1926
Mariani C, Spinnler H, Sterzi R, et al: Bilateral perysylvian softenings: bilateral anterior opercular syndrome (Foix-Chavany-Marie syndrome). J Neurol 223:269–284, 1980
Graff-Radford NR, Bosch EP, Stears JC, et al: Developmental Foix-Chavany-Marie syndrome in twins. Ann Neurol 20:632–635, 1986
Kuzniecky R, Andermann F, Guerrini R, et al: The epileptic spectrum in the congenital bilateral perisylvian syndrome. Neurology 44:379–385, 1994

FOIX-JEFFERSON

Synonyms. Foix-Chavany; Godtfredsen; cavernous sinus; hypophyseal-sphenoidal; lateral wall cavernous sinus; ophthalmoneurologic-nasopharyngeal; cavernous sinus thrombosis; sinonasopharyngeal tumor. Foix (when caused by pathology of lateral wall of cavernous sinus): Jefferson (when caused by pathology of cavernous sinus). See also Orbital apex.

Symptoms. Development of orbital and supraorbital pain. Involvement of oculomotor (III), trochlear (IV), trigeminal (V1 V2 but most severe over ophthalmic branch), and abducens (VI) nerve. Paralysis usually unilateral; if bilateral, asymmetric. Association with chiasma syndrome (later) relatively frequent. When thrombosis: fever cephalea, proptosis, and swelling of affected eye. Complete ophthalmoplegia and fixed pupil.

Etiology and Pathology. Pituitary tumors (chromophobe more frequent association; eosinophil more absolute incidence); fibrosarcoma of sphenoid bone; aneurysms of cavernous sinus (symptoms acute); metastatic carcinoma; cavernous sinus thrombophlebitis.

Diagnostic Procedures. *X-ray of skull. Angiography. CT scan. MRI. Electroencephalography. Hormonal studies:* for pituitary function.

Therapy. Depends on etiology: surgery; antibiotics.

Prognosis. According to etiology.

BIBLIOGRAPHY. Bartholow R: Aneurysms of the arteries at the base of the brain, their symptomatology, diagnosis, and treatment. Am J Med Sci 64:373–386, 1872
Foix C: Sindrome de la paroi externe du sinus cavernous. Rev Neurol (Paris) 37,38:827–832, 1922
Godtfredsen E: Ophthalmoneurological symptoms in malignant nasopharyngeal tumors. Br J Ophthalmol 31:78–100, 1947
Jefferson G: Cavernous sinus syndrome. Trans Ophthalmol Soc UK 73:117, 1953
Nelson DA, Holloway WJ, Kara-Eneff SC, et al: Neurological syndrome produced by sphenoid sinus abscess, with neuroradiologic review of pituitary abscess. Neurology 17:981–987, 1967
Ferrari G: Foix-Chavany Syndrome: CT study and clinical report of three cases. Neuroradiology 18:41–42, 1979
Adams RD, Victor M: Principles of Neurology, 5th ed, p 590. New York, McGraw-Hill, 1993

FOIX-THEVENARD

Synonyms. Tonic postural reflex.

Symptoms and Signs. Commonly seen in Wilson, in some cases of Parkinson, and in double athetosis: exaggerated shortening reaction. (When passive movement is made in the opposite direction of a previous movement, stretching the antagonist, some or all of the motor units in the first muscle cease discharge, followed by renewed discharge in some of them.)

Etiology. Dystonia owing to basal ganglia alteration.

BIBLIOGRAPHY. Foix C: Thévenard Les réflexes de posture. Rev Neurol 39:449–468, 1923

FOLATE METABOLISM, INBORN ERRORS

Synonyms. Methylmalonic acidemia—homocystinuria; vitamin B_{12} defect.

1. METHYLENETETRAHYDROFOLATE REDUCTASE DEFICIENCY

Synonyms. Mudd-Shih.

Symptoms. More than 30 cases reported. Sixty-six percent females. Variable clinical severity. Developmental delay. Motor and gait abnormalities; seizures; psychiatric manifestations. Moderate homocystinuria with homocystinemia constant findings. Three groups are distinguished according to time of onset; neonatal, childhood, and mild form. Very resistant to treatment. Relative success with combination of methionine, oral 5-formyltetrahydrofolic acid, vitamin B_{12}, cobolamin, and even better if betaine has been added. Differences in prognosis may be owing to type of therapy used.

2. FOLATE MALABSORPTION

Synonyms. Luhby, Lanzkowsky, Santiago-Borrero.

Symptoms. Few (13) cases, all but two girls, have been described. Onset few first months of life. All cases share as symptoms and signs—folate-responsive megaloblastic anemia and mental retardation. In some cases folinic-responsive peripheral neuropathy.

3. GLUTAMATE FORMIMINOTRANSFERASE DEFICIENCY

Synonyms. Arakawa I.

Symptoms. Mental and physical retardation, cortical atrophy, megaloblastic anemia. Massive urinary excretion of formiminoglutamic acid, 4-amino-5-imidazole-carboxamide, and hydantoin-5-propronate. Niederweiser-Perry reported: some cases with only massive excretion of formiminoglutamate without mental retardation.

4. FUNCTIONAL METHIONINE SYNTHASE DEFICIENCY

Synonyms. Methyl-H_4 folate.

Symptoms. Onset first few months of life. Megaloblastic anemia, developmental delay. Omocysthinuria.

Etiology. Methionine synthase deficiency owing to the cblE and cblG mutations. All these syndromes appear to have an autosomal recessive inheritance.

5. FOUR OTHER DISORDERS OF FOLATE INHERITED DISORDERS HAVE BEEN REPORTED AND WAIT CONFIRMATION

A. DIHYDROFOLATE REDUCTASE DEFICIENCY

Synonyms. DHFR deficiency; Walter.

Symptoms. Three cases described that share as symptoms and signs megaloblastic anemia and early death.

B. METHYLEN-H_4 FOLATE CYCLOHYDROLASE DEFICIENCY

C. CELLULAR UPTAKE DEFECTS

D. PRIMARY METHYL-H_4 FOLATE (HOMOCYSTEIN METHYLTRANSFERASE DEFICIENCY)

BIBLIOGRAPHY. Arakawa T, Ohara K, Kudo Z, et al: Hyperfolic acidemia with formiminoglutamic aciduria, following histidine loading. Suggested for a case of congenital deficiency in formiminotransferase. Tohoku J Exp Med 80:370–382, 1963

Luhby AL, Cooperman JM, Pesci Bourel A: A newborn error of metabolism: Folic acid responsive megaloblastic anemia, ataxia, mental retardation and convulsions. J Pediatr 67:1052, 1965

Arakawa T, Narisawa K, Tanno K, et al: Megaloblastic anemia and mental retardation associated with hyperfolicacidemia. Probably due to N5 methyltetrahydrofolate transferase deficiency. Tohoku J Exp Med 93:1–22, 1967

Lanzkowsky P: Congenital malabsorption of folate. Am J Med 48:580–583, 1970

Santiago-Borrero PJ, Santini R Jr, Perez-Santiago E, et al: Congenital isolated defect of folic acid absorption. J Pediatr 82:450–455, 1973

Rosenblatt DS: Inherited disorders of folate transport and metabolism. In Scriver CR, Beaudet AL, Sly WS, et al: The Metabolic and Molecular Bases of Inherited Disease, 7th ed, pp 3111–3128. New York, McGraw-Hill, 1995

FOLLING

Synonyms. Hyperphenylalanine type I; idiotia phenylketonuria; phenylpyruvic oligophrenia; classic phenylketonuria; classic PKU; phenylalanine hydroxylase deficiency; PAH.

Symptoms. Both sexes equally affected; normal at birth. Developmental landmarks reached at normal age or delayed. Frequent vomiting in early infancy (50%). "Mousy" odor. Seizures developing in first 18 months of life and stopping spontaneously before adulthood (in about 25%). Marked irritability; hyperactivity almost constant. Severe mental defect. Inability to talk; inability to walk (associated with incontinence).

Signs. In children, height and weight below normal; microcephaly (68%); skin deficient pigmentation; eczema; blond hair; blue eyes. Stance and gait often "stooping," "stamping." Muscular hypertonicity; tendon hyperreflexia; abnormal, voluntary, purposeless body movements; tremor.

Etiology. Disorders of phenylalanine hydroxylation. Autosomal recessive inheritance. Two conditions needed to promote clinical manifestations: mutation and exposure to L-phenylalanine.

Pathology. *Brain.* Weight two thirds of normal; deficient myelinization (not constant); normally pigmented brain areas may lack pigmentation.

Diagnostic Procedures. *Blood. Urine.* High level of phenylalanine. Peculiar "mousy" odor of urine; positive ferric chloride and Phenistix tests. Postprandial determination. Of phenylalanine tyrosine radiodiagnostic aids to recognize types I (classic) and II. Several types of hyperphenylalaninemia have been identified with variable clinical and etiologic characteristics, enzyme phenotypes in the different forms of hyperphenylalaninemia are associated with recognizable metabolic phenotypes (see Hyperphenylalaninemia syndromes). *Electroencephalography. CT scan. MRI.*

Therapy. Diet with phenylalanine limitation to minimal amount necessary for growth and repair. Preliminary trials with 5-hydroxytryptophan (and carbidopa) and L-l-Dopa promising. Supplements of folinic acid.

Prognosis. Treatment started as early as possible prevents or reduces development of expected defects.

BIBLIOGRAPHY. Folling A: Uber Ausscheidung von Phenylbrenztraubensäure in den Harn als Stoffwechselanomalie in Verbindung mit Imbezillität. Z Physio Chem 227:169–176, 1934

Scriver Cr, Kaufman S, Eisensmith RC, et al: The hyperphenylalaninemias. In Scriver CR, Beaudet AL, Sly WS, et al: The Metabolic and Molecular Bases of Inherited Disease, 7th ed, pp 1015–1075. New York, McGraw-Hill, 1995

FORBES

Synonyms. Amylo-1, 6-glucosidase deficiency; Cori type III glycogenosis, debrancher deficiency; glycogenosis type III limit dextrinosis.

Symptoms. Frequent in Israel. Both sexes affected; clinical onset in early childhood. Desire for sweets and carbohydrates; mild mental retardation; mild muscular weakness; Harris (see).

Signs. Doll facial features; marked hepatomegaly (not constant) that recedes as the child grows (after about 4 years). Occasionally, moderate splenomegaly.

Etiology. Amylo-1, 6-glucosidase (debrancher) deficiency leading to increase of glycogen in the liver, muscle, heart. Autosomal recessive inheritance. Lack of enzyme may be in muscle and/or in liver and relative clinical manifestations may become evident in one or both districts.

Pathology. In early stage, large accumulation of glycogen in liver and only a moderate accumulation in heart and muscle fibers. Later random scarring of liver and early cirrhosis.

Diagnostic Procedures. *Blood.* Deficiency of amylo-1, 6-glucosidase in leukocytes and erythrocytes; hypoglycemia; acetonemia; hyperlipemia. *Biopsy.* Of liver and muscle. Increased glycogen, absent amylo-1–6-glucosidase activity. *Electrocardiography. Ventricular hypertrophy. Electromyography.* Changes consistent with widespread myopathy. Nerve conduction abnormal.

Therapy. Diet rich in protein, protection from hypoglycemic crisis; trial with glucagon. In case of severe liver failure and heart failure transplantation of both organs.

Prognosis. Most patients survive into later life with persistence of altered glucose tolerance test and biochemical defect. Some cases at adolescence, may regain normal growth, decrease of hepatomegaly and normal glycemia. In others, possible progressive skeletal myopathy and, or cardiomyopathy. Good results with transplantations.

BIBLIOGRAPHY. Forbes GB: Glycogen storage disease: Report of a case with abnormal glycogen structure in liver and skeletal muscle. J Pediatr 42:645–653, 1953

Chen YT, Burchell A: Glycogen storage diseases. In Scriver CR, Beaudet AL, Sly WS, et al: The Metabolic and Molecular Bases of Inherited Disease, 7th ed, pp 949–950. New York, McGraw-Hill, 1995

FORDYCE

Synonyms. Pseudocolloid lip mucous membrane sebaceous milia. See also Steatocystoma multiplex.

Symptoms. Asymptomatic.

Signs. Small yellowish papules, distributed on oral mucosa, lips, occasionally, genital region, and breast.

Etiology. Unknown.

Pathology. Hypertrophic sebaceous glands free or connected by true sebaceous ducts.

Prognosis. Good.

BIBLIOGRAPHY. Fordyce J: A peculiar affection of the mucous membrane of the lips and oral cavity. J Cutan Dis NY 16:413–419, 1896

Ebling FJG, Cunlife WJ: Disorders of the sebaceous glands. In Champion RH, Burton JL, Ebling FJG (eds): Rook/Wilkinson/Ebling Textbook of Dermatology, 5th ed, p 1741. Oxford, Blackwell Scientific, 1992

FORESTIER-ROTES-QUEROL

Synonyms. Hyperostosic spondylosis; senile ankylosing—vertebral hyperostosis; spondylorheostosis.

Symptoms and Signs. Occurs in elderly people. Symptoms related to spine ossification of anterior ligaments. Degenerative changes of intervertebral disks (see Pulposus) and marginal osteophytosis leading to ankylosis.

Etiology. Unknown. It may represent a severe spondylosis (see Marie-Strumpell).

Pathology. See Symptoms. The cortex of vertebrae adjacent to ossified ligaments shows destructive changes.

Therapy. Physical therapy; calcium; vitamin D; testosterone derivatives.

Prognosis. Progressing condition leading to ankylosis.

BIBLIOGRAPHY. Forestier J, Rotés Querol J: Senile ankylosing hyperostosis of the spine. Ann Rheum Dis 9:321–330, 1950

Clinical pathologic osteoarthritis workshop (Queen's University, Kingston, Ontario, Canada). J Rheumatol 10 (suppl 9):1(complete issue), 1983

Hutton CW: Osteoarthritis. In Weatherall DJ, Ledingham JGG, Warrell DA (eds): Oxford Textbook of Medicine, 3rd ed, p 2979. Oxford, Oxford Med Pub, 1996

FORNEY

Symptoms and Signs. From birth. Congenital heart disease, deafness, and skeletal malformations.

BIBLIOGRAPHY. Forney WR, Robinson SJ, Pascoe DJ: Congenital heart disease, deafness and skeletal malformations: A new syndrome? J Pediatr 68:14–26, 1966

FORSIUS-ERIKSSON

Synonyms. Åland (refers to the island where the syndrome was discovered among natives); retina tapetal degeneration; tapetoretinal degeneration; 0A2.

Symptoms. Affects only males; females are carriers, usually asymptomatic, but may have, in some cases, slight latent nystagmus. Prematurity; mental retardation; epileptic attacks; impaired hearing; poor vision (myopia); defect in dark adaptation; dyschromatopsia.

Signs. Microphthalmia. Irregular latent nystagmus; astigmatism; tapetoretinal degeneration; localized pigment deficiency around macula and disk.

Etiology. X-chromosomal dominant type of inheritance or X-chromosomal recessive inheritance.

BIBLIOGRAPHY. Forsius H, Eriksson W: Ein neues Augensyndrome mit X-Chromosomaler Transmission. Eine Sippe mit Fundus Albinismus, Foveahypoplasie, Nystagmus, Myopie, Astigmatismus und Dyschromatopsie. Klin Monatsbl Augenheilkd 114:447–457, 1964

Witkop CJ, Quevedo WC, Fitzpatrick TB: Albinism and other disorders of pigment metabolism. In Stanbury JB, Wyngaarden JB, Fredrickson DS, et al: The Metabolic Basis of Inherited Disease, 5th ed, p 301. New York, McGraw-Hill, 1983

Schwartz M, Rosenberg T: Aland eye disease: linkage data. Genomics 10:327–332, 1991

Garner A, Klintworth GK (eds): Pathobiology of Ocular Disease: A Dynamic Approach, 2nd ed, pp 818, 828, 948, 950, 1224. New York, Marcel Dekker, 1994

FORSSELL

Synonyms. Nephrogenic erythrocytosis; nephrogenic polycythemia.

Symptoms and Signs. Increase of red cell mass, with or without other features of polycythemia vera (see Vaquez-Osler).

Etiology. Renal pathology of various types, most frequently hypernephroma, followed by (in order) cystic disease, hydronephrosis, carcinoma, other tumors, and renal ischemia owing to a disease of extrarenal vasculature. The association between renal pathology and erythrocytosis is inconsistent. The erythrocytosis seems to depend on the incretion of erythropoietin or a precursor formed by the tumor on the adjacent tissues compressed by it.

Pathology. See Vaquez-Osler and Etiology.

Diagnostic Procedures. *Blood and bone marrow.* Exclusion of polycythemia vera. *X-ray of kidney.*

Therapy. Removal of kidney lesions.

Prognosis. With removal of kidney lesions, cessation of erythrocytosis. With recurrence of lesion, recurrence of increased red cell production.

BIBLIOGRAPHY. Forssell J: Polycytemic vid hypernefrom. Nord Med 30:1415–1419, 1946
Athens JW, Lee GR: Polycythemia: erythrocytosis. In Lee GR, Bithel TC, Foerster J, et al (eds): Wintrobe's Clinical Hematology, 9th ed, p 1257. Philadelphia, Lea & Febiger, 1993

FOSTER KENNEDY

Synonyms. Gowers-Paton-Kennedy; Kennedy; basofrontal.

Symptoms. Reduction in visual acuity; headache; dizziness; vertigo; occasionally; forceful vomiting; psychic changes (moria); memory loss.

Signs. Papilledema of one eye; optical atrophy of the other, with central scotoma.

Etiology. Frontal lobe tumor or abscess producing homolateral optic atrophy and contralateral papilledema.

Pathology. Tumor (e.g., gliomas) or abscess of frontal lobe determining retrobulbar neuritis and increased intracranial pressure.

Diagnostic Procedures. *X-ray of skull. Angiography. Brain isotope scan. Electroencephalography. Spinal tap. CT scan. MRI.*

Therapy. If amenable to surgery, simple decompression (therapeutic or tapping) may partially relieve the symptomatology.

Prognosis. Poor, except if surgery is feasible.

BIBLIOGRAPHY. Kennedy F: Retrobulbar neuritis as an exact diagnostic sign of certain tumors and abscesses in the frontal lobes. Am J Med Sci 142:355–368, 1911
Frenkel RE, Spoor TC: Visual loss and intoxication. Survey Ophthalmol 30:391–396, 1986

FOTHERGILL

Synonyms. Trigeminal neuralgia; tic douloureux trifacial neuralgic.

Symptoms. Prevalent in females; onset usually after 45 years of age. Any division of trigeminal (V) nerve involved singly or in combination. Paroxystic attack of short, shooting pain, usually starting at a constant point (trigger point on the cheek, near lips or gums, side of tongue; and other locations) and diffusing to involve all territory of branch or branches affected. Ophthalmic branch less frequently involved. Peripheral stimulation of trigger point usually initiates attack. To avoid them, patient may not eat or drink and may become emaciated and dehydrated, or grow beard, and may not clean affected side. Usually, no night attacks, and little interference with sleep.

Etiology. Unknown; multiple types of sclerosis irritation around Gasser ganglion may produce attacks. Autosomal dominant inheritance reported in some kindred.

Pathology. No specific findings of Gasser ganglion.

Diagnostic Procedures. *X-rays of teeth, sinuses, skull. Angiography. CT scan. MRI brain scan.*

Therapy. Vitamin B_{12}; hydantoin; carbamazepine (Tegretol); alcohol infiltration; retrogasserian neurotomy. Other neurosurgical procedures in particular cases.

Prognosis. Attacks last a few moments, stop spontaneously. Paroxysmal attacks recur frequently with intervals of weeks or years.

BIBLIOGRAPHY. Fothergill J: Of a painful affection of the face. Med Obs Ing 5:129, 1773
Kirkpatrick DB: Familial trigeminal neuralgia: Case report. Neurosurgery 24:758–761, 1989
Zakrzewska JM: Trigeminal Neuralgia. London, WB Saunders, 1995

FOUNTAIN

Synonym. Mental retardation—sensoneural deafness—skeletal defects—coarse face—full lips.

Symptoms. Both sexes. From birth. Sensorineural type deafness; mental retardation.

Signs. Edematous facial changes; progressive swelling of the lips and in one case granulomatous mass in lower lip. Skeletal defects. Thickened calvaria, short stubby hands.

Etiology. Suggestion of autosomal recessive inheritance.

Diagnostic Procedures. *CT scan of head.* Congenital anomalies of cochlea.

BIBLIOGRAPHY. Fountain RB: Familial bone abnormalities, deaf mutism, mental retardation, and skin granuloma. Proc Roy Soc Med 67:878–879, 1974
Fryn J-P: Fountain's syndrome: mental retardation sensorineural deafness, skeletal abnormalities and coarse face with full lips. J Med Genet 26:722–724, 1989

FOURNIER

Synonyms. Gangrene, Fournier; scrotal idiopathic gangrene; necrotizing fascitis of male genitalia.

Symptoms and Signs. Often in diabetic patients; it may follow vasectomy or lower gut resection; it occurs suddenly, and progresses rapidly.

Etiology. Necrotizing cellulitis, disseminated intravascular coagulation, necrotizing fascitis-like, immunological defect. Group A streptococci or multiple organisms, bacteroides fragilis most frequently found organism. Frequent association with diabetes mellitus.

Pathology. Gangrene of scrotal region.

Diagnostic Procedures. See Etiology.

Therapy. Ample debridement, and general supporting care.

Prognosis. With proper treatment 55% survival.

BIBLIOGRAPHY. Fournier JA: Gangrene fuodroyante de la verge. Med Prat 4:459–497, 1883
Spirnak JP, Resnick MI, Hampel N, et al: Fournier's gangrene: Report of 20 cases. J Urol 132:289–291, 1984
Edmondson RA, et al: Fournier's gangrene: An aetiological hypothesis. Br J Urol 69:543–545, 1992

FOURNIER TIBIA

Synonyms. In congenital syphilis, fusiform thickening and anterior bowing of tibia.

BIBLIOGRAPHY. Fournier J: La syphilis héréditaire tardive. Paris Rueff, 1886

FOURTH VENTRICLE

Synonyms. Cerebellar line median; vermis.

Symptoms and Signs. Both sexes, all ages affected. Severe trunk ataxia; bilateral choked disks; coarse horizontal nystagmus in lateral terminal positions. Variable signs of fourth ventricle nuclei involvement: facial palsy; diminished corneal reflex; ocular dysmetria; vomiting; stiffness, and pain in neck and shoulders.

Etiology. Lesions of fourth ventricle.

Pathology. Neoplastic, vascular, or inflammatory lesion of floor of fourth ventricle, usually involving nuclei of trigeminal (V), abducens (VI), and facial (VII) nerves and medial longitudinal fasciculus.

Diagnostic Procedures. *CT brain scan. MRI. Angiography. Spinal tap.*

Therapy. According to Etiology.

Prognosis. Depends on Etiology.

BIBLIOGRAPHY. van Bogaert L, Marlin P: Les tumeurs du quatrième ventricule et le syndrome cérébelleux de la ligne médiane. Rev Neurol 2:431–483, 1928
Acers TE, Tenney R: Ocular symptomatology of posterior fossa tumors. Am J Ophthalmol 65:872–876, 1968
Adams RD, Victor M: Principles of Neurology, 5th ed, pp 685–686. New York, McGraw-Hill, 1993

FOVILLE I

Synonyms. Foville-Laehmung; Foville-Bruechen; Foville peduncular; alternating inferior hemiplegia; hemiplegia alternating inferior.

Symptoms and Signs. Hemiplegia; deviation of eye opposite side or paralysis of lateral gaze, in irritative lesions deviation toward hemiplegic side. Ipsilateral nuclear facial paralysis.

Etiology. Neoplastic, hemorrhagic, infective, degenerative lesions of pons involving longitudinal fasciculus.

Pathology. See Etiology.

Therapy. Conservative or surgical if indicated.

Prognosis. Depends on etiology.

BIBLIOGRAPHY. Foville A: Note sur une paralysie peu connue de certain muscles de l'oeil, et sa liaison avec quelques points de l'anatomie et la physiologie la protubérance annulaire. Bull Soc Anat 33:394–414, 1858
Schmidt D, Malin JP: Erkrankungen der Hirnnerven. Stuttgart, Thieme, 1986

FOVILLE II

Synonyms. Alternating inferior hemiplegia; pontine Foville.

Symptoms and Signs. Same symptoms and signs as in Foville I, but without facial nerve involvement.

BIBLIOGRAPHY. Foville A: Note sur une paralysie peu connue de certain muscles de l'oeil, et sa liaison avec quelques points de l'anatomie et la physiologie la protubérance annulaire. Gaz Hebd Med 6:146, 1859
Vick NA: Grinker's Neurology, 7th ed. Springfield, IL, Charles C Thomas, 1976

FOVILLE-WILSON

Symptoms and Signs. Impairment of lateral convergence of different degree in the two eyes; paralysis of adduction; abduction insufficient. Abducted eye: ample horizontal nystagmus, but the other eye does not adduct, does not show nystagmus, or shows only irregular, exhaustible jerks. Preservation of convergence.

Etiology. See Multiple sclerosis.

Pathology. See Multiple sclerosis.

Therapy. See Multiple sclerosis.

Prognosis. See Multiple sclerosis.

BIBLIOGRAPHY. Foville A: Note sure une paralysie peu connue de certain muscles de l'oeil, et sa liaison avec quelques points de l'anatomie et la physiologie de la protubérance annulaire. Bull Soc Anat 33:394–414, 1858
Wilson SAK: Case of disseminated sclerosis with weakness of each internal rectus et nystagmus. Brain 29:298, 1906
Klintworth GK: Ocular involvement in disorders of the nervous system. In Garner A, Klintworth GK (eds): Pathobiology of Ocular Disease: A Dynamic Approach, 2nd ed, pp 1712–1714. New York, Marcel Dekker, 1994

FOX

Obsolete. Comprises both Weber-Cockaine (see) and Goldscheider (see).

BIBLIOGRAPHY. Fox T: Notes on unusual or rare forms of skin disease. IV. Congenital ulceration of skin (two cases) with pemphigus eruption and arrest of development generally. Lancet 1:766–767, 1879

FOX-FORDYCE

Synonym. Montgomery-Fordyce; apocrine miliaris.

Symptoms. Onset after puberty; prevalent in women. Males and children less frequently affected. Recurrent episodes of severe pruritus in the axillae, anogenital region, and around breast.

Signs. Skin hyperpigmentation in the axillae, pubis, sternum, and nipples areolae; presence of dry papulae. Broken hair.

Etiology. Obstruction of sweat glands pori; rupture of duct and escape of the sweat into epidermis. Emotional factors precipitating the attack.

Pathology. Formation of vesicle around duct of sweat glands; dilatation and rupture of the ducts.

Therapy. Topical and systemic hormonal treatment (testosterone, corticosteroids, oral contraceptive). Roentgen irradiation in epilation dose. Topical retinoic acids and tretinoin: topical antibiotics successful, particularly clindamycin.

Prognosis. Recurrence; possible remission during pregnancy; spontaneous remission after menopause. Encephalitis possible complication.

BIBLIOGRAPHY. Fox G, Fordyce J: Two cases of a rare papular disease affecting the axillary region. J Cutan Dis 20:1–5, 1902
Pye RJ: Bullous Eruptions. In Champion RH, Burton JL, Ebling FJG (eds): Rook/Wilkinson/Ebling Textbook of Dermatology, 5th ed, pp 1761–1762. Oxford, Blackwell Scientific, 1992
Matthew L, Miller MC, Harford MC, et al: Fox Fordice disease treated with topical clindamycin solution. Arch Derm 131:1112–1113, 1995

FRAGA

See Addisonian syndromes. Chronic or acute Addison syndrome caused by malaria.

BIBLIOGRAPHY. Fraga A: Supra-renalite aguda no impaludismo. Brazil Med 31:349, 1917
Fraga C: La forma suprarenal del paludismo. Rev Iber Am Cien Med 40:9–19, 1918

FRAGILE X

Synonyms. Martin-Bell; FRAXA.

Symptoms and Signs. One per 1250 males and 1 per 2000 females is the single most common form of inherited mental retardation. IQ for males ranges 20–60. Long face and large prominent ears; macroorchidism; prognathism, large head circumference in early childhood; hyperextensible finger joints, mitral valve prolapse, aortic dilation, pectus excavatum, high-arched palate, myopia, flat feet, abnormal dermatoglyphics. Behavioral features: hand stereotypes; cluttered speech; hyperactivity; autism. Heterozygous females have a broad range of dysfunction: normal, mildly affected, or severely autistic.

Etiology. Initially thought to be inherited in X-linked manner, today inheritance has been redefined and the syndrome is considered to be the result of an unusual mutational mechanism, known as the "dynamic" mutation, only recently discovered in human genetics that consists of the amplification of a simple repeated DNA sequence. Male offspring of carrier females have 50% a priori risk of inheriting mutation but penetrance varies 18–100%. Daughters of carrier mothers have penetrance of 10–40%. In daughters of transmitting males penetrance is close to 0%. X chromosome has a fragile site in xg27 that can be evidenced only by pyrimidine nucleotide deprivation of culture medium.

Pathology. *Testes.* Edema and increased extracellular matrix. *Ovaries.* Ovarian cysts.

Diagnostic Procedures. *Lymphocyte cultures.* Affected patients demonstrate the defect in 5–50% (average 20%) of cells.

Therapy. Early speech and language therapy, occupational therapy, and special education assistance. Medical therapy: central nervous system stimulants, folic acid, and phenothiazines. Trimethoprim may lead to exacerbation of behavior problems, and this drug should be avoided.

Prognosis. With proper treatment decrease in the frequency and severity of autistic features and improvement in development performance.

BIBLIOGRAPHY. Martin JP, Bell J: A pedigree of mental defect showing sex-linkage. J Neurol Neurosurg Psychiatr 6:154–156, 1943
Mixon JC, Dev VG: Understanding the fragile X syndrome. Ala J Med Sci 21:284–286, 1984
Chludley AE, Hageiman RJ: Fragile X syndrome. J Paediatr 110:821–831, 1987
Nussbaum RL, Ledbetter DH: The fragile X syndrome. In Scriver CR, Beaudet AL, Sly WS, et al: The Metabolic and Molecular Bases of Inherited Disease, 7th ed, pp 795–810. New York, McGraw-Hill, 1995

FRAME

Synonym. Axial osteomalacia.

Symptoms. Both sexes. Caucasian and black. Diagnosed in middle age. Presenting symptoms: vague chronic axial pain, followed by back pain, fatigue in the extremities.

Signs. Mild tenderness to percussion over lumbar spine, no paravertebral muscle spasm, limited spinal range of motion possibly associated with polycystic kidney and liver disease.

Etiology. Bone cells enzyme defect leading to impaired bone formation. Disorder of vitamin D action (?). Autosomal dominant inheritance. It may fall into the various forms of osteogenesis imperfecta tarda (see).

Pathology. Bone: mean cortical width and cortical porosity increased; in medullary space: trabecular bone varies in thickness and forms a complicated branching network.

Diagnostic Procedures. *Blood.* Normal or negative results. Creatine phosphokinase increased; alkaline phosphatase activity increased. *Urine.* Normal. *X-rays.* From early adulthood. Coarsening of trabecular bone pattern of the axial, but not appendicular, skeleton. *Bone biopsy.* Osteomalacia of rib or iliac crest. *Tetracycline labeling to assess rate of bone formation.*

Therapy. Vitamin D + Ca: decreases unmineralized osteoid but no effect on symptoms.

Prognosis. Benign clinical course.

BIBLIOGRAPHY. Frame B, Frost HM, Ormond RS, et al: Atypical osteomalacia involving the axial skeleton. Ann Intern Med 55:632–639, 1961
White MP, Fallon MD, Murphy WA, et al: Axial osteomalacia: Clinical, laboratory and genetic investigation of an affected mother and son. Am J Med 71:1041–1049, 1981
Avioli LV, Krane SM: Metabolic Bone Disease, 2nd ed. Philadelphia, WB Saunders, 1990
Tsipouras P: Osteogenesis imperfecta. In Beighton P: McKusick's Heritable Disorders of Connective Tissue, 5th ed, p 282. St Louis, CV Mosby, 1993

FRANCESCHETTI

Synonyms. Fundus flavimaculatus. FF; see Stargardt.

Symptoms. Both sexes affected; onset between 10 and 25 years of age. Impairment of central vision with intact peripheral retinal function.

Signs. Irregular yellowish deposits in and around macula lutea forming a "garland."

Etiology. Unknown; autosomal recessive inheritance.

Pathology. In retinal pigment epithelium displacement of nucleus from base of cell to center or inner surface, variation in size of RPE cells, accumulation of mucopolysaccharides within inner half of cells.

Diagnostic Procedures. *Electroretinography.* Normal. *Fundoscopy.* Bilateral asymmetric, slowly progressive condition with yellow or yellowish white, round and linear pisciform flecks that vary in size, shape, and density. Borders of lesions are fuzzy with tendency to confluence. Limited to posterior pole, but may extend to equator.

Therapy. None.

BIBLIOGRAPHY. Franceschetti A, François J, Babel J: Les Héredo-Dégénérescenc chorio-rétiniennes, vol 1. Paris, 1963
Isashiki Y, Ohba N: Fundus flavimaculatus: Polymorphic retinal change in siblings. Br J Ophthalmol 69:522–524, 1985
Bottoni F, Fatigati, et al: Fundus flavimaculatus and subretinal neovascolarization. Graefes Arch Clin Exp Ophthal 230:498–500, 1992

FRANCESCHETTI-KAUFMAN

Synonyms. Franceschetti dystrophy; Kaufman; Valle, metaherpetic keratitis; posttraumatic keratitis; corneal erosion recurring; keratitis fugax hereditaria.

Symptoms. Pain when opening the eyes in the morning; diminishing as the day progresses. Photophobia. Mild fever.

Signs. Nondendritic corneal ulcer and stromal edema.

Etiology. Previous corneal trauma (virus; chemical; foreign bodies) that has damaged the epithelial basis. Or hereditary familial form (autosomal dominant).

Pathology. Ovoid nondendritic ulcer owing to poor attachment of new epithelial regrowth and accumulation of fluid in the stroma and corneal epithelium. Loss of desmosomes.

Diagnostic Procedures. *Virus culture.* Negative. Defects stain positively with fluorescein.

Therapy. Emollients and corticosteroids; not affected by chemical cautery or antiviral agents.

Prognosis. Good with proper treatment; improving with age.

BIBLIOGRAPHY. Franceschetti A: Hereditäre Rezidivierende. Erosion der Hornhaut. Z Augenheilkd 66:309–316, 1928
Kaufman HE: Epithelial erosion syndrome: Metaherpetic keratitis. Am J Ophthalmol 57:983–987, 1964
Valle O: Hereditary recurring corneal erosion: A family study with special reference to Fuch's dystrophy. Arch Ophthalmol 45:829–836, 1967
Klintworth GK: Degenerations depositions and miscellaneous reaction of the ocular anterior segment. In Garner A, Klintworth GK (eds): Pathobiology of Ocular Disease: A Dynamic Approach, 2nd ed, p 770. New York, Marcel Dekker, 1994

FRANCESCHETTI-KLEIN

Synonyms. Berry-Franceschetti-Klein; Franceschetti-Zwahlen-Klein; Treacher Collins-Franceschetti; mandibulofacial dysostosis. See Pierre Robin and Treacher Collins.

Symptoms and Signs. Evident at birth. Difficulty in sucking and swallowing; excessive mucus in mouth; cyanotic spells. Complete form includes antimongoloid obliquity of palpebral fissures, notching of lower eyelids, flattening of molar bones (Treacher Collins), small mandible, receding chin, considerable overbite, high arched palate, macrostomia, malformation of ears. Atypical hair growth. Incomplete, abortive, and unilateral forms described.

Etiology. See First arch syndrome. Autosomal dominant inheritance.

Pathology. Faulty development of multiple elements of first arch.

Diagnostic Procedures. *Chromosome studies.* Normal. *X-ray. Ultrasonography. Audiography.*

Therapy. Feeding major problem, use of feeder or gavage. If cyanosis attacks frequent, immobilization of tongue by stitching it to lower jaw.

Prognosis. Feeding trouble and cyanosis attacks disappear in a few weeks or months. The other congenital defects affect life and development according to severity.

BIBLIOGRAPHY. Berry GA: Note of congenital defect (coloboma) of lower lid. London Ophthalmol Hosp Rep 12:255–277, 1889
Collins ET: Cases with symmetrical congenital notches in the outer part of each lower lid and defective development of the molar bones. Trans Ophthalmol Soc UK 20:190–192, 1933
Franceschetti A: Un syndrome nouveau; La dysostose mandibulofaciale. Bull Schweiz Akad Med Wiss 1:60–66, 1944
Franceschetti A, Klein D: The mandibulofacial dysostosis, a new hereditary syndrome. Acta Ophthalmol (Copenh) 27:143–224, 1949
Peterson-Falzone S, Figueroa AA: Longitutinal changes in cranial base angulation in mandibulofacial dysostosis. Clef Palate J 26:31–35, 1989

FRANCESCHETTI-THIER

Synonyms. Corneal—cerebellar; spinocerebellar degeneration; corneal dystrophy.

Symptoms and Signs. Mental retardation; multiple lipomas; bilateral corneal opacification beginning in second year of life and progressing to visual impairment and slowly progressive cerebellar abnormalities with dorsal column and upper motor neuron deficiency.

Etiology. Unknown; autosomal recessive inheritance.

Pathology. Corneal edema. Thickened. Descemet membrane and degenerative pannus. Cerebellar, dorsal column and upper motor neuron damage.

Therapy. Penetrating keratoplasty.

BIBLIOGRAPHY. Franceschetti A, Thier CJ: Hornhautdystrophien bei Genodermatosen unter besonderen Berucksichtingung der Palmoplantarkeratosen. Albrecht von Graefes Arch Ophthalmol 162:610–670, 1961
Der Koloustian VM, Jarudi NI, Khoury MJ, et al: Familial spinocerebellar degeneration with corneal atrophy. Am J Med Genet 20:325–339, 1985

FRANÇOIS I

Synonyms. Jensen; chondrodermal corneal dystrophy; corneal–chondrodermal dystrophy; dermochondrocorneal dystrophy; arthropathic nodular fibromatosis.

Symptoms and Signs. Both sexes affected; normal at birth, onset at 1–2 years of age. Osteochondral deformities of hands and feet; subluxation and tendinous contractures may develop; concomitant development of xanthoma-like, small, yellowish, hard nodules in the skin. Later, appearance of bilateral peripheral or central corneal opacities and seizures.

Etiology. Unknown; possibly autosomal recessive inheritance. Related to lipid storage and possibly to mucopolysaccharidosis (not studied) disorders.

Pathology. *Skin.* Corium with large, round, or elongated cells with vacuolated cytoplasm (no lipids), dense connective tissue with some lymphatic space. Similar cells in the cornea. *Bone.* Defective endochrondral ossification involving short and long bones.

Diagnostic Procedures. *Blood.* Possibly, a hypercholesterolemic phase. *X-ray.* Skeleton survey. *EEG.* Abnormalities.

Therapy. Orthopedic correction.

Prognosis. Chronic progression.

BIBLIOGRAPHY. François J: Dystrophie dermochondrocornéene familiale. Ann Ocul 182:409–422, 1949
Jensen E: Retino-choroiditis justapapillaris. Abrecht Von Graefes Arch Ophthalmol 69:41–48, 1909
Caputo R, Sambvani N, Monti M, et al: Dermochondrocorneal dystrophy (François syndrome). Arch Dermatol 124:424–428, 1988

FRANÇOIS-EVENS

Synonym. Annular dystrophy of corneal endothelium.

Symptoms. Occurs at different ages. Vision and corneal sensitivity normal. Small flat granular opacity ring shaped at the level of corneal endothelium, peripheral zone of posterior side.

Etiology. Unknown.

Prognosis. Benign, nonprogressive condition.

BIBLIOGRAPHY. François J, Evens A: Hérédodystrophie anulaire de l'endothelium cornéen. Atti Congr Soc Oftalm Ital 18:352, 1959
Goldberg MF: Genetic and Metabolic Eye Disease, p 308. Boston, Little, Brown & Co, 1974
Rodrigues MM, Rajagopalan S, Jones KA: Anterior and posterior corneal dystrophy. In Garner A, Klintworth GK (eds): Pathobiology of Ocular Disease: A Dynamic Approach, 2nd ed. New York, Marcel Dekker, 1994

FRANÇOIS-HAUSTRATE

Synonym. Otomandibular dysostosis.

Symptoms and Signs. Hemifacial microsomia; microphthalmia, coloboma of uveal tract and optic disk.

Etiology. Consider a variant of hemifacial microsomia (see).

BIBLIOGRAPHY. François J, Haustrate L: Anomalies colobomatuses de globe oculaire et syndrome du prémièr arc. Ann Ocul 187:340–368, 1954

FRANÇOIS-NEETENS

Synonyms. Corneal dystrophy speckled, speckled dystrophy, spotted corneal degeneration; corneal dystrophy flecked; François dystrophy I; corneal dystrophy cloudy.

Symptoms. Both sexes affected; identified from 2 years of age or later. Vision normal; corneal sensation normal.

Signs. In the corneal stroma presence of small, semiopaque, flat opacities involving the centrum and the periphery. Opacities that may be of two different types: granular or homogeneous gray color and are neatly separated from each other by clear cornea or cloudy snowflakes with ill-defined margin concentrated mainly in the center of cornea.

Etiology. Autosomal dominant inheritance.

Pathology. Related abnormalities restricted to cornea; abnormalities restricted to fibroblast; they may contain large vacuoles reacting positively with Sudan black and oil red; between affected areas normal keratocytes.

Diagnostic Procedures. *Corneal reflexes.* May be depressed. *Retroillumination.* Shows opacities and their distribution, which does not involve Bowman layer and Descemet membrane.

Therapy. None.

Prognosis. Static disorders.

BIBLIOGRAPHY. François J, Neetens A: Nouvelle dystrophie hérédofamiliale du parenchyme cornéen (hérédodystrophie monchetée). Bull Soc Belg Ophthalmol 114:641–646, 1957
Nicholson DH, Green WR, Cross HE, et al: A clinical and histopathological study of François–Neetens speckled corneal dystrophy. Am J Ophthalmol 83:554–560, 1977
Klintworth GK: Disorders of glycosaminoglycans (mucopolysaccharides) and proteoglycans. In Garner A, Klintworth GK (eds): Pathobiology of Ocular Disease: A Dynamic Approach, 2nd ed, p 879. New York, Marcel Dekker, 1994

FRANKL-HOCHWART

Synonyms. Ophthalmic—neuropineal; von Frankl-Hochwart.

Symptoms and Signs. Bilateral deafness; ataxia; headache; vomiting; according to age of onset, various manifestations of hypopituitarism. Limitation of upward gaze; constriction of visual fields; choked disk; papilledema.

Etiology and Pathology. Tumor of pineal gland.

Diagnostic Procedures. *X-ray of skull. Angiography. CT scan. MRI. Blood and urine.* Demonstrate hypopituitarism (see Simmond).

Therapy. Surgery and X-ray treatment.

Prognosis. Poor.

BIBLIOGRAPHY. von Frankl-Hochwart L: Ueber Diagnose der Zirbeldrüsetumoren. Dtsch Z Nervenh 37:455, 1909; 38:309, 1910
Tassman I: The Eye Manifestations of Internal Disease, 3rd ed. St Louis, CV Mosby, 1951

Roy FH: Ocular Syndromes and Systemic Diseases. Orlando, Grune & Stratton, 1985

FRANKLIN

Synonyms. Heavy chain (gamma); gamma heavy chain; gamma HCD.

Symptoms and Signs. Occurs in both sexes (slight male predominance); onset in middle age. Abrupt onset of lymphadenopathy without fever. Edema and erythema of uvula and soft palate occasionally noticed. Spleen enlargement sometimes during course of disease; hepatomegaly not constant. Spontaneous regression of lymphadenopathy after some time. Pallor. Frequently associated with various conditions; lupus erythematosus; rheumatoid arthritis; Sjögren; Erb-Goldflam; hemolytic anemia.

Etiology. Unknown. Possible autoimmune disorder.

Pathology. *Lymph node.* Atypical and immature plasma cells; reticulum cells, atypical lymphocytes, eosinophils, and cells not easily classifiable. Lymph node pattern may suggest Hodgkin disease. *Bone marrow.* Similar cells to these described in lymph nodes. Erythroid hyperplasia. Liver biopsy normal.

Diagnostic Procedures. *Blood.* Normochromic anemia; hyperuricemia. Presence in the serum of large amount of IgG fragment. Abnormal and incomplete production of antibodies. *Urine.* Presence of IgG fragment. *X-ray.* Chest lymphadenopathy; normal skeleton. *Bone marrow.* Normal or increased plasma cells, lymphocytes, reticular cells; eosinophilia. *Biopsy.* Of lymph node. Cells similar to those mentioned in bone marrow.

Therapy. Trial with chemotherapy; corticosteroids. Alkylating agents; combination chemotherapy with MOPP. Radiotherapy not recommended.

Prognosis. Poor. Supervening infection or other effects of a malignant condition are frequent causes of death. Some patients have survived for several years.

BIBLIOGRAPHY. Franklin EC, Lowenstein J, Bigelow B, et al: Heavy chain disease: A new disorder of serum gamma globulins. Report of the first case. Am J Med 37:332–350, 1964
Osserman EF, Takatsuki K: Clinical and immunochemical studies of four cases of heavy (Htz 2) chain disease. Am J Med 37:351–373, 1964
Foerster J: Heavy chain diseases. In Lee GR, Bithel TC, Foerster J, et al (eds): Wintrobe's Clinical Hematology, 9th ed, pp 2266–2267. Philadelphia, Lea & Febiger, 1993

FRANZ

Indicates the cessation of the thrill that is observed after the proximal venous section of an arterovenous fistula.

BIBLIOGRAPHY. Franz CA: Klinische und experimentelle Beigrage betreffend das Aneurysma arteriovenosum. Arch Klin Chir 75:572–623, 1905

FRASER

Synonyms. Meyers-Schwickerath; Ullrich-Feichtiger; cryptophthalmos—syndactyly; deafness—cryptophthalmos—syndactyly. See Cyclopia.

Symptoms and Signs. Both sexes affected. Occasionally, stillborn. Cryptophthalmos (hidden eye) (85%), complete failure in development of lid folds, or subsequent destruction and absorption of lids. May be bilateral, monolateral, or cryptophthalmos on one side and microphthalmos on the other side. Associated defects: middle and external ear malformation; deafness; high or cleft palate; deformity of larynx; hoarse voice; wide separation of symphysis pubis; displacement of umbilicus and nipples; various digital malformations; meningoencephaloceles; anal stenosis; congenital cardiac malformations; renal hypoplasia or agenesis. Masculinization of external genitalia in females. Cryptorchidism, small penis, hypospadias in males.

Etiology. Unknown; autosomal recessive inheritance (?). Possibility of altered sex chromosomal pattern.

Pathology. Eye enophthalmos or various alteration; buphophthalmos; absence of trabeculae, Schlemm canal, and ciliary muscles; abnormal lens. See Signs.

Diagnostic Procedures. *Chromosome study. Endocrine studies.*

Therapy. Early surgical intervention may help in preserving adequate visual perception.

Prognosis. Survival depends on renal involvement and other malformations.

BIBLIOGRAPHY. Zehender W: Eine Missgeburt mit hautüberwachsenen Augen oder Kryptophthalmus. Klin Monatsbl Augenheilkd 10:225, 1872

Gupta SP, Saxena RC: Cryptophthalmos. Br J Ophthalmol 46:629–632, 1962

Fraser CR: Our genetic "load": A review of some aspects of genetical variation. Ann Hum Genet 25:387, 1962

Boyd PA, Keeling JW, Lindenbaum RH: Fraser syndrome (Cryptophtalmos-Syndactyly syndrome): A review of 11 cases with postmortem findings. Am J Med Genet 31:159–168, 1988

Ramsing M, Rehder H, Holzgreve W, et al: Fraser syndrome (cryptophthalmos with syndactyly) in the fetus and newborn. Clin Genet 37:84–96, 1990

FREEMAN–SHELDON

Synonyms. Craniocarpotarsal dystrophy; whistling face; windmill vane hand.

Symptoms. Present from birth. Prematurity. Vomiting; feeding difficulties; failure to thrive (secondary to feeding difficulties). Normal mental development. Nasal speech.

Signs. *Facies.* Mask-like; small mouth; whistling aspect; H-shaped dimple of chin. *Eyes.* Deep set. Epicanthus. *Nose.* Small; broad bridge; hypoplastic alae; long philtrum. *Mouth.* Small tongue; high palate. *Hands.* Ulnar deviation; thickening of skin of flexor aspect of proximal phalanges. *Feet.* Equinovarus. Associated abnormalities: small stature; scoliosis; strabismus; blepharophimosis. Generalized myopathy that is associated with the later development of kyphoscoliosis. In addition to intercostal myopathy, this can lead to restrictive lung disease.

Etiology. Sporadic, or autosomal dominant inheritance.

Diagnostic Procedures. *X-ray. Skeletal survey. Blood.* Normal. *Chromosome studies. Electromyography. Muscle biopsy.*

Therapy. Treatment consists of correcting malnutrition of the infant combined with corrective surgery in the child and adult for the wide range of musculoskeletal deformities, especially scoliosis.

Prognosis. Occasionally, failure to thrive. Normal intelligence. Possible reproduction. Early corrective surgery of the deformities can result in the patient leading a normal life with normal expectancy.

BIBLIOGRAPHY. Freeman EA, Sheldon JH: Cranio-carpo-tarsal dystrophy. An undescribed congenital formation. Arch Dis Child 13:277–283, 1938

Laishley RS, Roy WL: Freeman–Sheldon syndrome: Report of three cases and the anaesthetic implications. Can Anaesth Soc J 33:388–393, 1986

Marasovich WA, Mazaheri M, Stool SE: Otolaryngologic findings in

whistling face syndrome. Arch Otolaryng Head Neck Surg 115:1373–1380, 1989

FREIBERG INFRACTION

Synonyms. Freiberg; metatarsal head osteochondritis. See Epiphyseal ischemic necrosis.

Symptoms and Signs. Dull pain in anterior part of foot induced by walking. Swelling of metatarsal-phalangeal joint; overlying skin red.

Etiology. Epiphyseal ischemic necrosis of fourth or fifth metatarsal head.

Therapy. In acute stage, antiflammatory agents. Later if pain, deformity, or disability, surgery.

BIBLIOGRAPHY. Köhler A: Eine typische Erkrankung des 2 Metatarsophalangeal-gealaelenkes. MMW 67:1289–1290, 1920

Freiberg AH: The so-called infraction of the second metatarsal bone. J Bone Joint Surg 8:257–261, 1926

Klippel JH, Dieppe PA: Rheumatology, pp 5.13.9, 7.4.9. St Louis, CV Mosby, 1995

FRENKEL

Synonyms. Eyeball contusion; ocular contusion, anterior segment traumatic.

Symptoms. History of trauma of the anterior segment of eye. Visual disturbances.

Signs. D-shaped mydriasis (chord replacing the arc in a sector) observed in 85% of cases; single or multiple iris dehiscences (50%); lens lesions (opacities and subluxation) (60%); retrolenticular pigment particles (56%). Posterior segment lesions may also coexist.

Etiology. The syndrome consists of the variable sequelae observed after the trauma (sometimes months or, occasionally, years later).

Pathology. See Signs.

Diagnostic Procedures. *Slit lamp microscopic examination. Transillumination of iris.*

Therapy. As indicated by type of lesions.

Prognosis. Guarded.

BIBLIOGRAPHY. Frenkel H: Sur la valeur médicolégale du syndrome traumatique du segment antérieur. Arch Ophthalmol 48:5–27, 1931

Paton D, Goldberg MF: Injuries of the lids and the orbit. In Diagnosis and Management. Philadelphia, WB Saunders, 1976

Morris DA: Ocular trauma. In Garner A, Klintworth GK (eds): Pathobiology of Ocular Disease: A Dynamic Approach, 2nd ed. New York, Marcel Dekker, 1994

FREY (L.)

Synonyms. von Frey; Baillarger; Dupuy; auriculotemporal; salivo-sudoriparous; sweating gustatory. See also chorda tympani.

Symptoms and Signs. Unilateral localized flushing and hyperhydrosis of the pinna of ear and cheek, when eating hot, bitter, spicy substances or chocolate, or rinsing mouth, especially with acid substances; decreased sensitivity to the heat in the involved area. Flushing prevalent in females; sweating in males.

Etiology. Following injury or surgery of the parotid gland, or associated with infection of the gland in response to ingestion of acid food. Related to one of these mechanisms: regeneration of salivary fibers into sweat fiber; hypersensitivity of denervated sweat fibers.

Pathology. See Etiology.

Diagnostic Procedures. *Starch-iodine test.* Test the reflex with acid and substance on posterior third of tongue.

Therapy. Procaine injection of auriculotemporal nerve at the tragus level. Resection of parasympathetic tympanic plexus. Tympanic plexus resection.

Prognosis. Possible extension of area of involvement. In most patients symptoms tolerated. Ten percent of patients require surgery, 5% show spontaneous regression and disappearance of symptoms.

BIBLIOGRAPHY. Duphenix: Sur une playe compliquée à la joue, on le canal salivaire fut déchire. Néur Acad R Chir 3:431–437, 1757

Frey L: Le syndrome du nerf auriculotemporal. Rev Neurol (Paris) 2:97–104, 1923

Harper KE, Spievogel RL: Frey's syndrome. Int J Dermatol 25:524–526, 1986

Gorlin RJ, Cohen MM Jr, Levin LS: Syndromes of Head and Neck, pp 615–616. New York, Oxford Univ Press, 1990

FRIED

Synonyms. Tooth-nail Fried.

Symptoms and Signs. From birth. Hair: fine and short. Teeth: few, peg-shaped. Nails: thin and dystrophic.

Etiology. Autosomal recessive inheritance.

BIBLIOGRAPHY. Fried K: Autosomal recessive hydrotic ectodermal dysplasia. J Med Genet 14:137–139, 1977

FRIED-EMERY

Synonyms. Spino muscular atrophy Type II; S. M. A. II; spinal, intermediate muscular atrophy; see Werding-Hoffmann (type I) and Kugelberg (type II).

Symptoms and Signs. Onset between 3 and 12 months. Failure to achieve milestones of development. Patients barely reach ability to sit; weakness and wasting are symmetrical, and prevalently proximal, fasciculation may be present, no facial weakness, tendon reflexes absent or decreased, occasionally fine tremor of fingers, joint contractures typical at later age, scoliosis, normal intelligence.

Etiology. Autosomal recessive inheritance. It is likely that all three forms of SMA are allelic. Locus mapped to 5q12-q24.

Diagnostic Procedures. *Blood.* Creatinine kinase frequently normal.

Therapy. Symptomatic.

Prognosis. Survival into adolescence or adulthood.

BIBLIOGRAPHY. Fried K, Emery AEH: Spinal muscular atrophy type II. Clin Genet 2:203–209, 1971

Emery AEH: Muscular atrophy, spinal, intermediate. In Vinken PJ, Bruyn GW: Handbook of Clinical Neurology, vol 42, pp 89–90. Amsterdam, North-Holland,1981

Melki J, Abdelhak S, Sheth P, et al: Gene for chronic proximal spinal muscular atrophies maps to chromosome 5q. Nature 344:767–768, 1990

FRIEDMAN-ROY

Synonyms. Choroid plexus calcification; mental retardation.

Symptoms and Signs. From birth. Strabismus, hyperactive deep reflexes, positive Babinski, lolling speech, mental retardation.

Etiology. Autosomal recessive inheritance.

Pathology. Extensive calcification of choroid plexus.

Diagnostic Procedures. *X-ray. CT scan. MRI.* Choroid plexus diffuse calcification. CSF protein increased.

Therapy. Symptomatic.

BIBLIOGRAPHY. Friedman AP, Roy JE: An unusual familial syndrome. J Nerv Ment Dis 99:42–44, 1944

Lott IT, Williams RS, Schnur JA, et al: Familial amentia, unusual ventricular calcifications and increased cerebrospinal fluid proteins. Neurology 29:1571–1577, 1979

FRIEDREICH

Synonyms. Essential myoclonia; paramyoclonus multiplex, including myoclonus hereditary essential.

Symptoms and Signs. Onset usually in adult life. Sudden, brief, clonic jerks affecting single muscle part, entire muscle, or muscle group. With excitement contractions increase; stop during sleep.

Etiology. More a symptom than a syndrome. (1) Part of petit mal syndrome may initially be the only manifestation; (2) symptom of diffuse central nervous system degenerative diseases; (3) "sleep start," "night start," violent muscle contractions occurring in young healthy man; fatigue at time of waking. Familial occurrence reported with autosomal dominant type of inheritance.

Therapy. Clonazepam, valproic acid, and 5-hydroxytryptophan.

Prognosis. It persists with no practical changes throughout life.

BIBLIOGRAPHY. Friedreich N: Paramyoclonus multiplex. Arch Pathol Anat 86:421–430, 1881

Lance JW: Myoclonic jerks and falls: An etiology, classification and treatment. Med J Aust 1:113–119, 1968

Korten JJ, Notermans SLH, Frenken CWGM, et al: Familial essential myoclonus. Brain 97:131–138, 1974

Adams RD, Victor M: Principles of Neurology, 5th ed, p 993. New York, McGraw-Hill, 1993

FRIEDREICH ATAXIA

Synonyms. Spinocerebellar ataxia; FA. See spinocerebellar and Bassen-Kornzweig (in the past early cases of B-K considered among the variants of Friedreich ataxia).

Symptoms. Onset in first year of life; only deformity of feet (pes cavus; Friedreich foot; hammer toe). Onset between 7 and 15 years of age; clumsy gait that becomes more and more ataxic and broad-based, difficulty in turning arms, head, and trunk. Patients are affected later with tremor, dysmetria, asynergia, dysdiadochokinesia, slow ataxic speech, choreiform movement, and occasionally, pain and paresthesias. Blindness and deafness also reported.

Signs. Tendon reflexes decreased and then lost. Babinski sign. Nystagmus. Loss of position sense, vibratory sense, and two-point discrimination. Kyphoscoliosis in the thoracic column. Muscle wasting, more on lower extremity. High percentage of patients with signs of cardiac involvement.

Etiology. Unknown; autosomal recessive or dominant (rarely in this case associated with optic atrophy and sensineural deafness).

Pathology. Degeneration of spinocerebellar tracts, corticospinal tracts, and posterior columns of spinal cord. Optical and cochlear degeneration (possibly). Myocardial fibers degenerated and relaced by fibroblasts.

Diagnostic Procedures. *Spinal fluid.* Normal or occasionally moderate increase of protein and cells. *ECG.* Occasionally, bundle-branch block or complete heart block. *X-ray.* Marked scoliosis; pes cavus. *Blood.* Frequently, hyperglycemia (23%). *Motor and sensory nerve conduction.* Abnormalities. *CT scan. MRI.*

Therapy. Amantidine hydrochloride. Physostigmine, Thyrotropin-releasing hormone, 5-hydroxytryptophan benserazide. Claimed benefits from all these drugs have not been confirmed.

Prognosis. Progressive; occasionally, remission; possibly incapacitating by 20 years of age. Death from intercurrent diseases or cardiac failure.

BIBLIOGRAPHY. Friedreich N: Über degenerative Atrophie der spinalen, Hinterstränge. Arch Anat Physiol 26:391–419, 1863

Ackroyd RS, Finnegan JA, Green SH: Friedreich's ataxia: A clinical review with neurophysiological and echocardiographic findings. Arch Dis Child 59:217–221, 1984

Peterson PL, Saad J, Nigro MA: The treatment of Friedreich's ataxia with amantidine hydrochloride. Neurology 38:1478–1480, 1988

Keats BJB, Ward LJ, Shaw J, et al: "Acadian" and "classical" forms of Friedreich ataxia are most probably caused by mutations at the same locus. Am J Med Genet 33:266–268, 1989

Adams RD, Victor M: Principles of Neurology, 5th ed, pp 987–988. New York, McGraw-Hill, 1993

FRIEDREICH–AUERBACH

Synonym. Hypertrophic myopathy; hypertrophia musculorum vera.

Symptoms. Prevalent in males; onset usually in childhood, adolescence, or early adult life. Vague onset. Occasionally, poorly localized, vague, painful sensation in muscles affected.

Signs. Slow enlargement of the muscles of limbs more frequently than trunk. Any muscle of the body may be affected, however, including tongue. Different muscles may be involved at same time or successively. Strength of affected muscle usually increased. Myotonic phenomenon in 50% of cases. Reflexes normal. Hyperhidrosis of limb or side involved frequently observed. No visceral or skeletal involvement.

Etiology. Unknown. X-linked inheritance. In early reports includes several entities. See Kocher-Debrè-Semelaigne; Hoffmann; Becker; Masseter hypertrophy; Barnes; etc.

Pathology. Enlargement of muscle fibers. Nuclei may be found in central part of fibers; occasionally, vascular wall slightly thickened.

Diagnostic Procedures. *Electromyography.* Normal. *Biopsy.*

Therapy. None.

Prognosis. Spontaneous arrest.

BIBLIOGRAPHY. Auerbach L: Ein Fall von Waher Muskelhypertrophie. Virchows Arch (Pathol Anat) 53:397–417, 1817

Gardner-Medwin D: Hypertrophia musculorum vera. In Vinken PJ, Bruyn GW: Handbook of Clinical Neurology, vol 43, pp 83–85. Amsterdam, North-Holland, 1982

Adams RD, Denny-Brown D, Pearson CM: Diseases of the Muscle, 3rd ed, p 536. New York, Harper & Row, 1975

FRIEDRICH

Synonyms. Epiphyseal necrosis sternal ends; see Epiphyseal necrosis.

Symptoms and Signs. Asymptomatic or pain in the chest.

Etiology. See Epiphyseal necrosis.

BIBLIOGRAPHY. Friedrich H: Ueber ein noch nicht beschiriebenes der Perthesschen Enkrankung analoges, Krankheitsbild des sternalen Klaviclendes. Deut Zschr Chir 187:385–398, 1924

FROEHLICH

Synonyms. Babinski-Froehlich; Leaunois-Cléret; adiposogenital; hypothalamic infantilism-obesity; sexual infantilism.

Symptoms. Prevalent in males. Headache; retarded growth and sexual development; mental retardation; visual troubles; polyuria; polydipsia.

Signs. Prepubertal adiposity of breast, abdomen, femoral regions, large hips. Delayed appearance of secondary sexual characteristic, hair of pubis, axillae, face. Skin remains delicate. Dysonychia.

Etiology. Hypopituitarism; hypothalamic functional alterations; tumor compressing or involving anterior pituitary gland; idiopathic. Wilkins suggests limiting the diagnosis of Froehlich syndrome to only those cases in which the pituitary disturbance is proved.

Pathology. See above; occasionally, craniopharyngioma.

Diagnostic Procedures. *Urine.* Follicle-stimulating hormone (FSH), luteinizing hormone (LH), and 17-ketosteroid determinations. Vasopressin test for polyuria if diabetes insipidus. *X-ray.* Of skull. Suprasellar calcification or destructive lesion. Skeleton shows delayed ossification.

Therapy. If tumor, extirpation or X-ray, administration of pituitary extracts.

Prognosis. Depends on etiology.

BIBLIOGRAPHY. Froehlich A: Ein Fall von Tumor der Hypophysis Cerebri ohne Akromegalie. Wien Klin Rundshan 15:833–836; 906–908, 1901

Launois PE, Cléret M: Le syndrome hypophisaire adipose-génital. Gaz Hôp 83:57–64; 83–86, 1910

Bruch H: The Froehlich syndrome: Report of the original case. Am J Dis Child 58:1282–1289, 1939

Adams RD, Victor M: Principles of Neurology, 5th ed, p 486. New York, McGraw-Hill, 1993

FROIN

Synonyms. Lépine-Froin; Nonne-Froin; spinal fluid coagulation. Froin syndrome is the designation for the coagulation of spinal fluid shortly after being removed. Observed in tumor of spinal cord, in chronic arachnoiditis, and other conditions where a marked increase of protein occurs.

BIBLIOGRAPHY. Froin G: Inflammation méningées avec réactions chromatiques, fibrineuse et cytologique. Gaz Hôp 76:1005–1006, 1903

Nonne M: Weitere Erfahrungen zum Kapitel der Diagnose von Komprimirenden Rueckenmarks-tumoren. Dtsch Z Nervenheilk 47:436, 1913

Grinker RR: Chronic arachno-perineuritis with the syndrome of Froin, pseudotumor spinalis. J Nerv Ment Dis 64:616–628, 1926

Crook DWM, Phuapradit P, Warrell DA: Bacterial meningitis. In Weatherall DJ, Ledingham JGG, Warrell DA (eds): Oxford Textbook of Medicine, 3rd ed, p 4061. Oxford, Oxford Med Pub, 1996

FRUCTOSE 1,6-BISPHOSPHATASE, HEREDITARY DEFICIENCY

Synonyms. Baker-Winegrad; fructose 1, 6-Diphosphatase deficiency; FDPase deficiency.

Symptoms. Both sexes affected, slight prevalence in females; occurs in infants, usually before 6 months of age after ingesting food containing fructose or after infections, fatigue, fasting, and severe stress: hyperventilation, hypoglycemia (fits; seizures; coma) and acidosis frequently fatal or requiring hospitalization. Nausea and vomiting do not occur after fructose ingestion. At older age no aversion to sugar and sweets.

Signs. The child is not emaciated; frequently is obese and hepatomegalic.

Etiology. Autosomal recessive inheritance; deficiency of fructose 1,6-diphosphatase.

Pathology. Liver: hepatomegaly; fatty infiltration.

Diagnostic Procedures. *Blood.* In normal conditions, normal values of glucose and lactic acid; in stressful situation and after ingestion of fructose: hypoglycemia, lactic acidosis; aminoacidemia; hyperglycerolemia. *Biopsy of liver.* Lack of fructose 1,6-diphosphatase. *Caution.* Diagnostic measures such as administration of fructose, glycerol, dehydroxy-acetone are dangerous. After fasting, administration of glucagon (1 mg) is a less dangerous test. No rise of blood glucose.

Therapy. Prevention of stressful situation and of fructose administration. Glucose intravenous.

Prognosis. Severe in first months because of difficulty in recognizing the condition. Later on, if condition recognized, normal development and life span.

BIBLIOGRAPHY. Baker LI, Winegard AI: Fasting hypoglycemia and metabolic acidosis associated with deficiency of hepatic fructose 1,6-diphosphatase activity. Lancet 2:13–16, 1970
Gitzelmann R, Steinmann B, Van den Berghe G: Disorder of Fructose Metabolism. In Scriver CR, Beaudet AL, Sly WS, et al: The Metabolic and Molecular Bases of Inherited Disease, 7th ed, pp 920–924. New York, McGraw-Hill, 1995

FRUCTOSE INTOLERANCE, HEREDITARY

Synonyms. Chambers-Pratt; fructose intolerance; HFI.

Symptoms. Both sexes, even distribution. No symptoms as long as patients do not ingest food containing fructose. First symptoms in infancy when sucrose or fructose added to diet. Unconsciousness; convulsions; vomiting; failure to thrive; cachexia may result in death. In less severe case with true signs of hepatic cirrhosis. In older children and adults, strong aversion for fruit and sweets prevent other manifestations.

Signs. In infancy, hepatomegaly, jaundice, edema, ascites.

Etiology. Congenital absence of fructose phosphate-splitting liver aldolase. Autosomal recessive trait in most, but not all families. Defect of fructose-1-phosphate aldolase B of liver, kidney cortex, and small intestine. Autosomal recessive trait in most but not all families. Genetic heterogenecity owing to different genotype has been described.

Pathology. From diffuse steatosis to early cirrhosis of the liver in infants; kidney: discrete histological changes; granulation and vacuolization; intestine: submucosal or serosal hemorrhages.

Diagnostic Procedures. *Blood.* Anemia, thrombocytopenia, acanthocytes, fragmentocytes. Hypoglycemia following ingestion of fructose 1,6-diphosphate; aldolase, serum glutamic-oxaloacetic transaminase (SGOT), glutamic pyruvic transaminase (GPT) increase; fall of inorganic serum phosphorus. Hyperbilirubinemia; intravenous fructose tolerance test (200 mg/kg) typical signs. *Urine.* Albuminuria; aminoaciduria; fructosuria (after fructose ingestion).

Therapy. Diet without fructose. In case of cirrhosis, liver transplantation has been attempted with good results.

Prognosis. Good if no fructose ingested. Attacks do not seem to cause serious brain damage.

BIBLIOGRAPHY. Chambers RA, Pratt RTC: Idiosyncrasy to fructose. Lancet 2:340, 1956
Froesch ER, Prader A, Labhart A, et al: Die hereditare Fructoseintoleranz, eine bisher nicht bekannte kongenitale Stoffwechsel Störung. Schweiz Med Wochenschr 86:1168–1171, 1957
Gitzelmann R, Steinmann B, Van den Berghe G: Disorders of Fructose metabolism. In Scriver CR, Beaudet AL, Sly WS, et al: The Metabolic and Molecular Bases of Inherited Disease, 7th ed, pp 914–920. New York, McGraw-Hill, 1995

FRUCTOSURIA, ESSENTIAL

Synonyms. Hepatic fructokinase deficiency.

Symptoms and Signs. None.

Etiology. Autosomal recessive inheritance. Lack of hepatic fructokinase.

Diagnostic Procedures. After ingestion of food containing fructose: *Blood and urine.* Fructosuria; fructosemia of high level (over 25 mg/100 ml); normal glucose and galactose metabolism.

Therapy. Diet.

Prognosis. Harmless condition.

BIBLIOGRAPHY. Czapek F: Eine seltene Form von Diabetees mellitus. Prager Med Wochenschr 1:245–265, 1876
Zimmer K I: Levulose im harn eines Diabetikers. Dsch Med Wochenschr 1:329, 1976
Gitzelmann R, Steinmann B, Van Den Berghe G: Disorders of fructose metabolism. In Scriver CR, Beaudet AL, Sly WS, et al: The Metabolic and Molecular Bases of Inherited Disease, 7th ed, p 399. New York, McGraw-Hill, 1995

FRYNS

Symptoms and Signs. Both sexes. Broad and flat nasal bridge, receding mandible, misshapen ears, broad and short neck with additional skin folds; brachytelephalangy with hypoplastic nails of fingers and toes; cleft palate, hypoplasia and abnormal lobation of the lungs, diaphragmatic defects, uterus bicornis/duplex, malrotation of intestines. Less frequently, apparent heart defects, cystic dysplastic kidneys, and other abnormalities of the urinary tract, net-like form of tracheal and bronchial cartilage, and brain malformations.

Etiology. Autosomal recessive gene or sporadic.

Pathology. Cystic-adenomatoid malformations; total distortion of the architecture of the various organs; multiple glioneural heterotopias.

Diagnostic Procedures. *Prenatal ultrasonographic examination.*

Therapy. Symptomatic.

Prognosis. Lethal syndrome. After the birth of an affected child, the parents face a 25% recurrence risk for any further pregnancy.

BIBLIOGRAPHY. Fryns JP, Moerman F, Goddeeris P, Bossuyt C, Van den Berghe H: A new lethal syndrome with cloudy corneae, diaphragmatic defects and distal limb deformities. Hum Genet 50:65–70, 1979
Aymé S, Julian C, Gambarelli D, et al: Fryn's syndrome: Report of 8 cases. Clin Genet 35:191–201, 1989
Kerschisnik MM, Craven CM, Jung AL, et al: Osteochondroplasia in Fryn's syndrome. Am J Dis Child 145:656–660, 1991

FUCHS I

Synonyms. Cutaneous muco-oculoepithelial; mucocutaneous ocular; ocular mucocutaneous. Eponym indicates a nonfebrile Stevens-Johnson variant.

BIBLIOGRAPHY. Fuchs E: Herpes iris congiuntival. Klin Monatsbl Augenheilkd 14:333–351, 1876

FUCHS II

Synonym. Blepharochalasis. See Ascher.

Symptoms and Signs. Onset at young age with transient, recurrent edemas of angioneurotic type in both eyelids (usually, only the superiors; occasionally, also the inferiors). Then with the progress of the disease, prolapse of the orbital fat and lacrimal glands and blepharoptosis.

Etiology. Unknown. Localized atrophy of the eyelids, skin, and subcutaneous tissue.

Pathology. Histologic aspect depends on stage of disease, from simple edema of subcutis, lymphocytic perivascular infiltration to atrophy of dermis, and finally disappearance of elastic fibers.

Therapy. Plastic surgery.

Prognosis. Progressive condition.

BIBLIOGRAPHY. Fuchs E: Ueber Blepharochalasis (Erschlaffung der Lidhaut). Wein Klin Wochenschr 9:109, 1896
Schulze F: Beitrag zur heridetaeren Blepharocalasis. Klin Monatsbl Augenheilkd 14:863–877, 1965

FUCHS III

Synonyms. Fuchs heterochromia, heterochromic uveitis; heterochromic cyclitis.

Symptoms. Both sexes. Onset from puberty to fourth decade of life. Insidious onset; patient in most of the cases is unaware of condition until blurring of vision develops.

Signs. *Heterochromia:* Slight or marked difference in color between the two irides. Lighter in affected eye. One or both eyes may be involved (occasionally, heterochromia may be missing). *Cyclitis:* Mild, chronic, whitish keratic precipitates, not confluent, observed in pupillary area and lower part of cornea. *Cataract:* Develops only late in the disease. Peripheral choroiditis may be present.

Etiology. Iridocyclitis with loss of pigment in the iris of affected eye(s). Immunologic factors (humoral and cellular) may play a role.

Pathology. In iris, lower number of melanocytes, diffuse fibrosis, and lymphocyte and plasma cell infiltration. Ciliary body fibrosis; muscular atrophy. Focal cyclitis; peripheral choroiditis.

Diagnostic Procedures. *Ophthalmoscopy. Tonometry.*

Therapy. None; cataract removal once developed. Corticosteroids do not alter course of disease but decrease discomfort.

Prognosis. Relatively good for its slow chronic course. Possibility of glaucoma has to be kept in mind and eventually treated.

BIBLIOGRAPHY. Fuchs E: Uber Komplikationen der Heterochromie. Klin Monatsbl Augenheilk 15:191–212, 1906
Hart CT, Ward DM: Intraocular pressure in Fuchs' heterochromic uveitis. Br J Ophthalmol 51:739–743, 1967
Forster CS: Ocular manifestations of immune disease. In Garner A, Klintworth GK (eds): Pathobiology of Ocular Disease: A Dynamic Approach, 2nd ed, pp 165–166. New York, Marcel Dekker, 1994

FUCHS IV

Synonyms. Fuchs-Kraupa; Fuchs combined dystrophy; Kraupa; Groenouw-Fuchs; endothelial corneal dystrophy; corneal erosion.

Symptoms. Occurs in elderly persons; prevalent in females. Ocular pain; photophobia; disturbed vision.

Signs. Corneal vesicles and bullae, erosions, and scarring.

Etiology. Unknown. Most cases sporadic. Suggestion of autosomal dominant inheritance with greater expression in females, possibility of X-linked dominant inheritance also formulated. Etiopathogenesis owing to a decreased pumping and barrier function of the disordered endothelium.

Pathology. Descemet membrane presents hyaline deposits, endothelial erosions, edema; Bowman membrane shows degeneration features; on posterior corneal surface evidence of pigmentation.

Diagnostic Procedures. *Ophthalmoscopy.* See Signs and Pathology.

Therapy. Hypertonic solutions; irradiation of lacrimal glands; corneal transplantation.

Prognosis. Early in disease fair response to treatment. Corneal transplantation effective in 60% of cases.

BIBLIOGRAPHY. Fuchs E: Dystrophia epithelialis corneae. Albrecht von Graefes Arch Ophthalmol 76:478–508, 1910
Kraupa E: Pigmentierungen der Hornhauthinterflaeche bei "Dystrophia epithelialis (Fuchs)." Z Augenheilk Berlin 44:247, 1920
Rodrigues MM, Rajagopalan S, Jones KA: Anterior and posterior corneal dystrophy. In Garner A, Klintworth GK (eds): Pathobiology of Ocular Disease: A Dynamic Approach, 2nd ed. New York, Marcel Dekker, 1994

FUKUYAMA

Synonyms. Muscular dystrophy; mental retardation; epilepsy.

Symptoms and Signs. If not exclusive, prevalent in Japanese. In 20% of cases asphyxia at birth, and 50% show abnormal muscles in neonatal period (hypotonia, weak cry, and suck); slow motor development. Growing weakness becomes even more marked including all muscles (including face); atrophy or, in 40% of cases pseudohypertrophy develops; joint contractures, at 6 months in 30% and at 3 years in 65% of cases. Mental retardation with IQ 50 circa, with very limited vocabulary. Epilepsy in 40% circa. Tongue large; teeth small and irregular; palate arched; fingers short.

Etiology. Unknown. Autosomal recessive inheritance.

Diagnostic Procedures. *Blood.* Elevation of muscle enzymes. *Electromyography.* Slow conduction rate. *CT scan. MRI.* Ventricular dilatation. *Biopsy.* Muscle fiber degeneration, marked connective tissue infiltration rare, hypertrophic fibers, then fatty infiltration of motor endplates that are often ballooned or deformed. *Electroencephalography.*

Therapy. Symptomatic.

Prognosis. Premature death from respiratory infections, acute enteritis commonly before 12 years of age.

BIBLIOGRAPHY. Fukuyama Y, Kawazura M, Haruna H: A peculiar form of congenital muscular dystrophy. Paediatria Universitatis Tokio 4:5, 1960
Stevens DL: Muscular dystrophy, congenital with mental retardation and epilepsy (Fukuyama syndrome). In Vinken PJ, Bruyn GW: Handbook of Clinical Neurology, vol 43, pp 91–92. Amsterdam, North-Holland, 1982

FUNDUS ALBIPUNCTATUS

Symptoms. Both sexes affected; increasing constriction of visual fields; night blindness; and finally blindness.

Signs. White spots scattered on the retina, more concentrated at posterior pole.

Etiology. Unknown, autosomal recessive or dominant inheritance.

BIBLIOGRAPHY. Krill AE, Falk MR: Retinis punctata albescens: A functional evaluation of an unusual case. Am J Ophthalmol 53:450–454, 1962
Krill AE: Hereditary Retinal and Choroidal Diseases: Flecked Retina Diseases, vol 2, pp 739–819. Hagerstown, MD, Harper & Row, 1977
Garner A, Sarks S, Sarks JP: Degenerative and related disorders of the retina and choroid. In Garner A, Klintworth GK (eds): Pathobiology of Ocular Disease: A Dynamic Approach, 2nd ed. New York, Marcel Dekker, 1994

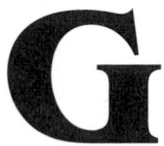

GAISBÖCK

Synonyms. Emotional polycythemia; stress erythrocytosis; benign polycythemia; polycythemia hypertonica; pseudopolycythemia; stress polycythemia.

Symptoms. Prevalent in men, usually in heavy smokers; onset at mean age 45. Tenseness; nervousness.

Signs. Moderate overweight; slight plethora; conjunctival congestion. Some patients have persistent blood hypertension. No splenomegaly.

Etiology. Constitutional disposition or association with emotional tension or both.

Diagnostic Procedures. *Blood.* Determination of blood volume; relative polycythemia (decreased plasma) or mild absolute polycythemia. High hematocrit. Leukocytes and platelets normal.

Therapy. None or diet; sedative; psychotherapy. Therapeutic value of phlebotomy not established.

Prognosis. Good; some develop or have associated vascular diseases.

BIBLIOGRAPHY. Gaisböck F: Die Bedeutung der Blutdruckmessung für die ärztliche Praxis. Dtsch Arch Klin Med 83:363–409, 1905

Russell RP, Conley CL: Benign polycythemia: Gaisböck's syndrome. Arch Intern Med 114:734–740, 1964

Avins LR, Krummenacher TK: Venous stasis retinopathy and Gaisböck's syndrome. Am J Ophthalmol 105:420–421, 1988

Athens JW, Lee GR: Polycythemia: Erythrocytosis. In Lee GR, Bithel TC, Foerster J, et al (eds): Wintrobe's Clinical Hematology, 9th ed, p 1250. Philadelphia, Lea & Febiger, 1993

GALACTOKINASE DEFICIENCY–GALACTOSEMIA

Synonyms. Gitzelmann; galactosemia II; galactose diabetes.

Symptoms and Signs. Both sexes affected; onset after a few weeks of life or in older age. Absence of inanition, gastrointestinal disorders, and jaundice. Irregularly progressing reduction of vision that may reach blindness. Normal intelligence. Hepatosplenomegaly only during the period of milk feeding (not consistently present). Recurrent cataract.

Etiology. Autosomal recessive inheritance. Deficiency of galactokinase activity. Cataracts caused by failure of galactose phosphorylation.

Pathology. Apparently limited to cataract formation.

Diagnostic Procedures. *Urine.* Galactosuria (especially after milk feeding). *Blood.* High galactosemia (after milk feeding); absence of galactokinase in red cells (normal galactose-1-phosphate uridyltransferase).

Therapy. Diet without milk and derivatives.

Prognosis. Variable degree of recurrence of cataracts and visual impairment.

BIBLIOGRAPHY. Fanconi G: Hochgrädige Galaktose-Intolleranz (Galaktose Diabetes) bei einem Kinde mit Neurofibromatosis Recklinghausen. Jahrb Klinderheilkd 138:1–8, 1933

Gitzelmann R: Hereditary galactokinase deficiency, a newly recognized cause of juvenile cataracts. Pediatr Res 1:14–23, 1967

Segal S, Berry GT: Disorders of galactose metabolism. In Scriver CR,

Beaudet AL, Sly WS, et al: The Metabolic and Molecular Bases of Inherited Disease, 7th ed, pp 987–989. New York, McGraw-Hill, 1995

GALACTORRHEA, BLACK

Synonyms. Black galactorrhea.

Symptoms and Signs. Excretion of black milk in lactating patient.

Etiology. Administration of minocycline or phenothiazine.

BIBLIOGRAPHY. Basler RSW, Lynch PJ: Black galactorrhea as a consequence of minocycline and phenothiazine therapy. Arch Dermatol 121:417–418, 1985

GALACTOSEMIA I

Synonyms. Mason-Turner; von Reuss; galactose-1-phosphate uridyltransferase deficiency; transferase deficiency galactosemia.

Symptoms. Both sexes affected; onset after few days or weeks of milk ingestion. Vomiting; diarrhea; dehydration; hypoglycemic crisis; failure to grow. In fulminating cases; death. In intermediate cases, hypotonia, lethargy, severe mental and neurologic manifestations. In mild cases, only milk intolerance.

Signs. Jaundice; ascites (found in infants who died); hepatomegaly between 4 and 8 weeks of life, formation of cataracts.

Etiology. Inability to metabolize galactose because of deficiency of galactose 1-phosphate uridyl transferase. Autosomal recessive inheritance. Various allelic types have been detected that cause intermediate syndromes. Negro, Duarte, Münster, Indiana, Rennes, Los Angeles, Chicago, variants.

Pathology. In liver, typical acinar formation, cirrhosis, galactose infiltration.

Diagnostic Procedures. *Blood.* Elevated galactose; decreased glucose (especially evident during crisis); abnormal galactose tolerance. Red cell screening test for determination of deficiency of galactose 1-phosphate uridyl transferase. Hemoglobinemia; immature red blood cells. *Bone marrow.* Erythroblastosis-like pattern (occasionally). *Urine.* Galactose; albumin; aminoaciduria (several amino acids).

Therapy. Galactose-free diet. Liver transplantation.

Prognosis. Continuation of administration of galactose-containing food leads to death. If galactose-free diet is started promptly, all symptoms and signs disappear. Cirrhosis and cataract also may regress. If mental retardation already established, no improvement. Preventable only by very early withdrawal of galactose from diet.

BIBLIOGRAPHY. von Reuss A: Zuckerausscheidung im Säuglingsalter. Wien Med Wochenschr 58:799–803, 1908

Mason HH, Turner ME: Chronic galactosemia: Report on a case with studies on carbohydrates. Am J Dis Child 50:359–374, 1935

Waggoner DD, Buist NRM, Donnell GN: Long term prognosis in galactosemia: Result of survey of 350 cases. J Inherit Metab Dis 13:802–818, 1990

Segal S, Berry GT: Disorders of galactose metabolism. In Scriver CR, Beaudet AL, Sly WS, et al: The Metabolic and Molecular Bases of Inherited Disease, 7th ed, pp 972–987. New York, McGraw-Hill, 1995

GALACTOSEMIA III

Synonyms. UDP-galactose-4-epimerase deficiency.

Symptoms and Signs. Both sexes affected. Benign form: usually asymptomatic and normal galactose tolerance. Malignant form resembles classic transferase deficiency, symptoms responding to galactose-free diet.

Etiology. Absence of UPD-galactose-4-epimerase in red cells and white cells without deranged metabolism in other tissues (in benign form) or systemic loss of enzyme activity also in liver and other tissue (in malignant form). Autosomal recessive inheritance.

Diagnostic Procedures. *Blood.* Elevated galactose; but normal uridltransferase and galactokinase levels. In red cell absence UDP-galactose-4-epimerase and increased galactose 1-phosphate. *Urine.* In malignant form albumin; aminoaciduria (several amino acids).

Therapy. Small amounts of dietary galactose (adequate for galacto-protein and galactolipid synthesis.)

Prognosis. Preventable only by very early marked reduction of galactose from diet.

BIBLIOGRAPHY. Gitzelmann R: Deficiency of uridine diphosphate galactose 4-epimerase in blood cells of an apparently healthy infant. Helv Paed Acta 28:49, 1973
Segal S, Berry GT: Disorders of galactose metabolism. In Scriver CR, Beaudet AL, Sly WS, et al: The Metabolic and Molecular Bases of Inherited Disease, 7th ed, pp 972–987. New York, McGraw-Hill, 1995

GALEAZZI

Synonyms. Radius fracture; dislocation ulnar head distally. See Monteggia.

Symptoms and Signs. Most frequent in children. Pain in the forearm. Fracture of the radius with disruption of the distal radioulnar joint.

Etiology. Blow on the forearm.

Diagnostic Procedures. *X-rays of forearm.*

Therapy. Closed reduction usually adequate.

Prognosis. Once the radius is restored to length and angulation corrected the distal radioulnar joint becomes stable.

BIBLIOGRAPHY. Galeazzi R: Di una particolare syndrome traumatica dello scheletro dell'avambraccio. Atti Mens Soc di Chir 2:12, 1934
Canale TS: Fractures and dislocation in children. In Crenshaw AH (ed): Campbell's Operative Orthopedics, 7th ed, pp 1853–1855. St Louis, CV Mosby, 1987

GALLAVARDIN

Synonyms. Blockypnea; inhibited respiration.

Symptoms and Signs. Exertion of various degrees or tension cause inhibition of breathing; rest brings relief. No wheezing or dyspnea. In some cases, alternating with typical angina symptoms.

Etiology. Equivalent of angina syndrome in patient with coronary arteriosclerosis and diseases central nervous system (spinothalamic tract to respiratory center in medulla stimulation). Increased susceptibility to stimulation of respiratory center.

Pathology. Coronary arteriosclerosis.

Diagnostic Procedures. All negative. *Electrocardiography.* May show anginal pattern, especially after effort.

Therapy. That of angina.

Prognosis. That of angina.

BIBLIOGRAPHY. Gallavardin L: Y a-t-il un equivalent non douloureux l'angine de poitrine d'effort? Lyon Med 134:345–358, 1924
Roesler H: Blockypnea (inhibited respiration), an equivalent of the angina syndrome. Am J Med Sci 244:85–87, 1962
Newsom-Davis J: Respiratory problems in neurological disease. In Weatherall DJ, Ledingham JGG, Warrell DA (eds): Oxford Textbook of Medicine, 3rd ed, pp 3887–3891. Oxford, Oxford Med Pub, 1996

GALLOWAY-MOWAT

Synonyms. Microcephaly; hiatus hernia, nephrotic.

Symptoms. Both sexes at birth. Microcephaly, large ears, vomiting from first feeding.

Etiology. Unknown. Possible autosomal recessive inheritance.

Pathology. Kidney. Focal glomerulosclerosis and microcystic dysplasia.

Diagnostic Procedures. *Urine.* Presence of albumin since birth or after a few days.

Prognosis. All cases died within 3 years.

BIBLIOGRAPHY. Galloway WH, Mowat AP: Congenital microcephaly with hiatus hernia and nephrotic syndrome in two sibs. J Med Genet 5:319–321, 1968
Shapiro LR, Duncan PA, Farnsworth PB, et al: Congenital microcephaly, hiatus hernia, and nephrotic syndrome: An autosomal recessive syndrome. Birth Defects XII (5):275–278, 1976
Shapiro LR: Microcephaly hiatus hernia and nephrotic syndrome (Galloway-Mowat). In Vinken PJ, Bruyn GW: Handbook of Clinical Neurology, vol 43, pp 431–432. Amsterdam, North-Holland, 1982

GAMEKEEPER THUMB

Synonym. Ulnar collateral ligament rupture.

Symptoms. Chronic pain and weakness of thumb–index finger grip.

Signs. Swelling, tenderness of ulnar margin of metacarpophalangeal joint. While pressing thumb and index forcefully together, the thumb drifts radially.

Etiology. Traumatic rupture of ulnar collateral ligament. In gamekeepers from repeated twisting of necks of wounded hares; frequently observed in skiers after trying to break a forward fall with the pole, or after a backward fall, by wedging thumbs in the snow.

Diagnostic Procedures. *X-ray.*

Therapy. Surgical correction or casting.

Prognosis. In untreated cases, chronic disability.

BIBLIOGRAPHY. Campbell CS: Gamekeeper's thumb. J Bone Joint Surg (Br) 37:148–149, 1955
Schultz RJ, Fox JM: Gamekeeper's thumb. Result of skiing injuries. NY J Med 73:2329–2331, 1973

GAMMA-CYSTATHIONASE DEFICIENCY

Synonyms. Cystathionase deficiency; CTH deficiency, cystathioninuria.

Symptoms and Signs. Rare condition. No clinical abnormalities are characteristically associated with this enzyme deficiency, but the following have been encountered: congenital defects (e.g., club foot, small ears); acromegaly; motor, and mental retardation; cataract; diabetes mellitus and insipidus.

Etiology. Gamma cystathionase deficiency. Genetic heterogeneity; autosomal inheritance. Relatives of those patients also had increased cystathionine level; however, they were asymptomatic. The relationship between metabolic defect and malformations may be coincidental.

Pathology. *Brain.* Diffuse atrophy. *Liver.* Smaller than normal; pale; fibrotic. *Heart.* Fatty degeneration (data based only on one autopsy).

Diagnostic Procedures. *Plasma, cerebrospinal fluid, and urine.* Marked increases of cystathionine (this finding "per se" does not establish diagnosis of gamma-cystathionase deficiency). *CT scan. MRI.*

Therapy. Pyridoxine reduces concentration of cystathionine, only in some patients (expression of genetic heterogeneity). Low methionine diet.

Prognosis. Relatives of patients with the metabolic defect remained completely asymptomatic.

BIBLIOGRAPHY. Harris H, Penrose LS, Thomas DHH: Cystathioninuria. Ann Hum Genet 23:442, 1959

Mudd SH, Levy HL, Skovby F: Disorders of transsulfuration. In Scriver CR, Beaudet AL, Sly WS, et al: The Metabolic and Molecular Bases of Inherited Disease, 7th ed, pp 1312–1313. New York, McGraw-Hill, 1995

GAMMOPATHY, BENIGN MONOCLONAL

Synonym. See Kahler-Bozzolo.

Symptoms and Signs. None or associated with a variety of other conditions. Only constant feature is the presence of monoclonal protein (M-component), which remains in a constant concentration over many years.

Etiology. Many conditions may be associated with this finding and the M-component increase could represent a response to antigen stimulation (infection; i.e., HIV seropositive patients, neoplasia); the increase may also represent a "premyeloma" condition. Hereditary factors have also been considered.

Diagnostic Procedures. *Blood.* Presence of M-component (similar to those of malignant plasma cell conditions). Normal levels of normal globulins. *Urine.* In rare cases, presence of Bence Jones proteins. *Bone marrow.* Less than 10% of plasma cells.

Therapy. None or that of associated condition.

Prognosis. Benign, however in 5% evolution into myeloma.

BIBLIOGRAPHY. Waldenström J: Studies on condition associated with disturbed gamma globulin formation (gammopathies). Harvey Lect 56:211–231, 1961

Foerster J: Multiple myeloma. In Lee GR, Bithel TC, Foerster J, et al (eds): Wintrobe's Clinical Hematology, 9th ed, p 2226. Philadelphia, Lea & Febiger, 1993

GAMSTORP

Synonyms. Westphals hyperkalemic; adynamia episodica hereditaria; hyperkalemic periodic paralysis; periodic paralysis II, includes periodic paralysis III.

Symptoms. Both sexes affected; more severe in males; onset during first decade. Patients may "walk off" attacks. (See Hypokalemic periodic paralysis.) Frequency of attacks is usually once a week. Between attacks patient is free of symptoms. Precipitating factors are rest after exertion, cold and dampness, and hunger. Attacks usually occur during the day. Attacks usually involve weakness of muscle, frequently localized at single muscle groups. May affect facial muscles also. Paresthesias frequent with cramping pain lasting 1 hour or longer. Mental faculties not affected.

Signs. Hyporeflexia of muscles involved. Percussion myotonia restricted to tongue in some cases, or to the eyelids or lips. Three types of adinamia episodica have been proposed: (1) clinical and electromyographic myotonia; (2) without myotonic manifestations; (3) combination of myotonia and paramyotonia (see Von Eulenberg). Periodic paralysis III thus has been classified according to the following data; attacks occur spontaneously or are induced by increasing serum potassium; percussion of tongue produces myotonia; normocalemia, and favorable response to Na chloride, dilatation of sarcoplasmatic reticulum of skeletal muscle (electron microscopy). Normokalemic and hyperkalemic are considered to be the same entity.

Etiology. Single autosomal dominant inheritance. Genetic defect linked to sodium channel alpha subunit (chromosome 17). In presence of high potassium concentration channels became inactive and muscle activation is defective. Gene defect is allelic to paramyotonia (see von Eulenberg) since many cases present both conditions. Reduction of muscle membrane potential considered as cause of paralysis. In addition it does not appear justifiable to separate a normokalemic form from the hyperkalemic because in both syndromes serum potassium levels do not always correlate with degree of muscle weakness.

Pathology. Not well established. Some muscle fibers present areas of accumulation of sarcoplasm on cross section. No degenerative changes.

Diagnostic Procedures. *Blood.* Hyperkalemia. *Induction of attack:* administration of 0.5 mg of potassium chloride per kg body weight or sodium bicarbonate.

Therapy. Prophylactic. Gentle exercise after exertion; carbohydrate intake. Avoid exposure to cold. Thiazide and acetazolamide effective in preventing attacks. Salbutamol (inhalatory) once a day is very effective. During attack. Calcium gluconate or Na chloride (see preceding).

Prognosis. Nonprogressive. Marked improvement during adult life. No muscle wasting occurs. Sudden death from bidirectional cardiac dysrhythmia reported.

BIBLIOGRAPHY. Buzzard EF: Three cases of family periodic paralysis with a consideration of the pathology of the disease. Lancet II:1564–1567, 1901

Gamstorp I: Adynamia episodica hereditaria. Acta Paediatr (Suppl) 108:1–126, 1956

Danowski TS, Fischer ER, Vidalon C, et al: Clinical and ultrastructural observations in kindred with normo-hyperkalemic periodic paralysis. J Med Genet 12:20–28, 1975

Harper PS: Myotonic dystrophy and other autosomal muscular dystrophies. In Scriver CR, Beaudet AL, Sly WS, et al: The Metabolic and Molecular Bases of Inherited Disease, 7th ed, pp 4227, 4242. New York, McGraw-Hill, 1995

GANSER

Synonyms. Balderdash; nonsense; prison psychosis; pseudodementia.

Symptoms. Usually appears suddenly, in young people in relation to circumstances by which it is precipitated. Approximate answers (which bear some relationship to the question but patient "passes by" the correct one and gives one near to it or says "I don't know") mixed with correct answer and absurd clouding of consciousness; apathetic indifference; lethargy; semistupor; disorientation. Somatic conversion features, manifested by motor and sensorial involvement, movements, tonus, flaccidity or rigidity, headache, backache, areas of anesthesia. Hallucination; visual or auditory.

Etiology. Unknown; hysterical dissociative reaction, unconscious or conscious, in the attempt to gain an advantage or escape responsibility. To be differentiated from malingering, true dementia, and some varieties of schizophrenia.

Therapy. During acute phase, hospitalization.

Prognosis. Relatively transient condition, spontaneous complete recovery; recurrences possible. Recovery from syndrome occurs also when other depressive symptoms persist.

BIBLIOGRAPHY. Ganser SJ: Ueber einen eigenartigen hysterischen Dammerzustand. Arch Psychiatr Nervkr 30:633–640, 1898

Peszke MA, Levin GA: The Ganser syndrome: A diagnostic and etiological enigma. Conn Med 51:79–83, 1987

Adams RD, Victor M: Principles of Neurology, 5th ed, p 1302. New York, McGraw-Hill, 1993

GÄNSSLEN I

An obsolete eponym used in the past to indicate the bone changes occurring with any chronic hemolytic syndromes. See Thalassemic, Widal-Ravaut, and Minkowski-Chauffard.

BIBLIOGRAPHY. Gänsslen M, Zipperlen E, Schuz E: Die Hämolytische Konstitution. Nach 105 Beobachtungen von hämolytischem Ikterus, 39 Beobachtungen von leichten hämolytischen Konstitutionen und 19 Milzexstirpationen. Arch Klin Med 146:1–46, 1925

GÄNSSLEN II

Synonym. Neutropenia familial benign chronic.

Symptoms. Family history. From completely asymptomatic to tendency toward chronic recurrent infections (especially periodontal), and occasionally severe generalized infections.

Signs. Frequent evidence of periodontal disease and scar of previous infections; no splenomegaly. Clubbing of fingers.

Etiology. Unknown; autosomal dominant or recessive (more frequent) transmission.

Diagnostic Procedures. *Blood.* Leukocyte count borderline low range; absolute neutropenia; relative lymphocytosis and monocytosis; irregular increase in eosinophils (40% circa). Hyperglobulinemia. *Bone marrow.* Erythroid and megakaryocytic series normal; myeloid series represented up to myelocytes, marked reduction of more mature elements; increase of lymphocytes and monocytes.

Therapy. Antibiotics.

Prognosis. Excellent; chronic lengthy course.

BIBLIOGRAPHY. Gänsslen M: Konstitutionelle familiäle Leukopenia (Neutropenie). Klin Wochenschr 20:922–925, 1941

Bousser J, Neyde R: La neutropénie familiale. Sang 18:521–529, 1947

Pincus SH, Boxer LA, Stossel TP: Chronic neutropenia in childhood: Analysis of 16 cases and a review of the literature. Am J Med 61:849–861, 1976

Holmes JA, Thompson PW: Expression of fra(10)(q25) in periferal blood and bone marrow in familial neutropenia. J Med Genet 25:238–242, 1988

Athens JW: Neutopenia. In Lee GR, Bithel TC, Foerster J, et al (eds): Wintrobe's Clinical Hematology, 9th ed, pp 1602–1603. Philadelphia, Lea & Febiger, 1993

G.A.P.O.

Synonyms. Andersen-Pindborg; growth retardation—alopecia—pseudoanadontia—optic atrophy.

Symptoms and Signs. Body length reduced with normal weight at birth. At sixth months full evidence of growth retardation. *Head.* Scalp hair present at birth but is lost within 1 year and does not regrow; both jaw bones crowned with nonerupting dentitions; frontal bossing, mild midfacial hypoplasia; variable in onset evidence of optic atrophy (not constant feature). *Variable changes.* Pectus excavatum; umbilical hernia; hypogonadism; polycystic kidneys; glaucoma.

Etiology. Autosomal recessive inheritance.

Diagnostic Procedures. *Skeleton X-rays.* Bone age significantly retarded; other bone changes not remarkable.

Prognosis. Survival up to fourth decade reported.

BIBLIOGRAPHY. Andersen TH, Pinborg JJ: Et tilgaelde of "pseudo anodonti" i forbindelse med kraniedeformitet, dvergvaekst og ektodermal displasi." Odont T 55:484–493, 1947

Wajuntal A, Kojffman CP, Mendonca BR, et al: GAPO syndrome (McKusick 23074) a connective tissue disorder: Report of two affected sibs and on pathologic findings in the other. Am J Med Genet 37:213–223, 1990

GARCIA*

Synonyms. See cyclic thrombocytemia.

Symptoms and Signs. Observed in a child 3 years of age and (platelet variation) in several members of family of both sexes. Petechiae, bruising, and repeated epistaxis requiring blood transfusion.

Etiology. Unknown. Autosomal dominant inheritance.

Diagnostic Procedures. *Blood.* Cyclic (21 days) variation of platelet counts. Negative search for antiplatelet auto-antibodies and for evidence of chronic intravascular coagulation.

Therapy. Prednisone.

Prognosis. Hemorrhagic manifestations on occasion of recurrent platelet variations.

BIBLIOGRAPHY. Aranda E, Dorandes S: Garcia's disease: Cyclic thrombocytopenic purpura in a child and abnormal platelets count in his family. Scand J Haematol 18:39–46, 1977

GARCIA-LURIE

Synonyms. Aprosencephaly; XK.†

Symptoms and Signs. Both sexes. From birth. Aprosencephaly, fused humerus and radius, and oligodactyly.

Etiology. Proposed autosomal recessive inheritance.

BIBLIOGRAPHY. Garcia CA, Duncan C: Atelencephalic microcephaly. Dev Med Child Neurol 19:227–232, 1977

Lurie LW, Nedzved MK, Lazjuk G, et al: Aprosencephaly-atelencephaly and aprosencephaly (XK) syndrome. Am J Med Genet 3:303–309, 1979

Townes Reuter K, Rosquete EE, et al: XK aprosencephaly and anencephaly in sibs. AM J Med Genet 29:523–528, 1988

GARDENER-DIAMOND

Synonyms. Autoerythrocyte sensitization; erythrocyte membrane sensitization; purpura; painful bruising. See David and Purpura, psychogenic.

Symptoms. Affects only women, not infrequently at various times after operations related to reproductive organs. History of bleeding episodes of different nature before onset of manifestations. Local sensation of tingling or burning preceding by several hours (18–24), the development of purpuric lesions that persist indolent for 5–7 days. Usually affecting extremities, face, and scalp; seldom the back. Frequently, these patients present particular psychologic manifestations.

---

*Name of family.

†Initials of patients' names.

Signs. Purpuric lesion frequently on areas not involved in trauma.

Etiology. Autosensitization to red cells or red cell stroma component, possibly phosphatidylserine (PPD) (proved in one case). Emotional factors of importance in the manifestation of symptoms.

Pathology. Data available from skin biopsy of lesion experimentally induced by the injection of PPD. Pattern in part resembling that of allergic vascular purpura.

Diagnostic Procedures. Injection into the skin of red cell or red cell stroma (positive reaction). For differential diagnosis, injection of deoxyribonucleic acid DNA (negative), histamine (negative), PPD (may be positive). *Blood.* Coagulation tests and platelet number: Normal.

Therapy. Corticosteroid; antihistamine; desensitization with erythrocyte unsuccessful. Chloroquine, primaquine, or hydroxychloroquine temporary benefit followed by immediate relapse.

Prognosis. Recurrent manifestation.

BIBLIOGRAPHY. Gardener RH, Diamond LK: Autoerythrocyte sensitization: A form of purpura producing painful bruising following autosensitization to red cells in certain women. Blood 10:675–690, 1955
Whitlock FA: Psychophysiological Aspects of Skin Diseases. London, WB Saunders, 1976
Bithell TC: Bleeding disorders caused by vascular abnormalities. In Lee GR, Bithel TC, Foerster J, et al (eds): Wintrobe's Clinical Hematology, 9th ed, pp 1384–1385. Philadelphia, Lea & Febiger, 1993

GARDNER

Synonyms. Bone tumor; epidermoid cyst; polyposis; multiple familial colon polyposis; epidermoid cyst; osteomatosis; polyposis; intestinal polyposis III; polyposis intestinal III; GRS.

Symptoms. Both sexes affected; average age of onset 20 years, but lesions have been found in 2-month-old children and a 70-year-old person. Early mild diarrhea and small amount of mucus and blood. Some patients with intestinal polyposis are asymptomatic. In 15–20 years after onset of intestinal symptomatology, multifocal malignant transformation of polyps.

Signs. *Soft tissue.* Multiple epidermoid cysts; dermoid tumors; fibromas; neurofibromas. *Bone.* Self-limited benign exostosis; osteomatosis mostly localized in face and skull; multiple impactions of supernumerary teeth (additional sign of the syndrome); long bones seldom involved. Frequently associated: retinal pigment epithelium hypertrophy (see).

Etiology. Unknown; autosomal dominant hereditary condition where soft tissue, bone tumors, and polyposis depend on same gene. Fifty percent of offspring affected. Chromosome mapping of gene has conducted to chromosome 5q.

Pathology. Benign cutaneous and subcutaneous tumors; benign bone tumor. Premalignant and eventually malignant transformation of multiple, scattered polyps most commonly in colon and rectum.

Diagnostic Procedures. *Biopsy of skin and intestine.*

Therapy. Subtotal colectomy with ileorectal anastomosis and fulguration of residual rectal adenomas. Followup to destroy reappearing polyps. If carcinoma develops, abdominoperineal resection and permanent ileostomy.

Prognosis. Death from cancer of colon occurs at an average age of 41–50 years.

BIBLIOGRAPHY. Cripps WH: Two cases of disseminated polyps of the rectum. Trans Path Soc London 33:165–168, 1882
Devic, Bussy: Un cas de polypose adénomateose; généralisée a tout l'intestin. Arch Mal Appar Dig 6:278–299, 1912
Gardner EJ, Stephens FE: Cancer of the lower digestive tract in one family group. Am J Hum Genet 2:41–48, 1950
Burn J, Chapman P, Delhanty J, et al: The UK northern region genetic

register for familial adenomatous polyposis coli: Use of age of onset, congenital hypertrophy of the retinal pigment epithelium, and DNA markers in risk calculations. J Med Genet 28:289–296, 1991
Lynch PM: Polyposis syndromes. In Haubrich WS, Schaffner F, Berk JE (eds): Bockus Gastroenterology, 5th ed, vol 2, pp 1731–1732. Philadelphia, WB Saunders, 1995

GARDNER-SILENGO-WACHTEL

Synonyms. Smith-Lemli-Optiz II; genito-palato-cardiac.

Symptoms. Phenotypic sex, nearly always female (one case hypospadia in male phenotype).

Signs. Pinnae low set, cheft palate and lips. Musculoskeletal defects: thumbs and great toe deformities, campodactyly, ribs dysplasic; clubfeet. Congenital heart defects: including tetrology of Fallot. Occasionally: cystic kidney urinary bladder dysgenesis, intestinal malrotation, gallbladder agenesis; hydrocephalus; dowslanting palpebrae.

Etiology. Autosomal recessive inheritance.

Diagnostic Procedures. Chromosomal sex 46 XY.

Therapy. Symptomatic.

Prognosis. Majority of patients die in neonatal period.

BIBLIOGRAPHY. Garder LI, Assemani SR, Neu RL: 46 xy female: antiandrogenic effect or oral contraceptive? Lancet II:667–668, 1970
Silengo M, Kaufman RL, Kissane JA: A46 XY infant with uterus, dysgenetic gonads and multiple anomalies. Humangenetik 25:65–68, 1974
Wachtel SS: X-Y antigen and biology of sex determination. New York, Grune and Stratton, 1983
Greenberg F, Gresik MV, Carpenter RJ, et al: The Gardner-Silengo-Wachtel or genito-palato-cardiac syndrome: Male pseudo hermaphroditism with micrognathia, cleft palate and frequent early lethality. Am J Med Genet 26:59–64, 1987

GARRÉ

Synonyms. Sclerosing nonsuppurative osteomyelitis; osteomyelitis sicca; Osteitis Garré.

Symptoms. Both sexes affected; onset in young adult, less frequently in late childhood. Fever. Moderate bone pain, especially during the night.

Signs. All bones may be affected, more frequently the tibia and femur; tenderness on palpation, and slow development of fusiform bone enlargement.

Etiology. Variable and frequently not clear: low grade infection (nonsuppurative acute or chronic of haversian canals); less frequently trauma; related to osteoid osteoma (see Bergstrand) or chronic renal failure; Hodgkin, sickle cell; systemic lupus erythematosis, on kidney transplant recipient.

Pathology. Scattered areas of necrosis; devascularization and fusiform thickening of cortex; and specific alteration of causing or associated conditions.

Diagnostic Procedures. *X-ray.* Subperiosteal calcification; cortex thickened with circumferential involvement and absence of nidus or rarefaction of focus.

Therapy. Guttering; drilling of multiple holes. Therapy of basic disorder.

Prognosis. Recurrences at interval of weeks or months. Recovery with subsidence of fever and persistence of described bone changes or according to basic condition.

BIBLIOGRAPHY. Garré C: Ueber besondere Formen und Folgezunstände der akuten intektiösen Osteomyelitis. Beitr Klin Chir 10:241–298, 1893
Mankin HJ: Nontraumatic necrosis of bone (osteonecrosis). N Engl J Med 326:1473–1479, 1992
Weatherall DJ, Ledingham JGG, Warrell DA (eds): Oxford Textbook of Medicine, 3rd ed, pp 3019, 3321, 3324, 3321, 3512, 3575. Oxford, Oxford Med Pub, 1996

GARRISON

Synonyms. Combat fatigue; battle fatigue; post-stress: See also old sergeant.

Symptoms and Signs. After withdrawing from battle and once sheltered in safety "falling apart" from complete exhaustion.

Etiology. Post-stress condition.

BIBLIOGRAPHY. Kettner B: Combat strain and subsequent mental health. Acta Psychiatr Scand (Suppl) 230, 1972
Ursano RJ, Holloway HC: Military psychiatry. In Kaplan HI, Sadock BJ: Comprehensive Textbook of Psychiatry, 4th ed, pp 1900–1909. Baltimore, Williams & Wilkins

GARROD

Synonyms. Alkaptonuria; ochronosis.

Symptoms. Both sexes affected; manifestation more severe in males; onset in first few days of life. (1) Passage of urine that becomes black on standing or if alkalinized (washed diapers become black). Black pigment excreted also with sweat. (2) Arthropathia; back pain; stiffness; onset in fourth decade; progressive involvement of several joints to complete disablement in 15–20 years. Severe pain over symphysis pubis. Extruded intervertebral disk frequent. (3) Renal and prostatic stones, usually during fifth decade. (4) Cardiovascular lesions; hoarseness; occasionally, deafness.

Signs. Pigmentation (blue black) of sclerae and ear cartilages (which also become stiff, a sign appearing in second decade), occasionally of tip of nose and tendons.

Etiology. Deficiency of homogentisic acid oxidase of liver and kidney. Autosomal recessive inheritance.

Pathology. Typical black pigmentation of cartilaginous structures, heart valves. Articular degenerative changes; accelerated arteriosclerotic changes. In kidney, black stones and secondary infections.

Diagnostic Procedures. *Urine.* Turns dark on standing and alkalination. Determination of homogentisic acid. *X-ray.* Narrowing of intervertebral space. Collapse and calcification of intervertebral disks. Degenerative changes in large joints.

Therapy. Ascorbic acid, dietary reduction of intake of tyrosine and phenylalanine. Kidney transplantation followed by recurrence of renal failure in years.

Prognosis. Arthropathy may make patient bedridden for years. Cardiovascular defects and uremia causes of death. Oldest patient reached 99 years.

BIBLIOGRAPHY. Boedeker C: Ueber das Alkapton; ein neuer Beitrug zur Frage Welche Stoff des Hanus können Kupferreduktion bewirken? Ztschr Rat Med 7:130–145, 1859
Garrod AF: About alkaptonuria. Lancet 2:1484–1486, 1901
Wolff JA, Barshop B, Nyhan WL, et al: Effects of ascorbic acid in alkaptonuria: alteration in benzoquinone acetic acid and oncogenic effect in infancy. Pediatr Res 2:140–144, 1989
La Du BN: Alcaptonuria. In Scriver CR, Beaudet AL, Sly WS, et al: The Metabolic and Molecular Bases of Inherited Disease, 7th ed, pp 1371–1386. New York, McGraw-Hill, 1995

GASS

Synonym. Epitheliopathy acute posterior placoid pigment; multifocal placoid pigment epitheliopathy acute posterior. APM, PPE.

Symptoms and Signs. Rapid loss of central vision acuity. Usually after influenza-like illness or in patients with erythema nodosum. Reported in some cases vasculitis, papillitis, serous retinal detachment, and anterior uveitis.

Etiology. Viral infection (?).

Diagnostic Procedures. Fundus: yellow-white placoid lesions at level of pigment, epithelium and choroid. *Fluorescin angiogram:* involvement of pigment epithelium and smaller choroidal vessels: in early arterial phase: yellow white lesions obscure underlying fluorescence from choroidal vessels. Later: localized hyperfluorescence in these areas.

Therapy. None.

Prognosis. Rapid resolution, with vision returning to normal or near normal state.

BIBLIOGRAPHY. Gass JDM: Acute posterior placoid pigment epitheliopathy. Arch Ophthalmol 80:177, 1968
Apple DJ, Rabb MF: Ocular Pathology, 337. St Louis, CV Mosby, 1991

GASSER-KARRER

Synonyms. Erythroblastopenia, acute, acquired. See pure red cell aplasia syndromes.

Symptoms and Signs. Both sexes affected; onset from first days of life. Jaundice progressing for a few days and then receding. As jaundice fades, anemia becomes evident (in second or third week). No splenomegaly.

Etiology. Exogenous toxin. Vitamin K analogues administration is frequently involved.

Pathology. Not specific.

Diagnostic Procedures. *Blood.* Anemia; reticulocytosis, hyperbilirubinemia. Presence of Heinz bodies in 9–45% of red cells. (Heinz bodies may be observed in many other conditions, such as inclusion body anemia-pigmenturia, after splenectomy, red cell enzymes defect. See Widal-Ravaut.) Negative Coombs test and absent cold-warm agglutinins.

Therapy. Transfusions.

Prognosis. Without treatment, infant deteriorates rapidly, becoming drowsy. Death may occur. If survival of hemolytic episode, the condition is self-limited.

BIBLIOGRAPHY. Gasser C, Karrer J: Delataere haemolytische Anaemie mit Spontan-innerkoerpe Bildung bei Fruehgeburt. Helv Paediatr Acta 3:387–403, 1948
Gasser C: Die hämolytische Frühgeburtenanamie mit spontaner Innenkörperbildung: Ein neues Syndrom, beobachtet an 14 Fallen. Helv Paediatr Acta 8:491–529, 1953
Sheehy TW: Inclusion body anemia with pigmenturia. Arch Intern Med 114:83–85, 1964
Williams: Pancytopenia, aplastic anemia, and pure red cell aplasia. In Lee GR, Bithel TC, Foerster J, et al (eds): Wintrobe's Clinical Hematology, 9th ed, p 914. Philadelphia, Lea & Febiger, 1993

GASSER II

Synonym. Hemolytic uremic; uremia hemolytica; HUS.

Symptoms. Occurs in seriously ill infants and children. Vomiting;

diarrhea; skin, gastrointestinal or urinary bleeding; pallor. Hemolytic anemia; acute renal failure.

Signs. Mild edema; ecchymosis and petechiae; jaundice; hepatomegaly; seldom, splenomegaly; hypertension in 50% of cases.

Etiology. Unknown; may represent one manifestation of autoimmune reaction. The syndrome has been also related to E. coli 0157:H7 infections. In Argentina the disorder seems unusually frequent and a viral etiology has been proposed. Other endemic areas are South Africa, the West Coast of the USA, and the Netherlands. Clinical and pathologic findings demonstrate sufficient correlation to define the hemolytic uremic syndrome as an entity separate from Moschcowitz, periarteritis nodosa, or necrotizing glomerulonephritis. Remuzzi suggested that deficiency of a vascular prostacyclin stimulator may underlie the disorder.

Pathology. Jaundice; edema; cutaneous hemorrhages; small serous effusions; variable submucosal hemorrhages throughout gastrointestinal tract. Liver enlarged and fatty. Kidney patchy to almost total cortical necrosis; in non-necrotic areas, glomerulitis, capillary microthrombi, and fibrinoid necrosis of efferent arterioles; casts of red cells and hemoglobin. Tubular necrosis without interstitial inflammation.

Diagnostic Procedures. *Blood.* Anemia with red cells showing morphologic alterations (fragmentation; anisopoikilocytosis; polychromasia). Reticulocytes high (10–20%). High sedimentation rate, Coombs test negative; lupus erythematosis (LE) test negative. Thrombocytopenia; increased blood urea nitrogen (BUN). *Bone marrow.* Erythroid hyperplasia. *Urine.* Proteinuria; hematuria; casts. *Biopsy of kidney.* (During recovery) specific changes (see Pathology).

Therapy. Blood transfusion. Fresh plasma for restoring the activity of prostacyclin may be tried. Electrolyte balance; peritoneal dialysis; antihypertensive therapy; steroids. Heparin (benefit not demonstrated). Streptokinase-streptodornase.

Prognosis. About 60% recovery; 10% residual hypertension; 30% death. Cases whose onset was within a short time of each other had a relatively good prognosis; those whose onset was more than 1 year apart had a poorer prognosis. This suggests an environmental agent in the first group and genetic factors in the second. Most of the first group of families came from an endemic area, whereas most of the second group came from a nonendemic area.

BIBLIOGRAPHY. Gasser C, Gantier E, Steck A, et al: Hämolytisch-urämische Syndrom: bilateral Nierenrindennenekrosen bei akuten erbworbenen hämolitisch Anä in mien. Schweiz Med Wochenschr 85:905–909, 1955

Neild G: The haemolytic uraemic syndrome: A review. Q J Med 63:367–378, 1987

Martin DL, MacDonald KL, White KE, et al: The epidemiology and clinical aspects of the hemolytic uremic syndrome in Minnesota. N Engl J Med 323:1161–1167, 1990

Foerster J: Red cell fragmentation syndromes. In Lee GR, Bithel TC, Foerster J, et al (eds): Wintrobe's Clinical Hematology, 9th ed, pp 1215–1219. Philadelphia, Lea & Febiger, 1993

GAS SYNDROMES

BELCHING, FREQUENT, REPETITIVE I

Synonym. Magenblase; Aerophagia I; including also Payr (see) and hepatic flexure.

Symptom. Usually in persons with exhibisionistic trait, or mentally retarded subjects; unabashed public belching. Sometimes pain in left (Payr) or right quadrant (hepatic flexure) with localized bloating and sensation of fullness.

Etiology. Air swallowing because of rapid food ingestion, sucking (cigarettes, straws, etc.), chewing gum, swallowing for uncomfortable dentures, asthma, stress, unimpaired swallowing (pseudo bulbar palsy).

Diagnostic Procedures. *Fluoroscopy.* Plain film, to see if air accumulates in flexures. Endoscopy to rule out esophagitis.

Therapy. Reassurance; tranquilizers; antacids without carbonates; training to recognize the act of swallowing air and repress belching; exhalation of air before swallowing.

Prognosis. Unlikely total abolition of condition.

BLOATING, FULLNESS, ABDOMINAL DISCOMFORT

Synonym. Phantom tummy; accordion abdomen; pseudoileus.

Symptoms. Episodic irregular exacerbations of abdominal bloating, fullness, and discomfort.

Signs. Slight abdominal protuberance, isolated slightly tender loop of gut.

Etiology. Double origin. Enteric pathology or "hysterical" condition.

Diagnostic Procedures. *Plain abdominal film. Barium film.* Digestive tract. Experimental Argon washout.

Therapy. Psychological help, antispasmodics, anticholinergics, prokinetics.

Prognosis. Prompt response to any treatment, but early relapses.

FLATUS, EXCESSIVE

Synonym. Bacterial fermentation.

Symptoms. Usually concurrent with various gastroenteric pathological conditions: chronic pancreatitis; enteritis; celiac disease; sprue; protein loosing enteropathies; intestinal bacterial overgrowth; Whipple; parasitic infections, etc., but observed also in healthy individuals. Excessive discharge of flatus (25 passages of gas a day are normal), occasionally also belching or bloating and abdominal distention. Occasionally Payr (see) or hepatic flexure syndrome. Exaggerated tympany in epigastric area, borborygmus.

Etiology. Dietary factors; bacterial overgrowth.

Diagnostic Procedures. *Stool culture.* For ova or parasites (exp Giardia lamblia). *Chemical analysis.* Of stool to assess adequacy of lactase activity. *X-ray.* Of G-I tract. *Endoscopy. Hydrogen breath test.*

Therapy. Dietary. Avoidance or reduction of fermentable food. Beta-D-galactosidase in drops or capsules; dimethicone, activated charcoal (subrevaluation) pancreatic enzymes, implantation of bacillus subtilis.

Prognosis. Good; but all treatments not fully resolutive.

In addition to these generic gas syndromes one may consider the following specific conditions characterized by excessive gas formation or retention.

GASTRIC ACID SECRETION I

Symptoms. Abdominal distention; flatulence.

Etiology. Gastric hypoacidity.

Diagnostic Procedures. *Gastric juice analysis. Bacterial examination.* Duodenal flora.

Therapy. Acid potions, specific for bacterial flora.

GASTRIC ACID SECRETION II

Symptoms. Epigastric pain; abdominal distention, flatulence.

Etiology. Gastric hyperacidity (with or without peptic ulcer); carbon dioxide production.

Diagnostic Procedures. *As above. Stool.* Occult blood and mucus.

Therapy. Antacids; anticholinergics; surgery.

INTESTINAL MOTILITY I

Symptoms. Occurs in elderly, aged patients; colonic distention; hepatic and splenic pressure complaints; delayed flatulence.

Etiology. Colonic hypomotility.

Diagnostic Procedures. *X-ray.* Motility from stomach to cecum normal; motility of cecum delayed.

Therapy. Betanechol chloride; reduction of carbohydrate intake.

INTESTINAL MOTILITY II

Symptoms. "Frothers"; borborygmi; occasional diarrhea; abdominal distention; flatulence.

Etiology. Hypermotility of intestine; mucus increase.

Diagnostic Procedures. *X-ray.* Small bowel gas (flat plate). Increased colonic motility; decreased transit time (carmine marker or barium or both).

Therapy. Dimethicone; pancreatic enzymes; anticholinergics.

MALDIGESTION

Synonyms. Pancreatic insufficiency; small intestinal hurry.

Symptoms. Borborygmi; abdominal distention; flatulence; occasionally, diarrhea.

Etiology. Pancreatic insufficiency; disaccharidase deficiency, small intestine accelerated motility.

Diagnostic Procedures. *X-ray.* Decreased transit time. *Stool.* Presence of undigested materials (protein; fat); duodenal enzymes, lactic acid decreased or increased according to etiology. *Disaccharide tolerance test.*

Therapy. Mecholyl; betanechol chloride.

REFLEX SMALL INTESTINE HYPOTONIA

Symptoms. Abdominal distention; delayed flatulence.

Etiology. Urologic instrumentation.

Diagnostic Procedures. *Fluoroscopy.* Increased gas in small bowel.

Therapy. Mecholyl; bethanechol chloride.

BIBLIOGRAPHY. Danhaf IE: The clinical gas syndromes, a pathophysiological approach. Ann NY Acad Sci 150:127–140, 1968
Berk JE: Gas. In Haubrich WS, Schaffner F, Berk JE (eds): Bockus Gastroenterology, 5th ed, pp 113–128. Philadelphia, WB Saunders, 1995

GASTROCUTANEOUS

Symptoms. From birth. Multiple lentigines; caffe-au-lait spots; hypertelorism; myopia; bleeding peptic ulcer, hiatal hernia. Other anomalies: ischemic heart condition; abnormal dermatogliphycs. At latter age development of diabetes.

Etiology. Autosomal dominant with high penetrance and variability.

BIBLIOGRAPHY. Halal F, Gervais MH, Baillargeon J, et al: Gastrocutaneous syndrome:peptic ulcer-hiatal hernia, multiple lentigines, cafe-au-lait spots, hypertelorism and myopia. Am J Med Genet 11:161–176, 1982

GASTRODUODENAL ULCERATION–CHRONIC PULMONARY DISEASE

Synonym. Chronic pulmonary disease-gastroduodenal ulceration. While the occurrence of gastroduodenal ulcer in the general population is in the 10% range, in patients with chronic pulmonary disease the incidence reaches 25%. This association is considered statistically significant, and the association considered as a syndrome.

BIBLIOGRAPHY. Green TP, Dundee VC: On the association of chronic peptic ulceration. Can Med Assoc J 67:438–439, 1952
West WO, Burns RO, Daniel JM, et al: The syndrome of chronic pulmonary disease and gastroduodenal ulceration. Arch Intern Med 103:897–901, 1959

GASTROINTESTINAL MILK ALLERGY (IN INFANTS)

Synonym. Cow milk allergy.

Symptoms. Onset in early infancy (2 days to 4–5 months) when cow milk feeding. Vomiting; chronic diarrhea; mucus and occult blood in the stool. Various degrees of severity from minimal to fulminating diarrhea, gastrointestinal bleeding, and collapse. Colic may precede diarrhea for months. Growth retardation.

Signs. Pallor; dehydration. Hypotension and tachycardia, and in some, shock (following milk challenge). On sigmoidoscopy, mucosa of rectum and colon from slight injection to red, ulcerated surface.

Etiology. Allergy to cow milk. Frequent family history of allergy and gastrointestinal diseases.

Pathology. Biopsy of rectum. From slight infiltrate of lymphocyte and plasma cells to granulocyte infiltrate and destruction of surface epithelium; abscesses.

Diagnostic Procedures. *Cow milk challenge (with caution).* Lactose tolerance normal. *Stool.* Precipitating antibodies against cow milk. *Studies of sugar-splitting enzymes.* For differential diagnosis.

Therapy. Change in formula (protein hydrolysate, soybean formula, or sheep milk formula).

Prognosis. Asymptomatic after starting change of formula. Usually obtain tolerance to cow milk at 2 years of age or later.

BIBLIOGRAPHY. Scholss OM, Worthen TW: The permeability of the gastroenteric tract of infants to indigest protein. Am J Dis Child 11:342, 1916
Gryboski JD: Gastrointestinal milk allergy in infants. Pediatrics 40:354–362, 1967
Lloyd ML, Olsen WA: Disaccharide malabsorption in Haubrich WS, Schaffner F, Berk JE (eds): Bockus Gastroenterology, 5th ed, vol 2, p 1095. Philadelphia, WB Saunders, 1995

GAUCHER

Synonyms. Gaucher-Schlagenhaufer; splenic anemia, familial; cerebroside lipidosis; glucosyl ceramide lipidosis; histiocytosis, lipid kerasin type; glucosidase deficiency.

TYPE I: NON-NEURONOPATHIC (ADULT) CHRONIC GAUCHER

Symptoms. Both sexes equally affected; high proportion of Ashkenazy Jews; onset at any age, usually as patient reaches the second part of second decade after an asymptomatic or paucisymptomatic period. Pains in extremities or trunk: episodic; severe; occasionally, accompanied by hyperthermia. In some cases, respiratory difficulties.

Signs. If symptoms appear early, stunted growth. Old patients have yellow pallor and pigmented face and legs. Abdominal distention. Splenomegaly; hepatomegaly (sometimes with later onset). Pathologic fractures. Pinguecula (brownish wedge-shaped thickening of subconjunctival fibrous tissue) first on nasal side, after also on temporal side.

Etiology. Autosomal recessive inheritance. Subnormal activity of glucocerebrosidase in organs and tissues, determining an accumulation of glucocerebroside (glucosylceramide). Gene for glucocerebrosidase has been mapped to chromosome 1q21.

Pathology. *Liver.* Enlarged; degree of infiltration by Gaucher cell variable (usually not in relation to size reached by the organ). Evidence of portal hypertension. *Spleen.* As above. *Lung.* Possibly, infiltration and pneumonia. *Bone.* Rarefaction of cortex, pathologic fractures.

Diagnostic Procedures. *Blood.* Mild microcytic anemia; leukopenia; thrombocytopenia; hyposideremia. Increased nontartrate inhibited acid phosphatase. *Bone marrow.* Infiltration by Gaucher cells. *X-ray.* Bone cortex reduced; pathologic fractures; expansion of cortex of lower end of femur; Erlenmeyer flasklike aspect. *Assay of glucocerebroside in tissue sample.* Possibility of prenatal diagnosis on amniocytes or chorionic villi.

Therapy. Splenectomy to correct hypersplenism (see); joint replacement. Administration of modified-glucosidase (alglucerase) glucocerebrosidase. Bone marrow transplantation curative.

Prognosis. Pain most severe in first 20 years; thereafter less intense. Hemorrhages, hematemesis, and pneumonia causes of death. Survival in relation to time of onset and severity of condition; poorer prognosis for early onset. Survival 6–80 years.

TYPE II: NEURONOPATHIC ACUTE (INFANTILE) GAUCHER

Symptoms. Panethnic. Both sexes affected; mild prevalence in male; onset between 6 months and 1 year of age; no racial prevalence. Progressive hepatosplenomegaly; strabismus; hyperextension of head; hypertonicity; rigidity of neck; dysphagia; apathy or catatonia; increased deep reflexes; laryngeal spasm; mental retardation.

Etiology. See Type I.

Pathology. *Liver, spleen, lymph nodes.* Enlargement, presence of characteristic Gaucher cells, large cells with reticular pattern (crumpled silk) of cytoplasm. *Bone.* Infiltration and eventual replacement of other marrow elements by Gaucher cells. Bone destruction by proliferating cells. *Central nervous system.* Focal, nonspecific, degenerative changes of neurons; active neurophagocytosis; Gaucher cell infiltration.

Therapy. See Type I.

Prognosis. Without treatment 80% fatality within second year of life.

TYPE III: SUBACUTE NEURONOPATHIC (JUVENILE) GAUCHER

Synonyms. Norrbottnian form of Gaucher.

Symptoms. In Sweden. Both sexes affected; onset at older age than Type II, up to adulthood. Seizures; occasionally, hypertonicity; strabismus, and lack of movement coordination; poor mentation.

Signs. Hepatosplenomegaly.

Etiology and Pathology. See Types I and II.

Diagnostic Procedures. See Type I. *Electroencephalography.* Abnormalities.

Therapy. As Type I.

Prognosis. Subacute course and longer survival than Type II second to fourth decade.

BIBLIOGRAPHY. Gaucher P: De l'epithelioma primitif de la rate (thesis) p 212. Paris, 1882

Beutler E, Grabowski GA: Gaucher disease. In Scriver CR, Beaudet AL, Sly WS, et al: The Metabolic and Molecular Bases of Inherited Disease, 7th ed, pp 2641–2670. New York, McGraw-HIll, 1995

GAUSTAD

Synonyms. Post-shunt encephalopathy; hepatocerebral; portal-systemic encephalopathy; transient hepatargy Gaustad.

Symptoms. Mental confusion; behavior disorders; apathy; drowsiness; delirium.

Signs. Precoma without loss of consciousness, as well as coma. Hyperreflexia; rigidity; flapping tremor (hands and wrists), fetor hepaticus, jaundice. In coma, flaccid extremities and areflexia.

Etiology. After portocaval shunt. Hepatic failure and toxic state (increased blood ammonia level). Precipitating causes: anoxia; intercurrent infections; exercise; pregnancy; abdominal paracentesis; gastrointestinal ammonia; blood transfusion; drugs; hypokalemia; shunts; alkalosis; cholemia.

Pathology. Liver cirrhosis. In brain, nonspecific changes in cerebral cortex, basal ganglia, thalamus, brain stem, and cerebellum. Increase of astrocytes.

Diagnostic Procedures. *Blood.* Bilirubin; prothrombin time; proteins; albumin, blood urea nitrogen (BUN), ammonia level; alkaline phosphatase. *EEG. Evoked potential. CT scan. MRI. Positron emission tomography. Intracranial pressure monitoring.*

Therapy. Recognition and treatment of precipitating causes. General supportive measures; avoidance of additional trauma to liver. Based on ammonia hypotesis: inibition of ammonia production increase removal. Based on false neurotransmitter hypotesis: modified aminoacid solutions, "coma" solutions, L-Dopa, bromocriptine. Based on GABA hypotesis. Flumazenil.

Prognosis. Reversible condition with appropriate therapy. That of severe liver cirrhosis. Mortality 60% circa.

BIBLIOGRAPHY. Hahn M, Massen O, Wencki M, et al: Die Eck'sche Fistel Zwischen der Unteren Holivene und der Pfortader und ihre Folgen fur den Organisms. Arch Exp Pathol 32:151, 1893

Baker AB: Interrelationship of diseases of the liver and brain. Arch Pathol 46:268–286, 1948

Gaustad V: Transient epatargia. Acta Scand 135:354–363, 1949

Langer B, Taylor BR, McKenzie DR, et al: Further report of a prospective randomized trial comparing distal splenorenal shunt with end-to-side portocaval shunt: An analysis of encephalopathy, survival, and quality of life. Gastroenterology 88:424–429, 1985

Ferenci P: Hepatic encephalopathy. In Haubrich WS, Schaffner F, Berk JE (eds): Bockus Gastroenterology, 5th ed, vol 2, pp 1988–2003. Philadelphia, WB Saunders, 1995

GAY BOWEL

Symptoms and Signs. In homosexual male. Enterocolitis.

Etiology. Result of oral-anal-genital sexual practices. Caused by a large variety of infective agents: virus (herpes, hepatitis), chlamydiae, bacteria (shigella, salmonella, neisseria, etc.), protozoa, etc.

Therapy. According to infective agents.

BIBLIOGRAPHY. Centers for Disease Control: Sexually transmitted diseases: Treatment guidelines, 1985. MMWR 34:755, 1985

GEE

Synonyms. Gee-Hertener-Heubner; Gee-Thoysen; Golden-Kantor; Heubner; Herter; infantile celiac; gluten-enteropathy; nontropical sprue, steatorrhea idiopathic; temperature sprue; celiac disease.

CHILDREN VARIETY

Symptoms and Signs. Both sexes affected; onset 6–9 months of age; prodromal signs may be present from birth. Celiac triad: diarrhea; weight loss; abdominal enlargement. Watery diarrhea (seen frequently in adult group) rare; vomiting frequent. Celiac crisis: dehydration with acidosis. Growth retardation.

Etiology. Autosomal dominant inheritance with incomplete penetrance. Deficiency of peptidases in intestinal mucosa and consequent inability to hydrolyze dietary gluten. This etiology presently is disputed and direct toxicity of gluten product on intestinal mucosa emphasized.

Pathology. Intestinal villi atrophic; surface epithelium degenerative changes. Bone osteoporosis.

Diagnostic Procedures. *Blood.* Variable degree of macrocytic anemia; hypoproteinemia; hypocalcemia; hypokalemia; hypolipemia. Prothrombin time prolonged. *Stool.* Steatorrhea. *X-ray of small bowel.* Segmentation and flocculation of barium meal; coarsening of jejunal folds, maulage sign. *Urine.* Measurement of d-xylose absorption; determination of urinary indoles. *Biopsy of jejuneum.*

Therapy. Gluten-free diet. Specific deficiencies must also be corrected (vitamin B$_{12}$, calcium, potassium, zinc). Corticosteroids.

Prognosis. Dramatic improvement in a few days with gluten-free diet. Occasionally, improvement only after 2–6 months of dietetic treatment. Have a late, increased incidence of abdominal lymphoma and carcinoma.

LATENT VARIETY (TEMPERATURE SPRUE)

All symptoms and signs of disease are not present, except for intermittent episodes of diarrhea (typical fatty stool) with intercurrent pulmonary infections. Presence of the condition may be demonstrated by diagnostic procedures. During adulthood the adult variety of the condition manifests itself (see).

ADULT VARIETY

Symptoms. Preponderant in females (2:1); at onset 25% of patients have history of childhood diarrhea that disappeared in later childhood, malabsorption persisting, however. Symptoms and signs between third and sixth decades, characterized by intermittent exacerbations and remissions. Stresses (psychological or physical) may trigger an acute phase with diarrhea, with foul smelling, bulky stools (during attacks may be watery), weakness, weight loss, bleeding phenomena, hypocalcemia manifestations, anorexia, skeletal disorders, hypotension.

Signs. Abdominal bloating, all degrees of malabsorption syndrome (see); muscle wasting; edema; glossitis or stomatitis; occasionally, clubbing of fingers; skin pigmentation (Addison-like).

Etiology. See Children variety.

Pathology. See Children variety.

Diagnostic Procedures. See Children variety.

Therapy. See Children variety.

Prognosis. See Children variety.

BIBLIOGRAPHY. Gee S: On the celiac affection. St Barth Hosp Rep 24:17–20, 1888
Golden R: The small intestine and diarrhea. Am J Roentgen 36:892–901, 1936
Kantor JL: The roentgen diagnosis of idiopathic steatorrhea and allied conditions. Practical value of the "maulage sign." Am J Roentgen 41:758–778, 1939
Tiwari JL, Betuel H, Gebuhrer L, et al: Genetic epidemiology of coeliac disease. Genet Epidemiol 1:37–42, 1984
Trier JS: Celiac sprue (medical progress). N Engl J Med 325:1209, 1991

GELFARD-HYMAN

Synonyms. Zayid-Farraj; histiocytic dermoarthritis. See also Multicentrix reticulohistiocytosis.

Symptoms. Both sexes affected; onset in childhood or adolescence. Joint pain, mainly on hands and wrists, but possible also on feet and elbows. Possibly, hearing loss and visual impairment. See Signs.

Signs. Multiple intracutaneous nodules and subcutaneous plaques with skin lichenification forming on face, ears, and limbs. Arthropathic changes of previously mentioned joints. Glaucoma; bilateral uveitis; cataracts. Hydronephrosis reported also.

Etiology. Unknown; autosomal dominant inheritance.

Pathology. Histology. Nodules of lipoidal histiocytoma type, characterized by the absence of multinucleated giant cells (differential element with multicentric reticulohistiocytosis).

Diagnostic Procedures. *Biopsy of skin.* See Pathology. *X-ray of skeleton.* Symmetric destructive arthritis of mentioned joints. *Kidney function evaluation.* Possible abnormalities.

Therapy. Symptomatic.

Prognosis. Progressive condition.

BIBLIOGRAPHY. Gerfarb M, Hyman AB: Multiple noduli cutanei. Arch Dermatol 85:89–94, 1962
Zayid I, Farraj S: Familial histiocytic dermatoarthritis: A new syndrome. Am J Med 54:793–800, 1973
Pastores GM, Michels VV, Stickler GB, et al: Autosomal dominant granulomatous arthritis, uveitis skin rash and synovial cysts. J Pediatr 117:403–408, 1990

GELINEAU

Synonym. Narcolepsy.

Symptoms. Onset in adolescence or early adulthood; male to female ratio, 6:1. Sudden attacks of sleep that cannot be resisted. Sleep from a few minutes to a half an hour. Intense concentration in activity may prevent attack; less concentrating activities, such as reading, facilitates attack. Driving a car does not prevent attack. Patients awake refreshed. Patients may easily be awakened by noises of different intensities depending on patient. Impossible to differentiate from normal sleep. Sleep paralysis and hypnagogic hallucinations are experienced in the early part or during REM (rapid eye movement) stage, especially when in a comfortable position. Sometimes syndrome is associated with somnambulism, and frequently (2/3) with cataplexy (attacks of weakness or paralysis), especially with strong emotions.

Signs. Patient tends to be obese. While asleep, normal deep reflexes, eyes in Bell position; sleep induces gentle muscle relaxation; normal breathing; slowing of pulse.

Etiology. Unknown (idiopathic type). Encephalitis; head injuries; systemic infections; polycythemia vera; multiple sclerosis; tumor of third ventricle. Familial cases with autosomal dominant trait. The 98–100% incidence of the HLA-DR2 and HLA-DQW1 antigens indicates a specific genetic substrate.

Pathology. None. It is assumed that disturbance of the reticular formation or of the hypothalamus may be responsible for this syndrome.

Diagnostic Procedures. *Blood.* Hematocrit; blood volume. *X-ray of skull. Angiography. CT scan. MRI. Electroencephalography. Electro-oculography. Electromyography.*

Therapy. Methylphenidate (Ritalin); amphetamine sulfate. Modafinil, Mazindol, and Selegiline improve daytime alertness and may have fewer side effects than amphetamine, but are no more effective. Naps (three or more 15–20-minute naps daily) often are used as an adjunct to medications.

Prognosis. Recurrent attacks for life (idiopathic); according to etiology (secondary).

BIBLIOGRAPHY. Gélineau E: De la narcolepsie. Gaz Hôp Paris 53:626–628; 635–637, 1880

Adie W: Idiopathic narcolepsy: A disease sui generis: with remarks on the mechanism of sleep. Brain 49:275–306, 1926

Aldrich MS: Narcolepsy. N Engl J Med 323:389–394, 1990

Adams RD, Victor M: Principles of Neurology, 5th ed, pp 345–347. New York, McGraw-Hill, 1993

GELLE

Synonyms. Crossed paralysis of VIIIth nerve.

Symptoms and Signs. Hemiparalysis that may precede or follow, usually contralateral seldom homolateral: tinnitus, dizziness, auricular pain deafness of rapid onset and gradual progression. Seldom V and VIIth nerves may be involved.

Etiology and Pathology. Infarction or ischemia of pons.

Diagnostic Procedures. *CT scan. MRI.*

Therapy. Symptomatic.

Prognosis. Guarded.

BIBLIOGRAPHY. Gellé ME: Paralisie alterne de l'acustique lésion protuberantial. CR Soc Biol (Paris) 53:997–1000, 1901

Loeb C, Meyer JS: Pontine syndromes. In Vinken PJ, Bruyn GW: Handbook of Clinical Neurology, vol 2, p 241. Amsterdam, North-Holland, 1969

GELOLEPSY

Synonyms. Gelastic epilepsy.

Symptoms and Signs. In epilepsy fits of automatic laughter and amnesia for such laughing.

Pathology. Questioned the need of this term since pathologic laughing can occur in any stage of epileptic attacks.

Diagnostic Procedures. *EEG.* There is not any specific characteristic (except for muscle artifacts).

BIBLIOGRAPHY. Martin JP: Fits of laughter (sham mirth) in organic cerebral disease. Brain 73:453–464, 1950

Curatolo PR, Cusmai G, Finocchi G, et al: Gelastic epilepsy and true precocious puberty due to hypothalamic hamartoma. Dev Med Child Neurol 26:509–527, 1984

GENEE-WIEDEMANN

Synonyms. Miller; Wildervanck-Smith; acrofacial postaxial dysostosis; postaxial acrofacial dysostosis.

Symptoms and Signs. In children. *Facies.* Hypoplastic malar bones; downslanting palpebral fissures; coloboma; usually ectropia of lower lid; cleft lip or palate; ear malformations; occasionally conical teeth. *Limbs.* Postaxial agenesis of digits; preaxial anomalies less frequently present. *Heart.* Possibly congenital defects. *Urogenital anomalies (occasional).*

Etiology. Possible autosomal recessive inheritance. Syndrome needs to be better delineated.

BIBLIOGRAPHY. Geneé E: Une forme de dysostose mandibulo-facial. J Genet Hum 17:45–52, 1969

Wiedemann H-R: Missbildungs-retardierungs-Syndrom mit Fehlen des 5 Strahls an Haenden und Fussen, Ganmenspalte, dysplastischen Ohren und Augenlidern und radioulnarer Synostose. Klin Paediatr 185:181–186, 1973

Wilderwanck LS: Case report 28. Syndrome Ident. 3:11–13, 1975

Miller M, Fineman R, Smith D: Postaxial acrofacial dysostosis syndrome. J Paediatr 95:970–975, 1979

Barbuti D, Orazi C, Reale A, et al: Postaxial acrofacial dysostosis or Miller syndrome: a case report. Eur J Pediatr 148:445–446, 1989

GEOGRAPHIC TONGUE

Synonyms. Erythema migrans tongue; exfoliatio aerata; glossitis areata exfoliativa; migratory glossitis; fissured tongue; lingua plicata.

Symptoms. Common condition 1–2% of general population. Children younger than 4 years most commonly affected. Usually, asymptomatic; occasionally, soreness or pain especially with some particular type of food. Occasionally association with atopic allergy.

Signs. Smooth patches on the dorsum of tongue, outlined by margin gray-yellow or whitish, constantly changing pattern, and coalescing in polycyclic map-like spots; occasionally, some lesions on lips and soft palate.

Etiology. Benign aspecific inflammation. Association with psoriasis and seborrheic dermatosis reported. A genetic factor suspected. Autosomal dominant inheritance.

Pathology. In dermis, acute inflammatory perivascular infiltrates of neutrophils and lymphocytes invading spongious epithelium; edema of rete; thickening of filiform papillae.

Diagnostic Procedures. HLA antigens (equivocal findings).

Therapy. Oral hygiene. If pain, gentian violet paint or mild anesthetic in tablet form. Treat associated conditions.

Prognosis. Spontaneous remission and relapses; years later may develop into "fissured tongue."

BIBLIOGRAPHY. Turpin R, Caretzali A: Contribution a l'etologie de la glossite exfoliatrice marginée. Presse Med 44:1273–1274, 1936

Rahaminoff P, Muhsauf HU: Some observations on 1246 cases of geographic tongue. Am J Dis Child 93:519–525, 1957

Seiler A: Zur Verbreitung und Vererbun der Faltenzunge (lingua plicata). Ach Klaus Stift Vererbungsforsch 11:541–569, 1963

Kullaa-Mikkonen A: Familial study of fissured tongue. Scand J Dent Res 96:366, 1988

Scully C: The oral cavity. In Champion RH, Burton JL, Ebling FJG (eds): Rook/Wilkinson/Ebling Textbook of Dermatology, 5th ed, pp 2740–2741. Oxford, Blackwell Scientific, 1992

GERBASI

See also Addison-Biermer; and Zuelzer.

Symptoms and Signs. Onset in neonatal period; both sexes affected. All symptoms and signs of megaloblastic anemia.

Etiology. Breast feeding from mother with marginal folate stores.

Diagnostic Procedures. See Zuelzer.

Therapy. Integration of alimentation with folate acid.

Prognosis. Prompt remission of symptoms and signs.

BIBLIOGRAPHY. Gerbasi M: Anemia perniciosiforme osservata in bambini ad allattamento materno esclusivo e protratto. Pediatria (Napoli) 48:505–526, 1940

Lee GR: Megaloblastic and non megaloblastic macrocytic anemias. In

Lee GR, Bithel TC, Foerster J, et al (eds): Wintrobe's Clinical Hematology, 9th ed, p 766. Philadelphia, Lea & Febiger, 1993

GERHARDT

Synonyms. Laryngeal adductor paralysis; LABD; vocal cord dysfunction, familial; lobster eye.

Symptoms and Signs. Impairment of phonation or severe inspiratory dyspnea leading to suffocation.

Etiology. Hemorrhage; infections; neoplasm in medulla oblongata; pons or exit from skull, or vagus (X) nerve determining paralysis of both pharyngeal adductor muscles. Autosomal dominant inheritance reported.

BIBLIOGRAPHY. Gerhardt C: Encephalitis; Stimmbandlähmung ohne Stimmveränderung. Arch Path Anat Berl 27:309, 1863
Gerhardt C: Ueber Diagnose und Behandlung der Stimmbandlähmung. Samml Klin Vortr (Leipzig) 36: (Inn Med 13:271–282); Allg Wien Med Stg 17:410–426, 1872
Cunningham MJ, Eavey RD, Shannon DC: Familial vocal cord dysfunction. Pediatrics 76:750–753, 1985

GERLIER

Synonyms. Kubisagari; "Le tourniquet"; paralytic vertigo; vertigo paralysant (fr).

Symptoms. Observed in epidemic form in Switzerland and Japan. During warm summer months, affects mainly young, healthy males who are in contact with cows (in Switzerland) or horses (Japan). Symptoms disappear if contaminated stables are abandoned and in the fall and winter. Attacks of palsies precipitated by severe exertion or bright light, warmth, hunger, or looking at a moving object (optokinetic irritation). Each attack lasts about 10 minutes, and they may follow each other at very short intervals. Mild form not incapacitating, severe form prevents any activity. Ptosis; dimness of vision; vertigo; diplopia; pains in the back of neck; nodding of head during attack.

Signs. Attack of temporary palsy of muscles: levator palpebrae superior; muscles of back of neck; extensor limbs; face; pharynx; larynx. During attack, hyperemia of fundus oculi; fundus normal and eyesight normal between attacks. Hyperreflexia in intervals.

Etiology. Infective agent suspected but not definitely provided. Small Gram-negative coccus from spinal fluid of patient, when injected in cats, gives multiple transient palsies. A similar syndrome may be observed in pellagra.

Pathology. Unknown; possibly brain stem lesion.

Therapy. Unknown; avoidance of contact with contaminated animals and stables.

Prognosis. Good; possible recurrence with reexposure.

BIBLIOGRAPHY. Gérlier E: Une épidémie de vertige paralysant. Rev Med Suisse Romande 7:5–29, 1887
Conchoud PL: Le Kubisagari, Maladie de Gerlier. Rev Med 34:241–296, 1914
De Raadt OLE: Paralytic vertigo (Gerlier's syndrome). Confin Neurol 8:312–320, 1947–1948

GERSTENBRAND

Synonyms. Pseudopsychopathic; temporo-basal, traumatic; traumatic temporo-basal.

Symptoms and Signs. Altered concentration: easy distraction, euphoria, reduced anxiety, flattening affects, inhibition loss (hypersexuality); altered social adjustment, vegetative disorders, occasionally seizures.

Etiology. Head trauma.

Diagnostic Procedures. *CT scan. MRI. EEG.*

Therapy. Treatment of seizures.

BIBLIOGRAPHY. Peters UH: Das pseudopsychopathische Affekt-syndrom der Temporallappepileptiker. Nerven Arzt 72:75–82, 1969
Gerstenbrand F: Organisches Psychosyndrom, Neurologie Vortrag Wiener Tagung der Gesellschaft Oesterr Nervenaerzte und Psychiater. Salzburg, April 1974
Binder H, Gerstenbrand F: Post-traumatic vegetative syndrome. In Vinken PJ, Bruyn GW: Handbook of Clinical Neurology, vol 24 p 582. Amsterdam, North-Holland, 1976

GERSTMANN

Synonym. Gerstmann-Badal; angular gyrus; bilateral somatognosia; asomatognosia bilateral.

Symptoms. Finger agnosia; right-left disorientation; dysgraphia; dyscalculia.

Etiology. Each of the symptoms component of the syndrome may be found isolated or in different combinations. The autonomous entity of this syndrome has been denied and considered an arbitrary selection of concurrent deficits. The fact that the concurrence of the four symptoms implies a localization of lesion on the angular gyrus of the dominant hemisphere has also been disproved (complete Gerstmann has been found to be extensive lesion of the posterior left hemisphere).

Prognosis. When the four components are found, severe impairment of brain function exists, and the underlying disease compromises the patient's life.

BIBLIOGRAPHY. Gerstmann J: Fingeragnosie: Eine umschreibene Storung der orientierung am eigenen Korper. Wien Klin Wochenschr 37:1010–1012, 1924
Gerstmann J: Some notes on the Gerstmann syndrome. Neurology 7:866–869, 1957
Benton AL: Gerstmann's syndrome. Arch Neurol 49:445–447, 1992
Orgogozo JM: Le syndrome de Gerstmann. Encéphale 2:41–43, 1976
Adams RD, Victor M: Principles of Neurology, 5th ed, pp 398, 421. New York, McGraw-Hill, 1993

GERSTMANN-STRAEUSSLER-SCHEINKER

Synonyms. Straussler; GSS; spongiform subacute; cerebellar ataxia–progressive dementia-amyloid dependent; amyloidosis cerebral-spongiform encephalopathy. See Prion syndromes.

Symptoms and Signs. Rare (less than ten per hundred million). Diversity of clinical manifestations. Onset in the fifth decade. Symptoms initially may be relapsing. Ataxia then dementia, accompanied by dysarthria, ocular dysmetria, hyporeflexia or areflexia in lower extremities with positive Babinski sign. Occasionally deafness, blindness, gaze palsy, extrapyramidal rigidity. Seldom seizures.

Etiology. Autosomal dominant inheritance. See Prion syndromes.

Pathology. Extensive amyloid plaques throughout central nervous system, and spongiform degeneration.

Prognosis. Death in 2–10 years (mean age of death 48 years).

BIBLIOGRAPHY. Heidenhain A: Klinische und anatomische Untersuchungen uber eine eigenartige organische des Zentralnervensystems im presenium. Z Gesamte Neurol Pschiatr 118:49, 1929
Gerstmann J, Straussler E, Scheinker I: Ueber eine eigenartige heredi-

taer-familiaere Erkrankung des Zentral Nerven Systems. Z Gensamte Neurol Psychiatr 154:736–762, 1936

Hudson AJ, Fanell MA, Calnins R, et al: Gerstmann-Straussler-Scheinker disease with coincidental familial onset. Ann Neurol 14:670–678, 1983

Prusiner SB: Prion diseases. In Scriver CR, Beaudet AL, Sly WS, et al: The Metabolic and Molecular Bases of Inherited Disease, 7th ed, pp 4526–4527. New York, McGraw-Hill, 1995

GESSLER

Synonym. Gold polishers. See Ulnar nerve compression.

Symptoms and Signs. Muscular atrophy in hands of gold polishers.

Etiology. Ulnar neuritis (not recognized by Gessler).

BIBLIOGRAPHY. Gessler H: Eine Egenartige Form von progressive muskelatrophie bei Goldpolirinner. Med Kor Bl J Württemerg Artstl 36:281, 1929

GIANNOTTI-CROSTI

Synonyms. Crosti-Giannotti; papular infantile acrodermatitis; infantile lichenoid acrodermatitis; eruptive papular infantile acrodermatitis. IPA; PAC.

Symptoms and Signs. Both sexes affected; onset in neonatal period or early infancy (highest frequency between 6 months and 12 years of age), seldom in adults. No seasonal predilection. Incubation period 15–29 days; few systemic manifestations; occasionally central nervous system irritative signs. Onset abrupt; erythematous-papular-lenticular eruption; occasionally, hemorrhagic; also with isolated elements on cheeks, chin, neck, extremities, buttocks. The trunk is rarely involved. No itching. In a few cases, mild fever; eruptions last 15–29 days. Modest lymphadenopathy (lasting 2 months). Splenomegaly (lasting a few days). Hepatomegaly. Jaundice in 9% of cases.

Etiology. Unknown. In some cases, may follow vaccination (smallpox or poliomyelitis). Hepatitis B virus (HBV), Epstein-Barr virus and Coxsackie virus have been suspected.

Pathology. *Skin.* Lymphomonocytic infiltration (histiocytic type of cells) of papillary and superficial derma; occasionally, red cell extravasation. *Lymph nodes.* Reactive intense follicular hyperplasia. *Liver.* Acute hepatitis.

Diagnostic Procedures. *Blood.* Transaminase, aldolase, phosphatase increased; sodium sulfobromophthalein (Bromsulphalein) increased retention (40%); increase of alpha-2 and beta globulins; hyperchromic anemia; monocytosis; presence of plasma cells; hepatitis B antigen. *Bone marrow.* Increase of reticular elements.

Therapy. None. Corticosteroids do not affect course of disease.

Prognosis. Spontaneous remission. Hepatopathy lasts 6–12 months; enzymatic increase may last longer.

BIBLIOGRAPHY. Crosti A: Contributo alla conoscenza della pityriasis rubra pilaris di Devergie e dei suoi rapporti con sindromi vicine. Gior It Dermatol Sif 71:305–340, 1930

Crosti A, Giannotti F: Dermatose eruptive acrosituée d'origine probablement virosique. Dermatologica 115:671–677, 1957

Giannotti F: L'acrodermatite papulosa infantile. Malattia. Gaz San 41:271–274, 1970

Draelos ZK, Hansen RC, James WD: Giannotti-Crosti syndrome associated with infections other than hepatitis B. JAMA 256:2386–2388, 1986

Highet AS, Kurtz J: Viral infections. In Champion RH, Burton JL, Ebling FJG (eds): Rook/Wilkinson/Ebling Textbook of Dermatology, 5th ed, pp 946–947. Oxford, Blackwell Scientific, 1992

GIANT CELL INTERSTITIAL PNEUMONIA

Synonym. GIP. See also Pneumonia lymphoid interstitial.

Symptoms. Both sexes affected; onset at all ages. Asthenia; cough; dyspnea; fever; weight loss.

Signs. Pulmonary rales and finger clubbing.

Etiology. Unknown. In children, defective immunologic system; in adults, intact immunologic system.

Pathology. Within alveoli, numerous bizarre, giant, multinucleated cells. Interstitial tissue thickened by fibrosis and plasma lymphocyte infiltrate.

Diagnostic Procedures. *Blood.* Usually, no defective immunologic findings in adults. *X-ray.* Streaked and mottled nodular density from hilum to periphery.

Therapy. Corticosteroids.

Prognosis. Good response to treatment.

BIBLIOGRAPHY. Reddy PA, Gorelich DG, Christianson CS: Giant cell interstitial pneumonia (GIP). Chest 58:319–325, 1970

Sokolowski JW, Cordray OR, Cantow EF, et al: Giant cell interstitial pneumonia. Report of a case. Am Rev Resp Dis 105:417–420, 1972

Fraser RS, Paré JAP, Fraser RG, Paré PD: Synopsis of Disease of the Chest, 2nd ed. Philadelphia, WB Saunders, 1994

GIBERT

Synonyms. Hebra herpes tonsurans maculosus; herpes tonsurans maculosus, pityriasis rosea.

Symptoms. Both sexes affected; onset at all ages; highest frequency 10–35 years of age. Malaise; mild pruritus; slight fever.

Signs. On thigh or upper arm, trunk or neck appearance of "herald patch": bright red; round or oval; covered by fine silvery gray scaling epidermis. The patch edge is slightly raised and patch rapidly reaches 2–5 cm in diameter or more. Usually after 5–15 days crops of smaller similar patches appear on the whole body with successive bursts, at 2–3 days' interval, for 4–7 weeks. Center of plaques clears and becomes wrinkled. Occasionally, lymphadenopathy.

Etiology. Unknown. Infective agent suspected.

Pathology. Not typical: edema, plus inflammatory changes.

Diagnostic Procedures. *Blood.* Negative. *Skin.* Mycelium search negative.

Therapy. In mild cases, none. In irritated cases, diluted corticosteroid ointments; ultraviolet light.

Prognosis. Self-limited condition of 1–2 months duration. Recurrences 2%.

BIBLIOGRAPHY. Gilbert CM: Traité Pratique des Maladies de la Peau, p 402. Paris, Plan, 1860

Highet AS, Kurtz J: Viral infections. In Champion RH, Burton JL, Ebling FJG (eds): Rook/Wilkinson/Ebling Textbook of Dermatology, 5th ed, pp 948–951. Oxford, Blackwell Scientific, 1992

GIBSON

Synonyms. Gibson-Scott-Griffith; hereditary methemoglobinemia with deficiency of nicotinamide adenine dinucleotide (NADH), cytochrome b5 reductase. See also Hoerlein-Weber. Enzymopenic hereditary methemoglobinemia; including Worster-Drought.

Symptoms and Signs. Both sexes affected; onset frequently from birth. Slate-gray cyanosis (patient more blue than sick); asymptomatic or fatigability and dyspnea after exercise. No evidence of pulmonary or cardiac condition; no finger clubbing. A minority of patients (10–15%) present lethal neurologic disability (see type II).

Today subdivided according to clinico-biochemical criteria in IV types. Type I: Erythrocyte reductase deficiency; deficit limited to erythrocyres, no hemolysis. Type II: Generalized reductase deficiency (Worster-Drought). Generalized cytochrome b5 reductase deficiency. Fully expressed: mental retardation, retarded growth, microcephaly, opisthotonus, athetosis, generalized hypertonia strabismus. Early death. Type III: Hematopoietic reductase deficiency. Deficiency demonstrated in red cell, platelets, leukocytes. No neurologic involvement. Type IV: Cytochrome b5 deficiency.

Etiology. Autosomal recessive inheritance. See clinico-biochemical classification. Gene coding for soluble NADH-cytochrome b5 reductase assigned to chromosome 22.

Pathology. Apparently, none. In type II, brain nonspecific alteration only reduced number of nerve elements and retarded myelinization.

Diagnostic Procedures. *Oxygen administration.* Does not reverse cyanosis. *Blood.* Shaking with air does not reduce the basic dark color. Spectral absorption peaks; qualitative and quantitative determination of methemoglobinemia. Hegesh reaction to assay NADH dehydrogenase.

Therapy. None necessary. Vitamin C and methylene blue reduce cyanosis.

Prognosis. Very good; normal life and longevity except in type II.

BIBLIOGRAPHY. Gibson QH: The reduction of hemoglobin in red blood cells and studies on the cause of idiopathic methemoglobinemia. Biochem J 42:13–23, 1948

Lukens JN: Methemoglobinemia and other disorders accompanied by cynosis. In Lee GR, Bithel TC, Foerster J, et al (eds): Wintrobe's Clinical Hematology, 9th ed, pp 1265–1267. Philadelphia, Lea & Febiger, 1993

Jaffé ER, Hultquist DE: Cytochrome b5 reductase deficiency and enzymopenic hereditary methemoglobinemia. In Scriver CR, Beaudet AL, Sly WS, et al: The Metabolic and Molecular Bases of Inherited Disease, 7th ed, pp 3399–3415. New York, McGraw-Hill, 1995

GIBSON (A.)

Obsolete.

Synonyms. Krabbe III; muscular hypoplasia, congenital, universal; muscular infantilism.

Symptoms and Signs. From birth. Severe generalized muscular hypoplasia.

Etiology. Possibly heterozygous group of conditions including cases of nemaline myopathy (see) and others without specific change except small muscle fibers.

Pathology. Small muscle fibers without pathologic changes.

Prognosis. Nonprogressive nature.

BIBLIOGRAPHY. Gibson A: Muscular infantilism. Arch Intern Med 27:338, 1921

Krabbe KH: Kongenit generaliseret muskelaplasi. Nord Med 35:1756, 1947

Pelias MZ, Thurmon TF: Congenital universal muscular hypoplasia: Evidence for autosomal recessive inheritance. Am J Hum Genet 31:548–554, 1979

GIGOGNOUX

Synonyms. See Schmidt.

Symptoms and Signs. Paralysis of the spinal part of 11th nerve and one vocal cord without paralysis of palate.

BIBLIOGRAPHY. Collet FJ: Les Troubles de L'innervation Pharygolaryngée et Oesophagienne. Paris, Masson, 1946

GILBERT-DREYFUS

Obsolete. See Pseudohermaphroditism male incomplete hereditary type I.

Symptoms and Signs. Male phenotype. Small phallus; hypospadias; gynecomastia; scanty body hair; absent beard; testis normal sized.

Etiology. X-linked inheritance. Considered as an incomplete form of androgen insensitivity syndrome

Pathology. Incompletely developed wolffian ducts.

Diagnostic Procedures. Male sex chromatin 46 XY karyotype; gonadotropin level elevated; testosterone and estradiol levels elevated.

Therapy. Resistance to the effects of testosterone.

Prognosis. Good for life; function poor.

BIBLIOGRAPHY. Gilbert-Dreyfus NI, Savoie NI, Sebaoun NI, et al: Etude d'un cas familial d'androgenoidisme avec hypospadias grave, gynécomastie et hypoestrenogénie. Ann Endocrinol (Paris) 18:93–101, 1957

Wilson JD, Harrod MJ, Goldstein JL, et al: Familial incomplete manifestations in a family with the Reifenstein syndrome. N Engl J Med 290:1097–1103, 1974

Josso N: Anatomy and endocrinology of fetal sex differentiation. In De Groot LJ (ed): Endocrinology, 3rd ed, p 1921. Philadelphia, WB Saunders, 1995

GILBERT (J.B.)

Synonyms. Choriogenic gynecomastia. See paraneoplastic syndromes.

Symptoms. Occurs in males. Tenderness and pain of nipples.

Signs. Unilateral or bilateral swelling, initially under areola, successive enlargement of breast.

Etiology. Excessive production of chorionic hormones from various types of hPL-producing malignant tumors (testes, lung, liver, lymphomas, pheochromocytoma, etc.).

Diagnostic Procedures. *Blood.* Elevated levels of hPL, estradiol, variously associated with the production of other placental proteins (hCG) and placental alkaline phosphatase. Studies of other more or less specific cancer markers. *X-rays. CT scan. MRI.*

Therapy. Surgery: orchidectomy or other types of tumor excision.

Prognosis. According to time of onset and therapy.

BIBLIOGRAPHY. Gilbert JB: Studies in malignant testis tumor II. Syndrome of coriogenic gynecomastia: Report of six cases and review of one hundred and twenty nine. J Urol 44:345–357, 1940

Sherwood LM: Paraneoplastic endocrine disorders (ectopic hormone syndromes). In De Groot LJ (ed): Endocrinology, 3rd ed, p 2777. Philadelphia, WB Saunders, 1995

GILBERT (N.A.)

Synonyms. Gilbert-Lereboullet. Meulengracht; unconjugated benign bilirubinemia; low-grade, chronic hyperbilirubinemia; icterus intermittens juvenilis; familial, nonhemolytic, nonobstructive jaundice; liver dysfunction constitutional.

Symptoms and Signs. Both sexes affected; male to female ratio 4:1; onset usually shortly after birth, but may not be recognized for many years. Scleral jaundice only abnormal finding. Usually after diagnosis is made, fatigue, nausea, abdominal pain in right quadrant (anxiety reaction?). Symptoms and jaundice become more pronounced after fasting, exertion, alcohol, intercurrent infections.

Etiology. Unknown; possibly autosomal dominant inheritance. Benign group of metabolic abnormalities. Attempts to determine impairment of bilirubin conjugation or decrease of glucuronyl transferase activity have failed. Slight reduction of red cell survival found in 50% of patients. Reduced bilirubin uridine diphosphate (UDP) glucuronyl transferase activity could possibly explain hyperbilirubinemia and impaired clearance of pigment, but it is not the only mechanism responsible for the syndrome.

Pathology. Normal hepatic histology.

Diagnostic Procedures. *Blood.* Unconjugated bilirubinemia (fasting increases hyperbilirubinemia); serum transaminases normal; serum alkaline phosphatase normal. No overt evidence of hemolysis or other conditions that may produce bilirubinemia. *Urine.* Bilirubinuria absent. *Biopsy of liver.* Normal. *Cholangiography.* Normal.

Therapy. Reassurance of the patient about benign prognosis to avoid anxiety-type symptoms. Phenobarbital administration reduces bilirubin level. Vitamin E.

Prognosis. Excellent; jaundice with fluctuation persisting through life.

BIBLIOGRAPHY. Gilbert NA, Castaigne J, Lereboullet P: De l'ictère familial. Contribution a l'étude de la diathèse bilaire. Bull Soc Méd Hop Lyon 17:948–959, 1900
Meulengracht E: Icterus intermittens iuvenilis. Klin Wschr 45:118–121, 1939
Chowdhury JR, Wolkoff AV, Chowdhury NR, et al: Hereditary jaundice and disorders of bilirubin metabolism. In Scriver CR, Beaudet AL, Sly WS, et al: The Metabolic and Molecular Bases of Inherited Disease, 7th ed, pp 2184–2187. New York, McGraw-Hill, 1995

GILCREEST

Synonym. Bicipital tendon.

Symptoms and Signs. Bicipital tendon dislocation.

Etiology. Trauma.

Diagnostic Procedures. *Specific test.* Dumbbell in each hand (2–3 kg), extension of arms, lifting to the overhead position in external rotation. Examiner finger on tendon of long head of the biceps; as the patient lowers the outstretched arms, at 90–100 degree angle a sharp pain occurs and a snap is palpable and audible.

Therapy. Surgery.

BIBLIOGRAPHY. Gilcreest EL: The common syndrome of rupture, dislocation and elongation of the long head of the biceps brachii: Analysis of 100 cases. Surg Gynecol Obstet 58:322–340, 1934
Justis EJ Jr: Traumatic disorders. In Crenshaw, AH (ed): Campbell's Operative Orthopedics, 7th ed, pp 2242–2243. St Louis, CV Mosby, 1987

GILFORD–BURNIER

Synonyms. Burnier; Hanhart (see for subtypes); ateliosis; pituitary dwarfism; prepuberal panhypopituitarism. ateliotic dwarfism–hypogonadism; pituitary dwarfism III.

Symptoms and Signs. Both sexes affected; age of onset variable. Characteristic diversity of appearance according to number of hormone deficiencies. All cases present delayed growth; symptomatic hypoglycemia is another almost constant feature; hypothyroidism features (52%); hypogonadism (88%); hypoadrenalism (56%).

Etiology. Idiopathic. Often secondary to pituitary adenoma or other destructive lesions of pituitary or other diencephalic pathology. Also possibly related to trauma at birth. Autosomal recessive inheritance also well described.

Pathology. According to etiology and type of hormone deficiencies.

Diagnostic Procedures. *Blood.* Determination of growth hormone; adrenocorticotropic hormone (ACTH); thyroid-stimulating hormone (TSH), gonadotropin, hypoglycemia. Other metabolic derangements according to hormones involved.

Therapy. Pituitary hormones, according to development of hormonal deficiencies (occasionally sequential).

Prognosis. Excellent response to hormone administration. That of primary lesion.

BIBLIOGRAPHY. Gilford H: Ateliosis: Form of dwarfism. Practitioner 70:797–819, 1903
Burnier R: A new hypophyseal syndrome; hypophyseal nanism. Ann Ophthalmol 21:263–273, 1912
Goodman GH, Grumbach MM, Kaplan SL: Growth and growth hormone. II. A comparison of isolated growth hormone deficiency and multiple pituitary-hormone deficiencies in 35 patients with idiopathic hypopituitary dwarfism. N Engl J Med 278:57–78, 1968
Wass JAH, Besser M: Tests of pituitary function. In De Groot LJ (ed): Endocrinology, 3rd ed, pp 487–494. Philadelphia, WB Saunders, 1995

GILLES DE LA TOURETTE

Synonyms. Brissaud II; Guinon; Tourette; coprolalia—generalized tic; myospasia impulsiva; compulsive tic; chorea variable de dégénérés (Fr.).

Symptoms. Occurs generally in boys (75% of patients are male); begins at age 7 or 8. Generalized tics limited preferably to facial muscles; inarticulate expiratory laryngeal noises at the beginning, spreading of tics to the shoulders and arms. With progression of the form, the patient begins to exclaim obscene words or short phrases (coprolalia) in a loud voice. Echolalia, pallilalia, echomimesia also may develop. Tics that may be very violent stop during sleep and are intensified by emotions. It has been reported that in some cases they may be suppressed by voluntary control. Coprolalia manifests only in presence of other people; it may, by some patients, be masked by coughing. Intelligence varies from superior to subnormal. In 43% observed self-mutilation.

Signs. In some cases, neurologic signs of doubtful significance.

Etiology. Unknown; not established if of organic or psychogenic origin. Emotional trauma frequently precipitating factor. Disturbed parent–child relation frequently encountered in history. Ten percent of patients have a family history of the condition, with possible transmission of autosomal semidominant (and or semirecessive) type.

Pathology. Only two autopsies: one normal; the second showed no gross pathology, but possibly an enlargement of large neurocytes of corpus striatum.

Therapy. Chlorpromazine; haloperidol; group psychotherapy (?); prefrontal leukotomy (in extremely severe cases). The proposed differentiation of Tourette syndrome subgroups according to the presence or absence of migraine and other serotonin-related associated symptoms may aid in predicting drug response to haloperidol, clonidine, L-5-hydroxytryptophan, and other agents and in the development of other drugs for the treatment of this disorder.

Prognosis. Course unpredictable. Spontaneous arrest with exacerbations; lifelong symptoms. Quoad vitam good.

BIBLIOGRAPHY. Gilles de la Tourette G: Étude sur une affection nerveuse caractérisée par de l'incoordination motrice accompagnée d'écholalie et de coprolalie. Arch Neurol 9:19–42; 158–200, 1885
Trousseau A: Clinique médicale de l'Hotel-Dieu de Paris, vol 1, p 855, 1873

Brissaud PE: La chorée variable de dégenerés. Rev Neurol 4:417–431, 1896

Shapiro AK, Shapiro ES, Brum RD, et al: Gilles de la Tourette Syndrome. New York, Raven Press, 1978

Comings DE, Comings BG: Clinical and genetic relationships between autism—pervasive developmental disorder and Tourette syndrome: A study of 19 cases. Am J Med Genet 39:180–191, 1991

Chase TN, Friedhoff AJ, Cohen DJ (eds): Tourette syndrome: Genetics, neurobiology and treatment. Adv Neurol 58, 1992

GILLESPIE

Synonyms. Aniridia; cerebellar ataxia; mental deficiency.

Symptoms and Signs. Both sexes. From birth. Bilateral aniridia; physical and mental retardation; hypotonia; normal tendon reflexes, normal sensitivity; gross incoordination, attention tremor, scanning speech.

Etiology. Unknown. Autosomal recessive inheritance proposed. Normal karyotype.

Diagnostic Procedures. All laboratory exams normal.

Prognosis. With age some improvement of motor performance. Persisting mental deficiency.

BIBLIOGRAPHY. Gillespie FB: Aniridia, cerebellar ataxia and oligophrenia in siblings. Arch Ophthalmol 73:338–341, 1965

Witting EO, Moreira CA, Freire-Maia N, et al: Partial aniridia, cerebellar ataxia and mental deficiency (Gillespie syndrome). Am J Med Genet 30:703–708, 1988

GILLIN AND PRYSE-DAVIS

Synonyms. Escobar; pterygium, multiple, lethal type I; pterygium colli; pterygium universale.

Symptoms and Signs. Those of pterygium in aborted fetuses. Varieties with bone fusion or spinal fusion described.

Etiology. Autosomal recessive inheritance.

BIBLIOGRAPHY. Hall JC: The lethal multiple pterygium syndromes (editorial). Am J Med Genet 17:803–807, 1974

Gillin ME, Pryse-Davis J: Pterygium syndrome. J Med Genet 13:249–251, 1976

Escobar V, Bixler D, Gleiser S, et al: Multiple pterygium syndrome. Am J Dis Child 132:609–611, 1978

Martin NJ, Hill JB, Cooper DH, et al: Lethal multiple pterygium syndrome: Three consecutive cases in one family. Am J Med Genet 24:295–304, 1986

Teebi AS, Daoud AS: Multiple pterygium syndrome: A relatively common disorder among Arabs (letter). J Med Genet 27:791, 1990

GILLUM-ANDERSON

Synonyms. Blepharoptosis; myopia inherited; ectopia lentis.

Symptoms and Signs. Both sexes. From birth bilateral ptosis. High grade myopia. Ectopia lentis. Dislocated lenses.

Etiology. Possibly autosomal dominant inheritance. Weakness of orbital connective tissue.

BIBLIOGRAPHY. Gillum WM, Anderson RL: Dominantly inherited blepharoptosis, high myopia and ectopia lentis. Arch Ophthalmol 100:282–284, 1982

GIROUX-BARBEAU

Synonyms. Erythrokeratodermia-ataxia; ataxia-erythrokeratodermia.

Symptoms and Signs. Both sexes. After birth. Papulosquamous erythematous plaques more evident in winter and disappear or are markedly reduced after 25 years of age. After a few years progressive neurologic alterations: decreased tendon reflexes, nystagmus, dysarthria, and ataxia.

Etiology. Unknown. Autosomal dominant inheritance.

Pathology. *Skin.* Centrifugal damage with spongiosis and necrosis of malpighian layer and absence of stratum granulosum.

Therapy. None specific. Temporal effacing by stripping of the lesions.

BIBLIOGRAPHY. Giroux JM, Barbeau A: Erythrokeratoderma with ataxia. Arch Dermatol 106:183–188, 1972

Warkang J: Syndromes associated with mental retardation. In Vinken PJ, Bruyn GW, Klawans HL (eds): Handbook of Clinical Neurology, vol 46, p 60. Amsterdam, Elsevier, 1985

GITELMAN

Synonyms. Renal tubular hypokalemic metabolic alkalosis; magnesium deficiency; hypocalciuria; Bartter variant, see Bartter and hyperprostaglandin E

Symptoms and Signs. Both sexes (M/F 1/1). Onset of symptoms at school age: febrile seizures and tetanic episodes (12/16), short stature (3/16). Chonic dermatitis (skin thickening with purple-red hue) seldom polyuria, polydipsia, or extracellular fluid volume contraction.

Etiology. Possibly a defective sodium-chloride carrier protein along the distal convoluted tubule since laboratory characteristics indicate a mechanism of binding to and inhibiting luminal sodium-chloride cotransporter in the distal convoluted tubule. Autosomal recessive inheritance.

Diagnostic Procedures. *Blood.* hypokalemic, metabolic alkalosis, Hypochloremia (with inappropriate chloruria), hypomagnesemia (with inappropiate magnesuria), hyponatremia, increased plasma renin activity. *Urine.* Calcium excretion reduced, impaired urinary concentration ability. *X-ray.* Nephrocalcinosis absent.

Therapy. Long-term correction of the potassuim deficit.

Prognosis. Benign as compared with Bartter.

BIBLIOGRAPHY. Gitelman HJ, Graham JB, Welt LG: A new familial disorder characterized by hypokalemia and hypomagnesemia. Trans Assoc Am Phys 79:221–235, 1966

Bettinelli A, Bianchetti MG, Girardin E, et al: Use of calcium excretion values to distinguish two forms of primary renal tubular hypokalemic alkalosis: Bartter and Gitelman Syndromes. J Pediatr 120:38–43, 1992

Editorial correspondence. Gitelman versus Bartter syndrome. J Pediatr 123:671–672, 1993

GJESSING

Synonym. Catatonia periodic.

Symptoms. Recurring periods of catatonic stupor and psychic excitement.

Etiology. Unknown. No further report on the syndrome. It may belong in the group of thyroid psychoses or manic depressive diseases; see also Catatonic schizophrenia.

Diagnostic Procedures. Increase of blood urea nitrogen (BUN) during episodes.

Therapy. Thyroid hormone.

Prognosis. Complete control with indicated treatment.

BIBLIOGRAPHY. Gjessing R: Disturbances of somatic function in catatonia with a period course, and their compensation. J Ment Sci 84:608–621, 1938

Adams RD, Victor M: Principles of Neurology, 5th ed, p 1335. New York, McGraw-Hill, 1993

GLANZMANN

Synonyms. Glanzmann-Naegeli; thromboasthenia; diacyclothrombopathia.

Symptoms and Signs. Both sexes affected; onset from birth. May be asymptomatic until trauma or surgical procedures make condition evident. Recurrent petechiae; epistaxis, menorrhagia, or metrorrhagia and other bleeding manifestations of different degrees of severity may spontaneously occur.

Etiology. Qualitative platelet defect. Characterized by deficient adenosine diphosphate (ADP)-induced platelet aggregation and deficient clot retraction causing lack of mechanism for viscous metamorphosis or clot retraction. Four different genotype changes apparently have been identified that lead to the phenotype of this syndrome. Several varieties of this condition have been identified to be inherited as autosomal recessive traits. Absence on platelet membrane of glycoprotein IIb-IIIa, which interacts with thrombin to form the clot. Absence of glycoprotein IIb-IIIa also is accompanied by absence of PL A1 antigen.

Diagnostic Procedures. *Blood.* Bleeding time prolonged; tourniquet test positive or negative. Platelets normal number (in some varieties of this condition decreased); may present normal morphology, or be small or large and bizarre; usually appear isolated rather than clumped. Usually, inability to be aggregated by ADP in one group: low platelet adenosine triphosphate (ADT), pyruvate kinase, and phosphoglyceraldehyde; in a second variety, only ATP low; in a third variety, ATPase deficient; in a fourth variety, absence of fibrinogen-like protein from surface of platelets.

Therapy. Allogenic bone marrow transplantation gives complete correction of defect. Fresh blood transfusion may temporarily modify defect.

Prognosis. Usually benign, but death from hemorrhage may occur. Usually hemorrhagic manifestation decreases with age.

BIBLIOGRAPHY. Glanzmann WE: Hereditäre hamorrhägische Thrombasthenie. Jahrb Kinderheilkd 88:1–42, 113–141, 1918

Newman PJ, Seligsohn U, Lyman S, et al: The molecular genetic basis of Glanzman thromboasthenia in the Iraqui-Jewish and Arab population in Israel. Proc Natl Acad Sci 88:3160–3164, 1991

Bithell TC: Qualitative disorders of platelets function. In Lee GR, Bithel TC, Foerster J, et al (eds): Wintrobe's Clinical Hematology, 9th ed, pp 1397–1400. Philadelphia, Lea & Febiger, 1993

GLANZMANN-RINIKER

Synonyms. Swiss type agammaglobulinemia; lymphocytosis–thymic alymphoplasia; thymic dysplasia; lymphopenic agammaglobulinemia; severe combined immunodeficiency; lymphocytophthisis. Including ADA deficiency, adenosine deaminase deficiency.

Symptoms and Signs. Male to female ratio, 3:1; onset from early infancy (3–6 months). Succession of debilitating infections (viral and bacterial); watery diarrhea; candidiasis; failure to thrive.

Etiology. Two different modes of inheritance: autosomal recessive and X-linked and sporadic cases reported. In 50% of autosomal recessive cases absence of adenosine deaminase (ADA). The pathogenesis in these cases is caused by ATP accumulation or S-adenosyl homocysteine toxicity on immunocompetent lymphocytes.

Pathology. *Thymus.* Small or almost absent; lack of Hassall corpuscles. *Bone marrow, spleen, lymph nodes.* Absence or small number of lymphocytes and plasma cells; lack of germinal centers.

Diagnostic Procedures. *Blood.* Leukopenia lower than 2000; marked lymphopenia (lack of both T- and B-types); lymphocytes unresponsive to phytohemoagglutinin or allogenic stimulation; many lymphocytes immature (lymphoblast types); granulocytes and platelets normal; moderate eosinophilia; negative adenosine deaminase in erythrocytes. *Protein electrophoresis.* Agammaglobulinemia. *Skin tests.* Negative response to Candida antigens; absence of sensitization to dinitrochlorobenzene; acceptance of heterologous skin grafts.

Therapy. Gammaglobulin injection of temporary and little effect. Bone marrow transplantation has been successful in cases without preexisting lung infection and for which a protected aseptic environment has been possible.

Prognosis. Overwhelming infections; fatal usually within first year of life.

BIBLIOGRAPHY. Glanzmann E, Riniker P: Essentielle Lymphocytophtise. Ein neues Krankheitsbild aus der Säugligspathologie. Ann Paediatr 175:1–32, 1950

Fischer A, Landais P, Friedrich W, et al: European experience of bone marrow transplantation for severe combined immunodeficiency. Lancet, 336:850–854, 1990

Lukens JN: Immune deficiency diseases: inherited and acquired. In Lee GR, Bithel TC, Foerster J, et al (eds): Wintrobe's Clinical Hematology, 9th ed, pp 1683–1684. Philadelphia, Lea & Febiger, 1993

GLASS-GORLIN

Synonyms. Deafness-oligodontia.

Symptoms and Signs. Both sexes. Profound deafness; oligodontia.

Etiology. Autosomal recessive inheritance (?).

BIBLIOGRAPHY. Glass L, Gorlin RJ: Congenital profound sensorineural deafness and olidontia: a new syndrome. Arch Otolaryng 105:621–622, 1979

GLENARD

Synonyms. Enteroptosis; spleneptosis; visceroptosis.

Symptoms. Female to male ratio, 4:1; onset at all ages. In erect position, abdominal discomfort, backache; fatigability; nausea; palpitation; occasionally, vomiting, and syncope; usually, chronic constipation.

Signs. Abdominal palpation reveals muscular atony, transverse colon in lower position, sagging, occasionally, to upper edge of pelvis, and epigastric pulsation. Tachycardia.

Etiology. Weakness of abdominal muscles; congenital or acquired condition, in the latter case after severe weight loss.

Diagnostic Procedures. *X-ray of gastrointestinal tract.* In various positions to evidentiate the displacement of diaphragm, hypochondrial organs, stomach, and intestinal sections. The heart too may appear elongated.

Therapy. Girdle; correction of severe weight loss; physical therapy to strengthen selected muscle groups. Surgery seldom indicated.

Prognosis. Worsening with age.

BIBLIOGRAPHY. Glénard F: Neurosthénie et entéroptose. Sem Med 6:211–212, 1886

GLOBUS

Synonyms. Includes bolus hystericus. See Plummer-Vinson and Schatzki.

Symptoms. Sensation of lump in throat, which interferes with swallowing.

Etiology and Pathology. Carcinomas; strictures; enlarged styloid process; pharyngeal pouch; pharyngeal paralysis; esophageal reflux (see); hypochromic anemia (see Plummer-Vinson) and cervical spine area pathology, especially osteoarthritis, psychoneurotic disorder (bolus hystericus).

Diagnostic Procedures. *Nose and throat examination. X-ray of cervical spine.* In different projections. *Blood.* Hemoglobin determination; red cell sedimentation rate.

Therapy. According to etiology; surgical; medical; psychotherapeutic.

Prognosis. Depends on etiology. Careful examination of the spine in cases with otherwise negative findings may reveal hidden pathology and significantly decrease the psychiatric group, and provides therapeutic means to cure these patients.

BIBLIOGRAPHY. Morrison LF: The cervical spine and the globus syndrome. Ann Otol 64:753–765, 1955
Lichtenstein GR: Esophageal rings, webs and diverticula. In Haubrich WS, Schaffner F, Berk JE (eds): Bockus Gastroenterology, 5th ed, vol 2, p 518. Philadelphia, WB Saunders, 1995

GLOBUS PALLIDUS NECROSIS

Symptoms. Patients who have suffered an episode of coma from carbon monoxide, nitrous oxide, carbon disulfide, or domestic gas inhalation. One to 3 weeks after recovering from initial coma, either with complete recovery, or with only residual slight confusion, patient relapses into coma a second time. Relapse may onset with akinetic mute state, with generalized rigidity and flexion of arm and extension of legs, with mental confusion, with visual agnosia, or catatonic postures. In a minority of cases, only a mild parkinsonian rigidity appears within 6 weeks of recovery of first episode of coma.

Etiology. Necrosis of globus pallidus associated, with major or minor cortical damage owing to coal gas toxicity (carbon monoxide) and hemorrhagic necrosis.

Pathology. When death occurs during first coma episode, usually the most anterior part of internal segments show symmetric hemorrhagic softening. When death occurs after delayed relapse, larger infarct involving external segments and even part of putamen. Patchy areas of cortical laminal necrosis are present.

Diagnostic Procedures. *CT scan. MRI.* Confirm damage of hippocampus and white matter.

Therapy. Symptomatic.

Prognosis. Very poor; death usually follows first or second episode of coma. In some cases, longer survival with development of astasia-abasia; then rigidity, and mutism.

BIBLIOGRAPHY. Meyer A: Ueber der Wirkung der Kohlenoxydvergiftung auf das Zentralnervensystem. Z Ges Neurol Psychiatr 112:172, 1926
Denny-Brown D: Basal Ganglia. London, Oxford Univ Press, 1962
Goldfrank's Toxicological Emergencies, 5th ed, pp 1204–1205. Norwalk, CT, Appleton-Lange, 1994

GLOMUS JUGULARE TUMOR

Symptoms. Prevalent in females; onset in second to sixth decade (average 48 years). Duration of symptoms before diagnosis 2–3 years.

Conduction deafness; fullness or pulsation in the ear; aural discharge; facial (VII) nerve paralysis; paralysis of IX through XII cranial nerves; paralysis of vocal cord.

Signs. Usually tumor behind tympanic membrane, less frequently in the external canal or cervical region.

Etiology. Unknown; tumor of glomus jugulare (including all chemodectomas arising in vicinity of ear).

Pathology. Circumscribed tumor reddish, friable, usually confined to middle ear, some extending into cochlea and eustachian tube and destroying temporal bone. No capsule submucosal involvement characteristic. Cells arranged in nest with vascular fibrous septa.

Diagnostic Procedures. *Angiography of carotid.*

Therapy. Surgical excision; total seldom possible. X-ray treatment.

Prognosis. Usually, cure with surgery; local recurrences or local invasion may develop; or metastasis in malignant type (rare).

BIBLIOGRAPHY. Rosenwasser H: Carotid body tumor of the middle ear and mastoid. Arch Otolaryngol 41:64–67, 1945
Oberman HA: Chemodectomas (nonchromaffin paraganglioma) of head and neck. Cancer 21:838–851, 1968
Horn KL, Creemley RL, Schindler RA: Facial neurolemmomas. Laryngoscope 91:1326–1331, 1981
Sabiston DC: Textbook of Surgery, 14th ed, p 1195. Philadelphia, WB Saunders, 1991
Adams RD, Victor M: Principles of Neurology, 5th ed, p 583. New York, McGraw-Hill, 1993

GLOSSODYNIA

Synonyms. Burning mouth.

Symptoms. Pain in the tongue without apparent causes.

Etiology. Multifactorial: psychic, mechanic, chemical, hormonal or owing to electrogalvanism from metallic tooth filling.

BIBLIOGRAPHY. Baurle G, Schonberger A: Glossodynie-Indikation zur Epikutantestung? Z Hautkr 61:1175–1184, 1986
Von der Ploeg HM, Von der Wal N, Eijkmann Maj: Psychological aspects of patients with burning mouth syndrome. Oral Surg. Oral Med Oral Pathol 63:664–668, 1987
Adams RD, Victor M: Principles of Neurology, 5th ed, p 1181. New York, McGraw-Hill, 1993

GLOSSOPALATINE ANKYLOSIS

Synonyms. Kettner. Kramer; ankyloglossia superior; glossopalatine ankylosis–microglossia hypodontia–limb anomalies. It may be included in the Oromandibular-limb hypogenesis spectrum (hypoglossia-hypodactyly; aglossia-adactyly; Moebius; Charlie M; facial limb disruptive spectrum).

Symptoms. Rare. Both sexes affected. Congenital symptoms related to signs and their association.

Signs. *Mouth.* Tongue small, with anterior part attached to hard palate or upper alveolar ridge or both; tip could be cleft. Upper lip and mandible hypoplastic. Palatal vault high; occasionally, hypodontia and ankylosing of temporomandibular joint. *Limbs.* Various anomalies both in the hands and feet, unilateral or bilateral syndactyly, clinodactyly, hypoplasia of digits, nail absence, lobster claw deformity. Occasionally, associated paralysis of abducens (VI) or facial (VII) nerve.

Etiology. Unknown. Possible alteration of environment between the eighth and twelfth week in utero. For simple ankyloglossia autosomal dominant inheritance reported

BIBLIOGRAPHY. Illera MD: Congenital occlusion of the pharynx. Lancet 1:724, 1887

Kettner H: Kongenitaler Zungendefekt. Dtsch Med Wochenschr 38:352, 1907

Kramer W: Zur Entstehung der angeborenen Gaumenspalte. Zentralbl Chir 38:385–387, 1911

Henderson JL: The congenital facial diplegia syndrome: Clinical features, pathology and etiology. Brain 62:381–403, 1936

Chicarelli ZN, Palayes IM: Oromantibular limb hypogenesis syndromes. Plast Reconstr Surg 76:13–24, 1985

GLUCAGONOMA

Synonyms. Alpha-2 cell carcinoma; pancreas alpha-2 cell carcinoma.

Symptoms and Signs. Prevalent in females (3:2); onset between second and seventh decade. Weight loss in 64% of cases; pallor; necrolytic migratory erythema (individual erythematous papules that blister, ooze, crust, and spread peripherally, while clearing in the center). Superinfections common; lesions evolve in 14 days and heal, leaving bronze discoloration, without scar formation. Stomatitis and glossitis (in 33% of cases). Susceptibility to deep veins thrombosis. Neuropsychiatric disturbances. Can be part of a pluriglandular syndrome.

Etiology. Alpha-2 cell tumor of the islets of Langerhans, producing excessive amount of glucagon. Rare instances of familial (autosomal dominant inheritance) hyperglucagonemia (high IRG 9000, and IRG 10–20,000)

Pathology. Tumor of pancreas. Metastasis in liver and other sites. Primary tumor averages 3 cm in diameter at time of surgery. Histologically. Alpha-2-type of islet cells.

Diagnostic Procedures. *Blood.* Normochromic anemia; plasma glucagon levels 0.3–96.0 ng/ml (normal less than 0.2 ng/ml); hyperglycemia or altered glucose tolerance test (or both); hypoaminoacidemia. Other procedures to identify presence of tumor and metastasis.

Therapy. Surgery whenever feasible. Chemotherapy by streptozocin (alone or in combination with 5-fluorouracil, chlorozotocyn, chlorozotocyn plus doxorubicin, and dacarbazine) gives good response; with diaminotriazenoimidazone carboximide as an alternative. The skin manifestation responds to amino acid infusions, zinc sulfate (IV and topical). In case of metastasized tumor; somatostatin analogue SMS 201–995.

Prognosis. Complete removal of tumor induces full remission of all symptoms. In inoperable cases, however, ungratifyng results (simple symptom control) obtained with medical treatment and chemotherapy.

BIBLIOGRAPHY. Becker SW, Kahn D, Rothman S: Cutaneous manifestations of internal malignant tumors. Arch Dermatol Syph 45:1069–1080, 1942

McGavran MH, Unger RH, Recant L, et al: A glucagon-secreting alpha-cell carcinoma of the pancreas. N Engl J Med 274:1408–1413, 1966

Bloom SR, Polak JM: Glucagonoma syndrome. Am J Med 82 (suppl 5B):25–35, 1987

Unger RH, Orci L: Glucagon secretion, alpha cell metabolism and glucagon action. In De Groot LJ (ed): Endocrinology, 3rd ed, pp 1348–1349. Philadelphia, WB Saunders, 1995

GLUCOCORTICOID-REMEDIABLE ALDOSTERONISM

Synonyms. Lifton; GRA; aldosteronism, glucocorticoid-remediable. See Liddle.

Symptoms and Signs. Severe hypertension (strong family history) and other features similar to Conn syndrome (see).

Etiology. Autosomal dominant inheritance. Chimeric gene duplication arising from unequal crossing over, fusing regulatory sequences of steroid 11 beta-hydroxylase to coding sequences of aldosterone synthase.

Diagnostic Procedures. *Urine.* Increased 18-OH-cortisol and 18-oxocortisol and absence of suppressed aldosterone excretion.

Therapy. Good response to spironolactone (high doses).

Prognosis. With treatment improvement of plasma electrolytes, but rarely patients become normotensive

BIBLIOGRAPHY. Lifton RP, Diuhy RG, Power M, et al: A chimeric 11 beta-hydroxylase/aldosterone synthase gene causes glucocorticoid-remedible aldosteronism and human hypertension. Nature 355:262–265, 1992

Rich G, Ulick S, Cook S, et al: Glucocorticoid-remediable aldosteronism in a large kindred: Clinical spectrum and and diagnosis using a characteristic biochemical phenotype. Ann Int Med 116:818–820, 1992

Waenock DG, Bubien JK: Liddle's syndrome: A public menace? Am J Kid Dis 25:924–927, 1995

GLUCOSE–GALACTOSE MALABSORPTION

Synonyms. See intestinal disaccharidase deficiency; and renal glycosuria.

Symptoms and Signs. Both sexes affected; onset with first milk feeding. Watery diarrhea following every milk intake. Failure to thrive; dehydration.

Etiology. Genetic hererogeneity of the disease. Intestinal Na+-d-glucose cotransporter (SGLT1) gene mapped to chromosome 22(22q13.1). Basic defect in absorption of both glucose and galactose confined to mucosal cells at brush border of intestine.

Pathology. Normal jejunal mucosa; accumulation of glucose in brush border of cells.

Diagnostic Procedures. *Stool.* Acid rich in glucose, galactose, lactic acid; disaccharides absent. *Urine.* Intermittent glycosuria. Elimination of lactose and galactose from diet. Relieves all symptoms. *Administration of fructose.* Well tolerated and increases plasma glucose. *Glucose-galactose oral tolerance test.* No rise in blood sugar. *Hydrogen breath test.*

Therapy. Omit milk and any carbohydrate, except fructose, from diet.

Prognosis. If defect readily identified and dietetic regimen instituted, good. Permanent damage if not treated early. Clinical remission with increased age.

BIBLIOGRAPHY. Laplane R, Polonovski C, Etienne M, et al: Intolerance to sugars of active intestinal transfer. Its relation to intolerance to lactose and the celiac syndrome. Arch Fr Pediatr 19:895–944, 1962

Wright RM, Turk E, Zabel B, et al: Molecular genetics of intestinal glucose transport. J Clin Invest 88:1435–1440, 1991

Desjeux J-F, Turk E, Wright E: Congenital selective Na+d-glucose cotransport defects leading to renal glycosuria and congenital selective intestinal malabsorption of glucose and galactose. In Scriver CR, Beaudet AL, Sly WS, et al: The Metabolic and Molecular Bases of Inherited Disease, 7th ed, pp 3563–3572. New York, McGraw-Hill, 1995

GLUCOSE-6-PHOSPHATE DEHYDROGENASE DEFICIENCY

Synonyms. G6PD. Cluster of syndromes owing to a congenital defect of normal glucose-6-phosphate dehydrogenase and presence of abnormal mutant enzymes (about 400 variants described), some of which may induce the different clinical manifestations.

DRUG-INDUCED HEMOLYTIC ANEMIA (G6PD)

Symptoms and Signs. Males affected; seldom seen in females, or mild symptoms; onset at all ages after exposure; to drugs (antimalarials; sulfonamides; sulfones; nitrofurans; antipyretics; analgesics; others). Hemolytic crises of mild degree; abdominal and back pains; hemoglobinuria.

EPISODIC HEMOLYTIC ANEMIA (G6PD) WITHOUT DRUG EXPOSURE

Symptoms and Signs. Whites, blacks of both sexes affected; onset at any age. Moderate or severe hemolytic crises spontaneous or in association with infections; metabolic alterations (ketoacidosis). Acute renal insufficiency may result from crises.

FAVISM

Symptoms and Signs. Occurs in population from Mediterranean areas (highest incidence in Sardinians); reported also in west China; male to female ratio 6.2:1; onset at 2–5 years of age. In a somewhat erratic fashion following ingestion of fava beans (2–3 days) or inhalation of pollen (few hours): headache, nausea, back pain, chills, and fever followed by hemoglobinuria and jaundice and anemia of variable degree.

NEONATAL JAUNDICE (G6PD)

Symptoms and Signs. Greeks, Thais, and other rates affected; onset in neonatal period. Severe hemolytic crisis, with possible kidney failure, spontaneous or after vitamin K, other drugs, or infections.

NONSPHEROCYTIC CONGENITAL HEMOLYTIC ANEMIA (G6PD)

Symptoms and Signs. Whites and blacks affected; onset in infancy or childhood. Symptoms and signs of chronic hemolytic anemia.

Etiology. X-linked inheritance. Glucose-6-phosphate deficiency and presence of various mutant enzymes. Different clinical syndromes precipitated by drugs, infections, other toxic factors (e.g., immunologic).

Pathology. Nonspecific.

Diagnostic Procedures. *Blood.* Anemia of various degree; hemoglobinemia. Identification of red cell deficiency and presence of various mutant enzymes. *Urine and stool.* Hemoglobin degeneration products.

Therapy. Avoidance of exposure to drugs or products that induce crises. Blood transfusions. Crisis may result in death. Usually, recovery after crisis and limited period of resistence to drug or product exposure.

BIBLIOGRAPHY. Fermi C, Martinetti P: Studio sul favismo. Ann Igiene Sper 15:76, 1905
Gasbarrini A: Il favismo. Policlinico Sez Prat 22:1505, 1915
Cordes W: Experiences with plasmochin in malaria: Preliminary reports, p 66. 15th Annual Report, United Fruit Company (Med Dept), 1926
Luisada A: Favism. Medicina (B Aires) 20:229–250, 1941
Lukens JN: Glucose-6-phosphate dehydrogenase deficiency and related deficiencies involving the pentose phosphate pathway and glutathione metabolism. In Lee GR, Bithel TC, Foerster J, et al (eds): Wintrobe's Clinical Hematology, 9th ed, pp 1006–1015. Philadelphia, Lea & Febiger, 1993
Luzzatto L, Metha A: Glucose 6-phosphate dehydrogenase deficiency. In Scriver CR, Beaudet AL, Sly WS, et al: The Metabolic and Molecular Bases of Inherited Disease, 7th ed, pp 3367–3398. New York, McGraw-Hill, 1995

GLUE EAR

Synonym. Otitis media, chronic exudative.

Symptoms and Signs. Affects children between the ages of 5 and 8; onset also in adulthood. Incidence about 3%. Deafness occasionally discovered in 5-year-old children by teachers, and routine testing, since patients are not aware of it. The conductive deafness usually has a threshold of 20 db or more. Detailed examination with binocular operating microscope often is required and sometimes also diagnostic myringotomy. At the onset, membrane appears normal, but at closer observation annular and radial vessels appear filled. Later, the membrane assumes yellowish color.

Etiology. Unknown. Have been considered: bacterial and viral infections, allergy; dysfunction of eustachian tubes owing to muscosal swelling in the tympanic orifice or other pathologic process at pharyngeal end.

Pathology. Accumulation in middle ear of sterile, highly viscous fluid containing cellular elements (neutrophils; lymphocytes; macrophages; plasma cells; rarely eosinophils).

Diagnostic Procedures. *Myringotomy.* Differential diagnosis with secretory otitis media (low-viscosity fluid).

Therapy. Aspiration of exudate by electrically driven suction through myringotomy; insertion of hourglass-shaped plastic tube to keep the middle ear at atmosphere pressure. Hearing aid needed in relapsing cases.

Prognosis. Inserted grommet is removed within 6 months and the membrane heals spontaneously. Susceptibility to this form of otitis media decreases with puberty.

BIBLIOGRAPHY. Jordan R: Chronic secretory otitis media. Laryngoscope 59:1002–1015, 1949
Glue ear (editorial). Br Med J 1:589, 1969
Eichenwald H: Development in diagnosis and treating otitis media. Am Fam Phys 31:155–164, 1985
Giebink GS: Otitis media update: pathogenesis and treatment. Ann Otol Rhinol Laryngol (Suppl) 155:21–23, 1992

GLUTARIC ACIDURIA I

Synonyms. Glutaricidemia I, GA I, glutaric-CoA dehydrogenase deficiency.

Symptoms and Signs. Both sexes. Microcephaly common at birth. Onset 6 months: opisthotonos, dystonia; athetoid posture; hepatomegaly; episodes of ketosis vomiting. Relative preservation of intellect.

Etiology. Autosomal recessive inheritance. Tissue deficiency of glutaryl-CoA dehydrogenase.

Pathology. Striatal degeneration in particular of putamen and caudate.

Diagnostic Procedures. *Blood.* Increased glutaric acid. Lysed leukocytes impairment to metabolize glutaryl CoA. *Urine.* Glutariciduria and 3-hydroxyglutaricaciduria (increased by L-lysine administration). *CT scan. MRI.* Dilatation of lateral ventricles and widening of cortical sulci.

Therapy. Trial with riboflavin, L-carnitine, restriction of dietary glutarigenic aminoacids (lysine, tryptophan, hydroxylysine) control of dehydration and acidosis.

Prognosis. Progressive dystonic cerebral palsy and usually death at early age with surviving intellect preserved even if severe spastic paralysis has developed.

BIBLIOGRAPHY. Goodman SI, Moc PG, Markey SP: Glutaric aciduria: A "new" inborn error of amino acid metabolism. Am J Hum Genet 26:36A, 1984
Stutchfield P, Edwards MA, Gray RGF, et al: Glutaric aciduria type I misdiagnosed as Leith's encephalopathy and cerebral palsy. Dev Med Child Neurol 27:514–521, 1985
Goodman SI, Frerman FE: Organic acidemias due to defects in lysine oxidation. 2-ketoadipic acidemia and glutaric acidemia. In Scriver CR, Beaudet AL, Sly WS, et al: The Metabolic and Molecular Bases of Inherited Disease, 7th ed, pp 1454–1458. New York, McGraw-Hill, 1995

GLUTARIC ACIDURIA IIB

Synonyms. Multiple acyl-CoA dehydrogenases deficiency (MAD); GA IIB; ethylmalonic-adidic aciduria, EMA, glutaricidemia II.

Symptoms and Signs. Both sexes. From birth: metabolic acidosis, hypoglycemia, sweaty feet odor. According to enzyme deficiency types distinctive congenital malformations owing to accumulation of toxic products not corrected by placental transfer; observed macrocephaly, flat nasal bridge, malformed ears, cerebral glyosis, hepatomegalia, polycystic kidneys, genital defects.

Etiology. Metabolic blocks in various pathways. Dehydrogenases for different acyl-CoAs. Autosomal recessive inheritance.

Diagnostic Procedures. *Urine.* (Glutarate is the principal component), various dicarboxylic acids, short chain fatty acids. *Blood.* Hypoglycemia, acidosis without ketosis.

Therapy. Bicarbonate infusion.

Prognosis. Usually death in early infancy, according to type and severity of enzyme defect.

BIBLIOGRAPHY. Przyrembel H, Wendel U, Becker K, et al: Glutamic aciduria type II: Report of a previously undescribed metabolic disorder. Clin Chim Acta 66:227–239, 1976

Jakobs C, Sweetman L, Wadman SK, et al: Prenatal diagnosis of glutaric aciduria type II by direct chemical analysis of dicarboxylic acids in amniotic fluids. Eur J Paediatr 141:153–157, 1984

Wilson GN, Chadarevian JP, Kaplan P, et al: Glutaric aciduria type II: Review of the phenotype and report of an unusual glomerulopathy. Am J Med Genet 32:395–401, 1989

Saudubray J-M, Charpentier C: Clinical phenotypes diagnosis/algorithms. In Scriver CR, Beaudet AL, Sly WS, et al: The Metabolic and Molecular Bases of Inherited Disease, 7th ed, pp 334–335. New York, McGraw-Hill, 1995

GLUTARIC ACIDURIA, NEONATAL FORM OF TYPE II

Synonyms. GA II A; Acyl-CoA dehydrogenase multiple deficiency; ACAD glutaricidemia IIA; GAIIB.

Symptoms and Signs. Males. From birth: Two forms, a mild one (GAIIB) recurrent hypoglycemia without ketosis and less severe evolution, and a more severe one (GAIIA) with metabolic acidosis hypoglycemia, hyperammonemia.

Etiology. X-linked inheritance.

Diagnostic Procedures. *Urine.* Large excretion not only of glutaric acid but also of lactic, ethylmalonic, butyric, isobutyric, 2-methylbutyric, and isovaleric acids.

Prognosis. Form GAIIA: early death. Form GAIIB patients known to survive at least 19 years.

BIBLIOGRAPHY. Mantagos S, Genel M, Tanaka K: Ethylmalonic adidic aciduria. J Clin Invest 64:1580–1589, 1979

Amendt BA, Rhead WJ: The multiple acyl-coenzyme A dehydrogenation disorders, glutaric aciduria type II and ethylmalonic-adidic aciduria: mitochondrial fatty acids oxidation, acetil coenzyme A dehydrogenase and electron transfer flavoprotein activities in fibroblast. J Clin Invest 78:205–213, 1986

Saudubray JM, Charpentier C: Clinical phenotypes diagnosis/algorithms. In Scriver CR, Beaudet AL, Sly WS, et al: The Metabolic and Molecular Bases of Inherited Disease, 7th ed, pp 334–335. New York, McGraw-Hill, 1995

GLUTATHIONE DEFICIENCIES

Synonyms. Hemolytic anemia—GSH deficiency; enzymopathy—GSH hemolytic anemia. GSH deficiency anemias are classified according to the enzyme deficiency.

1. GLUTATHIONE SYNTHETASE DEFICIENCY (see)

2. GLUTAMYLCYSTEINE SYNTHETASE DEFICIENCY

Symptoms and Signs. Hemolytic anemia, spinocerebellar degeneration, peripheral neuropathy, myopathy.

Etiology. Deficiency in synthesis of glutamyl cysteine and generalized glutathione deficiency.

Diagnostic Procedures. *Urine.* Aminoaciduria.

3. GLUTAMYL TRANSPEPTIDASE DEFICIENCY

Symptoms and Signs. Central nervous system involvement.

Etiology. Probably autosomal recessive inheritance.

Diagnostic Procedures. *Urine.* Glutathyonuria, and γ-glutamylcysteine and cysteine moieties. *Blood.* Glutathyonemia.

4. 4-OXOPROLINASE DEFICIENCY

Symptoms and Signs. From birth. Asymptomatic or enterocolitis, urolithiasis.

Etiology. Deficiency of 5-oxoproline level.

BIBLIOGRAPHY. Oort M, Loos JA, Prins HK: Hereditary absence of reduced glutathione in the erythrocytes. A new clinical and biochemical entity? Vox Sang 6:370–373, 1961

Konrad PN, Richards F II, Valentine VN, et al: Gamma glutamylcysteine synthetase deficiency. A cause of hereditary hemolytic anemia. N Engl J Med 286:557, 1972

Lukens JN: Glucose-6-phosphate dehydrogenase deficiency and related deficiencies involving the pentose phosphate pathway and glutathione metabolism. In Lee GR, Bithel TC, Foerster J, et al (eds): Wintrobe's Clinical Hematology, 9th ed. Philadelphia, Lea & Febiger, 1993

Meister A, Larsson A: Glutathione synthetase deficiency and other disorders of the glutamyl cycle. In Scriver CR, Beaudet AL, Sly WS, et al: The Metabolic and Molecular Bases of Inherited Disease, 7th ed, pp 1461–1477. New York, McGraw-Hill, 1995

GLUTATHIONE SYNTHETASE DEFICIENCY

Synonyms. Oxoprolinuria; pyroglutamicaciduria.

Symptoms and Signs. Two types of syndromes. (1) Congenital hemolytic anemia with slight reduction of leukocyte glutathione. Symptoms are not severe. Major predisposition to infections. (2) Hemolytic anemia accompanied by severe metabolic acidosis owing to high levels of 5-oxoproline in plasma and urine. Major predisposition to infections owing to impaired bactericidal activity of neutrophils.

Etiology. Autosomal recessive. Type 1 is caused by unstable glutathione synthetase enzyme. Type 2 is caused by absence of glutathione synthetase, which leads to overproduction of 5-oxoproline by glutamyl cysteine synthetase, the first enzyme of the glutathione synthetic pathway.

Diagnostic Procedures. Study of erythrocyte and leukocyte enzymes.

Therapy. In type 2, vitamin E administration. Sodium bicarbonate for metabolic acidosis.

Prognosis. Good quoad vitam.

BIBLIOGRAPHY. Oort M, Loos JA, Prins HK: Hereditary absence of reduced glutathione in the erythrocytes. A new clinical and biochemical entity? Vox Sang 6:370–373, 1961

Spielberg SP, Corash LM, Butler JD, et al: Biochemical heterogeneity in glutathione synthetase deficiency. J Clin Invest 61:1417, 1978

Lukens JN: Glucose-6-phosphate dehydrogenase deficiency and related deficiencies involving the pentose phosphate pathway and glutathione metabolism. In Lee GR, Bithel TC, Foerster J, et al (eds): Wintrobe's Clinical Hematology, 9th ed. Philadelphia, Lea & Febiger, 1993

Meister A, Larsson A: Glutathione synthetase deficiency and other disorders of the glutamyl cycle. In Scriver CR, Beaudet AL, Sly WS, et al: The Metabolic and Molecular Bases of Inherited Disease, 7th ed, pp 1461–1477. New York, McGraw-Hill, 1995

GLYCEROL INTOLERANCE

Symptoms and Signs. In both sexes. Possibly premature. Onset in first year episodes of pallor, sweating, inability to be aroused, vomiting, and seizures following milk ingestion.

Etiology. Suggested delayed maturation of enzymes of pathway of glycerol metabolism, or block of glycerol uptake owing to mutation of the carrier protein that mediates diffusion of glycerol across plasma membrane.

Pathology. *Liver biopsy.* Mitochondrial swelling and mitochondrial inclusion.

Diagnostic Procedures. *Blood.* Hypoglycemia. *IV glycerol tolerance test.* Rapid loss of consciousness.

Therapy. Low fat diet.

Prognosis. Fair with treatment.

BIBLIOGRAPHY. Maclaren NK, Cowles C, Ozand PT, et al: Glycerol intolerance in a child with intermittent hypoglycemia. J Ped 86:43, 1975

McKabe ERB: Disorders of glycerol metabolism. In Scriver CR, Beaudet AL, Sly WS, et al: The Metabolic and Molecular Bases of Inherited Disease, 7th ed, pp 1643–1644. New York, McGraw-Hill, 1995

GLYCEROLKINASE DEFICIENCY

Synonyms. Hyperglycerolemia; pseudo-hypertriglyceridemia; GK deficiency; GKD; GK1 deficiency; AGDCR phenotype; contiguous gene AGDCR.

Symptoms and Signs. In males (all but one). There are three different forms (by phenotypes) with late discovery or evident from birth. Infantile (complex glycerol kinase deficiency—CGKD) form presents adrenal hypoplasia, psychomotor retardation, growth delay, osteoporosis. Abnormal genitalia, characteristic facies with strabismus, and/or Duchenne muscular hypertrophy. Juvenile form (GK JUV) associated with vomiting, somnolence, or stupor and possibly coma. In adult form (GK BEN), incidental discovery of high levels of glycerol in blood or urine. Hyperlipidemia may be diagnostic.

Etiology. X-linked deficiency of glycerol kinase. GK locus maps to Xp21 region. Syndrome may be part of a contigous gene syndrome together with Duchenne (see), adrenal hypoplasia congenital (see).

Pathology. Muscle biopsy. Sometimes findings equal to those of Duchenne (see).

Diagnostic Procedures. Demonstration of deficiency of enzyme in blood cells and of high glycerol levels in blood and urine (pseudo hypertriglyceridemia).

Therapy. Low fat diet. If adrenal insufficiency glucocorticoid replacement and mineralocorticoids. If Duchenne, supportive treatment.

Prognosis. From death in first year in infantile to normal life span in adult forms.

BIBLIOGRAPHY. McCabe ERB, Fennessey PV, Guggenheim MA, et al:

Human glycerol kinase deficiency with hyperglycerolemia and glyceroluria. Biochem Biophys Res Comm 78:1327–1333, 1977

Schmickel RD: Contiguous gene syndromes: a component of recognizable syndromes. J Pediat 109:231–241, 1986

Matsymoto T, Kondoh T, Yoshimoto M: Complex glycerol kinase deficiency: molecular-genetic, cytogenetic, and clinical studies of five Japanese patients. Am J Med Genet 31:603–616, 1988

McKabe ERB: Disorders of glycerol metabolism. In Scriver CR, Beaudet AL, Sly WS, et al: The Metabolic and Molecular Bases of Inherited Disease, 7th ed, pp 1637–1643. New York, McGraw-Hill, 1995

GLYCOGEN STORAGE TYPE Ib

Synonyms. Includes also type Ic and Id. See von Gierke.

Symptoms and Signs. Identical to von Gierke, but also predisposition to infections (otitis, pneumonia, multiple abscesses, pyoderma, urinary tract infections). Possible evolution to myelogenous leukemia.

Etiology. Deficiency of glucose-6-phosphatase is owing to defect in G6P transport. Type Ic—defect in microsomal phosphate or pyrophosphate; type Id—defect in microsomal glucose transport.

Diagnostic Procedures. Only difference from von Gierke is presence of G-6-phosphatase activity in liver samples in vitro, but not in vivo because of lack of translocase responsible for transfer of glucose-6-phosphate into endoplasmic reticulum, indicating functional defect, but presence of the enzyme. *Blood.* Neutropenia. Impaired neutrophil function.

Therapy. See von Gierke.

Prognosis. See von Gierke.

BIBLIOGRAPHY. Narisawa K, Igarashi Y, Otomo H, et al: A new variant of glycogen storage disease type I probably due to a defect with glucose–6-phosphate transport system. Biochem Biophys Res Commun 83:1360–1364, 1978

Narisawa K, Ishizawa S, Okumura H, et al: Neutrophil metabolic dysfunction in genetically heterogenous patients with glycogen storage disease type Ib. J Inherited Metab Dis 9:297–300, 1986

Chen YT, Burchell A: Glycogen storage diseases. In Scriver CR, Beaudet AL, Sly WS, et al: The Metabolic and Molecular Bases of Inherited Disease, 7th ed, pp 947–949. New York, McGraw-Hill, 1995

GLYCOGEN STORAGE, TYPE IIb

Synonyms. Lysosomal glycogen storage disease without acid maltase deficiency; glycogen storage disease limited to the heart; GSDII deficiency. Antopol included.

Symptoms and Signs. All males. Proximal muscle weakness, hypertrophic cardiomiopathy, mental retardation and inconstant hepatomegaly.

Etiology. Autosomal recessive or X-linked recessive inheritance. Lysosomal glycogen storage disease without acid maltase deficiency.

Pathology. Glycogen storage limited to the miocardium. In Antopol also excessive deposits of glycogen in skeletal muscles.

Therapy. Death in second decade from cardiac failure.

BIBLIOGRAPHY. Antopol W, Boas EP, Levison W, et al: Cardiac hypertrophy caused by glycogen storage disease in a 15-year-old boy. Am Heart J 20:546–556, 1940

Danon MJ, Oh SJ, Di Mauro S, et al: Lysosomal glycogen storage disease with normal acid maltase. Neurology 31:51–57, 1981

Tripathy D, Coleman RA, Vidaillet HJ Jr, et al: Complete heart block with myocardial membrane-bound glycogen and normal peripheral alpha-glucosidase activity. Ann Intern Med 109:985–987, 1988

Hirschorn R: Glycogen storage disease type II: Acid-glucosidase (acid maltase) deficiency. In Scriver CR, Beaudet AL, Sly WS, et al: The Metabolic and Molecular Bases of Inherited Disease, 7th ed, pp 2457–2458. New York, McGraw-Hill, 1995

GLYCOGEN STORAGE, TYPE VIII

Synonyms. Hug; Huijing-Fernades; glycogenosis type VIII; glycogenosis type VIa; phosphorylase "b" kinase defect; PHK, PYK, glycogenosis VIIIa; glycogen storage disease IX.

Symptoms and Signs. Occurs in males. Asymptomatic except for hepatomegaly. Heterozygote females may show moderate symptoms. This is the mildest glycogenosis in men.

Etiology. X-linked inheritance. Deficient phosphorylase kinase activity.

Diagnostic Procedures. *Blood.* In leukocytes low activity of phosphorylase "b" kinase; SGPT, SGOT elevated; hypercholesterolemia, hypertriglyceridemia, hyperketosis after fasting. With age most of these findings disappear. *Biopsy of liver.* Increased glycogen storage; 90% deficit of phosphorylase "b" kinase activity.

Therapy. None.

Prognosis. Good.

BIBLIOGRAPHY. Huijing F, Fernandes J: X-chromosomal inheritance of liver glycogenosis with phosphorylase kinase deficiency. Am J Hum Genet 21:275–284, 1964
Hug G, Schubert WK, Chuck G: Deficient activity of dephosphorylase kinase and accumulation of glycogen in the liver. J Clin Invest 48:704–715, 1969
Willems PJ, Gerver WJM, Berger R, et al: The natural history of liver glycogenosis due to phosphorylase kinase deficiency: A longitudinal study of 41 patients. Eur J Pediat 149:268–271, 1990
Hers HG, van Hoof F, de Barsy T: Glycogen Storage Diseases. In Scriver CR, Beaudet AL, Sly WS, et al: The Metabolic and Molecular Bases of Inherited Disease, 7th ed, pp 425–452. New York, McGraw-Hill, 1995

GM1 GANGLIOSIDOSIS, ADULT

Synonym. GM1 gangliosidosis type III.

Symptoms and Signs. Early development is normal. From adolescence progressive cerebellar dysarthria spasticity and ataxia; occasionally action myoclonus; cherry-red spots and dysmorphism. Intellectual impairment progressive with time.

Etiology. Autosomal recessive inheritance. Diminished acid-β-galactosidase. Defect on chromosome 3.

Diagnostic Procedures. Intracellular-galactosidase activity low (10%); but plasma enzyme activity is normal

Pathology. Not known.

Therapy. None.

Prognosis. Good quoad vitam.

BIBLIOGRAPHY. Okada S O'Brien JS: Generalized gangliosidosis-galactosidase deficiency. Science 160:1002, 1968
Suzuki Y, Nakamara N, Fukuoka K, et al: Galactosidase deficiency in juvenile and adult patients: Report of six Japanese cases and review of the literature. Hum Gen 36:219, 1977
Wenger DA, Sattler M, Mueller OT, et al: Adult GM1 gangliosidosis: Clinical and biochemical studies of two patients and comparison to other patients called variant or adult GM1 gangliosidosis. Clin Genet 17:323, 1980
Suzuki Y, Sakuraba H, Oshima A: Galactosidase deficiency (galactosidosis): Gm1 gangliosidosis, and Morquio B disease. In Scriver CR, Beaudet AL, Sly WS, et al: The Metabolic and Molecular Bases of

Inherited Disease, 7th ed, pp 2789–2791. New York, McGraw-Hill, 1995

GM1 GANGLIOSIDOSIS, JUVENILE

Synonyms. Gangliosidosis type 2.

Symptoms and Signs. Both sexes. Psychomotor development normal during first year of life, developmental milestones within normal limits. Onset of symptoms from 6–20 months to 3–10 years: ataxia, strabismus, loss of hand movement coordination, choreoathetosis, loss of speech, muscular weakness of extremities; then progressing mental and motor deterioration, lethargy; blindness is reached, decerebrated spasticity. Macular cherry-red spots (pathognomonic). Seizures are an important clinical problem; recurrent infections. Hepatosplenomegaly and coarse facies are absent; corneas, retina, and macula initially are normal.

Etiology. See Normand-Landing.

Pathology. Neuronal lipidosis, visceral histiocytosis, glomerular epithelial ballooning.

Diagnostic Procedures. *Blood.* Vacuolated lymphocytes. *Bone marrow.* Foam cells. *X-ray.* Mild changes compared to infantile form. *Urine.* Mucopolysacchariduria.

Therapy. Symptomatic.

Prognosis. Life span 3–10 years.

BIBLIOGRAPHY. Derry DM, Fawcett JS, Andermann F, et al: Late infantile systemic lipidosis: Major monosialogangliosidosis. Delineation of two types. Neurology 18:340, 1968
Suzuki Y, Sakuraba H, Oshima A: Galactosidase deficiency (galactosidosis): Gm1 gangliosidosis, and Morquio B disease. In Scriver CR, Beaudet AL, Sly WS, et al: The Metabolic and Molecular Bases of Inherited Disease, 7th ed, p 2787. New York, McGraw-Hill, 1995

GODFRIED-PRICK-CAROL-PRAKKEN

Eponym used to indicate an association of Von Recklinghausen I and atrophoderma vermiculare, facies mongoloid, mental retardation, and congenital heart block.

BIBLIOGRAPHY. Carol WL, Godfried EG, Prakken MR, Prick JJ: Von Recklinghaussenische neurofibromatosis, atrophodermia vermiculata und kongenitale Herzanomalie als Haupkennizeichen eines familiaerhereditaere Syndromes. Dermatologica 81:345–346, 1940

GODIN

Symptoms and Signs. Consists of intermittent localized headache evoked by pressure on the arteries leading to the painful area.

Etiology. Claimed from capillary vasoconstriction and venous hypotension.

BIBLIOGRAPHY. Godin O: Algies cranio-faciales. Acta oto-rhino-laryngol 32:163–168, 1963

GOEBEL

Synonyms. Spheroid body myopathy; myopathy, spheroid body; cytoplasmic-spheroid body complex group (that includes cytoplasmic body myopathy, granulofilamentous myopathy; Mallori body-like inclusion; all forms belonging to a category of myopathies not sufficiently described and nosologically classified).

Symptoms and Signs. Both sexes. Onset in adolescence. Slowly developing myopathy causing motor incapacitation.

Etiology. Unknown. Autosomal dominant inheritance.

Diagnostic Procedures. *Muscle biopsy.* Presence of spheroid bodies (mainly type 1) in fibers, devoid of organelles. *Electromyography.*

Therapy. Symptomatic.

Prognosis. Progressive motor incapacitation up to degeneration. Life span normal.

BIBLIOGRAPHY. Goebel HH, Muller J, Gillen HV, et al: Autosomal dominant spheroid body myopathy. Muscle Nerve 1:14–26, 1978
Dickoff DJ: Adult onset of inherited myopathies. Prog Clin Neurosci 1:65–80, 1988
Helbig Goebel HH, Hop HC, et al: Spheroid cytoplasmic complexes in a congenital myopathy. Rev Neurol 147:300–307, 1991

GOEKAY-TUEKEL

Synonyms. Corticostriatocerebellar. See olivo cerebellar syndromes.

Symptoms and Signs. Onset in early childhood. Cerebellar ataxia, with dysarthria, dysmetria, and intention tremor; pyramidal signs and mental and motor retardation. Associated: myocardial and liver pathology may be found.

Etiology. Possibly autosomal recessive inheritance.

Pathology. Not available.

Diagnostic Procedures. *Urine.* Dysproteinuria and creatinuria.

Prognosis. Slow progression.

BIBLIOGRAPHY. Goekay FK, Tuekel K: Ueber Faelle von Familiaerem cortico-striato-cerebellaren. Syndrom Schweiz Med Wschr 78:1043, 1948
Salam M: Metabolic ataxias. In Vinken PJ, Bruyn GW (eds): Handbook of Clinical Neurology, vols 21, 22, p 575. Amsterdam, North-Holland, 1975

GOEMINNE

Synonym. Cryptorchidism—keloids—renal—torticollis; torticollis—keloids—cryptorchidism—renal dysplasia; TKCR.

Symptoms and Signs. Occurs in males; female carriers have less severe manifestations. Facial asymmetry; congential, progressive muscular torticollis; cryptorchidism; fever; multiple pigmented nevi. At puberty appearance of spontaneous keloids, varicose veins of legs; evidence of chronic pyelonephritis. None of affected males reproduced.

Etiology. X-linked inheritance (?). Gene for this syndrome mapped to Xq28, distal to G6PD.

BIBLIOGRAPHY. Geominne L: A new probably X-linked inherited syndrome: Congenital muscular torticollis, multiple keloids, cryptorchidism, and renal dysplasia. Acta Genet Med Gemellol (Rome) 17:439–467, 1968
Zuffardi O, Fraccaro M: Gene mapping and serendipidy. The locus for torticollis, keloids, cryptorchidism and renal dysplasia is at Xq28, distal to G6PD locus. Human Genet 62:280–281, 1982

GEOMINNE-DUJARDIN

Synonyms. Patella aplasia; coxa vera; tarsal synostosis. See Larsen-Johansson.

Symptoms and Signs. Patella aplasia; coxa vera; tarsal synostosis. Report of one family. Both sexes affected.

BIBLIOGRAPHY. Geominne L, Dujardin L: Congenital coxa vara, patella

aplasia and tarsal synostosis: a new inherited syndrome. Acta Genet Med Gemell 19:534–545, 1970

GOLDBERG-SHPRINTZEN

Synonyms. H-D; microcephaly; iris coloboma.

Symptoms and Signs. Hirschprung megacolon, microcephaly, hypertelorism, ptosis, submucous cleft palate, hypotonia, short stature, learning problems.

Etiology. Autosomal recessive inheritance.

BIBLIOGRAPHY. Goldberg RB, Shprintzen RJ: Hirschprung megacolon and cleft palate in two sibs. J Craniofac Genet Dev Biol 1:185–189, 1981
Yomo A, Taira T, Kondo I: Goldberg-Shprintzen syndrome: Hirschprung disease hypotonia and ptosis in sibs. Am J Med Genet 41:188–191, 1991

GOLDBERG-WENGER

Synonyms. Neuroaminidase-β-galactosidase deficiency; galactosialidosis; lysosomal protective protein, deficiency of; beta-galactosidase-2. Including juvenile galactosialidosis.

Symptoms. Both sexes. Three forms classified. Early infantile; late juvenile; juvenile adult. From birth or later (up to 15 years of age, one patient onset at 40 years). Clinical course variable broad and continuous spectrum of severity, usually according to age of onset, including delayed mental and physical development, seizures, visual defects, deafness.

Signs. Gargoyle facies. Dwarfism, corneal clouding; macular cherry-red spot; dyastasis multiplex; absence of hepatosplenomegaly.

Etiology. Autosomal recessive. Defect on chromosome 20q13.1. Defects in the processing mechanism that protects the two enzymes from enzymatic digestion by other enzymes in the lysosomes. A late infantile form has been described with slow progression and absence of mental retardation.

Pathology. See sialidosis.

Diagnostic Procedures. *Enzymatic studies.* In fibroblasts lack of galactosidase and neuraminidase. *Urine.* Mucopolysacchariduria. *Blood.* Absence of vacuolated cells.

Therapy. Symptomatic.

Prognosis. Long survival.

BIBLIOGRAPHY. Goldberg MF, Cottlier E, Fichenscher LG, et al: Macular cherry-red spot, corneal clouding and beta-galactosidase deficiency. Clinical, biochemical, and electron microscopic study of a new autosomal recessive storage disease. Arch Intern Med 128:387–398, 1971
Wenger DA, Tarby TJ, Wharton C: Macular cherry-red spots and myoclonus with dementia: Coexistent neuraminidase and β-galactosidase deficiencies. Biochem Biophys Res Commun 82:589–595, 1978
Strisciuglio P, Sly WS, Dodson WE, et al: Combined deficiency of beta-galactosidase and neuroaminosidase: Natural history of the disease in the first 18 years of an American patient with late infantile onset form. Am J Med Genet 37:573–577, 1990
d'Azzo A, Andria G, Strisciuglio P, et al: Galactosialidosis. In Scriver CR, Beaudet AL, Sly WS, et al: The Metabolic and Molecular Bases of Inherited Disease, 7th ed, pp 2825–2837. New York, McGraw-Hill, 1995

GOLDENHAR

Synonyms. Auriculovertebral; mandibulofacial dysostosis-epibulbar dermoids; oculoauriculovertebral spectrum; OAV; otofaciocervical; facioauriculovertebral anomaly; oculovertebral dysplasia; first-second brachial arch; hemifacial microsomia (definition used in the past for a clinical entity that was considered as autonomous with autosomal recessive inheritance).

Symptoms. Prevalent in males (70%), present at birth. Great variability of expression. Hearing defect of various degrees from near normal to severe hearing loss (conductive type); vision defect, including diplopia of various degrees. Feeding difficulty; moderate mental retardation in only 10% of cases.

Signs. Limited to one side in most cases. *Facies.* Marked facial asymmetry in 205, to a minor degree in 655. Asymmetry may become evident by age 4 years. *Ocular.* Epibulbar dermoid tumor; coloboma upper eyelids and eyebrows; ptosis of eyelid; antimongoloid obliquity. *Auricular.* Microtia; auricular appendices; atresia or stenosis of external auditory meatus; blind-ended fistula. *Oral.* Micrognathia; unilateral facial hypoplasia or hypoplasia of ramus and condyle; maxillary hypoplasia; high-arched palate; macrostomia; cleft palate; malocclusion. *Musculoskeletal.* Hemivertebrae; spina bifida; scoliosis; vertebral spinal fusion; supranumerary vertebrae; hypoplastic ribs; inguinal hernia; clubfoot; congenital heart defect. *Also lung, kidney and intestinal malformation have been reported.*

Etiology. Sporadic cases reported, also autosomal (recessive or dominant) inheritance. Embryonic malformation owing possibly to vascular abnormality involving first and second brachial arches, vertebrae, and eyes. To be differentiated from Treacher-Collins (see) and hemifacial microsomia (bilateral conditions usually without vertebral anomalies).

Pathology. See Signs.

Diagnostic Procedures. *X-rays. CT scan. MRI.* Hypoplasia of mandible; maxilla and temporal bones; vertebral anomalies; hypoplasia of external carotid artery; and altered cerebral flow; variable intracranial alterations: lipomas, dermoid; calcification, hydrocephalus, agenesis of vermis, corpus callosum. *Chromosome studies.* Negative.

Therapy. Early diagnosis important; hearing aid (very efficient); plastic surgery; combined effort of pediatrician, surgeon, dentist, orthodontist.

Prognosis. Good; only minority with mental retardation. Good result from plastic surgery.

BIBLIOGRAPHY. Canton E: Arrest of development of the left perpendicular ramus of the lower jaw, combined with malformation of the external ear. Tr Path Soc London 12:237–238, 1861
Arlt F von: Klinische Dortstellung der Krankheiten des Auges. Wien, Braunmüller, 1881
Van Duyse D: Bride dermoide oculo-palpebrale et coloboma partiel de la paupiere avec remarques sur la genese de cas anomalies. Ann Ocul 88:101–132, 1882
Goldenhar M: Associations malformatives de l'oeil et de l'oreille, en particulier le syndrome dermöide epibulbaire-appendices auriculaires-fistula auris congenita et ses relations avec la dysostose mandibulo-faciale. J Genet Hum 1:243–282, 1952
Mansour AM, Wang F, Henkind P, et al: Ocular findings in the facioauriculovertebral sequence (Goldenhar-Gorlin syndrome). Am J Ophthalmol 100:555–559, 1985
Cohen MM Jr, Rollnick BR, Kaye CI: Oculoauriculovertebral spectrum: An updated critique. Cleft Palate J 26:276–286, 1989

GOLDMANN-FAVRE

Synonym. Hyaloid-retinal degeneration; vitreoretinal dystrophy, recessive. See also Wagner hyaloid-retinal degeneration; retinoschisis, early hemeralopia.

Symptoms. Only a few cases reported. Severe night blindness from early childhood.

Signs. Extensive vitreoretinal dystrophy with bone corpuscle pigmentation; pattern of foveal retinoschisis coarse; occasionally cataract.

Etiology. Autosomal recessive inheritance.

Pathology. Liquified vitreous body with preretinal band-shaped structures, edema, macular changes, pigmentary degeneration of retina and hemeralopia.

Diagnostic Procedures. *Electroretinography.* Abolished b-wave (differential element to distinguish from Wagner and X-linked retinoschisis).

Therapy. Trials with cyclosporine A and bromocryptine under way.

BIBLIOGRAPHY. Goldmann H: Biomicroscopie du corps vitré et du fond d'oeil. Bull Neur Soc Fr Ophthalmol 70:265, 1957
Favre M: A propos de deux cas de dégénérescence hyaloidéorétinienne: Two cases of hyaloid-retinal degeneration. Ophthalmologica 135:604–609, 1958
Newsome DA: Retinal Dystrophies and Degenerations. Raven Press, New York, 1988
Nasr YG, Chefan GM, Michels RG, et al: Goldmann-Favre maculopathy. Retina 10:178–180, 1990

GOLDSTEIN-REICHMANN

Obsolete.

Synonym. Cerebellar, acquired.

Symptoms. Both sexes affected; onset at all ages. Tendency to fall; insecure ambulation with severe swaying. Intentional tremor; unilateral lack of normal arm movements; catalepsy.

Signs. Equilibrium disorders; posture abnormalities; adiadochokinesis; pendular knee reflex; choreiform hyperkinesia.

Etiology. Trauma; infection (ear); meningitis; encephalitis; neoplasia involving (directly or indirectly) the cerebellum.

Pathology. Cerebellar parenchymatous degeneration.

Diagnostic Procedures. *Spinal fluid. X-ray. Angiography. CT brain scan.* To show cerebellar involvement.

Therapy. According to etiology.

Prognosis. Variable.

BIBLIOGRAPHY. Goldstein K, Reichmann F: Beitraege zur Kasuistik und Symptomatologie der Kleinhirnerkrankung (in besondersen zu den Staerungen der Bewegungen der Gewichtsraum und Zeitschaetzung). Arch Psychiatr (Nevenkr) 56:466–521, 1915–1916

GOLLOP-WOLFGANG COMPLEX

Synonyms. Femur (unilateral bifid)—monodactylous ectrodactyly.

Symptoms and Signs. Both sexes. From birth. Unilateral, bifid femur, absent tibia, ectrodactyly.

Etiology. Developmental field defect. Autosomal dominant or recessive (not yet clearly established).

BIBLIOGRAPHY. Gallop TR, Lucchesi E, Martins RMM, et al: Familial occurrence of bifid femur and monodactylous ectrodactyly. Am J Med Genet 7:319–322, 1980
Kohn G, El Shawwa R, Grunebaum M: Aplasia of the tibia with bifurcation of the femur and ectrodactyly: Evidence of an autosomal recessive type. Am J Med Genet 33:172–175, 1989

GOLTZ

Synonyms. Goltz-Gorlin; Jessner-Cole; Liebermann-Cole; focal dermal hypoplasia; FDH; atrophoderma naeviform; ectodermal-mesodermal dysplasia, bone involvement.

Symptoms and Signs. Cases reported in females (90%). Shortness of stature and slight build. Mental retardation frequent. Cutaneous changes; poikiloderma (linear hypoplasia with pigmentation; telangiectasia). In some areas of the thinned skin, herniation of nodules of adipose tissue. Occasionally, angiofibromas around mouth, anus, and vagina (50%); dystrophic nails (50%); syndactylism and other finger and toe abnormalities (80%); usually third and fourth fingers. Eye defects (50%); microphthalmia; colobomas; strabismus; defective dentition (60%); malocclusion, malformation, absence of teeth. Lip, vulvar, and anal papillomas.

Etiology. X-linked dominant with lethality in males.

Pathology. Skin. Histologic examination of fatty deposit in skin reveals normal fat separated from epidermis by fragmented fibrillary collagen, absence of collagen bundles, decrease of normal elastic fibers. Nonaffected areas show normal skin.

Diagnostic Procedures. *Blood. Urine.* Normal. *X-ray.* Skeleton. Striated bones.

Therapy. Surgical correction of finger abnormalities.

BIBLIOGRAPHY. Naegeli O: Poikilodermie. Zbl Hautkrkh 23:638, 1927
Jessner M: Naeviforme, poikilodermieartige Hautveraenderungen mit Missbildungen. Zentralbl Haut Geschlkr 27:468, 1928
Goltz RW, Peterson WC, Gorlin RJ, et al: Focal dermal hypoplasia. Arch Dermatol 86:708–717, 1962
Temple IK, MacDowall P, Baraitser M, et al: Local dermal hypoplasia (Goltz syndrome). J Med Genet 27:180–187, 1990

G.O.M.B.O.

Synonyms. Growth retardation—ocular—microcephaly—brachydactyly—oligophrenia.

Symptoms and Signs. Both sexes. Microcephaly, microphtalmia, brachydactyly, clynodactyly 5, severe mental retardation. Delayed physical growth in puberty. Occasionally cyanotic heart defect.

Etiology. Unknown. Autosomal recessive inheritance.

BIBLIOGRAPHY. Verloes A, Delfortric J, Lambotte C: GOMBO syndrome of growth retardation, ocular abnormalities, microcephaly, brachydactyly and oligophrenia: a possible "new" recessively inherited MCA/MR syndrome. AM J Med Genet 32:15–18, 1989

GOMEZ-LOPEZ-HERNANDEZ

Synonyms. Cerebellotrigeminodermal dysplasia.

Symptoms and Signs. From birth. Both sexes. Short stature. Microcephaly, craniostenosis. Variable features. Ataxia; trigeminal anesthesia; mental deficiency; parietal alopecia; ocular hypertelorism; corneal opacities; midface hypoplasia, low set ears, clinodactyly, hypoplastic labia majora.

Etiology. Unknown.

Pathology. See Signs. Pons-vermis fusion.

BIBLIOGRAPHY. Kayser B: Ein Fall von augeborener Trigeminuslahmung und angeborenem totalem Tranenmangel. Klin Mbl Augenheik 66:652–654, 1921
Gomez MR: Cerebellotrigeminal and focal dermal dysplasia: A newly recognized neurocutaneos syndrome. Brain Dev 1:253–256, 1979
Lopez-Hernandez A: Craniosynostosis, ataxia, trigeminal anesthesia and parietal alopecia with pons-vermis fusion anomaly (atresia of fourth ventricle). Report of two cases. Neuropediatrics 13:99–102, 1982

Gomez MR: Cerebello-trigemino-dermal dysplasias. In Gomez MR (ed): Neurocutaneous Diseases I, pp 145–348. New York, Raven, 1987

GOOD

Synonyms. Thymoma-immunodeficiency; immunodeficiency-thymoma.

Symptoms and Signs. In adults 40–70 years of age. Evidence of thymoma and delayed and gradual onset of sinopulmonary infections, weight loss, and weakness; chronic diarrhea in approximately 33% of the patients. Seldom associated other autoimmune conditions.

Etiology. Unknown.

Pathology. Thymoma most cases spindle cell type; less frequently epithelial, lymphoepithelial, or lymphocytic. Germinal centers lacking in lymph nodes.

Diagnostic Procedures. *Blood.* Panhypogammaglobulinemia, relative number of T-cell subsets distorted, and reversal of T helper/T suppressor cell ratio. Organisms most frequently found: S. pneumoniae, H. influenza, klebsiella, candida, and cytomegalovirus. P. carini also frequently encountered.

Therapy. Antibiotics immunoglobulins.

Prognosis. Removal of thymoma does not change immunodeficient status. Immunoglobulin highly effective on clinical manifestations.

BIBLIOGRAPHY. Good RA, Pahwa RN, West A: Primary immunodeficiency diseases of man. In Safai B, Good RA (eds): Immunodermatology, pp 399–424. New York, Plenum, 1981
Lukens JN: Immunodeficiency diseases inherited and acquired. In Lee GR, Bithell TC, Foerster et al (eds): Wintrobe's Clinical Hematology, 9th ed, pp 1681–1682. Philadelphia, Lea & Febiger, 1993

GOODMAN

Synonyms. Acrocephalopolysyndactyly IV. ACPS IV.

Symptoms and Signs. From birth. Both sexes. Clinodactyly, camptodactyly, ulnar deviation. Congenital heart malformations. No mental retardation. Difficult clinical differentiation from Carpenter (see).

Etiology. Autosomal recessive.

Prognosis. Poor.

BIBLIOGRAPHY. Goodman RM, Steinberg M, Shem-Toy Y, et al: Acrocephalopolysyndactyly type IV: A new genetic syndrome in three sibs. Clin Genet 15:209–214, 1979
Hall JR, Reed SD, Sells CJ, et al: Autosomal recessive acrocephalosyndactyly revisited. Am J Med Genet 5:423–424, 1980
Cohen DM, Green JC, Miller J, et al: Achrocephalopolysyndactyly type II. Carpenter syndrome: Clinical spectrum and an attempt at unification with Goodman and Summit syndromes. AM J Med Genet 28:311–324, 1987

GOODPASTURE

Synonyms. Glomerulonephritis—pulmonary hemorrhages; lung purpura—glomerulonephritis; pneumorenal; reno-pneumonal; antibasement membrane antibody; ABMA. See Ceelen-Gellerstedt.

Symptoms. Prevalent in males; age of onset 16–61 years of age (median 21 years). Twenty percent of patients present preceding, nonspecific, viral respiratory infections. Hemoptysis, exertional dyspnea; cough; fatigue; occasionally, nausea and vomiting; weight loss; chest pains; hematuria.

Signs. Pallor; pulmonary rhonchi. Seldom, hypertension, edemas, skin rash, splenomegaly. Later in the disease hypertension and edemas more frequently observed.

Etiology. Autoimmune condition in which tissue damage is mediated by antibasement membrane antibodies, that bind to alpha 3 (IV) chain of type IV collagen and stimulate complement and tissue injury. Familial occurrence reported (autosomal recessive?). Noted in some cases previous inhalation of hydrocarbons.

Pathology. *Lung.* Mottled by areas of hemorrhage, especially lower lobes. Microscopically, intra-alveolar hemorrhage and siderophages, and thickening of alveolar septi with collagenization. Vasculitis absent; occasionally, infiltrate of polymorphonucleated cells. *Kidney.* Enlarged, pale, soft. Subcortical punctiform hemorrhages; capsule nonadherent. In cases of longer duration, kidney shrinks in size and capsule becomes adherent. Microscopically, diffuse involvement, capillary loops occluded by eosinophilic material PAS-negative. *Immunofluorescence.* Linear deposits of Ig G, deposits of C3. Epithelial cell proliferation; endothelial proliferation scarce or absent. Progressive glomerular fibrosis. Interstitial inflammatory infiltration mostly lymphocytes, and then fibrillar interstitial fibrosis and dilation and atrophy of tubules.

Diagnostic Procedures. *Blood.* Normocytic, normochromic anemia; normal or increased leukocytes; later in disease, hyperazotemia; immunofluorescence of circulating (and tissue) antibasement antibodies (anti GBM). *Urine.* Proteinuria; hematuria; increased leukocytes, casts. *Serum assay for ABMA by RIA ELISA and indirect immunofluorescence. X-ray of chest.* Infiltrates, especially lower lobes. *Biopsy of kidney.* Strongly positive linear staining for IgG along glomerular capillaries. *Lung biopsy:* Seldom indicated: IgG along glomerular capillaries. *Sputum.* Macrophages full of hemosiderin.

Therapy. Corticosteroids of limited value. Cytotoxic and immunosuppressant agents of potential value. Plasmapheresis and kidney transplantation: fair results.

Prognosis. With therapy, dialysis and kidney transplantation prognosis has ameliorated. More severe in cases of intraalveolar hemorrhages.

BIBLIOGRAPHY. Goodpasture EW: The significance of certain pulmonary lesions in relation to the etiology of influenza. Am J Med Sci 158:863–870, 1919

Carré P, Rakatoa-Rivony J, Didier A, et al: Actualité du syndrome de Goodpasture. Rev Mal resp 5:319–330, 1988

Glassock RJ: Goodpasture's syndrome. In Massry SG, Glassock RJ: Textbook of Nephrology, 3rd ed, pp 818–823. Baltimore, Williams & Wilkins, 1995

GORDAN-OVERSTREET

See Turner. Eponym to indicate the presence of mild virilization characteristics in cases of gonadal dysgenesis. It may not, in the light of present knowledge, be considered as an autonomous entity.

BIBLIOGRAPHY. Gordan GS, Overstreet EW, Traut HF, et al: A syndrome of gonadal dysgenesis: Variety of ovarian agenesis with androgenic manifestations. J Clin Endocrinol 15:1–12, 1955

GORDON-COOKE

Synonym. Chromosome-ring 1 "dwarfism."

Symptoms and Signs. Low birth weight; delayed mental and physical development; microcephaly; disproportionately tall for weight, although dwarfed. Cheerful and pleasant behavior.

Etiology. Large monocentric autosomal ring result of terminal deletion of chromosome 1.

Diagnostic Procedures. *Chromosome study.*

BIBLIOGRAPHY. Gordon RR, Cooke P: Ring 1 chromosome and microcephalic dwarfism. Lancet 2:1212–1213, 1964

Wolf CB, Peterson JA, Logrippo GA, et al: Ring 1 chromosome and dwarfism: A possible syndrome. J Pediatr 71:719–722, 1967

GORDON (H.)

Synonyms. Arthrogryposis multiplex congenita (distal type II A); camptodactyly—cleft palate—club foot.

Symptoms and Signs. Both sexes. From birth. Fixed camptodactyly (89%) sparing the thumb and affecting only the proximal interphalangeal joints (72%). Club feet (varus or valgus). Cleft palate (27%). Occasionally associated: short stature, nevus flammeus (see), dermatoglyphic anomalies, omphalocele.

Etiology. Autosomal dominant inheritance with variable expression.

BIBLIOGRAPHY. Gordon H, Davies D, Berman M: Camptodactyly, cleft palate and club foot. A syndrome showing the autosomal dominant pattern of inheritance. J Med Genet 6:266–274, 1969

Robinow M, Johnson GF: The Gordon syndrome: Autosomal dominant cleft palate, camptodactyly, and club feet. Am J Med Genet 9:139–146, 1981

Hall JG, Reed SD, Greene G: The distal arthrogryposes: Delineation of new entities: Review and nosologic discussion. Am J Med Genet 11:185–239, 1982

Reiss JA, Sheffield LJ: Distal arthrogypose type II: A family with varying congenital abnormalities. Am J Med Genet 24:255–267, 1986

GORDON (R.D.)

Synonyms. Pseudohypoaldosteronism, type II.

Symptoms and Signs. Detected in late childhood or early adulthood. Blood hypertension.

Etiology. Familial condition. Increased reabsorption of chloride in the distal nephron; decreased acid excretion and hyperchloremic acidosis; reduced renal cortical ammonia production by hyperkalemia are among the several pathophysiological mechanisms proposed.

Diagnostic Procedures. *Blood.* Hyperkalemia; hyperchloremic metabolic acidosis; hyporeninemia; very low aldosterone level; normal GFR; normal antinatriuretic and antichloruretic responses; subnormal kaliuretic response to exigenous mineralocorticoids.

Therapy. Low salt diet for 5 days then mineralocorticoids with either sodium sulfate or acetazolamide and bicarbonate. Diuretics: hydrochlorthiazide, furosemide. Antidiuretic hormone has been proposed.

BIBLIOGRAPHY. Gordon RD, Geddes RA, Pawsey CGK, et al: Hypertension and severe hyperkalemia associated with suppression of renin and aldosterone and completely reversed by dietary sodium restriction. Aust ANN Med 4:287–292, 1970

Melby JC, Azar ST: Hypoaldosteronism and milneralocorticoid resistance. In De Groot LJ (ed): Endocrinology, 3rd ed, pp 1808–1809. Philadelphia, WB Saunders, 1995

GORHAM

Synonyms. Gorham-Stout; disappearing bones; massive osteolysis; phantom bones; osteolysis massive; hemangio-lymphoangiomatosis of joints; osteolysis. See Haferkamp.

Symptoms and Signs. Both sexes affected; clinical onset from childhood to young adulthood. Almost constantly unilateral, focal hemangioma involving one or several contiguous bones, including adjacent vertebrae; massive osteolysis. Soft tissues near bone lesion usually involved. Diffuse muscle atrophy. Hemangiomas on overlying skin may or may not be present. Chylous or hematic pleural effusion. In some cases: paraplegia (caused by spinal cord transection).

Etiology and Pathology. Angioma of bone(s) with osteolysis and replacement of bone by fibrosis. Sporadic.

Diagnostic Procedures. *X-ray of skeleton.* In early stage patchy osteoporosis of one or more bones. Progressive bone resorption without evidence of reossification, pathological fractures. *Tc 99m pyrophosphate scan.*

Therapy. X-ray therapy.

Prognosis. Relatively benign condition, slowly progressing and self-limited. Seldom death from thoracic cage involvement. No therapy has changed the course of the disease significantly for its course to be predictable.

BIBLIOGRAPHY. Jackson JBS: Boneless arm. Boston Med Surg J 18:368–369, 1838

Gorham LW, Wright AW, Schurtz HH, et al: Disappearing bones: A rare form of massive osteolysis. Am J Med 17:674–682, 1954

Wallis LA, Asch T, Maisel BW: Diffuse skeletal hemangiomatosis: Report of two cases and review of literature. Am J Med 37:545–563, 1964

Choma ND, Biscotti CV, Bauer TW, et al: Gorham's syndrome: A case report and review of the literature. Am J Med 83:1151–1155, 1987

GORLIN-CHAUDHRY-MOSS

Symptoms and Signs. Present from birth. Craniofacial dysostosis; dental anomalies; microphthalmia; inability to close or open eyes completely; oblique palpebral fissures; horizontal nystagmus at lateral gaze; limited upper gaze. Astigmatism; hyperopia; corneal scars. Signs of patency of ductus arteriosus; hypertrichosis; hypoplastic labia majora.

Etiology. Autosomal recessive inheritance.

BIBLIOGRAPHY. Gorlin RJ, Chaudhry AP, Moss ML: Craniofacial dysostosis, patent ductus arteriosus, hypertrichosis, hypoplasia of labia majora, dental and eye anomalies: A new syndrome? J Pediatr 56:778–785, 1960

Gorlin RJ, Cohen MM Jr, Levin LS: Syndromes of Head and Neck, p 549. New York, Oxford Univ Press, 1990

GORLIN-COHEN

Synonyms. Gorlin-Holt; frontometaphyseal dysplasia; mephistophelean.

Symptoms. Present from birth. Deafness (conductive type). Impaired movements from ankylosis. Feeding troubles. Recurrent respiratory tract infections.

Signs. Generalized hirsutism. *Facies.* Coarse; nose with wide bridge; eyebrows prominent; teeth partially absent; mandible small; palate high. *Joints.* Ankylosis of main joints; arachnodactyly. *Bones.* Femur and tibia metaphyseal enlargement (Erlenmeyer flask type). *Heart.* Cardiac murmur. *Other.* Cryptorchidism. Uropathy.

Etiology. X-linked inheritance with severe manifestation in males and variable in females.

Diagnostic Procedures. *X-ray of skeleton (see Signs).* Vertebral interspaces widened; pelvis flared; carpal and tarsal bones partially fused; head thick; horn-like frontal ridge; absence of frontal sinuses; short maxilla; enlarged foramen magnum.

Prognosis. Progressive disability.

BIBLIOGRAPHY. Liachi G: Le torus sopraorbitalis variation cranienne rare. J Radiol Electrol 48:463–466, 1967

Gorlin RJ, Cohen MM: Frontometaphyseal dysplasia: A new syndrome. Am J Dis Child 118:487–494, 1969

Halt JF, Thompson GR, Arenberg IK: Frontometaphyseal dysplasia. Radiol Clin N Amer 10:225–243, 1972

Balestrazzi P: Herdite lièe au sexe dans la dysplasie fronto-metaphysaire. J Genet Hum 33:419–425, 1985

GORLIN-GOLTZ

Synonyms. Hermans-Herzberg; Sprengel anomaly; Ward basal cell nevus (carcinoma); multiple basal cell nevi; nevus epitheliomatosis multiplex; fifth phacomatosis; hydrocephalus—costovertebral.

Symptoms and Signs. No sex prevalence. *Skin.* Multiple nevoid basal cell carcinomas appearing in childhood or (especially) at puberty in exposed and unexposed areas. Other skin changes include palmar dyskeratosis, milia, cysts, fibromas and/or neurofibromas, especially on extremities. *Face.* Frontal and temporal bossing (pagetoid appearance); sunken appearance of eyes; broad nasal root; frequent strabismus; true hypertelorism; seldom, dystopia canthorum. Mild mandibular prognatism. *Mouth.* Multiple jaw cysts; fibrosarcoma jaws; ameloblastoma. *Skeletal system.* Rib: bifid; synostosis; partial agenesis. Vertebrae: scoliosis; cervical or thoracic fusion; deformed chest. Shortened metacarpals and distal phalanx of thumb. *Central nervous system.* Variable mental retardation; congenital hydrocephalus. *Eyes.* Congenital blindness; choroid and optic nerve coloboma. *Genitals.* Infantile genitals; female habit and hair distribution in boys; cryptorchidism. *Other.* Gastrointestinal disease also associated in some families.

Etiology. Unknown; autosomal dominant inheritance, determined by a highly penetrant gene.

Pathology. Basal cell nevus; wide diversity of histopathologic appearance giving rise to a spectrum of skin tumors from benign to aggressive ulcerating basal cell carcinoma. Ovarian fibroma; jaw fibroma; medulloblastoma and renal anomalies frequently found.

Diagnostic Procedures. *X-ray. CT scan. MRI.* Odontogexic cysts of maxilla and mandible; rib and vertebral anomalies; lamellar calcification of falx and other variable CNS calcifications. Limbs: anomalies; cyst-like osteolytic lesions. See Signs. *Biopsy. Chromosome study.* Normal.

Therapy. Curettage, electrodesiccation, X-radiation, and surgical excision of nevi. For resistant lesions, topical application of dichloroacetic acid and zinc chloride followed by shaving; process repeated until all tumor removed. Systemic chemotherapy produces only incomplete results. Topical chemotherapy (colchicine and methotrexate ointment, and 5-fluorouracil ointment). For all other manifestations of the syndrome use conventional means of treatment. These patients are hyporesponsive to parathyroid hormone.

Prognosis. Surgery and X-ray treatment results in a 5-year cure of nevi lesions in 90% of cases. Topical chemotherapy (colchicine and methotrexate) results in a 4-year cure in 70% of cases. 5-Fluorouracil effective in ulcerating basal cell tumor; recurrences, however, are frequent. It is not yet possible to evaluate the possible curative effect of high dose of 5-fluorouracil. Early fatality from medulloblastoma. Surviving male patients develop eunuchoid traits, whereas females develop ovarian fibromas and uterine calcifications.

BIBLIOGRAPHY. Jarisch A: Zur Lehre von den Hautgeschwuelsten. Arch J Dermatol Syph 28:163–222, 1894

Nomland R: Multiple basal cell epithelioma originating from congenital pigmented cell nevi. Arch Dermatol 25:1002–1008, 1932

Ward WH: Nevoid basal celled carcinoma associated with a dyskeratosis of the palms and soles. A new entity. Aust J Dermatol 5:204–207, 1960

Gorlin RJ, Goltz RW: Multiple nevoid basal cell epithelioma, jaw cysts and bifid rib: A syndrome. N Engl J Med 262:908–912, 1960

Gorlin RJ: Nevoid basal-cell carcinoma syndrome. Medicine 66:98–113, 1987

Stieler W, Plewig G, Kuester W: Basalzellnaevus-Syndrom mit Plattenepithelkarzinom des Larynx. Z Hautkr 63:113–120, 1988

Evans DGR, Sims DG, Donnai D: Family implications of neonatal Gorlin's syndrome. Arch Dis Child 66:1162–1163, 1991

GOSSELIN

Eponym used to indicate a V-fracture of lower end of tibia extending into ankle joint.

BIBLIOGRAPHY. Gosselin LA: Des fractures en V et de cours complications. Paris, Clayde, 1866

Sisk TD: Fractures of lower extremities. In Crenshaw AH (ed): Campbell's Operative Orthopedics, 7th ed, p 1637. St Louis, CV Mosby, 1987

GOTTRON (H.)

Synonyms. Acrogeria familial; familial acromicria. See Werner; acrogeria; acromicria and Ehler-Danlos IV.

Symptoms and Signs. Prevalent in females. From birth or soon afterward. Normal hair and eyes. Senile changes affecting prevalently skin and subcutaneous fat on distal extremities. Evident subcutaneous vascular pattern over the chest.

Etiology. Autosomal recessive inheritance.

Pathology. Absence of subcutaneous fat in most severely affected zones. Atrophia of dermis, abundant clumped elastin; sparse collagen bundles.

Prognosis. General health and life expectancy normal. Short stature.

BIBLIOGRAPHY. Gottron H: Familiaere Akrogerie. Arch Dermatol Syph 181:571–583, 1940

De Groot WP, Tafelkruyer J, Woerdman MJ: Familial acrogeria (Gottron). Br J Dermatol 103:213–223, 1980

Burton JL: Disorders of connective tissue. In Champion RH, Burton JL, Ebling FJG (eds): Rook/Wilkinson/Ebling Textbook of Dermatology, 5th ed, pp 1840–1841. Oxford, Blackwell Scientific, 1992

GOTTRON (H.A.)

Synonym. Erythrokeratoderma, symmetrical progressive.

Symptoms and Signs. Onset in childhood (4 months to 4 years) but occurs also in adult life. On hands, feet, and occasionally in other location (thighs, upper arms, neck, face), formation of strikingly symmetrical plaques of erythema with hyperkeratosis, margin frequently orange hue. Scarse pruritus.

Etiology. Unknown. Autosomal dominant inheritance with variable or sporadic expressivity.

Pathology. Hyperkeratosis, parakeratosis, acanthosis, and inflammatory changes.

Therapy. None or oral etretinate and acitretin therapy or PUVA.

Prognosis. Lesions reach greatest extent in puberty, then may persist or regress.

BIBLIOGRAPHY. Gottron HA: Congenital angelegte symmetrische progressive Erythrokeratodermie. Zentralbl Haut Geschlkrank 4:493–494, 1922

Ruiz-Maldonado R, Tamayo L, del Castillo V, et al: Erythrokeratodermia progressive simmetrica: Report of 10 cases. Dermatologica 164:133–141, 1982

MacFarlane AW, Chapman SJ, Verbov JL: Is erythrokeratoderma one disorder? A clinical and ultrastructural study of two siblings. Br J Derm 124:487–491, 1991

Griffiths WAD, Leigh IM, Marks R: Disorders of keratinization. In Champion RH, Burton JL, Ebling FJG (eds): Rook/Wilkinson/Ebling Textbook of Dermatology, 5th ed, pp 1350–1351. Oxford, Blackwell Scientific, 1992

GOUGEROT-BLUM

Synonym. Pigmented purpuric lichenoid dermatosis; prurigo pigmentosa; see Schamberg.

Symptoms. Rare in Western countries; more frequent in Japan. Both sexes affected (prevalent in females); onset in middle life (40–60 years of age). Itching at site of lesions. Occasionally found associated with porphyria.

Signs. Usually on lower extremities; seldom on upper extremities or trunk. Papules slightly elevated, clustered in irregular areas; round shape; smooth surface; evolving toward a reddish color; showing a fine desquamation in the center.

Etiology. Unknown. Capillaritis (?).

Pathology. Hyperkeratosis and parakeratosis; decreased papillae in the corium; fragmentation of elastic tissue; perivascular infiltration by lymphocytes, plasma cells, and fibroblasts; blood vessels show edematous walls, endoartheritic process.

Diagnostic Procedures. *Biopsy.* Immunofluorescence negative. *Blood.* Occasionally eosinophils increase.

Therapy. Systemic and topical cortisone treatment; keratolytics, and antihistamine with scarce response; 30% of cases respond to dapsone.

Prognosis. Chronic condition lasting for years.

BIBLIOGRAPHY. Gougerot H, Blum P: Purpura angioscléreux prurigineux avec éléments lichénoides. Présentation de malade. Bull Soc Fr Dermatol Syph 32:161–163, 1925

Champion RH: Purpura. In Champion RH, Burton JL, Ebling FJG (eds): Rook/Wilkinson/Ebling Textbook of Dermatology, 5th ed, p 1889. Oxford, Blackwell Scientific, 1992

GOUGEROT-CARTEAUD

Synonym. Papillomatosis, confluent, reticular. See Acanthosis nigricans.

Symptoms and Signs. Prevalent in females; onset after puberty. Appearance of flat warty papules, not larger than 0.5 centimeter in diameter, between the breasts and in the midline of the back; progressive extension of lesions, which become confluent to form an irregular network; extension proceeds in all directions, reaching neck, pubis.

Etiology. Unknown; usually isolated cases; however, probably a genetic condition. Autosomal dominant inheritance suggested. Amyloidosis also suggested. In some cases pityrosporum infection demonstrated.

Pathology. Hyperkeratosis and papillomatosis without acanthosis.

Diagnostic Procedures. *Biopsy of skin.*

Therapy. Topical and systemic retinoids; if pityrosporum demonstrated, treat as pityriasis versicolor: 2.5% selenium sulfate in a detergent base; 20% sodium hyposulfite in water/propilene glycol 50/50; topical or systemic antifungals.

Prognosis. Progression for a few years, then becomes stabilized. Good response to treatment; relapses frequent. In cases of pityrosporum infection repigmentation may take several months or hypopigmentation persists.

BIBLIOGRAPHY. Gougerot H, Carteaud A: Papillomatose pigmentée innominée. Bull Soc Fr Dermatol Syph 34:712–719, 1927

Gougerot H: Allé forme de transition entre la dermatite polymorphe douloureuse de Brock-Duhring et le pemphigus congénital familial héréditaire. Arch Derm Syph 5:255, 1933

Groh V, Schnyder VW: Nosologic der Papillomatose papuleuse confluente et reticulée (Gougerot-Carteaud). Hautarzt 34:81–86, 1983

Griffiths WAD, Leigh IM, Marks R: Disorders of keratinization. In Champion RH, Burton JL, Ebling FJG (eds): Rook/Wilkinson/Ebling Textbook of Dermatology, 5th ed, p 1390. Oxford, Blackwell Scientific, 1992

GOUGEROT-RUITER

Synonyms. Allergic vasculitis; arteriolitis allergica; leukocytoclastic angiitis; angiitis-urticarial vasculitis; pentasymptomatic Gougerot (papules, macules, petechiae, bullae, and ulcerations); Ruiter; tetrasymptomatic Gougerot (papules, macules, petechiae, and bullae); trisymptomatic Gougerot (papules, macules, and petechiae); Gougerot-Duperrat; Werther. (Dermatitis nodularis necroticans may be considered as a variant of this syndrome.)

Symptoms and Signs. Prevalent in females (3:2); onset at all ages. Pruritus; local pain. Frequently, fever, malaise, arthralgia, gastrointestinal manifestations. *Acute form.* Hemorrhagic, purpuric necrotic skin eruption on legs, arms, and buttocks; seldom other locations; erythema multiform-like lesions. Seldom, involvement of viscera with relative manifestations. *Subacute form.* Papules, maculoerythematous lesions, nodules; necrotic lesions usually confluent to form plaques; urticaria common. *Chronic form.* Papules, macules, petechiae, urticaria frequent. No systemic manifestations, except mild malaise.

Etiology. Common feature antigen-antibody reaction at vessel wall site. May be caused by a high number of underlying conditions initiated by various agents (drugs, bacteria, fungi, parasite, neoplasia, etc.) and modified by individual response.

Pathology. Dilatation and thrombosis of dermal capillaries and arterioles with fibrinoid and necrotic changes. Leukocytoclasis characteristic feature; erythrocyte extravasation.

Diagnostic Procedures. *Biopsy of skin. Blood.* Sedimentation rate normal or most frequently increased. Neutrophilia or eosinophilia possible. Frequently hypocomplementemia.

Therapy. Elimination of infective focus. Corticosterone, dapsone, or indomethacine: variable effects.

Prognosis. Removal of foci may be followed by cure.

BIBLIOGRAPHY. Gougerot H: Maladie trisymptomatique de H. Gougerot: Trisymptome associant petits nodules dermiques, cocardes d'erytheme polymorphe, purpura. Sem Hôp Paris 23:1311–1315, 1947

Ruiter M, Brandsman CH: Arteriolitis allergica. Dermatologica 97:265–271, 1948

Ryan TJ: Cutaneous vasculitis. In Champion RH, Burton JL, Ebling FJG (eds): Rook/Wilkinson/Ebling Textbook of Dermatology, 5th ed, p 1894. Oxford, Blackwell Scientific, 1992

GOULEY

Eponym is used to indicate the constriction of the pulmonary artery (partial or complete) in adhesive pericarditis. See Pick.

BIBLIOGRAPHY. Gouley BA: Constriction of the pulmonary artery by adhesive pericarditis. Am Heart J 13:470–482, 1937

GOUT SYNDROMES

Synonyms. "Disease of kings and king of diseases"; podagra; uric acid dysmetabolism.

Etiology. The gout disorder of purine metabolism may be classified according to etiology. *Primary.* There are various subtypes of primary gout, probably all with hereditary bases. There are two hypotheses as to the inheritance of gout: autosomal dominant or multifactorial. The gout syndrome appears to be associated also with other enzyme deficiencies: glucose-6-phosphatase deficiency (von Gierke, see); altered kinetics of phosphoribosyl pyrophosphate synthetase. (PP-ribose-P); hypoxanthine-guanine phosphoribosyl transferase deficiency (Lesch-Nyhan, see). *Secondary.* Hematologic disorders; myeloproliferative syndromes (including polycythemia); hemolytic disease; iatrogenic (administration of hyperuricacidemic drugs); obesity; starvation; chronic renal diseases; glycogen storage disease type 1; sarcoidosis; psoriasis; idiopathic. From a clinical point of view, this condition may manifest itself with several syndromes.

ACUTE GOUTY ARTHRITIS

Symptoms. Prevalent in adult males; peak of incidence, third to fifth decade. In women, appears postmenopause. Onset frequent during night. Severe, sharp gnawing pain in the great toe; less frequently other sites (instep, ankle, heel, knee, wrist, in order of frequency). Extreme discomfort; chills and shivers; no change in posture relieves the pain.

Signs. Skin overlying affected joint inflamed.

Diagnostic Procedures. *Blood.* Uric acid determination.

Therapy. Colchicine, phenylbutazone, oxyphenbutazone, indomethacin, allopurinol, adrenocorticotropic hormone (ACTH), or corticosteroids.

Prognosis. Pain lasts a few days or weeks if untreated. Complete recovery follows. Recurrent attacks at variable intervals (weeks or years), affecting the same or different joints.

CHRONIC GOUTY ARTHRITIS

Symptoms and Signs. Average time for development of this syndrome from first acute attack 11.6 years. Onset may be insidious or sequela of a repeated attack also affecting previously uninvolved joints. Usually, after chronic form develops, acute attacks disappear. Polyarthritic involvement with eventual evolution to grotesque, deforming, destructive, ulcerating changes. From ulcer of tophi, excretion of chalky material, usually painless. Tophi in ear cartilage, tendons, less frequently skin, nose cartilage, and eyes.

Pathology. Tophi are urate deposits with inflammation of foreign body reaction type of surrounding tissues. Predominantly located in cartilage, epiphyses, periarticular structures, and kidney. Necrotic changes of joint cartilage with synovial proliferation, bone destruction, and sometimes ankylosis. In kidney, uric acid crystal in interstitial tissue of pyramids; necrotic changes; urolithiasis.

Diagnostic Procedures. *Blood.* Hyperuricemia. *X-ray.* Punched-out lesion of bones; deformative changes of joints. *Biopsy.* Of joint or synovial fluid aspiration. Presence of uric acid crystals.

Therapy. Diet; anti-inflammatory (oral indomethacin, colchicine IV, nonsteroidal anti-inflammatory drugs, and intra-articular corticosteroids), antihyperuricemic and uricosuric agents (allopurinol, probenecid; sulfinpyrazone; zoxazolamine).

RENAL SYNDROME IN GOUT

Symptoms and Signs. Evidence of renal disease; albuminuria, hypertension, and urolithiasis with passage of stones.

Pathology. See Chronic gouty arthritis syndrome.

BIBLIOGRAPHY. Sydenham T: Tractatus de podagra et hydrope. London, G. Kettilby, 1783

Garrod AB: Observations on certain pathological conditions of the blood and urine in gout, rheumatism and Bright's disease. Trans Med Chir Soc Edinburgh 31:83, 1848

Becker MA, Roessler BJ: Hyperuricemia and gout. In Scriver CR,

Beaudet AL, Sly WS, et al: The Metabolic and Molecular Bases of Inherited Disease, 7th ed, pp 1655–1677. New York, McGraw-Hill, 1995

GOWERS PANATROPHY

Symptoms and Signs. Prevalent in women; onset in second to fourth decades. On the back, buttocks, thighs, or arms, occasionally forearms or lower legs, over a period of a few weeks without signs of preceding inflammation, development of clearly defined areas of atrophy of skin (otherwise normal) with disappearance of subcutaneous tissue. Single or multiple areas (usually quadrangular or triangular in shape, 2–20 cm in diameter).

Etiology. Unknown; to be differentiated from sclerotic panatrophy of scleroderma and forms of panniculitis.

Pathology. Atrophy of subcutaneous tissue and skin.

Diagnostic Procedures. Biopsy of skin.

Therapy. None.

Prognosis. Lesions progress for a few months, then remain unchanged indefinitely.

BIBLIOGRAPHY. Barnes S: Report on Sir William Gower's case of local panatrophy. Trans Clin Soc London 36:164–168, 1902–1903
Barnes S: Gower's case of local panatrophy. Br J Dermatol 51:377–380, 1939
Burton JL: Disorders of connective tissue. In Champion RH, Burton JL, Ebling FJG (eds): Rook/Wilkinson/Ebling Textbook of Dermatology, 5th ed, p 1780. Oxford, Blackwell Scientific, 1992

GOWER-WELANDER

Synonyms. Welander; distal muscular dystrophy; late distal hereditary myopathy; myopathy, late, distal, hereditary.

Symptoms and Signs. Observed in Sweden, occasionally in other areas; onset after second decade; peak at fifth decade. (Families with infantile and juvenile onset described also.) Initial symptom, weakness of thumb and first finger, then spreading to small muscles and extensors of hands and feet. Seldom, extension of moderate weakness to proximal muscles of extremities.

Etiology. Unknown; autosomal dominant inheritance. Proposed recessive inheritance may be explained instead by an unusual mechanism: germinal mosaicism in a parent.

Pathology. Muscle fiber degeneration fibrosis.

Diagnostic Procedures. *Electromyography.* No myotonia and compatible with myopathy (neurogenic atrophy). *Blood. Enzymes.* Normal.

Therapy. None.

Prognosis. Extremely slow progression; remains limited to distal parts.

BIBLIOGRAPHY. Gowers WR: A lecture on myopathy and distal form. Br Med J 2:89–92, 1902
Welander L: Myopathia distalis tarda hereditaria: 249 examined cases in 72 pedigrees. Acta Med Scand (Suppl) 141:1–115, 1951
Marksbery WR, Griggs RC, Herr B: Distal myopathy. Electron microscope and histochemical studies. Neurology 27:727–735, 1977
Buchman AS, Cochran EJ: Distal myopathies. In Rowland S, Mauro S: Handbook of Clinical Neurology, vol 18, p 197. Amsterdam, Elsevier, 1992

GOYER

Synonyms. Deafness—ichthyosis—renal.

Symptoms and Signs. Both sexes. Variable expression of symptoms. Only some isolated ones may be manifest in members of affected family. Significant hearing loss, since childhood. Renal disease. Ichthyosis.

Etiology. Autosomal dominant inheritance with variable expression. It falls in the spectrum of Alport (see). Not many reasons to keep it distinguished.

Pathology. Glomerulosclerosis (biopsy).

Diagnostic Procedures. *Audiogram.* Bilateral or monolateral hearing loss hight or middle frequency. *Urine.* Albuminuria, hematuria, prolinuria.

BIBLIOGRAPHY. Goyer RA, Reynolds J Jr, Burke J, et al: Hereditary renal disease with neurosensory hearing loss, polyuria, and ichthyosis. Am J Med Sci 256:166–179, 1968
Koenigsmark BW: Hereditary progressive cochloeovestibular atrophies. In Vinken PJ, Bruyn GW (eds): Handbook of Clinical Neurology, vol 22, p 490. Amsterdam, North-Holland, 1975

GRADENIGO

Synonyms. Lannois-Gradenigo; abducens nerve palsy—petrous osteomyelitis; temporal; petrosal. See Orbital apex.

Symptoms. Frontal headache (area of ophthalmic branch of nerve); acute otitis media with persistent diplopia.

Signs. Internal strabismus owing to homolateral abducens (VI) paralysis. Optic (II), trochlear (IV), trigeminal (V), and facial (VII) nerves occasionally may be involved.

Etiology. Localized meningitis over the tip of petrous pyramid, and perineuritis of trigeminal (V) and abducens (VI) nerve as they contact the bone. Neoplastic invasion of the petrous apex.

Pathology. Mastoiditis; purulent infection spreading from antrum to tip of petrous bone and localized pachymeningitis and perineuritis.

Diagnostic Procedures. *X-ray. CT scan. MRI of mastoid.* Haziness and then sclerosis of petrous apex.

Therapy. Antibiotics and surgery frequently required.

Prognosis. Recovery with adequate treatment.

BIBLIOGRAPHY. Gradenigo G: Sulla leptomeningite circoscritta e sulla paralisi dell' abducente di origine otitica. Gior R Accad Med Torino 10:59–84, 1904
Gillander DA: Gradenigo's syndrome revisited. J Otolaryngol 12:169–174, 1983
Cappina AH: Traumatic intracranial aneurysm and Gradenigo syndrome secondary to gunshot wound. Surg Neurol 22:263–266, 1984
Weatherall DJ, Ledingham JGG, Warrell DA (eds): Oxford Textbook of Medicine, 3rd ed, pp 3877, 3878. Oxford, Oxford Med Pub, 1996

GRAFT-VERSUS-HOST

Synonyms. Allogenic bone marrow; bone marrow transfusion; GVH; leukocyte transfusion; runt.

I. ACUTE

Symptoms. Occurs in patients who, after total irradiation, have received allogenic bone marrow transfusion or leukocyte transfusion. Onset 5–9 days after transfusion. Fever; asthenia; anorexia; nausea; vomiting; diarrhea; severe weight loss.

Signs. Exfoliative erythroderma; occasionally, jaundice and hepatomegaly, and transitory lymphoadenopathy.

Etiology. Graft against host reaction.

Pathology. Transient hyperplasia of lymphoid tissue (proliferation of hyperbasophilic cells), then aplasia of lymphatic tissue. Skin infiltration with lymphocytes and reticulum cells; epithelial vacuolization and dyskeratosis; area of acanthosis, hyperkeratosis, and parakeratosis. (These skin manifestations are concurrent with the myeloid repopulation).

Diagnostic Procedures. *Blood.* Transient lymphocytosis, followed by intense or moderate lymphocytopenia; anemia may be present. IgA, IgM, IgG decreased. Blood cultures: bacterial, viral, mycotic infections. Studies of immunoglobulin phenotype.

Therapy. Keep the patient in sterile environment to prevent infections. Antibiotics.

Prognosis. Complete remission of long duration of the primary leukemic condition may be obtained by the technique of total body radiation and bone marrow transplant. This secondary syndrome is one of the prices we pay for this drastic therapeutic procedure. Careful studies to establish maximum compatibility between host and graft marrow may reduce intensity of this reaction.

II. CHRONIC

Symptoms. Affects 25–45% of patients who survive longer than 180 days. Symptoms like those seen in various collagen diseases at skin, mucosal, and visceral levels. Significant weight loss (in 50% of cases).

Etiology. Suppressor T-cells and macrophages and B-cells appear involved in the immunosupression.

Therapy. Prednisone or prednisone plus cyclosporine and antibiotic prophylasis.

Prognosis. Good response to treatment. Therapy can be stopped in 1 year.

BIBLIOGRAPHY. Mathe G, Schwarzenberg L, de Vries MJ, et al: Les divers aspects du syndrome secondaire compliquant les transfusions allogéniques de moelle osseuse ou de leukocytes chez des sujects atteints d'hémopathies malignes. Eur J Cancer 1:75–113, 1965
Foester J: Bone marrow transplantation. In Lee GR, Bithel TC, Foerster J, et al (eds): Wintrobe's Clinical Hematology, 9th ed, pp 706–708. Philadelphia, Lea & Febiger, 1993

GRAHMANN

Synonym. Pituitary diencephalon.

Symptoms. Occurs in male adolescents. Periodic psychotic episodes with or without slight temperature elevation.

Signs. Obesity; underdevelopment; hypogonadism.

Etiology. Attributed to abnormality of diencephalon; secondary to intracerebral alterations; neoplastic, infectious, vascular, or granulomatous processes (see Engel-Aring and transient Cushing).

Pathology. Unknown.

Diagnostic Procedures. Not reported.

Therapy. Symptomatic.

Prognosis. Unknown.

BIBLIOGRAPHY. Grahmann H: Periodische Ausnahmezustände in der Reifezeit als diencephale Regulationstörung. Psychiatr Neurol 135:361–377, 1958
Wolff SM, Adler RC, Buskirsk ER, et al: A syndrome of periodic hypothalamic discharge. Am J Med 36:956–967, 1966
Melmed S: Tumor mass effects of lesions in the hypothalamus and pituitary. In De Groot LJ (ed): Endocrinology, 3rd ed, p 460. Philadelphia, WB Saunders, 1995

GRAM

Synonyms. Adiposalgia—arthritico—hypertonica; justoarticular adiposis dolorosa; postmenopausal triad. See Menopausal.

Symptoms and Signs. Occurs after menopause, usually in multiparae. Rheumatoid arthritis of knee; adiposis dolorosa; blood hypertension.

Etiology. See Menopause.

BIBLIOGRAPHY. Gram HC: A symptom-triade of the postclimateric period. (Adipositas dolorosa–arthritis genuum–hypertension arterialis). Acta Med Scand 73:139–207, 1930

G.R.A.N.D.D.A.D.

Synonyms. Growth retardation—aged facies—normal development—decreased subcutaneous fat—autosomal dominant.

Symptoms and Signs. Both sexes. From birth. Reduced intrauterine and postnatal growth; normal mental development; decreased subcutaneous fat. Aged facies: prominent forehead, absent hair (or thin) deep set eyes, midfacial and alar nasal hypoplasia, prominent nasal septum and ears; thin lips.

Etiology. Possibly autosomal inheritance.

BIBLIOGRAPHY. Marion RW, Goldberg RB, Young RS, et al: The GRAND-DAD syndrome: A disorder combining growth delay, aged facies, normal development and deficiency of subcutaneous fat (Abst). Am J Huma Genet 45:(Suppl)A 53, 1989

GRAND MAL

Synonyms. Epilepsia major; tonic or tonico-clonic seizures.

Symptoms. Prodromal.

1. Paroxysmal attacks of strangeness, short-lasting "dreamy states," giddiness, pain, isolated muscle contraction, palpitations.
2. Continuous irritability or lethargy 1 or 2 days preceding the attack; depression or euphoria; well being, bulimia; headache.
3. Auras immediately preceding the attack: epigastric, strange indefinable sensation in stomach, throat, nausea, or hunger, palpitation. Psychic terror, fright; cursive epileptic syndrome (the patient runs in terror before unconsciousness that follows). Dreamy states, with peculiar olfactory, gustative, visual, auditory sensations. Epileptic cry, and parrot scream are respectively forced expiration or inspiration that precede the convulsion.

Attack.

1. Sudden loss of consciousness following tonic spasm of all voluntary muscles almost equally bilaterally.
2. Cyanosis; fractures or dislocation from muscle contraction or fall. Release of sphincters with emission of feces or urine. Spastic relaxation and clonic contractions.
3. Finally, cessation of spasm and bubbling saliva emission.

Partial attack sometimes with only spastic phase or only loss of consciousness. Return of consciousness after a few minutes or hours, usually the patient falls asleep after regaining consciousness.

Signs. Typical loss of consciousness and convulsions; pupils dilated not reactive; reflexes abolished. Tachycardia; apnea during spastic phase. Increase in blood pressure.

Etiology and Pathology. Symptomatic. Cerebral injury; familial and congenital developmental defect; vascular occlusion; inflammatory disease or sequelae; tumor; paroxysmal diseases. Idiopathic.

Diagnostic Procedures. *EEG. X-ray. CT scan. MRI. Isotope brain scan.*

Therapy. Diphenylhydantoin; primidone; phenobarbital; methylphenylethylhydantoin. Neurosurgery (when indicated).

Prognosis. Recovery from single attacks. Possibility of status epilepticus (see). Psychic deterioration with repeated seizures.

BIBLIOGRAPHY. Temkin O: The Falling Sickness: A History of Epilepsy from the Greeks to the Beginning of Modern Neurology. Baltimore, Johns Hopkins Press, 1945

Adams RD, Victor M: Principles of Neurology, 5th ed, pp 273–297. New York, McGraw-Hill, 1993

GRANT*

Synonyms. See Beighton and osteogenesis imperfecta spectrum.

Symptoms and Signs. From birth. Bleu sclerae, mandibular hypoplasia, camptomelia, short stature, no tendency to fracture, no tooth alterations, tendency to shoulder dislocation.

Etiology. Autosomal dominant.

Pathology. Wormian bones prolonged persistence. Osteopenia in infancy, shallow glenoid fossae.

Diagnostic Procedures. *X-rays. CT scan. MRI.* See Pathology. *Blood.* Ca, P, alkaline phosphatase: normal.

Therapy. Symptomatic.

Prognosis. Improvement after infancy of bowing of long bones.

BIBLIOGRAPHY. McLean JR, Low RY RB, Wood BJ: The Grant syndrome. Persistent wormian bones, bleu sclerae, mantibular hypoplasia, shallow glenoid fossae and camptomelia. An autosomal dominant trait. Clin Genet 29:523–529, 1986

GRANT (R.T.)

Synonyms. Cholinergic urticaria; micropapular urticaria.

Symptoms. Both sexes affected; onset in adolescence or young adulthood. After exertion or emotional disturbances, itching irritable wheals (or both) appear on the skin. In some cases, accompanied by flushing and fainting.

Signs. Wheals 1–3 mm in diameter on all areas of the skin.

Etiology. Unknown. Sympathetic stimulation by heat, emotion, gustatory stimulus.

Diagnostic Procedures. Syndrome may be reproduced by intradermal administration of cholinergic drugs or intramuscular injection of nicotine or of sodium chloride solution (5–6%).

Therapy. No treatment required in most cases. Antihistaminic or anticholinergic drugs may prevent attacks. Exertion may relieve symptoms after induced attack for 24 hours.

Prognosis. Attacks last minutes or 1–2 hours. After attacks, for 24 hours, freedom from symptoms even if the patient exerts or is subject to emotional stress. Condition persists for months or years and usually regresses spontaneously.

BIBLIOGRAPHY. Grant RT, Pearson RSB, Comeau WS: Observations on urticaria provoked by emotion, by exercise and by warming the body. Clin Sci 2:253–272, 1936

Buckley RH, Mathews KP: Common "allergic" skin diseases. JAMA 248:2611–2622, 1982

Champion RH: Urticaria. In Champion RH, Burton JL, Ebling FJG (eds): Rook/Wilkinson/Ebling Textbook of Dermatology, 5th ed, pp 1875–1876. Oxford, Blackwell Scientific, 1992

GRANULOMA ANNULARE

Symptoms. All ages. Predominant in children and young adults. Both sexes, predominant in females. Symptomless and only occasionally pruritic lesions.

Signs. Usually localized lesion. Seldom three different patterns observed: generalized, perforating, and subcutaneous. All areas of skin may be involved, most frequently dorsal aspect of hands and feet. Rings of papules smooth and firm, 1–5 cm of diameter; mildly erythematous. Stretching of skin makes them more evident, scaling is rare. Lesions tend to enlarge.

Etiology. Unknown. Various hypothesis (not substantiated): insect bites; trauma; gold therapy; sun exposure; immunologic reactiod.

Pathology. Focal obstructive process of dermis with "palisading" granuloma.

Diagnostic Procedures. *Skin biopsy.* Direct immunofluorescence studies. *Blood.* Circulating immune complexes (60%); T-cell subtyping; macrophage inhibitory tests; glucose tolerance; insulin level; insulin antibodies.

Therapy. All useless or of scarce benefit.

Prognosis. Slow development for months or years, spontaneous regression without scar. Recurrences are common (40%) but regress faster than primary lesion.

BIBLIOGRAPHY. Prunty FC, Montgomery H: Granuloma annulare. Arch Dermatol Syph 46:394–413, 1942

Cunliffe WJ: Necrobiotic disorder. In Champion RH, Burton JL, Ebling FJG (eds): Rook/Wilkinson/Ebling Textbook of Dermatology, 5th ed, pp 2027–2033. Oxford, Blackwell Scientific, 1992

GRANULOSIS RUBRA NASI

Symptoms and Signs. Onset in early childhood (6 months to 10 years). Usually preceded by hyperhidrosis. Erythema starting on the tip of nose and progressively extending to cover nose and possibly cheeks, upper lip, and chin. Area of hyperhidrosis could be larger than that of erythema. Maculae, papules, and vesicles at sweat duct orifices. Associated symptomatology; coldness, hyperhidrosis of hands and feet.

Etiology. Unknown; possibly hereditary (undetermined mode of inheritance).

Diagnostic Procedures. Assess status of nutrition and general health.

Therapy. Usually disappointing. Improvement of nutrition and general care.

Prognosis. May recede spontaneously at puberty or after improvement of nutrition or persist complicated by cyst formation and telangiectasis.

BIBLIOGRAPHY. Maschkilleisson LN, Naeadow LA: 33 Fälle von Jodassohns Granulosis rubra nasi. Dermatol Z 71:79–84, 1935

Champion RH: Disorders of sweat glands. In Champion RH, Burton JL, Ebling FJG (eds): Rook/Wilkinson/Ebling Textbook of Dermatology, 5th ed, p 1756. Oxford, Blackwell Scientific, 1992

GRANULOVACUOLAR MYOPATHY

Synonyms. Myopathy granulovacuolar, lobular—myotonia; myotonia—granulovacuolar myopathy.

*Family surname.

Symptoms and Signs. In adults: muscle wasting (selective) weakness, difficulty in climbing stairs, etc.

Etiology. Possibly autosomal dominant inheritance.

Pathology. Muscle: vacuoles containing hematoxylinophilic granules and in 30% of type I fibers lobular reorganization.

Therapy. Symptomatic.

Prognosis. Good quod vitam.

BIBLIOGRAPHY. Juguilon A, Chad D, Bradley WG, et al: Familial granulo-vacuolar lobular myopathy with electric myotonia. J Neurol Sci 56:133–140, 1982
Walton J, Karpati G, Hilton-Jones D: Disorders of Voluntary Muscle, p 249. Edinburgh, Churchill-Livingstone, 1994

GRAVES OPHTHALMOPATHY

Synonyms. Includes euthyroid Graves disease. See Flajani.

Symptoms and Signs. Eyelid retraction, proptosis, periorbital edema, chemosis, and altered ocular motility. It may develop exposure keratitis with or without ulcerations and compressive optic neuropathy. Majority of patients manifest thyroid abnormality (see Flajani) and it appears at the same time (15% of patients with Graves ophthalmopathy have normal thyroid function).

Etiology. Unknown. Organ-specific autoimmune process.

Pathology. Orbital inflammation, exophthalmos, or proptosis of globe, retrobulbar soft tissue enlargement, with lymphocytic infiltration, glucosomanine deposition, and edema.

Diagnostic Procedures. *X-ray. CT scan. MRI.* Fundus oculi; visual evoked potentials; electrophysiologic studies. *Blood.* See Flajani, level of circulating antibodies particularly useful.

Therapy. Treatment of associated thyroid condition; if active, threatens vision ophthalmopathy (blurred vision, or ocular pain): high doses corticosteroids, irradiation; and surgical decompression

Prognosis. Self-limiting disease that runs a course of exacerbations and spontaneous remissions over several years. Possible residual damages: cosmetic disfiguration, visual loss, myopathy (diplopia).

BIBLIOGRAPHY. Graves RJ: Clinical lectures. London Med Surg J 7:516, 1835
Yeatts RP: Graves' ophthalmopathy. Med Clin N Am 79:195–209, 1995

GRAWITZ

Synonyms. Kidney adenocarcinoma; hypernephroma; renal cell carcinoma; RCC.

Symptoms. Both sexes affected; onset over 50 years of age. In 40% of cases asymptomatic. Dull pain in lumbar region; occasionally, colic. Later, anorexia, asthenia, nausea, weight loss, hematuria, hyperthermia.

Signs. Palpable mass in kidney; tenderness elicited at costovertebral angle. Occasionally, varicocele; blood hypertension.

Etiology. Unknown. Considered congenital malformation, embryonic residue; trauma; infections. Rarely, familial cases with possible autosomal dominant pattern reported.

Pathology. In kidney, spherical, 3–15 cm diameter, yellow gray encapsulated masses. Histologic examination shows tubular cells arranged in various patterns invading vessels.

Diagnostic Procedures. *Blood.* Normochromic anemia; occasionally, polycythemia. *Urine.* Hematuria; pyuria; presence of malignant cells. *X-ray.* Intravenous pyelography: presence of masses displacing and invading calyces. Of skeleton, possible metastases. *Biopsy.* See Pathology.

Therapy. Surgical excision. Chemotherapy. X-ray treatment.

Prognosis. Five-year survival in 30–50%.

BIBLIOGRAPHY. Grawitz PA: Die sogenannten Lipome der Niere. Arch Pathol 93:39–63, 1883
Goldman SM, Fishman EK, Abeshouse G, et al: Renal cell carcinoma diagnosed in three generations of a single family. South Med J 72:1457–1459, 1979
Levinson AK, Johnson DE, Strong LC, et al: Familial renal cell carcinoma: hereditary or coincidental? J Urol 144:849–851, 1990

GRAY

Synonym. Neonatal chloramphenicol toxicity; chloramphenicol toxicity.

Symptoms. In infants, occurs 3 or 4 days after starting administration of chloramphenicol. Vomiting, dyspnea; failure to suckle.

Signs. Skin grayish color; cyanosis; occasionally, jaundice; muscle flaccidity; abdominal distension; tachycardia; hypotension; cardiovascular collapse.

Etiology. Failure to metabolize (liver), excrete (kidney) chloramphenicol, possibly because of immature enzymes. Probably mitochondrial lack of resistance to chloramphenicol.

Diagnostic Procedures. *Blood.* Hyperbilirubinemia. *Stool.* Green.

Therapy. Symptomatic.

Prognosis. Shock and death. Severe shock and death frequent. Bone marrow cells from patients who survived chloramphenicol toxicity in vitro became more resistant.

BIBLIOGRAPHY. Burns LE, Hodgman JE, Cass AB: Fatal circulatory collapse in premature infants receiving chloramphenicol. N Engl J Med 261:1318–1321, 1959
Sutherland JM: Fatal cardiovascular collapse of infants receiving large amounts of chloramphenicol. Am J Dis Child 97:761–767, 1959
Poulton L: Mitochondrial DNA and genetic disease. Arch Dis Child 63:883–885, 1988

GRAYOUT

See also Blackout.

Symptoms. In fast acceleration or deceleration of vehicles (e.g., airplane). Gradual decrease of vision; misting; reduced peripheral vision area.

Etiology. Reduction of blood pressure of retina.

Diagnostic Procedures. For pilots or exposed persons: Testing the visual threshold. With progressive acceleration. *Ophthalmoscopy.*

GRAY PLATELET

Synonym. Raccuglia; platelet alpha granule deficiency.

Symptoms and Signs. Both sexes. Lifelong purpura.

Etiology. Unknown. Probably autosomal recessive inheritance.

Diagnostic Procedures. *Blood.* Bleeding time prolonged; clot retraction poor; platelet number normal; lack of granules, presence of vacuolization, and peculiar gray hue in Wright stained smears. Adenosine triphosphate (ATP) and extractable phosphatides from platelets reduced. Platelet aggregation with adenosine diphosphate (ADP), epinephrine, and collagen normal. Absence of alpha granules. Decrease of platelet fibrinogen, factor 4, β-thromboglobulin, growth factor, and protein sensitive to thrombin, glycoprotein Ig, or thromborespondine. *Bone marrow.* Cytoplasm of megakaryocytes vacuolated and lacking vacuoles in zones. Decrease of alpha granules in megacaryocytes and platelets. Sometimes observed myelofibrosis.

Therapy. Seldom required. Corticosteroids ineffective. DDAVP occasionally shortens bleeding time. Splenectomy reduces thrombocytopenia but fails to modify purpura and other clotting abnormalities.

BIBLIOGRAPHY. Raccuglia G: Gray platelet syndrome: A variety of qualitative platelet disorder. Am J Med 51:818–828, 1971

Greenberg-Sepersky SM, Simons ER, et al: Studies of platelets from patients with gray platelet syndrome. Br J Hematol 59:603–609, 1985

White JC: Inherited abnormalities of the platelet membrane and secretory granules. Hum Pathol 18:123–139, 1987

Bithell TC: Qualitative disorders of platelets function. In Lee GR, Bithel TC, Foerster J, et al (eds): Wintrobe's Clinical Hematology, 9th ed, p 1404. Philadelphia, Lea & Febiger, 1993

GRAYSON-WILBRANDT

Synonym. Anterior membrane dystrophy. See Reis-Bueckler.

Symptoms. Onset at end of first decade. Rare episodes of eye redness and pain; reduction of vision; normal corneal sensation.

Signs. Corneal changes variable from a mottled scarring (as in Reis-Bueckler syndrome, see) to small, macular, gray, raised opacities.

Etiology. Unknown; autosomal dominant trait. Considered as separated from Reis-Bueckler, because of (1) variable effect on vision, (2) partial corneal involvement, and (3) normal corneal sensation.

Pathology. See Reis-Bueckler.

Therapy. Corneal transplant if needed.

Prognosis. Progressive vision reduction of variable degree; in some cases vision not affected at all.

BIBLIOGRAPHY. Grayson M, Wilbrandt H: Dystrophy of the anterior limiting membrane of the cornea (Reis-Bückler type). Am J Ophthalmol 61:345–349, 1966

GREAT ARTERIES, COMPLETE TRANSPOSITION

Symptoms. Male prevalence (2–4:1); onset from birth. Feeding difficulty; dyspnea; growth retardation.

Signs. Higher weight at birth; squatting; syncopes; progressive cyanosis. Single accentuated first sound in second left interspace; tachypnea; digital clubbing; hepatomegaly; narrow pulse; pulmonary edema.

Etiology. Congenital malformation.

Pathology. Aorta originating from right ventricle and rotating forward to left; pulmonary artery from left ventricle and rotating backward to right. Associated various malformations (e.g., septal defects; ductus arteriosus). Arterial and venous thrombosis of gastrointestinal and cerebral, kidney, and pulmonary districts.

Diagnostic Procedures. *Electrocardiography.* Variable grade of right axis deviation according to type of abnormalities; right-left predominance. *X-ray.* Cardiomegaly; vascular pedicle narrow at the base; increased pulmonary vessels. *Angiography.* Evidence of vessel inversion at origin. *Blood.* Polycythemia. *Two-dimensional echocardiography with color flow imaging and spectral Doppler interrogation.*

Therapy. Surgery; interatrial transposition of venous returns, during cardiopulmonary bypass with hypothermia. In patients with an intact ventricular septum, the first step is to establish an adequate interatrial opening (balloon septostomy).

Prognosis. Death usually in infancy. Possible survival to adolescence and even to adulthood. Good results with surgery at the time of election (first year of age).

BIBLIOGRAPHY. Baillie M: Morbid Anatomy of Some of the Most Important Parts of the Human Body, 2nd ed. London, Johnson and Nicol, 1797

Farre JR: On malformations of the heart (essay I). In Pathological Researches, p 28. London, Longman, Hurst, Rees, Orme, Brown, 1814

Van Praagh R: The story of anatomical corrected malposition of the great arteries. Chest 69:2–4, 1976

Williams RG, Bierman FZ, Sanders SP: Echocardiographic Diagnosis of Cardiac Malformations, pp 165–169. Boston, Little, Brown & Co, 1986

Perloff JK: The Clinical Recognition of Congenital Heart Disease, 4th ed, p 663. Philadelphia, WB Saunders, 1994

GREBE

Synonyms. Quelce-Salgado. Achondrogenesis II (formerly); Brazilian achondrogenesis (limb malformation type). Nonlethal achondrogenesis.

Symptoms. Both sexes affected; evident from birth. Dwarfism. Obesity. Facies normal. Striking reduction of limbs, especially of distal part; legs shorter than arms; short digits (fingers similar to toes); valgus position of feet. Polydactyly (57% of cases). Mental development delayed, but mentality normal.

Etiology. Autosomal recessive inheritance.

Pathology. Missing or hypoplastic bones.

Diagnostic Procedures. *X-ray of skeleton.* Shortened forearms, greater reduction of ulnae with respect to radii. *X-ray of spine.* Clear spaces because of uncalcified vertebrae.

Therapy. Surgery to remove extra digits.

Prognosis. Stillborn; death in early infancy. Possible survival.

BIBLIOGRAPHY. Grebe H: Die Achondrogenesis ein einfach rezesives Erbmerkmal. Folia Hered Pathol (Milano) 2:23–28, 1952

Quelce-Salgado A: A new type of dwarfism with various bone aplasias and hypoplasia of the extremities. Acta Genet 14:63–66, 1964

Curtis D: Heterozygote expression in Grebe chondrodysplasia. Clin Genet 29:455–456, 1986

GREBE-MYLE-LOEWENTHAL

Synonyms. Lipomatosis, transition form.

Symptoms and Signs. Systemic lipomatosis (see) transition form with other phacomatosis (spina bifida, cafè-au-lait cutaneous spots, mental deficiency, myosclerosis).

Etiology. Unknown. Possible relation with myositis ossificans progressiva.

BIBLIOGRAPHY. Grebe H: Lipomatosis, psychische Anomalien und Missbildungen in einer Sippe. Erbartz 11:55, 1943

Myle G, Lowenthal A: Lipomatose et lymphangiomatose faciale—localisation trigéminale associées à des fragments de phacomatoses voisines. Acta Neurol Belg 51:473, 1950

Loewenthal A: Sur une forme congénitale et familale sclérose musculaire généralisée avec blépharoptose (Contribution a l'étude des maladies congénitales des muscles et de tissue conjontif). Acta Neurol Belg 52:151, 1952

Vuia O: Multiple lipomata Krabbe disease. In Vinken PJ, Bruyn GW (eds): Handbook of Clinical Neurology, vol 14. Amsterdam, North-Holland, 1972

GREEN NAIL

Symptoms. Prevalent in females. Occurs in patients whose occupation involves prolonged exposure of hands to soap, water, and detergents. Pain of involved fingers.

Signs. Green discoloration of the nail plate, entire nail, portion (proximally, distally, or laterally), or demarcated horizontal bands (in repeated episodes).

Etiology. Paronychial infections with Pseudomonas aeruginosa or some species of Aspergillus.

Pathology. Growth of Pseudomonas within nail and formation of pigment.

Diagnostic Procedures. Culture of infected material (beneath nail and shaving of colored portion of nail).

Therapy. Antimycotic agents (topical or systemic) for frequently associated Candida infection.

Prognosis. Recovery with treatment.

BIBLIOGRAPHY. Goldman L, Fox H: Greenish pigmentation of nail plates from Bacillus pyocyaneus infection: Report of two cases. Arch Dermatol Syph 49:136–137, 1944
Shellow WVR, Koplon BS: Green striped nails: Chromonychia due to Pseudomonas aeruginosa. Arch Dermatol 97:149–153, 1968
Samman PD: Management of disorders of the nails. Clin Exp Dermatol 7:189–194, 1982

GREEN STOOL

Symptoms. None.

Signs. Passage of green bile-stained stools without diarrhea.

Etiology. Unknown. Epidemic outbreak due to unknown agent that modifies intestinal flora and consequently urobilin metabolism.

Diagnostic Procedures. *Blood.* Low prothrombin level. *Urine.* Absence of bile and urobilinogen. *Stool.* Elevated bile; absent urobilinogen. *Culture.* Negative.

Therapy. Penicillin.

Prognosis. Stool becomes normal within 24 hours after administration of penicillin, prothrombin time is normal within 48 hours, and urobilinogen appears in urine and stool within that time.

BIBLIOGRAPHY. Greenblatt IJ, Bloch H, Turin RD, et al: "Green stool syndrome" of newly born infant. Pediatrics 5:180–183, 1950

GREEN URINE

Synonym. Pseudomonas toxemia.

Symptoms and Signs. In patient with infection of a large surface of body with Pseudomonas aeruginosa (e.g., extensive burn; empyema). One or 2 days before appearance of green urine, hemolytic crisis; followed by hypothermia, oliguria, dehydration, with or without shock.

Etiology. Massive infection with Pseudomonas aeruginosa determining massive hemolysis and formation of verdohemoglobin.

Pathology. That of Gram-negative sepsis complicating different conditions (of burn, lung, pleura, intestine).

Diagnostic Procedures. *Urine.* Presence of a dark bilious green pigment (verdohemoglobin) to be differentiated from other pigments produced by Pseudomonas infection. Fluorescence with ultraviolet. *Culture of pus. Blood.* Red cell volume; bilirubin; electrolytes.

Therapy. Gentamicin and other antibiotics effective against Pseudomonas plus general symptomatic treatment and prevention of development of other substituting flora.

Prognosis. Until now always fatal within 2–3 days, or if in intensive treatment, a few weeks.

BIBLIOGRAPHY. Stone HH: The green urine syndrome: An ominous manifestation of Pseudomonas toxemia. Bull Emory Univ Clin 3:81–86, 1964
Weatherall DJ, Ledingham JGG, Warrell DA (eds): Oxford Textbook of Medicine, 3rd ed, pp 550, 2437. Oxford, Oxford Med Pub, 1996

GREGG

Synonyms. Rubella embryopathy; postrubella.

Symptoms and Signs. Occurs in newborns of mothers exposed to rubella virus during first trimester of pregnancy. Hepatosplenomegaly; interstitial pneumonia; congenital heart defects (patent ductus arteriosus; stenosis of pulmonary trunk); low birth weight; congenital cataracts and visual disturbance with diplopia; purpura; hearing loss; inguinal hernias; mental retardation. Ataxia. Failure to thrive.

Etiology. Rubella virus affecting tissues during fetal development.

Pathology. Eye: Necrotizing iridocyclitis; retention of lens fiber nuclei within lens center, anterior chamber angle anomalies and infantile glaucoma; buphthalmos; "salt and pepper" fundus due to hyper and hypopigmentation of retina.

Diagnostic Procedures. Isolation of virus from throat swab, urine, and fecal material (positivity 63%). *Blood.* Anemia; hyperbilirubinemia; reticulocytosis; thrombocytopenia. *X-ray.* Changes in long bones; cerebral calcifications.

Therapy. Symptomatic. Keep infant isolated because he remains a carrier of the virus for a long time.

Prognosis. Severe mortality (14%) within a few months.

BIBLIOGRAPHY. Gregg NM: Congenital cataract following German measles in mother. Trans Ophthalmol Soc Aust 3:35–46, 1942
Singer DB, Rudolph AJ, Harvey S, et al: Pathology of the congenital rubella syndrome. J Pediatr 71:665–675, 1967
Pollock TM: Consequences of confirmed maternal rubella at successive stages of pregnancy. Lancet II:781–784, 1982
Atherton DJ: The neonate. In Champion RH, Burton JL, Ebling FJG (eds): Rook/Wilkinson/Ebling Textbook of Dermatology, 5th ed, pp 414–415. Oxford, Blackwell Scientific, 1992

GREIG I

Synonym. Ocular hypertelorism.

Obsolete. used in the past to indicate hypertelorism, complex of etiologic and pathogenetic heterogeneity. Suggested "eponym to be abandoned."

BIBLIOGRAPHY. Greig DM: Hypertelorism: A hitherto undifferentiated congenital cranio-facial deformity. Edinburgh Med J 31:560–593, 1924
Gorlin RJ, Cohen MM Jr, Levin LS: Syndromes of Head and Neck, 3rd ed. New York, Oxford Univ Press, 1990

GREIG II

Synonyms. Hootnick-Holmes; Marshall-Smith craniofacial; polysyndactyly, cephalopolysyndactyly Greigs; GCPS; frontodigital; oxycephaly; acrocephalopolysyndactyly. Noack type; frontonasal dysplasia; median cleft face.

Symptoms and Signs. Both sexes. From birth. Expanded cranial vault, high forehead, broad nose. Polysyndactyly of hands and feet. Normal intelligence. May be associated: ichthyosis, tapetoretinal degeneration, bilateral hip dislocation and acrofacial dystosis.

Etiology. Unknown. Autosomal dominant. Probably balanced translocation between chromosome 3p and 7p.

Diagnostic Procedures. *X-rays.* Markedly advanced bone age.

BIBLIOGRAPHY. Hoppe I: Eine angeborene Spaltung der Nase. Préss Med 2:164–165, 1859

Greig DM: Oxycephaly. Edinburgh Med J 33:189–218, 1928

Noack M: Ein Betrag zum Krankheitsbild der Akrozephalosyndaktylie (Apert). Arch Kinderh 160:168–171, 1959

Marshall RE, Smith DW: Frontodigital syndrome: A dominantly inherited disorder with normal intelligence. J Pediatr 77:129–133, 1970

Hootnick D, Holmes LB: Familial polysyndactyly and craniofacial anomalies. Clin Genet 3:128–134, 1972

Gorlin RJ, Cohen MM Jr, Levin LS: Syndromes of Head and Neck, p 799. New York, Oxford Univ Press 1990

GREITHER

Synonym. Palmoplantar progressive keratoderma. Including palmoplantar epidermatolytic variant; and keratosis palmoplantar striate. See Meleda; Hopf; Tylosis; keratosis Greither; Unna-Thost. Includes Bologna.

Symptoms. Both sexes affected, females experience less severe manifestations; onset in infancy and gradual progression. Asymptomatic or painful fissure on palms or soles.

Signs. Keratosis of palms and soles extending to all hands and feet and eventually to patches of arms and legs. Epidermolysis (in the PE variant). Family has been reported with lesions consisting of streaks of hyperkeratosis running along each finger to the palm (Bologna).

Etiology. Unknown; autosomal dominant inheritance.

Pathology. Keratoderma with scaling.

Therapy. Vitamin A in high doses; topical keratolytic agents and corticosteroids.

Prognosis. Progression and extension of lesions up to 40 years of age: then frequently, spontaneous, total regression in a few years.

BIBLIOGRAPHY. Greither A: Keratosis extremitatum hereditaria progrediens mit dominantem Erbgang. Hautarzt 3:198–203, 1952

Bologna EI: Durch vier generationen dominant vererblich geshlechtsgebundene keratosis palmaris striata (linearia). Dermatol Wochenschr 152:446–457, 1966

Gamborg Nielsen P: Two different clinical and genetic forms of hereditary palmoplantar keratoderma in the northernmost county of Sweden. Clin Genet 28:361–366, 1985

Griffiths WAD, Leigh IM, Marks R: Disorders of keratinization. In Champion RH, Burton JL, Ebling FJG (eds): Rook/Wilkinson/Ebling Textbook of Dermatology, 5th ed, p 1375. Oxford, Blackwell Scientific, 1992

GRENET

Synonyms. Crossed sensory paralysis.

Symptoms and Signs. Variable according to extension of lesion: global homolateral facial anesthesia for pain and temperature; patchy contralateral pain and anesthesia to temperature of the tunk; homolateral paralysis of masticatory muscles (with or without fasciculation or wasting); signs of lesion of fifth cranial nerve (indicating lesion of the pons); homolateral ataxia and tremor (if damage of superior cerebellar peduncle) crossed hemiparesis (if lesion extending to pyramidal tract).

Etiology and Pathology. Hemorrhage, thrombosis, neoplasia infection, involving of tegmentum of the middle third of pons, possible extension to sensory nucleus of fifth cranial nerve, spinothalamic tract, medial lemniscus motor nucleus of fifth cranial nerve, and superior cerebellar peduncle.

BIBLIOGRAPHY. Foville A: Note sur une paralysie peu connue de certains muscles de l'oeil et sa liaison avec quelques points de l'anatomie et la physiologie de la protubérance annulaire. Bull Soc Anat Paris (2)III 23:293–414, 1858

Loeb C, Meyer JS: Pontine syndromes. In Vinken PJ Bruyn GW: Handbook of Clinical Neurology, vol 2, p 239. Amsterdam, North-Holland, 1969

GRIERSON-GOPALAN

Synonyms. Gopalan; barashek; burning feet; chacalek; electric feet; nutritive melalgia.

Symptoms. Frequently observed in the Indian regions and in Africa. Prevalent in women; onset 20–40 years of age. Burning, pain, tingling, cramp-like pain on soles, occasionally in the palms; excessive sweating; tachycardia with exertion; amnesia; decreased vision; amblyopia.

Signs. Elevated skin temperature; vasomotor changes of feet; shuffling gait; reflexes decreased; sensory loss; ataxia; weight loss.

Etiology. Malnutrition; occurs in epidemic form in malnourished population of prisoner camps, jails. Observed in chronic alcoholism.

Pathology. Body wasting; trophic skin changes in affected part.

Diagnostic Procedures. *Blood.* Protein decreased; hypochromic anemia.

Therapy. Yeast extract; calcium pantothenate.

Prognosis. Rapidly fatal without treatment. Responds well to therapy.

BIBLIOGRAPHY. Grierson J: On the burning feet of natives. Trans Med Phys Soc Calcutta 2:275–280, 1826

Gopalan C: The "burning feet syndrome." Indian Med Gaz 81:22–26, 1946

Nuendoerfer B: Burning-feet syndrome. In Neundoerfer B, Schmrigk K, Soyka D (eds): Praktische Neurologic, vol 2, p 113. Polyneuriden und Polyneuropathien, p 394. Weinheim, Edit Medizin VCH, 1987

Adams RD, Victor M: Principles of Neurology, 5th ed, p 860. New York, McGraw-Hill, 1993

GRIESINGER

Synonyms. Ancylostoma duodenitis; Egyptian chlorosis; Gotthard tunnel; miner anemia; tunnel anemia.

Symptoms. Usually appears in barefoot workers operating in damp soil. Itching, usually on feet and between toes, later in perineal area. Cephalalgia; weakness; dizziness; palpitation; tinnitus, abdominal colic, and diarrhea. Possibly, cough and severe dyspnea. In some cases, duodenal ulcer symptomatology.

Signs. Early erythema and edematous change at site of invasion. Later, pallor; possibly, fever.

Etiology. Infestation with Ancylostoma duodenale or Necator americanus.

Pathology. *Jejunum.* Mucosal edema and inflammation with possible ulceration. *Liver.* Fatty infiltration.

Diagnostic Procedures. *Stool.* Parasites ova; Charcot-Leyden crystals. *Blood.* Microcytic anemia; hyposideremia; eosinophilia. *Gastric fluid.* Higher activity than in patients with duodenal ulcer. *X-ray.* Deformity of duodenal bulb; hyperperistalsis of duodenum; absence of ulcer niche.

Therapy. Mebendazole (Vermox); Pyrantel pamoate (Combantrin, Antiminth); Albendazole (Zentel); antianemic drugs.

Prognosis. Disappearance of duodenal symptoms within 24 hours and of radiologic findings in 10–24 days after treatment.

BIBLIOGRAPHY. Griesinger W: Kliniche und anatomiche Beobachtungen ueber die Krankheiten von Egypten. Arch Physiol Heilk 13:528–575, 1854

Yenikombistan H, Shehadi W: Duodenal ulcer syndrome caused by ankylostomiasis. Am J Roentgen 49:39–48, 1963

Monroe LS: Gastrointestinal parasites. In Haubrich WS, Schaffner F, Berk JE (eds): Bockus Gastroenterology, 5th ed, vol 2, pp 3151–3160. Philadelphia, WB Saunders, 1995

GRISCELLI

Synonyms. Chediack-Higashi-like; albinism-immunodeficiency.

Symptoms and Signs. Both sexes. Partial albinism; acute episodes of fever.

Etiology. Autosomal recessive inheritance.

Pathology. Large clumps of pigment in the shafts of hair; accumulation of melanosomes in the melanocytes.

Diagnostic Procedures. *Blood.* Recurrent neutropenia (with normal neutrophils) and thrombocytopenia (with normal bone marrow) specific protease activity; hypogammaglobulinemia; recurrent episodes of hypofibrinogenemia. *Skin.* Absence of delayed skin reaction and skin graft rejection.

Prognosis. Adulthood may be reached.

BIBLIOGRAPHY. Griscelli C, Durandy A, Guy-Grand D, et al: A syndrome associating partial albinism and immunodeficiency. Am J Med 65:691–702, 1978

Atherton DJ: The neonate. In Champion RH, Burton JL, Ebling FJG (eds): Rook/Wilkinson/Ebling Textbook of Dermatology, 5th ed, p 431. Oxford, Blackwell Scientific, 1992

GRISEL

Synonyms. Nasopharyngeal torticollis; atlantoaxial torticollis; torticollis atlanto-epistophealis.

Symptoms and Signs. Spastic contraction of sternocleidomastoid muscle, which pulls the head laterally. Condition may arise after tonsillectomy or infection of the nasal cavities.

Etiology. Synovial effusion that causes relaxation of the joint capsule of the atlas and its subluxation.

Therapy. Antibiotic, anti-inflammatory, and analgesic agents. Immobilization of the head.

Prognosis. Good with treatment.

BIBLIOGRAPHY. Grisel P: Enucleation de l'atlas et torticollis nasopharyngen. Presse Med 38:50–53, 1930

Parke WW, Rothman RH, Brown MD: The pharyngovertebral veins: An anatomical rationale for Grisel's syndrome. J Bone Joint Surg (Am) 66:568–674, 1984

GROB

Synonyms. Dysplasia linguofacialis II; Papillon-Léage and Psaume variant.

Symptoms. Mental deficiency. Feeding problems.

Signs. *Head.* Partial alopecia; epicanthus; cleft lip and palate; mucous membranes of mouth multiridged; fissured tongue; broad nasal bridge and small orifices. *Limbs.* Brachydactyly and clinodactyly.

Etiology. Unknown. See Papillon-Léage and Psaume.

BIBLIOGRAPHY. Grob M: Dysplasia linguo-facialis (Grob). Lehrbuch der Kinderchirurgie, Stuttgart, 1957

GROENBLAD-STRANDBERG-TOURAINE

Synonyms. Darier-Grönblad-Strandberg; Touraine; elastosis dystrophica; systemic elastorrhexis; pseudoxanthoma elasticum; PXE.

Symptoms and Signs. The complete syndrome or subsyndromes may be observed. Symptoms and signs may appear at any age. *Cutaneous.* Bands of small yellowish papules parallel to cutaneous grooves in the neck, axillae, flexor side of elbows, groin, popliteal area. Skin inelastic; when pinched retains folds for some time (opposite of Ehlers-Danlos). *Ocular.* Wide lines; reddish or greyish around optic disk in both eyes (angioid streaks). Occasionally, retinal and choroidal degeneration. *Cardiovascular.* Alteration of peripheral pulses; angina pectoris; hypertension; occasionally, visceral hemorrhages; hematemesis and melena. *Focal.* Cerebral symptoms.

1. Dominant type I: Flexures; orange skin pseudoxanthomatous rash, severe retinopathy; severe atheromatosis.
2. Dominant type II: Milder form: canary yellow macular rash and high skin extensibility; minimal vascular and retinal changes, blue sclerae and myopia may be present; mitral valve prolapse more common.
3. Recessive type I: Similar to dominant type I with milder vascular and retinal changes; common hematemeses, especially in females.
4. Recessive type II: Generalized skin laxity, no systemic manifestations.
5. Recessive type III: In Afrikaaner descent. Mild skin and cardiovascular manifestations. Occasionally telangiectasia of lips and cataracts. After 30 years of age: severe eye changes (angioid streaks, and retinal vessel neoformation with hemorrhages) causing severe vision impairment.

Etiology. Unknown; hereditary condition; autosomal dominant (two types) and recessive (three types) inheritance. Occasionally associated with Paget, Marfan, Herrick, Albers-Schönberg.

Pathology. *Skin.* Degeneration and fragmentation of elastic tissue with calcium accumulation. *Eyes.* Similar changes in the elastic Bruch membrane of the choroid. *Cardiocirculatory.* Generalized arteritis. Rupture of elastic vessel fibers with calcification of degenerated tissue. Proliferation of intima with occlusion of vessel. Necrotic lesions and secondary hemorrhages in gastrointestinal tract, kidney, brain. Renal angioma in one case responsible for hypertension.

Therapy. Symptomatic and plastic surgery to improve cosmetic aspect. Restriction of calcium intake, controversial benefit; laser photocoagulation for prevention retinal hemorrhages.

Prognosis. No effect on life span. Complicating hypertension or hemorrhages; visual impairment. In pregnancy, high incidence of gastrointestinal bleeding.

BIBLIOGRAPHY. Rigal D: Observation pour servir à l'histoire de la cheloide diffuse xanthélasmique. Ann Dermatol Syph 2:491–501, 1881

Darier J: Pseudoxanthoma elasticum. Monatssch Prakt Dermatol 23:609–617, 1896

Grönblad E: Angoid streaks: Pseudoxanthoma elasticum. Vorläufige Mitteilung. Acta Ophthalmol 7:329, 1929

Strandberg J: Pseudoxanthoma elasticum. Zentralbl Haut Ges Krkh 31:689, 1929

Touraine A: L'elastorrhexie systématisée. Bull Soc Fr Dermatol Syph 47:225–273, 1940

De Paepe A, Viljoen D, Matton M, et al: Pseudoxantoma elasticum: Similar autosomal recessive subtype in Belgian and Afrikaaner families Am J Med Genet 38:16–20, 1991

Burton JL: Disorders of connective tissue. In Champion RH, Burton JL, Ebling FJG (eds): Rook/Wilkinson/Ebling Textbook of Dermatology, 5th ed, pp 1782–1786. Oxford, Blackwell Scientific, 1992

GROENOUW I

Synonyms. Fleischer I; corneal granular dystrophy; see Reis-Bueckler.

Symptoms. Both sexes affected; onset during first 10 years of life. Visual reduction by 50–60 years of age.

Signs. Grayish-white opaque granules with sharp borders, mostly in central part of cornea. Cornea clear between opaque spots.

Etiology. Unknown; autosomal dominant inheritance. Sporadic cases also reported.

Pathology. Masses of hyaline substance between epithelium and Bowman membrane. Dehiscences in Bowman membrane. Disruption of nerve fiber.

Diagnostic Procedures. Biopsy of cornea.

Therapy. Corneal graft.

Prognosis. Deterioration becoming serious after fifth decade.

BIBLIOGRAPHY. Groenouw A: Knotchenformige Hornhauttrübungen. Arch Augenheilkd 21:281–289, 1890
Moller HU: Granular corneal dystrophy Groenouw type I: Clinical and genetic aspects. Acta Ophthalmol 69:(Supp 198)1–40, 1991
Klintworth GK: Proteins in ocular disease. In Garner A, Klintworth GK (eds): Pathobiology of Ocular Disease: A Dynamic Approach, 2nd ed, pp 1007–1013. New York, Marcel Dekker, 1994

GROENOUW II

Synonyms. Buckler II; macular corneal dystrophy Groenouw.

Symptoms. Both sexes affected; onset in early childhood. Corneal sensitivity may be reduced. Painful attacks, photophobia. Reduction of vision; significant reduction by age 30–40; then further progression.

Signs. Grayish opaque corneal spots; borders not sharply delimited; scattered over entire cornea, especially dense in central zone.

Etiology. Autosomal recessive inheritance. Deficiency of enzyme alpha-glactosidase or sulfotranferase in keratocytes and fibroblasts. Mucopolysaccharides accumulate in endoplasmic reticulum and not in lysosomes as in mucopolysaccharidoses.

Pathology. Accumulation of acid mucopolysaccharides in corneal corpuscles; mucoid degeneration of stromal lamellae; disappearance of stromal cells. Electron microscopy reveals no abnormality of skin or bulbar conjunctive.

Diagnostic Procedures. *Biopsy of cornea. Urine.* Absence of acid mucopolysaccharide.

Therapy. Corneal graft.

Prognosis. Patients may be blind by the age of 40, occasionally later.

BIBLIOGRAPHY. Groenouw A: Knötchenförmige Hornhaüttrubungen. Arch Augenheilkd 21:281–289, 1890
Hassel JR, Newsome DA, Krachmer JH, et al: Macular corneal dystrophy: Failure to synthesize a mature keratan sulfate proteoglycan. Proc Natl Acad Sci 77:3705–3709, 1980
Yang C: Immunohistochemical evidence of heterogeneity in macular corneal dystrophy. Am J Ophthalmol 106:65–71, 1988
Klintworth GK: Disorders of glycosaminoglycans (mucopolysaccharides) and proteoglycans. In Garner A, Klintworth GK (eds): Pathobiology of Ocular Disease: A Dynamic Approach, 2nd ed, pp 871–878. New York, Marcel Dekker, 1994

GROLL-HIRSCHOWITZ

Synonyms. Deafness—mesenteric diverticula—neuropathy. See Refsum.

Symptoms and Signs. In females. Onset at 3–24 years of age. Progressive deafness, normal vestibular function, peripheral sensory neuropathy, without trophic changes. Tachycardia; progressive impairment of digestive processes, steatorrhea (loss of gastric motility); diverticulosis.

Etiology. Autosomal recessive inheritance.

Pathology. Jejunoileal diverticula with ulceration. Peripheral nerves: demyelinization.

Diagnostic Procedures. *Feces.* Malabsorption with fat and protein loss. *Blood.* Hypocholesterolemia. *Electromyography. X-rays of intestine.* Diverticulosis of small bowel. *Electrocardiography. Biopsy.* Peripheral nerve: demyelinization.

Therapy. Symptomatic. Surgery.

Prognosis. Death in the end of second or third decade.

BIBLIOGRAPHY. Groll A, Hirschowitz BI: Steatorrhea and familial deafness in two siblings. Clin Res 14:47, 1966
Potasman I, Stermer E, Levy N, et al: The Groll-Hirschowitz syndrome. Clin Genet 28:76–79, 1985

GROSS-GROH-WEIPPL

Synonyms. Thrombocytopenia—radial aplasia; TAR.

Symptoms. Both sexes equally affected; present from birth.

Signs. Absence or hypoplasia of radius (usually bilateral). Frequent association of hypoplasia of ulna and hands or bones of the lower extremities. Tetraphocomelia in one case. Less frequent association of cardiac or renal defects; low stature; spina bifida and other bone involvement. Hemorrhagic tendency. Pallor out of proportion to blood loss.

Etiology. Unknown; probably, autosomal recessive inheritance.

Pathology. See Signs. Bone marrow. Absence (66%) or hypoplasia of megakaryocytes.

Diagnostic Procedures. *Blood.* Anemia out of proportion; white blood cells; leukemoid granulocytosis (62%); eosinophilia (53%). Thrombocytopenia and disorders of blood clotting secondary to platelet deficiency. *X-ray of skeleton.* See Signs. *Electrocardiography, heart catheterization, functional studies.* Different abnormalities possible.

Therapy. Corticosteroids have symptomatic action on hemorrhages, but do not affect thrombocytopenia. Orthopedic prosthesis.

Prognosis. Improvement of hematologic condition with advancing age.

BIBLIOGRAPHY. Gross H, Groh C, Weippl G: Kongenitale hypoplastische Thrombopenie mit Radialaplasie. Neue Osterr Zschr Kinderheilkd 1:574–582, 1956
Show S, Oliver RAM: Congenital hypoplastic thrombocytopenia with skeletal deformities in siblings. Blood 14:374–377, 1959
Gmyrek D, Otto FMG, Slym-Rapaport I: Über das familiare Auftreten von Fanconi-anamie und Thrombocytopenie mit Missbildungen (Bemerkungen zur Therapie der Fanconi-anaemie). Monatsschr Kinderheilkd 113:542–552, 1965
Ayane-Yeboa K, Jaramillo S, Nagel C, et al: Tetraphocomelia in the syndrome of thrombocytopenia with absent radii (TAR syndrome). Am J Med Genet 20:571–576, 1985
Donnenfeld AE, Wiseman B, Lavi E, et al: Prenatal diagnosis of thrombocytopenia absent radius syndrome by ultrasound and cordocentesis. Pren Diagn 10:29–35, 1990

GROSSHANS

Synonym. Cutaneous, amyloidpoikiloderma; poikiloderma, cutaneous, amyloid.

Symptoms and Signs. Two sisters affected; onset at 1 year of age.

Telangiectasia; skin atrophy; pigmentary poikiloderma-like alterations; at puberty, verrucous lesions on elbows and backs of feet and hands. Absence of cataract.

Etiology. Autosomal recessive inheritance proposed.

BIBLIOGRAPHY. Grosshans VE, Bergoend H, Khochnevis A: Die erbilichen Hand-amyloidosen: Die familiaere amyloide Poikilodermie. MMW 114:1183–1190, 1972

GROVER

Synonyms. Acantholytic, transient dermatosis; transient acantholytic dermatosis

Symptoms and Signs. Both sexes onset 40–50 years of age. In subjects with previous excessive exposure to sun. Eruption on the back or chest (extended successively to limbs) of mildly pruritic herpetiform papules and vesicles that erupt and crust.

Etiology. Unknown. Sun exposure?

Pathology. Typical acantolysis and clefting and vesicles within epidermis, round corps lacunae, and keratin plugs also may be observed.

Diagnostic Procedures. Skin biopsy.

Therapy. None significantly effective.

Prognosis. Self-limiting course within months from onset.

BIBLIOGRAPHY. Grover RW: Transient acantholytic dermatosias. Arch Dermatol 101:426–434, 1970
Pye RJ: Bullous eruptions. In Champion RH, Burton JL, Ebling FJG (eds): Rook/Wilkinson/Ebling Textbook of Dermatology, 5th ed, pp 1670–1671. Oxford, Blackwell Scientific, 1992

GRUND

Synonyms. Myokimia; myotonia; muscle atrophy; hyperhidrosis; neuromyotonia (misnomer). See Stiff-man.

Symptoms and Signs. Generalized or localized (shoulder or lower extremities) muscular stiffness with fine twitches (myokymia) and occasionally cramps accompanied by profuse sweating. Some patients do not manifest cramps, but rather an unusual sensitivity to stretching that is followed by rippling waves.

Etiology. Unknown. Distal motor neuropathy (?). Sporadic or autosomal dominant inheritance.

Diagnostic Procedures. *Blood.* Enzymes normal.

Therapy. Muscle stiffness reduced by phenytoin. Less consistent results with tocainide, or dantrolene.

Prognosis. Usually, recession after several years.

BIBLIOGRAPHY. Grund G: Ueber genetische Beziehungen zwischen Myotonie, Mustelkraempfen und Myokimie (Zugleich Beitrag zur Pathologie der neuralen Muskelatrophie). Dtsch Z Nervenheilk 146:3–14, 1938
Adams RD, Victor M: Principles of Neurology, 5th ed, p 1273. New York, McGraw-Hill, 1993

GRUNER-BERTOLOTTI

Combination of Parinaud (see) and von Monakow (see).

GUERIN

Eponym used to indicate a fracture of the maxilla.

BIBLIOGRAPHY. Guérin AF: Des fractures des maxillaires supérieures. Nouveau moyen de les reconnaitre dans les cas fréquents où elles ne l'accompagnent pas de déplacement. Arch Gen Med 2:5–13, 1866
Sabiston DC: Textbook of Surgery, 14th ed, p 288. Philadelphia, WB Saunders, 1991

GUERRY-COGAN

Synonyms. Cogan-Guerry; Cogan III; microcystic corneal dystrophy; corneal dystrophy, microcystic; map-out-fingerprint pattern.

Symptoms. Prevalent in middle-aged or elderly females, seldom in children. One or both eyes may be affected. Initially, vision not affected, then reduced according to degree of involvement of central cornea. Occasional pain.

Signs. Fine wavy lines (fingerprint-like) within corneal epithelium. In one third of cases recurrent epithelial erosions.

Etiology. Unknown. Probably nonspecific reaction to a variety of stimuli. Autosomal dominant inheritance reported.

Pathology. Intraepithelial cysts with pyknotic nuclei and debris. Basement membrane thickened or with multilaminar aspect (or both).

Diagnostic Procedures. *Binocular microscopy.* With retroillumination (see Signs). *Electromicroscopy.*

Therapy. None.

Prognosis. Progressive condition, eventually resulting in visual impairment.

BIBLIOGRAPHY. Guerry D: Fingerprint-like lines in the cornea. Am J Ophthalmol 33:724–726, 1950
Cogan DG, Donaldson DD, Kuwabara T, Marshall D: Microcystic dystrophy of the corneal epithelium. Trans Am Ophthalmol Soc 62:213–225, 1964
Werblin TP, Hirst LW, Stark WJ, et al: Prevalence of map-dot-fingerprint changes in the cornea. Br J Ophthalmol 65:401–409, 1981
Klintworth GK: Degenerations, depositions and miscellaneous reaction of the ocular anterior segment. In Garner A, Klintworth GK (eds): Pathobiology of Ocular Disease: A Dynamic Approach, 2nd ed, pp 771, 773. New York, Marcel Dekker, 1994

GUILLAIN-ALAJOUANINE-GARCIN

Synonyms. Garcin; Bertotti-Garcin; Hartmann; Schmincke tumor; unilateral cranial palsy; hemipolyneuropathy—cranial palsy; half base. See Foix I.

Symptoms and Signs. Hemilateral loss of function of all 12 cranial nerves. Primarily acoustic (VIII), glossopharyngeal (IX), vagus (X), spinal accessory (XI), and hypoglossal (XII). Seldom associated symptoms of pyramidal involvement or intracranial pressure.

Etiology and Pathology. Nasopharyngeal tumors; primary tumor of base of the skull; leukemic infiltrates (Schmincke) of basal meninges; trauma; metastases.

Diagnostic Procedures. *CT brain scan. MRI. X-ray. Blood. Bone marrow biopsy. Cerebrospinal fluid.* Normal or increased protein.

Therapy. According to etiology.

Prognosis. Poor; metastasis frequent.

BIBLIOGRAPHY. Guillain G, Alajonnaine R, Garcin R: Le syndrome paralitique unilateral global des nerfs cranieus. Bull Soc Med Hôp Paris 50:456–460, 1926
Garcin R: Le syndrome paralitique unilatèral global des nerfs cranieus. Paris (Thesis), 1927

Spiegal LA: Syndrome de Garcin–Unilateral total involvement of cranial nerves with report of one case. Ann Otol 52:706–712, 1943

Malin JP: Nervus facialis. In Schmidt D, Malin JP: Erkrankungen der Hirnnerven 2 auf. Stuttgart, Thieme, 1991

Adams RD, Victor M: Principles of Neurology, 5th ed, pp 1181–1182. New York, McGraw-Hill, 1993

GUILLAIN-BARRÉ

Synonyms. Guillain-Barré-Strohl; Glanzmann-Salaud; Kussmaul-Landry; Landry ascending paralysis; polyneuritis, acute, infective; radiculoneuropathy, postinfectious. Includes Fischer variant (ophthalmoplegia—ataxia—areflexia).

Symptoms. Affects all ages and both sexes. In 50% of cases, upper respiratory infection observed a few days or weeks before start of symptoms. Paresthesia; lower leg weakness initially (may begin in other part of body); progressive diffusion to trunk, upper extremities, neck, and cranial nerves. Pain in the back; muscle tenderness; mild stiffness of neck; fever (occasionally absent). Fischer variant: Frequently follows upper respiratory tract infection; acute external ophthalmoplegia, ataxia, hyporeflexia, occasionally also mild internal ophthalmoplegia.

Signs. Flaccid, atonic paralysis ascending (developing in hours or days [up to 7–10 days]). Motor involvement more evident than sensory involvement. Proximal muscles more prominently affected. Tendon reflexes decreased or absent. Plantar response absent. Lassègue sign present.

Etiology. Unknown; toxic, allergic, autoimmune mechanism. Observed following viral, bacterial, parasitic infections, leukemia and lymphoma, toxic condition, insect bite, surgery, vaccine injection.

Pathology. Early, fragmentation of cylinder axons in peripheral nerves, spinal ganglion, nerve roots. Later, inflammatory infiltrates and degeneration of medullary nerve sheaths.

Diagnostic Procedures. *Spinal fluid.* Increased proteins; normal or slightly elevated number of cells. *Blood.* Normal. Search for etiologic agent. *Serology.* Culture. Smears.

Therapy. Supportive; respirator necessary in some cases. Steroids are of no benefit; in severe cases (i.e., those requiring ventilation) plasmapheresis and immunosuppressants are indicated. Plasmapheresis.

Prognosis. The outcome has been graded as follows:

0. Healthy
1. Minor symptoms or signs
2. Able to walk 5 meters without help, walking frame or stick but unable to do manual work, including shopping or gardening
3. Able to walk 5 meters with help, walking frame, or stick
4. Chair or bed bound
5. Requiring assisted ventilation (for at least part of day or night)
6. Dead

Children seem to have a better prognosis than adults, and the need for ventilation is not necessarily to be considered a poor prognostic factor. Fisher variant usually benign with complete recovery.

BIBLIOGRAPHY. Landry JBO: Note sur la paralysie ascendante aigue. Gaz Hebd Med Chir 6:472–474; 486–488, 1859

Guillain G, Barré JA, Strohl A: Le réflexe médico-plantaire: Étude de ses caracteres graphiques et de son temps perdu. Bull Soc Med Hop Paris 40:1459–1462, 1915–1916

Fischer M: An unusual variant of acute idiopathic polyneuritis (syndrome of ophthalmoplegia, ataxia and areflexia). N Engl J Med 255:57–65, 1956

Cole GF, Matthew DJ: Prognosis in severe Guillain-Barré syndrome. Arch Dis Child 62:228–291, 1987

McKhann GM, Griffin JW, Cornblath DR, et al: Plasmapheresis and Guillain-Barré syndrome: Analysis of prognosis factors and the effects of plasmapheresis. Ann Neurol 23:347–353, 1988

Adams RD, Victor M: Principles of Neurology, 5th ed, pp 1126–1130. New York, McGraw-Hill, 1993

GUILLAIN-BERTRAND-LEREBOULLET

See Choreiform syndromes.

BIBLIOGRAPHY. Guillain G, Bertrand I, Lereboullet J: Myoclonies arythmiques unilaterales des membres par lésion du noyau dentlé du cervelet. Rev Neurol (Paris) 2:73–78, 1934

GULL

Synonyms. Adult myxedema; cachexia strumipriva. Includes myxedematous cachexia, adult myxedema.

Symptoms. Females more frequently affected than males; insidious onset in middle age. Decrease in sweating; cold hypersensitivity; decrease in activity; listlessness; lack of energy; easy fatigability. Mental dullness may follow or precede other symptoms. Progressive constipation; decrease of menstrual flow; deafness; thick speech; dizziness; headache may be another presenting symptom or follow in various orders. Decreased libido. In cases of more rapid onset (from surgery, radioiodine therapy), acute onset with the addition of anxiety or depression and severe skeletal symptoms.

Signs. Pallor; dry skin; falling hair; weight gain; facial puffiness. Pulse rate decreased; cardiomegaly; palpitations; muscles weak and flabby; arthropathy with effusion. Later; nonpitting edema (myxedema) remaining stable for years to end (if not treated) in myxedematous cachexia (intensification of described symptoms and signs).

Etiology. Autoimmune endemic iodine deficiency, genetic, iatrogenic infiltrative diseases, hypothalamic dysfunctions; Seabright-Bantam mechanism (see).

Pathology. *Thyroid.* Usually, dense fibrosis; infiltration by lymphocytes and plasma cells possible; follicle and active cells may persist in scattered fashion. *Pituitary.* Increase of gamma cells; decrease of acidophilic cells. *Skin.* Hyperkeratosis; plugging of sweat glands; edema; swelling and fraying of collagen fibers; deposition of intracellular material. *Muscles.* Edematous; swollen; pale. *Serous cavities.* Free fluid. *Brain.* Possibly; atrophy gliosis; foci of degeneration.

Diagnostic Procedures. *Metabolic rate.* Decreased. *Blood.* Free T3, T4, and protein-bound iodide reduced; 131I uptake reduced; thyroid-stimulating hormone (TSH) increased; antithyroid antibodies possibly increased; plasma creatinine phosphokinase, lactic dehydrogenase, uric acid, cholesterol increased. Anemia common. *ECG.* Low voltage; QT prolonged; T-wave abnormal.

Therapy. Thyroid or L-thyroxine per os.

Prognosis. Remission of all symptomatology and most of the body changes with treatment.

BIBLIOGRAPHY. Fagge CH: On sporadic cretinism occurring in England. Med Chir Trans 54:155, 1871

Gull WW: On a cretinoid state supervening in adult life in women. Trans Clin Soc 7:180–185, 1874

Utiger RD: Hypothyroidism. In De Groot LJ (ed): Endocrinology, 3rd ed, pp 752–768. Philadelphia, WB Saunders, 1995

GULLNER

Synonyms. Hypokalemia familial; hypokalemic alkalosis—renal tubulopathy.

Symptoms. Both sexes. From infancy. Weakness, muscle cramps, nausea, and intermittent vomiting. Normal blood pressure, in some cases asymptomatic.

Etiology. Unknown. Possibly autosomal recessive inheritance. Suggested abnormal magnesium metabolism as responsible for hypokalemia.

Pathology. *Kidney.* Changes in the proximal tubules: hypertrophy of basal membranes, intense staining of cells, pyknotic nuclei. *Juxtaglomerular apparatus, glomeruli, and distal tubule and Henle loops.* Normal.

Diagnostic Procedures. *Blood.* Inability to retain Na; elevated plasma K and renin levels or decreased plasma K levels. *Plasma.* Mg level normal. Hypokalemia corrected by Mg administration or high Na intake and triamterene. *Urine.* Prostaglandin increased.

Therapy. See Diagnostic Procedures. Hyperkalemia is corrected by Mg administration or high Na diet and triamterene.

BIBLIOGRAPHY. Potter WZ, Trygstad CW, Helmer OM, et al: Familial hypokalemia associated with renal interstitial fibrosis. Am J Med 57:971–977, 1974

Gullner HG, Gill JR Jr, Bartter FC, et al: A familial disorder with hypokalemic alkalosis hyperreninemia, aldosteronism, high urinary prostaglandins and normal pressure that is not Bartter's syndrome. Trans Assoc Am Phys 92:179–188, 1979

Gullner HG, Bartter FC, Gill JR Jr, et al: A sibship with hypokalemic alkalosis and renal proximal tubulopathy. Arch Intern Med 143:1534–1540, 1983

DuBose TD, Alpern RJ: Renal tubular acidosis. In Scriver CR, Beaudet AL, Sly WS, et al: The Metabolic and Molecular Bases of Inherited Disease, 7th ed, pp 3655–3689. New York, McGraw-Hill, 1995

GÜNTHER I

Synonyms. Congenital erythropoietic porphyria; photosensitive porphyria; CEP; uroporphyrinogen III synthetase deficiency.

Symptoms. No sex predominance; wide racial distribution; clinical onset at birth or during first year. (A milder form descibed with onset in adulthood.) Passage of red urine. This finding will persist showing considerable daily and seasonal variations. As exposure of the infant to sun increases, vesicular or bullous eruptions of areas exposed to sun appear (usually within first year); lesions heal slowly, leaving scars. Abdominal and neurologic symptoms absent. In some cases, poor somatic and mental development.

Signs. Acute manifestation (bullae) and scarring of different degrees of intensity, from mild to severely mutilating. Hypertrichosis (fine blond lanugo); slight chronic jaundice; erythrodontia (best visible with ultraviolet light). Splenomegaly (inconstant finding; variation in size during course of disease may occur). Normal blood pressure.

Etiology. Autosomal recessive inherited metabolic defect of porphyrin, with overproduction of porphyrin type I, confined to erythroid system. Autosomal recessive inheritance. Deficiency of uroporphyrogen III cosynthase activity that causes overproduction of porphyrin type I.

Diagnostic Procedures. *Blood.* Normochromic anemia seldom severe, intermittent in type; reticulocytes high; circulating normoblasts; decreased survival of an aliquot of red cell population. Deficiency of enzyme uroporphyrinogen III cosynthetase. *Bone marrow.* Erythroid hyperplasia; normoblasts may show central inclusion. Studies in unstained sample with fluorescent light microscope show intense fluorescence in one aliquot of nucleated red cell, maximal fluorescence in nuclear and perinuclear areas, and minor degree in some reticulocytes. *Urine.* Pale pink to deep red. Porphyrin type I dominating; small amount of porphyrin III: small amount of coproporphyrin. *Stool.* Large amount of coproporphyrin type I; only small amount of type III; increased fecal urobilinogen. *Amniotic cell culture* (for prenatal diagnosis). Deficiency of specific enzyme.

Therapy. Splenectomy (usually highly beneficial for hemolytic ane-

mia). Hypertransfusions of charcoal and cholestyramine to retard intestinal absoption of endogenous porphyrins; deferoxamine to decrease eventual iron overload. Avoid exposure to the sun; protect bullae from infection.

Prognosis. Following splenectomy, decrease of hemolytic process and of photosensitivity. Severe mutilation may result from scarring.

BIBLIOGRAPHY. Baumstark F: Zwei Pathologische Harnfarbstoffe. Arch Gesamte Physiol 9:568, 1984

Schultz JH: Ein fall von Pemphigus leprosus complicirt durch Lepra visceralis (thesis). Greifswald, 1874

Günther H: Die Hämatoporphyrie. Dtsch Arch Klin Med 105:89–146, 1911

Nordmann Y, Amram D, Deybach JC, et al: Coexistent hereditary coproporphyria and congenital erythropoietic porphyria (Gunter disease). J Inherit Metab Dis 13:687–691, 1990

Rank JM, Straka JG, Weimer MK, et al: Hematin therapy in late onset congenital erythropoietic porphyria. Br J Hematol 75:617–618, 1990

Lee GR: Porphyria. In Lee GR, Bithel TC, Foerster J, et al (eds): Wintrobe's Clinical Hematology, 9th ed, pp 1273–1276. Philadelphia, Lea & Febiger, 1993

GUSTATORY RHINORRHEA

Symptoms. Following parotid surgery or midface fracture: unilateral tearing, rhinorrhea, and sweating.

Etiology. Regeneration of damaged nerve fibers of lesser superficial petrosal nerve via the greater superficial petrosal nerve to the vidian nerve, spheropalatine ganglion, and long sphenopalatine nerve and finally to mucous gland.

BIBLIOGRAPHY. Doddie AW Jr, Guillamondegui OM, Byers RM: Gustatory rhinorrhea developing after radical parotidectomy: A new syndrome. Arch Otolaryngol 102:248–290, 1976

Stevens HE, Doyle PJ: Bilateral gustatory rhinorrhea following bilateral parotidectomy. A case report. J Othorynolaringol 17:191–193, 1988

Adams RD, Victor M: Principles of Neurology, 5th ed, pp 203–206. New York, McGraw-Hill, 1993

GUTIERREZ

Synonym. Horseshoe kidney.

Symptoms. Male to female ratio, 2:1. Frequently asymptomatic. Chronic gastrointestinal or urinary complaints (or both).

Signs. Hyperextension of body may elicit nausea and vomiting, signs that will be relieved by opposite movement (Rovsing signs).

Etiology. Congenital malformation: fusion of nephrogenic blastomas for mechanical reasons during fetal development.

Pathology. In great majority (90%) kidneys are fused on the inferior pole. Presence of solid mass (parenchymal fibrous) that joins the two kidneys across the midline.

Diagnostic Procedures. *Urography. Isotope scan. CT scan. Urine.* Variable changes in function. *Blood.* Features of chronic renal condition.

Therapy. Surgery according to entity of compression exerted on the ureters and technical feasibility of ureteral flow correction according to the associated malformation.

Prognosis. Variable.

BIBLIOGRAPHY. Gutierrez R: The clinical management of the horseshoe kidney. Am J Surg 15:132–165, 1932

Vaamonde CA, Oster JR: Renal involvement in heredofamilial and congenital disease. In Massry SG, Glassock RJ: Textbook of Nephrology, 3rd ed, p 886. Baltimore, Williams & Wilkins, 1995

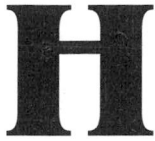

HAAB

Synonym. Macular retinal senile degeneration II. See age-related macular degeneration.

Symptoms. Onset in advanced age. Moderate decrease of visual function that usually remains fairly satisfactory for long time.

Signs. Bilateral, but usually asymmetric presence of drusen or small clumps of pigment or both; thickening of inner limiting membrane gives a "beaten bruise" aspect and gliotic glistening.

Etiology. Unknown; autosomal dominant inheritance suggested.

Pathology. See Signs. With evolution, destruction of cones.

Therapy. Symptomatic.

Prognosis. Benign course with fairly satisfactory vision for a long time; strong individual variability of speed of progression.

BIBLIOGRAPHY. Haab O: Erkrankungen der Macula Lutea Zentralbl Augenheilk 9:384–391, 1885
Garner A, Sarks S, Sarks JP: Degenerative and related disorders of the retina and choroid. In Garner A, Klintworth GK (eds): Pathobiology of Ocular Disease: A Dynamic Approach, 2nd ed, pp 631–632. New York, Marcel Dekker, 1994

HAAS

Synonym. Syndactyly type IV.

Symptoms and Signs. Syndactyly, complete and bilateral; six metacarpals and digits; fingers flexion. Teeth normal.

Etiology. Autosomal dominant inheritance.

Diagnostic Procedures. *X-ray.* Absence of bone fusion.

BIBLIOGRAPHY. Haas SL: Bilateral complete syndactylism of all fingers. Am J Surg 50:363–366, 1940
Gillesen-Kaesback G, Majevski F: Bilateral complete polysyndactyly (type IV Haas). Am J Med Genet 38:29–31, 1991

HABER

Synonym. Intraepidermal epithelioma; rosacea-like eruption.

Symptoms and Signs. Both sexes affected; onset in childhood. Rosacea-like eruption on the cheeks, nose, forehead, and chin. Erythema; telangiectasia; follicle papules; pitted areas. Later in life, appearance of warty lesions, scaly or keratotic (1 cm in diameter), not symmetric, on trunk and thighs.

Etiology. Unknown; autosomal dominant inheritance.

Pathology. Erythematous lesions: perivascular inflammation; fibrosis; acanthosis and parakeratosis; proliferation of sebaceous glands. Warty lesions: papillomatosis; acanthosis; dyskeratosis; mitotic figures.

Diagnostic Procedures. *Biopsy of skin.*

Therapy. For erythema, steroids. For warty lesions, X-ray treatment.

Prognosis. Good.

BIBLIOGRAPHY. Wilson HTH: Two cases of familial rosacea-like dermatosis with lanugo hair changes. Br J Dermatol 72:322, 1960
Sanderson KV, Wilson HTH: Haber's syndrome: Familial rosacea-like eruption with intraepithelial epithelioma. Br J Dermatol 77:1–8, 1965
MacKie RM: Epidermal skin tumors. In Champion RH, Burton JL, Ebling FJG (eds): Rook/Wilkinson/Ebling Textbook of Dermatology, 5th ed, pp 1468–1469. Oxford, Blackwell Scientific, 1992

HABITUATED HOARSENESS

Synonyms. Includes postoperative dysphonia.

Symptoms and Signs. Usually following acute episode of viral laryngitis, vocal cord surgery, or associated with reflux laryngitis (see esophageal reflux). Stable dysphonia or hoarseness persisting for months or years. Vocal fatigue and odynophonia are possibly related.

Etiology. Vocal misuse or abuse or lesion from surgery.

Diagnostic Procedures. *Laryngoscopy; frequency (pitch) analysis; waveform analysis; spectrography; laryngeal airway resistance.*

Therapy. Voice therapy. Refrain from smoking.

Prognosis. Over 50% of success from treatment.

BIBLIOGRAPHY. Koufman JA, Blalock PD: Functional voice disorders. Otolaryngol Clin N Am 24:1059–1073, 1991

HADEN

Obsolete. Hereditary nonspherocytic syndrome. See Enzymopathic hemolytic anemias.

BIBLIOGRAPHY. Haden RL: A new type of hereditary hemolytic jaundice spherocytosis. Am J Med Sci 214:255–259, 1947

HAENEL

Synonym. Ocular tabetic anesthesia.

Symptoms and Signs. Absence of pain on pressure applied on the eyes; associated with other symptoms of tabes dorsalis.

Etiology. Advanced stage of neurosyphilis.

BIBLIOGRAPHY. Haenel H: Eine neues Tabessymptom. Neurol Zentralbl 28:1199, 1909

HAFERKAMP

Synonyms. Gorham variant; hemoangiomatosis—malignant; osteolysis.

Symptoms and Signs. Related to generalized hemoangiomatosis and bone (incomplete) osteolysis (see Gorham).

Etiology. Unknown.

Pathology. Gorham syndrome plus a typical fatty degeneration of the tumor tissue and fatty infiltration of liver and kidney.

Diagnostic Procedures. *Blood.* Anemia; presence of immature cells, both erythroid and myeloid, in circulation. *X-ray.* See Gorham.

Therapy. Symptomatic.

Prognosis. Poor.

BIBLIOGRAPHY. Haferkamp O: Ueber das Syndrome generalisierte maligne Haemangiomatosis mit Osteolysis. Krebsforsch 64:418–426, 1962

Hardegger F, Simpson LA, Segmueller G: The syndrome of idiopathic osteolysis: classification, review and case report. J Bone Joint Surg 67B:89–93, 1985

HAFF*

Synonyms. Rhabdomyolysis; toxic myoglobinuria. Myoglobinuria following the ingestion of eel or fish poisoned by waste products of cellulose factory.

BIBLIOGRAPHY. Assmann H, Bielenstein H, Hobs H, et al: Beobachtungen and Untersuchungen bei der Haffkrankheit. Dtsch Med Wochenschr 59:122–126, 1933

Adams RD, Victor M: Principles of Neurology, 5th ed, p 1209. New York, McGraw-Hill, 1993

HAGEMAN FACTOR DEFICIENCY

Synonym. Factor XII deficiency.

Symptoms and Signs. Asymptomatic with few minor exceptions. Laboratory curiosity.

Etiology. Congenital deficiency of Hageman factor. Autosomal recessive inheritance. Families with autosomal dominant condition found.

Diagnostic Procedures. *Blood.* Normal bleeding time; prolonged clotting time; increased partial thromboplastin time corrected by absorbed plasma or aged serum; abnormal thromboplastin generation test when all reagents are from the patients; abnormal prothrombin consumption test; normal one-stage prothrombin time. *Radioimmunoassay of factor XII.* Lack of factor XII.

Therapy. None.

Prognosis. Excellent.

BIBLIOGRAPHY. Ratnoff OD, Colopy JE: Familial hemorrhagic trait associated with deficiency of clot-promoting fraction of plasma. J Clin Invest 34:602–613, 1955

Saito H, Ratnoff OD, Pensky J: Radioimmunoassay of human Hageman factor (factor XII). J Lab Clin Med 88:506, 1976

Bernardi F, Marchetti G, Volinia S, et al: A frequent factor XII gene mutation in Hageman trait. Human Genet 80:149–151, 1988

HAGLUND

Synonym. Calcaneus fracture. Eponym used to indicate a fracture of the nucleus calcaneus at the Achilles tendon insertion, without damage of cartilage or of the periostium. Occurs at a young age.

Etiology. Trauma, often preceding osteocondriotic lesions.

BIBLIOGRAPHY. Haglund P: Ueber Fractur des Epiphysenkerns des Calcaneus, nebst allgemeinen Bemerkungen über einige aehnliche juvenile Knochenkervverletzungen. Arch Klin Chir (Berlin) 82:922–930, 1907

Haglund P: Beitzag sur Klinik der Achillessehne. Z Orthop Chir 49:49–58, 1927

---

*From the name of a bay (Haff) in the area of Könisberg (Germany).

Perry JD: Sports medicine the clinical spectrum of injury. In Klippel JH, Dieppe PA: Rheumatology, p 5.21.8. St Louis, CV Mosby, 1995

HAILEY-HAILEY

Synonyms. Darier bullous variant; Gougerot; Hailey-Hailey; dyskeratosis bullosa hereditaria; pemphigus benign, familial.

Symptoms and Signs. Both sexes affected; high incidence among Jews. Onset usually with adolescence or early adulthood. Onset usually in hot, humid weather. Unilateral or bilateral lesions in zone of friction (neck, axillae, groin) and occasionally other areas (scalp, limbs). Recurrent eruption of cluster of small vesicles, first with clear fluid, becoming turbid; erythema of underlying skin, then breaking and crusting. Extending to periphery; center healing or moist vegetation.

Etiology. Unknown; unrelated to pemphigus vulgaris autosomal dominant inheritance with variable penetrance. A number of external stimuli precipitate manifestations.

Pathology. Similar to pemphigus vulgaris. Differences: (1) more extensive acantholysis; (2) less damage to acantholytic cells; (3) permanence of a few intercellular bridges.

Diagnostic Procedures. *Blood.* Circulating antibody to an intercellular cement substance (ICS). *Biopsy.* To differentiate histologically from Darier (see); presence of antibody to ICS (hallmark of the disease). *Bacteriologic examination.*

Therapy. Topical and systemic antibiotics. Cyclosporine. Topical steroids. Grenz rays. Excision and normal skin graft.

Prognosis. Spontaneous remission in cold weather. Chronic, recurrent condition. Long remission possible, becoming less severe at later age.

BIBLIOGRAPHY. Hailey H, Hailey H: Familial benign chronic pemphigus. Report of 13 cases in four generations of a family and report of 9 additional cases in 4 generations in a family. Arch Dermatol Syph 39:679–685, 1939

Gougerot H: La priorite du pemphigus chronique familial héréditaire benin. Ann Dermatol Syph 10:361–363, 1950

Alijotas J, Pedragosa R, Bosch J, et al: Prolonged remission after cyclosporine therapy in pemphigus vulgaris: Report of two young siblings. J Am Acad Derm 23:701–703, 1990

Burge SM, Millard PR, Wojnarowska F: Hailey-Hailey disease: A widespread abnormality of cell adhesion. Br J Dermatol 124:329–332, 1991

HAILEY-HAILEY, EPIDERMAL NEVUS

Synonyms. Acantolytic dermatosis, relapsing, linear; relapsing, linear acantholytic dermatosis.

Symptoms and Signs. Early onset. Epidermal nevus with well-defined linear erythematous plaques vesiculating, crusting, eroding (similar to Hailey-Hailey, see).

Etiology. Unknown.

Pathology. See Hailey-Hailey.

Prognosis. Spontaneous remissions and relapses.

BIBLIOGRAPHY. Vakilzadeh F, Kolde G: Relapsing linear acantholytic dermatosis. Br J Dermatol 112:349–355, 1985

HAIM-MUNK

Synonyms. Cochin Jewish; keratosis palmo plantaris—periodontopathia. See Keratoderma palmo-plantaris syndrome.

Symptoms and Signs. Inbred Jewish families from India and Indochina. Late onset palmo-plantar hyperkeratosis; progressive periodontal destruction; pes planus; recurrent skin infections; arachnodactyly.

Etiology. Autosomal recessive inheritance.

Diagnostic Procedures. *X-rays.* Tapering of phalangeal ends and claw-like volar curvature.

Therapy. Etretinate treatment.

BIBLIOGRAPHY. Haim S, Munk J: Keratosis palmo-plantaris congenita, with periodontosis, arachnodactyly and peculiar deformity of terminal phalanges. Br J Dermatol 77:42–54, 1965
Bergman R, Friedman-Birnbaum R: Papillon-Lefèvre syndrome: A study of the long-term clinical course, recurrent pyogenic infections and the effects of etretinate treatment. Br J Dermatol 119:731–736, 1988

HAIR-BRAIN

Synonyms. Amish brittle hair; brittle hair; intellectual impairment; decreased fertility; short stature; BIDS; Sabinas trichothiodystrophy. See Pollitt; and trichorrhexis nodosa.

Symptoms. Both sexes. Mild intellectual impairment; decreased fertility.

Signs. Short stature, brittle hair, nails break easily.

Etiology. Autosomal recessive inheritance. Possibly identical with Pollitt syndrome.

Pathology. *Hair.* Irregular grooved surface, lack of scales, reduction 50% of sulfur.

BIBLIOGRAPHY. Pollitt RJ, Jemer FA, Davis M: Sibs with mental and physical retardation and trichorrhexis nodosa with abnormal amino acid composition of hair. Arch Dis Child 43:211–216, 1968
King MD, Gummer CL, Stephenson JBP: Trichothiodystrophy-neurocutaneus syndrome of Pollitt: A report of two unrelated cases. J Med Genet 21:286–289, 1968
Jackson CE, Weiss L, Watson JHL: Brittle hair with short stature, intellectual impairment and decreased fertility: An autosomal recessive syndrome in Amish kindred. Pediatrics 54:201–212, 1974
Przedborski S, Ferster A, Goldman S, et al: Trichothiodystrophy, mental retardation, short stature, ataxia and gonadal dysfunction in three Moroccan siblings. Am J Med Genet 35:566–573, 1990

HAIRY ELBOWS

Synonyms. Hypertrichosis cubiti.

Symptoms and Signs. After birth. Hypertrichosis of the elbows.

Etiology. Unknown. Type of inheritance uncertain.

Prognosis. Increases up to 5 years of age then slowly regresses.

BIBLIOGRAPHY. Beighton P: Familial hypertrichosis cubiti: Hairy elbows syndrome. J Med Genet 7:158–160, 1970

HAJDU-CHENEY

Synonyms. Cheney; acro-osteolysis; osteoporosis; skull changes; arthrodento-osteodysplasia; dentoarthro-osteodysplasia; osteoarthro-dentodysplasia.

Symptoms. Both sexes affected; onset in early teens to sixth decade. Severe backache; occasionally, headache.

Signs. Both sexes. Short stature. Acro-osteolysis. Hypoplasia of terminal phalanges: short fingers and toes. Delayed closure of cranial sutures. Mild hypoplasia of mandibular ramus. Protuberance of occipital bone. In adult life, collapse of vertebral bodies with progressive loss of height.

Bone fractures from minor traumas. Early loss of teeth; lax joints; deep voice.

Etiology. Unknown; autosomal dominant inheritance.

Pathology. Generalized osteoporosis. Pseudosteolysis, disorder of development rather than destruction of tissue already formed. Multiple wormian bones and mast cells in affected tissues. Multiple fractures.

Diagnostic Procedures. *X-ray of skeleton. MR imaging.* Decalcification of bone; cranial changes; enlargement of sella turcica; basilar impression; spine; density of intervertebral disk greater than that of bones. *Blood.* Calcium, phosphorus, alkaline phosphatase normal or occasionally elevated; beta-glucoronidase elevated.

Therapy. Symptomatic.

Prognosis. Progressive alterations, mostly osteoporosis. Progressive loss of height. Fracture prone.

BIBLIOGRAPHY. Hajdu N, Kauntze R: Cranio-skeletal dysplasia. Br J Radiol 21:42–48, 1948
Van den Houten BR, Ten-Kate LP, Gerding JC: The Hajdu-Cheney syndrome: a review of literature and report of three cases. Int J Oral Surg 14:113–125, 1985
Udell J, Schumacher HR Jr, Kaplan F: Idiopathic familial acroosteolysis: Histomorphometric study of bone and literature review of the Hajdu-Cheney syndrome. Arthr Rheum 29:1032–1038, 1986
Kawamura J, Miki Y, Yamazaki S, et al: Hajdu-Cheney syndrome: MR imaging Neuroradiology 33:441–442, 1991

HALBAN

Synonyms. Secondary amenorrhea; persistent corpus luteum; functional ovarian disturbance.

Symptoms. Appears in young women. Amenorrhea, occasionally following cycles of decreasing frequency.

Signs. Absence of objective evidence of pregnancy.

Etiology. Benign tumor of the ovary with persistence of the corpus luteum activity. One of the many functional ovary disturbances responsible for secondary amenorrhea.

Diagnostic Procedures. Pregnancy test. Hormonal studies.

Therapy. Excision of tumor.

Prognosis. Good.

BIBLIOGRAPHY. Ascheim S, Varangot J: Verkante schwangershaft. Arch Gynecol 183:275–280, 1953
Kenigsberg Rosenwaks Z, Hodgen G: Ovarian follicular maturation, ovulation and ovulation induction. In De Groot LJ (ed): Endocrinology, 3rd ed, pp 2031–2045. Philadelphia, WB Saunders, 1995

HALF-AND-HALF NAIL

Synonym. Azotemic onychopathy.

Symptoms. Those of chronic nephropathy with hyperazotemia (25 cases of 1500 present nail findings).

Signs. Fingernail beds with red, pink brown, transverse, distal band, occupying at least 20–60% of nail length and with the remaining nail showing a dull, whitish aspect. Constriction of venous return does not affect the contrast between two zones. Lack of tendency of the pattern to grow out with the nail. No correlation between severity of azotemia and nail change.

Etiology. Unknown. This type of onychopathy observed in 20–40% of chronic hyperazotemic conditions; occasionally, in cases with cylindruria without azotemia. Association is also possible with liver cirrhosis (as an extension of the Terry syndrome).

Pathology. Chronic nephropathies. Pathology of onychopathy unknown.

Diagnostic Procedures. *Blood.* Determination of blood urea nitrogen in all patients exhibiting this type of onychopathy. Decreased creatinine clearance.

Therapy and Prognosis. That of chronic nephropathy.

BIBLIOGRAPHY. Bean WB: A discourse on nail growth and unusual fingernails. Trans Am Clin Climatol Assoc 74:152–167, 1963

Lindsay PG: The half and half nail. Arch Intern Med 119:583–587, 1967

Dawber RPR, Baran R: Disorders of the nails. In Champion RH, Burton JL, Ebling FJG (eds): Rook/Wilkinson/Ebling Textbook of Dermatology, 5th ed, p 2529. Oxford, Blackwell Scientific, 1992

HALL

Synonym. Anemic pseudohydrocephalus. Old eponym used to indicate a pseudohydrocephalic condition resulting from severe exhaustion or cachexia.

BIBLIOGRAPHY. Hall H: An Essay on a Hydrocephaloid Affection in Infants Arising from Exhaustion. London, Sherwood, 1836

HALLERMANN-DOERING

Synonyms. Band keropathy; deafness.

Symptoms and Signs. In senior individuals band keropathy (primary ribbon-like corneal degeneration, deafness).

Etiology. Unknown. Possibly autosomal dominant inheritance.

Diagnostic Procedures. *Blood.* Calcemia normal, reduction of calcium turnover.

BIBLIOGRAPHY. Hallermannn W, Doering P: Primaere bandfoermige Hornhautdegeneration, Schwrhoerigkeit und gestoerter Calciumsatz-ein hereditairer Symptomcomplex. Ber Dtsch Ophthal Ges 65:285–288, 1964

HALLERMANN-STREIFF

Synonyms. Audry I; Ullrich-Fremerey-Dohna; Fremerey-Dohna; François II; dyscephalia oculomandibularis-hypotrichosis; mandibulo-ocular dyscephaliahypotrichosis.

Symptoms and Signs. Affects both sexes equally. Teeth may be present at birth. Localized alopecia; beaked nose; microcornea; congenital cataracts with spontaneous rupture and absorption; occasionally, glaucoma. Proportionate nanism; atrophy of skin; retardation of psychomotor development.

Etiology. Unknown; sporadic occurrence, no chromosomal abnormalities detected. Both autosomal recessive and dominant inheritance considered (possible pseudodominance in apparently dominant cases).

Pathology. See Symptoms and Signs.

Diagnostic Procedures. *X-ray.* Reveals most distinctive features in the mandible: hypoplasia of rami; anterior displacement of temporomandibular joints. Condyles may be completely absent. Skull, brachycephalic, delayed closure of fontanelles. Face small; small orbits; gracile appearance of tubular bones.

Therapy. Surgical correcton of deformities.

Prognosis. Lesions may lead to respiratory insufficiency and cardiac complications up to failure and death in early infancy or childhood.

BIBLIOGRAPHY. Audry C: Variété singulière l'alopécie congenitale. Alopécie suturale. Ann Dermatol Syph 4:899–900, 1893

Hallermann W: Vogelgesicht und Cataracta congenita. Klin Monatsbl Augenheilkd 113:315–318, 1948

Streiff EB: Dysmorphie mandibulo faciale (tete d'oiseau) et alterations oculaires. Ophthalmologica 120:79–83, 1950

Ullrich O, Fremerey-Donna H: Dyskephalie mit Cataracta congenita und Hypotrichose als typischer Merkmalskomplex. Ophthalmologica 125:73, 1953

François J: A new syndrome. Dyscephala with birth face and dental anomalies, nanism, hypotrichosis, cutaneous atrophy, microphthalmia, and congenital cataract. Arch Ophth 60:842, 1958

Scharoff A, Eppley BL: Evaluation and surgical correction of the facial skeletal deformity in Hallermann-Streiff syndrome. Int J Oral Maxillofac Surg 16:738–744, 1987

Cohen MM Jr: Hallerman-Streiff syndrome: A review. Am J Med Genet 41:488–499, 1991

HALLERVORDEN

Synonyms. Poser dysmyelinating leukodystrophy; simple orthochromatic leukodystropy; see Pelizaeus-Merzbacher and Cockayne.

Symptoms and Signs. Rather heterogeneous group; age of onset varies greatly. Onset most frequently from first month to 15 years of age. Variable and aspecific. Neurologic and mental symptoms and signs of progressive loss of vision and speech, then hearing, down to decerebration.

Etiology. Unknown; possibly congenital. Autosomal recessive (?).

Pathology. Characterization of this syndrome is essentially on pathologic features. Central nervous system: no inflammation (except for simple reabsorption reaction); diffuse myelin disintegration, however, not excessively pronounced; large number of sudanophilic cells scattered throughout and not concentrated perivascularly; no metachromatic granules; nerve cells and axis well preserved.

Diagnostic Procedures. Rule out metachromatic leukodystrophy (see).

Therapy. Symptomatic.

Prognosis. Slow, progressive evolution.

BIBLIOGRAPHY. Hallervorden J: Die degenerative diffuse Sklerose. In Lubarsch O, Henke F, Rossle R (eds): Handbuch der speciellen pathologischen Anatomie und Histologie, vol 13, pp 716–782. Berlin, Springer-Verlag, 1957

Pfeiffer J: Differentiation of various types of leukodystrophies. World Neurol 3:580–601, 1962

Adams RD, Victor M: Principles of Neurology, 5th ed, pp 841–842. New York, McGraw-Hill, 1993

HALLERVORDEN-SPATZ

Synonyms. Globus pallidus pigmentary degeneration; pallidal degeneration, progressive; neuroaxonal dystrophy, late infantile. See Seitelberger and Schindler type I.

Symptoms. Onset at approximately 10 years of age. Gradually increasing stiffness of all extremities; dysarthria; dysphagia; cerebellar ataxia; visual impairment to blindness, mental deterioration, occasionally hyperkinesis.

Signs. Inversion of feet. Retinitis pigmentosa occasionally observed. Pigmentary changes of the skin; muscle atrophy.

Etiology. Autosomal recessive inheritance (some unrelated cases recorded). Considered one form of iron storage disease. The dopamine-neuromelanine system may be involved in the basic pathogenesis.

Pathology. Basal ganglia (occasionally also of the cortex) demyelination and less demyelination of nerve cells; deposit of iron in the globus pallidus and substantia nigra, in ganglion cells, and interstitial tissue.

Diagnostic Procedures. *X-ray of skull. CT scan. MRI. Electromyography.*

Therapy. Nonspecific. Symptomatic. Slight effect from L-dopa; chelating agents useless.

Prognosis. Progressive; death 10–20 years after onset of symptoms.

BIBLIOGRAPHY. Hallervorden J, Spatz H: Eigenartige Erkrankung im extrapyramidalen System mit besonderer Beteiligung des Globus pallidus und der Substantia nigra; ein Beitrag zu den Beziehungen zwischen diesen beiden Zentren. Z Neurol Psychiatr 79:254–302, 1922
Jankovic J, Kirkpatrick JB, Blonquist KA, et al: Late onset Hallervorden-Spatz disease presenting as familial parkinsonism. Neurology 35:227–234, 1985
Adams RD, Victor M: Principles of Neurology, 5th ed, pp 835–837. New York, McGraw-Hill, 1993

HALLGREN

Synonyms. Deafness—ataxia—pigmentary degeneration—mental abnormalities.

Symptoms and Signs. In Sweden frequency 3/100,000. Congenital deafness; visual impairment (nyctalopia, visual field restriction, nystagmus, etc., from primary pigmentary degeneration); gait disturbance, vestibulo-cerebellar type, seizures; mental deficiency; psychosis (25%).

Etiology. Autosomal recessive inheritance.

Diagnostic Procedures. *Blood. Urine. Cerebrospinal fluid.* Normal.

BIBLIOGRAPHY. Hallgren B: Retinitis pigmentosa combined with congenital deafness with vestibulo-cerebellar ataxia, and mental abnormality in a proportion of cases: A clinical and genetico-statistical study. Acta Psychiatr Scand 34:(Suppl) 138, 1959
Botermans CHG: Primary pigmentary retinal degeneration and its association with neurological diseases. In Vinken PJ, Bruyn GW: Handbook of Clinical Neurology, vol 13, pp 320–321. Amsterdam, North-Holland, 1972

HALLOPEAU I

Synonyms. Csilloag; von Zambusch; Zambusch guttate morphea; guttate scleroderma; lichen planus sclerosis atrophicus; white spot.

Symptoms. Prevalent in females (6:7.1); onset at any age, usually around menopause (average age in females 50, males 43). Soreness; pruritus; dyspareunia; mouth ulceration; asymptomatic skin lesions.

Signs. Skin eruption of small whitish round papules and macules, slightly raised; seldom bullae; horny plugs. Later; atrophy, wrinkling, and depression of skin involved. Lesions affect mostly trunk, neck, flexor areas. In females affect vulva, perineal areas, anus; whitish irritation; atrophy produces shrinkage of vulva and reduces vaginal introitus. In males, balanitis xerotica obliterans. Similar lesions in oral mucosa as described in the preceding.

Etiology. Unknown; hormonal factor may precipitate collagen disease; possibly, autoimmune type of reaction.

Pathology. Hyalinization of dermal collagen; thickening hyperkeratosis; dilation of capillaries. Secondary inflammatory changes.

Diagnostic Procedures. *Biopsy.* Immunoglobulins, complement, and fibrin in damaged skin.

Therapy. No effective treatment. Bland cream and corticosteroids. Excision of areas of leukoplakia.

Prognosis. Chronic condition; possibly spontaneous remission (especially in girls after puberty). Severe atrophy of vulva usually results.

BIBLIOGRAPHY. Hallopeau H: Du lichen plan, et particuliérement de sa forme atrophique. Union Méd 43:729–733, 1887
Rowell NR, Goodfield MJD: The connective tissue diseases. In Champion RH, Burton JL, Ebling FJG (eds): Rook/Wilkinson/Ebling Textbook of Dermatology, 5th ed, pp 2269–2271. Oxford, Blackwell Scientific, 1992

HALLOPEAU II

Synonyms. Hallopeau-Leredde; pemphigus vegetans (Hallopeau variety); pyodermite vegetante.

Symptoms and Signs. Both sexes affected; onset in middle age. Formation of pustules (not bullae) followed by warty vegetations that spread peripherally with erosions. Flexure zones most frequently affected. Mouth erosion frequent.

Etiology. Unknown; considered as a benign variant of pemphigus.

Pathology. Nonspecific granulomas with abscess formation and pseudoepitheliomatous hyperplasia; acanthosis; little hyperkeratosis.

Diagnostic Procedures. *Biopsy.* Positive intercellular immunofluorescence. *Blood.* Circulating antibodies to intercellular substance.

Therapy. Corticosteroids.

Prognosis. Chronic benign course of many years' duration. Spontaneous remissions; also complete healing.

BIBLIOGRAPHY. Hallopeau H: Nouvelle not sur la dermatose bulleuse hereditaire et traumatique. Arch Dermatol Syph 45:323–328, 1898
Pye RJ: Bullous eruptions. In Champion RH, Burton JL, Ebling FJG (eds): Rook/Wilkinson/Ebling Textbook of Dermatology, 5th ed, p 1647. Oxford, Blackwell Scientific, 1992

HALLOPEAU-SIEMENS

Synonyms. Polydysplastic epidermolysis bullosa; epidermolysis bullosa polydysplastic, recessive, generalized, dystrophic.

Symptoms and Signs. Both sexes affected, onset at birth or early infancy; especially later. Large, flaccid bullae developing spontaneously on any part of skin surface. Bullae heal, leaving scar and miliary cysts. Pseudowebbing may develop between fingers and toes. Mucosae frequently involved; tongue mobility may be limited by scarring, esophagous mucosa may be involved and strictures develop. Malformation of teeth and nail frequent. Hair may be sparse and alopecia develops. Physical and mental development impaired.

Etiology. Unknown; autosomal recessive inheritance. Increased and altered synthesis of immunoreactive skin collagenase. The lethal form is now considered on a histologic basis (electron microscopy) as a different entity, although clinically they overlap significantly.

Pathology. *Light microscopy.* Bullae in the upper dermal components attached to roof of blister. *Immunofluorescence study.* Antibodies pemphigoid antigen basement membrane in the roof blister. *Electron microscopy.* Dissolution of collagen fibrils (dermolysis).

Diagnostic Procedures. *Biopsy.* Of skin. *Electroencephalography.* May show abnormalities.

Therapy. Symptomatic; antibiotics; steroids.

Prognosis. Very poor; carcinoma frequently develops from scars in the skin and mucosae.

BIBLIOGRAPHY. Hallopeau FM: Sur une dermatose bulleuse infantile avec cicatrices indélébiles, kystes epidermiques et manifestations buccales. Ann Derrmatol Syph (Paris) 1:414, 1890
Gedde-Dahl T Jr: Epidermolysis bullosa: A clinical, genetic and epidemiological study. Universitetsforlaget Oslo. Baltimore, Johns Hopkins Press, 1971

Winberg JO, Gedde-Dahl T Jr, Bauer EA: Collagenase expression in the skin fibroblasts from families with recessive dysthrophic epidermolysis bullosa. J Invest Dematol 92:82–85, 1989

Hovnanian A, Duquesnoy P, Amselem S, et al: Exclusion linkage between the collagenase gene and generalized recessive dystrophic epidermolysis bullosa phenotype. J Clin Invest 88:1716–1721, 1991

HALL-RIGGS

Synonym. Mental retardation of Hall-Riggs.

Symptoms. From birth, both sexes. Sudden episodes of vomiting during infancy; severe mental retardation; lack of development of speech; retarded growth.

Signs. Microcephaly; depressed nasal bridge, anteverted nostrils, large lips; scoliosis; short limbs.

Etiology. Autosomal recessive inheritance.

Diagnostic Procedures. *X-ray of skeleton.* Flat femoral head and neck of femorus; flat epiphyses in the fingers and at the ankle.

BIBLIOGRAPHY. Hall BD, Riggs FD: A new familial metabolic disorder with progressive osseous changes, microcephaly, coarse severe mental retardation. Birth Defects Orig Art Ser XI (5):79–90, 1975

HAMMAN

Synonym. Mediastinal emphysema; emphysema, mediastinal.

Symptoms. Dyspnea; retrosternal pain accentuated on breathing; mediastinal crepitation noticed by patient.

Signs. Tachypnea; occasionally, subcutaneous emphysema of neck and upper thorax; cyanosis; hyperresonancy of chest; typical popping sounds synchronous with heart beat.

Etiology. Trauma; spontaneous from rupture of alveolus; secondary to air passage from various source (e.g., tracheostomy; trachea or esophagus perforation; retroperitoneal space); from rupture of viscus or diagnostic procedures (e.g., pneumoperitoneum; perineal air insufflation).

Diagnostic Procedures. *X-ray.* Streaks of radiolucency on lateral edges of mediastinum; outline of heart and major vessels.

Therapy. When needed, surgery.

Prognosis. Good. Spontaneous resolution in days if the air is removed.

BIBLIOGRAPHY. Hamman L: Spontaneous mediastinal emphysema. Bull Johns Hopkins Hosp 64:1–21, 1939

Fraser RS, Paré JAP, Fraser RG, Paré PD: Synopsis of Disease of the Chest, 2nd ed. Philadelphia, WB Saunders, 1994

HAMMAN-RICH

Synonym. See Idiopathic pulmonary fibrosis. This eponym is still used to indicate idiopathic pulmonary fibrosis and arthritis; but the original cases described by the authors are cases of organizing diffuse ear damage or cryptogenic organizing pneumonitis (see Bronchiolitis obliterans, idiopathic).

BIBLIOGRAPHY. Hamman L, Rich AR: Fulminating diffuse interstitial fibrosis of the lung. Trans Am Clin Climatol Assoc 51:154–163, 1935

Katzenstein ALA, Myers JL, Mazur MT: Acute interstitial pneumonia: A clinicopathologic ultrastructural, and cell kinetic study. Am J Surg Pathol 10:256–267, 1986

HAND-FOOT

Synonym. See Herrick.

Symptoms and Signs. Occurs in infants with sickle cell disease. Painful, symmetric (usually) swelling of hands and feet, persisting for 1–4 weeks, accompanied by fever.

Etiology. Unusual manifestation in Herrick syndrome (rare in the United States; more frequent in Africa). Report of hand-foot syndrome in Salmonella osteomyelitis and Herrick syndrome and in streptococcal infection without sickle cell disease.

Pathology. Metacarpals, metatarsals, and phalanges are thought to be infarcted by multiple small capillary red cell blocks in sickling crisis.

Diagnostic Procedures. *Blood.* Electrophoresis of hemoglobin: SS or SC pattern. Anemia; sickling phenomena; leukocytosis during attack. *X-rays. MRI or Scintigraphic techniques.* Destruction of involved bones; subperiosteal new bone formation.

Therapy. Analgesics.

Prognosis. Spontaneous recovery within 1–4 weeks. Attacks may recur until the patient reaches the age of 3 years.

BIBLIOGRAPHY. Danford EA, Marr R, Elsey EC: Sickle cell anemia, with unusual bone changes. Am J Roentgen 45:223–226, 1941

Koren A, Garty I, Katzuni E: Bone infarction in children with sickle cell disease: early diagnosis and differential from osteomyelitis. Eur J Pediatr 142:93, 1984

Lukens JN, Hemoglobinopathies S, C, D, E, and O and associated diseases. In Lee GR, Bithel TC, Foerster J, et al (eds): Wintrobe's Clinical Hematology, 9th ed, p 1069. Philadelphia, Lea & Febiger, 1993

HAND, FOOT, AND MOUTH

Synonyms. Exanthem—vesicularstomatitis—summer-term blains.

Symptoms. Especially affects children and farmers and people in contact with livestock. Incubation period 3–10 days. No distress or mild illness; painful stomatitis, fever; malaise; anorexia; diarrhea; sore throat.

Signs. Vesicular rash restricted to hands and feet. Oral enanthema or round or ovoid ulcers on mucosa, uvula, tonsillar pillars, tongue. Occasionally, hepatosplenomegaly and cervical lymphadenopathy.

Etiology. Coxsackie virus infection (Group A type 16 or B type or enterovirus).

Pathology. Gray vesicles on erythematous bases; some break. In the mouth, small ulcerative lesions. Histology: spongiosis, intraepithelial splits, necrosis of keratocytes.

Diagnostic Procedures. *Throat and rectal swabs. Blood. Fluid.* For isolation and identification of virus. *Serology.* During disease and convalescence. *Cytologic study.* With scrapings from lesions.

Therapy. Symptomatic.

Prognosis. Complete recovery, usually in 7 days.

BIBLIOGRAPHY. Robinson CR, Doane FW, Rhodes AJ: Report of an outbreak of febrile illness with pharyngeal lesions and exanthem: Toronto, Summer 1957: Isolation of group A coxsackie virus. Can Med Assoc J 79:615–621, 1958

Cherry JD, John CL: Hand, foot, and mouth syndrome: Report of six cases due to coxsackie virus, Group A type 16. Pediatrics 37:637–643, 1966

Highet AS, Kurtz J: Viral infections. In Champion RH, Burton JL, Ebling FJG (eds): Rook/Wilkinson/Ebling Textbook of Dermatology, 5th ed, pp 942–943. Oxford, Blackwell Scientific, 1992

HAND-FOOT-UTERUS

Synonym: HFU.

Symptoms. Present from birth.

Signs. *Hands.* Normal size or moderately smaller; moderate degree of clinodactyly of fifth finger; hypoplasia of thenar eminence; thumb incompletely rotated and in some cases angulated outward. No upper limb involvement. *Feet.* Markedly small; great toe short. *Urogenital tract.* Duplication of uterus; in some cases, associated with double cervix or subseptate vagina.

Etiology. Unknown; autosomal dominant inheritance. Full penetrance and variable expression.

Diagnostic Procedures. *X-rays of hands and feet.* Short first metacarpal (75%); pointed phalanx of thumb; clinodactyly of fifth finger; unusual fusion of wrist bones; short first metatarsal; in toe same changes as thumb; short calcaneus; seldom tarsal or middle-distal phalangeal bone fusion. *Hysterosalpingography.* See Pathology. *Chromosome studies.* Negative. *Dermatoglyphic studies.* Distal placed axial triradius; absence of pattern in thenar and hypothenar areas. Thumbs show low arches, no whorls or radial loops on the fingers; total ridge count reduced.

Therapy. Plastic surgery for genital malformation.

Prognosis. Good quoad vitam. Higher than normal incidence of stillbirth and of perinatal death.

BIBLIOGRAPHY. Stern AM, Gall JC, Perry BI, et al: The hand-foot-uterus syndrome. J Pediatr 77:109–116, 1970
Halal F: The hand-foot-genital (hand foot-uterus) syndrome: Family report and update. Am J Med Genet 30:793–803, 1988

HAND-SCHÜLLER-CHRISTIAN

Synonyms. Christian; Schüller-Christian; Hand-Rowland; Langerhans cell histiocytosis; craniohypophyseal xanthoma; xanthomatous granuloma; lipoid histiocytosis; lipoid granuloma; multifocal eosinophilic bone granuloma; nonlipoid reticuloendotheliosis; reticuloendothelial granuloma; xanthomatosis. See histiocytosis syndromes.

Symptoms. Both sexes affected (males slight predominance); onset mostly in children; may occur in young adults; seldom in elderly persons. Onset frequently with otitis media or externa; less frequently, with diabetes insipidus. Intermittent low-grade fever, occasionally. Seborrheic dermatitis of scalp, chest, neck, shoulders, occasionally becoming hemorrhagic. Lung involvement may be perihilar, central, or diffuse. Pulmonary fibrosis, honeycombing of the lungs, alveolocapillary block, cor pulmonale, and right heart failure are possible complications.

Signs. Lymphadenopathy; occasionally hepatomegaly; rarely, exophthalmos; rarely, splenomegaly.

Etiology. Unknown.

Pathology. Skeletal lytic lesions and visceral lesions. Proliferation of histiocytes in masses; vesicular nuclei, lobulated with phagocytic material. Rarely mitoses; large number of eosinophil aggregates, occasionally with necrotic changes. Foam cells; vacuolated histiocytes with sudanophilic material.

Diagnostic Procedures. *X-ray.* Osteolytic lesions with sharp borders (more frequently on ribs, femora, pelvic bones, skull). *Blood.* Anemia; normal cholesterol; changes due to diabetes insipidus (when present). *Biopsy of lesions.*

Therapy. Curettement or small doses of X-ray therapy to localized lesion. For widespread lesions: methotrexate, vinca alkaloids, corticotropin, adrenal steroids, cyclophosphamide, or nitrogen mustard. Etoposide appears as one of the most active agents and with minor toxicity. Allogenic bone marrow transplantation with recurrent progressive form.

Prognosis. Good response to treatment. Survival from onset variable from months to decades.

BIBLIOGRAPHY. Hand A Jr: Polyuria and tuberculosis. Arch Pediatr 10:673–675, 1893
Christian HA: Defects in membranous bones, exophthalmos, and diabetes insipidus: An unusual syndrome of dyspituitarism. Med Clin N Am 3:849–871, 1920
Hand A: Defects of membranous bones, exophthalmos and polyuria in childhood. Am J Med Sci 162:509, 1921
Schüller A: Dysostosis hypophysaria. Br J Radiol 31:156–158, 1926
Lukens JN: Langerhans cell histiocytosis. In Lee GR, Bithel TC, Foerster J, et al (eds): Wintrobe's Clinical Hematology, 9th ed, p 1643. Philadelphia, Lea & Febiger, 1993

HANEY-FALLS

Synonym. Keratoconus congenital posticus circumscriptus.

Symptoms. Mental retardation; stunted growth; visual alterations.

Signs. Sharply localized increase in curvature of posterior corneal surface; corneal nebulae; myopic astigmatism; corneal endothelial precipitate; mild hypertelorism; broad flat nose; upward displacement of lateral canthi; brachydactyly; ptergyium colli; barrel chest. Reported associated with congenital hip dislocation and as an occasional feature of mongolism. Keratoconus is also a feature of amaurosis congenita.

Etiology. Unknown; autosomal or (more likely) recessive inheritance reported.

Prognosis. Good quoad vitam.

BIBLIOGRAPHY. Van der Hoeve: Vererbbarkeit des Keratokonus Z Augenheilk 52:321–336, 1924
Butler TH: Keratoconus posticus. Trans Ophthalmol Soc UK 50:551–556, 1930
Haney WP, Falls HF: The occurrence of congenital keratoconus posticus circumscriptus in two siblings presenting a previously unrecognized syndrome. Am J Ophthalmol 52:57, 1961
Nucci P, Brancato R: Keratoconus and congenital hip dysplasia. Am J Ophthalmol 111:775–776, 1991
Klintworth GK: Degenerations, depositions and miscellaneous reaction of the ocular anterior segment. In Garner A, Klintworth GK (eds): Pathobiology of Ocular Disease: A Dynamic Approach, 2nd ed, pp 761–762. New York, Marcel Dekker, 1994

HANGMAN FRACTURE

Synonyms. Judicial hanging; spondylolisthesis, traumatic. See dashboard.

Symptoms and Signs. Tetraplegia. Marked retropharyngeal swelling, mechanical inability to swallow or breathe.

Etiology. Violent submental jerk, thrusting the head suddenly backward and snapping the arch of axis.

Diagnostic Procedures. *X-ray. CT scan. MRI.* Spondylolisthesis C2, C3, and damage of cord. Bilateral fracture of neural arch of axis, with detachment of the body of C3.

Therapy. Tracheotomy. Orthopedic immobilization.

Prognosis. If patient survives, neurological damage may be permanent or may regress.

BIBLIOGRAPHY. Wood JF: The ideal lesion produced by judicial hanging. Lancet 1:53, 1913
Schneider RCA, Livingstone KA, Cave JE, et a:l "Hangman fracture" of the cervical spine. J Neurosurg 22:141, 1965

Weiss MH, Kaufman: Hangman's fracture in an infant. Am J Dis Child 126:268–269, 1973

Brackman R, Penning L: Injuries of cervical spine. In Vinken PJ, Bruyn GW: Handbook of Clinical Neurology, vol 25, pp 326–329. Amsterdam, North-Holland, 1976

HANHART SYNDROMES

Synonyms. Hanhart dwarfism; Richner-Hanhart type IV; mandibular dysostosis-peromelia. See Gilford-Burnier. Part of a spectrum: The Oromantibular-limb hypogenesis syndromes.

TYPE I

Symptoms. Affect closely inbred group of people in Switzerland and one Adriatic island (Veglia); both sexes equally affected. Normal infancy and early childhood. Between 1e1/2 and 6 years of age growth retardation becomes evident that in following years results in a slow proportionate growth. Diminished or absent libido. Occasionally, mental retardation.

Signs. Typical facies; occasionally brachycephaly. Absence of secondary sexual characteristics. Adipose tissue hyperplasia on breast and abdominal regions; late development of gonads and of secondary sexual characteristics.

TYPE II

Onset from birth. Type I signs plus micrognathia hypoglossia, peromelia, and missing teeth.

TYPE III

Characterized by peromelia, micrognathia hypoglossia. Cleft palate, mental retardation (brain microgyrus); occasionally, symptoms related to kidney, genital, and uterine defects.

TYPE IV

Hyperkeratosis of palms and soles; anhydrosis; multiple lipoma in subcutaneous tissue (Richner). Excessive tears; photophobia; dendroid lesions of cornea. Periodontia; hypotrichosis. Absence of fingers and toes. Micrognathia. Mental retardation.

Etiology. Type I autosomal recessive inheritance. Multiple pituitary hormone deficiency. Types II–IV, non-Mendelian development disturbance.

Pathology. Absence of particular features; delayed epiphyseal closure.

Diagnostic Procedures. *Hormonal studies.* Growth hormone deficiency; adrenocorticotropic hormone or thyrotropic hormone deficiency or both. Protein-bound iodine level progressively falling. *X-rays.* Delayed closure of epiphyses.

Therapy. Correction of hormonal deficiency. Growth hormone, adrenocorticotropic, thyroid-stimulating hormone.

Prognosis. Good with treatment. If not treated, dwarfism with normal life expectancy.

BIBLIOGRAPHY. Hanhart E: Ueber heredodegenerativen Zwergwuchs mit Dystrophia adiposo-genitals und Hand von Untersuchungen bei drei Sippen von proportionierten Zwergen. Arch Julius Klaus 1:181–257, 1925

Richner H: Hornhaul affection bei Keratoma palmare et plantare hereditarium. Klin Monatsbl Augenheilkd 100:580–588, 1938

Hanhart E: Neuse Sonderformen von Keratosis palmoplantaris, u. a. eine regelmäss g-dominanten mit systematisierten Lipomen, ferner 2 einfach-rezessive mit Schwachsinn und Z. T. mit Hornhautveränderungen des Auges (Ektadermal syndrome). Dermatologica 94:286–308, 1947

Garner LD, Bixler D: Micrognathia, an associated defect of Hanhart's syndrome Types II and III. Oral Surg 27:601–606, 1969

Bokesoy I, Aksuyck C, Deniz E: Oromandibular limb hypogenesis, Hanhart's syndrome: Possible drug influence on the malformation. Clin Genet 24:47–49, 1983

Bar M: Amelia-splenogonadal fusion and Hanart syndrome: The same or different conditions? Proc Greenwood Genet Ctr: 180–181, 1987

HANOT

Synonyms. Cholangitis destructive, chronic nonsuppurative; primary biliary cirrhosis; hypertrophic primary cirrhosis; hypertrophic primary liver; cirrhosis hypertrophic primary.

Symptoms. Prevalent in middle-aged, elderly females; insidious onset (asymptomatic in 30% of diagnosed cases). Intense itching; steatorrhea; good general condition progressing to malnutrition, melena; coma.

Signs. Jaundice (72%); skin pigmentation (21%); palmar erythema (29%); spider angiomas (21%); xanthomas (31%); generalized lymphadenopathy; hepatomegaly (99%); moderate splenomegaly (50%); ascites (4%).

Etiology. An autoimmune disorder trigger unknown; considered infectious hepatitis, drug toxicity (chlorpromazine; methyl testosterone; arsenic preparations).

Pathology. Periportal inflammation and fibrosis; intracanalicular biliary obstruction; later, cirrhosis with granulation on periphery of lobules. Disruption of lobular pattern.

Diagnostic Procedures. *Blood.* Increased bilirubin, alkaline phosphatase level, lipid, globulins. Circulating antibodies against cells rich in mitochondria. *Urine.* Dark urobilinogen and biliary pigments increased. *Stool.* Discolored; increase in fatty acids. *X-rays.* Absence of extrahepatic obstruction; later osteomalacia. *Ultrasonography. Liver biopsy. Laparoscopy. Arteriography.*

Therapy. Correct malabsorption; fat-soluble vitamins; cholestyramine against pruritus; treatment of complication (portal hypertension; bleeding). Liver transplantation. Of partial utility and limited in time utilization. Corticosteroids; colchicine; cyclosporine; methotrexate, urusniol.

Prognosis. Death in approximately 10 years from onset of symptoms, survival of 20 years reported. Good results with transplantation.

BIBLIOGRAPHY. Addison T, Gull W: On a certain affection of the skin-vitiligo-idea alpha plana, beta tuberosa. Guys Hosp Rep 7(ser2):265–276, 1851

Virchow R: Ein Fall von Varix anastomoticus zwischen V. lienalis and azygos. Verh Physic-Med Ges Wuerzburg 7:21, 1857

Hanot V: Étude sur une forme de cirrhose hypertrophique du foie (cirrhose hypertrophique avec ictere chronique) (thesis). Paris, Medical Classic, 1875

Sherlock S: Primary biliary cirrhosis (chronic intrahepatic obstructive jaundice). Gastroenterology 37:574–586, 1959

Bodenheimer HC Jr: Primary biliary cirrhosis. In Haubrich WS, Schaffner F, Berk JE (eds): Bockus Gastroenterology, 5th ed, vol 2, pp 2276–2302. Philadelphia, WB Saunders, 1995

HANOT-ROESSLE

Obsolete.

Synonyms. Intrahepatic cholangitis; cholangitis lenta. See cholagitis, primary sclerosis and Charcot biliary fever.

Symptoms and Signs. Fever; jaundice; pruritus.

Etiology and Pathology. Intrahepatic suppurative cholangitis without extrahepatic duct cholangitis (Cholangitis lenta).

Diagnostic Procedures. *Blood.* Hyperbilirubinemia; sodium sulfobromophthalein retention; increase of enzymes; leukocytosis. *Urine.* Biliary pigments; hyperbilirubinemia. *Liver scan.*

Therapy. Antibiotics. Elimination of underlying causes of cholestasis.

Prognosis. With modern treatments this entity has almost disappeared.

BIBLIOGRAPHY. Albot G, Kopandji M: La cholangiolite obstructive ou course des cholangites diffuses non oblitérantes ou maladie de Hanot-Roessle. Semin Hôp 38:3213–3231, 1962
Wright R, Alberti KGMM, Karran S, et al: Liver and Biliary Disease, p 299. London, WB Saunders, 1979

HANSEN (K.B.)

Synonyms. Neutropenia autoimmune, autoimmune neutropenia.

Symptoms and Signs. Recurrent or persistent infections.

Etiology. Still confused group of a conditions characterized by presence of factors (autoimmune type) able to agglutinate otherwise normal leukocytes in the plasma.

Diagnostic Procedures. *Blood.* Elevated level of immunoglobulins: Positivity of various leukoagglutinin tests. *Bone marrow.* Variable pattern. Usually cellular with variable scarceness of mature neutrophils.

Therapy. Corticosteroids. Antibiotics according to need.

Prognosis. Variable.

BIBLIOGRAPHY. Hansen KB: Immunologic agranulocytosis? Acta Med Scand 145:169, 1953
Athens JW: Neutropenia. In Lee GR, Bithel TC, Foerster J, et al (eds): Wintrobe's Clinical Hematology, 9th ed, p 1603. Philadelphia, Lea & Febiger, 1993

HAPPLE

Synonyms. Chondrodysplasia punctata; X-linked recessive mosaic features consistent with lyonization I.

Symptoms and Signs. Higher ratio of female to males. Short stature; hypoplasia of distal phalanges; small nasal airway. Cerebral involvement. During early life severe respiratory distress, erythematous skin changes and striated ichthyosiform hyperkeratosis. Later patterned ichthyosis follicular atrophoderma, coarse, dull hair, and cicatricial alopecia.

Etiology. X-linked recessive inheritance. Steroid sulfatase deficiency?

Pathology. Chondrodysplasia punctata.

Diagnostic Procedures. *X-rays.*

Therapy. Symptomatic.

Prognosis. From cases stillborn to normal life span with persistence of specific features.

BIBLIOGRAPHY. Happle R. Matthas H-H. Macher E: Sex-linked chondtodysplasia punctata? Clin Genet 11:73–76, 1977
Ballabio A, Zollo M, Carrozzo R, et al: Deletion of the distal short arm of the X chromosome (Xp) in a patient with short stature, chondrodysplasia punctata, and X-linked ichthyosis due to steroid sulfatase deficiency. Am J Med Genet 41:184–187, 1991

HARADA

Now considered part of the Vogt-Koyanagi-Harada syndrome (see). Initially typified by retinal separation and absent or low-grade anterior uveal involvement. The poliosis and alopecia occasionally present in the Harada syndrome were considered as invariable features of the Vogt-Koyanagi syndrome.

BIBLIOGRAPHY. Harada E: Clinical study of nonsuppurative choroiditis: A report of acute diffuse choroiditis. Acta Soc Ophthalmol Japn 30:356, 1926

HARBITZ

Synonyms. Alveolar microlithiasis; pulmonary alveolar microlithiasis; microlithiasis alveolar.

Symptoms. Affects all races in familial form; found more often in females, but equal sex distribution in sporadic cases. Onset insidious in western countries at 30–50 years of age, in Japan at 6–9 years of age. Paucisymptomatic; moderate exertional dyspnea; late symptoms of cor pulmonale.

Signs. Right ventricular hypertrophy.

Etiology. Several etiologic factors and idiopathic forms; among them: (1) Familial form with suggestion of autosomal and recessive types of inheritance; (2) exposure to dust rich in calcium salt. This condition may result from alteration of unknown nature of alveolar lining membrane that predisposes to local calcification.

Pathology. Intra-alveolar calcific free deposits (microliths). No histologic abnormalities in alveolar membranes and capillaries.

Diagnostic Procedures. *Blood.* Moderate polycythemia may develop. *Calcium metabolism studies normal. Pulmonary function tests.* Decrease of alveolar ventilation; arterial hypoxia; lung volume reduced. *X-ray.* Typical radiologic pattern with numerous diffuse calcifications.

Therapy. Symptomatic.

Prognosis. Good; slow progressive course; cor pulmonale develops late.

BIBLIOGRAPHY. Harbitz F: Extensive calcification of the lungs as a distinct disease. Arch Intern Med 21:139, 1918
O'Neill RP, Cohn JE, Pellegrino ED: Pulmonary alveolar microlithiasis: A family study. Ann Intern Med 67:957–967, 1967
Prakash UBS, Barham SS, Rosenaw EC III, et al: Pulmonary alveolar microlithiasis: A review including ultrastructural and pulmonary function studies. Mayo Clin Proc 58:290–300, 1983
Fraser RS, Paré JAP, Fraser RG, Paré PD: Synopsis of Diseases of the Chest, 2nd ed. Philadelphia, WB Saunders, 1994

HARD-WATER

Synonym. Extracorporeal dialysis; hypercalcemia.

Symptoms and Signs. Onset during or after hemodialysis. Nausea; vomiting; warm skin; extreme weakness; lethargy; blood pressure changes. Occasionally, clotting within the arteriovenous cannula.

Etiology. Occurs when water softening process is abruptly discontinued while hemodialysis is being performed.

Diagnostic Procedures. *Blood.* Calcium and magnesium elevation. Analysis of water used for dialysis.

Prognosis. Good since the simultaneous increase of calcium and magnesium in plasma reciprocally neutralizes their pharmacologic effects.

BIBLIOGRAPHY. Freeman RM, Lawton RL, Chamberlain MA: Hard water syndrome. N Engl J Med 276:113–118, 1967
Schulten HK, Sieberth HG, Deck KA, et al: Das akute Hypercalcämiesyndrom als Dialysezwischenfall. Dtsch Med Wochenschr 93:387–340, 1968
Weatherall DJ, Ledingham JGG, Warrell DA (eds): Oxford Textbook of Medicine, 3rd ed, p 2316. Oxford, Oxford Med Pub 1996

HARE EYE

Synonyms. Gallop; frontofacionasal.

Symptoms and Signs. *Head.* Brachycephaly, bilateral blepharophymosis; widow's picking, ptosis, bilateral lower lid lagophthalmos, inability to close the eyes completely (hare eye); coloboma upper lid, bilateral cleft lip and palate, severe midface hypoplasia.

Etiology. Autosomal recessive inheritance.

BIBLIOGRAPHY. Gallop TR: Fronto-facio-nasal dystosis: A new autosomal recessive syndrome (letter). Am J Med Genet 10:409–412, 1981
Gallop TR, Kiota MM, Martins RMM, et al: Fronto-facio-nasal dysplasia evidence for autosomal recessive inheritance. Am J Med Genet 19:301–305, 1984

HARJOLA-MARABLE

Synonyms. Marable; celiac axis; celiac axis compression; median arcuate ligament; arcuate ligament. See Abdominal angina.

Symptoms. More frequent in young women. Epigastric crampy pain beginning 30 minutes to 4 hours after eating, not related to type of food. Moderate relief from knee-chest position. Occasionally, nausea, vomiting, diarrhea, eructation, flatulence.

Etiology and Pathology. External compression of celiac axis during its passage through the aortic hiatus by the median arcuate ligament.

Diagnostic Procedures. *X-ray.* Of gastrointestinal tract. *Angiography.*

Therapy. Incision of fibrous tissue of the anterior portion of aortic hiatus of diaphragm compressing celiac axis.

Prognosis. Following surgery, initial relief from symptoms in 83% of cases, but only 41% remained pain-free when followed for 3–11 years.

BIBLIOGRAPHY. Harjola PT: A rare obstruction of the celiac artery. Ann Chirur Gynecol Fenniae 52:547–549, 1963
Marable SA, Kaplan MF, Berman FM, et al: Celiac compression syndrome. Am J Surg 115:97–102, 1966
Jamieson CW: Celiac axis compression syndrome. Br J Med 193:159–160, 1986
Rogers AI, David S: Intestinal blood flow and diseases of vascular impairment. In Haubrich WS, Schaffner F, Berk JE (eds): Bockus Gastroenterology, 5th ed, pp 1231–1232. Philadelphia, WB Saunders, 1995

HARKAVY

Obsolete.

Synonym. Kussmaul-Maier variant.

Symptoms and Signs. Asthmatic crises associated with the symptoms of Kussmaul-Maier (see).

BIBLIOGRAPHY. Harkavy J: Vascular allergy. Pathogenesis of bronchial asthma with recurrent pulmonary infiltration and eosinophilic polyserositis. Arch Intern Med 67:709–734, 1941

HARLEQUIN COLOR CHANGE

Synonyms. Particolored infant; particolored baby.

Symptoms. None.

Signs. Reddening of one side of the body and blanching of the other half. Clear demarcation between the two halves from forehead through midline to legs (one red, one blanched).

Etiology. Unknown condition of no pathologic significance, caused by gravity (reddening and blanching revert with turning the infant from one side to the other).

Pathology. Unknown.

Prognosis. Color change lasts from a few minutes to hours; disappears no later than 3 weeks from birth; if still present beyond fourth week, possibly associated to hypoxia caused by cardiovascular defects.

BIBLIOGRAPHY. Neligan GA, Strang LB: "Harlequin" colour change in newborn. Lancet 2:1005–1007, 1952
Atherton DJ: The neonate. In Champion RH, Burton JL, Ebling FJG (eds): Rook/Wilkinson/Ebling Textbook of Dermatology, 5th ed, p 3884. Oxford, Blackwell Scientific, 1992

HARLEQUIN FETUS

Synonyms. Riecke type I and II ichthyosis congenita; ichthyosis congenita harlequin fetus. Keratoma malignum; see Collodion baby.

Symptoms and Signs. (1) Ichthyosis fetalis. At birth (often premature) encased in thickened skin (white armor). Difficulty in breathing and swallowing. Majority die in 3–4 days. (2) Ichthyosiform erythroderma. Present at birth or onset in first days of life, occasionally later. Generalized erythema; thickening of skin; scaling; crusting; edema; various degrees of severity from limited erythema to half of the body to encasing total body. Hair normal, hypertricosis, or alopecia. Nails normal.

Etiology. Unknown; autosomal recessive inheritance. Three phenotypes.

Keratine 6 and 16	Profilaggrin	Interfollicular epidermis
Type 1	Absent	Present
Type 2	Present	Present
Type 3	Present	Absent

Pathology. Skin thickening of all layers, increased mitotic rate, perivascular lymphocytic infiltrates. Early formation of clumps and perinuclear shells caused by an abnormal arrangement of tonofibrils (fibrillar structural proteins): Abnormal diffraction pattern of horn material points to a cross-beta-protein structure.

Diagnostic Procedures. *Skin biopsy.* See Pathology.

Therapy. Corticosteriods; antibiotics; careful nursing. Etretinate.

Prognosis. Extremely variable from death in first few days, to survival with circumscribed zones of hyperkeratosis, erythema, scaling, or return to normal skin after initial exfoliation.

BIBLIOGRAPHY. Seeligmann E: De Epidermis Imprimis Neonatorum Desquamatione. Inaugural Dissertation, Berlin, 1841
Thomson MS, Wakeley CPG: The harlequin fetus. J Obstet Gynecol Br Comm 28:190–203, 1921
Arnold ML, Lamprecht I: Problems in prenatal diagnosis of the ichthyosis congenita group. Hum Genet 71:301–311, 1985
Lawlor F: Progress of an harlequin fetus to nonbullous ichthyosiform erythroderma. Pediatrics 82:870–873, 1988
Griffiths WAD, Leigh IM, Marks R: Disorders of keratinization. In Champion RH, Burton JL, Ebling FJG (eds): Rook/Wilkinson/Ebling Textbook of Dermatology, 5th ed, pp 1333–1334. Oxford, Blackwell Scientific, 1992

HARRIS (S.)

Synonyms. Hyperinsulinoma; reactive, functional hypoglycemia; see McQuarrie. Neonatal hypoglycemic, Rabson-Mendeenhall and insulin autoimmune hypoglycemia.

Symptoms and Signs. Occurs at all ages, in both sexes during the course of wide variety of diseases and is the presenting sign of many other syndromes. Increasing nervousness; tachycardia; flushing; sweating; hunger (epinephrine response); headache; visual disturbances; twitching; thick speech; transitory hemiplegia; seizures (cerebral response). Personality alterations: negativism; maniacal behavior (psychiatric response).

Etiology and Pathology. Mutations in insulin receptor gene. *Organic.* Alteration of organs involved in keeping normal glucose level. Pancreatic and extrapancreatic tumors; hepatic diseases; endocrine diseases, toxic and metabolic conditions. *Functional.* When organic causes for hypoglycemia cannot be established.

Diagnostic Procedures. *Blood.* Determination of glucose level in blood; usually below 40 mg/100 ml during attack. *Provocative tests.* Prolonged fasting; tolbutamide (Orinase) tolerance tests. *Insulin assay.* Also, all tests indicated in different syndromes with hypoglycemia for differential diagnosis. It must be remembered that hypoglycemic symptoms may occur in presence of normal blood glucose concentration and in some individuals without symptoms, low glucose level may be found. *Pancreas selective arteriography. CT scan. MRI brain scan. Ultrasonography.*

Therapy. During attack; administration of glucose by mouth or intravenously; corticosteroids. Multiple feedings to prevent attack. Specific treatment according to diagnosis.

Prognosis. Depends on etiology.

BIBLIOGRAPHY. Harris S: Hyperinsulinism and dysinsulinism. JAMA 83:729–733, 1924
Taylor SI: Diabetes mellitus. In Scriver CR, Beaudet AL, Sly WS, et al: The Metabolic and Molecular Bases of Inherited Disease, 7th ed, pp 847–849. New York, McGraw-Hill, 1995
Service FJ: Hypoglycemia, including hypoglycemia in neonates and children. In Haubrich WS, Schaffner F, Berk JE (eds): Bockus Gastroenterology, 5th ed, vol 2, pp 1605–1623. Philadelphia, WB Saunders, 1995

HARTNUP

Synonyms. Hart; aminoaciduria—pellagra—cerebellar ataxia; H disease; tryptophan pyrrolase deficiency.

Symptoms. Intermittent and variable. From "disorders" without disease to itching rash on areas exposed to light from February to October. Headache; intermittent ataxia; pains in abdomen, chest, and extremities; emotional lability (crying spells); mental retardation; fainting attacks; psychotic reactions.

Signs. Skin thickened and scaling, hyperpigmented where exposed to light. Hair dry and hair of different color intermingled with normal hair. Nystagmus; deep tendon reflexes hyperactive; ataxic gait.

Etiology. Monogenic transport defect with polygenic and environmental factors; interaction of amino acid metabolism, in particular of defective tryptophan. Attacks precipitated by light exposure, drugs (sulfonamides), psychological stress, and inadequate or irregular diet. Autosomal recessive transmission. Genetic heterogeneity. At least two forms defined: (1) classic, with defect expressed in intestine and kidney; and (2) variant, with defect expressed only in kidney.

Pathology. Skin, pellagra-like lesions.

Diagnostic Procedures. *Blood.* Normal; glucose tolerance test followed by hypoglycemia after normal curve in some cases. Low concentration of amino acids. *Urine.* Normal at routine examination. Urinary chromatogram, aminoaciduria of renal origin with characteristic H-pattern. *Tryptophan loading test and neomycin and tryptophan loading test. Electroencephalography.* Altered in some cases. *Neuroimaging.*

Therapy. Nicotinamide and vitamin B complex. High protein diet.

Prognosis. Symptoms become milder with age, but without treatment mental deterioration may occur. Treatment effective for all symptoms except for aminoaciduria.

BIBLIOGRAPHY. Baron DN, Deut CE, Harris H, et al: Hereditary pellagralike skin rash with temporary cerebellar ataxia, constant renal aminoaciduria and other bizarre chemical features. Lancet II:421–428, 1956
Halvorsen K, Halvorsen S: Hartnup disease. Pediatrics 31:29–38, 1963
Scriver CR, Mahon B, Levy HL, et al. The Hartnup phenotype: Mendelian transport disorder, multifactorial disease. Am J Med Genet 40:401–412, 1987
Levy HL: Hartnup disorder. In Scriver CR, Beaudet AL, Sly WS, et al: The Metabolic and Molecular Bases of Inherited Disease, 7th ed, pp 3635–3639. New York, McGraw-Hill, 1995

HARTUNG

Synonyms. Hartung; epilepsy Hartung. See Myoclonic epilepsy; M.E.R.R.F.

Symptoms and Signs. From birth, those of Unverricht (see).

Etiology. Multiple etiology: X-linked and autosomal recessive. Virus, bacterial infections. Degenerative, toxic, or metabolic disorders.

Pathology. Brain diffuse atrophy, absence of Lafora bodies (see).

Therapy. Phenytoin.

Prognosis. Progressive evolution.

BIBLIOGRAPHY. Hartung E: Zwei Faelle von Paramyoclonus multiplex mit Epilesie. Z Ges Psychiatr 56:150–153, 1920
Vogel F, Hafner H, Diebald K: Zur Genetik der progressiven Myoklonusepilepsien (Unverricht-Lundberg). Humangenetik 1:437–475, 1965
Winkler TF, von Reutern GM, Ropers HH: Progressive myoclonus epilepsy: A variant with probable X-linked inheritance. Hum Genet 49:83–89, 1979
Adams RD, Victor M: Principles of Neurology, 5th ed, pp 90–91. New York, McGraw-Hill, 1993

HARVEY

Symptoms and Signs. Both sexes. From childhood. Fever, periodic attacks with loss of consciousness, followed by athetosis, hypotonia, absent tendon reflexes, usually upon awakening. Babinski sign positive. Mental retardation. Manifestations progress only after each febrile period and are stable between attacks.

Etiology. Unknown. Hereditary?

Pathology. Not available.

Diagnostic Procedures. *Spinal fluid. Blood. Urine.* Normal. *EEG.* High amplitude, synchronous, bilateral delta activity during febrile attacks, returning to normal in the interperiods.

Therapy. Symptomatic.

Prognosis. Progressive deterioration reching homogeneity of clinical pattern by age 4–5.

BIBLIOGRAPHY. Harvey CC, Haworth JC, Lorber J: A new hereditofamilial neurological syndrome. Arch Dis Child 30:338–344, 1955
Goetz CG: Harvey syndrome. In Vinken PJ, Bruyn GW: Handbook of Clinical Neurology, vol 42, pp 222–224. Amsterdam, North-Holland, 1981

HASHIMOTO

Synonyms. Lymphadenoid goiter; chronic lymphadenoid; struma lymphomatosa; chronic lymphocytic thyroiditis; autoimmune thyroiditis.

Symptoms. Incidence in females 15–20 times higher than in males; onset at any age; highest incidence 30–50 years of age. Initially, asymptomatic or vague discomfort in the neck; seldom, dysphagia or dyspnea. Periodic paralysis reported.

Signs. Gradual enlargement of thyroid, followed initially (in nearly 20% of cases) by signs of mild hypothyroidism and then by myxedema (see Gull). In 25% of cases, musculoskeletal symptoms and rheumatoid arthritis.

Etiology. Autoimmune reaction. Supported autosomal dominant inheritance defect in hormonogenesis; "forbidden clone" theory; abnormal exposure to thyroid antigens. Autosomal dominant inheritance observed in some families, possibly on the same basis of other autoimmune conditions (see Polymyalgia rheumatica, Horton, Lupus erythematosus, Addison-Biermer, etc.).

Pathology. Thyroid symmetric, rubbery consistency, pinkish to yellow color, nonadherent to perithyroid structures. Parenchymal atrophy; lymphoid infiltration and fibrosis; colloidal space reduced; colloid absent. Typically, all of the gland is involved.

Diagnostic Procedures. *Basal metabolic rate.* Normal or decreased. *Blood.* Thyroxine (T4) from low to high; free thyroxine iodide (FTI) normal or reduced; butanol, extractable iodine increased; antithyroid globulin diagnostic elevation. *Biopsy.* See Pathology. *Fluorescent thyroid scan.* High diagnostic value.

Therapy. None if situation is stable. Thyroid hormone useful, especially in early treatment of young person. Seldom, surgery may be considered. Cortisone of doubtful long-term utility.

Prognosis. Relatively benign condition; from long-term asymptomatic condition to severe, rapidly evolving hypothyroidism, associated more or less with other possible autoimmune conditions.

BIBLIOGRAPHY. Hashimoto H: Zur Kenntnis der lymphomatösen Verärderung der Schilddrüse (Strauma lymphomatosa). Arch Klin Chir 97:219–248, 1912
Leung AKC: Familial "hashitoxic" periodic paralysis. J Roy Soc Med 78:638–640, 1985
Hamburger JI: The various presentations of thyroiditis: Diagnostic considerations. Ann Int Med 104:219–224, 1986
Shuper A, LeathemT, Pertzelan A, et al: Familial Hashimoto's thyroiditis with kidney impairment. Arch Dis Child 62:811–814, 1987

HASHIMOTO-PRITZKER

Synonyms. Self-healing reticulohistiocytosis; reticulohistiocytosis, self-healing. See Langerhans cell histiocytosis.

Symptoms and Signs. Clinical and hematologic finding present at birth or developing a few days after. Pea-sized mobile nodules of dark brownish-blue color spreading over a period of two days on the face, scalp, trunk, and extremities; jaundice-hepatomegaly. No splenomegaly or lymphadenopathy.

Etiology. Unknown.

Diagnostic Procedures. *Blood.* Moderate anemia and thrombocytopenia; leukocytes normal range; lymphocytosis with atypical form. Hyperbilirubinemia, SGOT, SGPT increased. *X-ray.* Normal. *Bone marrow.* No specific pattern, few atypical cells. Surgical biopsy of nodules. Infiltrate of large lymphocytes and histiocytes. Histiocytes occasionally multinucleated with glassy eosinophilic cytoplasm or foamy cytoplasm and mitotic figures; PAS positive material. *CT scan. MRI.*

Prognosis. Self-healing within 1 month with complete recovery.

BIBLIOGRAPHY. Hashimoto K, Pritzker MS: Electron microscopy study of reticulohistiocytoma: An unusual case of congenital self-healing reticulohistiocytosis. Arch Derm 107:263–270, 1973

Hashimoto K, Griffin D, Kohsbaki M: Self-healing reticulohistiocytosis: A clinical, histologic and ultrastructural study of a fourth case in the literature. Cancer 49:331–337, 1982
Lukens JN: Langerhans cell histiocytosis. In Lee GR, Bithel TC, Foerster J, et al (eds): Wintrobe's Clinical Hematology, 9th ed, pp 1644–1645. Philadelphia, Lea & Febiger, 1993

HAVERHILL FEVER

Symptoms and Signs. Both sexes affected; onset at all ages. Abrupt onset. Fever; rubella-like rash on extremities; polyarthritis.

Etiology. Haverhillia multiformis (Streptobacillus). After rat bite or drinking contaminated milk.

Diagnostic Procedures. *Blood and synovial fluid.* Culture for demonstration of Streptobacillus. Specific agglutinin also found.

Therapy. Penicillin; streptomycin; tetracyclines.

Prognosis. Arthritis and functional joint limitation may last months.

BIBLIOGRAPHY. Willner O, Place EH, Sutton LE: Erythema arthriticum, epidemicum: Preliminary report. Med Surj J 194:285–287, 1926
Schmidt FR: Unusual features and special types of infectious arthritis. In Hollander JL, McCarty DJ: Arthritis and Allied Conditions, 8th ed, p 1268. Philadelphia, Lea & Febiger, 1972
Weatherall DJ, Ledingham JGG, Warrell DA (eds): Oxford Textbook of Medicine, 3rd ed, pp 687–688. Oxford, Oxford Med Pub, 1996

HAWKINSINURIA

Synonyms. Hawkin* disease.

Symptoms and Signs. Very rare condition. Both sexes (identical severity). Following weaning from breast milk: metabolic acidosis and failure to thrive, irritability, tachypnea; unusual body odor, "smell of swimming pool." Hepatomegaly. In one patient hemolytic anemia, in another microcephaly. Symptoms recede from administration of breast milk or other low-protein foods and vitamin C supplementation. Several asymptomatic members of family described, presenting same biochemical defect.

Etiology. Autosomal dominant inheritance (possible but unlike X-linked). Metabolic defect leading to accumulation and excretion of an abnormal metabolite of tyrosine the 2-L-cysteine-S-yl-1, 4-dihydroxy-cyclohex-5-en-L-yl-acetic acid (Hawkinsin). Exact molecular basis of condition still unknown.

Diagnostic Procedures. *Urine.* Presence of specific amino acid Hawkinsin (migrating on high voltage electrophoresis between urea and threonine).

Therapy. Breast milk and ascorbic acid for several weeks after symptoms subside and then slow progressive introduction of normal diet.

Prognosis. Very good with proper and early treatment. Unknown at longer term.

BIBLIOGRAPHY. Deanks DM, Tippett P, Rogers J: A new form of prolonged transient tyrosinemia presenting with severe metabolic acidosis. Acta Pediat Scand 64:209–214, 1975
Mitchell GA, Lambert M, Tanguay RM: Hypertyrosinemia. In Scriver CR, Beaudet AL, Sly WS, et al: The Metabolic and Molecular Bases of Inherited Disease, 7th ed, pp 1084–1085. New York, McGraw-Hill, 1995

HAXTHAUSEN I

Synonym. Keratoderma climactericum.

Symptoms and Signs. Occurs in menopausal women. Tenderness on

---

*Name of family in which it was first described.

walking; painful fissuring of feet, especially in winter. Hyperkeratosis of palms and soles appearing as discrete, sharply defined lesions, regular round or oval, lentil to pea size. Eczematous complication frequent. Obesity and hypertension and chronic arthritis frequently associated features.

Etiology. Unknown. There is no accepted evidence that this condition is caused by changes in endocrine incretion owing to the climatic condition.

Pathology. Horny layer slightly frayed and sometimes with superficial fissures. Eczematous lesions with miliary vesicles developing later.

Therapy. Hormonal treatment not indicated. Weight reduction; keratolytic ointments; paring of excessive horn.

Prognosis. After months of progression, stabilization of condition or improvement. Chronic condition refractory to treatment. Eczema and itching are complicating features.

BIBLIOGRAPHY. Haxthausen H: Keratoderma climactericum. Br J Dermatol Syph 46:161–167, 1934
Plouffe L Jr, Ravnikar VA, Speroff L, et al: Comprehensive Management of Menopause. New York, Springer, 1994

HAYDEN-GROSSMAN

Synonym. Familial rectal pain. See Painful ophthalmoplegia, McLennan and Frey.

Symptoms and Signs. Both sexes affected; onset in infancy. Brief excruciating pain in submandibular, ocular, and rectal zones, with flushing of the corresponding skin areas; followed by a normal bowel movement, buttock and leg flushing, and pain cessation. The orbital pain is accompanied by tears, squinting, and blurring of vision; the submandibular pain is followed by salivation.

Etiology. Autosomal dominant inheritance with variable penetrance. Dysautonomic nature (?).

Therapy. Symptomatic. See McLennan.

Prognosis. Pains occur once a day or once a week 5–10 times, then stop for some weeks or months. Cycles eventually recur.

BIBLIOGRAPHY. Thaysen TEH: Proctalgia fugax: A little known form of pain in the rectum. Lancet II:243–246, 1935
Hayden R, Grossman M: Rectal, ocular, and submaxillary pain: A familial autonomic disorder related to proctalgia fugax. Report of a family. Am J Dis Child 97:479–482, 1959
Mann TP, Cree JE: Familial rectal pain. Lancet I:1016–1017, 1972

HEAD-RIDDOCH

Synonyms. Autonomic hyperreflexia; high spinal myelomalacia; mass reflex.

Symptoms. Occurs in quadriplegic patients. Sweating; flushing; pilomotor activity; nasal stuffiness; blurred vision; headache; occasionally, generalized seizures.

Signs. Bradycardia; hypertension; dilated pupils.

Etiology. Distension of a viscus below the level of a spinal cord lesion or other type of nerve stimulation. More intense in patient with high cervical cord lesions than in the ones with low cervical or upper thoracic lesions. Lack of inhibitory impulses from high centers to control vasoconstrictor reflexes.

Pathology. High spinal myelomalacia.

1. Reduction of stimuli that precipitate symptoms, such as catheter obstruction, fecal impaction, bladder calculi, urinary infection, decubitus

2. Neurologic rhizotomy or pharmacologic destruction of spinal rootlets by intrathecal nerve block
3. Pharmacologic interruption of neuronal transmission by the use of ganglionic blockade with quaternary ammonium compounds or, better, by guanethidine

Prognosis. This syndrome occasionally ends in generalized seizures and death.

BIBLIOGRAPHY. Head H, Riddoch G: The automatic bladder, excessive sweating and some other reflex conditions in gross injuries of the spinal cord. Brain 40:188–263, 1917
Cole TM, Kottke FJ, Olson M, et al: Alterations of cardiovascular control of high spinal myelomalacia. Arch Phys Med Rehabil 48:359–368, 1967
Adams RD, Victor M: Principles of Neurology, 5th ed, pp 471, 1081. New York, McGraw-Hill, 1993

HEART DISEASE, CONGENITAL DEAFNESS–SKELETAL DEFECTS

Synonyms. Pulmonic stenosis—deafness; deafness—pulmonic stenosis. See Jervell-Lange-Nielsen.

Symptoms. Both sexes affected; onset in infancy. Deaf-mutism; dyspnea; feeding problems; growth retardation.

Signs. Hypertelorism; broad nasal root; low-set ears. Multiple variable skeletal malformations: acrocephaly; scoliosis; pectus excavatum; syndactyly; supernumerary digits. Signs of pulmonary stenosis in the heart or mitral insufficiency or both.

Etiology. Unknown; autosomal dominant inheritance with incomplete penetrance.

Pathology. Congenital heart defect (pulmonary stenosis in one family and mitral insufficiency in another family). *Skeletal malformations.* Malformation of stapes and other auricular bone defects (as cause of deafness).

Diagnostic Procedures. *Audiography. Electrocardiography. X-ray.* Of chest and skeleton. *Biochemical studies.* Negative. *Chromosome studies.* Negative. *Cardiac catheterization.*

Therapy. Surgery for cardiac malformation when indicated.

Prognosis. Nonprogressive condition, except for heart complications.

BIBLIOGRAPHY. Lewis SM, Sonnenblick BP, Gilbert L, et al: Familial pulmonary stenosis and deafmutism: Clinical and genetic considerations. Am Heart J 55:458–462, 1958
Koroxenidis GT, Webb NC Jr, Moschos CB, et al: Congenital heart disease, deaf-mutism and associated somatic malformation occurring in several members of one family. Am J Med 40:149–155, 1966
Forney WR, Robinson SJ, Pascoe DJ: Congenital heart disease, deafness and skeletal malformations: A new syndrome? J Pediatr 68:14–26, 1966

HEART TAMPONADE

Synonym. Cardiac tamponade.

Symptoms. Sudden chest pain; skin pale, sweating, cold; dyspnea; asthenia; syncope.

Signs. Jugular vein distended; paradoxical pulse; apex pulse absent. Tachycardia; cardiac sound faint; pericardial friction rub; blood pressure decreased. Central venous pressure increased; low cardiac output. Oliguria.

Etiology. Chest trauma; myocardial infarction; vessel rupture; intrapericardial bleeding causing an accumulation of pericardial fluid, which causes an increase of pressure and prevents cardiac filling.

Pathology.   See Etiology.

Diagnostic Procedures.   *Electrocardiography.* QRS low voltage; ST elevation; T-wave flattening. *X-rays.* Widening of heart shadow; obliteration of great vessels outlines. *Blood.* Anemia; elevated enzymes. *Echocardiography.* With spectral Doppler interrogation. *Analysis of the jugular pulsations.*

Therapy.   Pericardiocentesis or open drainage. Limited role of pharmacological intervention always to be considered as temporizing measures: intravascular volume expansion, venous and arterial pressure sustainment, and vasodilatation according to needs.

Prognosis.   Good with prompt and appropriate treatment, otherwise may be fatal.

BIBLIOGRAPHY. Lower R: Tractatus de Corde, Item de Motu et Colare Sanguinis et Chyli in Sum Transit r. London, J Allestry, 1669
Chevers N: Observation of diseases of the orifices and valves of aorta. Guy's Hosp Rep 7:387–439, 1842
Shabetai R: Diseases of pericardium. In Schlant RC, Alexander RW, et al: Hurst's The Heart, 8th ed, pp 1654–1662. New York, McGraw-Hill, 1994

HEBERDEN

Synonyms.   Master; Elsner; Rougnon de Magny; angina pectoris; initial angina; stable angina; stenocardia. See Preinfarction and Prinzmetal II.

Symptoms.   Sudden, mild, severe, or excruciating precordial dull pain, tightness, accompanied by anxiety. Radiation to left shoulder, arm, hand. Short duration (usually less than 3 minutes), precipitated by emotion, effort, cold exposure, heavy meal. Relieved by nitroglycerin (see also Gallavardin).

Signs.   Tachycardia or bradyarrhytmia, palpable left ventricular asynergy, new S4 or S3, reversed splitting of S2, murmur of papillary muscle dysfunction, bibasilar pulmonary rales.

Etiology.   Relative myocardial hypoxia owing to anatomic or functional coronary artery flow insufficiency.

Pathology.   Atherosclerosis of coronary vessels.

Diagnostic Procedures.   *Blood pressure.* Marked decrease of systolic. *Electrocardiography.* During attack S-T segment is depressed; in intermittent periods usually normal. Under effort (three-step test) alterations may appear. *X-ray.* Negative; cardiomegaly in advanced disease. *Catheterization with coronary angiography. Echocardiography. Left ventriculography.*

Therapy.   Management of underlying disease (atherosclerosis; syphilis; aortic valvular disease). Elimination of contributing factors (anemia; arrhythmias; gastrointestinal tract pathology). Avoidance of precipitating factors (e.g., heavy meals, cold). Nitroglycerin; isosorbide dinitrate; beta-adrenergic blockers; perhexiline maleate; digitalis (in specific cases); diuretics, long-acting nitrates, sedatives. Angioplasty or bypass grafting.

Prognosis.   Average survival 10 years from first attack.

BIBLIOGRAPHY. Lancisi GM: De Subitaneis Mortibus. Rome, 1707
Heberden W: Some account of a disorder of the breast. Med Tr R Coll Phys (London) 2:59–67, 1772
Anonymous: The Ebers Papyrus, XXVII, p 47 Ebbell B (trans). Copenhagen, Levin and Munksgaard, 1937
Caelius: In Drabkin IE (ed, trans): On Swift or Acute Disease, p 261. Chicago, Univ of Chicago Press, 1950
O'Rourke RA: Chest pain. In Schlant RC, Alexander RW, et al: Hurst's The Heart, 8th ed, pp 459–467. New York, McGraw-Hill, 1994

HEBERDEN NODES

Synonyms.   Rosenbach, Bouchard nodes (see Symptoms and Signs); interphalangeal distal osteoarthritis.

Symptoms and Signs.   More common in females; onset in middle life. Swelling at distal interphalangeal joints, which may develop unnoticed for years; or abrupt painful onset, with redness, paresthesia, and clumsiness. Followed by articular deformity and limitation of motion. When nodes are in juxtaphalangeal position, they are called Bouchard nodes.

Etiology.   Sex-linked inheritance; dominant in females; recessive in males or secondary to traumas.

Pathology.   Massive areas of necrobiosis, in subcutis, with degenerated collagen and surrounding palisading of histiocytes, fibrosis, and capillary hyperplasia. Marginal osteophytes of distal phalanges of fingers not distinguishable from osteoarthritic lesions of other joints.

Diagnostic Procedures.   *X-ray.* Typical osteoarthritic changes.

Therapy.   Analgesic and anti-inflammatory agents.

Prognosis.   Progressive condition.

BIBLIOGRAPHY. Heberden W: De Nodis Digitorum in His Commentarii de Morborum Historia et Curatione. London, Payne, 1802
Rosenback O: Die Anftreibung der Endphalangen der Finger eine bisher noch nicht beschriebene trophische Störung. Zentralbl Nervenh 13:191–205, 1890
Rowell NR, Goodfield MJD: The connective tissue diseases. In Champion RH, Burton JL, Ebling FJG (eds): Rook/Wilkinson/Ebling Textbook of Dermatology, 5th ed, p 2286. Oxford, Blackwell Scientific, 1992
Klippel JH, Dieppe PA: Rheumatology, pp 1.15.5, 7.4.8, 7.7.5. St Louis, CV Mosby, 1995

HEBRA PRURIGO

Synonyms.   Prurigo ferox; prurigo mitis.

Symptoms.   Both sexes affected; onset at 1–5 years of age. Itching of various intensities.

Signs.   Prevalent on extensor side of legs and arms, less frequently on trunk; appearance of small, numerous papules that rather rapidly ulcerate and crust. Thickening of interposed skin, but absence of lichenification. Regional lymphadenopathy.

Etiology.   Unknown; possible relation with atopic condition, malnutrition, poor hygiene.

Therapy.   Prevention of scratching. Avoidance of exposure to possible allergens. Identify allergens and treat by desensitization. Antihistamines: chlorpheniramine or promethazine for symptomatic relief. Topical corticosteroids or systemic (only to overcome acute phases). Ultraviolet light applications.

BIBLIOGRAPHY. von Hebra F: Traité Pratique des Maladies de la Peau. Paris, 1854
Burton JL: Eczema, lichenification, prurigo and erythroderma. In Champion RH, Burton JL, Ebling FJG (eds): Rook/Wilkinson/Ebling Textbook of Dermatology, 5th ed, p 583. Oxford, Blackwell Scientific, 1992

HECHT-BEALS

Synonyms.   Trismus-pseudocamptodactyly; TPS; Wilson; camptomelic trism; Dutch-Kentucky. Dutch-Kentucky.*

Symptoms and Signs.   Male to female ratio, 1:2. From birth, feeding problems from inability to open mouth completely; slow eaters. *Hand.* Handicaps caused by camptodactyly. Trismus with enlarged coronoid

---

*Eponym proposed in 1974 by Mabry et al. after performing an extensive pedigree of a Kentucky family. The earliest affected family member that they were able to trace was a young Dutch girl who immigrated to the southern United States circa 1780.

process of mandibula. When hands dorsiflexed, fingers partially flexed. *Feet.* Downturned toes; talipes equinovarus; metatarsus adductus; short gastrocnemius.

Etiology. Autosomal dominant inheritance.

Pathology. Short flexor tendons of hands and feet. Short muscles.

Therapy. Bilateral removal of the coronoid processes of the mandible has been performed in some cases.

BIBLIOGRAPHY. Hecht F, Beals RK: Inability to open the mouth fully: an autosomal dominant phenotype with facultative camptodactyly and short stature (preliminary note). Birth Defects Orig Art Ser 3:96–98, 1969

Wilson RV, Gaines DL, Brooks A, et al: Autosomal dominant inheritance of shortening of the flexor profundus muscle tendon unit with limitation of jaw excursion. Birth Defects Orig Art Ser 5:99–102, 1969

Mabry CC, Barnett IS, Hutcheson NW: Trismus pseudocamptodactyly syndrome: Dutch-Kentucky syndrome. J Pediatr 85:503–508, 1974

Tsukahara M, Shimozaki F, Kajii T: Trismus-pseudocampodactyly syndrome in a Japanese family. Clin Genet 28:247–250, 1985

Browder FH, Lew D, Shahbazian TS: Anesthetic management of a patient with Dutch-Kentucky syndrome. Anesthesiology 65:218–219, 1986

HECK

Synonyms. Focal epithelial hyperplasia.

Symptoms and Signs. In American Indians and Eskimos. Both sexes, especially in children. In Eskimos and Caucasians in the fourth decade. Asymptomatic. Multiple soft, sessile nodular masses of oral mucosa.

Etiology. Human papilloviruses (HPVs).

Pathology. Lesion areas show epithelial hyperplasia, acanthosis, elongated "bronze age axe" rete ridges, ballooning nuclear degeneration. Electron microscopy may show papovirus-like particles in epithelial cells.

Therapy. Reassurance of benignity of lesions.

BIBLIOGRAPHY. Achard HO, Heck WJ, Stanley HR: Focal epithelial hyperplasia: An unusual oral mucosal lesion found in Indian children. Oral Surg 20:201–212, 1965

Praetorius-Clausen F, Mogeltoft M, Roed-Petersen B, et al: Focal epithelial hyperplasia of the oral mucosa in a South-West Greenlandic population. Scand J Dent J 78:287–294, 1970

Scully C: The oral cavity. In Champion RH, Burton JL, Ebling FJG (eds): Rook/Wilkinson/Ebling Textbook of Dermatology, 5th ed, pp 2751–2752. Oxford, Blackwell Scientific, 1992

HEDBLOM*

Synonym. Acute primary diaphragmitis.

Symptoms. Sudden onset. Pain in the shoulder; upper abdominal pain.

Signs. Decreased lung expansion on inspiration. Deep inspiration prevented by pain.

Etiology. Unknown; aspecific myositis of one or both sides of diaphragm.

Pathology. Diaphragmatic leukocytic infiltration; swelling of muscle fibers; in some cases extension of inflammatory changes to pleura and peritoneum.

Diagnostic Procedures. *X-ray of chest. Fluoroscopy.*

___
*Nominated in honor.

Therapy. Antibiotic reported useful.

Prognosis. Self-limited condition; possible recurrences.

BIBLIOGRAPHY. Joannides M: Acute primary diaphragmitis (Hedblom's syndrome). Dis Chest 12:89–110, 1946

HEERFORDT

Synonyms. Uveoparotid fever; uveoparotic paralysis; uveoparotitis. Used also as synonym for Besnier-Boeck-Schaumann (see). See also Waldeström uveoparotitis.

Symptoms and Signs. Prevalent in females; onset in young adulthood. Bilateral uveitis; parotitis; mediastinal lymphadenopathy; splenomegaly, facial palsy; fever; skin nodules.

Etiology. Majority of cases affected by sarcoidosis. In some cases, Mycobacterium tuberculosis possibly may be the etiologic agent.

Pathology. Presence of tubercles that do not calcify; see Besnier-Boeck-Schaumann.

Diagnostic Procedures. See Besnier-Boeck-Schaumann.

Therapy. See Besnier-Boeck-Schaumann.

Prognosis. Swelling of parotid glands lasts from 6 weeks to 2 years. Paralysis disappears within a few months.

BIBLIOGRAPHY. Heerfordt CF: Ueber eine Febris uveoparotidea subchronica an der Glandula parotis und der Uvea des Auges lokalisiert und haufig mit Paresen cerebrospinaler Nerven kompliziert. Graefes Arch Ophthalmol 70:254–273, 1909

Dufour R, Bourquin A: Deux cas d'uveoparotidite histologiquement tuberculeuse. Ophthalmologica 120:50–56, 1950

Iwata K, Nanba K, Sobue K, et al: Ocular sarcoidosis: Evaluation of intraocular findings. Ann NY Acad Sci 278:445–454, 1976

James DG, Angi MR: Ocular sarcoidosis. In James DG (ed): Sarcoidosis and Other Granulomatous Disorders. New York, Marcel Dekker, 1994

HEIDE

Synonyms. Aortic stenosis; gastrointestinal bleeding; gastrointestinal angiodysplasia—aortic stenosis.

Symptoms and Signs. Those of aortic stenosis (see). Gastrointestinal bleeding in older age.

Etiology. Aortic stenosis very likely does not cause intestinal lesion but only bleeding of pre-existing lesions.

Pathology. See aortic valve stenosis. Abdominal lesions (angiodysplasia) may be present throughout the gastrointestinal tract, but they are most frequently located in the ascending colon.

Diagnostic Procedures. See Aortic stenosis. *X-ray of intestinal tract.*

Therapy. Symptomatic. Aortic valve replacement beneficial on the bleeding episodes.

Prognosis. Fair with treatment.

BIBLIOGRAPHY. Heide EC: Gastrointestinal bleeding in aortic stenosis. N Engl J Med 259:196–200, 1958

Scheffer SM, Leatherman LL: Resolution of Heide's syndrome of aortic stenosis and gastrointestinal bleeding after aortic valve replacement. Ann Thorac Surg 42:477–480, 1986

HEIDENHAIN

Synonym. Cortical blindness; presenile dementia; myoclonic dementia, subacute; spongiform encephalopathy; SSE; Creutzfeldt-Jakob (eponym inappropriately used for this condition since it is better to reserve it to indicate another pathological condition [see]).

Symptoms and Signs. Occurs in males; onset at 38–55 years of age. Progressive loss of vision; progressive mental deterioration of central type. Ataxia; dysarthria; athetoid movements and generalized rigidity.

Etiology. Unknown. Akin to Kuru (see) (transmissible agent). Iatrogenic transmission (transplantation, infected electrodes, etc.) demonstrated.

Diagnostic Procedures. *Electroencephalopathy.* Distinctive pattern. *Blood and cerebrospinal fluid.* Normal.

Pathology. Cortical degeneration prevalent in the occipital cortex and more or less generalized to other cortical zones. *Histology.* Altered architecture; protoplasmic and fibrous astrocyte proliferation; small nerve cell shrinkage and pigment atrophy.

Therapy. Symptomatic; antiviral agents ineffective.

Prognosis. Poor; death follows quite rapidly after onset.

BIBLIOGRAPHY. Heidenhain A: Klinische and anatomische Untersuchungen über eine eigenartige organische Enkrankung des Zentralnervensystems im Praesenium. Z Neurol Psychiatr 118:49–114, 1929
Meyer A, Leigh D, Bagg CE: Rare presenile dementia associated with cortical blindness (Heidenhain's syndrome). J Neurol Neurosurg Psychiatr 17:129–133, 1954
Bjoernsson J, Carp RI, Loeve A (eds): Slow infections of the central nervous system. Ann New York Acad Sci N 9334, 1994

HEINE-MEDIN

Synonyms. Infantile paralysis; paralytic spinal poliomyelitis, poliomyelitis.

Symptoms. Both sexes affected; onset most frequently between 6 months and 15 years of age. Symptoms appear from late spring to fall. In some cases, asymptomatic. Usually follows a prodromal phase characterized by fever, upper respiratory symptoms, or gastrointestinal symptoms: nausea; vomiting; diarrhea; stypsis; abdominal pain, or influenza-like symptoms (bone, muscle, and joint aches).

Signs. *Aborted type.* Initial vague signs of receding generic viral infection. *Nonparalytic type.* Prodromal signs acquiring consistency; possibly, meningeal irritation signs, then recession. *Paralytic type.* Onset of generalized or localized paralysis usually 3–5 days or less after onset of symptoms of nervous system involvement (onset may be later). In acute phase, irritability, tenderness, and spasm of affected muscles. Loss of corresponding tendon reflexes.

Etiology. Poliovirus (strain Brunhilde, Lansing, Leon).

Pathology. Necrosis of anterior horn cells of all segments of spinal cord with more frequent involvement of cervical and lumbar enlargements: hyperemia; then edema and softening. Medulla frequently affected. Cortex of brain and cerebellum more rarely involved. Mild inflammatory changes in subarachnoid space; infiltration by mononuclear cells; edema and hemorrhages of areas affected; when inflammation subsides, parenchymatous degeneration intervenes.

Diagnostic Procedures. *Oropharynx. Stool. Cerebrospinal fluid.* Demonstration of virus. *Cerebrospinal fluid.* Leukocytosis (initially polymorphs; later lymphocytes). Protein normal or slight elevation; chloride and sugar normal; pressure increased. *Blood.* Marked leukocytosis (polymorphonucleates). Complement fixing and neutralizing antibodies from first–second week from onset.

Therapy. Prophylaxis (vaccination). Symptomatic; gamma globulins. Strict bed rest at onset reduces paralysis. When needed, artificial ventilation.

Prognosis. Mortality 5–15%. Permanent paralysis rate of difficult esti-

mation. Recovery of muscle function possible within 3–4 months, then poorer outlook for complete recovery and residual atrophy.

BIBLIOGRAPHY. Heine J: Beobachtungen ueber Laehmungszustaende der untern Extremitaeten und deren Behandlung. Stuttgart, Köhler, 1840
Medin O: En epidemi af infantil paralysi. Hygiea (Stockh) 52:657–668, 1890
Agre JC, Rodriguez AA, Tafel TA: Late effects of polio: Critical review of the literature on neuromuscolar function. Arch Phys Med Rehabil 72:923–931, 1991
Srebel PM, Sutter RW, Cochi SL, et al: Epidemiology of poliomyelitis in the United States one decade after the last reported case of indigenous wild virus associated disease. J Infect Dis 14:568–579, 1992
Weatherall DJ, Ledingham JGG, Warrell DA (eds): Oxford Textbook of Medicine, 3rd ed, pp 385–386, 4067. Oxford, Oxford Med Pub, 1996

HEINER

Synonyms. Heiner-Sears; cow milk precipitins; pulmonary hemosiderosis; milk (bovine) precipitins pulmonary; bovine milk pulmonary sensitivity; hemosiderosis; pulmonary hypersensitivity cow milk. See Hemosiderosis idiopathic, pulmonary; allergic gastroenteritis.

Symptoms. Occurs in infants of both sexes. Failure to thrive; recurrent diarrhea; chronic respiratory distress.

Signs. Underweight; pallor; variable pulmonary findings.

Etiology. Not precisely delineated: delayed sensitivity to cow milk products; intravascular precipitation of antigen-antibody complexes; sensitivity reactions of blood vessel.

Pathology. Suppurative bronchitis with various degrees of atelectasis. Pulmonary hemosiderosis, secondary cor pulmonale, hypertrophic mesopharyngeal lymphoid tissue. Microhemorrhages in the intestinal mucosa.

Diagnostic Procedures. *Blood.* Hypochromic anemia; low sideremia; hypoproteinemia; high titer of circulating antibodies against cow milk; eosinophils may be present. *Stool.* Presence of milk coproantibodies and blood. In adults, however, cow milk sensitivity and the presence of antibodies may be associated with other diarrheal disorders (e.g., ulcerative colitis; regional enteritis; celiac disease; cystic fibrosis [has to be ruled out by specific tests]). *X-ray of lung.* Variable findings: patchy infiltrates; atelectasis; peribronchial infiltrated; enlarged lymph nodes.

Therapy. Discontinuation of cow milk feeding and substitution with carbohydrate solutions and with soybean-based or meat-based formulas. Pulmonary infections respond well to antibiotics. Iron if needed. Corticosteroids useful.

Prognosis. The syndrome is limited to newborn infants. The symptomatology recedes in older infants. Better than pulmonary hemosiderosis.

BIBLIOGRAPHY. Heiner DC, Sears JW: Chronic respiratory disease associated with multiple circulating precipitins to cow's milk. Am J Dis Child 100:500–502, 1960
Katz J, Spiro HM, Herskovic T: Milk precipitating substance in the stool in gastrointestinal milk sensitivity. N Engl J Med 278:1191–1194, 1968
Chang CH, Whitting HJ: Heiner's syndrome. Radiology 92:507–508, 1969
Simon RA: Allergic and other adverse reaction to foods. In Haubrich WS, Schaffner F, Berk JE (eds): Bockus Gastroenterology, 5th ed, vol 2, p 3273. Philadelphia, WB Saunders, 1995

HEINZ BODIES—CONGENITAL HEMOLYTIC ANEMIA

Synonyms. CHBA, Cathic; hemolytic anemia (Heinz bodies).

Symptoms and Signs. From birth. Congenital nonspherocytic hemolytic anemia; jaundice; splenomegaly; pigmenturia. Symptoms vary with different types of hemoglobin variants. Hemolytic crisis may be precipitated by sulfonamides.

Etiology. Autosomal dominant inheritance. Over 90 different types of unstable hemoglobin variants that precipitate spontaneously with physical or chemical insult to RBC causing hemolytic anemia.

Diagnostic Procedures. *Blood.* Punctate basophilia in red cells of the Heinz bodies (after splenectomy becomes evident). Heating the blood causes copious hemoglobin precipitates.

Pathology. Heinz bodies in RBC.

Therapy. None. Prevent rise of temperature and do not administer sulfonamides or other oxidative agents. Some authors advocate splenectomy.

Prognosis. Good.

BIBLIOGRAPHY. Cathic JAB: Apparent idiopathic Heinz body anemia. Creat Ormond St J 3:43, 1952

Dacie JV, Grimes AJ, Meisler A, et al: Hereditary Heinz body anemia: A report of studies on five patients with mild anemia. Br J Hematol 10:388–402, 1964

Bunn HF, Forget BG: Hemoglobin: Molecular, Genetic, and Clinical Aspects, p 565. Philadelphia, WB Saunders, 1986

Lee GR: Acquired hemolytic anemias resulting from direct effects of infectious, chemical or physical agents. In Lee GR, Bithel TC, Foerster J, et al (eds): Wintrobe's Clinical Hematology, 9th ed, p 1203. Philadelphia, Lea & Febiger, 1993

HELLER (J.)

Synonyms. Dystrophia unguis mediana canaliformis; dysonychia canaliformis; median nail dystrophy. Includes solenonychia.

Symptoms and Signs. Rare. Development of a split or true canal on one nail (usually of the thumb) or several nails.

Etiology. Unknown; possibly related to trauma or to some temporary defect in the nail matrix. Familial cases reported.

Therapy. Unnecessary. Emolient cream in the nail fold.

Prognosis. After months or years nail returns to normal; relapses may occur.

BIBLIOGRAPHY. Heller J: Zur Kasuistik seltener Nagelkrankheiten. XVIII. Dystrophia unguium (sic) mediana canali-formis. Dermatol Z 51:416–419, 1927

Sutton RJ: Solenonychia: canaliform dystrophy of the nails. So Med J 58:1143–1146, 1965

Dawber RPR, Baran R: Disorders of the nails. In Champion RH, Burton JL, Ebling FJG (eds): Rook/Wilkinson/Ebling Textbook of Dermatology, 5th ed, p 2509. Oxford, Blackwell Scientific, 1992

HELLER-NELSON

Synonym. Klinefelter variant (see).

BIBLIOGRAPHY. Heller CG, Nelson WO: Hyalinization of the seminiferous tubulus associated with normal or failing Leydig cell function. Discussion of relationship to eunuchoidism, gynecomastia, elevated gonadotropins, depressed 17-ketosteroids, and estrogens. J Clin Endocrinol 5:1–12, 1945

HELLERSTRÖM

Symptoms and Signs. Association between erythema chronicum migrans (Afzelius)and symptoms related to meningitic involvement.

Etiology. The same as Afzelius (see).

BIBLIOGRAPHY. Hellerström S: Erythema chronicum migrans afzelli. Acta Derm Venereol (Stockh) 11:315–321, 1930

HELLER (T.)

Obsolete.

Synonym. Aphonia; dementia infantilis.

BIBLIOGRAPHY. Heller T: Ueber Dementia infantilis. Z Kinderforsch 37:661–667, 1930

H.E.L.L.P.

Synonyms. Hemolysis; elevated serum enzymes; low platelets. Overlapping with liver, massive necrosis (see). See also Hepatorenal syndromes.

Symptoms and Signs. In approximately 10% of patients with preeclampsia. Cerebral disturbances, pulmonary edema, jaundice, oliguria, blood pressure over 160/110; hemorrhagic tendency.

Etiology. Unknown. See eclampsia.

Pathology. Liver fibrin deposits in the sinusoids, microvesicular fat (in some cases).

Diagnostic Procedures. *Urine.* Proteinuria over 5 g/24 h, oliguria less than 400 mm/24 h. *Blood.* Hemolysis, burr cells or schistocytes, thrombocytopenia, decreased prothrombin time, partial thromboplastin time, and fibrinogen, enzymes increased.

Therapy. See eclampsia.

Prognosis. Fetal and maternal mortality increased.

BIBLIOGRAPHY. Weinstein L: Preeclampsia/eclampsia with hemolysis, elevated liver enzymes and thrombocytopenias. Obstet Gynecol 66:657–660, 1985

Schaffner F: Nonalcoholic fatty liver. In Haubrich WS, Schaffner F, Berk JE (eds): Bockus Gastroenterology, 5th ed, vol 2, pp 2262–2263. Philadelphia, WB Saunders, 1995

HELMHOLTZ-HARRINGTON

Synonym. Corneal opacity; cranioskeletal dysostosis.

Symptoms and Signs. Both sexes affected; onset from birth. Zonular cataract; other ocular disorders owing to oxycephaly; various apical malformations (polydactyly; syndactyly; camptodactyly; lobster-claw type of dystrophy). Mental retardation; hepatosplenomegaly.

Etiology. Unknown.

BIBLIOGRAPHY. Appenzeller GFA: Ein Beitrag zur Lehre von der Erblichkeit des grauen Staars (these). Tübingen, 1884

Helmholtz H, Harrington EFR: Syndrome characterized by congenital clouding of cornea and by other anomalies. Am J Dis Child 41:793–800, 1931

François J: Syndromes with congenital cataract. Am J Ophthalmol 52:207–238, 1961

HELWEG-LARSEN-LUDVIGSEN

Synonym. Anhidrosis—neurolabyrinthitis—deafness; anhydrotic ectodermal dysplasia.

Symptoms. Both sexes affected; onset from birth. Temperature disturbances owing to anhydrosis or marked hypohydrosis. In fourth or fifth decade, vertigo (neurolabyrinthitis).

Signs. Normal skull configuration; no abnormalities of teeth or hair.

Etiology. Unknown; autosomal dominant inheritance.

BIBLIOGRAPHY. Helweg-Larsen HF, Ludvigsen K: Congenital familial anhydrosis and neurolabyrinthitis. Acta Dermatol Venereol (Stockh) 26:489–505, 1946
Brandt T: Vertigo: Its multisensory syndromes. London, Springer-Verlag, 1991

HELWIG

Synonyms. Inverted follicular keratosis; Follicular keratosis inverted.

Symptoms and Signs. In elderly. Single lesion in the face.

Etiology. Unknown.

Pathology. Invaginating, cup- or finger-shaped tumor. At periphery small basal cells, in the center squamoid cells that form different structures.

Diagnostic Procedures. *Biopsy.*

Therapy. Excision.

Prognosis. Benign.

BIBLIOGRAPHY. Helwig EB: Inverted follicular keratosis. Seminar on the skin. Int Cong Clin Pathol Washington DC, 1954
Mehregan AH: Inverted follicular keratosis. Arch Dermatol 98:229–235, 1964
MacKie RM: Tumors of the skin appendages. In Champion RH, Burton JL, Ebling FJG (eds): Rook/Wilkinson/Ebling Textbook of Dermatology, 5th ed, p 1506. Oxford, Blackwell Scientific, 1992

HEMATOMA, EPIDURAL

Synonym. Epidural hematoma.

Symptoms. Patient with trauma of the head, and temporary unconsciousness, who develops the following symptomatology after a more or less prolonged lucid interval (a few minutes or days). Symptoms may be subdivided in two groups: (1) Acute type with interval shorter than 7 days (82%); or (2) chronic type with longer interval (18%). The patient starts to grow sleepy, then stuporous, and then comatose. Symptoms progress rapidly once started.

Signs. Bradycardia; bradypnea; hypertension; pupil side of lesion dilated and fixed; occasionally, contralateral hemianopsia or hemiplegia may be observed.

Etiology. Hemorrhage between dura and inner table of skull, usually from middle meningeal artery.

Pathology. Fracture of skull and hematoma of the middle meningeal artery or laceration of dural sinuses; compression of cerebral hemisphere; occasionally cerebral infarction.

Diagnostic Procedures. *X-ray of skull. Spinal tap. CT brain scan. MRI.*

Therapy. Immediate surgery with decompression and ligation of bleeding artery.

Prognosis. Depends on degree of consciousness, patient's age, intensity of bleeding.

BIBLIOGRAPHY. Heyser J, Weber G: Die epiduralen Hämatome. Schweiz Med Wochenschr 94:2–7; 46–52, 1964
Adams RD, Victor M: Principles of Neurology, 5th ed, pp 760–761. New York, McGraw-Hill, 1993

HEMATURIA, ESSENTIAL

Synonyms. Benign recurrent hematuria; essential hematuria.

Symptoms. Prevalent in male children; onset 2–11 years of age. Asymptomatic.

Signs. Episodes of gross hematuria.

Etiology. Various conditions may cause the syndrome: 50% of cases, focal glomerulonephritis; some present the Berger syndrome (see), a smaller number, chronic progressive nephropathies.

Pathology. See Etiology. Usually, nonspecific changes.

Diagnostic Procedures. *Blood.* Normal. *Urine.* Gross recurrent hematuria. In some cases, persistent microscopic hematuria between episodes. *Biopsy of kidneys.* See Etiology. *X-ray.* Intravenous pyelography. *Renal arteriography. CT scan. MRI. Echography.*

Therapy. None, or according to etiology.

Prognosis. Generally good.

BIBLIOGRAPHY. Glassock RJ: Hematuria and pigmenturia. In Massry SG, Glassock RJ: Textbook of Nephrology, 3rd ed, pp 557–566. Baltimore, Williams & Wilkins, 1995

HEMI 3

Synonym. Hemihypertrophy subtype.

Symptoms and Signs. Observed in girls. Hemihypertrophy (see). Hemihyperesthesia, hemiareflexia, and scoliosis. In body, larger side (usually the left), increase of muscle size, strength, and bone thickness but not length.

Etiology. Neural tube defects with multifactorial inheritance.

Prognosis. Scoliosis progressive. Musculoskeletal and neurological defects stable.

BIBLIOGRAPHY. Nudleman K, Anderman E, Anderman F, et al: The hemi3 syndrome: hemihypertrophy-hemihypoesthesia, hemiareflexia and scoliosis. Brain 107:533–546, 1984

HEMIFACIAL MICROSOMIA

Synonyms. Unilateral mandibulofacial dysostosis. Definition substituted with oculo-auriculo-vertebral spectrum (see). See also Goldenhar, François-Haustrate; Nager Reyner, and Weyers-Thier.

BIBLIOGRAPHY. Gorlin RJ, Cohen MM Jr, Levin LS: Syndromes of Head and Neck. New York, Oxford Med Pub, 1990

HEMIFACIAL SPASM

Symptoms and Signs. In both sexes. Onset in fourth decade, with twitching of muscle orbicularis oculi and eventually extending to all muscles innervated by the VII cranial nerve.

Etiology. Microvascular compression of facial nerve. Reported familial occurrence with autosomal dominant pattern.

Pathology. Compression of VII cranial nerve root by anterior inferior cerebellar artery and its plexus.

Diagnostic Procedures. See Classic migraine.

Therapy. Carbamazepine, baclofen, botulin A toxin injected into affected muscles (4–5 months relief; injections may be repeated for years without damage or loss of effect).

Prognosis. Does not affect life expectancy.

BIBLIOGRAPHY. Campbell E, Keedy C: Hemifacial spasm: A note on the etiology in two cases. J Neurosurg 4:342–347, 1947

Coad JE, Wirtschafter JD, Haines SJ, et al: Familial hemifacial spasm associated with arterial compression of the facial nerve: A case report. J Neurosurg 74:290–296, 1991

Adams RD, Victor M: Principles of Neurology, 5th ed, p 1177. New York, McGraw-Hill, 1993

HEMIHYPERTROPHY

Synonyms. Friedriech; asymmetric lateral; hemigigantism; hemimacrosomia. See Bremer and Hemi 3.

Symptoms and Signs. Prevalent in males; present at birth in 40% of cases. Prevalent on the right side; varies in extent and severity in an extremely large spectrum. (Normal asymmetry exists, although not always apparent, and may be determined only by accurate measurements.) Syndrome has been divided into total (musculoskeletal and visceral organs of involved side), and limited, which has been subdivided into segmental and crossed. Numerous possible associated features, including skin, hand, and foot, vertebral column, genitourinary, and neurologic abnormalities. Occasionally, association with different tumors.

Etiology. Possibly more than one cause. Nervous system, vascular and lymphatic, endocrine, chromosomal abnormalities.

Pathology. Hypertrophy of muscle, bones, and viscera.

Diagnostic Procedures. *X-rays. Chromosome studies. Endocrine studies.*

Therapy. Symptomatic and orthopedic when needed.

Prognosis. Usually good; may be determined by associated conditions.

BIBLIOGRAPHY. Meckel JF: Ueber die Seitliche Asymmetrie im tierschen Körper. Anatomische physiologische Beobachtungen und Untersuchungen, p 147. Halle, Renger, 1822

Friedriech N: Ueber congenitale halbseitige Kopfhypertrophie. Virchows Arch (Pathol Anat) 28:474–481, 1863

Fraumeni JF Jr, Geiser CF, Manning MD: Wilms' tumor and congenital hemihypertrophy. Report of five new cases and review of literature. Pediatrics 40:886–899, 1967

Viljoen D, Pearn J, Beighton P: Manifestations and natural history of idiopathic hemihypertrophy: A review of eleven cases. Clin Genet 26:81–86, 1984

Mannens M, Slater RM, Heyting C, et al: Chromosome 11, Wilms tumor and associated congenital diseases. Cytog Cell Genet 46:655; 1987

HEMIPLEGIA, HEMIANESTHESIA, ALTERNATING, HYPOGLOSSAL

Symptoms. Hemiplegia of arm and leg (but not the face) and loss of position and vibration sensibility on the same side (without loss of pain or temperature sensibility). Paralysis (peripheral type) of the half of the tongue on opposite side.

Signs. Tongue hemiatrophy and twitching.

Etiology. Involvement of pyramidal tract and emergent fibers of hypoglossal nerve in the medulla. Basilar meningitis or other cause determining softening of pyramidal tract (rare).

BIBLIOGRAPHY. Alpers BJ: Clinical Neurology, 6th ed. Philadelphia, FA Davis, 1971

HEMIPLEGIA, INFANTILE

See Little (W.J.).

Symptoms. Both sexes affected; onset in infancy or early childhood. May develop suddenly as a complication of acute infection with high fever, or without associated illness. Generalized or focal seizures usually first symptom, followed by hemiplegia. Arms more severely affected than legs. Common, repeated uncontrollable convulsions and behavioral problems (disobedience, inattentiveness, hyperactivity, destructiveness).

Etiology. Injury to one hemisphere occurring at birth or later (e.g., encephalitis, cerebrovascular problem, developmental defects).

Diagnostic Procedures. *Scintigraphy. CT brain scan. MRI. Angiography. Electroencephalography.* Demonstration of nature and extension of lesion.

Therapy. Anticonvulsants. Removal of cerebral cortex of damaged hemisphere.

Prognosis. Little response to treatment; severe educational problems. Unilateral cerebral decortication results in striking improvement in behavior and reduction of number of seizures.

BIBLIOGRAPHY. Vick NA: Grinker's Neurology, 7th ed. Springfield, IL, Charles C Thomas, 1976

Adams RD, Victor M: Principles of Neurology, 5th ed, pp 1039–1040. New York, McGraw-Hill, 1993

HEMIPLEGIC MIGRAINE, FAMILIAL

Synonyms. See Classic migraine.

Symptoms and Signs. Recurrent attacks of migraine and hemiparesis. Additional manifestations reported in different families: cerebeller dysfunction, retinitis; deafness, nystagmus, coma, hypertermia, meningismus.

Etiology. Autosomal dominant inheritance.

Diagnostic Procedures. See Classic migraine.

Therapy. See Classic migraine.

BIBLIOGRAPHY. Clarke JM: On recurrent motor paralysis in migraine: With report of a family in which recurrent hemiplegia accompained the attacks. Br Med J 1:1534–1538, 1910

Munte TF, Muler-Vahl H: Familial migraine coma: A case study. J Neurol 237:59–61, 1990

Adams RD, Victor M: Principles of Neurology, 5th ed, p 156. New York, McGraw-Hill, 1993

HEMIPLEGIC, PURE

Synonyms. See Lacunar.

Symptoms and Signs. May evolve relatively slowly (2–3 days). Weakness involving face, arm, and leg and or pure dysarthria.

Etiology. Lacuna in the internal capsule or corona radiata.

Pathology. See Lacunar.

Diagnostic Procedures. *CT scan. MRI.*

Therapy. Symptomatic.

Prognosis. Recovery may initiate within hours or weeks and usually is complete.

BIBLIOGRAPHY. Fisher CM: Lacunar strokes and infarcts: A review. Neurology 38:871, 1982

Adams RD, Victor M: Principles of Neurology, 5th ed, p 696. New York, McGraw-Hill, 1993

HEMISENSORY, PURE

Synonyms. See Lacunar.

Symptoms and Signs. Pure hemisensory deficit, the neurologic defect evolves slowly.

Etiology. Lesion of the thalamus or parietal white matter owing to single or multiple lacunar infarction.

Pathology. See Lacunar.

Diagnostic Procedures. *CT scan. MRI.*

Therapy. Symptomatic.

Prognosis. Recovery may initiate within hours or weeks and usually is complete.

BIBLIOGRAPHY. Fisher CM: Lacunar strokes and infarcts: A review. Neurology 38:871, 1982
Adams RD, Victor M: Principles of Neurology, 5th ed, p 696. New York, McGraw-Hill, 1993

HEMOCHROMATOSIS

Synonyms. Hanot-Chauffard; Trousseau; Troisier-Hanot-Chauffard; Leschke; Recklinghausen-Applebaum; bronze diabetes; diabetes—hemochromatosis; iron storage. Includes Bantu siderosis.

Symptoms. Diagnosis more frequent in men (difference ranging from 2/1–18/1). Onset of symptomatology at 40–60 years of age. Lassitude; weakness; weight loss; palpitations; upper right abdominal quadrant sharp pain; dyspnea; loss of libido. Occasionally, specific progressive polyarthropathy.

Signs. Skin pigmentation of two types: (1) Addison-like or (2) grayish hue on genitals, face, arms, skinfolds (seldom mucosae, 15%); edema; ascites. Later, jaundice, loss of body hair, gynecomastia, hepatomegaly, splenomegaly, testicular atrophy; eventually, signs of heart failure.

Etiology. Idiopathic. Autosomal recessive inheritance. Mutant gene close to HLA-A locus on chromosome 6p. Complete expression only in males; females and sibs have only altered metabolism of iron or they compensate the iron overload by mentrual blood loss, pregnancy, etc. Various cell sites of anomalies of iron absorption: gut, plasma transferrin, liver, and reticuloendothelial system. Symptoms appear when iron overload reaches 15 gamma and hemosiderin deposits lead to organ impairment. Secondary forms owing to refractory anemia. Chronic defect of hemoglobin synthesis, ineffective erythropoiesis, hemolytic processes. Porphyria cutanea tarda. Iron loading. Medication; diet (Bantu siderosis); transfusions.

Pathology. *Skin.* Thin; melanin pigment in basal layer. *Liver.* Nodular cirrhosis; hemosiderin deposits. *Pancreas.* Nodular fibrosis. *Testes.* Atrophic. *Heart.* Deposit of hemosiderin.

Diagnostic Procedures. *Blood.* At onset high hemoglobin concentration; later macrocytic anemia, increased transferin saturation: threshold value 62%, serumferritin concentration. Hyperglycemia; hyperbilirubinemia; liver function test altered. *Biopsy of liver.*

Therapy. Diabetes treatment (insulin resistant in most cases). Vigorous phlebotomy (according to iron load up to 5 units per week). Chelate; desferrioxamine intramuscularly to be reserved for patients who do not tolerate agressive phlebotomy.

Prognosis. With adequate treatment; reversal of symptoms according to the amount of damage. Possible development of hepatomas (up to 29%).

BIBLIOGRAPHY. Trousseau A: Glycosurie diabete sucre. Clinque Med de l'Hotel de Paris, 2nd ed. 2:663, 1865
Troisier CE: Diabète sucré. Bull Soc Anat Paris 44:231, 1871
Hanot VC, Chauffard AM: Cirrhose hypertrophique pigmentaire dans le diabète sucrè. Rev Med 3:385–403, 1882
Edwards CQ: Hemochromatosis and other iron storage disorders. In Lee GR, Bithel TC, Foerster J, et al (eds): Wintrobe's Clinical Hematology, 9th ed, pp 872–884. Philadelphia, Lea & Febiger, 1993
Bothwell TH, Charlton RW, Motulsky AG: Hemochromatosis. In Scriver CR, Beaudet AL, Sly WS, et al: The Metabolic and Molecular Bases of Inherited Disease, 7th ed, pp 2237–2269. New York, McGraw-Hill, 1995

HEMOGLOBIN, CONSTANT SPRING

Synonym. HbCS. See also Hemoglobin H and Thalassemia syndromes.

Symptoms and Signs. In 50% of Asian subjects with HbH disease. Mild hemolytic anemia, splenomegaly.

Etiology. Mixed inheritance of hemoglobin H disease and anomalous hemoglobin. *Constant Spring.* Symptoms are apparent only in the homozygous state. Heterozygotes for HbCS are phenotypically similar to individuals with heterozygous alpha thalassemia 2.

Diagnostic Procedures. *Blood.* Reticulocytosis. No hypochromia and microcytosis.

Therapy. None.

Prognosis. Good.

BIBLIOGRAPHY. Milner PF, Clegg JB, Weatherall DJ: Hemoglobin H disease due to a unique hemoglobin variant with elongated chain. Lancet I:729, 1971
Clegg JB, Weatherall DJ, Milner PF: Hemoglobin Constant Spring: A chain termination mutant? Nature 234:337, 1971
Bunn HF, Forget BG: Hemoglobin Molecular Genetic and Clinical Aspects, p 331. Philadelphia, WB Saunders, 1986
Lukens JN: The thalassemias and related disorders: Quantitative disorders of hemoglobin synthesis. In Lee GR, Bithel TC, Foerster J, et al (eds): Wintrobe's Clinical Hematology, 9th ed, p 1112. Philadelphia, Lea & Febiger, 1993

HEMOGLOBIN C SYNDROMES

HEMOGLOBIN C HOMOZYGOUS (CC)

Symptoms. Mild recurrent bone and joint pains; recurrent abdominal pains of variable intensity; convulsions; hemorrhagic manifestations.

Signs. Frequently jaundice; splenomegaly; no skeletal abnormality.

Etiology. Hemoglobin abnormality (lysine for glutamic acid in the sixth position of the beta chain); homozygous, autosomal recessive inheritance.

Diagnostic Procedures. *Blood.* Normocytic or microcytic moderate anemia; microspherocytes; target cells; reticulocytosis: moderate. Hyperbilirubinemia, osmotic fragility: decreased. Thrombocytopenia frequent. Hemoglobin electrophoresis. Hemoglobin C represents the entire hemoglobin. *Bone marrow.* Hyperplasia.

Therapy. Symptomatic.

Prognosis. Good; normal life span.

SICKLE CELL, HEMOGLOBIN C

See Hemoglobin SC syndrome.

Symptoms. Milder than in Herrick (see).

Prognosis. Better than in Herrick.

HS-O ARABIA

See Hemoglobin S; Hemoglobin O.

Symptoms and Signs. Reported in Sudan, Jamaica, and the United States. See Sickle cell hemoglobin C.

Diagnostic Procedures. *Hemoglobin electrophoresis.* Migration of hemoglobin O to same position as hemoglobin C. Difficult to distinguish except for biochemical characteristic (hemoglobin O Arabia-beta 121 Glu[t402] = Lys).

HEMOGLOBIN C-THALASSEMIA

Synonym. Zuelzer-Kaplan.

Symptoms and Signs. Mild to severe bone pain; splenomegaly rare.

Diagnostic Procedures. *Blood.* Anemia; large, thin target cells; schistocytes; microspherocytes. Decreased osmotic fragility. *Bone marrow.* Hyperplasia.

BIBLIOGRAPHY. Itano HA: A third abnormal hemoglobin associated with hereditary hemolytic anemia. Proc Natl Acad Sci 37:775–784, 1951
Zeulzer WE, Kaplan E: Thalassemia-hemoglobin C disease: A new syndrome presumably due to the combination of the genes for thalassemia and hemoglobin C. Blood 9:1047–1054, 1954
Bunn HF, Forget BG: Hemoglobin: Molecular, Genetic, and Clinical Aspects. Philadelphia, WB Saunders, 1986
Lukens JN: Hemoglobinopathies S; C; D; E; and O and associated diseases. In Lee GR, Bithel TC, Foerster J, et al (eds): Wintrobe's Clinical Hematology, 9th ed. Philadelphia, Lea & Febiger, 1993

HEMOGLOBIN D SYNDROMES

(Beta 121 Glu [t402] = Gln). Hemoglobin D has subvariants in HbD-Punjab, HbD-Los Angeles, Ibadan, Iran, etc.

HEMOGLOBIN D TRAIT (AD)

Symptoms. Asymptomatic.

HEMOGLOBIN D HOMOZYGOUS (DD)

Symptoms. Mild hemolytic anemia; no splenomegaly or bone alterations.

SICKLE CELL HEMOGLOBIN D

Symptoms. Milder than in Herrick (see). Combination of hemoglobin D with other hemoglobinopathies also reported.

BIBLIOGRAPHY. Itano HA: A third abnormal hemoglobin associated with hereditary hemolytic anemia. Proc Nat Acad Sci 37:775–784, 1951
Chernoff AI: The hemoglobin D syndromes. Blood 8:116–127, 1958
Bunn HF, Forget BG: Hemoglobin: Molecular, Genetic, and Clinical Aspects, p 424. Philadelphia, WB Saunders, 1986
Lukens JN: Hemoglobinopathies S; C; D; E; and O and associated diseases. In Lee GR, Bithel TC, Foerster J, et al (eds): Wintrobe's Clinical Hematology, 9th ed. Philadelphia, Lea & Febiger, 1993

HEMOGLOBIN E SYNDROMES

(Alpha-2 beta-2 26 Glu [t402] = Lys). In Asians.

HEMOGLOBIN E TRAIT

Symptoms. Asymptomatic.

HEMOGLOBIN E HOMOZYGOUS

Symptoms. Anemia; occasionally, polycythemia; moderate or absent splenomegaly.

Diagnostic Procedures. *Blood.* Mild, microcytic normochromic anemia; target cells. Decreased osmotic fragility; mild hyperbilirubinemia.

HEMOGLOBIN E THALASSEMIA

Symptoms. Similar to Cooley (see Thalassemia syndromes).

SICKLE CELL, HEMOGLOBIN E

Symptoms. Milder than Herrick's (see).

BIBLIOGRAPHY. Itano HA, Bergren WR, Sturgeon P: Identification of a fourth abnormal human hemoglobin. J Am Chem Soc 76:2278, 1954
Bunn HF, Forget BG: Hemoglobin: Molecular, Genetic, and Clinical Aspects, p 426. Philadelphia, WB Saunders, 1986
Lukens JN: Hemoglobinopathies S; C; D; E; and O and associated diseases. In Lee GR, Bithel TC, Foerster J, et al (eds): Wintrobe's Clinical Hematology, 9th ed. Philadelphia, Lea & Febiger, 1993

HEMOGLOBIN H

Synonyms. Double heterozygous alpha thalassemia 1 + alpha thalassemia 2.

Symptoms and Signs. From birth. Some patients with mongoloid facies. Splenomegaly, hepatomegaly. Hemolytic anemia of variable severity. Anemia worsens during pregnancy and oxidative drug ingestion.

Etiology. Double heterozygous condition for alpha thalassemia 1 in one parent and alpha thalassemia 2 (silent carrier state) in the other parent. Presence of HbH (beta 4).

Diagnostic Procedures. *Hemoglobin electrophoresis.* In newborn 20–40% Hb Bart's (gamma-4); children and adults: HbH (beta) 5–30%. *Peripheral blood smear.* Hypochromia, microcytosis, poikilocytosis, polychromasia, targeting. *Bone marrow.* Erythroid hyperplasia.

Therapy. None. May require transfusions.

Prognosis. Good quoad vitam.

BIBLIOGRAPHY. Rigas DA, Koller RD, Osgood EE: New hemoglobin possessing a higher electrophoretic mobility than normal adult hemoglobin. Science 121:372, 1955, J Lab Clin Med 47:51–64, 1956
Bunn HF, Forget BG: Hemoglobin: Molecular, Genetic, and Clinical Aspects, p 329. Philadelphia, WB Saunders, 1986
Lukens JN The thalassemias and related disorders: quantitative disorders of hemoglobin synthesis. In Lee GR, Bithel TC, Foerster J, et al (eds): Wintrobe's Clinical hematology, 9th ed, p 1117. Philadelphia, Lea & Febiger, 1993

HEMOGLOBIN S-G (S-D)

Symptoms. Few individuals have symptomatic sickle cell disease.

Etiology. Double heterozygosity for HbS and HbD.

BIBLIOGRAPHY. Melurdy PR, Lorkin PA, Casey R, et al: Hemoglobin S-G (S-D) syndrome. Am J Med 57:665, 1974
Lukens JN: Hemoglobinopathies S; C; D; E; and O and associated diseases. In Lee GR, Bithel TC, Foerster J, et al (eds): Wintrobe's Clinical Hematology, 9th ed. Philadelphia, Lea & Febiger, 1993

HEMOGLOBIN S/HEMOGLOBIN LEPORE, BOSTON

Symptoms. Those of Herrick with hemolytic anemia and microcytes.

Etiology. Double heterozygosity for HbS and Hb Lepore Boston.

BIBLIOGRAPHY. Stevens MCG, Lehmann H, Mason KP, et al: Sickle cell-Hb Lepore Boston syndrome. Am J Dis Child 136:19, 1982

Lukens JN: Hemoglobinopathies S; C; D; E; and O and associated diseases. In Lee GR, Bithel TC, Foerster J, et al (eds): Wintrobe's Clinical Hematology, 9th ed. Philadelphia, Lea & Febiger, 1993

HEMOGLOBIN S/HEMOGLOBIN O, ARAB

Symptoms. Hand–foot syndrome (see) and symptoms of Herrick (see).

Etiology. Double heterozygosity for HbS and hemoglobin O, Arab.

BIBLIOGRAPHY. Gilman PA, Abel AS: Acute splenic sequestration in hemoglobin O, Arab disease. Bull Johns Hopkins Hosp Bull 146:285, 1980

Lukens JN: Hemoglobinopathies S; C; D; E; and O and associated diseases. In Lee GR, Bithel TC, Foerster J, et al (eds): Wintrobe's Clinical Hematology, 9th ed. Philadelphia, Lea & Febiger, 1993

HEMOGLOBIN SC

See Herrick.

Symptoms. In African blacks and Jamaicans. Milder than in Herrick. More frequent proliferative retinopathy.

Etiology. Double heterozygosity for HbS and HbC.

Prognosis. Better than in Herrick.

BIBLIOGRAPHY. Balls SK, Lewis CN, Noone AM, et al: Clinical, hematological and biochemical features of HbSC disease. Am J Hematol 13:37, 1984

Lukens JN: Hemoglobinopathies S; C; D; E; and O and associated diseases. In Lee GR, Bithel TC, Foerster J, et al (eds): Wintrobe's Clinical Hematology, 9th ed. Philadelphia, Lea & Febiger, 1993

HEMOLYTIC ANEMIA OF NEWBORN

Synonyms. Pfannestiel, Schridde; congenital newborn anemia; erythroblastosis fetalis; hemolytic disease newborn; HDN; hydrops fetalis; icterus gravis neonatorum.

Symptoms and Signs. From extremely severe form (stillbirth and hydrops fetalis) to simple serologic findings. In this vast spectrum fall clinical manifestations of variable severity; infants often born anemic, jaundiced, and edematous; or normal at birth and progressively developing jaundice and anemia. Liver and spleen usually palpable. Cutaneous purpura and bleeding from mucosa occasionally observed. Kernicterus syndrome (see) frequent sequela. In some cases the inspissated bile syndrome is observed (see).

Etiology. Isoimmunization of the mother by her fetus of different blood group. In 93% of cases caused by an Rh positive/negative infant carried by Rh positive/negative mother. Difference in ABO groups also may cause hemolytic disease and other antigens c, C, Cw, Cx, E, also, but seldom involved. If mother sensitized against fetus by previous incompatible blood transfusion, firstborn may be affected; otherwise, usually firstborn is normal and hemolytic disease appears in successive pregnancies.

Pathology. Jaundice; edema; effusions of serous cavities; occasionally, purpura; extensive extramedullary hematopoiesis and hemosiderin deposits in enlarged spleen and liver and several other organs (adrenal; genital organs). In macerated fetus, erythroblast in the lung is characteristic sign. Brain may show generalized or icteric stain localized in basal ganglia.

Diagnostic Procedures. *Blood.* Anemia; nucleated cells up to $100,000/mm^3$; polychromatophilia; reticulocytosis; leukocytosis (15,000–30,000); platelets normal or decreased. Hyperbilirubinemia increasing to a peak of 20 mg/100 ml on third day after birth. If infant survives, progressive decrease afterward. Prothrombin and fibrinogen deficiency, occasionally. If condition caused by Rh or some other group of antibodies, cord blood erythrocytes give a positive direct Coombs test. If caused by ABO incompatibility, the test is negative, or only slightly positive. Indirect reaction positive at birth. Prenatal testing of mother usually shows an increasing titer of anti-Rh antibodies. *Spectrophotometric examination of amniotic fluid.* Obtained transabdominally. *X-rays.* Bone within first week of life shows radiolucent metaphyseal bands.

Therapy. Prophylactic use of anti-Rh immunoglobulin for prevention of active immunization of Rh negative mother. Given intramuscularly in Rh negative mother with Rh positive baby in whom there are no antibodies detected within 48–72 hours. Repeated prophylaxis in successive pregnancies after each delivery. Exchange transfusions to remove antibodies and bilirubin.

Prognosis. Prior to advent of exchange transfusion, mortality up to 80% or severe sequelae. With modern treatment and prophylaxis, much improved.

BIBLIOGRAPHY. Schridde H: Die angeborene allgemeine Wassersucht. MM Wochen 57:397–398, 1910

Levine P, Stetson RE: An unusual case of intragroup agglutination. JAMA 113:126, 1939

Foerster J: Alloimmune hemolytic anemias. In Lee GR, Bithel TC, Foerster J, et al (eds): Wintrobe's Clinical Hematology, 9th ed, pp 1151–1164. Philadelphia, Lea & Febiger, 1993

HEMOPHAGOCYTIC REACTIVE

Synonyms. Reactive hemophagocytic; acquired hemophagocytic.

Symptoms. Age range 16–80 years (median 48). Male to female ratio 2:2/1. In patient with virus infections, AIDS, kidney transplantations, splenectomized, malignancy, collagen disorders, or under cortisone or immunosoppresive treatment, or apparently in healthy condition. Onset often insidious, course rapid. Fever (90%) chills, sweating (30%), fatigue (20%), anorexia (25%), gastrointestinal symptoms (30%), respiratory symptoms (20%)

Signs. Skin rash (20%). Splenomegaly (up to 90%). Lymphoadenopathy (48%). Hepatomegaly (48%). Weight loss (20%). Common disseminated intravascular coagulation or other thrombotic phenomena.

Etiology. Congenital, iatrogenic or acquired immunologic abnormalities.

Pathology. In several organs especially lymph node, spleen-liver, bone marrow, etc. Proliferation of benign histiocytes, with intense degree of hemophagocytosis. Lymph node and splenic pulp and myelofibrosis. Plasma cells in 30% of cases. Other procedures for underlying disease.

Diagnostic Procedures. *Blood.* Phagocytic mono and histiocytes. Pancitopenia, anemia; coagulopathy (up to 90% of cases), abnormal liver functions, BUN elevation, IgG increased. Antinuclear antibodies (0–50%). Coombs positivity (0–28%). *Bone marrow.*

Therapy. According to identified underlying disease: antibiotics, antineoplastic agents, etc.

Prognosis. Duration of illness 2–4 weeks. Mortality rate associated with infection 20–42%, if not 100% circa.

BIBLIOGRAPHY. Chandra P, Shaukat A, Chaudhery, Rosner F: Transient histiocytosis with striking phagocytosis of platelets, leukocytes, and erythrocytes. Arch Intern Med 135:989–991, 1975

Risdall RJ, McKenne RW, Nesbit ME: Virus-associated hemophagocytic syndrome: A benign histiocytic proliferation distinct from malignant histiocytosis. Cancer 44:993–1002, 1979

Hess CE: Hairy cell leukemia, malignant histiocytosis and related disorders. In Lee GR Bithel TC, Foerster J, et al (eds): Wintrobe's Clinical Hematology, 9th ed, pp 2189–2190. Philadelphia, Lea & Febiger, 1993.

HEMOPHILIA, CLASSIC

Synonyms. AHG deficiency; antihemophilic globulin deficiency; bleeder; factor VIII deficiency; hemophilia A.

Symptoms and Signs. Incidence, 60–80 per million. Occurs in males (with a few exceptions in homozygous females); onset from birth (umbilical hemorrhage; circumcision); more frequently when child begins to crawl and walk; occasionally later in childhood. Spontaneous, intramuscular, mucous membrane, gastrointestinal, pulmonary, pleural, intracranial, genitourinary tract, joint (with resultant hemarthrotic changes) hemorrhages. Spontaneous hemorrhages may have cyclic (3–6 week) character. A mild form of the disease exists where manifestations are less severe.

Etiology. Congenital deficiency of Factor VIII; X-linked recessive type of inheritance. Female carrier may have a decreased amount of Factor VIII. In hemophilia-like syndrome in female, circulating anticoagulant explains the hemorrhagic manifestations. Cases of females with hemophilia, without family history, are not explained. Possible mutation has been postulated; or Lyon hypothesis, which assumes that only one of the X chromosomes is functional.

Pathology. That of bleeding in different organs and tissues; hemarthrosis.

Diagnostic Procedures. *Blood.* Normal bleeding time; normal or prolonged clotting time; usually, increased partial thromboplastin time; usually, abnormal thromboplastin generation test; abnormal absorbed plasma reagent in Factor VIII deficiency; normal or abnormal prothrombin consumption test; Factor VIII assay is diagnostic; normal one-stage prothrombin time.

Therapy. Transfusion of fresh whole blood when blood loss; for prevention, fresh, frozen plasma, plasma concentrate, or concentrate antihemophilic globulin (AHG) preparation. Local therapy with topical thrombin. Corticosteroids also useful. Initially, good results with marrow transplantation.

Prognosis. Death in first 5 years of life in 57% of cases. Surgical procedures frequent cause of death. In mild form, prognosis relatively better.

BIBLIOGRAPHY. Otto JC: An account of an hemorrhagic disposition existing in certain families. M Repository 6:1, 1803

Epstein I (ed): The Babylonian Talmud, Yebamoth, sec 64B, vol 1, p 431. London, Soncino Press, 1936

Brocker-Vriends AHJ, Briet E, Dreesen JCFM, et al: Somatic origin of inherited hemophilia. A Human Genet 85:288–292, 1990

Green PM, Montandon AJ, Bentley DR, et al: Genetics and molecular biology of hemophilias A and B. Blood Coag Fibrin 2:239–256, 1991

HEMORRHAGIC, NEONATAL

Synonyms. Hemophilia neonatorum; neonatal hemorrhagic diathesis; melena neonatorum; morbus hemorrhagicus neonatorum; neonatal diathesis.

Symptoms and Signs. Both sexes affected; onset in first few days of life. Spontaneous (seldom massive; usually oozing type) external and internal hemorrhages: skin (30%), gastrointestinal tract (70%); umbilical cord (25%); brain; lungs. Signs according to site and extent of hemorrhage.

Etiology. *Maternal factors.* Dietary deficiency; poor absorption of vita-

min K. *Constitutional factors.* Functional immaturity of liver. More severe physiologic hypoprothrombinemia observed in between second and sixth day after birth. *Acquired factors.* Trauma or hemorrhage at delivery with depletion of coagulation factors. Not hereditary.

Pathology. According to site and extent of hemorrhage.

Diagnostic Procedures. *Blood.* Anemia; bleeding time and clotting time usually prolonged; prothrombin level low.

Therapy. Blood transfusion if needed; vitamin K parenterally immediately after delivery.

Prognosis. Cases with limited external hemorrhage not serious; internal hemorrhage, 70% mortality. Rapid course; death or complete recovery in 2–3 days.

BIBLIOGRAPHY. Lovegren E: Erfahrungen und Studien über Melaena neonatorum. Jahrb Kinderheilk 78:249, 1913

Bithell TC: Acquired coagulation disorders. In Lee GR, Bithel TC, Foerster J, et al (eds): Wintrobe's Clinical Hematology, 9th ed, pp 1474–1477. Philadelphia, Lea & Febiger, 1993

HEMORRHAGIC SHOCK AND ENCEPHALOPATHY

Synonym. HSES.

Symptoms. Loss of consciousness; cyanosis; agonal respiration; focal and generalized convulsions.

Signs. Hypotension; extreme hypothermia; diaphoresis; hypertonicity; brisk reflexes.

Etiology. Excessive wrapping and warming of infants (hyperpyrexial) for a mild upper respiratory tract infection.

Pathology. Cell loss, swelling and pyknosis in Purkinje cells of both cerebral as well as cerebellar cortex.

Diagnostic Procedures. Laboratory evidence of renal, hepatic, coagulation, and metabolic disfunction.

Prevention. Do not keep mildly ill children excessively warm.

Therapy. Resuscitation; lowering of body temperature; anticonvulsants: plasmapheresis.

Prognosis. Significant motor and intellectual deficits.

BIBLIOGRAPHY. Levine M, Kay JDS, Gould JD, et al: Hemorrhagic shock and encephalopathy: a new syndrome with a high mortality in young children. Lancet II:64–67, 1983

Whittington LK, Roscelli JD, Parry WH: Hemorrhagic shock and encephalopathy: further description of a new syndrome. J Pediatr 106:599–602, 1985

Sofer S, Phillip M, Hershkowits J, Bennet H: Hemorrhagic shock and encephalopathy syndrome: its association with hyperthermia. Am J Dis Child 140:1252–1254, 1986

Hervé F, Bakchine H, Le Loc'h H, et al: Le syndrome de choc hémorragique avec encéphalopathie. Arch Fr Pediatr 44:195–197, 1987

HEMORRHOIDAL PROSTATIC IMPOTENCE

Symptoms and Signs. Sexual impotence developing in patient with internal hemorrhoids.

Etiology. No detectable anatomic or physiologic mechanism. (Possible vascular prostatic congestion.) Psychic factors primary cause or component of etiology.

Therapy. Hemorrhoidectomy.

Prognosis. Good with therapy.

BIBLIOGRAPHY. Cantor AJ: Hemorrhoidal-prostatic-impotence syndrome. NY State J Med 46:1455–1456, 1946

HEMOSIDEROSIS IDIOPATHIC, PULMONARY

Synonyms. Pulmonary idiopathic hemosiderosis.

Symptoms and Signs. In children and young adults. Diagnosis of exclusion in case of alveolar hemorrhage in the absence of other systemic diseases. Pallor may be the initial and only symptom, hemoptysis frequent. After repeated episodes of dyspnea, clubbing, and signs of cor pulmonale.

Etiology. Unknown.

Pathology. Alveolar infiltrates. Later interstitial fibrosis.

Diagnostic Procedures. *Blood.* Iron deficiency; anemia. *X-ray.* Chest alveolar infiltrates.

Therapy. Symptomatic.

Prognosis. Fair.

BIBLIOGRAPHY. Kuhn MJ: Idiopathic pulmonary hemosiderosis: The importance of a chest radiograph in children with unexplained anemia. Mt Sinai J Med (NY)52:358–362, 1985

Lee GR: Iron deficiency and iron-deficiency anemia. In Lee GR, Bithel TC, Foerster J, et al: Wintrobe's Clinical Hematology, p 817. Philadelphia, Lea & Febiger, 1993

HENCH-ROSENBERG

Synonyms. Palindromic rheumatism.

Symptoms. Sudden attack of pain from moderate to very severe, and swelling of joints, reaching its peak in a few hours. Attacks occur at any time of day, but most often in late afternoon. Attack lasts and completely recedes in 1 or 2 days (occasionally lasts 7 days). Finger joint, usually of dorsum or hand, knees, wrists, shoulder, ankles, elbows, temporomandibular, sternoclavicular; cervical vertebra less frequently. Absence of constitutional effects. Occasionally, periarticular attacks, painful swelling involving periarticular or soft tissues (heel bottom; finger pads; flexor or dorsal surfaces of forearms; ankle tendon).

Signs. Swelling of periarticular tissue; skin discolored, reddish, or red. Variable degree of disability of articulation. Nonarticular attacks show brown discoloration, firm consistency, nonpitting, tenderness. Some patients show the sudden appearance of nodules that usually disappear within 1 week.

Etiology. Unknown. In some cases response to irritant or allergens.

Pathology. Acute nonspecific cellular exudates in synovial cavities, reverting to normal with cessation of attack. Nodules: nonspecific inflammation.

Diagnostic Procedures. *Blood.* Moderate lymphocytosis, moderate elevation of sedimentation rate during attack. All tests for rheumatoid arthritis or rheumatism negative. Occasionally, increase of blood lipids and fatty acids.

Therapy. None specifically indicated. Long remission reported with the use of gold salts. Corticosteroids only in severe forms. Prophylaxis of attack by indomethacin or phenylbutazone.

Prognosis. Repeated attacks 50%; complete remission 10%; evolution into rheumatoid arthritis or other collagen diseases 40%.

BIBLIOGRAPHY. Hench PS, Rosenberg EF: Palindromic rheumatism; "new" often recurring disease of joints (arthritis, periarthritis, para-arthritis) apparently producing no articular residues—report of 34 cases; its relation to "angioneural arthrosis," "allergic rheumatism" and rheumatoid arthritis. Arch Intern Med 73:293–321, 1944

Schumacher HR: Palindromic onset of rheumatoid arthritis: clinical, synovial fluid, and biopsy studies. Arthritis Rheum 25:361–369, 1982

Yousef W, Yan A, Russel AS: Palindromic rheumatism: A response to chloroquine. J Rheumatol 18:35–37, 1991

Zvaifler NJ: Cancer and miscellaneous arthropathies. In Klippel JH, Dieppe PA: Rheumatology, pp 3.38.1–3.38.2. St Louis, CV Mosby, 1995

HENNEBERT

Synonyms. Luetic—otitic—nystagmus; syphilitic—otitic—nystagmus; vertigo—nystagmus—luetic.

Symptoms and Signs. Occurs in children. Short, spontaneous attacks of giddiness and nystagmus. Fistula symptoms without fistula: compression with finger of external auditory meatus or pulling the tragus elicits spontaneous nystagmus. Tympanic membrane intact.

Etiology. Congenital syphilis.

Pathology. That of congenital syphilis.

Diagnostic Procedures. Serology.

Therapy. Penicillin; antisyphilitics.

Prognosis. This symptom complex is a transient phenomenon, occasionally encountered in congenital syphilis.

BIBLIOGRAPHY. Hennebert C: Réactions vestibularies dans les labyrinthites héredo-syphilitiques. Arch Int Laryngol Otol 28:93–96, 1909

Asherson N: Spontaneous nystagmus in congenital syphilis. Arch Dis Child 5:331–334, 1930

Brandt T: Vertigo: Its Multisensory Syndromes. London, Springer-Verlag, 1991

HENNEKAM

Synonyms. Lymphangiektasia—lymphedema.

Symptoms. At birth. Both sexes. Diarrhea. Mild growth and mental retardation. Seizures.

Signs. Lymphedema initially causes characteristic oriental facies; lymphedema then progress involving lower extremities and genitalia. Oozing lymph may become infected (Erysepelas).

Etiology. Autosomal recessive inheritance.

Pathology. Diffuse lymphagiectasis.

Signs. *Blood.* Hyperproteinemia. *Stool.* Protein losing enteropathy.

BIBLIOGRAPHY. Hennekam RCM, Geerdink RA, Hamel BCJ et al: Autosomal recessive intestinal lymphagiectasia and lymphedema with facial anomalies and mental retardation. Am J Med Genet 34:593–600, 1989

Gabrielli O, Catassi C, Coppa GV, et al: Intestinal lymphangiectasia, lymphedema, mental retardation and typical face: Confirmation of the Hennekam syndrome. Am J Med Genet 40:244–247, 1991

HENOCH

This eponym is sometimes used in place of the term Schönlein-Henoch (see) when abdominal manifestations are predominant.

HEPATIC FLEXURE

See Gas syndromes.

Symptoms. Feeling of abdominal fullness and desire to eructate. Pain in right renal zone, epigastrium, left upper abdominal hypochondrium, right shoulder.

Signs. Sometimes, increased tympansim, right hypochondrium.

Etiology. Collection of gas in hepatic flexure of colon. If gas collects in splenic flexure, called splenic flexure syndrome.

Diagnostic Procedures. *X-ray.* Flat plate of abdomen.

Therapy. Removal of anatomic or functional obstruction.

BIBLIOGRAPHY. Palmer ED, Deutsch DL, Scott NM Jr: Clinical experiences with the splenic flexure syndrome and the hepatic flexure syndrome. Am J Dig Dis 22:194–197, 1955

HEPATORENAL SYNDROMES

Synonyms. Flint; Heyd; HRS; functional renal failure; bile nephrosis; cholemic nephrosis; urohepatic. See also liver massive necrosis and HELLP.

Vague term that means any renal disease that occurs in patient with liver pathology. Laboratory evidence of renal involvement (oliguria-azotemia), frequently found in all types of liver pathology, the pathophysiologic interrelationships between liver and kidney have not yet been clarified completely. Deposition of pigment and other hemodynamic alterations (sensitivity of kidney tissue owing to an earlier stage of renal arterial vasocostriction) have been considered. Practical therapeutic considerations to be kept in mind in such conditions are to restrict salt in spite of hyponatremia and avoid administration of diuretics if at all possible.

Hepatorenal (HRS) term should be restricted to indicate a condition where, in absence of intrinsic renal failure, we observe a "progressive renal failure resulting from intense renal arteriolar constriction due to severe liver disease."

LIVER CIRRHOSIS

1. Cirrhosis associated with prerenal uremia—functional renal failure: minimal urine sodium concentration; absence of proteinuria; normal renal histology.
2. Cirrhosis associated with acute tubular necrosis: typical biochemical changes (high urine sodium concentration; isosmolality of urine); typical histologic pattern.
3. Alpha-1 antitrypsin deficiency.

Etiology. Cause of renal dysfunction has been uncertain for a long time. In some cases compression of inferior vena cava decreases renal blood flow, glomerular filtration rate, and sodium excretion. The compression of the inferior vena cava may precede the formation of ascites when caused by caudate lobe compression. Neurogenic vasoconstriction; false neurotransmitters; renin-angiotensin system role; possible role of endotoxins.

Pathology. A wide spectrum of alterations, from normal renal histology to tubular necrosis. Numerous glomerular lesions, papillary necrosis, pyelonephritis, interstitial nephritis have been described as well. Immunofluorescence: IgA in mesangium and capillary.

Diagnostic Procedures. *Hepatic function tests, enzyme studies, kidney function tests, determination of inferior vena cava pressure.* Strong correlation observed between caval pressure and glomerular filtration rate and urinary sodium excretion.

Therapy. That of cirrhosis. Demonstration of constriction of vena cava by caudate lobe is a necessary precautionary measure prior to portacaval surgery. Conservative management of renal failure.

Prognosis. Poor.

FULMINANT HEPATIC FAILURE

The association with renal failure (functional renal failure or acute tubular necrosis) is found in 80% of patients with fulminating hepatic failure in patients with eclampsia.

Etiology. Related to endotoxins.

Pathology. See Liver, massive necrosis.

Therapy. That of basic condition. Results with dialysis better than in cirrhosis. Treatment (including persevering with dialysis) may result in complete recovery in some cases. Liver transplantation.

Prognosis. Poor.

OBSTRUCTIVE JAUNDICE

Various degrees of kidney insufficiency occurring in association with any cause of obstruction of biliary tract (e.g., neoplastic; inflammatory; surgical).

Etiology. Enhanced absorption of endotoxin from intestine owing to lack of biliary salts; depression of reticuloendothelial function; sensitization of renal parenchyma to anoxia by bilirubin and bile salts.

Pathology. Fibrin deposits in kidney and tubular necrosis.

Therapy. Surgical. If needed, dialysis.

Prognosis. Fair.

SHOCK AND SEPSIS

In these conditions, frequent occurrence of jaundice and renal failure.

Etiology. Multifactorial (e.g., large transfusion; endotoxins; reticuloendothelial system insufficiency).

Pathology. *Liver.* From simple cholestasis to centrilobular necrosis (according to length of shock period). *Kidney.* Different degrees and types of lesions from none to tubular necrosis and glomerulonephritis.

Therapy. That of shock; once stabilized, prolonged dialysis until situation is overcome.

Prognosis. Seldom, progression to hepatic failure. Good results with intensive treatment.

INFECTIVE

Some particular infections affect both liver and kidney. Hepatitis B, especially in children of certain geographic areas (Asia, Eastern Europe, Africa). See also Yellow fever.

MISCELLANEOUS

1. Polycystic disease
2. Glomerulonephritis (immune complex type) associated with chronic hepatitis B and other conditions.
3. Drug reaction
4. Toxins

BIBLIOGRAPHY. Flint A: Clinical report on hydroperitoneum based on the analysis of 46 cases. Am J Med Sci 45:306–339, 1863
Heyd CG: The liver and its relation to chronic abdominal infection. Ann Surg 79:55–77, 1924
Helwig FC, Schutz CB: A liver-kidney syndrome. Surg Gynecol Obstet 55:570–580, 1932
Hoef JC: Hepatorenal syndrome. In Haubrich WS, Schaffner F, Berk JE (eds): Bockus Gasroenterology, 5th ed, pp 2023–2034. Philadelphia, WB Saunders, 1995

HEPATITIS, FULMINATING–HYPOGLYCEMIA, RECURRENT

Synonyms. Hemorrhage—hepatitis—hypoglycemia.

Spontaneous hypoglycemia in liver diseases is known to occur, although not too frequently. In one case of fulminating hepatitis with massive liver necrosis, the authors noticed an extreme degree of hypoglycemia not relieved by massive glucose administration (up to 2.5 kg of sugar/day). On theoretical grounds and with evidence of an increased insulin plasma level, the authors postulated the possible role of lack of insulin catabolism by the necrotic liver as responsible for the hypoglycemia in this case and in some of these conditions.

BIBLIOGRAPHY. Samson RI, Trey C, Tirune AH, et al: Fulminating hepatitis with recurrent hypoglycemia and hemorrhage. Gastroenterology 53:291–300, 1967

HERLITZ-PEARSON

Synonyms. Heinrichsbauer; epidermolysis bullosa hereditaria letalis; junctional, lethal, epidermolysis bullosa.

Symptoms and Signs. Present at birth. Bullous skin lesions. Fever; absence of residual scarring; bullous lesions of mucosae; loss of nails from toes and fingers.

Etiology. Unknown; recessive type of inheritance.

Pathology. Skin cleavage at the dermoepidermal junction with bulla formation present but not marked. Regeneration of basal cells at the edges of areas of ulceration; absence of inflammatory reaction and edema; characteristic vacuolization of basal part of germinal layer of epidermis. Other organs negative findings.

Diagnostic Procedures. *Biopsy of skin.* Blisters in junctional zone with hemidesmosomes reduced in number and showing abnormal structure. Exuberant granulation tissue considered the "hallmark" cutaneous feature of this form. *Blood.* Severe progressive hypoalbuminemia. *Amnion membranes. Biopsy.* For prenatal diagnosis.

Therapy. Symptomatic; antibiotics; steroids not effective.

Prognosis. Death within 1 year.

BIBLIOGRAPHY. Herlitz G: Kongenitaler nicht syphilitischer Pemphigus. Eine Übersicht nebst Beschreibung einer neuen Krankheitsform (Epidermolysis bullosa hereditaria letalis). Acta Paediatr 17:315–371, 1935
Roberts MH, Howell DRS, Bramhall JL, et al: Epidermolysis bullosa letalis. Pediatrics 25:283–290, 1960
Pearson RW, Potter B, Strauss F: Epidermolysis bullosa letalis. Clinical and histological manifestations and course of the disease. Arch Dermatol 109:394–355, 1974
Fine J-B, Bauer EA, Briggaman RA, et al: Revised clinical and laboratory criteria for subtypes of inherited epidermolysis bullosa: a consensus report by Subcommittee on diagnosis and classification of the National Epidermolysis Bullosa Registry. J Am Acad Dermatol 24:119–135, 1991

HERMAN

Not a well-defined entity, it represents the combination of possible neurologic symptomatology following a closed head injury. See Livedo reticularis.

BIBLIOGRAPHY. Herman E: Niezwyklyzespól oprazowy: livedo racemosa universalis u osobnika z objawami piramidwopozapiramidowymi i zaburzeniami psychicznymi. Warsz Czas Lek 14:107–109, 1973
Walt AJ, Wilson RF: Management of trauma. Pitfalls and Practice, p 201. Philadelphia, Lea & Febiger, 1979

HERMANN

Synonyms. Deafness—photomyoclonus—diabetes mellitus—nephropathy—cerebral dysfunction; photomyoclonus—deafness—diabetes mellitus—nephropathy—cerebral dysfunction. See Apert.

Symptoms and Signs. Both sexes. The different manifestations have variable age of onset and course from early childhood or adolescence with death from rapid neurologic deterioration and dementia, to onset in later age and slower progression: photomyoclonic seizures; progressive nerve deafness; progessive dementia, Bright syndrome rapidly progressing in the final stage.

Etiology. Unknown. Autosomal dominant inheritance of variable penetrance.

Pathology. *Kidney.* Small foci of interstitial chronic inflammation. *Brain.* Diffuse neuronal degeneration and astrocytosis; decrease of cerebellar cells and of indentate neurons or inferior olivary nucleus.

Diagnostic Procedures. *Blood.* Mild diabetes. *Audiogram.* Progressive cochlear degeneration. *CT scan. MRI. EEG.*

Therapy. Symptomatic.

Prognosis. Death after relatively short course or slowly progressing course. Death usually after few months of accelerated changes.

BIBLIOGRAPHY. Hermann C Jr, Aguilar MJ, Sacks OW: Hereditary photomyoclonus associated with diabetes mellitus, deafness, nephropathy and cerebral dysfunction. Neurology 14:212–221, 1964

HERMANSKI-PUDLAK

Synonyms. Albinism—hemorrhagic diathesis; albinism—thrombocytopathy; HPS; delta storage pool disease.

Symptoms and Signs. Prevalent in Puerto Ricans, but also in other ethnic groups. Both sexes affected; onset from birth. Pigment disorder with variable phenotypic expression of degrees of pigmentation affecting skin, hair, and eyes. Nystagmus; photophobia. Hemorrhagic episodes: usually, mild bleeding, seldom massive; easy bruisability; epistaxis; hemorrhages after tooth extraction and trauma (aspirin may intensify hemorrhages). Restrictive lung disease and ulcerative colitis may develop (see Diagnostic Procedures).

Etiology. Unknown. It is the combination of three defects (albinism, hemorrhagic diathesis, and storage of abnormal lipid-like material) attributed to a pleiotropic effect of a single autosomal recessive mutation. Suspected enzymatic defect.

Pathology. In skin, from no visible pigment to dermatization of granular melanin. Generalized infiltration by a yellow pigment (ceroid-lipofuscin-like) of spleen, liver, lungs, lymph nodes, and other organs. Electron microscopy. Presence of granules in circulating leukocytes and bone marrow full of pigment.

Diagnostic Procedures. *Blood.* Morphologic, chemical, and functional defects of platelets. Blood clotting abnormalities. Leukocytes with two types of cytoplasmatic inclusions: ceroid-like and fibrillar membrane-bound. *Bone marrow.* Presence of pigment-laden macrophages, which stain sea blue. *X-ray.* Changes similar to interstitial pulmonary fibrosis. *Hair incubation test.* Increased pigmentation after addition of L-tyrosine.

Therapy. Symptomatic. Avoid aspirin and nonsteroidal anti-inflammatory drugs. Vitamin E may be of some benefit.

Prognosis. Variable, from minor bleeding episodes to massive fatal hemorrhages.

BIBLIOGRAPHY. Hermanski F, Pudlak P: Albinism associated with hemorrhagic diathesis and unusual pigmented reticular cells in bone marrow. Blood 14:162–169, 1959
Depinho RA, Kaplan KL: The Hermansky-Pudlak syndrome: Report of three cases and review of pathophysiology and management considerations. Medicine 64:192–202, 1985
Wijermans PW, van Dorp DB, Hermansky-Pudlak syndrome: Correction of bleeding time by 1–desamino-8D-arginine vasopressin. Am J Hemat 30:154–157, 1989

HERMAPHRODITISM, TRUE

Synonyms. True hermaphroditism.

Symptoms and Signs. Present from birth. Incidence rarest of intersex disorders except in blacks of southern Africa. Four hundred patients have been reported. Most fetuses do not survive intrauterine life. External genitalia usually ambiguous or of apparently normal male or female aspect (20%); phallus usually bound in chordee; hypospadias; labioscrotal folds incompletely fused; cryptorchidism (see) and inguinal hernia frequent. At puberty, variable prevalence of one phenotypic functional features breast development, menses, some virilization characteristics.

Etiology. Genetic disorders (70% chromatin-positive; the majority with 46 XX karyotype; a lower percentage with 46 XY). Chimerism; hidden mosaicism. Mutant gene and environmental factors have been implicated. Underlying mutation could be transmitted by the father as an autosomal dominant trait. Autosomal recessive inheritance reported as well.

Pathology. Both ovarian and testicular tissue in the same gonad or opposite ones. The "ovotestis" with a fallopian tube in 65% and a vas in 45% of cases. Ovarian tissue must contain oocytes, the mere presence of ovarian stroma is not adequate criterion for diagnosis.

Diagnostic Procedures. *Hormonal studies. Karyotype. Biopsy of the gonads.*

Therapy. Planned according to the age of diagnosis. In newborn, after sex dominance assessment, removal of heterologous structures (e.g., either ovary or testis, mullerian duct) integrated with plastic surgery according to sex role decided upon. Eventual hormonal integration.

Prognosis. Variable according to degree of "confusion" and adequacy of treatment. Incidence of tumor higher than in people with normal gonads (Reason for preferring female sex rearing). In rare cases, ovulation and pregnancy described. Fertility in male not reported.

BIBLIOGRAPHY. Salèn E Ein Fall von Hermaphroditismus verus beim Menshen. Verh Dtschj Ges Pathol 2:241–243, 1899
Milner WA, Garlick WB, Fink AJ, et al: True hermaphrodite siblings. J Urol 79:1003–1009, 1958
Rosenberg HS, Clayton GW, Hsu TC: Familial true hermaphroditism. J Clin Endocrinol 23:203–206, 1963
Fraccaro M, Tiepolo L, Zuffardi O, et al: Familial XX true hermaphroditism in three siblings: Plasma hormonal profile and in vitro steroid biosynthesis in gonadal structures. J Clin Endocr 42:653–660, 1976
Josso N: Anatomy and Endocrinology of fetal sex differentiation. In De Groot LJ (ed): Endocrinology, 3rd ed, pp 1910–1912. Philadelphia, WB Saunders, 1995

HERPES GESTATIONIS

Synonyms. Dermatitis gestationis; prurigo gestationis; pemphigoid gestationis.

Symptoms. Less than 1 case every 60,000 pregnancies; onset during second trimester. Severe form recurring after delivery, during menstrual periods. Severe burning and itching on face, arms, legs, and trunk.

Signs. Multiform erythematous, vesicular, pustular, and bullous lesions that spread over the body centripetally, beginning around the umbilicus.

Etiology. High responsiveness of patient and possibly exposure to antigens derived from sexual consort or autoimmune condition. Condition hormonally modulated (balance of estrogen/progesterone responsible).

Pathology. Epidermal and papillary edema with (nonconstant) eosinophilic spongiosis subepidermal. Bullae.

Diagnostic Procedures. *Blood.* Eosinophilia up to 30%.

Therapy. Corticosteroids; adrenocorticotropic hormone (ACTH); in most severe cases, plasmapheresis. Dapsone and pyridoxine useless.

Prognosis. Good; disappears spontaneously a few weeks after delivery. May recur (in more severe form) during successive pregnancy. Severe form recurrent at menstrual cycles. Risk to fetus is minor (neonatal death reported, however).

BIBLIOGRAPHY. Milton JL: The Pathology and Treatment of Disease of the Skin, p 205. London, Hardwicke, 1972
Holmes RC, Black MM: Symposium on blistering diseases. Dermatol Clin 1:195, 1983
Pye RJ: Bullous eruptions. In Champion RH, Burton JL, Ebling FJG (eds): Rook/Wilkinson/Ebling Textbook of Dermatology, 5th ed, pp 1657–1658. Oxford, Blackwell Scientific, 1992

HERPETIFORM DERMATITIS, SENILE

Synonyms. Bullous pemphigoid; old-age pemphigus; parapemphigus; pemphigoid.

Symptoms and Signs. Both sexes affected; onset usually after 60 years of age (80%). Nonspecific urticarial or eczematous rash of extremities. In urticarial type, after 2–3 weeks, formation of bullae; in eczematous type, after months. Sudden generalization follows (erythema multiforme-like) bullae with clear serum, occasionally hemorrhagic. Reabsorption, without lesion or erosion, which heals rapidly, leaving hyperpigmentation. Mucosal lesions rare.

Etiology. Unknown. French authors consider it a variant of Stevens-Johnson syndrome.

Pathology. No acantholysis; subepidermal bullae. Inflammatory infiltrate with eosinophils, neutrophils, lymphocytes, and histiocytes

Therapy. Corticosteroids (oral, topical, or local infiltration), azathioprine, in few patients dapsone or sulfapyridine effective; tetracycline, niacinamide, plasma exchange, cyclophosphamide suggested also.

Prognosis. Spontaneous remission; good response to treatments, recurrences possible. Death from complications (pneumonia).

BIBLIOGRAPHY. Rook A, Waddington E: Pemphigus and pemphigoid. Br J Dermatol 65:425–431, 1953
Pye RJ: Bullous eruptions. In Champion RH, Burton JL, Ebling FJG (eds): Rook/Wilkinson/Ebling Textbook of Dermatology, 5th ed, pp 1647–1652. Oxford, Blackwell Scientific, 1992

HERRICK

Synonyms. African hemolytic anemia; sickle cell hemolytic anemia; hemoglobinopathy S; meniscocytosis; sickle cell; Chwechweechwe, Nwiiwii, Nuiduidui, Abotutuo (African tribe names); SS disease.

Symptoms. Occurs particularly in blacks, also in Greeks, Italians (especially Sicilians), and in Turkish families; more common in females. Increased fatigability. Subject to the occurrence and spontaneous remission of several symptoms. Sudden increase in weakness; severe pain in joints (in children, see Hand and Foot) and elsewhere in extremities. Abdominal cramps, epigastrium or right abdominal quadrant (simulating acute abdomen); fever (during crisis). Spontaneous hematuria; epistaxis; neurologic manifestations; headache; drowsiness; hemiplegia; aphasia; blindness (temporary or permanent).

Signs. Skin pale; mild subicterus of skin and mucosae; underweight; short trunk and long extremities; occasionally, dorsal kyphosis and lumbar lordosis; chest anteroposterior enlargement. Facial hair scanty. Heart enlarged; tachycardia; sinus arrhythmia, systolic thrill on precordium; diastolic tap in pulmonic area; accentuation of second sound. Abdominal or extremity tenderness or both (during crisis). Mild lymphadenopathy, as a rule; moderate hepatomegaly; seldom, splenomegaly. Chronic leg ulcers.

Etiology. Congenital hemoglobinopathy; autosomal intermediate inheritance. Presence of two hemoglobin S genes produce sickle cell anemia, whereas only one abnormal gene produces a sickle gene trait with only partial symptomatic manifestation.

Pathology. *Bone.* Deformities with abnormal calcifications. Generalized bone marrow hyperplasia and hemosiderosis except in smaller bones where fat substitution may be observed. Infarctions, necrosis, and hemorrhages of various tissues. *Liver.* Anoxic necrosis; hemochromatosis; erythrophagocytosis; in many cases micronodular cirrhosis. *Spleen.* Congestion with sickle cells; infarctions; eventually fibrosis and shrinkage (autosplenectomy). *Kidney.* Congestion; infarctions; necrosis and fibrotic calcific changes. *Nervous system.* Infarction and small hemorrhages.

Diagnostic Procedures. *Blood.* Anemia; anisopoikilocytosis; few drepanocytes; nucleated red cells; reticulocytes increased. Sickle cell test (drepanocytes developing for lack of oxygen). Leukocytosis with shift to the left; eosinophilia; increased monocytes. Platelets increased. Increased resistance to osmotic fragility. Low sedimentation rate. Hyperbilirubinemia. *Bone marrow.* Erythroid hyperplasia. *Urine.* Hematuria, decrease of kidney concentration ability after fluid deprivation. *X-ray of skeleton.* Abnormalities of bones; ground glass appearance of skull; peculiar radial striation, which may be noticed in other bones as well (vertebrae). Osteoporosis and osteosclerosis of long bones; pathologic fractures.

Therapy. Constant medical attention. Polyvalent pneumococcal vaccine. Folic acid administration. Hypertransfusion therapy. In crisis. Hydration, analgesics, antibiotics. Splenectomy in case of splenomegaly with hypersplenism. Antisickling agents are still in discussion. Bone marrow transplantation.

Prognosis. Good adaptation to anemic condition; partial remission of anemia occasionally observed, crisis of 4–6 days' duration recurrent at variable intervals (days or years). Majority die in first 10 years of life; few survive to fourth decade. Death from shock, intercurrent infections, cardiac and renal failure.

BIBLIOGRAPHY. Herrick JB: Peculiar elongated and sickle-shaped red corpuscles in a case of severe anemia. Arch Intern Med 6:517–521, 1910
Bunn HF, Forget BG: Hemoglobin: Molecular, Genetic and Clinical Aspects, p 502. Philadelphia, WB Saunders, 1986
Lukens JN: Hemoglobinopathies S; C; D; E; and O and associated diseases. In Lee GR, Bithel TC, Foerster J, et al (eds): Wintrobe's Clinical Hematology, 9th ed. Philadelphia, Lea & Febiger, 1993

HERRMANN

Synonyms. WL (initials of patient); facio-audio symphalangism; symphalangism—brachydactyly; synostoses—multiple brachydactyly; polysynphalangism.

Symptoms and Signs. Both sexes. Deafness, conductive type; facies peculiarities; broad nose; pectus carinatum; bilateral dysplasia and synostoses of elbow, wrist, fingers, and toes. Middle phalanges and metacarpals short. Nail malformations.

Etiology. Autosomal dominant inheritance.

BIBLIOGRAPHY. Herrmann J: Symphalangism-brachydactyly syndrome: report of the WL symphalangism brachydactyly syndrome: review of the literature and classification. Birth Defects Orig Art Ser 10(5):23–53, 1974
Hurvitz SA, Goodman RM, Hertz M, et al: The facio-audio-symphalangism syndrome: Report of case and review of the literature. Clin Genet 28:61–68, 1985

HERS

Synonyms. Cori type VI glycogenosis; glycogenosis type VI; glycogen storage defect type VI; hepatic phosphorylase kinase deficiency; phosphorylase kinase deficiency. Includes the rare variants: muscle phosphokinase deficiency and heart phosphokinase deficiency.

Symptoms. Both sexes affected, onset in infancy and early childhood. Symptoms may be so mild that syndrome may pass undetected. Moderate growth retardation; mild to moderate Harris (S.) syndrome (see).

Signs. Marked hepatomegaly.

Etiology. Includes at least three different genetic defects: (A) X-linked phosphorilase b kinase deficiency (muscle enzyme not affected) classified also as VIa; (B), autosomal phosphokinase b kinase deflciency (affecting muscle and liver); (C) complete or partial liver phosphorilase deficiency. Relationship between this biochemical defects and clinical manifestation not yet clearly established.

Pathology. Marked hepatomegaly. Glycogen accumulation. Biochemical study shows deficiencies of phosphorylase activity. Other enzymatic activity apparently normal. No accumulation of glycogen in heart or muscles (except for specific variants).

Diagnostic Procedures. *Blood.* In leukocytes, deficiency of phosphorylase activity. Glycogen in erythrocytes and leukocytes normal. Most patients respond normally to the hyperglycemic action of glucagone.

Therapy. Dietary management of hypoglycemia.

Prognosis. Excellent; normal growth and development with the exception of persisting hepatomegaly.

BIBLIOGRAPHY. Hers HG: Études enzymatiques sur fragments hepatiques application à la classification des glycogenoses. Rev Intern Hepatol 9:35–55, 1959
Newgard CB, Nakano K, Hwang PK, et al: Sequence analysis of the cDNA encoding human liver glycogen phosphorylase reveals tissue-specific codon usage. Proc Natl Acad Sci 83:8132–8136, 1987
Chen YT, Burchell A: Glycogen storage diseases. In Scriver CR, Beaudet AL, Sly WS, et al: The Metabolic and Molecular Bases of Inherited Disease, 7th ed, pp 953–954. New York, McGraw-Hill, 1995

HERSH (J.A.)

Symptoms and Signs. Both sexes. Craniosynostosis, sensineural hearing loss, craniofacial abnormalities: hypertelorism, nasal bridge: flat; nasal tip: broad; micrognathia; sparse curly hair. Intellectual abilities not impaired; in one case autistic-like behavior and language delay in one other.

Etiology. Autosomal recessive inheritance.

BIBLIOGRAPHY. Hersh JA, et al: Craniosynostosis, sensineural hearing loss and craniofacial abnormalities in siblings. Proc. Greenwood Genet Ctr 5:186, 1986

HERSMAN

Synonyms. Progressive hand growth; macrodactyly.

Symptoms and Signs. Progressive growth of hands without other signs of macroacromia or endocrine involvement.

BIBLIOGRAPHY. Hersman CF: A case of progressive enlargement of the hands. Intern Med Mag 3:662–665, 1894
Milford L: Congenital anomalies. In Crenshaw AH (ed): Campbell's Operative Orthopedics, 7th ed, pp 428–429. St Louis, CV Mosby, 1987

HERTWIG-MAGENDIE

Synonyms. Magendie-Hertwig; vertical diplopia; skew deviation.

Symptoms. Vertical diplopia. Various associated symptoms of neurologic nature. See Etiology.

Signs. Vertical deviation of one eye above the other, deviation possibly concomitant or variable (i.e., one eye faces down and the other one up and out).

Etiology and Pathology. Trauma or neurosurgery; atherosclerosis or neoplasia resulting in vascular brainstem lesions; primary cerebellar tumors; metastatic posterior fossa lesions; mesencephalic lesions; demyelinizing syndromes; syringobulbia; or as an isolated neurologic sign (vertical strabismus simulating skew deviation).

Diagnostic Procedures. *Screen and cover test.* Examination of old photographs to detect previous strabismus. *X-ray of skull. Angiography. CT scan. MRI imaging. Brain isotope scan.*

Therapy. According to etiology.

Prognosis. Depends on etiology.

BIBLIOGRAPHY. Hertwig H: Experimenta quaedam de effectibus laesionum in partibus encephali singularibus et de verosimili harum partium functione, Berolini, formis Feisterianis et Eiserdorffianis (1926). Ind Cat Surg Gen 1st series 6:185, 1885

Pötzl O, Sittig O: Klinische Befunde wit Hertwig–Magendiescher Augeneinstellung. Z Ges Neurol Psychiatr 95:701–730, 1925

Smith JL, David NJ, Klintworth G: Skew deviation. Neurology 14:96–105, 1964

Keane JR: Alternating skew deviation: 47 patients. Neurology 35:725–728, 1985

Adams RD, Victor M: Principles of Neurology, 5th ed, p 230. New York, McGraw-Hill, 1993

HERTWIG-WEYERS

Synonyms. Ulnae aplasia; multiple bone and visceral malformations; oligodactyly; ulnar hemimelia.

Symptoms and Signs. Present from birth. Ulnar aplasia associated with variable bone (sternum; jaw) or visceral (kidney; spleen) abnormalities.

Etiology. Unknown; possibly hereditary recessive or new mutation.

BIBLIOGRAPHY. Hertwig P: Sechs neue Mutationen bei der Hausmaus in ihrer Bedeutung für allgemeine Vererbungsfragen. Z Mensch Vereb 26:1–21, 1942

Weyers H: Das Oligodactylie-syndrome des Menschen und seine Parallelmutation bei der Hausmaus. Ann Paediatr (Basel) 189:351–370, 1957

HERVA

Synonyms. Salonen-Herva-Nario; cataract-cerebellar atrophy—mental retardation—myopathy; hydrolethalus.

Symptoms. and Signs. Congenital mental retardation; hypotonia; ataxia; cataracts.

Etiology. Autosomal recessive probable inheritance.

Pathology. Cerebellar atrophy myelin bodies. Muscle biopsy: vacular degeneration, fat infiltration, vacuolization.

Diagnostic Procedures. *X-rays. CT scan. MRI. Electromicroscopy. Muscle biopsy.*

BIBLIOGRAPHY. Herva R: A syndrome with juvenile cataract, cerebellar

atrophy, mental retardation and myopathy. Neuropediatrics 18:164–169, 1987

Salonen R, Herva R: Hydrolethalus syndrome. J Med Genet 27:756–7569, 1990

Camera G, Carbone LD, Centa A, et al: Diagnosi prenatale di "Hydrolethalus" (sindrome di Salonen-Herva-Nario) in donna a rischio sconosciuto: Presentazione di un caso con sopravvivenza prolungata. Pathologica 83:359–364, 1991

Muenke M, Ruchelli ED, Rake LB: On lumping and splitting: A fetus with clinical findings of the oral-facial-diastal syndrome type VII, the hydrolethalus syndrome, and the Pallister Hall syndrome. Am J Med Genet 41:548–556, 1991

HERXHEIMER

Synonyms. Pick-Herxheimer; Taylor; atrophic chronic acrodermatitis; acrodermatis chronica, atrophicans; Lyme boreliosis, late phase.

Symptoms. Insidious onset in country dwellers at 30–90 years of age; rare in childhood. Occurs mostly in north central European, Italian, and Spanish peoples. Insidious onset. Itching; burning; constitutional symptoms.

Signs. Reddish nodules or plaques appear on feet or legs, less frequently on forearms and hands, rarely affecting trunk or face. Slow, progressive peripheral inflammatory extension, whereas the central part of lesions shows hairless skin, pigmented or poikilodermatous. The nodules concentrate around knees and elbows, the fibrous bands along ulnar margins. Possible ulcerations on the legs.

Etiology. Unknown. Incriminated infective agents transmitted by *Ixodes ricinus.*

Pathology. *Skin.* Initially, dermal edema and perivascular inflammations; later, skin atrophy with destruction of appendages. Subdermal lymphocyte and histiocyte infiltration. *Lymph nodes.* Sinus catarrh; plasma cell infiltration.

Diagnostic Procedures. *Biopsy of skin.* See Pathology. *Blood.* High red cell sedimentation rate; hypergammaglobulinemia.

Therapy. Penicillin, tetracycline, doxocycline in standard doses for 1 month in initial stages.

Prognosis. Fair response to early treatment. Once atrophy established, no response. In some cases, involvement of joints with resulting limitation of functions of articulation (e.g., feet, hands, shoulders). Rare, squamous cell carcinoma development in atrophic cases.

BIBLIOGRAPHY. Pick PJ: Erythromelie. Festschr Kaposi Wien, p 919, 1900

Herxheimer K, Hartmann K: Ueber Acrodermatitis chronica atrophicans. Arch Dermatol Syph 61:57–76, 1902

Burton JL: Disorders of connective tissue. In Champion RH, Burton JL, Ebling FJG (eds): Rook/Wilkinson/Ebling Textbook of Dermatology, 5th ed, pp 1775–1776. Oxford, Blackwell Scientific, 1992

HESS

Synonyms. N syndrome (N initial of affected family).

Symptoms. One family described. Two brothers. Severe mental and physical retardation, visual and acoustic impairment.

Signs. Dolicocephaly, hypertelorism, large cornea, laterally overlapping upper eyelids, abnormal auricles, dental dysplasia, cryptorchidism, hypospadias, spasticity.

Etiology. X-linked inheritance. Mutation of DNA polymerase alpha considered responsible for the syndrome.

Diagnostic Procedures. *Blood.* Leukemia. *X-rays.* Distal long bones relatively shorter than proximal ones. Over tubulation of long bones.

Prognosis. Death for lymphoblastic leukemias in infancy.

BIBLIOGRAPHY. Hess RO, Kaveggia EG, Optiz JM: The new syndrome: A new multiple congenital anomaly—mental retardation syndrome. Clin Gene. 6:237–246, 1974

Hess RO, Hafez GR, Meisner LF: Updating the N syndrome: Occurrence of lymphoid malignancy and possible association with an increased rate of chromosomal breakage. Am J Med Genet 3:(Suppl) 383–388, 1987

Floy KM, Hess RO, Meisner LF: DNA polymerase alpha defect in the N syndrome. Am J Med Genet 35:301–305, 1990

HESSELBACH

Synonyms. Hernia of Hesselbach.

Symptoms and Signs. Those of a hernia with diverticula trough cribriform fascia.

Therapy. Surgery.

BIBLIOGRAPHY. Hesselbach FC: Anatomisch-chirurgische Abhandlung ueber den Ursprung der Leistenbrueche. Wuerzburg, Baumgaertner, 1806

Sabiston DC: Textbook of Surgery, 14th ed, p 1144. Philadelphia, WB Saunders, 1991

HIBERNOMA

Synonyms. Fetalocellulare lipoma; lipoma, granular cell.

Symptoms. Rare; occurs in both sexes; onset usually in early adult life. Asymptomatic.

Signs. On the cervical, axillary, or intrascapular regions (in order of incidence), appearance of a firm, nontender nodule, with vascular dilatation of the overlying skin.

Etiology. Vestiges of brown fat.

Pathology. Encapsulated, multilobular tumor of primitive fetal fat (tan to dark brown) histologically multiloculated masses of cells with fine sudanophilic granules and solitary central nucleus.

Therapy. Excision.

Prognosis. Good.

BIBLIOGRAPHY. Jennings RC, Behr G: Hibernoma (granular cell lipoma). J Clin Pathol 8:310–312, 1955

Burton JL, Cunlife WJ: Subcutaneous fat. In Champion RH, Burton JL, Ebling FJG (eds): Rook/Wilkinson/Ebling Textbook of Dermatology, 5th ed, p 2161. Oxford, Blackwell Scientific, 1992

HIDRADENOMA ERUPTIVUM

Synonym. Syringoma.

Symptoms. More frequent in females; onset usually in adolescence. Chest, face, eyelids, and neck areas mostly affected. Asymptomatic.

Signs. Small dermal papules (1–5 mm in diameter) yellowish in color, occasionally cystic; at onset, eruptive, then individual or group appearance. The lesions slowly expand to reach limited size (3–5 mm).

Etiology. Unknown; defective development of sweat ducts (?).

Pathology. Sweat ducts dilated and convoluted; lumina filled by amorphous debris. Characteristic strand of cells projecting from side of ducts like a comma.

Therapy. Diathermy for cosmetic reasons.

Prognosis. Partial removal followed by relapse.

BIBLIOGRAPHY. Daicker B: Das Lidsyringoma Studien über seinen geureblichen Bau und seine Histogenese. Dermatologica 128:417–463, 1964

MacKie RM: Tumors of the skin appendages. In Champion RH, Burton JL, Ebling FJG (eds): Rook/Wilkinson/Ebling Textbook of Dermatology, 5th ed, pp 1519–1520. Oxford, Blackwell Scientific, 1992

HIGH-ALTITUDE PULMONARY EDEMA

Synonyms. HAPE; noncardiac pulmonary edema.

Symptoms and Signs. Dyspnea; restlessness; cough. Rales heard diffusely or in an asymmetric pattern; mild fever.

Etiology. Not clear. Decrease of PO_2 causing marked nonuniform vasoconstriction of terminal pulmonary arterioles. Presence of preterminal arterioles emptying directly into venous side of pulmonary capillary bed and transmitting directly; elevated pulmonary pressure causing leakage of plasma or blood into parenchyma.

Pathology. See Etiology. Damage to arterial walls, microthrombi obstructing pulmonary vascular bed (occasionally).

Diagnostic Procedures. *Blood.* Mild leukocytosis. PO_2 decreased. *Chest x-ray.* Patchy irregular infiltrates.

Therapy. Bed rest and oxygen.

Prognosis. Good.

BIBLIOGRAPHY. Kliner JP, Nelson WP: High-altitude pulmonary edema: A rare disease? JAMA 234:491–495, 1975

Overland ES, Severinghaus JW: Noncardiac pulmonary edema. Ann Rev Med 23:307–311, 1978

Grover RF, Reeves JT, Rowell LB, et al: The influence of environmental factors on the cardiovascular system. In Schlant RC, Alexander RW: Hurst's The Heart, 8th ed, p 2122. New York, McGraw-Hill, 1994

HIGH-OUTPUT CIRCULATORY FAILURE

Synonym. Heart failure, high output. See Hyperkinetic heart.

Symptoms. Symptoms of right, or predominantly right, heart failure.

Signs. Cardiac enlargement and venous pressure elevation; diastolic pressure usually diminished; systolic and pulse pressure increased. All signs of congestive failure.

Etiology. Cardiac failure developing as complication of diminished circulatory resistance in various conditions. Arteriovenous fistula; hyperthyroidism; anemia; beriberi; severe pulmonary emphysema with hypoxemia; pregnancy; advanced Paget disease and Albright.

Pathology. See Etiology. Cardiac failure features. In this type of cardiac failure, initiating pathology is in the periphery not in the heart. Diminished peripheral resistance favors speeding of circulation.

Diagnostic Procedures. *Circulation time.* Rapid or normal. *Venous pressure.* Increased. *Cardiac catheterization. Echocardiography with spectral Doppler interrogation. Special laboratory study.* Evaluation of thyroid function, search for beriberi condition, anemia, hepatic condition. *X-ray.* Assess the possible presence of Paget disease of the bone (see).

Therapy. Control of heart failure; digitalis, sodium restriction, diuretics to correct failure and further increase cardiac output. Treatment of basic condition will restore the cardiac output to normal.

Prognosis. Depends on etiology.

BIBLIOGRAPHY. Ross J: Assessment of cardiac function and myocardial contractility. In Schlant RC, Alexander RW: Hurst's The Heart, 8th ed, pp 489, 490, 531. New York, McGraw-Hill, 1994

HILGER

Synonym. Carotodynia.

Symptoms. Cephalalgia and homolateral pain on the neck.

Etiology. Dilatation of carotid artery (?).

BIBLIOGRAPHY. Hilger JA: Carotid pain. Laryngoscope 59:829–838, 1949

HILL-SHERMAN

Synonyms. Cerebellar ataxia; helminthiasis.

Symptoms and Signs. In a large Negro family in Louisiana, in five generations. Both sexes. More common and severe in childhood. Attacks of sudden onset of gait and trunkal ataxia (usually upper limb ataxia), intention tremor, and dysarthria or aphonia. Occasionally headache, vomiting, nystagmus, seizures. In childhood, attacks lasted 4 weeks and there were no neurological sequelae. In adult (previous attacks in childhood) sudden attacks of ataxic gait, dysarthria and intention tremor cleared completely in 2 days. Patient completely well between attacks.

Etiology. Apparent autosomal dominant inheritance. The family attributed the attacks to ascariasis, that was found in several cases examined. Possibly a familiar predisposition with cerebellum vulnerability to ascariasis and/or to eosinophils, and/or to other noxious agents.

Diagnostic Procedures. *Blood.* Eosinophil increased. *Stool.* Presence of ova of ascaris lumbricoides.

Therapy. Disinfestation.

Prognosis. Attacks benign nature without apparent consequences.

BIBLIOGRAPHY. Hill W, Sherman H: Acute intermittent familial cerebellar ataxia. Arch Neurol (Chic) 18:350–357, 1968
Hill W, Dorsey D: Hereditary periodic ataxias. In Vinken PJ, Bruyn GW (eds): Handbook of Clinical Neurology, vol 21, pp 565–569. Amsterdam, North-Holland, 1975

HINMAN

Synonym. Beer; non-neurogenic bladder, NNNB; dysfunctional lazy bladder; lazy bladder; achalasia of urinary tract.

Symptoms and Signs. Usually males. Age of onset 5–7 years of age. In children, with particular personality, anxious, depressed, timid, quiet, shy, and with dominant fathers. Frequency, urgency, nocturia, enuresis. Sometimes encopresis. Urinary tract infections.

Etiology. Functional disorder. Failure to inhibit detrusor reflex and overcompensation by external sphincter that eventually may lead to incomplete voiding and vesico-ureteral reflex. Now viewed as a bad habit developed in children with certain personality types in unfavorable family settings.

Diagnostic Procedures. Interview with parents and children. *Neurological examination. Screening phenolsulfonphthalein test. IVP with voiding films. Voiding cystogram, panendoscopy. Cystometrogram:* uninhibited contractions. *Pressure flow cine studies, perineal electromyography.*

Pathology. Christmas tree bladder, vesicometeral reflex of variable degree.

Prognosis. Suggestion, including: (1) hypnosis; (2) retraining and bladder drill; (3) biofeedback; (4) drug administration (anticholinergics). No need for surgery (practice obsolete).

Prognosis. Optimal reversion of syndrome with adequate therapy.

BIBLIOGRAPHY. Beer E: Chronic retention of urine in children. JAMA 65:1709, 1915

Hinman F, Baimann FW: Vesical and ureteral damage from voiding dysfunction in boys without neurologic or destructive disease. J Urol 109:727–732, 1973
Hinman F Jr: Non neurogenic neurogenic bladder (The Hinman syndrome): 15 years later. J Urol 136:769–776, 1986
Weiss RM, Green DF: Physiology of ureter, bladder and urethra. In Massry SG, Glassock RJ: Textbook of Nephrology, 3rd ed, p 145. Baltimore, Williams & Wilkins, 1995

HIP, CONGENITAL DISLOCATION

Synonyms. Dislocation of hip, congenital.

Symptoms and Signs. Predominant in females. Dislocation of hip as an occasional feature of several conditions with joint laxity (Marfan, Ehler-Danlos, etc.).

Etiology. Complex genetics. Following under the autosomal inheritance group, prevalence in females could be accounted for by their greater degree of joint laxity.

BIBLIOGRAPHY. Perkins G: Signs by which to diagnose congenital dislocation of the hip. Lancet I:648–650, 1928
Peltier LF: The classic signs by which to diagnose congenital dislocation of the hip. Clin Orthop Rel Res 274:3–6, 1992

HIRANO

Synonyms. Dementia—parkinsonism complex; Guam parkinsonism—dementia; parkinsonism—dementia complex. See Creutzfeld-Jakob. See Prion.

Symptoms and Signs. Observed on the island of Guam, exclusively among members of Chamorro tribe; age of onset 32–64 years of age (mean 52 years); predominant in males (31%); insidious onset (no preceding history of encephalitis or other febrile illness). Akinesia; mask-like expressionless face; stooped posture; slow, shuffling gait; poor coordination of alternative movements and skilled actions. Generalized slowness of movements; mental deterioration; apathetic and indifferent depression. Tremor in mild or moderate degree (never major characteristic) or absent. Moderate or no appreciable rigidity; cogwheel phenomenon only in some cases. Generalized hyperreflexia in all cases. In some patients, symptoms and signs of amyotrophic lateral sclerosis. Cerebellar dysfunction not found.

Etiology. Unknown; autosomal dominant inheritance. This syndrome may be considered a clinical entity that represents a combination of Parkinson and presenile dementia and amyotrophic lateral sclerosis, without, however, having all the characteristic features of each one of them. Only difference from Creutzfeldt-Jakob is that this syndrome has a much faster course.

Pathology. Macroscopically, cerebral atrophy, pallidal atrophy, loss of pigmentation in the substantia nigra and locus ceruleus. Microscopically, severe neuronal alterations associated with fibroses, Alzheimer neurofibrillary changes, intracytoplasmatic granulovascular inclusion bodies, accumulation of intracytoplasmatic lipid granules. Loss of neurons most apparent in globus pallidus and substantia nigra.

Diagnostic Procedures. *Blood. Urine. Stool. Cerebrospinal fluid.* Normal. *Electroencephalography.* Background pattern shows generalized 8- to 9-cycle activity of moderate voltage, with superimposed occurrence of frequent, intermittent, moderate voltage. Slower activity present in all leads with accentuation over temporal areas. *CT scan. MRI.*

Therapy. Symptomatic.

Prognosis. Slow evolution but steady progression to death within 4–5 years from onset; 7% of deaths of Chamorro owing to this syndrome.

BIBLIOGRAPHY. Hirano A, Kurland LT, Krooth RS, et al: Parkinsonism-dementia complex, endemic disease on island of Guam. I. Clinical features. Brain 84:642–661, 1961

Malamud N, Hirano A, Kurland LT: Pathoanatomic changes in amyotrophic lateral sclerosis on Guam. Arch Neurol 5:401–415, 1961

Morris JC: Handbook of Dementing Illnesses. New York, Marcel Dekker, 1993

McKendal RR, Stroop WG: Handbook of Neurovirology. New York, Marcel Dekker, 1994

Ellenberg JH, Koller WC, Langston JW: Etiology of Parkinson's Disease. New York, Marcel Dekker, 1995

HIRSCHSPRUNG

Synonyms. Aganglionic megacolon; congenital megacolon.

Symptoms. Prevalent in males (3:1); prevalence 1/5000; onset from birth. Intensity of symptoms according to length of involved segment and age. Obstipation; bilious vomiting; rapid dehydration; small, narrow stool eventually passed. Infrequently, diarrhea may be the main symptom. If not treated, failure to thrive and weakness.

Signs. According to length and location of segment involved. Increased peristalsis; abdominal dilatation; elevation of diaphragm. Mass of feces palpated in lower abdomen, nontender and movable. Rectal examination shows normal anus and rectus, usually empty or with small, goaty fecal pellets. Impacted feces palpated anteriorly to the rectum. Complications are impaction, perforation, bleeding, and ulceration.

Etiology. Abnormal development of the neural crest. Inheritance heterogeneous. Autosomal dominant; autosomal recessive, and X-linked recessive cases reported. No definite hereditary pattern established (polygenetic).

Pathology. Colon dilatation with thickening of wall above the point of lesion. Sharp demarcation between dilated and normal part. Microscopically, all wall layer hypertrophic, absence of ganglia at end and in proximity of narrowing point.

Diagnostic Procedures. *Sigmoidoscopy.* Distal segment normal; dilated part filled with impacted feces; mucosa reddened and with small ulceration. *Biopsy of rectum.* Demonstration of aganglionosis. *X-ray.* Narrowed zone of colon with marked proximal dilatation. *Anorectal manometry.*

Therapy. Surgical removal of aganglionic zone. In mild case. With surgical treatment, 50% immediate recovery; 34% control within 5 years; 16% persistent mild symptoms.

Prognosis. If untreated, varies from development of megacolon in adult life to death in severe form.

BIBLIOGRAPHY. Hirschsprung H: Stuhlträgheit Neugeborener in folge von Dilatation und Hypertrophie des Colons, Jahrb Kinderheilk 27:1–7, 1888

Hirschsprung H: Erneiterung und Hypertrophie des Dickdarms. Berl Klin Wochenschr 36:977, 1899

Jayle F: La dilatation congenitale idiopathique du colon observee an XVII siecle. Presse Med 17:803, 1909

Garver KL, Law JC, Garver B: Hirschsprung disease: A genetic study. Clin Genet 28:503–508, 1985

Watier A, Feldman P, Martelli H, et al: Hirschsprung's disease. In Haubrich WS, Schaffner F, Berk JE (eds): Bockus Gastroenterology, 5th ed, vol 2, pp 1603–1618. Philadelphia, WB Saunders, 1995

HIRSCHSPRUNG-ASSOCIATED MALFORMATIONS

Hirschsprung disease may be associated with several malformations:

1. H-D; bilateral bicolored irides. Autosomal recessive inheritance.

BIBLIOGRAPHY. Liang JC, Juarez CP, Goldberg MF: Bilateral bicolored irides with Hirschsprung's disease: A neural crest syndrome. Arch Ophthalmol. 101:69–73, 1983

2. H-D; polydactyly; renal agenesis; deafness. Autosomal recessive inheritance.

BIBLIOGRAPHY. Santos H, Mateus J, Leal MJ: Hirschsprung's disease associated with polydactyly, unilateral renal agenesis, hypertelorism and congenital deafness: A new autosomal recessive syndrome. J Med Genet 25:204–208, 1988

3. H-D; ulnar polydactyly; polysyndactyly of big toes; ventricular septal defect.
Autosomal recessive inheritance

BIBLIOGRAPHY. Laurence KM, Prosser R, Rocker I, et al: Hirschsprung's disease associated with congenital heart malformation, broad big toes, and ulnar polydactyly in sibs: A case for fetoscopy. J Med Genet 12:334–338, 1975

4. H-D; hypoplastic nails; dysmorphic facial features. Autosomal recessive inheritance

BIBLIOGRAPHY. Al-Gazali LI, Donnai D, Mueller RF: Hirschsprung's disease, hypoplastic nails and minor dysmorphic features: A distinct autosomal recessive syndrome. J Med Genet 25:758–761, 1988

5. Goldberg-Shprintzen (see).
6. H-D; brachydactyly type D. X-linked recessive inheritance, however, the possibility of autosomal dominance with reduced penetrance cannot be excluded.

BIBLIOGRAPHY. Reynolds JF, Barber JC, Alford BA, et al: Familial Hirschsprung disease and type D brachydactyly: A report of four affected males in two generations. Pediatrics 71:246–249, 1983

7. H-D; Dawn.
8. H-D; Waardenburg.
9. H-D; Ondine.
10. H-D; Meckel diverticulum.
11. H-D; Sipple.

BIBLIOGRAPHY. Watier A, Feldman P, Martelli H, et al: Hirschsprung's disease. In Haubrich WS, Schaffner F, Berk JE (eds): Bockus Gastroenterology, 5th ed, vol 2, p 1603. Philadelphia, WB Saunders, 1995

HIRSUTISM, ESSENTIAL

Synonyms. Constitutional hirsutism (term restricted to androgen-dependent hair patterns); hypertrichosis (term restricted to other patterns of excessive hair growth).

Signs. Occurs in females. Increased amount of body hair (on face, chest, abdomen, and extremities) without changes of secondary sexual characteristics.

Etiology. Unknown; familial, racial.

Diagnostic Procedures. *Hormone study.* No underlying endocrine disorder. Dynamic alterations in the androgen metabolism evidentiated by repeated tests: increased production of testosterone, lower levels of SHBG (that bounds testosterone). See hypertrichosis syndromes for differential diagnosis.

Therapy. *Shaving.* In selected cases antiandrogenic drugs (cyproterone and spironolactone). Long-term effects of these drugs is unknown. Avoid pregnancy during their use, and consider that the effect is only temporary.

Prognosis. Permanent condition, temporarily relieved by treatments.

BIBLIOGRAPHY. Lipsett MB, Migeon CJ, Kirscher MA, et al: Physiologic basis of disorders of androgen metabolism. Combined Clinical Staff Conference at the National Institutes of Health. Ann Intern Med 68:1327–1344, 1968

Dawber RPR, Ebling FJG, Wojnarowska FT: Disorders of hair. In Champion RH, Burton JL, Ebling FJG (eds): Rook/Wilkinson/Ebling

Textbook of Dermatology, 5th ed, pp 2566–2567. Oxford, Blackwell Scientific, 1992

HISTIDINEMIA

Synonym. Hyperhistidinemia.

Symptoms. Both sexes affected; normal at birth. General physical and mental development normal. The slight retardation and speech retardation previously reported seems not supported by recent studies or could be attributed to a low frequency maladaptive variant.

Etiology. Unknown; probably autosomal recessive inheritance.

Pathology. None.

Diagnostic Procedures. *Blood and urine.* Increased plasma and urinary concentration of histidine and alanine (positive ferric chloride and phenystix test).

Therapy. None in 99% of cases or trial with low histidine diet; protected capsules of histidase suggested, but not tried in vivo yet.

Prognosis. All cases described alive. Mental retardation in some cases (see Symptoms).

BIBLIOGRAPHY. Ghadimi H, Partington MW, Hunter A: A familial disturbance of histidine metabolism. N Engl J Med 265:224, 1961
Ghadimi H: Diagnosis of inborn errors of amino acid metabolism. Am J Dis Child 114:433–439, 1967
De Braekeleer M: Hereditary disorders. In Saguenay-Lac-St-Jean (Quebec, Canada): Hum Hered 41:141–146, 1991
Levy HL, Taylor RG, McInnes RR: Disorders of histidine metabolism. In Scriver CR, Beaudet AL, Sly WS, et al: The Metabolic and Molecular Bases of Inherited Disease, pp 1115–1117. New York, McGraw-Hill, 1995

HISTIOCYTOSIS SYNDROMES

Synonyms. Histiocytosis X (discontinuation of this term suggested); Lichtenstein.

CLASS I: Langerhans-cell histiocytosis (LCH).

Inclusion of clinical syndromes that share the following diagnostic elements suggested:

A. For diagnostic confidence
   1. Positive stain for ATPase
   2. s-100 Protein
   3. Alpha-D-mannosidase or
   4. Characteristic binding of peanut lecithin

B. For definitive confidence
   1. Birbeck granules in lesional cells by electron microscopy, or
   2. Demonstration of T-6 antigenic determinants on the surface of lesional cells

Letterer-Siwe (see); Hand-Schüller-Christian (see); Lichtenstein-Jaffe (see); Hashimoto-Pritzker (see); Pure cutaneous histiocytosis, Langerhans-cell granulomatosis; Type II histiocytosis and the old term, nonlipid reticuloendotheliosis.

CLASS II: Histiocytoses of mononuclear phagocytes other than Langerhans cells. Hemophagocytic lymphohistiocytosis; infection-associated hemophagocytic; sinus histiocytosis reticulohistiocytoma.

CLASS III: Malignant histiocytic. Acute monocytic leukemia; malignant histiocytosis; histiocytic lymphomas; histiocytic sarcomas.

BIBLIOGRAPHY. Writing group of the Histiocyte Society. Histiocytosis syndromes in children. Lancet 1:208–209, 1987
Lukens JN: Langerhans cell histiocytosis. In Lee GR, Bithell TC,

Foerster J, et al: Wintrobe's Clinical Hematology, pp 1640–1649. Philadelphia, Lea & Febiger, 1993

HITZENBERGER

Obsolete.

Synonyms. Hereditary methemoglobinemia; idiopathic methemoglobinemia. Eponym used (mostly in past literature) to indicate Gibson (see) and Hoerlein-Weber (see).

BIBLIOGRAPHY. Hitzenberger K: Autotoxische Zyanose (Intraglobulaere Methämoglobinämia). Wien Arch Inn Med 23:85–96, 1932

HMG CoA LYASE DEFICIENCY

Synonyms. Leucine metabolism defect; 3-hydroxy-3-methylglutaric aciduria.

Symptoms and Signs. Normal at birth. Then vomiting, cyanosis, lypothymia, lethargy, metabolic acidosis, hypoglycemia. Recurrence of episodes.

Etiology. Autosomal recessive inheritance. Deficiency of HMG CoA lyase.

Pathology. Accumulation of lipid droplets in swollen hepatocytes; acute pancreatitis in 7% of autopsies.

Diagnostic Procedures. *Blood.* Hypoglycemia. Metabolic acidosis. *Urine.* Excretion of HMG, and related substances. *Biopsy.* Enzymatic analysis of fibroblast and lymphocytes.

Therapy. Leucine restriction and correction of hypoglycemia; carnetine administration appears useful.

Prognosis. If recovery from episodes: good, however, death occurs early.

BIBLIOGRAPHY. Faull K, Bolton P, Halpern B, et al: Patient with defect in leucine metabolism. N Engl J Med 294:1013, 1976
Wilson WG, Cass MB, Sovik O, McKusick, et al: A child with acute pancreatitis and recurrent hypoglycemia due to 3-hydroxy-3-methylglutaryl CoA lyase deficiency. Eur J Pediatr 142:289–291, 1984
Barash V, Mandel H, Sella S, et al: 3-Hydroxy-3-methylglutaryl-coenzyme A lyase deficiency: Biochemical studies and family investigation of four generations. J Inher Metab Dis 13:156–164, 1990
Sweetman L, Williams JC: Branched chain organic acidurias. In Scriver CR, Beaudet AL, Sly WS, et al: The Metabolic and Molecular Bases of Inherited Disease, 7th ed, p 1393. New York, McGraw-Hill, 1995

HNEVKOVSKI

Synonyms. Vastus intermedius contracture; progressive fibrosis vastus intermedius.

Symptoms and Signs. More common in females and in twins. Onset 1–7 years of age. Monolateral (occasionally bilateral). From mild to severe limitation of flexion of knee. No effusion. Occasionally, palpable dense band, tensing during knee flexion proximal to patella in the quadriceps. Mild proximal dislocation of patella occasionally subluxated.

Etiology. Unknown.

Pathology. Fascia of thigh adherent to quadriceps muscles and fibrosis and contraction of vastus intermedius. Increase of fibrosis tissue and fat decrease in muscle fibers.

Diagnostic Procedures. Muscle biopsy.

Therapy. Division of fascia and vastus intermedius. Conservative treatment ineffective.

Prognosis. Excellent with surgery.

BIBLIOGRAPHY. Hnevkovsky O: Progressive fibrosis of the vastus intermedius muscle in children: A cause of limited knee flexion of the patella. J Bone Joint Surg 43B:318–324, 1961
Justis EJ Jr: Nontraumatic disorders. In Crenshaw (ed): Campbell's Operative Orthopedics, 7th ed, pp 2247–2248. St Louis, CV Mosby, 1987

HOBAEK

Synonyms. Dreyfus; spondylo dysplasia; pure brachyolmia; brachyolmia recessive, type of Hobaek.

Symptoms and Signs. Both sexes. Short stature reduction limited to the trunk.

Etiology. Autosomal recessive inheritance.

Pathology. Histological changes on ilear crest. Biopsy typical: chondrocyte cluster at the growth plate and fibrosis cartilage matrix are combined with large lacunae of chondrocyte, excessive collagen aggregation and perilacunar loss of glycoaminoglycan.

Diagnostic Procedures. *X-rays.* Universal platyspondyly, lateral extension of vertebrae bodies beyond pedicle and irregular endplates.

BIBLIOGRAPHY. Dreyfus JR: Ueber ein neues mit allgemeiner wahrer oder scheinbarer Breitwirbligkeit (Platyspondylia vera aut spuria generalisata) einhergehendes Syndrom. Jahrb Kinderhk 150:42–49, 1938
Hobaek A: Problems of Hereditary Chondrodysplasias, pp 82–95. Oslo, Univ Press, 1961
Shohat M, Lachman R, Gruber HE, et al: Brachyolmia: Radiographic and genetic evidence of heterogeneity. Am Med Genet 33:209–219, 1989

HODGKIN

Synonyms. Bonfil; Hodgkin-Haltauf-Stemberg; Sternberg disease; HD; multiple lymphadenoma; lymphogranulomatosis malignant.

Symptoms. *Incidence rate:* 42:1 million in males; 32:1 million in females. Mixed incidence: three age periods 0–14, 15–34, 50 and over. *Sex:* 63% male; 37% female. Malaise; anorexia; weight loss; nausea; fever 30–50% (cyclic; continuous, intermittent or Epstein type); drenching sweats; pruritus; 10–15% early symptoms; 85% during course of disease. Lung involvement; brassy cough; dysphagia; alcohol intolerance 17–20% (not specific).

Signs. Painless; progressive enlargement of lymph nodes: cervical (60–80%); axillary (6–20%); inguinal (6–12%); mediastinal (6–12% initially, 60% in course of disease). Abdominal and peritoneal involvement frequent. *Lung.* Clinical involvement in 40%; simulation of various tumors or infections. *Pleura.* Effusion in 33% by clinical detection, 60% in autopsy findings. *Abdomen.* Bleeding, obstruction; infiltration of walls; extrinsic pressure from retroperitoneal mass. *Spleen.* Splenomegaly 30% initially, 80% during course of disease. Secondary hypersplenism (anemia; thrombocytopenia; leukopenia). *Liver.* Hepatomegaly 33%; jaundice. *Bone.* Clinical involvement 30%; at autopsy 60%. *Central nervous system.* 10%. *Skin.* Excoriation produced by response to pruritus, or direct involvement.

Initially, or at late stage, any organ may be involved. Association with herpes zoster frequent (13%), occasionally repeated episodes; fungus infection (Candida albicans 11%, Mucor; Aspergillus; Nocardia especially if treated with corticoid or chemotherapy). Association with active tuberculosis in only 2% of cases. Abnormalities in immune response, autoimmune hemolytic anemia, amyloidosis, collagen diseases should not be considered as complication, but, in some not yet explained way, connected with the pathogenesis of the disease.

Etiology. Unknown; malignant neoplasm or malignant inflammation. Possibly more than one disease included in this diagnosis. Infectious cause in young adults; environmental in older age? Recently demonstrated association with Epstein-Barr virus (20% of cases).

In differential diagnosis "great imitator" symptomatology may be confused with that of many diseases (other lymphomas; tuberculosis; brucellosis and other infections; neoplastic diseases).

Pathology. *Gross.* Lymph node involvement initially is usually confined to a single node or cluster of nodes. Nodes enlarged, well-defined, not adherent, firm. Cut surface shows nodular aspect with areas of dense, retracted, grayish-white (fish flesh) aspect. Different organ may be involved by the lymphomatous process in the form of extensive or nodular infiltration.

Microscopic. The morphologic expression of the disease is characterized by different combinations of the following features: lymphocytic or histiocytic proliferation (with the appearance of atypical, abnormal reticular elements: Reed-Sternberg cell) or both; diffuse or nodular fibrosis and variable degree of inflammatory reaction. In the past the different histologic patterns resulting from the combinations of the mentioned findings have been grouped into three main categories: paragranuloma; granuloma; sarcoma. More recently a finer classification, which better correlates the clinical aspects of the condition with the histologic patterns, has been proposed by Lukes (see Table).

Comparison Between Pathologic Classifications

Jackson Parker (1944)	Lukes (1963)
1. Paragranuloma	1. Lymphocytic and/or
	2. Nodular
2. Granuloma	3. Mixed
	4. Diffuse fibrosis
3. Sarcoma	5. Reticular hysticytic
	a. Diffuse
	b. Nodular

However, morphologic criteria of subtyping are not consistently reproducible and now it is recognized the distinct form of nodular sclerosis and a continuum of pathologic patterns subdivided into lymphocyte-predominant, mixed cellularity, and lymphocyte-depleted stages

Diagnostic Procedures. Biopsy of lymph nodes (see Pathology). and bone marrow (aspiration discloses HD in 9% of patients at time of diagnosis, on section two thirds demonstrable bone marrow involvement). *Blood.* Anemia; hemolytic anemia 80% (in late disease); Coombs test usually negative; leukocytosis with neutrophilia 50%; eosinophilia (may be seen); leukocyte alkaline phosphatase elevated during active phase, decreased in remission; sedimentation rate elevated in active disease. Hypercalcemia 30%; hypophosphatemia; high alkaline phosphatases in bone involvement. Serum albumin decreased; globulin alpha-1 increased, alpha-2 increased, beta-2 increased, gamma decreased; low zinc; high copper. *X-ray. Ultrasound scanning; CT scan. MRI. Bipedal lymphogram.* Lymph node enlargement or tissue infiltration. *Pyelography. Splenoportography. Gallium scan and technetium bone scan.*

Therapy. See Staging and Treatment.

Prognosis. Cure is possible in more than 80% of patients.

Complications Causing Death

Severe infections	21%
Failure of pulmonary function	20%
CNS involvement	11%
GI bleeding	10%
Liver failure	7%

BIBLIOGRAPHY. Hodgkin T: On some morbid appearances of the absorbent glands and spleen. Medico Chir Trans 17:68–114, 1832; republished in Can Res 26:1045–1311, 1966
Fuller LM, Hagemeister FB, Sullivan MP, et al: Hodgkin's disease and non-Hodgkin lymphomas in adults and children. New York, Raven, 1988
Eyre HJ: Hodgkin's disease. In Lee GR, Bithel TC, Foerster J, et al (eds):

Staging and Treatment

	Stage I	Stage II	Stage III	Stage IV
Lymph node group	Single	Multiple, all localized either above or below diaphragm	Above and below diaphragm	Decreased
Parenchymal involvement	None	None	None	Lesion in any of the following: bone; bone marrow; lung; skin; subcutaneous; gastrointestintal tract (considered secondary)
Systemic symptoms	None	A, none; B, +	A, none; B, +	+ + + +
Complications		None	±	+ + +
Treatments	X-ray (3500–4000γ) of local and contiguous nodes	X-ray, same as Stage I Chemotherapy	X-ray (palliative, 1000–2000γ) Chemotherapy* Coritsone and cortisonelike drugs Transfusion Antibiotics	

*Chemotherapy: MOPP (mechlorethamine, Oncovin, Procarbazine, prednisone). Resistant cases: ABVD (Adriamycin, bleomycin, vinblastine, dacarbazine); other combinations also indicated MVPP, ChVPP, MOPP/ABVD (alternating months of each), Mopp/ABV hybrid treatment

Wintrobe's Clinical Hematology, 9th ed, pp 2054–2081. Philadelphia, Lea & Febiger, 1993

HOFFA

Synonyms. Hoffa-Kaster; infrapatellar fat pad hypertrophy; patellar fat pad hypertrophy.

Symptoms. Usually, long history of pain in anterior compartment of knee related to exertion. Occasionally, sharp pain may cause the knee to "give way."

Signs. Swelling caused by the presence of enlarged fat pad. Mild effusion; forced extension reproduces pain; local tenderness with deep pressure.

Etiology. Hypertrophy of infrapatellar fat pad that causes nipping of synovial fringes between the condyles on extension of joint.

Pathology. Trauma of synovial membranes; hemorrhages; hypertrophy and fibrosis; occasionally, calcification.

Diagnostic Procedures. *X-ray and arthroscopy of knee.*

Therapy. *Conservative.* Addition of 25 mm (0.5 inch) to heel of shoes; quadriceps exercises. *Surgical.* In cases that do not respond to conservative treatment, excision of tags, reduction in size of fat pad.

Prognosis. Cured by surgical correction.

BIBLIOGRAPHY. Hoffa A: The influence of adipose tissue with regard to the pathology of knee joint. JAMA 43:795–796, 1904
Kaster J: Die Verwachsung des Kniegelenkfett Koeiers als selbastaengiges Krankheitsbild. Chirurg 24:390–394, 1953
Fulckerson JP, Hungerford DS: Imaging the patello femoral joint. In Disorders of the Patello Femoral Joint. Baltimore, Williams & Wilkins, 1990
Insall JN, Windsor RE, Scott WN, et al (eds): Surgery of the Knee. New York, Churchill Livingstone, 1993

HOFFMANN (E.)

Synonym. Projecting ear—everted lip—woolly hair.

Symptoms and Signs. Present from birth. Projecting ears; everted lower lip; sparse woolly hair.

Etiology. Unknown. Recessive inheritance.

BIBLIOGRAPHY. Hoffmann E: Ueber einen kräuselnaevus Innerhallo sonst glatten Kopfhaares im Vergleich zum erblichen Kraushaar und zur Lockenbildung näch Röntgenepilation. Dermatologica 107:281–291, 1953

HOFFMANN (J.) II

Synonyms. Myopathy—myxedema; myxedema myotonic dystrophy. This eponym is used to designate the muscular manifestations described in Kocker-Debré-Semelaigne (see) associated with myxedema in children. Most likely no fundamental difference between Hoffmann and Kocker-Debré-Semelaigne.

BIBLIOGRAPHY. Hoffmann J: Weiterer Beitrag zur Lehre von der Tetanie. Deutsch Z Nervenkr 9:278–290, 1897
Khaleeli AA, Griffith DG, Edwards RHT: The clinical presentation of hypothyroid myopathy and its relationship to abnormalities in structure and function of skeletal muscle. Clin Endocrinol 19:365–376, 1983

HOFFMANN-ZURHELLE

Synonym. Nevus lipomatosus cutaneous superficialis.

Symptoms. Rare. Both sexes affected; lesions present at birth or appearing later, up to adolescence. Asymptomatic.

Signs. Two principal presentations. (1) The buttocks, hips, lower trunk most frequent sites. Presence of soft, round papules and yellowish, usually smooth and less frequently orange skin-like nodes (domed, sessile, or pedunculated) that slowly grow to form a confluent plaque. Occasionally hairy, with comedo-like plugs. (2) Solitary, domed, or sessile papules, reported also in other sites.

Etiology. Unknown.

Pathology. Collection of ectopic fat cells in the dermis. Electron microscopy shows close association of lipocytes with capillaries (pericyte origin?).

Therapy. None. Excision for cosmetic reasons.

Prognosis. Good.

BIBLIOGRAPHY. Hoffman E, Zurhelle E: Ueber einen Naevus lipomatodes cutaneous superficialis der linken Glutäalgegend. Arch Dermatol Syph 130:227–333, 1921

Atherton DJ: Naevi and other developmental defects. In Champion RH, Burton JL, Ebling FJG (eds): Rook/Wilkinson/Ebling Textbook of Dermatology, 5th ed, pp 467–468. Oxford, Blackwell Scientific, 1992

HOLLENHORST

Synonym. Chorioretinal infarction.

Symptoms. Observed when the patient regains consciousness after surgery, when a headrest and faulty positioning of patient causes eye trauma. Unilateral blindness or only decrease of light perception.

Signs. Proptosis; lid edema; ecchymosis; dilated and fixed pupil; hazy cornea.

Etiology. Secondary eye trauma during surgery.

Pathology. See Signs. Retinal edema; pigmentary retinopathy.

Therapy. Symptomatic. Corticosteroids.

Prognosis. From persistent unilateral blindness to partial or total recovery of vision.

BIBLIOGRAPHY. Slocum HC, O'Neal KC, Allen CR: Neurovascular complications from malposition on the operating table. Surg Gynecol Obstet 86:729–734, 1948

Hollenhorst RW, Svien HJ, Benait CF: Unilateral blindness occurring during anesthesia for neurosurgical operations. AMA Arch Ophthalmol 52:819–830, 1954

Garner A: Vascular diseases. In Garner A, Klintworth GK (eds): Pathobiology of Ocular Disease: A Dynamic Approach, 2nd ed, p 1662. New York, Marcel Dekker, 1994

HOLMES I

Synonym. Marie; Foix; Alajouanine. Cortical familial cerebellar atrophy; cerebellar olivary degeneration; olivocerebellar degeneration. See olivopontocerebellar syndromes and Menzel.

Symptoms and Signs. Prevalent in males; onset gradual in sixth or seventh decade. Progressive disturbance of gait; eventual uncertainty of movements of arms; speech changes (hesitant scanning and explosive). Later, cerebellar tremor and nystagmus. Mild hyperreflexia; no ankle clonus.

Etiology. Unknown; sporadic cases and autosomic dominant inheritance.

Pathology. Progressive atrophy of cerebellar cortex; disappearance of Purkinje cells and preserved basket cells. Involvement of cerebellar white matter; cerebellar nuclei spared. No changes in remainder of nervous system.

Diagnostic Procedures. *Spinal tap. CT brain scan, MRI, and other brain imaging techniques.*

Therapy. Symptomatic.

Prognosis. Good for survival. Progressive evolution with severe neurologic impairment.

BIBLIOGRAPHY. Holmes G: A form of familial degeneration of the cerebellum. Brain 30:466–488, 1907

Dow RS, Moruzzi G: The Physiology and Pathology of the Cerebellum. Minneapolis, Univ of Minnesota Press, 1958

Adams RD, Victor M: Principles of Neurology, 5th ed, pp 989–990. New York, McGraw-Hill, 1993

HOLMES (A.F.)

Synonyms. Holmes heart; single ventricle; great arteries normally related. See Single ventricle. Variety of single ventricle characterized by single ventricle and aorta arising from left or primitive ventricle and pulmonary trunk from right ventricular infundibulum or rudimentary outlet chamber.

BIBLIOGRAPHY. Holmes AF: Case of malformation of the heart. Trans Med Chir Soc Edinburgh 1:252, 1824

Nugent EW, Plauth WH, Edwards JE, et al: The pathology, pathophysiology recognition and treatment of congenital heart disease. In Schlant RC, Alexander RW: Hurst's The Heart, 8th ed, pp 1816–1817. New York, McGraw-Hill, 1994

Perloff JK: The Clinical Recognition of Congenital Heart Disease, 4th ed, pp 638–639. Philadelphia, WB Saunders, 1994

HOLMGREN-CONNOR

Synonym. Semilethal short limb dysplasia. Glasgow type short-limb skeletal dysplasia; tanathophoric dysplasia, Glasgow type.

Symptoms. Most patients die within a few hours of birth from respiratory distress.

Signs. Micromelic dysplasia with incurvated limbs; hyperlaxity. *Head.* Large, flat nasal bridge. Occasionally heart defects.

Etiology. Autosomal recessive inheritance.

Pathology. *Cartilage:* irregular arrangement of cells; short primary trabeculae; bony bridge closing, some vascular lacunae.

Diagnostic Procedures. *X-rays.* Long bones: short and incurved. Enlarged metaphyses. Short irregular ribs.

BIBLIOGRAPHY. Holmgren G: Semilethal bone dysplasia in three sibs. A new genetic disorder. Clin Genet 26:249–251, 1984

Connor JM, Connor RA, Sweet EM, et al: Lethal neonatal chondrodysphasias in West of Scotland with a description of thanatophoric dysplasia like, autosomal recessive disorder Glasgow variant. Am J Med Genet 22:243–253, 1985

Maroteaux P, Stanescu R, Cousin S, et al: Recessive lethal chondrodysphasia "round femoral inferior epiphys's type." Eur J Pediatr 147:408–411, 1988

HOLOCARBOXYLASE SYNTHETASE DEFICIENCY

Synonyms. Multiple carboxylase deficiency (early onset).

Symptoms and Signs. Both sexes. Onset few hours after birth to 15 months of age. Tachypnea, breathing difficulty; hypothermia; feeding difficulties; hypotonia; tremor, seizures; lethargy; ataxia, coma; developmental delay; occasionally skin rash, alopecia. Odor of urine.

Etiology. Autososomal recessive inheritance. Disorder of biotinilation.

Diagnostic Procedures. *Prenatal diagnosis.* Cultured amniocytes holocarboxylase synthetase deficiency. *Amniotic fluid.* Demonstration of elevated concentration of hydroxyisovarate and/or methylcitrate. *Postnatal diagnosis. Biological fluids.* Reduced or absent biotinidase; ketolactic acidosis, organic aciduria; hyperammonemia. *Urine.* Presence of hydroxyisovaleric acid and other metabolites, including "methylcrotonylglycine" hydroxypropionate, methylcitrate, lactate, and triglylglycine. *Immunological studies.* Abnormalities of cellular immunity. *Blood.* Thrombocytopenia.

Therapy. Oral administration of free biotin (10 mg/d). Possible also prenatal therapy

Prognosis. Good with treatment; according to time of onset of treatment.

BIBLIOGRAPHY. Bonjour JP: Biotin-dependent enzymes in inborn errors of metabolism in humans. World Rev Nutr Diet 38:1, 1981
Wolf B: Disorders of biotin metabolism. In Scriver CR, Beaudet AL, Sly WS, et al: The Metabolic and Molecular Bases of Inherited Disease, 7th ed, pp 3151–3177. New York, McGraw-Hill, 1995

HOLT-ORAM

Synonyms. Atriodigital dysplasia; cardiac—limb; hand—heart.

Symptoms. Complete syndrome: Congenital heart defects and upper extremities defect. Either isolated heart or upper extremity defects observed in members of same family. May be asymptomatic or cardiac symptoms such as dyspnea and fatigue may be observed.

Signs. Congenital heart defects and upper extremity defects, including polydactyly and syndactyly. The association of radial defects (absence of a thumb on one side; hyperphalangeal thumb on the other side; manus vara; short radii; radioulnar synostosis) with heart defects are much more frequent than are ulnar defects.

Etiology. Idiopathic autosomal dominant inheritance with high degree of penetrance or secondary to antiepileptic drugs taken during first month of pregnancy.

Pathology. Secundum atrial septal defect and radial defect.

Diagnostic Procedures. *Evaluation of heart defect. X-ray.* Abnormalities of upper extremities. A large arteriovenous malformation with curvilinear calcification may be seen in the neck. *Chromosome studies.* Reported as normal or with suggested abnormalities of pair 16. *Dermatoglyphic studies.* Show only abnormalities secondary to the musculoskeletal defects, and do not appear to be genetically determined.

Therapy. Symptomatic; orthopedic correction if feasible.

Prognosis. Depends on heart defect.

BIBLIOGRAPHY. Holt M, Oram S: Familial heart disease with skeletal malformations. Br Heart J 22:236–242, 1960
Kaufman RL, Rimoin DL, McAlister WH, et al: Variable expression of the Holt-Oram syndrome. Am J Dis Child 127:21–25, 1974
Gladstone I Jr, Sybert VP: Holt-Oram syndrome: penetrance of the gene and lack of maternal effect. Clin Genet 21:98–103, 1982
Lin AE, Perloff JK: Upper limb malformations associated with congenital heart disease. Am J Card 55:1576–1583, 1983

HOLZBACH-SANDERS

Synonyms. Cholestasis, intrahepatic in pregnancy; recurrent intrahepatic cholestasis, pregnancy; pregnancy-related cholestasis.

Symptoms and Signs. During third trimester of pregnancy, pruritus, icterus (may be absent), biliary colics. Shortly after delivery, disappearance of all symptoms.

Etiology. Autosomal dominant inheritance.

Pathology. Liver normal.

Diagnostic Procedures. *Blood.* Hyperbilirubinemia. Trait can be demonstrated between pregnancies by the administration of oral contraceptive with reproduction of the symptoms.

Therapy. Symptomatic.

BIBLIOGRAPHY. Holzbach RT, Sanders JH: Recurrent intrahepatic cholestasis of pregnancy: observation on pathogenesis. JAMA 193:542–544, 1965

Holzbach RT, Sivack DA, Braun WE: Familial recurrent intrahepatic cholestasis of pregnancy: A genetic study providing evidence for transmission of a sex-limited dominant trait. Gastroenterology 85:175–179, 1983
Schaffner F: Cholestasis. In Haubrich WS, Schaffner F, Berk JE (eds): Bockus Gastroenterology, 5th ed, vol 2, p 1947. Philadelphia, WB Saunders, 1995

HOLZGREVE-WAGNER-REHDER

Symptoms and Signs. Potter sequence (see Potter) plus persistent buccopharyngeal membrane type II, postaxial, polydactyly, cleft palate, cardiac anomalies, intestinal nonfixation, growth retardation.

Etiology. See Potter.

BIBLIOGRAPHY. Holzgreve W: Bilateral renal agenesis with Potter phenotype, cleft palate, anomalies of cardiovascular system skeletal anomalies including hexadactyly and bifide metacarpal: A new syndrome? Am J Med Genet 18:177–182, 1984
Legius E, Moerman P, Fryns JP: Holzgreve-Wagner-Rehder syndrome: Potter sequence associated with persistent buchopharyngeal membrane. A second observation. Am J Med Genet 31:269–272, 1988

HOLZKNECKT

Eponym used to indicate a roentgenologic finding: the displacement of mediastinum to the right during inspiration occurring in patients affected by bronchial stenosis.

BIBLIOGRAPHY. Holzknekt G: Ein neues radioscopisches Symptom bei Bronchialstenose und Metodisches. Wein Klin Wehsch 13:785–787, 1899

HOMEN

Synonyms. Friedmann; repeated brain concussion; posttraumatic brain; boxer; postconcussion; post-traumatic personality; punch drunk; dementia pugilistica; vertigo posttraumatic; delayed hydrops included.

Symptoms and Signs. After head injury. Slurring of speech; rigidity of limbs and unsteady gait; poor memory; insomnia; irritability; headache; occasionally, vertigo; diminished intellectual faculties to progressive dementia. Chronic post-traumatic vertigo may also be of psychogenic origin, especially when accompanied by headache.

Etiology. Lesion of lentiform nucleus, frequently caused by chronic trauma (see Cerebral concussion), or as sequelae to a type of progressive subacute encephalitis caused by trauma (Friedmann). In the vertigo the cause may be the dislodgment of the otoconia that produces a type of benign paroxysmal vertigo (see Barany).

BIBLIOGRAPHY. Homen EA: Eine eigenthümliche Familien Krankheit unter der Form progressiven Dementia, mit besanteren anatomischen Befund. Neurol Zbb 9:514–518, 1890
Friedmann AP, Brenner C, Denny Brown D: Post-traumatic vertigo and dizziness. J Neurosurg 2:36–46, 1945
Brandt T: Vertigo: Its multisensory syndromes, pp 193–196. London, Springer-Verlag, 1991

HOMOCARNOSINOSIS

Synonym. Homocarnosinase deficiency.

Symptoms and Signs. In Norwegian pedigree. Both sexes. Only in some cases: progressive spastic paraplegia, retinal pigmentation, mental retardation. Majority of cases healthy.

Etiology. Autosomal recessive inheritance. Lack of homocarnosinase.

Possibly homocarnosine and carnosinase deficiency are one disorder. Association of clinical syndrome and metabolic disorder could be coincidental or caused by variables in genotype and/or environmental conditions.

Pathology. Cerebral biopsy. Atrophy of cortex.

Diagnostic Procedures. *Cerebrospinal fluid.* High homocarnosine content. *Blood and urine.* Normal. High excretion of carnosine in the urine on meat-free diet.

Therapy. Low histidine diet (of no benefit).

Prognosis. Progressive condition.

BIBLIOGRAPHY. Gjessing LR, Sjaastad O: Homocarnosinosis: a new metabolic disorder associated with spasticity and mental retardation. Lancet II:1028, 1974

Lemey JF, Pepper SC, Kucera CM, et al: Homocarnosinosis: lack of serum carnosinase is the defect probably responsible for elevated brain and CSF homocarnosine. Clin Chim Acta 132:157–165, 1983

Gibson KM, Nyhan WL, Jaeken J: Inborn errors of GABA metabolism. Bio Essays 4:24–27, 1986

Scriver CR, Gibson KM: Disorders of amino acids in free and peptide-linked forms. In Scriver CR, Beaudet AL, Sly WS, et al: The Metabolic and Molecular Bases of Inherited Disease, 7th ed, pp 1349–1350. New York, McGraw-Hill, 1995

HOMOLOGOUS BLOOD

Synonym. Sequestration; desequestration.

Symptoms and Signs. During extracorporeal circulation, the injection of a large volume of homologous blood results in decrease of effective circulating blood volume with significant hypotension, which, to be corrected, requires further blood infusion, far in excess of calculated blood balance. The hypotension is progressive and continues in the first postoperative day, during which tachypnea, cyanosis, hypoxemia, severe pulmonary congestion, and vascular stasis on nail bed compression are noted. Subsequently, there is a return to normal of plasma and red cell volume. However, if large volume of blood has been used to correct the postperfusion hypotension, hypervolemia develops.

Etiology. Intensity and severity of manifestations depend on body size of patient, amount of blood injected, and duration of injection. Blood sequestration (in lungs) induced by infusion of homologous blood, resembling the changes occurring with histamine shock.

Diagnostic Procedures. *Blood.* Metabolic acidosis and postperfusion anemia.

Therapy. Use of washed red cells; reduction of extracorporeal priming volume; substitution of electrolyte solutions for a part of homologous blood; reutilization of patient's own blood collected from pleural and precordial spaces during surgery. At the completion of perfusion, maintenance of normotension, but use of only minimum amount of blood and integration with cardiotonic and vasopressor agents. Maintenance of isotopic normovolemia should not be attempted; subsequent blood loss from oozing must be only partially replaced in anticipation of expected desequestration.

Prognosis. When pulmonary complications develop, poor (about 50% survival).

BIBLIOGRAPHY. Gadboys HL, Slonim R, Litwak RS: Homologous blood syndrome. I. Preliminary observations on its relationship to clinical cardiopulmonary bypass. Ann Surg 156:793–804, 1962

Gadboys HL, Jones AR, Slonim R, et al: The homologous blood syndrome. III. Influence of plasma, buffy coat and red cells in provoking its manifestation. Am J Cardiol 12:194–202, 1963

Connolly MW, Guyton RA: Cardiopulmonary bypass and intraoperative protection. In Schlant RC, Alexander RW: Hurst's The Heart, 8th ed, pp 2443–2450. New York, McGraw-Hill, 1994

HONEYCOMB ATROPHY

Synonyms. MacKee-Parounagian; atrophodermia reticulata; atrophodermia vermiculata; folliculitis ulerythematosa reticulata. See Scarring follicular keratosis.

Symptoms and Signs. Both sexes. Onset from 5 to 12 years of age. On the cheeks and preauricular areas typical symmetrical, skin lesion. Limited areas of skin atrophy causing a reticulate athrophy with pits with sharp edges and "wormeaten" or "honeycomb" appearance. Occasionally associated: oligophrenia, neurofibromatosis (see von Recklinghausen), cardiac defects.

Etiology. Sporadic and small pedigree of autosomal dominant and recessive inheritance.

Pathology. In early stage edema, perivascular infiltration with lymphocytes. Later dermal connective atrophy, hair follicle enlarging with horny plugs and attached epithelial cysts; small sebaceous glands.

Therapy. None successful. Retinoids potentially useful.

BIBLIOGRAPHY. MacKee GM, Parounagian MB: Folliculitis ulerythematosa reticulata. J Cutan Dis 36:339–352, 1918

Kooij R, Veuter J: Atrophodermia vermiculata with unusual localization and associated congenital anomalies. Dermatologica 118:161–167, 1959

Frosch PJ, Brumage MR, Schuster-Pavlovic C, et al: Atrophoderma vermiculatum. J Am Acad Dermatol 18:538–542, 1988

HONEYCOMB MYOPATHY

Synonyms. Myopathy honeycomb.

Symptoms and Signs. See tubular aggregate myopathy.

Etiology. X-linked recessive inheritance.

Pathology. Type I fibers atrophy, zebra bodies, honeycomb structures.

Diagnostic Procedures. *EMG.* Myopathic pattern. *Blood.* CK value elevated.

Therapy. Symptomatic.

Prognosis. Stable condition.

BIBLIOGRAPHY. Carrier H, Tommasi M, Kopp W, et al: Proliferation du systeme tubolaire transversal au cours d'une myopathie tardive et familiale. J Neurol Sci 27:499–512, 1976

Niakan E, Harati Y, Danon MJ: Tubular aggregates their association with myalgia. J Neurol Neurosurg Psychiatr 48:882–886, 1985

Goebel HH, Lenard HG: Congenital myopathies. In Handbook of Clinical Neurology 18th ed. Rowland P, DiMauro S (eds): The Myopathies, p 331. Amsterdam, Elsevier, 1992

HONEYMOON CYSTITIS

Synonyms. Honeymoon cystitis; honeymoon pyelitis; see dysuria-pyuria.

Symptoms. Occurs in females after frequent sexual intercourse. Dysuria; pollakiuria; perineal discomfort; chills; fever; flank pain. Occasionally, nausea, vomiting, abdominal pain, ileus; or only fever and chills.

Signs. Tenderness in upper or lower abdomen, frequently on costovertebral angle palpation.

Etiology. Cystitis. Gram-positive or more frequently Gram-negative bacteria.

Pathology. Inflammatory signs in bladder, ureter(s), kidney collecting system.

Diagnostic Procedures. *Blood.* Leukocytosis shift to the left. *Urine.*

Proteinuria; white cells and leukocyte casts. *Intravenous urography.* To be carried out in all patients.

Therapy. Antibiotics.

Prognosis. Recovery of acute phase in 5 days (90%).

BIBLIOGRAPHY. Stapleton A, Latham RH, Johnson C, et al: Postcoital antimicrobial prophylaxis for recurrent urinary tract infections. A randomized, double-blind, placebo controlled trial. Jama 264:703–706, 1990

Forland M: Dysuria and frequency. In Massry SG, Glassock RJ: Textbook of Nephrology, 3rd ed, p 553. Baltimore, Williams & Wilkins, 1995

HOOFT

Synonyms. Familial hypolipidemia; hypolipidemia—tryptophan abnormality.

Symptoms and Signs. Present from birth. *Hair.* Thin; singed; dry. *Teeth.* Abnormal. *Skin.* Squamous, erythematous rash, and opaque leukonychia. *Eye.* Tapetoretinal degeneration. *Mental retardation. Growth delay.*

Etiology. Unknown; autosomal recessive inheritance. Absence of coenzymes pyridine nucleotide for transformation of tryptophan into 5-hydroxylated derivatives and indolacetic acid.

Diagnostic Procedures. *Blood.* Cholesterol 90–115 mg/100 ml; low phospholipids; no acanthocytosis. *Urine.* Indoluria; hyperaminoaciduria. *Fat absorption test.* Normal.

Therapy. Symptomatic.

BIBLIOGRAPHY. Hooft C, De Lacy P, Herpal J, et al: Familial hypolipidemia and retarded development without steatorrhea. Another inborn error of metabolism? Helv Paediatr Acta 71:1–23, 1962

Herbert PN, Gotto AM, Fredrickson DS: Familial lipoprotein deficiency. In Stanbury JB, Wyngaarden JB, Fredrickson DS, et al: The Metabolic and Molecular Bases of Inherited Disease, 4th ed, p 569. New York, McGraw-Hill, 1978

HOOFT-BRUENS

Synonyms. Sudanophilic leukodystrophy; meningeal angiomatosis.

Symptoms and Signs. Apparent normal development in first months of life followed by rapid neurologic deterioration, with seizures, spasticity, hyperreflexia.

Etiology. Autosomal recessive inheritance.

Pathology. Noncalcifying meningeal angiomatosis and sudanophilic leukodystrophy. Necrosis of anoxic type in cerebral and cerebellar cortex areas.

Therapy. Not responsive to antiepileptic treatment.

Prognosis. Death at 2–4 years of age.

BIBLIOGRAPHY. Hooft C, Deloore L, Van Bogaert L, et al: Sudanophilic leucodystrophy with meningeal angiomatosis in two brothers: Infantile form of diffuse sclerosis with meningeal angiomatosis. J Neurol Sci 2:30–51, 1965

Bruens JH, Guazzi GC, Martin JJ: Infantile form of menigeal angiomatosis with sudanophilic leukodystrophy associated with complex abiotrophies: Study of a second family. J Neurol Sci 7:417–425, 1968

HOOFT-JONGBLOET

Symptoms and Signs. Oral frenula, ocular coloboma, microphthalmia, palatal malformations, part axial polydactyly. One case, tumor of brain.

Etiology. It may represent a variant of Varadi syndrome (see).

BIBLIOGRAPHY. Hooft C, Jongbloet P: Syndrome oro-digito-facial chez deux freres. Arch Fr Pediatr 21:729–740, 1964

HOPF

Synonym. Acrokeratosis verruciformis. See also Darier-White.

Symptoms and Signs. Both sexes affected; present at birth or appearing in early childhood. On back of hands and feet, knees or elbows, and forearms, presence of verrucous papules and colored skin. Occasionally, presence of crops of similar lesions on other skin areas; in some cases, diffuse thickening of palmar skin with small areas of hyperkeratosis. Friction may produce bullae formation. Nails are thicker, whitish, in some cases stripped.

Etiology. Unknown; Sporadic and autosomal dominant inheritance. Apparently, linkage with Darier-White (see) from which differs only histologically.

Pathology. Hyperkeratosis and acanthosis with thick granular layer resembling church spires. Absence of vacuolization.

Therapy. Topical application of keratolytic and emollient agents.

Prognosis. Chronic condition. Moderate response to treatment. Transformation to squamus cell carcinoma possible.

BIBLIOGRAPHY. Hopf G: Ueber eine bisher nicht beschriebene disseminierte Keratose (Acrodermatosis verruciformis). Dermatol Z 60:227–250, 1931

Blanchet-Bardon C, Durand Delorm M, Nazzaro V, et al: Acrokeratomatose verruciformis de Hopf ou maladie de Darier acrale. Ann Dermatol 115:1229–1232, 1988

Griffiths WAD, Leigh IM, Marks R: Disorders of keratinization. In Champion RH, Burton JL, Ebling FJG (eds): Rook/Wilkinson/Ebling Textbook of Dermatology, 5th ed, p 1367. Oxford, Blackwell Scientific, 1992

HOPPE-THURMAN

Synonym. Aneurysms of Valsalva sinuses congenital; aortic sinus aneurysm; Valsalva sinuses congenital aneurysms.

Symptoms and Signs. Three clinical patterns observed:

1. *Imperforate aneurysm.* Asymptomatic in most cases; or variable symptomatology according to size and location: continuous murmur (flow to and from aneurysm); right ventricular outflow obstruction; tricuspid regurgitation; various types of heart block; anginal pains.
2. *Small perforation of the aneurysm.* Occasionally, initially, asymptomatic. Minor dyspnea and continuous murmur may precede for years the onset of congestive failure.
3. *Large perforation of the aneurysm.* Predominant in males (4:1). Onset between puberty and 30 years of age and seldom out of this range. Severe retrosternal or abdominal pain, marked dyspnea, lasting hours or days, then receding with fair subsidence of symptoms. Wide pulse pressure; vigorous pulsation in the neck. After a variable period; congestive heart failure progressing to death.

Etiology. Congenital or acquired defect.

Pathology. Blind pouch originating from one of the Valsalva sinuses (right or noncoronary, 95%) and projecting finger-like into heart cavities. Rupture usually at the tip may communicate with right atrium or ventricle, pulmonary artery, left ventricle and atrium, or pericardial cavity. Crista supraventricularis septal defect frequently is associated.

Diagnostic Procedures. *Electrocardiography. Two-dimensional echocar-*

diography with color flow imaging and spectral Doppler interrogation. X-rays. Variable findings according to pathology. *Cardiac catheterization. Aortography.*

Therapy. Antibiotics if suspected endocarditis. Surgical correction in cardiopulmonary bypass. Heart transplantation.

Prognosis. Extremely variable according to pattern. Survival into old age or sudden death in early adulthood or sooner. Interval between sudden large rupture and death from immediate to 1 year.

BIBLIOGRAPHY. Hope J: A Treatise on the Diseases of the Heart and Great Vessels, 3rd ed. London, J. Churchill, 1839

Thurman J: On aneurysms, and especially spontaneous varicose aneurysms of the ascending aorta and sinuses of Valsalva, with cases. Med Chir Trans (London) 23:323–384, 1840

Burakovsky VI, Podsolkov VP, Sabirow BN, et al: Ruptured congenital aneurysm of the sinus of Valsava: Clinical manifestations, diagnosis and results of surgical correction. J Thor Cardivasc Surg 95:836–841, 1988

Nugent EW, Plauyh WH, Edwards JE, et al: The pathology pathophysiology, recognition and treatment of congenital heart disease. In Schlant RC, Alexander RW, et al: Hurst's The Heart, 8th ed, pp 1784–1785. New York, McGraw-Hill, 1994

Perloff JK: The Clinical Recognition of Congenital Heart Disease, 4th ed, pp 581–597. Philadelphia, WB Saunders, 1994

HORNER

Synonyms. Bernard-Horner; Claude Bernard-Horner; cervical sympathetic paralysis; sympathetic ophthalmoplegia; sympathetic cervical paralysis. See Bernard.

Symptoms and Signs. Miosis (paradoxical pupillary dilatation may occur after a few days from onset with emotional or physical stress). Ptosis; apparent or minimal exophthalmos; hypotonia oculi. Rise in temperature of homolateral side of face; lacrimation increased or decreased; hemifacial anhidrosis (lesion below bifurcation of common carotid artery). Occasionally, development of cataract. Depigmentation of iris (when syndrome occurs in children).

Etiology. Interruption of sympathetic chain in any part of its path. Trauma; surgery; neoplasm; thrombosis; aneurysm.

Pathology. See Etiology.

Diagnostic Procedures. *Ophthalmologic.* Failure of the pupil to dilate with cocaine. Supersensitivity to adrenergic amines (test for differentiation between preganglionic and postganglionic cervical lesions). *Angiography. CT brain scan. MRI. Spinal tap.*

Therapy. According to etiology.

Prognosis. Depends on etiology. Adrenergic supersensitivity may persist for many years.

BIBLIOGRAPHY. Bernard C: Des phénomènes oculopupillaires produits par la section du nerf sympathique cervical; ils son indèpendents des phénomènes vasculaires caloriques de la tête. C R Acad Sci (D) Paris 55:381–382, 1862

Horner F: Ueber eine Form von Ptosis. Klin Monatsbl Augenheilka 7:193–198, 1869

Van der Wiel HL, Van Gijn J: The diagnosis of Horner's syndrome: Use and limitations of the cocaine test. J Neurol Sci 73:311–316, 1986

Woodruff G, Buncic JR, Morin JD: Horner's syndrome in children. J Pediatr Ophthalmol Strabismus 25:40–44, 1988

Adams RD, Victor M: Principles of Neurology, 5th ed, pp 470–471. New York, McGraw-Hill, 1993

HORNOVÁ-DLUHOSOVÁ

Synonym. Oral conjunctival amyloidosis; mental retardation.

Symptoms. A brother and sister affected. Discovered within first year of life. Swelling of eyelids with nodular deposition of amyloid in the conjunctiva; congenital cataracts; ocular bulb atrophy; amaurosis; gingiva show amyloid deposits as well (icing-like). Mental retardation.

Etiology. Unknown.

BIBLIOGRAPHY. Hornová J, Dluhosová O: Primary amyloidosis of gingiva and conjunctiva and mental disorder, in a brother and sister. Oral Surg 25:451–466, 1968

HORTON

Synonyms. Horton-Gilmour; Horton-Magath-Brown; cranial arteritis; temporal arteritis; giant cell arteritis. See Polymyalgia rheumatica. Takayasu.

Symptoms. Occurs in old age group (seventh and eighth decade), seldom before age 55; affects both sexes equally. Unilateral or bilateral, localized, severe headache in region of temporal artery. Systemic manifestations: anorexia; insomnia; weight loss; low-grade fever. When process spreads to ophthalmic artery, blindness may result.

Signs. Swelling, tenderness over temporal artery area; arteries thickened, prominent, often pulseless.

Etiology. Unknown; included in the collagen diseases group. Autosomal dominant inheritance observed in some families, possibly on the same basis as other autoimmune conditions (see Polymyalgia rheumatica; Takayasu Hashimoto, lupus erythematoid, Addison-Biermer, etc.).

Pathology. Granulomatous arteritis and periarteritis changes: fragmentation of internal elastic membrane with infiltration of medial with granulocytes lymphocytes, plasmacells and the characteristic presence of giant multinucleated cells. The process often is diffuse and involves arteries in several organs.

Diagnostic Procedures. *Blood.* Increase of sedimentation rate; leukocytosis; increase of alpha-2 globulin fraction. Alkaline phosphatase increase. *Biopsy of artery.* See pathology

Therapy. Adrenocorticotropic hormone (ACTH) and corticosteroids; surgery in case of severe refractory pain.

Prognosis. Self-limited; course several months. Residual manifestation may be blindness.

BIBLIOGRAPHY. Hutchinson J: Diseases of arteries. Arch Surg (London) 1:323, 1890

Horton BT, Magath TB, Brown GE: An undescribed form of arteritis of temporal vessels. Proc Mayo Clin 7:700, 1932

Granato JE, Abben RP, May WS: Familial association of giant cell arteritis: A case report and brief review. Arch Intern Med 141:115–117, 1981

Gonzales-Gay MA, Alonzo MD, Aguero JJ, et al: Temporal arteritis in a northwestern area of Spain: Study of 57 biopsy proven patients. J Rheum 19:277–280, 1992

Ansaloni MC, Zizzi F, Giorgio M, et al: Quattro casi di arterite temporale di Horton. Rec Prog Med 85:22–28, 1994

Weatherall DJ, Ledingham JGG, Warrell DA (eds): Oxford Textbook of Medicine, 3rd ed, p 4026. Oxford, Oxford Med Pub, 1996

HOT DOG HEADACHE

Synonyms. Nitrates headache.

Symptoms and Signs. Headache after feeding with meats processed with nitrite as preservative.

Etiology. Vasodilating effect of sodium nitrite.

Pathology. None.

Prognosis. Cessation of headache within few hours.

BIBLIOGRAPHY. Haubrich WS: Food-borne diseases. In Haubrich WS, Schaffner F, Berk JE (eds): Bockus Gastroenterology, 5th ed, vol 2, p 1199. Philadelphia, WB Saunders, 1995

HOUSEMAID KNEE

Synonyms. Prepatellar bursitis; nun knee. See "Beat Knee."

Symptoms. Pain in the knee when kneeling.

Signs. Swelling of the anterior aspect of knee; palpable granules.

Etiology. Chronic or acute trauma of prepatellar bursa; secondary infection.

Pathology. Thickening of prepatellar bursa walls; loose bodies in the cavity.

Diagnostic Procedures. *X-ray.* Acute swelling of soft tissue; chronic radiopaque bodies in the bursa.

Therapy. Protection against further irritation. Injection of corticosteroids; X-ray therapy; ultrasonic treatment; surgical removal for refractory case.

Prognosis. Good with treatment.

BIBLIOGRAPHY. Insall JN, Windsor RE, Scott WN, et al (eds): Surgery of the Knee. New York, Churchill Livingstone, 1993
Hutton CW: Osteoarthritis. In Weatherall DJ, Ledingham JGG, Warrell DA (eds): Oxford Textbook of Medicine, 3rd ed, pp 2975–2983. Oxford, Oxford Med Pub, 1996

HOUSSAY

Synonyms. Houssay-Biasotti. Vanishing diabetes mellitus. See Pituitary apoplexy syndrome. Obsolete.

Symptoms and Signs. The symptoms and signs of diabetes disappear, whereas symptoms and signs of hypopituitarism become suddenly or progressively evident. Generally, there is a lack of clearly specific clinical features except in the fulminating type of hypopituitarism.

Etiology. Necrosis or infarction of pituitary in diabetic patients. (See Pituitary infarction.)

Pathology. Necrotic lesion of pituitary; according to duration of syndrome, adrenal atrophy, and other features of panhypopituitarism develop.

Diagnostic Procedures. *Blood.* Hypoglycemia. Persistence of abnormal tolerance curve. Decrease in urinary gonadotropin, corticoids, and 17-ketosteroids.

Therapy. Correction of hypoglycemia, and other features of hypopituitarism with adrenocorticotropic hormone (ACTH), corticoids.

Prognosis. Poor.

BIBLIOGRAPHY. Houssay BA, Biasotti A: La diabetes pancreatica de los perros hipofisoprivos. Rev Soc Argent Biol 6:251–296, 1930
Calvert RJ, Caplin G: The Houssay syndrome. Br Med J 2:71–74, 1957

HOWSHIP-ROMBERG

Synonyms. Romberg-Howship; von Romberg-Howship; obturator hernia

Symptoms. More common in women; onset especially in old age. Recurrent pain along thigh, radiating to the knee; if strangulation is generalized, abdominal pain.

Signs. Moving hip exacerbates pain in leg and abdomen. Palpation of abdomen reveals rigidity; rectal examination allows palpation of mass.

Etiology. Congenital abnormality of obturator canal.

Pathology. Sac passing through obturator foramen.

Therapy. Surgery.

Prognosis. High incidence of strangulation and irreducibility.

BIBLIOGRAPHY. Howship J: Practical Remarks on the Discrimination and Appearance of Surgical Disease. London, Churchill, 1840
Romberg MH: In Dieffenbach: Operative-Chirurgie. Leipzig, 1848
Arbman G: Strangulated obturator hernia: A simple method for closure. Acta Chir Scand 150:337–339, 1984
Tsubono Fukuda Muto: A case of bilateral obturator hernias: Image diagnosis and description of a retropubic operative approach. Surg Today 23:159–163, 1993

HSIEH-PIN

Synonyms. Possession by a deceased relative; Satanic possession; psychic possession. See Kandinskii-Clérambault.

Symptoms and Signs. Trance state (intrepreted as indicative of possession by a spirit) in which consciousness is greatly altered and attention greatly narrowed. These possession states are culturally accepted according to common beliefs.

Etiology. Delusional thinking.

BIBLIOGRAPHY. Gaines AD: Culture-specific delusions: Sense and nonsense in cultural context. In Sedler MJ (ed): The Psychiatric Clinics of North America, pp 294–295. June, 1995

HUFFER

Synonyms. Solvent mixture paralysis.

Symptoms and Signs. In individuals exposed to solvent mixtures (lacquer thinner) from clot imbibed by the agents. Severe, predominantly motor neuropathy that continues to develop also after cessation of exposure. Weakness involves distal and proximal muscles, respiratory facial and deglution muscles up to total paralysis of limbs, muscles; areflexia, mild involvement of sensory.

Etiology. Mixture includes xylene, 2-heptanone, acetone, isobutyl acetate, 2-nitropropanol, toluene, and small amount of alcohols, n-exane, and other volatile agents.

Pathology. From biopsy of sural nerve: depletion of myelinated axons, focal paranodal swelling with damage of myelin sheath, and accumulation of neurofilaments. Also CNS involvement reported.

Diagnostic Procedures. *Electromyography. Blood. Biopsy of nerve.*

Prognosis. Possible death. Survivors improve with persistent weakness for years.

BIBLIOGRAPHY. Prockop LD, Alt M, Tison J: Huffner's neuropathy. JAMA 229:1083–1084, 1974
Allen N: Solvents and other industrial organic compounds. In Vinken PJ, Bruyn GW: Handbook of Clinical Neurology, vol 36 p 374. Amsterdam, North-Holland, 1979

HUGHES

Synonyms. Acromegaloid; thickened oral mucosa; AFA; thick lips and oral mucosa.

Symptoms and Signs. Coarse, progressing facial acromegaloid features: thickened lips, overgrowth of oral mucosa; thickened palpebrae; large doughy hands with hyperextensive joints, no clubbing.

Etiology. Autosomal dominant inheritance.

BIBLIOGRAPHY. Hughes HE, McAlpine PJ, Cox DW, et al: An autosomal dominant syndrome with "acromegaloid" features and thickened oral mucosa. J Med Genet 22:119–125, 1985

HUGHES-STOVIN

Synonym. Pulmonary artery aneurysm—peripheral vein thrombosis.

Symptoms. Prevalent in males (all but one case reported); onset 14–37 years of age. Recurrent episodes of fever that do not respond to antibiotics; hemoptysis; symptoms from recurrent pulmonary, dural sinus, and peripheral vein thrombosis; frequently at onset, intracranial hypertension and/or optic neuritis.

Signs. Murmur or thrill over aneurysm of pulmonary artery.

Etiology. Unknown.

Pathology. Aneurysm of large and small pulmonary arteries and thrombosis of veins. Association with congenital cardiac defects.

Diagnostic Procedures. *Blood.* Clotting studies. *X-rays of chest.* Variable pattern. *Two-dimensional echography with color flow imaging and spectral Doppler interrogation. Electrocardiography. Angiography.* Similar findings on Behçet.

Therapy. None effective.

Prognosis. Poor. Terminal event; massive hemoptysis.

BIBLIOGRAPHY. Hughes JP, Stovin PGI: Segmental pulmonary-artery aneurysm with peripheral vein thrombosis. Br J Dis Chest 53:19–34, 1959
Durieux P, Bletry O, Huchon G, et al: Multiple pulmonary aneurysms in Behçet's disease and Hughes-Stovin. Am J Med 71:736–741, 1981

HUGUIER-JERSILD

Synonyms. Jersild; genitoanorectalis elephantiasis; genitoanorectal; penoscrotal lymphedema. See also Lymphedema.

Symptoms. Both sexes affected, but prevalent in females; more frequent onset in adult life. Pain; dysuria; stypsis.

Signs. Presence of initial ulcer, papula, or herpetiform lesion that causes lymphedema in the pelvic region. Edema, initially pitting, then becoming harder; hyperkeratosis may develop later as well as secondary infections.

Etiology. Lymphogranuloma venereum; syphilis; seldom, gonorrhea or other infections.

Pathology. Lymphatic obstruction; edema; secondary fibrosis; infection; hyperkeratosis.

Therapy. Antibiotics.

Prognosis. Good results with early treatment. Disappointing result in advanced forms.

BIBLIOGRAPHY. Huguier PC: Mémoire sur l'esthiomène ou dartre rongeante de la region vulvo-anale. Mem Acad Med (Paris) 14:501–514, 1849
Jersild O: Elephantiasis genito-anorectalis. Dermatol Wchnscr 96:433–438, 1933
Ryan TJ, Champion RH: Disorders of lymphatic vessels. In Champion RH, Burton JL, Ebling FJG (eds): Rook/Wilkinson/Ebling Textbook of Dermatology, 5th ed, p 2020. Oxford, Blackwell Scientific, 1992

HUNGRY BONES

Synonym. Postsurgical hypoparathyroidism; hypoparathyroidism postsurgical.

Symptoms and Signs. Follows parathyroidectomy. Those of hypocalcemia (see) associated with hypomagnesemia (see) and hypophosphatemia.

Etiology. Removal of hyperfunctioning parathyroids. The condition is determined by a great excess of bone formation over bone resorption. A mild form is seen during early healing of rickets or osteomalacia and with osteoblastic metastases from breast, prostate, and lung carcinoma.

Therapy. Aggressive treatment with calcium, vitamin D, calcitonin, etidronate disodium.

Prognosis. Good with treatment.

BIBLIOGRAPHY. Sackner MA, Spivak AP, Balian LJ: Hypocalcemia with presence of osteoblastic metastases. N Engl J Med 262:173–176, 1960
Krane SM, Schiller AL, Canalis E: Metabolic bone disease introduction and classification. In De Groot LJ (ed): Endocrinology, 3rd ed, p 1200. Philadelphia, WB Saunders, 1995

HUNNER

Synonyms. Bladder submucosae ulcer; interstitial cystitis; elusive ulcer; painful bladder (misnomer); detrussor mastocytosis (misnomer); see bladder neck and female prostate.

Symptoms and Signs. Occurs more frequently in women (6–11 females/1 male); onset insidious in middle age (at 30–60 years of age). Pollakiuria; stranguria.

Etiology. Unknown. Apparently related to hormonal imbalance, autoimmune pathology, infections, allergy, or psychological factors or combinations.

Pathology. Lack of uniformity of findings. Bladder contracted; wall edematous; epithelium thinned; ulcers of difficult identification. Ulcers shallow; increased vascularization with degenerative changes of vessels; submucosa infiltrated by mononucleated and polynucleated cells; fibrous tissue increased; involving all layers of bladder.

Diagnostic Procedures. *Cystoscopy. Biopsy (deep).*

Therapy. All unsatisfactory, of medical or surgical type; topical instillation with dimethylsulfoxide (DMSO), clorpactin (WCS-90), or silver nitrate produce some, temporary, symptomatic relief.

Prognosis. Symptoms seldom progress and frequently spontaneously regress. No risk for general health or life.

BIBLIOGRAPHY. Nitze M: Lehrbuch der Cystoskopie: Ihre Technik und Klinische Bedeutung, pp 205–210. Berlin, JE Bergman, 1907
Knorr R: Die Cystoskopie und Urethroskopie beim Weibe, p 211. Berlin, Urban & Schwarzenberg, 1908
Hunner GL: A rare type of bladder ulcer. JAMA 70:203, 1918
Messing EM: Interstitial cystitis and related syndromes. In Walsh PC, Gittes RF, Perlmutter AD, et al: Campbell's Urology, 5th ed, pp 1015–1040. Philadelphia, WB Saunders, 1992

HUNT (J.R.) I

Synonyms. Ramsay Hunt I; auricular herpes zoster; geniculate neuralgia; herpes zoster oticus.

Symptoms. Intense pain in the region of ear and mastoid process; paralysis of facial (VII) nerve; hearing loss; vertigo; tinnitus. Taste loss in two thirds of tongue; xerostomia and xerophthalmia.

Signs. Herpetic lesions over mastoid process, and around external auditory canal and ear drum that may extend to oral mucosa, face, neck, and scalp.

Etiology. Virus infection (herpes zoster) affecting the geniculate ganglion.

Pathology. Hyperemia and lymphocytic infiltration in perivascular spaces.

Therapy. Symptomatic; calamine lotion and protective dressing. Acyclovirus antibiotic to protect from secondary infections. Analgesic. Specific vaccine. Surgical measures and X-ray therapy of doubtful value.

Prognosis. Poor prognosis for recovery. Recovery of paresis occurs, but return of function is seldom complete. Intractable pain sometimes remains after recovery from herpetic lesions.

BIBLIOGRAPHY. Hunt JR: On herpetic inflammations of geniculate ganglion: A new syndrome and its aural complications. Arch Otol 36:371–381, 1907

Robillard RB, Hilsinger RL, Adour KK: Ramsay Hunt facial paralysis: clinical analyses of 185 patients. Otolaryngol Head Neck Surg 95:292–297, 1986

HUNT (J.R.) II

Synonyms. Ramsay Hunt II; Hunt ataxia; dentatorubro atrophy; dysynergia cerebellaris myoclonica; myoclonic dysynergia cerebellaris.

Symptoms and Signs. Average age of onset early adulthood. Convulsion and myoclonus; action tremor that begins locally in one of the extremities and then spreads to involve entire voluntary muscular system. Legs are disturbed less often than arms. Asthenia; dysarthria; dysmetria; hypotonia; adiadochokinesis. Mental deterioration (rare).

Etiology. Unknown; may be associated with Friedreich ataxia. Autosomal dominant inheritance with reduced penetrance suggested.

Pathology. Almost complete loss of cells in dentate nuclei; demyelinization of the brachium conjunctivum. Atrophy of column of Goll and ventral and dorsal spinocerebellar tracts.

Diagnostic Procedure. *Electroencephalographic brain mapping. CT scan. MRI. Cerebrospinal fluid.* Uric acid may be increased.

Therapy. Anticonvulsant therapy (see Epilepsy syndromes).

Prognosis. Slow progression of condition over 10 years or longer.

BIBLIOGRAPHY. Hunt JR: Dysynergia cerebellaris myoclonica: Primary atrophy of the dentate system, a contribution to the pathology and symptomatology of cerebellum. Brain 44:490–538, 1921

May DL, White HH: Familial myoclonus, cerebellar ataxia and deafness. Arch Neurol 19:331–338, 1968

Tanaka N, Ito K, Yoshimura J, et al: Familial chorea and myoclonus epilepsy. Neurology 28:913–919, 1978

Adams RD, Victor M: Principles of Neurology, 5th ed, p 833. New York, McGraw-Hill, 1993

HUNTER

Synonyms. Iduronate sulfatase deficiency; IDS; mucopolysaccharidosis (MPS) II; sulfoiduronate sulfatase deficiency. (In past literature referred to as mild Hunter gargoylism, or Hurler-Hunter.)

Symptoms. Males affected (cases in females rare but not unknown); clinical onset in infancy or childhood. A mild form (MPSIIB) and a severe form (MPS II A) distinguished; however, the severe one is less severe than Hurler. Symptomatology very similar in both conditions. Mental retardation (less severe than in Hurler); deafness (constant feature); no visual impairment (or appearing late in the course of the disease). Chronic diarrhea in many cases. Hoarseness in a limited number of cases.

Signs. Dwarfism; grotesque facial features; joint stiffness; dorsal gibbus (less evident than in Hurler); nodular lesions on posterior thorax and arms (unique to this type of mucopolysaccharidosis). Corneal clouding (evident only on slit lamp examination). In some cases, atypical retinitis pigmentosa. Hepatosplenomegaly. In adult rosy cheeks and plethoric facies.

Etiology. Autosomal; X-linked recessive inheritance; about 33% of cases represent a new mutation. Gene has been mapped to Xq 26–27. Deficiency of iduronate sulfatase.

Pathology. Identical to those of Hurler.

Diagnostic Procedures. *Serum and cells.* Test directly and indirectly for assay of iduronate sulfatase. *Urine.* Equal amount of dermatan sulfate and heparan sulfate, but high rate of the latter is frequent. *X-ray.* Dysostosis multiplex.

Therapy. Experimental evaluation of normal plasma and lymphocyte infusion.

Prognosis. In severe form, death in adolescence, usually from heart failure after progressive mental deterioration; in mild forms, survival into old age with several degrees of manifestation, from minimal (allowing a normal life) to relatively severe with marked impairment.

BIBLIOGRAPHY. Hunter C: A rare disease in two brothers. Proc R Soc Med 10:104–116, 1917

Machill G, Barbujani G, Danieli GA, et al: Segregation and sporadic cases in families with Hunter's syndrome. J Med Genet 28:398–401, 1991

Neufeld EF, Muenzer J: The mucopolysaccharidoses. In Scriver CR, Beaudet AL, Sly WS, et al: The Metabolic and Molecular Bases of Inherited Disease, 7th ed, pp 2472–2474. New York, McGraw-Hill, 1995

HUNTINGTON

Synonyms. Lund-Huntington; Mount; chorea, chronic progressive; microcellular—striatal.

Symptoms. Insidious onset 30–45 years of age (20–60 extreme ages of reports). Gradual increase of choreiform movements in early stages. Patient may be mistaken for drunk. Muscle movements become very violent and finally in later stage decrease to akinesia. Mental deterioration, usually concurrent with chorea progressing to dementia. Death from coronary artery disease is frequent and may occur before 10 years from onset.

Etiology. Biochemical defect underlying the condition is unknown (neurotoxic effect of glutamate or other neuroexitatory compounds?). Autosomal dominant programmed, premature selective neural cell death. Recently a gene containing a CAG trinucleotide that is expanded on HD chromosome has been identified.

Pathology. Brain small; degenerative changes in nucleus caudatus, putamen, and cerebral cortex; neuroglia proliferation; ventricles enlarged.

Diagnostic Procedures. *Electroencephalography. CT brain scan. MRI.*

Therapy. Haloperidol; chlorpromazine; choline chloride 150–230 mg/kg + lecithin 350 mg/kg. Ayres and Mihan suggested that a fault in vitamin E metabolism may be at the root of the syndrome, and recommended vitamin E therapy for its antioxidant effect.

Prognosis. Death within 18 years circa; suicidal tendency.

BIBLIOGRAPHY. Waters CO: Description of chorea. In Dunglison R, Practice of Medicine, vol 2, p 312. Philadelphia, Lea & Blanchard, 1842

Huntington G: On Chorea. Med Surg Reporter Philadelphia 26:317–321, 1872

Lund JC: Chorea Sti Viti i Saetersdalen Uddrag of Distrikslaege. JC Lunds Medicinalberetuig for 1860. Norges officielle Statistikk 1882C N. 4

Gilliam TC, Tanzi RE, Haines JL, et al: Localization of the Huntington's disease gene to a small segment of chromosome 4 flanked by D4S10 and the telomere. Cell 50:565–571, 1987

Hayden MR, Kremer B: Huntington disease. In Scriver CR, Beaudet AL, Sly WS, et al: The Metabolic and Molecular Bases of Inherited Disease, 7th ed, pp 4483–4509. New York, McGraw-Hill, 1995

HURIEZ

Synonyms. Keratoderma; scleroatrophic Huriez.

Symptoms and Signs. Both sexes affected; onset from birth. Keratoderma of palms, and less of the soles; scleroderma-like changes of fingers; atrophy back of the hands. Not Raynaud phenomenon.

Etiology. Unknown; autosomal dominant inheritance. Gene located on chromosome 2 and linked to MNS blood groups.

Prognosis. Squamous epitheliomas developing during adolescence.

BIBLIOGRAPHY. Huriez C, Desmons F, Bombart M: Plasmocytomes dermiques malins de la fesse. Bull Soc Fr Dermatol Syph 70:743, 1963
Griffiths WAD, Leigh IM, Marks R: Disorders of keratinization. In Champion RH, Burton JL, Ebling FJG (eds): Rook/Wilkinson/Ebling Textbook of Dermatology, 5th ed, p 1382. Oxford, Blackwell Scientific, 1992

HURLER

Synonyms. Hunter-Hurler; Johnie; Pfaundler-Hurler; Hurler-Pfaundler; Sheldon-Ellis; Thompson; alpha-L-iduronidase deficiency (H); dysostosis multiplex; gargoylism; MCL; lypochondrodystrophy (misnomer); mucopolysaccharidosis IH; MPSH. See Hunter.

Symptoms. Both sexes affected; clinical onset in infancy or early childhood. After a few months of normal growth, physical and mental abilities show progressive deterioration. Troubles of vision.

Signs. Hydrocephalus; grotesque facial features; macroglossia; lumbar gibbus; stiff joints; chest deformities; dwarfism; clouding of cornea and retinal degeneration; hepatosplenomegaly. Thickened skin and nodules over scapulae; hirsutism.

Etiology. Homozygous for mucopolysaccharidosis (MPS) IH gene. Deficiency of alpha-L-iduronidase blocking the degradation of both dermatan sulfate and heparan sulfate.

Pathology. Cellular deposition of mucopolysaccharides in cartilage, periosteum, fasciae, tendons, heart valves, meninges, cornea. Hepatic cells show diffuse discrete vacuolization. Brain may contain bodies of abnormal lipid material.

Diagnostic Procedures. *Urine.* Mucopolysacchariduria: dermatan sulfate and heparan sulfate. *Blood.* Reilly (Alder) bodies (metachromatic inclusions) in polymorphonuclear leukocytes. Direct measurement of alpha-L-iduronidase activity in leukocytes. *Bone marrow.* Reilly bodies in histiocytes and lymphocytes. *X-ray. CT scan. MRI.* Enlargement of shafts of long bones; convex vertebra; backward displacement of one or two upper lumbar bodies; coxa valga. Skull thickening restricted to vault. Frontal sinuses may be absent. Pituitary fossa deformed. Jaw and teeth alteration and dental cysts. Prenatal diagnosis is possible now.

Therapy. Some improvement reported with fresh plasma infusion.

Prognosis. Death by 10 years of age. Respiratory infections; cardiac failure.

BIBLIOGRAPHY. Hurler G: Ueber einen Typ multipler Abartungen, vorwiegend am Skelettsystem. Z Kinderheilkd 24:220–234, 1919
Neufeld EF, Muenzer J: The mucopolysaccharidoses. In Scriver CR, Beaudet AL, Sly WS, et al: The Metabolic and Molecular Bases of Inherited Disease, 7th ed, pp 2471–2472. New York, McGraw-Hill, 1995

HURLER-SCHEIE

Synonyms. Alpha-L-iduronidase deficiency H/S; mucopolysaccharidosis IH/S; MPS H/S. Hurler-Scheie "compound" alpha-L-iduronidase deficiency.

Symptoms and Signs. A combination of symptoms less severe than Hurler, more severe than the Sheie. A unique feature seems represented by the dimension and consequence of presence of arachnoid cysts, which probably have the time to grow because of the longer survival of the patient with this genetic combination. Distinctive micrognathism.

Etiology. Autosomal inheritance. Genetic compound of MPS IH and I/S genes.

Pathology. See Hurler and Scheie.

Diagnostic Procedures. See Hurler and Scheie. Differential diagnosis on clinical basis only. Prenatal diagnosis is possible now.

Therapy. Symptomatic.

Prognosis. May reach adult life. All the features of the two basic conditions evolving with less severity.

BIBLIOGRAPHY. Kajii T, Matsuda K, Osawa T, et al: Hurler/Scheie genetic compound (mucopolysaccharidosis IH/IS) in Japanese brothers. Clin Genet 6:394–400, 1974
Neufeld EF, Muenzer J: The mucopolysaccharidoses. In Scriver CR, Beaudet AL, Sly WS, et al: The Metabolic and Molecular Bases of Inherited Disease, 7th ed, p 2472. New York, McGraw-Hill, 1995

HURST

Symptoms and Signs. Short stature, microcephaly, craniosynostosis, small ears, atretic external meatus; microstomia, small mantible, slender bones, dislocated radial heads, campodactyly.

Etiology. Unknown. Sporadic.

Diagnostic Procedures. *X-rays.* See Signs. Delayed bone age.

BIBLIOGRAPHY. Hurst JA, Winter RM, Baraitser M: Distinctive syndrome of short stature, craniosynostosis, skeletal changes and malformed ears. Am J Med Genet 29:107–115, 1988

HUTCHINSON-GILFORD

Synonyms. Gilford; Souques-Charcot; premature senility; progeria.

Symptoms and Signs. Occurs in children of both sexes. Normal appearance at birth and during first year. Then, lack of weight gain, retardation of growth become evident, with height and weight below third percentile. Baldness; absence of eyelashes; loss of subcutaneous fat; appearance of dwarfism; small face; prominent eyes and beaked nose; irregular teeth; senile aspect; parchment skin with brownish pigmentation; infantile sex organs; protruding abdomen; poor muscle development.

Etiology. Unknown; possibly heterogenic phenotype, autosomal dominant or recessive type germinal mosaicism. The primary source of multiple defects unknown.

Pathology. Absence of subcutaneous fat; senile features; atherosclerosis; occlusion of coronary vessel.

Diagnostic Procedures. *Blood.* Increased lipids. Erythrocytes heat lability of G6PD and 6-phosphogluconate dehydrogenases. *Urine.* Seldom, aminoaciduria. *X-ray.* Premature fusion of epiphyses; long thin bone with decalcification; poorly developed mandible; crowding of teeth. *Chromosome study.* Pattern normal.

Therapy. Symptomatic.

Prognosis. Death by the middle of second decade.

BIBLIOGRAPHY. Hutchinson J: Congenital absence of hair and mammary glands with atrophic conditions of skin and its appendages. Med Chir Trans 69:473–477, 1886
Gilford H: Progeria: A form of senilism. Practitioner 73:188–217, 1904
Badame AJ: Progeria. Arch Dermatol 540–544, 1989
Harjacek M, Batini D, Sarnavka V, et al: Immunological aspects of progeria (Hutchinson-Gilford syndrome) in a 15 month old child. Eur J Pediatr 150:40–42, 1990
De Busk FL, Brown WT: Progeria. In Behrman RE: Kliegman Arvin Nelson Textbook of Pediatrics, 15th ed, pp 1996–1997. Philadelphia, WB Saunders, 1995

HUTCHINSON (J.)

Synonyms. Choroiditis guttata senilis; Tay choroiditis (see Age-related retinopathy).

Symptoms. Both sexes affected; onset in advanced age. Gradual and progressive visual loss.

Signs. Large colloidal deposit in and about macula.

Etiology. Unknown; possibly, autosomal dominant inheritance.

BIBLIOGRAPHY. Hutchinson J: Illustration of Clinical Surgery, pp 49–52. London, J. Churchill, 1875
Garner A, Sarks S, Sarks JP: Degenerative and related disorders of the retina and choroid. In Garner A, Klintworth GK (eds): Pathobiology of Ocular Disease: A Dynamic Approach, 2nd ed. New York, Marcel Dekker, 1994

HUTCHINSON MELANOTIC WHITLOW

Synonyms. Hutchinson III; melanotic whitlow; subungual melanotic whitlow.

Symptoms. Rare; onset in middle to advanced age. Pain.

Signs. Three modes of presentation:

1. Pigmented band in the nail followed by granulation at the edge of nail bed
2. Chronic paronychia (single finger) with pigmentation in contiguous cutaneous area
3. Warty growth on nail bed with loss of nail

Etiology. Unknown.

Pathology. Malignant melanotic tumor.

Diagnostic Procedures. *Biopsy.* Must be performed as soon as syndrome suspected. Performed after application of a tourniquet. Frozen section analysis.

Therapy. If positive histology, immediate amputation at the metacarpophalangeal joint level.

Prognosis. Depends on the results of early surgery and prevention of metastases.

BIBLIOGRAPHY. Hutchinson J: Melanotic disease of the great toe following a whitlow of the nail. Trans Pathol Soc London 8:404–405, 1857
MacKie RM: Melanocytic naevi and malignant melanoma. In Champion RH, Burton JL, Ebling FJG (eds): Rook/Wilkinson/Ebling Textbook of Dermatology, 5th ed, p 1553. Oxford, Blackwell Scientific, 1992

HUTCHINSON (R.)

See Parker.

Symptoms and Signs. Those of Parker (see) plus multiple bone metastases that confer at the bones a "moth eaten" aspect.

BIBLIOGRAPHY. Hutchinson R: On suprarenal sarcoma in children with metastases to the skull. Q J Med 1:33–38, 1907

HUTCHINSON TRIAD

Synonym. Deafness-interstitial keratitis-Hutchinson teeth. Eponym indicates the association of the three signs occurring in congenital syphilis.

Symptoms and Signs. (1) Hutchinson teeth: permanent teeth; dirty gray color; widely separated; upper incisor narrowed; small, bowed at sides; central depression of cutting edge. Lower incisors peg-shaped, center notched. First molar maldeveloped. (2) Deafness. (3) Interstitial keratitis.

Etiology. These symptoms, together with others, develop during infancy and early childhood in cases of late congenital syphilis. The Hutchinson teeth may be observed also in rickets and traumatic lesions.

BIBLIOGRAPHY. Hutchinson J: On the different forms of inflammation of the eye consequent on inherited syphilis. Ophthalmol Hosp Rep 1:191–203; 226–244, 1858; 2:54–105, 1859
Hutchinson J: Med Class 5:138–146, 1940
Morton RS: The treponematoses. In Champion RH, Burton JL, Ebling FJG (eds): Rook/Wilkinson/Ebling Textbook of Dermatology, 5th ed, p 1101. Oxford, Blackwell Scientific, 1992

HYALINE MEMBRANE

Synonyms. Perinatal respiratory distress; pulmonary hypoperfusion; respiratory distress; RDS.

Symptoms and Signs. Most frequently in premature infants, infants born of diabetic mothers, infants delivered by cesarean section, or infants of mothers with antepartum hemorrhages or toxemia. Less frequently in full term, normally delivered infants. Onset within a few hours from birth. Tachypnea; poor chest excursion, inspiratory retraction; expiratory grunting; weak cry; rales; frothing at lips; often, cyanosis and edema.

Etiology. Unknown; genetically determined RDS predisposing factor; high risk mothers. Possibly decreased surface activity agent in lung; damage to alveolar cells by asphyxia; toxic product or effect of reflex vasoconstriction owing to hypoxemia, acidemia, hypothermia, hypovolemia.

Pathology. Lung voluminous, purplish red; poor stability of expansion; extensive atelectasis; alveolar septa vascular congestion; hemorrhages; homogeneous eosinophilic lining on bronchial epithelium and alveolar ducts (hyaline membranes). Right heart dilatation.

Diagnostic Procedures. Findings of inadequate oxygenation and carbon dioxide removal. Respiratory and metabolic acidosis. *X-ray.* Granular appearance of lung fields.

Therapy. Supportive care; oxygen, avoid oxygen toxicity to the retina (see Terry syndrome) and the lungs with a careful monitoring of arterial PO_2. Treatment in a neonatal intensive care unit by skilled personnel.

Prognosis. Mortality of low birth weight infants referred to proper intensive unit is steadily declining. About 50% of those under 1000 gm survive, and over 95% of those weighing more than 2500 gm survive.

BIBLIOGRAPHY. Swyer PR: The respiratory distress syndrome of the newly born. Chicago Med 70:12–17, 1967
Klaus MH, Fanaroff AA: Care of the High-Risk Neonate, 2nd ed. Philadelphia, WB Saunders, 1979

Civetta JM, Taylor RW, Kirby RR (eds): Critical Care, 2nd ed. Philadelphia, JB Lippincott, 1992

Fraser RS, Paré JAP, Fraser RG, Paré PD: Synopsis of Disease of the Chest, 2nd ed. Philadelphia, WB Saunders, 1994

HYDATIDIFORM MOLE

Synonyms. Hydatid mole; vesicular mole; pregnancy molar. Part of a spectrum that incudes also Invasive mole and Choriocarcinoma (see).

Symptoms. Incidence 1:1500 pregnancies in the Western world; more frequent in some Far East areas. 1:125 bleeding (spotting or profuse); nausea and vomiting. (33%) Pain owing to rapid uterine enlargement. Seldom preclampsia-eclampsia.

Signs. Enlargement of uterus beyond the size for the estimated period of gestation (20%). Bilateral adnexal enlargement owing to the lutein cysts of ovary. Grape-like clusters or enlarged villi may be passed through vagina. Hypertension during the second trimester.

Etiology. Complete moles from androgenetic conception almost always euploid. Partial moles from conception where sets of paternal chromosomes excede maternal sets.

Pathology. Hydatidiform mole is placental tissue in which chorionic villi are converted to vesicles of varying sizes (a few mm to 2–3 cm in diameter) arranged in grape-like clusters. The contents usually distend the uterus to the size of a gestation of 6 months. Microscopically, villi show hydropic degeneration and swelling, scanty blood vessels, proliferation of chorionic epithelium, especially syncytial trophoblasts. Ovaries very often exhibit multiple lutein cysts, produced by overstimulation by chorionic gonadotropin.

Diagnostic Procedures. *Serum.* hCG-beta subunit above 40,000 IU/ml. *Urine.* hCG above 100,000 IU/24 hour. *Echography.*

Therapy. Once diagnosed, immediate evacuation of the uterus, either vaginally, by dilatation and curettage, or by abdominal hysterectomy (the latter for selected multiparas). Supportive measures: blood, antibiotics, nutrition. Because of the danger of chorionepithelioma, the patient should be followed for 1 year: look for abnormal bleeding; make serial biologic pregnancy tests. No chorionic gonadotropin should be detected 30 days after evacuation of the uterus. A persistent or rising hormone titer is an indication for exploratory laparotomy and hysterectomy. Antitumor chemotherapy. *Low risk patients.* Methotrexate 0.4 mg/kg im 5-day period, or dactinomycin 10–12, μg/kg/d IV over 5-day period. *High risk patients.* Refer for multiple agent chemotherapy. If acceptable prescribe oral contraceptives to avoid hazard or confusion because of a rising titer in case of pregnancy.

Prognosis. Hydatidiform mole destroys the fetus. Prognosis of mother depends chiefly on the amount of bleeding, infection, or perforation of the uterine wall. Risk of abortion and fetal anomaly not greater in patients who have had hydatiform mole. After courses of chemotherapy (even when metastases) 5-years' arrest can be expected in 85% of cases of choriocarcinoma.

BIBLIOGRAPHY. Szulman AE, Surti U: The syndromes of partial and complete molar gestation. Clin Obstet Gynecol 27:172–180, 1984

Cunningham FG, MacDonald PC, Gant NF, et al (eds): Williams Obstetrics, pp 748–755. Englewood Cliffs, NJ, Prentice-Hall, 1993

HYDE

Synonyms. Lailler-Brocq lichen obtusus corné; nodular lichenification; nodular prurigo.

Symptoms. Rare. Both sexes. Onset 20–60 years of age. Intense crisis of pruritus lasting minutes or 1–2 hours, daily or more frequent intervals.

Signs. On the back of forearms, but also, less frequently, on thighs and legs. Few, widespread, nodular lesions 1–3 cm of diameter, with hard and warty surface. Initially red in color, they become pigmented, crust, and scale. Halo of hyperpigmentation around nodules.

Etiology. Unknown. Emotional stress (?). Considered also as a variant of lichen simplex. 80% of patients are atopic even without eczema; 20% after insect bite. Gluten enteropathy in a few patients.

Pathology. Thickening of horny layer. Chronic inflammatory infiltrates; schwannomas.

Therapy. Infiltration with corticosteroids. Tranquilizers; psychiatric counseling. PUVA; Benaxaprofen useful in some cases.

Prognosis. New nodules may appear; old ones remain pruriginous, seldom regressing with a residual scar.

BIBLIOGRAPHY. Hyde JN: A Practical Treatise on Diseases of the Skin for the Use of Students and Practictioners, 3rd ed. Philadelphia, Lea & Febiger, 1883

Burton JL: Eczema, lichenification, prurigo and erytroderma. In Champion RH, Burton JL, Ebling FJG (eds): Rook/Wilkinson/Ebling Textbook of Dermatology, 5th ed, pp 583–584. Oxford, Blackwell Scientific, 1992

HYDROARTHROSIS INTERMITTENS

Synonyms. Perrin; intermittent hydroarthrosis; periodic arthritis.

Symptoms. Prevalent in females; onset after puberty or in old age. Usually, single joint pain (knee most frequently affected, less frequently ankle). Functional limitation lasting 7–20 days. In some cases, symptoms parallel menses.

Signs. Swelling and distension of affected joint. Absence of systemic manifestation and local signs of inflammation.

Etiology. Unknown; familial (?). In many cases, history of allergy.

Pathology. No specific changes.

Diagnostic Procedures. *Blood. Urine. Synovial fluid. Negative. X-ray.* Soft tissue swelling.

Therapy. None satisfactory.

Prognosis. Length of recurrences unpredictable (months, lifetime).

BIBLIOGRAPHY. Perrin ER: J Med 3:82, 1845

Ehrlich GE: Intermittent and periodic arthritic syndromes. In Hollander JL, McCarty DJ: Arthritis and Allied Condition, 8th ed, p 822. Philadelphia, Lea & Febiger, 1972

Burssens AD, Dequeker J: Regional bone diseases. In Klippel JH, Dieppe PA: Rheumatology, 7.43.9, 7.43.10. St Louis, CV Mosby, 1994

HYDROA VACCINIFORME

Synonym. Hydroa aestivale (term is best reserved for a variant of polymorphic light eruption).

Symptoms. Male to female ratio, 2:1; onset in infancy or early childhood; onset after exposure to sun. Malaise; light hyperthermia; restlessness; pruritus absent; after 12 hours, skin eruption.

Signs. On the face, arms, and any other area exposed to light, red papules that evolve into bullae and then into crusted lesions and, finally, into scars. Various developmental anomalies may be associated.

Etiology. Unknown; type of inheritance not established; possibly, autosomal recessive.

Pathology. Early stage: epidermal spongiosis with dermal perivascular mononuclear cells infiltration; then epi and dermal necrosis and ulceration.

Diagnostic Procedures. *Blood and urine.* To exclude porphyria.

Therapy. Sunscreen of little effect. Chloroquine possibly useful; estrogen (in a girl) and gonadotropin (in a boy) claimed useful. Prophylactic low-dose UVB or PUVA occasionally useful.

Prognosis. Attacks last about 2 weeks; become milder and less frequent in early adult life (at 20–30 years of age), but they may persist.

BIBLIOGRAPHY. Schiff M, Jillson OF: Photoskin tests in hydroa vacciniforme. Arcg Dermatol 82:812–815, 1960
Hawk JLM: Cutaneous photobiology. In Champion RH, Burton JL, Ebling FJG (eds): Rook/Wilkinson/Ebling Textbook of Dermatology, 5th ed, pp 860–861. Oxford, Blackwell Scientific, 1992

HYDROLETHALUS

See Herva.

Symptoms and Signs. The syndrome is lethal and is characterized by polydactyly and central nervous system malformation, as observed in the Meckel-Gruber syndrome (see), but unlike the latter disorder does not show cystic kidney and liver and the central nervous system derangement is hydrocephalus not encephalocele. Other possible malformations in this syndrome are heart defects, stenosis of the airway, and abnormal lobation of the lungs.

Etiology. Recessive inheritance.

Diagnostic Procedures. *Prenatal diagnosis by ultrasonography. CT brain scan. MRI.*

Therapy. None. Cerebrospinal fluid shunt for hydrocephalus as palliative treatment.

Prognosis. Poor.

BIBLIOGRAPHY. Salonen R, Herva R, Norio R: The hydrolethalus syndrome: delineation of a "new" lethal malformation syndrome, based on 28 patients. Clin Genet 19:321–330, 1981
Toriello HV, Bauserman SC: Bilateral pulmonary agenesis: association with the hydrolethalus syndrome and review of the literature from a developmental field prospective. Am J Med Genet 21:93–103, 1985
Salonen R, Herva R: Hydrolethalus Syndrome. J Med Genet 27:756–759, 1990

HYDROPS FETALIS-Hb BART

Synonym. Homozygous alpha thalassemia 1; Bart Hb-Hydrops fetalis.

Symptoms and Signs. Individuals from Southeast Asia, Greece, and Cyprus. Premature delivery with stillborn fetus or death few hours after birth. Hydrops fetalis.

Etiology. Autosomic recessive. Absence of alpha chain synthesis.

Diagnostic Procedure. *Peripheral blood smear.* Large hypochromic RBC, reticulocytosis. Hb electrophoresis: Hb Bart's (gamma 4) prevalent; absence of alpha chains.

Pathology. Hydrops fetalis. Hepatosplenomegaly.

Therapy. Cesarean section. Exchange transfusions.

Prognosis. Poor.

BIBLIOGRAPHY. Lie-Injo LE, Jo BH: A fast-moving hemoglobin in hydrops fetalis. Nature 185:698, 1960
Bunn HF, Forget BG: Hemoglobin Molecular Genetic and Clinical Aspects, p 332. Philadelphia, WB Saunders, 1986
Lukens JN: The thalassemias and related disorders: quantitative disorders of hemoglobin synthesis. In Lee GR, Bithel TC, Foerster J, et al (eds): Wintrobe's Clinical Hematology, 9th ed, p 1115. Philadelphia, Lea & Febiger, 1993

HYPERALGESIC PSEUDOTHROMBOPHLEBITIS

Symptoms and Signs. In male homosexuals. Frequent association with Kaposi sarcoma (see). Painful swelling in the legs, with overlying skin showing erythematous and intensely tender reactions. Hyperthermia.

Etiology. Unknown. Unusual manifestation of AIDS (see).

Diagnostic Procedures. *Venography.* No evidence of venous occlusion.

Therapy. Diagnosis needed to prevent unnecessary anticoagulation. Nonsteroidal anti-inflammatory agents.

Prognosis. Erythema and pain persisting for 1 month.

BIBLIOGRAPHY. Abramson SB, Odajnyk CM, Grieco AJ, et al: Hyperalgesic pseudothrombophlebitis: new syndrome in male homosexuals. Am J Med 78:317–320, 1985

HYPERCALCEMIA

Symptoms. Malaise; muscular weakness; polyuria; polydipsia; constipation; dehydration; nausea; vomiting; anorexia. Mental derangement from depression to delirium.

Signs. Cardiac arrhythmias; muscle hypotonia, areflexia; band keratopathy.

Etiology and Pathology. Increase of calcium in circulation observed in many different conditions: malignancy of bones; myeloma; sarcoidosis; hypervitaminosis D; primary and secondary hyperparathyroidism; Burnett; hypophosphatasia. In patients subject to prolonged immobilization, and patients treated with estrogen or testosterone. Idiopathic.

Diagnostic Procedures. *Blood.* Elevation of calcium level; associated with other findings typical of various pathologic entities. *Electrocardiography.* Short Q-T interval.

Therapy. In crisis. Electrocardiographic monitoring; sodium chloride 0.9% infusion and potassium as needed; vasopressor agents; furosemide or etiodronate intravenously. If inadequate response, phosphate infusion, then per os; mithramycin. If no response (renal failure), corticosteroids and calcitonin. Treatment of underlying condition by specific measures.

Prognosis. Depends on etiology.

BIBLIOGRAPHY. Goldsmith RS, Ingbar SH: Inorganic phosphate treatment of hypercalcemia of diverse etiologies. N Engl J Med 274:1–7, 1966
Mundy GR: The hypercalcemia of cancer. Clinical implication and pathogenesis mechanisms. N Engl J Med 310:1718–1727, 1984
Ryzen E, Martodam RR, Troxeu M, et al: Intravenous etiodronate in the management of malignant hypercalcemia. Arch Intern Med 145:449–452, 1985
Marx SJ: Vitamin D and other calciferols. In Scriver CR, Beaudet AL, Sly WS, et al: The Metabolic and Molecular Bases of Inherited Disease, 7th ed, pp 3103–3104. New York, McGraw-Hill, 1995

HYPERCALCEMIA, INFANTILE IDIOPATHIC

Comprehensive designation to indicate a constant complication of the SAS syndrome (Williams-Beuren) and to designate a variant of this syndrome that presents all symptoms and signs except the presence of supravalvular aortic stenosis and peripheral pulmonary stenosis.

Etiology. Possibly defect concerning vitamin D inactivation. A later onset of the process (hypercalcemia) has been considered responsible for the absence of these particular vascular injuries.

BIBLIOGRAPHY. Smith DW, Blizzard RM, Harrison HE: Idiopathic hypercalcemia: a case report with assay of vitamin D in the serum. Pediatrics 24:258–269, 1959

Wiltse HE, Goldbloom RB, Antia AU, et al: Infantile hypercalcemia syndrome in twins. N Engl J Med 275:1157–1160, 1966

Marx SJ: Familial hypocalciuric hypercalcemia. N Engl J Med 303:810–811, 1980

Marx SJ: Vitamin D and other calciferols. In Scriver CR, Beaudet AL, Sly WS, et al: The Metabolic and Molecular Bases of Inherited Disease, 7th ed, p 3103. New York, McGraw-Hill, 1995

HYPERCALCIURIA, FAMILIAL IDIOPATHIC

Symptoms and Signs. Urolithiasis; hematuria; urinary tract infections; abnormal urinary concentrating ability; enuresis. Hypercalciuria is defined as 24-hour urine excretion of calcium greater than 0.094 mmol/kg/d (4 mg/kg/d) and/or a calcium/creatinine ratio greater than 0.56 mmol/mmol (0.2 mg/mg).

The condition has been classified into three different pathogenic types based on response to changes in dietary calcium and sodium.

Group I. Absorptive hypercalciuria. Low calcium excretion on low-calcium diet (400–600 mg/day) with sodium excretion 2.5 mmol/kg/d.

Group II. Renal hypercalciuria. Low calcium excretion only when hydrochlorothiazide (HCT) is administered.

Group III. Sodium-dependent hypercalciuria. Low calcium excretion only if sodium excretion (#2.5 mmol/kg/d).

Etiology. Idiopathic. Sporadic and autosomal dominant inheritance.

Therapy. Varies according to the response to dietary manipulation described in the preceding. A high fluid intake is recommended to all patients. Patients belonging to group II should receive HCT 1–2 mg/kg/d. Excessive sodium intake can block HCT effect. Patients belonging to groups I and III should follow a low-calcium, low-sodium diet.

Warning. A severely calcium-restricted diet can produce a negative calcium balance, which may be harmful in childhood.

Prognosis. Good if early institution of treatment.

BIBLIOGRAPHY. Berlin LJ, Clayton BE: Idiopathic hypercalciuria in a child. Arch Dis Child 39:409–414, 1964

Moore ES: Hypercalciuria in children. Contr Nephrol 27:20–32, 1981

Cervera A, Corral MJ, Gomez JM, et al: Idiopathic hypercalciuria in children: Classification, clinical manifestations, and outcome. Acta Pediatr Scand 76:271–278, 1987

Prien EL, Curhan GC: Calcium nephrolithiasis. In De Groot LJ (ed): Endocrinology, 3rd ed, p 1180. Philadelphia, WB Saunders, 1995

HYPERCHOLESTEROLEMIA, FAMILIAL

Synonyms. Harbiz-Mueller; LDL receptor defect; familial hyperbetalipoproteinemia; hyperlipoproteinemia IIa: xanthomatosis—hypercholesterolemia; xanthoma tuberosum simplex.

Symptoms. Both sexes affected; age of detection from infancy to third or fourth decade. Anginal pain; symptoms of arterial obstruction in different organs. Possibly, recurrent attacks of polyarthritis and tenosynovitis without temperature elevation.

Signs. Xanthoma tendinosum or tuberosum, especially elbows, knees, hands, feet; arcus senilis; no hepatosplenomegaly.

Etiology. Autosomal dominant inheritance. Autosomal dominant inheritance with gene dosage effect. Mutant alleles for LDL receptors (Rb0, Rb–, Rb+10) (all inactive), do not allow LDL uptake from plasma and as a consequence low density proteins accumulate in arteries and macrophages.

Pathology. Diffuse atheromatosis.

Diagnostic Procedures. *Blood.* Subtype a: plasma aspect clear, increased LDL; normal very low-density lipoproteins (VLDL); increased cholesterol and normal triglycerides. Subtype b: aspect clear or slightly turbid; increased LDL and VLDL; increased cholesterol and triglycerides. Sedimentation rate frequently increased; fibrinogen marked increase. Normal glucose tolerance test. *Electrocardiography. X-ray.* Calcification of vascular atheromas. Prenatal diagnosis possible on amniotic cells.

Therapy. Diet: cholesterol intake below 300 mg/day for adult; reduction of saturated fats and increase of polyunsaturated fats. Cholestyramine, preferably in combination with nicotinic acid. Lovastatin-Simvastatin. Three new experimental approaches: (1) Intravenous hyperalimentation; (2) end-to-side portocaval anastomosis; (3) use of continuous-flow blood-cell separator for repeated plasma exchange.

Prognosis. Vast spectrum of possibilities, from simple increase of beta-lipoprotein without limitation of life span to fatality from atheromatosis during first year of life.

BIBLIOGRAPHY. Fagge CH: General xanthelasma or vitiligoidea. Trans Pathol Soc London 24:242–250, 1872

Rayer PFO: Traite theorique et pratiques des maladies de la peau. Paris, 1836

Harbitz F: Svulster indeholdende xanthomaev I. Sarkomer utgaaende fra sense-skeder og ledkapler. II. Multiple symmetriske xanthomer III Xantosarkomer. Norsch Mag Laegevid 86:321–348, 1925

Mueller C: Xanthomate hypercholesterolemia, angina pectoris. Acta Med Scand (Suppl) 89:75–84, 1938

Schettler G, Habenicht AJR (eds): Principles and Treatment of Lipoprotein Disorders. New York, Springer, 1994

Havel RJ, Kane JP: Introduction: Structure and metabolism of pasma lipoproteins. In Scriver CR, Beaudet AL, Sly WS, et al: The Metabolic and Molecular Bases of Inherited Disease, 7th ed, pp 1849–1850. New York, McGraw-Hill, 1995

HYPEREMESIS GRAVIDARUM

Synonyms. Emesis gravidarum; pregnancy pernicious vomiting; pernicious vomiting, pregnancy

Symptoms. Begins as simple vomiting around sixth week, gradually increasing in spite of treatment, so that no food or water can be retained. Nervousness and insomnia; polyneuritis, coma.

Signs. Dehydration; starvation; emaciation.

Etiology. Not known; some metabolic change is the fundamental factor, but psychoneurosis plays a role also. Thyreotoxicosis may be associated.

Pathology. Most marked morbid changes occur in liver: fatty degeneration of central portion of lobule extending to acute yellow atrophy; liver glycogen is depleted. Kidney lesions.

Diagnostic Procedures. *Urine.* High concentration; albuminuria; casts. *Blood.* Electrolyte imbalance; hyperbilirubinemia; increased blood urea nitrogen. In case of thyreotoxicosis up to 70% increased TSH, 50% increased FT 4, FT3, and T3.

Therapy. *Prophylaxis.* Good antenatal care; differentiation between neurotic and toxic type. *Curative.* Complete rest in bed; intravenous fluid medication with maintenance of electrolyte balance. *Sedation.* Sodium phenobarbital; thorazine as central nervous system depressant. Consider antithyroid treatment in selected cases. If intractable, therapeutic abortion.

Prognosis. Can be prevented by proper antenatal care; even death if inadequate therapeutic measures. Prompt resolution after delivery.

BIBLIOGRAPHY. Becks GP, Burrow GN: Diagnosis and treatment of thyroid disease during pregnancy. In De Groot LJ (ed): Endocrinology, 3rd ed, p 806. Philadelphia, WB Saunders, 1995

HYPEREOSINOPHILIC

Synonyms. See also individual eosinophilic syndromes.

Symptoms and Signs. The term idiopathic hypereosinophilic syndrome is applied when the following criteria are fulfilled: (1) eosinophilia $1.5 \times 10/1$; (2) persists for at least 6 months or fatal in a shorter time; (3) results in organ system dysfunction; (4) absence of a recognized cause for the eosinophilia. Three different forms have been recognized: (a) hypereosinophilia with lung involvement and angioedema; (b) severe cardiac and central nervous system complications; (c) eosinophilic cytogenic abnormalities and other features of a leukemic disease.

Etiology. Unknown. Various theories have been put forward: autoimmune disease; neoplastic disease; exaggerated response to a parasite or allergic disease.

Pathology. *Lung.* Eosinophilic infiltration; signs of pulmonary hypertension. *Myocardium.* Increase of collagen connective tissue and eosinophilic infiltration. Other organs. Mature eosinophil infiltration and proliferation of collagen tissue.

Therapy. Corticosteroids. Hydroxyurea is used in patients who do not respond to steroids and also to allow the steroid dosages to be reduced. Vincristine has been used in patients with aggressive disease. Anticoagulants are required in most patients. Leucophoresis and plasma exchange are useful in cases with increased blood viscosity and widespread vessel occlusions.

Prognosis. Favorable prognostic factors are high IgE concentrations, the presence of angioneurotic edema, and eosinopenia within a few hours after the first dose of prednisone. Unfavorable signs are leucocytosis and myeloblasts in peripheral blood and congestive heart failure.

BIBLIOGRAPHY. Chusoil MJ, Dale DC, West BC, et al: The hypereosinophilic syndrome: analysis of fourteen cases with review of literature. Medicine 54:1–27, 1975

Alfaham MA, Ferguson SD, Sihna B, Davies J: The idiopathic hypereosinophilic syndrome. Arch Dis Child 62:601–613, 1987

Athens JW: Variation of leukocytes in disease. In Lee GR, Bithel TC, Foerster J, et al (eds): Wintrobe's Clinical Hematology, 9th ed, p 1576. Philadelphia, Lea & Febiger, 1993

HYPERHIDROSIS

Synonyms. Asymmetric hyperhidrosis; gustatory hyperhidrosis; mental sweating; thermoregulatory hyperhidrosis. Four clinical variants of this condition recognized.

ASYMMETRIC HYPERHIDROSIS

Symptoms and Signs. Both sexes affected; onset at all ages. Localized excessive sweating occurring in any area of the body. Usually associated with various neurologic or visceral symptoms and signs.

Etiology. Neurologic or visceral lesion producing an abnormal stimulation of selected sympathetic pathway.

Therapy. Topical atropine-like drugs; aluminum salts; ethanol glycerine of little effect. Atropine-like drugs have limited effect. Sympathectomy of temporary utility; removal of area with affected sweat gland could be beneficial.

Prognosis. That of main neurologic condition.

GUSTATORY HYPERHIDROSIS

See also Bogorad and Von Frey.

Symptoms and Signs. Both sexes affected; onset in childhood. It also appears frequently (50–80%) 4–7 months after surgery on the parotid glands. Localized sweating on lips, nose, and forehead or, seldom, on other areas of the body (e.g., knee) after eating, especially hot or spicy foods.

Etiology. In most cases, unknown reflex mechanism; in others, lesion within central nervous system or damage to sympathetic and parasympathetic systems of face or neck.

Therapy. See Asymmetric hyperhidrosis.

Prognosis. Form of no clinical significance and lifelong persistence, or symptomatic, where the syndrome may wane after 3–5 years.

MENTAL SWEATING

Symptoms and Signs. Both sexes affected; onset in childhood or early puberty. Following emotions or mental activity sweating (usually very profuse) on palms, soles, axillae, groin, and face. Hands usually cold and show tendency to acrocyanosis (see). Sweating could also be continuous. Pompholyix (see) and contact dermatitis possible complications.

Etiology. Unknown; overactivity of endocrine glands.

Therapy. See Asymmetric hyperhidrosis.

Prognosis. Persistent condition; tendency to improvement after the 25th year of life.

THERMOREGULATING HYPERHIDROSIS

Synonym. Sweating sickness.

Symptoms. Bouts of persistent sweating, not related to exogenous heating and without fever. More frequent during sleep.

Etiology. Extremely variable. Following infective processes or as presenting manifestation; intoxications (e.g., alcohol) or metabolic disorders (e.g., diabetes; endocrinopathies; obesity) or malignancies.

Therapy. See Asymmetric hyperhidrosis.

Prognosis. Variable.

BIBLIOGRAPHY. Guttmann L, List CF: Zur Topik und Pathophysiologie der Schweiss-Secretion. Ztschr Neurol Psychiatr 116:504–536, 1928

Sulzberger MB, Hermann F: The clinical significance of disturbances in the delivery of sweat. Springfield, IL, CC Thomas, 1954

Champion RH: Disorders of sweat glands. In Champion RH, Burton JL, Ebling FJG (eds): Rook/Wilkinson/Ebling Textbook of Dermatology, 5th ed, pp 1752–1756. Oxford, Blackwell Scientific, 1992

HYPERHYDROXYPROLINEMIA

Synonym. Hydroxyprolinemia 4-hydroxy-l-proline oxidase deficiency.

Symptoms and Signs. Only a trait. Some cases with association of mental retardation reported.

Etiology. Autosomal recessive. Probably absence of 4-hydroxy-L-proline oxidase.

Diagnostic Procedures. *Urine.* Hyperhydroxyprolinuria. Microscopic hematuria

Prognosis. Good.

BIBLIOGRAPHY. Efron ML, Bixby EM, Palattao LG, et al: Hydroxyprolinemia associated with mental deficiency. N Engl J Med 267:1193, 1962

Phang JM, Yeh GC, Scriver CR: Disorders of proline and hydroxyproline metabolism. In Scriver CR, Beaudet AL, Sly WS, et al: The Metabolic and Molecular Bases of Inherited Disease, 7th ed, pp 1135–1136. New York, McGraw-Hill, 1995

HYPER IgM

Synonyms. Hyperimmunoglobulin M immunodeficiency; hypergammaglobulinemia IgM, dysgammaglobulinemia IgM; IgM hyperglobulinemia.

Symptoms and Signs. From birth frequent various infective episodes. Tonsils and lymph nodes enlarged, possible spleno-hepatomegaly. See diagnostic procedures for other possible symptoms. Occurrence of sclerosing cholangitis and neurological complications.

Etiology. Sex-linked but autosomal dominant and recessive and sporadic cases reported. Also may be a complication of rubella. Considered impaired transformation of IgM in IgG, IgA, IgE.

Pathology. Lymph nodes show few follicles and absence of germinal centers, with decreased plasma cells.

Diagnostic Procedures. *Blood.* Normal lymphocytes B and T; IgM (polyclonal, with both kappa and lamda chains and IgD increased); IgG, IgA and IgE absent or decreased. Cyclic neutropenia may be associated or described as well hemolytic anemia thrombocytopenia nephritis evidence. *X-rays.* Possible arthritis.

Therapy. Immunoglobulin. IgG regular infusions. Antibiotic at need.

Prognosis. Good protection against recurrent infections. Frequent development of lymphoma.

BIBLIOGRAPHY. Rosen FS, Kevy SV, Merler E, et al: Recurrent bacterial infections and dysgammaglobulinemia: A deficiency of 7S gamma-globulins in the presence of 19 S gamma-globulins. Pediatrics 28:182–195, 1961

Goldman AS, Ritzniann SE, Houston EW, et al: Dysgammaglobulinemic antibodies deficiency syndrome increased gamma M-globulin and decreased gamma-G and gamma-A globulins. J Pediatr 70:16–27, 1967

Banatvala N, Davis J, Kanariou M, et al: Hypergammaglobulinemia associated with normal or increased IgM (the hyper IgM syndrome): A case series review. Arch Dis Child 71:150–152, 1994

HYPERKALEMIC

Synonym. Potassium intoxication.

Symptoms. None in mild form. In severe attack (potassium 6 mEq/liter), nausea, vomiting, abdominal pain, weakness, flaccid paralysis, dysarthria, oliguria, respiratory arrest, syncope.

Signs. Earliest sign is provided by the electrocardiographic changes: tall tent-shaped T-waves; decreased P-wave amplitude; and finally atrial systole. Hypotension; arrhythmias; ileus; cardiac arrest.

Etiology. Renal damage: acute tubular necrosis; chronic renal failure; diabetic coma; postsurgical electrolyte imbalance. As component of Addison, Conn syndromes. Iatrogenic: spironolactone; triamterene; blood transfusion; excessive potassium administration.

Diagnostic Procedures. *Blood.* Total serum. Determination of serum potassium. *Urine.* Urinary potassium excretion; pH; base excess; osmolarity. *Electrocardiography.* See Signs.

Therapy. Interdiction of all intake of potassium. If there is trauma and necrosis, removal of necrotic tissue. Infusion of glucose and insulin. Administration of sodium bicarbonate, calcium gluconate to counteract potassium effect on myocardium. Cation exchange resin in sodium cycle (per os or per rectum) to remove potassium from body. Hemodialysis (if other therapeutic approach unsuccessful). Pacemaker if there are severe arrhythmias.

Prognosis. According to etiology. Good response to treatment.

BIBLIOGRAPHY. Schwartz WB: Fluid, electrolyte, and acid-base balance. In Beeson PB, McDermott W (eds): Cecil-Loeb Textbook of Medicine, 12th ed. Philadelphia, WB Saunders, 1967

Tanner RL (ed): Symposium on potassium homeostasis. Kidney Int 11:389 (whole issue), 1977

Du Bose TD, Alpern RJ: Renal tubular acidosis. In Scriver CR, Beaudet AL, Sly WS, et al: The Metabolic and Molecular Bases of Inherited Disease, 7th ed, pp 3656, 3667, 3670–3673. New York, McGraw-Hill, 1995

HYPERKINETIC HEART

Synonyms. Athletic heart; circulatory hyperkinetic; hyperdynamic heart.

Symptoms. Occurs in patients of all ages. Less than 50% have cardiorespiratory symptoms (dyspnea; orthopnea; chest discomfort); about 20% are participating in athletic activities. Occurs in young or early middle age.

Signs. Overactivity of heart and great vessels; thrusting ventricles; pulse full and quick; basal or left parasternal ejection-like systolic murmur, up to grade 4 in intensity. Systolic ejection click and split second pulmonic sound (50%). Over femoral vein, in the inguinal trigone, venous murmur increasing with lifting of leg or on exertion. Labile blood pressure (50%).

Etiology. Unknown; possibly, psychic pressure; anxiety, prehypertensive condition, superficial similarities to the effects of catecholamine stimulation. Time used for ejection shorter than normal; volume per beat not necessarily increased. Unknown. Related to hyperstimulation of beta-adrenergic system.

Diagnostic Procedures. *Electrocardiography.* Left ventricular hypertrophy; in some patients completely normal tracing. *X-ray.* Usually normal. Pulmonary plethora only in minority of patients. *Echocardiography.* Normal thickness of walls.

Therapy. Beta-adrenergic reception blockade.

Prognosis. This syndrome, usually observed in hypertensive or prehypertensive patients, may lead to circulatory failure.

BIBLIOGRAPHY. Starr I, Jonas L: Supernormal circulation in resting subjects (hyperkinemia) with a study of the relation of the kinetic abnormalities to the basal metabolic rate. Arch Intern Med 71:1–22, 1943

Gorlin R: The hyperkinetic heart syndrome. JAMA 182:823–829, 1962

Gillium RF, Teichholz LE, Herman MV, et al: The idiopathic hyperkinetic heart syndrome: clinical course and long term prognosis. Am Heart J 102:728, 1981

Fowler NO: High-cardiac-output states. In Schlant RC, Alexander RW: Hurst's The Heart, 8th ed, pp 509–510. New York, McGraw-Hill, 1994

HYPERLEUCINE ISOLEUCINEMIA

Synonym. Branched-chain amino transaminase.

Symptoms and Signs. Only one description of this rare abnormality. Both sexes. From 2–3 months of age: seizures, failure to thrive, mental retardation. Retinal degeneration, hearing loss.

Etiology. Unknown. Defective metabolism of leucine, isoleucine, and proline.

Diagnostic Procedures. *Blood.* High leucine, isoleucine, and proline. *Urine.* Leucine, isoleucine normal; increased glycine and delta-pyrolidine-5-carboxylic acid.

Therapy. Low-protein diet (apparently of no benefit).

Prognosis. Death in early age.

BIBLIOGRAPHY. Jeune M, Collombel E, Michel M, et al: Hyperleucine isoleucinemie par defaut partial de transamination associée a une hyperprolinemie de type 2: observation familiale d'une double aminoacidopathie. Ann Pediatr 17:85–99, 1970

Chuang DT, Shih VE: Disorders of branched chain aminoacid and ketoacid metabolism. In Scriver CR, Beaudet AL, Sly WS, et al: The Metabolic and Molecular Bases of Inherited Disease, 7th ed, p 1250. New York, McGraw-Hill, 1995

HYPERLEXIA

Synonyms. Words recognition; words decoding; compulsive reading.

Symptoms and Signs. In children with otherwise reduced mental abilities: unexpected easiness in reading; we observed not an accelerated, fluent reading but a peculiar ability to match orthographic characters with phonological segments without actually recognizing the meaning of the words.

Etiology. Autosomal recessive inheritance reported. Autism has been considered as the prototypic pervasive developmental disorder.

BIBLIOGRAPHY. Silberberg NE, Silberberg MC: Hyperlexia: Specific word recognition skills in young children. Except Chil 34:41–42, 1967
Hutterlocher RR, Hutterlocker A: A study of children with hyperlexia. Neurology 23:1107–1116, 1973
Burd L, Kerbeshian J: Familial pervasive disorder: Tourette disorder and hyperlexia. Neurosci Biobehav Rev 12:233–234, 1988

HYPERLIPEMIC RETINITIS

Adult form of Coats (see). Same findings as in childhood form, with the exception of constant history of some preceding uveal inflammation and constant findings of hypercholesterolemia.

Therapy. This form does not respond to diathermy or photocoagulation. Dietary treatment and anticholesterolemic agents are indicated.

BIBLIOGRAPHY. Garner A: Vascular diseases. In Garner A, Klintworth GK (eds): Pathobiology of Ocular Disease: A Dynamic Approach, 2nd ed, pp 1690–1699. New York, Marcel Dekker, 1994

HYPERLIPOPROTEINEMIA TYPE III

Synonyms. Broad beta; remnant hyperlipemia β-VLDL; carbohydrate-induced hyperlipemia; dysbetalipoproteinemia; familial type III hyperlipoproteinemia; floating beta; xanthoma tuberosum.

Symptoms. Both sexes affected; age of detection third to fourth decade. Anginal pain and symptoms of arterial obstruction in different organs. Attacks of abdominal pain may occur.

Signs. Appearance, during third or fourth decade, of nodules in tendons in various locations, and other xanthomas, both planar (xanthoma striata palmaris) and tuberous types. Hepatosplenomegaly.

Etiology. Autosomal dominant inheritance (?); pathogenesis unknown. Possibly, aberrant synthesis and direct release of the unusual lipoproteins into the blood. Uncertain relationship with hyperlipoproteinemia type II since, to the features of this form is added the increase of prebetalipoprotein that is carbohydrate-dependent. Homozygosity for the Ed allele, which determines synthesis of an inactive type of apoprotein (E-3) combined with other factors elevating blood cholesterol (i.e., other inherited hyperlipidemias or thyroid deficiency, obesity, glucose intolerance). The necessary presence of two cofactors causes a pseudodominant inheritance. It is hypothesized that deficiency of normal E-3 causes altered degradation of chylomicrons and VLDL determining the appearance of β-VLDL. The β-VLDL alone among lipoproteins rich in cholesterol have the capacity of accumulating in macrophages, determining foam cells and xanthomas.

Pathology. Diffuse atheromatosis; gallstones, and cholecystitis frequent. Foam cells in various organs.

Diagnostic Procedures. *Blood.* Plasma aspect usually turbid, often

faint cream layer; presence of beta very low-density lipoproteins (VLDL) (floating beta; low-density lipoproteins [LDL] of abnormal composition). *Abnormal glucose tolerance test; frank diabetes in some cases.* Hyperuricemia in 50% of cases. *Electrocardiography. X-ray.* To demonstrate calcification of atheromas.

Therapy. Diet: low calorie intake; 40% carbohydrates; 40% fats; cholesterol below 300 mg/day; alcohol restriction. Clofibrate; nicotinic acid; d-thyroxine; cholestyramine not indicated.

Prognosis. Wide variation, from death in early infancy or in fifth or sixth decade. Good with therapy.

BIBLIOGRAPHY. Gofman JW, De Lalla O, Glazier F, et al: The serum lipoprotein transport system in health metabolic disorders, atherosclerosis and coronary artery disease. Plasma 2:413–484, 1954
Fredrickson DS, Levi RI, Lees RS: Fat transport in lipoproteins: An integrated approach to mechanisms and disorders. N Engl J Med 276:32, 94, 148, 251, 273, 1967
Schettler G, Habenicht AJR (eds): Principles and Treatment of Lipoprotein Disorders. New York, Springer, 1994
Havel RJ, Kane JP: Introduction structure and metabolism of plasma lipoproteins. In Scriver CR, Beaudet AL, Sly WS, et al: The Metabolic and Molecular Bases of Inherited Disease, 7th ed, pp 1849–1850. New York, McGraw-Hill, 1995

HYPERLIPOPROTEINEMIA, TYPE IV

Synonym. Carbohydrate-inducible hyperlipemia; endogenous; VLDL.

Symptoms and Signs. Early atherosclerotic changes, eruptive xanthoma may be present.

Etiology. It represents a phenotype including many conditions: hypertriglyceridemia (see); combination of III and V hyperlipoproteinemias (see); uremia; hypopituitarism, anticonceptional steroids, von Gierke (see). Carbohydrate and ethanol consumption strongly influence the degree of biochemical alterations.

Diagnostic Procedures. *Plasma.* High VLDL and triglycerides, normal cholesterol, and phospholipids.

Therapy. Diet. Antilipid agents.

Prognosis. Variable. Early atherosclerosis and increased incidence of myocardial infarction.

BIBLIOGRAPHY. Sprinz N: Carbohydrate-induced lipemia: report of a familial occurrence. N Engl J Med 271:291–293, 1964
Schettler G, Habenicht AJR (eds): Principles and Treatment of Lipoprotein Disorders. New York, Springer, 1994
Havel RJ, Kane JP: Introduction structure and metabolism of plasma lipoproteins. In Scriver CR, Beaudet AL, Sly WS, et al: The Metabolic and Molecular Bases of Inherited Disease, 7th ed, pp 1849–1850. New York, McGraw-Hill, 1995

HYPERLIPOPROTEINEMIA, TYPE V

Synonyms. Essential hyperlipemia; familial hyperlipoproteinemia type V; fat-carbohydrate-induced hyperlipemia; lipoprotein lipase deficiency mixed hyperlipemia; VLDL + chylomicrons.

Symptoms and Signs. Occurs in both sexes; onset in adulthood. Recurrent abdominal pain related to high fat intake; symptoms and mild diabetes (occasionally). Seldom, eruptive xanthomas; no tuberous or tendinous lesions. No striking history of heart ischemia. Hepatosplenomegaly. Mild paresthesias of extremities. Gout in 10–20% of cases.

Etiology. Dominant inheritance (?); familial inheritance of undetermined type, probably carrying mutations different from those of other reported hyperlipoproteinemias (see); can also be secondary to diabetes, alcoholism, nephrotic syndrome, hypothyroidism.

Pathology. Nonspecific changes.

Diagnostic Procedures. *Blood.* Plasma, cream layer on top, turbid below; presence of chylomicrons; increased very low-density lipoproteins VLDL cholesterol and triglycerides. Removal of fat from diet causes temporary fall in triglyceride concentration. Abnormal glucose tolerance tests (80%). Hyperuricemia almost constant. Postheparin lipoprotein lipase; and hepatic triglyceride lipase activities in plasma are normal.

Therapy. Restriction of dietary fat to 50 g/d to prevent abnormal attacks. Reduction of carbohydrates. Nicotinic acid 1.0 to 1.5 g/d and clofibrate induce only a moderate reduction of blood hyperlipemia. Steroid hormones more effective in women.

Prognosis. Myocardial ischemia not abnormally prevalent in this condition.

BIBLIOGRAPHY. Malmros H, Swahn B, Truedsson E: Essential hyperlipaemia. Acta Med Scand 149:91–108, 1954
Schettler G, Habenicht AJR (eds): Principles and Treatment of Lipoprotein Disorders. New York, Springer, 1994
Havel RJ, Kane JP: Introduction structure and metabolism of pasma lipoproteins. In Scriver CR, Beaudet AL, Sly WS, et al: The Metabolic and Molecular Bases of Inherited Disease, 7th ed, pp 1849–1850. New York, McGraw-Hill, 1995

HYPERLYSINEMIA, PERIODIC

Synonyms. Colombo; hyperlysinemia—hyperammonemia; lysine intolerance; hyperlysinuria—hyperammonemia. See Hyperlysinemia, persistent.

Symptoms and Signs. Present from birth. Episodes of vomiting; abdominal pain; diarrhea; dehydration; spasticity; episodes of convulsions and comas. Severe motor retardation; hepatosplenomegaly; protein aversion; intelligence retarded or normal.

Etiology. Partial defect in L-lysine nicotinamide adenine dinucleotide (NAD) oxidoreductase activity; incapacity of degrading lysine. Since this amino acid inhibits arginase, it most likely interferes with urea synthesis and leads to ammonia intoxication.

Diagnostic Procedures. *Blood.* Increased plasma lysine and arginine level. Extremely high blood ammonia during attacks. Protein intake (3 g/kg/d) precipitates crisis lasting weeks. Dietary protein restriction and fluid therapy correct and prevent crisis.

Therapy. Diet with reduced amount of lysine. Attacks always follow an excessive protein ingestion.

Prognosis. Poor; treatment prevents acute attacks. If treatment started early enough, may also prevent brain damage.

BIBLIOGRAPHY. Colombo JP, Richterich R, Spahr DA, et al: Congenital lysine intolerance with periodic ammonia intoxication. Lancet I:1014–1015, 1964
Colombo JP, Bürgi W, Richterich R, et al: Congenital lysine intolerance with periodic ammonia intoxication: a defect in L-lysine degradation. Metabolism 16:910–925, 1967
Cox RP, Dancis J: Errors of lysine metabolism. In Scriver CR, Beaudet AL, Sly WS, et al: The Metabolic and Molecular Bases of Inherited Disease, 7th ed, pp 1233–1238. New York, McGraw-Hill, 1995

HYPERLYSINEMIA, PERSISTENT

Synonyms. Ghadimi-Woody; Woody-Ghadimi; lysine-ketoglutarate reductase deficiency. See Hyperlysinemia, periodic.

Symptoms. Both sexes; age of detection from infancy to early adulthood. Severe mental retardation; occasionally, convulsions. Physical development variable from retardation to normality.

Signs. Absence of secondary sex characteristics; strabismus, hepato-splenomegaly; altered facial features. Occasionally, laxity of joints and synophrys.

Etiology. Inherited condition; autosomal recessive.

Diagnostic Procedures. *Blood.* Mild anemia; persistent hyperlysinemia with absence of hyperammonemia, even under lysine loading. Lysine loading abnormal response. *Urine.* Hyperlysinuria; usually absence of other basic amino acids. *Electroencephalography.* From normal to petit mal pattern.

Therapy. Symptomatic. Low protein diet not warranted.

Prognosis. Poor.

BIBLIOGRAPHY. Woody NC: Hyperlysinemia (abstr). Proc Am Pediatr Soc VII Ann Meeting (Seattle): p 33, 1964
Ghadimi H, Bimington VL, Pecora F: Hyperlysinemia associated with retardation. N Engl J Med 273:723–729, 1965
Cox RP, Markovitz PJ, Chuang DT: Familial hyper lysenemia: Multiple enzyme deficiencies associated with the bifunctional aminoadipic semialdehyde synthetase. Trans Am Clin Chem Assoc 97:69–81, 1985
Cox RP, Dancis J: Errors of lysine metabolism. In Scriver CR, Beaudet AL, Sly WS, et al: The Metabolic and Molecular Bases of Inherited Disease, 7th ed, pp 1233–1238. New York, McGraw-Hill, 1995

HYPERMAGNESEMIA

Symptoms. Nausea; vomiting; malaise; micturition; central nervous system depression (drowsiness; lethargy; slight slurring of speech); ataxic gait. Coma (with very high concentration). Cardiac arrest.

Signs. Blood hypotension (if high magnesium plasma concentration); absent tendon reflexes; bradypnea.

Etiology. In newborn (if mother received large doses of magnesium intravenously prior to delivery); in patients who ingest high doses of magnesium, antacids, or receive parenteral administration of magnesium salts, and in patients with renal disease where ability to excrete magnesium is seriously impaired.

Pathology. Unknown.

Diagnostic Procedures. *Blood.* Serum magnesium determination. *Electrocardiography.* P-R prolongation; slight reduction of P-waves and QRS duration; nodal rhythm with branch block; Q-T interval increased.

Therapy. Calcium administration; avoidance of magnesium administration in patients with reduced renal function. In severe intoxication, hemodialysis or peritoneal dialysis.

BIBLIOGRAPHY. Randall RE, Cohen MD, Spray CC, et al: Hypermagnesemia in renal failure: Etiology and toxic manifestations. Ann Intern Med 61:73–88, 1964
Beck LH (ed): Symposium on body fluid and electrolyte disorders. Med Clin No Am 65:249 (whole issue): 1981
De Groot LJ (ed): Endocrinology, 3rd ed, pp 1023, 1033, 1126. Philadelphia, WB Saunders, 1995

HYPERMEDULLIPIN

Symptoms and Signs. Observed in a 46-year-old female who had left nephrectomy for nephrolytiasis complicated by several abscesses, and with right kidney failure. Hypertension, hemodialysis, and later peritoneal dialysis. Blood pressure drop after 18 months without orthostatic changes, no response to IV norepinephrine.

Etiology. Medullipinoma (benign neoplasm secreting medullipin MED I).

Diagnostic Procedures. See Symptoms.

Therapy. No response to drugs for raising blood pressure.

Prognosis. The patient died from peritonitis.

BIBLIOGRAPHY. Muirhead EE, Streeten DPh, Byers LV, et al: Lipomedullipinoma: A source of hypermedullipinemia. Blood Pressure 1:138–148, 1992; 2:183–188, 1993

HYPERMOBILE CECUM

Obsolete.

Synonym. Mobile cecum.

Symptoms and Signs. Lower right quadrant pain; symptoms mimicking partial bowel obstruction and acute appendicitis. (No real evidence to relate the reported symptomatology to the anatomic condition.)

Etiology. Large range of mobility of cecum and lower half of ascending colon.

Diagnostic Procedures. *X-ray.* Cecum located in midline with dilatation and stasis.

BIBLIOGRAPHY. Rogers RL, Hartford FJ: Mobile cecum syndrome. Dis Colon Rectum 27:399–402, 1984
Cywes S, Millar AJW: Embriology and anomalies of the intestine. In Haubrich WS, Schaffner F, Berk JE (eds): Bockus Gastroenterology, 5th ed, vol 2, p 919. Philadelphia, WB Saunders, 1995

HYPERMOBILITY

Symptoms. Pain localized to the knees, hands, and fingers.

Signs. The diagnosis of the syndrome is made if the patient is able to perform at least three of the following maneuvers: (1) extension of the wrists and metacarpal phalanges so that the fingers are parallel to the dorsum of the forearm; (2) passive apposition of thumbs to the flexor aspect of the forearm; (3) hyperextension of knees (to 10 degrees); (4) hyperextension of elbows (to 10 degrees); (5) flexion of trunk with knees extended so palms rest on the floor. The absence of easy bruising, lens dislocation, and characteristic skin changes makes posssible the differential diagnosis with Ehlers-Danlos syndrome (see). The hypermobility syndrome also may be seen in association with rheumatic diseases and does not seem to affect the course of these conditions.

Diagnostic Procedures. *Blood and X-ray examinations to rule out rheumatic diseases.*

Therapy. Reassurance, physical therapy, and symptomatic therapy (nonsteroid anti-inflammatory agents).

BIBLIOGRAPHY. Kirk JA: The hypermobility syndrome. Am Rheum Dis 26:419, 1967
Biro F, Gewanter HL, Baum J: The hypermobility syndrome. Pediatrics 72:701–706, 1983
Bulbena A, Duno JC, Matero A, et al: Joint hypermobility syndrome and anxiety disorders. Lancet 2:694, 1988

HYPERORNITHINEMIA–HYPERAMMONIEMIA–HOMOCITRULLINURIA

Synonyms. HHH; Shih.

Symptoms and Signs. Both sexes. After breast feeding is stopped, vomiting, lethargy, delayed milestones. After infancy, spontaneous selection of low-protein diet. From moderate to severe mental retardation. Occasionally onset of symptoms may be delayed to childhood or even adulthood. No hepatosplenomegaly.

Etiology. Autosomal recessive. Suggested defect of ornithine entry in mitochondria, which decreases urea cycle and impairs ammonia detoxification.

Pathology. Liver light microscopy normal, ultrastructural elongation of mitochondria some containing crystalloid structures.

Diagnostic Procedures. *Blood.* Postprandial hyperammonemia, hyperornithinemia. *Urine.* Homocitrullinuria.

Therapy. Protein restriction initiated early in life permits normal development.

Prognosis. Some patients survive to adulthood with few symptoms. Usually lethargy, ataxia, choreoathetosis, delayed development, muscle hypotonia, seizures, characterize the evolution of this condition.

BIBLIOGRAPHY. Shih VE, Efron ML, Moser HW: Hyperornithinemia, hyperammonemia and homocitrullinuria: a new disorder of amino acid metabolism associated with myoclonic seizures and mental retardation. Ann J Dis Child 117:83–92, 1969
Dionisi-Vici C, Bachman C, Gambarara M, et al: Hyperornithinemia–hyperammoniemia–homocitrillinuria syndrome: Low creatinine excretion and effect of citrulline, arginine or ornithine supplement. Pediatr Res 22:364–367, 1987
Tuchman M, Knopman DS, Shih VE: Episodic hyperammoniemia in adult siblings with hyperornithinemia, hyperammoninemia and homocitrillinuria syndrome. Arch Neurol 47:1134–1137, 1990
Valle D, Simel O: The hyperornithinemias. In Scriver CR, Beaudet AL, Sly WS, et al: The Metabolic and Molecular Bases of Inherited Disease, 7th ed, pp 1173–1176. New York, McGraw-Hill, 1995

HYPEROSMOLALITY SYNDROMES

1. Part of classic diabetes insipidus (traumatic, see) syndrome (with sodium increase)
2. Intracranial lesions with hypernatremia
3. Essential hypernatremia
4. Asymptomatic hypovolemic hypernatremic (Goldberg variant)
5. Pure water depletion (with sodium increase)
6. Part of renal failure and urea retention (without sodium increase)
7. As part of uncontrolled diabetes (without sodium increase).

BIBLIOGRAPHY. Bartter FC: Hyper- and hypoosmolality syndromes. Am J Cardiol 12:650–655, 1963
Goldberg M, Weinstein G, Adesman J, et al: Asymptomatic hypovolemic hypernatremia: A variant of essential hypernatremia. Am J Med 43:804–810, 1967
Foster DW, McGarry JD: Diabetes mellitus: Acute complications, ketoacidosis, hyperosmolar coma, lactic acidosis. In De Groot LJ (ed): Endocrinology, 3rd ed, pp 1516–1518. Philadelphia, WB Saunders, 1995

HYPEROSTOSIS CRANIALIS INTERNA

Synonyms. See van Buchem and Morgagni-Stewart-Morel.

Symptoms and Signs. Both sexes. Recurrent facial palsy, variable contemporary involvement of smell, taste, vision, and cochleovestibular functions.

Symptoms. See Diagnostic Procedures.

Etiology. Autosomal dominant inheritance.

Diagnostic Procedures. *X-rays.* Intracranial hyperostosis and osteosclerosis of calvaria and base of skull. Mandibal and rest of skeleton: Normal.

Prognosis. Relatively benign evolution.

BIBLIOGRAPHY. Manni JJ, Scaf JJ, Huygen PLM, et al: Hyperostosis corticals interna: A new hereditary syndrome with cranial nerve entrapment. N Engl J Med 322:450–454, 1990

HYPEROSTOSIS–HYPERPHOSPHATEMIA

Symptoms and Signs. Rare. In the Middle East. Female prevalence. Onset in childhood. Recurrent episodes of swelling and pain of long bones (especially tibia).

Etiology. Two hypothesis: selective defect of phosphatemic action of parathyroid hormone on renal tubules causing increased phosphate absorption or specific defect of proximal tubules causing increased phosphate absorption independently from parathyroid hormonal activity.

Pathology. Bone biopsy. New normal periosteal bone formation.

Diagnostic Procedures. *X-rays.* Of involved bones: periosteal reaction, cortical thickening, sclerosis. ^{99m}Tc *bone scan.* Increased uptake.

BIBLIOGRAPHY. Melhem RE, Najjar SS, Katchandurian AK: Cortical hyperostosis with hyperphosphatemia. J Pediatr 77:986–990, 1970
Mikati MA, Mechem RE, Najjar SS: The syndrome of hyperostosis with hyperphosphatemia. J Pediatr 99:900–941, 1981
Talab YA, Mallouh A: Hyperostosis with hyperphosphatemia: A case report and review of literature. J Pediatr Orthop 8:338–341, 1988

HYPERPARATHYROIDISM, FAMILIAL

Symptoms. Variable manifestation of hyperparathyroidism in members of same family. Frequent association with glandular pathology. Most frequent association with peptic ulceration, pancreatitis, and renal calculi. See multiple endocrine neoplasia.

Etiology. Unknown; autosomal dominant inheritance.

Pathology. Most common finding is primary chief-cell hyperplasia.

Diagnostic Procedures. *Blood.* Calcium; phosphorus; alkaline phosphatase. *X-ray of gastrointestinal tract. Intravenous pyelogram.*

Therapy. Excision of enlarged parathyroid gland. Abdominal operation for gastrointestinal hemorrhage and for calculi of kidney.

Prognosis. Depends on complications.

BIBLIOGRAPHY. Goldmann L, Smith FS: Hyperparathyroidism in siblings. Ann Surg 104:971–981, 1936
Cutler RE, Reiss E, Ackerman LV: Familial hyperparathyroidism: A kindred involving eleven cases with a discussion of primary chief cell hyperplasia. N Engl J Med 270:859–865, 1964
Segre GV, Potts JT Jr: Differential diagnosis of hypercalcemia. In De Groot LJ (ed): Endocrinology, 3rd ed, pp 1082–1083. Philadelphia, WB Saunders, 1995

HYPERPARATHYROIDISM SYNDROMES

Synonyms. Primary hyperparathyroidism; parathyroid—hyperfunction. Prevalent in female; onset usually in adulthood. The full blown, complete syndrome is seldom seen initially. A cluster of different syndromes with various degrees of overlapping is the rule.

MYOPATHY

Symptoms. Rare condition (3:76 cases of hyperparathyroidism). Fatigue; muscle weakness (subjective weakness frequent symptom of primary hyperparathyroidism, but presence of objective weakness and atrophy characterize this syndrome).

Signs. Objective muscle weakness; atrophy suggesting diagnosis of primary muscle disease.

Etiology. Unknown; adenoma of parathyroid.

Pathology. Scattered areas of muscle fiber degeneration and neutrophilic infiltration. Presence of functioning adenoma in parathyroid.

Diagnostic Procedures. *Blood.* Typical finding of hyperparathyroidism (see). *Urine.* Increased creatine excretion. *Biopsy of muscle. Electromyography.* High percentage of polyphasic potentials.

Therapy. Surgery to excise adenoma.

Prognosis. Removal of adenoma results in complete recovery of muscle function.

BIBLIOGRAPHY. Vicale CT: The diagnostic features of a muscular syndrome resulting from hyperparathyroidism, osteomalacia, owing to renal tubular acidosis and perhaps to related disorders of calcium metabolism. Trans Am Neurol Assoc 74th Meeting, p 143, 1949
Frame B, Heinze EG, Block MA, et al: Myopathy in primary hyperparathyroidism. Ann Intern Med 68:1022–1027, 1968
Segre GV, Potts JT Jr: Differential diagnosis of hypercalcemia. In De Groot LJ (ed): Endocrinology, 3rd ed. Philadelphia, WB Saunders, 1995

SKELETAL SYNDROME OF HYPERPARATHYROIDISM

See von Recklinghausen.

Symptoms. Seldom seen in pure form (without urologic syndrome). Fifteen percent of cases of hyperparathyroidism. Bone or articular discomfort; fractures and vertebral collapse.

Signs. Cystic formation in various bones (frequent site: mandible or maxilla).

Etiology. Unknown; sporadic adenoma hyperplasia or cancer of parathyroid; familial form of hyperparathyroidism. Adenomas also found in association with multiple different endocrine adenomas (see Wermer).

Pathology. *Parathyroid.* Edema usually limited to one gland (in 90–95% of cases); size of gland, from pea to large egg. The gland may be ectopically found in mediastinum or embedded in thymus; orange brown mass; necrosis and hemorrhage into the gland frequent; water-clear cells. Carcinoma rare. *Bones.* Increased osteoclastic and osteoblastic activity; generalized reabsorption and rarefaction; cyst formation and fibrous tissue replacement of marrow space.

Diagnostic Procedures. *Blood.* Increased calcium and decreased phosphorus; increased alkaline phosphatase activity. *Urine.* Hypercalcuria. *X-ray of skeleton.* Evidence of generalized osteoporosis; coarse trabeculation; increased size; partial fractures; cyst formation.

Therapy. Exploration and excision of parathyroid tumor.

Prognosis. Good; recovery of bone defects of calcification once tumor is removed.

UROLOGIC SYNDROME OF HYPERPARATHYROIDISM

Symptoms and Signs. Most common manifestation in 75% of hyperparathyroid patients. It is almost constantly associated with major or minor degree of skeletal changes. Symptoms of renal calculosis. Pain in lumbar region with radiation along the ureters to testes or groin.

Etiology. See Skeletal syndrome section.

Pathology. Parathyroid, see Skeletal syndrome. Kidneys more frequently present definite concretions; seldom, generalized nephrocalcinosis. Associated inflammatory changes. Tubular damage from calcium deposition.

Diagnostic Procedures. *Blood.* See Skeletal syndrome, plus increase of blood urea nitrogen. *Urine.* Abnormality of urine-concentrating ability. *X-ray.* Demonstration of kidney lesions.

Therapy. See Skeletal syndrome.

Prognosis. Depending on time of surgical excision of tumor. If process too advanced, irreversible kidney changes and death from uremia. If early treatment, good recovery.

HYPERCALCEMIC SYNDROME IN HYPERPARATHYROIDISM

See Hypercalcemic.

Symptoms and Signs. Occurs usually in mild form with other manifestations of hyperparathyroidism.

PEPTIC ULCER SYNDROME IN HYPERPARATHYROIDISM

See Wermer.

Symptoms and Signs. The association of peptic ulcer symptoms and hyperparathyroidism is higher than incidence of peptic ulcer in general population. Symptoms and signs are those of peptic ulcer. Distinctive features are (1) preponderance of duodenal ulcer in females; (2) relative high frequency of gastric ulcer in males; (3) absence of gastric hypersecretion; (4) more refractoriness to direct medical and surgical treatment; (5) prompt healing after removal of parathyroid tumor (but not in Wermer, see).

ACUTE PANCREATITIS IN HYPERPARATHYROIDISM

Symptoms and Signs. Those of acute pancreatitis.

Etiology. Calcium precipitate in alkaline pancreatic ducts.

CENTRAL NERVOUS SYSTEM

Symptoms and Signs. Apathy, depression, malaise, fatigue. Mental depression or other psychiatric manifestations (occasionally, anxiety or psychiatric behavior). Mental obtundation up to coma when severe hypocalcemia.

Diagnostic Procedures. *Electroencephalography.* No specific abnormalities.

BIBLIOGRAPHY. von Recklinghausen FD: Die Fibröse oder Deformirende Ostitis, die Osteomalacie und die Osteoplastische Carcinose in Ihren Gegenseitigen Beziehungen. Festschrift Rudolf Virchow (Berlin), 1891

Ellis C, Nicoloff DM: Hyperparathyroidism and peptic ulcer disease. Arch Surg 96:114–118, 1968

Segre GV, Potts JT Jr: Differential diagnosis of hypercalcemia. In De Groot LJ: Endocrinology, 3rd ed, pp 1082–1083. Philadelphia, WB Saunders, 1995

HYPERPATHIA

Synonym. Thalamic hyperpathia. See Dejerine-Roussy.

Symptoms. Hemilateral disagreeable sensations caused by different stimuli (heat; cold; touch; vibration) but usually with a raised threshold to stimulation. Seldom, sensations may give a pleasurable effect that may be isolated or associated with other symptoms of Dejerine-Roussy (see).

Etiology. Release of thalamic activity from cortical control (?); observed also with peripheral nerve diseases.

Therapy. Painful sensations unresponsive to analgesics.

BIBLIOGRAPHY. Head H, Holmes G: Sensory disturbances from cerebral lesions. Brain 34:102–254, 1911

Adams RD, Victor M: Principles of Neurology, 5th ed, p 685. New York, McGraw-Hill, 1993

HYPERPHENYLALANINEMIA SYNDROMES

TYPE 1

See Foelling.

TYPE 2 PERSISTENT HYPERPHENYLALANINEMIA

Asymptomatic.

TYPE 3 TRANSIENT MILD HYPERPHENYLALANINEMIA

Asymptomatic.

TYPE 4 DIHYDROPTERIDINE REDUCTASE DEFICIENCY

Symptoms and Signs. Normal at birth. Within 1 year of life; seizures, abnormal mental development; at 18 months, voluntary movements and social awareness have stopped.

Etiology. Dihydropteridine reductase deficiency. Autosomal recessive inheritance.

Diagnostic Procedures. *Electroencephalography.* Gross abnormalities.

Therapy. Dopa, 5-OH-tryptophan, carbidopa.

Prognosis. Physical growth fair in spite of severe cerebral damage.

TYPE 5

Symptoms. Myoclonus, tetraplegia, recurrent hyperthermia, greasy skin.

Etiology. Dihydrobiopterin synthesis defect.

Diagnostic Procedures. *Urinalysis.* Abnormal biopterin metabolites.

Therapy. DOPA, 5-OH-tryptophan, carbidopa.

TYPE 6 PERSISTENT HYPERPHENYLALANINEMIA AND TYROSINEMIA

Symptoms and Signs. Progressive ataxia and seizures appearing at 12–18 months.

Etiology. Perhaps defect of catabolism of tyrosine.

Diagnostic Procedures. *Urinalysis.* Phenylethylamine, mandelic acid, p-OH mandelic acid.

Therapy. Diet.

TYPE 7 TRANSIENT NEONATAL TYROSINEMIA

Asymptomatic.

Therapy. Vitamin C.

TYPE 8 HEREDITARY TYROSINEMIA (see)

BIBLIOGRAPHY. Smith J: Atypical phenylketonuria accompanied by a severe progressive neurological illness unresponsive to dietary treatment. Arch Dis Child 49:245–250, 1974

Kaufman S, Helzman NA, Milstein S, et al: Phenylketonuria due to a deficiency of dehydropteridine reductase. N Engl J Med 293:785, 1979

Scriver CR, Kaufman S, Eisensmith RC, et al: The hyperphenylalaninemias. In Scriver CR, Beaudet AL, Sly WS, et al: The Metabolic and Molecular Bases of Inherited Disease, 7th ed, pp 1015–1075. New York, McGraw-Hill, 1995

HYPERPHOSPHATASIA, MENTAL RETARDATION

Symptoms and Signs. Severe mental retardation; seizures, neurologic abnormalities.

Etiology. Possibly autosomal recessive inheritance.

Diagnostic Procedures. *Blood.* Alkaline phosphatase greatly elevated.

BIBLIOGRAPHY. Mabry CC, Bautista A, Kirk RFH, et al: Familial hyperphosphatasia with mental retardation, seizures and neurological deficits. J Pediat 77:74–85, 1970

HYPERPROLINEMIA

Synonyms. Joseph; iminoglycinuria, renal, familial. Two types described.

Type I is caused by proline oxidase deficiency. Benign disorder that may be completely asymptomatic. Association of this type of hyperprolinemia with renal disease mental retardation, convulsions, ocular disease, and facial malformation is not clear.

Type II is caused by delta-pyrrolidine 5-carboxylate dehydrogenase deficiency. In this type there is no kidney disease, and patients may present causal association with mild mental retardation or other neurologic manifestations.

Etiology. Autosomal recessive inheritance for both types. Different loci involved in the two phenotypes, not yet mapped to particular chromosomes. Clinical manifestations seem not related to hyperprolinemia per se, but to increased operation of the metabolic interlock.

Diagnostic Procedures. *Blood.* Plasma proline value higher in type II homozygotes than in type I homozygotes. In heterozygotes one third of type I have hyperprolinemia, wheareas type II have normal plasma proline values.

Therapy. Treatment for basic derangement not indicated because apparently not responsible for clinical manifestations. Symptomatic.

Prognosis. Basically benign disorder, often limited to metabolic findings without clinical consequences.

BIBLIOGRAPHY. Joseph R, et al: Maladie familiale associant des convulsions à début très précoce, une hyperaminoacidurie. Arch Fr Pediatr 15:374–387, 1958

Berlow S, Efron ME: A new cause of hyperprolinemia associated with the excretion of [A5]D pyrrolidine-5-carboxylic acid. Proc Soc Pediatr Res, 34th Annual Meeting, Seattle, WA 1974, p 43

Phang JM, Yeh GC, Scriver CR: Disorders of proline and hydroxyproline metabolism. In Scriver CR, Beaudet AL, Sly WS, et al: The Metabolic and Molecular Bases of Inherited Disease, 7th ed, pp 1125–1146. New York, McGraw-Hill, 1995

HYPERPROSTAGLANDIN E

Synonyms. HPGES; Bartter neonatal variant. See Bartter and Gitelman.

Symptoms and Signs. Prenatal onset with polyhydramnios and prematurity. Polyuria, polydypsia, diarrhea, normal blood pressure (despite high renal activity). Failure to thrive.

Etiology. Unknown. Complex congenital tubular disorder with excessive renal and systemic prostaglandin E_2 synthesis. Relationship between increased PGE_2 synthesis and biochemical variation of calcium homeostasis not completely clarified.

Pathology. Significant hypertrophy of juxtaglomerular apparatus, focal tubular, and interstitial calcification with interstitial fibrosis and tubular atrophy.

Diagnostic Procedures. *Blood.* PGE_2 increased. Plasma renin activity increased; secondary hyperaldosteronism. Base excess increased; hypokalemia. *Urine.* Polyuria; hypercalciuria; FE Na decreased; FEK increased; creatinine clearance decreased; Tamm-Horsfall protein reduced. *X-ray.* Nephrocalcinosis; osteopenia.

Therapy. Indomethacin, long course.

Prognosis. Indomethacin to decrease calcium wasting.

BIBLIOGRAPHY. Fanconi A, Schachenmann GG, Nuessli R, et al: Chronic

hypokalemia with growth retardation, normotensive hyperrenin-hyperaldosreronism (Bartter's syndrome) and hypercalciuria. Helv Paedi Acta 26:144–163, 1971

Leonhardt A, Timmermanns G, Roth B, et al: Calcium homeostasis and hypercalciuria in hyperprostaglandin E syndrome. J Pediatr 120:546–553, 1992

Schroeter J, Timmermans G, Seyberth HW, et al: Marked reduction of Tamm-Horsfall protein synthesis in hyperprostaglandin-E syndrome. Kidney Int 44:401–410, 1993

HYPERREACTION LUTEINALIS

Synonyms. Human chorionic gonadotropin-related hyperandrogenism. See adrenogenital syndromes.

Symptoms and Signs. Maternal virilization signs appearing in 25% of patients with this condition.

Etiology. Androgen hypersecretion by hyperaction luteinalis (or luteoma).

BIBLIOGRAPHY. Ehrmann DA, Barnes RB, Rosenfield RL: Hyperandrogenism, hirsutism, and the polycystic ovary syndrome. In De Groot LJ (ed): Endocrinology, 3rd ed, p 2103. Philadelphia, WB Saunders, 1995

HYPERSARCOSINEMIA

Synonym. Sarcosinemia.

Symptoms and Signs. Originally reported: mild motor and mental retardation and few morphological abnormalities, now considered as a benign metabolic state without clinical manifestations.

Etiology. Autosomal recessive. Deficiency of sarcosine dehydrogenase activity.

Diagnostic Procedures. *Liver biopsy.* Deficiency of sarcosine dehydrogenase.

BIBLIOGRAPHY. Gerritsen T, Waisman HA: Hypersarcosinemia: An inborn error of metabolism. N Engl J Med 275:66–69, 1966

Kang ES, Seyer J, Tood TA, et al: Variability in the phenotypic expression of the abnormal sarcosine metabolism in a family. J Hum Genet 64:80–85, 1983

De Braekeleer M: Hereditary disorders in Saguenay-Lac-St-Jean (Quebec, Canada). Hum Hered 41:141–146, 1991

Scott CR: Sarcosinemia. In Scriver CR, Beaudet AL, Sly WS, et al: The Metabolic and Molecular Bases of Inherited Disease, 7th ed, pp 1329–1335. New York, McGraw-Hill, 1995

HYPERSOMNIA

Synonyms. Somnosis, includes idiopathic hypersomnia. See Gélineau, Kleine-Levin, pickwickian, Von Economo, and Elpenor.

Symptoms. Gradual onset of irresistible desire to sleep, which allows the patient enough time to withdraw and go to bed; prolonged sleep (not associated with cataplexy, sleep paralysis, or hypnagogic hallucination, as in narcolepsy). Sleep is prolonged for hours, days, or weeks. Difficult to arouse; irritable; drowsy; slow mentation after awaking. Introverted; slightly anxious; mildly depressed.

Etiology and Pathology. Multiple conditions are responsible for this syndrome: idiopathic, trauma; brain tumors; destructive lesions or inflammation of brain stem; menarche or menstrual cycle; psychogenic basis; diencephalic dysfunction. The syndrome of Kleine-Levin may be considered a particular form of hypersomnia, as well as pickwickian and Elpenor.

Diagnostic Procedures. *Electroencephalography.* Normal sleep stage pattern. Cyclic regularity of (no rapid eye movement) NREM-REM (rapid eye movement) stages for all periods of sleep. *X-ray of skull. CT brain scan. Angiography of skull. Basal metabolism.*

Therapy. Stimulant drugs useful.

Prognosis. According to etiology.

BIBLIOGRAPHY. Bonkalo A: Hypersomnia: A discussion of psychiatric implication based on three cases. Br J Psychiatr 114:69–75, 1968
Hartmann E: Sleep requirements: long sleepers, short sleepers, variable sleepers and insomniacs. Psychosomatics 14:95–103, 1973
Adams RD, Victor M: Principles of Neurology, 5th ed, p 343. New York, McGraw-Hill, 1993

HYPERSPLENISM SYNDROMES

Symptoms and Signs. All clinical manifestations associated with any combination of anemia, thrombocytopenia, and leukopenia. In patient with enlarged spleen, bone marrow not primarily involved. According to some authors, all cases in which there is a return to normal values of blood elements after splenectomy. See Doan-Wright, Doan-Wiseman, Felty, Hodgkin syndromes, Banti, Besnier-Boek-Schaumann.

Etiology. Sequestration and increased rate of destruction of blood cells owing to idiopathic or secondary splenomegaly. Splenic suppression of bone marrow cell production postulated but not confirmed.

BIBLIOGRAPHY. Doan CA: Hypersplenism. Bull NY Acad Med 25:625–650, 1949
Cooney DP, Smith BA: The pathophysiology of hypersplenic thrombocytopenia. Arch Intern Med 121:332–337, 1968
Athens JW: Disorders primarily involving the spleen. In Lee GR, Bithel TC, Foerster J, et al (eds): Wintrobe's Clinical Hematology, 9th ed. Philadelphia, Lea & Febiger, 1993

HYPERSTIMULATION

Synonym. Secondary Meigs; Meigs, secondary.

Symptoms. Occurs in patients receiving human menopausal gonadotropins for treatment of amenorrhea and infertility. Abdominal pain and distension; acute abdominal crisis; tachycardia; oliguria; hematuria; chest pain; dyspnea.

Signs. Ascites; ovarian enlargement; hydrothorax.

Etiology. Administration of human menopausal gonadotropins, clomiphene.

Pathology. Ovarian enlargement, necrosis. Ascites; hydrothorax; in some cases; intra-abdominal hemorrhages.

Diagnostic Procedures. *Blood. Urine.* Electrolytes. Nonprotein nitrogen. *Electrocardiography.*

Therapy. Discontinuation of administration of drug; rest; fluid therapy. If surgery necessary, wedge resection indicated rather than castration, except in uncontrollable hemorrhage.

Prognosis. Generally good. Cases of death reported.

BIBLIOGRAPHY. Vandiest L, DeBast A: Syndrome adbominal aigü par dégénirescence kystique massive et totale des ovaires due a l'administration des gonadotrophines. Brux Med 38:1636–1642, 1958
Neuwirth RS, Turksoy RN, Vande Wiele RL: Acute Meig's syndrome secondary to ovarian stimulation with human menopausal gonadotropins. Am J Obstet Gynecol 91:977–981, 1965
Baird DT: Amenorrhea, anovulation, and dysfunctional bleeding. In De Groot LJ (ed): Endocrinology, 3rd ed, pp 2069–2071. Philadelphia, WB Saunders, 1995

HYPERTRICOSIS, CONGENITAL ANTERIOR CERVICAL–PERIPHERAL SENSORY, MOTOR NEUROPATHY

Symptoms and Signs. Both sexes. Painless ulcer of foot, osteomyelitis of feet, hypertrichosis localized in the anterior cervical region.

Etiology. Autosomal dominant inheritance suggested.

BIBLIOGRAPHY. Trattner A, Hodak E, Sagie-Lerman T, et al: Familial congenital anterior cervical hypertrichosis associated with peripheral sensory and motor neuropathy: A new syndrome? J Am Acad Dermatol 25:767–770, 1991

HYPERTRICHOSIS, CONGENITAL GENERALIZED

Symptoms and Signs. Males more severe form; females only patchy hirsutism.

Etiology. X-linked dominant inheritance.

BIBLIOGRAPHY. Marcias-Flores MA, Garcia-Cruz D, Rivera H, et al: A new form of Hypertrichosis inherited as an X-linked dominant trait. Hum Genet 66:66–70, 1984

HYPERTRICHOSIS "FIBROMATOSIS, GINGIVAL"

Synonyms. Gingival fibromatosis—hypertrichosis; fibromatosis—hypertrichosis.

Symptoms and Signs. Both sexes affected; onset from infancy to ninth year. Progressive growth of gingiva (especially anterior upper region of jaw), eventually to cover teeth completely, sometimes to such extent that lips may not be closed. (This may be the only manifestation.) Marked hypertrichosis, progressive from infancy. Mental retardation; cranial deformities; gynecomastia (not constant features).

Etiology. Unknown; autosomal dominant inheritance, and recessive forms with generalized and focal types.

Pathology. Hyperplasia of gingiva with thick bundles of hyalinized collagen; few fibroblasts; little or no inflammatory changes (except when secondary).

Therapy. Surgery.

Prognosis. Recurrences also after extensive surgery.

BIBLIOGRAPHY. Waterman T: Diseases of the jaws. Boston Med Surg J 81:165–168, 1869
Weski H: Elephantiasis gingival hereditaria. Dtsch Mschr Zahnheilk 38:557–584, 1920
Horning GM, Fisher JG, Barker BF, et al: Gingival fibromatosis with hypertrichosis: A case report. J Periodontol 56:344–347, 1985
Anavy Y: Idiopathic familial gingival fibromatosis associated with mental retardation, epilepsy and hypertrichosis. Develop Med Child Neurol 31:538–542, 1989

HYPERTRICHOSIS LANUGINOSA, CONGENITAL

Synonyms. Hypertrichosis universalis.

Symptoms and Signs. Present at birth. Overgrowth of lanugo hair and precocious teeth.

Etiology. Autosomal dominant with varying expressivity.

Therapy. Dental care; counseling; shaving; bleaching the hair; chemical and electrical epilation.

Prognosis. Good. In some cases, hypertrichosis diminishes later in childhood. Shaving does not increase the profusion or rate of regrowth of hair.

BIBLIOGRAPHY. Broster LR: Hypertrichosis: A report of three cases. Br Med J 1:1171–1174, 1950
Felgenhauser WR: Hypertrichosis lanosa universalis. J Genet Hum 17:1–44, 1969
Partridge JW: Congenital hypertrichosis lanuginosa: Neonatal shaving. Arch Dis Child 62:623–625, 1987

HYPERTRICOSIS–OSTEOCHONDRODYSPLASIA

Synonym. Osteo—chondro—dysplasia—hypertrichosis.

Symptoms and Signs. Both sexes. At birth: macrosomy; marked hypertrichosis; cardiomegaly; wide ribs; narrow thorax, coxa valga; platyspondyly.

Etiology. Suggested autosomal recessive inheritance.

Pathology. Generalized osteopenia.

BIBLIOGRAPHY. Cantu JM, Garcia-Cruz D, Sanchez-Corona J, et al: A distinct osteochondrodysplasia with hypertrichosis. Individualization of a probable autosomal recessive entity. Hum Genet 60:36–41, 1982

HYPERVALINEMIA

Synonym. Valinemia.

Symptoms and Signs. Present from early infancy. Vomiting; diarrhea; failure to thrive; mental retardation; hyperkinesia; muscular hypotonia; nystagmus.

Etiology. Deficiency of enzyme converting valine to corresponding keto-acid.

Diagnostic Procedures. *Plasma. Urine.* Increased valine concentration. *Electroencephalography. Electromyography.*

Therapy. Low-protein diet. Plasmapheresis of questionable benefit: Penicillamine, corticosteroids and azathioprine.

Prognosis. Poor.

BIBLIOGRAPHY. Wada Y, Tada K, Minagawa A, et al: Idiopathic hypervalinemia: Probably a new entity of inborn error of valine metabolism. Tohoku J Exp Med 81:46, 1963
Chuang DT, Shih VE: Disorders of branched aminoacid and ketoacid metabolism. In Scriver CR, Beaudet AL, Sly WS, et al: The Metabolic and Molecular Bases of Inherited Disease, 7th ed. New York, McGraw-Hill, 1995

HYPERVENTILATION

Synonyms. Carbonic acid deficit; psychophysiologic hyperventilation; respiratory alkalosis.

Symptoms. Rare; most often females 20–40 years of age. Precipitating factor nervous tension accompanied by headache, apprehension, indigestion, irritable colon. Presyncopal symptoms: palpitation; weakness; dizziness; trembling; sweating; paresthesias in extremities and perioral region; flushed face; chest pain; shortness of breath; sighing respiration. Attack occurs with patient standing or sitting, not lying down. Syncope (there may be short loss of consciousness or just brief dimming of consciousness as only manifestation). Dimming of consciousness may sometimes last hours because, after losing and regaining consciousness, the patient hyperventilates again for a few seconds. Tetany is rarely associated. Postsyncopal: weakness; apprehension for hours.

Symptoms and Signs. Tetany (rare); sweating; tachycardia.

Etiology. (1) Fast breathing and susceptibility to syncope. Combination of factors: emotion, tension, drop of Pco_2; reduced cerebral flow and decreased oxygen release by oxihemoglobin. (2) Central nervous lesions. (3) Salicylate, sulfonamides administration. (4) Compensatory reaction in respiratory acidosis (tracheotomy or sudden increase in ventilation).

Pathology. According to etiology.

Diagnostic Procedures. Rule out other causes of syncope (see Syncope syndromes). Many patients may reproduce voluntary syncope by overbreathing. *Blood.* Pco_2 low; pH high; carbon dioxide content, actual bicarbonate low, carbon dioxide capacity and standard bicarbonate normal. Chloride high; serum sodium low or normal.

Therapy. Correct the tension and advise the patient about the mechanism precipitating the syncope; correct other causes when different etiology.

Prognosis. Good.

BIBLIOGRAPHY. Maytum CK: Tetany caused by functional dyspnea with hyperventilation: Report of case. Proc Staff Meet Mayo Clin 8:282–284, 1933
Magarian GJ: Hyperventilation syndromes: Infrequently recognized common expression of anxiety and stress. Medicine 61:219–236, 1982
Lewis RP, Budoulas H, Schaal SF, et al: Diagnosis and management of syncope. In: Schlant RC, Alexander RW: Hurst's The Heart, 8th ed. New York, McGraw-Hill, 1994

HYPOALPHALIPOPROTEINEMIAS

Synonyms. Vergani-Battalle; Familial hypoalpha proteinemia FHA.

Symptoms and Signs. Rare condition. No typical clinical signs. Not constant association with premature atherosclerosis.

Etiology. Not definitely established type of inheritance, suggested sex-linked. Probably this disorder represents a group of conditions of different etiologies.

Diagnostic Procedures. *Blood.* Normal total cholesterol and TG values, low serum HDL-C cholesterol (below the 10% percentile), apo A-1 levels usually are less markedly decreased.

BIBLIOGRAPHY. Vergani C, Bettalle A: Familial hypoalphalipoproteinemia. Clin Chim Acta 114:45–82, 1981
Steiner G, Shafrir E: Primary Hyperlipoproteinemias, p 281. New York, McGraw-Hill, 1991

HYPOBETALIPOPROTEINEMIA

Synonym. Beta-lipoprotein deficiency.

Symptoms and Signs. Similar to Bassen-Kornzweig (see) in the homozygous state. In the heterozygotes only, hypolipidemia. In homozygous state neurological symptoms are less severe than in the Bassen-Kornzweig.

Etiology. Autosomal dominant inheritance. Defects involving the gene for apo B in most cases.

Diagnostic Procedures. *Blood.* LDL low but present; HDL normal.

Therapy. Vitamin E.

Prognosis. Good for heterozygotes. For homozygotes, see Bassen-Kornzweig.

BIBLIOGRAPHY. Salt HB, Wolff OH, Lloyd JK, et al: On having no beta-lipoprotein: A syndrome comprising abetalipoproteinemia, acanthocytosis and steatorrhea. Lancet 2:325, 1960
Van Buchem FSP, Pol G, De Grier J, et al: Congenital beta-lipoprotein deficiency. Am J Med 40:794, 1966

Schettler G, Habenicht AJR (eds): Principles and Treatment of Lipoprotein Disorders. New York, Springer, 1994

Kane JP, Havel RJ: Disorders of the biogenesis and secretion of lipoproteins containing the B apolipoproteins. In Scriver CR, Beaudet AL, Sly WS, et al: The Metabolic and Molecular Bases of Inherited Disease, 7th ed, pp 1866–1870. New York, McGraw-Hill, 1995

HYPOCALCEMIA

Symptoms. Tetany. In infants, laryngospasm, facial muscle spasm, paresthesia, change of mood, asthmatic attacks, convulsions.

Signs. Trousseau, Chvostek signs. Skin dry, coarse; absent or patchy scalp hair; scant body hair. Other signs associated with basic condition (see Etiology).

Etiology. As part of (1) rickets and osteomalacia; (2) malabsorption syndromes; (3) Balser-Fitz (see); (4) hypoparathyroidism; (5) pseudohypoparathyroidism; (6) renal insufficiency; or (7) Epstein. As result of use of chelating agent in administration of large amount of citrated blood.

Pathology. According to etiology.

Diagnostic Procedures. *Blood.* Hypocalcemia; potassium normal, low, or high. *Urine.* Absence of calcium. *Ellsworth-Howard test. Electrocardiography.* Q-T interval prolonged; normal RS-T segment and T-wave. *X-ray.* According to etiology. *Stool.*

Therapy. If tetany, calcium gluconate or calcium lactate intravenously. High calcium, low phosphorus, vitamin D in diet. Specific treatment of basic condition (see Etiology).

Prognosis. Depends on etiology.

BIBLIOGRAPHY. Rabin D, McKenna TJ: Calcium and phosphate homeostasis. In Clinical Endocrinology and Metabolism, vol 9. Science and Practice of Medicine, pp 324–371. Philadelphia, Grune & Stratton, 1982

Fitzpatrick LA, Arnold A: Hypoparathyroidism. In De Groot LJ (ed): Endocrinology, 3rd ed, pp 1123–1135. Philadelphia, WB Saunders, 1995

HYPOFIBRINOGENEMIA, HEREDITARY

Synonyms. Factor I deficiency; fibrinogen synthesis, partial deficiency. See Dysfibrinogenemias and Rabe-Salomon.

Symptoms. Both sexes affected; onset not as early as the preceding. Same hemorrhagic manifestations as the preceding; both less severe and infrequent.

Etiology. Deficient synthesis of fibrinogen or molecular fibrinogen variants; possibly autosomal dominant with different degree of penetration; or "autosomal codominant" (presence of normal and abnormal molecules of fibrinogen).

Diagnostic Procedures. Fibrinogen markedly reduced; poor clot formation.

Therapy. Fibrinogen during bleeding episodes.

Prognosis. All patients reach adulthood.

BIBLIOGRAPHY. Revol L: Les grandes hypofibrinémies costitutionalles hémorrhagiques. Étude clinique, hématologique, génetique et thérapeutique. Hemostase 2:243–254, 1962

Gilabert J, Regañon E, Vila V, et al: Congenital hypofibrinogenemia and pregnancy: Obstetric and hematological management. Gynecol Obstet Invest 24:171–176, 1987

Vila V, Regañon E, Aznar J, et al: Congenital dysfibrinogenemia characterized by defective release of fibrinopeptide A and fibrinogen degradation products. Thrombs Res 45:437–449, 1987

Bithell TC: Hereditary coagulation disorders. In Lee GR, Bithel TC, Foerster J, et al (eds): Wintrobe's Clinical Hematology, 9th ed, p 1439. Philadelphia, Lea & Febiger, 1993

HYPOGAMMAGLOBULINEMIA, X-LINKED, COLLAGEN DISORDERS

Synonyms. Bruton-collagen disorders (see Bruton); agammaglobulinemia collagen disorders.

Symptoms and Signs. Appears in males; present from early age. Weakness; rash over extensor areas of joints; edema; induration of muscle; infections.

Etiology. See Bruton. This represents a variant of collagen vascular disorder that becomes associated particularly with patients who have not received optimal replacement: dermatomyositis-like; juvenile rheumatoid arthritis-like; scleroderma; diffuse vasculitis; etc.

Pathology. See Bruton. Also lymphorrhages (normal lymphocytes) around small blood vessels of skin and in the muscles and occasionally in the central nervous system.

Diagnostic Procedures. *Blood.* See Bruton. *Biopsy of skin and muscle.* See Pathology.

Therapy. None. Steroids, antimetabolites, and gammaglobulins of minor utility at this stage

Prognosis. Fatal.

BIBLIOGRAPHY. Gitlin D, Janeway CA, Apt L, et al: Agammaglobulinemia in Cellular and Humoral Aspects of Hypersensitivity States: Symposium. New York, Hoeber-Harper, 1959

Good RA, Roystein J: Rheumatoid arthritis and agammaglobulinemia. Bull Rheum Dis 10:203, 1960

Stewart SR, Gershwin ME: The association and relationships of congenital immune deficiency states and autoimmune phenomena. Semin Arthritis Rheum 9:95, 1979

Lukens JN: Immune deficiency diseases: Inherited and acquired. In Lee GR, Bithel TC, Foerster J, et al (eds): Wintrobe's Clinical Hematology, 9th ed. Philadelphia, Lea & Febiger, 1993

HYPOGLOBULINEMIA, TRANSIENT INFANTILE

Symptoms and Signs. Both sexes affected. After a few months of normal life, severe irritability, mild gastrointestinal disturbance. Edema in periorbital region; pallor. Moderate liver enlargement. Lineal growth continues at normal rate.

Etiology. Transitory deficiency that develops because of delayed onset of production of immunoglobulin, after catabolism of placental transferred maternal IgG.

Diagnostic Procedures. *Blood.* Anemia; hypoglobulinemia; absence of gamma globulin. Liver function. Minor alterations. *Urine.* Normal.

Therapy. Injection of gamma globulin.

Prognosis. Cases with early onset more severe manifestation. Recovery with normalization of protein; disappearance of hepatomegaly in 3–5 months.

BIBLIOGRAPHY. Ulstrom RA, Smith NJ, Heimlich EM: Transient dysproteinemia in infants: A new syndrome. Am J Dis Child 92:219–253, 1956

Sell S: Immunological deficiency diseases. Arch Pathol 86:95–107, 1968

Tiller TL, Buckley RH: Transient hypoglobulinemia of infancy: Review of the literature, clinical and immunological features of 11 new cases: A long-term follow-up. J Pediatr 92:347–353, 1978

Lukens JN: Immune deficiency diseases: Inherited and acquired. In Lee

GR, Bithel TC, Foerster J, et al (eds): Wintrobe's Clinical Hematology, 9th ed, p 1682. Philadelphia, Lea & Febiger, 1993

HYPOGLYCEMIA, TRANSIENT HEMIPLEGIA

Symptoms. No sex preference; all age groups affected. Usually, attacks precipitated by fasting or exercise. Transient flaccid or spastic paralysis, with various degrees of muscle weakness, involving the right side more frequently. Attack may last a few hours or a few days, recurring frequently about three times within a period of a few days.

Signs. Babinski sign, often bilateral; sensory change inconstant. Tachycardia; profuse sweating usually precedes the paralysis and convulsions (often coma). Occasionally, however, hemiplegia may be an isolated manifestation.

Etiology. Hypoglycemia of endogenous or exogenous origin. Insulin administration; adrenal tumor; pancreatic adenomas; idiopathic hypoglycemia.

Pathology. Damage from hypoglycemia usually is transient, and no data are available.

Diagnostic Procedures. *Blood.* Hypoglycemia. Functional studies (see Hypoglycemia). *X-ray.* To determine cause of hypoglycemia.

Therapy. Glucose intravenous infusion.

Prognosis. Easily reversible if treated promptly.

BIBLIOGRAPHY. Miller WL, Trescher JH: Amnesia, epileptiform convulsive seizures and hemiparesis as manifestations of insulin shock. Am J Med Sci 174:453, 1927
Montgomery BM, Pinner CA: Transient hypoglycemic hemiplegia. Arch Intern Med 114:680–684, 1964
Koivisto M, Blenco-Sequiros M, Krause V: Neonatal symptomatic hypoglycemia: A follow-up of 151 children. Dev Med Chil Neurol 14:603, 1972
Service FJ: Hypoglycemia including hypoglycemia in neonates and children. In De Groot LJ (ed): Endocrinology, 3rd ed, pp 1605–1623. Philadelphia, WB Saunders, 1995

HYPOGLYCEMIA, TRANSIENT NEONATAL

Synonym. Neonatal hypoglycemia.

Symptoms. Predominant in males born of mothers reported to have had pre-eclampsia (50% of cases); in normal newborn infants who breathed and cried spontaneously, symptoms beginning from 2 hours to 7 days after birth. Tremor; cyanosis; convulsion; apnea or respiratory distress; eye rolling; limpness; apathy; weak or high-pitched cry; difficulty in feeding.

Signs. Usually underweight; below the 10th percentile. When twin birth, the syndrome usually is present in the lower weight twin. Prompt response to intravenous administration of glucose.

Etiology. Several causes: malnutrition in intrauterine environment; small for gestational age infants; primary brain defect; faulty glycogenolytic mechanism (see glutaric aciduria II; fructose intolerance; cobolamin A disease, acyl-CoA dehydrogenase deficiencies; ETF deficiency; pyruvate carboxylase deficiency; diabetes); erythrobastosis; infant of diabetic mother, Beckwith-Wiedemann (see).

Pathology. Unknown.

Diagnostic Procedures. *Blood.* Blood sugar level lower than 20 mg/100 ml; calcium usually low; polycythemia. *Spinal fluid.* Normal except for hypoglycorrhachia. Glucagon, tolbutamide, leucine tolerance tests. *Glucose tolerance test. Epinephrine and glucagon combined tolerance test. MRI of head.*

Therapy. Glucose intravenously. Adrenocorticotropic hormone (ACTH) or corticosteroids.

Prognosis. Self-limited course within days in healthy term infants, whereas preterm infants require weeks. Dramatic improvement after glucose administration.

BIBLIOGRAPHY. Cornblath M, Odell GB, Levin EY: Symptomatic neonatal hypoglycemia associated with toxemia of pregnancy. J Pediatr 55:545–562, 1959
Koivisto M, Benco-Sequiros M, Krause V: Neonatal symptomatic and asymptomatic hypoglycemia: A follow-up of 151 children. Dev Med Chil Neurol 14:603–614, 1972
Polk DH, Fischer DA: Fetal and neonatal endocrinology. In De Groot LJ (ed): Endocrinology, 3rd ed, pp 2252–2253. Philadelphia, WB Saunders, 1995
Darmaun D, Haymond MW, Bier DM: Metabolic aspects of fuel homeostasias in the fetus and the neonate. In De Groot LJ (ed): Endocrinology, 3rd ed, pp 2269–2273. Philadelphia, WB Saunders, 1995
Service FJ: Hypoglycemia including hypoglicemia in neonates and children. In De Groot LJ (ed) Endocrinology, 3rd ed, pp 1605–1623. Philadelphia, WB Saunders, 1995

HYPOKALEMIA

Synonyms. Hypopotassemia; potassium deficiency. See also Siegal-Cattan-Manou.

Symptoms. Anorexia; nausea; vomiting; abdominal distention; paralytic ileus; generalized weakness; mental depression. Thirst and polyuria (occasional). Tetany may also occur.

Signs. Abdominal tympanism; tendon hyporeflexia.

Etiology. (1) Excessive fluid administration. (2) As part of the metabolic alkalosis or of several other syndromes: Aldosteronism, mineralocorticoid excess, Bartter, Cushing, ectopic ACTH secretion, Fanconi, Flajani, Liddle, etc. (3) Loss of potassium from gastrointestinal tract or through urine. (4) Chronic malnutrition. (5) Potassium redistribution in the body (i.e., into liver, muscles).

Pathology. *Kidney* (in chronic deficiency). Degenerative changes of tubules; no glomerular vascular changes. *Heart.* Degeneration of myocardium; loss of muscle cell striation; karyorrhexis; karyolysis; infiltration with neutrophils and monocytes, progressing to fibrosis.

Diagnostic Procedures. *Blood.* Potassium low; calcium normal, low, or high; features of metabolic alkalosis (see). *Urine.* Potassium may be increased, normal, or low. *Electrocardiography.* Best diagnostic tool for this condition. Lowering and broadening of T-wave; prolongation of Q-T interval; with more severe hypokalemia, progression of those findings up to downward shifting of T-wave, appearance of a prominent U-wave, depression of RS-T segment.

Therapy. Potassium through a peripheral IV line can be given at rates up to 40 mEq/h. It is better not to exceed 100–200 mEq/daily. Correct the underlying cause (alkalosis, gastrointestinal pathology, etc.).

Prognosis. Severe condition that may result in death if not efficiently corrected.

BIBLIOGRAPHY. Du Bose TD, Alpern RJ: Renal tubular acidosis. In Scriver CR, Beaudet AL, Sly WS, et al: The Metabolic and Molecular Bases of Inherited Disease, 7th ed, pp 3667, 3680. New York, McGraw-Hill, 1995
De Groot LJ (ed): Endocrinology, 3rd ed, pp 1605–1623; 1699–1700; 1779; 1795–1796. Philadelphia, WB Saunders, 1995

HYPOKALEMIC PERIODIC PARALYSIS

Synonyms. Shakhonovich; Cavaré-Romberg; Westphal; periodic paralysis I; paroxysmal myoplegia; paralysis periodic hypokalemic. See Albright-Hadorn and Hypokalemia.

Symptoms. Prevalent in males in most affected families and in sporadic cases; age of onset from first year to fifth decade (7–21 years in 90% of cases). Between attacks, patients are free of symptoms; occasionally, slight decrease of muscle strength. Attacks of migraine may precede for years the onset of the muscular syndrome. Precipitating factors: stresses (infection; surgery; emotions; menstruation; cold); large meal rich in carbohydrates; rest after intense exercise; various drugs (epinephrine; adenocorticotropic hormone [ACTH]; desoxycorticosterone; thyroid; licorice). Prodromal symptoms: Most of the time attacks occur in early hours of the morning upon awaking. During the day stiffness, cramps, paresthesia, irritability, severe thirst may warn of attack. Exercise may "work out" the attack. Attack: onset in the legs, spreading to the rest of the body of a flaccid type of paralysis. Limited paralysis also reported. Eye movement, speech, swallowing, respiration, mental faculties, and sensory acuity unaffected during attack. Occasionally, nausea, vomiting, or constipation. Recovery in 1 hour or 1 day, or later, following diuresis and sweating; strength returns first in neck and arms.

Signs. Between attacks, increased muscular size (in some cases suggesting pseudohypertrophic muscular dystrophy). During attacks muscles may have firmer consistency and increased circumference. Tendon reflexes are diminished or absent. In some cases, bradycardia, cardiomegaly during attack. In these cases, tachycardia precedes attack.

Etiology. Unknown. Maybe linked to a defect of a subunit of the sodium channel gene that leads to impairment of sodium-potassium pump and unexitability of muscle. Primary defect of muscle. Autosomal dominant in most families; sporadic cases reported.

Pathology. Mainly normal muscle fiber; some fiber degenerative changes (especially after years of attacks). Typical lesion observable with light and electron microscope, consisting of small subsarcolemmic vacuolization.

Diagnostic Procedures. *Blood.* During attack, neutrophilia, leukocytosis, and eosinopenia; followed, after recovery, by lymphocytosis and eosinophilia. Between attacks, potassium normal or low; during attack, low. Sodium retention preceding the attacks; slight serum elevation preceding and during attack. Phosphorus (inorganic) falls during attack. Cholesterol rises during attack. *Urine.* Potassium excretion falls simultaneously with serum value fall; after end of attack, potassium diuresis for 1–2 days. Sodium increases at termination of attack. During attack mild proteinuria, glycosuria, acetonuria, and cylindruria. *Electromyography.* Normal between attacks; during attack, progressive increase in latent period, action potential more prolonged in duration and reduced in amplitude. *Electrocardiography.* Changes typical of hypokalemia. *Biopsy muscle.* See Pathology.

Therapy. Primary treatment: avoid all situations that promote attacks (those that cause alkalosis especially) and rich carbohydrate meals. Acetazolamide chromalym. During attack 10g of KCl (or other salt). Exceptionally intravenous K+ administration (40 mEq/h). Prophylactic treatments abandoned.

Prognosis. Severity and frequency of attacks increasing up to 20 years, stable up to 30 years, and declining or disappearing afterward, especially in females. In some patients, especially males, severe attacks may continue in middle and later life. Progressive muscular atrophy may supervene in elderly patients. The control of acute attacks by potassium appears to slow or halt the progress of myopathy. Death may be caused by respiratory arrest or aspiration during attacks followed by pneumonia.

BIBLIOGRAPHY. Musgrave W: A periodical palsy: The phylosophical transactions and collections to the end the year 1700. London 2:33, 1727

Shakhnovitch: On a case of intermittent paraplegia. Russk Vratch 32:537, 1882; London M Rec 12:130, 1884 (abstr by Idelson V)

Westphal KFO: Ueber einen merkwuerdingen Fall Von peridischer Lahmung aller 4 Extremitaeten mit gleichzeitigem Erloschensein der elektrischen Erregbarkeit waehrend der Laehmung. Berlin klin Wschr 22:489–491, 509–511, 1855

Schipperheyn JJ, Wintzen AR, Buruma OJJ: Periodic paralysis. In Handbook of Clinical Neurology, vol 18. Rowland LP, DiMauro S (eds): The Myopathies, p 457. Amsterdam, Elsevier, 1992

HYPOMAGNESEMIA

Synonym. Magnesium deficiency; includes hypomagnesemic tetany.

Symptoms. Tremor and twitching; liability to severe potentially fatal epileptiform seizures. Occasionally, mental disturbance, confusion, agitation, hallucination.

Signs. Chvostek sign; no Trousseau sign.

Etiology. Magnesium deficiency in severe gastroenteritis, malnutrition, and diarrhea. Increased calcium intake after prolonged severe diarrhea, after parathyroidectomy or parathyroid hormone deficiencies; in Flajani; in altered phosphate reabsorption. Primary forms with autosomal, recessive (both sexes owing to renal magnesium wasting), and X-linked (hypomagnesemic tetany with secondary hypocalcemia only in males) inheritance.

Diagnostic Procedures. *Blood.* Determination of magnesium, calcium, protein levels.

Therapy. Administration of magnesium.

Prognosis. Symptoms respond rapidly to treatment with magnesium deficient diet, children deteriorate rapidly, developing neurologic complications; recovery is rapid with treatment.

BIBLIOGRAPHY. Flink EB, McCollister R, Prasad AS, et al: Evidences for clinical magnesium deficiency. Ann Int Med 47:956–968, 1957

Albertson PD, Krauss M (eds): The pathogenesis and clinical significance of magnesium deficiency. Ann NY Acad Sci 162:705–984, 1969

Dudin KI, Teebi AS: Primary hypomagnesemia: A case report and literature review. Eur J Pediatr 146:303–305, 1987

Pronicka E, Gruszczynska B: Familial hypomagnesemia with secondary hypocalcemia: autosomal or X-linked inheritance? J Inherit Metab Dis 14:397–399, 1991

De Groot LJ (ed): Endocrinology, 3rd ed, pp 690, 1033, 1119, 1126. Philadelphia, WB Saunders, 1995

HYPONATREMIA SYNDROMES

Synonyms. Dehydration (also used as synonym of "pure water depletion syndrome"); desalting water loss; hypo-osmolality; low sodium; pure salt depletion; sodium loss.

Symptoms. In acute loss, shock. In chronic loss; weakness, apathy, faintness, no thirst, anorexia, nausea, muscle cramps, orthostatic hypotension, cold extremities. Progression to confused state, brain syndrome, acute (see).

Signs. Eyeballs sunken and soft; glassy stare, tongue shrunken, longitudinal wrinkling; skin lacks elasticity and when pinched, remains folded. Tachycardia; low blood pressure; small pulse; absent peripheral pulse; vein collapse. In severe form; clammy, sweating skin.

Etiology. Sodium loss: from vomiting, diarrhea, gastrointestinal or biliary fistula, intestinal tubing and lavage, intense sweating (and drinking); in aging; burns; as part of mucoviscidosis. Small bowel obstruction: salt loss into and from serous cavities. In immediate postoperative period, as component of Addisonian syndromes (see), Thorn (see), Schwartz-Bartter (see). Iatrogenic: administration of diuretics or forced fluid, in syndromes of secondary hyperaldosteronism, and sodium retention (see Schroeder), and after hypodermoclysis of dextrose in water.

Diagnostic Procedures. *Blood.* Hemoconcentration, with high mean corpuscular volume of red cells. Blood volume low; sodium low; chloride and bicarbonate low; potassium usually high; blood urea nitrogen high;

serum osmolality low.* *Urine.* Volume low; specific gravity normal; sodium and chloride very low.

Therapy. Treatment of shock. Arrest of further sodium loss and replacement of sodium to compensate for loss; addition of other electrolytes as necessary. Plasma transfusion indicated. Treatment of basic pathology.

Prognosis. Severe outcome according to severity of form and etiology.

BIBLIOGRAPHY. Schroeder HA: Renal failure associated with low extracellular sodium chloride; the low salt syndrome. JAMA 141:117–124, 1949
Bartter FC: Hyper and Hypo-osmolality syndromes. Am J Cardiol 12:650–655, 1963
Flear CT, Gill GU: Burn J: Hyponatremia mechanisms and management. Lancet II:26–31, 1981
Anderson RJ, Chung HM, Kluge R, et al: Hyponatremia: A prospective analysis of its epidemiology and the pathogenetic role of vasopressin. Ann Intern Med 102:164–168, 1985
De Groot LJ (ed): Endocrinology, 3rd ed. Philadelphia, WB Saunders, 1995. See hyponatremia.

HYPOPARATHYROIDISM, ISOLATED SYNDROMES

Synonyms. Hypoparathyroidism acquired; hypoparathyroidism isolated (autosomal dominant); hypoparathyroidism isolated (autosomal recessive); hypoparathyroidism isolated (X-linked).

Symptoms. *Acquired.* Onset at all ages, both sexes. *Congenital.* Onset in first year of life in X-linked, only in males. Muscle spasm and tetany; nervousness; weakness; paresthesia of hands; blurred vision; headache; memory loss. In congenital forms, edema in neonatal period.

Signs. Chvostek, Trousseau signs. Papilledema; teeth and nail disorders; dry, coarse skin; patchy hair; alopecia; cataracts. Absence of candida infection and other endocrine gland deficiencies. Differentiate these syndromes from Multiple endocrine neoplasia (see).

Etiology. *Acquired.* Surgery; miscellaneous pathologic processes. *Congenital.* Autosomal (late onset) dominant, or recessive, and X-linked inheritance (most of the cases of early onset).

Pathology. Absence or hypoplasia of parathyroid.

Diagnostic Procedures. *Blood.* Hypocalcemia; hyperphosphatemia; no circulating antibodies antiparathyroid; subnormal level of immunoreactive PTH. *X-ray.* Absence of rickets, osteomalacia, or kidney calcification. *Electrocardiography. Urine.* Absence of signs of renal insufficiency. After parathyroid hormone administration, acute phosphate diuresis.

Therapy. Parathyroid hormone; vitamin D; dihydrotachysterol (DHT); calcium; low-phosphorous diet; dihydroxycholecalciferol (1–25 [OH$_2$]); acetazolamide (to increase phosphate excretion).

Prognosis. Good with treatment.

BIBLIOGRAPHY. Buchs S: Familial hypoparathyroidism. Ann Paediatr 188:124–127, 1957
Ahn TG, Autonarakis SE, Kronenberg HM, et al: Familial isolated hypoparathyroidism: a molecular genetic analysis of 8 families with 23 affected persons. Medicine 81, 65:73–84, 1986
McLeod DR, Hanley DA, McArthur RG: Autosomal dominant hypoparathyroidism with intracranial calcification outside the basal ganglia. Am J Med Genet 32:32–35, 1989

Fitzpatrick LA, Arnold A: Hypothyroidism. In De Groot LJ (ed): Endocrinology, 3rd ed, pp 1123–1135. Philadelphia, WB Saunders, 1995

HYPOPHOSPHATASIA, ADULT

Synonyms. See Acid phosphatase deficiencies.

Symptoms and Signs. Onset in middle age. Anamnestic memory of premature loss of deciduous teeth and good health in adolescence and younger age. Pain in the feet and discomfort in the lower limbs from stress fractures and pseudofractures. Attacks of pseudogout (see); calcific periarthritis.

Etiology. Deficiency of acid phosphatase in all cell lines. Autosomal recessive inheritance. Mild forms may be transmitted as autosomal dominant trait.

Diagnostic Procedures. *X-ray.* Osteopenia; pseudofractures (Looser zone, see); periarticular calcium deposition and ligaments ossification; spinal hyperostosis (resembling Forestier-Rotes-Querol, see).

Therapy. No medical treatment. Avoid traditional therapies for rickets or osteomalacia. Enzyme replacement and ALP infusion offer some clinical benefits. Cortisone occasionally useful. Nonsteroid antiinflammatory agents used for periarticular calcium deposition. Antibiotic in case of infections. Supportive treatments: dental care, orthopedic measures for fractures, craniotomy in premature synostosis.

BIBLIOGRAPHY. Fraser D: Hypophosphatasia. Am J Med 22:730–746, 1957
Bethune JE, Dent CE: Hypophosphatasia in the adult. Am J Med 28:615–622, 1960
White MP, Teitelbaum SL, Murphy WA, et al: Adult hypophosphatasia: Clinical, laboratory, and genetic investigation of a large kindred and review of the literature. Medicine (Baltimore) 58:329–347, 1979
Whyte MP: Hypophosphatasia. In Scriver CR, Beaudet AL, Sly WS, et al: The Metabolic and Molecular Bases of Inherited Disease, 7th ed, pp 4095–4111. New York, McGraw-Hill, 1995

HYPOPHOSPHATASIA, CHILDHOOD

Synonyms. See Acid phosphatase deficiencies. Includes Mabry.

Symptoms and Signs. Earlier than 5 years loss of deciduous teeth (aplasia, hypoplasia, and dysplasia of cementum); pain, stiffness, and weakness of muscles, short stature, waddling gait, rachitic deformities. In Mabry seizures, neurologic defects and mental retardation.

Etiology. Deficiency of acid phosphatase in all cell lines. Autosomal recessive inheritance. Mild forms may be transmitted as autosomal dominant trait.

Diagnostic Procedures. *X-ray.* Characterizing sign. In metaphyseal areas of long bones tongues of radiolucency, premature closure of cranial sutures, skull "beaten-copper" appearance. *Dental radiography.* Enlarged pulp chambers and root canals, "shell teeth."

Therapy. No medical treatment. Avoid traditional therapies for rickets or osteomalacia. Enzyme replacement and ALP infusion offer no significant benefits. Cortisone occasionally useful. Nonsteroid antiinflammatory agents used for periarticular calcium deposition. Antibiotic in case of infections. Supportive treatments: dental care, orthopedic measures for fractures, craniotomy in premature synostosis.

Prognosis. May spontaneously improve in adolescence.

BIBLIOGRAPHY. Macey HB: Multiple pseudofractures: Report of a case. Proc Staff Meet Mayo Clin 15:789–791, 1940
Mabry CC, Bautista A, Kirk RFH, et al: Familial hypophosphatasia with mental retardation, seizures and neurologic deficits. J Pediatr 77:74–85, 1970
Whyte MP: Hypophosphatasia. In Scriver CR, Beaudet AL, Sly WS, et

---

*Hyponatremia without hypo-osmolality may be seen in hyperlipemia (where serum lipid displaces serum water and produces low sodium concentration) and hyperglycemia, and when mannitol is given for therapeutic use in patient with defective mannitol excretion. In those cases, asymptomatic and no treatment is necessary if primary sodium loss has been ruled out.

al: The Metabolic and Molecular Bases of Inherited Disease, 7th ed, pp 4095–4111. New York, McGraw-Hill, 1995

HYPOPHOSPHATASIA, INFANTILE

Synonyms. Fraser (D), hypophosphatemic, nonrachitic bone disease. See Acid phosphatase deficiencies.

Symptoms and Signs. Both sexes. Onset before sixth month of age. Postnatal development apparently normal, then failure to thrive and features of rickets. Bulging of anterior fontanella, papipilledema, proptosis, mild hypertelorism, brachycephaly, blue sclerae (occasionally). Predisposition to pneumonia.

Etiology. Deficiency of acid phosphatase in all cell lines. Autosomal recessive inheritance. Mild forms may be transmitted as autosomal dominant trait.

Diagnostic Procedures. *Blood. Urine.* Hypercalcemia, hypercalciuria, and evidence of kidney functional impairment. *X-ray.* Characteristic, less marked than those of of perinatal form. *Skeletal scintigraphy.*

Therapy. No medical treatment. Avoid traditional therapies for rickets or osteomalacia. Enzyme replacement and ALP infusion offer no significant benefits. Cortisone occasionally useful. Nonsteroid anti-inflammatory agents used for periarticular calcium deposition. Antibiotic in case of infections. Supportive treatments: dental care, orthopedic measures for fractures, craniotomy in premature synostosis.

Prognosis. Variable course after a period of deterioration improvement. Fifty percent of patients die from respiratory infections.

BIBLIOGRAPHY. Fraser D: Hypophosphatasia. Am J Med 22:730, 1957
Whyte MP: Hypophosphatasia. In Scriver CR, Beaudet AL, Sly WS, et al: The Metabolic and Molecular Bases of Inherited Disease, 7th ed, pp 4095–4111. New York, McGraw-Hill, 1995

HYPOPHOSPHATASIA, PERINATAL

Synonyms. Nadler-Egan; hypophosphatasia perinatal (lethal). See Acid phosphatase deficiencies.

Symptoms and Signs. It is expressed in utero, frequent stillbirth. Caput membranaceum, short limbs, ostheochondral spurs may protrude from midportion of forearms and legs. If surviving to delivery: vomiting; hypotonia; lethargy; opisthotonus; seizures; bleeding; recurrent respiratory infections.

Etiology. Deficiency of acid phosphatase in all cell lines. Autosomal recessive inheritance.

Diagnostic Procedures. *Assay of lysosomal acid phosphatase in cultured fibroblast and multiple tissues.* No activity. Prenatal diagnosis possible. *X-ray.* Skeleton almost completely demineralized, fractures often present.

Therapy. No medical treatment. Avoid traditional therapies for rickets or osteomalacia. Enzyme replacement and ALP infusion offer no significant benefits. Cortisone occasionally useful. Nonsteroid anti-inflammatory agents used for periarticular calcium deposition. Antibiotic in case of infections. Supportive treatments: dental care, orthopedic measures for fractures, craniotomy in premature synostosis.

Prognosis. Death a few days after birth.

BIBLIOGRAPHY. Nadler HL, Egan TJ: Deficiency of lysosomal acid phosphatase: A new familial metabolic disorder. N Engl J Med 282:303–307, 1970
Whyte MP: Hypophosphatasia. In Scriver CR, Beaudet AL, Sly WS, et al: The Metabolic and Molecular Bases of Inherited Disease, 7th ed, pp 4095–4111. New York, McGraw-Hill, 1995

HYPOPHOSPHATEMIA, X-LINKED

Synonyms. Hypophosphatemic rickets; X-linked hypophosphatemia; rickets; X-linked hypophosphatemia; XLH.

Symptoms. Occurs in males; in females, only hypophosphatemia or less severe clinical manifestations. Normal at birth. Onset when beginning to walk. Waddling gait. Absence of tetany, convulsion and myopathy.

Signs. Mild growth deficiency; bowing of legs; coxa vara.

Etiology. X-linked inheritance. Defect of proximal tubular phosphate transport coupled with rate of 1, 25–(OH)2 D3 synthesis. It has been mapped to Xp22.1–p22.2.

Pathology. See Rickets.

Diagnostic Procedures. *Blood.* Hypophosphatemia; hyperphosphatasemia alkaline; calcium and urea normal elevated parathormone. *Urine.* Hyperphosphaturia; amino acid excretion normal. Occasionally, renal glycosuria; reduced TmP/GFR. *X-ray.* Typical changes of rickets.

Therapy. Phosphate supplement (1–4 g); vitamin D (25,000–75,000 IU); careful monitoring.

Prognosis. Partially responsive to combined phosphate-vitamin D treatment. Deformities may progress into adult life. Final adult height 130–160 cm.

BIBLIOGRAPHY. Winters RW, Graham JB, Williams TF, et al: A genetic study of familial hypophosphatemia and vitamin D-resistant rickets. Trans Assoc Am Physicians 70:234–242, 1957
Glorieux FH: Rickets, the continuing challenge (editorial). N Engl J Med 325:1875–1877, 1991
Rasmussen H, Tenenhouse HS: Mendelian Hypophosphatemias. In Scriver CR, Beaudet AL, Sly WS, et al: The Metabolic and Molecular Bases of Inherited Disease, 7th ed, pp 3732–3739. New York, McGraw-Hill, 1995

HYPOPHYSEAL, SENILE (SYNDROMES)

According to Herman, based on Kretschmer types of physical constitution, analysis of senile signs occurring in Cushing syndrome makes it possible to establish two types of physiologic senescence: (1) Asthenic (leptosome), corresponding to the Simmonds syndrome; and (2) pyknic, type corresponding to Cushing.

BIBLIOGRAPHY. Kretschmer E: Körperbau und Charakter Untersuchungen zun Konstitutionsproblem und zur Lehre von den Temperamenten. Berlin, Springer, 1921
Herman E: Senile hypophyseal syndromes. J Neurol Sci 4:101–110, 1966

HYPOPLASTIC LEFT HEART

Synonyms. HLHS; aortic arch atresia or interruption; aortic arch hypoplasia; aortic valve atresia; mitral valve atresia. See Mitral valve atresia.
    This definition has been used interchangeably with hypoplasia of aortic tract complex including coexistent aortic and mitral atresia or stenosis, preductal coarctation, hypoplasia of ascending aorta, and hypoplasia of transverse aortic arch. Considering the functional and anatomic adequacy of the left ventricle as the basic factor in these lesions, Sinha prefers the term hypoplastic left ventricle syndrome and excludes from the entity the conditions where a functionally adequate left ventricular chamber exists.

Symptoms and Signs. Sudden onset of severe respiratory distress and slate-gray cyanosis; moist rales; severe hepatomegaly.

Etiology. Multifactorial inheritance. Subtype with autosomal recessive type possible.

Diagnostic Procedure. *X-ray.* Cardiac enlargement, pulmonary arterial and venous engorgement. *Electrocardiography.* Right axis deviation and marked right catheterization. Ventricular hypertrophy. *M-mode and two-dimensional echocardiography.*

Therapy. Palliative operations cause only temporary benefit. Heart replacement by allotransplantation is a potential definitive form of treatment.

Prognosis. Inexorably progressive and fatal without transplant.

BIBLIOGRAPHY. Lev M: Pathology, anatomy and interrelationship of hypoplasia of the aortic tract complex. Lab Invest 1:61–70, 1952
Baily LL, Nehlsen-Cannarella SL, Doroshow RW, et al: Cardiac allotransplantation in newborns as therapy for hypoplastic left heart syndrome. N Engl J Med 315:949–951, 1986
Towbin JA, Roberts R: Cardiovascular diseases due to genetic abnormalies. In Schlant RC, Alexander RW: Hurst's The Heart, 8th ed, p 1730. New York, McGraw-Hill, 1994
Perloff JK The Clinical Recognition of Congenital Heart Disease, 4th ed, pp 727–737. Philadelphia, WB Saunders, 1994

HYPOPLASTIC RIGHT HEART

This definition is used to designate a group of congenital cardiac anomalies that share anatomic atresia or stenosis on right hemicardium, with hypoplasia of right ventricle and hypertrophy of left ventricle and functionally a right-to-left shunt (usually) at atrial level. In this group are included tricuspid atresia, pulmonary atresia, severe pulmonary stenosis with intact ventricular septum, and congenital isolated hypoplasia of right ventricle (rare).

BIBLIOGRAPHY. Peacock TB: On Malformation of the Human Heart, 2nd ed. London, J. Churchill, 1866
Perloff JK: The Clinical Recognition of Congenital Heart Disease, 2nd ed, p 605. Philadelphia, WB Saunders, 1978
Towbin JA, Roberts R: Cardiovascular diseases due to genetic abnormalies. In Schlant RC, Alexander RW: Hurst's The Heart, 8th ed, p 1730. New York, McGraw-Hill, 1994

HYPOTENAR HAMMER

Synonyms. Ulnar artery, traumatic thrombosis; post-traumatic digital ischemia; digital ischemia, post-traumatic.

Symptoms and Signs. Following single or repeated trauma. Pain, paresthesias, and Raynaud phenomenon on ulnar side of hand. Ring and little fingers may be cold. Allen test abnormal.

Etiology. Blant trauma(s) of ulnar artery at wrist. Especially from baseball, karate, judo, hockey, and handlebar injuries.

Pathology. Damage of intima and of tunica media often associated with thrombosis.

Diagnostic Procedures. *Doppler digital plethysmography. Radionuclide studies.* Arteriography better not used.

Therapy. Conservative treatment, if failure and especially if poor backflow, excision of thrombosed segment of artery with or without reconstruction. In case of good backflow, ligation of vessel alone relieves complaints.

Prognosis. Good with complete regression if detected early. If prolonged, secondary ischemic changes.

BIBLIOGRAPHY. Conn J, Bergan JJ, Bell JJ, et al: Hypotenar hammer syndrome: Post traumatic digital ischemia. Surgery 68:1122–1128, 1970
Zemel N: Neurovascular disorders. In Jobe FW: Operative Techniques in Upper Extremity Sport Injuries. St Louis, CV Mosby, 1996

HYPOTENSION, ORTHOSTATIC

Synonyms. Postural hypotension; orthostatic hypotension. See Bradbury-Eggleston and Sly-Dragger.

Symptoms. Prevalent in men (4:1); slow progression of symptoms; sometimes years before patient seeks medical attention. Impotence (usually first symptom). Episodic feelings of exhaustion, lightheadedness, blurring of vision, slow mentation, and faintness in upright position. Syncope common, preceded by the described premonitory symptoms. Convulsive seizures may occur (especially if bystander helps the patient up after he falls). Chronic diarrhea; nocturnal polyuria; intolerance to heat.

Signs. Usually, youthful appearance. Pallor precedes the attack. Decrease in systolic and diastolic pressure in erect position. Valsalva maneuver results in marked fall of arterial blood pressure and the characteristic "overshoot" and bradycardia (that are present in normal individual) are absent. Various degrees of anhidrosis can be demonstrated by sweating tests.

Etiology. Unknown; autonomic dysfunction: impaired arteriolar constriction; anhidrosis; xerostomia; heat intolerance; impotence. It is distinguished from a primary form (see Bradbury-Eggleston and Sly-Dragger) and secondary form owing to impairment of autonomic function from peripheral neuropathy caused by infections, toxins, malnutrition, amyloidosis, age.

Pathology. Unknown.

Diagnostic Procedures. *Blood pressure.* Vasopressin increases systolic and diastolic pressure in patients (and not in normal individuals). *Sweat tests. Basal metabolism rate,* low. *Blood.* Moderate increase in blood urea nitrogen; mild anemia.

Therapy. Various therapeutic measures usually fail or present several disadvantages, such as vasopressin (water intoxication and myocardial ischemia). Best treatment appears to be wearing a special custom-fitted counterpressure suit, made of elastic mesh, which allows adequate ventilation (Jobst garment).

Prognosis. In early stage of disease, patients are able to work. With progression of disease, wearing the described special suit becomes necessary. Fluctuation of intensity of symptoms. Progression of neurologic symptoms. General debility and sudden death reported.

BIBLIOGRAPHY. Bradbury S, Eggleston C: Postural hypotension: A report of three cases. Am Heart J 1:73–86, 1925
Lanbry C, Doumer E: L'hypotension orthostatique. Presse Med 1:17–20, 1932
Lewis RP, Budoulas H, Schaal SF, et al: Diagnosis and management of syncope. In Schlant RC, Alexander RW: Hurst's The Heart, 8th ed, pp 930–931. New York, McGraw-Hill, 1994

HYPOTHALAMIC CARREFOUR

Symptoms. Occurs in middle-aged females with blood hypertension; sudden onset. Hemiplegia; hemianesthesia; astereognosis; apraxia; asynergy.

Etiology. Unknown.

Therapy. Symptomatic.

Prognosis. Tendency to regression.

BIBLIOGRAPHY. Ramirez F, Iniguez A: Sindrome de la encrucijada hipotalamica. An Fac Med Montevideo 37:109–116, 1952

HYPOTHALAMIC POSTINFECTIVE

Synonym. Hyperphagia—hyperthermia—hypothyroidism.

Symptoms and Signs. Occurs following infections, trauma, or without preceding causes. Development of hyperthermia with good appetite and weight gain, with or without secondary hypothyroidism symptoms and signs.

Etiology and Pathology. Lesion of hypothalamus owing to infection (viral), trauma, or leukemia.

Diagnostic Procedures. *Blood.* Cultures; complete blood count. *Basal metabolic rate. Thyroid function tests. Adrenal function tests. X-ray of skull.*

Therapy. Symptomatic.

Prognosis. Poor; sudden death.

BIBLIOGRAPHY. Grossman M: Late results of epidemic encephalitis. Arch Neurol Psychiatr 5:580, 1921

Lipsett MB, Dreifuss FE, Thomas LB: Hypothalamic syndrome following varicella. Am J Med 32:471–475, 1962

HYSTERICAL SYNCOPE

Symptoms. In young adult with severe emotional illness. Attacks always in presence of public. Slumping is gentle and graceful, may last long time (1 hour or longer).

Signs. Unresponsive to verbal stimulation. Skin color, pulse, blood pressure normal. Changing position (recumbency) does not modify symptoms.

Etiology. Emotional imbalance.

Therapy. Psychotherapy.

Prognosis. Good. Possible conversion to other hysterical symptoms.

BIBLIOGRAPHY. Lewis RP, Budoulas H, Schaal SF, et al: Diagnosis and management of syncope. In Schlant RC, Alexander RW: Hurst's The Heart, 8th ed. New York, McGraw-Hill, 1994

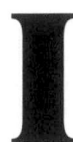

IATROGENIC HYPOTHYROIDISM

Synonym. Iodide-induced hypothyroidism. See Gull.

Symptoms and Signs. Onset following prolonged iodine administration for treatment of thyroid disorders or for any other therapeutic reason (e.g., for chronic bronchitis or for radioiodine therapy and other drugs, such as lithium carbonate).

Etiology. Probably depending on pre-existing defect in thyroid metabolism.

Pathology. Varies; cases studied histologically showed colloid storage goiter; thyroid hyperplasia with tendency to colloid depletion.

Diagnostic Procedures. *Basal metabolic rate.* Low. *Blood.* Serum cholesterol; butanol extractable iodine determination. *Radioiodine uptake.* Rapid thyroidal uptake in first few hours; followed by decline to low value within 24 hours; enlarged thyroidal iodide space; discharge of ^{131}I with thiocyanate. Rebound phenomena following discontinuation of iodide.

Therapy. Discontinuation of treatment and then thyroid administration.

Prognosis. Good with therapy.

BIBLIOGRAPHY. Thompson WO, Thompson PK, Brailey AG, et al: Myxedema during the administration of iodide in exophthalmic goiter. Am J Med Sci 179:733–749, 1930
Oppenheimer JH, McPherson HT: The syndrome of iodide-induced goiter and myxedema. Am J Med 30:281–288, 1961
Utiger RD: Hypothyroidism. In De Groot LJ (ed): Endocrinology, 3rd ed, p 756. Philadelphia, WB Saunders, 1995

ICE CREAM HEADACHE

Symptoms and Signs. Pain in anterior temporal region, sometimes encroaching on the orbit, elicited by eating ice cream. The pain spreads to surrounding regions and is rapidly relieved by cessation of stimulus and rapidly reinduced by a new bowl of ice cream.

Etiology. Unknown. Noxious stimulation of tissue of palate, stimulation of sensory ends, vascular changes (?).

BIBLIOGRAPHY. Smith RO: Ice cream headache. In Vinken PJ, Bruyn GW: Handbook of Clinical Neurology, vol 5, pp 188–191. Amsterdam, North-Holland, 1968

ICHTHYOSIFORM ERYTHRODERMA, UNILATERAL

Synonym. Congenital hemidysplasia—ichthyosiform erythroderma—limb deformity (CHILD); ectromelia unilateral—psoriasis—central system anomalies—ichthyosis—limb reduction.

Symptoms and Signs. Prevalent in females (19:1). From birth. Unilateral ichthyosis and limb malformations accompanied by hypoplasia of several organs on the same side (lung, thyroid), as well as psoas muscle, central nervous system, and cranial nerves. Impaired hair growth and linear areas of alopecia on affected side; onychorrhexis.

Etiology. X-linked inheritance.

Diagnostic Procedures. *X-rays. CT scan. MR imaging.* Punctate epi-

physeal calcification. Unilateral hypoplasia or aplasia of a limb; hypoplasia: calvaria, mandible scapula, clavicle, ribs; vertebral defects. Visceral anomalies: heart, kidney, lung, thyroid, adrenal, ovary.

Prognosis. Males, stillbirth or early death.

BIBLIOGRAPHY. Falek A, Heath CW Jr, Ebbin AJ, et al: Unilateral limb and skin deformities with congenital heart disease in two siblings: A lethal syndrome. J Pediatr 73:910–913, 1968
Hebert AA, Esterly NB, Holbrook KA, et al: The CHILD syndrome: Histologic and ultrastructural studies. Arch Dermatol 123:503–509, 1987
Traupe H: The Ichthyoses: A Guide to Clinical Diagnosis, Genetic Counseling and Therapy. New York, Springer-Verlag, 1989

ICHTHYOSIS BULLOSA SIEMENS

Synonyms. Siemens III.

Symptoms and Signs. Both sexes; all ages. Unusual peeling and moulting aspect in localized areas on flexures; no erythema.

Etiology. Unknown. Autosomal dominant inheritance suggested.

Pathology. *Skin.* Vacuolar degenerative change throughout epidermis confined to granular-cell layer.

Therapy. Retinoid drugs.

Prognosis. Fair results with treatment.

BIBLIOGRAPHY. Siemens HW: Dichtung und Wahrheit ueber die "Ichthyosis bullosa" mit Bemerkungen zur Sistematik der Epidermolysen Arch Dermatol Syphil 175:590–608, 1937
Traupe H: The Ichthyoses: A Guide to Clinical Diagnosis, Genetic Counseling and Therapy. New York, Springer-Verlag, 1989
Murdoch ME, Leigh IM: Ichthyosis bullosa of Siemens and bullous ichthyosiform erythroderma—variants or same disease? Clin Exper Dermatol 15:53-56, 1990

ICHTHYOSIS-CHEEK-EYEBROW

Synonym. ICE (not to be confused with Irido-corneo-endothelial, see).

Symptoms and Signs. Both sexes, Ichthyosis vulgaris, prominent and full cheeks, sparse lateral eyebrow, high arched palate, kyphoscoliosis, chest deformities, pes planus.

Etiology. Autosomal dominant inheritance suggested.

BIBLIOGRAPHY. Sidransky E, Feinstein A, Goodman RM: Ichthyosis-cheek-eyebrow (ICE) syndrome: A new autosomal dominant disorder. Clin Genet 31:137–142, 1987
Begas AM, Delleman JW: ICE syndrome (letter). Clin Genet 33:63, 1988

ICHTHYOSIS FOLLICULARIS–
ATRICHIA–PHOTOPHOBIA

Synonyms. IFAP; McLeod.

Symptoms and Signs. Occurs in males. In infancy. Alopecia; ichthyosis follicularis; photophobia.

Etiology. X-linked inheritance.

BIBLIOGRAPHY. MacLeod JMH: Three cases of ichthyosis follicularis associated with baldness. Br J Derm 21:165–189,1909

Hamm H, Meinecke P, Traupe H: Further delineation of the ichthyosis follicularis, atrichia and photophobia syndrome. Eur J Pediat 150:627–629, 1991

ICHTHYOSIS HEPATO-SPLENOMEGALY-ATAXIA

Synonym. Dykes.

Symptoms and Signs. See ichthyosis vulgaris dominant. Hepatosplenomegaly and dysarthria and ataxia begin after age 50.

Etiology. Suggested storage disease, nature not yet evident. Autosomal recessive inheritance. X-linked inheritance excluded on the basis of biochemical studies showing steroid sulfatase activity in the fibroblasts.

BIBLIOGRAPHY. Dykes PJ, Markes R, Harper PS: A syndrome of ichthyosis, hepatosplenomegaly and cerebellar degeneration. Br J Derm 100:585–590, 1979

Dikes PJ, Markes R, Harper PS: Syndrome of ichthyosis, hepatosplenomegaly and cerebellar degeneration. Steroid sulphatase activity. Br J Dermatol 102:353–354, 1980

Traupe H: The Ichthyoses: A Guide to Clinical Diagnosis, Genetic Counseling and Therapy. New York, Springer-Verlag, 1989

ICHTHYOSIS HYSTRIX

Etiology.

1. Spriegler-Fendt (see)
2. Lambert (see)
3. Ichthyosis hystrix Curth-Macklin type (see)
4. Ichthyosiform erythroderma (BIE) (see) and localized form warty linear nevus
5. Ichthyosis hystrix gravior of Rheydt

Pathology. The different forms mentioned in the etiology are difficult to distinguish by light microscopy. Only electron microscopy provides the differential characteristics.

Therapy. Specific. Emollients and topical, keratolytic retinoic acid or etretinate per os or isotretinoid also are helpful in some cases.

BIBLIOGRAPHY. Anton-Lamprecht I: Hereditaire ichthyosen. In Herzberg JJ (ed): Paediatrische Dermatologie, p 161. Stuttgart, Schattauer, 1978

Kanerva L, Kardonen J, Oikarinen A, et al: Light and electronic microscopic studies performed before and after etretinate treatment. Arch Dermatol 120:1218–1223, 1984

Griffiths WAD, Leigh IM, Marks R: Disorders of keratinization. In Champion RH, Burton JL, Ebling FJG (eds): Rook/Wilkinson/Ebling Textbook of Dermatology, 5th ed, pp 1340–1341. Oxford, Blackwell Scientific, 1992

ICHTHYOSIS HYSTRIX, CURTH-MACKLIN TYPE

Symptoms and Signs. See Ichthyosis hystrix, Curth-Macklin.

Etiology. Autosomal dominant inheritance.

Pathology. Continuous perinuclear tonofibril shell in spinous and granular cell layers and absence of tonofilament clumps (typical of ichthyosiform erythroderma).

BIBLIOGRAPHY. Curth HO, Macklin MT: The genetic basis of the various types of ichthyosis in a family group. Am J Hum Genet 6:377–381, 1954

Curth HO, Allen FH Jr, Schneider VW, et al: Follow-up of a family

group suffering from ichthyosis hystrix, type Curth-Macklin. Hum Genet 17:37–48, 1972

Kanerva L, Kardonen J, Oikarinen A, et al: Light and electron microscopic studies performed before and after etretinate treatment. Arch Dermatol 120:1218–1223, 1984

Traupe H: The Ichthyoses: A Guide to Clinical Diagnosis, Genetic Counseling and Therapy. New York, Springer-Verlag, 1989

ICHTHYOSIS HYSTRIX, GRAVIOR OF RHEYDT

Synonyms. Nevus linear; nevus verrucosus; porcupine man; Rheydt-Lambert type ichthyosis.

Symptoms and Signs. Both sexes affected; present from infancy. Marked hyperkeratosis with quill-like projection involving entire body with the exception of face, palms, soles, and genitalia.

Etiology. Unknown; autosomal dominant inheritance. Variant of harlequin fetus (see).

Pathology. Extreme hyperkeratinization of skin.

Therapy. Specific. Emollients and keratolytic topical retinoic or etretinate per os or isotretinoid also are helpful in some cases.

Prognosis. No change with age.

BIBLIOGRAPHY. Penrose LS, Stern C: Reconsideration of the Lambert Pedigree (ichthyosis hystrix gravior). Ann Hum Genet 22:258–283, 1957

Anton-Lamprecht I: Electron microscopy in the early diagnosis of genetic disorders of the skin. Dermatologica 157:65–85, 1978

Traupe H: The Ichthyoses: A Guide to Clinical Diagnosis, Genetic Counseling and Therapy. New York, Springer-Verlag, 1989

ICHTHYOSIS, MALE HYPOGONADISM

Synonym. Lynch. See Rud syndrome.

Symptoms and Signs. Occurs in males. Very rare. Those related to congenital ichthyosis and secondary hypogonadism. Anosmia could be an additional feature.

Etiology. X-linked inheritance.

Diagnostic Procedures. *Blood.* Low titer of pituitary gonadotrophic hormones.

Prognosis. Males do not reproduce.

BIBLIOGRAPHY. Lynch HT, Ozer FL, Mevutt CW, et al: Secondary male hypogonadism and congenital ichthyosis: An association of two rare genetic diseases. Am J Hum Genet 12:440–447, 1960

Dodinval PA, Husquinet HA, Legros JS: Ichthyosis, hypogonadotrophic hypogonadism and mild epilepsy in two young male sibs, p 260. Sixth Int Cong Hum Genet, Jerusalem, 1981

Traupe H: Ichthyosis and Hypogonadism: Reflections on the so-called Rud's syndrome. In The Ichthyoses: A Guide to Clinical Diagnosis, Genetic Counseling and Therapy, pp 91–97. New York, Springer-Verlag, 1989

ICHTHYOSIS VULGARIS, DOMINANT

Synonyms. Ichthyosis nitidus; ichthyosis simplex; xeroderma; ADI.

Symptoms. Both sexes affected; onset at 1–4 years of age. No symptoms except irritation of skin in cold weather. High percentage of patients manifest asthma and eczema.

Signs. From dryness and roughness of skin in cold weather (milder form: xeroderma) to dryness with small, white, shiny scales, progressively becoming more severe over a few years. Affected are extensor areas of limbs and sometimes the trunk, the back more severely than abdomen or anterior chest; axillae and groin always unaffected. Face affected in childhood, usually clears at later age. Seasonal variations with enhancing of manifestation during winter and remission during summer.

Etiology. Unknown; autosomal dominant inheritance.

Pathology. Horny layer slightly thickened, reduced or absent granular layer, low mitotic count, dermal and perivascular lymphocytic infiltrates.

Therapy. Moving to warm climate regions. Salicylic acid (3%) in emulsifying ointment. Bath oil in bath water. Ultraviolet light application; vitamin A.

Prognosis. Chronic condition never too severe; tendency to improve with age.

BIBLIOGRAPHY. Felsher Z, Rothman S: Insensible perspiration of skin in hyperkeratotic conditions. J Invest Dermatol 6:271–278, 1945

Wells RS: Ichthyosis. Br Med J 2:1504–1506, 1966

Sybert VP, Dale BA, Holbrook KA: Ichthyosis vulgaris: evidentiation of a defect in synthesis of filaggrin correlated with an absence of keratohyaline granules. J Invest Dermatol 84:191–194, 1985

Williams ML, Elias PM: Ichthyosis: Genetic heterogeneity, genodermatoses and genetic counseling. Arch Dermat 122:529–531, 1986

Griffiths WAD, Leigh IM, Marks R: Disorders of keratinization. In Champion RH, Burton JL, Ebling FJG (eds): Rook/Wilkinson/Ebling Textbook of Dermatology, 5th ed, pp 1330–1332. Oxford, Blackwell Scientific, 1992

ICHTHYOSIS VULGARIS, SEX-LINKED, DOMINANT

Synonyms. Chondrodysplasia punctata, X-linked dominant.

Symptoms and Signs. Only in females; lethal in male fetus. In infancy generalized erythema and scaling that improves after a few months (I component). Persistent linear hyperkeratoses (reminiscent of Bloch-Sulzberger, see). Cataracts (II component). Occasionally localized scalp hair loss and generalized follicular atrophoderma; stature shorter than normal; kyphoscoliosis, normal intelligence.

Etiology. Sex-linked dominant inheritance.

Diagnostic Procedures. *X-rays.* Chondrodysplasia punctata (frequently unilateral in the epiphyses) (III component of syndrome).

Therapy. Symptomatic.

Prognosis. Normal life expectancy.

BIBLIOGRAPHY. Happle R: X-linked dominant chondrodysplasia punctata: Review of literature and report of a case. Hum Genet 53:65–73, 1979

Traupe H: The Ichthyoses: A Guide to Clinical Diagnosis, Genetic Counseling and Therapy. New York, Springer-Verlag, 1989

ICHTHYOSIS VULGARIS, SEX-LINKED, RECESSIVE

Synonyms. Ichthyosis negricans; ichthyosis nigricans; steroid sulfatase deficiency placental steroid sulfatase deficiency; arylsulfatase C.

Symptoms. Only males (1 in 6000 male births); onset at birth. Lesions may be troublesome and disfiguring.

Signs. Scattered, large, brownish scales, affecting all areas of skin, including axilla, groin, antecubital and popliteal fossas; front of trunk more markedly affected than back. Tendency to shed in autumn and spring. Alopecia may develop. Corneal opacities. Palms and soles are spared; nails are normal. Possible association with mental retardation, skeletal abnormalities, hypogonadism. Mothers of affected males may have trouble in parturition.

Etiology. X-linked recessive inheritance. Deficiency of steroid sulfatase with probable accumulation of cholesterol esters in skin.

Pathology. Horny and granular layer thickened with acanthosis; constant dermal lymphocytic infiltrates.

Diagnostic Procedures. *Maternal urine.* Low estrogens. *Fibroblast culture.* Absence of steroid sulfatase.

Therapy. Specific. Emollients and keratolytic topical retinoic or etretinate per os or isotretinoid are also helpful in some cases.

Prognosis. Chronic condition; no improvement with age.

BIBLIOGRAPHY. Kerr CB, Wells RS: Sex-linked ichthyosis. Ann Hum Genet 29:33–50, 1965

Lake BD, Smith VV, Judge MR, et al: Hexanol dehydrogenase activity shown by enzyme histochemistry on skin biopsies allows differentiation of Sjogren-Larsson syndrome from other ichthyoses. J Inherit Metab Dis 14:338–340, 1991

Griffiths WAD, Leigh IM, Marks R: Disorders of keratinization. In Champion RH, Burton JL, Ebling FJG (eds): Rook/Wilkinson/Ebling Textbook of Dermatology, 5th ed, pp 1342–1344. Oxford, Blackwell Scientific, 1992

IDIOPATHIC, DIFFUSE, CRESCENTIC, GLOMERULONEPHRITIS, TYPE I

Synonyms. Antiglomerular basement membrane antibody mediated; glomerulonephritis (crescentic) type I, without pulmonary hemorrhage.

Symptoms and Signs. Usually young or middle-aged males. Sometimes preceded by exposure to hydrocarbon fumes or respiratory illness. Onset like acute glomerulonephritis (see Bright) but more insidious, with fever, myalgia, or abdominal pain.

Etiology. Unknown. Antiglomerular basement membrane antibodies (IgG) are probably the pathogenetic mechanism. This may be a partial type of Goodpasture syndrome (see).

Pathology. *Light microscopy.* Accumulation of cells (crescents) in Bowman space in 50% of glomeruli; in time, glomerular sclerosis. *Electron microscopy.* Widened zones in subendothelial space with detachment gaps in basement membrane. *Immunofluorescence.* Glomeruli with linear deposits of IgG (rarely IgA); C3 deposits are rare. Pattern similar to Goodpasture syndrome

Diagnostic Procedures. *Urine.* Dysmorphic RBC, casts. Decreased glomerular filtration rate. *Blood.* Circulating antiglomerular basement membrane antibodies; signs of uremia. HLA-DR2 in 85% of patients. Fibrin degradation products high in urine and serum.

Therapy. Plasmapheresis; steroids; cyclophosphamide; azathioprine.

Prognosis. Without therapy, progression to renal insufficiency in 6 months. With therapy, better prognosis. Renal transplantation is followed by a 10–30% recurrence of disease.

BIBLIOGRAPHY. Brenner BM, Rector FC Jr: The Kidney, 3rd ed, p 940. Philadelphia, WB Saunders, 1986

Weatherall DJ, Ledingham JGG, Warrell DA (eds): Oxford Textbook of Medicine, 3rd ed, pp 3153–3167. Oxford, Oxford Med Pub, 1996

IDIOPATHIC, DIFFUSE, CRESCENTIC, GLOMERULONEPHRITIS, TYPE II

Synonym. Immune complex-mediated crescentic glomerulonephritis; glomerulonephritis, diffuse, crescentic, idiopathic type II.

Symptoms and Signs. Middle-aged patients, no sex predominance. Fever; malaise; hypertension. Occult visceral sepsis or necrotizing vasculitis may be present.

Etiology. Unknown. Basement membrane lesion caused by immune complex deposition. The antigen is occult but infection usually is the cause (virus).

Pathology. *Light microscopy.* Lesions similar to type I. *Electron microscopy.* Electron-dense deposits in mesangium and subendothelial space. *Immunofluorescence.* Scattered deposits (mesangial and capillary) of IgG and IgM often with C3.

Diagnostic Procedures. *Urine.* Hematuria; proteinuria. *Serum.* C3 decreased; cryoimmunoglobulins and circulating immune complex.

Therapy. Plasma exchange; cortisone (pulses of corticosteroid). Quadruple therapy (anticoagulant, antithrombotic, glucorticoid, immunosuppressive).

Prognosis. Better than in type I. Spontaneous resolution is possible; response to therapy is good.

BIBLIOGRAPHY. Brenner BM, Rector FC Jr: The Kidney, 3rd ed, Philadelphia, WB Saunders, 1986 p 944
Weatherall DJ, Ledingham JGG, Warrell DA (eds): Oxford Textbook of Medicine, 3rd ed, pp 3153–3167. Oxford, Oxford Med Pub, 1996

IDIOPATHIC, DIFFUSE, CRESCENTIC, GLOMERULONEPHRITIS, TYPE III

This syndrome is disputed.

Symptoms and Signs. Older patients, predominantly males. Fever, arthralgias, abdominal pain.

Etiology. Unknown.

Pathology. *Light microscopy.* Absence of proteinaceous deposits. *Electron microscopy.* Absence of electron-dense deposits. *Immunofluorescence.* Absence of IgG deposits.

Diagnostic Procedures. See types I and II. No antiglomerular basement membrane antibodies, immune complexes, or rheumatoid factors.

Therapy. Pulses of corticosteroids.

Prognosis. Better than in type I. In case of chronic renal failure, kidney transplantation gives good results.

BIBLIOGRAPHY. Brenner BM, Rector FC Jr: The Kidney, 3rd ed, p 945. Philadelphia, WB Saunders, 1986
Weatherall DJ, Ledingham JGG, Warrell DA (eds): Oxford Textbook of Medicine, 3rd ed, pp 3153–3167. Oxford, Oxford Med Pub, 1996

IDIOPATHIC, HYPERTROPHIC, SUBAORTIC STENOSIS

Synonyms. Bernheim-Schmincke; Schmincke-Bernheim; IHSS; subvalvular aortic stenosis; familial cardiomyopathy; obstructive cardiomyopathy; noncoronary cardiopathy; hypertrophic obstructive cardiomyopathy; hypertrophic cardiomyopathy, HC.

Symptoms. Both sexes affected; familial form: 1:1; male to female ratio: 1:1; sporadic: 4:1. Onset from birth to late age, most common in third or fourth decade. Exertional dyspnea; angina pectoris; dizziness especially in assuming upright position.

Signs. Patients are physically well-developed; many may have practiced athletic activities before onset of symptomatology. Heart enlarged; left ventricular lift. Findings suggesting ventricular defect or mitral regurgitation. Protodiastolic gallop in 50% of cases; systolic murmur (100%); second sound single. Friedreich ataxia (see) frequently associated.

Etiology. Variable sporadic cases and autosomal dominant inheri-

tance. Several etiologic causes under this heading. "Aberration of catecholamine function" in the embryo heart proposed.

Pathology. Hypertrophy of left ventricle, with marked hypertrophy in the septal region, centimeters below the aortic valve, septum bulges into right ventricle. Muscle bundles arranged into whorls, separated; bizarre nuclei of fibers.

Diagnostic Procedures. *ECG.* Left ventricular hypertrophy; Wolf-Parkinson (see) in 25% of cases; abnormal Q-waves. *X-ray.* In 50% of cases, abnormally large cardiothoracic ratio. *Angiocardiography.* Thickening of left ventricle walls. *Hemodynamic studies.* Variable results. *Echocardiography.* Radionuclide imaging. *Phonocardiogram.* Systolic time intervals. *Apex cardiogram.*

Therapy. In case of syncope, antishock position and phenylephedrine or methoxamine. Basic treatment: propranolol and other beta-blocking agents (symptoms of failure may be enhanced). Calcium blocking agents; Amiodarone. Surgical treatment. Laser myoplasty.

Prognosis. Sudden death frequent occurrence.

BIBLIOGRAPHY. Frank S, Brunewald E: Idiopathic hypertrophic subaortic stenosis: Clinical analysis of 126 patients with emphasis on natural history. Circulation 37:759–788, 1968
Michels VV, Moll PP, Miller FA, et al: The frequency of familial dilated cardiomyopathy in a series of patients with idiopathic dilated cardiomyopathy. N Engl J Med 326:77–82, 1992

IDIOPATHIC PULMONARY FIBROSIS (IPF)

Synonym. Hamman-Rich (misnomer because usually associated with rheumatoid arthritis, see); cryptogenic fibrosing alveolitis, usual interstitial pneumonitis, desquamative interstitial pneumonitis, fibrosing alveolitis, diffuse alveolar fibrosis, honeycomb lung; idiopathic pulmonary fibrosis.

Symptoms and Signs. Affects 3–5/100,000. Age 40–70 years, prevalent in males. Breathlessness with excertion, dry nonproductive cough, occasionally after flu-like illness. Successive malaise and weight loss. Rarely arthralgias and myalgias. Thorax: bibasilar end-inspiratory dry crackles. Clubbing, rarely pulmonary osteoarthropathy. Later cor pulmonale and cyanosis.

Etiology. Unknown. Genetic basis is suggested by HLA linkage, association with other inherited syndromes (Hermansky-Pudlak, Gaucher, neurofibromatosis, Nieman-Pick, tuberous sclerosis), and a familial form (Sandoz, see). A viral etiology also has been suggested.

Pathology. *Open lung biopsy:* Three patterns described: one with increased number of macrophages and lymphocytes (desquamative interstitial pneumonia, DHP); one with intense interstitial infiltration of lymphocytes, eosinophils, monocytes with fibrotic pattern (usual interstitial pneumonitis, UIP); one with replacement of parenchyma by irregular cysts (1–2 mm in diameter) and septa thickened and lined by metaplastic epithelium (honeycomb end-stage pattern). Bronchoalveolar lavage shows variable patterns of neutrophilia, eosinophilia, and lymphocytosis. *Immune histochemistry of lung.* Shows immune complex deposition on alveolar surfaces.

Diagnostic Procedures. *Bronchoalveolar lavage, open lung biopsy* (see). *Blood.* Hypergammaglobulinemia (17–20%), cryoglobulins (41%), ESR elevated (60–90%), antinuclear antibodies (7–25%), RF (14%), decreased complement levels (6%), elevated circulating immune complexes. *Blood gases.* O_2 normal at onset, then decreased and $P(A-a)$ O_2 widens, resting hypoxiemia. *Immunological studies.* On alveolar lavage shows B- and T-cell activation. *Radiology:* Chest normal (14.8%), ground glass appearance, reticular pattern with nuclear opacities. *CT scan.* Lower lung predominant reticular pattern honeycomb. *Gallium-67 scintillation scanning. Physiological studies.* Pulmonary function testing, reduced VC, as with restrictive process. FEV1 and FVC reduced, FEV1/FCV normal or increased.

Therapy. Corticosteroids (Prednisone 1–2 mg/kg), cyclophosphamide, azatoprine, chlorambucil, vincristine. Oxygen therapy. Hydralazine to improve pulmonary hemodynamics. Lung transplantation.

Prognosis. Mean life span 3–5 years. Death caused by respiratory failure (40%), cardiovascular complications (25%), bronchogenic carcinoma, spontaneous pneumothorax. Lung transplantation is the only therapy offering hope of long-term survival.

BIBLIOGRAPHY. Panos RJ, King TE: Idiopathic pulmonary fibrosis. In Lynch JP, De Reeme RA: Immunologically Mediated Pulmonary Diseases. Philadelphia, Lippincott, 1991

IgA SELECTIVE DEFICIENCY

Synonym. Gamma-A-globulin selective deficiency; immunoglobulin A selective deficiency.

Symptoms and Signs. Incidence 1/700 individuals. Asymptomatic. Infections of upper respiratory and/or intestinal tract. Associated allergic manifestations.

Etiology. Unknown. Sporadic and familial cases (autosomal dominant phenotype) reported. In some cases association with deletion of chromosome 18 (18q-).

Diagnostic Procedures. *Blood.* Selective decrease of IgA1 and A2. In some cases increased IgE in a group presence of anti-A antibodies.

Therapy. No treatment. Immunoglobulin administration not advised.

Prognosis. Good.

BIBLIOGRAPHY. Goldberg LS, Barnett EV, Fudenberg HH, et al: Selective absence of IgA: A family study. J Lab Clin Med 72:204–212, 1968
Stocker F, Ammann P, Rossi E: Selective gamma-A-globulin deficiency with dominant autosomal inheritance in a Swiss family. Arch Dis Child 43:585–588, 1968
de Laat PCJ, Weemaes CMR, Bakkeren JAJM, et al: Familial selective IgA deficiency with circulating anti-IgA antibodies: a distinct group of patients? Clin Immunol Immunopathol 58:92–101, 1991

ILIOCAVAL COMPRESSION

Symptoms and Signs. More frequent in females. Classic form on the left side; rarely on the right. Characteristic lower extremity pains, moderate to severe swelling, varicosities.

Etiology. Left common iliac vein compressed between right common iliac artery and lumbar spine. Occasionally, other sources of compression that may cause the manifestation on the right side (e.g., metastatic nodes, bone spur).

Diagnostic Procedures. *Doppler venous survey.* Exercise strain gauge venous plethysmography. Ambulatory venous pressure. Descending and ascending venography.

Therapy. Surgical. Direct operative repair of the iliocaval junction, rerouting of the iliac artery, and excision of ileocaval webs with vein patch angioplasty.

Prognosis. Long-term sequelae of venous insufficiency.

BIBLIOGRAPHY. McMurrich JP: The occurrence of congenital adhesion in the common iliac veins and their relation to thrombosis of the femoral and iliac veins. Am J Med Sci 135:342, 1908
Cockett B, Thomas ML: The iliac compression syndrome. Br J Surg 51:816–821, 1965
Toheri SA, Williams J, Powell S, et al: Iliocaval compression syndrome. Am J Surg 154:169–172, 1987

ILLIG

Synonym. See Isolated growth hormone deficiency.

Symptoms and Signs. Features more severe than in the isolated growth hormone deficiency (see): shorter at birth; more marked dwarfism; puppet facies.

Etiology. Unknown. Autosomal recessive inheritance.

Diagnostic Procedures. *Blood.* Hypoglycemia; total absence of growth hormone; presence of growth hormone antibodies after treatment characterizing feature of the syndrome.

Therapy. Growth hormone. Increased antibodies response to hormone administration makes treatment more difficult. Recent availability of synthetic hormone preparations reduces antibody formation.

Prognosis. Good response to hormonal treatment

BIBLIOGRAPHY. Illig R: Growth hormone antibodies in patients treated with different preparations of human growth hormone (HGH). J Clin Endocr Metab 31:679–688, 1970
Matsuda I, Hata A, Jinno Y, et al: Heterogeneous phenotypes of Japanese cases with growth hormone gene delection. Jpn J Hum Genet 32:227–235, 1987
Ranke MB: Growth hormone insufficiency: Clinical features, diagnosis and therapy. In De Groot LJ (ed): Endocrinology, 3rd ed, pp 330–340. Philadelphia, WB Saunders, 1995

ILIO-INGUINAL

Symptoms and Signs. Pain in area of inguinal nerve and hyperesthesia of cutaneous area of thigh aggravated by the erect position and by hip movements, producing a type of intermittent claudication.

Etiology. Caused by tight abdominal muscles and pressure on the nerve passing through muscle and fascial edge. Tightness of muscles is a reflex to derangements of lower spine.

Diagnostic Procedures. *X-ray. CT scan. MRI of column.*

Therapy. Orthopedic correction of spine derangement.

BIBLIOGRAPHY. Kopel HP, Thompson WAL: Peripheral Entrapment Neuropathies. Baltimore, Williams & Wilkins, 1963
Dowson DM, Hallett M, Millender LH: Entrapment Neuropathies, 2nd ed. Boston, Little, Brown, 1990

ILLUM

Synonyms. Arthrogryposis multiplex congenita—whistling face. Fetal hypokinesia. See Arthrogryposis distal type II.

Symptoms and Signs. Both sexes. Contractures of joints. Mental and physical retardation, scialorrhea, apneic crisis, temperature instability, bradycardia.

Etiology. Possibly autosomal recessive inheritance.

Pathology. Calcium deposit in brain and muscles.

Prognosis. Few days or months survival.

BIBLIOGRAPHY. Illum N, Reske-Niesen E, Skovby F, et al: Lethal autosomal recessive arthrogryposis multiplex congenital with whistling face and calcification of the nervous system. Neuropediatrics 19:186–192, 1988
Schander-Trumpel C, Fryus JP, Beemer FA, et al: Association of distal arthrogryposis, mental retardation, whistling face and Pierre Robin sequence: evidence of nosologic eterogeneity. Am J Med Genet 38:557–561, 1991

ILLUSION OF FREGOLI

Synonyms. Fregoli illusion; hyperidentification. See Capgras.

Symptoms. Patient identifies persecutors in several persons (e.g., doctor, nurse, aide, postman) accusing them of being the same person and changing faces to persecute him.

Etiology. Considered an extension of Capgras syndrome (see). Form of illusion of positive doubles as contrasted with the Capgras syndrome illusion of negative doubles or hypoidentification. To be differentiated also from Illusion of Intermetamorphosis (see).

BIBLIOGRAPHY. Courbon P, Fail G. Syndrome d' "illusion de Frégoli" et schizophénie. Bull Soc Clin Med Ment 15:121–125, 1927
Kaplan HI, Sadock BJ: Comprehensive Textbook of Psychiatry, 6th ed, p 1044. Baltimore, Williams & Wilkins, 1995

ILLUSION OF INTERMETAMORPHOSIS

Synonyms. Intermetamorphosis illusion.

Symptoms. Patient has the illusion that the persons with whom he is in contact change one with another: A becomes B; B becomes C; C becomes A.

Etiology. Considered an extension of Capgras (see). Differs from illusion of Fregoli. In the intermetamorphosis, physical resemblance is claimed in addition to false identification.

BIBLIOGRAPHY. Courbon P, Tusques J: Illusions d'intermétamorphose et de charme. Ann Med Psychol 90:401–406, 1932
Kaplan HI, Sadock BJ: Comprehensive Textbook of Psychiatry, 4th ed, p 1231. Baltimore, Williams & Wilkins, 1985

IMERSLUND-GRAESBECK

Synonyms. Addison-Biermer, infantile, megaloblastic juvenile hereditary anemia; pernicious anemia juvenile; enterocyte cobolamine malabsorption; pernicious infantile anemia; intrinsic factor congenital malabsorption; familial selective vitamin B_{12} malabsorption.

Symptoms. Both sexes affected; clinical onset in early childhood (1 year of age), occasionally later fatigue; weakness.

Signs. Pallor.

Etiology. Autosomal recessive inheritance. Defect in the process of vitamin B_{12} transport through the ileum.

Pathology. Gastric, jejunal mucosa normal. Kidney, in some cases glomerular changes suggestive of mild subacute glomerulonephritis.

Diagnostic Procedures. *Blood.* Megaloblastic anemia. No evidence for serum antibodies to intrinsic factor and gastric parietal cells. *Bone marrow.* Typical megaloblastic changes. *Gastric fluid.* Normal free acid and intrinsic factor. *Urine.* Proteinuria; in some cases aminoaciduria. *Biopsy of kidney.* See Pathology.

Therapy. Vitamin B_{12}.

Prognosis. Administration of vitamin B_{12} corrects anemia but does not affect albuminuria or aminoaciduria. No progression of renal lesion.

BIBLIOGRAPHY. Graesbeck R, Gordin R, Kantero I, et al: Selective vitamin B_{12} malabsorption and proteinuria in young people: A syndrome. Acta Med Scand 167:289–296, 1960
Imerslund O: Idiopathic chronic myeloblastic anemia in children. Acta Paediat (Suppl 119) 49:1–115, 1960
Lee GR: Megaloblastic and non megaloblastic macrocytic anemias. In Lee GR, Bithel TC, Foerster J, et al (eds): Wintrobe's Clinical Hematology, 9th ed, p 765. Philadelphia, Lea & Febiger, 1993

IMINOGLYCINURIA

Symptoms and Signs. Benign condition associated with other pathologies and syndromes but not pathological per se.

Etiology. Deficiency of tubular carriers for amino acids. Autosomal recessive inheritance.

Diagnostic Procedures. *Urine.* Excessive amounts of proline, hydroxyproline, and glycine.

Therapy. Symptomatic.

Prognosis. Good.

BIBLIOGRAPHY. Joseph R, Ribierre M, Job J, et al: Maladie familiale associante des convulsions a debut tres precoce, une hyperalbuminorachie et une hyperamminoacidurie. Arch Fr Pediatric 15:374, 1948
Chesney RW Iminoglycinuria. In Scriver CR, Beaudet AL, Sly WS, et al: The Metabolic and Molecular Bases of Inherited Disease, 7th ed, pp 3643–3653. New York, McGraw-Hill, 1995

IMMERSION FOOT

Synonyms. Paddy foot; swamp foot; trench foot; tropical immersion foot. See Pernio.

Symptoms and Signs. Occurs in individuals (e.g., soldiers; hunters) subjected to prolonged exposure of lower extremities to cold and moisture as well as dependency and immobility.

1. *Initial vasospastic, ischemic phase.* Edema; pallor; cyanosis of feet; followed by petechiae, shallow ulcerations. Anesthesia of patchy type.
2. *Postimmersion, hyperemic phase.* After removal from cold exposure, feet red and hot; peripheral pulsation full (changes similar to erythromelalgia syndrome). Bullae filled by hemorrhagic fluid. Ecchymosis; ulcerations; gangrene. Burning paresthesia starts at the 10th day. Condition lasts about 2 weeks if gangrene complication does not supervene.
3. *Late vasospastic, ischemic phase.* (In mild case properly treated, this stage is absent.) Coldness, pain, stiffness, and paresthesia of lower extremities. Exposure to cold results in Raynaud phenomenon, hyperhidrosis.

Etiology. Changes of peripheral circulation owing to prolonged exposure to cold and dampness.

Pathology. In early stage similar to Pernio (see). In later stages fibrosis, intimal thickening of small arteries, mild periarterial fibrosis. Secondary damage to veins, perivenous fibrosis, thrombosis, muscle fiber degeneration.

Therapy. Prevent by minimizing exposure to moisture (silicone grease most effective) and heat dispersion; avoid constriction. Practice movement and avoid prolonged dependency of legs (standing or sitting, especially with feet immersed in the water). During hyperemic phase: avoid trauma and infections; elevate feet to reduce edema; warm body, cool feet. During vasospastic phase: avoid cold exposure; passive exercises; mild heat application; fever treatment (may be tried); stop smoking. Sympathectomy in selected cases.

Prognosis. According to stage reached. In full course, patient cannot work in cold climate; also reduced ability in warmer climate.

BIBLIOGRAPHY. Wright IS, Allen EV: Frostbite, immersion foot, and allied conditions. Army Med Bull 65:136–150, 1943
Killian H: Cold and frost injuries. Berlin, Springer, 1981
Sabiston DC: Textbook of Surgery, 14th ed, pp 206–207. Philadelphia, WB Saunders, 1991
Keatinge WR: Cold, drowning and seasonal mortality. In Weatherall DJ, Ledingham JGG, Warrell DA (eds): Oxford Textbook of Medicine, 3rd ed, p 1183. Oxford, Oxford Med Pub, 1996

IMMUNOGLOBULIN DEFICIENCY, ADDISON-BIERMER

Synonyms. Anemia pernicious—immunoglobulin deficiency; pernicious anemia—immunoglobulin deficiency; transcobalamine II deficiency, hereditary. See also Addison-Biermer.

Symptoms and Signs. Prevalent in males (70%); onset at mean age of 34 years. Recurrent bacterial infection (predominantly pneumococcal) preceding other symptoms. Episodic diarrhea. All symptoms of Addison-Biermer (see). In some cases, rheumatoid arthritis, idiopathic ulcerative colitis, allergic manifestations.

Etiology. Unknown. The pernicious anemia and the immunoglobulin deficiency are independent consequences of single defect, based (or not based) on genetic abnormality. Gastric atrophy (responsible for pernicious anemia) resulting from delayed-type cellular immune hyperactivity, host hypersensitivity, or both, role of giardiasis to be considered. Autosomal recessive inheritance deficiency of transcobalamine 2.

Pathology. Gastric mucosal atrophy, with infiltrates of lymphocytes and lack of plasma cells. Typical pattern of pernicious anemia, deficiency in plasma cells of bone marrow. Biopsy of small intestine mucosa normal. Findings typical of recurrent infections and of pernicious anemia.

Diagnostic Procedures. *Blood.* Hyperchromic anemia and other findings of pernicious anemia; Coombs test negative; absence of serum antibodies against parietal cell, thyroid antigens, or against binding of B_{12} to intrinsic factor. *Gastric fluid.* Achlorhydria, absence of intrinsic factor in gastric juice; vitamin B_{12} malabsorption, not corrected by exogenous intrinsic factor. Presence of Giardia infestation in majority of cases. *Immunologic studies.* IgG, IgA, IgM strongly decreased or absent. Positive delayed cutaneous response; positive mitotic response to phytohemoagglutinin (PHA).

Therapy. That of Addison-Biermer; antibiotics; gamma globulins.

Prognosis. Not reported. According to chronic nature of disease: poor. Possibility of development of gastric adenocarcinoma, and of different immunologically based (?) disorders (e.g., rheumatic arthritis; ulcerative colitis).

BIBLIOGRAPHY. Twomey JJ, Jordan PH, Jarrold T, et al: The syndrome of immunoglobulin deficiency and pernicious anemia. Am J Med 47:340–350, 1969
Hitzig WH, Dohmann H, Pluss HJ, et al: Hereditary transcobalamine II deficiency: Clinical findings in new family. J Pediatr 85:622–628, 1984
Lukens JN: Immune deficiency diseases: Inherited and acquired. In Lee GR, Bithel TC, Foerster J, et al (eds): Wintrobe's Clinical Hematology, 9th ed. Philadelphia, Lea & Febiger, 1993

IMMUNOPROLIFERATIVE SMALL-INTESTINAL

Synonyms. Mediterranean lymphoma; IPSID; heavy chain disease.

Symptoms and Signs. Common in the Middle East and generally in the Mediterranean areas, in low socioeconomic class. Age: second-third decades. Fever, vomiting, abdominal pain, diarrhea, steatorrhea, general debilitation.

Etiology. Unknown, frequent association with parasite infestation.

Pathology. Lymphoplasmacitic infiltrate with IgA producing B-cells located usually along the jejunum, duodenum, and seldom in the stomach or colorectum. Lymph nodes are involved early in the disease.

Diagnostic Procedures. *X-ray. CT scan. MRI. Endoscopy. Biopsy. Stool analysis. Blood.* Normal white cell count and differential, presence of circulating heavy chains (present also in duodenal juice without light chain).

Therapy. Often responds initially to broad spectrum antibiotic ther-apy. In more advanced stages surgical excision, chemotherapy, and adjuvant therapies.

Prognosis. Runs a prolonged course over many years till high grade transformation occurs. Reported cases cured by early antibiotic treatment.

BIBLIOGRAPHY. Ramot B, Shahin N, Bubis JJ: Malabsorption syndrome in lymphoma of small intestine: A study of 13 cases. Isr J Med Sci 1:221–226, 1965
Isaacson PG, Norton AJ: Extranodal Lymphomas, pp 45–50. Edinburgh, Churchill Livingstone, 1994

IMMUNOTACTOID GLOMERULOPATHY

Synonyms. Fibrillary glomerulopathy; nonamyloidotic fiblillary glomerulopathy; amyloid-like glomerulopathy; amyloid stain negative; microfibrillary glomerulopathy.

Symptoms and Signs. Slight prevalence in males; presentation ranges from 10–80 years of age (average 44 years). Hypertension and hematuria. Absence of systemic manifestations.

Etiology. Unknown. Immunoglobulin disorder.

Pathology. Light microscopy mesangial expansion by PAS-positive material with mild increase of cells; glomerular capillary walls focal or diffuse alterations. Congo stain: negative. Fluorescence microscopy. Reflect distribution of fibrils in areas decribed in the light, presence of immunoglobulins (IgG and C3 other less frequently). Ultrastructural: glomerular deposition of fibrils with larger diameter than amyloid.

Diagnostic Procedures. *Biopsy.* See Pathology. *Blood.* Absence of cryoglobulinemia, paraproteinemia, or systemic lupus erythematosus features (see). *Urine.* Proteinuria (presenting feature), hematuria.

Therapy. Scarce or no response to glucocorticoids, plasma exchange, cyclophosphamide. With transplantation frequent recurrences of lesions similar to those of native kidney.

Prognosis. End-stage renal disease in 50% of cases in 4 years.

BIBLIOGRAPHY. Duffy JL, Khurana E, Susin M, et al: Fibrillary renal deposits and nephritis. Am J Pathol 113:279–290, 1983
Glassock RJ: Glomerular Diseases. In Massry SG, Glassock RJ: Textbook of Nephrology, 3rd ed, pp 746–749. Baltimore, Williams & Wilkins, 1995

INAPROPPROPIATE FALSETTO

Synonyms. Falsetto voice.

Symptoms and Signs. In males developmental (failure of deepening of voice at puberty); in female sudden manifestation. Stable defect (nonfluctuant).

Etiology. In male hormonal; in female possible variant of psychophonoasthenia (see).

Diagnostic Procedures. *Laryngoscopy. Frequency (pitch) analysis; waveform analysis; spectrography; laryngeal airway resistance.*

Therapy. Voice therapy; refrain from smoking. Psychotherapy.

Prognosis. High percentage of good response to treatment.

BIBLIOGRAPHY. Koufman JA, Blalock PD: Functional voice disorders. Otolaryngol Clin N Am 24:1059–1073, 1991

INCLUSION BODY ENCEPHALITIS

Synonyms. Bodechtel-Guttmann; Dawson; Pette-Doering; Bogaert van; Van Bogaert; subacute sclerosing leukoencephalitis; encephalitis subacute sclerosing; leukoencephalitis subacute sclerosing.

Symptoms. History of measles, before 2 years of age; for 6–8 years asymptomatic then gradual manifestations. Predominant in children younger than 12 years of age. *Early.* Intellectual deterioration; jerky movements of trunk and extremities. *Later.* Bilateral spasticity; decerebrate rigidity; cachexia and dementia. Possibly, cranial nerve palsies; vision and hearing usually spared until last stage.

Etiology. Unknown. Delay in the development of immune response, unable to clear the infection. Failure of the brain cells to synthesize "M" protein and lack of protection from seeding of virus in the brain during first infection in early age.

Pathology. Brain. Fibrillary gliosis; infiltration by lymphocytes and plasma cells. Inclusion bodies in neurons.

Diagnostic Procedures. *Cerebrospinal fluid.* Pressure and cells normal; gammaglobulins increased, measles-virus specific antibodies. *EEG.* High-voltage slow complexes; initial spike or sharp wave.

Therapy. Measles vaccination has reduced the incidence. Amantadine or inosiplex may prolong survival.

Prognosis. In younger children, death within months. In adolescents, from many months to years survival.

BIBLIOGRAPHY. Spielmeyer W: Histopathologie des Nervensystems. Springer, Berlin, 1922

Bodechtel G, Guttmann E: Diffuse Encephalitis mit Sklerosierender. Entzundung des Hemispharenmarkes. Z Ges Neur Psychiat 1133:601–619, 1931

Dawson JR Jr: Cellular inclusions in cerebral lesions of lethargic encephalitis. Am J Pathol 9:7–15, 1933

Bogaert van L, De Busscher J: Sur la sclérose inflammatoire de la substance blanche des hémisphères (Spielmeyer) (Contribution a l'étude des scléroses diffuses non familiales). Rev Neurol 71:679–701, 1939

Pette H, Doring G: Uber einheimische Panencephalomyelitis vom Charakter der Encephalitis japonica. Dtsch Z Nervenheilk 149:7–44, 1939

Sigurdsson B, Carp RI, Loeve A (eds): Slow infections of the central nervous system. Proc NY Ac Sci N 9434, 1993

INCLUSION BODY MYOSITIS

Synonyms. IBM; myositis inclusion body.

Symptoms and Signs. In adults. Progressive (insidious and slow) symmetrical weakness of proximal muscles, in more than 50% of cases also distal muscles are involved (especially foot extensor and finger flexors). Selective weakness and atrophy of flexor digitorum profundus (flexors for third, fourth, and fifth finger) is specific sign for IBM. Prominent dysphagia. Association with systemic autoimmune or connective tissue diseases in 15% of cases.

Etiology. Autoimmune disorder. Families with autosomal dominant inheritance described. Otherwise sporadic occurrence.

Pathology. Muscle. Endomysial inflammation similar to polymyositis (see). Histologic hallmarks: (a) basophilic granular inclusions around edges of rimmed vacuoles; (b) small, round, or angulated fibers in small groups; (c) eosinophilic cytoplasmic inclusions.

Diagnostic Procedures. *Electromyography Blood.* CK levels. *Muscle biopsy.*

Therapy. Empirical: steroids; azathioprine, methotraxate, cyclophosphamide; cyclosporine; plasmapheresis; total lymphoid irradiation; intravenous Ig administration. All treatment tried with no definitive assessment of real benefit. Cricopharingeal myotomy from dysphagia.

Prognosis. Condition generally resistant to present treatment attempts. Usually progressive that may lead to death from interstitial lung diseases.

BIBLIOGRAPHY. Banker BQ, Engel AG: The polymyositis and dermatomyositis syndrome. In AG Engel, BQ Banker (eds): Myology, pp 1385–1422. New York, McGraw-Hill, 1986

Dalakas MC: Polymyositis, dermatomyositis and inclusion body myositis. N Engl J Med 325:1487–1498, 1991

INDIAN CHILDHOOD CIRRHOSIS

Synonyms. Sen; liver cirrhosis of Indian children.

Symptoms and Signs. Occurs on Indian subcontinent; both sexes equally affected; onset usually 1–3 years of age. In some cases asymptomatic. *First stage.* Gastrointestinal symptoms; abdominal distension; hepatosplenomegaly; fever. *Second stage.* Marked hepatosplenomegaly; ascites; jaundice (75%). *Third stage.* Liver size reduction; gastrointestinal bleeding; other signs of liver failure up to hepatic coma and death.

Etiology. Unknown. No consistent association with foods, viruses; possibly multifactors including genetic predisposition.

Pathology. Liver swelling and vacuolization of hepatocytes followed by necrosis; lymphocytes and polymorphonuclear infiltration; later fibrotic changes; in advanced stages cholestasis. Characteristic lack of regeneration and presence of deposits of hepatocellular hyaline material.

Diagnostic Procedures. *Blood.* Hypoalbuminemia; presence of alphafetoprotein in the serum. Complement fractions low. *Urine.* Standard liver function test. Abnormal.

Therapy. Symptomatic.

Prognosis. Very severe. Cases with milder course have been reported.

BIBLIOGRAPHY. Chaudhuri A, Chaudhuri KC: The karyotype in Sen's syndrome (infantile cirrhosis of liver). Ind J Pediatr 31:309–311, 1964

Behrman RE: Kliegman Arvin Nelson Textbook of Pediatrics, 15th ed, p 1141. Philadelphia, WB Saunders, 1996

INFANTILE

Synonym. Coronary artery origin from pulmonary artery.

Symptoms and Signs. Rare. Onset within 4 months of life in 80% of patients with defect; angina pectoris or congestive heart failure, with mitral regurgitation. In the remaining 20%, onset during childhood or adult life; asymptomatic murmur, mitral insufficiency, angina pectoris, and sudden death.

Etiology. Unknown.

Pathology. Origin of coronary artery from pulmonary artery. Origin of left coronary artery from left posterior pulmonary sinus, 90%; origin of right coronary artery or both, rare. Patients surviving develop large intercoronary collateral flow with vessel dilatation.

Therapy. Early surgical correction to eliminate left to right shunt and establish good flow to anomalous vessel or to reimplant anomalous vessel into aortic root.

Prognosis. See Symptoms. High morbidity and mortality.

BIBLIOGRAPHY. Levin DC, Fellows KE, Abrams HC: Hemodynamically significant primary anomalies of the coronary arteries. Ang Aspects Circ 58:25–32, 1978

Fyler DC (ed): Nadas' Pediatric Cardiology. Philadelphia, Hanley-Belfus, 1992

Perloff JK: The Clinical Recognition of Congenital Heart Disease, 4th ed, p 738. Philadelphia, WB Saunders, 1994

INFECTIOUS CRYSTALLINE KERATHOPATHY

Synonym. Kerathopathy infectious crystalline, corneal post-bacterial infiltration.

Symptoms and Signs. In patients with corneal transplants or recurrent herpes infections receiving corticosteroids. Opacities of vision. Discrete anterior stromal opacities that appear white, branching and proceed insidiously to create distinct lesion associated with little or no corneal inflammation.

Etiology. Infection of graft by bacteria, usually streptococcus viridans or Hemophilus aphorophilus. Role of local immunosuppression.

Diagnostic Procedures. *Eye.* Progressive branching, needle-like stromal opacities. *Light microscopy.* Analysis of corneal button: localized epithelial ingrowth into stromal at suture tract, accompanied by intrastromal pockets of Gram-positive cocci. Lamellar keratectomy is necessary for recovering organisms. *Gram stain. Electromicroscopy.* Characteristic trilamellar structure of bacterial cell wall.

Therapy. Discontinuation of steroids and broad spectrum antibiotics.

Prognosis. Infection often progressive.

BIBLIOGRAPHY. Gorovoy MS: Intrastromal noninflammatory bacterial colonization of a corneal graft. Arch. Ophthalmol 101:1749–1752, 1983

Reiss GR, Campbell RJ, Bourne WM: Infectious crystalline keratopathy. Surv Ophthalmol 31:69–72, 1986

Garner A: Specific ocular manifestations of immunological processes. In Garner A, Klintworth GK (eds): Pathobiology of Ocular Disease: A Dynamic Approach, 2nd ed, pp 169–170. New York, Marcel Dekker, 1994

INFECTIOUS MONONUCLEOSIS

Synonyms. Filatov; Pfeiffer (misnomer, see); Sprunt; Türck; kissing disease; mononucleosis infectiva.

Symptoms. Both sexes equally affected; onset at all ages, but higher frequency in the 20–25 year bracket. Epidemics in young communities. Incubation 33–49 days. Symptoms variable: malaise and fatigue (100%); increased sweating (80–95%); dysphagia and throat angina (80–85%); anorexia (50–80%); cephalalgia (50–70%); chills (50%); cough (40%); myalgia (35%); ocular muscle pain (15%); photophobia (10%); diarrhea (10%); epistaxis (5%). Seldom at third to fourth week, spleen rupture.

Signs. Adenopathy (100%); hyperthermia (90%); splenomegaly (50%); bradycardia (40%); periorbital edema (35%); palatal enanthema (30%); hepatosplenic tenderness (20%); hepatomegaly (20%); rhinitis (20%); jaundice (5–10%); skin rash (5%).

Etiology. Caused by the Epstein-Barr (EB) virus.

Pathology. Generalized and marked perivascular infiltration with normal and abnormal lymphocytes. *Lymph nodes.* Lymphocytic and reticular hyperplasia with moderate simple distortion of normal architecture; diminished follicular prominence; focal proliferation of macrophages and presence of atypical lymphocytes (Downey cells-virocytes). *Spleen.* Hyperplastic and markedly infiltrated by equal type of cells. *Liver.* Minimal cellular damage, infiltration with lymphocytes and virocytes. Other organs (including brain, spine, and meninges). May show moderate, scanty, similar cell infiltrations.

Diagnostic Procedures. *Blood.* Increase of white blood cells (10,000–20,000, seldom up to 60,000–80,000). Presence (60–90%) of abnormal lymphocytes (Downey cells), which vary in size and shape and show peculiar characteristics. Decrease of red cells and platelets seldom observed; coagulation abnormalities frequently observed (suggesting thrombocytopathia). Hyperbilirubinemia 5–10%. Heterophil antibodies present, a variety of anti-EBV antibodies almost always observed. Throat washing. Isolation of EBV up to 18 months after onset of infection.

Therapy. No therapy is indicated in majority of cases. Salicylates and/or other symptomatic drugs for treatment of fever, headache, and sore throat. (Careful use, since in patients treated with aspirin reported longer course). Antibiotics are employed only if throat cultures are positive for group A- or B-hemolytic streptococci. Corticosteroids are indicated in severe tonsillitis with pharyngeal edema and impending respiratory obstruction; acute hemolytic anemia and thrombocytopenia; neurological complications; myocarditis, and pericarditis. Specific antiviral chemotherapy is under evaluation, but with negative results till now: Adenine arabinoside, acyclovir, human interferon. Gammaglobulin in large doses is useful in immune thrombocytopenia associated with the condition.

Prognosis. Condition usually benign, hepatitis, myocarditis, and encephalitis possible complications. Complete recovery within 2 months, followed by a period of variable length of asthenia and easy fatigability. Observed cases with lengthy course and persistent thrombocytopenia; seldom, fulminating cases (fatal complication 1:3000 cases). Recurrences nonexistent or extremely rare. From even minor abdominal trauma possible rupture of spleen (glass spleen).

BIBLIOGRAPHY. Filatov N: Leksii ob ostrykh infeksionnykh bolezniakh u detei. Moska, 1887

Türck W: Vorlesungen ueber klinische Haematologie, vol 2. Wien, 1904

Sprunt TPV, Evans FA: Mononuclear leukocytosis in reaction to acute infection (infectious mononucleosis). Bull Johns Hopkins Hosp 31:410–417, 1920

Betts RF: The infectious mononucleosis syndromes in hematology and oncology. In Lichtman MA (ed): The Science and Practice of Clinical Medicine. New York, Grune & Stratton, 1980

Audiman WA: Epstein-Barr virus associated syndromes. Pediatr Infec Dis 3:198–203, 1984

Foerster J: Infectious mononucleosis. In Lee GR, Bithel TC, Foerster J, et al (eds): Wintrobe's Clinical Hematology, 9th ed, pp 1650–1675. Philadelphia, Lea & Febiger, 1993

INSPISSATED BILE

Synonym. Jaundice obstructive infantilis.

Symptoms and Signs. Occurs in newborns. Jaundice developing within first 2 days of life and lasting about 3 weeks. Anemia; splenomegaly; hepatomegaly.

Etiology. Bile inspissation caused by excessive hemolysis. See Hemolytic anemia of newborn.

Pathology. Distortion of bile canalculi caused by massive hepatic hematopoiesis, bile thrombosis, and liver necrotic changes.

Diagnostic Procedures. See Hemolytic anemia of newborn. *Blood.* Direct and indirect bilirubin in blood and urine markedly increased, negative flocculation tests.

Therapy. See Hemolytic anemia of newborn syndrome.

Prognosis. That of hemolytic anemia of newborn, progression to liver cirrhosis as sequela considered.

BIBLIOGRAPHY. Hsia DY, Patterson P, Allen FH Jr, et al: Prolonged obstructive jaundice in infancy. I. General survey of 156 cases. Pediatrics 10:243–252, 1952

Schaffner: Jaundice. In Haubrich WS, Schaffner F, Berk JE (eds): Bockus Gastroenterology, 5th ed, vol 2, p 131. Philadelphia, WB Saunders, 1995

INSTITUTIONALISM

Synonym. Attachment disorder, reactive.

Symptoms. Psychological changes developing in people kept in segregated communities. Apathy; resignation; dependence; depersonalization, and reliance on fantasy.

BIBLIOGRAPHY. Bettelheim B, Sylvester E: A therapeutic milieu. Am J Orthopsychiatr 18:191–206, 1948
Wing JK: Institutionalism in mental hospitals. Br J Soc Clin Psychol 1:38–51, 1963
Kaplan HI, Sadock BJ: Comprehensive Textbook of Psychiatry, 6th ed, pp 2354–2355. Baltimore, Williams & Wilkins, 1995

INSULINOPATHIES

Synonyms. See also organic hyperinsulinism.

Symptoms and Signs. Six families with this type of disorder identified. Not all affected individuals present symptoms and signs of overt diabetes; those are generally limited to mild diabetes or glucose intolerance, eventually evolving into frank diabetes similar to Type II (or non-insulin dependent [NIDDM]).

Etiology. Autosomal dominant inheritance. Single nucleotide substitution in only one of the two alleles leading to a single amino acid replacement within the insulin molecule.

Diagnostic Procedures. *Blood.* Insulin level elevated; circulating A chain-C peptide linked intermediate cleavage form of (AC) proinsulin.

BIBLIOGRAPHY. Tager H, Given B, Baldwin D, et al: A structurally abnormal insulin causing human diabetes. Nature 281:122–125, 1979
Haneda M, Polonsky KS, Bergenstal RM, et al: Familial hyper-insulinemia due to a structurally abnormal insulin: Definition of an emerging new clinical syndrome. N Engl J Med 310:1288–1294, 1984
Nanjo K, Sanke T, Miyano M, et al: Diabetes due to secretion of a structurally abnormal insulin (insulin Wakayama) clinical and functional characteristics of (Leu A3) insulin. J Clin Invest 77:514–519, 1986
Steiner DF, Tager HS, Nanjo, et al: Familial syndromes of Hyperinsulinemia and hyperinsulinemia with mild diabetes. In Scriver CR, Beaudet AL, Sly WS, et al: The Metabolic and Molecular Bases of Inherited Disease, 7th ed, pp 901–903. New York, McGraw-Hill, 1995

INSULIN RESISTANCE, POLYCYSTIC OVARY

Symptoms and Signs. In adolescent subjects obese and lean. Combination of symptoms and signs of Stein-Leventhal (see), insulin resistance similar to that observed with patients with type II diabetes (other signs of insulin resistance: hypertension, dyslipidemia, and coronary artery disease are absent, however); occasionally acanthosis nigricans (see).

Etiology. Unknown. Signal transduction via phosphorylation cascade.

Diagnostic Procedures. See Stein Leventhal; diabetes with insulin resistance and compensatory hyperinsulinism.

Therapy. See Stein-Leventhal and diabetes.

BIBLIOGRAPHY. Dunaif A: Insulin resistance and ovarian hyperandrogenism. Endocrinologist 2:248–260,1992
Davidson MB: Clinical implications of insulin resistance syndromes. Am J Med 99:420–426, 1995

INTENSIVE CARE

Synonym. ICU.

PATIENTS

Symptoms. Acute disorganization of behavior occurring in many patients when exposed to a variety of intense diagnostic and therapeutic procedures (monitoring; infusion; contact with other acutely ill patients). Observed in particular in coronary care units and intensive care units.

Etiology. Incapacity to handle stress plus basic pathologic conditions.

Diagnostic Procedures. Monitoring of signs and symptoms of organic brain syndromes.

Therapy. Prevention by establishing personal relationship with attendant involved in care, active participation, physical presence, visits, and explanations of procedures by personal physician. Avoid or minimize delirifacient drugs. Make environment look as familiar as possible.

STAFF

Symptoms. Complex psychological reactions that may go through phases from enthusiasm to discouragement; in some cases, with acquired tendency to become less attentive to hygienic prophylactic measures. From intense, disturbing participation in patient fate, to indifference and resentment. Conflict and tension between nurses and physicians.

Etiology. Life under stressful physical and psychological situation.

Therapy. Rotation through different departments and avoid excessively lengthy period in intensive care unit. Psychological evaluation before assignment of personnel to the unit. Recognize the inevitability of conflict and tension. Maximize communication between and within professional groups in the unit and with other groups in the hospital.

BIBLIOGRAPHY. Nahum LH: Madness in the recovery room from open heart surgery or "They kept waking me up." Conn Med 29:771–772, 1965
McKegney FP: The intensive care syndrome. Conn Med 30:633–639, 1966
Harrell RC, Othmer E: Postcardiotomy confusion and sleep loss. J Clin Psychiatr 48:445–446, 1987
Civetta JM, Taylor RW, Kirby RR (eds): Critical Care, 2nd ed. Philadelphia, Lippincott, 1992

INTERMITTENT VERTEBRAL COMPRESSION

Synonyms. Bärtschi Rochain; cervical-vertigo; vertebral artery compression; vertigo head extension. See Barré-Lieou.

Symptoms. Onset unpredictable. Precipitating factors include emotional tension, rotation or extension of head. Vertigo; dizziness; decreased hearing; tinnitus (which may persist when vertigo is over and in some patients is continuous); headache. Gastrointestinal symptoms: nausea; vomiting; explosive diarrhea. Visual disturbances; paresthesia; numbness; coldness of ipsilateral arm.

Signs. Diminution or obliteration of radial pulse with Adson maneuver; supraclavicular bruit may be heard (30% of cases) or appear with change of position of head.

Etiology and Pathology. Anomaly of vertebral artery system, which results in intermittent compression at the origin or at site of cervical course of the artery. Defect of cervical spine that intermittently compresses the artery. Vertebrobasilar aneurysm.

Diagnostic Procedures. *X-ray. Arteriography. CT scan. MRI.*

Therapy. According to etiology, different surgical procedures: surgical mobilization of the artery with stripping of vertebral plexus; fusion of vertebrae; correction of aneurysm.

Prognosis. Good response to surgery.

BIBLIOGRAPHY. Pratt-Thomas HR, Berger KE: Cerebellar and spinal injuries after chiropractic manipulation. JAMA 133:600–603, 1947
Bärtschi-Rochain W: Migrain cervicale (Das encephale Syndrome nach halswirbel Trauma). Berne, Huber, 1949
Morley JB: Unruptured vertebro-basilar aneurysms. Med J Austr 2:1024–1027, 1967

Brandt T: Vertigo: Its Multisensory Syndromes, pp 167–169. London, Springer-Verlag, 1991

INTERPEDUNCULAR

Synonyms. Ventral peduncular.

Symptoms and Signs. Palsy of both III cranial nerves variously associated with limb palsy of one side or both, symptoms appearing slowly and progressively, additional cranial nerves may also be compromised.

Etiology and Pathology. Disease process extending across cerebral midline.

BIBLIOGRAPHY. Sachsenweger: Clinical localization of ocular disturbances. In Vinken PJ, Bruyn GW: Handbook of Clinical Neurology, vol 2, p 298. Amsterdam, North-Holland, 1969

INTERSTITIAL KERATITIS I

Synonyms. Keratitis infectiva, syphilitic keratitis, see also Cogan I.

Symptoms and Signs. Corneal lesions absent at birth, occur late in teenage years. Photophobia, lacrimation, progressive loss of vision.

Etiology. May be due to different agents: (1) allergic sequela of bacterial infection (syphilis, tuberculosis, leprosy); (2) virus infections like herpes simplex, disciform keratitis, herpes zoster, varicella, lymphogranuloma venereum, or mumps; (3) onchocerciasis; (4) sarcoidosis, mycosis fungoides, Hodgkin; (5) foreign body induced (ophthalmia nodosa and nummular keratitis); (6) after long-term heavy metal therapy (arsenic and gold).

Pathology. Infiltration of inflammatory cells into corneal stroma in absence of overlying ulceration, separation of corneal lamellae and vascularization (ghost vessels). In syphilitic interstitial keratitis red areas in cornea ("salmon patches") indicates vascularization.

Therapy. Symptomatic.

Prognosis. Evolution to opacification of deeper layers of cornea, secondary band keratopathy, lipid deposition in stroma, secondary glaucoma.

BIBLIOGRAPHY. Friedewold JS: Ocular lesions in fetal syphilis. Bull John Hopkins Hosp 46:185, 1930
Patterson A: Interstitial keratitis. Br J Ophthalmol 50:612–613, 1966
Garner A, Klintworth GK (eds): Pathobiology of Ocular Disease: A Dynamic Approach, 2nd ed, pp 268, 1007, 1064, 1194. New York, Marcel Dekker, 1994

INTESTINAL ATRESIA

Synonyms. Polyatresia intestinalis.

Symptoms and Signs. Clinical manifestations vary according to site and number of obstructions.

Etiology. Possibly autosomal recessive inheritance (French Canadian group more affected). It represents a distinguished entity to be separated from duodenal and jejunal atresia, because of wide dissemination of the obstruction from stomach to anus.

Diagnostic Procedures. *X-rays.* According to site and degree of obstruction. Intraluminal calcifications have been reported.

Therapy. Surgery.

Prognosis. Variable according to treatment.

BIBLIOGRAPHY. Blank CE, Okmian L, Robbe H: Mucoviscidosis and intestinal atresia: A study of four cases in the same family. Acta Paediat Scand 54:557–569, 1969

Shen-Schwarz S, Fitks R: Multiple gastrointestinal atresias with imperforate anus: pathology and pathogenesis. Am J Med Genet 36:451–459, 1990

INTESTINAL CARBOHYDRATE DYSPEPSIA

Synonym. Carbohydrate dyspepsia. See Irritable bowel.

Symptoms. Prevalent in middle-aged females with depressive tendency, anxiety, nervousness. Characteristic intermittent attacks following emotional stress. Attacks are extremely variable in length (days or many years). Abdominal pains, usually after meals; nocturnal distress; abdominal fullness; distension; flatus; belching; intolerance to certain foods (starches, vegetables, milk). Constipation or diarrhea; asthenia; fatigability.

Signs. In some patients, weight loss, chronic choroidoretinitis (in 25% of patients), hypotension (30%), tachycardia.

Etiology. Alteration of intestinal flora; deficiency of diastatic enzymes; intestinal hypermotility; dietary disorders; sensitivity to carbohydrates, aerophagia.

Pathology. No constant pathologic changes; chronic state of congestion and increased mucosal desquamation reported.

Diagnostic Procedures. *Blood.* Moderate anemia. *Stool.* Rich in undigested carbohydrates; increased mucus and gas bubbles. *Sigmoidoscopy.* Normal. *X-ray.* Colon dilatation, spasm, accelerated transit (in some cases).

Therapy. Difficult. Psychotherapy to correct emotional factors; correction of aerophagia; dietary measures; vitamin supplementation; pancreatic enzymes; atropine in diarrhea; modification of flora with short course of antibiotic also useful.

Prognosis. Periodic recurrence with period of freedom from symptoms.

BIBLIOGRAPHY. Althausen TL, Gunnisin JB, Marshall MD, et al: Carbohydrate intolerance and intestinal flora: A clinical study based on sixty cases. Tr Am Gastroenterol A 36:143–174, 1935
Semenza G, Auricchio S: Small-intestinal disaccharidases. In Scriver CR, Beaudet AL, Sly WS, et al: The Metabolic and Molecular Bases of Inherited Disease, 7th ed, pp 4463–4470. New York, McGraw-Hill, New York, 1995

INTESTINAL IDIOPATHIC PSEUDO-OBSTRUCTION

Synonym. IIP; argyrophil myenteric plexus deficiency. See Diffuse esophageal spasm. See Megaduodenum–Megacystis.

Symptoms and Signs. Both sexes affected; onset insidious in childhood or young adulthood. Recurrent signs of esophageal obstruction and, later, recurrent signs of small and large bowel dysfunction: pain; distension; diarrhea; constipation; steatorrhea. History of repeated laparotomies.

Etiology. Variable in same cases failure of development of argyrophil myenteric plexus. It represents a miscellanous group with variable clinical manifestations and sporadic or autosomal dominant inheritance with variable penetrance.

Pathology. In some cases autopsy reveals degeneration of myenteric plexus in the esophagus small intestine and colon.

Diagnostic Procedures. *Manometry.* Lower esophageal sphincter pressure in the normal range with incomplete relaxation. *X-rays. Barium swallow.* Small bowel involment frequent: megaduodenum; dilatation of variable length and location; colon atonic; high incidence of volvulus; malrotation pyloric hypertrophy.

Therapy. Medical management. Nifedipine and isosorbide dinitrate (modest results). If unsuccessful, surgical myotomy; pneumatic dilatation.

Prognosis. Good. From few months to many years: possible death from starvation.

BIBLIOGRAPHY. Schuffer MD, Pope CH II: Esophageal motor dysfunction in idiopathic intestinal pseudo-obstruction. Gastroenterology 70:677–682, 1976

Vargas JH, Sacho P, Ament ME: Chronic intestinal pseudo-obstruction syndrome in pediatrics. Results in a national survey by Members of the North American Society of Pediatric Gastroenterology and Nutrition. J Pediatr Gastroenterol Nutr 7:323–332, 1988

Malagelata JR, Camilleri M: Motility disorders of the stomach. In Haubrich WS, Schaffner F, Berk JE (eds): Bockus Gastroenterology, 5th ed, vol 2, p 622. Philadelphia, WB Saunders, 1995

INTESTINAL KNOT

Synonyms. Compound volvulus; double volvulus.

Symptoms and Signs. Prevalent in males (85%); maximal incidence in fifth and sixth decades. Relatively rare. Sudden, severe, abdominal pain and nausea. Abdomen board-like with generalized tenderness. Chest examination normal.

Etiology and Pathology. Knotting strangulation of both cecal and sigmoid segments. Variations reported such as appendiceal knot and subsequent closed loop, ileal obstruction, and others. No precipitating factor identified. Possibly, underlying mesenteric inflammatory change with shortening of proximal and distal sigmoid segments. Intestinal parasites a predisposing factor in some cases.

Diagnostic Procedures. *Blood.* White blood cells increased. *Abdominal paracentesis.* Cloudy fluid with low amylase content. *X-ray of abdomen.* Oval loop of dilated bowel in right lower quadrant. With patient erect, no free air, several gas-filled and dilated loops of small bowel. Classical "breaking" of barium column at site of sigmoid volvulus.

Therapy. Immediate surgical intervention. When possible, separation and unwinding of loops; resection with end-to-end anastomoses of both ileum and colon, with decompressing cecostomy.

Prognosis. Determined by promptness of surgical intervention.

BIBLIOGRAPHY. Parker E: Case of intestinal obstruction: sigmoid flexure strangulated by the ileum. Edinburgh Med Surg J 64:306, 1845

Boyden FM, Tappan WM: The intestinal knot syndrome. JAMA 211:662–663, 1970

Gumbs MA, Kashan F, Shumofsky E, et al: Volvulus of the transverse colon: Report of cases and review of literature. Dis Colon Rectum 26:825–828, 1983

Livingstone AS, Sosa JL: Ileus and obstruction. In Haubrich WS, Schaffner F, Berk JE (eds): Bockus Gastroenterology, 5th ed, vol 2, p 1245. Philadelphia, WB Saunders, 1995

INTESTINAL NODULAR HYPERPLASIA

Synonyms. Steatorrhea—immunoglobulin A deficiency.

Symptoms. Cases reported in adults. Steatorrhea; general fatigue; bone pain.

Signs. Moderate abdominal distention; pitting edema of ankle.

Etiology. Unknown.

Pathology. Diffuse nodules in the intestinal mucosa consisting of enlarged lymphoid follicles within lamina propria. Intense mitotic activity; large germinal center. Plasma cells almost absent.

Diagnostic Procedures. *Blood.* Anemia; hypogammaglobulinemia (absence of IgA; moderate depression of IgG). *X-ray.* Lymphoid hyperplasia diffuse in all intestinal tract, evident as multiple mucosal nodules. *D-xylose absorption test.*

Therapy. Some cases will improve on gluten-free diet and vitamin supplementation.

Prognosis. Long-range prognosis not established.

BIBLIOGRAPHY. Hermans PE, Huizenga KA, Hoffman HN, et al: Dysgammaglobulinemia associated with nodular lymphoid hyperplasia of the small intestine. Am J Med 40:78–89, 1966

Sell S: Immunological deficiency diseases. Arch Pathol 86:95–107, 1968

Lukens JN: Immune deficiency diseases: Inherited and acquired. In Lee GR, Bithel TC, Foerster J, et al (eds): Wintrobe's Clinical Hematology, 9th ed, p 1680. Philadelphia, Lea & Febiger, 1993

INTESTINAL POLYPOSIS, FAMILIAL

Symptoms. Onset before the age of 40, usually in late childhood or young adulthood. Symptoms not specific; occasionally, diarrhea and weakness, with development of malignant changes. Change in bowel habits. Pain; obstruction; malnutritional findings.

Signs. Pallor; pain over colon.

Etiology. Familial autosomal dominant trait (about half of offspring of person with disease affected).

Pathology. Benign adenomas, small usually sessile, densely packing the entire colon mucosal surface; frequent malignant transformation at early age; adenocarcinomas enlarge and spread rather rapidly.

Diagnostic Procedures. *Barium enema. Sigmoidoscopy.* Appearance pathognomonic.

Therapy. Subtotal colectomy with ileoproctostomy and careful follow-up for possible development of carcinoma on remaining stump. Fulguration of remaining polyps also recommended.

Prognosis. Guarded; occasionally, remission of remaining polyps.

BIBLIOGRAPHY. Cripps H: Two cases of disseminated polyps of rectum. Trans Med Soc Lon 33:165, 1882

Lynch HT, Krush AF: Heredity and adenocarcinoma of the colon. Gastroenterology 53:517–527, 1967

Lee RG: Benign tumors of the colon. In Haubrich WS, Schaffner F, Berk JE (eds): Bockus Gastroenterology, 5th ed, vol 2, pp 1715–1724. Philadelphia, WB Saunders, 1995

INTESTINAL PRIMARY LYMPHOMA OF ADULT, WESTERN

Synonyms. MALT type intestinal lymphoma (Western).

Symptoms and Signs. Worlwide, although most cases from developed countries. Age: sixth decade. Abdominal pain, acute abdomen (perforation, obstruction). Frequent bleeding if colorectal localization.

Etiology. Unknown.

Pathology. Large tumors in 75%. B-cell localized in small intestine, less frequently in the colonrectum. Lymph node involvement frequent.

Diagnostic Procedures. *X-ray. CT scan. MRI. Endoscopy. Biopsy. Stool analysis. Blood.* Normal white cell count and differential.

Therapy. Surgery in early stages followed by chemotherapy, radiotherapy, and adjuvant therapies.

Prognosis. According to staging colon worse than small intestine localization.

BIBLIOGRAPHY. Dawson IMP, Cornes JS, Morson BC: Primary malignant lymphoid tumors of the intestinal tract: report of 37 cases with a study of factors influencing prognosis. Br J Surg 49:80–89, 1961

Turowski GA, Basson MD: Primary malignant lymphoma of the intestine. Am J Surg 169:433–441, 1995

INTESTINAL PRIMARY LYMPHOMA OF CHILDHOOD

Symptoms and Signs. Worldwide distribution. Children 7–11 years. Usual onset acute abdomen, tender abdominal mass, intussusception.

Etiology. Unknown.

Pathology. Mostly Burkitt type, small noncleaved B-cell, almost no low-grade tumors. Most commonly in ileocecal zone, seldom in stomach and colorectum. Lymph nodes usually are involved.

Diagnostic Procedures. *X-ray. CT scan. MRI. Endoscopy. Biopsy. Stool analysis. Blood.* Normal white cell count and differential.

Therapy. Surgery in early stages followed by chemotherapy and adjuvant therapies.

Prognosis. Good in stage I and II.

BIBLIOGRAPHY. Turowski GA, Basson MD: Primary malignant lymphoma of the intestine. Am J Surg 169:433–441, 1995

INTRAMURAL CORONARY ARTERY ANEURYSM

Synonyms. Coronary artery aneurysm, intramural. See Coronary artery steal.

Symptoms. Angina pectoris, dyspnea, and fatigue on exertion.

Signs. Harsh systolic and diastolic murmur along left sternal border and on apex.

Etiology and Pathology. Intramural coronary artery aneurysm.

Diagnostic Procedures. *ECG.* Suggests posterior myocardial infarction. *X-ray.* Heart normal size. *Heart catheterization.* Normal output; normal pressure; no shunt. *Left ventricular angiography and aortography.* Left ventricle normal size and normal contraction. Right coronary normal. Left descending coronary dilated to 1 cm in diameter; tortuous emptying into an aneurysmal sac at the apex of heart; aneurysm large in diastole, contracted in systole.

Therapy. Closure of aneurysmal neck and approximation of walls. Anticoagulant or antiplatelet therapy.

Prognosis. Variable; good result with surgery.

BIBLIOGRAPHY. Björk VO, Björk L: Intramural coronary artery aneurysm: A coronary artery steal syndrome. J Thorac Cardiovasc Surg 54:50–52, 1967
Baue AE, Baum S, Blakemore WS, et al: A large stage of anomalous coronary circulation with origin of the left coronary artery from pulmonary artery-coronary artery steal. Circulation 36:878–885, 1967
Waller BF: Nonatherosclerotic coronary heart disease. In Schlant RC, Alexander RW: Hurst's The Heart, 8th ed, pp 1247–1248. New York, McGraw-Hill, 1994

IRIDO CORNEAL ENDOTHELIAL

Synonyms. I.C.E. See Chandler, Cogan-Reese. Encopasses: Essential iris atrophy, Chandler, and Cogan-Reese.

Symptoms and Signs. Visual disturbance: halos, blurred vision.

Etiology. X-linked phenotype inheritance or primary proliferation of endothelial membrane over anterior chamber and on the iris.

Therapy. That of glaucoma and then enucleation.

Diagnostic Procedures. *Slit lamp.* Abnormality of posterior cornea. *Ultramicroscopy.* Substitution of posterior corneal epithelium by Descemet membrane.

In iris atrophy: peripheral anterior synechiae with displacement of the pupil, mild to moderate ectropion. In Cogan-Reese: see Chandler, intermediate changes

Prognosis. Evolution toward angle closure glaucoma. Enucleation.

BIBLIOGRAPHY. Frank-Kamenetzki SG: Eine eigenartige hereditaere Glaukomform mit Mangel des Irisstromas und geschlechtsgebundener. Vererbung Klin Mbl Augenheilk 74:133–150, 1925
Yanoff M: Irido corneal endothelial syndrome: Unification of a disease spectrum. Surv Ophthalmol 24:1–2, 1979
Klintworth GK: Degenerations depositions and miscellaneous reaction of the ocular anterior segment. In Garner A, Klintworth GK (eds): Pathobiology of Ocular Disease: A Dynamic Approach, 2nd ed, pp 777–779. New York, Marcel Dekker, 1994

IRRITABLE BOWEL

Synonyms. IBS; adaptive colitis; mucous colitis; colonic neurosis; spastic colitis; dyssynergia colon; irritable colon; unstable colon; neurogenic mucous colitis.

Symptoms. In 15% of Western population. More frequent in women. From adult age. *Precipitating factors.* Psychogenic: cancer phobia; emotional tension; fatigue; weakness; menstrual periods; tobacco; diet; bowel irritants. Constipation alternated with normal bowel movement and diarrhea (in about 25% of cases); epigastric pains; turbulence feeling of incomplete evacuation. *Associated symptoms.* Aerophagy; anxiety; insomnia; nervousness; fatigue. *Vasomotor symptoms.* Flushing, faintness; sweating, cardiac arrhythmias, headache; urinary frequency; dysuria; dysmenorrhea; pruritus ani and vulvae.

Signs. Symptoms during attack: palpation of spastic colon (lower descending portion), tenderness over ascending and transverse parts; absence of muscle guarding (except for excessive reaction of patient). Mucus in the stools. Rectal examination negative.

Etiology. Functional disorder. Emotional tension, as manifestation of numerous endocrinopathies or small intestinal disaccharidases, deficiencies. Probably owing to alteration of vagus nerve function. May be part of autonomic failure syndrome. Lately have been demonstrated alteration of motility of esophagus, gallbladder, visica, small intestine, ileocecal area.

Diagnostic Procedures. *Stool.* Abnormal, small, hard, narrow cylindrical or fragmented; mucus. *Sigmoidoscopy.* Colon irritability and spasm; absence of organic lesion or dilatation. *X-ray.* Barium enema and barium meal reveal increased speed of transit; smooth narrowing of lumen of colon; other spastic features. Gastric secretory response to insulin hypoglycemia impaired.

Therapy. Corrections of psychologic factors by psychotherapy; anti-anxiety, antidepressant, anticholinergic agents of food related factors by gas reducing agents and poorly tolerated foodstuff, symptomatic treatment of constipation and diarrhea. The relationship of patient to physician is important.

Prognosis. Recurrence in most patients. Gratifying result may be obtained by adequate treatment.

BIBLIOGRAPHY. Da Costa JM: Mucus enteritis. Am J Med Sci 89:321–335, 1871
Ryle JA: Chronic spasmodic affections of the colon. Lancet II:1115–1119, 1928
Bockus HL, Bank J, Wilkinson SA: Neurogenic mucous colitis. Am J Med Sci 176:813–829, 1928
Snape WJ Jr: Irritable bowel syndrome. In Haubrich WS, Schaffner F, Berk JE (eds): Bockus Gastroenterology, 5th ed, pp 1619–1636. Philadelphia, WB Saunders, 1995

IRVINE-GASS

Synonyms. Cataract extraction; vitreous cataract extraction; vitreous tug; vitreous wick; pseudopathic cystoid macular edema.

Symptoms. Posttraumatic or onset 2–3 weeks after intraocular surgery. Sensation of light flashes. Decreasing vision.

Signs. Irregular pupils. Vitreous strand passing through pupil attached to corneal scar. Possibly, vitreous detachment.

Etiology. It is not entirely clear whether cystoid macula edema occurs because of (1) an increased permeability of perifoveolar capillaries; (2) an ischemic tissue injury; (3) a secondary response to intraocular inflammation; or (4) a direct traction on the macula following vitreous shifts.

Diagnostic Procedures. *Ophthalmoscopy.* Loss of foveal reflex; localized edema retinae; occasionally, posterior retinal detachment.

Therapy. Surgical repair.

Prognosis. Good with surgery.

BIBLIOGRAPHY. Irvine SR: Newly defined vitreous syndrome following cataract surgery: Interpreted according to recent concepts of structure of vitreous wick (Seventh Francis P Proctor Lecture). Am J Ophthalmol 36:599–619, 1953

Stainer GA, Binder PS: Vitreous wick syndrome following a corneal relaxing incision. Ophthal Surg 12:567–570, 1981

Apple DJ, Rabb MF: Ocular Pathology, p 155. St Louis, Mosby Year Book, 1991

Garner A, Klintworth GK (eds): Pathobiology of Ocular Disease: A Dynamic Approach, 2nd ed, pp 411, 653, 657, 720. New York, Marcel Dekker, 1994

ISAACS-MERTENS

Synonym. Continuous muscle fiber activity. See Moersch-Waltmann; and myokymia.

Symptoms and Signs. Both sexes. Persistent myokymia from first months, then diminishing motor activity with flexion, contractures of lower limbs. Increased muscular tone persists during sleep. Cyanotic episodes. At later age persistence of myokymia and transient stiffness after initiation of movements.

Etiology. Autosomal dominant inheritance.

Diagnostic Procedures. *Electromyography.* Continuous motor activity that persists in spite of peripheral nerve blockade or anesthesia. *X-rays.* Thoraco-abdominal. *CT scan. Sonography.* Eventration of diaphragm with poor motion.

Therapy. Phenytoin sodium.

Prognosis. Considerable improvement with therapy.

BIBLIOGRAPHY. Isaac HA: A syndrome of continuous muscle fiber activity. J Neurol Neurosurg Psychiatr 24:319–325, 1961

Martens HG, Zschocke S: Neuromyokymia. Klin Wchnsch 43:917–925, 1965

McGuire SA; Tomasovic JJ, Ackermann N Jr: Hereditary continuous muscle fiber activity. Arch Neurol 41:395–396, 1984

Adams RD, Victor M: Principles of Neurology, 5th ed, p 1273. New York, McGraw-Hill, 1993

ISCHEMIC COLON

Synonym. Transient intestinal ischemic attack. See Abdominal angina.

Symptoms. In patients of both sexes over 50. Average age 70. Acute onset. Cramping lower or left side abdominal pain; urge to defecate, nausea, vomiting. Occasionally fever, bloody diarrhea.

Signs. Abdominal tenderness and/or rigidity of abdominal wall.

Etiology. Occlusion spontaneous, use of vasoconstricting drugs, methamphetamine, "crack" cocaine, or following surgery of branches of interior mesenteric artery with transient ischemia of portion of colon. In younger patients association with diabetes mellitus, lupus erythematosus, sickle cell crisis. Usually without intestinal infarction.

Pathology. See Etiology. Minor atherosclerotic changes of vessels, intestinal lesions, edema, and then necrotic changes leading to strictures.

Diagnostic Procedures. *X-ray. Gentle barium enema (colonoscopy preferable).* Mass lesion or edema of mucosa (pseudotumor). In advanced cases lesions similar to ulcerative colitis and strictures splenic flexure; descending colon most frequent location. *Mesenteric arteriography. Blood.* Leukocytosis. *Stool.* Blood.

Therapy. Symptomatic: general supporting measures (no corticosteroids). Immediate surgery not required and reserved only for severe form.

Prognosis. Usually self-limited condition; Most episodes mild, transient, and reversible (24–48 h). May heal in 2 weeks without permanent lesion. Fair also for severe form.

BIBLIOGRAPHY. Boley SJ, Scgwartz S, Lash J, et al: Reversible vascular occlusion of the colon. Surg Clin North Am 72:203–229, 1963

Williams LF, Nittenberg J: Ischemic colitis: A useful clinical diagnosis. But is it ischemic! Ann Surg 182:439–448, 1975

Rogers AI, David S: Intestinal blood flow and diseases of vascular impairment. In Haubrich WS, Schaffner F, Berk JE (eds): Bockus Gastroenterology, 5th ed, vol 2, pp 1228–1230. Philadelphia, WB Saunders, 1995

ISOLATED GROWTH-HORMONE DEFICIENCY

Synonyms. Ateliosis; pituitary dwarfism I; growth hormone deficiency isolated. See Gilford-Burnier, Illig and Larson.

Symptoms and Signs. Both sexes affected; birth weight and gestational age usually normal. Usually, normal growth during first year, then continuing at markedly diminished rate. Occasionally, later onset (up to 10 years) of slowed growth. Normal or delayed pubertal development; height more retarded than weight. Symptomatic Harris syndrome (see).

Etiology. Isolated deficiency of secretion of growth hormone. Usually sporadic cases. Familial cases reported with autosomal dominant inheritance.

Diagnostic Procedures. *Plasma.* Low or absent growth hormone; lack of increase after insulin stimulation. Normal level of thyroid-stimulating hormone (TSH), adrenocorticotropic hormone (ACTH), gonadotropins. Hypoglycemia. *X-ray.* Markedly retarded bone age. No lesions of sella turcica.

Therapy. Growth hormone.

Prognosis. Striking growth with administration of hormone. Pubertal development may also be accelerated by treatment.

BIBLIOGRAPHY. Gilford H: Ateliosis: form of dwarfism. Practitioner 70:797–819, 1903

Antonin JMF: Hypothalamo-hypophysarer Zwergwuchs mit spontaner Pubertat. Helv Paediat Acta 16:267–276, 1961

Van Gelderen HH, Van der Hoog CE: Familial isolated growth hormone deficiency. Clin Genet 20:173–175, 1981

Ranke MB: Growth hormone insufficiency: Clinical features, diagnosis and therapy. In De Groot LJ (ed): Endocrinology, 3rd ed, pp 330–340. Philadelphia, WB Saunders, 1995

ISOVALERIC ACIDEMIA

Synonyms. Isovaleryl-CoA dehydrogenase deficiency.

Symptoms and Signs. Both sexes affected. Normal at birth; after a few days, attacks of vomiting, acidosis, coma, strong objectionable body odor (sweaty feet) that increases with recurrence of symptoms. During attacks, ataxia and tendon hyperreflexia. Mild psychomotor retardation;

aversion to protein-rich foods. Two clinical forms, possibly allelic, are recognized: acute severe type and chronic intermittent type.

Etiology. Inborn error of leucine metabolism with accumulation of isovaleric acid in serum; defect of isovaleric coenzyme A (CoA) dehydrogenase. Autosomal recessive inheritance. The gene for the enzyme has been assigned to chromosome 15q14–q15.

Pathology. Changes related to hematologic findings; bone marrow hypoplastic; viscera with diffuse hemorrhages and signs of terminal septicemia.

Diagnostic Procedures. *Blood.* High accumulation of isovaleric acid and inability of leukocytes to degrade 214C leucine normally. Pancytopenia, thrombocytopenia and neutropenia. Ketonemia during crisis. *Bone marrow.* Hypoplastic *Urine.* Excretion of isovaleric acid (typical odor). *Leucine tolerance test.*

Therapy. Low-protein diet. Glycine and carnitine supplementation.

Prognosis. Neonatal death may be associated with this condition. Cause of death: severe metabolic acidosis, cerebral edema, hemorrhages, or infections. Patients have survived since syndrome identified and further development may be normal.

BIBLIOGRAPHY. Holmes LB, Tanaka K, Budd MA, Isselbacher KJ, et al: Isovaleric acidemia (abstr). Soc Pediat Res 69:961, 1966

Naglak M, Salvo R, Madsen K, et al: The treatment of isovaleric acidemia with glycine supplement. Pediatr Res 34:9–13, 1988

Vockley J, Parimoo B, Tanaka K: Molecolar characterization of four different classes of mutations in isovaleryl-CoA dehydrogenase gene responsible for isovaleric acidemia. Am J Hum Genet 49:147–157, 1991

Sweetman Williams JC: Branched chain organic acidurias. In Scriver CR, Beaudet AL, Sly WS, et al: The Metabolic and Molecular Bases of Inherited Disease, 7th ed, pp 1387–1393. New York, McGraw-Hill, 1995

ISRAEL

Synonym. Hyperbilirubinemia shunt.

Symptoms and Signs. Prevalent in males; onset at 16–40 years of age. Modest signs of anemia and jaundice; 50% with splenomegaly, without hepatomegaly.

Etiology. Autosomic recessive inheritance. Primitive increase of early labeled bilirubin diphasic or multiphasic. The first (diphasic) deriving from nonerythropoietic source; the second (multiphasic) from premature destruction of newly formed erythrocytes.

Pathology. *Spleen.* Enlarged, no remarkable changes; little deposit of iron pigment. *Liver.* Heavy infiltration of brown pigment in granules of irregular size and shape into parenchymal cells. Kupffer cells increased and pigment loaded. *Bone marrow.* Erythroblastic hyperplasia.

Diagnostic Procedures. *Blood.* Anemia; reticulocytosis (2–5%). Occasionally, spherocytosis. Autohemolysis and mechanical fragility of red cells normal. Red cell survival normal or reduced. Moderate hyperbilirubinemia (2–7 mg/100 ml); prevalent nonconjugated form. *Liver function test.* Normal. *Urine.* Urobilinogen increased. *Stool.* Stercobilinogen markedly increased.

Therapy. Hemolysis when present, corrected by splenectomy.

Prognosis. Persistent benign condition, hyperbilirubinemia persists after splenectomy and consequent correction of hemolysis and bone marrow hyperplasia.

BIBLIOGRAPHY. Kalk H, Wildhirt E: Die posthepatitische Hyperbilirubinaemie. Z Klink Med 153:354–387, 1955

Israel LG, Suderman HJ, Ritzmann SE: Hyperbilirubinemia due to an alternate path of bilirubin production. Am J Med 27:693–702, 1959

Berk PD, Noyer C: Hereditary hyperbilirubinemias. In Haubrich WS,

Schaffner F, Berk JE (eds): Bockus Gastroenterology, 5th ed, vol 2, p 1906. Philadelphia, WB Saunders, 1995

I.S.S.D.

Synonyms. Infantile free sialic acid storage disease. See Salla and sialiduria.

Symptoms. No ethnic predilection. Onset at birth. Failure to thrive; hypotonia; marked psychomotor delay.

Signs. Facial dysmorphism; edema and ascites; visceral enlargement; hypopigmentation of skin and hair; skeletal changes.

Etiology. Genetic defect of lysosomal membrane transport of free sialic acid.

Pathology. Widespread neuronal storage with myelin loss, axonal spheroids, and gliosis. Direct evidence for sialic acid accumulation in neuronal cells. Clear vacuoles in various visceral organs.

Therapy. Symptomatic.

Prognosis. Early death (within first year).

BIBLIOGRAPHY. Pueschel SM, O'Shea PA, Alroy J, et al: Infantile sialic acid storage disease associated with renal disease. Ped Neurol 4:207–212, 1988

Gahl WA, Schneider JA, Aula PP: Lysosomal transport disorders: Cystinosis and sialic acid storage disorders. In Scriver CR, Beaudet AL, Sly WS, et al: The Metabolic and Molecular Bases of Inherited Disease, 7th ed, pp 3787–3789. New York, McGraw-Hill, 1995

ITAI-ITAI

Synonyms. "Ouch-ouch."

Symptoms and Signs. In Japanese populations. Bone pains. Signs of chronic nephropathy and hyperuricemia and gout (see).

Etiology. Cadmium intoxication.

Pathology. Chronic tubulointerstitial nephritis; osteomalacia.

Diagnostic Procedures. *Blood.* Hyperuricemia. *Urine.* Hypercalciuria. *X-ray.* Osteomalacia.

Therapy. Tubular acidosis correction by sodium bicarbonate; chelating agents not useful in this situation. Only useful measure removal from exposure. Kidney transplantation may be considered.

Prognosis. According to degree of lesions and therapy.

BIBLIOGRAPHY. Thun MJ, Osorio AM, Shober S, et al: Nephropathy in cadmium workers: Assessment of risk from airborne occupational exposure to cadmium. Br J Ind Med 46:689–697, 1989

ITCHING PURPURA

Synonyms. Pruritic angiodermatitis; angiodermatitis pruriginosa, disseminata; eczematoid-like purpura. See Schamberg.

Symptoms. Prevalent in males; onset in adulthood. Pruritus around ankles, extending to entire legs and also, occasionally, elsewhere.

Signs. Purpuric lesions appearing on lower part of body. Typical orange color.

Etiology. Unknown.

Pathology. Perivascular inflammatory reaction in upper corium; endothelial swelling and lymphohistiocytic-red cell infiltration.

Therapy. None specific. Topical steroids with or without polyethylthene exclusion.

Prognosis. Spontaneous improvement in months. Frequent recurrences.

BIBLIOGRAPHY. Davis E: Schoenlein-Henoch syndrome of vascular purpura. Blood 3:129–136, 1948

Champion RH: Purpura. In Champion RH, Burton JL, Ebling FJG (eds): Rook/Wilkinson/Ebling Textbook of Dermatology, 5th ed, p 1889. Oxford, Blackwell Scientific, 1992

ITO

Synonym. Nevus depigmentosus systematicus bilateralis; incontinentia pigmenti achromians; hypomelanosis Ito. Confused with Naegeli syndrome.

Symptoms and Signs. Onset early in life and persisting for years. Progressive pigment loss without preceding inflammation. Sharply demarcated, linear or band-like, depigmented, bizarre macules. (Negative picture of pigmentation observed in patient with Bloch-Sulzburger.) Frequently associated: mental retardation; teeth abnormalities strabismus; alopecia; congenital dislocation of the hip.

Etiology. Highly heterogenic disorder association between pigmentary anomaly and chromosomal mosaicism. Autosomal dominant inheritance suggested in some families.

Pathology. Biopsy of lesion shows absence of inflammatory changes, decreased amount of granules of melanin in basal layer, epidermal melanocytes weaker in dopa reaction.

Prognosis. Lesions may disappear or remain for undetermined time.

BIBLIOGRAPHY. Blaschko A: Die Nervenveteilung in der Haut in ihrer Beziehung zu den Erkrankungen der Haut. Vienna, Leipzig Braumuller, 1901

Ito M: Studies on melanin. XI. Incontinentia pigmenti achromians: A singular case of nevus depigmentosus systematicus bilateralis. Tohoku J Exp Med (Suppl) 55:57–59, 1952

Rosemberg S, Arita FM, Campos C, et al: Hypomelanosis of Ito: Case report with involvement of the central nervous system and review of the literature. Neuropediatrics 15:52–55, 1984

Lungarotti MS, Martello C, Calabro A, et al: Hypomelanosis of Ito associated with chromosomal translocation involving X p11. Am J Med Genet 40:447–448, 1991

ITO NEVUS

Synonyms. Nevus of Ito; nevus fusco-caeruleus deltoideus.

Symptoms and Signs. Common in Japanese. Increased pigmentation in the shoulder area and upper chest.

Etiology. Unknown.

Pathology. See Ota.

Therapy. Cosmesis; short application of CO_2 snow may reduce hyperpigmentation.

BIBLIOGRAPHY. Ito M: Studies on melanin: XXII Naevus fusco-caeruleus acromio-deltoidus. Tohoku J Exper Med 60:10–20, 1954

IVE

Synonym. Actinic reticuloid.

Symptoms and Signs. Only males, elderly subjects. History of contact dermatitis and mild photosensitivity. Progressively increasing photosensitivity: erythema, edema, "leonine" aspect of areas exposed to light.

Etiology. Enhanced sensitivity to light: entire spectrum. Relationship to allergy to plants (particularly composite); light sensitivity and reticulosis not yet clarified.

Pathology. *Skin.* Intense superficial and deep infiltration of lymphocytes (some atypical). Collagen damaged.

Therapy. Light avoidance; sun screens; systemic mild steroid or azathioprine.

Prognosis. Recovery difficult (lifelong condition). Few cases evolve into frank Alibert-Bazin (see) or into squamous cell carcinoma (see Bowen).

BIBLIOGRAPHY. Ive FA, Magnus IA, Warin RP, et al: "Actinoid reticuloid": A chronic dermatosis associated with severe photosensitivity and the histological resemblance to lymphoma. Br J Dermat 81:469–485, 1969

Campbell RJ: Tumors of the eyelids, conjunctiva and cornea. In Garner A, Klintworth GK (eds): Pathobiology of ocular disease: A dynamic approach, 2nd ed, pp 1370–1371. New York, Marcel Dekker, 1994

IVEMARK

Synonyms. Asplenia; congenital spleen absence; splenic agenesis.

Symptoms. Prevalent in males. Maternal pregnancy history and familial history occasionally significant. Dyspnea; retardation of growth.

Signs. Cyanosis from neonatal period; clubbing of fingers and toes in oldest patients. Systolic cardiac murmur diffuse along left sternal border in about 50% of patients. Symptoms and signs are of no value in differentiating this form from other types of cyanotic heart diseases.

Etiology. Unknown. Most cases sporadic. Maternal virus infection during pregnancy and familial form reported with autosomal recessive inheritance.

Pathology. Asplenia or hypoplasia of spleen; pulmonary stenosis or atresia (100%); ostium primum atrial septal defect (100%); transposition of great vessels (95%); persistent complete atrioventricular canal (95%); bilateral superior venae cavae (85%); infundibular inversion (85%); common atrium (80%); anomalous pulmonary venous connection (75%). Cases may be subdivided as follows: Those with two ventricles and large ventricular septal defect; those with common ventricle.

Diagnostic Procedures. *Spleen scan.* Absence of spleen. *Blood.* Signs of asplenia; normoblast and presence of Howell-Jolly and normoblast and presence of Howell-Jolly and Heinz bodies. *ECG.* Features of persistent common atrioventricular canal. *X-ray.* Hepatic symmetry; diminished pulmonary blood flow; transposed blood vessels. *CT scan. MRI. Ultrasonography.*

Prognosis. For patient with these lesions, no indication for surgery. Death at young age from heart failure, overwhelming bacterial infections; in oldest patient (19 years) multiple systemic thrombosis was cause of death.

BIBLIOGRAPHY. Martin MG: Observation d'une deviation organique de l'estomac, d'une anomalie dans la situation, dans la configuration du coeur et des vaisseaux qui en partent on qui s'y rendent. Bull Soc Anat Paris 1:39, 1826

Ivemark BI: Implications of agenesis of the spleen on the pathogenesis of conotruncus anomalies in childhood: An analysis of the heart malformations in the splenic agenesis syndrome with fourteen new cases. Acta Paediatr 44 (Suppl 104):1–110, 1955

Van Praagh S, Santini F, Sanders SP: Cardiac malposiitions with special emphasis on visceral heterotaxy (asplenia and polysplenia syndromes). In Fyler DC (ed) Nadas' Pediatric Cardiology. Philadelphia, Hanley-Belfus, 1992

IVEMARK II

Synonyms. Asplenia—kidney, liver, pancreas dysplasia. See Polycystic, prevalent renal cystic syndrome, infantile type.

Symptoms and Signs. See Ivemark I and Polycystic, prevalent renal cystic syndrome, infantile type.

Etiology. Autosomal recessive lethal disorders.

BIBLIOGRAPHY. Ivemark BI, Oldfeld V, Zetterstrom R: Familial dysplasia of kidneys, liver, and pancreas: A probable genetically determined syndrome. Acta Paediatr 48:1–11, 1959
Crawford MDA: Renal dysplasia and aplasia in two sibs. Clin Genet 14:338–344, 1978
Van Praagh S, Santini F, Sanders SP: Cardiac malpositions with special emphasis on visceral heterotaxy (asplenia and polysplenia syndromes). In Fyler DC (ed): Nadas' Pediatric Cardiology. Philadelphia, Hanley-Belfus, 1992

IVEMARK III

Symptoms and Signs. Polyasplenia. Associated with caudal deficiency including imperforate anus, ambiguous external genitalia, contractures of lower limbs with short femura and neurological symptoms owing to agenesis of corpus callosum.

Etiology. May be a variant of Ivemark or represent a distinct autosomal recessive entity.

BIBLIOGRAPHY. Rodriguez JI, Palacios J, Omenaka F, et al. Polyasplenia caudal deficiency and agenesis of corpus callosum. Am J Med Genet 38:99–102, 1991
Van Praagh S, Santini F, Sanders SP: Cardiac malpositions with special emphasis on visceral heterotaxy (asplenia and polysplenia syndromes). In Fyler DC (ed): Nadas' Pediatric Cardiology. Philadelphia, Hanley-Belfus, 1992

IVES-HOUSTON

Synonyms. Microcephaly; micromelia.

Symptoms and Signs. In Cree-Indians (Canada). Stillborn or severe recurrent apneic episodes. Intrauterine growth retardation. Severe microcephaly. Short palpebral fissures, microphthalmia, prominent nose, micrognathia, microstomia. *Limbs.* Fixed elbows, short forearms; hands abnormalities; legs less severely affected. Variable additional skeletal anomalies.

Etiology. Autosomal recessive inheritance.

Pathology. *Brain.* Small with only primary sulci and gyri. Absence of corpus callosum.

Prognosis. Usually, stillborn or early death for apnea.

BIBLIOGRAPHY. Ives EJ, Houston CS: Autsomal recessive microcephaly and micromelia in Cree Indians. Am J Med Genet 7:351–360, 1980

I.V.I.C.

(Acronym for Istituto Venezolano Investigationes Cientificas)

Synonyms. Radial ray defects; deafness; internal ophthalmoplegia; thrombocytopenia.

Symptoms and Signs. From birth. In most cases strabismus, deafness, and occasional upper limb radial ray defect (from almost normal thumbs to thumbs with longer metacarpal and shorter phalanx). Radial bone always affected. In a few cases imperforated anus.

Etiology. Autosomal dominant inheritance.

Diagnostic Procedures. *Blood.* Thrombocytopenia (mild); leukocytosis (mild).

Prognosis. Fair.

BIBLIOGRAPHY. Arias S, Penchaszadeh VB, Pinto-Cisternas J, et al: The IVIC syndrome: A new autosomal dominant complex pleiotropic syndrome with radial ray hypoplasia, hearing impairment, internal ophthalmoplegia, thrombocytopenia. Am J Med Genet 6:25–29, 1980
Sammito V, Motta D, Capodieci G, et al: IVIC syndrome: Report of a second family. Am J Med Genet 29:875–881, 1988
Czeizel A, Goblyos P, Kodaj I: IVIC syndrome: Report of a third family. Am J Med Genet 33:282–283, 1989

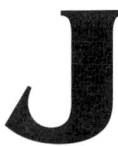

JABS-BLAUS

Synonym. Granulomatous synovitis—uveitis—cranial neuropathies, familial; synovitis—granulomatous—uveitis—cranial neuropathies. See Rotenstein.

Symptoms and Signs. Onset; childhood. Granulomatous synovitis; symmetric, boggy polysynovitis of the hands and wrists, resulting in boutonniere deformities. Recurrent nongranulomatous acute iridocyclitis. *Cranial neuropathies.* Bilateral neurosensory hearing loss; 6th cranial nerve palsy.

Etiology. Hereditary syndrome with an autosomal dominant inheritance pattern.

Diagnostic Procedures. *Synovectomy specimens.* Granulomatous inflammation with giant cells. *X-rays of hand.* No erosions or joint destruction.

Therapy. Corticosteroids (both local and systemic administration). Mydriatics.

Prognosis. The major long-term problems are iritis and joint contractures.

BIBLIOGRAPHY. Jabs DA, Honk JL, Bias WB, et al: Familial granulomatous synovitis, uveitis and cranial neuropathies. Am J Med 78:801–804, 1985
Blaus EB: Familial granulomatous arthritis, iritis and rash. J Pediatr 107:689–693, 1985
Pastores GM, Michels VV, Stickler GB, et al: Autosomal dominant granulomatous arthritis, uveitis skin rash and synovial cysts. J Pediat 117:403–408, 1990

JACCOUD (S.)

Synonym. Arthritis deforming, not erosive; post-rheumatic fever arthritis, systemic lupus arthritis.

Symptoms and Signs. After severe repeated attacks of rheumatic fever, development of articular changes, especially of metacarpophalangeal joints: ulnar deviation, followed by subluxation with little pain and minor mobility loss.

Etiology. Unknown; possibly, consequence of rheumatic fever or rheumatoid arthritis (see Diagnostic Procedures).

Pathology. Progressive periarticular fibrosis of selected joints.

Diagnostic Procedures. *Blood.* Rheumatoid factor seldom present. All features of acute rheumatic fever.

Therapy. Antibiotics; anti-inflammatory agents.

Prognosis. Long course. Characteristically, joint deformities may be voluntarily corrected by the patient.

BIBLIOGRAPHY. Jaccoud S: Leçons de Clinique Médicale Faites à l'Hôpital de la Charitaé, 2nd ed. Paris, Delahaye, 1869
Beausang E, Barnett E, Goldstein S: Jaccoud's arthritis. Ann Rheum Dis 26:239–245, 1967
Bittle JA, Perloff JK: Chronic post-rheumatic fever arthropathy of Jaccoud. Am Heart J 105:515–517, 1983
Gladman DD, Urowitz MB: Systemic lupus erythematosus. In Klippel JH, Dieppe PA: Rheumatology, p 6.2.4. St Louis, CV Mosby, 1994

JACKSON II

Synonyms. Hughlings Jackson; McKenzie; Jackson paralysis; vago-accessory-hypoglossal.

Symptoms and Signs. Paralysis of half of soft palate and larynx, sternocleidomastoid and trapezius muscles; hemiatrophy of tongue. Tachycardia.

Etiology and Pathology. Paralysis of vagus (X), spinal accessory (XI), and hypoglossal (XII) nerves usually owing to vascular lesion, seldom neoplasia, trauma, or infections; affecting one lateral half of medulla oblongata at the level of the hypoglossus, ambiguous and spinal nuclei or pathways of the above-mentioned cranial nerves.

BIBLIOGRAPHY. Jackson JH: Paralysis of tongue, palate, and vocal cord. Lancet I:689–690, 1886
Adams RD, Victor M: Principles of Neurology, 5th ed, pp 1180–1181. New York, McGraw-Hill, 1993

JACKSON-BARR

Synonyms. Deafness (conductive)—ptosis—skeletal anomalies.

Symptoms and Signs. Two sisters. Atresia of external auditory canal and middle ear space; chronic infection, ptosis. Nose: thin and pinched; delayed hair growth; dysplastic teeth; skeletal abnormalities.

Etiology. Autosomal recessive inheritance (?).

BIBLIOGRAPHY. Jackson LG, Barr MA: Conductive deafness with ptosis and skeletal malformations in sibs: A probable autosomal recessive disorder. Birth Defects Orig Art Ser 14(6B):199–204, 1978

JACKSON CEREBELLAR

Synonyms. Wurffbain; cerebellar seizures; cerebellar epilepsy.

Symptoms and Signs. Both sexes affected; onset at all ages. Seizure occasionally preceded by a loud cry. Head drawn back and back curved; no twitching of face or deviation of eyeballs. Hands clenched; forearms flexed; upper arm (usually) kept to the sides; legs extended; feet arched backward. Urine and fecal loss (occasional). Between attacks, persistent hyperextended posture remains (cerebellar attitude).

Etiology. Midline cerebellar tumor. Brain stem lesions are also considered necessary for occurrence of these seizures.

Pathology. Neoplastic, inflammatory, vascular lesions with cerebellar involvement and brain stem lesions.

Diagnostic Procedures. *Angiography. EEG. CT brain scan. MRI.*

Therapy. According to etiology.

Prognosis. Depends on etiology.

BIBLIOGRAPHY. Jackson JH: Case of tumor of the middle lobe of the cerebellum: Cerebellar paralysis with rigidity (cerebellar attitude), occasional tetanus-like seizures. Brain 29:425–440, 1906
Fulton JF: A case of cerebellar tumor with seizures of head retraction described by Wurffbain in 1691. J Nerv Ment Dis 70:577–583, 1929
Dow RS, Moruzzi G: The Physiology and Pathology of the Cerebellum. Minneapolis, Univ of Minnesota Press, 1958

JACKSONIAN

Synonyms. Jackson I; Bravais-Jackson; focal epilepsy.

Symptoms. Contraction starts from a focus such as tip of toe, finger, corner of mouth, and then gradually spreads to other muscles. If it remains hemilateral, consciousness is preserved.

Etiology and Pathology. Organic brain diseases are usually recognized as responsible for this type of epilepsy (e.g., neoplastic, vascular lesion).

Therapy. Surgical removal of lesion; diphenylhydantoin; phenobarbital; carbamazepine; felbamate.

Prognosis. Depends on etiology.

BIBLIOGRAPHY. Bravais LF: Recherches sur les symptomes et le Traitement de l'Épilepsie Haemiplégique, Paris (thesis), 1827
Jackson JH: Epileptiform convulsions from cerebral disease. Trans Int Med Congr 2:6–15, 1881
Faught E, Sachdeo RC, Remler MP, et al: Felbamate monotherapy for partial onset seizures: An active control trial. Neurology 43:688–692, 1993

JACKSON-LAWLER

Synonyms. Murray; pachyonychia congenita. See Jadassohn-Lewandowsky.

Symptoms and Signs. Both sexes affected, male predilection (9:5); present from birth. Hoarse voice; natal teeth (poor calcification; occasionally, erupted at birth). Pachyonychia; palmoplantar hyperkeratosis and hyperhydrosis; follicular keratosis; large epidermoid cysts on the head, neck, upper chest (onset at puberty); corneal dystrophy; absence of oral leukokeratosis. During warm weather bullae appear on feet; painful and easily infected.

Etiology. Unknown; autosomal dominant inheritance.

Pathology. Skin thickened, acanthosis, parakeratosis follicles and pores dilated and plugged with horny material. Electron microscopy shows findings consistent with defect in keratinization.

Diagnostic Procedures. Skin biopsy.

Therapy. Kerotolytic agents.

Prognosis Permanent condition.

BIBLIOGRAPHY. Murray FA: Four cases of hereditary hypertrophy of the nail bed associated with a history of erupted teeth at birth. Br J Dermatol 33:409–411, 1921
Jackson ADM, Lawler SD: Pachyonychia congenita: A report of six cases in one family. Ann Eugen 16:142–146, 1951
Gorlin RJ, Cohen MM Jr, Levin LS: Syndromes of the Head and Neck, 3rd ed, pp 445–448. New York, Oxford Univ Press, 1990

JACKSON-WEISS

Synonyms. See Apert, Crouzon, Pfeiffer; Saethre-Chotzen.

Symptoms and Signs. Both sexes. From birth. *Facies:* Midfacial hypoplasia, craniosynostosis. *Limbs.* Abnormalities of feet (cutaneous syndactyly between second and third and great toes).

Etiology. Autosomal dominant inheritance with high penetrance and variability in expression.

Diagnostic Procedures. *X-rays.* Of feet: most consistent finding: short, broad first metatarsal, abnormal tarsal bone, calcaneocuboid fusion, and occasionally fusion of II and I metatarsal and/or II and III.

BIBLIOGRAPHY. Jackson CE, Weiss L, Reynold WA: Craniosynostosis, mid-

facial hypoplasia, and foot abnormalities: An autosomal dominant phenotype in a large Amish kindred. J Pediatr 88:963–968, 1976
Cohen MM Jr: Craniosynostosis: Diagnosis evaluation and management. Raven Press, New York, 1986
Gorlin RJ, Cohen MM Jr, Levin LS: Syndromes of Head and Neck, 3rd ed, pp 529–531. New York, Oxford Univ Press, 1990

JACOB-DOWNEY

Synonyms. Arthropathy—camptodactyly; E family arthritis; hypertrophic synovitis congenita familial. Including campodactyly; arthropathy—pericarditis; CAP; PAC: arthropathy—campodactly—pericarditis.

Symptoms and Signs. Both sexes. At birth, flexor contracture of fingers, camptodactyly; polyarticular large joint arthritis in early infancy.

Etiology. Autosomal recessive inheritance. Manifestation of pericarditis.

Pathology. Synovial membrane: hyperplasia, necrotic villi deposits of eosinophilic and periodic acid-Schiff positive material, presence of multinucleated giant cells.

Therapy. Synovectomy when needed.

Prognosis. Spontaneous tendency to regression in older age.

BIBLIOGRAPHY. Jacob JC, Downey JA: Juvenile rheumatoid arthritis. In Downey JA, Low NL: The Child with Disabling Illness, p 524. Philadelphia, WB Saunders, 1974
Di Liberti JM, McKean R, Hecht F: Progressive tenosynovitis with contractures and possible systemic involvement: A new heritable disorder of connective tissue? Birth Defects Orig Art Ser 11(6):81–82, 1975
Laxer RM, Cameron BJ, Chaisson D, et al: The campodactyly-arthropathy-pericarditis syndrome: Case report and literature review. Arthritis Rheum 29:439–444, 1986

JACOB (J.C.)

Synonym. Brachial plexus neuritis; cleft palate.

Symptoms and Signs. Both sexes affected; present from birth. Facial asymmetry; mongoloid slant of palpebrae; hypotelorism; cleft palate (similarity with a Modigliani portrait). At 3 years of age, often after a minor infection: sudden pain in the shoulder, radiating to arm and hand and gradually subsiding; leaving paresthesia and weakness; after repeated attacks, sensory loss, limitation of elbow extension. The legs are involved only in case of severe arm compromise.

Etiology. Autosomal dominant inheritance with hight penetrance. Palsy precipitated by exogenous factors because of abnormalities of Schwann cells.

Pathology. Nerve biopsy; tomaculous neuropathy.

Diagnostic Procedures. *Electromyography.* Partial denervation of some arm and hand muscles.

BIBLIOGRAPHY. Jacob JC, Andermann F, Robb, JP: Heredofamilial neuritis and brachial predilection. Neurology (Minneapolis) 11:1025–1033, 1961
Erickson A: Hereditary syndrome consisting in recurrent attacks resembling brachial plexus neuritis, special facial features and cleft palate. Acta Paediatr Scand 63:855–888, 1974
Araksinen EM, Iivanainen M, Karli P, et al: Hereditary recurrent brachial plexus neuropathy with dysmorphic features. Acta Neurol Scand 71:309–316, 1985
Phillips LH II: Familial long thoracic nerve palsy: A manifestation of brachial plexus neuropathy. Neurology 36:1251–1253, 1986

JACOBS (E.C.)

Synonyms. Genital oculo oral; oculogenital; oro-oculogenital.

Symptoms. Intense burning and itching of the scrotum; conjunctivitis; stomatitis; fissuring of alae nasi.

Signs. Scrotal dermatitis and pigmentation with scaling and superficial ulceration.

Etiology. Riboflavin deficiency and other vitamin B complex components and zinc. Local inflammation may play a role. (In prisoners of war, also other causes of malnutrition.) Prolonged antibiotic treatment.

Diagnostic Procedures. *Blood.* Anemia; other signs of malnutrition.

Therapy. Diet and vitamin B complex.

Prognosis. Complete recovery with treatment.

BIBLIOGRAPHY. Jacobs EC: Oculo-oro-genital syndrome: a deficiency disease. Ann Intern Med 35:1049–1054, 1951

Klintworth GK: Vitamin deficiency and excesses. In Garner A, Klintworth GK (eds): Pathobiology of Ocular Disease: A Dynamic Approach, 2nd ed, p 1153. New York, Marcel Dekker, 1994

JACOBSEN

Synonyms. SED tarda; X-linked; spondyloepiphyseal dysplasia tarda; X-linked spondyloepiphyseal dysplasia.

Symptoms and Signs. Occurs only in males. Changes become evident at 5–10 years of age. Pain in the back and hip. Dwarfish short trunk variety. Limbs relatively long. Female may present arthritic complaints.

Etiology. Unknown; sex-linked inheritance. SED tarda locus on Xq28 band or Xp22.

Pathology. Degenerative changes of cartilage.

Diagnostic Procedures. *X-ray of spine.* Posterior portion of superior plate of vertebrae is "humped" (distinctive feature). Osteoarthrosis of other joints (hips, knees, shoulders) is precocious.

Therapy. Symptomatic.

Prognosis. Progressive condition. Disabling polyarthrosis in the fourth to fifth decade.

BIBLIOGRAPHY. Nilsonne H: Eigentuemliche Wirbelkorper-veraenderungen mit familiaerem Auftreten. Acta Chir Scand 62:550–554, 1927

Jacobsen AW: Hereditary osteochondrodystrophia deformans: A family with 20 members affected in 5 generations. JAMA 113:121–124, 1939

Iceton JA, Horne G: Spondilo-epiphyseal dysplasia tarda: The X-linked variety in three brothers. J Bone Joint Surg 68b:616–619, 1986

Rimoin DL, Lachman RS: Genetic disorders of the osseous skeleton. In Beithon P (ed): McKusick's Heritable Disorders of Connective Tissue, 5th ed, p 615. St Louis, CV Mosby, 1993

JACOBSEN-BRODWALL

Synonyms. Oculo-oto-reno anemia; reno-oculo-oto-oro anemia; oculo-oto-oro-reno anemia; oro-oculo-oto-reno anemia; oto-oculo-oro-reno anemia.

Symptoms. One case in female reported; present from birth. Dizziness; weakness; hearing loss (neurogenic); progressive visual loss up to blindness. Abdominal colic.

Signs. Pallor. Atypical development of periodontium and caries; high arched palate. Glaucoma; iridocyclitis; cataract. Genu valgum and pes excavatus.

Etiology. Has not been classified. Possibly, genetic defect.

Pathology. Renal biopsy shows dysplasia with smooth muscle in parenchyma and absent Henle loops.

Diagnostic Procedures. *Blood.* Hypochromic anemia; anisocytosis; and few target cells. *Urine.* Lack of concentration. *Bone marrow.* Increased erythropoiesis. *X-ray of skull.* Enlargement of lateral and third ventricles. *EEG.* Possible changes in medial structures; generalized dysrhythmia. *Kidney function test.* Altered. *Ophthalmoscopy.* Mild macular changes, hemorrhages, and exudates.

Therapy. Symptomatic; blood transfusion.

Prognosis. Slowly progressive to blindness and severe kidney insufficiency (patient age 28 at time of report).

BIBLIOGRAPHY. Jacobsen CD, Brodwall EK: A clinical syndrome with inborn defect in erythropoiesis, dysplastic kidneys, eye lesions, malformation of the teeth and impaired hearing: a new syndrome in a 28-year-old woman. Acta Med Scand 195:231–235, 1974

Geeraets AJ: Ocular Syndromes, 3rd ed. Philadelphia, Lea & Febiger, 1976

JACOD

Synonyms. Jacod-Rollett, Silvio Negri; Negri-Jacod; petrosphenoidal carrefour; retrosphenoidal paralysis; retrosphenoidal space; see orbital apex and Rochon-Davigneau (often confused with).

Symptoms and Signs. Unilateral trigeminal neuralgia (second branch area, then third branch) and optic tract lesion (unilateral amaurosis); total unilateral ophthalmoplegia; sometimes optic (II), oculomotor (III), and trochlear (VI) nerves may escape. Then deafness (middle ear type) and palatal muscle paralysis. Unilateral or bilateral cervical nodes involved in 30% of cases.

Etiology and Pathology. Neoplastic lesion, primary or metastatic beginning at medial part of medial cranial fossa, near cavernous sinus; expanding to foramen rotundum, foramen ovale, superior orbital fissure (optic foramen) to the base of skull, involving eustachian tubes and palatal muscles; total loss of function of optic (II), oculomotor (III), trochlear (IV), trigeminal (V), and abducens (VI) nerves.

Diagnostic Procedures. *X-ray. CT brain scan. MRI.*

Therapy. Deep X-rays.

Prognosis. Extremely poor.

BIBLIOGRAPHY. Jacod M: Sur la propagation intracranienne de sarcomes de la trompe d'Eustache, syndrome du carrefour pétrosphenoidal paralysie des 2e, 3e, 5e, et 6e pairs craniennes. Rev Neurol 28:33–38, 1921

Adams RD, Victor M: Principles of Neurology, 5th ed, p 1172. New York, McGraw-Hill, 1993

JACQUET

Synonyms. Alopecia reflex; circumscribed congenital alopecia. Includes alopecia oerata; vertical alopecia; triangular alopecia (or Sabouraud alopecia). See also Christ-Siemens-Touraine.

Signs. Circumscribed alopecia occurring in association with several other ectodermal dysplasias (e.g., nail, dental, see Hallermann-Streiff, Pseudopelade, Bloch-Sulzberger, and others), or associated with epidermal nevi (most common form). Alopecia may be present at birth, or develop in first month of life not preceded by apparent inflammatory changes.

Etiology. Autosomal dominant inheritance reported; autoimmune mechanism suggested.

BIBLIOGRAPHY. Jacquet L: Les rapports de la pelade avec lésions dentaires. Presse Med 8:327, 1900

Valsecchi R, Vicari O, Frigeni A, et al: Familial alopecia areata—genetic susceptibility or coincidence? Acta Derm Venereol 65:175–177, 1985

Zlotogorski A, Weinrauch L, Brautbar C: Familial alopecia aerata: No linkage with HLA. Tiss Ant 35:40–41, 1990

Dawber RPR, Ebling FJG, Wojnarowska FT: Disorders of hair. In Champion RH, Burton JL, Ebling FJG (eds): Rook/Wilkinson/Ebling Textbook of Dermatology, 5th ed, p 2580. Oxford, Blackwell Scientific, 1992

JACQUET

Synonyms. Diaper papular rash; nappy rash of neglect; papulo-ulcerative rash.

Symptoms and Signs. In infants, in diaper area papular rash.

Etiology. Long contact with urine and feces causing skin maceration and promoting secondary infections.

Therapy. Hygienic measures.

Prognosis. Cure with preventive measures; possible scars.

BIBLIOGRAPHY. Jacquet L: Des érythémes papuleux fessiers post-érosifs. Rev Mal Enf 4:208–218, 1886

Cooke JV: Dermatitis of the diaper region in infants. Arch Dermatol 14:539–546, 1926

Ive FA: The umbilical, perianal and genital regions. In Champion RH, Burton JL, Ebling FJG (eds): Rook/Wilkinson/Ebling Textbook of Dermatology, 5th ed, p 2883. Oxford, Blackwell Scientific, 1992

JADASSOHN

Synonym. Solomon; Schimmelpennig; Feuerstein-Mims; epidermal nevus; nevus phacomatosis; nevus sebaceus linear; choristoma—convulsions; mental retardation, linear nevus sebaceus; organoid nevus; including Comedo-cataract. See CHILD.

Symptoms. Onset at birth. Nevus sebaceous on scalp or face (midline); convulsion and mental retardation developing during early childhood; failure to thrive. Symptoms related to association with various malignancies, endocrine disorders, cardiac, vascular (coarctation of aorta), urogenital malformations, and ocular abnormalities (33%).

Signs. Nevus sebaceus: smooth, yellowish papules and nodules in well-delimited patches. In the first stage: alopecia with small hypoplastic sebaceus glands that later (during puberty) became verrucous with hyperplastic sebaceus glands. Occasionally hydrocephalus, and the variable, mentioned abnormalities and deformities.

Etiology. Unknown; congenital abnormality. Normal chromosomal studies. In some instances inherited autosomal dominant inheritance.

Pathology. Microscopic examination of skin lesion: thickening and hyperkeratosis of epidermis and hyperplasia of sebaceous glands (normal in appearance) increased in vascularity of dermis.

Diagnostic Procedures. *Biopsy of skin.* See Pathology. *EEG.* Focal abnormalities. *X-ray of skull.* Normal. *CATscan. MRI.* Lateral ventricular enlargement.

Therapy. Treatment of epilepsy (see).

Prognosis. Repeated infections; occasionally, seizures, failure to thrive. Skin lesion subject to malignant transformation.

BIBLIOGRAPHY. Jadassohn J, Lewandowsky F, Neisser A, et al: Ikonographia Dermatologica. Berlin, Urban Schwarzenburg, 1906

Feuerstein RC, Mims LC: Linear nevous sebaceus with convulsions and mental retardation. Am J Dis Child 104:675–679, 1962

Marden PM, Venters HD: A new neurocutaneous syndrome. Am J Dis Child 112:79–81, 1966

Monahan RH, Hill CW, Venters HD: Multiple choristomas, convulsions and mental retardation as a new neurocutaneous syndrome. Am J Ophthalmol 64:529–532, 1967

Sahl WJ Jr: Familial nevus sebaceus of Jodassohn: Occurrence in three generations. J Am Acad Dermatol 22:853–854, 1990

Atherton DJ: Naevi and other developmental defects. In Champion RH, Burton JL, Ebling FJG (eds): Rook/Wilkinson/Ebling Textbook of Dermatology, 5th ed, pp 460–462. Oxford, Blackwell Scientific, 1992

JADASSOHN-LEWANDOWSKY

Synonyms. Jackson-Lewandowsky; pachyonychia congenita. See Jackson-Lawler (possible variant expression of same condition).

Symptoms and Signs. Both sexes affected; evident at birth or developing in early infancy. Nails of fingers and toes. A yellow wedge-like thickening and prominent transverse curve, inflammatory changes, and nail shedding occur frequently. Teeth may be already erupted at birth; occasionally corneal dyskeratosis. Keratoderma of palms and soles appear in second or third year. Hyperhidrosis with bullae, occasionally developing on toes, edges of foot, and ankles. Horny papules in the extremities, face. Leukoplakia of oral and anal mucosa frequently develop in second decade. Hair normal or abundant, or hypotrichosis. Subdivided into four clinical types.

Etiology. Unknown; autosomal dominant inheritance with variable penetrance. Cases with recessive forms also described.

Pathology. Subungual keratosis; various dyskeratosis features.

Therapy. None. Watch for possible malignant changes of leukoplakias.

Prognosis. If nails are removed, they regrow abnormally. Slowly progressing condition.

BIBLIOGRAPHY. Jadassohn J, Lewandowsky F, Neisser A, Jacobi E: Ikonographia Dermatologica, pp 29–31. Berlin, Urban & Schwarzenburg, 1906

Young LL, Lenox JA: Pachyonychia congenita: a long term evaluation. Oral Surg 36:663–666, 1973

Stieglitz JB, Centerwall WR: Pachyonychia congenita (Jadassohn-Lewandowsky syndrome): A seventeen member, four generation pedigree with unusual respiratory and dental involvement. Am J Med Genet 14:21–28, 1983

Dawber RPR, Baran R: Disorders of the nails. In Champion RH, Burton JL, Ebling FJG (eds): Rook/Wilkinson/Ebling Textbook of Dermatology, 5th ed, pp 2530–2531. Oxford, Blackwell Scientific, 1992

JADASSOHN-PELLIZZARI

Obsolete.

Synonyms. Pellizzari-Jadassohn; macular atrophy; dermatitis atrophicans maculosa. See Anetoderma and Schweninger-Buzzi.

Symptoms and Signs. Characterizing feature is that the specific lesions are preceded by erythema or urticaria. Predominant in women; onset usually in second to fourth decade. Crops of round-oval, pink, small maculae usually on trunk and extremities, seldom on face or neck. Larger erythema plaques may be present.

Etiology. Focal elastolysis owing to release of elastase from inflammatory cells. Inflammatory onset that distinguishes this syndrome from Schweninger-Buzzi, in which there is no such sequence. Distinction between the two forms today seems of historical interest only.

Pathology. Early edema and perivascular lymphocytic infiltrates of dermis. Later, flattening of epidermis, fragmentation, and disappearance of elastic fibers, leaving cone-shaped areas.

Diagnostic Procedures. *Biopsy.*

Therapy. Some cases respond to penicillin during the inflammatory stage, later no treatment effective.

Prognosis. Slow fading with residual maculae of atrophic skin, yielding to pressure, admitting finger in a sort of ring; defect remaining for life.

BIBLIOGRAPHY. Pellizzari C: Eritema orticato atrofizzante; atrofia parziale idiopatica della pelle. Gior Ital Mal Ven 19:230–243, 1884
Jadassohn J: Ueber eine eigenartige Form von Atrophia maculosa cutis. Verh Dtsch Dermatol Ges, pp 342–358, 1891
Burton JL: Disorders of connective tissue. In Champion RH, Burton JL, Ebling FJG (eds): Rook/Wilkinson/Ebling Textbook of Dermatology, 5th ed, p 1773. Oxford, Blackwell Scientific, 1992

JAFFE-CAMPANACCI

Synonyms. Non-ossifying fibromas; von Recklinhausen; von Recklinghausen—nonosteogenic fibromas.

Symptoms. Both sexes. History of pathologic fractures before puberty. Localized pain; possible mild mental retardation.

Signs. Localized swelling; multiple café-au-lait spots; neurofibromas. Occasionally, eye anomalies, hypogonadism or precocious puberty; alopecia, and congenital heart malformations.

Etiology. Possibly related to type VII neurofibromatosis (see), genetically heterogeneous.

Pathology. Biopsy of bone lesion: cellular fibrous tumor with a whorled pattern and focal collection of foamy histiocytes, giant cells and hemosiderin.

Diagnostic Procedures. *X-rays. CT scan.* Multiple osteolytic lesions involving cortex and medulla of long bones and pelvis, fractures and kiphoscoliosis.

Therapy. Orthopedic treatment, bone grafting.

Prognosis. Fractures heal with routine treatment. Possible residual deformities.

BIBLIOGRAPHY. Jaffe HL: Tumors and Tumorous Conditions of Bones and Joints, pp 83–91. London, H Kimpton, 1958
Campanacci M, Lans M, Boriani S: Multiple nonossifying fibromata with extra skeletal anomalies: A new syndrome? J Bone Joint Surg (Br) 65:627–632, 1983
Steinmetz JC, Pilon VA, Lee JK: Jaffe-Campanacci syndrome. J Pediatr Orthop 8:602–604, 1988

JAFFE-LICHTENSTEIN

Synonyms. Jaffe II; Jaffe-Lichtenstein-Uehlinger; polyostotic fibrous dysplasia; monostotic fibrous dysplasia. See McCune-Albright.

Symptoms and Signs. Occurs in healthy children. Usually unilateral swelling, tenderness, and pain in one long bone or ribs, facial bone, or skull; leontiasis ossea appearance may be present; occasionally skin ulceration in overlying area; pathologic fractures; absence of systemic endocrine or other skeletal manifestations.

Etiology. Unknown; congenital anomaly or possibly disturbance of normal reparative process after trauma. Few instances of familial occurrence, autosomal dominant. Disorder owing to a mosaic state of an activating mutation in the GNAS 1 gene, which codes for a stimulatory adenosine triphosphate-dependent G protein.

Pathology. Solitary bone cyst usually affecting metaphyseal end of long bones; however, each single bone may be involved. Lacunar absorption of bone and fibrous replacement. Giant cells.

Diagnostic Procedures. *X-ray.* Cystic area in the bone cortex.

Shepherd crook deformity of femoral neck. *Blood.* Slight elevation of calcium and alkaline phosphatase occasionally observed.

Therapy. Osteotomy indicated to prevent fracture. Bone grafting indicated.

Prognosis. Excellent with treatment.

BIBLIOGRAPHY. Jaffe HL, Lichtenstein L: Non-osteogenic fibroma of bone. Am J Pathol 18:205–215, 1942
Ross DW, Vitale CC: Monostotic fibrous dysplasia of the metacarpal. J Bone Joint Surg (Am) 37:196–200, 1955
Rimoin DL, Lachman RS: Genetic disorders of the osseous skeleton. In Beithon P (ed): McKusick's Heritable Disorders of Connective Tissue, 5th ed, pp 672–673. St Louis, CV Mosby, 1993

JAFFE-LICHTENSTEIN-SUTRO

Synonyms. Jaffe I; pigmented villonodular synovitis; tendon sheath xanthogranuloma.

Symptoms. Pain in one or several of the large joints with functional limitation of articulation (knee most frequently affected). Absence of systemic symptoms.

Signs. Mild to moderate limitation of movement in joint affected by pain.

Etiology. Unknown. Aspecific inflammation, neoplasm, trauma have been suggested as causes.

Pathology. Formation of brownish moss-like villi or nodular proliferation of synovial membrane, localized or diffuse, in one joint or several articulations. Hyperplasia and proliferation of synovial lining cells. Large spindle-shaped stromal cells and multinuclear giant cells. Dark serohemorrhagic synovial fluid.

Diagnostic Procedures. *X-ray.* Biopsy synovial membrane. *Blood.* Rheumatoid arthritis (RA) test; sedimentation rate.

Therapy. Debridement of joint and arthroplasty.

Prognosis. Very benign process; good response to treatment.

BIBLIOGRAPHY. Jaffe HL, Lichtenstein L, Sutro CJ: Pigmented villonodular synovitis, and bursitis, tenosynovitis. A discussion of the synovial and bursal equivalents of the tenosynovial lesion commonly denoted as xanthoma, xanthogranuloma, giant-cell tumor, or myeloplaxoma of the tendon sheath, with some consideration of this tendon sheath lesion itself. Arch Pathol 31:731–765, 1941
Chung SMK, Jones JM: Diffuse pigmented villonodular synovitis of hip joint. J Bone Joint Surg (Am) 47:293–303, 1965
Richardson EG: Miscellaneous non traumatic disorders. In Crenshaw AH (ed): Campbell's Operative Orthopedics, 7th ed, pp 1006–1007. St Louis, CV Mosby, 1987

JAKE PARALYSIS

Symptoms and Signs. 1–3 weeks after injestion of contaminated products (see Etiology), soreness of lower leg muscle, numbness of toes and fingers few days later bilateral foot-drop and later bilateral wrist drop, no sensory changes.

Etiology. Drinking of extract of Jamaican ginger "jake" contaminated with triorthocresylphosphate (TOCP) (15,000 cases). Other epidemics have been reported in Morocco (10,000 cases from contaminated olive oil) and other regions of the world (grain, cooking oil, etc.). TOCP is toxic if ingested, inhaled, or contacted with skin.

Pathology. "Dying back" from terminal ends of largest medullated motor nerve fibers; degeneration of pyramidal tract anterior horn cells and peripheral motor nerves.

Diagnostic Procedures. *Blood.* Acetylcholinesterase level.

Therapy. Atropine; pralidoxime mesylate.

Prognosis. Recovery slow; residual paralysis depends on extent of neurological damage. Complete recovery possible.

BIBLIOGRAPHY. Smith MI, Elvove Frazier WH: The pharmacological actions of certain phenol esters with specific reference to the etiology of so called ginger paralysis. Publ Health Rep (Wash) 45:2509–2524, 1930
Nambe IT, Nalte CT, Jackerel J, et al: Poisoning due to organophosphate insecticides: acute and chronic manifestations. Am J Med 50:475, 1971
Gosselin RE, Smith RP, Hodge HC: Clinical Toxicology of Commercial Products, 5th ed. Baltimore, Williams & Wilkins, 1984

JAKSCH

Synonyms. Jaksch-Hayem-Luzet; von Jaksch; pseudoleukemic anemia infantilis.

Symptoms. Occurs in young children (under 3 years of age). Listlessness; weakness; gastrointestinal troubles; irregular fever.

Signs. Pallor; hepatosplenomegaly; lymphadenopathy.

Etiology and Pathology. Represents a symptom complex with a large variety of etiologic factors from malnutrition to infections, thalassemia, hemolytic diseases of newborn. This eponym, in view of better understanding of pathology of anemia in childhood, has become obsolete.

Diagnostic Procedures. Anemia; anisopoikilocytosis; leukocytosis with relative lymphocytosis.

Therapy and Prognosis. Depends on etiology.

BIBLIOGRAPHY. von Jaksch R: Ueber Leukämie und Leukocytose im Kindesalter. Wien Klin Wochenschr 2:435–437; 456–458, 1889

JALILI-SMITH

Synonyms. Cone rod dystrophy—amelogenesis imperfecta. Amelogenesis imperfecta—cone-rod dystrophy.

Symptoms. First years of life photophobia and nystagmus. Altered color vision. No night blindness.

Signs. Discoloration and abnormal shape of teeth.

Etiology. Autosomal recessive inheritance.

Pathology. Unknown.

Diagnostic Procedures. *Fundoscopy.* Characteristic bull-eye macula, spotty clumping of pigment in macula and posterior pole.

Therapy. None.

Prognosis. Achromotopsia; eventually blindness.

BIBLIOGRAPHY. Jalili IK, Smith NJD: A progressive cone-rod dystrophy and amelogenesis imperfecta: A new syndrome. J Med Genet 25:738–740, 1988

JAMAICAN VOMITING SICKNESS

Synonyms. Ackee fruit intoxication; intoxication ackee fruit.

Symptoms and Signs. Predominant in children, but also in adults. After ingestion of unripe ackee fruit, vomiting, convulsions, coma, and death.

Etiology. Intoxication by toxins (hypoglycins A and B) from unripe ackee fruit.

Pathology. Liver. Fatty infiltration.

Diagnostic Procedures. *Blood. Urine.* Findings, like those of glutaric aciduria type II (see).

Therapy. Supportive.

Prognosis. Death.

BIBLIOGRAPHY. Hill KR: The vomiting sickness of Jamaica: A review. W Ind Med J 1:243, 1952
Billington D, Osmundsen H, Sherratt HSA: The biochemical basis of Jamaican ackee poisoning. N Engl J Med 295:1482, 1976
Sherratt HSA, Al-Bassan SS: Glycine in ackee poisoning. Lancet II:1243, 1976
Cooper MR, Johnson AW: Poisonus plants and fungi. In Weatherall DJ, Ledingham JGG, Warrell DA (eds): Oxford Textbook of Medicine, 3rd ed, p 1159. Oxford, Oxford Med Pub, 1996

JANETTA

Synonyms. Disabling positional vertigo; vestibular paroxysmia; neurovascular compression—vertigo; octavus nerve neurovascular compression syndrome.

Symptoms and Signs. Constant positional vertigo or disabling lack of equilibrium and nausea (malignant vertigo) and occasionally vomiting, no hearing impairment (50%), no loss of vestibular function. Staggering, clumsiness, bumping into objects. Worsening of symptoms with physical activity with reduction or disappearance of symptoms with bed rest. Most of the drugs such as meclizine, dimenidrinate, scopolamine worsen symptoms. Occasionally tinnitus, more pronounced in one ear; ear pain. In 50% abnormal or absent acoustic middle ear reflexes. Spontaneous or positional nystagmus and reduced calori irrigation response.

Etiology and Pathology. Neurovascular compression of the eighth cranial nerve owing to vascular malformation or aneurysm of arterial fossa.

Diagnostic Procedures. *CT scan. MRI imaging. Cerebral arteriography. Caloric irrigation testing. Audiometry.*

Therapy. Carbamazepine may be effective. Surgery should be restricted to well diagnosed cases: microvascular decompression.

Prognosis. Good with surgery.

BIBLIOGRAPHY. Janetta PJ: Neurovascular cross-compression in patients with hyperactive dysfunction symptoms of the eighth cranial nerve. Surg Forum 26:467–468, 1975
Moeller MD: Controversy in Meniere's disease. Results of microvascular decompression of the eighth nerve. Ann J Otol 9:60–63, 1988
Brandt T: Vertigo: Its multisensory syndromes, pp 159–163. London, Springer-Verlag, 1991

JANEWAY LESIONS

Symptoms and Signs. Reddish macular spots in thenar and hypothenar areas observed in bacterial endocarditis.

BIBLIOGRAPHY. Janeway EG: Certain clinical observations upon heart disease. Med News 75:257–262, 1899

JANSEN

Synonyms. Murk Jansen; dysostosis enchondralis metaphysaria (type C-I); metaphyseal chondrodysplasia Jansen; spondylometaphyseal dysostosis (type C-I).

Symptoms and Signs. Both sexes affected. Dwarfism evident from childhood; variable deafness. Mental deficiency. Mild supraorbital frontonasal hyperplasia; micrognathia. Metaphysis of all bones affected with marked widening. Hands and feet not spared; short diaphysis. Squatting stance from flexion deformities of knee.

Etiology. Unknown; autosomal dominant inheritance. Most cases sporadic.

Pathology. Metaphysis enlarged, sponge-like and granite in appearance; epiphysis normal.

Diagnostic Procedures. *X-ray.* Abnormalities described; condyles and glenoid appear irregular. Vertebrae irregular, some cuneiform or with irregular contours. Hyperostosis of calvaria; thick dense skull base. *Blood.* Hypercalcemia, hypophosphatemia.

Therapy. Orthopedic.

Prognosis. Severe articular dysfunction.

BIBLIOGRAPHY. Jansen M: Ueber atypische Condrodystrophie (Achondroplasie) und über eine noch nicht beschriebene angeborene Wachstumsstöring des Knochensystems: Metaphysare Dysostosis. Orthop Chir 61:253–286, 1934

Silverthorn KG, Houston CS, Duncan BP: Murk Jansen's metaphyseal chondrodyplasia with long term follow-up. Pediatr Radiol 17:119–123, 1987

Rimoin DL, Lachman RS: Genetic disorders of the osseous skeleton. In Beithon P (ed) McKusick's Heritable Disorders of Connective Tissue, 5th ed, pp 627–630. St Louis, CV Mosby, 1993

JANSKY-BIELSCHOWSKY

Synonyms. Bielschowsky; Dollinger-Bielschowsky; amaurotic idiocy late infantile type; ceroid lipofuscinosis late infantilis; neuronal ceroid; lipofuscinosis, late infantilis; see ceroid lipofuscinosis.

Symptoms and Signs. Both sexes affected; onset at 2–4 years of age. Slightly retarded early development rather than mental development arrest. Early symptoms seizures, myoclonic jerks; then hypotonia, ataxia, visual impairment (not constant). Fundus oculi hypopigmentation, atrophy, discoloration of macula with yellow-gray areas (not constant). Liver and spleen not enlarged and no bone abnormalities. Later stage, severe dementia, muscle wasting. In early onset cases, microcephaly.

Etiology. Autosomal recessive inheritance. Disturbance of linoleic acid metabolism.

Pathology. Deposits of autoflourescent lipopigments in all tissues, predominant in the brain. *Brain.* Small, loss of nerve cells and status spongiosus; various sizes and structures of lipopigment deposits (lamellar, granular, "fingerprint" aspect), with acid phosphatase activity. *Retina.* Loss of cones and rods; degeneration of epithelial cells; lipoid pigment accumulation.

Diagnostic Procedures. *ERG.* Waveforms lost when retina compromised. *EEG.* High voltage; triphasic waves; later only delta waves. *CT scan. MRI.* Lateral ventricles slighly dilated. *Electron microscopy.* Of endocrine glands of skin. No enzyme deficiency has been yet demonstrated. *Bone marrow and other tissue biopsy.* Presence of lipopigments. *Urine.* Presence of lipopigments in sediment. *Blood.* Lipopigments in lymphocytes; azurophilic hypergranulation in neutrophils and lymphocyte vacuolization (only in homozygotes).

Prognosis. Survival to 4–8 years of age.

BIBLIOGRAPHY. Jansky J: Dosud nepopsany pripad familiàrni amaurotické idiotie komplicovanè hypoplasii mozeckovou Sborn lék 13:165–196, 1908

Bielschowsky M: Ueber spaetinnfantile amaurotische Idiotie mit Kleinhirnsymptomen. Dtsch Zschr Nervenheilk 50:7–29, 1914

Dollinger A: Zur Klinik der infantilen Form der familiaeren amaurotischen Idiotie (Tay-Sachs). Einige neue Symptome. Ein Beitrage zu den von Magnus beschrieben tonischen "Hals-und Labyrinthreflexen." Zsch Kinderh 22:167–194, 1919

Hassin GB: Amaurotic family idiocy: Late infantile type (Bielschowsky) with the clinical picture of decerebrate rigidity. Arch Neurol Pschiatr 16:708–727, 1926

Rosenberg RN, Prusiner SB, Di Mauro S, et al: The Molecular and Genetic Basis of Neurological Disease. Oxford, Butterworth-Heinemann, 1993

JANZ

Synonyms. Myoclonic epilepsy juvenile; impulsive petit mal; see Unverricht-Lundborg; Baltic myoclonus; Cherry-red spot-myoclonus; Ford.

Symptoms and Signs. Onset in early adolescence. Usually in the morning isolated myoclonic jerks not followed by seizure.

Etiology. Unknown autosomal recessive inheritance.

Diagnostic Procedures. *EEG.* Characteristic changes. Typical 4–6 Hz multispike and wave complex.

Therapy. Valproate control of seizures.

Prognosis. Good control with proper treatment.

BIBLIOGRAPHY. Dreifuss FE: Juvenile myoclonic epilepsy: Characteristics of a primary generalized epilepsy. Epilepsia 30(Suppl 4): s1–s7, 1989

Panayiotopoulos C, Obeid T: Juvenile myoclonic epilepsy: An autosomal recessive disease. Ann Neurol 25:440–443, 1989

Adams RD, Victor M: Principles of Neurology, 5th ed, pp 90–91. New York, McGraw-Hill, 1993

JARCHO

Synonyms. Carcinoma disseminated; thrombocytopenic purpura; paraneoplastic thrombocytopenic purpura; disseminated carcinoma.

Symptoms. Purpura and hemorrhagic manifestations in patients with carcinoma and hematologic malignancies.

Etiology. Autoimmune destruction of platelets.

Diagnostic Procedures. Platelet-bound IgG has been demonstrated in some patients.

Prognosis. The time of onset of the purpura bears little relation to the duration, severity, or state of activity of the neoplasm, and, except for the hazard posed by thrombocytopenia itself, has no adverse prognostic implications.

Therapy. Prednisone, splenectomy, platelet transfusion.

BIBLIOGRAPHY. Jarcho S: Diffusely infiltrative carcinoma. A hitherto undescribed correlation of several varieties of tumor metastasis. Arch Pathol 22:674–696, 1936

Kim HD, Boggs DR: A syndrome resembling idiopathic thrombocytopenic purpura in 10 patients with diverse forms of cancer. Am J Med 67:371–377, 1979

JARCHO-LEVIN

Synonyms. Lavy-Palmer-Merritt; dysostose condrovertebrale; spondylocostal dysostose; costovertebral dysostosis; spondylothoracic dysplasia.

Symptoms. Predominant in Spanish families. From birth. Both sexes. Occasionally, severe respiratory insufficiency.

Signs. *Head.* Prominent occiput; broad forehead; mongoloid slant eyes; wide nasal bridge; short neck (with limited mobility); short thorax; rib anomalies (chest anteroposterior diameter: increased), winged scapulae; skoliosis or kyphoscoliosis. *Limbs.* Long, thin; syndactyly, kampodactyly;

abdomen protuberant; genitourinary malformations and several variable changes secondary or tertiary to primary change of the spine.

Etiology. Autosomal recessive or dominant inheritance.

Diagnostic Procedures. *X-rays.* Typical "crab-like" appearance of thoracic skeleton. Characteristic vertebrae (hemivertebral and block vertebrae) and ribs fan shaped. The rest of skeleton normal.

Therapy. Symptomatic. Antibiotics; respiratory assistance.

Prognosis. From lethality in first year of life for respiratory infections to normal survival (seldom).

BIBLIOGRAPHY. Jarcho S, Levin PM: Hereditary malformations on the vertebral bodies. Bull J Hopkins Hosp 62:216–226, 1938
Aymé S, Preus M: Spondylocostal/spondylothoracic dysostosis: The clinical basis for prognosticating and genetic counseling. Am J Med Genet 24:599–606, 1986
Roberts AP, Conner AN, Tolmie JL, et al: Spondylocostal dysostosis: Hereditary forms of spinal deformity. J Bone Surg (Br) 70:123–126, 1988

JAUNDICE, BREAST MILK

Synonyms. Breast feeding hyperbilirubinemia, transient nonhemolytic unconjugated hyperbilirubinemia associated with breast feeding; maternal milk hyperbilirubinemia; breast milk jaundice.

Symptoms. Jaundice associated with breast feeding, becoming maximal during first 10–20 days of life and disappearing after 30–60 days, in spite of continuation of breast feeding.

Etiology. Presence of inhibitor of UDP-glucuronyl transferase in maternal milk: 3(alpha), 20(beta) pregnanediol.

Diagnostic Procedures. *Blood.* Unconjugated hyperbilirubinemia. *Maternal milk.* 3(Alpha), 20(beta) pregnanediol.

Therapy. Discontinuation of breast feeding.

Prognosis. Recession of jaundice with artificial feeding. Usually no kernicterus develops.

BIBLIOGRAPHY. Arias IM, Gardner LM, Seifter S, et al: Prolonged neonatal unconjugated hyperbilirubinemia associated with breast feeding and a steroid pregnane-3(alpha),20(beta)-diol in maternal milk, that inhibits glucoronide formation in vitro. J Clin Invest 43:2037–2047, 1964
Chowdhury JR, Wolkoff AW, Chowdhury NR, et al: Hereditary jaundice and disorders of bilirubin metabolism. In Scriver CR, Beaudet AL, Sly WS, et al: The Metabolic and Molecular Bases of Inherited Disease, 7th ed, p 2187. New York, McGraw-Hill, 1995

JAYLE-OURGAUD

Synonym. Internuclear ophthalmoplegia; ophthalmoplegia internuclear.

Symptoms and Signs. Paresis of internal rectus muscles, becoming apparent in attempted lateral gaze, while convergence is usually preserved; nystagmus of abducted eye (?).

Etiology. Lesion in the median longitudinal fasciculus. Usually observed in multiple sclerosis (see).

BIBLIOGRAPHY. Hugonnier R, Magnard P: Paralysie internucléaire antérieure. Bull Soc Ophthalmol Fr 71:265–268, 1958
Klinworth GK: Ocular involment in disorders of the nervous system. In Garner A, Klintworth GK (eds): Pathobiology of Ocular Disease: A Dynamic Approach, 2nd ed, pp 1713, 1714. New York, Marcel Dekker, 1994

JEJUNITIS, CHRONIC ULCERATIVE

Synonym. Regional nongranulomatous enteritis. See Crohn and ulcerative colitis.

Symptoms and Signs. All symptoms and signs of malabsorption syndromes of differing degrees.

Etiology. Unknown; distinct from (1) nontropical sprue, (2) lymphoma, and (3) dysgammaglobulinemia because of lack of response to gluten-free diet and type of pathologic lesions, and return to normal of protein after treatment.

Pathology. Ulceration of jejunum with adjacent atrophic and normal mucosa.

Diagnostic Procedures. See Gee. Biopsy of jejunum.

Therapy. Corticosteroids.

Prognosis. Temporary remission or unremitting course with no response to treatment.

BIBLIOGRAPHY. Jeffries GH, Steinberg H, Sleisenger MH: Chronic ulcerative (nongranulomatous) jejunitis. Am J Med 44:47–59, 1968
Meyers S: Clinical features and diagnosis. In Haubrich WS, Schaffner F, Berk JE (eds): Bockus Gastroenterology, 5th ed, pp 1411–1412. Philadelphia, WB Saunders, 1995

JENNETTE

Synonyms. Clq nephropathy; chloroquine nephropathy.

Symptoms and Signs. Most common in blacks. In older children and young adults.

Etiology. Asymptomatic proteinuria or features of nephrotic syndrome.

Pathology. By light microscopy no glomerular changes, focal mesangial hypercellularity or focal segmental sclerosis. Immunostaining mesangial presence of Clq-containing immune complex.

Diagnostic Procedures. *Blood.* Possibly alteration of nephrotic syndrome. *Urine.* Proteinuria.

Therapy. Poor response to glucocorticoids.

Prognosis. Possible spontaneous remission. Life table analysis shows renal survival of 84% at 3 years.

BIBLIOGRAPHY. Jennette JC, Hipp CG: Clq nephropathy: A distinct pathologic entity usually causing nephrotic syndrome. Am J Kidney Dis 6:103–110, 1985
Jennette JC, Wilman AS, Hogan SL, et al: Clinical and pathologic features of Clq nephropathy (ClqN). J Am Soc Nephrol 4:681, 1993

JENSEN

Synonym. Opticoacoustic nerve atrophy—dementia.

Symptoms and Signs. In males. Onset in infancy; sensineural deafness; in adolescence, optic nerve atrophy; in adulthood, progressive dementia.

Etiology. Unknown. X-linked recessive inheritance.

Pathology. Extensive calcification in entire central nervous system, including nerves vessels and meninges. Moderate wasting of skeletal muscles.

Prognosis. Death at 40 years of age in general deterioration.

BIBLIOGRAPHY. Jensen PKA: Nerve deafness, optic nerve atrophy and dementia: A new X-linked recessive syndrome. Am J Med Genet 9:55–60, 1981

Jensen PKA, Reske-Nielsen E, Hein Sorensen O: The syndrome of opticoacoustic nerve atrophy with dementia: A new X-linked recessive syndrome with extensive calcifications of the central nervous system. Clin Genet 35:222–223, 1989

JERVELL AND LANGE-NIELSEN

Synonym. Cardioauditory; surdo-cardiac; long QT—deafness.

Symptoms and Signs. Occurs in children (prevalence at 4–15 years of age) of either sex with bilateral conduction type deafness; and repeated attacks of syncope. Seizures may begin with a piercing scream followed by pallor and then cyanosis and loss of consciousness of short duration, followed by deep sleep. Attack may result in sudden death. Seizures precipitated by exertion or emotional strain.

Etiology. Unknown; autosomal recessive condition.

Pathology. No gross or pathologic cardiac abnormality. In two cases infarction of sinoatrial node, abnormality of Purkinje fibers. Stiking anomaly: PAS-positive hyaline nodules in both cochlear and vestible of membranous labyrinth or adjacent structures.

Diagnostic Procedures. *ECG.* Prolongation of Q-T interval. *Audiography.* Bilateral perceptive hearing loss. *Blood.* Moderate hypochromic anemia. Other changes (electrocardiographic, electroencephalographic, and biochemical) not constant features of condition.

Therapy. Beta-blocking drugs, left sympathetic atelectomy with or without beta-blockade therapy. Denervation of heart attempted without benefit; possibly allotransplantation useful.

Prognosis. Most cases terminate fatally during childhood. Sudden death follows a syncopal attack. In surviving cases, it seems that attacks may become less frequent as patients grow older.

BIBLIOGRAPHY. Meissner F: Taubstummheit and Taubstummenbildung. Leipzig, Wenter 120, 1856

Locati E, Moss AJ, Schwartz PJ, et al: The long Q-T syndrome. J Am Cardiol 3:516, 1948

Jervell A, Lange-Nielsen F: Congenital deaf mutism, functional heart disease with prolongation of Q-T interval and sudden death. Am Heart J 54:59–68, 1957

Till JA, Shinebourne EA, Pepper J, et al: Complete denervation of the heart in a child with congenital long QT and deafness. Am J Cardiol 62:1319–1321, 1988

Jeffery S, Jamieson R, Patton MA, et al: Long Q-T and Harvey-ray. Lancet 339:255, 1992

JERVIS

Synonym. Scherer; early familial cerebellar degeneration; cerebello-parenchymal disorder III; cerebellar granular cell hypoplasia; mental retardation, early, familial. See Marinesco-Sjögren.

Symptoms and Signs. Both sexes affected. Present from birth. Inconspicuous and nonprogressive cerebellar signs; mental deficiency, delayed motor and language development.

Etiology. Unknown. Autosomal recessive inheritance. Possible genetic linkage with albinism.

Pathology. Shrinking of all divisions of cerebellum, cerebellar cortex site of primary involvement, granular cells rather than Purkinje cells affected. Some Purkinje cells show "torpedoes" in the axon and "cactus-like" formation on their dendrites. Several "basket cells."

Diagnostic Procedures. *CT brain scan. MRI. EEG.*

Therapy. None.

Prognosis. Death in first year of life, or in less severe form, some improvement in walking and talking.

BIBLIOGRAPHY. Scherer HJ: Beitrege zur pathologischen Anatomie des Kleinhirns: genuine Kleinhirnathrophien. Z Neurol Pschiatr 145:335–405, 1933

Jervis GA: Early familial cerebellar degeneration (report of three cases in one family). J Nerv Ment Dis 111:398–407, 1950

Wichman A, Frank LM, Kelly TE: Autosomal recessive congenital cerebellar hypoplasia. Clin Genet 27:337–382, 1985

Bamezai R, Husain SA, Misra S, et al: Cerebellar ataxia and total albinism. Clin Genet 31:178–181, 1987

JESSNER-KANOF

Synonym. Lymphocytic benign skin infiltration.

Symptoms and Signs. Occurs predominantly (almost exclusively) in men; onset between second and eighth decades. Seasonal variability (more winter than summer exacerbations). Usually asymptomatic occasionally burning or pruritus. Single or multiple flat, reddish papules, occasionally circinate, becoming firm. Face (molar region) usually affected; any other body region may be involved. Sun exposure may irritate or aggravate lesion. No systemic symptoms or visceral involvement.

Etiology. Unknown. Familial cases reported,

Pathology. Normal epidermis; diffuse lymphocytic infiltration of dermis, perivascular and periadnexal, without follicular pattern (see Spiegler-Fendt). Basophilic degeneration of dermis; no germinal center.

Diagnostic Procedures. *Biopsy. Blood.* Occasionally, lymphocytosis. *Immunopathological studies.* Majority of cells are T-lymphocytes and bear CD4 T-helper/inducer marker. Lymphocytic cells are Leu 8 positive.

Therapy. Trials with antimalarial agents; topical steroids; gold; PUVA X-rays; carbon dioxide.

Prognosis. Improvement with treatment. Condition persists for years, spontaneous remission, and relapses. No systemic effect; no progression of lesion to skin atrophy (lupus erythematosus).

BIBLIOGRAPHY. Jessner M, Kanof NB: Lymphocytic infiltration of the skin. Arch Dermatol Syph 68:447–449, 1953

Willemze R, Dijkstra A, Meijer CJ: Lymphocytic infiltration of the skin (Jessner): a T-cell lymphoproliferative disease. Br J Dermatol 110:523–529, 1984

MacKie RM: Cutaneous lymphocytic infiltrates and pseudolymphomas. In Champion RH, Burton JL, Ebling FJG (eds): Rook/Wilkinson/Ebling Textbook of Dermatology, 5th ed, pp 2103–2104. Oxford, Blackwell Scientific, 1992

JEUNE

Synonyms. Asphyxiating thoracic dystrophy; infantile thoracic dystrophy; suffocating thoracic dystrophy; thoracic-pelvic-phalangeal dystrophy.

Symptoms. The syndrome is thought to be genetically heterogeneous because it occurs in both a neonatal form, with life-threatening thoracic deformity, and a late form that develops in childhood, mainly manifested as renal dysfunction.

Signs. Hypoplastic horizontal ribs; elevated clavicles; reduced growth and motility of thorax. Long bones wide and short; fraying of epiphyses; distal bones more severely affected. Pelvic changes: "squaring" of iliac wings; "saw-toothing" of acetabular roofs. Occasionally, lacunar skull.

Etiology. Unknown; autosomal recessive condition. Variant of Ellis-van Creveld (see) characterized by lower incidence of ectodermal dysplasia, and by more severe thoracic deformity. Suggested also autosomal dominant inheritance with incomplete penetrance.

Pathology. See Ellis-van Creveld.

Diagnostic Procedures. *X-ray of chest and skeleton.* Multiple ossification centers in body of sternum; shortened ulnae and fibulae; notches at the ends of metacarpal and metatarsal bones; lacking typical knee alterations (distinctive characteristic from Ellis-van Creveld).

Therapy. Antibiotics and prevention of pulmonary infections. Corrective thoracoplasty; long-term ventilatory support; renal transplantation.

Prognosis. Some patients die from asphyxia when pulmonary infection occurs. Pulmonary complication tends to decrease with age. Early high incidence of liver cirrhosis reported.

BIBLIOGRAPHY. Jeune M, Carron R, Beraud C, et al: Polychondrodystrophie avec blocage thoracique d'evolution fatale. Pediatrie 9:380–392, 1954

Langer LO: Thoracic-pelvic-phalangeal dystrophy, asphyxiating thoracic dystrophy of the newborn, infantile thoracic dystrophy. Radiology 91:447–456, 1968

Giorgi PL, Gabrielli O, Bonifazi V, et al: Mild form of Jeune syndrome in two sisters. Am J Med Genet 35:280–282, 1990

Hudgins L, Rosengren S, Treem W, et al: Early cirrhosis in survivors with Jeune thoracic dystrophy. Am J Med Genet 47:A61, 1990

JEUNE-TOMMASI

Synonym. Ataxia; deafness; cardiomyopathy.

Symptoms and Signs. In gypsies. Onset circa 6 years of age. Cerebellar ataxia; sensineural deafness; mental deficiency. Diffuse lentigines. Cardiomegaly.

Etiology. Autosomal recessive inheritance.

Diagnostic Procedures. Heart block frequently develops.

BIBLIOGRAPHY. Jeune M, Tommasi M, Freycon F, et al: Syndrome familial associant ataxia, surdité et oligophrenie: Sclerose myocardique d'evolution fatale chez l'un des enfants. Pediatrie 18:984–987, 1963

Koenigsmark BW, Gorlin RJ: Genetic and Metabolic Deafness, pp 306–307. Philadelphia, WB Saunders, 1976

JOB

Synonyms. Buckey; granulomatous disease variant; hyper IgE; hyperimmunoglobulin E—recurrent infection; HIE.

Symptoms and Signs. No sex or race predilection, onset from birth. Recurrent suppurative infections of the skin involving more than 50% of the body. Pulmonary infections (45%), lymphadenitis, and conjunctivitis (20%) may be features. Coarse facies with hypoplastic midface and prominent nose (50%), occasionally craniosynostosis, osteoporosis, osteogenesis imperfecta, and other skeletal anomalies. As part of the syndrome (to justify its name) a feeling of depression, guilt, and rejection from relatives and friends may also be present.

Etiology. Unknown. It appears that this syndrome is not an isolated entity, but part of the spectrum of chronic granulomatous diseases. Agent responsible for infections is usually Staphylococcus.

Pathology. Not reported for original cases. Biopsy material from other cases does not show granuloma formation.

Diagnostic Procedures. *Blood.* Low-grade eosinophilia (10%). Serum IgE 10 times normal vaue. High sedimentation rate. Leukocytes chemotactic defect (in 50% of cases). *Culture for determination of bacteria.* Staphylococcus aureus (90%), candidosis (40%).

Therapy. Antibiotics. Attempt with isotretinoin.

Prognosis. Various degrees of disability according to extent and type of infections.

BIBLIOGRAPHY. The Bible, Job 2:7–8, 19:1–29

Davis SD, Schaller J, Wedgewood RJ: Job's syndrome recurrent "cold" staphylococcal abscesses. Lancet I:1013–1015, 1966

Dreskin SC, Goldsmith PK, Gallin JI: Immunoglobulin in the hyperimmunoglobulin E and recurrent infection (Job's) syndrome: Deficiency of anti-Staphylococcus aureus immunoglobulin A. J Clin Invest 75:26–34, 1985

Leung PDYM, Geha RS: Clinical and immunologic aspects of the Hyperimmunoglobulin E syndrome. Hematol Oncol Clin N Am 2:81–100, 1988

Athens JW: Qualitative disorders of leukocytes. In Lee GR, Bithel TC, Foerster J, et al (eds): Wintrobe's Clinical Hematology, 9th ed, p 1622. Philadelphia, Lea & Febiger, 1993

JOHANSON-BLIZZARD

Synonyms. Blizzard. Deafness—hypothyroidism—hypoplasia alae nasi—oligodontia; hypoplasia alae nasi—mental retardation.

Symptoms and Signs. Prenatal onset. Both sexes. Generalized edema. From normal to severe mental (60%) and growth deficiencies. Sensorineural hearing loss (60%). Microcephaly (35%). Sparse hair. Hypoplasia alae nasi. Hypoplastic deciduous; absent permanent teeth. Imperforate anus (50%); septate or double vagina (30%); severe hypotonia and joint hyperextensibility (80%). Heart malformations (15%).

Etiology. Unknown. Sporadic and autosomal recessive inheritance.

Pathology. Small thyroid filled with colloid, replacement with fat of the pancreas, abnormalities in central nervous system (cortex).

Diagnostic Procedures. *Blood.* Cholesterol normal; macrocytic anemia. Hypoproteinemia hypocalcemia. *Stools.* Fat, foul, bulky. *Thyroid studies.* Hypothyroidism (30%). *Gastrointestinal enzymes study.* Complete absence of trypsin, chymotrypsin, amylase, carboxypeptidase, and lipase. *Fat and nitrogen balance.* Evidence of malabsorption. *X-ray kidney.* From dilatation of calix of ureters to hydronephrosis; bone delay of bone age (80%).

Therapy. Thyroid and pancreatic extracts.

Prognosis. Poor because of scarce response to treatment of growth and mental deficiencies. Need for institutionalization in some cases. Death from pancreatic exocrine insufficiency reported.

BIBLIOGRAPHY. Grand RJ, Rosen SN, di Sant'Agnese PA, et al: Unusual case of XXY Klinefelter's syndrome with pancreatic insufficiency, hypothyroidism, deafness, chronic lung disease, dwarfism and microcephaly. Am J Med 41:478–485, 1966

Johanson A, Blizzard RA: A syndrome of congenital aplasia of alae nasi, deafness, hypothyroidism, dwarfism, absent permanent teeth, and malabsorption. J Pediatr 79:982–987, 1971

Hurst JA, Baraitser M: Johanson "Blizzard" syndrome. J Med Genet 26:45–48, 1989

Harper J: Genetics and genodermatoses. In Champion RH, Burton JL, Ebling FJG (eds): Rook/Wilkinson/Ebling Textbook of Dermatology, 5th ed, p 345. Oxford, Blackwell Scientific, 1992

JOHNSON

Synonyms. Adherence; ocular rectus muscles; pseudoparalysis; synkinesis of rectus muscle.

Symptoms and Signs. Observed in children under 3 years of age, occasionally 3–5 years, and seldom later. Strabismus simulating bilateral lateral rectus paralysis. Four possible variants of this syndrome, depending on anomalous adhesions simulating paralysis of (1) lateral rectus (usually bilateral); (2) inferior oblique (theoretical); (3) superior rectus; (4) superior oblique (manifest when tilting head).

Etiology. Congenital anomalous development, possibly autosomal dominant inheritance.

Diagnostic Procedures. "Fixed muscle" deduction test.

Therapy. Adherent area separated by closed lysis or open lysis.

Prognosis. Normal rotation re-established by surgery. Spontaneous recovery also observed.

BIBLIOGRAPHY. Johnson LV: Adherence syndrome: Pseudoparalysis of lateral or superior rectus muscles. Arch Ophthalmol 44:870–878, 1950
Pang MP, Zweifach PH, Goodwin J: Inherited levator-medial rectus synkinesis. Arch Ophthal 104:1489–1491, 1986

JOHNSON NEUROECTODERMAL

Synonyms. Anosmia—alopecia—deafness—hypogonadism; AADH.

Symptoms and Signs. From birth, deafness; anosmia; occasionally, mental retardation; microtia; protruding ears or aural atresia (external ear canal); alopecia; occasionally undeveloped secondary sexual characteristics; dental caries; congenital heart defect; cleft palate.

Etiology. Autosomal dominant inheritance. Involvement of ectoderm and neuroectoderm of the first two brachial arches, Rathke pouch and diencephalon.

BIBLIOGRAPHY. Johnson VP, McMillin JM, Aceto T Jr, et al: A newly recognized neuroectodermal syndrome of familial alopecia, anosmia, deafness, hypogonadism. Am J Med Genet 15:497–506, 1983
Johnston K, Golabi M, Hall B, et al: Alopecia-anosmia-deafness-hypogonadism syndrome revisited: Report of a new case. Am J Med Genet 26:925–927, 1987

JOLLIFFE

Synonyms. Nicotinic acid deficiency encephalopathy. See Jacob.

Symptoms and Signs. Clouding of consciousness; cogwheel rigidities; grasping and sucking reflexes. Association with polyneuritis features and oculomotor signs of central neuritis.

Etiology. Complete nicotinic acid deficiency as part of the pellagra syndrome, where a partial nicotinic acid deficiency is present.

Pathology. Focal demyelination and ganglion cell degeneration in the cerebrum.

Therapy. Nicotinic acid and other vitamins of the B group as indicated by associate symptomatology.

Prognosis. If treatment of nicotinic acid given before irreversible stage is established, mortality of 14% in contrast to a mortality of nearly 100% without treatment or with treatment with hydration and thiamine only.

BIBLIOGRAPHY. Jolliffe N, Bowman KM, Rosenblum LA, et al: Nicotinic acid deficiency encephalopathy. JAMA 114:307–312, 1940
Adams RD, Victor M: Principles of Neurology, 5th ed, p 863. New York, McGraw-Hill, 1993

JONES

Synonyms. Cherubism; fibrous jaw dysplasia (misnomer); mandibular cystic dysplasia. See Ramon, Noonan; Noonan like; von Reklinghausen; Jaffe-Lichtenstein-Sutro (where cherubism may be associated).

Symptoms and Signs. Both sexes affected. Onset 18 months of age to 4 years. Rounded cheeks and jaw fullness; submandibular region swelling and narrow V-shaped palate. On sclera, beneath the iris, presence of a white line. Abnormal dentition; proliferation of tissue after tooth extraction. Occasionally lymphoadenopathy.

Etiology. Unknown. Autosomal dominant inheritance, with variable penetrance ranging 80–100% in male patients and 50–70% in female patients.

Pathology. In affected bones, presence of multinucleated giant cells of osteoclastic type, small hemorrhages and fibroblasts. In the bone cortex lacunar absorption and replacement by connective tissue.

Diagnostic Procedures. *X-ray. CT scan. MRI. Sonography.* Symmetric or unilateral expansion of mandible, with well-defined bubbles of radiolucency. In adults residual granular and sclerotic changes. *Biopsy of bone.* Three stages: (1) osteolytic with giant cells rich in acid phosphatases; (2) connective tissue rich in fibroblastic cells; (3) bone formation.

Therapy. Symptomatic.

Prognosis. Permanent condition. The syndrome generally regresses during puberty and on into adult life. Maxillary regression generally precedes mandibular regression.

BIBLIOGRAPHY. Jones WA: Familial multilocular cystic disease of the jaw. Am J Cancer 17:946–950, 1933
Hille JJ, Buch B, Evans M: Cherubism: Two case reports and a review of literature. J Dent Assoc S Afric 41:461–466, 1986
Gorlin RJ, Cohen MM Jr, Levin LS: Syndromes of Head and Neck, 3rd ed, pp 529–531. New York, Oxford Univ Press, 1990

JOUBERT

Synonyms. Joubert-Boltshauser; famlal cerebellar vermis agenesis; cerebello-parenchymal disorder IV; CPD IV.

Symptoms and Signs. Both sexes affected; onset congenital. Episodic hyperpnea, alternating with periods of apnea, with occasional single deep inspiration; episodes initiated or intensified by stimulation (e.g., emotional upsets; crying). Abnormalities of eye movements (e.g., conjugate; irregular jerky movements; rotatory nystagmus). Ataxia; psychomotor retardation. Associated nonspecific malformations.

Etiology. Unknown. Frequently related to other midline malformations (see Dandy-Walker and Bailey-Cushing). Autosomal recessive with pleotropic manifestations or variable expressivity. Sporadic cases also reported.

Pathology. Agenesis of vermis (partial or complete); more widespread cerebral involvement suggested by clinical findings has not been histologically confirmed yet. Retinitis pigmentosa.

Diagnostic Procedures. *CT brain scan. MRI.* Findings suggesting agenesis of vermis. *Ultrasonography. Blood.* Negative. Rule out metabolic causes for altered respiration. *Electroretinogram.*

Therapy. Symptomatic.

Prognosis. The respiratory abnormality tends to improve with age. Quoad vitam fair; quoad functionem poor.

BIBLIOGRAPHY. Joubert M, Eisenring JJ, Robb JP, et al: Familial agenesis of the cerebellar vermis. Neurology 19:813–825, 1969
King MD, Dudgeon J, Stephenson JBP: Joubert's syndrome with retinal dysplasia: Neonatal tachypnea as the clue to a genetic brain-eye malformation. Arch Dis Child 59:709–718, 1984

JOUSSEF

Synonyms. Vesicovaginal postcesarean fistula; menstrual hematuria.

Symptoms. Occurs after cesarean section or after prolonged labor. Urinary incontinence; vaginal irritation. Odor of decomposing urine.

Signs. Urinary incontinence. Hematuria at period of menses.

Etiology. Vesicovaginal fistula owing to surgical lesion or possibly infection, irradiation, neoplasia.

Diagnostic Procedures. Methylene blue injected into vagina passes into urine. *Cytoscopy.* Evidence of fistula. *Urine.* Features of cystitis.

Therapy. Surgical.

Prognosis. Good.

BIBLIOGRAPHY. Joussef AF: "Hemouria" following lower segment cesarean section: A syndrome. Am J Obstet Gynecol 73:759–767, 1957
Cunningham FG, MacDonald PG, Gant NF, et al (eds): Williams Obstetrics, p 533. Englewood Cliffs, NJ, Prentice-Hall, 1993

JUBERG-HAYWARD

Synonyms. Orocraniodigital; cleft lip; palate; abnormal thumbs; microcephaly.

Symptoms and Signs. Both sexes. From birth. Cleft lip and palate; microcephaly; hypoplasia or absence of thumbs; elbow deformity; occasionally, toe anomalies; short stature.

Etiology. Unknown. Autosomal recessive inheritance.

Diagnostic Procedures. *X-ray.* Sella turcica normal or absent. No endocrine dysfunction; in one case deficiency of growth hormone.

BIBLIOGRAPHY. Juberg RC, Hayward JR: A new familial syndrome of oral, cranial and digital anomalies. J Pediatr 74:755–762, 1969
Kingston HM, Hughes IA, Harper PS: Orocraniodigital (Juberg-Hayward) syndrome with growth hormone deficiency. Arch Dis Child 57:790–792, 1982

JUBERG-HOLT

Synonyms. Multiple epiphyseal dysplasia tarda; MEDT type Ie.

Symptoms and Signs. Present from birth. Dwarfism. Waddling gait; limited motion of hips and elbows; short fingers; abnormal position of thumbs.

Etiology. Autosomal recessive inheritance.

Diagnostic Procedures. *X-ray.* Flattening of epiphyses of all bones; clefting of patellae.

BIBLIOGRAPHY. Juberg RC, Holt JF: Inheritance of multiple epiphyseal dysplasia tarda. Am J Hum Genet 20:549–563, 1968
Beighton P: McKusick's Heritable Disorders of Connective Tissue, 5th ed, pp 622–625. St Louis, CV Mosby, 1993

JUBERG-MARSIDI

Synonyms. Mental and growth retardation; deafness; microgenitalism, X-linked.

Symptoms and Signs. *In males.* Microcephaly, deafness, flat nasal bridge, variable ocular anomalies, microgenitalism, mental retardation. *Heterozygous females.* Microcephaly and mild mental retardation.

Etiology. X-linked inheritance.

Prognosis. In males death in early age, oldest at 9 years.

BIBLIOGRAPHY. Juberg RC, Marsidi I: A new form of X-liked mental retardation with growth retardation, deafness and microgenitalism. Am J Hum Genet 32:714–72,2 1980
Mattei JF, Collignon P, Ayme S, et al: X-liked mental retardation, growth retardation deafness and microgenitalism: A second family report. Clin Genet 23:70–74, 1983

JUERGENS

Obsolete.

Synonyms. Hemorrhagic diatesis.

BIBLIOGRAPHY. Juergens R: Beitrag zur Pathologie und Klinikder Blutungsbereitschaft. Zschr Klin Med 123:649–686, 1933

JUHLIN-MICHÄLSSON

Synonym. Basophils; eosinophils absence.

Symptoms. Repeated infections; asthma; vasomotor rhinitis; hemolytic anemia; alopecia totalis; scabies; extensive warts.

Signs. Those of repeated infections; burrows of scabies on several areas of the body; warts on hands, resistant to treatment.

Etiology. Unknown. Possibly immunologic destruction of eosinophils and basophils.

Pathology. Bone marrow. Normal erythropoiesis. Scarce plasma cells. Absence of eosinophils and basophils.

Diagnostic Procedures. *Blood.* Absence of eosinophils and basophils, differential counts otherwise normal. Immunoglobulin levels low, but within normal limits. Demonstration of an eosinophil-basophil destruction factor in plasma. *Sputum.* Absence of eosinophils and basophils. *Biopsy of bone marrow.* See Pathology.

Therapy. Antibiotic or surgical treatment (or both) of infections and infestations.

Prognosis. Fair.

BIBLIOGRAPHY. Juhlin L, Michälsson G: A new syndrome characterized by absence of eosinophils and basophils. Lancet I:1233–1235, 1977
Nakahata T, Spicer SS, Leary AG, et al: Circulating eosinophil colony forming cells in pure eosinophil aplasia. Ann Inter Med 101:321–324, 1984

JUMPER KNEE

Synonyms. Patellar tendonitis.

Symptoms and Signs. All ages, but more frequently young sportsmen. Pain in inferior pole of patella, on climbing, running, jumping.

Etiology and Pathology. Mucoid degeneration of patellar tendon at its insertion into inferior pole of patella.

Therapy. Rest and nonsteroidal anti-inflammatory agents. Cortisone injection into tender area. Surgery seldom required

BIBLIOGRAPHY. Graham GP, Fairclough JA: The knee. In Klippel JH, Dieppe PA: Rheumatology, p 5.12.5. St Louis, CV Mosby, 1995

JUMPING FRENCHMEN OF MAINE

Synonyms. Myriachit (Russian: to act foolishly) Beard; startle; hyperexplexia; see also Kok.

Symptoms and Signs. Both sexes. Observed among French-Canadian lumbermen in Maine (in 19th and early 20th century) or their offspring. In response to a sudden stimulation, occurrence of an abnormal reaction: response to a quick, sudden command with asked action, often echoing the words of command, if addressed in foreign language simple repetition of the same, response to the command executed also if illogical or dangerous.

Etiology. Possible autosomal recessive inheritance. Doubts about nature of the condition. Neurological or psychological conditioning.

BIBLIOGRAPHY. Beard GM: Remarks upon "jumpers or jumping Frenchmen." J Ment Dis 5:526, 1878

Andermann F, Keene DL, Andermann E, et al: Startle disease or hyperexplexia: Further delineation of the syndrome. Brain 103:985–997, 1980

Saint-Hilaire MH, Saint-Hilaire JM, Granger L: Jumping Frenchmen of Maine. Neurology 36:1269–1271, 1986

JUNG

Symptoms and Signs. Recurrent and persistent pyoderma, folliculitis, and atopic folliculitis.

Etiology. Unknown. Hypotheses include (1) defects of histamine metabolism resulting in raised histamine levels; (2) increase in histamine receptor expression on cell surfaces, leading to increased sensitivity to histamine.

Diagnostic Procedures. *Immunological studies.* Abnormalities of lymphocyte function, including defective proliferative responses to phytomitogens, and subnormal response in immunoglobulin production after stimulation of the lymphocytes by pokeweed mitogen; defective leucocyte chemilluminescence responses, associated with defective ability for intracellular killing of microbial organisms.

Therapy. Chlorpheniramine (histamine-1 antagonist).

Prognosis. Good with lifelong treatment.

BIBLIOGRAPHY. Jung LKL, Kapoor N, Engelhard D, et al: Pyoderma eczema and folliculitis with defective leucocyte and lymphocyte function: A new familial immunodeficiency disease responsive to a histamine-1 antagonist. Lancet II:185–187, 1983

Burton JL: Eczema lichenification, prurigo and erythroderma. In Champion RH, Burton JL, Ebling FJG (eds): Rook/Wilkinson/Ebling Textbook of Dermatology, 5th ed, pp 574–575. Oxford, Blackwell Scientific, 1992

JUNIUS-KUHNT

Synonyms. Kuhnt-Junius; macula senile disciform degeneration; macula lutea juvenile degeneration; degeneration maculae lutae disciformis; disciformis macular degeneration; senile disciform macular degeneration. See age-related macular degeneration.

Symptoms and Signs. Macula lutea senile disciform degeneration. Usually bilateral, after 60, male–female ratio 1:1. Often antecedent signs of nondisciform degeneration with drusen. Reduction of visual acuity, central scotoma.

Macula Lutea Juvenile Degeneration. Onset in juvenile period. Same symptoms. Exudative and atrophic reaction with deposit in and about macula.

Etiology and Pathology. Unknown; possibly autosomal dominant or recessive inheritance. A variety of age-related macular degeneration and not a separate entity. The mass of connective tissue (overdescribed) seems to result from organization of hemorrhage under the RPE owing to choriocapillary insufficiency, leading to subpigment epithelial neovascularization or caused by detachment of pigment epithelium and sensory retina and diseases of choroid. Drusen determine defects in degenerated Bruch membrane, through which neovascularization from choroid leads to subpigment epithelial neovascularization. Eventually macular hole.

Diagnostic Procedures. Important differential diagnosis with tumor of posterior pole. Fundoscopy: subretinal pigment epithelial neovascular membrane, exudative neurosensory detachment with circinate deposition of lipids surrounding the lesion.

Pathology. In the end, disciform pigmented plaque.

Therapy. Photocoagulation arrests the process.

Prognosis. Usually, improvement of visual acuity of temporary nature and then relapse, up to ultimate degeneration; however, usually, the patient remains able to manage his daily activities.

BIBLIOGRAPHY. Junius P, Kuhnt H: Die scheibenformige Entartung der Netzhaumitte (Degeneratio maculae lutae disciformis). Berlin 1926 S. Karger

Apple DJ, Rabb MF: Ocular Pathology, p 346. St Louis, CV Mosby, 1991

Garner A, Sarks S, Sarks JP: Degenerative and related disorders of the retina and choroid. In Garner A, Klintworth GK (eds): Pathobiology of Ocular Disease: A Dynamic Approach, 2nd ed, p 631. New York, Marcel Dekker, 1994

JUVENILE XANTHOGRANULOMA

Synonyms. Xanthogranuloma, juvenile.

Symptoms and Signs. Both sexes, male to female ratio 4:1. In infancy and childhood. *Skin.* Macular or nodular reddish brown lesions 1 mm to 5 cm on the head and neck. *Eyes.* Usually unilateral lesion. The iris is commonly affected but ciliary body, choroid, retina, and optic nerve may be involved. Hepatosplenomegaly.

Etiology. Unknown. No familial tendency.

Pathology. In the skin and eyes and more seldom in the viscera (lung, pleural space, liver, testicle, lymph node, spleen, and kidney). Nodular histiocytic infiltrates with xanthomatous cells, Touton-type giant cells, and eosinophils.

Diagnostic Procedures. *X-rays. Ultrasonography. CT scan.* Echogenic nodules, hypodense mass. *Biopsy of lesion.* See Pathology.

Therapy. None.

Prognosis. Regression of lesion in 6–12 months. Occasionally persistent. May also result lesion of the eye from repeated hemorrhages and secondary glaucoma.

BIBLIOGRAPHY. Diard F, Cadier L, Billaud C, et al: Neonatal juvenile xanthogranulomatosis with pulmonary, extrapleural and hepatic involvement: One case report. Ann Radiol (Paris) 25:113–118, 1982

Gupta AK, Bahargava S: Juvenile xanthogranuloma with pulmonary lesions. Pediatr Radiol 18:70, 1988

Grossniklaus HE, Green WR: Uveal tumors. In Garner A, Klintworth GK (eds): Pathobiology of Ocular Disease: A Dynamic Approach, 2nd ed, pp 1459–1462. New York, Marcel Dekker, 1994

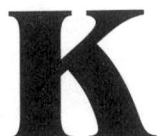

K

KABUKI MAKEUP

Synonym. Niikawa-Kuroki; KMS.

Symptoms and Signs. Prevalent in Japanese. Both sexes. Moderate mental retardation. Recurrent otitis (60%), deafness (25%). Reduced physical development leading to dwarfism. *Facies*. Long palpebral fissures; eversion of lateral third of lower eyelids *Kabuki mask*: broad, depressed nose; large ears; high arched or cleft palate. *Limbs*. Short fifth finger (90%). Abnormal dermatoglyphic patterns (70%). *Spine*. Scoliosis (50%). Congenital heart anomalies (30%).

Etiology. Unknown. Suggest both autosomal dominant and X-linked inheritance.

Diagnostic Procedures. *X-ray*. Abnormalities of vertebrae, joints, hands.

BIBLIOGRAPHY. Kuroki Y, Suzuki K, Chyo H, et al: A new malformation syndrome of long palpebral fissures, large ears, depressed nasal tip and skeletal anomalies associated with postnatal dwarfism and mental retardation. J Pediatr 99:570–573, 1981
Niikawa N, Kuroki Y, Kajii T, et al: Kabuki Make-Up (Niikawa-Kuroki) Syndrome: A study of 62 patients. Am J Med Genet 31:565–589, 1988
Clarke LA, Hall JG: Kabuki make-up syndrome in three Caucasian children. Am J Hum Genet 47:A52, 1990

KAESER

Synonym. Scapuloperoneal dystrophy; spinal scapuloperoneal atrophy.

Symptoms and Signs. Both sexes. At onset, bilateral foot drop and talipes equinovarus; however, only peroneal muscles are affected whereas feet muscles are spared. Then years later, in a second phase, the shoulder girdle and finally bulbar involvement may occur.

Etiology. Autosomal dominant inheritance.

Pathology. All muscles below the knee except the intrinsic foot muscles undergo atrophy. Involvement of caudal cranial nerves. In one autopsy observed degeneration of anterior horn motoneurons.

Diagnostic Procedures. *Electromyography*. Suggestion of anterior horn cell pathology. *Blood serum*. Enzymes increased. *Biopsy*.

Therapy. Symptomatic.

Prognosis. Progressive condition.

BIBLIOGRAPHY. Kaeser HE: Die familiaere scapulo-peroneale Muskelatrophie. Dtsch Z Nervenheilk 186:379–394, 1964
Kazakov VM, Bogorodiusky DK, Skorometz AA: The myogenic scapuloperoneal syndrome. Muscular dystrophy in the K kindred: Clinical study and genetics. Clin Genet 10:41–50, 1976
Munsat TL, Serratrice G: Facioscapulohumeral and scapuloperoneal syndromes. In Rowland LP, Di Mauro S (eds): Handbook of Clinical Neurology, vol 18. Myopathies, p 161. Amsterdam, Elsevier, 1992

KAHLER-BOZZOLO

Synonyms. Bence Jones; Huppert; McIntyre; von Rustitski; myelopathic albuminuria; myeloma multiple; multiple myeloma; plasma cell myeloma; multiple plasmacytoma; sarcomatous osteitis.

Symptoms and Signs. Incidence 2/100,000 in whites, 3/100,000 in blacks per year. Prevalent in males; incidence increasing with age (mean age 62). Asthenia; anorexia; weight loss; weakness; bone pains (at onset wandering and intermittent; usually at the back, less frequently chest and extremities; then at site of bone tumefactions and spontaneous fractures). Usually, later hepatomegaly, seldom splenomegaly. Neurologic complications frequent.

Etiology. Unknown. Genetic factors, oncogenes, chronic stimulation of the reticuloendothelial system, viruses considered. Transforming event that involves a hematopoietic precursor cell that produces lineages of various pathologic types with uncontrolled and progressive proliferation of mature and immature plasma cells. Clinical manifestations caused by consequent overproduction of particular proteins and their constituent polypeptide chains.

Pathology. *Bones*. Thinning of shell; cortex may be reabsorbed; in marrow presence of gelatinous reddish substance. Microscopically, plasma cells, hemorrhages. *Kidney*. Atypical nephritis. *Liver, spleen, and various organs*. Para-amyloid deposition (10%).

Diagnostic Procedures. *Blood*. Moderate normocyte anemia. Leukocytes usually normal; occasionally, presence of plasma cells in peripheral blood. Platelets usually normal; coagulation test usually abnormal. Hyperproteinemia; typical electrophoretic patterns; cryoglobulinemia; hypercalcemia; hyperuricemia; frequently high blood urea nitrogen; usually normal phosphorus; alkaline phosphatase normal or slightly elevated. Immunological studies; various immunologic classes of myeloma have been established: IgG myeloma; IgA myeloma; IgD myeloma; light chain disease; nonsecretory myeloma; biclonal gammopathies (with variable clinical manifestations and courses). *Urine*. Albumin; casts; Bence Jones protein; abnormal kidney function test. *Bone marrow*. Characteristic infiltration with myeloma cells. Hemogenic series usually normal. *X-ray of skeleton*. Rounded punched-out lesions; diffuse osteoporosis may also be observed.

Therapy. Encourage an increase of physical activity with the use of analgesics, corsets, and walkers. Radiation therapy for bone pain from pathological fractures, and for areas of spinal cord compression. Adequate hydration to prevent and control renal complications from the precipitation of Bence Jones protein. Hemodialysis. Antibiotics against bacterial infections. Treatment of hypercalcemia: prednisone, calcitonin, bisphosphonates, gallium nitrate (strong nephrotoxicity). Polychemotherapy with various combinations: MP: melphalan, prednisone; VBCMP: vincristina, BCNU, cyclophosphamide, melphalan, prednisone; VCPM vincristine, cyclophosposphamide, melphalan prednisone; VBAP vincistine, BCNU adriamicine, prednisone VAD: vincistine adriamicine desametazone intervals. Other agents: androgens, interferon, vindesine. Allogenic bone marrow transplantation.

Prognosis. Wide variation in severity of manifestation and survival.

BIBLIOGRAPHY. Dalrymple J: On the microscopical character of mollities ossium. Dublin Q J Med Sci 2:85–95, 1846
Jones HB: On a new substance occurring in the urine of a patient with mollities ossium. Philosoph Trans R Soc Lond 138:55–62, 1848
Kahler O: Zur Symptomatologie des multiplen Myeloms; Beobachtung von Albumosurie. Prag Med Wochenschr 14:33–45, 1889
Bozzolo: Sulla malattia di Kahler. Archochen Internat Med Chir (Napoli) 409, 1897
Nadeau LA, Magalini SI, Stefanini M: Familial multiple myeloma. Arch Path 61:101–106, 1956
Durie BG: Cellular and molecular genetic features of myeloma and related disorders. Hematol Oncol Clin No Am 6:463–477, 1992

Bataille R: Plasmacytomes humaines: etude clinique, diagnostic et prognostic Edit. thecniques Encyclo Méd Chir (Paris France) Hématologie 13–1014–C-10 1994

KALLIN*

Synonyms. Epidermolysis bullosa simplex localisata; anadontia hair and nail disorders.

Symptoms and Signs. Considered a variant of Weber-Cockaine (see).

Etiology. Possibly autosomal recessive inheritance.

BIBLIOGRAPHY. Nielsen PG, Sjoelund E: Epidermolysis bullosa simplex localisata associated with anadontia, hair and nail disorders. Acta Derm Venerol 65:526–530, 1985

KALLMANN

Synonyms. Anosmia eunuchoidism; olfactogenital dysplasia; hypogonadism anosmia; De Morsier III.

Symptoms and Signs. Both sexes affected; prevalent in males (3:1); possibility of female carrier. Body proportions and lack of development of secondary sexual characteristics consistent with gonadotropic hypogonadism. Anosmia; hypertension; mental retardation; occasionally, color blindness.

A patient with this syndrome was found to have an atrial septal defect, mitral valve prolapse, and a large intracranial cyst.

Other clinical abnormalities observed include obesity, cryptorchidism, osteopenia, mild neurosensory hearing loss, gynecomastia, diabetes mellitus, cleft lip, or palate.

Etiology. Unknown. Condition appears to be X-linked or of autosomal recessive or dominant (most likely) inheritance. Dysfunction of hypothalamus and pituitary.

Pathology. *Male.* In testis, absence of spermatogenesis and Leydig cells; abiotrophy of tubules. *Female.* Hypoplastic ovary and uterus. Nasal mucosa. Agenesis of olfactory nerve cells. Slight atrophy of part of telencephalon.

Diagnostic Procedures. *Blood.* Hyposecretion of gonadotropin and lack of response to LHRH. Evaluation of loss of sense of smell. *Biopsy of the testis.*

Therapy. Gonadotropins. Testosterone or estrogen for 4–6 months.

Prognosis. Treatment corrects eunuchoidism also in the adult age, but not the anosmia.

BIBLIOGRAPHY. Maester de San Juan A: Falta total de los nervios olfactorios con anosmia en un individuo en quien existia una atrofia congenita de los por el Dr. M. de San Juan, p 211. Madrid, El Siglo Medico, 1856
Kallmann FJ: The genetic aspects of primary eunuchoidism. Am J Ment Defic 48:203–236, 1943–1944
De Morsier G: Median cranioencephalic dysraphias and olfactogenital dysplasia. World Neurol 3:485–506, 1962
Winters SJ: Clinical disorders of the testis. In De Groot LJ (ed): Endocrinology, 3rd ed, pp 2379–2380. Philadelphia, WB Saunders, 1995
Weatherall DJ, Ledingham JGG, Warrell DA (eds): Oxford Textbook of Medicine, 3rd ed, pp 1670–1671. Oxford, Oxford Med Pub, 1996

KANDINSKII-CLÉRAMBAULT

Synonym. Clérambault II.

Symptoms and Signs. Confusing clinical entity characterized by automatism of mental apparatus: automatic obedience to any command or suggestion as well as echolalia, echopraxia, and waxy muscle flexibility; feeling of being possessed by dissociated forces, internal (e.g., fluid; humors; spirits) or external (e.g., metereologic; magnetic).

Etiology. Part of schizophrenia or expression of organic cerebral (i.e., hypophysiodiencephalic) disturbance. The frequency of the occurrence of these symptoms and their indistinct nature suggest the discontinuation of the use of this eponym.

BIBLIOGRAPHY. Kandinskii VK: Opsevdogalliutsinatsiiakh. Kritiko-klinicheskii étud. St. Petersburg, 1890
de Clérambault CG: Syndrome mécanique et conception mécaniciste des psychoses hallucinatoire. Ann Med Psychol 85:398–413, 1927
Kaplan HI, Sadock RJ: Comprehensive Textbook of Psychiatry, 4th ed, p 1332. Baltimore, Williams & Wilkins, 1985

KANDORI

Synonym. Flecked retina; night blindness.

Symptoms. Both sexes affected; onset at young age. Mild anomaly of dark adaptation; no changes in visual acuity or field.

Signs. Large, irregular, yellowish, well-outlined flecks under retinal vessels, especially in midperipheral area.

Etiology. Unknown; possibly hereditary autosomal recessive (?). Toxic causes also considered.

Pathology. Unknown.

Diagnostic Procedures. *Ophthalmologic examination.* To differentiate from fundus flavimaculatus and drusen. *Functional studies and angiography.* Focal alteration of retinal pigment epithelium. Prolonged interval of dark adaptation to reach scotopic potentials. *Electro-oculography.* Normal.

Therapy. None.

Prognosis. Nonprogressive condition.

BIBLIOGRAPHY. Kandori F: Very rare cases of congenital non-progressive night blindness with flecked retina. Jpn J Ophthalmol 13:386–394, 1959
Bullock JD, Albert DM: Flecked retina. Arch Ophthalmol 93:26–31, 1975
Bird AC, Jay B, Hussain AA: Retinal photoreceptor disorders. In Garner A, Klintworth GK (eds): Pathobiology of Ocular Disease: A Dynamic Approach, 2nd ed, p 1226. New York, Marcel Dekker, 1994

KANNER

Synonyms. Autistic child; infantile autism; "wild boy of Aveyron." See also Asperger.

Symptoms. Frequency 4.5:10,000; more frequent in males; no special birth order. In mother, increased incidence of pregnancy complications or perinatal complications. Parents in above average occupation and intelligence bracket. Siblings normal. Onset in first years of life (usually before second birthday). Lack of responsiveness to other human beings. Insistence on preservation of sameness in environment. The child appears alert and attractive in spite of odd behavior. Usually not intellectually subnormal; 50% show marked delay in motor milestones. Speech development abnormality very frequent.

Etiology. Unknown; organic causes suspected, possibly derangement in tryptophan metabolism. Genetic predisposition proposed: Fragile X (see) has been found in autistic boys (16%) but not in girls.

Therapy. Early psychiatric treatment. These children are highly vulnerable to understimulating environment.

Prognosis. With early treatment, good results possible. If inadequately treated in institution, development of institutionalism syndrome.

BIBLIOGRAPHY. Stard JMG: The Wild Boy of Aveyron. Humphrey G, Humphrey M (trans). New York, 1932

Kanner L: Autistic disturbances of affective contact. Nerve Child 2:217–250, 1943

Strayhorm JM, Rapp N, Donina W, Strain PS: Randomized trial of methylphenidate for an autistic child. J Am Acad Child Adolesc Psychiatr 27:244–247, 1988

Weatherall DJ, Ledingham JGG, Warrell DA (eds): Oxford Textbook of Medicine, 3rd ed, p 4108. Oxford, Oxford Med Pub, 1996

KANZAKI

Synonyms. Schindler II, lyposomal glycoaminoacid storage; angiokeratoma corporis diffusum; angiokeratoma corporis diffusum; glycopeptiduria.

Symptoms and Signs. Disseminated angiokeratoma and symptoms of Schindler I (see) but milder, since evidence of neurodegeneration or neuroaxonal dystrophy is absent.

Etiology. Deficiency of an allelic form of alpha-galactosidase B. Basic defect: Substitution of tryptophane for arginine 329.

Pathology. Cytoplasmic vacuoles on cells of skin and kidney.

Diagnostic Procedures. *Urine.* Large amount of sialylglycoaminoacids, predominant excretion of O-glycoside-linked glycoaminoacid. *Blood.* Enzyme activities in leukocytes and fibroblast are normal.

BIBLIOGRAPHY. Kanzaki T, Yokota M, Mizuno N: Clinical and ultrastructural studies of novel angiokeratoma corporis diffusum. Clin Res 36:377A, 1988

Kanzaki T, Waug AM, Desnick RJ: Lysosomal alpha-*N*-acetylgalactosaminoacidose deficiency. The enzymatic defect in angiokeratoma corporis diffusum with glycopeptiduria. J Clin Invest 88:707–711, 1991

KAPOSI I

Synonyms. Endotheliosarcoma; multiple idiopathic hemorrhagic sarcoma; hemoangiosarcoma, multiple pigmented.

Symptoms and Signs. Predominant in males (10:1); occurs with major frequency in European Jews, Italians, and blacks. Onset in Europeans at late age; in blacks at all ages, or in subjects with AIDS (see). (Endemic cases observed in Zaire, Uganda, and Rwanda). Dark, bluish macular skin lesions, usually on extremities, enlarging to 1–3 cm in diameter. Adjacent maculae may fuse and form a plaque. Edema may develop. Lesions may involute, leaving scar, or ulcerate and fungate. Progressive invasion, along course of superficial vein to involve both limbs symmetrically. Lymph node enlargement; occasionally, visceral involvement (e.g., liver; spleen). Association with diabetes, lymphomas.

Etiology. Unknown. Possible correlation with acquired cellular immunodeficiency (HTLV III) and opportunistic infections (Pneumocystis carinii). Sporadic; endemic; associated with nonhuman immunodeficiency virus (induced secondary immunosupression); HIV-related.

Pathology. At onset, invasion of mid-dermis by bands of spindle cells in a network of reticulin and vascular spaces; around spindle bands, macrophages and inflammatory changes are found. Invasion proceeds along course of vein. Proliferative endarteritis of vessel surrounding tumor. Similar features in lymph node and visceral organs when involved.

Diagnostic Procedures. *Blood.* Humoral and cellular immune response may be impaired. *Biopsy.* See Pathology.

Therapy. Palliation considering status of immunodeficiency that must not be further compromised. If localized, excision and radiotherapy. If diffuse, single and rotating vinblastine, vincristine, etoposide, doxorubicin, or multiagent chemotherapy. Interferons (beneficial), radiation therapy, provides effective palliation.

Prognosis. Course of progression extremely variable. When initial lesion excised, recurrences in other sites. Death usually owing to complcations from opportunistic infections complicating immunodepression.

BIBLIOGRAPHY. Kaposi M, Kohn M: Idiopathisches, multiples Pigmentsarkom der Haut. Arch Dermatol Syph 4:265–273, 1872

Warner LC, Fisher BK: Cutaneous manifestations of the acquired immunodeficiency syndrome. Int J Dermatol 25:337–350, 1986

Lukens immune deficiency diseases: Inherited and acquired. In Lee GR, Bithel TC, Foerster J, et al (eds): Wintrobe's Clinical Hematology, 9th ed, pp 1693–1694. Philadelphia, Lea & Febiger, 1993

KAPOSI II

Synonyms. Atrophoderma pigmentosum; progressive melanosis lenticularis; xeroderma pigmentosum (XP); xeroderma pigmentosum types C, E, F, and "variant"; xeroderma pigmentosum, non-neurologic form. See De Sanctis-Cacchione.

Symptoms. Occurs in many races; both sexes affected; onset in first year, in early life (75%), or later. Increased sensitivity to sunlight; photophobia; opacification of cornea with cloudiness of vision.

Signs. Freckling and dryness of skin areas exposed to light, followed by sunburn and persistent erythema. Freckles tend to enlarge and become confluent to form patches. Initially they fade in winter; later, remain unchanged year round. Successive formation of telangiectasis, small angiomas, white atrophic spots, and warty keratosis. Sunburned areas are followed by ulcerations, crustings, scarrings, and contractions. From third and fourth year or later malignant transformation (basal cells; squamous cells; melanoma). Teeth are occasionally defective. Neoplasms of eyes.

Type C. Most common. Classic XP only skin disorders.

Type D. Skin disorders plus late-developing neurologic signs of group A (see De Sanctis-Cacchione)

Type E. Slight skin lesions

Type F. Mild skin involvement; in Japanese variant (pigmented xerodermoid). Mild to severe symptoms starting in old age

Etiology. Increased sensitivity to sunlight. Autosomal recessive inheritance. Defective capacity for excision repair of damaged DNA at pyrimidine dimers because of enzyme deficiency. All the various forms have different enzymatic alterations in the fibroblasts. Fibroblasts from one group of patients may correct defects of another group when hybridized. In the variant form post-replication repair in altered.

Pathology. Skin of senile type; lack of special characteristics. Malignant transformation (see Signs).

Diagnostic Procedures. *Biopsy.* Identification of malignancies. *Blood.* In some cases increased serum glutamic-oxaloacetic transaminase (SGOT), serum glutamic-pyruvic transaminase (SGPT), and alpha-2-globulin. *Urine.* In some cases, aminoaciduria. *Cell culture studies.*

Therapy. Protection from sunlight (physical and cosmetic). Early excision of tumors. Oral retinoids as prophylasis. Artificial tears, contact lens or corneal transplant. Genetic counseling, patient and family education.

Prognosis. Frequently, fatal before 10 years of age; 66% die before age 20 from metastases. With adequate protection and treatment, prognosis highly improved. High variability of course and possibility of longer survival even in the same family.

BIBLIOGRAPHY. Kaposi M: Xeroderma pigmentosum. Med Jahrb 619–633, 1882

Cleaver JE, Kraemer KH: Xeroderma pigmentosum. In Scriver CR, Beaudet AL, Sly WS, et al: The Metabolic and Molecular Bases of Inherited Disease, 6th ed, p 2949. New York, McGraw-Hill, 1989
Harper J: Genetics and genodermatoses. In Champion RH, Burton JL, Ebling FJG (eds): Rook/Wilkinson/Ebling Textbook of Dermatology, 5th ed, pp 348–351. Oxford, Blackwell Scientific, 1992

KAPOSI III

Synonyms. Dermatitis, Kaposi-Juliusberg; eczema herpeticum; varicelliform eruption.

Symptoms. Unexplained prevalence in males; highest incidence in infancy. Usually affects patients with active or recently suppurated atopic manifestation of other type of dermatitis. Incubation period from time of exposure to virus (herpes simplex or vaccinia). Severe itching. Severe constitutional symptoms in many cases.

Signs. Sudden appearance of crops of vesicles-pustules (varicelliform) in areas already affected by dermatitis, or generalized. After 1 week new crop eruption may follow. Pustules crust in 4–5 days, then heal with moderate scarring. Lymphadenopathy.

Etiology. Infection usually primary to virus (herpes simplex or vaccinia) and other viruses (Coxsackie A16, etc.) in patients with skin affected by atopic condition.

Pathology. Necrosis of epidermis; presence of intranuclear (herpes) or intracytoplasmic (vaccinia) bodies in corium cells. In addition, in the herpes condition multinucleated giant cells.

Diagnostic Procedures. Cytologic examination of lesion smears.

Therapy. Isolation. Acyclovir. Antibiotics for secondary infections. Corticosteroids contraindicated. Hyperimmune gammaglobulins: vaccinal or herpetic Lupidion; inosine p-acetaminobenzoate 1-dimethylamino-2-propanole (1:3).

Prognosis. Fever subsides in 4–5 days. Majority of patients recover completely. Possibly, encephalitis, transverse myelitis. Mortality for vaccine form 6%; for herpetic form not known.

BIBLIOGRAPHY. Kaposi M: Pathologie und Therapie der Hautkrankheiten, p 483. Wien, Urban-Schwarzenberg, 1887
Juliusberg F: Ueber Pustulosis acuta varioliformis. Arch Dermatol Syph 46:21–28, 1898
Highet AS, Kurtz J: Viral infections. In Champion RH, Burton JL, Ebling FJG (eds): Rook/Wilkinson/Ebling Textbook of Dermatology, 5th ed, pp 895–897. Oxford, Blackwell Scientific, 1992

KAPOSI-IRGANG

Synonyms. Lupus erythematosus profundus; lupus panniculitis.

Symptoms. Male to female ratio, 1:2. Onset in females usually in the fourth decade; in males, the fifth decade. Good general health.

Signs. Under normal skin, appearance of firm nodules (1–10 cm in diameter) most frequent on the cheeks, less frequent in other areas of face, arms, hands, trunk, or legs. In 20% of patients, telangiectasis of face.

Etiology. Unknown. Genetic factors (?); somatic mutation (?). Environmental factors (coagent?). Autoimmune etiology suggested. Considered an unusual clinical variant of lupus erythematosus, systemic (see).

Pathology. Epidermal atropy; basal layer hydropic degenerative changes; dermal collagen degenerated; foci of lymphocytes; occasionally, vasculitis and panniculitis.

Diagnostic Procedures. *Blood.* Anemia; leukopenia; thrombocythemia (33%); hypergammaglobulinemia (30%); erythrocyte sedimentation rate increased in 20% of cases. Rheumatoid arthritis (RA) test positive (17%); lupus test positive (2%). *Biopsy.* See Pathology.

Therapy. Antimalarial drugs. Intralesional injection of corticosteroids. Thalamidone oral.

Prognosis. Chronic and relapsing. Healing results in depressed scarring and pigmentation. Risk of systemic lupus development less than 5%.

BIBLIOGRAPHY. Kaposi M: Pathologie und Therapie der Hautkrankheiten, 2nd ed, p 642. Urban & Schwarzenberg, 1883
Irgang S: Lupus erythematosus profundus: Report of example with clinical resemblance to Darrier-Roussy sarcoid. Arch Dermatol Syph 42:97–108, 1940
Rowell NR, Goodfield MJD: The connective tissue diseases. In Champion RH, Burton JL, Ebling FJG (eds): Rook/Wilkinson/Ebling Textbook of Dermatology, 5th ed, pp 2178–2179. Oxford, Blackwell Scientific, 1992

KAPUR-TORIELLO

Synonyms. Long columella—cleft lip/palate; eye, heart, intestinal anomalies.

Symptoms and Signs. Brother and sister. Severe mental retardation. *Facies.* Cleft lip/palate, nose flat tipped and bulbous with long columella; microphthalmia, iris coloboma. Evidence of congenital heart defects, intestinal malrotation, displaced kidney.

Etiology. Unknown.

Diagnostic Procedures. See Signs. Chromosomal studies normal.

BIBLIOGRAPHY. Kapur S, Toriello HV: Apparently new MCA/MR syndrome in sibs with cleft lip and palate and other facial, eye, heart and intestinal anomalies. Am J Med Genet 41:423–425, 1991

KARPATI

Synonym. Carnitine deficiency, systemic, SCD.

Symptoms and Signs. In children. Attacks of encephalopathy with vomiting; stupor; coma; weakness of proximal muscles, also of head and neck; cardiomyopathy.

Etiology. Autosomal dominant inheritance. Deficit of carnitine synthesis or metabolism.

Pathology. *Muscle biopsy; liver biopsy; neutral lipid droplets.*

Diagnostic Procedures. *Urine.* Carnitine above normal levels. *Blood.* Hyperglycemia, ketosis absent during fasting, hypoprothrombinemia, hyperammoniemia, elevation of transaminases. *Tissues.* Low carnitine in liver rather than in the muscle.

Therapy. Administration of L-carnitine not always beneficial. During attacks, glucose administration. A diet low in fat and high in carbohydrate.

Prognosis. Half of affected patients die before 20 years of age. Improved with treatment.

BIBLIOGRAPHY. Karpati G, Carpenter S, Engel AG, et al: The syndrome of systemic carnitine deficiency: Clinical, morphologic, biochemical, and pathophysiologic features. Neurology 25:16–24, 1975
Stanley CA, DeLeeuw S, Coates PM, et al: Chronic cardiomyopathy and weakness or acute coma in children with a defect in carnetine uptake. Ann Neurol 30:709–716, 1991
Ferrari R, Di Mauro S, Sherwood G (eds): L-carnitine and its role in medicine: From function to therapy. London, Academic Press, 1992

KARSCH-NEUGENBAUER

Synonyms. Split hand; congenital nystagmus; fundal changes; cataracts; nystagmus; split hand.

Symptoms and Signs. From birth. Both sexes. Split hand and foot deformities. Nystagmus (modulatory); fundal changes; cataracts (possibly at later age).

Etiology. Autosomal dominant inheritance.

BIBLIOGRAPHY. Karsch J: Erbliche Augenmissbildung in Verbindung mit Spalthand und-Fuss. Z Augenheilk 89:274–279, 1936
Neugenbauer H: Spalthand und-fuss mit familiaerer Besonderheit. Z Orthop 95:500–506, 1962
Piparski RT, Pauli RM, Bresnick GH, et al: Karsch-Neugenbaur syndrome: Split foot, split hand, and congenital nystagmus. Clin Genet 27:97–101, 1985

KARTAGENER

Synonyms. Siewert; Kartagener triad, bronchiectasis—dextrocardia—sinusitis; situs inversus—sinusitis—bronchiectasis; dextrocardia—bronchiectasis—sinusitis; immotile cilia. See dyskinetic cilia.

Symptoms. Onset in early infancy (90% before 15 years of age). Dyspnea; productive cough; recurrent respiratory infections; palpitation; otitis media; nasal speech; conductive hearing loss; anosmia.

Signs. Clubbing of fingers. In chest, diffuse crepitant rales, dextrocardia (right-sided apical beat and sounds). Features of sinusitis. Hepatic dullness on left side.

Etiology. Unknown; autosomal recessive inheritance with incomplete penetrance. See Immotile cilia.

Pathology. Dextrocardia alone or situs inversus totalis; bronchiectasis; maldevelopment of frontal paranasal sinuses; edema; hyperemia of nasal mucosa; nasal polyposis (frequent). See dyskinetic cilia.

Diagnostic Procedures. *X-ray of skull and chest. ECG. Sputum.* Culture and bacterial sensitivity. *Blood.* In infancy transient immunoglobulin deficiency. See Dyskinetic cilia.

Therapy. Antibiotics for recurrent pulmonary infections. Lobectomy or lung resection when indicated.

Prognosis. Relatively good. Recurrent pulmonary infections and asthma. Congestive heart failure and infection causes of death.

BIBLIOGRAPHY. Siewert AK: Ueber einen Fall vor bronchiectasie bei einem Patieten mit situs inversus viscerum. Berl Klin Wochr 41:139–141, 1904
Kartagener M: Zur Pathogenese der Bronchiektasien: Bronchiektasien bei Situs viscerum inversus. Beitr Klin Tuberk 83:489–501, 1933
Afzelius BA: A human syndrome caused by immobile cilia. Science 193:317–319,1976
Aitken J: A clue to Kartagener's. Nature 353:306, 1991
Afzelius BA, Bjoern Mossberg: Immotile-cila syndrome (primary ciliary dyskinesia) including Kartagener syndrome. In Scriver CR, Beaudet AL, Sly WS, et al: The Metabolic and Molecular Bases of Inherited Disease, 7th ed, pp 3943–3945. New York, McGraw-Hill, 1995

KARYOMEGALIC INTERSTITIAL NEPHRITIS

Synonyms. Interstitial, karyomegalic nephritis; nephritis interstitial karyomegalic.

Symptoms and Signs. Both sexes. Asymptomatic progressive renal failure in the third decade, and recurrent infections, mostly in upper respiratory tract.

Etiology. Unknown. Possibility of genetic defect on chromosome 6, inherited and linked to HLA locus.

Pathology. Markedly enlarged and hyperchromic nuclei in many tubular epithelial cells in the nephrons with interstitial fibrosis in the surrounding atrophic tubules. Karyomegaly may be observed also in

many other organs, however, further histologic damage observed only in kidneys.

Diagnostic Procedures. *Blood.* Those of interstitial nephritis. *Urine.* Proteinuria and presence of karyomegalic tubular cells cells. *Biopsy.*

Therapy. Conservative or kidney transplantation. Antibiotics for infections.

Prognosis. Sepsis or uremia may be causes of death.

BIBLIOGRAPHY. Burry AF: Extreme dysplasia in renal epithelium of a young woman dyng from hepatocarcinoma. J Pathol 113:147–150, 1974
Mihatsch MJ, Gudat F, Zollinger HU, et al: Systemic karyomegaly associated with chronic interstitial nephritis: A new disease entity? Clin Nephrol 12:54–62, 1979
Spoendling M, Moch H, Brunner F, et al: Karyomegalic interstitial nephritis: Further support for a distinct entity and evidence for a genetic defect. Am J Kid Dis 25:242–252, 1995

KASABACH-MERRITT

Synonyms. Capillary angioma—thrombocytopenia; hemangioma—thrombocytopenia; thrombocytopenia—purpura—hemangioma.

Symptoms. Occurs in infants. Purpura and bleeding.

Signs. Large capillary angioma; pallor; petechiae and ecchymosis.

Etiology. Angioma causes sequestration of platelets and platelet deficiency.

Pathology. Capillary angioma containing platelet thrombi.

Diagnostic Procedures. *Blood.* Thrombocytopenia; injected 51Cr tagged platelets collect in the tumor. Anemia; increased fibrinolytic activity (release of plasmin from clotting into the tumor).

Therapy. X-ray or radium treatment of the tumor. Surgical excision. Antifibrinolytic agents (epsilon-aminocaproic acid) have been used, with success for almost 1 year, allowing the possibility of natural involution of the hemangioma.

Prognosis. Recovery (platelet number returns to normal) following destruction of tumor.

BIBLIOGRAPHY. Kasabach HH, Merritt KK: Capillary hemangioma with extensive purpura: Report of a case. Am J Dis Child 59:1063–1070, 1940
Shulkin BL, Argenta LC, Cho KJ, et al: Kasabach-Merritt syndrome: Treatment with epsilon-aminocaproic acid and assessment by indium 111 platelet scintigraphy. J Pediatr 117:746–749, 1990
Bithell TC: Acquired coagulation disorders. In Lee GR, Bithel TC, Foerster J, et al (eds): Wintrobe's Clinical Hematology, 9th ed, pp 1483, 1492, 1493. Philadelphia, Lea & Febiger, 1993

KASHIN-BECK

Synonyms. Aso; Lin Kuatang-tz'w; Tokut-ze; Urov; osteochondrorthrosis deformans endemica.

Symptoms. Example of regional disease occurring principally in childhood; endemic in Korea, northern China, and Siberia. Onset asymptomatic or ache, muscular weakness, cramps, paresthesias, fatigability. After 6 months to 1 year, joint stiffness. Clinical classification of three degrees according to degree of joint involvement and clinical findings: *First degree.* Mild form; initial stage moderate involvement and few symptoms. *Second degree.* Increased involvement of joints; pain and systemic symptoms. *Third degree.* Chronic deforming arthritis and general manifestations. Reduction of height; involvement of vertebral column; chronic gastritis.

Signs. Most often wrist and interphalangeal joint deformities; crepitation; no inflammation or effusion. Symmetric involvement; slow progression of osteoarthrosis to other joints. Atrophy of muscles adjacent to joints involved.

Etiology. Toxic origin following ingestion of a cereal grain infected with the fungus Fusarium sporotrichiella.

Pathology. Necrobiotic degenerative changes of the aseptic focal necrosis type, involving those parts of the growing skeleton associated with hyaline cartilage. Abnormalities most marked in epiphyses and metaphyses. Muscle atrophy; no pathology of viscera except chronic gastritis during the third stage.

Diagnostic Procedures. *X-ray.* Narrowness and rarefaction of zone of preliminary calcification; dystrophic process of growth of tubular bones and shortening of extremities; vertebral bodies flatten with beak osteophytes. *Blood.* Normal; in third degree, anemia with lymphocytosis. Calcium and phosphorus always normal.

Therapy. Avoidance of use of contaminated bread, and importation of "healthy" food in regions where disease occurs. Some improvement with sodium selenite.

Prognosis. Slow progression. Emigration or change of diet prevents further development of the disease.

BIBLIOGRAPHY. Kashin NI: The description of the endemic and other disease, prevailing in the Urov-river area. The records of physico-medical scientific society attached to the Moscow University, 1859
Beck EB: To the problem of deforming endemic osteoarthritis in the Baikal area. Russ Phys 5:74–75, 1906
Nesterov AI: The clinical course of Kashin-Beck disease. Arthritis Rheum 7:29–40, 1964
Weatherall DJ, Ledingham JGG, Warrell DA (eds): Oxford Textbook of Medicine, 3rd ed, pp 2976–2977. Oxford, Oxford Med Pub, 1996

KATAYAMA

Synonyms. Bilharziasis (invasive phase); cardiopulmonary schistosomiasis; schistosomiasis japonica. See Marchand and Manson schistosomiasis—pulmonary artery obstruction.

Symptoms. Usually not seen in natives. Fever; headache; angioneurotic edema; urticaria; abdominal pain; diarrhea; melena (later massive hematemesis). Pulmonary migration: dry cough, dyspnea. Cerebral migration: disorientation; coma; aphasia; paraplegia; jacksonian epilepsy and other neurologic manifestations.

Signs. *Early.* Hepatomegaly; pain on palpation of liver edge; splenomegaly. *Later.* Smaller liver; ascites; caput medusae; progressive weight loss.

Etiology. Infestation with Schistosoma japonicum; katayama snails intermediate host. Infestation with S. mansoni and S. haematobium gives a similar clinical pattern, and the term Katayama syndrome may be applied to all three conditions. The syndrome primarily is owing to an allergic response to developing schistosomes.

Pathology. Eggs of parasite in different tissues surrounded by eosinophils. *Colon.* Rigid, mucosa edematous and congested; hemorrhages; ulcerated polyps. *Liver.* Early, enlarged and congested; later, cirrhosis; periportal fibrosis. *Spleen.* Enlarged.

Diagnostic Procedures. *Blood.* Marked eosinophilia; anemia; leukopenia; thrombocytopenia; hypoproteinemia. *Stool.* Ova.

Therapy. Nutritional; correction of anemia; improvement of general condition prior to chemotherapy. Praziquantel metrifonate; oxamniquine; niridazole; antimonial trivalent compounds. Surgery (filtering worms from the portal system).

Prognosis. Good in early moderate infestation if adequate treatment. Severe in chronic infestation and from complications.

BIBLIOGRAPHY. Walt F: The Katayama syndrome. South Afr Med J 28:89–93, 1954

Capron A, Dessaint JP: Immunologic aspects of schistosomiasis. Ann Rev Med 43:209–218, 1992
Weatherall DJ, Ledingham JGG, Warrell DA (eds): Oxford Textbook of Medicine, 3rd ed, pp 971, 975, 2004. Oxford, Oxford Med Pub, 1996

KAUFMAN

Synonym. Mental retardation; microcornea; microcephaly.

Symptoms. Present from birth. Mental and physical retardation; myopia; congenital hypotonia; respiratory distress; constipation.

Signs. Microcephaly; hypertelorism; epicanthus, eyelid ptosis; mongoloid slant of palpebral fissures; microcornea; eyebrows sparse and brooding laterally; flat filtrum; high and narrow palate; lordosis; flat feet.

Etiology. Autosomal recessive or dominant inheritance or sporadic.

BIBLIOGRAPHY. Kaufman RL, Rimoin DL, Prensky AL, et al: An oculocerebrofacial syndrome. Birth Defects 7:135–138, 1971
Jureka SB, Evans J: Kaufman oculocerebrofacial syndrome: Case reported. Am J Med Genet 3:15–19, 1979

KAUFMAN-McKUSICK

Synonyms. McKusick-Kaufman; hydrometrocolpos—postaxial polydactyly—congenital heart malformations.

Symptoms. Onset in newborn. Respiratory embarassment; urinary, intestinal, circulatory obstruction.

Signs. Abdominal mass; transvaginal membrane (vaginal atresia) or imperforate hymen; accumulation of fluid in upper vagina and uterus. Occasionally, swelling of breast and "witches' milk" production. Postaxial polydactyly (may be limited to one limb) and/or congenital heart malformation.

Etiology. Lack of patency of vaginal canal; excessive secretion from uterus and cervical glands in response to maternal hormone. Presence of transvaginal membrane transmitted as female-limited autosomal recessive inheritance in members of the Amish community; occasionally, associated with other somatic malformations.

Pathology. Accumulation of fluid proximal to vaginal obstruction. See Signs.

Diagnostic Procedures. Hydrometrocolpos fluid. Presence of glycogen-containing vaginal cells.

Therapy. Surgical removal of obstruction.

Prognosis. Marked variation of intensity of manifestation from minimal to very severe; it may even be lethal if treatment is not instituted. Cases with minimal symptomatology that escape diagnosis will manifest hematocolpos at age of menarche. Possibly infection (pyocolpos).

BIBLIOGRAPHY. McKusick VA, Bauer RL, Koop CE, et al: Hydrometrocolpos as a simply inherited malformation. JAMA 189:813–816, 1964
Kaufman RL, Hartman AF, McAlister WH: Family studies in congenital heart disease II: A syndrome of hydrometrocolpos, postaxial polydactyly and congenital heart disease. Birth Defects Orig Art Ser VIII(5):85–87, 1972
Vince JD, Martin NJ: McKusick Kaufman syndrome: Report of an instructive family. Am J Med Genet 32:174–177, 1989

KAWASAKI

Synonym. Mucocutaneous lymph node, MLN.

Symptoms. Observed in Japan. Higher incidence in summer. Male to female ratio 1:5.1; occurs in infants and children 2 months to 9 years.

Hyperthermia (1–2 weeks duration). Dry lips; pharyngeal angina; stomatitis; arthralgia; dyspnea; diarrhea. In some cases, symptoms related to meningitis.

Signs. "Strawberry tongue" and oral and pharyngeal hyperemia; polymorphic exanthema; indurative edema; red palms and soles; and (during convalescence) desquamation of fingertips. Cervical adenopathy. Signs of myocardial involvement. Occasionally, icterus and signs of meningitis. Coronary aneurysms.

Etiology. Unknown. Considered an allergic reaction or unusual reaction to various types of infections. Possible connection with Stevens-Johnson (see).

Diagnostic Procedures. *Blood.* Leukocytosis; erythrocyte sedimentation rate increased; alpha-2–globulin and C-reactive protein increased, moderate anemia. Bilirubin increased (occasionally). *ECG.* Myocarditis (70%). *CSF.* Aseptic meningitis (occasionally). *Urine.* Proteinuria.

Therapy. Salicylate and high-dose intravenous gamma globulin. Steroids and antibiotic of no value.

Prognosis. Self-limited. Clinical, electrical, radiological, echographic cardiac surveillance did not show any sign of aneurysms more than 6 months after the onset of the disease. Possible sudden death from coronary thrombosis (1–2%).

BIBLIOGRAPHY. Kawasaki T: Acute febrile mucocutaneous syndrome with lymphoid involvement with specific desquamation of fingers and toes in children. Jpn J Allergol 16:178–222, 1967

Rowley AH, Duffy E, Shulman ST: Prevention of giant coronary artery aneurysms in Kawasaki disease by intravenous gamma globulin therapy. J Pediatr 113:290–294, 1988

Weatherall DJ, Ledingham JGG, Warrell DA (eds): Oxford Textbook of Medicine, 3rd ed, pp 3047–3050. Oxford, Oxford Med Pub, 1996

KBG*

Synonyms. Herman.

Symptoms and Signs. From birth. Mental retardation. *Head and Facies.* Brachycephaly, telecanthus, wide eyebrows, macrodontia. *Skeleton.* Abnormal vertebrae; short metacarpals and femoral necks. Pectus excavatum.

Etiology. Autosomal dominant with variable penetrance.

BIBLIOGRAPHY. Hermann J, Pallister PD, Tiddy W, et al: The KBG syndrome—a syndrome of short stature, characteristic facies, mental retardation, macrodontia and skeletal anomalies. Birth Defects 11:7–18, 1975

Fryus JP, Haspeslagh M: Mental retardation, short stature, minor skeletal anomalies, craniofacial dysphormism and macrodontia in two sisters and their mother: Another variant example of the KBG syndrome? Clin Genet 26:69–72, 1984

KEARNS-SAYRE

Synonyms. Kearns-Sayre-Daroff; Kearns-Shy; heartblock; retinitis pigmentosa—ophthalmoplegia; ophthalmoplegia—retina pigmentary degeneration—cardiomyopathy; KSS; oculocraniosomatic; ophthalmoplegia plus. See Barnard-Scholz, and Pearson.

Symptoms and Signs. Prevalent in females. Onset before 20 years of age. Progressive external ophthalmoplegia (see Barnard-Scholz); pigmentary degeneration of retina; deafness symptoms and signs related to heart block. Limb weakness, in some cases encephalopathy. Less common features: dementia, sensorineural deafness, short stature, diabetes, hypoparathyroidism.

Etiology. Mitochondrial cytopathy reduced level of coenzyme Q(10) in serum and in the mitochondrial fraction of skeletal muscle. Genetic heterogeneity sporadic (mytochondrial DNA deletions that are not present in the mother) and familial forms (autosomal dominant and recessive) reported.

Pathology. See Barnard-Scholz. Abnormal mitochondria with paracrystalline inclusion in muscle cells.

Diagnostic Procedures. *ECG.* Heart block. *Spinal fluid.* Elevated proteins. Study of intact mitochondria from skeletal muscle. Deficiency of mitochondrial protein synthesis, and absence of a translation product with the mobility of a 5 KDa protein. *Evaluation of intracellular respiration.* Shows that the absent protein is not a functional subunit of a respiratory chain complex.

Therapy. Pacemaker frequently required. Coenzyme Q(10) 60–120 mg daily for 3 months produced reduced cardiac and ocular deficiencies. Cardiac transplantation.

Prognosis. Heart involvement may cause sudden death.

BIBLIOGRAPHY. Kearns TP, Sayre GP: Retinitis pigmentosa, external ophthalmoplegia and complete heart block. Arch Ophthalmol 60:280–289, 1958

Berenberg RA, Pellock JM, Di Mauro S, et al: Lumping or splitting? "Ophthalmoplegia plus" or Kearns-Sayre syndrome. Ann Neurol 1:37–54, 1977

Holt IJ, Harding AE, Petty RKH, et al: A new mitochondrial disease associated with mitochondrial DNA heteroplasmy. Am J Hum Genet 46:428–433, 1990

Di Mauro S: Mitochondrial encephalopathies. In Rosenberg RN, Prusiner SB, Di Mauro S, et al (eds): Molecular and Genetic Basis of Neurologic Diseases, pp 665–694. Stoneham, CT, Butterworth, 1993

KEIPERT

Synonyms. Nasodigitoacoustic. See Rubinstein.

Symptoms. Male siblings affected. Sensorineural deafness.

Signs. *Facies.* Large nose; high bridge; prominent alae. *Mouth.* Upper lip protruding; cupid bow laterally overlapping the lower lip. *Extremities.* Broad terminal phalanges of all toes and of thumbs and first, second, and third fingers; fifth fingers show shortness and clinodactyly.

Etiology. Autosomal recessive (?) or X-linked inheritance.

Diagnostic Procedures. *X-ray.* Bifid terminal phalanges (one case) of both indexes.

BIBLIOGRAPHY. Keipert JA, Fitzgerald MG, Damks DM: A new syndrome of broad terminal phalanges and facial abnormalities. Austr Paediatr J 9:10–13, 1973

KELLEY-SEEGMILLER

Symptoms and Signs. Early adult-onset gout-arthritis; urolithiasis; occasionally mild neurologic manifestations.

Etiology. X-linked inheritance. Partial deficiency of hypoxanyhine-guanine phosphoribosyltransferase.

Diagnostic Procedures. *Blood.* Hyperuricemia. *Urine.* Massive crystalluria. *Echography.* Renal urolithyasis. *X-rays.* Arthritic changes.

Therapy. That of gout.

Prognosis. After alkalnization and allopurinol, regression of symptoms and laboratory findings.

BIBLIOGRAPHY. Kelley WN, Rosenbloom FM, Henderson JF, et al: A specific enzyme defect in gout associated with overproduction of uric acid. Proc Natl Acad Sci USA 57:1735–1739, 1967

---

*Initials of prototype family's surname.

Becker MA, Roessier BJ: Hyperuricemia and gout. In Scriver CR, Beaudet AL, Sly WS, et al: The Metabolic and Molecular Bases of Inherited Disease, 7th ed, p 1670. New York, McGraw-Hill, 1995

KEMP-ELLIOT-GORLIN

Synonym. Angina pectoris; normal coronary arteriography. See Heberden and anterior chest.

Symptoms. Represents 9% of patients with angina pectoris. Prevalent in females (66% of cases). Typical angina pectoris symptoms.

Etiology. Unknown. Possibly, disease of small heart arteries beyond resolution of coronary arteriography; regional functional small artery constriction.

Pathology. Unknown.

Diagnostic Procedures. *ECG*. Normal or abnormal after effort. *Cineangiocardiography*. Normal. *Blood*. Normal. Lactate myocardial production during isoproterenol infusion or tachycardia induced by right atrial pacing (in 30% of cases).

Therapy. That of classic angina (see Heberden).

Prognosis. Much better than that for other patients with other forms of angina.

BIBLIOGRAPHY. Kemp HG, Elliott WC, Gorlin R: The anginal syndrome with normal coronary arteriography. Trans Assoc Am Phys 80:59–70, 1967
O'Rourke RA: Chest pain. In Schlant RC, Alexander RW: Hurst's The Heart, 8th ed, pp 459–463. New York, McGraw-Hill, 1994

KENNEDY

Synonyms. Kennedy-Alter-Sung; bulbospinal muscular atrophy, X-linked; spinal–bulbar muscular atrophy; muscular atrophy, spinal bulbar. See Kugelberg-Welander.

Symptoms and Signs. In males. Onset in third to fourth decade. Muscle weakness, facial fasciculation, and atrophic changes. First reduced sexual potency then impotence. *Bulbar signs*. Dysphagia. Absent pyramidal (negative Babinsky) sensory and cerebellar signs. Occasionally, gynecomastia.

Etiology. Unknown. X-linked recessive inheritance.

Pathology. Muscle involvement prevalent in the limbs. Distal sensory neuropathy. Marked involution of Leydig cells in testis.

Diagnostic procedures. *Nerve conduction study*. Decreased sensory response amplitude. *Blood*. Hypobetalipoglobulinemia (clear relationship not established).

Prognosis. Slow progression. Compatible with long life.

BIBLIOGRAPHY. Kennedy WR, Alter M, Sung JH: Progressive proximal spinal and bulbar muscular atrophy of late onset: A sex-linked recessive trait. Neurology 18:671–680, 1968
Nagashima T, Seko K, Hirose K, et al: Familial bulbo-spinal muscular atrophy and sensory neuropathy (Kennedy-Alter-Sung syndrome): Autopsy case report of two brothers. J Neurol Sci 87:141–152, 1988
La Spada A, Fischbeck KH: Androgen receptor gene defect in X-linked spinal and bulbar muscular atrophy. Am J Hum Genet 49:20, 1991
Weatherall DJ, Ledingham JGG, Warrell DA (eds): Oxford Textbook of Medicine, 3rd ed, pp 3988, 4089. Oxford, Oxford Med Pub, 1996

KENNEY-CAFFEY

Synonym. Dwarfism; tubular bone stenosis; transient hypocalcemia.

Symptoms. Both sexes with equal severity. Onset a few days after birth. Tetanic convulsions; delayed physical development; activity and intelligence normal. Myopia; nanophthalmos with hyperopia. Papilledema; vascular tortuosity; macular crowding.

Signs. Proportionate dwarfism; large anterior fontanelle; occasionally hypoplastic nails.

Etiology. Unknown. Autosomal dominant (and recessive) inheritance suggested, but X-linked variants not excluded.

Pathology. Narrow long-bone shafts with stenosed medullary cavities; lack of differentiation of calvaria into a diploic space; relative craniofacial disproportion. Only one autopsy report: absence of parathyoid, calcification of basal ganglia, cerebrum and cerebellum.

Diagnostic Procedures. *Blood*. Transient hypocalcemia; hyperphosphatemia; microcytic anemia. Parathyroid hormone and calcitonine determination. Occasionally neutropenia, abnormal T-cell function, and evidence of neonatal liver disease. *X-ray of skeleton*. See Pathology.

Therapy. Convulsions and hypocalcemia and hyperphosphatemia fully corrected by vitamin D and calcium. Anemia corrected by iron administration.

Prognosis. Skeletal configuration persists unchanged. Proportionate dwarfism results.

BIBLIOGRAPHY. Kenney FM, Linarelli L: Dwarfism and cortical thickening of the tubular bones: Transient hypocalcemia in mother and son. Am J Dis Child 111:201–207, 1966
Caffey J: Congenital stenosis of medullary spaces in tubular bones and calvaria in two proportionate dwarfs' mother and son; coupled with transitory hypocalcemic tetany. Am J Roentgen 100:1–11, 1967
Franceschini P, Testa A, Bogetti G, et al: Kenney-Caffey syndrome in two sibs born to consanguineous parents: Evidence for an autosomal recessive variant. Am J Med Genet 42:112–116, 1992

KERATITIS FUGAX HEREDITARIA

Synonym. Valle. See Francescetti-Kauffman.

Symptoms. Both sexes affected; onset at 2–12 years of age. Pain; photophobia; impairment of vision; recurrent attacks two to eight times a year.

Signs. Corneal bullae and vescicles; edema; erosions.

Etiology. Unknown; hereditary dominant inheritance.

Pathology. Acute, subacute, and then chronic keratitis.

Diagnostic Procedures. *Ophthalmoscopy*. See Pathology.

Therapy. Hypertonic fluids; irradiation of lacrimal glands.

Prognosis. Recurrent, becoming milder after 50 years of age.

BIBLIOGRAPHY. Valle D: Keratitis fugax hereditaire. Duodecim 80:659–664, 1964
Pouliquen Y: Précis d'opthalmologie. Masson, Paris, 1984

KERATODERMA PALMO-PLANTAR (K.P.P.) SYNDROMES

Synonym. Palmo-plantar keratoderma.

K.P.P.–CLINODACTYLY

Synonym. See Greither.

Symptoms and Signs. In Mexican families palmo-plantar hyperkeratosis with radial curvature of fifth finger.

Etiology. Autosomal dominant inheritance.

BIBLIOGRAPHY. Anderson IF, Klinworth GK: Hypovitaminosis A in a family with tylosis and clinodactyly. Br Med 1:1293–1297, 1961

Hernandez A, Aguirre-Negrete MG, Gonzales-Mendoza A, et al: Autosomal dominant keratosis palmaris et plantaris with clinodactyly. Birth Defects Orig Art Ser 18(3B):207–210, 1982

K.P.P.–DEAFNESS

Association of KPP and hearing loss in two families. Possibly autosomal dominant inheritance.

BIBLIOGRAPHY. Bititci OO: Familial hereditary, progressive sensori-neural hearing loss with keratosis palmaris and plantaris. J Laryng Otol 89:1143–1146, 1975

Hatamochi A, Nakagawa S, Ueki H, et al: Diffuse palmo-plantar keratoderma with deafness. Arch Dermatol 118:605–607, 1982

K.P.P–ESOPHAGEAL CANCER

Synonyms. Leukoplakia—Tylosis—esophageal carcinoma.

Symptoms and Signs. Both sexes. Clinical leukoplakia as early as 4 years of age. Tylosis usually second decade (occasionally earlier). Cancer of esophagus usually at 65 years of age, possibly as early as fifth decade.

Etiology. Autosomal dominant inheritance.

Pathology. Leukophasic lesions. Gray-whitish lesion. Parakeratosis, spongiosis of superficial layer, and acanthosis. Skin: lesions may be yellow, see Greither carcinoma. Typical findings. Characteristic intranuclear electron-dense particles in nuclei.

BIBLIOGRAPHY. Howel-Evans W, McConnell RB, Clarke CA, et al: Carcinoma of aesophagus with keratosis palamaris and plantaris (tylosis): A study of two families. Quat J Med 27:413–429, 1958

Yesudian P, Preuralatha S, Thambiah AS: Genetic tylosis with malignancy: A study of South Indian Pedigree. Br J Dermatol 102:597–600, 1980

K.P.P.–NAIL DYSTROPHY—NEUROSENSORY NEUROPATHY

Synonyms. Charcot-Marie-Tooth—palmo-plantar keratoderma; axonal neuropathy—palmo-plantar keratoderma.

Symptoms and Signs. Nail dystrophy. Present at birth or developing during early childhood. Palmo-plantar keratoderma in later childhood. Clinical evidence (see Charcot-Marie-Tooth syndrome).

Etiology. Type of inheritance debated: genetic heterogeneity.

Diagnostic Procedures. *Electrophysiology.* Evidence of axonal neuropathy.

BIBLIOGRAPHY. Rabbiosi G, Borroni G, Pinelli P et al: Palmo-plantar keratoderma and Charcot-Marie-Tooth disease. Arch Dermatol 116:789–790, 1980

Talmie JL, Wilcox De, McWilliam R, et al: Palmo-plantar keratoderma, nail dystrophy, and hereditary motor and sensory neuropathy an autosomal dominant trait. J Med Genet 25:754–757, 1988

Outshoorn Skin (see).
Greither keratosis (see).
Buske-Fischer-Brauer (see).

K.P.P., FOCAL–GINGIVAL

Synonym. Fred; focal palmo-plantar—gingival hyperkeratosis.

Symptoms and Signs. Prevalent in males. Onset around puberty. Painful hyperkeratosis of the soles especially over weight-bearing areas. Trauma related hyperkeratosis of palms. Hyperhidrosis in hyperkeratotic areas. Nails of all digits: sub and circum-ungual keratin deposit. Starting at toes (4–5 years of age) and extending to fingers (8–9 years). *Facies.* Follicular keratosis. *Mouth.* Labial and lingual attached gingive: sharply marginated areas of hyperkeratosis (appears in early childhood).

Etiology. Autosomal dominant inheritance.

Pathology. Condensation of tonofilaments appearing as paranuclear bodies in keratocytes.

Therapy. See Papillon-Lefevre.

Prognosis. Progressive condition.

BIBLIOGRAPHY. Fred HL, Gieser RG, Berry WR, et al: Keratosis palmaris et plantaris. Arch Int Med 113:866–871, 1964

Young WG, Newcomb GM, Daley TJ: Focal palmoplantar and gingival hyperkeratosis syndrome: report of a family, with cytology syndrome ultrastructural and histochemical findings. Oral Surg 53:473–482, 1982

Olmsted (see).
Papillon-Lefèvre (see).
Hain-Munch (see).
Schoepf (see).
Scoe (see).
Meleda (see).
Mendez da Costa (see).
Spanlang-Tappeiner (see).
Schaefers (see).

KERATOSIS PILARIS ATROPHICANS

Synonyms. Ulerythema ophryogenes. See scarring follicular keratosis.

Symptoms and Signs. Onset: present at birth or developing soon after. Erythema and small horny pugs in the external halves of eyebrows, slowly extending toward center: nonconstant follicular plugs on the cheeks. Erythema is followed by atrophy. Seldom associated congenital malformation and, or mental retardation.

Etiology. Sporadic or autosomal dominant inheritance.

Pathology. In early stage edema, perivascular infiltration with lymphocytes, later dermal connective atrophy, hair follicle enlarging with horny plugs and attached epithelial cysts; small sebaceous glands.

Therapy. None satisfactory.

Prognosis. Scarring alopecia of eyebrows.

BIBLIOGRAPHY. Davenport DD: Ulerythema ophryogenes. Review and report of a case. Discussion of relationship to cerain other skin disorders and association with internal abnormalities. Arch Dermatol 89:74–80, 1964

Burnett JDW, Schwartz MF, Berberian BJ: Ulerythema ophryogenes with multipe congenital anomalies. Arch Dermatol 18:437–440, 1988

KERATOSIS PILARIS DECALVANS

Synonyms. Siemen; Taenzer; Unna (PG) II; Quinquaud; Arnozan; Brocq lupoid sycosis; Little; Feldman; acne decalvans; folliculitis decalvans; ulerythema sycosiformis; keratosis follicularis spinulosa decalvans. Includes follicular ichthyosis. See Scarring follicular keratosis and Lasseur-Graham-Little. According to old classification: Quinquaud: predominant involvement of scalp; Brocq and Unna: of beard; Arnozan: of legs.

Symptoms and Signs. Complete picture only in males; in heterozygous females, partial expression. Onset in infancy or early childhood (in males) in females from third to sixth decade. First manifestation usually on the face with possible extension to other areas, over years, especially in the extensor surfaces of extremities. Variable occurrence of associated symptoms and signs. Complete pattern includes follicular hyperkeratosis, loss of hair in round, oval patches (scar), surrounded by perifollicular pustules. Pruritus occasionally succeeded by atrophy; generalized alopecia on head (particularly under occipital protuberances), face, axillae, pubic area, and lanugo; sparse eyelashes and eyebrows (particularly on the later portion); photophobia; lacrimation; corneal abnormalities (punctate lesions). Associated findings: blepharitis; ectropion; telangiectasis in the cheeks; hypoplasia of mandible. Follicular ichthyosis: similar condition, noninflammatory that does not progress to atrophy.

Etiology. Unknown; X-linked transmission. Autosomal dominant trait also reported.

Pathology. In early stage edema, perivascular infiltration with lymphocytes. Later dermal connective atrophy, hair follicle enlarging with horny plugs and attached epithelial cysts; small sebaceous glands.

Diagnostic Procedures. *Skin biopsy. Slit-lamp examination.* Corneal lesions. *Urine.* Altered amino acid excretion pattern. *Culture.* Rule out ringworm infections and lupus vulgaris.

Therapy. None successful. Retinoids theoretically potentially useful.

Prognosis. Quoad vitam good. Severe disfiguration may result.

BIBLIOGRAPHY. Quinquaud CS: Folliculite destructive des régions vellues. Bull Soc Med Hop 5:95–98, 1888

Taenzer P: Uber das Ulerythema ophryogenes, eine noch nicht beschriegene Hautkrankheit. Mschr Prak Derm 8:197–208, 1889

Unna PG: The Histopathology of the Diseases of the Skin, p 1086. New York, Clay, 1896

Lameris: Ichthyosis follicularis. Ned Tijdschr Geneeskd 41:1524, 1905

Siemens HW: Ueber einen in der menschlichen Pathologie noch nicht beobachteten. Vererbungsmodus: Dominant-geschlechsgebundene Vererbung. Arch Rass U Ges Biol 17:47–61, 1925

Siemens HW: Keraton; follicularis spinulosa decalvans. Arch Dermatol Syph 151:384–386, 1926

Knops HJ: Siemens's syndrome I (keratosis follicularis spinulosa decalvans). Br J Dermatol 100:611, 1979

Griffiths WAD, Leigh IM, Marks R: Disorders of keratinization. In Champion RH, Burton JL, Ebling FJG (eds): Rook/Wilkinson/Ebling Textbook of Dermatology, 5th ed, p 1354. Oxford, Blackwell Scientific, 1992

KERNICTERUS

Synonyms. Bilirubin encephalopathy; nuclear jaundice; neonatal hyperbilirubinemia.

Symptoms and Signs. Occurs in icteric infant during first 2 or 3 weeks of life. Hypotonia; lethargy and diminution of sucking reflex; spasticity; opisthotonos; convulsions; fever; high-pitched cry. If surviving, neurologic signs develop: seizures; mental deficiency; ataxia; bilateral choreoathetosis.

Etiology. Hyperbilirubinemia with deposition of pigment in the brain and damage of cells. Hemolytic diseases of newborn: Rh, ABO incompatibility; administration of vitamin K water-soluble analogue; congenital hyperbilirubinemic conditions (see Crigler-Najjar).

Pathology. Edema and enlargement of brain; yellowish, orange stain of nuclear masses, especially basal ganglia; degenerative changes of ganglion cells. In patients who survive the acute phase, the brain loses the brilliant stain and shows only loss of ganglion cells and gliosis.

Diagnostic Procedures. *Blood.* Hyperbilirubinemia (indirect); anemia; nucleated red cells.

Therapy. Exchange transfusion with Rh-negative blood. Keep the bilirubin below 20 mg/100 ml. Phototherapy.

Prognosis. Usually fatal in first days when patient survives development of clinical manifestations from neurologic damage.

BIBLIOGRAPHY. Van Praagh R: Diagnosis of kernicterus in the neonatal period. Pediatrics 28:870–876, 1961

Weatherall DJ, Ledingham JGG, Warrell DA (eds): Oxford Textbook of Medicine, 3rd ed, pp 2054, 2058, 3545, 4121. Oxford Med Pub, 1996

KERSHNER-ADAMS

Obsolete.

Synonym. Eponym used to indicate a nonspecific suppurative pneumonitis.

BIBLIOGRAPHY. Kershner RD, Adams WE: Chronic nonspecific suppurative pneumonitis. J Thorac Surg 17:495–511, 1948

KERSTING-HELLWIG

Synonyms. Werther; Stokes spiroadenoma; spiradenoma; eccrine spiradenoma; syringoadenomatosus papilliferus.

Symptoms. Male to female ratio, 2:1; onset at 15–35 years of age. Pain at location of lesion.

Signs. On any area of skin, appearance of a usually solitary, well-defined nodule, diameter 0.5–3.0 cm, overlying skin of normal color or various colors (e.g., blue, yellow).

Etiology. Unknown. Autosomal dominant inheritance possible.

Pathology. Diagnosis is made by histologic examination. Cells of two kinds: around lumina, larger, paler cells; in the periphery, smaller and darker (mioepithelial) cells forming the edges of the lobulated mass. Possibly, cystic spaces in the centers of masses.

Diagnostic Procedure. *Biopsy.*

Therapy. Excision.

Prognosis. Slow growth for years; removal curative. Recurrence if excision incomplete.

BIBLIOGRAPHY. Kersting DW, Helwig B: Eccrine spiradenoma. Arch Dermatol 73:199–227, 1956

Yesudian P, Thambiah A: Fam Syring Dermatol 150:32–35, 1975

MacKie RM: Tumors of the skin appendages. In Champion RH, Burton JL, Ebling FJG (eds): Rook/Wilkinson/Ebling Textbook of Dermatology, 5th ed, p 1518. Oxford, Blackwell Scientific, 1992

KESAREE-WOOLEY

Synonyms. Penta-X.

Symptoms and Signs. Present from birth. Postnatal growth deficiency (65%); failure to thrive (35%); mental deficiency of variable degrees (80%). *Head.* Small (55%); moderate mongoloid slant (60%); low nasal bridge (55%); low ears (65%); dental abnormalities (50%). *Neck.* Short (45%). *Extremities.* Campodactyly/clinodactyly (75%), and arms and feet malformations (radio-ulnar synostosis [45%], micromelia [30%]; joint hyperflexion and dislocations [35%]; etc.). *Congenital heart defects.* Mainly patency of ductus arteriosus (40%).

Diagnostic Procedures. *Chromosome studies.* Presence of five X chromosomes. *Blood.* Reported ketotic hypoglycemia.

Prognosis. Variable. Failure to thrive.

BIBLIOGRAPHY. Kesaree N, Wooley PV Jr: A phenotypic female with 49 chromosomes presumably: A case reported. J Pediatr 63:1099–1103, 1963

Varella J, Alvesalo L: Taurodontism in females with extra X chromosomes. J Craniofac Genet Dev Biol 9:129–133, 1989

KESHAN

Symptoms and Signs. Occurs in the East, particularly in China. Muscle weakness and myalgia.

Etiology. Not defined. Selenium deficit (?), genetic deficiency of selenium dependent enzyme (?), interaction with virus (?).

Pathology. Cardiomyopathy with multifocal necrosis and fibrosis of myocardium.

Therapy. Protection claimed from prophylactic doses of selenomethionine. Improvement with sodium selenite.

BIBLIOGRAPHY. Chen X, Yang G, Chen J, et al: Studies on the relations of selenium and Keshan disease. Biol Trace Elem Res 2:91–107, 1980
Simmer K, Thompson RPH: Trace elements. In Cohen RD, Lewis B, Allberti KGMM, et al: The Metabolic and Molecular Basis of Acquired Disease, vol 1, pp 670–683. London, Baillère Tindall, 1990

KESTENBAUM

Synonyms. Sylvian aqueduct.

Symptoms and Signs. Includes Parinaud (impaired vertical gaze), retraction nystagmus, pupillary abnormalities, convergence and vertical nystagmus, convergence spasm and extraocular palsies.

Etiology and Pathology. Various affections, most of vascular origin, involving periaqueductal gray matter.

BIBLIOGRAPHY. Kestenbaum A: Clinical Methods of Neuro-ophthalmologic Examination. New York, Grune & Stratton, 1946, 1961
Fog M, Hein-Srensen O: Mesencephalic syndromes. In Vinken PJ, Bruyn GW: Handbook of Clinical Neurology, vol 2, p 279. Amsterdam, North-Holland, 1969

KETOTIC HYPERGLYCINEMIA

Obsolete.

This denomination is obsolete because the syndrome may be seen in a number of different disorders (e.g., propionic acidemia; methylmalonic acidemia; isovaleric acidemia). Crisis precipitated by infections or protein intake in majority of cases. Defect of oxidation of propionate and deficiency of propionylcoenzyme A (CoA) carboxylase, and defect of glycine oxidation.

Synonyms. Glycinemia infantilis; secondary hyperglycinemia; hyperglycinuria-hyperglycinemia.

BIBLIOGRAPHY. Fenton WA, Rosenberg LE: Disorders of propionate and methylmalonate metabolism. In Scriver CR, Beaudet AL, Sly WS, et al: The Metabolic and Molecular Bases of Inherited Disease, 7th ed, pp 1423–1449. New York, McGraw-Hill, 1995

KETRON-GOODMAN

Synonyms. See Woringer-Kallopp.

Symptoms and Signs. Generalized pagetoid reticulosis: hyperkeratotic verrucous plaques with prominent epidermatropism (relatively sparing the dermis) with enlarged atypical cutaneous T-cells.

Etiology. Considered a variant of mycosis fungoid (see Alibert-Bazin) or a discrete entity in the light of immunological studies.

Therapy. According to various factors: age, stage of condition, toxicity of therapeutic agents, etc.

BIBLIOGRAPHY. Ketron LW, Goodman MH: Multiple lesions of the skin apparently of epithelial origin resembling clinically mycosis fungoides. Arch Dermatol 24:758, 1931
Bithell TC: Hereditary coagulation disorders. In Lee GR, Bithell TC, Foerster J, et al (eds): Wintrobe's Clinical Hematology, 9th ed. Philadelphia, Lea & Febiger, 1993

Isaacson PG, Norton AJ: Extranodal Lymphomas, p 152. Edinburgh, Churchill Livingstone, 1994

KEUTEL

Synonyms. Pulmonic stenosis; brachytelephalangism; cartilage calcification.

Symptoms. Both sexes. Neural hearing loss. Respiratory difficulty.

Signs. *Facies.* Midface hypoplasia, depressed nasal bridge, small alae nasi. *Other.* Calcification and ossification of cartilage in the ears, nose, larynx, trachea, ribs. *Limbs.* Short terminal phalanges.

Etiology. Autosomal recessive inheritance.

Pathology. Same as in multiple peripheral pulmonary stenosis: multiple peripheral pulmonary stenosis; calcification, and/or ossification of cartilage (external ears, nose, larynx, trachea, and ribs).

Diagnostic Procedures. *X-rays.* Tracheobronchial and other cartilage calcification noted at 13 months as well as stippled epyphyses at knees and elbows. Pulmonary and cardiologic functional studies.

BIBLIOGRAPHY. Keutel J, Jorgensen G, Gabriel P: A new autosomal recessive syndrome: Peripheral pulmonary stenosis, brachytelephalangism, neural hearing loss, and abnormal cartilage calcification-ossification. Birth Defects Orig Art Ser 8(5):60–68, 1972
Fryus JP, Van Fleteren A, Mattalaer P, et al: Calcification of cartilages, brachytelephalangy, and peripheral pulmonary stenosis: confirmation of the Keutel syndrome. Eur J Pediatr 142:201–203, 1984
Khosroshahi HE, Uluoglu O, Olgunturk R, et al: Keutel syndrome: A report of four cases. Eur J Pediatr 149:188–191, 1989

KHALIFEH-ZELLWEGER-PLANCEREL

Synonyms. Pyramidal acropathy mutilant; acro-mutilant neuropathy, pyramidal. See Thévenard.

Symptoms and Signs. Spastic paraplegia and late onset sensory neuropathy with mutilating acropathy.

Etiology. Hereditary condition.

BIBLIOGRAPHY. Kalifeh RR, Zellweger H: Hereditary sensory neuropathy. Neurology (Minneapolis) 13:405–411, 1963
Plancerel AC: Un cas atypique d'acropathie ulcéro-mutilante avec syndrome pyramidal de caractére familial. Schweiz Arch Neurol Neurochir Psych 94:305–347, 1964
Wells CEC: Hereditary sensory radicular neuropathy. In Vinken PJ, Bruyn GW: Handbook of Clinical Neurology, vol 21, p 76. Amsterdam, North-Holland, 1975

K.I.D.

Synonyms. Senter; keratosis—ichtyosis deafness; ichthyosiform erythroderma; sensineural deafness.

Symptoms and Signs. Those of Ichthyosiform erythroderma (see), plus sensineural deafness; vascularized corneas; cryptorchidism; variable flexion joints contraction. In some cases in middle age: hepatomegaly, hepatic cirrhosis, glycogen storage.

Etiology. Unknown. Possibly autosomal recessive inheritance.

Prognosis. May reach middle age.

BIBLIOGRAPHY. Burns FS: A case of generalized congenital keratoderma. J Cutan Dis 33:255–260, 1915
Desmond F, Bar J, Chevillard Y: Erythrodermic ichthyosiforme congenitale seche, surdimutite, hepatomegalie de transmission recessive autosomique. Bull Soc Franc Dem Syph 78:585, 1971

Senter TP, Jones KL, Sakati N, et al: Atypical ichthyosiform erythoderma and congenital sensorineural deafness: A distinct syndrome. J Pediatr 92:68–72, 1978

Griffiths WAD, Leigh IM, Marks R: Disorders of keratinization. In Champion RH, Burton JL, Ebling FJG (eds): Rook/Wilkinson/Ebling Textbook of Dermatology, 5th ed, pp 1331–1332. Oxford, Blackwell Scientific, 1992

KIDNEY ARTERIOVENOUS FISTULA

Symptoms. Headache and other common symptoms of blood hypertension, and early symptoms of cardiac failure.

Signs. Blood hypertension; bruit heard best over upper part of abdomen, anteriorly or posteriorly; palpable thrill. Cardiac enlargement, edema, and other signs of cardiac failure.

Etiology. Arteriovenous fistula of the kidney.

Pathology. See Etiology.

Diagnostic Procedures. *Blood.* Polycythemia. *Excretory urography. Aortography. CT scan.*

Therapy. Surgery.

Prognosis. Early cardiac failure; good response to surgery with remission of all signs.

BIBLIOGRAPHY. Kirby CK, et al: Arteriovenous fistula of renal vessels: case report. Surgery 37:267–271, 1955

Scheifley CH: A new clinical syndrome producing hypertension–arteriovenous fistula of the kidney. JAMA 174:1625–1627, 1960

Morton MJ, Charboneau JW: Arteriovenus fistula after biopsy of renal transplant: detection and monitoring with color flow and duplex ultrasonography. Mayo Clin Proc 64:531–534, 1989

KIENBÖCK

Synonyms. Lunatomalacia; lunate bone osteochondrosis. See Epiphyseal ischemic necrosis.

Symptoms and Signs. More common in males. Onset at young age (15–40 years), usually after severe trauma with wrist in dorsiflexion (75% of cases). Symptoms become manifest 18 months prior to X-ray-shown lesions. Recurrent pain, stiffness, and limitation of extension of wrist. Swelling over lunate bone area, with thickening of skin and tenderness on palpation.

Etiology. See Epiphyseal ischemic necrosis.

Therapy. Not standardized. Surgical based on ulnar lengthening. Conservative; early casting (4 months, with uncertain results).

Prognosis. According to success of treatment.

BIBLIOGRAPHY. Kienböck R: Ueber traumatische Malazie des Mondbeins und ihre Folgezustaende: Entartungsformen und Kompressions-frakturen. Forschr Roentgen 16:77–103, 1910

Klippel JH, Dieppe PA: Rheumatology, p 7.4.8. St Louis, CV Mosby, 1995

KIENBÖCK SYRINGOMYELIA

Eponym used to indicate the traumatic form of Morvan I (see).

BIBLIOGRAPHY. Kienböck R: Kritik der sogennanten Traumatischen syringomyelie. Jahrbuch Psychiatr 21:50–110, 1910

Kienboeck's disease. In Vastamaeki M: Current Trends in Hand Surgery, pp 99–124. Netherlands, Excerpta Medica, 1995

KIFAFA SEIZURES

Symptoms and Signs. In an isolated tribe in Tanzania. In children, head nodding preceding seizures. Parkinson-like manifestation associated with the other neurological abnormalities; mental retardation and psychotic attacks. Severe burns because of lack of coordination and sensibility.

Etiology. Possibly autosomal recessive inheritance.

BIBLIOGRAPHY. Jilek-Aall L, Jilek W, Miller JR: Clinical and genetic aspects of seizure disorders prevalent in an isolated African population. Epilepsia 20:613–222, 1979

KIKUCHI

Synonyms. Lymphoadenitis cervical subacute necrotizing; necrotizing subacute cervical lymphoadenitis.

Symptoms and Signs. Fever and exanthema. Painful cervical lymphoadenopathy.

Etiology. Unknown. Viral (?). Toxoplasma (?).

Pathology. *Lymph nodes.* Necrotic changes with histiocytes and immunoblastic cells and absence of neutrophils or granulomas.

Diagnostic Procedures. *Blood.* Neutropenia. *Lymph node biopsy.*

Prognosis. Remission after 3–6 weeks.

BIBLIOGRAPHY. Kikuchi M: Lymphadenitis showing focal reticulum cells hyperplasia with nuclear debris and phagocytosis. Acta Haemat Jpu 35:379–380, 1972

Ali MH, Horton LWL: Necrotising lymphoadenitis without neutrophilic infiltration (Kikuchi's disease). J Clin Pathol 38:1252–1257, 1985

KILOH-NEVIN II

Synonyms. Anterior interosseous nerve; interosseus neuritis. See Parsonage-Turner.

Symptoms and Signs. Spontaneous onset or following injury of bones. Isolated paralysis of flexor pollicis longus and flexor digitorum profundus; absence of sensory involvement (may be combined with partial medium nerve paresis). Square pinch sign. Contact between pulps of thumb and index (impossible).

Etiology. Idiopathic or associated with fracture or injury of forearm bones or nerve entrapment of median nerve by tendons, arteries; thrombosis of vessels; Volkmann (see) contracture.

Pathology. Lesion of anterior interosseous nerve.

Diagnostic Procedures. *Electromyography. Triketohydrindene hydrate test.*

Therapy. Surgery to free the nerve in all cases if traumatic nature; and in spontaneous cases when there is no improvement after 12 weeks.

Prognosis. Within 2 years, almost complete recovery in idiopathic cases.

BIBLIOGRAPHY. Parsonage MJ, Turner JWA: Neurologic amyotrophy: The shoulder-girdle syndrome. Lancet I:973–978, 1948

Kiloh LG, Nevin S: Isolated neuritis of anterior interosseous nerve. Br Med J 1:850–851, 1952

Chan KM, Lamb DW: The anterior interosseous nerve syndrome. J Roy Coll Surg Edinburgh 29:350–353, 1984

Weatherall DJ, Ledingham JGG, Warrell DA (eds): Oxford Textbook of Medicine, 3rd ed, pp 4094–4096. Oxford, Oxford Med Pub, 1996

KIMMELSTIEL-WILSON

Synonym. Diabetic glomerulosclerosis; intercapillary glomerulosclerosis.

Eponym used in the past to indicate the various forms of diabetic glomerulopathies. It is better to restrict its use to the anatomic-pathologic finding of nodular glomerular sclerosis. This lesion is characterized by tubular atrophy and dilatation, ball-like hyaline acidophilic masses situated at the periphery of glomerular tuft containing nuclei, and thickening of basal membrane. Kimmelstiel himself writes: "We have learned that this correlation is much closer to nonspecific glomerular changes which were carefully excluded in the original presentation. The term Kimmelstiel-Wilson syndrome is, therefore, not justified."

BIBLIOGRAPHY. Kimmelstiel P, Wilson C: Benign and malignant hypertension and nephrosclerosis: A clinical and pathological study. Am J Pathol 12:45–48, 1936
Friedman EA: Diabetes mellitus: Late complications, nephropathy. In De Groot LJ (ed): Endocrinology, 3rd ed, p 1574. Philadelphia, WB Saunders, 1995
Ritz E, Fliser D, Siebel M: Diabetic nephropathy. In Weatherall DJ, Ledingham JGG, Warrell DA (eds): Oxford Textbook of Medicine, 3rd ed, pp 3167–3172. Oxford, Oxford Med Pub, 1996

KIMURA

Synonyms. Angiolymphoid hyperplasia—eosinophils; epithelioid hemangioma; hemangioma epithelioid; eosinophilic lymphofolliculosis of skin; E.L.S.

Symptoms and Signs. More common in Japan in young male adults. Cluster of translucent nodules (2–3 cm) around ear. Frequent renal involvement (membranous glomerulonephritis).

Etiology. Unknown. Possibly antigenic stimulation after insect bite.

Pathology. Proliferating capillaries lined with swollen endothelial cells and surrounded by lymphocytes and eosinophils.

Diagnostic Procedures. *Blood.* Eosinophilia; evidence of nephrotic syndrome may be present. *Urine.* Proteinuria may be found.

Therapy. None and observation or surgery or radiotherapy (both effective).

Prognosis. Spontaneous regression after variable period of time.

BIBLIOGRAPHY. Kimura T, Yoshimura S, Ishikawa E: On the unusual granulation combined with hyperplastic changes of lymphatic tissues. Trans Jap Path Soc 37:179, 1948
Wells GC, Whimster IW: Subcutaneous angiomatous hyperplasia with eosinophilia. Br J Dermatol 81:1–15, 1969
Yamada A: Membranous glomerulonephritis associated with eosinophilic lymphofolliculosis of the skin (Kimura's disease): A report of a case and review of the literature. Clin Nephrol 18:211–215, 1982
MacKie RM: Soft tissue tumors. In Champion RH, Burton JL, Ebling FJG (eds): Rook/Wilkinson/Ebling Textbook of Dermatology, 5th ed, pp 2085–2086. Oxford, Blackwell Scientific, 1992

KINDLER

Synonyms. Weary-Kindler; poikiloderma, acrokeratoic, hereditary; bullous acrokeratotic poikiloderma.

Symptoms and Signs. Both sexes. Pigmentary anomalies in majority of cases; tendency to blister following mild trauma. Four clinical expressions identified.

1. *Onset 1–3 months.* Vescico-pustule on hands and feet resolving in late childhood.
2. *Onset 3–6 months.* Eczematoid diffuse dermatitis resolving at age 5 years.
3. *Onset in first month.* Gradual diffuse poikiloderma striate and reticulate atrophy (sparing face and ears) persisting into adulthood.
4. *Onset before age 5.* Keratotic papules on hands, feet, elbows, knees. Persisting into adulthood.

Etiology. Unknown. Autosomal dominant inheritance; recessive also suggested (with photosensitivity in addition to other symptoms). The nosologic status of the congenital poikiloderma cluster of syndromes is under revision.

BIBLIOGRAPHY. Kindler T: Congenital poikiloderma with traumatic bulla formation and progressive cutaneous atrophy. Br J Derm 66:104–111, 1954
Weary PE, Manley WF Jr, Graham GF: Hereditary acrokeratotic poikiloderma. Arch Derm 103:409–422, 1971
Hacham-Zadeh S, Garfunkel AA: Kindler syndrome in two related Kurdish families. Ann Med Genet 20:43–48, 1985
Burton JL: Disorders of connective tissue. In Champion RH, Burton JL, Ebling FJG (eds): Rook/Wilkinson/Ebling Textbook of Dermatology, 5th ed, p 1777. Oxford, Blackwell Scientific, 1992

KING-DENBOROUGH

Synonym. Malignant hyperthermia—myopathy—multiple anomalies.

Symptoms and Signs. Almost all males—one female. From childhood. Short stature; delayed motor development; malar hypoplasia; micrognathia; ptosis or blepharophimosis; downslanting of palpebral fissures; malignant hyperthermia; pectus carenatum; cryptorchidism.

Etiology. Unknown. Apparently nonfamilial. Increase of creatinine phosphokinase in some cases in healthy members of family may suggest an autosomal dominant trait.

Pathology. *Fresh muscle biopsy.* Increased contracture on exposure to halotane. *Muscle histologic examination.* Predominance of type 2 fibers.

Diagnostic Procedures. *Muscle biopsy. Electromyography. Blood.* Creatine phosphokinase level occasionally increased.

Therapy. Physical therapy with some improvement of muscle strength. Surgery for the correction of kyphoscoliosis, pectus carinatum, and cryptorchidism. Prior to surgical operation, pretreatment with dantrolene for the prevention of malignant hyperthermia (MH). Avoid drugs like halothane and succinylcholine that can trigger an MH episode.

Prognosis. Relatively mild, slowly progressing course. High risk for malignant hyperthermia (usual cause of death in reported cases).

BIBLIOGRAPHY. King JO, Denborough MA: Anesthetic-induced malignant hyperpyrexia in children. J Pediatr 83:37–40, 1973
Steenson AJ, Torkelson RD: King's syndrome with malignant hyperthermia: Potential outpatient risks. Am J Dis Child 141:271–273, 1987

KINGSTON

Synonym. Cleft lip/palate; uveal colobomata; mental retardation.

Symptoms and Signs. Eye anomalies (uveal colobomata, cataracts, microphthalmia, retina detachment, posterior embryotoxon, glaucoma, pstosis); cleft lip/palate.

Etiology. Autosomal dominant.

BIBLIOGRAPHY. Kinston HM, Harper PS, Jones PW: An autosomal dominant syndrome of uveal colobomata, cleft lip and palate and mental retardation. J Med Genet 19:444–446, 1982

KINSBOURINE

Synonyms. Dancing eye; oculogyric crisis. See also West.

Symptoms and Signs. Occurs in children 1–3 years old. Irregular jerky eye movements; twitching of eyelids and eyebrows, enhanced or promoted by activity. Occasionally, lateral nystagmus. Lack of coordination; ataxia; irritability; generalized myoclonic attacks; mental retardation.

Etiology. Unknown.

Diagnostic Procedures. *Electromyography. Myoclonic action potentials.*

Therapy. See West.

BIBLIOGRAPHY. Kinsbourine M: Myoclonic encephalopathy of infants. J Neurol Neurosurg Psychiatr 27:271–276, 1962
Adams RD, Victor M: Principles of Neurology, 5th ed, p 230. New York, McGraw-Hill, 1993

KIRMAN

Synonyms. Idiocy; ectodermal dysplasia.

Symptoms and Signs. In one female. Anhidrosis, alopecia, severe mental retardation; normal nails, teeth, and breasts.

BIBLIOGRAPHY. Kirman BH: Idiocy and ectodermal dysplasia. BR J Dermatol 67:303–307, 1953

KIRNER

Synonym. Dystelephalangy.

Symptoms. Lesion not manifest before five years of age. Male to female ratio, 1:2. *Females.* More frequently bilateral. *Male.* Monolateral. Becomes evident from fifth year of life. Asymptomatic.

Signs. Painless soft tissue swelling of the tip of fifth fingers that progressively point toward the tenar eminence.

Etiology. Unknown; autosomal dominant inheritance.

Diagnostic Procedures. *X-ray of hand.* Metaphyses of distal phalanx of fifth finger angulated. No bone deformity.

Therapy. Orthopedic surgery.

BIBLIOGRAPHY. Kirner J: Doppelseitge Verkuemmungen des Kleinefingerendgliedes als selbstaendiges Krankheitbild. Fortschr Roengenstr 36:804, 1927
Brailsford JF: Radiology of Bones and Joints, 5th ed, p 64. Baltimore, Williams & Wilkins, 1953
David TJ, Burnwood RL: The nature and inheritance of Kirner's deformity. J Med Genet 9:430–433, 1972
Kerboul B, LeSaout J, Lefevre C: La déformation de Kirner. A propos de 3 nouveaux cas. Revue de la littèrature. J Radiol 67:523–527, 1986

KITAMURA

Synonym. Periodic thyrotoxic paralysis; thyrotoxic paralysis, periodic.

Symptoms. Occurs more often in males; onset in third or fourth decade. Occurs mostly in people of Japanese extraction. (Two to eight percent of hyperthyroid Japanese patients suffer from this syndrome.) Usually occurs in the early morning; episodes during the day occur when resting after either heavy exertion or large meals. Painless episodes of paroxysmal symmetric muscle weakness that make the patient unable to rise or move. Eye movements, speech, swallowing, respiration unimpaired. Attacks last from 1 to several hours. Between attacks, completely normal. When attack occurs during the day, initial weakness announces attack. This may be prevented by activity. All symptoms of hyperthyroidism (see Flajani). Clinical manifestation of hyperthyroidism may appear after months of muscle syndrome. In some cases, thyroid may be enlarged without other signs of hyperthyroidism.

Signs. During attack; reflexes of group of muscles involved reduced or absent; in unaffected muscles, normal reflexes. No myotonia. Signs of hyperthyroidism.

Etiology. Shift of extracellular potassium into cells causing paralysis in patients in whom a latent defect has been unmasked by the hyperthyroid condition.

Pathology. *Muscle biopsy.* Shows mainly normal, rare fibers undergoing degenerative changes. *Light and electron microscopy.* Disclose in affected muscles small, central subsarcolemmal vacuolization.

Diagnostic Procedures. Paralytic attack induced by 10 U of insulin. *Electromyography.* During attack, myopathic type paresis. *Blood.* Glucose tolerance test altered. Lymphocytosis during attack. Hypokalemia accompanies every induced attack. All tests for hyperthyroidism.

Therapy. Treatment of hyperthyroidism. Episodes aborted by potassium administration or propranolol. Prophylaxis by avoiding precipitating causes or heavy meals.

Prognosis. Correction of thyroid function induces complete remission of periodic paralysis and associated findings.

BIBLIOGRAPHY. Shinosaki T: Klinische Studien ueber die periodischen Paralyse der Extremitaten. Zt Ges Neurol Psychiatr 100:564–611, 1926
Norris FH, Panner BJ, Stormont JM: Thyrotoxic periodic paralysis; metabolic and ultrastructural studies. Arch Neurol 19:88–98, 1968
McKenzie JM, Zakarija M: Hyperthyroidism. In De Groot LJ (ed): Endocrinology, 3rd ed, p 689. Philadelphia, WB Saunders, 1995

KITAMURA

Synonyms. Angiolymphoid hyperplasia, eosinophils.

Symptoms and Signs. More frequent in Japan. In young adults. Small (2–3 cm), translucent nodules around hairline.

Etiology. Unknown: possibly antigenic response to insect bites. Possible difference between Kitamura (deeper sited lesions) and angiolymphoid hyperplasia, eosinophils (smaller papullar lesions).

Pathology. Proliferating blood vessels surrounded by lymphocytes and eosinophils infiltrate.

Diagnostic Procedures. *Blood.* Eosinophilia.

Therapy. Wait and observe. Surgery and radiotherapy effective.

BIBLIOGRAPHY. Vàzquez-Botet M Sàncez JL: Angiolymphoid hyperplasia with eosinophilia: Report of a case and review of literature. J Derm Surg Oncol 4:931–936, 1978
Chan JKC, Hui PK, Ng CS, et al: Epithelioid haemangioma (angiolymphoid hyperplasia with eosinophilia) and Kitamura's disease. Chin Histopathol 15:557–574, 1989

KJELLIN

Synonyms. Spastic paraplegia, retinal degeneration; optic athophy, spastic paraplegia. See Barnard-Scholz.

Symptoms and Signs. Both sexes. Mental retardation (stationary), later onset and (onset at 25 years of age) progressive course of spastic paraplegia, atrophy of small muscles of hands (onset apparent at 35 years of age), amyotrophic changes. Visual reduction with slow progression from central retinal degeneration with small atrophic foci and pigment displacement in the macula and immediate vicinity (late onset); striking resemblance in appearance, speech, facial expression, and symptoms and signs of subjects within same family ("double" phenomenon). If olphthalmoplegia is added to these signs, it is called Barnard-Scholz (see).

Etiology. Possibly autosomal dominant inheritance, also X-linked family reported.

BIBLIOGRAPHY. Kjellin KG: Hereditary spastic paraplegia and retinal degeneration (Kjellin syndrome and Barnard-Scholz syndrome). In Vinken PJ, Bruyn GW (eds): Handbook of Clinical Neurology, vol 22, pp 467–473. Amsterdam, North-Holland, 1975

Kjellin KG: Hereditary spastic paraplegia and retinal degeneration (Kjellin syndrome and Barnard-Scholz syndrome). In Vinken PJ, Bruyn GW: Handbook of Clinical Neurology, vol 22, pp 467–473. Amsterdam, North-Holland, 1975

Rothner AD, Yahr F, Yahr MD: Familial spastic paraparesis, optic atrophy and dementia: Clinical observations of affected kindred. New York, J Med 76:756–758, 1976

Adams RD, Victor M: Principles of Neurology, 5th ed, p 999. New York, McGraw-Hill, 1993

KJER OPTIC ATROPHY

Synonyms. Optic atrophy, infantile.

Symptoms and Signs. Loss of vision, beginning in infancy and becoming manifest insidiously in childhood, with a highly variable pattern. Nystagmus in severe cases. Bitemporal pallor of the nerve head, seldom macula shoes, fine pigment stippling. Visual fields: cecocentral scotoma, particular poor perception for color blue. No systemic or neurologic abnormalities associated.

Etiology. Autosomal dominant inheritance. Less frequently recessive. Linked to chromosome 2p.

Diagnostic Procedures. *ERG.* Normal. *VER.* Abnormal.

Prognosis. Often remains stationary beyond a certain degree of impairment or progresses during childhood.

BIBLIOGRAPHY. Snell S: Diseases of the optic nerve I. Hereditary or congenital optic atrophy and allied cases. Trans Ophthalmol Soc UK 17:66–81, 1897

Kjer P: Infantile optic atrophy with dominant mode of inheritance. Acta Ophthalmologica Suppl 54. 1959

Vinken PJ, Bruyn GW: Handbook of Clinical Neurology, vol 42, p 408. Amsterdam, North-Holland, 1981

Kivlin JD, Lovrin EW, Bishop DT, et al: Linkage analysis in dominant optic atrophy. Am J Hum Genet 35:1190–1195, 1983

KLEINE-LEVIN

Synonyms. Bulimia; hypersomnia; morbid hunger; periodic somnolence; hibernation. See Gelineau syndrome.

Symptoms. Usually affects adolescent males. Attacks of somnolence lasting several days or weeks; ravenous appetite when awake. Sometimes attacks accompanied by motor unrest, irritability, incoherent speech, hallucination, absence of nocturnal disturbance of sleep.

Etiology. Unknown; occasionally appearing after acute illness (suggesting postencephalitic condition) or following trauma. A family with autosomal inheritance reported.

Pathology. Unknown; possibly lesion of prefrontal zone or hypothalamus or both.

Diagnostic Procedures. *Electroencephalography.* Occasional spiking as in epilepsy.

Therapy. Amphetamine; lithium.

Prognosis. Interval of months or years between attacks. Patient normal in the interval. Attacks tend to disappear as full adulthood is reached.

BIBLIOGRAPHY. Kleine W: Periodische Schlafsucht. Mschr Psychiatr Neurol 57:285–320, 1925

Levin M: Narcolepsy (Gelineau's syndrome) and other varieties of morbid somnolence. Arch Neurol Psychiatr 22:1172–1200, 1929

Levin M: Periodic somnolence and morbid hunger: A new syndrome. Brain 59:494–504, 1936

Giannini AJ, Slaby AE: The Eating Disorders. Ijmuiden, The Netherlands, Springer, 1993

KLEINSCHMIDT

Obsolete. Eponym used to indicate the respiratory distress secondary to laryngeal stenosis, dyspnea, tachycardia, hyperthermia, associated with nucal rigidity, observed as complications of influenza.

BIBLIOGRAPHY. Kleinschmidt H: Ein charakteristisches Syndrom durch Influenzabazilleninfektion. Kinderaerztl Prax 10:52–58, 1939

KLEINST

Synonyms. Mayer-Gross; apraxia; constructional apraxia.

Symptoms. Inability to assemble elements to form a significant or correct whole (arranging; building; drawing). The fourth form of apraxia (see Liepmann).

Etiology. Resulting from lesions of right hemisphere in left-handed persons.

BIBLIOGRAPHY. Kleinst K: Gehirnpathologie. Vornehmlich Aufgrund der Kriegerfahrungen. Aus: Handboch der Artzlichen Weltkriege, Band IV, TL 9. Leipzig, Clothbarth, 1934

Mayer-Gross W: Some observations on apraxia. Proc R Soc Med 28:1203–1212, 1935

Adams RD, Victor M: Principles of Neurology, 5th ed, p 406. New York, McGraw-Hill, 1993

KLEIN-WAARDENBURG

Synonym. Waardenburg III, WS III.

Symptoms and Signs. Those of Waardenburg (see) with associated limb anomalies: hypoplasia of musculoskeletal system; flexion contractures, fusion of carpal bones; syndactyly; without dystopia canthorum but unilateral ptosis.

Etiology. Autosomal dominant inheritance.

BIBLIOGRAPHY. Klein D: Albinism partial (leucisme) avec surdi-mutism, blepharophimosis et dysplasie myo-osteo-articulaire. Helv Paediatr Acta 5:38–58, 1950

Klein D: Historical background and evidence for dominant inheritance of the Klein-Waardenburg syndrome (type III). Am J Med Genet 14:231–239, 1983

Sheffer R Zlotogora J Autosomal dominant inheritance of Klein Waardenburg syndrome. Am J Med Genet 42:320–322, 1992

Zoghbi HY, Ballabio A: Waardenburg syndrome. In Scriver CR, Beaudet AL, Sly WS, et al: The Metabolic and Molecular Bases of Inherited Disease, 7th ed, pp 4575–4580. New York, McGraw-Hill, 1995

KLINEFELTER

Synonyms. Reifenstein-Albright; aspermatogenesis; gynecomastia; seminiferous tubule dysgenesis; XXY; XXXY; XXYY; XXXXY.

Symptoms. Occurs in 1/500 to 1/2000 male births. Manifestations become evident at adolescence. Infertility; usually asymptomatic except for a decrease of libido in about 30% of cases and many psychopathologic manifestations: immaturity; shyness; lack of judgment; assertive unrealistic activity.

Signs. Testes small and firm. Gynecomastia (usually minimal); tendency toward obesity; secondary sex characteristics well developed except in some patients, who may present sparsity of facial hair and other eunuchoid characteristics (arm span that exceeds body length by more than 4 inches). Frequently associated with this syndrome are asthma, chronic pulmonary diseases, hypothyroidism, diabetes mellitus (8%).

Etiology. Syndrome caused by chromosomal polysomy. Presence of 47 chromosomes, including two X and one Y. Other patterns of chromosomal aberration, such as XXXY, XXYY, and some mosaic patterns may result in the same syndrome.

Pathology. Testes: variable degree of hyalinization of tubules; absence of elastic fibers around tunica propria; Leydig cells adequate number, frequently clumped.

Diagnostic Procedures. *Urine.* Follicle-stimulating hormone (FSH) levels usually elevated; 17-ketosteroids and 17-hydroxycorticoids low, normal, or diminished. *Buccal smears.* Sex chromatin positive. *Blood.* Drumsticks in smears. *Chromosome studies.* Forty-seven chromosomes or other abnormal patterns. *Biopsy of testes.* See Pathology.

Therapy. Androgens when secondary sex characteristics do not develop properly (Also improve the mood, school performance, and work capacity.) For gynecomastia, plastic surgery.

Prognosis. Good; infertility; normal life span.

BIBLIOGRAPHY. Klinefelter HR Jr, Reifenstein EC Jr, Albright F: Syndrome characterized by gynecomastia, aspermatogenesis without A-leydigism, and increased excretion of follicle-stimulating hormone. J Clin Endocrinol 2:615–627, 1942

Bandmann HJ, Breit R (eds): Klinefelter's Syndrome. Berlin, Springer Verlag, 1984

Netley C: Personality in 47, XXY males during adolescence. Clin Genet 39:409–418, 1991

Winters SJ: Clinical disorders of the testis. In De Groot LJ (ed): Endocrinology, 3rd ed, pp 2386–2388. Philadelphia, WB Saunders, 1995

KLINTWORTHE

Synonyms. Myoclonic ataxia, acute.

BIBLIOGRAPHY. Salam M: Metabolic ataxias. In Vinken PJ, Bruyn GW: Handbook of Clinical Neurology, vol 21, p 583. Amsterdam, North-Holland, 1975

KLIPPEL

Eponym used to indicate motion incapacitation owing to severe osteoarthritic ankylosing changes in elderly people also suffering from arteriosclerotic changes. A generalized arthritic pseudoparalysis results.

BIBLIOGRAPHY. Klippel M: De la pseudoparalysie générale arthritique. Rev Med 12:280–285, 1892

KLIPPEL-FEIL

Synonyms. Brevicollis, congenital cervicothoracic vertebrae synostosis; congenital osseous; torticollis. Including K-F and conductive deafness; K-F and absent vagina.

Symptoms. Females prevalently affected (65%). Difficulty in breathing and swallowing. Occasionally, associated neurologic disturbance caused by congenital myeloid dysplasia. Convergent strabismus; horizontal nystagmus; deafness. "Mirror movements" syndrome may be said to be present in the condition where voluntary movements of one arm are involuntarily mimicked by the other one.

Signs. Shortening of neck; lowering of hairline on back of neck; platybasia; limited neck motion; occasionally associated, torticollis;

facial asymmetry; scoliosis and kyphosis; Sprengel (see) deformity of scapula (congenital displacement upward) sometimes also associated. This syndrome may be subdivided into four types:

Type 1. Extensive anomalies with elements of several vertebrae incorporated into a single block.

Type 2. Failure of complete segmentation of one or two cervical interspaces.

Type 3. Includes type 1 or type 2 with coexisting abnormalities of lower dorsolumbar spine.

Type 4. Includes type 1 with sacral agenesis.

Etiology. Unknown; autosomal dominant or recessive disorder with various degrees of penetrance. Congenital fusion of two or more cervical vertebrae. Particular features may be associated as conductive deafness or absent vagina. Those features allow the separation of distinct disorders.

Pathology. See Signs. Webbed trapezius muscle.

Diagnostic Procedures. *X-ray.* Cervical spine shortened and vertebrae fused; associated malformation. *Complete radiological evaluation.* Including a metrizamide-enhanced computerized tomography scan with sagittal reconstruction. Magnetic resonance imaging can be useful, particularly if an associated syringomyelia is suspected.

Therapy. Various surgical approaches. Posterior cervical fusion with autogenous bone graft is indicated in presence of unstable fusion pattern. Anterior or posterior decompression if there is cranio-cervical anomaly and radiological evidence of a compression area. Decompressive laminectomy in presence of cervical spine stenosis, symptomatic.

Prognosis. Malformation static during life. Progressive paraplegia possible later in life.

BIBLIOGRAPHY. Klippel M, Feil A: Un cas d'absence des vertebres cervicales avec cage thoracique remontant jusqua à la base du crane (cage thoracique cervicale). Nouv Icon Salpetrière 25:223–250, 1912

Naguib MG, Maxwell RE, Chou SN: Klippel-Feil syndrome in children: Clinical features and management. Child Nerv Syst 1:255–263, 1985

Raas-Rothschild A, Goodman RM, Grunbaum M, et al: Klippel-Feil anomaly with sacral agenesis: An additional subtype, Type IV. J Cranio Fac Genet Dev Biol 8:297–301, 1988

KLIPPEL-TRENAUNAY-WEBER

Synonyms. Ollier-Klippel; Parkes-Weber I; Trenaunay; Weber Leschke; angio-osteohypertrophy; hemangiectasia hypertrophicans; osteohypertrophic nevus flammeus; nevus verucosus hypertrophicans (P.F.).

Symptoms and Signs. Nevi unilaterally located; varicose veins; hypertrophy of soft tissue and bones of affected extremity (usually upper), which makes it longer and warmer than the unaffected one. (If hypertrophy secondary to arteriovenous aneurysm is present the syndrome is called Parkes-Weber or Leschke.) Varicose veins and osteohypertrophy not always present at birth but develop during first few months or years of life. Syndactyly and polydactyly frequently associated. Other internal anomalies also associated.

Etiology. Unknown; possibly, hereditary weakness of mesenchymal tissue of vascular walls. Autosomal dominant inheritance.

Pathology. Nevi with dilated capillaries, lined with single layer of endothelial cells; in some cases arteriovenous fistula. Hypertrophy of muscles and bones of affected limb (see Signs).

Diagnostic Procedures. *X-ray.* (Not diagnostic.) Thickening of bone cortex.

Therapy. Some vascular lesions can be defined and their feeding vessel ligated; in some cases it is possible to extirpate the entire lesion.

Prognosis. Very rapid period of enlargement, then sudden cessation of growth; residual deformity.

BIBLIOGRAPHY. Klippel M, Trenaunay P: Naevus variqueux osteohypertrophique. Arch Gen Med (Paris) 3:641–642, 1900

Weber PF: Angioformation in connection with hypertrophy of limbs and hemihypertrophy. Br J Derm 19:231–235, 1907

Viljoen DL: Klippel-Trenaunay-Weber syndrome (angio-osteohypertrophy syndrome). J Med Genet 25:250–252, 1988

Atherton DJ: Nevi and other developmental defects. In Champion RH, Burton JL, Ebling FJG (eds): Rook/Wilkinson/Ebling Textbook of Dermatology, 5th ed, pp 498–500. Oxford, Blackwell Scientific, 1992

KLÜVER-BUCY

Synonym. Temporal lobectomy behavior.

Symptoms. Symptoms appear soon after bilateral removal of temporal lobes. Loss of recognition of people, including close relatives; loss of fear and rage reaction; hypersexuality, also hypersexuality in the form of masturbation; homosexual tendency; bulimia; hypermetamorphosis (response by motor action to every object or event); marked memory deficiency.

Etiology. Surgery attempting removal of bilateral epileptogenic foci. In humans this operation in some cases reproduces the syndrome experimentally induced by Klüver and Bucy in rhesus monkeys. The syndrome has been observed also after treating herpes encephalitis.

Pathology. Bilateral removal of anterior portion of temporal lobes, uncus, anterior part of the hippocampus, and amygdaloid nucleus.

Diagnostic Procedures. *X-ray of skull.* Atrophy of temporal lobe. *Angiography. CT brain scan.*

Therapy. Carbamazepine.

Prognosis. Result of the operation for treatment of the epileptic attacks arising from temporal lobes is poor. In the postencephalitic syndrome, improvement can occur over an extended period, and chronic residual sequelae may be relatively mild.

BIBLIOGRAPHY. Klüver H, Bucy PC: An analysis of certain effects of bilateral temporal lobectomy in the rhesus monkey, with special reference to "psychic blindness." J Psychol 5:33–54, 1938

Bucy PC, Klüver H: Anatomic changes secondary to temporal lobectomy. Arch Neurol Psychiatr 44:1142–1146, 1940

Hart RP, Kwentus JA, Frazier RB, et al: Natural history of Klüver-Bucy syndrome after treated herpes encephalitis. S Med J (Birmingham) 79:1376–1378, 1986

Adams RD, Victor M: Principles of Neurology, 5th ed, p 391. New York, McGraw-Hill, 1993

KNEE JOINT, INTERNAL DERANGEMENT

Synonyms. IDK; internal knee derangement; knee locking; weak knee. See plica.

Symptoms. Pain on movement of knee; locking, buckling, snapping.

Signs. Local tenderness; thigh atrophy; joint swelling; special maneuvers to reproduce symptoms.

Etiology and Pathology. IDK is a loose term that includes many etiologic causes: tears of menisci; cyst of menisci; discoid meniscus; calcified meniscus; ligament tears; incomplete tears; fractures of tibial plateaus; tears of patellar tendons; fracture of patella; chondromalacia of patella; traumatic synovial effusions; plica articularis syndrome; Pellegrini-Stieda, osteochondritis dissecans; Osgood-Schlatter; Baker cyst; osteoarthritis; pigmented villonodular synovitis rheumatoid arthritis. (Many of these syndromes have been described under proper headings.)

Diagnostic Procedures. *X-ray. Aspiration of fluid. Biopsy of synovial membrane.*

Therapy. Rest; immobilization, surgical correction, or repair according to etiology or systemic medication.

Prognosis. Depends on etiology.

BIBLIOGRAPHY. Hey W: Practical Observations in Surgery. London, Cadell and Davis, 1803

Insall JN, Windsor RE, Scott WN, et al (eds): Surgery of the Knee. New York, Churchill Livingstone, 1993

Graham GP, Fairclough JA: The knee. In Klippel JH, Dieppe PA: Rheumatology. St Louis, CV Mosby, 1995

KNIEST

Synonyms. Dwarfism Kniest; metatrophic dwarfism II; Swiss cheese cartilage dysplasia.

Symptoms and Signs. Present from birth. Moon facies with prominent eyes; saddle nose; short arms and legs. Incapacity to make a fist; violaceous hue of the palms. Swelling of joints; lack of full elbow extension. Reduced length; variable weight. Delay of motor milestones. Poor vision; decreased hearing; muscle weakness. Frequently, cleft palate. Intelligence normal. First and second cervical nerve irritability with secondary myelopathy signs.

Etiology. Autosomal dominant inheritance. Abnormal proteoglycan synthesis suggested.

Pathology. Swiss cheese cartilage; intracytoplasmatic accumulation of metachromatic material. Hiatal hernia.

Diagnostic Procedures. *Urine.* High excretion of keratan sulfate. *X-rays.* General skeletal hypoplasia (that of odontoid process of greatest clinical significance). See Atlantoaxial-spinal dislocation. Characteristic pelvic changes (wineglass deformity). *Cartilage biopsy.* Soft resistance at needle penetration. See Pathology.

Therapy. Stabilization of unstable atlantoaxial joint. Prevention of joint contractures. Total joint replacement.

Prognosis. Poor. Bony fusion between anterior arch of atlas and odontoid and posterior arch of atlas and cranial base.

BIBLIOGRAPHY. Kniest W: Zur Abgrenzung der Dysostosis enchondralis von der Chondrodystrophie. Z Kinderheilkd 70:633–640, 1952

Dobin SM, Daniel CA: Further delineation of the natural history of Kniest syndrome. March of Dimes Clinical Genetics Conference. Baltimore, July 10–13, 1988

Sayli U, Brooker AF Jr: Kniest disease and total joint replacement for functional salvage. Adv Orthop Surg 13:85–87, 1989

Klippel JH, Dieppe PA: Rheumatology, pp 7.44.8, 7.45.3. St Louis, CV Mosby, 1995

KNIEST-LIKE, LETHAL

Synonyms. Silverman-Handmaker; dyssegmental dysplasia I; see Rolland-Desbuquois.

Symptoms and Signs. Stillborn or death within 48 hours; severely hydropic, encephalocele, or occipital defects, micrognathia, ear abnormalities, orbital hypoplasia, short neck, narrow chest, severe microcampomelia.

Etiology. Autosomal recessive inheritance.

Pathology. Bone and cartilage lesion similar to those of Kniest (Swiss cheese appearance) with other distinctive changes in cartilage and growth plate. Electron microscopy shows stronger differences from Kniest lesions.

Diagnostic Procedures. *X-ray.* Dumbbell-shaped long bones (as in Kniest), but with noticeably shortened diaphyseal and metaphyseal changes.

BIBLIOGRAPHY. Stevenson RE: Micromelic chondrodysplasia: further evidence for autosomal recessive inheritance. Proc Greenwood Genet Center 1:52–57, 1982

Scouyers SM, Rimoin DL, Lachman RS, et al: A distinct chondrodysplasia resembling Kniest dysplasia: Clinical, roentgenographic, histologic, and ultrastructural findings. J Pediatr 103:898–904, 1983

Rimoin DL, Lachman RS: Genetic disorders of the osseous skeleton. In Beithon P (ed): McKusick's Heritable Disorders of Connective Tissue, 5th ed, pp 601–602. St Louis, CV Mosby, 1993

KNOBLOCH-LAYER

Synonym. Retinal detachment; occipital encephalocele.

Symptoms and Signs. Myopia; vitreoretinal detachment; and occipital encephalocele (meningocele?). Normal mental development.

Etiology. Autosomal recessive inheritance.

BIBLIOGRAPHY. Knobloch WA, Layer JM: Retinal detachment and encephalocele. J Ped Ophthalmol 8:181–184, 1971

Pagon RA, Handler JW, Collie W, et al: Hydrocephalus, agyria, retinal dysplasia, encephalocele (HARD E) syndrome: An autosomal recessive condition. Birth Defects Orig Art Ser 14(6B) 233–241, 1978

Cohen MM Jr, Lemire RJ: Syndromes with cephaloceles. Teratology 25:161–172, 1982

KOBBERLING-DUNNIGAN

Synonyms. Dunnigan; lipoatrophic diabetes; lipodystrophy, reverse partial; see Lawrence-Seip and symmetric adenolipomatosis.

Symptoms and Signs. Full syndrome only in females. Fat accumulation on the neck, shoulder, buffalo hump area, and genitalia. *Limbs.* Typical loss of subcutaneous fat; lean muscles. Phlebectasia. Occasionally: symptoms of diabetes mellitus and gout. Acanthosis nigricans. Two types described: one with loss of fat limited to limbs and a second involving also the trunk with the exception of the vulva.

Etiology. Unknown. Sporadic and familial cases. Possibly autosomal dominant trait and X-linked (lethality in hemizygous males?).

Diagnostic Procedures. *Blood.* Hyperglycemia (insulin-resistant), hyperlipoproteinemia (type IV, see). Hyperuricemia.

BIBLIOGRAPHY. Greene ML, Gheck CJ, Fujimoto WY, et al: Benign symmetric lipomatosis (Lannois-Bensaude adenolipomatosis) with gout and hyperlipoproteinemia. Am J Med 48:239–246, 1970

Dunnigan MG, Cochrane M, Kelly A, et al: Familial lipodystrophic diabetes with dominant transmission: A new syndrome. Q J Med 43:33–48, 1974

Kobberling J, Willms B, Kattermann R, et al: Lipodystrophy of extremities: a dominantly inherited syndrome associated with lipoatrophic diabetes. Hum Genet 29:111–120, 1975

Kobberling J, Dunnigan MG: Familial partial lipodystrophy: Two types of an X-linked dominant syndrome, lethal in the hemizygotous state. J Med Genet 23:120–127, 1986

Reardon W, Temple IK, Mackinnon H, et al: Partial lipodystrophy syndromes: A further male case. Clin Genet 38:391–395, 1990

Flier JS: Syndromes of insulin resistance and mutant insulin. In De Groot LJ (ed): Endocrinology, 3rd ed, p 1599. Philadelphia, WB Saunders, 1995

KOBY

Synonym. Floriform cataract; includes also: pisciform cataract, spirochetiform cataract, spear cataract, dilacerated cataract.

Symptoms. Both sexes affected. Asymptomatic or visual impairment.

Signs. Multiple opacities of different shapes (anular, floriform, and of different colors), found especially around structures of embryonic nucleus.

Etiology. Unknown. Possibly autosomal dominant inheritance.

Therapy. Cornea transplantation.

Prognosis. Usually static.

BIBLIOGRAPHY. Koby FE: Cataracte familiale d'un type particulier, se transmettant apparentent suivant le mode dominant. Arch Ophthalmol 40:492–503, 1923

Tosch C: Beitrag zur Stammbaumforschung der Cataracta floriformis. Klin Monatstbl Augenheilkd 133:60–66, 1958

Klintworth GK, Garner AR: The causes, types, and morphology of cataracts. In Garner A, Klintworth GK (eds): Pathobiology of Ocular Disease: A Dynamic Approach, 2nd ed, p 493. New York, Marcel Dekker, 1994

KOCKER-DEBRÉ-SÉMÉLAIGNE

Synonyms. KDS; cretinism; muscular hypertrophy; Debré-Sémélaigne; myxedema; muscular hypertrophy. See Hoffmann syndrome.

Symptoms. Occurs in children and adults. Typical clinical manifestations of cretinism, associated with a sense of stiffness and discomfort in large muscles; some movements painful. Slow muscle contractions and slow clumsy gait; cold weather enhances slowness of movements (paramyotonia); dysarthria (caused by big tongue).

Signs. Firm, large, well-developed muscles (true hypertrophy). Prolongation of tendon reflexes.

Etiology. Unknown. Association with clinical manifestations of cretinism and the muscular disorder that constitutes KDS; the combination of myxedema and myotonoid muscular disorder constitute Hoffmann; most likely no fundamental difference between the two conditions. Familial occurrence reported.

Pathology. No consistent pathologic changes have been found in skeletal muscles, except a volumetric increase of muscle fibers (presence of large fibers or increase in small fibers and slight distension of sarcoplasmic reticulum and subsarcolemmal glycogen).

Diagnostic Procedures. *Electromyography.* "Worm-like" contraction persisting for nearly a second after stimulation. No evidence of true myotonia. *Urine.* Lack of creatinuria; high creatine tolerance. *Blood.* Elevated serum cholesterol, lowered iodine uptake transaminase normal, CK elevated; globulin increased; and other thyroid functional studies.

Therapy. Thyroxine.

Prognosis. Complete recovery may follow the administration of thyroxine.

BIBLIOGRAPHY. Kocker T: Zur Verhüntung des Cretinismus und cretinoider Zustände nach neuen Forschungen. Dtsch Z Chir 34:556–626, 1892

Hoffmann J: Weiterer Beitrag zur Lehre von der Tetanie. Dtsch Z Nervenkr 9:278–290, 1896

Debré R, Sémélaigne G: Syndrome of diffuse muscular hypertrophy in infants causing athletic appearance: Its connection with congenital myxedema. Am J Dis Child 50:1351–1361, 1935

Adams RD, Victor M: Principles of Neurology, 5th ed, p 1235. New York, McGraw-Hill, 1993

KOEBNER

Synonyms. Acantholysis bullosa; epidermolysis bullosa hereditaria simplex. See Fox; Hurliers, Hallopeau-Siemens, epidermolysis bullosa hyperplastic; and Goldscheider.

Symptoms and Signs. Present from infancy. No symptoms, except pain and discomfort when bullae rupture. Bullous elevations on the hands and feet. (There is involvement of other areas of the body. This wider extension differentiates it from the epidermolysis bullosa hyperplastic type Cockaine Touraine [see].) Develops after minor trauma (e.g., walking, using tools). Associated hyperhidrosis of hand and feet. The bullae appear especially in warm weather and frequently are hemorrhagic. Scars frequently may be so severe as to affect growth of the patient.

Etiology.   Autosomal recessive inheritance.

Pathology.   Subepidermal bullae, containing usually clear fluid, little or no inflammatory reaction unless infection supervenes. Elastic tissue may be frayed and splintered but not destroyed.

Diagnostic Procedures.   *Biopsy.* Differentiate from porphyria drug reactions and other forms of epidermolysis bullosa.

Therapy.   Nonspecific. Protection from secondary infections and damage owing to extensive scar retraction.

Prognosis.   Chronic persistence of the condition that may result in various growth disorders up to dwarfism.

BIBLIOGRAPHY. Goldscheider A: Hereditäre Neigung zur Blasebildung. Mhefte Prakt Dermatol 1:163–174, 1882

Koebner H: Hereditaere Anlage zur Blasenbildung (Epidermolysis bullosa hereditaria). Dtsch Med Wochenschr 12:21–22, 1886

Elliot GT: Two cases of epidermolysis bullosa. J Cutan Genitourin Dis 13:10–18, 1895

Fine JD, Bauer EA, Briggaman RA, et al: Revised clinical and laboratory criteria for subtypes of inherited epidermolysis bullosa: A consensus report by the subcommittee on diagnosis and classification of the National Epidermolysis Bullosa Registry. J Am Acad Dermatol 24:119–135, 1991

Pye RJ: Bullous eruptions. In Champion RH, Burton JL, Ebling FJG (eds): Rook/Wilkinson/Ebling Textbook of Dermatology, 5th ed, p 1625. Oxford, Blackwell Scientific, 1992

KOENEN

Synonyms.   Kothe Koenen.

Symptoms and Signs.   Frequently observed in tuberous sclerosis (which are considered typical lesions). Develop at puberty as isolated or multiple firm, flesh-colored, with conical swelling (diameter up to 5 cm) protuding from the groove of the nailbed into the nail and ending in a firm pink or brown tip. More frequent in toenails than fingernails.

Etiology.   See Bourneville.

BIBLIOGRAPHY. Koenen J: Eine familaere, herditaere Form von Tuberoeser Sklerose. Acta Psychiat (Kbl) 1:213–821, 1932

Donegani G, Grattarola F-R, Wildi E: Tuberous sclerosis: Bourneville disease. In Vinken PJ, Bruyn GW (eds): Handbook of Clinical Neurology, vol 22, p 343. Amsterdam, North-Holland, 1972

KOENIG I

Synonyms.   Paget (quiet bone necrosis); arthrolithiasis; joint loose body; joint mice; osteochondrolysis; osteochondritis dissecans.

Symptoms.   Both sexes affected; onset at all ages. Usually after trauma. Asymptomatic for a long time; occasional or persistent sharp pain in joint caused or exacerbated by pressure. Occasionally, locking of joint (transitory).

Signs.   Usually the knee involved. Crepitus; swelling; inflammatory signs. Occasionally loose bodies may be palpated.

Etiology.   It is now established that this condition is caused by trauma causing subchondral fracture that then fragments into loose bodies. In case of associated conditions such as hemoglobinopathies, Gaucher, hyperuricemia, alcoholism, or corticosteroid therapy. It may depend on fat embolism and chondral necrosis.

Pathology.   In cartilage cavity, round, smooth, cartilagineous or fibrous loose bodies; secondary synovial inflammatory changes.

Diagnostic Procedures.   *X-ray.* Visibility of bodies according to their degree of calcification.

Therapy.   Arthroscopic removal when interfering with motion; debridement of cartilagineous tabs, spurs.

Prognosis.   Good with removal; frequent consequence: chronic persistent synovitis.

BIBLIOGRAPHY. Paget J: On production of some of the loose bodies in joints. St Bartholomews Hosp Rep 6. 1870

Koenig F: Lehrbuch der allgemeinen Chirurgie fuer Ärzte und Studierente, p 751. Berlin, 1889

Aichroth P: Osteochondritis dissecans of the knee. In Insall JN, Windsor RE, Scott WN, et al: Surgery of the Knee. New York, Churchill Livingstone, 1993

KOENIG II

Synonym.   Ileocecal valve.

Symptoms and Signs.   Alternating diarrhea and constipation. Recurrent abdominal pain; meteorism; borborygmi in right iliac fossa. A mass may or may not be palpated in right lower abdominal quadrant.

Etiology.   Tuberculous lesion at the level of ileocecal valve or other conditions interfering with ileocecal valve function. See Ischemic colon.

Diagnostic Procedures.   *X-ray.* Of intestinal tract, chest. *Sputum. Stool.* Microscopic examination and culture. *Mantoux test.*

Therapy.   Antitubercular chemotherapy.

Prognosis.   Good with treatment.

BIBLIOGRAPHY. Koenig F: Die stricturirende Tuberculose des Darmes und ihre Behandlung. Dstch Z Chir 34:65–81, 1892

KOFFERATH

Synonym.   Diaphragmatic obstetric paralysis.

Symptoms and Signs.   Occurs in newborn, especially when forceps has been used in delivery. Dyspnea; cyanosis, unilateral edema of the neck; asymmetric thoracic movements on breathing. Frequently associated, Duchenne-Erb paralysis (see).

Etiology.   In some cases, lesion of one phrenic nerve also associated with lesions of cervical nerves.

Therapy.   Symptomatic. Protection from respiratory infections.

Prognosis.   Good quoad vitam. Nerve function may return according to extent of lesion.

BIBLIOGRAPHY. Kofferath W: Ueber eine Fall von rechtsseitigen erbscher Lähmung und Phrenikuslaehmung nach Zangenextraktion. Mschr Geburtshecol 55:33–38, 1921

Robotham JL: A physiological approach to hemidiaphragm paralysis. Crit Care Med 7:563–566, 1979

KOGOJ

Synonyms.   Spongiform pustules.

Symptoms and Signs.   Characteristic lesions formed by spongiform pustules caused by accumulation of masses of neutrophils. Usually observed in psoriasis.

BIBLIOGRAPHY. Kogoj F: Un cas de maladie de Hallopeau. Acta Derm Venerol 8:1–12, 1927

Champion RH, Burton JL, Ebling FJG (eds): Rook/Wilkinson/Ebling Textbook of Dermatology, 5th ed, pp 213, 1402, 1403, 1451. Oxford, Blackwell Scientific, 1992

KÖHLER I

Synonyms. Köhler-Mouchette; Panner I. See Epiphyseal ischemic necrosis.

Symptoms and Signs. More common in males; onset at 3–10 years of age. Asymptomatic or pain on medial side of foot. Tenderness on palpation and swelling over area of navicular bone. Slight, usually unilateral, limp.

Etiology. See Epiphyseal ischemic necrosis.

BIBLIOGRAPHY. Köhler A: Ueber eine häufige, bisher anscheinen unbekannte Erkrankung inzelner kindlicher knochen. MMW 55:1923–1925, 1908

Canale ST: Osteochondrosis or epiphysitis? In Crenshaw AH (ed): Campbell's Operative Orthopedics, 7th ed, p 989. St Louis, CV Mosby, 1987

KÖHLMEIER-DEGÓS

Synonyms. Degós; Degós-Delort-Tricot; cutaneo intestinal; atrophic dermatitis papulo squamosa; malignant atrophic papulosis; arteriolar cutaneogastrointestinal thrombosis.

Symptoms and Signs. Predominant in males; onset in third decade of life. *Stage 1. Skin.* Of varying duration from weeks to years; affecting trunk, proximal extremities, neck, occasionally face. Palms and soles spared. Appears as circular erythematous papules that enlarge and assume irregular form, umbilicate, and ulcerate leaving depressed atropic scar. At any time, different degrees of evolution. *Ocular manifestations.* White avascular plaque on bulbar conjunctiva; chorioretinal lesions. *Stage 2.* Abdominal symptoms and signs of peritonitis.

Etiology. Unknown; possibly clinical variation of polyarteritis; immune or autoimmune process.

Pathology. *Skin.* Vascular changes affecting both arteries and veins; inflammatory changes mostly in intima. Elastica and media rarely involved. Endothelial proliferation; fibrinoid degeneration; thrombosis. Epithelial changes appear as secondary. *Small bowel.* White subserous plaque; shallow ulcers; perforation followed by peritonitis. *Stomach and colon.* May be similarly affected.

Diagnostic Procedures. *Biopsy. X-rays.* Intestine: bowel infarction; perforation; peritonitis. Chest: pleural and pericardial effusion and calcification. *Arteriography.* Occlusion of interlobar renal artery; multiple intracerebral and visceral occlusious.

Therapy. None; exploratory laparotomy. Does not respond to corticosteroids. Trials with phenylbutazone, aspirin, dipyridamole, and fibrinolytics.

Prognosis. Fatal. Few cases with only skin lesions reported to have survived.

BIBLIOGRAPHY. Köhlmeier W: Multiple Hautnekrosen bie Thromboangiitis obliterans. Arch Dermatol Syph 181:783–792, 1941

Degós R, Delort J, Tricot R: Dermatitie papulo-squameuse atrophiante. Bull Soc Fr Dermatol Syph 49:148–150, 1942

Civatte J: Robert Degos (1904–1987). Presse Med 16:1214–1215, 1987

Ryan TJ: Cutaneous vasculitis. In Champion RH, Burton JL, Ebling FJG (eds): Rook/Wilkinson/Ebling Textbook of Dermatology, 5th ed, pp 1951–1953. Oxford, Blackwell Scientific, 1992

KOHLSCHUTTER

Synonyms. Amelogenesis imperfecta; epilepsy; mental deterioration; epilepsy; yellow teeth.

Symptoms. Occurs in males; normal at birth; onset at 1–4 years of age. Sudden and generalized epileptic attacks, followed by progressive mental deterioration.

Signs. Amelogenesis imperfecta; associated with hypohidrosis and myopia.

Etiology. Unknown. Autosomal recessive (?) or X-linked (?) inheritance.

Diagnostic Procedures. *Sweat test. Blood.* Mild hypernatremia and chloremia; marked hyperkalemia. *Electroencephalography.*

BIBLIOGRAPHY. Kohlschutter A, Chappuis D, Meier C, et al: Familial epilepsy and yellow teeth: A disease of the central nervous system associated with enamel hypoplasia. Helv Paediatr Acta 29:283–294, 1974

Witkop CJ Jr, Sank JJ Jr: Heritable defects of enamel. In Stewart RE, Prescott GH (eds): Oral Facial Genetics, pp 200–202. St Louis, CV Mosby, 1976

Christodolou J, Hall RK, Menaham S, et al: A syndrome of epilepsy, dementia and amelogenesis imperfecta: Genetic and clinical features. J Med Genet 25:827–830, 1988

KOK

Synonyms. Startle; hyperexplexia; hyperekplexia, stiff baby; startle disease. See also Moersch-Woltmann.

Symptoms and Signs. Both sexes. At birth. Hypertonia in flexion; exaggerated startle response to minor stimuli (e.g., light touch of the nose, light hand clapping), which may cause generalized hypertonia and falling "like a log" to the ground; exaggerated brainstem reflexes; and, occasionally, seizures. Symptoms disappear during sleep (in one family reported nocturnal myoclonic jerks); occasionally congenital hip dislocation and inguinal hernia.

Etiology. Hyperactive long-loop reflexes proposed as mechanism for exaggerated startle. Autosomal dominant inheritance.

Diagnostic Procedures. *Electrophysiological studies.* Prominent C response after nerve stimulation.

Therapy. Barbiturates, clonazepam usually effective in reducing symptoms. Some resistant cases reported.

Prognosis. After 1 year usually reduction of intensity of symptoms, which may, however, persist for life.

BIBLIOGRAPHY. Kok O, Bruyn GW: An unidentified hereditary disease (letter). Lancet I:1359, 1962

Suhuren O, Bruyn GW: Tuynman hyperexplexia: A hereditary startle syndrome. J Neurol Sci 3:577–605, 1966

Cook W, Kaplan RF: Neuromuscular blockade in a patient with stiff baby syndrome. Anesthesiology 55:525–528, 1986

Hayashi T, Tachibana H, Kaji T: Hyperekplexia: Pedigree studies in two families. Am J Med Genet 40:138–143, 1991

KOLLER

Synonyms. Bone thickening—ichthyosis; ichthyosis—bone thickening.

Symptoms and Signs. Both sexes. From infancy. Ichthyosis. Weakness in the legs, waddling gait, bowing on weight of bearing bones (femor-tibia).

Etiology. Autosomal dominant inheritance.

Prognosis. Tendency to fracture.

BIBLIOGRAPHY. Koller ME, Mauseth K, Haneberg B, et al: A familial syndrome of diaphyseal thickening of long bones, bowed legs tendency to fracture and ichthyosis. Pediatr Radiol 8:179–182, 1979

KONIGSMARK

Synonyms. Deafness, progressive low tone; low frequency hearing loss, hereditary; LFHL1.

Symptoms and Signs. Hearing loss from birth or during infancy. Later onset has also been reported. Absence of physical and mental symptoms and signs.

Etiology. Autosomal dominant inheritance. Probably caused by alterations in the strie vascularis or from labyrinthine otosclerosis.

Diagnostic Procedures. *Audiometry.* Low frequency deafness of sensorineural type. Normal or near normal findings over 2000 cycles per second.

Prognosis. Deafness.

BIBLIOGRAPHY. Konigsmark BW, Menge MC, Berlin CI: Dominant low frequency hearing loss: Report of three families. Laryngoscope 81:759–771, 1971
Parving A: Inherited low frequency hearing loss: A new conductive sensorineural entity. Scand Audiol 13:47–56, 1984

KOREAN HEMORRHAGIC FEVER

Synonyms. Hemorrhagic epidemic fever; hemorrhagic nephroso nephritis fever.

Symptoms. Reported in Manchuria, Siberia, Korea, Eastern Russia, Czechoslovakia, and Hungary. Two seasonal peaks of incidence, but endemic cases during the entire year. Onset at all ages; both sexes affected. Abrupt onset. Headache; fever; chills; anorexia; nausea; vomiting; backache. In Scandinavia and the rest of Europe less severe form, epidemic nephropathy, without hemorrhagic phenomena.

Signs. *Day 1.* Conjunctival congestion; skin flushed; especially face and neck. *Day 2.* Petechiae on the face, oral mucosa, conjunctiva, axillar areas. *Day 4.* Periorbital edema. *Day 5.* Fever stops; hypotension, oliguria. *Day 10.* Diuretic phase lasting days or weeks with fluctuation between shock and hypertension and with pulmonary edema according to fluid balance. Convalescence 3–12 weeks, with gradual recovery.

Etiology. The disease is caused by Hantaan virus, first recovered from the striped field mouse, Apodemus agrarius excreta in Korea. Sometimes arthropod vector.

Pathology. *Kidney.* Pallor of cortex; congested pyramids. *Heart.* Hemorrhagic lesions of right atrial wall. *Anterior pituitary.* Intense congestion; various degrees of necrosis. *Capillaries.* Generalized dilatation. *Small vessels.* Lack of inflammatory changes.

Diagnostic Procedures. *Blood.* High hematocrit; leukocytosis up to 50,000 with immature elements. Thrombocytopenia. Electrolyte imbalance. In oliguric phase, high blood urea nitrogen and creatinine. *Urine.* Proteinuria. Specific diagnosis is made by immunofluorescent techniques, using lung sections from Apodemus rodents as source of antigen.

Therapy. Limit fluid intake; human serum albumin; treatment of the acute renal failure, with careful control of the electrolytes; if necessary, hemodialysis. Trials with antiviral agents.

Prognosis. Oriental, including Russia form, overall mortality with proper treatment seldom surpasses 5%. In Europe and the United States mild symptoms and rapid recovery.

BIBLIOGRAPHY. Symposium on epidemic hemorrhagic fever. Am J Med 16:617, 1954
Myhrman G: Nephropathia epidemica: A new infectious disease in Northern Scandinavia. Acta Med Scand 140:52–56, 1951
PHLS Report. Febbre emorragica con interessamento renale: Infezione da Hantaan virus. Br Med J (Italian ed) 5:177–179, 1986
Weatherall DJ, Ledingham JGG, Warrell DA (eds): Oxford Textbook of Medicine, 3rd ed, pp 425–427. Oxford, Oxford Med Pub, 1996

KORO

Synonyms. Depersonalization; depersonalization psychosis.

Symptoms. Occurs mostly in people of Malayan archipelagos. Prevalent in males, who are possessed by fear of penis shrinking and disappearing inside the abdomen, with death to follow. Usually patients try to secure penis by putting a ribbon around it or clamping in a wooden box. In females, fear of shrinkage of vagina and breast.

Etiology. Unknown. Type of depersonalization syndrome resulting from cultural-social and psychologic factors. Sexual excess or physical injuries, including cold exposure of penis, may be precipitating factors.

Therapy. Psychotherapy; tranquilizer.

Prognosis. Only 30% recover completely.

BIBLIOGRAPHY. Yap PM: Koro's culture-bound depersonalization syndrome. Br J Psychiatr 111:43–50, 1965
Gaines AD: Culture-specific delusions: Sense and nonsense in cultural context. In Sedler MJ (ed): Psychiatr Clin N Am 292–293, 1995

KORSAKOFF

Synonyms. Amnestic; amnestic confabulatory. See Wernicke-Korsakoff.

Symptoms. Retrograde amnesia. Impaired capacity to recall events and information that were known before onset. Anterograde amnesia. Impaired capacity to acquire new information; concentration, spatial organization, visual and verbal abstraction partially affected. Confabulation. Fabrication of stories of recent events occasionally present. Remote memory and immediate memory (digit repetition) intact.

Etiology. Not well defined. Medial temporal lobe and median thalamic regions lesion. Can be observed in several clinical conditions, atherosclerosis, trauma, hemorrhages, CO_2 poisoning, concussion, Wernicke-Korsakoff (see), virus encephalitis, tuberculous meningitis, tumor and brain degenerative disorders (e.g., Alzheimer).

Pathology. Critical structures damaged seem to be the hippocampus and mostly the underlying temporal stem.

Diagnostic Procedures. *CT scan. MRI. EEG. Cerebrospinal fluid.*

Therapy. General care. Symptomatic to reduce restlessness, anxiety, and aggressive symptoms or to stimulate.

Prognosis. Poor.

BIBLIOGRAPHY. Korsakoff SS: Ob alkogol'nom paraliche Vest. Psychiatr (Moskva) 4, 1887
Adam RD, Victor M: Principles of Neurology, 5th ed, pp 915–916. New York, McGraw-Hill, 1993

KOSTMANN

Synonyms. Infantile genetic agranulocytosis; agranulocytosis, infantile genetic; neutropenia, hereditary.

Symptoms. Onset usually in early infancy. Recurrent infections.

Signs. According to localization of infections; no splenomegaly.

Etiology. Unknown; autosomal recessive inheritance. Possibility of sporadic occurrence suggested. Possible deficiency of a growth factor considered as responsible for this syndrome.

Pathology. Necrotic ulceration of oral and genital mucosae. Diffuse inflammatory reactions with lymphocytes, plasma cells, and histiocytes, and without neutrophils, in various tissue. Liver and spleen moderately congested. Extramedullary hematopoiesis in various tissues.

Diagnostic Procedures. *Blood.* Leukocytes in normal number with absolute or very marked neutropenia. Absolute and relative eosinophilia and monocytosis. No anemia or only secondary at later stage of the disease. *Bone marrow.* Variable cellularity. Erythropoiesis and megakaryocytes normal; myeloid series—absence of myeloid precursors beyond early myelocyte stage. *Epinephrine stimulation test. Window test (Rebuck).* Reveals absence of neutrophils. Addition of sulfur-containing aminoacids to tissue cultures leads to maturation of neutrophils.

Therapy. Antibiotics. All types of treatment fail, both medical and surgical (splenectomy). Intravenous or subcutaneous rhG-CSF increases the concentration of neutrophils and stops recurrent infections.

Prognosis. Poor, death a few months after discovery of condition (usually before age 3 years) because of severe infections. Meningitis frequent. In cases with sporadic disorder survival into late teens because monocyte may partially compensate for neutrophil deficiency.

BIBLIOGRAPHY. Kostmann R: Infantile genetic agranulocytosis (agranulocytosis infantilis hereditaria): New recessive lethal disease in man. Acta Paediatr (suppl 105) 45:1–78, 1956

Iselius L, Gustavson KH: Spatial distribution of the gene for infantile genetic agranulocytosis. Hum Hered 34:358–363, 1984

Athens JW, Neutropenia. In Lee GR, Bithel TC, Foerster J, et al (eds): Wintrobe's Clinical Hematology, 9th ed, pp 1600–1601. Philadelphia, Lea & Febiger, 1993

KOWARSKI

Synonym. Biodefective growth hormone; pituitary dwarfism, type IV.

Symptoms and Signs. Growth retardation and delayed bone age.

Etiology. Presumably mutation in the growth hormone (GH) on chromosome 17, causing a biologically ineffective GH molecule, unable to stimulate somatomedin.

Diagnostic Procedures. *Blood.* Normal immunoreactive GH after stimulation and low level of somatomedin.

Therapy. Exogenous GH administration induces normal level of somatomedin and increases growth rate.

BIBLIOGRAPHY. Kowarski AA, Schneider JJ, Ben Galim E, et al: Growth failure with normal serum RIA–GH and low somatomedin activity: Somatomedin restoration and growth acceleration after exogenous GH. J Clin Endocrinol 47:461–464, 1978

Valenta LJ, Sigel MB, Lesnik MA, et al: Pituitary dwarfism in a patient with circulating abnormal growth hormone polymers. N Engl J Med 312:214–217, 1985

Ranke MB: Growth hormone insufficiency: Clinical features, diagnosis and therapy. In De Groot LJ (ed): Endocrinology, 3rd ed, pp 330–340. Philadelphia, WB Saunders, 1995

KOZHEVNIKOV

Synonyms. Kojewnikoff; Koshewnikow; epilepsia partialis continua.

Symptoms. At onset, high fever, delirium, localized muscular spasms, and generalized convulsions; then clonic twitching of one group of muscles (face, upper [more frequently] or lower limbs) at regular intervals (a few seconds) lasting for hours or months, always remaining localized. May be reduced but not abolished during sleep and enhanced by passive or active movements.

Etiology. Focal motor status epilepticus. (Kozhevnikov reported it on the occasion of an encephalitis epidemic in Russia in the spring.) May be caused by acute or chronic brain lesions. Cortical origin favored.

Pathology. Lesion of opposite side of brain cortex and involvement of deeper structures.

Diagnostic Procedures. *Electroencephalography. CT scan. MRI.*

Therapy. Same as for epilepsy.

Prognosis. Difficult treatment. Partial recovery from acute stage; paralysis recedes, but after some time, continuous muscular contractions persisting for years only in affected limbs. Major seizures may occur.

BIBLIOGRAPHY. Kozhevnikov A: Ia Osobyi vid Kortical no: épilepsii. Moskva, 1952

Thomas JE, Regan TJ, Klass DW: Epilepsie partialis continua: A review of 32 cases. Arch Neurol 34:266, 272, 1977

Adams RD, Victor M: Principles of Neurology, 5th ed, p 89, 279. New York, McGraw-Hill, 1993

KOZLOWSKI

Synonym. Spondylometaphyseal dysplasia (type GII).

Symptoms. Both sexes affected; onset at 1 year of age. Reduction of growth (especially of trunk) between 1 and 4 years of age. Waddling gait; limitation of joint mobility.

Signs. Dwarfism (adult height 130–165 cm). Short neck and trunk. Kyphosis; dorsal kyphoscoliosis; platyspondylisis; pectus carinatum; bowed legs; irregular metaphyses.

Etiology. Autosomal recessive inheritance (?).

Pathology. Cellular reduction in proliferation cartilage zone; vacuolization of cells and reduction of calcification of bony precursors.

Diagnostic Procedures. *X-ray. CT scan. MRI of spine and pelvis.* Evident at age 2. Platyspondylisis in "tongue" form; anterior deformity in spine. In infancy, horizontal and trident acetabular roof.

Therapy. Control of evolution of hypoplastic odontoid process (see Atlantoaxial spine dislocation).

Prognosis. Limited growth; joint degeneration producing pain and limiting motion.

BIBLIOGRAPHY. Kozlowski K, Maroteaux P, Spranger G: Le dysotose spondylo-metaphysaire. Presse Med 75:2769–2774, 1967

Kozlowski K, Beemer FA, Bens G, et al: Spondylometaphyseal dysplasia: Report of 7 cases and assay of classification. In Papadatos CJ, Bartsocas CS (eds): Skeletal Dysplasias. New York, Alan R Liss, 1982

Onadfel Meziane A, Ksiyer M, et al: Spondilometaphyseal dysplasia: Report of three familial cases. Ann Genet 30:216–220, 1987

KRABBE I

Synonyms. Globoid cell brain sclerosis; galactocerebroside beta-galactosidase deficiency; galactosylceramide lipoidosis; globoid cell leukodystrophy; galactosyl ceramide lipoidosis.

Symptoms and Signs. Both sexes affected; onset usually in childhood (first year of life); described also in adults. Ambiguous onset: irritability or hypersensitivity to stimuli, followed rapidly by mental and motor deterioration and visual and hearing disorders. Hypertonicity in early phase, then hypotonicity. Variable clinical pattern according to areas of cerebral lesions, prevalent involvement of internal capsule (abnormal reflexes, paralysis, contractures), optic nerve, optic tract. Systemic manifestations are rare.

Etiology. Autosomal recessive inheritance. Deficiency of galactocerebroside beta-galactosidase and accumulation of galactocerebroside and psychosine in macrophages, which causes degeneration of oligodendroglia (the cells that produce myelin). Human galactosylceramidase gene mapped to chromosome 14.

Pathology. Demyelinization of central nervous system areas. In demyelinized areas, appearance of globoid cells, giant cells with peripherally displaced nucleus and homogeneous cytoplasm, clustering around small blood vessels or diffuse in border areas of demyelinization areas. Similar cells may be found also in lung, spleen, and lymph nodes. Absence of metachromatic leukodystrophy nodes. Absence of metachromatic breakdown product (see Metachromatic leukodystrophy).

Diagnostic Procedures. *Blood.* Galactocerebroside beta-galactoside assay in white cells (and fibroblasts) decreased. *Spinal tap.* Protein elevation. *EEG.* Nonspecific slowing without spikes. *Electromyography.* Evidence of denervation and decreased motor nerve conduction velocity. *X-ray of skull. Angiography. CT scan. MRI.* Progressive brain atrophy. *Brain biopsy.* Final resort for definite diagnosis. Prenatal diagnosis: assay of galactosyl ceramidase activity on amniotic cells.

Therapy. None specific; symptomatic.

Prognosis. In infantile form death within second year. In later onset (2–6 years) possible survival up to 5 years. Most surviving infants show early slowing and then arrest of growth, leading progressively to microcephaly and severe failure to thrive. In adult type, 2–10 years survival from onset.

BIBLIOGRAPHY. Krabbe KH: A new familial; infantile form of brain sclerosis. Brain 39:74–114, 1916
Zlotogora J, Regev R, Hadar S, et al: Growth pattern in Krabbe's disease. Acta Paediatr Scand 75:251–254, 1986
Suzuki K, Suzuki Y, Syzuki K: Galactosylceramide lipidosis: Globoid cell leukodystrophy (Krabbe's disease). In Scriver CR, Beaudet AL, Sly WS, et al: The Metabolic and Molecular Bases of Inherited Disease, 7th ed, pp 2671–2692. New York, McGraw-Hill, 1995

KRABBE II

Synonyms. Sturge-Weber-Krabbe facial-meningeal angiomas. See also Sturge-Weber.

Symptoms and Signs. Both sexes affected; present from birth, develops more or less rapidly. Mental deterioration; hemiplegia; epileptic attacks; facial hemiatrophy and flat angioma in the distribution area of the trigeminal V nerve.

Etiology. Unknown; congenital malformation with irregular dominant inheritance.

Pathology. *Skin.* Nevus flammeus (see). *Brain.* Atrophy; cerebral angiomas.

Diagnostic Procedures. *X-rays of skull.* Presence of calcium deposits that follow cerebral gyri. *Angiography. CT brain scan. MRI Brain biopsy.* Final resort for definitive diagnosis. Prenatal diagnosis: assay of galactosyl ceramidase activity of amniotic cells.

Therapy. Surgery and X-rays.

Prognosis. Variable, but generally poor.

BIBLIOGRAPHY. Krabbe KH: Facial and meningeal angiomas associated with calcification of the brain cortex: A clinical and anatomopathologic contribution. Arch Neurol Psychiatr 32:737–755, 1934
Chomette G, Auriol M: Classification des angiodysplasics et tumeurs vasculaires. Rev Stom Clin Maxillo Fac 87:1–5, 1986

KRAEMER

Synonyms. Metastatic furunculiformi episcleritis; suppurative scleritis.

Symptoms. Severe ocular pain; lacrimation; photophobia.

Signs. Abscess in scleral vessels.

Etiology. Septic embolus, especially staphylococcal.

Therapy. Systemic and topical antibiotics.

Prognosis. Good.

BIBLIOGRAPHY. Kraemer R: Episkleritis metastatic furunculiformis. Klin Monatstbl Augenheilkd 66:441–450, 1921

KRAMER-POLLNOW

Eponym indicating an entity of doubtful individuality consisting in a sudden onset, at 1–4 years of age, of progressive hyperkinesia, followed by retardation of mental development, anxiety, and regression of expressive capacities. See Little.

BIBLIOGRAPHY. Kramer F, Pollnow H: Ueber eine hyperkinetische Erkrankung in Kindersalter. Mschr Psychiatr Neur 82–83:1–40, 1932

KRAUSE

Synonyms. Yudkin; Krause-Reese; encephalo-ophthalmic dysplasia; ophthalmo-encephalic dysplasia. See Reese-Blodi and Patau.

Symptoms. Usually discovered months after birth in premature infants. Ocular symptoms of variable degrees from minimal vision trouble in only one eye to total vision loss. Cerebral symptoms also of variable degrees from mild symptoms of mental deficiency to cerebral agenesis.

Signs. Ocular signs range from small areas of retinal atrophy and slight structural eye anomaly to ptosis, enophthalmos, strabismus, glaucoma, microphthalmia, retinal and choroid optic nerve malformation. Microcephaly; hydrocephalus. Visceral malformations possibly associated.

Etiology. Unknown; neuroectodermal congenital defect. Autosomal recessive inheritance (?); chromosomal basis.

Pathology. Microphthalmia; retinal dysplasia of hyaloid artery, intraocular hemorrhages. Brain hyperplasia; hypoplasia and aplasia of cerebrum and cerebellum.

Therapy. Symptomatic.

Prognosis. Poor; death in early infancy or mental retardation.

BIBLIOGRAPHY. Yudkin AM: Congenital bilateral microphthalmos accompanied by other malformations of the body. Am J Ophthalmol 11:128–131, 1928
Krause AC: Congenital encephalo-ophthalmic dysplasia. Arch Ophthalmol 36:387–444, 1946
Reese AB, Blodi FC: Retinal dysplasia. Am J Ophthalmol 33:23–32, 1950
Matthes A, Stenzel K: Familiaere, encephalo-retinale Dysplasie (Krause-Reese Syndrome) mit myoklonischastatischem petit mal. Z Kinderheilk 103:81–89, 1968

KRAUSE-KIVLIN

Synonyms. Peters anomaly; Peters-plus; short limb dwarfism.

Symptoms and Signs. Both sexes. Peters anomaly (see) and short limb dwarfism. Severe mental retardation (not constant). *Facies.* Thin upper lip, cleft lip/palate (in several cases) hypoplastic columella, round face, mild micrognathia, abmormal ears. Hydrocephalus, failure to thrive. *Hands.* Short fifth finger and clinodactyly.

Etiology. Autosomal recessive inheritance.

BIBLIOGRAPHY. Peters A: Ueber angeborene Defekbildung der descemetschen Membran. Klin Mbl Augenheilk 44:27–40, 105–119, 1906

Krause U, Koivisto M, Rantakallio P: A case of Peter's anomaly with spontaneous corneal perforation. J Paediat Opthalmol 6:145–149, 1969

Kivlin JD, Fineman RM, Crandallas AS, et al: Peter's anomaly as a consequence of genetic and non genetic syndromes. Arch Ophthal 104:61–64, 1986

Frydman M, Weinstock AL, Cohen HA et al: Autosomal recessive Peter's anomaly, typical facial appearance, failure to thrive, hydrocephalus and other Krause-Kivlin syndrome. Am J Med Genet 40:34–40, 1991

KREIBIG

Synonym. Opticomalacia atherosclerotica.

Symptoms. Usually occurs in people past middle age; onset acute. Unilateral vision disturbance, which progresses up to unilateral blindness.

Signs. Irregular narrow arteries, with wide light reflex and nicking of crossing veins. Hemorrhages (if associated with hypertension).

Etiology. Atherosclerosis.

Pathology. Degeneration of optic nerve.

Diagnostic Procedures. *Ophthalmoscopy.*

Therapy. None.

Prognosis. Progressive condition.

BIBLIOGRAPHY. Hruby K: Ueber einige neue Krankheitsbilder in der Angenheilkunde. Wien Klin Wochenschr 61:693–695, 1949

Garner A Vascular diseases. In Garner A, Klintworth GK (eds): Pathobiology of Ocular Disease: A Dynamic Approach, 2nd ed, pp 1666–1667. New York, Marcel Dekker, 1994

KRETSCHMER I

Synonyms. Apallic syndrome; locked-in; de-efferented state; akinetic mutism; coma vigile. (The two latter definitions have been used also to define another clinical condition where the patient is awake, but unresponsive.)

Symptoms. Patient is mute and immobile; eyes may follow people's movements or may be diverted by sound. Pain reflexes are present, but no emotional change accompanies them. If fed, patient swallows but does not always chew. Sleep is prolonged; arousal by normal stimuli. Catatonia may be present during recovery period.

Etiology. Diffuse bilateral degeneration of cerebral cortex, sometimes following anoxia, head injury, or encephalitis.

Diagnostic Procedure. *CT brain scan. Nuclear magnetic resonance. Angiography. Cerebral blood flow measurements. EEG. Evoked potentials.*

Therapy. According to etiology. General assistance. Levodopa and cytidine diphosphate choline seem to shorten the recovery period.

Prognosis. Poor. Variable according to etiology and entity of lesions.

BIBLIOGRAPHY. Kretschmer E: Das apallishe Syndrom. Z Ges Neurol 169:576–579, 1940

Dalle Ore G, Gerstenbrand F, Lucking CH (eds): The Apallic Syndrome. New York, Springer-Verlag, 1977

Inguar DH, Brun A, Johansson L: Survival after severe cerebral anoxia with destruction of the cerebral cortex: The apallic syndrome. In Koscin J (ed): Brain death: Interrelated Medical and Social Issues. Ann NY Acad Sci 315:184–214, 1978

Adams RD, Victor M: Principles of Neurology, 5th ed, p 303. New York, McGraw-Hill, 1993

KRETSCHMER II

Synonyms. Fronto-basal, traumatic; traumatic fronto-basal.

Symptoms and Signs. In the acute stage includes restlessness, frontal symptoms, loss of vegetative inhibition; in the subacute stage changes in higher brain function, loss of emotion control, motor overactivity, hypersexuality, bulimia, changes in circulation temperature and sweating, sleeping.

Etiology. Head trauma.

Diagnostic Procedures. *CT scan. MRI. EEG.* Basal metabolic rate increased. *Blood.* Increased BUN and cathecolamine.

Therapy. Sedatives for neurovegetative symptoms; neurosurgery.

Prognosis. According to severity of lesion and treatment.

BIBLIOGRAPHY. Kretschmer E: Das Orbitalhirn-und Zwischenhirn-syndrome nach Schaedelbasisfracturen. Arch Psuchiat Nervenkr 182:454–477, 1949

Binder H, Gerstenbrand F: Post-traumatic vegetative syndrome. In Vinken PJ, Bruyn GW: Handbook of Clinical Neurology, vol 24, p 582. Amsterdam, North-Holland, 1976

KRISHABER

Synonym. Cerebrocardiac.

Symptoms. Both sexes affected; predominant in females; onset at all ages. Patient complains of "empty head," vertigo, or dizziness, and insomnia.

Signs. Tachycardia. No other objective signs.

Etiology. Form of psychoneurosis. Diagnosis of exclusion after ruling out all other possibilities, especially Barré-Liéou (see).

Therapy. Psychotherapy and mild tranquilizers.

Prognosis. Difficult to cure. Possible conversion into other symptoms.

BIBLIOGRAPHY. Krishaber M: De la Néuropathie Cérébrocardiaque. Paris, Masson, 1873

KRUKENBERG

Synonym. Ovary carcinoma mucocellulare.

Symptoms. Occurs in elderly women. In early stage asymptomatic. Weight in lower abdomen; fatigue.

Signs. Ascites. Palpation in adnexal zones of abdominal masses.

Etiology. Unknown. Metastatic tumor from gastrointestinal tract or breast, occasionally of primary ovarian origin.

Pathology. Metastatic tumor of the ovary, usually bilateral. Histologically, signet ring cells (mucin pushing and flattening nucleus at periphery). Stroma areas of hypercellularity and edema.

Diagnostic Procedures. *Vaginal smear.* Presence of malignant cells. *X-ray.* Of gastrointestinal tract, for identification of primary tumor.

Therapy. Surgery; chemotherapy; X-rays.

Prognosis. Poor.

BIBLIOGRAPHY. Krukenberg F: Ueber das Fibrosarcom Ovarii mucocellulare (carcinomatodes). Arch Gynecol (Berlin) 50:287–321, 1896

McGuire WP: Primary treatment of epithelial ovarian malignancies. Cancer 7:(Supp 4)1541, 1993

KUBISAGARI

Symptoms and Signs. In nutritonally deprived children or prisoners of war, ptosis and bulbar weakness (myasthenic-like symptoms).

Etiology. Lack of vitamins; neurotoxin (?).

Therapy. Effect of neostigmine on symptoms not clearly reported; claimed resolution from thiamine parenteral administration.

Prognosis. Recovery with proper nutrition and vitamin supplement.

BIBLIOGRAPHY. Denny-Brown D: Neurological conditions resulting from prolonged and severe dietary restriction. Medicine 26:41, 1947
Walton J, Karpati G, Hilton-Jones D: Disorders of Voluntary Muscle, pp 681–682. Edinburgh, Churchill Livingstone, 1994

KUESS

Synonym. Constipation.

Symptoms. Complaints of small-caliber stools, difficult and unsatisfactory evacuation frequently accompanied by pain or bleeding.

Etiology. Stenosis of rectum and sigmoid caused by inflammatory process (e.g., fissure) or secondary to habitual use of laxatives.

Diagnostic Procedures. Proctoscopy.

Therapy. Cortisone and antibiotic suppository or ointment. Surgical division of fibrotic strictures usually needed; mobilization of normal epithelium to cover defect.

Prognosis. Good with treatment.

BIBLIOGRAPHY. Kuess G: Les retrécissements pseudocancéreux pericoliques pelviens. Bull Acad Natl Med 134:377–380, 1950
Koch TR: Constipation. In Haubrich WS, Schaffner F, Berk JE (eds): Bockus Gastroenterology, 5th ed, pp 102–112. Philadelphia, WB Saunders, 1995

KUFS

Synonyms. Ceroid lipofuscinosis, adult type; neuronal ceroid-lipofuscinosis, adult type.

Symptoms. Onset in adolescence (15–25 years). Normal intelligence at onset. Progressive gait and postural deterioration; and dysarthria, personality changes, seizures, and some degree of myoclonus. After ataxia, spasticity and rigidity or athetosis, finally dementia. Normal vision.

Signs. Ascending muscular atrophy; pes cavus. Normal fundus oculi.

Etiology. Autosomal recessive inheritance. No clear biochemical definition.

Pathology. Deposits of autoflourescent lipopigments in all tissues, predominant in the brain. *Brain.* Small, loss of nerve cells and status spongiosus; various sizes and structures of lipopigment deposits (lamellar, granular, "fingerprint" aspect), with acid phosphatase activity.

Diagnostic Procedures. *Blood, urine, spinal fluid, tissue, and cell cultures.* No deficiency of hexosaminase activity in the serum. *Bone marrow and other tissue biopsy.* Presence of lipopigments. *Urine.* Presence of lipopigments in sediment. *Blood.* Lipopigments in lymphocytes; azurophilic hypergranulation in neutrophils and lymphocyte vacuolization (only in homozygotes).

Therapy. Symptomatic.

Prognosis. Slow progression. Death within 19–20 years of onset.

BIBLIOGRAPHY. Kufs H: Ueber eine Spätform der amaurotishchen Idiotie und ihre heredofamiliaren Grundlagen. Z Neurol Psychiatr 95:169–188, 1925

Rapin I, Suzuki K, et al: Adult (chronic) GM2 gangliosidosis: Atypical spinocerebellar degeneration in a Jewish sibship. Arch Neurol 33:120–130, 1976
Adams RD, Victor M: Principles of Neurology, 5th ed, p 832. New York, McGraw-Hill, 1993

KUGELBERG-WELANDER

Synonyms. KWS; Wohlfart-Kugelberg-Welander; juvenile spinal muscular atrophy; spinal muscular atrophy, juvenile; spinal muscular atrophy III.

Symptoms and Signs. Both sexes affected; onset from 2–17 years of age. Weakness and atrophy of proximal muscles (muscular dystrophy-like); frequently, fasciculation (important differentiating sign). Normal reflexes; sphincters seldom affected. Slow progression. Later onset and milder course distinguish it from Strümpell-Lorrain.

Etiology. Unknown; autosomal recessive in 90% of cases (more severe in males than females), or dominant inheritance (equal severity in both sexes).

Pathology. In muscle; neurogenic type of atrophy and hypertrophic hyalinized fibers with central nuclei. Degeneration of anterior horn cells of spinal cord and motor nuclei of brain stem and Betz cells in the cortex. Degeneration of anterior spinal roots and peripheral nerves.

Diagnostic Procedures. *Electromyography.* Lower motor neuron disease. *Biopsy of muscle. Blood.* Serum enzymes. Creatine phosphokinase (CPK) normal or slight elevation.

Therapy. Symptomatic.

Prognosis. Slow progression; subject can still walk 20 years after onset.

BIBLIOGRAPHY. Strümpell A: Ueber spinale, progressive, muskelatrophic und amyotrophische Seitenstrangsklerose. Dtsch Arch Klin Med 42:230–260, 1888
Wohlfart G, Fex J, Eliasson S: Hereditary proximal spinal muscular atrophy: Clinical entity simulating progressive muscular dystrophy. Acta Psychiatr Neurol Scand 30:395–406, 1955
Kugelberg E, Welander L: Heredofamilial juvenile muscular atrophy simulating muscular dystrophy. Arch Neurol Psychiatr 75:500–509, 1956
Hausmanowa-Petrusewicz I, Zaremba J, et al: Chronic proximal spinal muscular atrophy of childhood and adolescence: Problems of classification and genetic counseling. J Med Genet 22:350–353, 1985
Adams RD, Victor M: Principles of Neurology, 5th ed, p 997. New York, McGraw-Hill, 1993

KUGEL-STOLOFF

Obsolete. See Cardiomegaly, idiopathic. Eponym denoting onset in children in first year of life. Dyspnea; progressive cardiomegaly; cyanosis, and sudden death; no temperature elevation.

BIBLIOGRAPHY. Kugel MA, Stoloff EG: Dilatation and hypertrophy of the heart in infants and young children, with myocardial degeneration and fibrosis (so-called congenital idiopathic hypertrophy). Am J Dis Child 45:828–864, 1933

KULENKAMPFF-TORNOW

Synonyms. Cervico-linguo-masticatory; chlorpromazine toxicity; neck/face.

Symptoms and Signs. Occurs in patients during first days of chlorpromazine therapy. Spasmodic contraction of neck, mouth floor, pharynx, and tongue muscles that causes speech alterations; respiratory disorders. Tachycardia and hypotension.

BIBLIOGRAPHY. Kulenkampff C, Tornow G: Ein eigentümliches Syndrom in oralen Bereich bei Magaphenapplikation. Nervenarzt 27:178–180, 1956

AHFS 95: Drug Information. Bethesda (MD), p 1510. Am Hosp Formulary Service, 1995

KÜMMELL

Synonyms. Kümmell-Verneuil; osteoporotic vertebra collapse.

Symptoms and Signs. Occurs months after trauma, direct or indirect, of major or minor entity of vertebrae, especially in patient with osteoporosis. Formation of gibbus and kyphosis associated or not associated with neurologic symptoms: pain; paralysis of legs; sphincter disturbances.

Etiology. Degenerative change of vertebrae following trauma.

Pathology. Rarefaction of vertebral structure without inflammatory signs and with deformation and collapse of body.

Diagnostic Procedures. *X-ray of spine. Biopsy. Myelogram. Electromyography.*

Therapy. Orthopedic correction.

Prognosis. Good.

BIBLIOGRAPHY. Kümmell H: Ueber traumatische Ezkrankungen der Wirbelsäuld. Dtsch Med Wochenschr 21:180–181, 1895

Alpers BJ: Clinical Neurology, 6th ed. Philadelphia, FA Davis, 1973

Weatherall DJ, Ledingham JGG, Warrell DA (eds): Oxford Textbook of Medicine, 3rd ed, p 3066. Oxford, Oxford Med Pub, 1996

KURU

Synonym. Laughing death. See Prion diseases.

Symptoms. Restricted to the "Fore" tribe of Eastern New Guinea; prevalent in children and adult women. Afebrile; ataxia, trembling of leg muscles; abnormal extraocular movements; incoordination spreading to the arms; exaggeration of voluntary movements; jerks; slurred speech; fecal incontinence. Finally, aphonia and dysphagia.

Signs. Ataxia. Typical apprehensive facial expression remaining unchanged for long period, interrupted by laughter with other members of tribe. No muscular wasting or diminished strength. Increased resistance to passive movements, or mild rigidity; no hypotonia; no choreiform movements. Hyperactive tendon reflexes of the lower limbs; ankle clonus. Sensory examination: normal responses to pinprick, temperature, touch, and vibration; nystagmus and strabismus rarely associated.

Etiology. Unknown. Possibly prior infection affecting only members of tribe (transmitted experimentally to chimpanzees with inoculation from brain of patients). It is common in this tribe because cannibalism was practiced.

Pathology. Changes widespread through brain; demyelinization; loss of neuron; microglia proliferation; perivascular infiltration.

Diagnostic Procedures. *Blood.* High level of globulins; all other tests normal.

Therapy. Symptomatic.

Prognosis. Death in 3–6 months from onset. In the past in 70% of females in the tribe, death was caused by this condition. Today this syndrome is gradually disappearing because of cessation of cannibalism.

BIBLIOGRAPHY. Gajdusek DC, Zigas V: Degenerative disease of the central nervous system in New Guinea: The endemic occurrence of "Kuru" in the native population. N Engl J Med 257:974–978, 1957

Gajdusek DC, Gibbs CJ, Alpes M: Experimental transmission of a Kuru-like syndrome to chimpanzees. Nature 209:794–796, 1966

Adams RD, Victor M: Principles of Neurology, 5th ed, pp 658–659. New York, McGraw-Hill, 1993

Prusiner SB: Prion diseases. In Scriver CR, Beaudet AL, Sly WS, et al: The Metabolic and Molecular Bases of Inherited Disease, 7th ed, pp 4525–4526. New York, McGraw-Hill, 1995

KURZ

Eponym used to indicate a confusing condition of congenital blindness, high grade of axial hyperopia; enophthalmos; wandering eye movements. In second stage, a delay of mental development becomes noticable.

BIBLIOGRAPHY. Kurz J: Syndrom Vrozené slepoty. Cesk Oftalmol 7:377–387, 1951

KUSKOKWIM*

Synonym. Arthrogryposis variant. See also Guerin.

Symptoms. Found in Alaskan Eskimos; more males than females affected. From birth, impaired movements, especially of the limbs because of joint contractures. Propensity to walk on knees or develop duck-like waddle. Normal mental development.

Signs. Multiple joint contractures especially affecting the knee and ankles; muscle atrophy or hypertrophy (compensatory). Deep tendon reflexes normal. Absent or diminished corneal reflex, pigmented nevi may be associated.

Etiology. Unknown; autosomal recessive inheritance suggested.

Pathology. Abnormal muscle attachment, involving primarily the extensor muscles.

Diagnostic Procedures. *Blood.* Normal. *Urine.* Normal. *X-rays.* Cyst formation in proximal part of long bone (occasional). *Electromyography.* Normal. *Biopsy of muscle.* Normal. *Enzyme study.* Normal.

Therapy. Standard orthopedic procedure and physiotherapy manipulation as soon as possible, at 15–18 months fitting with long leg braces and surgical shoes.

Prognosis. Good quoad vitam. Function according to degree of lesions and treatment.

BIBLIOGRAPHY. Patjan JH, Momberg GL, Aasc J, et al: Arthrogryposis syndrome (Kuskokwim disease) in the Eskimo. JAMA 209:1481–1486, 1969

KUSSMAUL-MAIER

Synonyms. Necrotizing arteritis; nodosa panarteritis; periarteritis nodosa; polyarteritis nodosa.

Symptoms. Male to female ratio, 2.4:1; onset at all ages. Respiratory infection (21%) or drug reaction (24%). During preceding years protean features: fever (50%); malaise; weight loss; myalgia and arthralgia; abdominal pain; anginal pain; polyneuritis (motor and sensory changes); hemiplegia; convulsion; acute brain syndrome; visual troubles.

Signs. Skin lesion (25%), polymorphic manifestation: diffuse erythema; purpura; urticaria; various types of rash; ulcers; painful, tender, occasionally pulsating, cutaneous or subcutaneous nodules; Raynaud phenomenon (frequent); gangrene in acute cases. Blood hypertension (67%); tachycardia (out of proportion with temperature elevation),

---

*Named for the river delta where original cases were found.

edema (50%); pericarditis; aoritis. Fundus oculi exudates; uneven caliber of vessels; retinal detachment.

Etiology. Idiopathic. Belongs to collagen disease (autoimmune) group. See also Zeek and Strauss-Churg-Zak.

Pathology. Widespread inflammatory necrotizing panangiotis in small elastic arteries, arterioles, and veins; aneurysm formation. Ischemia and infarction of organs involved. Limited to selected organs or widespread. Renal involvement (87%). Usually, absence of vasculitis in pulmonary circulation and splenic follicular arteries (see Zeek).

Diagnostic Procedures. *Blood.* Anemia; neutrophil leukocytosis; leukopenia in some cases; eosinophilia up to 75%; high sedimentation rate; protein increase of gamma globulin, lupus erythematosis (LE) test negative; high blood urea nitrogen. *Urine.* Albumin; red cell; casts. *Biopsy of nodules and muscles.*

Therapy. Adrenocorticotropic hormone (ACTH) or corticosteroids in high doses, then maintenance doses. Elimination of septic foci. Antibiotics (rule out sensitivity first).

Prognosis. Severe; survival variable: from fulminating cases dying in a few days, to complete recovery. Before steroids, 50% spontaneous remission. If renal involvement, poor prognosis. Cutaneous variety (Lindberg) better prognosis.

BIBLIOGRAPHY. Kussmaul A, Maier R: Ueber eine bisher nicht beschriebene eigenthumliche Arterienerkrankung (Périarteritis nodosa), die mit Morbus Brightii und rapid fortschreitender allgemeiner, Muskellähmung einhergeht. Dtsch Arch Klin Med 1:484–518, 1866
Moskowitz RW, Baggenstoss AH, Slocumb CH: Histopathologic classification of periarteritis nodosa: a study of 56 cases confirmed at necropsy. Proc Staff Meet Mayo Clinic 38:345–357, 1963
Ryan TJ: Cutaneous vasculitis. In Champion RH, Burton JL, Ebling FJG (eds): Rook/Wilkinson/Ebling Textbook of Dermatology, 5th ed, pp 1946–1951. Oxford, Blackwell Scientific, 1992

KWASHIORKOR–DISPLACED CHILD

Synonyms. Nutritional dystrophy; malignant malnutrition; mehlährschaden; nutritional edema; plurideficiency; polycarential.

Symptoms. Prevalent in infants and young children (rarely observed in full-blown form in adults, except as complication of alcoholism); onset after child has been weaned and kept for some time on any diet very poor in protein. Failure to grow; apathy; irritability; weak cry; diarrhea.

Signs. The child appears well nourished (because fat is still present, more or less in normal amount). Edema (that further contributes to hide muscle wasting). Skin pigmentation, desquamation, oozing areas, dryness that may give a particular aspect called "crazy pavement skin." Hair changes colors from black to brown, and then to red. If hair curly before onset, it becomes straight. Marked hepatomegaly; no tenderness of liver.

Etiology. Protein deficiency.

Pathology. Fatty liver; atrophy of pancreas; muscle wasting.

Diagnostic Procedures. *Blood.* Anemia; hypoproteinemia; all fractions, including albumin, markedly decreased.

Therapy. Milk or protein-rich preparation providing 1–1.5 mg/kg body weight daily. Multivitamin preparation; potassium, if depleted and good excretion observed.

Prognosis. If treated, reversal of symptoms. Fatty liver, infiltration recedes without sequelae. Lack of treatment results in death.

BIBLIOGRAPHY. Williams CD: Kwashiorkor. JAMA 153:1280–1285, 1953
Adams EB, Scragg JN, Naidoo BT, et al: Observation on the aetiology and treatment of anaemia in Kwashiorkor. Br Med J 3:451–454, 1967

Weatherall DJ, Ledingham JGG, Warrell DA (eds): Oxford Textbook of Medicine, 3rd ed, pp 1281, 3498–3499. Oxford, Oxford Med Pub, 1996

KYLE-LINMAN

Synonyms. Neutropenia, chronic idiopathic. Benign chronic neutropenia.

Symptoms and Signs. Recurrent or persistent mild infection. Gengivitis is prominent. No splenomegaly.

Etiology. Unknown.

Diagnostic Procedures. *Blood.* Neutropenia of different degree from moderate to severe. No other cellular changes. Leukoagglutinins usually absent. *Bone marrow.* Normal myeloid maturation, absence of segmentation of neutrophils.

Therapy. None needed. No response to corticosteroids or splenectomy.

Prognosis. Condition lasting from 1 year to decades.

BIBLIOGRAPHY. Kyle RA, Linman JW: Chronic idiopathic neutropenia. N Engl J Med 279:1015, 1968
Kyle RA: Natural history of chronic idiopathic neutropenia. N Engl J Med 302:908–909, 1980

KYRLE

Synonym. Hyperkeratosis follicularis penetrans. See Flegel.

Symptoms and Signs. Age of onset 20–63 years; no sex difference. Bilateral, asymptomatic, chronic, scattered, generalized papular eruptions having hyperkeratotic cone-shaped plugs. Lesions may coalesce into hyperkeratotic verrucous plaques. Mucous membranes, palmar and plantar surfaces are consistently respected. Symptoms and signs of hepatic insufficiency or diabetes mellitus frequently associated.

Etiology. Unknown; association in siblings suggests autosomic dominant inheritance. Frequent association with diabetes mellitus suggests that this syndrome belongs in the diabetic syndromes.

Pathology. Histologic criteria for diagnosis: keratotic plug filling epithelial invagination; parakeratosis in part of plug, basophilic cellular debris not staining with elastic tissue stains in the plug; epidermal disruption with keratinized cells in dermis and surrounding granuloma reaction.

Diagnostic Procedures. *Biopsy of skin.* (See Pathology.) *Blood.* Glucose tolerance test, Liver function test. *Urine.* Albuminuria (frequent); glycosuria.

Therapy. High doses of vitamin A. Topical keratolytics improve appearance. Topical isotretinoin. Large lesions: cautery or CO_2 snow.

Prognosis. Good response to vitamin A administration after 1 month of treatment. No patients reported cured. Correction of systemic disease when associated, accompanied by clearing of Kyrle lesions.

BIBLIOGRAPHY. Kyrle J: Hyperkeratosis follicularis and parafollicularis in cutem penetrans. Arch Dermatol Syph 123:466–493, 1916
Carter VH, Costantine VS: Kyrle's disease I. Arch Dermatol 97:624–632, 1968
Costantine VS, Carter VH: Kyrle's disease II. Arch Derm 97:633–639, 1968
Griffiths WAD, Leigh IM, Marks R: Disorders of keratinization. In Champion RH, Burton JL, Ebling FJG (eds): Rook/Wilkinson/Ebling Textbook of Dermatology, 5th ed, p 1367. Oxford, Blackwell Scientific, 1992

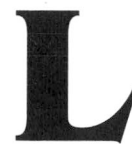

LABAND

Synonyms. Zimmermann-Laband; acrodefects—gingival fibromatosis; hepatosplenomegaly; fibromatosis gingival; abnormal fingers, nose, ears; splenomegaly.

Symptoms and Signs. Both sexes affected; present from birth. Nose and ears poorly structured; gingival fibromatosis (present at birth or appearing in first months of life); generalized hirsutism. Hypoplasia of thumb and other digits; hypoplasia or absence of nails; occasionally absence of terminal phalanges; joint hypermobility; hepatosplenomegaly and splenomegaly. (Zimmermann denies these features.) Occasionally, mental retardation.

Etiology. Possibly, autosomal dominant inheritance.

Diagnostic Procedures. *X-ray.* See Symptoms and Signs. Spina bifida occulta; third thoracic vertebra may be sagittally divided and the fourth flattened.

BIBLIOGRAPHY. Zimmermann KW: Ueber Anomalien des Ektoderms (Cases 1 und 2). Vjschr Zahnh 44:419–434, 1928
Laband PF, Habib G, Humphreys OS: Hereditary gingival fibromatosis: Report of an affected family with associated splenomegaly and skeletal and soft tissue abnormalities. Oral Surg 17:339–351, 1964
Pina-Neto JM, Martelli-Soares LR, Oliveira-Souza AH, et al: A new case of Zimmerman-Laband syndrome with mild mental retardation, asymmetry of limbs and hypertrichosis. Am J Med Genet 31:619–695, 1988

LABBÉ

Eponym used to indicate the hypertensive paroxysmal crisis in pheochromocytoma (see).

BIBLIOGRAPHY. Labbé M, et al: Crises solaires et hypertension paroxystique en rapport avec une tumeur surrénale. Bull Soc Med Hôp 46:982–990, 1922

LABYRINTHINE APOPLEXY

Synonyms. Vertigo paroxysmal.

Symptoms and Signs. Single abrupt attack of vertigo, nausea, vomiting, no tinnitus or hearing loss; permanent loss of labyrinthine function of one side.

Etiology. Occlusion of labyrinthine division of internal auditory artery (?).

Pathology. No report.

BIBLIOGRAPHY. Brandt T: Vertigo: Its Multisensory Syndromes. London, Springer-Verlag, 1991

LACTASE DEFICIENCY, CONGENITAL

Synonym. Alactasia hereditary; lactase malabsorption, congenital; disaccharide intolerance II; CLD; Lactase phlorizin hydrolase.

Symptoms and Signs. After first feeding of breast milk: severe diarrhea, dehydration, failure to thrive.

Etiology. Absent lactase in duodenal mucose. Autosomal recessive inheritance.

Diagnostic Procedures. *Feces.* Large amounts of lactose. *Intestinal biopsy.* Lactase present at trace level much lower than in adult hypolactasia.

Therapy. Lactose and cellobiose free diet (sucrose, maltose, and starch well tolerated).

Prognosis. Good with therapy.

BIBLIOGRAPHY. Holzel A, Schwarz V, Sutcliffe KW, et al: Defective lactose absorption causing malnutrition in infants. Lancet 1:1126–1128, 1959
Semenza G, Auricchio S: Small intestinal disaccharidases. In Scriver CR, Beaudet AL, Sly WS, et al: The Metabolic and Molecular Bases of Inherited Disease, 7th ed, p 4467. New York, McGraw-Hill, 1995

LACTATE DEHYDROGENASE DEFICIENCY

Synonyms. LDH deficiency; glycogenosis, type XI.

Symptoms and Signs. Rare. Cases described in Japanese and Brazilians. Excercise intolerance, desquamating erythematosquamous lesion on extensor surface of extermities.

Etiology. Autosomal recessive (?) inheritance. Defect of H-subunit of LDH that appears composed only of H subunits. No hemolysis with deficiency of H subunit; myopathy with lack of M subunit.

Diagnostic Procedures. *Urine.* Myoglobinuria. *Blood.* Lack of LDH H-subunit in red blood cells. No hemolytic anemia. After ischemic work of forearm: nonlactate increase in blood lactate.

Therapy. Usually not necessary.

Prognosis. Good.

BIBLIOGRAPHY. Boyer SH, Fainer DC, Watson-Williams ES: Lactate dehydrogenase variant from human blood: Evidence for molecular subunits. Science 141:642–643, 1963
Kanno T, Sudo K, Mackewa M, et al: Lactate dehydrogenase H-subunit deficiency: A new type of hereditary exertional myopathy. Clin Chim Acta 173:89–78, 1988
Takayasu S, Fujiwara S, Waki T: Hereditary lactate dehydrogenase H-subunit deficiency: Lactate dehydrogenase activity in skin lesions and in hair follicles. J Am Acad Derm 24:339–342, 1991

LACTIC ACIDOSIS, IDIOPATHIC

Synonym. Acidosis of infancy idiopathic. Includes several errors of metabolism:

1. Glycogen storage disease (type 1)
2. Pyruvate carboxylate or pyruvate dehydrogenase deficiency
3. Branched chain ketonuria (maple syrup disease)
4. Isovaleric acidemia
5. Beta-ketathiolase deficiency
6. Propionic acidemia
7. Methylmalonic acidemia

BIBLIOGRAPHY. Intensive Care World 4, no. 4 (whole issue), 1987
Robinson BH: Lactic acidemia (Disorders of pyruvate carboxylase, pyruvate dehydrogenase). In Scriver CR, Beaudet AL, Sly WS, et al:

The Metabolic and Molecular Bases of Inherited Disease, 7th ed, pp 1479–1499. New York, McGraw-Hill, 1995

LACUNAR

Synonyms. Cerebral atherosclerosis; état lacunaire; arteriopathic dementia; multi-infarct dementia; including état criblé. See C.A.D.A.S.I.L.; pseudobulbar palsy and Binswanger.

Symptoms. Onset usually past middle age. Mental symptoms always present. Impairment of memory for recent events; usually, vivid recall of past events; repetition of facts or repeated requests for some information in a more or less monotonous tone. Lack of grasp and storage of recent facts. Altered mental processing of facts and manifestations of paranoid tendencies that may lead to foolish acts. Headache; vertiginous attacks, or, more commonly, giddiness; occasionally, convulsions.

Signs. Several clinical syndromes may be recognized in this condition, which derives its name from anatomic-pathologic findings: homolateral cerebellar ataxia, with pyramidal tract signs; isolated hemiplegia; pure sectorial sensory stroke; the dysarthria–clumsy hand syndrome.

Etiology. Cerebral atherosclerosis or systemic hypertension or both, causing occlusion of small arteries.

Pathology. Brain microinfarctions that produce a number of lacunae (irregular cavities 0.9–15.0 mm in diameter) irregularly distributed in all cerebral nervous system structures. In these areas, ganglion cells are degenerated or necrotic, little increase of fibrous glial elements and microglial stimulation. Lacunae are located in the periphery of sclerosed and occluded arterioles. Etat criblé alleged different condition where lesions are owing to a fine loosening of tissue around thickened vessels entering anterior and posterior perforated spaces (Marie). Distinction abandoned.

Diagnostic Procedures. *Angiography.* Not necessary because clinical symptoms are so evident. *CT scan. MRI.*

Therapy. Antihypertensive agents; mild sedatives; some success reported with the use of vincamine and phosphocholine.

Prognosis. Progressive mental deterioration, although in many cases with abrupt onset the situation may become stabilized and remain at the same level for years.

BIBLIOGRAPHY. Marie P: Des foyers lacunaires de désintégration et de différents autres états cavitaires du cerveau. Rev Méd 21:281–298, 1901
Fisher CM: Lacunar strokes and infarct: A review. Neurology 38:871–876, 1982
Adams RD, Victor M: Principles of Neurology, 5th ed, p 692, 694, 696. New York, McGraw-Hill, 1993

LADD

Synonyms. Duodenal stenosis; includes Weyer I.

Symptoms and Signs. Occurs in newborn within a few hours of birth or after first feeding. Usually bilious, continuous vomiting indicates complete obstruction; distension of epigastrium; meconium may be excreted; jaundice in 30% of cases. Intermittent vomiting at variable times after birth (days, weeks, months, or years) indicates partial obstruction.

Etiology. Not well defined. In atresia, possibly autosomal recessive inheritance. In atresia or stenosis, vascular defects in embryo, lack of relief of normal temporary obstruction occurring during fetal life (sixth or seventh week of embryonic development). If multiple zones of intestinal atresia; also called Weyer I.

Diagnostic Procedures. *X-ray, plain film.* Evidence of gastric and duodenal gas distension proximal to the "double bubble" sign. Presence or absence of gas in intestinal lumen indicates partial or total obstruction; rule out extrinsic compression (annular pancreas).

Therapy. Duodenojejunostomy or gastrojejunostomy (if atresia of first part of duodenum).

Prognosis. Related to the time of intervention and, eventually, to complications.

BIBLIOGRAPHY. Ladd WE: Congenital obstruction of the duodenum in children. N Engl J Med 206:277–283, 1932
Best LG, Wiseman NE, Chudley AE: Familial duodenal Atresia: A report of two families and review. Am J Med Genet 34:442–444, 1989

LADD-GROSS

Synonym. Bile duct atresia.

Symptoms and Signs. Both sexes affected; present from birth or onset at 2–3 weeks of life. Jaundice of progressive intensity. Hepatosplenomegaly. Fetor hepaticus.

Etiology. Arrest of canalization of biliary ducts in fetal life. Intrauterine infection by Listeria Monocytogenes Sporadic reported as possible cause. Autosomal recessive inheritance possible in some cases.

Pathology. Lack of canalization at extrahepatic or intrahepatic level or both.

Diagnostic Procedures. *Urine.* Bilirubin increased. *Stool.* Alcoholic. *Blood.* Hyperbilirubinemia over 6 mg/100 ml; prothrombin time increased; alkaline phosphatases increased.

Therapy. Surgical correction (possible in 16%). Chemotherapy. Vitamin K. Liver transplantation in patients with end-stage liver disease.

Prognosis. Good with surgery. If surgery not feasible, fatal within 1 year. Longer survival with defect limited to intrahepatic region. Many patients develop recurrent cholangitis after correction. Re-exploration and surgical revision may be needed.

BIBLIOGRAPHY. Ladd WE, Gross RE: Abdominal Surgery in Infancy and Childhood, pp 260–275. Philadelphia, WB Saunders, 1971
Cunningham ML, Sybert VP: Idiopathic extrabiliary atresia: Recurrence in sibs in two families. AM J Med Genet 31:421–426, 1988
Cywes S, Millar AJW: Embryology and anomalies of the intestine. Haubrich WS, Schaffner F, Berk JE (eds): Bockus Gastroenterology, 5th ed, vol 2, p 920. Philadelphia, WB Saunders, 1995

LAENNEC

Synonyms. Morgagni-Laennec; alcoholic cirrhosis (obsolete and wrong); fatty nutritional cirrhosis; portal liver cirrhosis; portal cirrhosis; septal cirrhosis. See also Zieve.

Symptoms. Prevalent in males. Asymptomatic in 10–20% of patients. Onset insidious; becomes symptomatic usually at 50 years of age. Anorexia; fatigability; later nausea; emesis; diarrhea; abdominal pain.

Signs. Initially, progressive hepatomegaly with smooth surface; then reduction of size and firm edge becoming sharp, then nodular. Initially, liver tender on palpation; weight loss; jaundice (in two-thirds of patients) of variable degree and progression; ascites, leg edema; spider nevi; caput medusae; gynecomastia and loss of axillary and pubic hair; splenomegaly. Frequently, low-grade and continuous fever. Encephalopathy with asterixis; bleeding tendency and interstitial hemorrhages from esophageal or gastric varices.

Etiology. Direct action of ethanol on the liver plus (more important) dietary insufficiency. Increased peripheral fat mobilization; enhanced hepatic lipogenesis; decreased lipid oxidation; altered hepatic protein production and release.

Pathology. Early, presence on the surface of gold yellow micronodules

(Laennec cirrhosis). Size variable, from 4 kg to a small hard mass. Later, increase in nodule size and appearance of scars. Early nodules are regular in size and shape, then they become irregular and "relobulized"; scar tissue distorts architecture of parenchyma. Bands of connective tissue between portal and central zones; changes in hepatic circulation, limited by neovascularization of connective tissue septae. Fat deposits; inflammatory changes; cholestasis; iron deposits.

Diagnostic Procedures. *Blood.* Sodium sulfobromophthalein retention; hyperbilirubinemia; hypoalbuminemia; hyperglobulinemia (beta and gamma); IgA and to lesser degree IgG and IgM elevated; esterified fraction of cholesterol decreased, serum glutamic-oxaloacetic transaminase (SGOT), serum glutamic pyruvic transaminase (SGPT), and alkaline phosphatase moderately elevated. Impaired glucose tolerance. Anemia; leukocytosis. *Biopsy of liver.* See Pathology. *Echography.*

Therapy. Alcohol abstension; correction of diet. Silimarin; colchicine: corticosteroids of little benefit. Portacaval shunting (does not improve survival). Vegetable protein diet; branched-chain amino acids; removal of fecal material from the colon, using oral or rectal lactulose; oral or rectal neomycin; treatment of infections; correction of electrolyte abnormalities; salt restriction; bed rest; diuretics and/or dopamine if needed; propanolol to decrease risk of first bleeding episode. In patients with ascites refractory to medical therapy, peritoneovenous shunt (Le Veen or Denver shunt). Present treatment liver transplantation.

Prognosis. Five-year survival for patients without jaundice, ascites, and hematemesis is 88.9% in abstainers and 62.8% in drinkers. If mentioned signs are present, 50% in abstainers and 33% in drinkers.

BIBLIOGRAPHY. Laennec RT: Traité de l'auscultation médical et des maladies du poumon et du coeur. Paris, 1819
Crabb DW, Lumeng L: Alcoholic liver cirrhosis. In Haubrich WS, Schaffner F, Berk JE (eds): Bockus Gastroenterology, 5th ed, vol 2, pp 2234–2240. Philadelphia, WB Saunders, 1995

LAFORA BODIES

Synonyms. Myoclonus epilepsy; Lafora body. See Unverricht; Hartung.

Symptoms and Signs. Onset in the second decade in previously normal subject. Progressive seizures; myoclonus; dementia; ataxia; dysarthria; visual troubles. Symptoms and signs of extrapyramidal and bulbar musculature involvement.

Etiology. Unknown; autosomal recessive inheritance. On the basis of presence of bodies considered different from Unverricht; although it presents similar clinical features and evolution.

Pathology. Presence of Lafora bodies (bodies resembling plant starch formed by insoluble polyglucosan) in ganglion cells (substantia nigra and dentate nuclei predilected), retina, and axons of spinal nerves. Little demyelinization. Lafora bodies' presence may be demonstrated also in heart, liver, and striated muscles.

Diagnostic Procedures. *Blood.* Decreased mucoprotein content. *EEG.* Diffuse slow waves and spikes and focal or multifocal discharges. *Muscle and liver biopsy.*

Therapy. Anticonvulsants.

Prognosis. Death 2–10 years from onset of symptoms.

BIBLIOGRAPHY. Lafora GR, Gluck G: Beitrag zur Histologie der myoklonischen Epilepsie. Z Neurol Psychiatr 6:1–14, 1911
Noris R, Koskiniemi M: Progressive myoclonus epilepsy: genetic and nosological aspects with special reference to 107 Finnish patients. Clin Genet 15:382–398, 1979
Busard HLSM, Gabreels-Festen AAWM, Renier WO, et al: Axilla skin biopsy: a reliable test for the diagnosis of Lafora's disease. Ann Neurol 21:599–601, 1987
Adams RD, Victor M: Principles of Neurology, 5th ed, pp 831–832. New York, McGraw-Hill, 1993

LAGER

Synonyms. Concentration camp I; persecution victim; postdetention, survived. See also Todeserwartung.

Symptoms and Signs. Observed in victims who have survived prolonged detention in concentration camps, or mental and psychological stresses caused by persecution (hiding and fighting for survival). Chronic state of tension; alertness; irritability; depression; restlessness and tremor; sleep disturbed; nightmares; cephalalgia; prostration; excessive sweating. Patients usually avoid company and in most severe cases seek complete isolation. They have a feeling of guilt because of their survival, especially when they are the only survivers of a family or a group. Frequent also are memory defects and parapraxia.

Etiology. After effect of severe psychological traumas.

Prognosis. Difficult treatment and generally poor results.

BIBLIOGRAPHY. Niederland WG: Psychiatric disorder among persecution victims: A contribution to the understanding of concentration camp. Pathology and its after-effects. J Nerv Ment Dis 139:458–474, 1964
Ochberg F (ed): Post-traumatic Therapy and Victims of Violence. New York, Brunner/Mazel, 1988

LAHEY

Eponym used to indicate the thyroid crisis in its two main forms: "agitating" Lahey I (see also Waldenström II) and "apathetic" Lahey II (see Apathetic thyrotoxin storm).

BIBLIOGRAPHY. Lahey FH: The crisis of exophthalmic goiter. N Enlg J Med 199:235–257, 1928
McKenzie JM, Zakarija M: Hyperthyroidism. In De Groot LJ (ed): Endocrinology, 3rd ed, pp 704–705. Philadelphia, WB Saunders, 1995

LAIGNEL-LAVASTINE-VIARD

Mitchell II (see) with hypertrophy of subcutaneous fat of the lower part of the body.

BIBLIOGRAPHY. Laignel-Lavastine M, Viard M: Adipose segmentaire des membres inférieurs. Nouv Icon Saltpétrière 25:473–482, 1912
Perrot H, Delaup JP, Chouvet B: Partial lipodystrophy, complement abnormalities and cutaneous leukocytoclastic vasculitis. Ann Dermatol 114:1083–1091, 1987
Flier JS: Syndromes of insulin resistance and mutant insulin. In De Groot LJ (ed): Endocrinology, 3rd ed, p 1599. Philadelphia, WB Saunders, 1995

LAMBERT

Lambert is the name of a family affected by ichthyosis hystrix and exhibited at fairs in Suffolk, at the end of the 19th century.

Synonyms. Porcupine man. See Ichthyosis hystrix.

LAMBERT-EATON

Synonyms. Eaton-Lambert; bronchial carcinoma-myasthenia. See Erb-Goldflam and paraneoplastic.

Symptoms and Signs. In cases reported by Eaton and Lambert prevalence in males. Onset in middle life. Those of Erb-Goldflam (see), plus muscular pain and tenderness, depression of tendon reflexes, before bulbar muscles are affected.

Etiology. Bronchial carcinoma of small cell or oat cell type.

Pathology. Bronchial carcinoma (oat cell or anaplastic).

Diagnostic Procedures. *Neostigmine (Prostigmine and edrophonium chloride (Tensilon) tests.* Negative or feebly positive. *Electromyography.* Increase in amplitude on repetitive stimulation (allows the distinction of this syndrome from myastenia gravis). *X-ray of chest. Bronchography. Bronchoscopy.*

Therapy. High voltage radiation, chemotherapy for carcinoma or both; or surgery if feasible. Treatment of Erb-Goldflam (see). Response to intravenous neostigmine usually slight or moderate. Tumor removal causes some improvement.

Prognosis. According to degree of diffusion or metastasis of carcinoma. Usually, rapid deterioration and death.

BIBLIOGRAPHY. Anderson JH, Churchill-Davidson HD, Richardson AT: Bronchial neoplasm with myasthenia. Lancet 2:1291–1293, 1953

Lambert EH, Eaton LM, Rooke ED: Defect of neuromuscular conduction associated with malignant neoplasm. Am J Physiol 187:612–613, 1956

O'Neill JH: The Lambert-Eaton myasthenic syndrome: A review of 50 cases. Brain III:577–586, 1988

Lisak RP: Handbook of Myasthenia Gravis and Myasthenic Syndromes. New York, Marcel Dekker, 1994

LAMBERT (J.C.)

Synonyms. Branchial dysplasia; club foot; inguinal hernia; biliary atresia. See Alagille.

Symptoms and Signs. Both sexes. From birth. Branchial dysplasia; club foot; inguinal hernia; jaundice. *Facies.* Malar hypoplasia; macrostomia; preauricular tags, meatal atresia. Hypospedias. Mental deficiency.

Etiology. Autosomal recessive inheritance.

Pathology. Intrahepatic biliary atresia from complete to paucity of bile ducts.

Prognosis. From death in neonatal period to longer survival.

BIBLIOGRAPHY. Lambert JC, Ayraud N, Marin J, et al: Familial occurrence of a syndrome with branchial dysplasia, mental deficiency; club feet, and inguinal herniae. J Med Genet 19:214–215, 1982

Lambert JC, Saint-Paul MC, Bastiani F, et al: Branchial dysplasia, mental deficiency; club feet and inguinal herniae: A report of two further cases associated with paucity of interlobular bile ducts. J Med Genet 27:330–332, 1990

LAMBLING

Synonym. Postgastrectomy malabsorption. See also Postgastrectomy, dumping syndromes.

Eponym used to indicate the symptom complex owing to malabsorption appearing in variable combinations in a percentage of patients after gastrectomy: diarrhea (postprandial); weight loss; specific nutritional deficiencies; mild anemia; bone disease; metabolic neuropathy. Diarrhea occurs particularly when a total or selective vagotomy was performed.

BIBLIOGRAPHY. Lambling A: Syndrome carentiel complexe chez des gastrectomisés: Étude biologique. Bull Soc Med Hôp 65:161–164, 1949

Ammon HV: Diarrhea and constipation. In Haubrich WS, Schaffner F, Berk JE (eds): Bockus Gastroenterology, 5th ed, vol 2, p 93. Philadelphia, WB Saunders, 1995

LAMBOTTE

Synonyms. Microcephaly; holoprosencephaly; intrauterine growth retardation.

Symptoms and Signs. Arabic race. Intrauterine growth retardation. Microcephaly; large soft pinnae; hypertelorism with squint; looked nose; retrognathia; mental retardation. Occasionally preaxial polydactyly of feet; cardiac malformations; atresia of auditory meatus.

Etiology. Autosomal recessive inheritance.

Pathology. Cerebral malformations, compatible with holoprosencephaly.

Prognosis. Stillborn or death in early infancy (second year) from cachexy.

BIBLIOGRAPHY. Verloes A, Dodinval P, Beco L, et al: Lambotte syndrome; microcephaly holoprosencephaly, intrauterine growth retardation facial anomalies and early lethality: A new sublethal multiple congenital anomaly/mental retardation syndrome in four sibs. Am J Med Genet 37:119–123, 1990

LANCE-ADAMS

Synonyms. Intention myoclonus; action myoclonus; myoclonus intentional; posthypoxic myoclonus.

Symptoms and Signs. Sequel of hypoxic encephalopathy, when patient is relaxed no symptoms; fast movements, especially if finalized, induce series of irregular myoclonic contractions (different in speed and rhythm from intention tremor) limited to the moving limb; speech may be affected; cerebellar ataxia.

Etiology. Irregular discharges via corticospinal tracts; cortical reflex and/or reticular relex mechanism postulated.

Therapy. Clonazepam, mebaral, valproic acid.

BIBLIOGRAPHY. Lance JW, Adams RD: The syndrome of intention or action myoclonus as a sequel to hypoxic encephalopathy. Brain 86:111–136, 1963

Adams RD, Victor M: Principles of Neurology, 5th ed, pp 91–92. New York, McGraw-Hill, 1993

LANCE-ANTHONY

Synonyms. Neck-tongue.

Symptoms and Signs. Attacks of pain and sudden turning of the head and numbness of tongue.

Etiology. Lesion at level of C2.

Diagnostic Procedures. *X-rays. CT scan. MRI.*

Therapy. According to nature of lesion.

BIBLIOGRAPHY. Lance JW, Anthony M: Neck-tongue syndrome on sudden turning of the head. J Neurol Neurosurg Psychiatr 43:97–101, 1980

LANDAU-KLEFFNER

Synonyms. Aphasia—epilepsy, acquired.

Symptoms and Signs. In children, who have normally acquired speech with convulsive disorders. Early and/or predominant difficulties of comprehension, fluctuating with time and occasionally disappearing. Associated: hyperkinesia, attention disorders, and others behavioral changes. Seizures of various types usually are sporadic.

Etiology. Unknown. Metabolic alteration (?).

Pathology. No relevant findings reported.

Diagnostic Procedures. *CT scan. MRI.* Normal. *EEG.* Abnormalities, predominantly of paroxysmal character, generalized, bilateral synchronous, focal, or multifocal.

Therapy. Seizures, usually easily controlled by anti-epileptic drugs.

BIBLIOGRAPHY. Landau WM, Kleffner FR: Syndrome of acquired aphasia with convulsive disorder in children. Neurology 7:523–530, 1957

Maquet P, Hirsch E, Dive D, et al: Cerebral glucose utilization during sleep in Landau-Kleffner syndrome: A PET study. Epilepsia 31:778–783, 1990

LANDOUZY I

Eponym used to indicate the secondary muscular atrophy caused by sciatica. See Cotugno.

BIBLIOGRAPHY. Landouzy JT: De la sciatique et de l'atrophie musculair qui peut la compliquer. Arch Gen Med 25:303–325, 1875

LANDOUZY-DEJERINE

Synonyms. Facioscapulohumeral muscular dystrophy, FSH, FSHD; muscular dystrophy, facioscapulohumeral.

Symptoms. Onset at 12–14 years of age, to as late as 30–40 years; males and females equally affected. Preclinical condition presents compromission limited to face muscles, resulting in difficulty in closing the eyes, sucking through straw, blowing cheeks, whistling. Patient then develops weakness in the use of shoulder muscles (in female, noticed while combing hair). Later on involvement of pelvic muscles and legs.

Signs. Typical pouting of lips; "ironing out" of facial expression; pectus excavatum may be present. Scapulae winging; muscular hypertrophy very rare in this form.

Etiology. Unknown; usually autosomal dominant inheritance, but hereditary autosomal recessive and X-linked transmission also observed. Locus probably on end of chromosome 4.

Pathology. Atrophic muscles; loss of striation in swollen fibers; increased number of sarcolemma nuclei; increase of endomysial collagen and fat.

Diagnostic Procedures. (1) Review of old photographs to identify changes in facial expression. (2) Observation of face during smiling and asking to blow the cheeks. (3) Checking of resistance to eye closure. (4) Observation of arm movement and scapule winging. (5) Invite the patient to walk on heels (impossible). *Electromyography.* Interference to mixed pattern. *Urine.* Slight creatinuria. *Blood.* Elevated serum creatinine kinase, glutamic oxaloacetic transaminase (SGOT), aldolase; decreased creatinine.

Therapy. None specific; steroids, surgery to stabilize scapulae; keep the patient ambulatory; passive and active physical therapy. Treatment of cardiac condition, digitalis.

Prognosis. Normal life span, with incapacitation at late age.

BIBLIOGRAPHY. Landouzy L, Déjérine J: De la Myopathie Atrophique Progressive; Myopathie Héréditaire, sans Neuropathie, debutant d'Ordinaire dans l'Enfance par la Face sans alteration du systeme nerveux. Paris, F Alcan, 1885

Lunt PM, Harper PS: Genetic counseling in facioscapulohumeral muscolar dystrophy. J Med Genet 28:655–664, 1991

Munsat TL, Serratrice G: Facioscapulohumeral and scapuloperoneal syndromes. In Rowland LP, Di Mauro S (eds): Handbook of Clinical Neurology, vol 18. Myopathies, p 161. Amsterdam, Elsevier, 1992

LANE (J.E.)

Synonyms. Acroerythema symmetricum naeviforme; erythema palmare hereditarium; palmoplantar erythema; red palms.

Symptoms and Signs. Evident at birth or onset in early infancy or during adult life. Symmetric, stable, permanent erythema of the palms (localized especially on thenar, hypothenar eminences, and pads of fingers) and soles (talon, lateral margin of foot, and plantar surface). No signs of sympathetic excitability (changes with temperature or emotion). Pregnancy may cause appearance of hereditary erythema.

Etiology. Unknown; hereditary autosomal dominant condition, isolated form also observed. Mildest form of keratoderma may be considered in the group of palm and sole dyskeratosis syndromes. One family with autosomal recessive inheritance reported with associated clubfoot and dental anomalies.

Pathology. Uniform thickening of all layers of epidermis; hyperkeratosis; but epidermis normal appearance (except for the change in color). No parakeratosis, no evidence of spongiosis or inflammation. Normal architecture respected; increased number of capillaries.

Therapy. None.

Prognosis. Stable, permanent; no evolving lesions; no functional troubles.

BIBLIOGRAPHY. Lane JE: Erythema palmare hereditarium (red palms). Arch Dermatol Syph 20:445–448, 1929

Poinso R, Calas E, Stahl A, et al: Le "syndrome" des paumes rouges. Presse Med 61:275–278, 1953

Champion RH: Disorder of blood vessels. In Champion RH, Burton JL, Ebling FJG (eds): Rook/Wilkinson/Ebling Textbook of Dermatology, 5th ed, p 1834. Oxford, Blackwell Scientific, 1992

LANE (W.A.)

Synonyms. Chronic ileal obstruction; intestinal stasis.

Eponym used to indicate the intestinal stasis resulting from congenital or acquired obstructive ileum.

BIBLIOGRAPHY. Lane WA: The kink of the ileum in chronic intestinal stasis. Nisbet, 1910

LANGE-AKEROYD

Synonyms. Hemolytic anemia—congenital Heinz body; CIBHA infuscuria; unstable hemoglobin; Heinz bodies—hemolytic anemia.

Symptoms. Both sexes affected; onset within first year of life for some variants, in others is delayed until late childhood or adolescence. Variable jaundice, cholelithiasis, and splenomegaly. Symptoms are of variable degrees of severity. Classified according to intensity of hemolysis in four groups, from I (very severe hemolysis) to IV (not associated with signs of hemolysis).

Etiology. Autosomal dominant inheritance or spontaneous mutations. Presence of one type of unstable hemoglobin (Hb); (over 125 variants have been identified and named according to towns where discovered, e.g., Hb Zurich, Hb Torino, Hb Saint Louis, Hb Sidney); the most common is Hb Koeln. Variable clinical manifestations occur according to type of hemoglobin (see groups in Symptoms and Signs).

Pathology. Nonspecific. According to severity of form.

Diagnostic Procedures. *Hemoglobin electrophoresis.* To identify type. Presence of Heinz body in red cells of all groups, increased after splenectomy. *Blood.* Group I: Hemoglobin from below 4–8 g/100 ml; reticulocytes, hyperbilirubinemia very high. Group II: episodic hyperbilirubinemia; hemoglobin 6–9 g/100 ml; reticulocytes 4–20%. Group III: normal hemoglobin level; reticulocytes 4–10%. Group IV: normal findings. Heat denaturation test; isopropanol precipitation test. *Urine.* Groups I, II, III: dark urine. Presence of pigmenturia in almost all patients; pigment appears to be a dipyrrole related to mesobilifuscin. *Bone marrow.* Erythroid hyperplasia.

Therapy. Mildly affected patients require little therapy. Avoid sulfonamides and other oxidant drugs. Prompt treatment of infections. (Infections can precipitate hemolytic crisis.) Blood transfusions in cases of severe anemia. Splenectomy is beneficial in some variants.

Prognosis. Variable according to Hb type.

BIBLIOGRAPHY. Lange RD, Akeroyd JH: CIBHA infuscuria: a new clinical syndrome. Clin Res Proc 4:234, 1946
Lange RD, Akeroyd JH: Congenital hemolytic anemia with abnormal pigment metabolism and red cell inclusion bodies: A new clinical syndrome. Blood 13:950–958, 1958
Lukens JN, Lee GR: Unstable hemoglobin disease. In Lee GR, Bithell TC, Foerster J, et al (eds): Wintrobe's Clinical Hematology, 9th ed, pp 1054–1060. Philadelphia, Lea & Febiger, 1993

LANGER

Synonyms. Leri-Weill; homozygous dyschondrosteosis; mesomelic dwarfism Langer; ulna—fibula—mandible hypoplasia.

Symptoms and Signs. Present at birth. Short upper and lower limbs, especially of the middle segments. Hands and feet rarely involved. Lack of Madelung deformity. Mandible with mesomelic micromelia. Trunk normal.

Etiology. Autosomal recessive inheritance (?).

Pathology. Hypoplasia of ulna (minor hypoplasia of radius), fibula, and mandible.

Diagnostic Procedures. *X-ray. Ultrasonography.* Lack of ossification in distal half of ulna and proximal half of fibula; increased lumbar lordosis.

BIBLIOGRAPHY. Braisford JF: Dystrophies of the skeleton. Br J Radiol 8:533–569, 1935
Langer LO Jr: Mesomelic dwarfism of the hypoplastic ulna, fibula, mandible type. Radiology 89:654–660, 1967
Goldblatt J, Wallis C, Viljoen D, et al: Heterozygous manifestations of Langer's mesomelic dysplasia. Clin Genet 31:19–24, 1987
Evans MI, Zador IE, Qureshi F, et al: Ultrasonographic prenatal diagnosis and fetal pathology of Langer mesomelic dwarfism. Am J Med Genet 31:915–920, 1988

LANGER II

Synonyms. Spondylometaphyseal dysplasia, corner fracture type.

Symptoms and Signs. Both sexes. Disorder identified at two years of age. Short stature, developmental coxa vara.

Etiology. Autosomal dominant.

Diagnostic Procedures. *X-ray.* Changes in long tubular bone simulating corner fractures (large triangular fragments lateral to distal tibial metaphyses, on ulnar aspect of distal radius and proximal humerus). Typical vertebral changes of the condition (see Spondylometaphyseal dysplasia).

Therapy. Surgical correction.

BIBLIOGRAPHY. Langer LO Jr, Brill PW, Ozonoff MB, et al: Spondylometaphyseal dysplasia, corner fracture type: A heritable condition associated with coxa vara. Radiology 175:761–766, 1990

LANGER-GIEDION

Synonyms. Klingmüller; acrodysplasia V; trichorhinophalangeal II; LG. See also Trichorhinophalangeal I.

Symptoms. Both sexes affected majority males; present from birth. Moderate mental deficiency; growth deficiency; hypotonia; delayed speech, occasionally; recurrent respiratory infections (in first 5 years of life) and delayed speech development.

Signs. Redundance of skin, nevi; scalp and body hair scarce. *Head.* Mild microcephaly; full, bushy eyebrows; large nose, less bulbous than in trichorhinophalangeal syndrome; elongated philtrum; thin upper lips; recessed mandible, protruding large ears. *Skeleton.* Multiple exostoses (for onset and distribution, see Ehrenfried); tendency to fractures. Occasionally hyperextensible joints.

Etiology. Unknown. Sporadic. Autosomal dominant inheritance discussed. A variety of chromosomal abnormalities have been reported (8q24.11 to 8q24.13).

Diagnostic Procedures. *X-ray of skeleton.* Multiple exostoses.

Prognosis. After fifth year, good health except for tendency to fractures.

BIBLIOGRAPHY. Langer LO Jr: The thoracic-pelvic-phalangeal dystrophy. Radiology 91:447–456, 1968
Giedion A: Autosomal dominant transmissions of the tricorhinophalangeal syndrome. Helv Pediatr Acta 28:249–259, 1973
Buhler EM, Malik NJ: The tricho-rhinophalangeal syndrome(s): Chromosome 8 long arm deletion: Is there a shortest region of overlap between reported cases? TRP I and TRP II syndromes: Are they separate entities? Am J Med Genet 19:113–119, 1984
Brenholz P, Swayne L, Twersky S, et al: Dominant inheritance of the Langer-Giedion syndrome. Am J Hum Genet 45:A41, 1989
Ludecke H-J, Johnson C, Wagner MJ, et al: Molecular definition of the shortest region of deletion overlap in the Langer-Giedion syndrome. Am J Hum Genet 49:1197–1206, 1991

LANGER-SALDINO

Synonyms. Spranger type II; achondrogenesis type Ib (formerly) achondrogenesis type II; achondrogenesis—hypocondrogenesis type II; thanatophoric dysplasia type II; chondrogenesis imperfecta; pseudochondrogenesis with fractures. See Achondrogenesis I, II, IV.

Symptoms and Signs. Fewer stillbirths, longer survival, and less marked features than Parenti-Fraccaro (see). Characteristic craniofacial signs. Prominent forehead; flat face; micrognathia. Short trunk; prominent abdomen; hydropic aspect; marked micromelia. Cleft palate.

Etiology. Autosomal recessive inheritance. It represents the most severe end of the SED spectrum (see Spranger-Weidemann), that range from the mildest precocious osteoarthropathy through hypochondrogenesis, Stickler (see) etc; all disorders that share defects in type II collagen secondary to mutation in the COL2A1 gene.

Pathology. Increased vascularity in proliferative zones; enlarged lacunae with normal cells; irregular columns; bone spurs; reduced cartilage matrix; molecular defect type II cartilage.

Diagnostic Procedures. *X-ray of skeleton.* Thin ribs with multiple fractures, lack of mineralization of vertebral bodies; shortness of long and tubular bones; enlarged calvaria with normal calcification. *Ultrasound for prenatal diagnosis (second month).*

BIBLIOGRAPHY. Saldino RM: Lethal short limb dwarfism: achondrogenesis and thanotophoric dwarfism. Am J Roentgen 112:185–197, 1971
Borochowitz Z, Ornoy A, Lachman R, et al: Achondrogenesis II-hypochondrogenesis. Variability vs heterogeneity. Am J Med Genet 24:273–288, 1986
Rimoin DL, Lachman RS: Genetic disorders of the osseous skeleton. In Beithon P (ed): McKusick's Heritable Disorders of Connective Tissue, 5th ed, pp 642–644. St Louis, CV Mosby, 1993

LANGE-SHADE

Synonyms. Myogelosis; occupational myalgia; painful myosis.

Symptoms. Pain in one or several muscles.

Signs. Nodular change in texture of affected muscles. The nodules persist during sleep and anesthesia.

Etiology. Unknown; possibly, localized cramps owing to exertion or posture. According to most authors, it cannot be distinguished from muscle cramps.

Pathology. Biopsy of nodules does not show microscopic abnormalities or shows only minor changes of doubtful significance.

Diagnostic Procedures. *Electromyography.*

Therapy. Rest and massage.

Prognosis. Good.

BIBLIOGRAPHY. Lange M: Die Muskelhaerten (Myogelosen). Munich, Lehmann, 1931

Jordon HH: Myogeloses: the significance of pathologic conditions of musculature in disorders of posture and locomotion. Arch Phys Ther 23:36–41, 1942

Adams RD, Victor M: Principles of Neurology, 5th ed, pp 1195, 1279. New York, McGraw-Hill, 1993

LANZIERI

Synonym. Craniofacial malformation; dwarfism; fibula absence.

Symptoms and Signs. Present from birth. Dwarfism. *Head.* Dyscephalia; microphthalmia; anophthalmia; congenital cataracts; coloboma (iris and optic nerve); dental anomalies. *Skin.* Atrophic changes; hypertrichosis. *Skeleton.* Absence of fibula and some tarsal and metatarsal bones.

Etiology. Unknown. Developmental anomaly.

BIBLIOGRAPHY. Lanzieri M: Su una rara associazione di una sindrome malformativa cranio facciale e assenza congenita della fibula. Ann Ital Clin Ocul 87:667–673, 1961

LARON

Synonyms. Dwarfism Laron; GH-resistance: Growth hormone insensitivity. See Seabright-Bantam.

Symptoms and Signs. Both sexes. More than 50% from Middle East. Acrohypoplasia blue scleras; high-pitched voice. Menarche usually delayed. Normal body proportion in chilhood, but childlike proportion in adulthood. Head size normal, contrasting with smaller body. Limited elbow extension. From reduced to normal or even superior intelligence.

Etiology. Autosomal recessive. Anomalies of growth hormone (GH) receptor, caused by gene deletions or point mutations

Diagnostic Procedures. *Blood.* Low IGF-1 and IGF-binding protein 3 elevated GH concentration; exaggerated GH response to stimuli; no response to exogenous human (pituitary) growth hormone (h-GH); serum somatomedin low.

Therapy. Long-term IGF-1 treatment could be of benefit.

Prognosis. Height of patients ranges 10.0–6.7 SD below normal mean height for age in the United States.

BIBLIOGRAPHY. Laron Z, Pertzelan A, Mannheimer S: Genetic pituitary dwarfism with high serum concentration of growth hormone: A new inborn error of metabolism? Isr J Med Sci 2:152–155, 1966

Laron Z: Laron syndrome: from description to therapy. Endocrinologist 3:21–28, 1993

Rosenfeld RG, Albertsson-Wikland K, Cassorla F, et al: Diagnostic controversy: The diagnosis of childhood growth hormone deficiency revisited. J Clin Endocrinol Metab 80:1532–1540, 1995

Rosenfeld RG: Broadening the growth hormone insensitivity syndrome (editorial). N Engl J Med 333:1145–1146, 1995

LARSEN

Synonyms. McFarland; flat facies; short fingernails; multiple joint dislocation; dish face.

Symptoms. Present at birth. Prevalent in females. Mentally normal; occasionally, respiratory difficulty at young age.

Signs. *Facies.* Flat; depressed nasal bridge; bossed forehead; hypertelorism. *Joints.* Laxity causing bilateral dislocation of tibia and femur, elbows, and hip; feet equinovalgus or equinovarus. *Fingers.* Long and cylindrical; spatulate thumbs. Short metacarpals. Occasionally associated, palatoschisis (50%); teeth abnormalities, abnormal vertebral segmentation, congenital cardiac defects, hydrocephalus, laryngotracheomalacia.

Etiology. Unknown; autosomal recessive and; in some families dominant inheritance.

Diagnostic Procedures. *X-rays.* See Signs.

Prognosis. Fair quoad vitam; reported familiar occurrence of a rare lethal form.

BIBLIOGRAPHY. McFarland BL: Congenital dislocation of the knee. J Bone Joint Surg II:281–285, 1929

Larsen LJ, Schottstaedt ER, Bost FC: Multiple congenital dislocations associated with characteristic facial abnormality. J Pediatr 37:574–581, 1950

Houston CS, Reed MH, Desansch JEL: Separating Larsen's syndrome from the "arthrogryposis basket." J Can Assoc Radiol 32:206–214, 1981

Mostello D, Hoechstetter L, Bendon R, et al: Recurrence and prenatal diagnosis of lethal Larsen syndrome. Am J Hum Genet 45:A56, 1989

LARVA VISCERAL MIGRANS

Synonyms. Eosinophilia—hepatomegaly; toxocariasis. See Loeffler.

Symptoms. Occurs in children, predominantly in boys. Pica; cough; wheezing; fever; convulsions; vision impairment (in order of frequency).

Signs. Hepatomegaly; pulmonary rales or wheezes; malnutrition; skin lesions; lymphadenopathy; eye ground lesion (in order of frequency).

Etiology. Visceral infiltration with larvae of *Toxocara canis* or *T. cati. Capillaria hepatica, Ascaris suis, A. hominis,* and Strongyloides may also produce this syndrome.

Pathology. Hepatic and cerebral infestation with parasites. Eosinophilic granulomas with necrotic centers containing larvae; lymphoplasmocytic and giant cell halo.

Diagnostic Procedures. *Blood.* Hypochromic anemia; leukocytosis; chronic peripheral blood and bone marrow eosinophilia (over 30%); hypoalbuminemia; increase gamma globulins and IgM globulin. Precipitating antibodies to A and B blood group substances or helminth antigens or both. Isohemoagglutinion titers elevated; sheep cell agglutination titers slightly elevated; presence of heat-stable antiglobulins. *Biopsy of liver.* Presence of larvae. *X-ray of chest.* Bilateral peribronchial infiltration. *Stool.* Presence of intestinal parasites.

Therapy. No specific treatment. Trials with thiabendazole, levamisole, mebendazole. Symptomatic. Cortisone antibiotics, analgesics, antihistamines.

Prognosis. Depends on spread of infestation and specific organ involvement (e.g., brain, eyes). Usually clears in 1–2 years.

BIBLIOGRAPHY. Beaver PC, Snyder CH, Carrera GM, et al: Chronic eosinophilia due to visceral larva migrans, report of 3 cases. Pediatrics 9:7–19, 1952

Danis P, Parmentier N, Maurus R, et al: Syndrome de "visceral larva migrans" et atteinte oculaire. Bull Soc Belge Ophthalmol 144:899–908, 1966

Molk R: Ocular toxocariasis: A review of literature. Ann Ophthal 15:216–219, 1983

Monroe LS: Gastrointestinal parasites. In Haubrich WS, Schaffner F, Berk JE (eds): Bockus Gastroenterology, 5th ed, vol 2, pp 3153–3154. Philadelphia, WB Saunders, 1995

LARYNGEAL NEURALGIA, SUPERIOR

Symptoms. Evoked by coughing, yawning, sneezing, or talking. Severe, lancinating paroxysmal pain of larynx, usually localized unilaterally or bilaterally to small area over hypothyroid membrane.

Etiology. Unknown.

Therapy. Relieved by carbamazepine.

BIBLIOGRAPHY. Smith LA, Moersch HJ, Love JG: Superior laryngeal neuralgia. Proc Staff Meet Mayo Clin 16:164–167, 1941

Browstone PK, Ballanger JJ, Vick NA: Bilateral superior laryngeal neuralgia. Arch Neurol 37:525, 1980

Adams RD, Victor M: Principles of Neurology, 5th ed, p 1180. New York, McGraw-Hill, 1993

LASEGUE I

Synonym. Persecution mania; delusion persecutory.

Symptoms and Signs. Delusion of being persecuted by a particular person, by groups of people (e.g., police, army, organized groups), or by everybody. Manifestation may vary from a feeling of unexpressed discomfort to complaints limited to relatives, friends, doctors, or public authorities with minor or major emphasis on violence. Reaction may vary from aggression to suicide.

Etiology. Unknown.

Therapy. Psychotherapy and pharmacotherapy.

Prognosis. Variable. Tendency to chronicity or conversion to other psychotic delusions.

BIBLIOGRAPHY. Lasègue CE: Du Délire des Persécutions. Arch Gen Med (Paris) 28:129–159, 1852

Kaplan HI, Sadock BJ: Comprehensive Textbook of Psychiatry, 6th ed, p 1128. Baltimore, Williams & Wilkins, 1995

LASEGUE II

Synonyms. Amblyopic hysteric paralysis. See Briquet.

Symptoms. Prevalent in females. Anesthesia and paralysis of an extremity appearing when the patient closes eyes. Accompanied by other hysterical symptoms.

Signs. Reflexes normal; the patient can move and feel as long as the part involved can be seen.

Etiology. Unknown.

Therapy. Psychotherapy.

Prognosis. Good recovery; relapse possible or substitution with other hysteric manifestation.

BIBLIOGRAPHY. Lasègue C: Anesthésie et ataxie hystériques. Arch Gen Med (Paris) 3:385–402, 1864

Lasègue C: Des hysteriques périphériques. Arch Gen Med (Paris) 1:641–656, 1878

Kaplan HI, Sadock BJ: Comprehensive Textbook of Psychiatry, 6th ed, p 1128. Baltimore, Williams & Wilkins, 1995

LASEGUE-FALRET

Synonyms. Association psychosis; double insanity; folie a deux; folie communiquée; paranoid disorder(s), shared.

Symptoms and Signs. Prevalent among women living more or less confined. (1) Coincidental appearance of psychotic symptoms in members of a family while living together; (2) appearance of psychotic symptoms in two closely associated persons and retention of symptoms once initiated, in spite of separation; (3) transmission of psychotic symptoms from a sick person to one person or several healthy individuals who elaborate on the induced delusions.

Etiology. Unknown; hereditary factors frequently involved.

Therapy. Separation frequently results in recovery of the secondary (usually less affected) person. Psychiatric treatment for primarily affected one.

BIBLIOGRAPHY. Lasègue C, Falret J: La Folie à deux ou folie communiquée. Ann Med Psychol 18:321–355, 1877

Kaplan HI, Sadock BJ: Comprehensive Textbook of Psychiatry, 6th ed, pp 538, 1044. Baltimore, Williams & Wilkins, 1995

LASSUER-GRAHAM-LITTLE

Synonyms. Brocq pseudopelade; Graham-Little; Piccardi; folliculitis decalvans et atrophicans; lichen planopilaris.

Symptoms and Signs. Prevalent in females, age range 30–70. Cicatricial alopecia of pubes and less frequently of scalp, trunk, and limbs; follicular plugging and keratosis pilaris. Occasionally, alopecia of axillae and trunk.

Etiology. Unknown. Distinctive syndrome, suggestion of relationship with lichen planopilaris. Possibility of autosomal inheritance in some families.

Pathology. Destruction of follicles. No scarring.

Diagnostic Procedures. *Skin biopsy. Immunofluorescence studies.*

Therapy. Keratolytics. Surgical treatment as in other cicatritial alopecia.

BIBLIOGRAPHY. Brocq L: Alopecia. J Cutan Venereol Dis 3:49–51, 1885

Piccardi G: Cheratosi spinulosa del capillizio e suoi rapporti con la pseudo-pelada di Brocq. Gior Ital Malad Vener Pelle 35:416–422, 1914

Graham-Little EG: Folliculitis decalvans et Atrophicans. Br J Dermatol 27:183–190, 1915

Dawber RPR, Ebling FJG, Wojnarowska FT: Disorders of hair. In Champion RH, Burton JL, Ebling FJG (eds): Rook/Wilkinson/Ebling Textbook of Dermatology, 5th ed, pp 2602–2603. Oxford, Blackwell Scientific, 1992

LATAH

Symptoms. Mostly observed in Malaysian people, predominantly in women. Patterns of manifestation: (1) Following a sudden stimulus, all normal activities stop and inappropriate uncontrollable motor and verbal manifestations occur. (2) Following a sudden stimulus, person exhibits a complete echolalia, echopraxia, and automatic obedience. The person remains aware of situation, but in spite of his protestation against unacceptable actions, performs them as commanded.

Etiology. Disorganization of ego and ego boundaries following sudden fright.

Therapy. Psychotherapy; tranquilizers. If associated with chronic mental disorders, pharmacotherapy and electroconvulsive therapy may be indicated.

Prognosis. If it becomes chronic, leads to automatic obedience and echo reaction with severe personality deterioration.

BIBLIOGRAPHY. Yap PM: The Latah reaction: Its pathodynamics and nosological position. J Ment Sic 98:515–564, 1952
Kaplan HI, Sadock BJ: Comprehensive Textbook of Psychiatry, 6th ed, p 1056. Baltimore, Williams & Wilkins, 1995

LATERAL SINUS THROMBOSIS

Synonym. Sigmoid sinus thrombosis.

Symptoms. Children more frequently affected than adults; onset acute or secondary to chronic otitic infections. Fever; pain behind the eye; temporal headache; nausea; vomiting; muscle palsies; possible lesions of glossopharyngeal (IX), vagus (X), spinal accessory (XI) nerves (involvement of jugular bulb). Occasionally, swelling over mastoid region; tenderness of homolateral jugular vein; symptoms and signs of intracranial hypertension. Papilledema (50%). Seldom, seizures and hemiplegia.

Etiology. Any microorganism may be responsible for infection and secondary thrombosis.

Pathology. Thrombosis of lateral sinus and venous congestion of perimastoid area.

Diagnostic Procedures. *Cerebrospinal fluid.* Cloudy; leucocytes, proteins, and pressure increased. Tobey-Ayer test negative on affected side. Queckenstedt sign on affected side. *Blood.* Leukocytosis; culture positive in 50% of cases. *X-ray. Angiography. CT brain scan. MRI.*

Therapy. Antibiotics. Thrombolytics. Surgery if indicated.

Prognosis. High mortality without treatment.

BIBLIOGRAPHY. Goldberg RA: Lateral sinus thrombosis: medical or surgical treatment? Arch Otolaryngol 3:56–58, 1985
Adams RD, Victor M: Principles of Neurology, 5th ed, p 611. New York, McGraw-Hill, 1993

LATHYRISM

Synonym. Neurolathyrism.

Symptoms. Still common in some zones of India and Africa. Prevalent in males, in persons who consume large amounts of Lathyrus peas; onset sudden, preceded by exposure to cold or dampness. On awakening, pain in lumbar region, weakness of legs, slight fever (occasionally), paresthesias, weakness progressing slowly to spastic paralysis; then loss of control of bladder and rectum and impotence. Arms may become involved successively. Later, loss of sensation to pain and thermal changes.

Signs. Tendon hyperreflexia; Babinski sign.

Etiology. Toxic effect of Lathyrus sativus (grass pea), owing to a toxinbeta-N-oxalylaminoalanine (BOAA). In some cases, nutritional deficiencies may result in similar manifestations (lathyrism-like syndrome).

Pathology. Sclerosis of anterior and posterior part of spinal cord, particularly corticospinal and direct spinocerebellar tracts.

Diagnostic Procedures. *Spinal tap. Electromyography. Biopsy of muscle. Chemical analysis. Identification of BOAA.*

Therapy. Symptomatic.

Prognosis. Neural lesions permanent; however, nonconstantly progressive patients may live normal life span.

BIBLIOGRAPHY. Minchin R: Primary lateral sclerosis of South India. Lathyrism without lathyrus. Br Med J 1:253–255, 1940
Gopalan C: Lathyrism syndrome. Trans Roy Soc Trop Med Hyg 44:333–338, 1950

Arya LS, Qurescima, Jabor A, Singh M: Lathyrism in Afghanistan. Indian J Pediatr 55:440–442, 1988
Adams RD, Victor M: Principles of Neurology, 5th ed, pp 1109–1110. New York, McGraw-Hill, 1993

LATISSIMUS DORSI

Symptoms. Pain in lower back and lower extremities (sclerotomes of second lumbar and first sacral nerves) with occasionally associated pain of upper back, shoulder, upper extremities, neck, and chest.

Signs. Diagnostic injection of local anesthetic on the lumbodorsal fascia produces remission of pain within minutes.

Etiology. Irritation of sensory fibers in aponeurosis of latissimus dorsi muscle owing to fibrosis of subfascial fat, adhesion of tissue to fascia, and defect of the fascia. See also fibrositis.

Diagnostic Procedures. See Signs. *X-ray of spine.*

Therapy. Resection portion of aponeurosis of latissimus dorsi (narrow strip that arises from lumbodorsal fascia).

Prognosis. Good with treatment.

BIBLIOGRAPHY. Copeman WSC, Ackerman WL: Edema or herniations of fat lobules as a cause of lumbar and gluteal "fibrositis." Arch Intern Med 79:22–35, 1947
Dittrich RJ: The latissimus dorsi syndrome. Ohio Med J 51:973–975, 1955

LAUBER

Synonyms. Retinitis punctata albescens, stationary; fundus albipunctatus—hemeralopia. See also Punctata albescens, progressive.

Symptoms. Both sexes affected. Usually bilateral. Static or slowly progressing hemeralopia.

Signs. Minute white spots scattered on all retinal area, with some concentration at the posterior pole that became more numerous over years. Macula may or not be involved.

Etiology. Abnormal photopigment kinetics; both autosomal recessive and dominant inheritance have been proposed.

Diagnostic Procedures. *Fluorescein angiography. Scotopic ERG, delayed.*

Prognosis. Slowly progressing.

BIBLIOGRAPHY. Lauber H: Die sogenannte Retinitis punctata albescens. Klin Monatsbl Augenheilkd 48:133–148, 1910
Marmor MF: Defining fundus albipunctatus. Doc Ophthalmol 13:227–234, 1977
Bird AC, Jay B, Hussain AA, et al: Retinal photoreceptor disorders. In Garner A, Klintworth GK (eds): Pathobiology of Ocular Disease: A Dynamic Approach, 2nd ed, p 1225. New York, Marcel Dekker, 1994

LAUBRY-PEZZI

Synonym. Aortic valve regurgitation; ventricular septal defect; ventricular septal defect; aortic regurgitation.

Symptoms. Male to female ratio, 2:1; onset of symptoms in childhood, 2–10 years of age. Pulsation in the neck; precordial movements, especially when lying on left side. Eventually, chest pain, diaphoresis, sudden death.

Signs. Good general development and normal health during first years of life. Bounding water-hammer pulse; capillary pulsation (nails); head shocks; left ventricular pulsation; holosystolic and early diastolic murmurs. Cardiomegaly.

Etiology. Congenital heart defect.

Pathology. Supracristal ventricular defect and fault in aortic valve leaflet support, or infracristal ventricular defect and previously mentioned aortic valve lesion. Infundibular pulmonic stenosis occasionally coexisting.

Diagnostic Procedures. *ECG.* Left ventricular hypertrophy of marked degree. *X-ray.* Disproportion between large left ventricle and aspect of pulmonary trunk and vasculature. Aorta prominent. *Two-dimensional echocardiography with color flow imaging and spectral Doppler interrogation.*

Therapy. Prevention of bacterial endocarditis. Surgical correction.

Prognosis. Slowly developing clinical pattern. Survival into adulthood possible; cardiac failure develops and is cause of death. Accelerated course in case of complicating subacute bacterial endocarditis.

BIBLIOGRAPHY. Laubry C, Pezzi C: Traite de Maladies Congenitales de Coeur. Paris, JB Baillière et Fils, 1921
Rhodes L, Keane JF, Keane JP, et al: Long follow-up (up to 43 years) of ventricular septal defect with audible aortic regurgitation. Am J Cardiol 66:340–345, 1990
Fyler DC (ed): Nadas' Pediatric Cardiology. Philadelphia, Hanley-Belfus, 1992
Perloff JK: The Clinical Recognition of Congenital Heart Disease, 4th ed, pp 422–428. Philadelphia, WB Saunders, 1994

LAUGIER

Synonyms. Hernia Laugier, Velpeau.

Symptoms and Signs. Femoral hernia, passing trough Gimbernat ligament.

Therapy. Incision of ligament frequently needed to free incarcerated mass.

BIBLIOGRAPHY. Laugier Note sur une nouvelle espèce de hernie de l'abdomen à travers le ligament de Gimbernat. Arch Gén Méd Paris 2:27–37, 1833
Sabiston DC: Textbook of Surgery, 14th ed, p 1145. Philadelphia, WB Saunders, 1991

LAUGIER-HUNZIKER

Symptoms and Signs. Rare. Onset in adult life Macular pigmentation of lips and oral mucosa; black, linear streaks of nails. No systemic changes.

Etiology. Unknown. No genetic basis.

BIBLIOGRAPHY. Laugier P, Hunziker N: Pigmentation melaniques lenticulaire essentielle de la muqueuse jugale et de lèvres. Arch Belg Derm Syph 26:391–399, 1970
Koch SE, LeBoit PE, Odom RB: Laugier-Hunziker syndrome. J Am Acad Dermatol 16:431–434, 1987

LAUNOIS

Synonyms. Neurath-Cushing; acromegaloid gigantism; pituitary gigantism; fractional hypopituitarism-gigantism.

Symptoms. Onset in adolescents who show retarded skeletal growth, delayed puberty, muscle weakness. Headache; perspiration; joint pain. At approximately 18–20 years of age abnormal growth starts and continues until 27–30 years of age. Possibly, mental retardation.

Signs. Pallor; smooth skin; youthful appearance; broad face; scanty facial and body hair; small penis and testes; eunuchoid aspect; high-pitched voice; large limbs, hands, and feet; slipped epiphysis. In one case, hypothyroidism and hypoadrenalism.

Etiology. Idiopathic or chromophobe adenoma; craniopharyngioma with diminished production of gonadotropic hormones and occasionally thyroid-stimulating hormone (TSH) and adrenocorticotropic hormone (ACTH). Increase of secretion of growth hormone.

Diagnostic Procedures. *Blood.* Determination of gonadotropins, 17-ketosteroids, 11-desoxicortisol metabolites, protein-bound iodine. Thyroidal ^{131}I uptake. *X-ray. CT scan. MRI.* Sella turcica normal or signs of tumor; bone age determination.

Therapy. Correction of hormonal deficiency. If tumor, surgery, X-ray radiation, or radium implantation.

Prognosis. Determined by etiology and time of diagnosis.

BIBLIOGRAPHY. Launois PE, Roy P: Études biologiques sur les Géants, p 50. Paris, Masson, 1904
Goldman JK, Cahill GF Jr, Thorn GW: Gigantism with hypopituitarism. Am J Med 34:407–416, 1963
Daughaday WH: Growth hormone, insulin-like growth factors and acromegaly. In De Groot LJ (ed): Endocrinology, 3rd ed, pp 319–326. Philadelphia, WB Saunders, 1995

LAUNOIS-BENSAUDE

Synonyms. Madelung; adenolipomatosis; cephalothoracic lipodystrophy; symmetric adenolipomatosis.

Symptoms and Signs. Male to female ratio, 4:1. Masses developing in lymphatic stations neck, axillae, groin.

Etiology. Autosomic dominant inheritance (?). Alcohol intoxication (?).

Pathology. Fat infiltration into lymph nodes.

Diagnostic Procedures. *CT scan. Echograhy. Biopsy.*

Therapy. Surgery. Consider possibility of deturpating scars.

Prognosis. Benign condition.

BIBLIOGRAPHY. Brodie BC: Clinical lectures on surgery delivered at St George's hospital, pp 201–202. Philadelphia, Lea-Blanchard, 1846
Madelung OW: Ueber den Fetthals (diffuses Lipom des Halses). Arch Klin Chir Berlin 37:106–130, 1888
Launois-Bensaude PEL: Adenolipomatose symetrique. Bull Soc Med Hop Paris 15:298–318, 1898
Mc Poland PR, Garrigie NN, Cupp CK: Subcutaneous masses of the head and neck. Arch Dermatol 126:235–240, 1990

LAURENCE-MOON

Synonym. Incorrectly called Laurence-Moon-Bardet-Biedl. See Bardet-Biedl and also Kearns-Sayre (possibly same condition).

Symptoms. Higher incidence in the population of Kuwait. Twice as frequent in males; onset in childhood. Mental deficiency. Initially, problem of night vision; then central vision and then peripheral vision loss progressing to blindness. Spastic paraplegia.

Signs. All or only some of the characteristic features may be present: hypogenitalism; pigmentary degeneration of retina; cataract; strabismus; microphthalmia; body hair scanty or absent. In male, pseudogynecomastia, azoospermia. In female, amenorrhea, lack of breast development.

Etiology. Unknown; single recessive autosomal gene, or two genes in same chromosome, acting early in embryologic life producing secondary manifestations according to variable degrees of penetrance.

Pathology. Most remarkable lesions observed in kidney (chronic glomerulonephritis or hydronephrosis), pituitary, testicles, eyes (retinitis pigmentosa); features of secondary hypogenitalism.

Diagnostic Procedures. *Electroretinography. Hormonal studies. Chromosome studies.*

Therapy. Symptomatic.

Prognosis. Usually fatal at early age with infection. If adulthood reached, eye lesions progress to blindness at 20 years of age (73%); other signs stay stationary. A great proportion of the patients with this syndrome have significant renal abnormalities with risk of progression to renal insufficiency.

BIBLIOGRAPHY. Laurence JZ, Moon RC: Four cases of "retinitis pigmentosa," occurring in the same family, and accompanied by general imperfections of development. Ophthalmol Rev 2:32–41, 1866
Biedl A: Retinitis pigmentosa: Ein Geschwisterpaar mit adiposogenitaler Dystrophie. Dtsch Med Wochenschr 48:1630, 1922
Cheng IKP, Chan KW, Chan MK, et al: Glomerulopathy of Laurence-Moon-Biedl syndrome. Postgrad Med J 64:621–625, 1988
Williams B, Jenkins D, Walls J: Chronic renal failure: An important feature of the Laurence-Moon-Biedl syndrome. Postgrad Med J 64:462–464, 1988
Farag TI, Teebi AS: Bardet-Biedl and Laurence-Moon syndromes in a mixed Arab population. Clin Genet 33:78–82, 1988

LAZZARONI-FOSSATI

Synonym. Fibrochondrogenesis; fibrodyschondrogenesis.

Symptoms and Signs. Rare. Both sexes. From birth. Chondrodysplasia rhizomelic (dwarfism). *Head.* Normal size, frontal bossing; flat nose; small palpebral fissures. *Neck.* Short. *Thorax.* Narrow, bell-shaped. *Abdomen.* Protuberant. *Limbs.* Short, bowed. *Joints.* Markedly enlarged *Hands and feet.* Normal. *Occasionally.* Cleft palate; patent foramen ovale.

Etiology. Sporadic and autosomal recessive inheritance.

Pathology. Cartilage: Characteristic interwoven fibrous septa and fibroblastic dysplasia of chodrocytes often clustered two to four cells per lacuna.

Diagnostic Procedure. *X-ray of skeleton.* Tubular bones short and dumbell. Vertebral bodies flattened and pear shaped on lateral view, ribs short, capped anteriorly, clavicle long and thin, ischia and pubic bones short and broad.

Prognosis. Neonatal death.

BIBLIOGRAPHY. Lazzaroni-Fossati F, Stanescu V, Stanescu R, et al: La fibrochondrogenese. Arch Fr Pediatr 35:1016–1104, 1978
Eteson DJ, Adomian GE, Ornoy A, et al: Fibrochondrogenesis: Radiologic and histologic studies. Am J Med Genet 19:277–290, 1984
Bankier A, Fortune D, Duke J, et al: Fibrochondrogenesis in male twins at 24 weeks gestation. Am J med Genet 38:95–98, 1991

LAZY LEUKOCYTE

Synonym. Neutrophils motility impaired.

Symptoms and Signs. Both sexes affected; onset in early childhood. Recurrent stomatitis, gingivitis, and various infections.

Etiology. Deficiency of response of granulocytes to chemotactic stimuli, believed to be related to a structural/functional abnormality of actomycin-like microfilaments of cytoplasma. Autosomal dominant inheritance possible.

Diagnostic Procedures. *Blood.* Neutropenia; few granulocytes released into blood after epinephrine or endotoxin injection. Random mobility and chemotactic function: defective. Phagocytic activity, opsonin activity, complement-mediated chemotaxis: normal. *Bone marrow.* Normal number of mature neutrophils.

BIBLIOGRAPHY. Miller ME, Oski FA, Harris MB: Lazy leukocyte syndrome: A new disorder of neutrophil function. Lancet I:665–669, 1971
Goldman JM, Foroozanfar N, Gazzard BG, et al: Lazy leukocyte syndrome. J Roy Soc Med 77:140–141, 1984
Grange M-J, Hakim J: Physiologie du polynucléaire neutrophile Ed Tech. Encycl. Mèd chir (Paris, France). Hèmatologie 13-009-F-10, 1993

LEAKING DUODENAL STUMP

Symptoms. Onset 3–6 days after gastric resection. Severe, constant pain in the right upper abdomen, initially remaining localized. If condition not recognized, peritonitis spreads slowly. Eventually, abscess or fistula develops.

Signs. Tenderness and moderate muscle spasm; progressive rise of pulse and temperature.

Etiology. Leaking duodenal stump.

Therapy. Prompt surgical treatment.

Prognosis. If not recognized, mortality 85%.

BIBLIOGRAPHY. Larsen BB, Foreman RC: Syndrome of leaking duodenal stump. Arch Surg 63:480–485, 1951
Nance FC: Diseases of the peritoneum, retroperitoneum, mesentery and omentum. In Haubrich WS, Schaffner F, Berk JE (eds): Bockus Gastroenterology, 5th ed, vol 2, pp 3087–3088. Philadelphia, WB Saunders, 1995

LEAKY RED CELL

Synonym. Jaffe-Gottfried-Bradley; hemolytic nonspherocytic anemia-lipid membrane abnormality; high red cell phosphatidylcholine hemolytic anemia, HPCHA; phosphatidylcholine red cell membrane disorder.

Symptoms and Signs. Both sexes affected; onset in infancy. Chronic moderate hemolysis that is worsened during infections or stress. Increased incidence of gallstone formation.

Etiology. Altered phospholipid composition of erythrocyte; autosomal dominant inheritance.

Pathology. Not specific.

Diagnostic Procedures. *Blood.* Moderate anemia; reticulocytosis (6–15%); mild hyperbilirubinemia; osmotic fragility decreased, and less increase in fragility after 24 hours incubation than normal cells. Autohemolysis slightly increased. Correction with addition of glucose. Increased erythrocyte membrane phosphatidylcholine and cholesterol and decrease of phosphatidylethanolamine. Normal red cell enzymes. Plasma lipids: normal.

Therapy. None.

Prognosis. Relatively benign condition.

BIBLIOGRAPHY. Jaffe ER, Gottfried EL, Bradley TB Jr: Hereditary nonspherocytic hemolytic disease associated with altered phospholipid composition of erythrocytes. J Clin Invest 45:1027, 1966
Jaffe ER, Gottfried EL: Hereditary nonspherocytic hemolytic disease associated with an altered phospholipid composition of the erythrocytes. J Clin Invest 47:1375–1388, 1968
Lukens JN: Hereditary spherocytosis and other hemolytic anemias associated with abnormalities of the red cell membrane and the cytoskeleton. In Lee GR, Bithell TC, Foerster J, et al (eds): Wintrobe's Clinical Hematology, 9th ed, p 982. Philadelphia, Lea & Febiger, 1993

LEBER I

Synonyms. Optic neuritis hereditary; optic atrophy, Leber; neuroretinopathy.

Symptoms. Occurs usually in males in Europe 85%, in Japan 59%; acute onset usually at 15–25 years of age (in Europe). Unilateral or bilateral visual loss; affecting primarily central vision. Association with hereditary-familial ataxia frequent.

Signs. At onset, optic disk normal or swelling of optic (II) nerve head; later, atrophy of disks. Signs of widespread central nervous system damage may be associated (protean clinical manifestations).

Etiology. Unknown; possibly, sex-linked recessive. Possibly a toxic metabolic disorder, or an abnormality of cyanide metabolism, or related to smoking. Cytoplasmic inheritance and vertical transmission of an infectious agent (a slow virus) also have been considered.

Pathology. Neuronal degeneration of the retina and optic (II) nerve with secondary degenerative changes of optic system, except for calcarine cortex.

Diagnostic Procedures. *Neurologic examination. Spinal fluid. Urine. Culture.*

Therapy. Avoiding exposure to cyanide is theoretically advisable: no smoking; prevention and treatment of infection, particularly urinary (formation of cyanide by Escherichia coli, Pseudomonas pyocyanea). Hydroxocobalamin in massive doses; sodium thiosulfate (both yet untried).

Prognosis. Marked visual loss.

BIBLIOGRAPHY. Leber T: Beitrage zur Kenntniss der Atrophischen Veranderungen des Sehnerven nebst Bemerkungen uber die normale Structur des Nerven. Arch Ophthalmol 14:164–176, 1868
Nikoskelainen E, Hassinen IE, Palijarvi L, et al: New aspects of the genetic, etiologic, and clinical puzzle of Leber's disease. Neurology 34:1482–1484, 1984
Vikki J, Ort J, Savontaus ML, et al: Optic atrophy in Leber hereditary optic neuroretinitis is probably determined by an X-chromosomal gene closely linked to DXS7. AM J Med Genet 48:486–491, 1991
Klintworth GK: Ocular involvement in disorders of the nervous system. In Garner A, Klintworth GK (eds): Pathobiology of Ocular Disease: A Dynamic Approach, 2nd ed, pp 1731–1732. New York, Marcel Dekker, 1994

LEBER II

Synonyms. Amaurosis, congenital; neuroepithelial dysgenesis of retina; congenital amaurosis I and II; congenital retinal blindness (CRB). See Alstroem-Olsen.

Symptoms. Both sexes affected; may be present at birth, but usually onset at 15–30 years (most frequent in younger years). Decreased visual acuity; psychiatric disorders in some patients. Mental retardation.

Signs. Microcephaly; mongoloid-like face; oculodigital reflex. Nystagmus of various types, keratoconus (20–40%). Initially, normal appearing retina, then narrowing of retinal arteries (67%). Macular lesions, "salt and pepper"; retinal pigment changes or "bone corpuscle."

Etiology. Two types of amaurosis congenita have been described. Type I limited to the eye, and type II with possible associated mental disorders. Both have autosomal recessive inheritance.

Diagnostic Procedure. *Electroretinography.* Extinguished or decreased response.

Therapy. None.

Prognosis. Progressive visual loss.

BIBLIOGRAPHY. Leber T: Ueber Retinitis pigmentosa und angeborene Amaurose. Arch Ophthalmol 15:1–25, 1869
Leber T: Ueber hereditare und kongenitalangelegte Sehnervenleiden. Arch Ophthalmol 17:249–291, 1871
Nickel B, Houyt CS: Leber's congenital amaurosis: Is mental retardation a frequent associated defect? Arch Ophthalmol 100:1089–1092, 1982

Adams RD, Victor M: Principles of Neurology, 5th ed, pp 1017–1018. New York, McGraw-Hill, 1993

LEBER MILIARY ANEURYSMS

Synonyms. See Coats.

Symptoms and Signs. In circumscribed areas of retinal capillary bed, telangiectasis or varicosity, causing intra- and subretinal exudation leading eventually to Coats (see).

Etiology. Unknown.

Pathology. Telangiectasic vessels initially have thin walls, later they become thickened.

Prognosis. Leading to retinal detachment or Coats.

BIBLIOGRAPHY. Tripathi RC, Ashton N: Electron microscopical study of Coats disease. Br J Ophthalmol 55:289–301, 1971
Garner A: Vascular disease. In Garner A, Klintworth GK (eds): Pathobiology of Ocular Disease: A Dynamic Approach, 2nd ed, p 1648. New York, Marcel Dekker, 1994

LEDDERHOSE

Synonym. Plantar fibromatosis. See Dupuytren; fibromatosis juvenile; fibromatosis, congenital, generalized.

Symptoms. Both sexes affected; onset usually in young age. Asymptomatic; then pain on walking.

Signs. Multiple fibrous nodules, adherent to the plantar aponeurosis, localized in the medial region of the plantar arch. In some cases, nodules cause retraction of the tendons of last four toes (hammer toes).

Etiology. Unknown. Frequent association with other varieties of fibromatosis suggests a common etiology. Familial occurrence (hereditary pattern not yet established).

Pathology. In different areas formation of bands of connective tissue with variable cellular density and discrete hyaline component. In some areas, polymorphic nuclei with hyperchromic scarce mitotic figures.

BIBLIOGRAPHY. Ledderhose G: Ueber Zerreisungen der Plantarfascie (Langenbeeks). Arch Klin Chir 48:853–856, 1894
Burton JL: Disorders of connective tissue. In Champion RH, Burton JL, Ebling FJG (eds): Rook/Wilkinson/Ebling Textbook of Dermatology, 5th ed, p 1803. Oxford, Blackwell Scientific, 1992

LEGAL

Obsolete.

Synonyms. Cephalalgia pharyngotympanica; pharyngotympanic neuralgia. See Hunt syndrome.

BIBLIOGRAPHY. Legal E: Ueber eine öftere Ursache des Schlaefen und hinterhapts Kopfschmerzes (Cephalagia pharyngotympanica). Dtsch Klin Med 40:201–216, 1886–1887

LE FORT FRACTURES

Symptoms and Signs. Fractures with dento-alveolar component. Horizontal maxillary fracture (Le Fort I). Pyramidal maxillary fracture (Le Fort II). Craniofacial dysjunction.

BIBLIOGRAPHY. Le Fort R: Etude expérimental sur les fractures de la machoire supérieure. Rev Chir (Paris) 23. 1901
Sabiston DC: Textbook of Surgery, 14th ed, pp 288–289. Philadelphia, WB Saunders, 1991

LEGG-CALVÉ-PERTHES

Synonyms. Calvé-Perthes; Perthes; capital femoral epiphysis coxa plana; femoral osteochondrosis.

Symptoms. Both sexes. Sudden or gradual onset at 6–12 years of age. Moderate pain in the hip; limitation of motion and limp of involved leg that become progressively more intense. In familial cases bilateral involvement more likely.

Signs. Tenderness and muscular spasm in the hip. Eventually atrophy of muscles and shortening of leg.

Etiology. Idiopathic ischemia of ossification centers. Trauma. Occasionally associated with Herrick (see). Polygenic inheritance suggested (risk from affected parent 3%).

Pathology. Osteocyte disappearance; reactive hyperemia; osteoclast and osteoblast invasion; replacement with normal bone.

Diagnostic Procedures. *Blood.* Sedimentation rate slightly elevated. *X-ray.* Initially, bone resorption; then sclerosis; indentation of subchondral tissue; fragmentation of epiphysis; joint irregularity.

Therapy. Bed rest; relative immobility for 2 or 3 years.

Prognosis. Self-limiting; may persist for years; heals with residual deformity (30% good recovery; 30% fairly normal; 25% continuous pain, limited movements).

BIBLIOGRAPHY. Legg AT: The cause of atrophy in joint disease. Am J Orthop Surg 6:84–90, 1908–1909
Calvé F: Sur une forme particulière de pseudocoxalgie greffée sur des deformations caractéristiques de l'extrémite supérieure du fémur. Rev Chir (Paris) 42:54–84, 1910
Perthes G: Ueber arthritis deformans juvenilis. Dtsch Z Chir 107:111–159, 1910
Hall DJ: Genetic aspects of Perthes' disease: A critical review. Clin Orthop 209:100–114, 1986
Wenger DR: Legg-Perthes-disease. In Klippel JH, Dieppe PA: Rheumatology, pp 7.42.1–7.42.4. St Louis, CV Mosby, 1994

LEIGH

Synonyms. Wernicke infantilis (misnomer). Subacute necrotizing encephalopathy (SNE); necrotizing encephalopathy, infantile. See Pyruvate carboxylase deficiency.

Symptoms and Signs. Both sexes affected; onset in early infancy. Occasionally in adults. Lack of evidence of primary dietary deficiency or hepatic-gastroenteric diseases. Slow develpment, "mild hypotonia," brief "spasms," moderate tendon hyporeflexia, evolving through progressive deterioration to terminal stupor, hypertonia, myoclonic spasms, or severe hypotonia, and areflexia.

Etiology. Apparently, autosomal recessive inheritance; X-linked inheritance and sporadic cases also reported. A common expression of several genetic defects involving pyruvate metabolism. Most common known biochemical cause is a mutation in a nuclear regulatory gene that controls stability of complex IV of mitochondria, rather than to mutation of a gene that encodes a specific cox subunits.

Pathology. In brain, rarefaction of interstitial neuroglia or "ground substance" proceeding to vacuolization and parenchymal cavitation, associated with mesoglial proliferative reaction. Tendency to preserve nerve cell bodies. Changes affecting primarily pons, globus pallidus, optic nerve, chiasm tract, and spinal cord. Mammillary bodies are spared.

Diagnostic Procedures. *Blood.* Leukocytosis; mild metabolic acidosis; increased lactate, pyruvate, and alanine; cytochrome *c* oxidase deficiency. *CSF.* Increase in protein. *CT brain scan. MRI.* Ventricles ditated. Prenatal diagnosis possible from cultured fibroblasts.

Therapy. Thiamine and lipoic acid.

Prognosis. Death within few years; a few patients have survived to midteens.

BIBLIOGRAPHY. Leigh D: Subacute necrotizing encephalomyelopathy in an infant. J Neurol Neurosurg Psychiatr 14:216–221, 1951
Richter RB: Infantile subacute necrotizing encephalopathy (Leigh's disease): Its relationship to Wernicke's encephalopathy. Neurology 18:1125–1132, 1968
Van Coster R, Lombes A, De Vivi DC, et al: Cytochrome *c* oxidase-associated Leight syndrome phenotypic features and pathogenetic speculations. J Neurol Sci 104:97–111, 1991
Robinson BH: Lactic acidemia (Disorders of pyruvate carboxylase, pyruvate dehydrogenase). In Scriver CR, Beaudet AL, Sly WS, et al: The Metabolic and Molecular Bases of Inherited Disease, 7th ed, pp 1483–1484. New York, McGraw-Hill, 1995

LEINER

Synonym. Erythroderma desquamativum. Includes: Leiner-C5 dysfunction; erythroderma—failure to thrive—diarrhea; EFD; yeast opsonization defect.

Symptoms and Signs. Prevalent in infant females; onset in second to fourth month of life. Rapid onset. Severe seborrheic dermatitis of scalp and flexures associated with maculae or plaques of erythema with scaling on trunk and limbs. Severe diarrhea, recurrent local and systemic infections; fever; wasting lymphadenopathy (mild).

Etiology. Confused entity possibly owing to a variety of abnormalities of immune function, nutritional deficiency (specific or aspecific). Differential diagnosis on fundamental etiology. Sporadic cases as well as familial occurences reported (autosomal recessive inheritance suggested).

Pathology. Seborrheic dermititis, plus superimposed infection (Staphylococcus and Candida 66%). Autopsy: Lymph nodes—Lymphatic hypoplasia, increased reticular cells.

Diagnostic Procedures. *Blood.* Anemia; hypoproteinemia; changes in immunoglobulin levels; complement defects; yeast opsonization defect. *Culture and biopsy of skin.*

Therapy. Incubator control of heat loss; control of fluid and food intake; antibiotics; vitamins, transfusion if needed. Corticosteroids if other measures insufficient.

Prognosis. Without careful management, 50% mortality (from pneumonia, meningitis, nephritis). With good management, 10% mortality.

BIBLIOGRAPHY. Leiner C: Erythrodermia desquamativa (universal dermatitis of children at the breast). Br J Dis Child 5:244–251, 1908
Simon C, Becker V, Wiedemann H-R: Ueber ein unter dem Bilde der Erythrodemia desquamativa Leiner verlaufenes toedliches Leiden bei drei Bruedern. Z Kinderheilk 94:12–24, 1965
Atherton DJ: The neonate. In Champion RH, Burton JL, Ebling FJG (eds): Rook/Wilkinson/Ebling Textbook of Dermatology, 5th ed, pp 441–442. Oxford, Blackwell Scientific, 1992

LEIRI

See Choreiform syndromes.

BIBLIOGRAPHY. Leiri F: Ueber Tremor bei Kleinhirnaffektionen. J Psychol Neurol 29:429–433, 1923

LEISHMANIOSIS, NEW WORLD

Synonyms. American Leishmaniosis; bush yaws; Chichero ulcer (Guatemala, Honduras, Mexico); Espundia (Peru); Pian bois (Guiana); Picatura de Pinto; Uta (Peru).

Symptoms and Signs. Distinct clinical patterns according to different species of Leishmanias. *Primary lesion.* In exposed parts; small papula, then red nodule, and finally ulceration. In Central America frequently affects the ear. *Secondary infection.* Regional adenitis and lymphangitis. *Secondary lesions.* Mucosae of nose, mouth, and nasopharynx eroding the cartilage and forming necrotic ulcers.

Etiology. Phlebotomus bite transmitting various species of Leishmanias.

Pathology. Central necrotic infected areas surrounded by edema and epithelial hyperplasia. Secondary mucosal lesions. Macrophages with leishmanias; inflammatory signs; capillary blockage, necrosis.

Therapy. Sodium antimony gluconate; pentamidine isothionate; stilbamidine isothionate (in antimony-resistant cases); allopurinol (under clinical trial in antimony-resistant cases); amphotericin B; antibiotics for secondary infection. Cauterization in some cases.

Prognosis. Good with early treatment. If untreated or late treatment, death from secondary infection.

BIBLIOGRAPHY. Pessoa SB, Barretto MP: Leishmaniose Tegumentar Americana. Rio de Janeiro Imprensa National, 1948

Bryceson ADM, Hay RJ: Worms and protozoa. In Champion RH, Burton JL, Ebling FJG (eds): Rook/Wilkinson/Ebling Textbook of Dermatology, 5th ed, pp 1258–1260. Oxford, Blackwell Scientific, 1992

LEITNER

Synonyms. Eosinophilia; pulmonary tuberculosis. Loeffler syndrome associated with tubercular infection. Used occasionally as synonym for Loeffler (see).

BIBLIOGRAPHY. Leitner J: Ueber flüchtige hyperergische Lungeninfiltrate mit Eosinophilie bei Tuberkulose. Beitr Klin Tuberk 88:388–420, 1936

LE MERRER

Synonyms. Gloomy face; dwarfism; gloomy face.

Symptoms and Signs. Both sexes. Very short stature. Typical facial dysmorphism (gloomy). Normal mental development.

Etiology. Autosomal recessive inheritance.

Diagnostic Procedures. *X-rays.* Skeleton: normal. *Blood.* No hormonal level alterations.

Prognosis. Good quoad vitam.

BIBLIOGRAPHY. Le Merrer M, Brauer R, Maroteaux P: Dwarfism with gloomy face: a new syndrome with features of 3–M syndrome. J Med Genet 28:186–191, 1991

LEMIEUX-NEEMEH

Synonym. Charcot-Marie-Tooth deafness. See Rosenberg-Chutorian.

Symptoms and Signs. Both sexes. In childhood. Progressive weakness of peroneal muscles; poor balance; steppage gait; legs; hypoesthesia and absent reflexes, then muscle atrophy, clubfoot, and muscle involvement. In second decade, deafness (severe to deep) becomes apparent. The nephropathy of the original cases of Lennieux-Neemeh has not been reported in other families.

Etiology. Autosomal dominant trait; a family with possible recessive trait also reported (Cornell).

Diagnostic Procedures. *Electromyography. Audiography. Blood.* To exclude amyloidosis and uremic polyneuropathy.

BIBLIOGRAPHY. Lemieux G, Neemeh JA: Charcot-Marie-Tooth disease and nephritis. Can Med Assoc J 97:1193–1198, 1967

Lemieux G, Neemeh JA: Charcot-Marie-Tooth disease with sensorineural hearing loss: An autosomal dominant trait, p 241. Sixth Cong Hum Genet Jerusalem, 1981

Cornell J, Sellar S, Beighton P: Autosomal recessive inheritance of Charcot-Marie-Tooth disease associated with sensorineural deafness. Clin Genet 25:163–165, 1984

LENEGRE

See Lev.

Symptoms and Signs. Both sexes affected; onset over 50 years of age. Those of progressive heart block.

Etiology. Obscure degenerative process limited to the heart conductive system.

Pathology. Sclerodegenerative process limited to the conduction system.

Diagnostic Procedures. *Electrocardiography.* Right bundle heart block, left anterior hemiblock, or other varieties or combinations of conductive defects.

Therapy. After pharmacologic trials; pacemaker as last resort.

Prognosis. Slow progression (in years) toward complete heart block.

BIBLIOGRAPHY. Lenègre J: Etiology and pathology of bilateral bundle branch block in relation to complete heart block. Prog Cardiovasc Dis 6:409–444, 1964

Rosenbaum MB: Interventricular trifascicular block. Heart Lung 1:216, 1972

Myerburg RJ, Kessler KM, Castellanos A: Recognition clinical assessment and management of conduction disturbances. In Schlant RC, Alexander RW: Hurst's The Heart, 8th ed, pp 748–750. New York, McGraw-Hill, 1994

LENNERT

Synonyms. Lymphoma Lennert; lymphoepithelioid lymphoma.

Symptoms and Signs. Usually in old women. Onset lymphoadenopathy of cervial region (particularly in the palatine tonsil then generalized usually characterized by recurrent relapses). Seldom cutaneous involvement.

Etiology. Unknown. Problematic classification among lymphomas.

Pathology. Lymph nodes. Sheets of loosely clustered epitheliod cells with an intervening infiltrate of small pleomorphic helper/inducer (CD4–positive) lymphocytes and rare transformed cells.

Diagnostic Procedures. Lymphonode biopsy; bone marrow.

Therapy. Combination chemotherapy.

Prognosis. Tends to behave as a low-grade lymphoma.

BIBLIOGRAPHY. Lennert K, Messdagh J: Lymphogranulomatosen mit kostant lohem. Epitheloidzellgehaer Virchows Arch A 344:1–20, 1968

Greer JP, Macon WR, List AF, et al: Non-Hodgkin's lymphomas. In Lee GR, Bithell TC, Foerster J, et al: Wintrobe's Clinical Hematology, 9th ed, p 2119. Philadelphia, Lea & Febiger, 1993

LENNOX-GASTAUT

Synonyms. Doose (when genetic basis); Gastaut; astatic petit mal-hemiconvulsion; hemiplegia; epilepsy, HHE; Lennox variant; petit mal variant.

Symptoms. It is a form of epilepsy that usually appears in the preschool age. Several seizure types, with atypical absences, head nodding, and drop attacks particularly prominent, in association with mental retardation and brain damage caused by a diverse group of conditions.

Etiology. Diverse conditions. Doose described a group of patients with a similar syndrome, but a strong familial disposition to convulsive diseases, normal development, and good response to treatment with sodium valproate.

Diagnostic Procedures. *Electroencephalography.* In the awake patient slow spike and wave pattern; tonic seizures associated with low-amplitude, fast activity are common during sleep. *Positron-emission tomographic scan.* Hypometabolism.

Therapy. Nitrazepam, clorazepam, valproate, felbamate.

Prognosis. Poor.

BIBLIOGRAPHY. Lennox WG: Clinical correlates of the fast and slow spikewave electroencephalogram. Pediatrics 5:626, 1950

Gastaut H, Vigoroux M, Trevisan C, et al: Le syndrome hemiconvulsion-hémiplégie-épilepsie (syndrome HHE). Rev Neurol (Paris) 97:37–52, 1957

Lennox WG: Epilepsy and Related Disorders. Boston, Little, Brown, 1960

Hopkins IJ: The Lennox Gastaut Syndrome. Aust Paediatr J 22:269–270, 1986

Felbamate study group: Efficacy of felbamate in childhood epileptic encephalopathy (Lennox-Gastaut syndrome). N Engl J Med 328:29–33, 1993

LENOBLE-AUBINEAU

Synonym. Myoclonia; nystagmus.

Symptoms and Signs. Prevalent in males; manifested in first years of life. Lateral nystagmus; myoclonic movements of extremities and trunk. Cold or tapping muscles enhances the symptoms. Patient partially controls them. Tendon hyperreflexia. Frequently associated, abnormalities of teeth, hypospadias, facial asymmetry, local hyperhidrosis, and localized edema.

Etiology. Unknown; possibly congenital and familial.

Pathology. Nonspecific meningovascular and glial changes in brain.

Therapy. Symptomatic. Ethosuximide; phenobarbital may be associated; ACTH or corticosteroid are also effective.

Prognosis. Incurable, but not progressive.

BIBLIOGRAPHY. Lenoble E, Aubineau E: Une variété nouvelle de myoclonie congénitale pouvant être héréditaire et familiale á nystagmus constant. Rev Med 26:471–515, 1906

Adams RD, Victor M: Principles of Neurology, 5th ed, p 89. New York, McGraw-Hill, 1993

LENTICULO-OPTIC

Synonyms. See other thalamic syndromes.

Symptoms and Signs. Predominant motor disorders, variable hemianesthesia, no pains.

Etiology and Pathology. Vascular end degenerative or neoplastic origin, with a more discrete participation of thalamus compared with other thalamic syndromes.

BIBLIOGRAPHY. Martin JJ: Thalamic syndromes. In Vinken PJ, Bruyn GW: Handbook of Clinical Neurology, vol 2, p 486. Amsterdam, North-Holland, 1969

LENZ-MAJEWSKI

Synonym. Braham-Lenz; osteosclerosis; syndactyly; hyperostotic dwarfism.

Symptoms. Rare. Advanced paternal age. Both sexes; from birth. Mental retardation (IQ 20–40) sensineural hearing loss.

Signs. *Head.* Enlarged with large fontanels and sutures; prominent veins especially in the scalp. *Ear.* Large and floppy. Enamel hypoplasia. Choanal atresia or stenosis. Hypertelorism. *Trunk and limbs.* Reduced. Joint hyperextension. *Hands and feet.* Syndactyly. *Muscle.* Hypotonia. *Skin.* Loose, wrinkled (progeriod aspect). *Genitourinary.* Cryptorchidism, hypospadia. Inguinal hernia.

Etiology. Unknown. Sporadic. Possible autosomal inheritance considered.

Diagnostic Procedures. *X-rays.* Increased density of skull base, mandible, clavicles, ribs, and long bones diaphyses. Tetracycline kinetics: increased bone formation and defective coupling. *Blood.* Alkaline phosphatase elevated. *Chromosomes.* Normal.

BIBLIOGRAPHY. Braham RL: Multiple congenital anomalies with diaphyseal dysplasia (Camurati–Engelmann's syndrome). Oral Surg 27:20–26, 1969

Lenz WD, Majewski FA: A generalized disorder of the connective tissue with progeria, choanal atresia, symphalangism, hypoplasia of dentine and craniodiaphyseal hyperostosis. Birth Defects 10:133–136, 1974

Chrzanoska KH: Skeletal dysplasia syndrome with progeroid appearance, characteristic facial and limb anomalies, multiple synostoses and distinct skeletal changes. A variant example of the Lenz-Majewsky syndrome. Am J Med Genet 32:470–474, 1989

LENZ (W.)

Synonym. Mycrophthalmos Lenz; anophthalmos Lenz.

Symptoms and Signs. From birth. In males microphthalmos or anophthalmos; Physical and mental retardation; ear malformations; dental anomalies; urogenital anomalies. Occasionally: heart defects; skeletal malformations; intestinal anomalies.

Etiology. X-linked inheritance.

BIBLIOGRAPHY. Lenz W: Recessiv-geschlechtsgebundene Mikrophthalmie mit multiplen Missbildungen. Z Kinderheilk 77:384–390, 1955

Graham CA, McCleary BG, Malcom S, et al: Linkage analysis in a family with X-linked anophthalmos. J Med Genet 25:643, 1988

Merin S: Inherited Eye Diseases: Diagnosis and Clinical Management, p 121–136. New York, Marcel Dekker, 1991

LEOPARD

Synonyms. Cardiocutaneous; cardiomyopathic lentiginosis; lentigo-electrocardiographic changes; multiple lentigines. (Leopard achronym for lentigines—electrocardiographic; ocular; pulmonary; abnormal genitalia; retardation; deafness).

Symptoms and Signs. Both sexes affected; present from birth. Generalized freckling (not related to sunlight exposure), especially on neck and trunk, increasing with time. Systolic murmur that diffuses, more intense at heart base. Mild sensorineural deafness; mild growth deficiency; hypertelorism; prominent ears; scapula alata; pectus carinatum or excavatum. Delayed sexual development. Occasionally, mental deficiency, hypospadias, hypogonadism.

Etiology. Autosomal dominant inheritance with variable expression (incomplete syndrome a possibility).

Pathology. Pulmonary stenosis. Occasionally, unilateral kidney agenesis, subaortic stenosis, unilateral gonadal agenesis.

Diagnostic Procedures. *EEG.* Prolonged PR and QRS; abnormal P-waves; first degree AV block; left anterior hemiblock or complete heart block. *Hormonal studies.* Hypopituitarism and primary or secondary hypogonadal hormones. *X-ray of lung.* Vascular engorgement.

Therapy. Hormone replacement, if indicated.

Prognosis. Fair.

BIBLIOGRAPHY. Walther RJ, Polansky BJ, Crotis IA: Electrocardiographic abnormalities in family with generalized lentigo. N Engl J Med 275:1220–1225, 1966

Senn M, Hess OM, Krayenbuhl HP: Hypertrophe Kardiomyopathic und Lentiginose. Schweiz Med Wochenschr 114:838–841, 1984

Peter JR, Kemp JS: LEOPARD syndrome: Death because of chronic respiratory insufficiency. Am J Med Genet 37:340–341, 1990

LEPOUTRE

Synonyms. Oxalosis; hyperoxaluria primary; hyperoxaluria secondary.

Symptoms and Signs. Clinical onset in early adulthood. Those of nephrolithiasis and nephrocalcinosis progressing to chronic renal insufficiency. Some cases of congenital type: Onset in early childhood. Nausea; vomiting; dry, burning mouth; abdominal pain; renal colic; passage of calculi in urine; occasionally, tetany.

Etiology. Congenital form: Autosomal recessive inheritance. Acquired forms: Metabolic disorders with accumulation in tissues of oxalic acid. *Type I.* Glycolic aciduria; defect of 2-oxoglutarate/glyoxylate carboligase. *Type II.* L-glyceric aciduria; defect of D-glyceric dehydrogenase. Numerous other acquired conditions exist where calcium oxalate accumulates in tissues: oxalate poisoning; ethylene glycol poisoning; glyoxylate administration; pyridoxine deficiency; liver cirrhosis; renal tubular acidosis syndrome.

Pathology. In kidneys, deposits of crystal of calcium oxalate, calculi formation. Fibrosis; necrotic changes in tubules and glomeruli. Deposits of crystals observed in other tissues as well.

Diagnostic Procedures. *Blood.* Increase of oxalates; hypocalcemia. *Bone marrow.* Crystals of calcium oxalate may be observed. *Urine.* Oxalate excretion three to five times normal; albuminuria; hematuria; casts and stones of calcium oxalate. *X-ray of kidney.* Bilateral kidney calculosis. Osteoporosis.

Therapy. Magnesium oxide; sodium bicarbonate, mandelic acid. Alkalinization of urine, especially during night, and keeping volume abundant; diet low in calcium, high in phosphate. If specific cause such as pyridoxine deficiency, correction of deficiency. Lithotripsy and surgery. Renal transplantation is followed by recurrence of the disease. Liver transplantation for reversal of metabolic defect. Ideal candidate for gene therapy.

Prognosis. Progressive course. Death in early adulthood (in congenital form), from various causes according to etiology, from renal failure in acquired forms. Presently brighter than before; future very promising.

BIBLIOGRAPHY. Lepoutre C: Calculs multiples chez un enfant: Infiltration du parenchyme rénal par des depots cristallins. J Urol (Paris) 20:424, 1925

McDonald JC, Landrenau MD, Rohr MS, et al: Reversal by liver transplantation of the complication of primary hyperoxaluria as well as the metabolic defect. N Engl J Med 321:1100–1103, 1989

Seargeant LE, deGroot GW, Dilling LA, et al: Primary oxaluria type 2 (L-glyceric aciduria): A rare case of nephrolithiasis in children. J Pediat 118:912–914, 1991

Danpure CJ, Purdue PE: Primary hyperoxaluria. In Scriver CR, Beaudet AL, Sly WS, et al: The Metabolic and Molecular Bases of Inherited Disease, 7th ed, pp 2385–2424. New York, McGraw-Hill, 1995

LEPTOMENINGEAL ADHESIVE THICKENING

Synonyms. Chronic adhesive arachnoiditis; circumscribed serum meningitis. See also Spinal chronic arachnoiditis.

Symptoms and Signs. Onset insidious. According to localization of process: headache; diplopia; nausea; vomiting; vertigo; epileptic seizures.

Etiology. Follows a chronic leptomeningeal infection, trauma, or after spontaneous subarachnoid hemorrhages. Occasionally, unknown.

Pathology. Fibrous tissue proliferation in limited areas of leptomeninge with chronic inflammatory cellular reaction.

Diagnostic Procedures. *Blood.* Leukocytosis. *Cerebrospinal fluid.* Increased proteins; xanthochromia. *X-ray. Angiography. Scintigraphy. CT scan. MRI.*

Therapy. If infections demonstrated, antibiotics; corticosteroid of relative benefit. Surgery when indicated.

Prognosis. Progressive condition.

BIBLIOGRAPHY. Adams RD, Victor M: Principles of Neurology, 5th ed, p 601. New York, McGraw-Hill, 1993

LERICHE

Synonyms. Abdominal thrombosis of aorta; aortic bifurcation; aorto-iliac obstruction (chronic).

Symptoms. Occurs in males. Intermittent claudication; pain and discomfort at high level (thighs, hips, buttocks); impotence.

Signs. Arterial pulses in the legs decreased or absent; bruits occasionally heard over abdominal aorta and iliac and femoral arteries. Muscle atrophy; in skin, usually good perfusion (high obstruction and fair collateral circulation) or coldness, pallor, cyanosis, trophic changes, and gangrene. Hypertension.

Etiology. Atheromatous plaques at bifurcation of aorta; segmental arteritis; gradual thrombosis at terminal portion of aorta.

Pathology. Thrombus (red, white, or mixed), eventually organized.

Diagnostic Procedures. *Doppler studies.* Absence or deplete reduced pulsation. *X-ray. CT scan. MRI. Ultrasonography.* Basket-like calcification at bifurcation of aorta. *Aortography.* To determine site and extent of obstruction.

Therapy. Conservative therapy or surgery.

Prognosis. Cerebral and coronary arteriosclerosis cause of death.

BIBLIOGRAPHY. Leriche R: De la résection du carrefour aortico-iliaque avec double sympathectomie lombaire pour thrombose artéritique de l'aorte. Le syndrome de l'oblitération terminoaortique par arterite. Presse Méd 48:33–604, 1940

Lindsay J, De Backey ME, Beals AC: Diagnosis and treatment of diseases of the aorta. In Schlant RC, Alexander RW, Hurst's The Heart, 8th ed, p 2177. New York, McGraw-Hill, 1994

LERI-JOANNY

Synonyms. Flowing hyperostosis; monomelic hyperostosis; melorheostosis; osteosis eburnisans; monomelic periostitis. See Ollier.

Symptoms and Signs. Both sexes affected; onset in infancy. Severe pain of difficult localization, involving one bone or several. In 75% of cases, only the bones of a single extremity (monomelic) affected; side of pelvis or shoulder contiguous to affected limbs also involved. If condition has an early onset, premature closure of epiphysis and dwarfism may result. Limb motion may be reduced, because of ankylosis (from extension of changes across joints) or muscle sclerosis or both.

Etiology. Unknown; congenital. No mendelian basis established. Melorheostosis may be a feature of Albright; Sturge-Weber; Klippel-Trenaunay-Weber; and others syndromes. Postulated an aquired postnatal neuropathy of sensory nerves (?).

Pathology. Along shaft of long bones growth of bone that protrudes externally, beneath periostium (melorheostosis: like melted candle wax) and internally into medulla. Microscopically, normal bone structure.

Diagnostic Procedure. *X-ray.* Peculiar bone malformation with long asymmetical irregular streaks in a flowing pattern.

Therapy. Symptomatic benefit from vasodilators.

Prognosis. Severe incapacitation and dwarfism may result according to area affected and time of onset.

BIBLIOGRAPHY. Léri A, Joanny: Une affection non décrite des os: hyperostose "en coulée" sur toute la longuer d'un membre ou "melorhéostose." Bull Soc Méd Hôp 46:1141–1145, 1922
Maroteaux P: Les désordres de la transparence osseuse. Encycl Méd Chir, p 3. Appareil Locomoteur 14023 B10, 1982
Rimoin DL, Lachman RS: Genetic disorders of the osseous skeleton. In Beithon P (ed): McKusick's Heritable Disorders of Connective Tissue, 5th ed, p 657. St Louis, CV Mosby, 1993

LERI PLEONOSTEOSIS

Synonyms. Premature bone ossification; pleonosteosis.

Symptoms. Both sexes affected; onset in early infancy. Usually, normal mental development. Some cases of impaired intelligence reported. Physical disabilities; limited motion of joints, including spine. Carpal tunnel syndrome. Morton metatarsalgia (see) may result.

Signs. Mongoloid facies (inconstant). Broadening and deformity of thumbs and great toes; hands short, thick. Flexion contractures of interphalangeal articulations; semiflexed internal rotation of upper limbs. Semiflexed external rotation of lower limbs.

Etiology. Unknown; autosomal dominant inheritance.

Pathology. Thickening of bones; joint deformities; capsular contraction; capsule formed by dense fibrous fibrocartilaginous tissue without elastic fibers.

Diagnostic Procedure. *X-ray.*

Therapy. Orthopedic treatment of complications.

Prognosis. Life expectancy not affected. Progressive articular impairment.

BIBLIOGRAPHY. Lèri A: Une dystrophie osseuse géneralisée et hereditaire la pleonosteose familiale. Presse Med 30:13–16, 1922
Metcalfe RA: Spinal cord compression in Lèri's plenosteosis. Br J Radiol 58:1117–1119, 1985
Beighton P: Other heritable and generalized disorders of connective tissue. In Beithon P (ed): McKusick's Heritable Disorders of Connective Tissue, 5th ed, pp 523–524. St Louis, CV Mosby, 1993

LERI-WEILL

Synonyms. Leri-Weill mesomelic dwarfism; Leri-Weill dyschondrosteosis; Lamy-Bienefeld. See Madelung.

Symptoms and Signs. Both sexes affected, but prevalent in females (4:1); detection at birth to end of growing period. Bilaterality of lesions characterizing element (unilateral lesions, see Madelung). Wrist pain when lifting objects. Forearms shorter with respect to hands and upper arm; distal ulna dorsal dislocation; dislocation easily reduced but unstable. Limited motion of elbows and wrists; legs shorter with respect to thighs.

Etiology. Autosomal dominant inheritance (sex influenced?).

Diagnostic Procedures. *X-ray of limbs.* Shortening of radius; triangularity of the distal radius epiphyses; wedging of carpal bones between radius and ulna.

Therapy. Splinting; orthopedic intervention for cosmetic reasons.

Prognosis. Pain stops with growth cessation. Mild dwarfism results.

BIBLIOGRAPHY. Leri A, Weill J: Une affection congénitale et symétrique du développement osseaux. La dyschondrostéose. Bull Soc Med Hôp 53:1491–1494, 1929
Lamy M, Bienefeld C: La Dyschondrosteose. In Gedda (ed): Analecta Genetica, pp 153–164. Rome, Mendel Institute, 1954
Jackson LG: Dyschondrosteosis: clinical study of a sixth generation family. Proc Greenwood Genet Cent 4:147–148, 1985
Rimoin DL, Lachman RS: Genetic disorders of the osseous skeleton. In Beithon P (ed): McKusick's Heritable Disorders of Connective Tissue, 5th ed, pp 637–639. St Louis, CV Mosby, 1993

LERMOYEZ

Synonyms. Deafness; tinnitus; vertigo. Vertigo; deafness; tinnitus; allergic vestibulitis; labyrinthitis, nonsuppurative.

Symptoms and Signs. Onset in the thirties and forties (as opposed to Ménière syndrome's onset in the fifties and sixties). The sequence of tinnitus and deafness, which diminishes or disappears after vertigo becomes established (as opposed to the sequence of vertigo followed by tinnitus and deafness, characteristic of Ménière). Allergic manifestations, especially urticaria, sometimes preceding the syndrome.

Etiology. Vasospasm of internal auditory artery. Allergic origin, especially urticaria. Some think that this syndrome is merely a transient phenomenon during an attack of Ménière caused by a transitory improvement of hearing.

Pathology. Unknown.

Diagnostic Procedures. *Otologic examination. Audiography. Skin tests.*

Therapy. See Ménière.

Prognosis. Excellent; recovery of normal health and disappearance of tinnitus and deafness (as opposed to Ménière, which causes a more or less permanent disability).

BIBLIOGRAPHY. Lermoyez M: La Vertige qui fait entendre (angiospasme labyrinthique). Presse Med 27:1–3, 1919
Eagle WW: Lermoyez's syndrome-an allergic disease. Ann Otol 57:453–464, 1948
Eckhardt J, Claussen CF: Ein Beitrag zum Lermoyez-Syndrom. Arch Klin Exp Ohr Nas Kehlk Heilk 201:159–171, 1972
Bandt T: Vertigo: Its Multisensory Syndromes, p 42. London, Springer-Verlag, 1991

LEROY I-CELL

Synonyms. Mucolipidosis II, ML II; I-cell.

Symptoms and Signs. High frequency in Arab communities. Both sexes affected; present at birth or onset in early postnatal period. Lack of striking corneal clouding; mild retinopahy; hyperopic astigmatism; minimal hepatomegaly; dislocation of hips; thoracic deformities; hyperplastic gums; hernia; restricted joint mobility; retarded psychomotor development; recurrent respiratory infections.

Etiology. Autosomal recessive inheritance. Defect of phosphorylation of hydrolases that prevents them from entering lysozomes and thus prevents their becoming active. Many mucopolysaccharides are not metabolized. Enzyme defective is UDP-N-acetylglucosamine: lysosomal enzyme N-acetylglucosaminyl-1-phosphotranspherase that adds mannose-6 phosphate to lysosomal enzymes.

Pathology. Subepithelial connective tissue, hypercellular with numerous vacuolated histiocytes and fibroblasts. Contains numerous inclusion cells (I-cells). Also affected: chondrocytes, Schwann cells, glomerular epithelial, vascular parietal cells, and peripheral neurons. Lipid content of I-cell three times above normal.

Diagnostic Procedures. *Fibroblast culture.* See Pathology. High levels of lysosomal enzymes in medium of culture. *Urine.* Moderate mucopolysacchariduria or normal level. *X-ray.* Radiologic features suggest Hurler syndrome. *Blood.* No metachromatic granules in leukocytes; increased lysosomal enzyme values. Ten- or 20-fold increase of beta-hexosaminidase; presence of iduronate sulfatase and aryl sulfatase A in serum is diagnostic. Prenatal diagnosis is possible from amniotic fuid.

Therapy. Bone marrow transplantation, benefits not clearly determined.

Prognosis. Most patients die by age 5 or 6 from infections or heart failure.

BIBLIOGRAPHY. Leroy JG, De Mars RI: Mutant enzymatic and cytological phenotypes in cultured human fibroblasts. Science 158:1097–1103, 1968

Leroy JG, O'Brien JS: Mucolipidosis II and III: Differential residual activity of beta-galactosidase in cultured fibroblasts. Clin Genet 9:533–539, 1976

Kornfeld S, Sly WS: I cell disease and pseudo-Hurler polydystrophy: Disorders of lysomal enzyme phosphorylation and localization. In Scriver CR, Beaudet AL, Sly WS, et al: The Metabolic and Molecular Bases of Inherited Disease, 7th ed, p 2498. New York, McGraw-Hill, 1995

LESCHKE-ULLMANN

Synonyms. Parkes Weber II; Webber II; dystrophia pigmentosa.

Symptoms and Signs. Asthenia, adynamia, hypotonia. Multiple pigmented skin maculae, physical and mental retardation, somatic deformities notably dwarfism, obesity of pituitary type, genital dystrophy (sexual hypoplasia and hypofunction), abnormalities of autonomic nervous system

Etiology. Possibly a variant of Von Recklinghausen, lacking skin tumors. Autonomy of this syndrome denied by modern literature.

Diagnostic Procedures. *Blood.* Frequently altered sugar metabolism; variable multihormonal alterations.

Therapy. Symptomatic.

Prognosis. Variable according to type and degree of endocrine involvement.

BIBLIOGRAPHY. Weber FP: Patches of deep pigmentation of oral mucous membrane not connected with Addison's disease. Quart J Med 12:404–408, 1919

Leschke E: Ueber Pigmentierung bei Funktions-stoerungen der Nebenniere und des sympathischen Nervensystems bei der Recklinghausenschen Krankheit Berl. Med Ges Klin Wschr 28:1433, 1922

Lesche E: Ullmann H Pigmentation und endocrine Dystrophie. Z Klin Med 102:388–411, 1926

Liebald GP, Leiber B: Cutaneous dysplasia associated with neurological disorders. In Vinken PJ, Bruyn GW: Handbook of Clinical Neurology, vol 14, p 117. Amsterdam, North-Holland, 1972

LESCH-NYHAN

Synonyms. Nyhan; choreoathetosis—self-mutilation—juvenile gout; hyperuricemia—oligophrenia; uric acid disorder—hypoxanthine guanine phosphoribosyl transferase deficiency; HGPRT deficiency.

Symptoms and Signs. Major manifestation in affected males; onset at 3–4 months of age. Extensor spasm of the trunk; generalized muscular weakness; athetoid or clonic movements; hypotonia when at rest; occasionally seizures; increased deep tendon reflexes; Babinski sign. No sensory disturbances. Self-destructive behavior usually starts at 2 years of age. Lip, thumb, and foot biting; dislocation of eyes; face scratching; head banging. Mental retardation, usually severe. If speech develops, it remains extremely limited; dysarthria. Growth severely impaired.

Etiology. Sex-linked recessive type of inheritance. Several independent mutations have been identified. Deficient activity of hypoxanthine guanine phosphoribosyltransferase (HGPRT) demonstrated. In some patients complete deficiency of hypoxanthine guanine phosphoribosyltransferase. Patients with partial deficiency of HGPRT have severe gout (see). Growth retardation is related to testicular atrophy and partial failure of 11-hydroxylation of steroids.

Pathology. Lesions from biting and trauma. In brain, no characteristic pathologic changes; unidentified homogeneous substance and mild brownish pigmentation may be associated with lesions. Kidneys bilaterally shrunken and changes associated to obstructive uropathy.

Diagnostic Procedures. *Blood.* Hyperuricemia. Anemia (usually macrocytic type). *Erythrocytes.* HGPRT absence and increased adenine phosphoribosyl-transferase. *Urine.* Yellow staining of diaper from uric acid from first days of life. High uric acid excretion. *X-ray.* Negative. Tophaceus deposits in some older patients. *CT brain scan. MRI.* Ventricular dilatation and cortical atrophy.

Therapy. Allopurinol; alkalinization of urine (sodium citrate/citric acid) prevents complication from uric acid stones and renal damage. Restraints to prevent biting and self-inflicted damage. L-5–hydroxytryptophan plus imipramine and carbidopa to reduce self mutilating behavior. Attempt somatic gene therapy and bone marrow transplantation.

Prognosis. Poor. Treatment does not affect neurologic defect, which appears not to be progressive. Death in second or third decade from infections or renal failure.

BIBLIOGRAPHY. Catel W, Schmidt J: Ueber familiare gichtische Diathese in Verbindung mit zerebralen und renalen Symptomen bei einem Kleinkind. Dtsch Med Wochenschr 84:2145–2147, 1959

Lesch M, Nyhan WL: A familial disorder of uric acid metabolism and central nervous system function. Am J Med 36:561–570, 1964

Davidson BL, Tarle SA, Van Antwerp M, et al: Identification of 17 independent mutations responsible for human Hypoxantine-guanine phosphoribosyl-transferase (HPRT) deficiency. Am J Med Genet 48:941–958, 1991

Rossiter BJJF, Caskey CT: Hypoxanthine-guanine phosphoribosyltransferase deficiency: Lesch-Nyhan syndrome and gout. In Scriver CR, Beaudet AL, Sly WS, et al: The Metabolic and Molecular Bases of Inherited Disease, 7th ed, pp 1679–1708. New York, McGraw-Hill, 1995

LETTERER-SIWE

Synonyms. Abt-Letterer-Siwe; Siwe; aleukemic reticulosis; aleukemic reticuloendotheliosis; see Histiocytosis syndromes.

Symptoms. Occurs in infants and growing children (under 3 years of age); onset occasionally later, up to young adulthood. Fatigue; anorexia; irritability; wasting; chronic otitis media. Low-grade, persistent fever.

Signs. On the scalp (primarily), face, and trunk, cutaneous maculopapular lesions, yellowish brown papules with red edge and yellow center. Weeping erosion on skin folds, ecchymoses, and petechiae. Edema; generalized lymphadenopathy and hepatosplenomegaly.

Etiology. Unknown; Autosomal recessive trait reported. Disseminated condition of histiocytosis syndromes (see). Differentiation from Hand-Schueller-Christian clinically irrelevant.

Pathology. Histiocytic proliferation resembling generalized reticular cell sarcoma or monocytic leukemia. Generalized eosinophilia, hepatomegaly, and splenomegaly. Histiocytic infiltration of lungs.

Diagnostic Procedures. *Blood.* Leukocytosis, anemia, thrombocytopenia. *X-ray.* Destructive lesions of bones, especially skull.

Therapy. Corticosteroids; vinblastine; vincristine; cyclophosphamide; antibiotics; and other chemotherapeutic agents.

Prognosis. Acute form: rapidly fatal; possibility of chronicity or remission; variable duration from weeks to years.

BIBLIOGRAPHY. Letterer E: Aleukämische Retikulose. Frank Z Pathol 30:377–394, 1924
Siwe S: Die Reticuloendotheliose-ein neues Krankheitsbild unter den Hepatosplenomegalien. Z Kinderheilkd 55:212–247, 1933
Schoeck VW, Peterson RDA, Good RA: Familial occurrence of Letterer-Siwe disease. Pediatrics 32:1055–1063, 1963
Lukens JN: Langerhans cell histiocytosis. In Lee GR, Bithell TC, Foerster J, et al (eds): Wintrobe's Clinical Hematology, 9th ed, p 1643. Philadelphia, Lea & Febiger, 1993

LEUKOCYTE ADHESION DEFICIENCY

Synonyms. LAD; leu-cam; LFA-1 immununodeficiency; intergrin beta-2; CD18.

Symptoms and Signs. Both sexes. Age range in severe form 1–14 years; in milder form 11–44 years. Recurrent necrotic and indolent infections of soft tissue (skin, mucosae, intestine, etc.). Small, erythematous, nonpustular lesions progressing to craters healing slowly and with dysplastic scars, occasionally rapidly progressing to gas gangrene or septicemia, perirectal abscess; recurrent invasive candidiasis of gastrointestinal tract, necrotizing enterocolitis; peritonitis; pneumonitis. In patients who survive infancy, gingivitis and/or periodontitis.

Etiology. Autosomal recessive inheritance. Broad spectrum of functional abnormalities of myeloid and lymphoid cells from heterogenous mutations of subunit of CD18 (2) integrins leading to defective biosynthesis of three glycoproteins. The beta subunit is coded by chromosome 21.

Pathology. Extravascular inflammatory, totally devoid of neutrophils, sites displaced in various organs.

Diagnostic Procedures. *Blood.* Granulocytosis (15,000–160,000 mm³). *Skin windows.* Absence of migrating neutrophils. *Culture of material.* Wide spectrum of Gram-positive and -negative bacteria and fungi.

Therapy. Allogenic bone marrow transplantation. Attempt of cell gene therapy.

Prognosis. Patients with severe form die in infancy or demonstrate susceptibility to severe recurrent infections. In cases with moderate deficiency only infrequent severe infections.

BIBLIOGRAPHY. van der Meer JWM, Zwet TL, van Furth R, et al: New familial defect in microbicidal function of polymorphonuclear leukocytes. Lancet II:630–632, 1975
Anderson DC, Kishimoto TK, Smith CW: Leukocyte adhesion deficiency and other disorders of leukocyte adherence and motility. In Scriver CR, Beaudet AL, Sly WS, et al: The Metabolic and Molecular Bases of Inherited Disease, 7th ed, pp 3955–3973. New York, McGraw-Hill, 1995

LEUKOCYTE GLUCOSE-6-PHOSPHATE DEHYDROGENASE DEFICIENCY

Synonym. G6PDH deficiency; glucose-6-phosphate dehydrogenase deficiency of leukocytes.

Symptoms and Signs. Very rare. Both sexes. From birth, severe infections. Congenital nonspherocytic hemolytic anemia (owing to G6PDH deficiency also in erythrocytes).

Etiology. X-linked. Associated to erythrocyte G6PDH deficiency.

Diagnostic Procedures. Neutrophil function tests. Normal particle ingestion and degranulation. Defective killing of catalase positive and catalase negative infection in females and catalase-positive in males.

Therapy. Prevention and treatment of infections.

Prognosis. Patients described have reached adulthood.

BIBLIOGRAPHY. Cooper MR, De Chatelet LR, McCall CE, et al: Complete deficiency of leukocyte glucose-6-phosphate dehydrogenase with defective bactericidal activity. J Clin Invest 51:769–772, 1972
Mallouh AA, Abu-Osba YK: Bacterial infections in children with glucose-6-phosphate dehydrogenase deficiency. J Pediat 111:850–852, 1987
Athens JW: Qualitative disorders of leukocytes. In Lee GR, Bithel TC, Foerster J, et al (eds): Wintrobe's Clinical Hematology, 9th ed, p 1622. Philadelphia, Lea & Febiger, 1993

LEV

Synonym. Atrio-ventricular block; AV block. See Lenegre.

Symptoms and Signs. Usually occurs in elderly persons. Those of atrioventricular (AV) block of various degrees up to complete.

Etiology. Exogenous invasion of heart conduction system. See Pathology.

Pathology. Fibrosis or calcification spreading into conducting system from adjacent fibrous structures: e.g., calcification of aortic valve; fibrosis of summit of muscular septum; fibrosis or calcification of mitral ring.

Diagnostic Procedure. *ECG. Heart block.*

Therapy. Pharmacological trials. Permanent pacemaker.

Prognosis. Variable according to basic condition. Optimal results with pacemaker implantation.

BIBLIOGRAPHY. Lev M: The pathology of complete atrioventricular block. Am J Med 37:742–748, 1964
Myerburg RJ, Kessler KM, Castellanos A: Recognition, clinical assessment and management of arrhytmias and conduction disturbances. In Schlant RC, Alexander RW: Hurst's The Heart, 8th ed, pp 748–751. New York, McGraw-Hill, 1994

LEVIN II

Synonym. Osteogenesis imperfecta; skeletal lesions, unusual.

Symptoms and Signs. Those of osteogenesis imperfecta. Normal teeth; frequent infection of jaws.

Etiology. Autosomal dominant inheritance.

Diagnostic Procedures. *X-ray of maxilla and mandible.* Multiocular radiolucent-radiopaque lesions. Coarseness of trabecular and osteopenia of skeleton.

Prognosis. Good.

BIBLIOGRAPHY. Levin LS, Wright JM, Byrd DL, et al: Osteogenesis imperfecta with unusual skeletal lesions: Report of three families. Ann J Med Genet 21:257–259, 1985

LEVINE-CRITCHLEY

Synonyms. Acanthocytosis; neurologic disease; choreo-acanthocytosis; neuroacanthocytosis.

Symptoms and Signs. More frequent in Japan. Both sexes. From infancy. Various patterns of neurologic conditions reminiscent of Gilles de la Tourette (see); Huntington (see); Friedreich (see); chorea syndromes (see); self-mutilation of tongue, lips, and cheeks; parkinsonism.

Etiology. Unknown. Heterogenous inheritance (autosomal dominant and recessive).

Pathology. *Brain.* Neural loss, gliosis, and degeneration of basal ganglia.

Diagnostic Procedures. *Blood.* Acanthocytosis. Normal serum lipoproteins. *CT brain scan. MRI. EEG.*

Therapy. Symptomatic.

Prognosis. Survival into adulthood.

BIBLIOGRAPHY. Critchley EMR, Clark DB, Wikler A: An adult form of acanthocytosis. Trans Am Neurol Assoc 92:132–137, 1967

Levine IM, Estes JW, Looney JM: Hereditary neurological disease with acanthocytosis: A new syndrome. Arch Neurol 19:403–409, 1968

Spitz MC, Jankovic J, Killian JM: Familial tic disorder, parkinsonism motor neuron disease, and acanthocytosis: a new syndrome. Neurology 35:366–370, 1985

Villegas A, Moscat J, Vazquez A, et al: A new family with hereditary choreoacanthocytosis. Acta Haemat 77:215–219, 1987

LEVY-HOLLISTER

Synonyms. Lacrimo—auriculo—dento—digital, LADD; lacrimo—auriculo—radio—digital (LARD) (see EEC).

Symptoms and Signs. Both sexes. From birth. Lack of lacrimation; conjunctivitis; cupped pinnas; mixed hearing defects. Small peg-shaped teeth and enamel dysplasia. *Hands.* Variable malformations; clinodactyly, syndactyly, duplication of phalanx; radial aplasia. Other variably associated features of EEC.

Etiology. Sporadic cases and autosomal dominant inheritance. Incomplete expression of EEC (?) (see).

Pathology. Aplasia or hypoplasia of puncta of lacrimal ducts. See Signs.

BIBLIOGRAPHY. Levy WJ: Mesoectodermal dysplasia: A new combination of anomalies. Am J Ophthalmol 63:978–982, 1967

Hollister DW, Klein SH, Dejager HL, et al: The lacrimo-auriculo-dento-digital syndrome. J Pediatr 83:438–444, 1973

Wiedemann HR, Drescher J: LADD syndrome: Report of new case and review of the clinical spectrum. Eur J Pediatr 144:579–582, 1986

Kreutz JM, Hoyme HE: Levy-Hollister syndrome. Pediatrics 82:96–99, 1988

LEWANDOWSKY I

Synonym. Periporitis staphylogenes.

Symptoms and Signs. Occurs in infants of both sexes. Inflammation of sweat glands evolving into small abscesses.

Etiology. In miliaria profunda: pyogenic microorganisms associated with variable systemic conditions depressing immune response and defenses. Secondary infection by Staphylococcus aureus; miliaria progresses to abscesses of the sweat glands.

Pathology. Abscesses and pustules associated with sweat glands.

Diagnostic Procedures. Screening for identification of possible systemic condition.

Therapy. Antibiotics and correction of basic disorder.

Prognosis. Good with adequate treatment.

BIBLIOGRAPHY. Lewandowsky F: Zur Pathogenese der multiplen Abszesse im Säuglingsalter. Arch Dermatol Syph 80:179–191, 1906

Champion RH: Disorders of sweat glands. In Champion RH, Burton JL, Ebling FJG (eds): Rook/Wilkinson/Ebling Textbook of Dermatology, 5th ed, p 1758. Oxford, Blackwell Scientific, 1992

LEWANDOWSKY II

Synonyms. Lupoid rosacea; rosacea-like eruption.

Symptoms and Signs. Predominant in women. Onset age 20–50. Eruption of numerous tiny, reddish-blue or brown micropapules on the cheeks and forehead, seldom entire face, with erythematous background.

Etiology. Variant of rosacea. Once attributed to tuberculosis.

Pathology. Epitheliod cell tubercles with perifollicular tendency; few giant cells; perivascular inflammation with edema and disorganization.

Therapy. Tetracycline.

Prognosis. Slow spontaneous resolution.

BIBLIOGRAPHY. Lewandowsky BF: Ueber rosacea A ha liche Tuberkulidedes Gesichtes. Schweiz Aerzte 47:1280–1282, 1917

Marks R: Rosacea, flushing and perioral dermatitis. In Champion RH, Burton JL, Ebling FJG (eds): Rook/Wilkinson/Ebling Textbook of Dermatology, 5th ed, p 1862. Oxford, Blackwell Scientific, 1992

LEWANDOWSKY-LUTZ

Synonyms. Lutz; epidermodysplasia verruciformis; verrucosis, generalized.

Symptoms. More frequent in Asians. Both sexes affected; onset at any age; develops more rapidly in infancy.

Signs. On the face, neck, back of hands, and feet; more rarely on trunk. Development of flat, verrucous warts (2 cm in diameter). The warts on the face (most frequent site) are the flat type, whereas those on the trunk and extremities are larger and firmer. In some cases, they present a pink or violet color. The confluence of neighboring lesions forms lines or large plaques.

Etiology. Wart virus (papova). To develop this syndrome, a special hereditary predisposition is needed. Autosomal recessive or dominant and X-linked inheritance.

Pathology. Typical histologic changes observed in common warts.

Diagnostic Procedures. *Biopsy.* Electron and fluorescent microscopic examination to show presence of virus.

Therapy. Unsatisfactory. Role of etretinate not clear with temporary benefit in majority of cases. Frequent recurrence, even after large excision.

Prognosis. The lesion may remain static for decades. In nearly 20% development of squamous epithelioma in one or more lesions. Malignancy only in cases affected with HPV4.

BIBLIOGRAPHY. Lewandowsky F, Lutz W: Ein Fall einer bisher nicht beschriebenen Hauterkrankung (Epidermodysplasia verruciformis). Arch Dermatol Syph 41:193–202, 1922

Jablonka S, Orth G, Jarzabel-Chorzelske M, et al: Twenty-one years of follow-up studies of familial epidermodysplasia verruciforms. Dermatologica 158:309–327, 1979

Androphy EJ, Dvoretzky I, Lowy DR: X-linked inheritance of epidermodysplasia verruciforms: genetic and virologic studies of a kindred. Arch Derm 121:864–868, 1985

Highet AS, Kurtz J: Viral infections. In Champion RH, Burton JL, Ebling FJG (eds): Rook/Wilkinson/Ebling Textbook of Dermatology, 5th ed, p 914. Oxford, Blackwell Scientific, 1992

LEWIS (C.S.)

Synonym. Symphalangism, Lewis type; stiff thumbs.

Symptoms and Signs. Presumed synostosis involving the first metacarpophalangeal joint. Lewis described his own condition. The same type of lesion accompanied by brachydactyly and mental retardation has been also described (see Piussan).

Etiology. Autosomal dominant inheritance.

Prognosis. Manual clumsiness (which the eponymous author says drove him to become a writer).

BIBLIOGRAPHY. Lewis CS: Surprised by Joy: The Shape of My Early Life, p 12. New York, Harcourt, Brace and World, 1955
Piussan C, Lenaerts C, Mathieu M, et al: Dominance reguliere d'une ankilose des pouces avec retard mental se transmettant sur trois generations. J Genet Hum 31:107–114, 1983
Barber C, Carpenter NJ, Say B: Bilateral ankylosed thumbs and mental retardation. Am J Med Genet 36:367, 1990

LEWIS (F.)

Synonyms. Heart—hand II; cardiovascular—arm; ventriculo—radial dysplasia. See Holt-Oram.

Symptoms. Present from birth. Association of multiple heart and upper limb defects:

1. Atrial septal defect; ventricular septal defect; great vessel transposition; single coronary artery; retroesophageal right subclavian artery
2. Absence or deformity of thumbs; phocomelia; deformed long bones (humerus, radius, and ulna) and metacarpal bones

Etiology. Autosomal dominant inheritance very likely does not differ from that of Holt-Oram.

BIBLIOGRAPHY. Lewis F: High defects of atrial septum. J Thorac Cardiovasc Surg 36:1–11, 1958
Harris LC, Osborne WP: Congenital absence or hypoplasia of the radius with ventricular septal defect: ventriculo-radial dysplasia. J Pediatr 68:265–272, 1966

LEWIS (R.A.)

Synonym. Ocular albinism; lentigines; sensorineural deafness. See Nettleship Falls and albinism ocular autosomal recessive.

Symptoms and Signs. Both sexes. From birth. Reduced visual acuity; photophobia nystagmus; translucent irides; refractive errors. Sensorineural deafness. with vestibular hypofunction. Lentigines.

Etiology. Autosomal dominant inheritance.

Pathology. *Skin.* Macromelanosomes. *Eyes.* Optic nerve dysplasia.

Diagnostic Procedures. *Fundus.* Albinotic with hypoplasia of fovea.

Therapy. None.

BIBLIOGRAPHY. Lewis RA: Ocular albinism and deafness. Twenty-ninth Annual Meeting, American Society of Human Genetics, Vancouver. Am J Hum Genet 30:57(abstr), 1978

LEYDEN II

Symptoms and Signs. Tetraparesis with fatal evolution following an epileptic attack.

Etiology. Hemorrhage in the pons or bulb.

BIBLIOGRAPHY. Leyden E: Klinik der Rueckenmarks-Krankheiten, vol. 2, p 64. Berlin, Hirschwald, 1875

LEYDEN-MÖBIUS

Synonyms. Femoral dystrophy; limb-girdle inferior dystrophy; pelvifemoral muscular dystrophy; limb girdle muscular dystrophy 2; LGMD2.

Symptoms and Signs. Muscular dystrophy of lumbosacral muscles. Later onset and more benign course than Erb III (see).

BIBLIOGRAPHY. Leyden E: Klinik der Rueckenmarks-Krankheiten, vol 2. Berlin, Hirschwald, 1876
Jerusalem F, Sieb JP: The limb girdle syndromes. In Rowland LP, Di Mauro S: Handbook of Clinical Neurology, vol 18: Myopathies, p 179. Amsterdam, Elsevier, 1992

LHERMITTE-CORNIL-QUESNEL

Synonym. Extrapyramidal—pyramidal degeneration, operculum.

Symptoms and Signs. Appears in middle age or later. Periods of excitation and depression. Gradual onset and slow progression; absence of sudden vascular accidents that usually are at the onset of pseudobulbar palsy. Pain and paresthesia and rigidity of lower limbs. Dysarthria; aphonia; dysphagia; involuntary laughing and crying. Further retrograde mental changes; apathy and negativism. Muscular hypertonia, more marked in proximal muscles. Hand posture similar to that observed in paralysis agitans: extended wrist; fingers flexed at metacarpophalangeal joints and extended at other joints. Lower limb posture not particularly characteristic. Good muscular power (slowness of movement associated with extrapyramidal hypertonia). Tendon hyperreflexia; presence of ankle clonus; Babinski sign. Normal fundus oculi.

Etiology. Unknown; observed in cases of epidemic encephalitis. Considered by the authors a distinct entity from very similar conditions: Parkinson; pseudobulbar palsy; Creutzfeld-Jakob; amyotrophic lateral sclerosis; paralysis agitans.

Pathology. In putamen reduction of cells, neuroglial overgrowth, degeneration of fibers originating in the putamen. Globus pallidus shows similar pattern, but less severe. Pyramidal tract degeneration below level of medulla. In the cord, degeneration of crossed pyramidal tracts.

Diagnostic Procedures. *Blood and cerebrospinal fluid.* Normal.

Therapy. Symptomatic.

Prognosis. Rapid evolution; death within 1 year.

BIBLIOGRAPHY. Magnus A: Fall von Aufhebung des Willenseinflussens auf einige Hirnnerven. Muellers Arch Physiol Wissensch Med 258–266, 1837
Lhermitte J, Cornil L, Quesnel: Le syndrome de la dégénération pyramidopallidale progressive. Rev Neurol 27:262–269, 1920
Lhermitte J, McAlpine D: A clinical and pathological résumé of combined disease of the pyramidal and extrapyramidal systems, with special reference to a new syndrome. Brain 49:157–181, 1926
Bruyns GW, Gothier JC: The operculum syndrome. In Vinken PJ, Bruyn GW: Handbook of Clinical Neurology, vol 2, pp 776–783. Amsterdam, North-Holland, 1969

LHERMITTE-DUCLOS

Synonyms. Spiegel; cerebellar hypertrophy, diffuse; cerebellar hamartoma; gangliocytoma dysplasticum; gangliocytoma myelinicum; Purkinjenoma.

Symptoms and Signs. Those of cerebellar tumor. Intracranial hypertension ataxia. Frequent association with other tumors and hamartomas.

Etiology. Unknown.

Pathology. Cerebellar enlargment, widening and distortion of the folia: Thickened molecular layer and replacement of the Purkinje and granular layers by disorganized proliferation of abnormal neurons (some granule-like, some Purkinje-like). Hypertrophy, amartoma, or benign neoplasia (?).

Diagnostic Procedures. *CT scan. MRI.*

Therapy. Surgery.

Prognosis. Long-term (over 10 years) postoperative survival reported.

BIBLIOGRAPHY. Lhermitte J, Duclos P: Sur un Ganglioneurome diffus du cortex de cervelet. Bull Assoc Fran Cancer 9:99–107, 1920
Spiegel E: Hyperplase des Kleihirns Beitr. Pathol Anat 67:539–548, 1920
Albrecht S, Haber RM, Goodman JC, et al: Cowden syndrome and Lhermitte-Duclos disease. Cancer 70:869–876, 1992

LHERMITTE-LEVY

Synonyms. Lhermitte-Delthil-Garnier; hallucinosis; red nucleus; peduncular hallucinosis.

Symptoms. Occurs in elderly people. Slowly progressing paralysis after a stroke. Incessant choreiform movement of arms and legs (rhythmic trembling). Visual and auditory hallucinations.

Etiology. The combination of movements and hallucination attributed by the authors to a lesion of unknown nature in the upper portion of peduncle and subthalamic region.

BIBLIOGRAPHY. Lhermitte MJ, Levy G: Phenomenes d'allucinose chez une malade presentant une torsion et une contracture athetoides intentionnelles du bras. Soc Neurol May 7, 1931
Lhermitte MJ, Delthil, Garnier: Syndrome controlateral du noyau rouge avec hallucinations visuelles et auditives. Rev Neurol 70:623–628, 1938
Adams RD, Victor M: Principles of Neurology, 5th ed, p 685. New York, McGraw-Hill, 1993

LIAN-SIGUIER-WELTI

Eponym used to indicate a venous thrombosis complicating eventration or diaphragmatic hernia.

BIBLIOGRAPHY. Lian G, Siguier F, Welti JJ: Le syndrome "hernia diaphragmatique ou éventration diaphragmatique et thrombose veineuses." Presse Med 61:145–146, 1953

LIBMAN-SACKS

Synonyms. Kaposi-Besnier-Libman-Sacks; Osler-Libman-Sacks; atypical verrucous endocarditis; nonbacterial verrucous endocarditis; nonrheumatic endocarditis; see Lupus erythematosus, systemic.

Symptoms. Those of lupus erythematosus.

Signs. Systolic and diastolic apical murmurs.

Etiology. Associated with lupus erythematosus, systemic (see).

Pathology. Mucoid degeneration of cardiac valves; fibrinoid necrosis; necrotic fibrinoid vegetation without bacteria.

Diagnostic Procedures. Those of lupus erythematosus, systemic.

Therapy. Same as for lupus erythematosus, systemic.

Prognosis. Same as for lupus erythematosus, systemic.

BIBLIOGRAPHY. Libman E, Sacks B: A hitherto undescribed form of valvular and mural endocarditis. Arch Intern Med 33:701–737, 1924
Healy BP, Schlant RC, Gonzales EB: The heart and connective tissue disease. In Schlant RC, Alexander RW: Hurst's The Heart, 8th ed, pp 1922–1923. New York, McGraw-Hill, 1994

LICHEN PLANUS

Synonyms. Wilson (E.), including lichen planus familial and Hebra.

Symptoms. More common in men; onset in young adulthood (recorded in infancy and old age as well). Pruritus; malaise. Familial form earlier onset, tendency to chronicity, more severe and atypical manifestations that are classified under different name according to specific features: hypertrophic; follicular; linear; actinic; annular; atropic; guttate; palms and soles; pigmentosum; mucus membrane; symptomatic (toxic).

Signs. Usually, insidious onset (chronic type) or less frequently (5%) sudden (acute). On inner side of thighs, knees, back, less frequently on genitalia and mucosae, appearance of papules varying in shape (polygonal), size (pinpoint to over 1 cm), and distribution (widely scattered or aggregated). Papular surface is shining, flat; the color is violet with dots and striae.

Etiology. Unknown. Toxic, viral, psychogenic factors blamed without proof or confirmation. Families with autosomal dominant inheritance reported.

Pathology. Moderate increase of horny layer; increase of granular layer; irregular acanthosis; liquefaction necrosis of basal layer. Dermis is infiltrated by lymphocytes and histiocytes. Presence of colloid bodies.

Therapy. Corticosteroids; adrenocorticotropic hormone (ACTH) in severe cases. Antipruritic drugs also useful. Symptomatic; topical fluorinated steroid creams or ointments; in hypertrophic form, occlusive dressing with tar, ichthammol, or cream with salicyclic acid added. Retinoic acid. Photochemotherapy. (Warning: danger of carcinogenesis.)

Prognosis. Acute form: average duration 8 months (from weeks to years). Chronic form: average duration 3 years (up to 20). May leave areas of atrophy or hyperpigmentation.

BIBLIOGRAPHY. Wilson E: On lichen planus: The lichen ruber of Hebra. Br Med J 2:399–402, 1866
Mahood JM: Familial lichen planus: A report of nine cases from four families with a brief review of the literature. Arch Derm 119:292–294, 1983
Black MM: Lichen planus and lichenoid disorders. In Champion RH, Burton JL, Ebling FJG (eds): Rook/Wilkinson/Ebling Textbook of Dermatology, 5th ed, pp 1675–1695. Oxford, Blackwell Scientific, 1992

LICHTENSTEIN-JAFFE

Synonyms. Unifocal eosinophilic bone granuloma; eosinophilic granuloma. See Histiocytosis syndromes.

Symptoms and Signs. Males more frequently affected (3:2); onset all ages. At onset, asymptomatic or low-grade fever (intermittent), pain, tenderness, and, occasionally, tumor on affected bone site. Most frequently affected are the head and femur in children and the ribs in adults. Moderate shotty cervical lymphadenopathy; no otitis media; cutaneous manifestation or exophthalmos at onset (see Hand-Schüller-Christian). Seldom (after years), diabetes insipidus may develop.

Etiology. Unknown.

Pathology. Single or multiple lytic lesions in bone. Histiocytic proliferation with eosinophilia.

Diagnostic Procedures. *X-ray. Biopsy.*

Therapy. Curettement of the lesion, simultaneously with the biopsy. Modest doses of X-ray therapy (500–1500 rads).

Prognosis. Relatively benign condition; long survival; spontaneous remission observed.

BIBLIOGRAPHY. Lichtenstein L, Jaffe HL: Eosinophilic granuloma of bone, with report of case. Am J Pathol 16:595–604, 1940

Oberman HA: Idiopathic histiocytosis: a clinico-pathologic study of 40 cases and review of the literature on eosinophilic granuloma of bone. Hand-Schüller-Christian disease and Letterer-Siwe disease. Pediatrics 28:307–327, 1961

Lukens JN: Langerhan's cell histiocytosis. In Lee GR, Bithell TC, Foerster J, et al (eds): Wintrobe's Clinical Hematology, 9th ed, p 1643. Philadelphia, Lea & Febiger, 1993

LICHTENSTEIN (J.R.)

Symptoms and Signs. In newborns (in one couple of female twins) frequent infections; tendency to fractures; subluxation of C1–C2 (long tract signs) campodactyly (ulnar deviation); simian crease, unusual facies.

Etiology. Unknown. Possibly autosomal recessive inheritance.

Diagnostic Procedures. *Blood.* Neutropenia, IgA deficiency. *X-rays.* Peripheral osteoporosis; failure of fusion of posterior spinal arches; giant cysts of the lungs.

BIBLIOGRAPHY. Lichtenstein JR: A new syndrome with neutropenia, immunoglobulin deficiency, peculiar facies, and bony anomalies. Birth Defects 8:178–190, 1972

LICHTENSTEIN-KNORR

Synonyms. Deafness—ataxia; ataxia—deafness.

Symptoms and Signs. Onset in childhood of progressive sensorineural hearing loss. In adolescence slow progressive ataxia; depression of joint reflexes: dysarthric speech; hypotonia; pes cavus; kiphoscoliosis. Occasionally cataract. Vestibular function: normal.

Etiology. Autosomal recessive inheritance.

Diagnostic Procedures. No test reported.

Prognosis. See Symptoms and Signs.

BIBLIOGRAPHY. Lichtenstein H, Knorr A: Ueber einige Faelle von fortschreitender Schwerhoerigkeit bei hereditaerer Ataxie. Dtsch Z Nervenheilkd 114:1–28, 1930

LICHTENSTERN

Eponym used to indicate an association of pernicious anemia (see Biermer-Addison) and tabes dorsalis.

BIBLIOGRAPHY. Lichtenstern O: Ueber progressive perniziöse Anaemie bei Tcabeskranken. Dtsch Med Wochenschr 10:849–850, 1884

LICHTHEIM I

Synonyms. Word deafness; pure word deafness; perisylvian temporal (posterior) variety. See Broca aphasia.

Symptoms and Signs. Defective auditory verbal comprehension amnestic aphasia (nominal) where the patient is unable to say words but may indicate (indirectly) the number of syllables or letters of the word in question, repetition, and writing under dictation. Defective repetition differentiates it from the transcortical sensory aphasia, and preservation of reading, writing, and spontaneous speech from Wernicke (see). No deafness. Mental status evaluation: normal attentiveness, orietation, memory, calculation, and visuospatial skills.

Etiology. Cerebrovascular accidents from presumed cardiac embolization, with bitemporal cortico-subcortical lesions.

Pathology. Bilateral perisylvian damage.

Diagnostic Procedures. *CT scan. MRI. EEG.* Hearing evaluation: normal or near normal; pure tone. Audiometric findings: normal. Language evaluation: occasional literal paraphasias and word finding difficulty. Nonverbal environmental sounds: normal perception.

Therapy. Symptomatic, teaching special communication techniques: nonverbal cues, writing things out or spelling words.

Prognosis. According to damage. Usually nonprogressive.

BIBLIOGRAPHY. Lichtheim L: On aphasia. Brain 7:433–484, 1885

Buchman AS, Garron DC, Trost-Cardamone JE, et al: Word deafness: One hundred years later. J Neurol, Neurosurg Psych 49:489–499, 1986

Mendez MF, Rosenberg S: Word deafness mistaken for Alzheimer's disease: Differential characteristics. J Am Ger Soc 39:209–211, 1991

LICHTHEIM II

Synonyms. Dana II; Putnam-Dana II; ataxic paraplegia; combined system; spinal funicular; neuroanemic; posterolateral sclerosis; spinal cord degeneration; subacute combined degeneration (SCD). See Addison-Biermer.

Symptoms. Condition widely disseminated, but more common in blond Nordic races; male and female same incidence. Onset most commonly in fourth decade. Great variability of symptoms, onset subacute or chronic. Slowly progressing: paresthesias that cannot be rubbed away; aggravated by cold; relieved by heat. Ataxia of various degrees. Motor symptoms may be present (weakness and easy fatigability). Spasticity or flaccid paralysis of various degrees; sphincter disturbances. Sensory symptoms rare; visual disturbances; mental changes (not specific).

Signs. Position and vibration senses lost. Babinski sign; hyperreflexia initially, then areflexia. Eyes may present retinal hemorrhage, changes in visual field. If pernicious anemia, pallor and typical tongue. This syndrome may precede the blood changes for a long time.

Etiology. Pernicious anemia most frequent cause; chronic alcoholism, sprue, and other conditions may be responsible; lack of intrinsic factor in gastric secretion.

Pathology. If limited to spinal cord, thoracic and lumbar tracts most frequently affected. Degeneration of posterior columns, pyramidal tract, spinocerebellar tract, and anterior portion. Loss of myelin and axis cylinders; glyosis in old lesion. Spongy appearance. Cerebral cortex may show evidence of damage and infarcts.

Diagnostic Procedures. *Blood.* If associated with pernicious anemia, macrocytic anemia. *Bone marrow.* Megaloblastosis. *Gastric fluid.* Achlorhydria.

Therapy. Vitamin B_{12} and thiamine. Curare and intensive care for spasms.

Prognosis. Poor; improvement with treatment. Complete regression with early treatment.

BIBLIOGRAPHY. Lichtheim: Zur Kenntniss der perniciösen Anämia. Verh Cong Innere Med 6:84–96, 1889

Dana C: The degenerative diseases of the spinal cord with a description of a new type. J Nerv Ment Dis 205–216, 1891

Adams RD, Victor M: Principles of Neurology, 5th ed, pp 864–867. New York, McGraw-Hill, 1993

LIDDLE

Synonyms. Inappropriate excessive renal sodium conservation; pseudoaldosteronism; apparent mineralocorticoid excess. See also Glucocorticoid-remediable aldosteronism.

Symptoms and Signs. See Conn.

Etiology. Unknown; Autosomal dominant inheritance. Primary intrinsic renal defect in the regulation of salt absorption rather than the effects on distal tubule of some unidentified mineralocorticoid other than aldosterone.

Diagnostic Procedures. As in primary hyperaldosteronism except lower level of aldosterone and the patients do not respond to spironolactone administration. Excessive renal reabsorption of sodium; potassium depletion; plasma renin and angiotensin activity suppression and inhibition of aldosterone secretion.

Therapy. Hypertension, potassium loss, and hypokalemia are corrected by restriction of dietary salt intake and triamterene administration. Renal transplantation seems to cure the condition.

Prognosis. Death in the forties from hypertensive vascular disease.

BIBLIOGRAPHY. Liddle GW, Bledsoe T, Coppage WS Jr: A familial renal disorder simulating primary aldosteronism, but with negligible aldosterone secretion. Trans Assoc Am Phys 76:199–213, 1963
Gadallah MF, Abreo K, Work J: Liddle's syndrome: An underrecognized entity: A report of four cases, including the first report on black individuals. Am J Kid Dis 25:829–835, 1995
Warnock DG, Bubien JK: Liddle's syndrome: A public menace? Am J Kid Dis 25:924–927, 1995

LIEBENBERG

Synonym. Brachydactyly; joint dysplasia; synostosis carpal; dysplastic elbow joints; brachydactyly.

Symptoms and Signs. Flexion deformity simulating anterior dislocation of elbow. Wrist slight flexion and radial deviation. Fingers short, club form of distal phalanges. Grooved nails. Absence of other bone fusions.

Etiology. Autosomal dominant inheritance.

Diagnostic Procedures. *X-rays.* Of hand: multiple anomalies. Of wrist: triquetrous-pisiform fusion; small capitate; trapezium; and trapezoid; enlarged tetriquetum and hammate. Aplasia of bones at elbow.

BIBLIOGRAPHY. Liebenberg F: A pedigree with unusual anomalies of elbow, wrists and hands in five generations. S Afr Med J 47:745–747, 1973

LIEBOW-CARRINGTON

Synonym. Wegener lymphomatoid variant (noncorrect); LYG; lymphomatoid granulomatosis; angiocentric immunoproliferative lesions (AIL); polymorphic reticulosis. See Carrington-Liebow and Angioimmunoblastic lymphoadenopathy; Midline granuloma (possibly same nature).

Symptoms and Signs. Those of Wegener (see) involving also upper respiratory tract, skin, central and peripheral nervous system, kidneys, gastrointestinal tract.

Etiology. Unknown. Probably a low-grade T-cell lymphoma.

Pathology. Lack of true granulomas. Vessels show dense lymphoid infiltrate with plasma cells polymorphonuclear leukocytes, large bizarre atypical cells, conspicuous necrosis. Lymph nodes are not involved. Grading I–III is used to indicate progressive atypia. A predominance of CD4 T-cells is observed.

Therapy. Corticosteroids of uncertain benefit. Cyclophosphamide: benefits in few cases.

Prognosis. Some cases have subsequently developed malignant lymphoma. Seventy percent die within 5 years from onset.

BIBLIOGRAPHY. Liebow AA, Carrington CB: The lymphomatoid variant of limited Wegener's granulomatosis (abstr). Am J Pathol 55:78–83, 1969
Friedman PJ: Idiopathic and autoimmune type III-like reactions: interstitial vasculitis and granulomatosis. Semin Roentgenol 10:43–51, 1975
Katzenstein AL, Carrington CB, Liebow AA: Lymphomatoid granulomatosis: A clinicopathological study of 152 cases. Cancer 43:360–373, 1979
Jaffe ES, Travis WD: Lymphomatoid granulomatosis and lymphoproliferative disorders of the lung. In Lynch JP, Deremee RA: Immunologically Mediated Pulmonary Diseases, p 274. Philadelphia, Lippincott, 1991

LIEPMANN

Synonym. Apraxia.

Symptoms and Signs. Inability to carry out purposeful or skilled actions, although general mental capacity and motor power are present. Varieties of the condition are recognized:

1. *Kinetic or motor.* Usually one hand or arm affected
2. *Ideational.* Inability to program a plan of action
3. *Ideokinetic.* Lack of coordination between ideation and motor pattern
4. *Constructional.* Inability to assemble objects (see Kleinst)

Etiology. Organic brain lesions.

1. Focal lesion of precentral contralateral cortex
2. Bilateral diffuse lesions or toxic state
3. Supramarginal gyrus: unilateral or bilateral lesion
4. Right hemisphere lesion (usually)

BIBLIOGRAPHY. Liepmann H: Das Krankheitsbild der Apraxie ("motorischen Asymbolye") auf Grund eines Falles von einseitiger Apraxie. Mschr Psychiatr Neurol 8:15–44; 10–32; 182–197, 1900
Adams RD, Victor M: Principles of Neurology, 5th ed, pp 48–51. New York, McGraw-Hill, 1993

LI-FRAUMENI

Synonyms. Sarcoma family Li-Fraumeni; LFS; Germline P53 mutation: SBLA (Sarcoma-brain, breast-leukemia, laryngeal, lung-adrenal).

Symptoms and Signs. Familial occurrence of a spectrum of cancers: breast, soft tissue sarcomas, brain, bones, leukemia, adrenocortical carcinoma, and other types and location. Development of malignant changes at early age.

Etiology. Autosomal dominant inheritance. Incidental finding: germ line mutation in P53 gene.

Prognosis. Risk of malignant evolution 50% for age 30; 90% for age 70.

BIBLIOGRAPHY. Li FP, Fraumeni JF: Rhabdomyosarcoma in children: An epidemiologic study and indentification of a familial cancer syndrome. J Noct Cancer Inst 43:1364–1373, 1969
Li FP, Fraumeni JF Jr, Mulvihill JJ, et al: A cancer family syndrome in twenty four kindreds. Cancer Res 48:53–58, 1988
Birch JM, Hartley AL, Blair V, et al: Identification of factors associated with high breast cancer risk in the mother of children with soft tissue sarcoma. J Clin Oncol 8:583–590, 1990

LIGAND-DEFECTIVE APO B, FAMILIAL

Synonyms. Familial defective apo B.

Symptoms and Signs. Asymptomatic.

Etiology. Defects of the ligand in apo B for LDL receptor.

Diagnostic Procedures. *Blood.* Hyperlipidemia, moderate hypercholesterolemia, and only LDL and not VLDL remnants accumulate.

Therapy. Restriction of dietary fats with adequate amount of fatty acids, vitamin E and A.

BIBLIOGRAPHY. Vega GL, Grundy SM: In vivo evidence for reduced binding of low density lipoproteins to receptors as a cause of primary moderate hypercholesterolemia. J Clin Invest 78:1410–1414, 1986
Kane JP, Havel RJ: Disorders of the biogenesis and secretion of lipoproteins containing the B apolipoproteins. In Scriver CR, Beaudet AL, Sly WS, et al: The Metabolic and Molecular Bases of Inherited Disease, 7th ed, p 1871. New York, McGraw-Hill, 1995

LIGHT ERUPTION, POLYMORPHOUS

Synonyms. Solar dermatitis; solar eczema; polymorphic light eruption. See Magnus and Solar elastosis.

Symptoms. All races, both sexes affected; onset at any age; it becomes manifest in spring and early summer and diminishes later in the year. After exposure to the sun, the latent period ranges from hours to a week. Itching.

Signs. In areas exposed to the sun, usually on the face, triangle of neck, and arms, formation of small papules or vescicular papules (hydroa aestivalis) or large diskoid plaque resembling those observed in erythema multiforme or lupus erythematosus.

Etiology. Phototoxicity (most active wavelength, 290–320 μ).

Pathology. Dermal inflammatory response.

Diagnostic Procedures. *Skin test.* With light to assess active wavelength.

Therapy. Avoidance of sun exposure during season. Antimalarial drugs intermittently; protection with topical cream and lotions. Severe forms: systemic corticosteroids; in case of disabling, unremitting forms azathioprine.

Prognosis. Tendency to yearly recurrence without improvement or increase in severity. Severe unremitting forms reported.

BIBLIOGRAPHY. Anderson D, Wallace HJ, Howes EIB: Juvenile spring eruption. Lancet I:755–756, 1954
McGrae JDV, Perry HO: Chronic polymorphic light eruption: A review. Arch Dermatol 43:364–379, 1963
Norris PG, Murphy GM, Hawk JL, et al: A histological study of the evolution of solar urticaria. Arch Dermatol 124:80–83, 1988
Hawk JLM: Cutaneous photobiology. In Champion RH, Burton JL, Ebling FJG (eds): Rook/Wilkinson/Ebling Textbook of Dermatology, 5th ed, pp 856–857. Oxford, Blackwell Scientific, 1992

LIGHTWOOD-ALBRIGHT

Obsolete.

Synonyms. Albright III; Butler-Albright; renal tubular acidosis (I, II, and IV). Old eponym for renal tubular acidosis (see individual syndromes).

BIBLIOGRAPHY. Lightwood R: Calcific infarction of the kidneys in infants. Communication. Proc Br Paediatr Soc Arch Dis Child 10:205–206, 1935
Albright F, et al: Metabolic studies and therapy in a case of nephrocalcinosis with rickets and dwarfism. Bull Johns Hopkins Hosp 66:7–33, 1940

LIJO PAVIA

Synonym. Retinohypophyseal (obsolete).

Symptoms. Onset at all ages, more frequent in women. Headache; psychic disturbances; vertigo and diminution of vision. Atypical alteration of visual field.

Signs. Narrowing of retinal vessel; optic neuritis; optic atrophy.

Etiology and Pathology. Unknown.

Diagnostic Procedures. *Urine.* Glycosuria. *X-ray of skull.* Alteration of bone structure of sella turcica with decalcification and osteolysis of posterior clinoid processes.

Therapy. Gonadotrophic hormone injection.

Prognosis. With treatment, vision only slightly improved, but increase of well-being remarkable.

BIBLIOGRAPHY. Lijo Pavia J: Sindrome retinohipofisario tratado por la gonadotropina suérica: Cuatro neuvas observaciones. Rev Oto Neuro Oftal 22:5–9, 1947
Lijo Pavia J, Lis M: Sindrome retinohipofisario binigno. Sobre 30 observaciones. Rev Oto Neuro Oftal 24:41–45, 1949; 73–76, 1949

LILLIPUTIAN

Synonym. Leroy; micropsia.

Symptoms and Signs. Occurs in patients suffering from acute infection, toxic delirium (from drugs or alcohol), dementia, or traumatic brain injuries. Visual aura, where little people appear, usually with offensive attitude. Left-sided hemianopia; transient deviation of head and eyes to the left.

Etiology. Psychovisual phenomenon correlated to brain alteration. The Bonnet Syndrome (see) is similar to the Lilliputian hallucination.

BIBLIOGRAPHY. Kauders O: Drehbewegungen um die Körperlangsachse, Hallucination im hemianopischen Gesichtsfeld als Folge eines Schädeltraumas. Z Ges Neurol Psychiatr 98:602–614, 1925
Leroy E: Les Visions du Demi-Sommeil. Paris, Alcan, 1926
Brown JW: Hallucinations Imagery and microstructure of perception. In Vinken PJ, Bruyn GW (eds): Handbook of Clinical Neurology, vol 45, p 358. Amsterdam, North-Holland, 1984

LINGUA NIGRA

Synonym. Black hairy tongue.

Symptoms. Occurs only in adults. Usually, asymptomatic; in some cases tickling of mouth and retching.

Signs. Proliferation of papillae on the dorsum of tongue, assuming colors that vary from yellow brown to black.

Etiology. Unknown. In some cases, related to antibiotics; in others, to poor oral hygiene or smoking.

Pathology. Hyperplasia of filiform papillae (up to 2 cm) with increased pigmentation.

Therapy. Oral hygiene; gentle brushing with soft toothbrush, after application of strong (long-steeped) tea or 40% solution of urea, or sucking a peach stone.

Prognosis. Condition may persist for months or years.

BIBLIOGRAPHY. Tomaszewski W: Incidence of black tongue in antibiotic treatment. Br Med J I:1249–1251, 1953

Scully C: The oral cavity. In Champion RH, Burton JL, Ebling FJG (eds): Rook/Wilkinson/Ebling Textbook of Dermatology, 5th ed, p 2742. Oxford, Blackwell Scientific, 1992

LIPOMATOSIS, MULTIPLE

Synonyms. Roch-Léri; Blascko; lipomatosis mesosomatic; systemic multicentric lipoblastosis; metastasizing lipoma.

Symptoms and Signs. Onset from puberty to 40 years of age. Slow development of subcutaneous masses. Occasionally gastrointestinal tract may be involved. From personal observations: Usually the development may be accompanied by local prurigo, that with time subsides, and some hardening and volume reduction may be observed. Final dimension is variable, but usually contained at a maximum to that of a large egg.

Etiology. Autosomal dominant inheritance. Chromosomal abnormalities have been observed. Four main cytogenetic subtypes recognized: normal kariotype; rearrangement of 12q13–q14; ring chromosomes; other clonal changes.

Pathology. Nonencapsulated fat growth, affecting (in scattered and disordered pattern) subcutaneous tissue, internal cavity, organs, and bones. Predominance of mature fat cells with transitional forms; lack of cellular anarchy and mitotic figures suggesting neoplastic process.

Diagnostic Procedures. *Biopsy.* Lipid biochemical studies.

Therapy. Excision of masses, affecting function or for esthetic reasons.

Prognosis. Long duration; years of the process. Tendency of fat tissue to regrow after excision.

BIBLIOGRAPHY. Blascko H: Eine seltene erbliche Lipombildung. Virchows Arch Path ANAT 124:175, 1891

Rabbiosi G, Borroni G, Scuderi N: Familial multiple lipomatosis. Acta Dermatol Venerol 57:265–267, 1977

Sreekantaiah C, Leong SPL, Karakousis CP, et al: Cytogenetic profile of 109 lipomas. Cancer Res 51:422–433, 1991

Burton JL, Cunlife WJ: Subcutaneous fat. In Champion RH, Burton JL, Ebling FJG (eds): Rook/Wilkinson/Ebling Textbook of Dermatology, 5th ed, p 2162. Oxford, Blackwell Scientific, 1992

LIPOPROTEIN LIPASE INHIBITOR, FAMILIAL

Symptoms and Signs. Both sexes, From asymptomatic to cases with recurrent abdominal pain following the ingestion of fat and eruptive xanthomas. Symptoms respond to severe fat ingestion restriction.

Etiology. Autosomal dominant inheritance.

Diagnostic Procedures. *Blood.* Presence of chilomicronemia. Triglycerides very elevated. Inhibitor of LPL activity in plasma. Normal apoC-II does not correct lipid defect in protheparin plasma. Adipose-tissue LPL activity elevated.

Therapy. Fat restriction.

Prognosis. Good with treatment.

BIBLIOGRAPHY. Brunzell JD, Miller NE, Alaupovic P, et al: Familial chylomicronemia due to a circulating inhibitor of lipoprotein lipase activity. J Lipod Res 24:12, 1983

Brunzell JD: Familial lipoprotein lipase deficiency and other causes of the chylomicronemia syndrome. In Scriver CR, Beaudet AL, Sly WS, et al: The Metabolic and Molecular Bases of Inherited Disease, 7th ed, pp 1924–1925. New York, McGraw-Hill, 1995

LIPSCHUTZ

Synonyms. Ulcus vulve acutum.

Symptoms and Signs. Fifty percent of cases in adolescent girls. Onset acute, In the vulva single or sparse ulceration surrounded by reddish area with a dirty, adherent membrane, that detaches in a few days. Lymphoadenopathy.

Etiology. Associated with infections: typhoid, paratyphoid, infectious mononucleosis, etc.

Diagnostic Procedures. *Bacterial and viral tests. Blood. Immunological studies.*

Therapy. That of basic disease and local symptomatic.

Prognosis. Good.

BIBLIOGRAPHY. Lipschuetz B: Ueber Ulcus vulvae acutum. Wien Klin Wschr 31:461–464, 1918

Ive FA: The umbilical perianal and genital regions. In Champion RH, Burton JL, Ebling FJG (eds): Rook/Wilkinson/Ebling Textbook of Dermatology, 5th ed, pp 2848–2849. Oxford, Blackwell Scientific, 1992

LISCH

Synonyms. Iris; nystagmus (with or without) fundus flavimaculatus.

Symptoms and Signs. Both sexes. Isolated perlucid iris; horizontal nystagmus; fundus flavimaculatus (not constant).

Etiology. Autosomal dominant inheritance.

BIBLIOGRAPHY. Lisch K: Das syndrom des mit perluzider Iris gekoppelten hereditaeren Nystagmus. Ber Dtsch Ophthalmol Ges 77:795–797, 1980

LISKER

Synonym. Motor neuropathy (peripheral) autonomic dysfunction.

Symptoms and Signs. Distal, slowly progressive muscle weakness and hypotrophy beginning in childhood; evidence of autonomic dysfunction starting a few years later and consisting of profuse sweating, distal cyanosis related to cold weather, orthostatic hypotension, and achalasia appearing in the third decade of life.

Etiology. Autosomal recessive/dominant inheritance with reduced penetrance. The disease results from an abnormality of cholinergic innervation.

Pathology. Light and electron microscopic studies of a nerve specimen show nonspecific demyelinization.

Diagnostic Procedures. *Electromyography. Muscle biopsy. Upper gastrointestinal. X-ray.*

Therapy. Surgical correction of achalasia; symptomatic medical therapy.

Prognosis. Good quoad vitam; variable for the various disturbances.

BIBLIOGRAPHY. Lisker R, Garcia G, de la Rosa-Laris C, et al: Peripheral motor neuropathy associated with autonomic dysfunction in two sisters: New hereditary syndrome? Am J Med Genet 9:255–259, 1981

LISSAUER

Synonym. Paralysis of Lissauer. See Dementia paralytica.

Symptoms. Occurs in patients affected by dementia paralytica (see). Mild or severe strokes, usually following convulsive attacks and leaving hemiplegia, monoplegia, cranial nerve palsy, which after a short period partially or totally recede and leave only mild permanent defects.

Etiology and Pathology. See Dementia paralytica.

BIBLIOGRAPHY. Storch E: Ueber einige Fälle atypischer progressiver. Paralyse. Nach einem hinterlassenen Manuscript Dr. H. Lissauer. Mschr Psychiatr 9:401–434, 1901

Weitbrecht HJ: Psychiatrie im Grundriss 3. Aufl. Berlin, Springer, 1973

Adams RD, Victor M: Principles of Neurology, 5th ed, pp 623–627. New York, McGraw-Hill, 1993

LIST

Synonyms. Foraminal impaction; tonsillar herniation. See Arnold-Chiari and Klippel-Feil.

Symptoms. Recurrent headache; dizziness, tinnitus; nausea; stiffness of neck on exertion and after coughing; sneezing.

Signs. Absent or few neurologic signs.

Etiology and Pathology. Congenital malformation. Transitory tonsillar herniation because of minor foraminal malformation.

Diagnostic Procedures. *Spinal tap. X-ray. CT scan. MRI.*

Therapy. Surgical.

Prognosis. Good.

BIBLIOGRAPHY. Cushing H: Some experimental and clinical observations concerning states of increased intracranial tension. Am J Med Sci 124:375, 1902

List CF: Neurologic syndromes accompanying developmental anomalies of occipital bone, atlas, and axis. Arch Neurol Psychiatr 45:577–616, 1941

Michie I, Clark M: Neurological syndromes associated with cervical and craniocervical anomalies. Arch Neurol 18:241–247, 1968

Adams RD, Victor M: Principles of Neurology, 5th ed, p 560. New York, McGraw-Hill, 1993

LITTLE (W.J.)

Synonyms. Cerebral palsy; cerebral diplegia; infantile cerebral diplegia; cerebral paralysis infantilis. See Hemiplegia, infantile.

Symptoms. Both sexes affected; firstborn more frequently affected. Prematurity frequent. Onset at 6 months of age or later. Slow and delayed first motor milestones and speech development; paucity of voluntary movements; scissor-like gait.

Signs. Spasticity, sometimes limited to the legs. Tendon reflexes exaggerated; Babinski, Oppenheim, Gordon signs; clonus; spared abdominal reflexes. In double hemiplegia, bilateral paresis and spasticity more severe in upper extremities. Focal damage signs possibly present. Athetosis and chorea may be present; frequently generalized seizures; frequently mental deficiency (however, remarkable intelligence possible).

Etiology. Widely differing. Prenatal, natal, and postnatal factors (see Pathology). Encephalitis; toxic defect in development.

Pathology. *Brain.* Small defects in individual gyri. Diffuse degenerative process or atrophic lobar sclerosis; gross malformations or developmental defects; grossly normal but pathologic alteration in neurons and cellular architecture.

Diagnostic Procedures. *X-ray. Angiography. Scintigraphy. CT brain scan.* Variable patterns of degenerative processes and primitive or secondary malformations.

Therapy. Pharmacologic control of convulsion. Antispastics (little effect). Orthopedic measures. Special schooling.

Prognosis. Poor.

BIBLIOGRAPHY. Little WJ: On the influence of abnormal parturition, difficult labour, premature birth, and asphyxia neonatorum on the mental and physical condition of the child, especially in relation to deformities. Trans Obstet Soc 3:293–344, 1862

Adams RD, Victor M: Principles of Neurology, 5th ed, pp 1037–1039. New York, McGraw-Hill, 1993

LITTRE

Synonyms. Hernia, Littre.

Symptoms and Signs. More common in men and on the right side. Hernia (50% inguinal, 20% femoral, 20% umbilical, 10% miscellaneous). When strangulation occurs: pain, fever while small bowel obstruction symptoms and signs are delayed.

Etiology. Hernia sac containing a Meckel diverticulum.

Therapy. Repair of hernia and excision of diverticulum.

Prognosis. Good with appropriate treatment.

BIBLIOGRAPHY. Littre A: Observation sur la nouvelle espace de hernia. Hist Acad Roy d Sc 1700, Paris 1719, pp 300–310

Zuniga D, Zupanec R: Littre's hernia. JAMA 237:1599, 1977

Cywes S, Millar JW: Embryology and anomalies of the intestine. In Haubrich WS, Schaffner F, Berk JE (eds): Bockus Gastroenterology, 5th ed, p 913. Philadelphia, WB Saunders, 1995

LIVEDO RETICULARIS

Synonyms. Feldacker-Hines-Kirland; O'Leary-Montgomery-Brunsting; asphyxia reticularis multiplex; dermatopathia pigmentosa reticularis; inflammatio cutis racemosa; livedo annularis; livedo racemosa; purple toes. Includes cholesterol microembolization (or multiple cholesterol emboly syndrome). See also Cutis marmorata and Sneddon.

Symptoms. Manifestation different according to etiology. Hereditary. Present from birth. Idiopathic. Occurs in young adults and middle-aged females. Secondary. Onset at all ages. In all forms, usually no symptoms except tingling or numbness on cold exposure.

Signs. Dilation of small vessels; reticular, blotchy red bluish discoloration of the skin of extremities (legs in particular); ulcerations; scaling.

Etiology. Variable: congenital; idiopathic; secondary to collagen and infective process; from chronic close exposure to heating sources, charcoal containers, or hot water bottles (ab igne); cold intensifies manifestations. Microcholesterol embolization; warfarin and related compounds.

Pathology. Pigmentary changes; scaling; ulcers.

Therapy. None satisfactory. Severe cases with ulceration are helped by anticoagulants.

Prognosis. Changes initially reversible when cause may be abolished, but subsequently vessel dilatation and skin changes become permanent. Congenital form may improve with growth.

BIBLIOGRAPHY. Unna PG: The Histopathology of the Diseases of the Skin. Walker N (trans). Edinburgh, Clay, 1896

O'Leary PA, Montgomery H, Brunsting LA: Livedo reticularis: Recurring ulcerations of the ankles in the summer. Arch Dermatol Syph 50:213, 1944

Champion RH: Reactions to cold. In Champion RH, Burton JL, Ebling FJG (eds): Rook/Wilkinson/Ebling Textbook of Dermatology, 5th ed, pp 837–839. Oxford, Blackwell Scientific, 1992

Hauben M: Letter. N Engl J Med 332:959, 1995

LIVER, MASSIVE NECROSIS

Synonyms. Acute fatty metamorphosis of the liver; parenchymatous hepatitis acute; microvesicular fat disease of liver; microsteatosis; icterus gravis; pregnancy, fatty metamorphosis of the liver; yellow liver atrophy;

includes acute fatty liver of pregnancy (AFLP). See Reye (R.K.D.) II; hepatorenal syndromes and H.E.L.L.P.

Symptoms. Occurs in young women in third trimester of pregnancy, earlier in case of eclampsia (or pre-eclampsia). Epigastric and right upper quadrant pain. Excessive fatigue; fainting episodes; nausea and vomiting. Later, confusion, disorientation, stupor, coma.

Signs. Jaundice.

Etiology. Unknown, but among possible etiologic agents: (1) Medications given to pregnant woman during third trimester of pregnancy, e.g., tetracyclines, especially intravenously; chlorothiazides; (2) overwhelming viral hepatitis during pregnancy; (3) lipotropic deficiency; (4) hepatotoxins.

Pathology. At autopsy, the main findings are in liver: centrolobular fatty metamorphosis; occasionally, hepatocellular necrosis.

Diagnostic Procedures. *Blood.* Total serum bilirubin increased. *Liver profile.* Liver function deterioration. Liver biopsy contraindicated.

Therapy. Liver transplant.

Prognosis. Fatal outcome in majority of cases.

BIBLIOGRAPHY. Peters RL, Edmondson HA, Kunelis CT: Acute fatty metamorphosis of the liver in pregnancy. JAMA 180:767, 1962
Czernobilsky B, Bergnes MA: Acute fatty metamorphosis of the liver in pregnancy with associated liver cell necrosis. Obstet Gynecol 26:792–798, 1965
Pockros PJ, Esrason KT: Microvesicular fat diseases of liver (microsteatosis). In Haubrich WS, Schaffner F, Berk JE (eds): Bockus Gastroenterology, 5th ed, vol 2, pp 2254–2275. Philadelphia, WB Saunders, 1995

LIVER PELIOSIS

Synonyms. Liver angiomatosis; hepatic peliosis; peliosis hepatis; purpura hepatis; sinusoidal ectasia (closely related condition).

Symptoms and Signs. Markedly variable. Hepatomegaly and jaundice main features.

Etiology. In the past associated mainly with neoplastic marasmus or tuberculosis; today associated with contraceptive pill and prolonged androgenic steroid treatment; attributed also to azathioprine treatment in a patient with kidney transplant. Possibly, direct toxic mechanism acting on lining cells of sinusoids.

Pathology. In liver; cavernous cysts filled with blood in continuity with the sinusoids. Minor changes of the hepatocytes contiguous to the cysts.

Diagnostic Procedures. *Biopsy of liver.* Caution: danger of hemorrhagic complication. *Liver scan.* Isotopes; ultrasound.

Therapy. Symptomatic. Discontinuation of previous therapy.

Prognosis. Related mainly to basic condition, possibility, however, of progression to hepatic failure.

BIBLIOGRAPHY. Zak FG: Peliosis hepatis. Am J Pathol 26:1–15, 1950
Zafrani ES, Pinaudeau Y, Dhumeaux D: Drug induced vascular lesions of the liver. Arch Int Med 143:495–503, 1983
Sabiston DC: Textbook of Surgery, 14th ed, p 1007. Philadelphia, WB Saunders, 1991
Waters B, Riely CA, Drug- and chemical-induced liver disease. In Haubrich WS, Schaffner F, Berk JE (eds): Bockus Gastroenterology, 5th ed vol 2, pp 2177–2178. Philadelphia, WB Saunders, 1995

LLOYD

Eponym used to indicate the association of pituitary, parathyroid, and pancreatic adenomas. See Wermer.

BIBLIOGRAPHY. Lloyd PC: A case of hypophyseal tumor with associated tumorlike enlargement of the parathyroides and islands of Langerhans. Bull John Hopkins Hosp 45:1–14, 1929

LOBAR EMPHYSEMA

Synonyms. Congenital lobar emphysema, including Hislop-Reid syndrome.

Symptoms and Signs. Male predominance (3:1); onset at birth in 30% of cases, in the remainder, onset after some weeks, occasionally months, of life. Respiratory distress; cyanosis in severe forms; thoracic asymmetry (unilateral overinflation); breath sounds reduced; rales and local wheeze; tachypnea.

Etiology. Lobar emphysema caused by congenital malformations; vascular type; idiopathic (e.g., unrecognized infection); absence or hypoplasia or bronchial cartilage; gigantism of pulmonary acini (Hislop-Reid syndrome). Familial cases, autosomal dominant inheritance.

Pathology. Severe overinflation of pulmonary lobe with predilection for left upper lobe and, slightly less, for right middle lobe.

Diagnostic Procedures. *X-ray.* Overinflation of a particular lobe; depression of corresponding hemidiaphragm and mediastinum displacement; vascular markings in the lobe are separated. Usually hyperlucency of affected lobe; occasionally, increased density (impaired fluid drainage). *Cardiac catheterization. Angiography.*

Therapy. Surgery according to evolution, or supportive therapy.

Prognosis. Usually, course rapid and progressive; in many cases, spontaneous regression.

BIBLIOGRAPHY. Sloan H: Lobar obstructive emphysema in infancy treated by lobectomy. J Thorac Cardiovasc Surg 26:1–20, 1953
Wall MA, Eisenberg JD, Campbell JR: Congenital lobar emphysema in a mother and daughter. Pediatrics 70:131–133, 1982
Weatherall DJ, Ledingham JGG, Warrell DA (eds): Oxford Textbook of Medicine, 3rd ed, p 2768. Oxford, Oxford Med Pub, 1996

LOCKED-IN SYNDROME

Synonym. De-efferentation. See Krestschemer.

Symptoms. Paralysis of all four extremities and the lower cranial nerves without interference with consciousness. Possibility of maintaining the capacity to use vertical eye movements and blinking to communicate awareness of internal and external stimuli.

Etiology. Midbrain infection, pontine tumor, or hemorrhage; myelinolysis; head injury; polyneuritis; myasthenia gravis.

Pathology. Lesions of ventral and paramedian pontine tegmentum.

Diagnostic Procedures. *CT scan. Angiography. Transcranial Doppler. MRI.*

Prognosis. Poor.

Therapy. Same as for Krestschemer (see).

BIBLIOGRAPHY. Hawkes CH: Locked-in syndrome: Report of seven cases. Br Med J 4:379–382, 1976
Feldam MH: Physiological observation in a chronic case of locked-in syndrome. Neurology 21:459–478, 1978
Adams RD, Victor M: Principles of Neurology, 5th ed, pp 451, 3903. New York, McGraw-Hill, 1993

LOCKED LUNG

Synonym. Paradoxical bronchospasm; iatrogenic asthma.

Symptoms and Signs. Status asthmaticus unresponsive to adrenalin, steroids, aminophylline, and intermittent positive pressure treatment occurring in patients who use an excess of nebulized isoproterenol or analogs.

Etiology. Excessive exposure to nebulized isoproterenol determining a cumulative irritating effect on respiratory tract mucous membranes. No allergic factor seems involved, but a direct effect of the drug is responsible for the syndrome.

Therapy. Discontinuation of use of isoproterenol. Asthmatic patient should be advised to use only isoproterenol spray, as little as possible, preferably less than seven times a day. Other bronchodilator drugs have become available with beta-2-adrenergic selectivity, to be used alone or in combination, with prolonged action compared to isoproterenol.

Prognosis. Death may result from abuse of isoproterenol. Discontinuation of drug cures the condition. Reexposure to the drug in usual therapeutic doses after recovery does not induce discomfort.

BIBLIOGRAPHY. Keighley JF: Iatrogenic asthma associated with adrenergic aerosols. Ann Intern Med 65:985–995, 1966
Death from asthma (Annotation). Lancet I:1412–1413, 1968
Whitsett TL, Manion CV: Cardiac and pulmonary effects of therapy with albuterol and isoproterenol. Chest 74:251–255, 1978
Szefler Leung DYM (eds): Severe Asthma. New York, Marcel Dekker, 1995

LOEFFLER I

Synonyms. Idiopathic eosinophilic lung disease; transient eosinophilic pneumonia; ascaris lumbricoides infestation.

Symptoms. Malaise; anorexia; fever; cough; pain in the chest and dyspnea. Occasionally asymptomatic.

Signs. Pleural rales; pericardial effusion; prolonged expiration and wheezing.

Etiology. Infestation from ascaris lumbricoides or other parasites (Ancylostoma duodenale; Necator americanus; Toxocara canis; Toxocara cetis; Strongiloides stercoralis; Schistosoma species; Trichinella spiralis). Parasite eggs hatch in the intestine. Immigratory larval stage: travel through lung where eosinophilic inflammatory host response ensues. Larvae are ingested and mature parasites live in the intestine.

Pathology. Lung infiltration with eosinophils, giant cells, interstitial proliferation, serous exudation, and vascular alterations.

Diagnostic Procedures. *Blood.* Leukocytosis: 20,000 white blood cells, in great part eosinophils. *Sputum.* Rich in eosinophilis careful search may yield larvae. *X-ray of lung.* Migratory patchy infiltration.

Therapy. For ascaris lumbricoides mebendazole 100 mg b.i.d. for 3 days. In some cases short courses of corticosteroids.

Prognosis. Acute, self-limited form with benign outcome.

BIBLIOGRAPHY. Loeffler W: Zur Differential-diagnose der Lungeninfiltrierungen: ueber flüchtige Succedaninfiltrate (mit Eosinophilie). Beitraege Klin Tubercolose 79:338–367, 1932
Lynch JP, Flint A: Sorting out the pulmonary eosinophilic syndromes. J Respir 5:61, 1984
Lopez M, Salvaggio JE: Eosinophilic pneumonias. In Lynch JP, De Remmee RA: Immunologically Meditated Pulmonary Diseases, p 413. Philadelphia, Lippincott, 1991

LOEFFLER ENDOCARDITIS

Synonyms. Loeffler II; eosinophilic endomyocarditis; endomyocardial eosynophilia; obliterative myocardial.

Symptoms. Malaise; anorexia; fever; cough; pain in the chest and dyspnea. Occasionally asymptomatic.

Signs. Those of diastolic heart failure: pulmonary congestion, edema (eventually anasarca), pericardial effusion; murmurs of mitral and tricuspid regurgitation.

Etiology. Immunologic disorder caused by clones of abnormal eosinophils.

Pathology. Endocardial eosinophilic infiltration with adjacent necrosis, fibrosis, and successive occlusion of ventricles by scars and thrombi.

Diagnostic Procedures. *X-ray.* Biatrial enlargement pericardial and pleural effusion. Two-dimensional echocardigraphy: decreased volume of ventricles restrictive cardiomyopathy. *Biopsy.* Endomyocardial. Typical infiltration and pathological changes. *Blood.* Hypereosinophilia.

Therapy. Corticosteroids. Resection of endocardium.

Prognosis. Poor.

BIBLIOGRAPHY. Rindfleisch Inaugural Dissertation. Koenigsberg, 1898
Loeffler W: Endocarditis fibroplastica mit Bluteosinophilie. Ein eingenartiges Krankheitsbild Schw Med Wschr 66:817–820, 1936
Spry CJ, Tai PC: Studies on blood eosinophilia: 11 patients with Loeffler's cardiomyopathy. Clin Exp Immunol 24:423–434, 1976
Shabetai R: Restrictive cardiomyopathy. In Schlant RC, Alexander RW: Hurst's The Heart, 8th ed, p 1645. New York, McGraw-Hill, 1994

LOEHR-KINDBERG

Synonyms. Loeffler variant; subacute allergic pneumonia; eosinophilic pneumonia chronic (or subacute); pulmonary eosinophilia chronic.

Symptoms. Predominantly in women. High fever; malaise; dyspnea; occasionally, hemoptysis.

Signs. All features of pneumonia with slow resolution. Weight loss.

Etiology. Unknown; atopic background common, but not always demonstrated.

Pathology. Massive infiltration of alveolar walls by polymorphonuclear leukocytes, especially eosinophils and macrophages, histiocytes, lymphocytes. In some cases, mild angitis and granulomas.

Diagnostic Procedures. *Blood.* Eosinophilia (frequently, but not always). Pulmonary function test. Nonconstant reduced diffusing capacity. *X-ray.* See Loeffler.

Therapy. Corticosteroids.

Prognosis. Prompt and dramatic response to treatment. Clinical resolution in 3–10 days of onset of therapy. Chronic evolution without specific treatment.

BIBLIOGRAPHY. Loehr H: Ueber flöchtige Lungeninfiltrierungen mit und ohne Eosinophilie des Blutes. Z Klin Med 137:297, 1940
Kindberg LM: Pneumopathie à eosinophiles. Presse Med 48:277–278, 1940
Christoforidis AJ, Molnar W: Eosinophilic pneumonia: Report of two cases with pulmonary biopsy. JAMA 173:157–161, 1960
Lynch JP, Flint A: Sorting out of pulmonary eosinophilic syndromes. J Respir Dis 5:61, 1984
Weatherall DJ, Ledingham JGG, Warrell DA (eds): Oxford Textbook of Medicine, 3rd ed, pp 2804–2808. Oxford, Oxford Med Pub, 1996

LOEWENTHAL

Synonym. Myosclerosis of Loewenthal. See artrogryposis multipla.

Symptoms and Signs. Present from birth. Hyperhidrosis; atony of limbs; flaccidity or poorly developed muscles; joint hyperextension; rhizomelic contractures; reduced movements; blepharoptosis.

Etiology. Unknown. Congenital hereditary condition. Entity discussed. Manifestation may be attributed to trauma.

Diagnostic Procedures. *Biopsy of muscle.* Sclerosis of connective tissue and of subcutaneous fat as well. *X-ray.* Kyphoscoliosis; spurs on calcaneus.

Therapy. Orthopedic.

Prognosis. Gradual spontaneous improvement from birth.

BIBLIOGRAPHY. Loewenthal A. Une groupe heredodegenerative nouveau: le myoscleroses heredofamiliales. Acta Neurol Belg 54:155–165, 1954
Loewenthal A: Étude sur les myosites. IV. Sur une forme congénitalisée avec blépharoptose (contribution à l'étude des maladies congénitales des muscles et du tissue conjonctif). Acta Neurol Belg 52:141–145, 1952
Walton J, Karpati G, Hilton-Jones D: Disorders of Voluntary Muscle, p 794. Edinburgh, Churchill Livingstone, 1994

LÖFGREN

Synonym. Hilar bilateral lymphadenopathy. BHI. See Besnier-Boeck-Schaumann and erythema nodosum.

Symptoms and Signs. Prevalent in females, especially during pregnancy or puerperium. Fever; erythema nodosum; signs of bilateral enlargement of mediastinal lymph nodes.

Etiology. Sarcoidosis leading cause. In Hodgkin syndrome, viral, bacterial, or atypical tuberculosis infections.

Diagnostic Procedures. *X-ray of chest.* Bilateral enlargement of mediastinal lymph nodes, sometimes, also right paramediastinal glands. *Kveim test.* Frequently positive. *Tuberculin test.* Negative or weak. *Biopsy of lymph node and liver.*

Therapy. According to Etiology.

Prognosis. Benign course, that subsides in 3 weeks (mild) or 6 weeks (severe). Exceptionally, recurrences after these periods. Fatigue and general depression may continue for months.

BIBLIOGRAPHY. Löfgren S: Erythema nodosum: Studies on etiology and pathogenesis in 185 adult cases. Acta Med Scand (suppl) 174:1–197, 1946
Weatherall DJ, Ledingham JGG, Warrell DA (eds): Oxford Textbook of Medicine, 3rd ed, p 2821. Oxford, Oxford Med Pub, 1996

LOIN PAIN, HEMATURIA

Symptoms. Occurs in young women (19–34 years of age). Repeated attacks of unilateral or bilateral (nonradiating) intense, and usually incapacitating, loin pain of variable duration, from 2 days to 2 weeks, followed by hematuria. Low-grade fever.

Signs. Loin tenderness.

Etiology. Unknown. Relationship to treatment with estrogen compounds, and to consistent renal angiographic abnormalities (intravascular coagulation within the kidneys).

Pathology. *Kidney biopsy.* Normal glomeruli. Thickening of interlobular arteries with deposit of C3 but not Ig. *Arteriography.* Narrowing of intrarenal vessels.

Diagnostic Procedures. *Urine.* Mild proteinuria. *Blood.* Platelet factor 3 availability increased and platelet life span diminished; heparin-thrombin clotting time reduced. *X-ray.* Renal arteriography shows abnormalities of smaller vessels and local variations in the rate and flow of contrast.

Therapy. Suspension of estrogens or warfarin or both.

Prognosis. Good with treatment.

BIBLIOGRAPHY. Little PJ, Sloper JS, de Wardener HE: A syndrome of loin-pain and hematuria associated with disease of peripheral renal arteries. Q J Med 36:253–259, 1967
Burden RP, Dathan JR, Etherington MD, et al: The loin pain syndrome. Lancet I:897–900, 1974
Glassock RJ: Hematuria and pigmenturia. In Massry SG, Glassock RJ: Textbook of Nephrology, 3rd ed, pp 557–566. Baltimore, Williams & Wilkins, 1995

LONDSDALE-BLASS

Synonyms. Pyruvate dehydrogenase complex deficiency; PDHC deficiency, PDC deficiency; pyruvate decarboxylase deficiency; ataxia intermittent lactic acidosis I; thiamine responsive lactic acidemia; cerebellar ataxia, intermittent; hyperalaninemia—hyperpyruvatic acidemia.

Symptoms. Both sexes. Attacks of intermittent ataxia, and choreoathetosis precipitated by acute infections; carbohydrate intolerance; failure to thrive; severe psychomotor retardation; blindness

Signs. Microcephaly, optic atrophy, hypotonia.

Etiology. Autosomal recessive inheritance. Deficiency of pyruvate dehydrogenase complex in all tissue.

Pathology. At autopsy, brain with reduced white and gray matter.

Diagnostic Procedures. *Blood.* Lactate acidosis. Assay for PDHC.

Therapy. Low carbohydrate diet; thiamine in large doses; sodium benzoate in neonate with hyperammoniemia.

Prognosis. In severe cases, death in first decade. In less severe cases, normal life expectancy.

BIBLIOGRAPHY. Lonsdale D, Faulkner WR, Price DL, et al: Intermittent cerebellar ataxia associated with hyperpyruvic acidemia, hyperphenylalaninemia and hyperalaninuria. Pediatrics 43:1025–1034, 1969
Blass JP, Avigan J, Uhlendorf BW: A defect in pyruvate decarboxylase in a child with intermittent movement disorder. J Clin Invest 49:423–432, 1970
Robinson BH: Lactic acidemia. In Scriver CR, Beaudet AL, Sly WS, et al: The Metabolic and Molecular Bases of Inherited Disease, 7th ed, p 1490. New York, McGraw-Hill, 1995

LONG CHAIN 3-HYDROXYACYL COA DEHYDROGENASE DEFICIENCY

Synonyms. LCHAD deficiency; hydroxyacyl CoA dehydrogenase deficiency.

Symptoms and Signs. From birth. Encephalopathy; feeding difficulties; failure to thrive; lowered consciousness; myopathy; cardiomyopathy.

Etiology. Deficiency of long chain 3-hydroxyacyl CoA dehydrogenase that does not allow metabolization of long chain fatty acid. Autosomal dominant inheritance, may be defect on chromosome 7.

Pathology. *Muscle.* Myopathy with carnitine deficiency and lipid storage.

Diagnostic Procedures. *Blood.* Hypoketosis, hypoglycemia. Serum signs of hepatic dysfunction. *Urine.* Long chain urinary decarboxylic acids with hydroxyl group in 3 position.

Therapy. Diet enriched medium chain tryglicerides.

Prognosis. Sudden infant death. Better with therapy.

BIBLIOGRAPHY. Glasgow AM, Engel AG, Bier DM, et al: Hypoglycemia, hepatic dysfunction, muscle weakness, cardiomyopathy free carnitine deficiency and long chain acylcarnitine excess responsive to medium chain triglyceride diet. Pediatr Res 17:319–326, 1983

Jackson S, Bartlett K, Land J, et al: Long-chain 3–hydroxyl acyl CoA dehydrogenase deficiency. Pediatr Res 29:406–411, 1991

Scriver CR, Beaudet AL, Sly WS, et al: The Metabolic and Molecular Bases of Inherited Disease, 7th ed, pp 1501–1502. New York, McGraw-Hill, 1995

LONGER LEG

Synonyms. Leg discrepancy; lower limb length discrepancy. See hemihypertrophy.

Symptoms. Fifteen percent of population have a leg length disparity of 1 cm or more. Patients with 0.5–1 cm usually present no symptoms or may have the same symptoms as patients with larger disparity. Pain in buttock, thigh, sometimes low back, knee, occasionally calf.

Signs. Leg length disparity. Five types of discrepancies have been classified according to slope pattern versus age, from continuous increase to various patterns of deceleration.

Etiology. Various causes. Idiopathic congenital short femur; coxa vara; proximal femoral focal deficiency; epiphyseal destruction; Ollier (see) anisomelia; hemihypertrophy (see); hemoangiomatosis; poliomyelitis; juvenile rheumatoid arthritis; neurofibromatosis syndromes (see); Legg-Calvé-Perthes (see); septic arthritis of hip; fractures.

Diagnostic Procedures. Serial observation at 6-month intervals initially and later at 12-month intervals. Teleoroentgenograms (before 5 years of age) and orthoroentgenograms at older age.

Therapy. According to diagnosis of basic disorder and age of patients.

Prognosis. Variable according to basic disorder and stage of evolution.

BIBLIOGRAPHY. Codivilla A: On the means of lengthening in the lower limbs, the muscle and tissues which are shortened through deformity. Am J Orthop Surg 2:353–370, 1905

Beaty JH: Congenital anomalies of lower extremities. In Crenshaw AH (ed): Campbell's Operative Orthopedics, 7th ed, pp 2683–2703. St Louis, CV Mosby, 1987

LONG Q-T SYNDROMES

Congenital. See Jervell-Lange-Nielsen (1) and Romano-Ward (2).

Acquired (1) due to class 1 antiarrhythmic drugs, tricyclic antidepressants, and phenothiazines. (2) Electrolyte abnormalities; myocarditis; acute ischemia; cardiomyopathies; mitral valve prolapse syndrome (rarely).

BIBLIOGRAPHY. Locati E, Moss AJ, Schwartz PJ, et al: The long Q-T syndrome. J Am Coll Cardiol 3:516, 1984

Towbin JA, Roberts R: Cardiovascular diseases due to genetic abnormalities. In Schlant RC, Alexander RW: Hurst's The Heart, 8th ed, p 1745. New York, McGraw-Hill, 1994

LONG THUMB, BRACHYDACTYLY

Synonym. Brachydactyly; long thumb.

Symptoms and Signs. Both sexes. From birth. Limitation of hand motion (inability to form fist). Symmetric brachydactyly; long thumbs; fifth finger clinodactyly. Shoulders (limitation of rotation), pectus excavatum. Rhizomelic shortness of limbs. Murmur of pulmonic stenosis; apparent cardiomegaly, possible cardiac conduction defects.

Etiology. Consistent with autosomal dominant inheritance.

Therapy. Symptomatic.

Prognosis. Rhizomelic shortness does not produce shortness of stature, but only reduced length of arms.

BIBLIOGRAPHY. Hollister DW, Hollister WG: The "long-thumb" brachydactyly syndrome. Am J Med Genet 8:5–16, 1981

LORAIN-LEVI

Synonyms. Brissaud III; Brissaud-Meigs; Levi; Nebecourt; snubnosed dwarfism; dwarfism snubnosed; essential microsomia. See also Gilford-Burnier.

Symptoms. History of normal growth with successive periods of impaired growth; delayed puberty; precocious senility; hypoglycemic attacks.

Signs. Relatively normal proportions; face childish; skin dry, loose, wrinkled; sparse subcutaneous fat; dwarfism.

Etiology. Lack or deficient secretion of growth hormone; lesions involving pituitary (cyst; craniopharyngioma; idiopathic fibrosis). The distinction between sexual ateleiosis and primordial short stature is not clear. Possibly autosomal recessive inheritance.

Pathology. Craniopharyngioma (most common lesion); suprasellar cysts; fibrosis of pituitary gland.

Diagnostic Procedures. *Urine.* Absence of gonadotrophin. *Blood.* Reduced protein-bound iodine; hypoglycemia; subnormal elevation of plasma corticoid level after intravenous adrenocorticotropic hormone (ACTH) injection. *X-ray.* Delayed fusion of epiphyses; destruction of sella turcica by tumor or cyst.

Therapy. Growth hormone, thyroid hormone, and gonadal steroid.

Prognosis. Spectacular results with growth hormone treatment. Some results with thyroid and gonadal steroids alone. Depends on etiology.

BIBLIOGRAPHY. Lorain PJ quoted in Faneau de la Cour, Ferdinand-Valére: Du féminisme et de l'infantilisme chez les tuberculeux, No 1 Paris, 1871

Levi E: Contribution à l'étude de l'infantilisme du type Lorain. Nouv Icon Saltpetriére 21:297–324;421–471, 1908

Soyka LF, Ziskind A, Crawford JD: Treatment of short stature in children and adolescents with human pituitary growth hormone. N Engl J Med 271:754, 1964

Bailey JA: Disproportionate Short Stature: Diagnosis and Management. Philadelphia, WB Saunders, 1973

LORTAT-JACOB-DEGÓS

Synonyms. Duhring-Brocq variant; mucosynechial dermatitis; mucosynechial atrophic bullous dermatitis; ocular pemphigus; cicatricial pemphigoid; benign pemphigoid mucosal.

Symptoms and Signs. Prevalent in women (2:1); onset (on average) over 65 years of age. Recurrent bullae of mucosal and skin zones adjacent to body orifices. Conjunctivae affected in 75% of patients. Bullae eventually break and leave erosions slow to heal. No severe discomfort.

Etiology. Unknown. Gluten-sensitive enteropathy in majority of patients. Its role on the dermopathy, however, has not been established yet.

Pathology. Subepidermal bullae; no acantholysis. Infiltration of derma by lymphocytes, plasma cells, and eosinophils leading to fibrosis.

Therapy. Dapsone, sulfapyridine, if dapsone not tolerated; gluten-free diet; corticosteroids of little use; skin grafting for persistent erosions.

Prognosis. Scar formation after healing; adhesions may develop.

BIBLIOGRAPHY. Lortat-Jacob E: Benign mucosal pemphigoid: Dermatite bulleuse muco-synéchante et atrophiante. Br J Dermatol 70:361–367, 1958

Mitchell RD, Smith NH: Cicatricial pemphigoid: A review of 11 cases. Austr Dent J 24:260–265, 1979

LOUIS-BAR

Synonyms. Border-Sedgwick; ataxia-telangiectasia syndrome I; cephalo—oculocutaneous—telangiectasia; cerebello—cutaneous—telangiectasia; teleangiectasia—ataxia I. See Paine-Efron.

Symptoms. Affects both sexes equally. Choreoathetosis beginning at early age; progressive ataxia; apraxia of ocular movement; seldom mental retardation (50%); repeated respiratory infections.

Signs. Telangiectasia of bulbar conjunctivae, zygomatic areas, palate, ears, and neck; antecubital and popliteal fossas showing at 4–6 years of age. (Patients without this sign are not uncommon.) Growth deficiency.

Etiology. Autosomal recessive inheritance. Basic defects involve immune mechanism, hypoplasia of thymus, and one or more enzymes involved in DNA reappearing or processing.

Pathology. Loss of Purkinje cells; degenerative lesions in cortex of cerebellum; venules dilated in cerebellar leptomeninges and white matter. Association of bronchiectasis. Thymus atrophic or absent. Lymphoid tissues devoid of lymphocytes.

Diagnostic Procedures. *CT brain scan. MRI.* Atrophy of cerebellum. *Blood.* Hypogammaglobulinemia; IgA low (50%); rarely, IgG low (5%); IgM normal; IgE low; 80–85% decrease in insulin receptor activity of circulating monocytes. Lymphopenia. *Urine.* Presence of unusual substance reported by Pelc and Vis.

Therapy. Symptomatic. X-ray treatment of malignancies may be fatal.

Prognosis. Slowly progressing; treatment of recurrent respiratory infection. High incidence of malignancy (reticuloendothelial system) with this condition.

BIBLIOGRAPHY. Louis-Bar D: Sur an syndrome progressif comprenant des télangiectasies capillaires cutanées et conjonctivales symétriques a disposition naevode et des troubles cérébelleux. Confin Neurol 4:32–42, 1941
Pelc S, Vis H: Ataxia familiale avec Telangiectasies oculaires. Acta Neurol Belg 60:905–922, 1960
Gatti RA, Boder E, Vinter HV, et al: Ataxia-telangiectasia: An interdisciplinary approach to pathogenesis. Medicine 70: 99–117, 1991
Adams RD, Victor M: Principles of Neurology, 5th ed, pp 821–822. New York, McGraw-Hill, 1993

LOUTIT

Obsolete eponym used to indicate autoimmune hemolytic anemia.

BIBLIOGRAPHY. Loutit FJ, Mollison PL: Hemolytic icterus (acholuric jaundice): Congenital and acquired. J Path Bact 58:711–728, 1946

LOWE

Synonyms. Lowe-Bickel; Lowe-Terrey-MacLachlan; organic aciduria; ammonia, reduced renal production; cerebro-oculorenal dystrophy; oculocerebrorenal dystrophy; renal-oculocerebrodystrophy.

Symptoms. Males affected (a few cases reported in females); symptoms apparent in very early infancy. Mental retardation; generalized hypotonia; hyperactivity with bizarre choreoathetoid movements and screaming. Blindness; no deafness; difficulty in feeding and thriving.

Signs. Striking resemblance of all affected children. Blond (except one Mexican patient). At younger age, chubby, then emaciation. Hypotonic; flabby musculature; areflexia or severe hyporeflexia. Cataracts, and in some congenital glaucoma. Joint hypermobility; cryptorchidism.

Etiology. Inherited metabolic error affecting only males and transmitted by heterozygous female (X-linked trait). Renal lesions appear as

secondary manifestation. Gene defect on X q25–q26. Renal lesions appear as secondary manifestations.

Pathology. No common features from general observation at autopsy. Histologically, kidney tubule dilatation, protein casts, interstitial fibrosis, glomeruli hyalinized, no inflammatory components. *Testes.* Increased interstitial fibrous tissue; diminution of size of tubules. *Eye.* Lenses are small (microphakia) and with wart-like excrescences of the capsule; small size of lens creates glaucoma through traction on ciliary processes and retards of poorer cleavage of anterior chamber. Suprachoroidal layer; prominence of vessels (dilatation); retinal abnormalities of ganglion cells. *Brain.* Diffuse alteration of cortex; tendency for vacuolization of subpial parenchyma; perivascular rarefaction. Proliferation of endothelial elements of arterioles with formation of granulation.

Diagnostic Procedures. *Blood.* Normal or slightly elevated nonprotein nitrogen; variable metabolic acidosis; serum chloride elevated, sodium and potassium normal or low. *Urine.* Usually dilute, but good concentration with fluid restriction. Intolerance to acid stress; organic aciduria; hyperaminoaciduria; proteinuria.

Therapy. Cataract extraction, control of glaucoma, speech and physical therapy. If needed anticonvulsant and control of acidosis and prevention of bone disease.

Prognosis. Poor; mental retardation and metabolic defects. The result of cataract surgery poor. Renal failure can occur in second to fourth decade.

BIBLIOGRAPHY. Lowe CU, Terrey M, MacLachlan EA: Organic aciduria, decreased renal ammonia production, hydrophthalmos and mental retardation. Am J Dis Child 83:164–184, 1952
Charnas LR, Nussbaum RL: The oculocerebrorenal syndrome of Lowe (Lowe syndrome). In Scriver CR, Beaudet AL, Sly WS, et al: The Metabolic and Molecular Bases of Inherited Disease, 7th ed, pp 3705–3716. New York, McGraw-Hill, 1995

LOWENBERG-HILL

Synonym. Pelizaeus-Merzbacher (adult type); leukodystrophy adult onset; multiple sclerosis-like; type IV Pelizaeus-Merzbacher. See Pelizaeus-Merzbacher.

Symptoms. Both sexes affected; onset in adulthood (fourth to fifth decades). Progressive, increasing tremor of head, jaw, extremities. Transitory attacks (not well definable) during which the patient becomes helpless. Mild depression.

Signs. Absence of abdominal reflexes; tendon hyperreflexia.

Etiology. Unknown; autosomal dominant or recessive.

Pathology. Incomplete patchy demyelinization (similar to carbon monoxide poisoning); dense fiber gliosis; perivascular sudanophilic microglia cells.

Diagnostic Procedures. *EEG. Spinal tap. CT brain scan. MR imaging.* Symmetric decrease of white matter density.

Therapy. Symptomatic.

Prognosis. Slow progression to complete incapacitation. Usually 20 year survival.

BIBLIOGRAPHY. Lowenberg K, Hill TS: Diffuse sclerosis with preserved myelin islands. Arch Neurol Psychiatr 29:1232–1245, 1933
Norman RM, Tingey AH, Harvey PW, et al: Pelizaeus-Merzbacher disease: A form of sudanophil leukodystrophy. J Neurol Neurosurg Psychiatr 29:521–529, 1966
Eldridge R, Anayotos CP, Schlesinger S, et al: Hereditary adult-onset leukodystrophy simulating chronic progressive multiple sclerosis. N Engl J Med 311:948–953, 1984
Zoghbi HY, Ballabio A: Pelizaeus-Merzbacher disease. In Scriver CR,

Beaudet AL, Sly WS, et al: The Metabolic and Molecular Bases of Inherited Disease, 7th ed, p 4581. New York, McGraw-Hill, 1995

LOWER LEG STASIS

Synonym. Gravitational leg; gravitational eczema.

Symptoms. Four times more frequent in women than in men. Burning; itching; pain; muscle cramps in the legs.

Signs. Dilatation and tortuosity of leg veins. Chronic edema; induration; ulceration; pigmentation; stasis; eczema, secondary contact dermatitis.

Etiology. Venous antigravitational failure resulting from incompetence of venous valves, a familial trait; postphlebitic lesions; increase in venous pressure.

Pathology. Elongation, tortuosity of veins; medial fibrosis; fragmentation of tunica elastica; disappearance or atrophy of valves.

Therapy. Bed rest; elastic stockings; sponge rubber dressing; injection of sclerosing solutions; high ligation or excision; skin grafting.

Prognosis. Good response to treatment.

BIBLIOGRAPHY. Bauer G: Pathophysiology and treatment of the lower leg stasis syndrome. Angiology 1:1–8, 1950
Burton JL: Eczema, lichenification, prurigo and erythroderma. In Champion RH, Burton JL, Ebling FJG (eds): Rook/Wilkinson/Ebling Textbook of Dermatology, 5th ed, pp 571–572. Oxford, Blackwell Scientific, 1992

LOWER NEPHRON NEPHROSIS

Of historical interest only. See acute tubular insufficiency.

BIBLIOGRAPHY. Strauss MB: Acute renal insufficiency due to lower nephron nephrosis. N Engl J Med 239:693–700, 1948

LOWN-GANONG-LEVINE

Synonyms. LGL; Clerc-Levy-Cristeco, CLP; coronary nodal rhythm; short P-R interval; short P-Q interval. Eponym used to indicate an electrocardiographic pattern: right P waves in leads II, III and a VF with short P-Q interval, and normal QRS complex. Clinically, this pattern may be observed in paroxysmal tachycardia. Experimentally, this pattern can be obtained by a stimulating electrode in the right atrium, in front of coronary sinus, close to the AV node.

Symptoms and Signs. Young patients. Both sexes. Paroxysmal supraventricular tachycardia or atrial fibrillation flutter. Sometimes ventricular tachycardia.

Etiology. Anomalous atrioventricular conduction pathways. Either reentry using the AV node or reentry using slow AV nodal pathways anterograde and a fast AV nodal pathway retrograde.

Diagnostic Procedures. *ECG.* Short P-R interval, narrow QRS complexes, various and/or arrhythmias.

Therapy. Antiarrhythmic drugs. Special precautions in using verapamil, diltiazem, or beta adrenergic blockers in patients with an accessory bypass tract.

Prognosis. In a small percentage sudden cardiac death.

BIBLIOGRAPHY. Clerc A, Levy R, Cristesco C: A propos du raccourcissement permanent de l'espace P-R de l'electrocardiogramme sans déformation du complexe ventriculaire. Arch Mal Coeur 31:569–582, 1938
Lown B, Ganong W, Levine S: The syndrome of short PR interval, normal QRS complex and paroxysmal rapid heart action. Circulation 8:693–706, 1952
Weiner I: Syndromes of Lown-Ganong-Levine and enhanced atrioventricular nodal conduction. Am J Cardiol 52:637–639, 1983
Gifford RW: Treatment of patients with systemic arterial hypertension. In Schlant RC, Alexander RW: Hurst's The Heart, 8th ed, p 1442. New York, McGraw-Hill, 1994

LOW OUTPUT

Synonyms. Heart forward failure; heart power failure.

Symptoms and Signs. Recognition from clinical data alone impossible. Diagnosis reached with the aid of monitoring equipment. Usually observed following cardiac surgery. Oliguria.

Etiology and Pathology. Inadequate cardiac output to meet the needs of tissues for oxygen and other nutrients. Increase of the vascular systemic resistences. Reductions of the cardiac pumping ability.

Diagnostic Procedures. Hemodynamic measurements; oxygen consumption. *Blood.* Lactic acid production; plasma catecholamine; pH. Cardiac index (CI): 2.2 $L/min/m^2$. Systemic vascular resistance (SVR): 1500 dyne sec/cm^3. Mixed venous O_2 saturation (SVO_2): 55%. O_2 consumption index (VO_2J): 100 $ml/mn/m^2$. Lactic acid 20 mg%.

Therapy. Digitalis; vasopressors; inotropes, vasodilators. Correction metabolic acidosis. Mechanical circulatory support.

Prognosis. Usually poor. If not given early after onset, vasopressors are frequently ineffective in preventing death.

BIBLIOGRAPHY. Lillehei RC, Dietzman RH, Block JH: Hypotension and low output syndrome following cardiopulmonary bypass. In Norman JC (ed): Cardiac Surgery, pp 437–456. New York, Appleton-Century-Crofts, 1967
Dietzman RH, Ersek A, Lillehei CW, et al: Low output syndrome, recognition and treatment. J Thorac Cardiovasc Surg 57:138–150, 1969
Ross J Jr: Assessment of cardiac function and myocardial contractility. In Schlant RC, Alexander RW, Hurst's The Heart, 8th ed, pp 487–502. New York, McGraw-Hill, 1994

LOWRY

Synonyms. Craniosynostosis—fibula aplasia.

Symptoms and Signs. Aplasia of fibulae in two brothers; craniosynostosis.

Etiology. Autosomal recessive inheritance.

BIBLIOGRAPHY. Lowry RB: Congenital absence of the fibula and craniosynostosis in sibs. J Med Genet 9:227–229, 1972

LOWRY-WOOD

Synonyms. Epiphyseal dysplasia—microcephaly—nystagmus.

Symptoms and Signs. Both sexes. At birth small babies; microcephaly; multiple epiphyseal dysplasia; nystagmus; short stature; mental retardation.

Etiology. Unknown. Autosomal recessive inheritance (?).

Diagnostic Procedures. *X-rays.* Small irregular epiphyses; square iliac bones; flattened acetabula.

BIBLIOGRAPHY. Lowry RB, Wood BJ: Syndrome of epihyseal dysplasia, short stature, microcephaly and nystagmus. Clin Genet 8:269–274, 1975
Nevin NC, Thomas PS, Hutchinson J: Syndrome of short stature,

microcephaly mental retardation and multiple epiphyseal dysplasia. Lowry-Wood syndrome. Am J Med Genet 24:33–39, 1986

LOW SALT

Synonyms. Cellular hypo-osmolality; essential hyponatremia.

Symptoms and Signs. Occurs in patient with advanced congestive heart failure (treated as well as untreated), protracted wasting diseases, malnutrition, or severe chronic infection in hospitalized and ambulatory elderly people (observed in 22.5% of chronically institutionalized patients). Muscle cramps; hyporeflexia; lethargy and seizures; laboratory diagnosis of hyponatremia; or same symptoms and signs as Schroeder. Lethargy; anorexia; disorientation; edema; ascites; pleural cavity fluid accumulation.

Etiology. Aging where a decline in hypothalamic-neurohypophyseal function is present is considered among the most frequent causes. Continuous potassium release from the cells with replacement by sodium ions. Not to be confused with Schroeder (see), which occurs in intensively treated congestive heart failure and presents the same clinical features. Observed also in: vasopressin disorders, aldosterone deficiency, pseudohypoaldosteronism, myxedema, 21-hydroxylase deficiency.

Pathology. *Kidney.* Decrement in nephron mass. Cells in hypothalamic paraventricular and supraoptic nuclei may exibit changes typical of hormonal enhanced synthesis.

Diagnostic Procedures. *Blood.* Low serum sodium and potassium; blood urea nitrogen normal; anemia, with decreased mean corpuscular red cell volume. *Hypoproteinemia.* Estimation of total body water and electrolytes reveals normal sodium values. *Urine.* May show increase in potassium. Decreased ability to maximally concentrate or dilute urine after challenges.

Therapy. Treatment of underlying disease and complication. Administration of sodium contraindicated; continuation of salt restriction; limitation of fluid intake. Ammonium chloride and potassium chloride; mercurial diuretics at long intervals, and with caution.

Prognosis. That of associated condition; persisting indefinitely in chronically ill patients.

BIBLIOGRAPHY. Vogl A: The low-salt syndrome in congestive heart failure. Am J Cardiol 3:192–198, 1959
La Rotonda ML, Grace WJ: The low salt syndrome: An extreme example in heart failure. Am J Cardiol 6:676–677, 1960
Packer M, Medina N, Yushak M: Correction of dilutional hyponatremia in severe chronic heart failure by converting enzyme inhibition. Ann Int Med 100:782–789, 1984
Schrier RW: Treatment of hyponatremia: Editorial retrospective. N Engl J Med 312:1121–1122, 1985
Blackman MR, Elahi D, Harman SM: Endocrinology and aging. In De Groot LJ (ed): Endocrinology 3rd ed, pp 2704–2705. Philadelphia, WB Saunders, 1995

LUBARSCH-PICK

Eponym used to indicate the association of macroglossia with primary amyloidosis, or amyloidosis syndromes (see).

BIBLIOGRAPHY. Königstein H: Ueber Amyloidose der Haut. Arch Dermatol Syph 148:330–383, 1925
Lubarsch O: Zur Kenntnis ungewöhnlicher Amyloidablagerungen. Virchows Arch (Pathol Anat) 271:867–889, 1929

LUBINSKY

Synonyms. Enamel—renal; amelogenesis imperfecta—nephrocalcinosis.

Symptoms and Signs. Amelogenesis imperfecta; lifelong nocturnal enuresis activity.

Etiology. Autosomal recessive inheritance.

Pathology. Punctate nephrocalcinosis.

Diagnostic Procedures. *Urine.* Calcium and phosphates excretion decreased over 24 hours and after acute load; decreased urine carboxyglutamic acid. *Blood.* Increased serum osteocalcin.

Therapy. That of renal failure.

Prognosis. Progressive deterioration of renal function

BIBLIOGRAPHY. Lubinsky M: Syndrome of amelogenesis imperfecta, nephrocalcinosis, impaired renal concentration and possible abnormality of calcium metabolism. Am J Med Genet 20:233–243, 1985
Taybi H, Lachman RS: Radiology of Syndromes, Metabolic Disorders, and Skeletal Dysplasias, 3rd ed. Chicago, Year Book, 1990

LUBS

Synonyms. Male pseudohermaphroditism, familial; male familial pseudohermaphroditism; androgen insensitivity; testicular feminization; dihydrotestosterone receptor deficiency. See pseudohermaphroditism, male, incomplete hereditary (type I).

Symptoms and Signs. Male pseudohermaphrodites. Signs variable with age. Enlarged clitoris; labia with scrotal characteristics containing testes; pseudohernia; urogenital sinus containing urethra. Female breast development and hair distribution. Phenotype voluptuously feminine.

Etiology. X-linked inheritance. Represents the most severe form in terms of changes among the variants toward the feminine end of the spectrum of male pseudohermaphroditism, hereditary (Type I). Endorgan unresponsiveness to androgen (see Seabright-Bantam). Autonomous recognition of this syndromic presentation should no longer be made; it is now considered as part of the group of incomplete androgen insensitivity syndromes.

Pathology. Presence of testicular tissue bilaterally with marked degree of Leydig-cell hyperplasia. Tubules appearance variable, usually with almost normal spermatogenesis. Epididymis; rete testis; vas deferens normal.

Diagnostic Procedures. *Biopsy of testis. Endocrine studies.* Lack of significant abnormalities. *Sex chromatin studies.* No chromatin positive cells. *Chromosome studies.*

Therapy. Removal of testes.

Prognosis. Good quoad vitam.

BIBLIOGRAPHY. Pallaillon NI: Observation d'hermaphroditisme. Bull Neur Soc Obstet Gynec (Paris) 123–130, 1891
Dieffenbach H: Familiarer Hermaphroditism. Inaugural Dissertation Stuttgart, 1912
Lubs HA, Vilar, O, Bergenstal DM: Familial male pseudohermaphroditism with labial testes and partial feminization: Endocrine studies and genetic aspects. J Clin Endocrinol Metab 19:1110–1120, 1959
Wilson JD, Carlson BR, Weaver DD, et al: Endocrine and genetic characterization of cousins with male pseudohermaphroditism: Evidence that the Lubs phenotype can result from a mutation that alters the structure of the androgen reception. Clin Genet 26:363–370, 1984
Forest MG: Diagnosis and treatment of disorders of sexual development. In De Groot LJ (ed): Endocrinology, 3rd ed, p 1921. Philadelphia, WB Saunders, 1995

LUCEY-DRISCOL

Synonyms. Lucey-Arias; hyperbilirubinemia, transient familial neonatal; breast feeding, jaundice included.

Symptoms and Signs. Both sexes; from birth. Rapidly progressive jaundice; after 7th–10th day, kernicterus. In some cases, sudden death.

Etiology. Unidentified inhibitor of uridine diphosphate (UDP) glucuronosyltransferase (probably arogestional steroid or presence in milk of other steroids that inhibit bilirubin conjugation). Reported families with possible autosomal recessive inheritance.

Pathology. At autopsy, kernicterus.

Diagnostic Procedures. *Blood.* Unconjugated hyperbilirubinemia up to 60–65 mg/dl. Maternal serum. Inhibitor of UDP glucuronosyltransferase.

Therapy. Phototherapy; exchange transfusion.

Prognosis. Death in some cases; in others, survival with or without neurological sequelae.

BIBLIOGRAPHY. Lucey JF, Arias IM, McKay RJ Jr: Transient familial neonatal hyperbilirubinemia. Am J Dis Child 100:787–789, 1960

Lucey JF, Driscol JJ: Physiological jaundice re-examined. In Saal-Korttsak A (ed): Kernicterus, p 29. Toronto, Univ of Toronto Press, 1961

Arias IM, Wolfson S, Lucey JF, et al: Transient familial neonatal hyperbilirubinemia. J Clin Invest 44:1442–1450, 1965

Grunebaum E, Amir J, Merlob P, et al: Breast mild (sic) jaundice, natural history, familial incidence and late neurodevelopmental outcome of the infant. Eur J Pediatr 150:267–270, 1991

LUDWIG

Synonym. Parapharyngeal abscess.

Symptoms and Signs. Most frequent in males; onset in childhood. Dysphagia; dyspnea; trismus; fever; malaise. Pharyngeal and laryngeal edema; cellulitis of the submaxillary region and oral cavity floor and tongue, and possibly extending to anterior part of neck. Tachycardia; occasionally, cyanosis.

Etiology. Severe pharyngitis usually caused by streptococci, less frequently by other infective agents; usually, secondary to tooth extraction, trauma of interior of mouth, dental caries, or paradental infections.

Pathology. Cellulitis with possible pus formation involving submaxillary ducts, sublingual space, fascial neck spaces.

Diagnostic Procedures. *Blood.* Polymorphonuclear leukocytosis. *Swab culture.* Streptococcus pyogenes frequently identified. *Ultrasonography.*

Therapy. Antibiotics. Surgery if needed.

Prognosis. Good with treatment. Possible complications: jugular thrombosis; mediastinitis; pneumonia; metastatic infection of myocardium; cavernous sinus; meninges.

BIBLIOGRAPHY. Ludwig D, et al: Ueber eine in neuere Zeit wiederholt beier vorgkommene Form von Halsentzündung. Med Corresp Wuertt Aerztl Vereims 6:21–25, 1836

Fliacher I, Peleg H, Joackims HZ: Mediastinitis and bilateral pneumothorax complicating a parapharyngeal abscess. Head Neck Surg 3:438, 1981

Weatherall DJ, Ledingham JGG, Warrell DA (eds): Oxford Textbook of Medicine, 3rd ed, pp 572, 1847. Oxford, Oxford Med Pub, 1996

LUEERS-SPATZ

Synonyms. Frontal atrophy, total.

Symptoms and Signs. Occurrence of spastic paraplegia in cases of Pick (see) in whom the absence of anterior horn lesions makes impossible the diagnosis of amyotrophic lateral sclerosis.

Etiology. See Pick.

Pathology. Extension to the motor area of the cortical atrophy.

BIBLIOGRAPHY. Lueers Th, Spatz H: Pickshe Krankheit. In Henke F, Lubarsch O, Roessle R, eds: Handbuch der speziellen pathologischen. Anatomie und Histologie, vol 13, p 636. Berlin, Springer, 1957

Bonduelle M: Amyotrophic lateral sclerosis. In Vinken PJ, Bruyn GW: Handbook of Clinical Neurology, vol 22, p 314. Amsterdam, North-Holland, 1975

LUETSCHER I

Synonyms. Fever dehydration; pure dehydration; dehydration; hypertonicity; dessication; transitory fever newborn; water depletion.

Symptoms. Thirst (this symptom may be missing in patient with cerebral lesions); inability to swallow dry food; weakness; weight loss; fever; change in personality (forced vivacity); hallucination; delirium.

Signs. Skin flushed; sweating decreased; xerostomia; lack of tears; tongue dry and fissured; skin doughy-feeling. Tachycardia, hyperpnea, and then coma (terminal signs).

Etiology and Pathology. (1) Lack of water; (2) difficulty in swallowing; (3) adipsia in debilitated infants because of cerebral lesions; (4) diabetes insipidus neurohypophyseal (see); (5) water-losing nephritis; (6) diarrhea (mild, especially in infants and young children); (7) hyperventilation or tracheostomy; (8) burns; (9) sudden water loading; (10) diabetes insipidus syndromes, antidiuretic hormone (ADH)-resistant (see).

Diagnostic Procedures. *Blood.* Early stage normal, then hemoconcentration (high hematocrit, serum electrolytes, and protein); high blood urea nitrogen. *Urine.* Small volume; high specific gravity (except if previous inability to concentrate); hematuria; proteinuria; casts.

Therapy. Water alone (if ion deficiency has been ruled out), orally or rectally, or intravenous isotonic solution, or intravenous 10% dextrose in water. One half replacement water and daily requirement given on first day; the remainder the second day. If diabetes insipidus, vasopressin; if vasopressin-resistant diabetes, drug of chlorothiazide group.

Prognosis. According to amount of water loss and pathogenetic mechanism; cases of 12% water loss, inability to swallow: 12–25% mortality.

BIBLIOGRAPHY. Luetscher JA Jr, Blackman SS Jr: Severe injury to kidneys and brain following sulfathiazole administration: High serum sodium and chloride levels and persistent cerebral damage. Ann Int Med 18:741–756, 1943

Schoolman HM, Dubin A, Hoffman WS: Clinical syndromes associated with hypernatremia. Arch Int Med 95:15–23, 1955

Opas LM, Lieberman E: Fluid and electrolyte disorders in infants and children. In Massry SG, Glassock RJ: Textbook of Nephrology, 3rd ed, pp 530–535. Baltimore, Williams & Wilkins, 1995

LUJAN-FRYNS

Synonyms. Mental retardation, X-linked, marfanoid habitus; marfanoid habitus-mental retardation, X-linked. See Marfan.

Symptoms and Signs. In males. Marfanoid habitus, mental retardation; possible psychotic behavior.

Etiology. Suggested X-linked dominant inheritance with high penetrance and greater expressivity in males.

BIBLIOGRAPHY. Lujan JE, Carlis ME, Lubs HA: A form of X-linked mental retardation with marfanoid habitus. Am J Med Genet 17:311–322, 1984

Fryus JP: X-linked mental retardation with Marfanoid habitus. Am J Med Genet 38:253, 1991

LUNDBAEK

Synonyms. Stiff hand.

Symptoms and Signs. In longstanding diabetic patients. Pain and parasthesia of the hands, followed by stiffness contractures of fingers and finally atrophy of muscles of hands.

Etiology. Vascular degeneration owing to diabetes mellitus.

Diagnostic Procedures. *X-rays.* Sclerosis of arteries of hands.

BIBLIOGRAPHY. Lundback K: Stiff hands in long-term diabetes. Acta Med Scand 158:447, 1975

LUNDBERG I

Symptoms and Signs. Both sexes from childhood optic atrophy, ataxia, pyramidal tract signs; absence of Achilles reflex and pes cavus.

Etiology. Autosomal dominant inheritance.

BIBLIOGRAPHY. Lundberg PO, Wranne I, Brun A: Family with optic atrophy and neurologic symptoms. Acta Neurol Scand 43:87–105, 1967

LUNDBERG II

Synonyms. Myopathy—cataract—hypogonadism.

Symptoms and Signs. Both sexes. Mental retardation; from childhood dense cataract. Myopathy affecting mainly proximal muscles and facial (masticatory, external ocular) signs of hypogonadism.

Etiology. Autosomal recessive inheritance.

Diagnostic Procedures. *Blood. Urine.* Hypergonadotropic hormones increase.

Therapy. Symptomatic.

Prognosis. Confinement to wheelchair.

BIBLIOGRAPHY. Lundberg PO: Hereditary myopathy, oligophrenia, cataract, skeletal abnormalities and hypergonadotropic hypogonadism: A new syndrome. Acta Genet Med Gemellol 23:245–247, 1974

LUPUS ERYTHEMATOSUS, DISCOID

Synonyms. Discoid lupus erythematosus; cutaneous lupus erythematosus.

Symptoms. Female to male ratio, 2:1; onset at any age; however, usually, it begins in the fourth decade in females and slightly later in males. Onset may occur coincidentally with trauma of different types: mechanical; sun; cold; psychological (e.g., worry). Frequently, history of Raynaud phenomenon (see) and pernio (see). Itching or tenderness of affected areas may be present.

Signs. Facial areas more frequently involved; extremities and trunk less frequently. Unilateral or bilateral lesions represented by erythematous plaques, sharply circumscribed, covered by adherent grayish scales of variable diameter (a few millimeters to 10–19 cm). Under the scales, in the pilosebaceous canals, horny plugs are present. Regional lymph node enlargement.

Etiology. Unknown. Genetic factor plus somatic mutations may be implicated, plus environmental factors that precipitate the onset by interfering with defense mechanisms.

Pathology. Degeneration of basal cell layer; degenerative changes of connective tissue (hyalinization, edema, fibrinoid changes); lymphocyte infiltration; keratotic plugs in follicular openings.

Diagnostic Procedures. *Biopsy.* See Pathology. *Blood.* Erythrocyte sedimentation rate increased in 20% of cases; antinuclear factor in 35%; leukopenia in 13%. Hypergammaglobulinemia.

Therapy. Screening from sun. Protective topical creams and corticosteroid creams (or intralesional injection of corticosteroid). Oral antimalarial agents (e.g., chloroquine sulfate; hydroxychloroquine).

Prognosis. Tendency toward persistence of lesions. Good response to treatment, determined, however, by type and duration of lesion. Scarring and pigmentation frequent. Relapses with trauma, sun, cold. General good health is maintained.

BIBLIOGRAPHY. Kaposi M: Pathologie und Therapie der Hautkrankheiten, 2nd ed, p 642. Vienna, Urban & Schwarzenberg, 1883
Rowell NR, Goodfield MJD: The connective tissue diseases. In Champion RH, Burton JL, Ebling FJG (eds): Rook/Wilkinson/Ebling Textbook of Dermatology, 5th ed, pp 2166–2177. Oxford, Blackwell Scientific, 1992

LUPUS ERYTHEMATOSUS, SYSTEMIC

Synonyms. SLE; Dubois; disseminated lupus erythematous.

Symptoms. Predominantly in women in childbearing age. Malaise; weakness; anorexia; migratory joint pains; intermittent abdominal pleuritic pains; "anaphylactoid" pneumonitis (tachypnea, dyspnea, and cyanosis); mental reaction; anxiety; hallucination; convulsions; recurrent fever. Exposure to sunlight may induce manifestations.

Signs. Butterfly face eruption (in 50%), and maculopapular erythematous eruptions on neck, extremities; telangiectasis; chronic leg ulcers; scarring of nail bed and fingertips; frequently cottonwool retinal exudates. Enlargement of lymph nodes; splenomegaly; hepatomegaly. Signs of involvement of cardiovascular system (pericarditis, endomyocarditis in 50% of cases) and of kidney (in 75%).

Etiology. Unknown; alteration of immune mechanism. Congenital susceptibility. Primary lesion appears to be cellular breakdown releasing cellular antigens. Antigens combine with anti-DNA and are phagocytized, resulting in release of lysosomal products. These cause further tissue breakdown and a continuous cycle.

Pathology. *Kidney biopsy.* Various histological patterns are seen: mesangeal glomerulonephritis, chronic (see), focal and segmental proliferative glomerulonephritis, diffuse proliferative glomerulonephritis, membranous GNF, glomerular sclerosis.

Diagnostic Procedures. *Blood.* Leukopenia; eosinophils reduced; anemia; thrombocytopenia; lupus erythmatosus cell; hypergammaglobulinemia; presence of anticoagulant in plasma. A chronic false-positive serology test for syphilis may antedate the onset of clinical manifestations of SLE by many years. Antinuclear antibodies (IgG, but also IgM, IgA, and IgE), antibodies to double-stranded DNA (ds DNA), antibodies to ribonuclear antigens, serum complement depression, circulating immune complexes. Association with HLA B7 and B8. Rheumatoid factor, cryoglobulins, abnormalities of T4/T8 ratio. *Urine.* Albuminuria.

Therapy. Corticosteroids; adrenocorticotropic hormone; immunosuppressant agents (azanthioprine; mercaptopurine). Transplantation.

Prognosis. Periods of activity of different durations. Hypertension, cardiac and renal failure, hemorrhages causes of death. Recurrence in transplanted kidney is rare.

BIBLIOGRAPHY. Kaposi MK: Neue Beiträge zur Kenntniss des Lupus Erythematosus. Arch Dermatol Syph 4:36–78, 1872
Lehman TJA, McCurdy DK, Bernstein BH, et al: Systemic lupus erythematosus in the first decade of life. Pediatrics 83:235–239, 1989
Miescher PA (eds): Systemic Lupus Erythematosus. Berlin, Springer, 1995

LUTEMBACHER

Synonyms. Atrial septal defect; mitral stenosis.

Symptoms. Predominantly in women; onset in young adulthood. History of rheumatic fever; cardiac disease; slow growth; congestive heart failure. Varying hemodynamic patterns depending on the size of the atrial septal defect and the severity of the mitral stenosis.

Signs. Left atrial enlargement; systolic murmur on the apex; atrial fibrillation at older age.

Etiology. Congenital atrial septal defect with mitral stenosis.

Pathology. Interatrial septal defect; mitral stenosis; dilated pulmonary artery. This syndrome makes up 6% of all general atrial defects.

Diagnostic Procedures. *Electrocardiography.* P-waves broadened, notched; right ventricular hypertrophy; right bundle branch block; possibly, atrial fibrillation or flutter. *X-ray.* Small aorta; dilated pulmonary artery; large pulmonary trunk; hypertrophy, right side. *Angiocardiography. Cardiac catheterization. Two-dimensional echocardiography with color flow imaging and spectral Doppler interrogation.*

Therapy. Surgical treatment when symptoms and systemic manifestation indicate.

Prognosis. Average life span 35 years; longevity possible.

BIBLIOGRAPHY. Lutembacher R: De la stenose mitrale avec communication interauriculaire. Arch Mal Coeur 9:237–250, 1916
Gaasch O'Rourke RA, Cohn LH, et al: Mitral valve disease. In Schlant RC, Alexander RW, et al: Hurst's The Heart, 8th ed, p 1483. New York, McGraw-Hill, 1994
Perloff JK: The Clinical Recognition of Congenital Heart Disease, 4th ed, pp 323–328. Philadelphia, WB Saunders, 1994

LUTZ-JEANSELME

Synonyms. Jeanselme; Steiner; periarticular nodosities.

Symptoms and Signs. Mobile, periarticular, nodular formations appearing during treponemic infections.

Etiology. Syphilis and pinta.

Therapy. Antibiotics.

Prognosis. Regression with therapy.

BIBLIOGRAPHY. Lutz A: Mhefte Prakt Derm 14:30, 1892
Jeanselme E: Nodosités juxtarticulaires. Cong, p 15. Colonial, Paris, Sect Med Hyg Colon, 1904

LUTZ-MIESCHER

Synonyms. Miescher; elastosis perforans serpiginosa; keratosis follicularis serpiginosa; elastoma intrapapillare perforans serpiginosa.

Symptoms and Signs. Prevalent in males; onset before 30 years of age in 90% of cases (youngest patient 5 years old; oldest patient 84); all races. Usually, localized to the neck; less frequently to upper extremities, face, lower extremities, trunk (in this order). Asymptomatic or slight pruritus. Slight erythematous keratotic papules (2–5 mm in diameter), with small central scaling arranged in diffuse, serpiginous, or circular pattern; satellite lesions usually appear. Frequently, symmetric distribution on both sides of neck, both forearms. Also, frequently associated with various disorders of Van Der Hoeve, Grönblad-Strandberg-Touraine, Marfan, and Rothmund, Ehlers-Danlos, Down.

Etiology. Unknown; familial incidence has been reported; autosomal dominant (?).

Pathology. Areas of skin perforation in the form of narrow canals, whose openings are plugged with keratinous corium, which shows foreign body granulomas. Peripheral canal part: loose parakeratinous flakes; central part: mixture of degenerated epithelial cells, inflammatory cells, and eosinophilic fibers. Staining for elastic fibers reveals increase of these fibers in the corium, thicker than those seen in normal skin.

Therapy. Dry ice; electrosurgery (may induce formation of keloid scar). Best treatment: cellophane tape and stripping of keratinous material.

Prognosis. Difficult to predict. From spontaneous regression without scar, to persistence and recurrences up to 5 years with or without scar. Very good results with cellophane tape technique; recurrences are possible, however.

BIBLIOGRAPHY. Jones PE, Smith DC: Porokeratosis, review and report of cases. Arch Dermatol 56:425–436, 1947
Lutz W: Keratosis follicularis serpiginosa. Dermatologica 106:318–320, 1953
Miescher G: Elastoma intrapapillare perforans verruciforme. Dermatologica 110:254–266, 1955
Patterson JW: The perforating disorders. J Am Acad Dermatol 10:561–581, 1984
Burton JL: Disorders of connective tissue. In Champion RH, Burton JL, Ebling FJG (eds): Rook/Wilkinson/Ebling Textbook of Dermatology, 5th ed, pp 1821–1822. Oxford, Blackwell Scientific, 1992

LUTZ-RICHNER

Synonyms. Biliary malformation, renal tubular insufficiency, cholestatic jaundice.

Symptoms and Signs. Neonatal jaundice. Failure to thrive. Repeated infections. Occasionally micrognathia, low-set ears, highly arched palate, barrel chest, club feet, hypotonia.

Etiology. Autosomal recessive inheritance.

Pathology. *Liver.* Intrahepatic biliary hyperplasia. *Kidney.* Normal structure with calcification of some distal tubules.

Diagnostic Procedures. *Blood.* Hyperbilirubinemia; defect of polymorphonucleates cell migration and intracellular killing. *Blood gas.* Metabolic acidosis. *Urine. Aminoaciduria, proteinuria, glycosuria.*

Therapy. Symptomatic.

Prognosis. Death within few months.

BIBLIOGRAPHY. Lutz-Richner AR, Landolt RF: Familiaere Gallengangmissbildungen mit tubolaerer Niereninsuffizienz. Helv Paediatr Acta 28:1–12, 1973
Mikati MA, Barakat AY, Suhl HB, et al: Renal tubular insufficiency, cholestatic jaundice, and multiple congenital anomalies: A new multisystem syndrome. Helv Paediatr Acta 39:463–471, 1984
Norslen Quarrell: Tanner Liver histology in the arthrogryposis multiplex congenita: Renal dysfunction and cholestasis (ARC) syndrome: Report of 3 new cases and review. J Med Genet 31:62–64, 1994

LUXURY-PERFUSION

Synonyms. Lassen I; cerebral hypoxia; relative hyperemia.

This designation is used to indicate the dissociation between overabundant cerebral blood flow and cerebral oxygen uptake and arterial carbon dioxide tension. It is observed in many acute brain diseases, such as apoplexy, acute neurosurgical conditions, tumor, head injury, encephalitis; and in patients with severe diabetic acidosis, sickle cell anemia, other chronic anemias, severe ethanol intoxication, and prolonged hypoglycemia. The diminution of cerebral oxygen uptake is the main feature; arterial-jugular venous oxygen difference is small. Aphasiaproducing lesions appear as areas of low flow with a "luxury perfusion" of high flow surrounding them in the acute stage.

Etiology. Acute metabolic acidosis (probably owing to increased cerebral lactic acid concentration) of the whole (or part) of brain is the most likely mechanism responsible for this syndrome.

Pathology. Cerebral hyperemia; edema; plus specific lesions according to the etiology.

Diagnostic Procedures. *X-ray. CT scan. MRI. Serial angiography (with special attention to capillary phase and early filling of vein).* Regional cerebral blood flow measurements: Arteriovenous oxygen difference; arterial pH, cerebrovascular resistance, cerebral oxygen uptake. Blood-brain barrier, using radioisotope scanning. *Cerebrospinal fluid.* Bicarbonate content.

Therapy. Hyperventilation that may normalize local pH at expense of alkalosis in other parts of the body.

Prognosis. Extremely poor, depends on etiology.

BIBLIOGRAPHY. Lassen NA: The luxury-perfusion syndrome and its possible relation to acute metabolic acidosis localized within the brain. Lancet II:1113–1115, 1966

Shapiro W, Eisenberg S: Cerebral blood flow and metabolism in the coma of St Louis encephalitis. JAMA 202:145–147, 1967

Davis S, Ackerman R: Cerebral blood flow and cerebrovascular CO_2 reactivity in stroke age normal controls. Neurology 33:391–399, 1983

Kertesz A: Aphasia. In Vinken PJ, Bruyn GW (eds): Handbook of Clinical Neurology, pp 297–298. Amsterdam, North-Holland, 1984

LYLE

Synonyms. Variant of Bickers-Adams.

Symptoms and Signs. Bilateral nerve palsy with bilateral mydriasis. In some cases somnolence, and/or vertical gaze palsy or vertical gaze nystagmus and sometime miosis and convergence spasms.

Etiology and Pathology. A lesion extending to the vicinity of cerebral aqueduct, warping or occluding the aqueduct

BIBLIOGRAPHY. Lyle TK: A discussion of ocular motor apraxia with a case presentation. Trans Am Ophthal Soc 59:274–285, 1962

Sachsenweger R: Clinical localization of oculomotor disturbances. In Vinken PJ, Bruyn GW: Handbook of Clinical Neurology, vol 2, p 302. Amsterdam, North-Holland, 1969

LYME*

Synonyms. Afzelius (B).

Symptoms and Signs. Oligoarticular arthritis with the unique skin lesion erythema chronicum migrans. May be accompanied by headache, stiff neck, fever, arthralgias, and meningoencephalitis.

Etiology. A tick believed to transmit the disease has been identified, and recently spirochetal etiology has been proposed (Borrelia burgdorferi).

Pathology. A round papule, which expands peripherally to form an erythematous ring with central clearing.

Diagnostic Procedures. Circulating immune complexes; specific test for Borrelia burgdorferi; high titers of complement.

Therapy. Penicillin.

Prognosis. Good.

BIBLIOGRAPHY. Afzelius BA: Afzelius disease: Or is it Lyme? Curr Contents 32(49):9, 1989

Steere AC, Malawista SE, Hardin JA, et al: Erythema chronicum migrans and Lyme arthritis: The enlarging clinical spectrum. Ann Intern Med 86:685–698, 1977

Seligmann J, Hager M, Drew L, et al: Tiny tick, big worry. Newsweek, May 22, 1989

Weber K, Burgdorfer W: Aspects of Lyme. The Netherlands, Borreliosis Ijmuiden, 1993

LYMPHADENOSIS BENIGNA ORBITAE

Synonyms. Baefverstedt II.

Symptoms and Signs. Onset reported at 18–66 years of age; possibly, higher incidence in women. Exophthalmos (may be absent); tumor-like swelling in the orbita, growing slowly, well circumscribed, painless. Affecting one eye or both eyes; if both, developing symmetrically and simultaneously. Not adherent to the skin; eye movements slightly restricted; no palsy; no papilledema. In one case development of glaucoma (lymphadenoglaucomatous syndrome). Absence of lymphadenopathy.

Etiology. Localized inflammatory process of undetermined origin. Individual reaction to different stimulation: trauma; insect bite; malignant tumor in another part of organism. Localized manifestation of Spiegler-Fendt (see).

Pathology. In lymphoreticular tissue, mature lymphocytes, plasma cells, eosinophils, leukocytes; absence of Langhans or Sternberg cells.

Diagnostic Procedures. *Biopsy.* Blood. *Bone marrow.* Normal.

Therapy. X-ray therapy.

Prognosis. Duration of disease 2–12 months, occasionally years. Prompt response to X-ray treatment; recurrence seldom.

BIBLIOGRAPHY. Bäfverstedt B, Lundmark C, Mossberg H, et al: Lymphadenosis benigna orbitae. Acta Ophthalmol 34:367–376, 1956

Orlowski WJ, Korobowicz J: The lymphadenoglaucomatous syndrome. Am J Ophthalmol 52:101–106, 1961

MacKie RM: Cutaneous lymphocytic infiltrates and pseudolymphomas. In Champion RH, Burton JL, Ebling FJG (eds): Rook/Wilkinson/Ebling Textbook of Dermatology, 5th ed, p 2101. Oxford, Blackwell Scientific, 1992

LYMPHANGIECTASIA INTESTINAL

Synonyms. Homburger-Petermann; Gordon (RS); protein-losing; enteropathy lymphangiectatic; exudative enteropathy; hypercatabolic-hypoprotein; familial hypoproteinemia—lymphangiectatic enteropathy; intestinal lymphangiectasia; lymphangiectatic enteropathy; neonatal lymphedema—exudative enteropathy.

Symptoms and Signs. Both sexes affected; onset from infancy to early adulthood. Initially, intermittent bilateral or unilateral edema, usually preceding diarrhea; then persistent edema and hydrothorax; ascites. Repeated infections, malnutrition, and wasting late stage.

Etiology. Unknown. With onset at birth, possibly congenital malformation of lymphatic system. With onset in early adulthood, acquired, secondary to several conditions, including Ormond (see), infective, collagen, neoplastic, cardiovascular disorders. Familial form reported (autosomal recessive).

Pathology. Small intestine shows edema of affected areas; serosa covered with fibrinous exudate; dilatation of lymphatic vessels; yellowish nodules along their course. Mesenteric lymph nodes enlarged with yellowish foci. No mucosal atrophy; villi swollen; red brownish pigmentation in external muscular layer. Absence of inflammatory reaction.

Diagnostic Procedures. *Blood.* Moderate anemia. Hypoproteinemia;

---

*First recognized in Lyme, Connecticut, in 1975 in an epidemic.

albumin and gammaglobulin decreased. Cholesterol usually normal. *Bone marrow.* Slight hyperplasia. *Absorption studies.* Steatorrhea; abnormal fat and vitamin A tolerance; normal carbohydrate and D-xylose test. Rapid degradation of radioactive iodine labeled albumin, with decreased normal half-life; increased fecal excretion of ^{131}I labeled polyvinylpyrrolidone. *Biopsy of jejunum.* (See Pathology.) *X-ray.* Thickening and coarsening of jejunal fold.

Therapy. Protein administration; reduction of alimentary fat; medium-chain triglycerides provide a good fat substitute; parenteral nutrition when indicated. Surgery if disease confined to limited intestinal area.

Prognosis. Immunologic deficiency (hypogammaglobulinemia) may develop. Excellent response to treatment depending, in secondary forms, on basic condition.

BIBLIOGRAPHY. Homburger F, Petermann ML: Studies on hypoproteinemia II: Familal idiopathic dysproteinemia. Blood 4:1085–1108, 1949
Gordon RS Jr: Exudative enteropathy: Abnormal permeability of the gastrointestinal tract demonstrable with labeled polyvinylpyrrolidone. Lancet 1:325–326, 1959
Goldberg RI, Calleja A: Protein-losing gastroenteropathy. In Haubrich WS, Schaffner F, Berk JE (eds): Bockus Gastroenterology, 5th ed, vol 2, pp 1077–1082. Philadelphia, WB Saunders, 1995

LYMPHOCYTE INTERSTITIAL PNEUMONIAE

Synonyms. LIP.

Symptoms and Signs. Common in Haitians with HIV infection. Idiopathic (from birth or childhood) or complicating dysproteinemias (monoclonal and polyclonal gammapathies, macroglobinemia, hypogammaglobulinemia), pernicious anemia, autoerythrocyte sensitization syndrome, collagen vascular disease, immunodeficiences, viral infection, bone marrow transplantation and drug therapies with dilantin. Dyspnea, cough, fever, joint stiffness.

Etiology. Pulmonary infiltrate from B lymphocytes. A familiar autosomic recessive instance reported.

Pathology. *Lung biopsy.* Diffuse lymphoplasmacytic interstitial infiltrate with lymphocytes and plasma cells. Occasionally epitheliod granulomas or multinucleated giant cells.

Diagnostic Procedures. *Chest X-rays.* Fine, coarse, reticular, or nodular interstitial infiltrates. *Pulmonary function tests.* Restrictive defect. *Blood.* Hypergammaglobulinemia or hypogammaglobulinemia.

Therapy. Corticosteroids.

Prognosis. Generally good. Some may progress to end-stage interstitial fibrosis or develop malignant lymphoma.

BIBLIOGRAPHY. Liebow AA, Carrington CB: Diffuse pulmonary lymphoreticular infiltrations associated with dysproteinuria. Med Clin North Am 57:809–843, 1973
Tierstein AS, Rosen MJ: Lymphocyte interstitial pneumoniae. Clin Chest Med 9:467–471, 1988

LYMPHOCYTIC COLITIS

Synonyms. Microscopic colitis; see also collagenous colitis.

Symptoms and Signs. Male to female ratio, 1:1. Usually affects sixth decade (range 28–82 years). Stronger association with autoimmune disorders than collagenous colitis.

Etiology. Unknown.

Pathology. *Colon.* Usually normal macroscopic aspect, seldom polyps or diverticula. *Biopsy.* Lymphocytic infiltration in surface epithelial layer and crypts. No subepithelial collagen deposits.

Diagnostic Procedures. *Haplotype.* High incidence HLA-A1, mild increase HLA-DRW 53. *Blood.* Elevated antinuclear antibody 83359 and antiparietal cell antibodies (22%), ESR elevated (50%) mild eosinophilia. *Colonic biopsy.* See Pathology.

Therapy. Antidiarrheal agents. Fiber supplements. Sulfasalazopirine, and prednisone.

Prognosis. Spontaneous remission and generally good response to treatment.

BIBLIOGRAPHY. Read NW, Kregs GJ, Read MG, et al: Chronic diarrhea of unknown origin. Gastroenterology 78:264–271, 1980
Maxson CJ, Klein HD, Rubin W: Atypical forms of inflammatory bowel disease. Med Clin N Am 78:1259–1273, 1994
Schiller LR: Microscopic and collagenous colitis. In Haubrich WS, Schaffner F, Berk JE (eds): Bockus Gastroenterology, 5th ed, p 1700. Philadelphia, WB Saunders, 1995

LYMPHOHISTIOCYTOSIS, FAMILIAL

Synonyms. Farquhar, Omenn (could be a distinct entity); reticulosis FEL; erythrophagocytic familial lymphohistiocytosis; hemophagocytic reticulosis; familial reticulendotheliosis; familial histiocytic.

Symptoms and Signs. Both sexes. Onset in infancy or early childhood. Two phases: (1) *Chronic.* Eczema, failure to thrive, multiple abscesses, chronic otitis media, frequent respiratory tract infections, fever. (2) *Fulminating.* Progressing lymphadenopathy, hepatosplenomegaly, jaundice, pulmonitis. Neurological symptoms (47%).

Etiology. Unknown; possibly autosomal recessive inheritance or virus or both. Possibly includes several entities that share a genetically determined faulty T-cell differentiation and forms a nosologically confused group. Other etiologic hypothesis: genetic defect in cytokine regulation.

Pathology. Generalized reticular cell infiltration of all body tissue, including central nervous system, disruption of lymphoid architecture, and increased presence of plasma cells and eosinophils. Absence of granulomatous formation, necrosis, erythrophagocytosis, and storage-laden histiocytes.

Diagnostic Procedures. *Blood.* Anemia; moderate reticulocytosis; leukopenia. Platelets increased in number in a family report. Hypergammaglobulinemia terminally; hyperbilirubinemia. *Bone marrow.* Reticular cell infiltration; erythroid hyperplasia.

Therapy. Stable remission obtained with chemotherapy, associated or not with bone marrow transplantation.

Prognosis. Death 2–6 weeks after onset; pneumonia; bacteriemia; candidiasis. Longest survival 2 years.

BIBLIOGRAPHY. Farquhar JW: Claireaux, a familial haemophagocytic reticulosis. Arch Dis Child 27:519, 1952
Nelson P, Santamaria A, Olson RL, et al: Generalized lymphohistiocytic infiltration: A familial disease not previously described and different from Letterer-Siwe disease and Chediak-Higashi syndrome. Pediatrics 27:931–950, 1961
Omenn GS: Familial reticuloendotheliosis with eosinophilia. N Engl J Med 273:427–432, 1965
Miller DR: Familial reticuloendotheliosis: Concurrence of disease in five siblings. Pediatrics 38:986–995, 1966
Martin VJ, Cras P: Familial erythrophagocytic lymphohistiocytosis: A neuropathologic study. Acta Neuropath 66:140–144, 1985
Henter JI, Elinder G: Familial hemophagocytic lymphohistiocytosis: Clinical review based on the finding in seven children. Acta Paediatr Scand 80:269–277, 1991
Nespoli L, Locatelli F, Bonetti F, et al: Familial haemophagocytic lymphohistiocytosis treated with allogenic bone marrow transplantation. Bone Marrow Transplant 7:139–142, 1991

LYNCH

Synonyms. Site-specific familial colonic cancer; colonic cancer site specific familial; colorectal cancer; cancer family.

Symptoms and Signs. *Type I:* Early age. Diarrhea or stipsy. Abdominal distension. *Type II:* See Type I plus cancer of female genital tract and/or other sites, reported also carcinoma of pancreas, stomach, and atrophic gastritis with intestinal metaplasia.

Etiology. Autosomal dominant inheritance.

Pathology. Colon: mucinous or colloidal malignancies (nonpolyposis) located in proximal segment.

Diagnostic Procedures. *X-rays. CT scan. MR imaging.*

Therapy. Colon resection.

Prognosis. Malignant transformation if not removed.

BIBLIOGRAPHY. Lynch HT, Shaw MW, Magnuson CW, et al: Hereditary factors in cancer: Study of two large midwestern kindreds. Arch Int Med 117:206–212, 1966

Lynch HT, Lynch P: The cancer-family syndrome: A pragmatic basis for syndrome identification. Dis Colon Rectum 22:106–110, 1979

Abusamra H, Maximova S, Bar-Meir S, et al: Cancer family syndrome of Lynch. Am J Med 83:981–983, 1987

Delattre O, Olshwang S, Law DJ, et al: Multiple genetic alteration in distal and proximal colorectal cancer. Lancet 2:353–356, 1989

Salomon E: Colorectal cancer genes. Nature 340:412–414, 1990

Ellis A: Genetics in gastroenterology. In Haubrich WS, Schaffner F, Berk JE (eds): Bockus Gastroenterology, 5th ed, vol 2, pp 3295–3296. Philadelphia, WB Saunders, 1995

LYSOSOMAL GLYCOGEN STORAGE DISEASE WITHOUT GLUCOSIDASE DEFICIENCY

Synonyms. GSDIIB.

Symptoms and Signs. Both sexes. Onset usually in adolescence. Minimal clinical signs of skeletal muscle myopathy; frequent mental retardation, hypertrophic cardiomyopathy; arrhythmias; including Wolff-Parkinson-White; absent other organomegaly.

Etiology. Different modes of inheritance considered. May encompass more than one disease.

Pathology. Muscle. Vacuolar storage of glycogen, prevalent in the myocardium.

Diagnostic Procedures. *Blood.* CK enzyme elevated up to tenfold. *Muscle biopsy and cultured fibroblasts.* Studies of enzymes.

Therapy. Symptomatic.

BIBLIOGRAPHY. Rigs JE, Schochet SS, Di Mauro S, et al: Lysosomal glycogen storage disease without normal acid maltase deficiency. Neurology 33:873–877, 1983

Hirschhorn R: Glycogen storage disease type II acid-glucosidase (acid maltase) deficiency. In Scriver CR, Beaudet AL, Sly WS, et al: The Metabolic and Molecular Bases of Inherited Disease, 7th ed. New York, McGraw-Hill, 1995

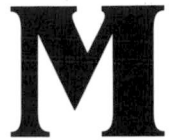

MACROAMYLASEMIA

Symptoms and Signs. Men prevalence or equal sex distribution both reported. Onset in later life. Usually no particular symptom complex per se (in type I and II an obscure abdominal pain may be present). Associated condition malabsorption symptoms and signs as determining cause.

Etiology. "A biochemical aberration in search of a disease." Abnormal or unusual protein (particularly immunoglobulins) developing during illness of any type linking with normal amylase. Usually a temporary condition accompanying evolution of the disease and disappearing with recovery. Persistent macroamylasemia usually associated with a variety of disorders, but prevalently with malabsorptive conditions.

Pathology. According to type of basic disease.

Diagnostic Procedures. *Blood. Urine.* Chrotographic studies, ultracentrifugation, electrophoresis, polyethylene glycol precipitation, immunological procedures. Three types recognized. *Type I.* Persistent hyperamilasemia, reduced amylase in the urine. *Type II.* Hyperamilasemia, ratio of macroamylase to normal amylase in serum lower than in type I, in the urine amylase concentration not uniformly diminished. *Type III.* Normal serum amylase activity, and low ratio of macroamylase to normal amylase, in the urine normal value.

Therapy. Treatment of associated or concurrent conditions.

Prognosis. According to basic condition. Per se the macroamylasemia, presently is viewed as a relatively benign condition.

BIBLIOGRAPHY. Wilding P, Cooke WT, Nicholson GI: Globulin-bound amylase: A cause of persistently elevated levels in serum. Ann Intern Med 60:1053–1059, 1964
Levitt MD, Goetzl EJ, Cooperband SR: Two forms of macroamylasaemia. Lancet I:957–958, 1968
Berk JE: Macroamylasemia. In Haubrich WS, Schaffner F, Berk JE (eds): Bockus Gastroenterology, 5th ed, pp 2851–2860. Philadelphia, WB Saunders, 1995

MADELUNG I

Synonyms. Carpus curvus; manus valga. See Lèri-Weill (different type of the same condition?).

Symptoms. Females more frequently affected (4:1); diagnosed usually in adolescence. Moderate stature shortness (failure of growth of tibia and resulting genu varum); typical wrist pain and deformity: fork deformity because of backward subluxation of distal end of ulna, owing to failure of growth in distal radial growth plate.

Etiology. Autosomal dominant inheritance. Isolated Madelung deformity occurs as a distinct genetic trait, when associated with shortening of tibia it is better to consider the diagnosis of Lèri-Weill.

Diagnostic Procedures. *X-ray.*

Therapy. Orthopedic measures. Ulnar subluxation may be reduced, but only temporarily.

Prognosis. Short stature; limitation of wrist and elbow motion.

BIBLIOGRAPHY. Madelung OW: Die spontane Subluxation der Hand nach Vorne. Verh Dent Ges Chir 7:259–276, 1878
Jackson LG: Dyschondrosteosis: Clinical study of a sixth generation family. Proc Greenwood Genet Center 4:147–148, 1985

Rimoin DL, Lachman RS: Genetic disorders of the osseous skeleton. In Beithon P (ed): McKusick's Heritable Disorders of Connective Tissue, 5th ed, pp 637–638. St Louis, CV Mosby, 1993

MADIDA

Symptoms and Signs. Hypersecretion of hypotonic tears (as contrasted to the sicca syndrome).

Etiology. Supposed response to central nervous system lesion owing to toxic irritation of hypothalamus.

Pathology. Unknown.

BIBLIOGRAPHY. Prinz CW: Das Madida-Syndrom bei Akrodinie als gegensatz sum Sicca syndrom. Klin Monatsbl Augenheilkd 141:749–463, 1932

MAFFUCCI

Synonyms. Kast; chondrodystrophy hemangiomas; dyschondroplasia hemangiomas; multiple enchondromatosis; hemangimatosis chondrodystrophica; enchondromatosis hemoangimaotosis; vascular hamartoma—dyschondroplasia. See Ollier.

Symptoms. Both sexes affected. Normal at birth; bone and cartilage deformities may appear at all ages, even during childhood. Usually, no history of pain; orthostatic hypotension in sitting or standing position (pooling of blood in dependent hemangiomas). Normal intelligence. Fracture of bones (26%) following minimal trauma; slow reunion.

Signs. Before puberty a hard nodule appears on finger or toe, followed by other tumors with asymmetric distribution in the cylindrical bones. In the subcutaneous and soft tissue, bluish hemangiomas appear. Deformities and inequality of bones (large and grotesque because of tumors and fractures). Tumor of flat bones less common. No visceral involvement.

Etiology. Unknown; combination of enchondromatosis and hemangiomatosis. Does not appear to be hereditary. Chromosomal abnormalities have not been found.

Pathology. *Bone.* Areas of dyschondroplasia. Sarcomatous degeneration of bone lesion frequent (18%). *Skin.* Vascular malformation; hemangioma. No relation between the two types of lesions.

Diagnostic Procedures. *X-ray. CT scan. MRI of skeleton. Arteriography. Venography. Biopsy of skin and bones.*

Therapy. Surgical removal of sarcomatous transformation; orthopedic measures and corrective surgery when indicated.

Prognosis. Progression of lesions to the end of second decade, then stabilization. Malignant transformation or association with various different malignancies may be cause of death.

BIBLIOGRAPHY. Maffucci A: Di un caso di encondroma ed angioma multiplo. Contribuzione alla genesi embrionale dei tumori. Movimento Medico-Chirurgico Nap 13:399–342, 565–575, 1881
Kast A, von Recklinghausen F: Ein Fall von Enchondrom mit ungewoehnlicher Multiplikation. Virchows Arch Pathol Anat 118:1–18, 1889
Ben-Itzhak I, Denolf F, Versfeld GA, et al: The Maffucci syndrome. J Pediatr Orthoped 8:345–348, 1988
Rimoin DL, Lachman RS: Genetic disorders of the osseous skeleton. In Beithon P (ed): McKusick's Heritable Disorders of Connective Tissue, 5th ed, pp 670–671. St Louis, CV Mosby, 1993

M.A.G.I.C.

Synonyms. Behçet-relapsing polycondritis. Mouth—genital—ulcers—inflamed—cartilage (M.A.G.I.C.). See Overlap.

Symptoms and Signs. Those of Behçet (see) and relapsing polychondritis (see).

Etiology. Unknown. Suggested autoantibodies against elastic tissue.

BIBLIOGRAPHY. Firestein GS, Gruber HE, Weisman MH, et al: Mouth and genital ulcers with inflamed cartilage: MAGIC syndrome. Am J Med 79:69–72, 1985

Orme RL, Nordlung JJ, Barich L, et al: The MAGIC syndrome (mouth and genital ulcers with inflamed cartilage). Arch Dermatol 126:940–944, 1990

MAGNUS

Synonyms. Erythropoietic protoporphyria, EPP; hydroa aestivale; PP.

Symptoms. Both sexes affected; onset in childhood or adolescence. Various intensities of manifestations, from minimal to relatively severe, with fluctuation of intensity also in the same individual. After exposure to sun, from a few minutes to a prolonged time (according to individuals), intense pruritus, erythema, edema of areas exposed. Usually, receding completely in 12–24 hours without sequelae. Exceptionally, formation of chronic eczema persisting for days and leaving scars. Frequently associated, cholelithiasis symptoms at early age.

Signs. Erythrodontia; abnormal mechanical fragility of skin; hirsutism; pigmentation absent. Occasionally, splenomegaly.

Etiology. Unknown. Autosomal dominant inheritance. Excessive production of protoporphyrin in bone marrow and possibly in other organs. Generalized deficiency of ferrochelatase activity.

Pathology. Fluorescence of skin. No particular pathologic findings in liver.

Diagnostic Procedures. *Blood.* Mild hypochromic anemia; seldom, hemolysis; frequently, evidence of liver insufficiency. *Urine.* Normal. Only positive findings are increased concentration of protoporphyrin in circulating erythrocytes (isomer type III [9a] protoporphyrin) and increase of same pigment in the feces. *Stool.* Large excretion of protoporphyrin. *Bone marrow.* Increased fluorescence limited to cytoplasm of erythroid cells.

Therapy. Avoidance of exposure to sun; topical sunscreens effective in the 400-nm portion of spectrum (containig oxidates of zinc or titanium). Prolonged treatment with cholestyramine; beta-carotene ameliorates skin symptoms; iron (carbonyl iron or ferrousulfate) decreases porphyrin formation and improves liver function. Liver transplantation if severe liver damage has occurred.

Prognosis. Relatively mild condition with possible severe hepatic damage leading to cirrhosis and liver failure.

BIBLIOGRAPHY. Magnus IA, Jarrett A, Prankerd TAJ, et al: Erythropoietic protoporphyria: A new porphyria syndrome with solar urticaria due to protoporphyrinaemia. Lancet II:448–451, 1961

Lee GR: Porphyria. In Lee GR, Bithel TC, Foerster J, et al (eds): Wintrobe's Clinical Hematology, 9th ed, pp 1280–1282. Philadelphia, Lea & Febiger, 1993

MAJEWSKI

Synonyms. Short rib; polydactyly II; SRP-2; polydactyly; neonatal chondrodystrophy; polydactyly II.

Symptoms and Signs. At birth. Hydrops; prominent forehead; low set malformed ears; short flat nose; median cleft lip and palate; lobulated tongue; micrognathia (features similar to those of Mohr, see); larynx malformed; narrow and short thorax; protuberant abdomen; micromelia; pre- and postaxial polysyndactyly; short limbs; ambiguous genital and visceral (pulmonary, glomerular, tubular renal, cerebral, and cerebellar) anomalies. Distinguishing feature: disproportionate short tibia.

Etiology. Autosomal recessive inheritance.

Pathology. Cartilage: stunted and disorganized endochondral calcifications (kidneys, lungs, heart, epiglottis, genitals, pachygiria, and cerebellar).

Diagnostic Procedures. *X-rays. CT scan. MRI. Ultrasonography.* Prenatal diagnosis. See Signs.

Prognosis. Death in perinatal period.

BIBLIOGRAPHY. Majewski F, Pfeiffer RA, Lenz W, et al: Polysyndaktylie, verkuerzte Gliedmassen und Genitalfehlbildungen: Kennzeichen eines selbstaendigen Syndrome? Z Kinderheilk 111:118–138, 1971

Pauli RM: Short rib polydactyly type Majewski. Proc Greenwood Genet Cent 7:168–169, 1988

Rimoin DL, Lachman RS: Genetic disorders of the osseous skeleton. In Beithon P (ed): McKusick's Heritable Disorders of Connective Tissue, 5th ed, pp 589–590. St Louis, CV Mosby, 1993

MAJOCCHI

Synonyms. Purpura annularis telangiectoides; telangiectasia follicularis annulata.

Symptoms and Signs. Both sexes affected; onset usually in adolescence or early adulthood. Any site of body skin may be affected. Small annular plaques (1–3 cm in diameter), purple, yellow-brownish, with or without "cayenne spots." Centrifugal extension; slight atrophy in the center of lesion.

Etiology. Unknown.

Pathology. Hemosiderin deposit; telangiectases.

Therapy. None.

Prognosis. Persistence for months or years.

BIBLIOGRAPHY. Majocchi D: Sopra una dermatosi telangettode non ancora descritta "purpura annularis" "telangiectasia follicularis annulata." Studio clinico Giorn Ital Mal Venereol 37:242–250, 1896

Champion RH: Purpura. In Champion RH, Burton JL, Ebling FJG (eds): Rook/Wilkinson/Ebling Textbook of Dermatology, 5th ed, p 1889. Oxford, Blackwell Scientific, 1992

MALABSORPTION SYNDROMES

Symptoms. Both sexes affected; onset at all ages. One or more frequently severe attacks of diarrhea with passage of gray or yellowish, soft, greasy stools; anorexia; weight loss; borborygmi; muscle tenderness; bone pain; weakness; fatigue; dyspnea; paresthesias.

Signs. Abdominal bloating; muscle wasting; dehydration; hyperkeratosis; folliculitis; bleeding manifestations; glossitis; cheilosis.

Etiology and Pathology. Numerous hereditary and acquired conditions may be responsible for these syndromes. On the basis of clinical features and diagnostic procedures they may be subdivided under different headings.

Group 1. Inadequate digestion. Postgastrectomy syndromes; pancreatic exocrine insufficiency; biliary insufficiency.

Group 2. Metabolic defects. Sprue; sugar-splitting enzyme deficiency.

Group 3. Inadequate absorptive area. Fistulas; resection; gastroileostomy; jejuneal exclusion.

Group 4. Intestinal wall pathology or lymphatic obstruction. Radiation syndromes; amyloidosis; enteritis (bacterial; viral; parasitic); scleroderma; carcinoid syndrome; pneumatosis cystoides intestinalis; lymphomas; Whipple; tuberculosis; Crohn; chronic ulcerative jejunitis (nongranulomatous).

Group 5. Altered bacterial flora. Blind loop syndrome; multiple jejunal diverticula; antibiotic enterocolitis.

Group 6. Endocrinopathies. Diabetes mellitus; hypoparathyroidism; hyperparathyroidism; islet cell tumor of pancreas (Zollinger-Ellison; watery diarrhea; hypokalemia associated with pancreatic islet cell adenoma).

Group 7. Protein abnormalities. Dysgammaglobulinemia; Bassen-Kornzweig; intestinal lymphangiectasia; intestinal lymphangiectasia; hypobetalypoproteinemia.

Group 8. Vascular. Superior mesenteric artery syndrome; congestive heart failure; Pick I, tricuspid regurgitation; protein-losing enteropathy.

Diagnostic Procedures. See specific condition.

Therapy. According to etiology.

Prognosis. Depends on etiology.

BIBLIOGRAPHY. Kalser MH: Malabsorption syndromes. In Haubrich WS, Schaffner F, Berk JE (eds): Bockus Gastroenterology, 5th ed, vol 2, pp 996–1026. Philadelphia, WB Saunders, 1995

MALAMUD-COHEN

Synonyms. Cerebellar ataxia, extrapyramidal.

Symptoms and Signs. From early infancy. Onset only cerebellar signs, later addition of extrapyramidal signs.

Etiology. X-linked inheritance.

Pathology. Cerebellar and extrapyramidal involvement.

BIBLIOGRAPHY. Malamud N, Cohen P: Unusual form of cerebellar ataxia with sex linked inheritance. Neurology 8:261–266, 1958

MALE CLIMACTERIC

Synonym. Climacterium male.

Symptoms and Signs. Diminished libido; impotence; fatigue; hot flashes; nervousness; depression; memory and concentration decreased; sleep disturbed; generic loss of interest in sex.

Etiology. Rare disorder, usually caused by emotional disturbances.

Pathology. Variable degrees of decreased spermatogenesis and of parenchymal atrophy.

Diagnostic Procedures. *Blood.* Plasma level of testosterone, follicle-stimulating hormone (FSH), luteinizing hormone (LH). *Semen analysis.* Normal or variable degree of decreased number and mobility of spermatozoa. *Urine.* 17-ketosteroids usually normal; gonadotropins usually normal. In rare cases, positive findings make a legitimate climacteric condition.

Therapy. Psychotherapy; androgen may be beneficial.

Prognosis. Good in many cases if psychological block is removed.

BIBLIOGRAPHY. Heller CG, Myers GB: The male climacteric, its symptomatology, diagnosis and treatment. Use of urinary gonadotropins, therapeutic tests with testosterone proprionate and testicular biopsies in delineating the climacteric from psychoneurosis and psychogenic impotence. JAMA 126:472–477, 1944

Ryan RJ: Uncertain and hypothetic disorders; unclassifiable syndromes. Dis Mon 27–36, 1961
Blackman MR, Elahi D, Harman SM: Endocrinology and aging. In De Groot LJ (ed): Endocrinology, 3rd ed, pp 2716–2719. Philadelphia, WB Saunders, 1995

MALHERBE

Synonyms. Malherbe-Chenantais; calcified epithelioma; benign calcifying epithelioma; pilomatrixoma.

Symptoms. Females more frequently affected; onset at any age (majority of cases under 30 years). Frequently associated with myotonic dystrophy.

Signs. On the head, neck, or upper extremities, solitary dermal tumor, which on palpation feels smooth or lobulated and of stone-hard consistency; overlying skin normal. Frequent and repeated associated infections.

Etiology. Hamartoma of hair matrix. Familial autosomal dominant cases reported.

Pathology. Encapsulated tumor, well defined, surrounded by inflammatory cells; tumoral peripheral cells small and dark; rarely, mitotic figures; scanty cytoplasm; intracellular connections; internal zone calcified and surrounded by cells with larger eosinophilic cytoplasm.

Diagnostic Procedures. *Biopsy.*

Therapy. Excision.

Prognosis. No recurrence if completely excised. Possibility of malignant degeneration.

BIBLIOGRAPHY. Malherbe A, Chenantais J: Note sur l'epithéliome calcifié des glandes sébacées. Prog Med 8:826–828, 1880
MacKie RM: Tumors of the skin appendages. In Burton JL, Cunlife WJ: Subcutaneous fat. In Champion RH, Burton JL, Ebling FJG (eds): Rook/Wilkinson/Ebling Textbook of Dermatology, 5th ed, pp 1509–1510. Oxford, Blackwell Scientific, 1992

MALI

Synonyms. Acroangiodermatitis; pseudokaposi, see Favre-Chaix.

Symptoms and Signs. Male prevalence. Onset at 30–40 years of age. In patients with chronic venous insufficiency. Purple maculae and plaques on the extensor side of the digits and the foot that may develop ulceration. Mostly on the I and II digits, the extensor side, other digits, the triangular region with ground phalanges at the base and tarsus at the top. Edema of ankle and foot with or without reticular pigmentation.

Etiology. Complication of chronic venous insufficiency. Special form of chronic venous insufficiency.

Pathology. Small lesions from pinpoint to lentile-plaques the size of a hand on back of foot with central ulceration. "Kaposiform" lesion.

Diagnostic Procedures. *Arterovenous Doppler. Phlebography, arteriography, and measure of venous pressure at different site of limbs.*

Therapy. Therapy resistant lesions.

BIBLIOGRAPHY. Mali JWH, Kuiper JP, Hamers AA: Acroangiodermatitis of the foot. Arch Derm 92:515–518, 1965
Ruedinger R: Kaposiform Akroangiodermatiten (Pseudokaposi). Hautartz 36:65–68, 1985

MALIGNANT HYPERTHERMIA*

Synonym. Pharmacogenic myopathy. See King.

---

*The Malignant Hyperthemia Association of the United States has a hotline number (209-634-4917) that is available 24 hours a day for information.

Symptoms. Both sexes affected; onset at any age. Induced by general anesthesia or triggered by various pharmacologic agents or environmental stresses (temperature, infection, emotion, injuries, exercise).

Signs. *Early manifestations.* Rapid multifocal ventricular arrhythmias; unstable blood pressure; rapid and deep respiration; excessive heat; mottled cyanosis. In 80% of cases, skeletal muscle rigidity (especially after injection of succinylcholine). *Later manifestations.* High fever, rapidly rising to 44°C to 46°C and not controllable by physical or pharmacologic means. Oliguria; anuria; pupils fixed and dilated; deep tendon reflexes absent; convulsions. Milder reaction (fever without muscle rigidity) may also occur, because of minor defect (see Etiology) or weaker agents.

Etiology. Autosomal dominant inheritance or weaker recessive gene. Crisis caused by sudden rise in concentration of myoplasmic calcium induced by the administration of several drugs. Several syndromes appear possibly related: Duchenne; King; myoadenylate deaminaser deficiency; other myopathies.

Pathology. Muscle contraction, rigor that may precede death.

Diagnostic Procedures. *Blood.* Metabolic acidosis; hypoxia; electrolytes, enzymes, and myoglobin alterations. *Urine.* Myoglobinuria. *Muscle biopsy.* Vigorous in vitro contracture of the specimen in presence of halothane, and reduced contracture threshold to caffeine.

Therapy.

1. Stop anesthesia and surgery immediately.
2. Hyperventilate patient with 100% oxygen.
3. Administer dantrolene (Dantrium) 2.5 mg/kg IV and procainamide (up 15 mg/kg IV slowly if required for arrhythmias) as soon as possible.
4. Initiate cooling.
5. Correct acidosis.
6. Secure monitoring lines: electrocardiograph, temperature, Foley catheter, arterial pressure, central venous pressure.
7. Maintain urine output.
8. Monitor patient until danger of subsequent episodes is past (48–72 hr).
9. Administer oral or IV dantrolene for 48 to 72 hr.

Prognosis. With constant vigilance and proper, aggressive treatment, the syndrome can be treated adequately for a successful outcome.

BIBLIOGRAPHY. Denborough MA, Forster JFA, Lovell RRH, et al: Anaesthetic deaths in a family. Br J Anaesth 34:395–396, 1962
Britt BA: Malignant Hyperthermia. Boston, Martinus Nijhoff, 1987
Williams CH (ed): Experimental Malignant Hyperthermia. New York, Springer-Verlag, 1988
Kalow W, Grant DM: Pharmacogenetics. In Scriver CR, Beaudet AL, Sly WS, et al: The Metabolic and Molecular Bases of Inherited Disease, 7th ed, pp 301–303. New York, McGraw-Hill, 1995

MALLORY-WEISS

Synonym. Gastroesophageal laceration.

Symptoms. Prevalent in males, usually onset after 30 years of age. Vomiting; severe retching, and then hematemesis and melena.

Signs. Pallor; tachycardia; in some patients shock.

Etiology. Longitudinal laceration of mucosa and submucosa of gastroesophageal junction following severe retching. Usually following large ingestion of alcohol.

Pathology. See Etiology. Acute and chronic gastritis; pancreatitis; liver cirrhosis may or may not be associated.

Diagnostic Procedures. *Blood.* Blood cell count; liver function test; serum amylase; blood urea nitrogen; glucose; clotting studies. *Esophagogastroscopy.* As soon as condition of patient allows it, followed by X-ray of upper gastrointestinal tract. Arteriographic demonstration of the site of lesion in case of active bleeding.

Therapy. Stomach emptied and washed with iced saline. Blood replaced. Coagulants, atropine, and sedative. Laceration identified and injection with adrenaline (1:10,000) or cautery with coagulation device effective in 90% of cases. If bleeding does not stop, angiographic arterial embolization or high gastrotomy. Sengstaken-Blakemore tube and blind gastric resection in these cases not useful.

Prognosis. Fair with adequate treatment; affected by pre-existing general conditions (e.g., liver cirrhosis).

BIBLIOGRAPHY. Quincke H: Ulcus oesophagi ex digestione. Arch Klin Med 24:72, 1879
Mallory GK, Weiss S: Hemorrhages from lacerations of the cardiac orifice of the stomach due to vomiting. Am J Med Sci 178:506–515, 1929
Sugawa C, Benishek D, Walt AJ: Mallory-Weiss syndrome: A study of 224 patients. Am J Surg 145:30–33, 1983
Harris JM, Di Palma JA: Clinical significance of Mallory-Weiss tears. Am J Gastroenterol 88:2056–2058, 1993

MALPUECH

Synonyms. Facial clefting, gypsy type.

Symptoms. In gypsy family: mental and physical retardation.

Signs. Facial clefting; hypertelorism. Urogenital anomalies: micropenis, hypospadias, ectopic testis.

Etiology. New autosomal recessive syndrome (?).

BIBLIOGRAPHY. Malpuech G, Demeocq F, Palcoux JB, et al: A previously underscribed autosomal recessive multiple congenital anomalies/mental retardation (MCA/MR) syndrome with growth failure, lip/palate cleft(s) and urogenital anomalies. Am J Med Genet 16:475–480, 1983

MANCALL-ROSALES

Synonyms. Paraneoplastic myelitis.

Symptoms and Signs. Loss of motor and successively of sensory function, sphincter disorder. No pains.

Etiology. Association with solid visceral lymphomas or other tumors (ovarian, bronchogenic, etc.); in some cases no tumor found.

Pathology. Necrotic lesion affecting both gray and white matter. Lack of evidence of inflammatory or ischemic lesions. Absence of neoplastic cells in CSF.

Diagnostic Procedures. *X-rays. CT scan. MRI* Negative for cord compression. Presence of abdominal tumor. *Spinal fluid.* Negative or modest increase of mononuclear cells and proteins.

Therapy. Steroids and plasmapheresis not effective.

Prognosis. Fatal condition.

BIBLIOGRAPHY. Mancall EL, Rosales RK: Necrotizing myelopathy associated with visceral carcinoma. Brain 87:639, 1964
Adams RD, Victor M: Principles of Neurology, 5th ed, p 1092. New York, McGraw-Hill, 1993

MAN-IN-THE-BARREL

Synonyms. MIB; Mohr (J.P.); brachial diplegia—intact motor function of legs.

Symptoms and Signs. In comatose patients. Lack of movement of either arm following any stimulus (as if arms and trunk constrained into a barrel). Intact motor functioning of legs (spontaneously or from stimulus, brain stem reflexes functionally intact).

Etiology and Pathology. Hemorrhage, cardiac arrest, sedative or hypotensive drugs, postmyocardial infarction, airway obstruction. Neurological consequence of systemic hypotension and global cerebral hypoperfusion of rapid onset.

Pathology. Not clearly assessed, possible bilateral prerolandic cerebral damage.

Diagnostic Procedures. *EEG.* Variable alterations not modified by anticonvulsivants. *CT scan. MRI.* Normal or variable alteration according to etiology.

Therapy. According to etiology. Symptomatic.

Prognosis. According to etiology. Poor. Death in 66% of cases.

BIBLIOGRAPHY. Mohr JP: Distal Field infarction. Neurology 12:279, 1969
Sage JI, Van Uiter RL: Man in the barrel syndrome. Neurology 36:1102–1103, 1986
Olejhiczek PG, Ellenberg MR, Eilender LMet al: Man in the barrel syndrome in a non comatose patient: A case report. Arch Phys Med Rehabil 72:1021–1023, 1991

MANSON SCHISTOSOMIASIS, PULMONARY ARTERY OBSTRUCTION

Synonyms. Cardiopulmonary bilharziasis; pulmonary schistosomiasis; protopulmonary bilharziasis; cardiopulmonary schistosomiasis. See Katayama.

Symptoms. Occurs in young adults living (or who have lived) in areas with endemic schistosomiasis. Progressive dyspnea; pain in upper abdomen.

Signs. Cyanosis; engorgement of neck vessels; edema of legs; scanty pulmonary findings (contrasted with severe dyspnea); hepatosplenomegaly. In heart, loud S2, systolic and diastolic murmurs.

Etiology. Manson Schistosoma infestation.

Pathology. Widespread pulmonary obliterative arteriolitis owing to repeated emboli; ova of Schistosoma; granulomas; para-arterial angiomatosis arteritis with fibrinoid necrosis; hyaline thrombi. Right ventricular hypertrophy.

Diagnostic Procedures. *Stool.* Demonstration of Schistosoma. *Biopsy of rectum. Blood.* Moderate anemia; normal white blood cells. *ECG.* Cor pulmonale pattern. *X-ray of chest.* Right ventricular hypertrophy; dilated pulmonary arteries. *Ultrasound.*

Therapy. Praziquantel (or Metifonate, not available in the United States). Digitalis; oxygen and salt restriction; diuretics.

Prognosis. Poor; death usually within 1 year. These patients do not tolerate surgical procedures well.

BIBLIOGRAPHY. Belelli V: Les oeufs de Bilharzia haematobia dans les poumons. Unione med Egiz Alessandria 1: No. 22–23, 1884–1885
Macieira-Coelho E, Duarte CS: The syndrome of portopulmonary schistosomiasis. Am J Med 43:944–950, 1967
Weatherall DJ, Ledingham JGG, Warrell DA (eds): Oxford Textbook of Medicine, 3rd ed, pp 970–981. Oxford, Oxford Med Pub, 1996

MANUBRIOSTERNAL

Synonyms. Pseudoangina; thoracic pain. See S.A.P.H.O. and Tieze.

Symptoms. Occurs in patients with rheumatoid arthritis or without any joint changes. Sharp pain over or on either side of manubrium; pain induced or aggravated by exercise (walking, climbing stairs, bending, or straightening), coughing and sneezing.

Signs. Tenderness; occasionally, slight swelling of manubriosternal joint. Relief by procaine infiltration.

Etiology. Unknown; part of rheumatoid arthritis syndrome or isolated inflammatory condition.

Diagnostic Procedures. *X-ray.* Occasionally, slight changes of manubriosternal joint; usually no changes. *ECG.* Normal.

Therapy. Relief by procaine or corticoid infiltration.

Prognosis. Symptoms may persist and recur for years.

BIBLIOGRAPHY. Söderstrom N: Manubrial pain and angina pectoris. Svensk Lakartidn 48:1845–1847, 1951
Fisher CM, Light W: Manubriosternal arthralgia. N Engl J Med 256:799–801, 1957

MAPLE SYRUP

Synonyms. Menkes I; branched chain ketoaciduria I; ketoaciduria; maple syrup urine disease (MSUD); thiamine-responsive MSUD; ketoacid decarboxylase deficiency.

Symptoms and Signs. Both sexes affected; onset in first week of life. Vomiting; difficulty in feeding; failure to thrive; absence of grasping reflex; irregular gaspy breathing. Later, generalized rigidity and opisthotonos. Hypoglycemic crisis may occur. Severe mental retardation. Maple syrup odor in the urine. Five different phenotypes recognized: (1) classic; (2) intermittent; (3) intermediate; (4) thiamine-responsive; and (5) E3 deficiency.

Etiology. Deficient activity in various components of branched-chain 2-ketoacid dehydrogenase (BCKADH). Classic type is autosomal recessive; other types, present genetic heterogeneity.

Pathology. In central nervous system, marked deficiency in myelin, and astrocytosis.

Diagnostic Procedures. *Blood.* Investigation of enzymatic activity of leukocytes. Shows block of branched chain ketoacid metabolism. Elevation of plasma level of leucine, isoleucine, valine, and presence of alloisoleucine. Immunological studies to define mutations with immunologically altered proteins. *Urine. Cerebrospinal fluid.* Presence of ketoacids (identifiable at bed side with a solution of 2 N HCl saturated with 2,4-dinitrophenylhydrazine). Confirmed diagnosis by *thin-layer chromatography; gas chromatography and mass spectroscopy.*

Therapy. Long-term diet in which branched amino acids are omitted. After level of these amino acids falls to normal, resumption of administration without exceeding minimum requirement, but providing sufficient amount for growth requirement. Liver transplantation. Indication for future somatic gene therapy.

Prognosis. Death occurs early; if not in first week, then usually within first year. If patient survives long enough, mental damage becomes evident. Therapeutic approach, if instituted before 10 days of age, may result in prevention of mental complications. The difficulty of this treatment has to be pointed out.

BIBLIOGRAPHY. Menkes JH, Hurst PL, Craig JM: A new syndrome: Progressive familial infantile cerebral dysfunction associated with an unusual urinary substance. Pediatrics 14:462–466, 1954
Chuang DT, Shih VE: Disorders of branched chain aminoacid and ketoacid metabolism. In Scriver CR, Beaudet AL, Sly WS, et al: The Metabolic and Molecular Bases of Inherited Disease, 7th ed, pp 1250–1264. New York, McGraw-Hill, 1995

MARAÑON I

Symptoms and Signs. Flatfoot, scoliosis, and various spinal disorders associated with ovary insufficiency.

BIBLIOGRAPHY. Marañon G: Syndrome ostéomusculaire douloureux de l'insuffisance ovarique juvénile. Paris Med 1:414–419, 1930

MARAÑON II

Eponym used to indicate the particular aspect of a wrestler that may be conferred by generalized symmetric muscle lipomas.

BIBLIOGRAPHY. Jablonski S: Illustrated Dictionary of Eponymic Syndromes and Diseases and Their Synonyms. Philadelphia, WB Saunders, 1969

MARAÑON III

Association of a thyrotoxic status (see Flajani), fever, and adiposity.

BIBLIOGRAPHY. Marañon G: Vei Sindrome adiposidad-Basedow-distermia (ABD). Med Espan 30:509–516, 1953

MARAÑON IV

Eponym used to indicate a clinical association of hypertrophy of testicle (?) and gynecomastia.

BIBLIOGRAPHY. Marañon G: Contribution casuistica al sindrome ambihipergenital hipertesticulismo con ginecomastia. Bull Inst Pat Med 12:237–240, 1957

MARBLE BRAIN

Synonyms. Guibaud-Vainsel; carbonic anhydrase II deficiency syndrome; osteopetrosis (recessive); renal tubular acidosis; cerebral calcification; carbonic anhydrase B deficiency. See Albert-Schonberg.

Symptoms. Prevalent in families of Saudi Arabian descent. From birth. mental retardation (90%); growth failure. Moderate to severe lung disease. Increased susceptibility to fractures (that heal normally, however).

Signs. Typical facial features: broad head, prominent forehead, prominent narrow nose, slight epicanthal folds, small philtrum, micrognathia, teeth abnormalities.

Etiology. Inborn error of metabolism consisting of carbonic anhydrase II deficiency. Autosomal recessive inheritance.

Pathology. Osteopetrosis; cerebral calcification.

Diagnostic Procedures. *Blood.* Deficiency of carbonic anhydrase II; metabolic acidosis; hyperchloremia; normal anion gap. Analysis of carbonic anhydrase II in fetal blood or amniotic cells might prove to be of value in this syndrome for antenatal diagnosis. *X-rays of skull.* Intracranial calcifications; osteopetrosis; stiff and deformed rib cage. *EEG.* Abnormal for age. *Urine.* Alkaline, pH 6.0.

Therapy. Symptomatic; sodium bicarbonate until after adolescence; orthopedic management. Bone marrow transplantation is not indicated.

Prognosis. Variable.

BIBLIOGRAPHY. Guibaud P, Larbre F, Freycon MT: Osteopetrose et acidose renale tubulaire deux cas de cette association dans une fraterie. Arch Fr Pediatr 29:269–286, 1972
Vainsel M, Fondu P, Cadranel S, et al: Osteopetrosis associated with proximal and distal tubular acidosis. Acta Paediatr Scand 61:429–434, 1972
Venta PJ, Welty RJ, Johnson TM, et al: Carbonic anhydrase II deficiency syndrome in a Belgian family is caused by a point mutation at an invariant histidine residue (107his-to-tyr): Complete structure of the normal human CA II gene. Am J Med Genet 49:1082–1090, 1991
Sly WS, Hu PY: The carbonic anhydrase II deficiency syndrome: Osteo-petrosis with renal tubular acidosis and cerebral calcification. In Scriver CR, Beaudet AL, Sly WS, et al: The Metabolic and Molecular Bases of Inherited Disease, 7th ed, pp 4113–4124. New York, McGraw-Hill, 1995

MARCHAND

Synonyms. Postnecrotic liver; cirrhosis; toxic cirrhosis; posthepatitic cirrhosis. See Posthepatitis. Includes Cryptogenic cirrhosis.

Symptoms and Signs. Those of liver cirrhosis (see Laennec). Pathologic pattern (see) distinguishes it and seems to represent a common end-stage cirrhosis evolving from other less advanced stages.

Etiology. Difficult to assess, except when clear anamnesis or specific microscopic features are present: e.g., hepatitis B; alpha-antitrypsin deficiency (see); iron storage. Various factors are implicated in the passage from chronic hepatitis to cirrhosis

Pathology. In liver, nodules are separated by large bands of dense collagen; bile ductal proliferation and lymphocyte infiltration into the band may be observed. In some areas the hepatic parenchyma is missing and the fibrotic area includes different portal tracts. Nodules appear encapsulated by concentric collagen fiber; bile retention in hepatocytes and canaliculi may be observed; all forms of hepatocyte degeneration may be present, up to uniform coagulation necrosis of entire nodules.

Diagnostic Procedures. *Blood.* See Laennec. *Biopsy of liver.* (See Pathology.)

Therapy. See Laennec.

Prognosis. Variable according to different authors; may be better or worse than for Laennec.

BIBLIOGRAPHY. Gordon BL, Barclay WR, Rogers HC (eds): Current Medical Information and Terminology, 4th ed. Chicago, American Medical Association, 1971
Davis GL, Lau JYN: Hepatis C: In Haubrich WS, Schaffner F, Berk JE (eds): Bockus Gastroenterology, 5th ed, p 2097. Philadelphia, WB Saunders, 1995

MARCHAND (E.J.)

Synonyms. Hepatosplenic bilharziasis; cyanosis in schistosomiasis; hepatosplenic schistosomiasis; portal hypertension; cyanosis in schistosomiasis. See Katayama.

Symptoms and Signs. Chronic severe cyanosis. Clubbing of fingers; hepatosplenomegaly. No significant signs of pulmonary and cardiac abnormalities.

Etiology. Hepatosplenic schistosomiasis with portal hypertension. (See Manson schistosomiasis; pulmonary artery obstruction.)

Pathology. Hepatosplenic schistosomiasis with or without complicating portal cirrhosis. Evidence of portal hypertension and abnormal ramification of both pulmonary arteries and veins; increase of vascular bed of lung parenchyma; presence of arteriovenous fistula.

Diagnostic Procedures. *Stool.* Ova of schistosoma. *ECG.* No evidence of cardiac disease. *Blood.* Liver function test. Moderate liver impairment or cirrhosis. *Right heart catheterization.* Normal pressure of right side of heart and associated vessels. *Pulmonary function test.* Demonstration of lack of arterial oxygen saturation even after administration of 100% oxygen.

Therapy. Treatment of infestation. In some cases, portal shunt and splenectomy.

BIBLIOGRAPHY. Marchand EJ, De Jesus M, Biascoechea ZA: Cyanotic syndrome of portal hypertension in hepatosplenic schistosomiasis and portal cirrhosis. Am J Cardiol 10:496–506, 1962

Boros DL: Schistosomiasis mansoni: a granulomatous disease of cell-mediated immune etiology. Ann NY Acad Sci 278:36–46, 1976
Weatherall DJ, Ledingham JGG, Warrell DA (eds): Oxford Textbook of Medicine, 3rd ed, pp 970–981. Oxford, Oxford Med Pub, 1996

MARCHIAFAVA-BIGNAMI

Synonyms. Corpus callosum degeneration; demyelinating callosal encephalopathy.

Symptoms. Observed in middle-aged or old people who have consumed large quantities of wine. Gradual mental changes from excitement to apathy. Convulsions; tremors; dysarthria; ataxia; sphincter alteration; remission and exacerbations.

Etiology. Alcohol abuse and/or nutritional disorder.

Pathology. Symmetric demyelinization of central part of corpus callosum; involvement of white matter and anterior commissure.

Diagnostic Procedures. *EEG. Spinal fluid. Liver function tests. Brain CT scan. MRI. Other imaging techniques.*

Therapy. Vitamins, correct diet.

Prognosis. Death 4–6 years after onset.

BIBLIOGRAPHY. Marchiafava E, Bignami A: Sopra un alterazione del corpo calloso osservata in soggetti alcoolisti. Riv Patol Nerv Ment 8:544–549, 1903
Poser CM: Central pontine myelinolysis and Marchiafava-Bignami disease. Ann NY Acad Sci 215:373–381, 1973
Adams RD, Victor M: Principles of Neurology, 5th ed, pp 870–871. New York, McGraw-Hill, 1993

MARCHIAFAVA-MICHELI

Synonyms. Strübing-Marchiafava; hemolytic anemia; paroxysmal nocturnal hemoglobinuria; paroxysmal nocturnal hemoglobinuria.

Symptoms. Onset usually between the third and fourth decade in both sexes; rarely in childhood or old age. Frequently asymptomatic. Abdominal, lumbar, substernal pain; Dysphagia (worse in the morning), malaise, and fever. Urine passed during night or in the morning is dark; day urine has normal appearance. Atypical forms common (chronic hemolysis; pancytopenia; thrombotic episodes).

Signs. Pallor with yellowish discoloration of skin and mucosae; sometimes, bronzing discoloration. Functional cardiac murmur; splenomegaly; occasionally, hepatomegaly.

Etiology. Intracorpuscular defect makes red cells abnormally susceptible to lytic action of complement. Nature of abnormality unknown; not a familial condition.

Pathology. Venous thrombosis in systemic or portal circulation. Splenomegaly; hepatomegaly (central zone necrosis). In bone marrow, erythroid hyperplasia.

Diagnostic Procedures. *Blood.* Anemia; reticulocytosis. Icterus index high, free hemoglobin in plasma; leukopenia; low neutrophil alkaline phosphatase; moderate thrombocytopenia; iron deficiency; Ham test or acidified serum test. Sucrose hemolysis test; sugar-water test;. clotting test; tendency to thrombosis. *Urine.* Urobilinuria; hemosiderinuria; free hemoglobin. *Bone marrow.* Normoblastic hyperplasia (seldom megaloblastic changes), possible hypoplasia.

Therapy. There is no specific therapeutic agent for the erythrocyte membrane abnormality. In cases with severe anemia, frequent hemolytic crisis, thromboses, and infection: bone marrow grafts; adrenal steroids; blood transfusions; iron; anticoagulants; dextran.

Prognosis. Chronic condition; great variability of survival time (median survival 10 years). The severity of the disease is reflected in the degree of anemia. In some patients the severity lessens with time. Median survival time approximately 10 years, with occasional survival over 40 years. In 50% of cases venous thrombosis cause of death. Possibility of development of acute nonlymphocytic leukemia.

BIBLIOGRAPHY. Strübing P: Paroxysmale Haemoglobinurie. Dtsch Med Wochenschr 8:17–21, 1882
Marchiafava E, Nazari A: Nuovo contributo allo studio degli itteri cronici emolitici. Policlinico (Sez Prat) 18:241–254, 1911
Micheli F: Uno caso di anemia emolitica con emosideriuria perpetua. Accad Med Torino 7:148, 1928
Bell WR, Zerhouni E, Spitz R: Paroxysmal nocturnal hemoglobinuria. Johns Hopkins Med J 142:218–223, 1978
Lee GR: Paroxysmal nocturnal hemoglobinuria. In Lee GR, Bithel TC, Foerster J, et al (eds): Wintrobe's Clinical Hematology, 9th ed, pp 1232–1244. Philadelphia, Lea & Febiger, 1993

MARCUS GUNN

Synonyms. Gunn; jaw-winking. See Marin Amat.

Symptoms and Signs. Present from birth. Moderate ptosis of one eyelid when opening mouth. Jaw has lateral deviation toward the opposite side of the ptosis and results in elevation of upper lid and widening of palpebral fissure. When acquired, condition may appear at any age.

Etiology. Unknown; inherited (irregular dominant), congenital, or acquired condition.

Therapy. Surgery.

Prognosis. Usually remains constant for life; may also be transient, may progress, or may disappear, whereas only the ptosis remains.

BIBLIOGRAPHY. Gunn RM: Congenital ptosis with peculiar associated movements of the affected lid. Trans Ophthalmol Soc UK 3:283–286, 1883
Doucet TW, Crawford JS: The quantification, natural course and surgical results in 57 eyes with Marcus Gunn (jaw-winking) syndrome. Am J Ophthalmol 92:702–707, 1981
Bossen EH: Muscular disorders. In Garner A, Klintworth GK (eds): Pathobiology of Ocular Disease: A Dynamic Approach, 2nd ed, pp 1772–1773. New York, Marcel Dekker, 1994

MARDEN-WALKER

Synonyms. Blepharophimosis—joint contractures—muscular hypotonia—generalized connective tissue.

Symptoms and Signs. Present at birth. Fixed facial expression; micrognathia; cleft soft palate and uvula; blepharophimosis; pectus carinatum; kyphoscoliosis; arachnodactyly. Myotonia and contractures limiting adduction of hips and extension of elbows and knees that disappear during first year of life. Failure to thrive. Decreased deep tendon reflexes.

Etiology. Unknown; very similar to Schwartz-Jampel. Claimed to be different by Marden and Walker on the basis of the presence of cardiac and renal abnormalities, lack of respiratory system abnormalities, and presence of lesions at birth. Autosomal recessive (?) inheritance.

Pathology. *Heart.* Inferior vena cava common opening with superior vena cava. *Kidney.* Microscopically revealed diffuse dilation of large collecting tubules and hydropic degeneration of proximal and distal tubules (microcystic disease). *Skeletal muscles.* Atrophic without infiltrates. *Liver.* Mild fatty degeneration. *Other organs.* Normal.

Diagnostic Procedures. *Chromosome studies.* Normal. *X-rays of skull.* Small frontal region of skeleton. Metacarpal phalanges, metatarsal longer than normal. Bilateral talipes equinovarus. *Dermatoglyphic study.* Simian creases. *CT scan. MRI.* Partial or complete agenesis of cerebellum and brainstem. *Electromyography*. No myotonia or myotonic discharge on percussion. *Blood and urine*. Normal.

Prognosis.   Death in 3 months.

BIBLIOGRAPHY. Marden PM, Walker WA: A new generalized connective tissue syndrome. Am J Dis Child 112:225–228, 1966

Jaatoul NY, Haddad NE, Khoury LF, et al: The Marden-Walker syndrome. Am J Med Genet 11:259–271, 1982

Gossage D, Perrin JM, Butler MG: Brief clinical report and review: A 26-month-old child with Marden Walker syndrome and pyloric stenosis. Am J Med Genet 26:915–919, 1987

MARFAN I

Synonyms.   Marfan-Achard; arachnodactyly—dolichostenomelia; dolichostenomelia—arachnodaktyly; mesodermal dystrophy, congenital.

Symptoms.   Both sexes affected. Variable symptoms according to type and extent of organs involved (see Signs).

Signs.   Slender elongated body; dolichocephalic skull; prominent ears; arched palate; long arms and legs; hands with long slender fingers (arachnodactyly); kyphoscoliosis; pectus excavatum; flat feet; hammer toes. Subcutaneous fat scanty; hyperextensibility and dislocation of articulations; muscles hypotonic. Eyes involved in 50% of cases: myopia; strabismus; myosis; nystagmus; subluxation of lens; tremulous irides; cataract; coloboma. Heart and vascular system involved in 40–60% of cases: valvular deformities; septal defects; dilatation of aortic root and ascending aorta leading to aorta valve incompetence and eventually to aortic dissection, occasionally aneurism of pulmonary arteries as well. Pulmonary and kidney defects. A rare case of Marfan syndrome presenting as intrapartum death has been described. Recognizable mitral valve lesions were present.

Etiology.   Unknown; congenital disorder of connective tissue; biochemical incompetence of microfibrillar fibers may be responsible of some clinical manifestations. Autosomal dominant inheritance.

Pathology.   Mesodermal dystrophy; loss of elastic fibers; hyperplasia, dilatation of vessel; valvular defects of heart; fusion of vertebrae.

Diagnostic Procedures.   *Blood*. Decreased mucoprotein in serum. *X-ray*. Aorta dilatation and dissection or other cardiovascular defects. *Metacarpal index*. Greater length-to-width ratio than normal. *ECG*.

Therapy.   Prophylactic or early repair of cardiovascular defects with composite graft when indicated (surgery difficult because of poor consistency of tissues). Pharmacologic blockade of beta-adrenergic receptors: propanolol and now atenolol.

Prognosis.   Long life possible according to degree of heart involvement, which can be markedly reduced by pharmacologic treatment.

BIBLIOGRAPHY. Marfan AB: Un cas de déformation congénitale des quatre membres, plus prononcée aux extrémités, caracterisée par l'allongement des os avec un certain degre d'amincissement. Bull Soc Med Hôp Paris 13:220–226, 1896

Hollister DW, Godfrey M, Sakay LY, et al: Immunohistologic abnormalities of the microfibrillar-fiber system in the Marfan syndrome. N Engl J Med 323:152–159, 1990

Francke U, Furthmayr H: Marfan's syndrome and other disorders of fibrillin. N Engl J Med 330:1384–1385, 1994

MARFANOID HYPERMOBILITY

Symptoms and Signs.   Patients present some features of Marfan: increased height and slenderness; arachnodactyly; fibrous tendon contractures in hand; sparse subcutaneous fat; pectus excavatum; genu recurvatum; scoliosis; abnormalities of external ear; skin striae; and features of Ehlers-Danlos (skin hyperextensibility and joint laxity far

exceeding the degree occasionally observed in Marfan). Valvular heart disease reported in some cases.

Etiology.   Considered only by some authors a separate clinical entity within the heterogeneous Marfan group of conditions.

Pathology.   *Biopsy of skin*. No abnormalities.

Diagnostic Procedures.   *X-ray*. Bone alteration reported earlier; mild generalized osteoporosis; absence of calcified subcutaneous spheroids. *Urine*. Absence of abnormal excretion of amino acids.

Therapy.   Symptomatic.

Prognosis.   Not reported.

BIBLIOGRAPHY. Roederer C: Syndrome d'Ehlers-Danlos atypique coincidant avec une dolichostenomélie. Arch Fr Pediatr 8:192–195, 1951

Daneshwar A, Tavakoli D, Nazarian J: Marfanoid hypermobility syndrome associated with coarctation of the aorta. Br Health J 41:621–623, 1979

Godfrey M: The Marfan syndrome. In Rimoin DL, Lachman RS: Genetic disorders of the osseous skeleton. In Beithon P (ed): McKusick's Heritable Disorders of Connective Tissue, 5th ed, p 99. St Louis, CV Mosby, 1993

MARIE I

Obsolete.

Synonyms.   Fraser; Nonne; Sanger Brown; Klippel-Durante; cerebellar heredoataxia; ataxia cerebellar hereditary. See Déjerine-Thomas, Friedreich, Holmes and olivopontocerebellar atrophy (OPCAI).

Symptoms and Signs.   Both sexes. From early infancy. Ataxia: Persistence of tendon reflexes (alien to Friedreich ataxia) and occasionally ophthalmoplegia, retinal degeneration, optic atrophy.

Etiology.   Hereditary ataxia (autosomal dominant or recessive inheritance). Attempt to classify by P. Marie describes a cluster of syndromes, recognizing in the etiology a predominance of cerebellar lesions.

Pathology.   Lack of agreement on typical features, so that no specific anatomic findings may be assigned. In some of the cases considered, not even cerebellar lesions were found at autopsy.

Diagnostic Procedures.   *Brain. CT scan. MRI. Electromyography. Biopsy of muscle. Spinal tap.*

Therapy.   Symptomatic.

Prognosis.   Variable

BIBLIOGRAPHY. Brown S: On hereditary ataxia, with a series of twenty-one cases. Bain 15:250–258, 1892

Marie P Sur L'hérédo-atasie cerebelleuse. Semin Med 13:444–447, 1893

Pedersen L, Platz P, Ryder LP, et al: A linkage study of hereditary ataxias and related disorders: Evidence of heterogeneity of dominant cerebellar ataxia. Hum Genet 54:371–383, 1980

Adams RD, Victor M: Principles of Neurology, 5th ed, p 989. New York, McGraw-Hill, 1993

MARIE II

Synonyms.   Acromegalic; anterior pituitary adenoma; growth hormone hypersecretion; pituitary eosinophilic adenoma; somatotropic growth hormone hypersecretion. From a clinical point of view, it is useful to distinguish two syndromes: (1) The endocrine syndrome owing to the hormonal secretion; and (2) the neurologic syndrome owing to the mechanical compression of the growing tumor.

ENDOCRINE SYNDROME

Symptoms.   Slow gradual onset, usually at 30–50 years of age. Headache; backache; pain in limbs; sweating; hypomenorrhea or anemorrhea in women; loss of libido and potency in men (early symptoms). Sometimes temporary increase of libido at the onset of disease; polyuria; polydipsia; later muscular weakness.

Signs. *Facial changes.* Prognathism and separation of teeth; coarsening of nose; prominence of supraorbital ridges; enlargement of lips and tongue. *Skin changes.* Fibroma; pigmentation; hirsutism, increased sebaceous secretion. *Trunk and limb changes.* Enlargement of hands and feet (changing size of shoes impresses the patient). *Thoracic cage changes.* Kyphosis, muscle and joint hypertrophy. *Genitalia changes.* Testes become small and flabby. *Other changes.* Enlargement of heart size; tachycardia; hypertension.

Etiology. Excessive secretion of growth hormone (GH) after puberty. Can be secreted by (1) hypothalamus (growth hormone releasing hormone [GH-RH]-producing gangliocytoma; hyperfunctioning neuronal hamartoma/adenohypophyseal choristoma with pituitary GH cell hyperplasia, with pituitary GH cell hyperplasia adenoma); (2) anterior pituitary (GH adenomas; GH cell adenomas; mixed GH-prolactin adenoma; plurihormonal adenoma; mammosomatotropic adenoma; acidophilic stem cell adenoma; ectopic adenomas [GH cell]); (3) ectopic neoplasms (GH-producing; GHRH-producing).

Pathology. Hyperplasia or adenoma of pituitary, splanchnomegaly (liver, spleen, heart, kidney, intestine); enlargement of terminal parts of bones. Metachromatic material in muscles, which are atrophic. Frequently, goiter; adrenal enlarged; thymus usually large.

Diagnostic Procedures. *Blood.* Glucose tolerance curve; increased alkaline phosphatase and phosphorus level; increased follicle-stimulating hormone (FSH). *Urine.* Decreased FSH; increased 17-ketosteroids; glycosuria; increased creatine; occasionally, elevated basal metabolic rate. *MRI. CT scan.* Skull thickened; enlargement of sella turcica; paranasal sinus. Osteolytic process together with cortical periosteal thickening; conspicuous excrescences of muscle insertion. Osteoarthritis; tufted distal phalanges.

Therapy. *Surgery.* Total or partial hypophysectomy; radiation therapy; 90yttrium implantation. *Medical treatment.* Pergolide, bromocriptine, somatostatin analogs after surgery or radiation therapy to compensate for deficient secretion.

Prognosis. Progressive evolution usually in several years, but variable. Stabilization at later stage.

NEUROLOGIC SYNDROMES

Different syndromes may develop according to direction of adenoma expansion. For instance, see Chiasma and Cavernous sinus.

BIBLIOGRAPHY. Marie P: In Major RH: Classic Descriptions of Diseases, 2nd ed. Springfield, IL, Charles C Thomas, 1939
Brennan MD, Jackson IT, Keller EE, et al: Multidisciplinary management of acromegaly and its deformities. JAMA 253:682–683, 1985
Bauman G: Acromegaly. Endocrin Metab 16:685–705, 1987
Daughaday WH: Growth hormone, insulin-like growth factors and acromegaly. In De Groot LJ (ed): Endocrinology, 3rd ed, pp 303–329. Philadelphia, WB Saunders, 1995

MARIE-BAMBERG

Synonyms. Bamberg III; Von Bamberger; Hagner hypertrophic osteoarthropathy; Mankowsky hypertropic pulmonary osteoarthropathy; pachydermoperiostosis secondary.

Symptoms. Warm sensation at fingertips; sweating of hands and feet; arthralgia.

Signs. Clubbing of fingers; swelling of joints; followed by enlargement of epiphyses of long bones. Deformity of cyanotic nails.

Etiology. Unknown. See Dysacromelias. This particular syndrome may

be hereditary (autosomal dominant), idiopathic, or secondary to chronic pulmonary, cardiac, gastrointestinal, hepatic, endocrine, infective, or neoplastic conditions.

Pathology. Chronic inflammatory changes of synovial membranes; articular capsules; and adjacent tissues; infiltration of periosteum with round cells.

Diagnostic Procedures. *X-ray.* Osteoporosis; thickening of periosteum along shaft of long bones; thinned cortex; enlargement of terminal phalanges.

Therapy. With treatment of primary condition, pain ceases and periostitis is decreased.

Prognosis. That of primary condition. The appearance of this syndrome may serve as the only clue to a silent lesion.

BIBLIOGRAPHY. Marie P: De l'osteo-arthropathie hypertrophiante pneumique. Rev Med 10:1–36, 1890
Kuhlewein H: Hyppocratis opera quae feruntur omnia. Leipzig, 1894–1902
von Bamberger E: Ueber Knochenveranderungen bei chronischen Lungenund Herzkrankheiten. Zschr Klin Med 18:193–217, 1891
Fischer DS, Singer DH, Feldman SM: Clubbing: A review with emphasis on hereditary acropachy. Medicine 43:459–479, 1964
Harper J: Genetics and genodermatoses. In Champion RH, Burton JL, Ebling FJG (eds): Rook/Wilkinson/Ebling Textbook of Dermatology, 5th ed, p 362. Oxford, Blackwell Scientific, 1992

MARIE-LERI

Synonyms. Acro-osteolysis, rheumatoid; trophopathy myelodysplastica. See Hajdu-Cheney and acro-osteolysis.

Symptoms. Peculiar hand alteration; the fingers may be extended and shortened like a telescope. Syndrome seen in congenital indifference to pain; in congenital sensory neuropathy, in Thevenard syndrome.

Etiology. The authors attributed the syndrome to a peculiar form of rheumatoid arthritis causing acro-osteolysis. Likely related to Ehlers-Danlos. A toxic acro-osteolysis has been reported owing to exposure to vinylchloride.

BIBLIOGRAPHY. Marie P, Leri A: Une varieté de rheumatisme chronique: la main en largnette (présentation de pièces et de coupes). Bull Soc Ed Hôp 36:104–107, 1913
Dodson VN, Dinman BD, Whitehous WN, et al: Occupational arteriosclerosis: A clinical study. Arch Environ Health 22:83–91, 1971
Largauer-Lewowicka H: Nailford capillari abnormalities in polyvinyl chloride production workers. Int Arch Occup Environ Health 51:337–340, 1983
Klippel JH, Dieppe PA: Rheumatology, pp 6.8.7.–6.8.8. St Louis, CV Mosby, 1994

MARIE-SAINTON

Synonyms. Hulkcrantz anosteoplasia; Scheuthaurer; cleidocranial dysplasia; cleidocranial dysostosis; "Arnold head."

Symptoms and Signs. Widespread racial, ethnic, and regional occurrence; family history; also cases of spontaneous occurrence. Varying degrees of aplasia of clavicles that allow unusual mobility of shoulders. Neurologic and vascular symptoms from compression of clavicular stumps. Excessive development of head (brachycephaly). Metopic suture remains open in childhood and adulthood. Incomplete closure of fontanelles. Facial bones small, poorly developed; mastoid air cells absent or small. Hyptertelorism may be present; frequently, dwarfism; kyphosis; scoliosis; lordosis; spina bifida. Also, frequently, pathologic fractures. Epilepsy, schizophrenia, and mental retardation also reported in association.

Etiology. Disorder of ossification primarily affecting bones that ossify earliest in life. Autosomal dominant inheritance; also cases of spontaneous occurrence.

Pathology. Tendency for ossification to proceed slowly in skull, hands, pelvis; concurrent osteosclerosis also noticed.

Diagnostic Procedures. *X-ray of skeleton.* See Signs.

Therapy. Surgical correction of defect when feasible.

Prognosis. Disability rarely severe; normal activities and life span.

BIBLIOGRAPHY. Marie P, Sainton P: Sur la dysostose cléido-crânienne héréditaire. Bull Mém Soc Méd Hôp Paris 15:436, 1898
Scheuthauer G: Kombination rudimentärer. Schlüssel beine mit Anomalien des Schädels beim erwachsen Menschen. All Weir Med Ztg 16:293–295, 1871
Jackson WPU: Osteo-dental dysplasia (cleidocranial dysostosis): The "Arnold Head." Acta Med Scand 139:292–307, 1951
Arvystas MG: Familial generalized delayed eruption of dentition with short stature. Oral Surg 41:235–243, 1976

MARIE-SEE

Synonyms. Julien Marie-See; hydrocephalus—hypervitaminosis pseudotumor cerebri; liver lover headache.

Symptoms. Occurs in infants within 24 hours of receiving a massive doses of vitamin A and D. Vomiting; somnolence.

Signs. Brusque and intense fontanelles bulging. All other findings negative.

Etiology. Acute vitamin A toxicity. Equivalent of cephalalgia reported in adult receiving massive doses of vitamin A.

Pathology. Hydrocephalus.

Diagnostic Procedures. *CT scan.* Of fundus oculi.

Therapy. Spinal tap (with caution).

Prognosis. Within 24 hours all signs and symptoms disappear spontaneously.

BIBLIOGRAPHY. Marie J, See G: Hydrocéphalie aiguë bénigne du nourrisson apres ingestion d'une dose massive et unique de vitamines A et D. Arch Fr Pediatr 8:563–565, 1951
Selhorst JB, Waybright EA, Jennings S, et al: Liver Lover's headache: pseudotumor cerebri and vitamine A intoxication. JAMA 252:24, 33, 65, 1984
Weatherall DJ, Ledingham JGG, Warrell DA (eds): Oxford Textbook of Medicine, 3rd ed, p 4042. Oxford, Oxford Med Pub, 1996

MARIE UNNA

Synonyms. Unna (M.); hereditary hypotrichosis.

Symptoms and Signs. Very rare. Both sexes affected; onset in childhood. Eyebrows and eyelashes could be missing from birth or fall out shortly later; usually, however, they eventually grow back to normal. Later in childhood, loss of hair; hair loss progressively extends from the vertex to produce a partial or complete bald vertico-occipital patch by adulthood. Scanty growth of nails and of axillary and pubic hair; limited growth of teeth and nails. Mental development and health are normal. In women, hair is thick and abundant but seldom exceeds 20 cm in length.

Etiology. Autosomal dominant inheritance.

Pathology. Hairs show several irregularities of caliber, pigmentation, and are rotated 180 degrees on their axis.

Therapy. None.

Prognosis. See Signs.

BIBLIOGRAPHY. Unna M: Ueber hypotricosis congenita hereditaria. Derm Wochenschr 81:1167–1178, 1925
Bentley-Phillips B, Grace HJ: Hereditary hypotrichosis: A previously undescribed syndrome. Br J Derm 101:331–339, 1979
Dawber RPR, Ebling FJG, Wojnarowska FT: Disorders of hair. In Champion RH, Burton JL, Ebling FJG (eds): Rook/Wilkinson/Ebling Textbook of Dermatology, 5th ed, pp 2579–2580. Oxford, Blackwell Scientific, 1992

MARIN AMAT

Synonyms. Mueller-Kannberg; Marcus Gunn inverted; inverted Marcus Gunn; pterygo corneal reflex; winking-jaw; corneo-mandibular reflex.

Symptoms. Automatic, involuntary, or reflex closure of the eye.

Signs. With pressure on the cornea (with eye open) to produce winking, and quick movement of the mandible of contralateral side, sometimes mandible moves slightly forward. Movement very rapid and minimal; easily overlooked.

Etiology. Unknown; not found in normal subject. It can be demonstrated best a few weeks after hemiplegic attacks, and in cases of amyotrophic lateral sclerosis. Considered an associated movement between orbicularis oculi and external pterygoid muscles; release phenomenon owing to supranuclear lesion.

BIBLIOGRAPHY. Mueller-Kannberg: Eigentumliche Mitbewegung eines ptotischen Lides bei Unterkiefer–Bewegungen. Der Artz Prack, 7:1177–1180, 1894
Marin Amat M: Contribution al estudio de la curabilidad de la paralisis oculares de origen traumatico substitution functional del VII por el V par craneal. Arch Oftalmol Hip-Amer 18:70–99, 1918
Marin Amat M: Sur le syndrome ou phenomene de Marcus Gunn. Ann Ocul 156:513–528, 1919
Wartenberg R: Winking-jaw phenomenon. Arch Neurol Psychiatr 59:734–753, 1948
Adams RD, Victor M: Principles of Neurology, 5th ed, p 242. New York, McGraw-Hill, 1993

MARINESCO-SJÖGREN I

Synonyms. Garland-Moorhause; Sjögren II; Torsten; ataxia—cataract—dwarfism; hereditary oligophrenic cerebellolental degeneration; oligophrenic cerebellolenticular degeneration; MMS.

Symptoms and Signs. Both sexes affected; clinical onset when child learns to walk. Ataxia; rotary and horizontal nystagmus; dysarthria; physical and mental development retarded, weakness with or without muscle hypotonia; association with variable skeletal defects (short stature; kyphoscoliosis; genu valgum; reduced extensibility of the knee; digital defects). Hair sparse, short, fine, usually poor in pigment. Congenital cataract. Hypersalivation.

Etiology. Autosomal recessive inheritance. Possibly a lysosomal storage disorder.

Pathology. Degenerative process in the cortical areas of the cerebellum. Biopsy suggests chronic atrophy of nerve cells rather than inflammation. Electron microscopy shows enlarged lysosomes containing whorled lamellar or amorphous inclusion bodies.

Diagnostic Procedures. *X-ray. EEG. Biopsy of muscle. Electromyography. Ophthalmoscopy.*

Therapy. Symptomatic.

Prognosis. Normal life expectancy.

BIBLIOGRAPHY. Marinesco G, Draganesco S, Vasiliu D: Nouvelle maladie

familiale, caractérisée par une cataracte congenitale et un arrêt du
dévelopement somatoneuro-psychique. Encéphale 26:97–109, 1931
Sjögren T: Hereditary congenital spinocerebellar ataxia accompanied by
congenital cataract and oligophrenia. Confinia Neurol 10:293–308,
1950
Walker PD, Blitzer MG, Shapira E, et al: Sjögren syndrome: Evidence
for a lysosomal storage disorder. Neurology 35:415–419, 1985
Adams RD, Victor M: Principles of Neurology, 5th ed, p 830. New
York, McGraw-Hill, 1993

MARJOLIN

Synonym. Marjolin ulcer.

Symptoms and Signs. Occurs in both sexes, usually in elderly persons;
onset a few months after burn. Cicatricial scar; then 30–40 years later,
pruritus, hyperesthesia, pain, malodorous discharge.

Etiology. Carcinomatous degeneration of burn scar, or of lesions owing
to lupus vulgaris or erythematosus.

Pathology. On margin of ulcer or scar, epidermoid carcinoma, dense
fibrosis, reduced vascularization; seldom, basal cell carcinoma type.

Diagnostic Procedures. *Biopsy.*

Therapy. Surgery; radiotherapy; local destruction.

Prognosis. Poor.

BIBLIOGRAPHY. Marjolin Ulcère. Dictionnaire de Médecine 2nd ed, vol 30,
pp 10–31. Paris, 1846
Sabiston DC: Textbook of Surgery, 14th ed, pp 202–203. Philadelphia,
WB Saunders, 1991
Ryan TJ, Burnand K: Diseases of the veins and arteries, Leg ulcers. In
Champion RH, Burton JL, Ebling FJG (eds): Rook/Wilkinson/Ebling
Textbook of Dermatology, 5th ed, p 200. Oxford, Blackwell Scien-
tific, 1992

MARKOVITS

Synonym. Ophthalmodynia hypertonica copulationis.

Symptoms. Ocular pain during copulation in prone position.

Etiology. Prone position enhancing the closure of a narrow-angle
glaucoma.

BIBLIOGRAPHY. Markovits AS: Ophthalmodynia hypertonica copulationis.
Can J Ophthalmol 9:484–485, 1974

MAROTEAUX

Obsolete.*

Synonyms. Metaphyseal dysplasia (type A-III); metaphyseal dysostosis
(type A-III). See Pyle and Schmid.

Symptoms and Signs. Present from birth. Metaphyseal dysostosis limited to knees.

Etiology. Autosomal recessive inheritance.

Diagnostic Procedures. X-ray. Limited metaphyseal abnormalities.

BIBLIOGRAPHY. Maroteaux P, Savart P, Lefebvre J, et al: Les formes parti-
elles de la dysostoses metaphysaire. Presse Med 71:1523–1526, 1963
Sutcliffe J: Metaphyseal dysostosis (dysostosis methaphysaire). Ann
Radiol 9:215–223, 1966

*According to International Nomenclature of constitutional disorders of bone. Eur J
Pediatr 151:407–415, 1992

MAROTEAUX-LAMY I

Synonyms. Polydystrophic dwarfism; mucopolysaccharidosis VI; MPS
VI; N-acetylgalactosamine-4-sulfatase deficiency; arylsulfatase B deficiency.

Symptoms. Both sexes affected; clinical onset (growth retardation) at
2–3 years of age (severe form) or later. Visual impairment; deafness
(owing to recurrent otitis) restriction of articular movements; dyspnea;
neurologic manifestations (spastic paraplegia from compressive myelopathy and complication of hydrocephalus). Normal intelligence (rare
mental retardation).

Signs. Short stature; hydrocephalus (in some cases); coarse facies (not
as severe as in Hurler). Clouding of cornea; glaucoma; pigmented retinopathy. Progressive sternal protrusion. Murmurs indicating valvulopathies. Lumbar kyphosis. Genu valgum. Atlantoaxial subluxation (see)
(in some cases). Hips severely involved.

Etiology. Autosomal recessive inheritance. Two or more alleles producing, respectively, more or less severe clinical patterns. Inability to
hydrolyze the sulfate group from N-acetylgalactosamine-4-sulfate (arylsulfatase B).

Pathology. Striking amount of abnormal metachromatic inclusion in
many tissues and leukocytes. Glycosaminoglycan accumulation in the
cornea, in fibrous tissue in cartilages; and in central nervous system.
Thickening of heart valves and endocardium, fibrosis of bundle of His.
Reduction of vertebral canal.

Diagnostic Procedures. *Urine.* Excretion of dermatan sulfate only.
Measurement of arylsulfatase activity. *X-ray.* See Hurler. Prenatal diagnosis now is possible.

Therapy. Symptomatic: keratoplasty (repeated) early decompression of
cervical myelopathy, ventriculoperitoneal shunting for hydrocephalus,
cardiosurgery; and for systemic treatment bone marrow transplantation.

Prognosis. Variable according to severity of the condition. In severe
cases, maximal survival to the late twenties. In mild cases, longer survival reported.

BIBLIOGRAPHY. Maroteaux P, Lamy M: Hurler's disease, Morquio's disease
and related mucopolysaccharidoses. J Pediatr 67:312–323, 1965
Maroteaux P, Levéque B, Marie J, et al: Une nouvelle dysostose avec
élimination urinaire de chondroitine-sulfate. B Presse Med 71:1849–
1852, 1969
Whitley CB: The Mucopolysaccharidoses. In Beithon P (ed): McKusick's
Heritable Disorders of Connective Tissue, 5th ed, pp 442–450. St
Louis, CV Mosby, 1993
Neufeld EF, Muenzer J: The mucopolysaccharidoses. In Scriver CR,
Beaudet AL, Sly WS, et al: The Metabolic and Molecular Bases of
Inherited Disease, 7th ed, pp 2477–2478. New York, McGraw-Hill,
1995

MAROTEAUX MEDT

Obsolete.*

Synonyms. Multiple epiphyseal dysplasia tarda (type Id), MEDT (type Id).

Symptoms and Signs. Both sexes affected. Usually normal at birth
Moderate dwarfism (mainly trunk shortness). Normal length of extremities, mildly curved varus, with hands and feet short. Frequently,
arthrosis of hips. Occasionally scoliosis or kyophosis or both. Cranio-
facies normal.

Etiology. Autosomal dominant or recessive inheritance.

Pathology. Short, irregular columns and wide septa in chondro-osseous tissue, metachromatic inclusions.

Diagnostic Procedures. *X-ray of spine.* Platyspondyly. Vertebral irregularity and increased intervertebral disk height; corpus spongiosum

hernial changes. Extremities, alteration of femoral epiphyses; minor alteration of proximal epiphyses of umeri. Metaphyses widened, sclerotic and irregular. Iliac bones short and flared, coxa vara.

BIBLIOGRAPHY. Maroteaux P: Spondiloepiphyseal dysplasias and metatropic dwarfism. Birth Defects 5:35–41, 1969

Maroteaux P, Spranger J: The spondylometaphyseal dysplasias: A tentative classification. Pediatr Radiol 21:293–297, 1991

MARSDEN

Synonyms. Dystonia, familial; visual failure; striatal lucencies.

Symptoms and Signs. Initially pure dystonia, then subacute visual loss or asymptomatic optic atrophy.

Etiology. Unknown autosomal recessive inheritance. Mitochondrial disease (?).

Diagnostic Procedures. *CT scan. MRI.* Bilateral symmetric lucencies, especially in the putamen.

BIBLIOGRAPHY. Miyoshi K, Matsuoka T, Mizushima S: Familial holotopistic striatal necrosis. Acta Neuropath 13:240–249, 1969

Marsden CD, Lang AE, Quinn NP, et al: Familial dystonia and visual failure with striatal CT lucencies. J Neurol Neurosurg Psychiatr 49:500–509, 1986

MARSHALL (D.)

Synonym. Atypical ectodermal dysplasia. Possibly part of a spectrum, including Stikler, Wagner, Weissenbacher-Zweymuller, Walden, Pierre Robin, Kniest, SED congenita.

Symptoms. Both sexes affected; present from birth. Partial (usually) deafness; myopia; hypohidrosis.

Signs. Facial malformation with saddle nose. Cataract; fluid vitreous.

Etiology. Autosomal dominant inheritance.

Therapy. Symptomatic.

Prognosis. Frequently, spontaneous absorption of cataract; in some cases; luxation. Permanent condition.

BIBLIOGRAPHY. Marshall D: Ectodermal dysplasia: Report of kindred and ocular abnormalities and hearing defect. Am J Ophthalmol 45:143–156, 1958

Gorlin RJ, Cohen MM Jr, Levin LS: Syndromes of the Head and Neck, 3rd ed, p. 288–290. New York, McGraw-Hill, 1990

MARSHALL (J.)

Synonyms. Cutis laxa, aquired; elastolysis postinflammatory. PECL; postinflammatory elastolysis; cutis laxa.

Symptoms and Signs. Reported in Afro-european children in South Africa; onset before the age of 3 years. Eruption of red edematous papules, slowly progressing up to 2–10 cm, followed by successive sporadic new eruptions for 1 year. During eruptive phase, some patients develop pneumonia.

Etiology. Unusual reaction to arthropod bite (?).

Pathology. Reduction and degenerative changes of elastic fibers in affected areas.

Therapy. None.

Prognosis. Papules disappear to leave areas of cutis laxa.

BIBLIOGRAPHY. Marshall J: Alopecia after tick bite. S Afr Med J 40:1555–1556, 1966

Lewis PG, Hood AF, Barnett NF: Post-inflammatory elastolysis and cutis laxa. J Am Acad Dermatol 22:40–48, 1990

MARSHALL (R.E.)

Synonyms. Marshall-Smith; see Weaver.

Symptoms. Present from birth. Noisy breathing; repeated respiratory infections; failure to thrive; mental retardation; accelerated skeletal growth.

Signs. Underweight for length. Long cranium; prominent forehead; head hyperextension. Bulging eyes; blue sclerae; megalocornea; thick eyebrows; small upturned nose, small mandible. Broad middle and maximal phalanges.

Etiology. Unknown; sporadic.

Diagnostic Procedures. *X-ray.* Bone age markedly advanced; mandibular rami hypoplastic; absence of normal angle of chest. Frequently pneumonia.

Therapy. Prevention of respiratory infections. Feeding.

Prognosis. All patients died with pneumonia before the 20th month of age.

BIBLIOGRAPHY. Marshall RE, Graham CB, Scott CR, et al: Syndrome of accelerated skeletal maturation and relative failure to thrive: A newly recognized clinical growth disorder. J Pediatr 78:95–101, 1971

Fitch N: Update on the Marshall-Smith-Weaver controversy. Am J Med Genet 20:559–562, 1985

Charon A, Gillerot Y, van Maldergem L, et al: The Marshall-Smith syndrome. Eur J Pediat 150:54–55, 1990

MARSHALL-WHITE

Synonym. Bier.

Symptoms. Sporadic periods of insomnia and tachycardia, with the appearance of spots in the palms that are colder and paler than surrounding skin.

Etiology. Unknown; vasospastic phenomenon.

BIBLIOGRAPHY. Bier A: Die Entstehung des Collateral-kreisedlaufs. II Der Rüeckfluss des Bluts aus ischaemichen Koerperteilen. Virchows Arch (Pathol Anat) 153:306–334, 1898

Marshall W, White C: Localized area of ischemia of the hands. J Lab Clin Med 18:386–388, 1932–1933

MARTIN

Synonym. Bosviel-Martin; apoplexia uvulae; staphylohematoma.

Symptoms and Signs. Hemoptysis.

Etiology. Hemorrhage from hematoma of uvula.

BIBLIOGRAPHY. Martin A: Ueber das Staphylohaematoma. Neue Med Chir Ztg 225–227, 1846

MARTIN-ALBRIGHT

Synonyms. Albright IV; Albright hereditary osteodystrophy; AHO; pseudohypoparathyroidism. See also Pseudo-pseudohypoparathyroidism.

Symptoms. Female to male ratio 2:1; onset of symptoms at about 8 years of age. Headache; weakness; lethargy; numbness; paresthesia; dyspnea; laryngeal stridor; photophobia and blurred vision. Muscular cramps; abdominal pain; convulsion. Some degree of mental deficiency.

Signs. Short stature; round face; thick neck; shortness of limbs in relation to trunk. Hands fat; stubby short fingers; short metacarpal and metatarsal bones. Chvostek and Trousseau signs.

Etiology. Hereditary condition with diminished end-organ responsiveness (Seabright-Bantam syndrome) to parathyroid hormone, which is secreted in normal amount. Genetic heterogeneity. Different forms are described according to the pathogenesis.

Pseudohypoparathyroidism type 1a: Deficiency in a guanine nucleotide-binding protein (Gs) that couples hormone receptors to stimulation of adenylate cyclase. These patients may show other endocrinopathies because of generalized hormone resistance. Autosomal dominant inheritance.

Type 1b: Absence of physical signs, resistence limited to parathyroid hormone. Also here defect is located proximal to cAMP formation, but it appears to involve a specific signal transduction componenent: parathyroid hormone receptor. Sporadic or familial of not defined type of inheritance.

Type II: Resistance limited to parathyroid hormone and owing to a defect distal to cAMP formation. Sporadic; seldom if ever inherited.

Pathology. Normal or hyperplastic parathyroid glands. Subcutaneous calcification; calcification of basal ganglia of brain.

Diagnostic Procedures. *Blood.* Normal serum phosphatase activity; low calcium; increased serum phosphate. *Urine.* Decreased urinary excretion of calcium and phosphate. *Ellsworth-Howard test.* No response of kidneys to parathyroid hormone. Patients with pseudohypothyroidism show no change of urinary excretion of adenosine 3':5'-cycle phosphate (cyclic AMP), whereas normals and patients with true hypoparathyroidism show a tenfold to 20-fold increase. *X-ray.* Early epiphyseal closure; subcutaneous and basal ganglia of brain calcifications.

Therapy. Large dose of parathyroid hormone has little or no effect on serum calcium and phosphorus and urinary phosphate excretion. Fair response to large dose of vitamin D (or 1, 25 [OH]2D3 or 1 [OH]D) and calcium salts (monitoring to avoid hypercalciuria).

Prognosis. Satisfactory response to treatment indicated.

BIBLIOGRAPHY. Martin D, Bourdillon J: Un cas de tétanie idiopathique chronique. Échec thérapeutique de la graffe d'un adénome parathyrodien. Rev Med Suisse Rom 60:1166–1177, 1940
Albright F, Burnett CH, Smith PH, et al: Pseudo-hypoparathyroidism—example of "Seabright-Bantam syndrome": Report of three cases. Endocrinology 30:922–932, 1942
Levine MA, Spiegel AM: Pseudohypoparathyroidism. In De Groot LJ (ed): Endocrinology, 3rd ed, pp 1142–1144. Philadelphia, WB Saunders, 1995

MARTIN DU PAN-RUTISHAUSER

Synonym. Laminar osteochondritis. See Epiphyseal ischemic necrosis.

Symptoms and Signs. Prevalent in males; onset in adolescence. Pain; progressive motion reduction, due to ankylosis of a single joint.

Etiology. Unknown.

Pathology. Destruction of cartilage from infiltration of connective tissue between cartilage and spongious tissue.

BIBLIOGRAPHY. Martin du Pan C, Rutishauser E: Un type d'hartrose infantile nouvelle: Ostéochondrite laminaire. Schweiz Med Wochenschr 75:955–956, 1945

MARTORELL I

Synonym. Hypertensive ischemic ulcer.

Symptoms and Signs. Predominant in women, onset in middle or old age. Painful ulceration of the leg (frequently bilateral) above the ankle. Other symptoms and signs of blood hypertension.

Etiology. Blood hypertension.

Pathology. Arteries present accumulation of hyalin material between elastica and endothelium.

Therapy. Firm, nonelastic bandage; Heparin i.m.; triamcinolone intralesion; excision; control of pressure and sympathectomy. Stop smoking and avoid beta-blockers. Grafting valid quick method.

Prognosis. Weeks before necrosis completes, necrotic crust separates and granulation occurs, good response to treatments, fundamental blood pressure control.

BIBLIOGRAPHY. Martorell R: Ulcera hypertensiva. Barcellona Ediciones BTP, 1953
Ryan TJ, Burnand K: Diseases of the veins and arteries leg ulcers. In Champion RH, Burton JL, Ebling FJG (eds): Rook/Wilkinson/Ebling Textbook of Dermatology, 5th ed, pp 2005–2006. Oxford, Blackwell Scientific, 1992

MARTSOLF

Synonym. Cataract; mental retardation; hypogonadism.

Symptoms and Signs. Prevalent in males. From infancy. Severe mental retardation; cataract, short stature; features of primary hypogonadism; minor cephalic (microcephaly, maxillary retrusion, pointing mouth, nonaligned teeth) and digital anomalies (short metacarpals and short phalanges). In one case reported cardiomyopathy.

Etiology. Possibly autosomal recessive inheritance.

BIBLIOGRAPHY. Cuendet JF, Netter C, Catti A, et al: Association de congenitale et oligophrenie. Bull Mem Soc Fr Ophthal 87:164–168, 1976
Martsolf JT, Hunter AGW, Haworth JC: Severe mental retardation, cataracts, short stature, and primary hypogonadism in two brothers. Am J Med Genet 1:291–299, 1978
Hennekam RCM, Van de Meeberg AG, Van Doorne JM, et al: Martsolf syndrome in a brother and sister: Clinical features and pattern of inheritance. Eur J Pediatr 147:539–543, 1988
Harbord MG, Baraitser M, Wilson J: Microcephaly, mental retardation, cataracts, and hypogonadism in sibs: Martsolf's syndrome. J Med Genet 26:397–408, 1989

MASSETERIC HYPERTROPHY

Synonym. Includes benign masseteric hypertrophy and Poch.

Symptoms and Signs. Benign form: Unilateral or bilateral masseter muscle hypertrophy manifesting itself as a painless swelling below and anterior to the ear, with or without earache or temporomandibular arthralgia. Habitual grinding of teeth during sleep. Usually, tense personality. Congenital form (Poch): enlargement of masseter and calf muscles without generalized muscular hypertropy; no symptoms or cramps and paresthesia in the calves.

Etiology. Acquired condition owing to different mechanisms: primary or secondary malocclusion; displacement of the mandible by "cracking" jaw while reading; tension and teeth grinding; or congenital in three generations considered an anomaly of muscular development rather than a truly pathological condition.

Pathology. Masseter hypertrophy; wearing of teeth surfaces; temporomandibular joint changes.

Diagnostic Procedures. *X-ray.* When unilateral condition, severe distortion of mandible. *Blood.* Enzymes normal. *Dental consultation.* Malocclusion; *Electromyography.* Normal. *Biopsy.*

Therapy. Restoration of normal bite; frequently, simple explanation of nature of condition reassures the patient and cures associated complaints arising from fear of cancer or incurable infections. Sedative may be useful in particularly tense patients to break the habit.

Prognosis.   Good with proper treatment.

BIBLIOGRAPHY. Gurney GE: Chronic bilateral benign hypertrophy of masseter muscles. Am J Surg 73:137–139, 1947
Barton RT: Benign masseteric hypertrophy: A syndrome of importance in the differential diagnosis of parotid tumors. JAMA 164:1646–1647, 1957
Gardner-Medwin D: Hypertrophia musculorum vera. In Vinken PJ, Bruyn GW: Handbook of Clinical Neurology, vol 43, pp 83–85. Amsterdam, North-Holland, 1982

MASSIVE ASPIRATION

Synonyms.   Massive fetal aspiration; atelectasia neonatorum; fetal aspiration. See Meconium aspiration.

Symptoms.   Occurs in newborn: they may be stillborn, die in a few hours after birth, or survive. Tachypnea; wheezing; apnea; flaccidity; rigidity; convulsions in more severe cases. In milder form, dyspnea soon after birth, lasting 2 or 3 days followed by rapid recovery.

Signs.   Intercostal retraction; asphyxia pallida; brain damage in severe cases; chest percussion diminished resonance; generalized or localized area of hyperresonance possible. Rales may or may not be present; temperature normal (except when infection develops); no cough.

Etiology.   Fetal asphyxia causes the fetus to gasp in the uterus or birth canal (postmaturity may also play an important role) and to inhale amniotic, vaginal, or oropharyngeal fluids.

Pathology.   Lung firm, poorly aerated; bronchi full of mucus or fluid; alveoli collapsed; some expanded; squamae and amniotic debris elements recognized. Edema and hemorrhages present. Brain hemorrhages and edema may coexist. Right heart dilatation in many cases.

Diagnostic Procedures.   *X-ray of chest.* Coarsely granular pattern with irregular aeration.

Therapy.   Bronchoscopic suction; oxygen; humidity control; antibiotic prophylaxis.

Prognosis.   Brief course unless complications develop (hours or days later). Severe form lethal.

BIBLIOGRAPHY. Farber S, Wilson JL: Atelectasis of the newborn: A study and critical review. Am J Dis Child 4b:572–589, 1933
Civetta JM, Taylor RW, Kirby RR (eds): Critical Care, 2nd ed. Philadelphia, Lippincott, 1992

MASSON

Synonym.   Glomus tumor multiple; angio-endothelioma arterial; glomangioma, multiple.

Symptoms and Signs.   Soft blue-black, painful, usually raised skin lesions. Present at birth, or usually appearing before age 20, on forearm, thighs and buttocks, head, neck, penis. Isolated. Tumors that vary from few mm to several cm. Appears later (33 years of age) and usually in subungueal zone. History of trauma preceding tumor has been reported. Possible association of malformation of affected limbs.

Etiology.   Autosomal dominant inheritance.

Pathology.   Lesion reminiscent of cavernous hemangiomas. Presence of multiple layers of glomus cells and nerve fibers lining blood-filled cavities.

Therapy.   Surgical excision (if total nonrecurrence).

Prognosis.   Malignant changes do not occur. They may, however, be associated with other malignancies.

BIBLIOGRAPHY. Wood W: On painful subcutaneous tubercle. Edinburgh Med J 8:283, 1812
Masson P: Hémangioendothéliome végétant intra-vasculaire. Bull Soc Anat (Paris) 93:517–523, 1923
Masson P: Le glomus neuro-myo-artérial des regions tactiles et ses tumeurs. Lyon Chir 21:257, 1924
Baesley SW, Mel J, Chow CW, et al: Hereditary multiple glomus tumors. Arch Dis Child 61:801–802, 1986
McKie RM: Soft tissue tumors. In Champion RH, Burton JL, Ebling FJG (eds): Rook/Wilkinson/Ebling Textbook of Dermatology, 5th ed, p 2090. Oxford, Blackwell Scientific, 1992

M.A.S.S. PHENOTYPE

Synonyms.   Mitral valve prolapse, aortic; skeletal, skin manifestation; mitral valve prolapse.

Etiology.   It may represent a phenotypic continuum with Marfan syndrome (see).

BIBLIOGRAPHY. Salomon J, Shah PM, Heinle RA: Thoracic skeletal abnormalities in idiopathic mitral valve prolapse. Am J Cardiol 36:32–36, 1975
Glebsby MJ, Pyeritz RE: Association of mitral valve prolapse and systemic abnormalities of connective tissue: A phenotypic continum. JAMA 262:523–528, 1989

MATERNAL–FETAL TRANSFUSION

Synonym.   See Neonatal polycythemia.

Symptoms and Signs.   Neonatal polychythemia (see).

Etiology.   Maternal–fetal transfusion.

Pathology.   Plethora.

Diagnostic Procedures.   *Blood.* High hemoglobin and hematocrit values. Demonstration of maternal erythrocytes in newborn (Ashby differential agglutination method). Presence in the newborn blood of beta-2-M-globulin.

Therapy.   See Neonatal polycythemia.

Prognosis.   Usually good.

BIBLIOGRAPHY. Hedenstedt S, Naeslund J: Investigations of the permeability of the placenta with the help of elliptocytes. Acta Med Scand 170(Suppl):126–134, 1946
Michael AF, Mauer AM: Maternal-fetal transfusion as a cause of plethora in neonatal period. Pediatrics 28:458–461, 1961
Rosenkrantz TS, Oh W: Neonatal polycythemia and hyperviscosity. In Milunsky A, Friedman EA, Gluck L, et al: Advances in Perinatal Medicine, vol 5, p 93. New York, Plenum, 1986
Van der Zee DC, Poelmann RE, Vermeij-Keers C, et al: Materno-embryonic transfusion and congenital malformations: An experimental study using rat embryos. J Pediatr Surg 23:266–269, 1988

MATERNALLY INHERITED SENSORINEURAL DEAFNESS

Synonyms.   MISD; deafness, sensorineural, maternally inherited

Symptoms and Signs.   Female transmission. Both sexes. Onset during first few years of life, seldom later. Diabetes and profound sensorineural deafness.

Etiology.   Hypothesis: Cosegregation of the mtDNA with an autosomal recessive mutation.

Diagnostic Procedures.   OXPHOS enzymology on mitochondria-enriched lysate of lymphoblastoid cells interpreted to represent an increased OXPHOS activity (complexes III and V).

Therapy. See OXPHOS syndromes.

BIBLIOGRAPHY. Jaber L, Shohat M, Bu X, et al: Sensorineural deafness inherited as a tissue specific mitochondrial disorder. J Med Genet 29:86–90, 1992
Shoffner JM, Wallace DC: Oxidative phosphorylation diseases. In Scriver CR, Beaudet AL, Sly WS, et al: The Metabolic and Molecular Bases of Inherited Disease, 7th ed, p 1571. New York, McGraw-Hill, 1995

MATHES

Synonym. Puerperal mastitis.

Symptoms. Occurs 10 days after delivery, or later (parenchymatous type). Fever; chills; malaise; breast pain, initially slight, then progressive, accentuated by nursing.

Signs. Two types distinguished. *Interstitial.* Inflammatory area tense and hard, from nipple to breast margin. *Parenchymatous.* Localized, tender masses in breast lobe, evolving into abscesses.

Etiology. Infections. Most common agent responsible is *Micrococcus aureus.*

Pathology. Interstitial inflammatory features, extending among septa between lobes; parenchymatous infection, involving lactiferous ducts and glands.

Diagnostic Procedures. *Blood.* Leukocytosis.

Therapy. Antibiotics; breast support; nursing interruption; oral stilbestrol. If abscess formation, surgery.

Prognosis. Good with adequate therapy.

BIBLIOGRAPHY. Mathes P: Eine typische Form der Brustentzündung im Wochenbett. Munch Med Wochenschr 68:15, 1921
Cunningham FG, MacDonald PC, Gant NF, et al (eds): Williams Obstetrics, pp 647–648. Englewood Cliffs, NJ, Prentice-Hall, 1993

MATSOUKAS

Synonym. Articulo-oculo-cerebro-skeletal dysplasia.

Symptoms. Both sexes affected; present from birth. Mental retardation; myopia.

Signs. Small stature; multiple joint dislocation. Small mouth; high palate; microphthalmia; reduced palpebral fissures. Senile cataract; corneal sclerosis. In-curved little finger.

Etiology. Autosomal dominant inheritance. Not well differentiated from Larsen, Schwartz, Hallermann-Streiff, Mieter, and Stickler.

BIBLIOGRAPHY. Matsoukas J, Liarikos S, Giannikas A: A newly recognized dominantly inherited syndrome: Short stature, ocular and articular anomalies, mental retardation. Helv Pediatr Acta 28:383–386, 1973

MATZENAUER-POLLAND

Synonym. Dermatitis symmetrica dysmenorrhoica.

Symptoms and Signs. Includes the periodic activation or exacerbation of many existing dermatoses during premenstrual and menstrual periods. Associated with the dermatologic manifestation are emotional tension, headache, and abdominal, articular, and urinary symptoms (see Premenstrual).

Etiology. Part of premenstrual syndrome (see); no reason to separate this dermatologic syndrome from premenstrual. Some of the derma-

tologic manifestations have been attributed to autoimmune mechanism or hypersensitivity to progesterone.

BIBLIOGRAPHY. Matzenauer R, Polland R: Dermatitis symmetrica dysmenorrhoica Beitrag zur Angioneurosefrage. Arch Dermatol Syph 111:385–394, 1912
Graham-Brown RAC, Ebling FJG: The ages of man and their dermatoses. In Champion RH, Burton JL, Ebling FJG (eds): Rook/Wilkinson/Ebling Textbook of Dermatology, 5th ed, p 2885. Oxford, Blackwell Scientific, 1992

MAUGERI

Synonym. Silicotic mediastinitis; mediastinal silicosis.

Symptoms. Onset after chronic (10–30 years) exposure to silicates. Frequently asymptomatic. Dyspnea; congestive heart failure symptoms; cough.

Signs. Evidence of thoracic deformity; pleural effusion; basal crepitations; finger clubbing. Broadbent sign; systolic retraction of apex during inspiration; pulsus paradox; frequently, hepatosplenomegaly.

Etiology. Chronic exposure to silicate products.

Pathology. Silicates, usually in fibrous forms (asbestos, talc), in bronchioles and alveoli of lungs with typical formation of reacting bodies and secondary fibrosis; distortion; microcysts and honeycombing formations. Striking pleural thickening, in this case fibrous attachment with pericardium and other mediastinal structures. Congestive heart failure features.

Diagnostic Procedures. *X-ray.* Pleural changes: plaques; calcifications; effusion. Pulmonary changes: small or large opacities. *ECG.* Low voltage, especially of QRS complex; T-waves flattened or inverted. Right axis deviation. *Blood.* Polycythemia; hypercapnia.

Therapy. Symptomatic.

Prognosis. Progressive evolution. Possibly, development of mesothelial neoplasm of pleura.

BIBLIOGRAPHY. Maugeri S: La mediastinite silicotica. Folia Med 36:136–143, 1953
Thurlbeck WM, Churg MA: Pathology of lung, pp 879–884. New York, Thieme, 1995

MAUMENEE

Synonym. Harboian; Stocker-Hol; congenital, hereditary corneal dystrophy, CHCD; corneal dystrophy congenital deafness; deafness, congenital dystrophy.

Symptoms and Signs. Both sexes affected; corneal edema present at birth. Corneas show diffuse milky or ground-glass opacity and thickening. Opacity may be central or peripheral. Vision variously impaired, sometimes worse at wakening. Progressive sensineural deafness. Occasionally, nystagmus.

Etiology. Autosomal dominant or recessive inheritance.

Pathology. Corneal endothelial cells reduced or atrophic, pigmented or absent pigment; increased thickness in Descemet membrane, replacement by a mixture of long-spacing and regular collagen.

Diagnostic Procedures. *Biopsy. Blood. Urine.* Normal.

Therapy. Penetrating keratoplasty; corneal transplant; hearing aid.

Prognosis. Some cases static; in others slow progression of visual impairment.

BIBLIOGRAPHY. Maumenee AE: Congenital hereditary corneal dystrophy. Am J Ophthalmol 50:1114–1124, 1960
Harboyan G, Mamo J, Der Kaloustian V, et al: Congenital corneal dystrophy. Arch Ophthal 85:27–32, 1971
Kirkness CM, McCartney A, Rice NSC, et al: Congenital hereditary

corneal edema of Maumenee: Its clinical features, management and pathology. Br J Ophthalmol 71:130–144, 1987

Rodrigues MM, Rajagopalan S, Jones KA: Anterior and posterior corneal dystrophies: In Garner A, Klintworth GK (eds): Pathobiology of Ocular Disease: A Dynamic Approach, 2nd ed, pp 1200–1201. New York, Marcel Dekker, 1994

MAURIAC (C.)

Synonym. Syphilitic erythema nodosum.

Symptoms and Signs. Those of erythema nodosum (see), among other manifestations of tertiary syphilis.

BIBLIOGRAPHY. Mauriac C: Pathologie générale de la syphilis terziarie. Paris, Capiomont et Renault, 1886

Goldin D, Rook A, Gairdner D: Granuloma annulare in Mauriac's syndrome. Br J Dermatol 93:(Supp 11)31, 1975

MAURIAC (P.)

Synonym. Diabetes; dwarfism; obesity. See Wolcott-Rallison.

Symptoms. Slowly developing in diabetic children of the "brittle" type. Hard to manage diabetes; slow growth; abdominal colic.

Signs. Dwarfism; obesity with moon facies; hepatomegaly, splenomegaly, hypersensitivity to quick-acting insulin; favorable response to slow-acting types.

Etiology. Nutritional deficiencies; lack of insulin. Possibly, metabolic derangement owing to diabetes or associated conditions.

Pathology. Liver fat infiltration; lesion typical of diabetes (see).

Diagnostic Procedures. *Blood. Urine* Evaluation of diabetes, adrenal cortex, and pituitary functions. Rule out storage diseases. *X-ray.* Retarded ossification; osteoporosis.

Therapy. Slow-acting insulin; adequate diet.

Prognosis. That of juvenile diabetes.

BIBLIOGRAPHY. Mauriac P: Gros ventre, Hépatomégalie. Troubles de la croissance cher les enfants diabétiques, traités depuis plusieurs années par l'insuline. Gaz Hebd Sci Med Bordeaux 51:402–404, 1930

Guest GM: The Mauriac syndrome. Diabetes 2:415–417, 1953

Tulzer W, Ploier R: Untersuchungen zur Pathogenese des Mauriac Syndroms. Paediat Paedol 11:356–363, 1976

Kasa-Vubu JZ, Kelch RP: Precocious and delayed puberty diagnosis and treatment. In Haubrich WS, Schaffner F, Berk JE (eds): Bockus Gastroenterology, 5th ed, vol 2, p 1960. Philadelphia, WB Saunders, 1995

MAYER-ROKITANSKY-KÜSTER-HAUSER

Synonyms. Rokitansky-Küster-Hauser, RKH; non-Rokitansky-Küster-Hauser; vaginal congenital absence; uterus bipartitus solidus rudimentarius cum vagina solida; absent uterus.

Symptoms and Signs. Incidence statistics differ from 1:4000 (at birth) to 1:20,000 at female hospital admissions. Recognized usually at time of expected menarche. Primary amenorrhea; congenital absence of vagina; uterus normal or rudimentary; bicornate cords or complete absence; normal ovulation; normal breast development; normal body and hair. Abdominal pain if rudimentary uterine anlage that has enough tissue to desquamate. Frequent association with urinary tract anomalies (34%); skeletal abnormalities (12%); congenital heart conditions (4%); inguinal hernia (7%).

Etiology. Usually sporadic. Possibly, karyotype abnormalities. Normal initial phases of Müller duct development and impairment of subse-

quent development; defect in organization of mesoderm. Familial form consistent with autosomal recessive trait. Cases with vertebral anomalies cosidered as part of VATER syndrome (see).

Pathology. See Symptoms and Signs.

Diagnostic Procedures. *Chromosome studies.* Karyotype 46XX. *Basal body temperature.* Biphasic. *Hormone studies.* Normal ovulation pattern. *X-rays.* Evaluation of urinary tract anatomy. *Laparoscopy. Sonography. CT scan. MRI.*

Therapy. Nonsurgical. Repeated application of pressure against vaginal dimple with a dilator (Frank or Ingram technique). Surgical: Construction of a functional vagina by McIndoe technique.

Prognosis. High success rate with nonsurgical technique (95%). Surgery is necessary only in patients that do not respond to nonsurgical technique. Pregnancy possible with in vitro fertilization and surrogate mother.

BIBLIOGRAPHY. Mayer CAJ: Ueber Verdoppelungen des Uterus und ihre Arten, nebst Bemerkungen über Hasenscharte und Wolfsrachen. J Chir Augenheilked 13:525–564, 1829

Rokitansky KF: Ueber die sogenannten Verdoppelungen des Uterus. Med Jahrb Ostet Staat 26:39–77, 1838

Las Casas dos Santos NI: Missbildungen des Uterus, 2 Geburtsh Gynaeck 14:140–84, 1888

Küster H: Uterus bipartitus solidus rudimentarius cum vagina solida. Z Gebur Gynaekol 67:692–718, 1910

Hauser GA, Keller M, Koller T, et al: Das Rokitansky-Küster-Syndrom. Uterus bipartitus solidus rudimentarius cum vagina solida. Gynaecologia 151:111–112, 1961

Rock JA, Keenan DL: Surgical correction of uterovaginal anomalies. In Sciarra HH ed: Gynecology and Obstetrics, vol 1, pp 1–20. New York, Harper & Row, 1992

Forest MG: Diagnosis and treatment of disorders of sexual development. In De Groot LJ (ed): Endocrinology, 3rd ed, p 1925. Philadelphia, WB Saunders, 1995

MAY-HEGGLIN

Synonyms. Döhle bodies; myelopathy; Hegglin.

Symptoms and Signs. Both sexes affected; detection possible from birth. Usually asymptomatic; seldom, minor hemorrhagic manifestation.

Etiology. Autosomal dominant inheritance.

Pathology. Inclusion bodies may be paracrystalline arrays of depolymerized ribosomes.

Diagnostic Procedures. *Blood.* Mild leukopenia; increased percentage of polymorphonuclear leukocytes. These cells show in the cytoplasma fusiform or semilunar basophilic inclusion bodies (same features as Döhle or Amato bodies). Mild thrombocytopenia; platelets giant and poorly granulated. *Clotting tests.* Tourniquet: frequently positive; increased time of clot retraction. *Bone marrow.* Megakaryocytes clamping (impaired fragmentation?).

Therapy. None.

Prognosis. Good.

BIBLIOGRAPHY. May R: Leukocytenanschlüfsse. Kausistiche Mitteilung. Dtsch Arch Klin Med 96:1–6, 1909

Hegglin R: Gleichzeitige konstitutionelle Veränderungen an Neutrophilen und Thrombozyten. Helv Med Acta 12:439–440, 1945

Cabrera JR, Fontan G, Lorente, F, et al: Defective neutrophil mobility in the May-Hegglin anomaly. Br J Haemat 47:337–343, 1981

Athens JW: Qualitative disorders of leukocytes. In Lee GR, Bithel TC, Foerster J, et al (eds): Wintrobe's Clinical Hematology, 9th ed, pp 1615–1616. Philadelphia, Lea & Febiger, 1993

MAY-THURNER

Synonyms. Including unilateral left leg edema.

Symptoms and Signs. Persistent edema of left leg.

Etiology. "Spur" of the left common iliac vein at the crossover with right common iliac artery or compression by tortuous left common iliac artery.

Pathology. Hypertrophy of the intima of left common iliac vein.

Diagnostic Procedures. *Hemodynamic study.* Marked increase of differential pressure between external iliac vein and lower inferior cava. *CT scan. Ultrasonography. Venography.* Doppler obstruction of the vein.

Therapy. Surgical.

Prognosis. Good with treatment.

BIBLIOGRAPHY. May R, Thurner J: Ein Gefsspornin der v. iliac com. sin. als wahrscheinliche Ursache der uberwiegend liknsseitigen Beckenvenenthrombose. Z Kreislforsch 45:912, 1956

Hassell DR, Reifsteck JE, Harshfield DL, et al: Unilateral left leg edema: A variation of the May-Thurner syndrome. Cardiovasc Intervent Radiol 10:89–91, 1987

MAY-WHITE

Synonyms. Cerebellar ataxia—deafness—myoclonus; myoclonus—cerebellar ataxia—deafness; including Latham-Munro.

Symptoms and Signs. Both sexes affected; onset at various ages, usually in adolescence. Progressive cerebellar ataxia; myoclonic seizures and neural hearing loss. In some members of the affected family, forme fruste may be present.

Etiology. Unknown; autosomal dominant inheritance. One family with autosomal recessive inheritance reported (Latham) in which manifestation occurred at 10–12 years of age.

Diagnostic Procedures. *EEG.*

Therapy. Attacks controlled by phenytoin and valproic acid.

Prognosis. Chronic progressive condition. Life expectancy may be within normal limits.

BIBLIOGRAPHY. Latham AD, Munro TA: Familial myoclonus epilepsy associated with deaf-mutism in a family showing other psychobiological abnormalities. Ann Eugen 8:166–175, 1937

May DL, White HH: Familial myoclonus, cerebellar ataxia and deafness. Arch Neurol 19:331–338, 1968

Chayasirisobhon S, Walters B: Familial syndrome of deafness, myoclonus and cerebellar ataxia. Neurology 34:78–79, 1984

MAZAR

Synonyms. Short dura matter; dura matter, short.

Symptoms and Signs. Painful manifestation in occipital region in patients suffering from malformation of Arnold-Chiari (see) type, or platibasia or atlanto-occipital malformation.

Etiology and Pathology. Notable tension of dura matter, contracted by a transverse bridge passing from one cerebellar lobe to the contralateral and joining the lateral sinuses with a fibrous strap.

Diagnostic Procedures. *X-ray. CT scan. MRI.*

Therapy. Opening of dura, leaving subjacent arachnoid intact to abolish the pain.

BIBLIOGRAPHY. Mazar Physiopathologie de la douleur Thése. Paris, 1948

Sigwald J, Janet F: Occipital neuralgia. In Vinken PJ, Bruyn GW: Handbook of Clinical Neurology, vol 5, p 372. Amsterdam, North-Holland, 1972

McARDLE

Synonyms. McArdle-Schmid-Pearson; Cori type V glycogenosis; glycogenosis, type V; myophosphorylase deficiency; muscle phosphorylase deficiency.

Symptoms. Onset usually in childhood, although diagnosis may be made later. First pain; then stiffness following exercise of any muscle, including masseter. Rest makes symptoms disappear. Transient myoglobinuria may appear in some cases.

Signs. Size and initial power tone of muscle normal at outset of exercise. No fasciculation or fibrillation; no myoclonia; reflexes normal. After three decades, some muscle atrophy and permanent weakness may be noted.

Etiology. Myophosphorylase deficiency. Autosomal recessive inheritance. Dominant form also reported. Gene for muscle phosphorylase has been cloned and mapped to chromosome 11q13–11qter.

Pathology. Increased glycogen deposits in muscle; no detectable phosphorylase with diphosphopyridine nucleotide (DPNH) stain.

Diagnostic Procedures. *Routine laboratory analyses.* All normal. Venous return: from exercised muscle, poor in concentration of lactate and pyruvate (opposite of that in normal). *Epinephrine test.* Reduced lactate response than normal. *Biopsy of muscle.* Usually no immunologic cross reacting material to normal phosphorylase; biochemical study. *Electromyography.* Normal prior to exercise; no activity after. *Urine.* myoglobinuria (90%).

Therapy. Avoidance of extreme exercise (frequently sufficient). Oral fructose and glucose and injection of glucagon (not reccomended for long-term treatment). Ubiquinone and protein-rich diet also reported as inducing prolonged improvement.

Prognosis. Usually, stable condition, progression to atrophy according to reduction of amount of exercise. Longevity nonaffected.

BIBLIOGRAPHY. McArdle B: Myopathy due to a defect in muscle glycogen breakdown. Clin Sci 10:13–35, 1951

Schmidt B, Servidei S, Gabbai AA, et al: McArdle's disease in two generations: Autosomal recessive transmission with manifesting heterozygote. Neurology 37:1558–1561, 1987

Chen YT, Burchell A: Glycogen storage diseases. In Scriver CR, Beaudet AL, Sly WS, et al: The Metabolic and Molecular Bases of Inherited Disease, 7th ed, pp 951–953. New York, McGraw-Hill, 1995

McCUNE-ALBRIGHT

Synonyms. Albright I; Albright-McCune-Stenberg; Fuller Albright; fibrous dysplasia; osteitis fibrosa disseminata; osteodystrophia fibrosa; polyostotic fibrous dysplasia. See Jaffe-Lichtenstein.

Symptoms. Occurs in children or young adults; predominantly in females (3:2). Difficulty in walking; pain in the legs; pathologic fractures; in both sexes sexual precocity with early development. Deafness and blindness from lesions involving cranial nerves foramina.

Signs. Bone deformities and pathologic fractures especially of lower extremities and pelvic ring; cutaneous brownish pigmentations (absent in some cases) of various sizes ("Maine coast like"), more frequently observed on head, neck, sacrum, thighs. In monostotic variety, unilateral exophthalmos, unilateral optic atrophy, loss of hearing, convulsions, mental retardation. Signs of precocious development (genitals, breasts, early menarche). In some cases, associated with hyperthyroidism (19%). Differential diagnosis with hyperparathyroidism and adrenocortical and ovarian tumors.

Etiology. Sporadic conditions. Families with autosomal dominant trait reported. Identification of activating mutations in the GNAS1 gene. Excessive secretion of hypothalamic releasing hormone or multipe embryonic changes in various tissues (abnormal response to normal stimuli).

Pathology. No bone is spared: bone cysts; avascular fibrous tissue replacing normal medullary structure. Pigmented spots on the skin with melanin in the inner layer of epidermis. Possible multinodular changes in adrenals and/or thyroid.

Diagnostic Procedures. *X-ray.* Reveals fusiform enlargement of bone with thin cortex; translucent foci. *Blood.* Serum phosphatase elevated; calcium, phosphorus normal. *Urine.* 17-ketosteroids and follicle-stimulating hormone (FSH) excretion normal.

Therapy. Treatment of fractures and orthopedic correction of deformities.

Prognosis. Disease progressive until growth stops.

BIBLIOGRAPHY. McCune DJ: Osteitis fibro-cystica: The case of a nine year old girl who also exhibits precocious puberty, multiple pigmentation of the skin and hyperthyroidism. Am J Dis Child 52:743–747, 1936

Albright F, Butler AM, Hampton AO, et al: Syndrome characterized by osteitis fibrosa disseminata, areas of pigmentation and endocrine dysfunction with precocious puberty in females. N Engl J Med 216:727–746, 1937

McCune DJ, Bruch H: Osteodystrophia fibrosa. Am J Dis Child 54:806–848, 1937

Kasa-Vubu JZ, Kelch RP: Precocious and delayed puberty diagnosis and treatment. In Haubrich WS, Schaffner F, Berk JE (eds): Bockus Gastroenterology, 5th ed, vol 2, p 1967. Philadelphia, WB Saunders, 1995

McDERMOT

Synonyms. Spondoloepiphyseal dysplasia; myopia; sensory neural deafness. See: David-Stickler and spondiloepiphyseal dysplasia, congenital.

Symptoms and Signs. Described in four females. Short stature, epiphyseal dysplasia (of femoral heads), mild vertebral changes, sensineural deafness. In adult life, in some members of the family, also myopia and retinal detachment.

Etiology. Autosomal dominant inheritance.

BIBLIOGRAPHY. MacDermot KD, Roth SC, Hall C, et al: Epiphyseal dysplasia of the femoral head, mild vertebral abnormality, myopia and sesineural deafness: Report of a pedigree with autosomal dominant inheritance. J Med Genet 24:602–608, 1987

McDUFFIE

Synonyms. Hypocomplementemic urticarial vasculitis; urticarial vasculitis; hypocomplementemia.

Symptoms and Signs. Prevalent in females. In a high percentage smokers. Age of onset of urticaria 19–62; age of onset of dyspnea 31–55. Criteria for diagnosis: Chronic urtical vasculitis with chronic hypocomplementemia and the *presence* of at least two of the following minor criteria: arthralgias (transient and migratory), or arthritis, uveitis, or episcleritis; recurrent abdominal pains; and venulitis of dermid (by biopsy); evidence of glomerulonephritis; positive C1 precipitin test (by immunodiffusion); and the *absence* of: significant cryoglobulinemia; elevated antibodies to native SNA; high titer of antinuclear antibodies; hepatis B antigenemia; depressed C1 esterase inhibitor; or presence of congenital complement deficiency.

Etiology. Unknown. Suggested relationship with lupus erythematosus (?). Autosomic recessive inheritance (?).

Pathology. Biopsy of urticarial lesion. Inflammation of superficial venules, predominant neutrophilic, high percentage of fibrinoid necrosis. Direct immunofluorescence positive in majority of cases. Kidney diffuse necrotizing glomerulonephritis, focal proliferative glomerulopathy, or other types of glomerulopathies.

Diagnostic Procedures. *Blood.* Total hemolytic complement decreased in all patients; low levels of C4 and C3, all other complement components generally decreased. *Urine.* In about 50% of patients microhematuria and proteinuria. *Biopsy of lesion.* See Pathology. *X-ray of chest.* Normal or hyperinflation.

Therapy. Antihitamines, chloroquine, dapsone, and indomethacin have no effect on urticaria. Corticosteroids relieve urticaria, uveitis, abdominal pain, arthritis (large doses needed). Corticosteroids and cytotoxins stabilize renal condition. Bronchodilators when needed.

Prognosis. Benign course.

BIBLIOGRAPHY. McDuffie FC, Sams WM Jr, Maldonado JE, et al: Hypocomplimentemia with cutaneous vasculitis and arthritis: Possible immune complex syndrome. Mayo Clin Proc 48:340–348, 1973

Schwartz HR, McDuffie FC, Black LF, et al: Hypocomplementemic urticarial vasculitis: Association with chronic obstructive pulmonary disease. Mayo Clin Proc 57:231–238, 1982

Weatherall DJ, Ledingham JGG, Warrell DA (eds): Oxford Textbook of Medicine, 3rd ed, p 3770. Oxford, Oxford Med Pub, 1996

McKINDER

Synonym. Brachydactyly type B; symbrachydactyly.

Symptoms and Signs. Short middle phalanges. Absence or rudimentary distal phalanges of fingers and toes. Thumb and hallux often involved. Symphalangism and mild syndactyly may be present.

Etiology. Autosomal dominant inheritance.

Prognosis. The most disabling of brachydactylies.

BIBLIOGRAPHY. McKinder D: Deficiency of fingers transmitted through six generations. Br Med J 1:845–846, 1857

McArthur JW, McCullough E: Atypical dystrophy as inherited defect of hands and feet. Hum Biol 4:179–207, 1932

Battle HI, Walker NF, Thompson MW: MacKinder's hereditary brachydactyly: Phenotypic, radiological, dermatoglyphic and genetic observations in an Ontario family. Ann Hum Genet 36:415–424, 1973

McKITTRICK-WHEELOCK

Symptoms and Signs. Eponym used to indicate severe electrolyte imbalance, caused by the presence of a large villous adenoma in the colon or rectum.

Therapy. Correction of electrolyte imbalance and surgery.

Prognosis. Good with treatment.

BIBLIOGRAPHY. McKittrick LS, Wheelock FC Jr: Carcinoma of the Colon, 3rd ed. Springfield, IL, Charles C Thomas, 1954

McKUSICK-CROSS

Synonyms. Achondroplasia, Swiss type agammaglobulinemia; lymphopenic agammaglobulinemia, dwarfism; ataxia telangiectasia III.

Symptoms. Present from birth. Failure to thrive. Repeated infections. Diarrhea.

Signs. Growth deficiency; short limbs; small thorax. Redundant skin; erythema; dyskeratosis; hair loss.

Etiology. Unknown; possibly, autosomal recessive inheritance. In the two original sibs described: one presented Louis-Bar syndrome (see) and the other Swiss-type agammaglobulinemia (see), thus suggesting possible relationship between these two disorders.

Diagnostic Procedures. *Blood.* Anemia; lymphopenia; agammaglobulinemia; *X-ray.* Radial and ulnar metaphyseal cusping. Hypoplastic thymus. *Bone marrow.* Occasionally, aplasia of all erythropoietic elements.

Prognosis. Death in early infancy.

BIBLIOGRAPHY. McKusick VA, Cross HE: Ataxia-telangiectasia and Swiss-type agammaglobulinemia: Two genetic disorders of the immune mechanism in related Amish. JAMA 195:739–745, 1966
Gatti RA, Platt N, Pomerance HH, et al: Hereditary lymphopenic agammaglobulinemia associated with a destructive form of short-limbed dwarfism and ectodermal dysplasia. J Pediatr 75:679–684, 1969
MacDermot KD, Winter RM, Wigglesworth JS, et al: Short stature/short limbs: Skeletal dysplasia with severe combined immunodeficiency and bowing of the femora: Report of two patients and review. J Med Genet 28:10–17, 1991

McLENNAN

Synonyms. Proctalgia fugax; Thaysen includes anal sphincter myopathy. See Hayden-Grossman.

Symptoms. In the area of rectal sphincter: attacks of sharp, severe, brief pain (about 1 minute)—elicited by micturition, coitus, or local trauma—that may shoot down both legs. After the pain, a red flush spreads over the buttocks and down the back of one or both legs seldom extending to the soles, lasting approximately 1 hour. Frequently associated with generalized pallor, sweating, precordial oppression, ocular pain (with or without conjunctival suffusion and erythema) and fainting.

Etiology. Unknown. Sporadic or autosomal dominant inheritance (Hayden-Grossman). Attributed to contraction of levator ani muscle. Usually neurotic nature of patients describing these symptoms.

Diagnostic Procecures. To exclude other causes of anal pain. *Sigmoidoscopy; manometry.*

Therapy. Pain may be relieved by bowel movement, flatus, or heat. Upward pressure against perineum, inhalation of salbutamol, sublingual nitroglycerine; quinine. Masturbation or abstinence have also been suggested. Defecation, forceful anal dilatation. Elimination of factors suspected of precipitating attacks. The effectiveness of oral clonidin has been reported. Reassurance and explanation.

Prognosis. Harmless, unpleasant, and incurable.

BIBLIOGRAPHY. Myrtle AS: Some common afflictions of the anus often neglected by medical men and patients. Br Med 1:1061–1062, 1883
MacLennan A: A short note on rectal crises of nontabetic origin. Glasgow Med J 88:129–131, 1917
Thaysen TE: Proctalgia fugax. Lancet II:243–246, 1935
Schuster MM: Rectal pain. In Bayless T: Current Therapy in GI and Liver Diseases. Toronto, BC Decker, 1990
Kamm MA, Hoyle CHV, Burleigh DE, et al: Hereditary internal anal sphincter myopathy causing proctalgia fugax and constipation. Gastroenterology 100:805–810, 1991

McLEOD*

Synonyms. McLeod phenotype. Contiguous gene syndrome with chronic granulomatous disease (see) and sometimes also with Duchenne (see) and glycerol kinase deficiency (see).

*Name from patient Hugh McLeod.

Symptoms and Signs. In boys from asymptomatic to muscle weakness with or without symptoms and signs of chronic granulomatous disease (see) and mild hemolytic anemia.

Etiology. X-linked. Females are carriers. Deletion of X-linked locus codifing for K x antigen (part of Kell) that determines hemoluytic anemia and acanthocytosis and disturbance of white blood cell adhesion (may be responsible for CGD).

Pathology. Muscle biopsy, similar to Duchenne (see).

Diagnostic Procedures. *Blood.* Acanthocytosis, anisocythosis, polychromasia mild anemia (female dual population). *Serum.* Elevated creatinine phosphokinase activity. Anti KL antibodies after transfusion.

Therapy. Usually none required.

Prognosis. Good if no contiguous gene syndrome present.

BIBLIOGRAPHY. Allen FH, Krabbe SMR, and Corcoran PA: A new phenitype (McLeod) in the Kell blood group system. Vox Sang 6:555–560, 1961
Danek A, Witt TN, Stockman HBAC, et al: Normal dystrophin. In McLeod syndrome. Ann Neurol 28:720–722, 1990
Ledbetter DH, Ballabio A: Molecular cytogenetics of contiguous gene syndromes: Mechanisms and consequences of gene dosage imbalance. In Scriver CR, Beaudet AL, Sly WS, et al: The Metabolic and Molecular Bases of Inherited Disease, 7th ed, pp 819–820. New York, McGraw-Hill, 1995

McQUARRIE

Synonym. Hypoglycemia; infantile, familial. See Cochrane.

Symptoms and Signs. Onset in early infancy (84% under 2 years); prevalent in males. Vague clinical signs of hypoglycemia usually attributed to hunger, teething, fatigue, or environmental changes. Generalized convulsions recurring at specific times, without fever or evidence of other illness.

Etiology. Unknown. Possibly, familial or hereditary character. Today the condition may be attributed to one of the following metabolic derangements: defects in amino acid; defects in fatty acid; various hepatic enzyme deficiencies of carbohydrate.

Pathology. Unknown. In two original cases, biopsy of pancreas showed absence of alpha cells and in other two cases, normal pattern.

Diagnostic Procedures. *Blood.* Fasting sugar; glucose tolerance curve; epinephrine test; glucagon test; adrenocorticotropic hormone (ACTH) and cortisone administration test. *Biopsy of pancreas.*

Therapy. Glucose stops convulsion. ACTH and corticosteroids.

Prognosis. Normal physical and mental growth if treated. Permanent improvement possible following prolonged treatment and Kell blood group antigen K (KI) transfusion ACTH treatment. Possible brain damage if condition goes unrecognized and maltreated (i.e., with antiepileptic drugs).

BIBLIOGRAPHY. McQuarrie I: Idiopathic spontaneously occurring hypoglycemia in infants. Am J Dis Child 87:399–428, 1954
Koh THH, Eyre JA, Anysley-Green A: Neonatal hypoglycaemia: The controversy regarding definition. Arch Dis Child 63:1386–1398, 1988
Darmaun D, Haymond MW, Bier DM: Metabolic aspects of fuel homeostasis in the fetus and the neonate. In De Groot LJ (ed): Endocrinology, 3rd ed, p 2269. Philadelphia, WB Saunders, 1995

MEADOWS

Synonyms. Postpartum myocardiopathy; puerperium myocardiopathy; peripartum cardiopathy. See Cardiomegaly, idiopathic.

Symptoms. Occurs in mothers between second week and second month after delivery. Cough; nocturnal paroxysmal dyspnea; hemoptysis; chest pain. Gastrointestinal symptoms: nausea; vomiting. Symptoms of cerebral embolism with hemiplegia or pulmonary embolism.

Signs. The physical findings are those of congestive heart failure: left-sided first; then right-sided. Diastolic hypertension; pulsus alternans; gallop rhythm; cyanosis; liver enlargement; fundus oculi abnormal.

Etiology. Unknown. Myocarditis or myocardiopathy, possibly of viral origin or autoimmune disease; familial occurrence has been reported.

Pathology. Heart dilated, soft and flabby, average weight 500 g. Left and right ventricular mural thrombi. Microscopically, focal and diffuse areas of degeneration of myocardial fibers with occasional hemorrhages; lymphocytic and fat droplet infiltration.

Diagnostic Procedures. *X-ray.* Enlargement of transverse diameter of heart. *ECG.* T-wave inversion; significant Q-wave and conduction defects.

Differential Diagnosis. Clinical or subclinical toxemia of pregnancy; specific infections; unrecognized pre-existing renal or cardiac disease; autoimmune condition.

Therapy. Bed rest until diameter of heart returns to normal. Control of symptoms of congestive heart failure with digitalis, diuretics. Anticoagulation if embolization occurs. Azathioprine and prednisone may be of benefit.

Prognosis. Approximately two-thirds of cases make complete recovery; syndrome tends to recur.

BIBLIOGRAPHY. Hull E, Hafkesbring E: Toxic post-partal heart disease. New Orleans Med Surg J 39:550–557, 1937
Woolford RM: Post-partum myocardosis. Ohio Med J 48:924–930, 1952
Meadows WR: Idiopathic myocardial failure in the last trimester of pregnancy and the puerperium. Circulation 15:903–914, 1957
Elkayam U, Ostrzega EL, Shotan A: Peripartum cardiomyopathy. In Gleicher N (ed): Principles and Practice of Medical Therapy in Pregnancy, 2nd ed. Norwalk, CT, Appleton and Lange, 1992

MEALEY

Synonyms. Head injury pediatric.

Symptoms and Signs. After mild head trauma in children. Temporary dazing or unconsciousness, followed by a period of well-being and a successive (1 hour or longer) onset of somnolence or lethargy, irritability, and/or vomiting. When examined they cry, tend to withdraw and promptly return to a sleep-like state, retaining the position in which they are placed or curling up on their sides.

Etiology. Brain concussion in children (see).

BIBLIOGRAPHY. Mealey J: Pediatric Head Injuries, p 243. Springfield, IL, Charles C Thomas, 1968

MECKEL-GRUBER

Synonyms. Gruber; von Hippel-Lindau, lethal form; Simopoulos; splanchnocystic dyscephalia; dysencephalia splanchnocystic.

Symptoms. Prevalent in females; present from birth. Symptoms related to signs.

Signs. *Head.* Microcephaly; posterior encephalocele; sloping forehead; micrognathia; cleft lip and palate; olfactory hypoplasia; cryptophthalmos; mongoloid slant of lids; sclerocornea; cataract; retinal dysplasia. *Neck.* Short. *Limbs.* Polysyndactyly; clubfeet. *Heart.* Congenital defects. *Urogenital tract.* Cryptorchidism. *Other.* Spina bifida.

Etiology. Unknown; autosomal recessive inheritance.

Pathology. See Signs. Polycystic kidney; occasionally, absence of adrenal glands; intestinal malrotation; accessory spleen; imperforate anus; hydrocephalus; absent olfactory lobes and pituitary; incompletely developed forebrain, basal and hypothalamic areas. Septal heart defect; patent ductus; coarctation of aorta; pulmonary stenosis. Lung hypoplasia. Liver cysts; fibrosis.

Diagnostic Procedures. See Signs. *Chromosome studies.* Normal.

Prognosis. Early death (in days or weeks).

BIBLIOGRAPHY. Meckel JF: Beschreibung zweier durch sehr ähnliche Bildungsabweichungen entstellter Geschwister. Dtsch Arch Physiol 7:99–172, 1822
Gruber GB: Beiträge zur Frage "gekoppelter" Missbildung (Akrocephalo-Syndactylie und Dysencephalia splanchnocystica). Beitr Pathol Anat 93:459–476, 1934
Simopoulos AP, Breunan GC, Alwan A, et al: Polycystic kidneys, internal hydrocephalus, and polydactylism in newborn siblings. Pediatrics 39:931–934, 1967
Farag TI, Usha R, Uma R, et al: Phenotypic variability in Meckel-Gruber syndrome. Clin Genet 38:176–179, 1990

MECONIUM ASPIRATION

See Massive aspiration.

Symptoms and Signs. Occurs in newborns, usually with weight over 2500 g, shortly after birth. Tachypnea and mild cyanosis, resolving in 24–72 hours, or worsening, respiration becoming irregular and gasping, cyanosis deeper, and appearance of gross, diffuse rales.

Etiology. Aspiration of meconium-stained amniotic fluid at moment of delivery.

Diagnostic Procedures. *Apgar score.* Below 6 at 1 and 5 minutes (predisposing factor). *X-rays.* Nonuniform, coarse, patchy infiltrates of the lungs; areas of atelectasis and of emphysema; chest hyperexpansion; diaphragm flattening.

Therapy. Aspiration of all traces of meconium fluid first from airways as soon as possible, and, then from pharynx and trachea under laryngoscopic vision. Gastrolysis. Intubation and repeated aspiration and, if needed, ventilatory assistance (expiratory pressure) and general intensive care assistance. Hydrocortisone therapy is not of benefit. For severe cases, extracorporeal membrane oxygenation (ECMO) has been tried with success.

Prognosis. Mortality 4.6%.

BIBLIOGRAPHY. Bacsik RD: Meconium aspiration syndrome. Pediatr Clin N Am 24:463–477, 1977
MacFarlane PI, Heaf DP: Pulmonary function in children after neonatal meconium aspiration syndrome. Arch Dis Child 63:368–372, 1988
Wiswell TE, Tuggle JM, Turner BS: Meconium aspiration syndrome have we made a difference? Pediatrics 85.715–721, 1990

MECONIUM PLUG

Synonyms. Meconium ileus; meconium peritonitis; distal intestinal obstruction; DIOS.

Symptoms. Occurs in newborns. Inability to defecate within 48 hours from birth. Nausea; vomiting; abdominal distention.

Signs. Rectal examination reveals meconium plug.

Etiology. Impaction of the meconium plug into the sigmoid flexure of colon, lower ileum, or ileocecal valve. Causes of impaction; deficiency of biliary secretion; deficiency of pancreatic secretion; diminution of amniotic fluid swallowed during intrauterine life. Associated with aganglionosis (see Hirschsprung) or mucoviscidosis (10%).

Pathology. Meconium plug formed by solidly packed material. Aganglionosis of segment of rectum demonstrated in some cases.

Diagnostic Procedures. Insertion of rectal catheter. *X-ray.* Flat plate of abdomen. Intraluminal or extraluminal calcification in 10–25% of cases. *Sweat test.* Later.

Therapy. Enema and meconium plug removal and concurrent intravenous fluid therapy to counteract the hyperosmolar effect of enema. If aganglionosis demonstrated, colostomy, and Swenson pull-through procedure and later, colostomy closure.

Prognosis. Survival in both complicated and uncomplicated cases about 50%. Patient with this syndrome must be followed, and aganglionosis and cystic fibrosis ruled out.

BIBLIOGRAPHY. Van Leeuwen G, Riley WC, Glenn L, et al: Meconium plug syndrome with aganglionosis. Pediatr 40:665–666, 1967

Shwachman H: Meconium ileus: Ten patients over 28 years of age. J Pediatr Surg 18:570–575, 1983

Cywes S, Millar AJW: Embriology and anomalies of the intestine. In Haubrich WS, Schaffner F, Berk JE (eds): Bockus Gasroenterology, pp 914–916. Philadelphia, WB Saunders, 1995

MEDITERRANEAN FEVER

Synonyms. Reimann; Siegal-Cattan-Mamou; Armenian; benign paroxysmal peritonitis; familial Mediterranean fever; Mediterranean fever; FMF; periodic amyloid; periodic peritonitis; recurrent polyserositis.

Symptoms. Peculiar ethnic distribution in people of Mediterranean ancestry (Armenian and sephardic Jews); more frequent in males. Onset most frequently in late adolescence, also in early age, seldom after 40 years of age. Complete syndrome of subsyndromes may represent the clinical manifestation of this disease. Paroxysmal attacks, most frequently accompanied by fever, are the common feature for this condition. Frequency of attack variable from once a year to once a week. Cycles of repeated attacks with periods of complete remission. In women, attack may be largely limited to the menstrual periods. *Abdomen.* Pain most frequently in right lower quadrant, lower left quadrant, upper left quadrant, with stooped posture. *Thorax.* Stabbing unilateral pain; chest or shoulder dyspnea. *Joints.* Arthralgias (2–3 days duration); occasionally monoarthralgia of big articulations. *Skin.* Urticaria or erysipelas-like erythema (rare). Occasionally orchitis and meningitis.

Signs. *Abdomen.* Tenderness, spasm, and guarding; distention; occasionally, moderate splenomegaly. Occasionally signs of needless laparotomies. *Chest.* No function sound; tenderness of chest wall; decreased sound transmission of minor degree. *Joints.* Local erythema; swelling.

Etiology. Unknown; congenital familial autosomal recessive trait; R (recessive inheritance also reported especially from Armenian families) possibly, inherited error in metabolism of one or more steriod hormones; lipocortin deficiency (?) and or presence of an inhibitor of neutrophil chemotaxisis causing inappropriate inflammatory reaction.

Pathology. Transient peritonitis with simple hyperemia of peritoneum or extended to abdominal organs; scattered deposit of fibrinous material. Small amount of free fluid. In microscopic study of exudate, fibrin mesh with neutrophils. Typical lack of peritoneal adhesions in spite of recurrent attacks. Liver and spleen may show adhesions. In kidney, progressive lesion consistent with amyloidosis or in some cases, with chronic glomerulonephritis.

Diagnostic Procedures. Symptoms may be elicited by 10 mg metaraminol bitartrate. *Blood.* During attack mild leukocytosis (15,000, seldom higher); neutrophilia; moderate anemia. Sedimentation rate; glycoprotein, serum amyloid A; α_2-globulin; fibrinogen: increased. Evanescent minimal signs of hepatic involvement may be recorded; bilirubin; flocculation test. *Urine.* Occasionally proteinuria and deterioration of renal function. *Peritoneal and pleural fluid.* Serofibrinous, predominantly polymorphonuclear or mixed response. *Joint fluid.* Polymorphic cytology. *X-ray.* During attack, presence of fluid in abdomen or chest or both. Gastrointestinal tract may show transient abnormalities of mucosa of small bowel.

Therapy. Attack dramatically responds to adrenal steroid. Low-fat diets seem to benefit a number of patients. Rest, treatment of tension also effective in number of cases. Colchicine (preventive in 95% of cases).

Prognosis. Essentially benign condition, despite the recurrence of attacks with intervals of symptom-free period from days to years. Amyloidosis and renal failure possible complications.

BIBLIOGRAPHY. Siegal S: Benign paroxysmal peritonitis. Ann Intern Med 23:1–21, 1945

Mamou H, Cattan R: La maladie périodique (sur 14 cas personnels dort 8 compliqués de néphropathies). Sem Hop Paris 28:1062–1070, 1952

Barakat MH, EI, Chawad AO, Gumaa KA, et al: Metaraminol provocative test: A specific diagnostic test for familial Mediterranean fever. Lancet 656–657, 1984

Majeed HA, Barakad M: Familial mediterranean fever (recurrent hereditary polyserositis) in children: Analysis of 88 cases. Eur J Pediatr 148:636–641, 1989

Eliakim M: Recurrent polyserositis (familial Mediterranean fever), periodic disease. In Weatherall DJ, Ledingham JGG, Warrell DA (eds): Oxford Textbook of Medicine, 3rd ed, pp 1525–1527. Oxford, Oxford Med Pub, 1990

MEESMANN

Synonym. Meesmann-Wilke; Stocker-Holt; dystrophia epithelialis cornea; juvenile epithelial dystrophy, corneal dystrophy juvenile, epithelial.

Symptoms and Signs. Both sexes affected; onset in first 2 years of life. Slight corneal irritation; slight, but progressive visual impairment. Multiple punctiform opacities on the cornea, extending in some cases to Bowman membrane.

Etiology. Unknown; autosomal dominant inheritance.

Pathology. Corneal dystrophy, characterized by vacuoli full of glycogen and cysts containing degenerated cells.

Therapy. Corneal transplant.

BIBLIOGRAPHY. Meesmann A: Ueber eine bisher nicht beschriebene, dominant vererbte Dystrophia epithetelialis Cornae. Ber Dtsch Ophthalmol Ges 52:154–158, 1938

Meesmann A, Wilke F: Klinische und anatomische Untersuchungen ueber eine bisher unbekannte, dominant vererbrate Epitheldystrophia der Hornhaut. Klin Monatsbl Augenheilkd 103:361–391, 1939

Fine BS, Yanoff M, Pitts E, et al: Meesmann's epithelial dystrophy of the cornea. Am J Ophthalmol 83:633–642, 1977

Rodrigues MM, Rajagopalan S, Jones KA: Anterior and posterior corneal dystrophy. In Garner A, Klintworth GK (eds): Pathobiology of Ocular Disease: A Dynamic Approach, 2nd ed, pp 1189–1190. New York, Marcel Dekker, 1994

MEGADUODENUM AND/OR MEGACYSTIS

Synonyms. MMHI, Megacystis—microcolon—intestinal pseudo-obstruction; visceral familial myopathy. See Pseudo-obstruction, intestinal childhood.

Symptoms and Signs. Both sexes affected; onset from infancy, or later. Symptoms related to dilated duodenum possibly associated with megacystitis (see). Subjects with marfanoid habitus (see Marfan syndrome). Within families, high variability of severity.

Etiology. Unknown; sporadic or autosomal dominant inheritance.

Pathology. *Biopsies.* Duodenum, jejunum, ileum, colon, urinary bladder. Thinning and collagen replacement of muscle layer, normal ganglion cells.

Diagnostic Procedures. *Sonography. X-rays. Biopsy. Silver stain.*

Therapy. Avoid unnecessary laparatomy for presumed obstruction. Metoclopramide non effective.

Prognosis. Variable, from asymptomatic cases to severe impairment owing to recurrent gastrointestinal symptoms and urinary retention. Good life expectancy.

BIBLIOGRAPHY. Weiss W: Zur Aetiologie des Megaduodenums. Dtsch Z Chir 251:317–330, 1938
Schuffler MD, Rohrmann CA, Chaffee RG, et al: Chronic intestinal pseudoobstruction: a report of 27 cases and review of literature. Medicine 60:173–196, 1981
Camilleri M, Carbone LD, Schuffler MD: Familial enteric neuropathy with pseudoobstruction. Digest Dis Sci 36:1168–1171, 1991

MEGASIGMOID

Symptoms. Observed in elderly patients, and also in young patients, when neurologic damage is present. Psychotic reaction preceding or following manifestation of this syndrome. Mental deterioration (that may mask symptoms of megasigmoid even in progressed stage). Long-standing constipation, masked by fluid fecal incontinence; loss of tone of sphincter. Abdominal pain; fever, nausea; vomiting.

Signs. Abdominal distension; sudden peritonitis or intermittent or recurring volvulus. Occasionally; liver dislodged medially.

Etiology. It is always acquired (as contrasted with megacolon, which may be acquired or congenital). Neurogenic disorder of sigmoid in association with mental deterioration, cerebral concussion or arteriosclerosis, Parkinson syndrome, multiple sclerosis, tabes.

Pathology. Only sigmoid enlarged; it may fill entire peritoneal cavity and also push diaphragm into chest cavity. Feces from semiliquid to very compact; deep ulcers with embedded fecaliths. Histologic features of acute and chronic inflammation. Mucosal atrophy; necrosis; hemorrhages of sigmoid walls; hypertrophic ganglion cells preserved.

Diagnostic Procedures. *X-ray of abdomen.* According to amount of gas and location of fecal material three well-defined radiodiagnostic patterns may be obtained. *Barium enema.* Very informative, but difficult to perform.

Therapy. Difficult because of anal sphincter relaxation. Digital removal of feces; tube inserted to remove gas. Cholinergic drug to stimulate peristalsis. Surgical intervention difficult; emergency operation for stercoraceous ulcer. Sigmoidoscopic management for removal of impaction.

Prognosis. Permanent localized and irreversible condition (as opposed to megacolon, which is reversible or changed into total megacolon).

BIBLIOGRAPHY. Kraft E, Finby N: Megacolon and megasigmoid syndrome. GP 36:104–114, 1967

MEIGE

Synonyms. Brueghel; oral—facial—oromantibolar spasms.

Symptoms and Signs. In adult life major incidence in sixth decade. Forceful opening of jaw; lip retraction; platisma spastic contractions; tongue protrusion or jaw contracted with pursed lips. Frequently associated spastic dysphonia and blepharospasm; occasionally torticollis, or dystonia of trunk and limbs.

Etiology. Unknown. Syndrome may be produced also with neuroleptics administration.

Pathology. Scanty reports. Many foci of neuron loss in the striatum.

Diagnostic Procedures. *CT scan. MRI. EEG. EMG.*

Therapy. Success with botulin toxic injection in affected muscles. Other drugs practically useless except for minor symptomatic effects.

Prognosis. Persistent condition.

BIBLIOGRAPHY. Meige H: Les convulsions de la face: Une forme clinique de convulsion faciale, bilatèrale et médiane. Rev Neurol (Paris) 10:437–443, 1910
Jancovic J, Ford J: Blepharospasm and orofacial-cervical dystonia: Clinical and pharmaceutical findings in 100 patients. Ann Neurol 13:402–411, 1983
Adams RD, Victor M: Principles of Neurology, 5th ed, p 94. New York, McGraw-Hill, 1993

MEIGS

Synonyms. Demons-Meigs; Meigs-Cass; ascites, pleural effusion, ovarian.

Symptoms. Abdominal distension; pain in the chest; dyspnea; edema of legs not uncommon; weight loss; urinary incontinence.

Signs. Ascites; hydrothorax (62% left side; 11% right side; 24% both sides); adnexal mass; uterine prolapse.

Etiology and Pathology. Solid ovarian tumor, usually benign fibroma, thecoma, granulosa cell tumor, or Brenner tumor. Mechanism of formation of ascites and hydrothorax is unknown. Removal of tumors eliminates fluid effusions.

Diagnostic Procedures. *Ascitic and pleuric fluid.* Transudates (SG 1015 clear, amber, or yellowish). Nonprotein nitrogen (NPN) normal; total serum proteins normal. Carbon particles injected into ascitic fluid pass rapidly and irreversibly into thoracic cavity.

Therapy. Removal of tumor.

Prognosis. Good. If malignant, disease according to histologic grade and extent.

BIBLIOGRAPHY. Meigs JV, Cass JW: Fibroma of the ovary with ascites and hydrothorax, with a report of 7 cases. Am J Obstet Gynecol 33:249–267, 1937
O'Flanagan SJ, Tighe BF, Egan TJ, et al: Meigs' syndrome and pseudo-Meigs syndrome. J R Soc Med 80:252–253, 1987
Sabiston DC: Textbook of Surgery, 14th ed, p 1721. Philadelphia, WB Saunders, 1991

M.E.L.A.S.

Synonyms. Mitochondrial encephalopathy; lactic acidosis; stroke-like episodes. See OXPHOS syndromes.

Symptoms and Signs. Sporadic presentation or as members of maternal pedigrees. Onset variable: In infancy variety of motor and cognitive developmental abormalities or normal development until first stroke-like episode, that occurs usually between 5 and 15 years of age seldom. A stroke-like episode may resolve in a few hours or months, along with the conseguent neurologic defects: seizures, hemiparesis, etc. Different combination of additional clinical manifestations: myopathy; myalgias, ophthalmoplegia, cardiomyopathy, respiratory insufficiency, visual troubles (pigmentary retinopathy), deafness (neurosensory), ataxia, migraine, acquired dementia, various endocrinopathies, short stature, occasionally purpura, etc.

Etiology. Falls under Class II mutations of OXPHOS (see). mtDNA mutation: Brain infarcts, hypothetically, considered as nonvascular but owing to OXPHOS dysfunctions of parenchyma (increased production of free radicals damaging vascular endothelium and determininig areas of vasoconstrition).

Pathology. Brain infarctions most frequently observed in the cortical areas supplied by large vessels of the posterior temporal, parietal, and occipital regions. Mitochondrial changes in vascular smooth muscle and endothelial cells.

Diagnostic Procedures. *SPECT (single photon emission computed tomography).* Better than CT and MTI to evidenciate brain lesion. *CSF.* Elevated lactate levels. *Blood.* Lactic acidemia. OXPHOS enzymology, often associated diabetes. *MtDNA analysis. Biopsy.* Proliferation of ragged red muscle fibers.

Therapy. See OXPHOS syndromes.

Prognosis. Varible but overall poor. Stroke-like episodes may either resolve completely or are followed by permanent neurologic deficits.

BIBLIOGRAPHY. Pavlakis SG, Phillips PC, Di Mauro S, et al: Mitochondrial myopathy, encephalopathy, lactic acidosis, and stroke-like episodes: A distinctive clinical syndrome. Ann Neurol 16:481–488, 1984
Shoffner JM, Wallace DC: Oxidative phosphorylation diseases. In Scriver CR, Beaudet AL, Sly WS, et al: The Metabolic and Molecular Bases of Inherited Disease, 7th ed, pp 1562–1564. New York, McGraw-Hill, 1995

MELEDA

Synonyms. Siemens; mal de Meleda; Mljet; keratosis palmoplantaris transgradiens.

Symptoms. Both sexes affected; onset in first month of life. Redness of palms and soles, followed by scaling and thickening, localized or diffuse, extending progressively to dorsal surface. Erythema remains. Hyperhidrosis is frequently associated; frequently, eczematization; continuous patchiform progression of new lesions on extremities. Poor physical development and mental retardation. Occasionally cardiac abnormalities.

Etiology. Autosomal recessive inheritance.

Pathology. Different from tylosis: marked acanthosis; irregular hyperkeratosis and parakeratosis and perivascular lymphohistiocyte infiltration.

Diagnostic Procedures. *Biopsy. Electroencephalography.* Frequently, abnormalities.

Therapy. None.

Prognosis. Progresses through life.

BIBLIOGRAPHY. Neuman NI: Ueber das keratoma hereditarism. Arch Derm Syph 42:163–174, 1898
Kogoj F: Die Krankheit von Mljet ("Mal de Meleda"). Acta Dermatovener (Stockh) 15:264–299, 1934
Protonotarius N, Tsatsopoulou A, Patsourakos P, et al: Cardiac abnormalities in familial palmoplantar keratosis. Br Heart J 56:321–326, 1986
Griffiths WAD, Leigh IM, Marks R: Disorders of keratinization. In Champion RH, Burton JL, Ebling FJG (eds): Rook/Wilkinson/Ebling Textbook of Dermatology, 5th ed, p 1376. Oxford, Blackwell Scientific, 1992

MELENA NEONATORUM

Synonyms. Hemorrhagic newborn; morbus hemorrhagicus neonatorum; newborn hemorrhagic disease; swallowed blood. Clinically important in the newborn. Differentiate (1) maternal blood swallowed by the newborn; (2) intrinsic bleeding in the gastrointestinal tract of the newborn. Differentiation between the two conditions is of utmost importance. If the blood in the stools is proved to be of maternal origin, the newborn must be spared all the elaborate laboratory tests, X-rays, and even surgical exploration that should be done instead if blood is suspected to be of fetal origin.

Diagnostic Procedures. *Blood.* Fetal hemoglobin is resistant to denaturation by alkalis. Adult hemoglobin is readily denaturalized by alkaline solution. Comparison between clinical findings in both conditions.

EXTRINSIC BLEEDING

Onset. Bloody stools are passed within the first 12 hours. *Anemia.* No anemia found in the newborn. No change in bleeding time, clotting time, or prothrombin time. Usually associated with complications of labor: e.g., placenta previa or premature separation of placenta. The general clinical condition of newborn is good.

INTRINSIC BLEEDING

Onset. Bloody stools are passed usually after first 24 hours. *Anemia.* Gradual and proportionate decrease in the hemoglobin level of the newborn. Change may be found. No associated complications of labor. The clinical condition of the newborn is poor.

Pathology. If the bleeding is intrinsic: (1) evidence of severe infection in the newborn; (2) evidence of bowel pathology (e.g., volvulus); (3) evidence of hepatitis; (4) evidence of upper gastrointestinal tract pathology (e.g., esophageal ulcer). For extrinsic causes of bleeding, no pathology is found.

Therapy. Therapy is needed if bleeding is of fetal origin. Depending on the etiology, from medical management to surgical exploration.

Prognosis. If detected early, the prognosis is good for those patients with intrinsic bleeding.

BIBLIOGRAPHY. Singer K, Chernoff AI, Singer L: Studies on abnormal hemoglobins; I. their demonstration in sickle cell anemia and other hematologic disorders by means of alkali denaturation. Blood 6:413–428, 1951
Apt L, Downey WS: "Melena" neonatorum: The swallowed blood syndrome. A simple test for the differentiation of adult and fetal hemoglobin in bloody stools. J Pediatr 47:6–12, 1955
Bithell TC: The diagnostic approach to the bleeding disorders. In Lee GR, Bithell TC, Foerster J, et al (eds): Wintrobe's Clinical Hematology, 9th ed, pp 1304–1305. Philadelphia, Lea & Febiger, 1993

MELKERSSON

Synonyms. Melkersson-Rosenthal; Rossolino cheilitis granulomatosis. See Miescher II.

Symptoms and Signs. No sex or racial preference; onset in childhood or youth. Facial paralysis (unilateral or bilateral); facial edema (nonpitting, involving one or both lips, chin, cheeks, or tongue) appearing in association with the paralysis or spaced by as long as 25 years. Lingua plicata (scrotal tongue). Episodes of facial paralysis and edema associated or independently recurrent (formes fruste). Migraine, corneal ulcers, parotitis may be associated occasionally.

Etiology. Autosomal dominant inheritance with variable expressivity.

Pathology. Intracellular edema; nonspecific round cell infiltration, of lymphohistiocytic, sarcoidal, or tuberculoid type. Thickening of epithelium; dilated lymph vessels in corium.

Therapy. During the stage of acute facial paralysis, moisture chamber eye shields, artificial tears, and analgesics. Facial massage, electrical stimulation, and warm compresses may be helpful. Possible benefit from corticosteroid therapy. If the bouts of facial palsy are frequent, consider surgical decompression of the facial nerve. If the lip swelling becomes unsightly, a cheiloplastic reduction is indicated. Cheiloplasty plus continuously repeated injection of triamcinolone into the lips. Dapsone reported beneficial.

Prognosis. Recurrent episodes with complete remission initially; then tendency to become chronic.

BIBLIOGRAPHY. Rossolimo GJ: Recidivirende Facialislähmung bei Migräne. Neurol Zenbl 20:744–749, 1901
Melkersson E: Ett fall av recidiverande facialispares i samband med angioneurotiskt odem. Hygiea 90:737–741, 1928

Rosenthal C: Klinisch-erbbiologischer Beitrag zur Konstitutions-Pathologie: Gemeinsames Auftreten von (rezidivierender familiairer) Facialislähmung, angioneurotischem Gesichtsödem und Lingua plicata in Arthritismus-Familien. Z Neurol Psychol 131:475–501, 1931

Wadlington WB, Riley HD, Lowbeer L: The Melkersson-Rosenthal syndrome. Pediatrics 73:502–506, 1984

Burton JL: The lips. In Champion RH, Burton JL, Ebling FJG (eds): Rook/Wilkinson/Ebling Textbook of Dermatology, 5th ed, p 2767. Oxford, Blackwell Scientific, 1992

MELNICK-NEEDLES

Synonym. Osteodysplasty.

Symptoms and Signs. Both sexes affected. Male to female ratio, 1:7. Present from birth. Facial abnormalities; micrognathia; malocclusion. Recurrent respiratory and ear infections. Generalized bone dysplasia (see Diagnostic Procedures).

Etiology. Suggested autosomal dominant and/or recessive inheritance; strong possibility for X-linked inheritance. Male cases reported possibly are new mutations since the form is lethal in male.

Diagnostic Procedures. *X-rays of head.* Delayed closure of anterior fontanelle; sclerosis of skull base and mastoids; underdevelopment of paranasal sinuses. *X-rays of spinal column.* Vertebral bodies tall (more so axis, atlas, and occipital condyles); thoracic vertebrae show anterior concavity and beaking. *X-rays of sternum.* Delayed ossification. *X-rays of ribs.* Ribbon-like. *X-rays of pelvis.* Flaring of the crest of iliac bones and constriction in superacetabular area; tapering of ischial bones. *X-rays of long bones.* Bowing of tibia and radius; flaring of ends of humerus, fibia, and tibia; coxa valga.

BIBLIOGRAPHY. Melnick JC, Needles CF: An undiagnosed bone dysplasia: A 2 family study of 4 generations and 3 generations. Am J Roentgenol 97:39–48, 1966

Wettke-Schaeffer R, Kantner G: X-linked dominant inherited diseases with lethality in homozygous males. Hum Genet 64:1–23, 1983

van der Lely H, Robben SGF, Meradji M, et al: Melnick-Needles syndrome (osteodysplasty) in an older male: Report of a case and review of the literature. Br J Radiol 64:852–854, 1991

MELZER

Synonym. Cryoglobulinemia, familial mixed; essential mixed cryoglobulinemia.

Symptoms and Signs. Both sexes. In adolescence, evidence of progressive deterioration of renal function: hematuria, edema, anasarca, blood hypertension.

Etiology. Described in association with lymphoproliferative, autoimmune, hepatic, diseases or in cases with autosomal dominant inheritance.

Diagnostic Procedures. *Blood.* Mixed IgG and IgM cryoglobulins and blood urea nitrogen and creatinine increase. Other kidney functions altered.

BIBLIOGRAPHY. Meltzer M, Franklin EC: Cryoglobulinemia: a clinical and laboratory study. Ann J Med 40:837–856, 1966

Nightingale SD, Pelley RP: A shared cryoglobulin antigen in familial cryoglobulinemia. Ann J Hum Genet 33:722–734, 1981

Foerster J: Cryoglobulins and cryoglobulinemia. In Lee GR, Bithell TC, Foerster J, et al (eds): Wintrobe's Clinical Hematology, 9th ed, p 2285. Philadelphia, Lea & Febiger, 1993

MEMBRANEOUS APLASIA CUTIS

Synonyms. Hair collar sign, aplasia cutis—hair collar. See Aplasia cutis congenita.

Symptoms and Signs. In perinatal period, membraneous aplasia in the scalp, often appearing as translucent, soft cysts, that with time change into flat, atrophic scars with the surrounding area forming hair collars.

Etiology. Suggestion that the lesion represents a mild manifestation of cranialneural tube closure defect and not the result of external trauma.

Diagnostic Procedures. *Spinal column X-ray. CT scan.*

BIBLIOGRAPHY. Commens C, Rogers M, Kan A: Heterotopic brain tissue presenting as bald cysts with collar of hypertrophic hair: The hair collar sign. Arch Dermatol 125:1253–1256, 1989

Drolet B, Prendiville J, Golden J, et al: Membraneous aplasia cutis with hair collar: Congenital absence of skin or neuroectodemal defect? Arch Dermatol 131:1427–1431, 1995

MENDE

Synonyms. See Klein-Waardenburg.

Symptoms and Signs. Partial albinism (hair and skin); persistent lanugo type of hair, congenital deafness; mongoloid facies; chronic blepharitis; stunted growth; cleft lip; occasionally mental deficiency; brachycephaly.

Etiology. Considered today a variant of Klein-Waardenburg.

BIBLIOGRAPHY. Mende I: Ueber eine Familie hereditaer-degenerativer Taubstummer mit mongoloidem Einschlag und teilweisem Leukismus der Haut und Haare. Arch Kinderheilk 79:214, 1926

MENDELSON

Synonyms. Acid—pulmonary—aspiration; aspiration pneumonitis; chemical pneumonitis; acid aspiration pneumonitis.

Symptoms and Signs. The syndrome has been described in association with obstetric anesthesia. Can occur also in states of altered consciousness, neuromuscular disease, gastrointestinal disease, and with the use of medical devices such as nasogastric tubes or uncuffed tracheostomy tubes. Aspiration may be liquid or solid. Two distinct clinical pictures are present, depending upon the nature of the aspiration. *If liquid.* Cyanosis; tachycardia; tachypnea; hypotension; acute asthma-like syndrome in form of wheeze, rales, and bilateral rhonchi. *If solid.* Laryngeal or bronchial obstruction with atelectasis; mediastinal shift; signs of consolidation; decreased breath sounds; cyanosis; tachycardia.

Etiology. Aspiration of acid gastric content during general anesthesia. It has been demonstrated experimentally that the acidity of the gastric contents is responsible for the whole clinical and pathologic picture. The critical pH is 2.5 or below. Experimentally, in cats and rabbits, injection into trachea of distilled water, normal saline, 11.3% sodium bicarbonate solution; did not give rise to the preceding pathologic changes, whereas the injection of an acid solution reproduced the typical syndrome.

Pathology. At autopsy the pathologic findings are limited to the lung. The heart may show cardiac enlargement if cardiac failure supervenes. Trachea and bronchi are infarcted with areas of necrosis. Pleural cavities contain serum and hemorrhagic fluid. Peribronchiolar hemorrhage and exudate; bronchiolar epithelium is necrotic and sloughed into lumen. Alveolar walls are hyaline, and edema around the blood vessels is noticed.

Diagnostic Procedures. *Blood.* Signs of hypoxia and sometimes acidosis. *X-ray.* Homogeneous density with mediastinal shift. In liquid aspiration, usually irregular soft, mottled densities in both lungs.

Therapy. Prompt establishment of an adequate airway; suction of the airway; single lavage with 10 ml of saline; avoid lavage with larger volumes and intratracheal instillation of sodium bicarbonate and steroid. Fluid replacement with crystalloid or colloid solutions; oxygen and positive-pressure ventilation with PEEP; aminophylline; avoid diuretics. (The pulmonary edema in this syndrome is not cardiogenic and usually is associated with intravascular volume depletion.) Avoid systemic corticosteroids. Intensive care.

Prognosis. High mortality (28–62%).

BIBLIOGRAPHY. Mendelson CL: Aspiration of stomach contents into the lungs during obstetric anesthesia. Am J Obstet Gynecol 52:191–205, 1946

Mimmo WS: Aspiration of gastric contents. Br J Hosp Med 34:76–179, 1985

James FM: Anesthetic complications in obstetric anesthesia. American Society of Anesthesiologists. 37th Annual Refresher Course: Lectures and Clinical Update Program, Las Vegas, Nevada, 1986

Civetta JM, Taylor RW, Kirby RR (eds): Critical Care, 2nd ed. Philadelphia, Lippincott, 1992

MENDES DA COSTA

Synonyms. Da Costa (M.); erythrokeratodermia variabilis, EKV; keratitis rubra figurata.

Symptoms and Signs. Both sexes affected; onset usually at early infancy up to 3 years; occasionally, much later. Trunk and buttocks most common sites; may occur, however, in any other site: (1) plaques of erythema and hyperkeratosis, polycyclic, occasionally darker edges; (2) plaques of erythema that vary in intensity and location.

Etiology. Unknown; autosomal dominant inheritance.

Pathology. Edema; cellular infiltration; hyperkeratosis; acanthosis of variable degree.

Diagnostic Procedures. *Biopsy of skin.*

Therapy. Vitamin A (of temporary benefit); oral retinoic acid; etretinate: good results.

Prognosis. Condition persisting for life; general health not affected.

BIBLIOGRAPHY. Mendes da Costa S: Erythrodermia and keratodermia variabilis in mother and daughter. Acta Dermvenereol 6:255–261, 1925

Brown J, Kierland RR: Erythrokeratodermia variabilis. Arch Dermatol 93:194–201, 1966

Van der Schroeff JG, Nijenhuis LE, et al: Genetic linkage between erythrokeratodermic variabilis and Rh locus. Hum Genet 68:165–168, 1984

Macfarlane AW, Chapman SJ, Verbov JL: Is erythrokeratoderma one disorder? A clinical and ultrastructural study of two siblings. Br J Dermatol 124:487–491, 1991

MENETRIER

Synonyms. Giant hypertrophic gastritis; protein-losing gastroenteropathy.

Symptoms. Onset at all ages; prevalent in males. Epigastric distress; ulcer-like pain relieved by alkali. Anorexia; nausea and vomiting; weight loss. Food may relieve or enhance symptoms. Occasionally, diarrhea, melena, hematemesis, and steatorrhea.

Signs. Usually none; occasionally, epigastric tenderness, edema, ascites.

Etiology. Unknown. Suggested possibility of autosomal dominant inheritance in some families.

Pathology. Stomach with large swollen folds, separated by deep sulci; mucosal erosions; hemorrhagic effusions; covered by abundant mucus; hyperplasia of epithelium; mucous cysts. Eosinophils abundant; edema of muscularis; lack of inflammatory or neoplastic changes.

Diagnostic Procedures. *Blood.* Hypoproteinemia. *X-ray. CT scan. Ultrasonography. Gastroscopy. Biopsy of stomach.*

Therapy. High-protein diet if hypoproteinemia; alkai for relief of pain. Partial or total gastrectomy as last resort. Postoperative course difficult, especially if hypoproteinemia not previously corrected.

Prognosis. Severe; occasionally, uncontrollable ulcer. Malignant transformation possible. Reported duration from 2 months to 22 years.

BIBLIOGRAPHY. Menétrier P: Des polyadénomes gastriques et des leurs rapports avec le cancer de l'estomac. Arch Physiol Norm Pathol 1:32–55, 236–262, 1888

Jeffries GH, Holman HR, Sleisenger MH: Plasma proteins of the gastrointestinal tract. N Engl J Med 266:652–660, 1962

Baker A, Volberg F, Sumner T, et al: Childhood Ménétrier: Four new cases and discussion of the literature. Gastrointest Radiol 11:131–134, 1986

Heatley RV, Wyatt JI: Gastritis and duodenitis. In Haubrich WS, Schaffner F, Berk JE (eds): Bockus Gastroenterology, 5th ed, vol 2, p 651. Philadelphia, WB Saunders, 1995

MÉNIÈRE

Synonyms. Labyrinthine; recurrent aural vertigo; labyrinthine hydrops; cochlear Ménière (episodic deafness without vertigo).

Symptoms. Onset usually between third and fifth decade. Initial stage. Unilateral (90%) hearing loss, fluctuating inner ear type, affecting first only low tones, then both low and high. Tinnitus, first low-pitched, then high-pitched tone. Sudden appearance of vertigo: violent; totally incapacitating, lying still in bed to minimize symptoms is all that the patient can do. Nausea and vomiting frequently accompany vertigo. Possible loss of consciousness. Repeated attacks.

Signs. Nystagmus (may be present); psychological maladjustment.

Etiology. Endolymphatic hydrops of the labyrinth owing to insufficient fluid resorption in the endolymphatic sac or blockage of longitudinal endolymph flow. Attacks are caused by periodic rupture of endolymph membrane with potassium palsy of ampullary nerves. Conditon may be acquired because of viral, bacterial infections; traumatic, embriopathy. Mondini dysplasia (see) or idiopathic.

Pathology. Dilatation of endolymph spaces of cochlea and saccule; degenerative changes of vestibular sense organs.

Diagnostic Procedures. *Audiometry.* Hearing severely reduced in affected ear; caloric response not much affected. *CT scan. MRI. X-ray of skull.*

Therapy. Medical low-salt diet; nicotinic acid; dimenhydrinate to control attacks; best results with betahistine hydrochloride; instillation ototic agents (gentamycin). If medical management fails, surgical selective destruction vestibular nerve section or cryo techniques; surgical destructive: vestibularectomy, labirinthectomy.

Prognosis. Recurrent progressive condition. After years progressive involvement of opposite ear (about 50%). Less than 5% require surgery. Complete hearing loss is frequently followed by cessation of vertigo spells.

BIBLIOGRAPHY. Ménière P: Maladie de l'oreille interne offrant les symptömes de congestion cérébrale apoplectiforme. Gaz Med Paris 3:16:88, 1861

Ménière P: Mémoire sur des lésions de l'oreille interne donnant lieu è des symptömes de congestion cérébrale apoplectiforme. Gaz Med J Paris 16:597–601, 1861

Brandt T: Vertigo: Its multisensory syndromes, p 41. London, Springer-Verlag, 1991

MENINGOCOCCEMIA

Symptoms and Signs. Occurs in relatively healthy appearing individual. Fever; malaise; joint pain. A few days after onset of fever; rash, ill-defined erythematous macules in dependent parts of the body (frequently sparing palms and soles) developing in irregular hemorrhagic areas. Most characteristic element: pink lesions with central petechial element. Splenic enlargement.

Etiology. Chronic meningococcemia; allergic basis for the skin rash suggested; individual with partial immunity to meningococcus.

Pathology. Biopsy of the skin lesion at 36–48 hours after appearance shows perivascular infiltrate of lymphocytes and macrophages, few granulocytes, no fibrin or thrombus occlusion, vascular wall intact, no endothelial swelling, edema in upper dermis, normal epithelium. Absence of bacteria (pattern strikingly differing from that of acute meningococcemia).

Diagnostic Procedures. *Blood culture.* Meningococcus. Inability to agglutinate meningococci isolated from blood. White blood cells increased. *Spinal fluid.* Normal.

Therapy. Penicillin; streptomycin; sulfonamides.

Prognosis. Afebrile within 24–48 hours of onset of treatment; skin lesion and splenomegaly disappear in a few days.

BIBLIOGRAPHY. Salomon H: Ueber Meningokokkenseptikämie. Klin Wochenschr 39:1045–1048, 1902
Ognibene AJ, Dito WR: Chronic meningococcemia. Arch Intern Med 114:29–32, 1964
Baxter P, Priestley B: Meningococcal rash. Lancet 1:1166–1167, 1988
Highet AS, Hay RJ, Roberts SOB: Bacterial infections. In Champion RH, Burton JL, Ebling FJG (eds): Rook/Wilkinson/Ebling Textbook of Dermatology, 5th ed, p 990. Oxford, Blackwell Scientific, 1992

MENKES II

Synonyms. Kinky hair; steely hair; trichopolydystrophy; X-linked copper deficiency; pili torti; copper transport; MK; MNK.

Symptoms. Only males affected; present from early infancy. Spasticity; refractary motor seizures; dementia; retarded growth; decreased visual function.

Signs. Small at birth; lack of facial expression; skin thick and dry. Transient jaundice. Hair normal at birth; at 6 weeks begins to lose pigmentation and assumes the typical aspect: twisting and breaking. A mild form described with less severe neurologic effects.

Etiology. X-linked recessive inheritance. Gene location Xp13. Malabsorption of copper and sequestration of the metal in tissues where it cannot be accessible for copper enzyme synthesis. Deficiency of lysyl oxydase activity that creates disulfide bond in hair (pili torti).

Pathology. *Brain.* Small, diffuse degenerative changes of both gray and white matter in cerebrum and cerebellum. *Hair.* Monilethrix. *Bones.* Wormian bones of the skull; ribs and femur, metaphyseal widening with spur formation. Arterial elongation and tortuosity with fragmentation and reduplication of the internal elastic lamina.

Diagnostic Procedures. *X-ray.* Arteriopathic and skeletal changes. *Blood.* Decreased copper and ceruloplasmin levels.

Therapy. Parenteral administration of copper salts.

Prognosis. Death in infancy. Treatment reverses clinical features. One case survived (decerebrated) for 12 years. With the mild form longer survival.

BIBLIOGRAPHY. Menkes JH, Alter M, Steigeeder GK, et al: A sex-linked recessive disorder with retardation of growth, peculiar hair, and focal cerebral and cerebellar degeneration. Paediatrics 29:764–769, 1962
Gupta A, Arora NK, Desai N, et al: Menkes disease. Indian J Pediatr 55:445–447, 1988
Danks DM: Disorders of copper transport. In Scriver CR, Beaudet AL, Sly WS, et al: The Metabolic and Molecular Bases of Inherited Disease, 7th ed, pp 2223–2230. New York, McGraw-Hill, 1995

MENOPAUSAL

Synonym. Female climacteric.

Symptoms. Experienced by some women during climacteric. Hot facial flashes; chills; sweats, tachycardia; palpitations; nervousness; insomnia; irritability; depression; headaches; lost or increased libido; abnormal uterine bleeding; pruritus valvae; atrophic vaginitis; breast pain; hypertrophy of breasts; bursitis and bone pains; hypertension. Local regressive changes in the urogenital tract.

Etiology. Waning ovarian function and deficiency of estrogen secretion.

Pathology. Changes associated with decreased estrogen secretion: climacteric changes of ovary, genital tract, uterus, cervix, vagina, external genitalia, breasts.

Diagnostic Procedures. *Blood.* Increased follicle-stimulating hormone (FSH), increased cholesterol. *X-ray.* Bone density. Osteoporosis; arthritic changes.

Therapy. Sedation, barbiturate and benzodiazepines. If depression, amphetamine or bromazepam. Hormonal therapy: cyclic estrogen administration (3 weeks therapy and 1 week rest) for several months.

Prognosis. Condition tends to disappear spontaneously, after months, sometimes years. With treatment, symptoms may be well controlled.

BIBLIOGRAPHY. Greenblatt RB, Emperaire JC: Changing concepts in the management of the menopause. Med Times 98:153, 1970
Odell WD: The menopause and hormonal replacement. In De Groot LJ (ed): Endocrinology, 3rd ed, pp 2128–2139. Philadelphia, WB Saunders, 1995

MENOPAUSAL MUSCULAR DYSTROPHY

Synonyms. "Late life" muscular dystrophy; necrotizing myopathy. See Polymyositis, Group I.

MENSTRUAL PERIOD, UNEXPLAINED DELAY

Synonym. Psychosexual menstrual period.

Symptoms. Usually associated with beginning of sexual life or a change in its pattern. Menstrual delay of 10–60 days followed by abnormal uterine bleeding.

Signs. Normal anatomic and functional capacities.

Etiology. Psychogenic origin: beginning of sexual relations; change in its patterns; fear of or desire for pregnancy. To be differentiated from (1) incomplete abortion, (2) incipient abortion, (3) extrauterine pregnancy.

Pathology. Endometrial curettage: Proliferative endometrium or early secretory endometrium or both. Puncture of Douglas pouch: 5–20 ml of serohematic fluid.

Diagnostic Procedures. *Pregnancy tests.* Negative (see Pathology).

Therapy. Psychotherapy.

Prognosis. Good; condition will spontaneously correct itself.

BIBLIOGRAPHY. Soferman N, Haimov M: The syndrome of unexplained delayed menstrual period. Am J Obstet Gynecol 91:137–141, 1965
Baird DT: Amenorrhea, anovulation, and dysfunctional uterine bleeding. In De Groot LJ (ed): Endocrinology, 3rd ed, p 2072. Philadelphia, WB Saunders, 1995

MENZEL

Synonyms. Olivopontocerebellar-spinocebellar degeneration. See Déjerine-Thomas, Friedreich and olivopontocerebellar atrophy (OPCAI).

Symptoms and Signs. Both sexes affected; onset after 20 years of age. Cerebellar ataxia with moderate or severe coordinative disturbances; dysarthria, dysphagia. Deep reflexes normal or exaggerated. (Hyperreflexia as contrasted with hyporeflexia observed in Friedreich ataxia is one of the main differentiating features.) Spasticity. In individual cases varible associated findings. Hemiballismus, athetosis, leg contractures, ophthalmoplegia, fixed pupils, ptosis, retinal degeneration; seizures; parkinsonism; mental retardation or dementia, scoliosis; claw foot, etc.

Etiology. Possibly, heterogeneous group; autosomal dominant or (in some cases) recessive forms (?). This syndrome is subject of intense discussion and disagreement. Considered similar or identical to Déjerine and Friedreich ataxia.

Pathology. Lack of agreement on typical features, so that no specific anatomic findings may be assigned. Importance of ponto-olivocerebellar atrophy emphasized by certain authors. In general less involvement of Purkinje cells of cerebellar cortex. Involvement of spinal cord relatively frequent. In the original case: marked atrophy of the middle cerebellar peduncles, pontine and olivary nuclei and minor changes in the superior cerebellar peduncles and dentate nuclei; degeneration of dorsal columns and spinocerebellar and corticospinal tracts with minor changes in the anterior horns of spinal cord and motor nuclei of brain stem.

Diagnostic Procedures. *Brain CT scan. MRI. EMG. Biopsy of muscle. Spinal tap.*

Therapy. Symptomatic.

Prognosis. Death in middle age.

BIBLIOGRAPHY. Menzel P: Beitrage zur Kenntnis der hereditaren Ataxie und Kleinhirnatrophie. Arch Psychiatr Nervenkr 22:160–190, 1891
Pedersen L, Platz P, Ryder LP, et al: A linkage study of hereditary ataxias and related disorders: Evidence of heterogeneity of dominant cerebellar ataxia. Hum Genet 54:371–383, 1980
Adams RD, Victor M: Principles of Neurology, 5th ed, p 990. New York, McGraw-Hill, 1993

MERETOJA

Synonym. Amyloidosis V; Finland type amyloidosis; see also Meesmann; Biber-Haab-Dimmer and Melkersson.

Symptoms and Signs. Both sexes equally affected; onset in third decade. Cranial neuropathies (facial palsy or other manifestations). Corneal lattice degeneration. Occasionally kidney and/or cardiac involvement.

Etiology. Autosomal dominant inheritance. Deposition of gelsolin in various tissues.

Therapy. Corneal transplant.

Pathology. Widespread amyloid degeneration.

BIBLIOGRAPHY. Meretoja J: Genetic aspects of familial amyloidosis with corneal lattice dystrophy and cranial neuropathy. Clin Genet 4:173–185, 1973
Haltia M, Ghiso J, Prelli F, et al: Amyloid in familial amyloidosis, Finnish type, is antigenically and structurally related to gelsolin. Am J Pathol 136:1223–1228, 1990
Starck T, Kenion KR, Hanninen LA, et al: Clinical and histopathologic studies of two families with lattice corneal dystrophy and familial systemic amyloidosis (Meretoja syndrome). Ophthalmology 98:1197–1206, 1991
Benson MD: Amyloidosis. In Scriver CR, Beaudet AL, Sly WS, et al: The Metabolic and Molecular Bases of Inherited Disease, 7th ed, p 4178. New York, McGraw-Hill, 1995

MERMAID

Synonyms. Caudal dysplasia; caudal regression; sirenomelia. See Townes-Brocks.

Symptoms and Signs. Variable anomalies:

1. Lower limbs. Symmelia; flexion and turning of independent leg into external rotation; atrophy; clubfoot; defective motion of joints
2. Rectum. Imperforate anus
3. Kidney and urinary tract. Bilateral or unilateral agenesis
4. Genital organ. Agenesis with exception of gonads
5. Lumbosacral spine. Agenesis or increase in number of vertebrae epistasis
6. Other visceral or somatic anomalies also may be associated. Some anomalies incompatible with life.

Etiology. Genetic (autosomal and X-linked inheritance) and nongenetic teratogenic mechanisms. Of great interest is the presence of the syndrome in infants born from diabetic mothers.

BIBLIOGRAPHY. Feller A, Sternberg H: Zur Kenntnis der Fehlbildungen der Wirbelsäule. III. Mitteilung. Ueber den vollständigen Mangel der unteren Wirbelsäulenabschinitte und seine Bedeutung für die formale Genese der Defektbildungen des hinteren Körperendes. Virchows Arch Pathol Anat 280:649–692, 1931
Welch J P, Aterman K: The syndrome of caudal dysplasia: A review, including etiologic considerations and evidence of heterogeneity. Pediatr Phatol 2:213–327, 1984
Jones KL: Smith's Recognizable Patterns of Human Malformations, p 72. Philadelphia, WB Saunders, 1988

M.E.R.R.F.

Synonyms. Myoclonus epilepsy; ragged; red fibers. See Ophthalmoplegia.

Symptoms and Signs. See Unverricht plus mitochondrial myopathy.

Etiology. Unknown. Mutation in mitochondrial DNA. Inheritance of any type excluded for the time being.

BIBLIOGRAPHY. Rosing HS, Hopkins LC, Wallace DC, et al: Maternally inherited mitochondrial myopathy and myoclonic epilepsy. Ann Neurol 17:228–237, 1985
Yoveda M, Tanno Y, Horai S, et al: A common mitochondrial DNA mutation in the tRNA-lys of patients with myoclonus epilepsy associated with rugged-red fibers. Biochem Int 21:789–796, 1990

MERWARTH

Synonym. Rolandic vein occlusion.

Symptoms. Progressively developing hemiplegia, starting and affecting particularly the foot and leg. Sensory and motor disturbances. Arm weakened; hand usually not affected.

Signs. Leg tendon hyperreflexia; mucle tone varies from spasticity (usually) to hypotonia.

Etiology. Idiopathic thrombosis of cortical veins.

Pathology. Cerebral venous thrombosis. Areas of hemorrhage and softening of variable degrees.

Diagnostic Procedures. *Clotting studies. Spinal tap. Venography. EEG.*

Therapy. Anticoagulants.

Prognosis. Complete recovery seems to be the rule. Function returns progressively in the arm first, then eventually to leg, and last in the foot.

BIBLIOGRAPHY. Merwarth HR: Hemiplegia of cortical or venous origin (occlusion of rolandic veins). Brooklyn Hosp J 2:193–212, 1940

Sudarsky L: An overview of neurological diseases causing gait disorders. In Spivack BS: Evaluation and management of gait disorders. New York, Marcel Dekker, 1995

Crawford SC, Digri KB, Palmer CA, et al: Thrombosis of the deep venous drainage of the brain in adults. Arch Neurol 52:1101–1108, 1995

MESENTERIC ARTERY, SUPERIOR

Synonym. SMA; including cast chronic forms (Wilkie syndrome). See Dorph.

Symptoms. Usually begins in early childhood. The syndrome may also appear in patients with chronic illness or after surgery when remaining for prolonged period in supine position. Postprandial fullness; abdominal cramps and pains; nausea; vomiting; failure to gain weight.

Signs. Height to weight ratio with tendency toward slender habitus seems to be of significance. Prone or knee chest position may relieve pain.

Etiology and Pathology. Many structural abnormalities that reduce the angle formed by the aorta and vertebrae posteriorly, and the root of superior mesenteric artery and vein anteriorly. Reduction of this angle compresses the duodenum. Kyphoscoliosis; lordosis; weight loss with decrease of fat; lymphadenopathy; tumors in the retroperitoneum; rotation of intestine with abnormal fibrous bands; wearing constrictive girdles or body cast.

Diagnostic Procedures. *Fluoroscopy. Echography.* Permanence of barium in obstructed areas.

Therapy. Medical: small feedings with bland, low-residue, high-calorie food. Removal of extrinsic obstruction (e.g., girdle, cast). If failure, surgery: division of ligament of Treitz and freeing the duodenum, or, if needed, bypass of obstruction by gastrojejunostomy or duodenojejunostomy.

Prognosis. In many cases, good response to conservative treatment, and child may grow out of the situation (gain weight). In incapacitating cases (vomiting; dehydration, failure to grow), surgery indicated and good results obtained.

BIBLIOGRAPHY. Von Rokitansky C: Lehrbuch der pathologischen Anatomie, p 187. Vienna, Braumüller, 1861

Wilkie DPD: The blood supply of duodenum: With special reference to the supraduodenal artery. Surg Gynec Obstr 13:399–405, 1911

Hyde JS, Swarts CL, Nicholas EE, et al: Superior mesenteric artery syndrome. Am J Dis Child 106:25–34, 1963

Gondos B: Duodenal compression defect and the superior mesenteric artery syndrome. Radiology 123:575–580, 1977

Weatherall DJ, Ledingham JGG, Warrell DA (eds): Oxford Textbook of Medicine, 3rd ed, p 2367. Oxford, Oxford Med Pub, 1996

MESIAL TEMPORAL-LOBE EPILEPSY

Synonyms. Epilepsy—mesial temporal—lobe.

Symptoms and Signs. Common familial history of epilepsy. High incidence of complicated febrile convulsions. Seizures begining in the latter half of first decade of life lasting 1–2 minutes. An aura of several seconds usually is present and postrictal phase (lasting several minutes) with disorientation, recent memory defects, amnesia and dysphasia, if seizures begin in the language-dominant hemisphere. Rare secondary generalized seizures. Seizures often may remit for several years up to adolescence or early adulthood. Neurologic examination usually normal. Depression in the interictal period frequently present. Seizures characteristically become intractable as early as adolescence.

Etiology and Pathology. Hippocampal sclerosis.

Diagnostic Procedures. *EEG.* Unilateral or bitemporal independent anterior temporal spikes with mx amplitude in basal electrodes. *Positron-emission tomography with fluorodeoxyglucose.* Temporal-lobe hypometabolism often involving ipsilateral portion of thalamus and basal ganglia. *MRI.* Hippocampal atrophy.

Therapy. Neurosurgery, anterior mesial lobe resection.

Prognosis. Surgery offers a 70–80% chance of cure.

BIBLIOGRAPHY. Wieser H-G, Engel J Jr, Willamson PD, et al: Surgically remediable temporal lobe syndromes. In Engel J Jr (ed): Surgical Treatment of the Epilepsies, 2nd ed, pp 49–63. New York, Raven, 1993

Engel J Jr: Surgery for seizures. N Engl J Med 334:647–652, 1996

METACHONDROMATOSIS

Synonym. Different from multiple exosostosis; Ollier and Langer-Giedon.

Symptoms and Signs. Both sexes. Lumps and bumps on hand, feet. Knees: painless swelling that may enlarge or regress. Exostosis typically point toward the epiphysis.

Etiology. Autosomal dominant inheritance.

Pathology. Combination of classic changes of exostosis and enchondromas.

Diagnostic Procedures. *X-rays.* Osteocartilagineous exostoses. Most common in tubular bone of hands and feet; encondromatous lesions of iliac crest and femur; same lesions may involve vertebrae.

Therapy. Symptomatic.

Prognosis. Evolution not predictable, may regress spontaneously.

BIBLIOGRAPHY. Maroteaux P: La metachondromatose. Z Kinderheilk 109:246–261, 1971

Bassett GS, Cowell HR: Metachondromatosis: Report of four cases. J Bone Joint Surg 67:811–814, 1985

Klippel JH, Dieppe PA: Rheumatology, p 7.43.5. St Louis, CV Mosby, 1994

METACHROMATIC LEUKODYSTROPHY

Synonyms. MLD; Greenfield; Scholz; Scholz-Bielschowsky-Henneberg; sulfatide lipoidosis; Van Bogaert-Nyssen-Pfeiffer; diffuse brain sclerosis; cerebroside sulfatase deficiency, arylsulfatase A.

CONGENITAL

Symptoms and Signs. Apnea, cyanosis, general weakness, seizures.

Etiology. Autosomal recessive inheritance. Arylsulfatase activity: unknown. It may represent an early state of late infantile MLD; existence of this form is still conjectural.

Prognosis. Death after a few weeks.

LATE INFANTILE FORM

Symptoms. Both sexes affected. Usually recognized in second year of life. Early development normal (locomotion and speech at normal age); then progressive weakness and hypotonia of legs; ataxia or spastic paralysis; seizures (in 50% of cases); optic atrophy (30%); dementia; urinary incontinence.

Signs. *Stage 1.* Muscle tone decreased, reflexes absent, decreased, or increased. Stage lasts from a few months to 1 year or longer. *Stage 2.*

Patient can sit up but can no longer stand. Muscle tone is increased only in the legs (arms remain hypotonic); Babinski sign; reflexes absent or increased; mental regression is obvious; speech deteriorates, optic atrophy and a gray discoloration of macula; nystagmus; ataxia, intermittent pains in arms and legs. Stage lasts few months. *Stage 3.* Muscle tone is variable. Bedridden and quadriplegic, decerebrated, decorticaded or dystonic posture; bulbar and pseudobulbar palsy; speech no longer distinct, mental deficit more severe, still present ability to smile to parents. *Stage 4.* Unreactive to visual and auditory stimuli. Feeding through tube. This stage lasts months or years.

Etiology. Autosomal recessive inheritance. Deficiency of arylsulfatase A (cerebroside sulfatase). Sulfatides accumulate mainly in nervous tissue and to a smaller extent in other organs.

Pathology. In brain; white matter symmetric diffuse involvement, increased consistency, grayish or brown discoloration, sometimes cavitation. Loss of normal myeline sheaths; accumulation of lipoid granular masses that are typically stained (metachromatic). Certain group of neurons and peripheral nerves also involved. Kidney, gall-bladder (mucosa contains macrophages with some granules), liver, pancreas, pituitary, adrenal cortex, and testes are also involved.

Diagnostic Procedures. *Urine.* Direct examination of urine sediment with the addition of toluidine blue reveals metachromatic bodies; application of lipid extracted from urine to filter paper and staining with toluidine blue; arylsulfatase test, absence of the enzyme. *Spinal fluid.* Proteins elevated. *Nerve conduction.* Velocity: slowed. *Biopsy.* Of sural nerve.

Therapy. Trials with low vitamin A diet and thiosulfate are under study.

Prognosis. Death occurs 5 months to 10 years after onset.

JUVENILE FORM

Symptoms. Subdivided in two subgroups early juvenile and late juvenile with onset respectively at 4–6 and 6–12 years of age. First symptoms: failure in schoolwork; emotional disturbances; visual trouble, frequently evolving in blindness. Other signs: loss of speech, quariparesis, peripheral neuropathy and seizures.

Etiology. Autosomal recessive inheritance. Deficiency of arylsulfatase A (cerebroside sulfatase). Sulfatides accumulate mainly in nervous tissue and to a smaller extent in other organs.

Diagnostic Procedures. See preceding.

Prognosis. Progression slower than preceding.

ADULT FORM

Symptoms. Both sexes. Onset after 16th year of life (higher age of onset recorded, 62). Change in personality and poor school or job performance as first symptoms followed by defective visual spatial discrimination, loss of memory and mental alertness, depression, appearance of psychosis, depersonalization or paranoia, hallucinations, ataxia, progressive spastic quadraparesis, incontinence. In final stage mutism, blindness, unresposiveness, patient becomes bedridden. Occasionally seizures.

Etiology. Autosomal recessive inheritance. Deficiency of arylsulfatase A (cerebroside sulfatase). Sulfatides accumulate mainly in nervous tissue and to a smaller extent in other organs.

Diagnostic Procedures. See preceding.

Prognosis. Survival 5–10 years. In few cases much more rapid or longer (over several decades).

MLD WITHOUT ARYLSULFATASE A DEFICIENCY

Synonyms. Cerebroside sulfatase activator deficiency; sphingolipid activator protein 1; SPA 1.

Symptoms and Signs. Onset 4–6 years of life. Clinical course of adolescent form but without arysulfatase A deficiency or with mild reduc-

tion. What is probably lacking is an activator protein for arylsulfatase activity.

MLD WITH MULTIPLE SULFATASE DEFICIENCY

Symptoms and Signs. Onset over 1 year of age, signs as in late infantile form, plus coarse facies, deafness, ichthyosis hepatosplenomegaly, skeletal anomalies.

Diagnostic Procedures. *Urine.* Increased sulfatide and mucopolysaccharide excretion. *Blood.* In white cells presence of Alder-Reilly granules, multiple sulfatase deficiency. *Spinal fluid.* Protein elevated. *Nerve conduction.* Slowed velocity.

ARYLSULFATASE A DEFICIENCY WITHOUT MLD

Synonyms. Pseudoarylsulfatase A deficiency. This defect without clinical manifestations is sometimes present in relatives of people with MLD or in patients with neurological disabilities different from MLD.

Etiology. It has been suggested that autosomal dominant inheritance, sex-linked factors, and mutation are genetic possibilities to be considered in different families.

Pathology. While in the infantile form, metachromatic material may be demonstrated only in frozen section; in adult form, it also may be demonstrated in paraffin- or celloidin-treated material.

Prognosis. Long course.

BIBLIOGRAPHY. Alzheimer A: Beitrage zur Kenntnis der pathologischen Neurologie und ihren Beziehung zu den Abbauvorgangen im Nervengewebe Nissl-Alzheimer's. Histol Histopathol Arb 3:493, 1910

Perusini G: Ueber klinisch und histologisch eigenartige psychische Enkrankungen des spaeteren Lebensalters Nissl-Alzheimer's. Histol Histopathol Arb 3:297, 1910

Witte F: Ueber pathologische Abbauvorgange im Zentralnervensystem. Munch Med Wochenschr 68:69, 1921

Scholz W: Klinische, patologischanatomische und erbbiologische Untersuchungen bei familiaer, diffuser Hirnsklerose im Kindersalter. Z Neurol Psychiat 99:651–717, 1925

Dewji N, Wenger D, Fujibayashi S, et al: Molecular cloning of sphingolipid activator protein 1 (SAP1): The sulfatide sulfatase activator. Am J Hum Genet 37:A150, 1985

Kolodny EH, Fluharty: Metachromatic leukodystrophy and multiple sulfatase deficiency: Sulfatide lipidosis. In Scriver CR, Beaudet AL, Sly WS, et al: The Metabolic and Molecular Bases of Inherited Disease, 7th ed, pp 1721–1750. New York, McGraw-Hill, 1995

METATROPIC DYSPLASIA

Synonyms. Maroteaux-Spranger-Weidemann; hyperchondrogenesis; metatrophic dwarfism I; hyperplastic achondroplasia.

Symptoms. Both sexes affected; evident at birth and progressing during infancy. Motor milestones delayed. Birth length normal or slightly decreased (long trunk, especially thorax, and short limbs). Linear fold that overlies the coccyx and may extend as a tail-like process. Waddling gait. Knobby and lax joints. Elbow may not fully extend. Occasionally, inguinal hernia and cleft palate. In infancy and childhood, retarded growth, severe kyphoscoliosis, short neck, upward displacement of sternum, generalized weakness. In adolescence, progressive disability. Dyspnea.

Etiology. Unknown; both autosomal dominant and recessive (lethal) types of inheritance.

Pathology. Lack of endochondral ossification in growth areas and irregular arrangement of trabeculae.

Diagnostic Procedures. *X-rays.* Delayed ossification; kyphoscoliosis; pelvic supraacetabular notch; squared iliac wings; bell-shaped ends of long bones. *Blood.* Phosphorus elevated.

Therapy. Mainly orthopedic.

Prognosis. Few survive beyond adulthood because of cardiopulmonary complications and atlantoaxial instability.

BIBLIOGRAPHY. Kaufmann E: Untersuchungen ueber die sogenanulte foetale Rachitis Chondrodystrophia foetalis. Berlin, G Reimer, 1892

Maroteaux P, Spranger J, Weidemann HR: Der metatropische Zwergwuchs. Arch Kinderheilkd 173:211–226, 1966

Maroteaux P, Spranger J: The spondylometaphyseal dysplasias: A tentative classification. Pediatr Radiol 21:293–297, 1991

Beighton P: McKusick's Heritable Disorders of Connective Tissue, 5th ed, pp 583–587. St Louis, CV Mosby, 1993

METHEMOGLOBINEMIAS, HEREDITARY

Synonyms. Hoerlein-Weber; Tamyra-Takahashi; methemoglobininemia congenital; M hemoglobin.

Symptoms and Signs. Both sexes affected; onset of cyanosis at birth (alpha-substituted M hemoglobin) or at 6–12 months of age (beta chain mutants). In alpha-substituted, asymptomatic, no exercise intolerance. In beta-substituted, usually pallor, splenomegaly.

Etiology. NADH-cytochrome-b5-reductase deficiency (autosomal recessive inheritance). Cytochrome-b5 deficiency; hemoglobin M disorders (autosomal dominant inheritance).

Diagnostic Procedures. *Blood.* Color chocolate brown; color does not change with shaking in air; hemoglobin electrophoresis (better after oxidation with potassium ferrocyanide).

Therapy. Methylene blue or ascorbic acid.

Prognosis. Normal longevity and health.

BIBLIOGRAPHY. Hoerlein H, Weber G: Ueber chronische familiäre Methämoglobinemia und eine neue Modifikation des Methämoglobins. Dsch Med Wochenschr 73:476–478, 1947

Bunn HF, Forget BG: Hemoglobin: Molecular Genetic, and Clinical Aspects, p 623. Philadelphia, WB Saunders, 1986

Lukens JN: Methemoglobinemia and other disorders accompanied by cyanosis. In Lee GR, Bithel TC, Foerster J, et al (eds): Wintrobe's Clinical Hematology, 9th ed, pp 1265–1267. Philadelphia, Lea & Febiger, 1993

METHYLMALONIC ACIDEMIA

Synonym. Ketotic hyperglycinemia (see).

Symptoms and Signs. Includes at least five biochemical derangments (see Etiology) with similar but not identical clinical features. The four etiologic groups (1, 2, 3, and 4) show a common clinical pattern. Both sexes affected; onset within first months (50%) or within first year of life (50%). Failure to thrive; vomiting; lethargy; developmental retardation; recurrent infections (50%). A fifth group (5) shows instead variable manifestation from asymptomatic to critical illness from birth. Manifestations include seizures; failure to thrive, psychosis, and abnormal cerebellar and spinal cord function.

Etiology.

1. Methylmalonyl coenzyme A (CoA) racemase deficiency
2. Methylmalonyl CoA mutase apoenzyme deficiency
3. AdoCbl synthesis defect I
4. AdoCbl synthesis defect II
5. Combined synthesis defect of AdoCbl and MeCbl.

Pathology. Groups 1, 2, 3, 4. Osteoporosis; absence of megaloblastic changes. Features secondary to overwhelming infection. Group 5. Brain and spinal cord abnormalities similar to that of Lichtheim (see).

Diagnostic Procedures. *Blood (1, 2, 3, 4).* Neutropenia and thrombocytopenia (in 50% of cases) absence of megaloblastic changes; hyperglycinemia; severe ketoacidosis (pH 6.9–7.1). *Urine.* (1) Hyperglycinemia. *Bone marrow.* Absence of megaloblastic change. *Blood.* (5) Absence of ketoacidosis; occasionally, megaloblastic anemia.

Therapy. Groups 1, 2, 3, 4. Fifty percent of cases respond to cobalamine administration.

Prognosis. Extremely severe. Death between 40 days and 3 years (40%); survival 2–8 years, 60%.

BIBLIOGRAPHY. Oberholzer VG, Levin B, Burgess EA, et al: Methylmalonic aciduria: An inborn error of metabolism leading to chronic metabolic acidosis. Arch Dis Child 42:492–504, 1967

Ledley FD, Crane AM, Lumetta M: Heterogeneous alleles and expression of methylmalonyl Co A mutase in methylmalonic acidemia. Am J Med Genet 46:539–547, 1990

Saudubray J-M, Charpentier C: Clinical phenotypes: Diagnosis/algorithms. In Scriver CR, Beaudet AL, Sly WS, et al: The Metabolic and Molecular Bases of Inherited Disease, 7th ed, pp 338–340. New York, McGraw-Hill, 1995

MEYER-BETZ

Synonyms. Guenther II; myoglobinuria type II; paroxysmal idiopathic myoglobinuria; exercise intolerance; recurrent hemiglobinuria.

Symptoms and Signs. Predominant in males (4:1). Clinically divided into two types. (1) Onset at puberty to early adulthood, few hours after exertion. (2) Onset in childhood, associated with an infection. Sudden severe pain and cramping in the muscle; usually followed by temporary weakness or paralysis. Chills; vomiting; pallor; abdominal pain; fever and shock may also occur at time of attack.

Signs. After a few hours, urine becomes first pink, then deep red brown. Oliguria and anuria in some cases. Urine coloration persists for 72 hours. Affected muscles, swollen "woody" consistency, tender. After repeated attacks, muscles may become atrophic.

Etiology. Usually sporadic appearances; some familial cases reported. Fatty acid oxidation disorders; glycolytic disorders; respiratory chain disorders; myopathies.

Pathology. Muscle biopsy obtained after attack shows coagulative muscle necrosis and necrotic discolored fibers dispersed among normal fibers. In kidney, myoglobin casts.

Diagnostic Procedures. *Urine.* After attack, color red to chocolate brown; presence of myoglobin. *Blood.* Serum, normal color; leukocytosis; CPK and other sarcoplasmic enzymes elevation. *Biopsy of muscle.*

Therapy. Force fluid to prevent anuria.

Prognosis. Attack usually recurs with major and minor episodes, with differing frequency, sometimes at intervals of years. Renal failure may follow an attack; muscular atrophy may result from repeated attacks.

BIBLIOGRAPHY. Meyer-Betz F: Beobachtungen an einem eigenartigen mit Muskellahmungen verbundenen Fall von Hämoglobinurie. Dtsch Arch Klin Med 101:85–127, 1911

Guenther H: Myositis myoglobinuria. 70:517, 1913

Knochel JP: Rhabdomyolysis and myoglobinuria. Ann Rev Med 33:435–443, 1982

Saudubray J-M, Charpentrier C: Clinical phenotypes: Diagnosis/algorithms. In Scriver CR, Beaudet AL, Sly WS, et al: The Metabolic and Molecular Bases of Inherited Disease, 7th ed, pp 350–352. New York, McGraw-Hill, 1995

MEYER DYSPLASIA FEMORAL HEAD

Synonyms. Epiphyseal capitis femoris dysplasia.

Symptoms and Signs. Prevalent in males. Usually before age 5 years. Asymptomatic or limp and pain at the lip.

Etiology. Unknown.

Pathology. Delay in development of epiphyseal ossification of femoral heads.

Therapy. Symptomatic.

Prognosis. Ossification normalizes at 6 years of age (circa) in some cases; aseptic necrosis of femoral head.

BIBLIOGRAPHY. Karup Pedersen E: Dysplasia epiphysealis capitis femoris. J Bone Joint Surg (Br) 42:663–667, 1960

Meyer J: Dysplasia epiphysealis capitis femoris: a clinical radiological syndrome and its relationship to Legg-Calvé-Pathès disease. Acta Orthoped Scand 34:183–187, 1964

Maroteaux P, Hedon C: Dysplasies bilatérale isolées de la hanche chez le jeune enfante. Ann Radiol (Paris) 24:181–197, 1981

Funnery L, Timmermans J, Leroy JG: Dysplasia epiphysealis capitis femoris? Eur J Pediatr 140:345–347, 1983

Klippel JH, Dieppe PA: Rheumatology, p 349. St Louis, CV Mosby, 1995

MEYERSON

Synonyms. Nevus Meyerson.

Symptoms and Signs. In young adults. Multiple, papulosquamous lesions prurigo, around melanocytic nevi.

Etiology. Unknown.

Pathology. Around benign nevus dermal infiltration (with lymphocytes and eosinophils) and acanthosis, spongiosis and parakeratosis.

Prognosis. Spontaneous resolution within few months. Nevus is not involved.

BIBLIOGRAPHY. Meyerson LB: A peculiar papulosquamous eruption involving pigmented naevi. Arch Dermatol 103:510–512, 1971

Nichols DSH, Mason GH: Halo dermatitis around a melanocytic naevus: Meyerson's naevus. Br J Dermatil 118:125–129, 1988

MIBELLI

Synonyms. Porokeratosis isolated; hyperkeratosis eccentrica; keratoderma eccentrica; including Mantoux or Guss (porokeratosis palmoplantaris et disseminate), porokeratosis disseminated superficial; linear porokeratosis; giant porokeratosis and actinic porokeratosis.

Symptoms and Signs. Both sexes affected. Male to female ratio, 3:1. Onset usually in young adulthood. On limbs, eruption of a single or few lesions in crops of miliary translucent papules, slowly enlarging and forming a dark center. Shedding after weeks, leaving small pits that eventually fade away.

Etiology. Sporadic or autosomal dominant type of inheritance with lower penetrability in females. (Guss claims a separate entity for prevalent localization on palm and soles and with possible autosomal or X-linked dominant inheritance.) A photosensitive variety also has been recognized, affecting areas exposed to the sun, with particular histologic pattern (Chernosky-Freeman).

Pathology. Typical changes seen in the edge of lesions. Hyperkeratosis of stratum corneum with parakeratosis, spongiosis shrunken nuclei, and mild infiltration with lymphocytes. Atrophy and hyperkeratosis of central area.

Therapy. Keratolytics of scarce benefit. 5-fluorouracil ointment and cryotherapy beneficial in some cases. Etetrinate also effective but not justified because of risk.

Prognosis. Recurrences for years; occasionally, short duration. Seven percent of patients develop skin cancer. Especially in patients with giant and linear forms.

BIBLIOGRAPHY. Mibelli V: Di una nuova forma di cheratosi "angio-cheratoma." Giorn Ital Mal Vener 30:285–301, 1889

Mantoux C: Porokératose pokillomateuse palmaire et plantaire. Ann Dermatol Syph 4:15–31, 1903

Chernosky ME, Anderson DE: Disseminated superficial actinic porokeratosis: Clinical studies and experimental production of lesions. Arch Derm 99:401–407, 1969

Guss SB, Osbourn RA, Lutzner MA: Porokeratosis plantaris, palmaris et disseminate: A third type of porokeratosis. Arch Derm 104:366–373, 1971

Griffiths WAD, Leigh IM, Marks R: Disorders of keratinization. In Champion RH, Burton JL, Ebling FJG (eds): Rook/Wilkinson/Ebling Textbook of Dermatology, 5th ed, pp 1388–1390. Oxford, Blackwell Scientific, 1992

MICHELIN TIRE BABY

Synonyms. Generalized folded skin; lipomatous nevus.

Symptoms and Signs. Onset from birth. In otherwise healthy babies. Various features may be associated with this syndrome widespread stellate scarring; microcephaly and mental retardation; generalized smooth muscle hamartomatomatosis; hypertrichosis; etc.

Etiology. It represents a nonspecific clinical feature reflecting a variety of pathologic conditions. Chomosomal alterations reported in some cases, autosomal dominant inheritance in others.

Pathology. Lipomatous chages from absence in some cases to lipomatous hypertrophy in others.

Prognosis. Gradual improvement spontaneous in some cases.

BIBLIOGRAPHY. Ross CM: Generalised folded skin with underlying lipomapous nevus "the Miochelin tyre baby." Arch Dermatol 100:320–323, 1969

Atherton DJ: Naevi and other developmental defects. In Champion RH, Burton JL, Ebling FJG (eds): Rook/Wilkinson/Ebling Textbook of Dermatology, 5th ed, pp 468–469. Oxford, Blackwell Scientific, 1992

MICHELS

Synonym. Oculopalatoskeletal; craniosynostosis—lid anomalies (see).

Symptoms and Signs. Both sexes. Blepharophimosis, blepharoptosis, and epicanthus inversus, corneal opacities, limitation of upward gaze, cleft lip palate. Minor skeletal defects: spina bifida occulta, cranial asymmetry, radioulnar synostosis. Fifth finger short.

Etiology. Unknown. Considered autosomal recessive inheritance.

BIBLIOGRAPHY. Michels VV, Hittner HM, Beaudet AL: A clefting syndrome with ocular anterior chamber defect and lid anomalies. J Pediatr 93:444–446, 1978

Cunniff C, Jones KL: Craniosynostosis and lid anomalies: Report of a girl with Michel's syndrome. Am J Med Genet 37:28–30, 1990

MICROMYOMAS UTERI

Synonym. Uterine adenomyoma uterus.

Synonym. Menorrhagia, unresponsive to hormone therapy, curettage, or oxytocics, with normal timing of menstrual periods.

Signs. Rectovaginal examination. Uterus slightly enlarged and firm without irregular nodules on the surface.

Etiology. Unknown. Micromyomas interfere with contractile power of myometrium so that bleeding results.

Pathology. Myometrium of uterus with muscular hypertrophy resembling diffuse miliary fibroid process; increased tortuosity of vessels with hyalinized walls.

Diagnostic Procedures. *Curettage. Biopsy. Blood clotting studies. Doppler.*

Therapy. Total hysterectomy.

Prognosis. Benign condition.

BIBLIOGRAPHY. Hiller RI: Micromyomas of the uterus with severe menorrhagia: A syndrome. Am J Obstet Gynecol 87:163–165, 1963
Cunningham FG, MacDonald PC, Gant NF, et al (eds): Williams Obstetrics, pp 302, 533. Englewood Cliffs, NJ, Prentice-Hall, 1993

MICTURITION SYNCOPE

Symptoms. Syncope occurring during or after termination of voiding urine. Usually, attacks occur at night, when arising after some hours of sleep. Pallor; lightheadedness may precede the syncope or occasionally not progress to it. Attacks may be aborted by sitting down promptly.

Signs. Bradycardia; hypotension.

Etiology. Unknown. Represents one form of the vasovagal syndrome (see).

Diagnostic Procedures. *Electroencephalography.* To differentiate from epilepsy. *Valsalva maneuver.* Occasionally, may reproduce the syndrome.

BIBLIOGRAPHY. Gastaut H, Gastaut Y: Etude électroencéphalographique des syncopes. III. Formes cliniques des syncopes vasovagales: Differentiation d'avec l'épilepsie. Rev Neurol (Paris) 95:547–549, 1956
Godec CJ, Cass AS: Micturition syncope. J Urol 126:551, 1981
Lewis RP, Budoulas H, Schaal SF, et al: Diagnosis and management of syncope. In Schlant RC, Alexander RW: Hurst's The Heart, 8th ed, p 934. New York, McGraw-Hill, 1994

MIDLINE GRANULOMA

Synonym. Stewart type of malignant granuloma; lethal midline granulomatosis; nonhealing midline granuloma. Stewart; idiopathic midline destructive disease (IMDD); lymphomatoid granulomatosis. See Liebow-Carrington.

Symptoms and Signs. Affects all ages, most common 30–50 years of age; prevalent in men and whites. Prodromal. For 1 year or longer nasal stuffiness with serous or serous-hemorrhagic discharge. Disease. Increased discharge, which becomes purulent; areas of necrotic tissue in the nasal cavity that spread to involve entire nose and pharynx; production of fistula through skin. Tongue not involved. Eye involved directly by granulomatous process or because of involvement of adnexum. Pain minimal; episodes of high spiking fever only late in the course.

Etiology. Unknown. Manifestation of malignant lymphoma (?); possible essential role of infections and/or autoimmune condition; relation with Wegener granuloma discussed.

Pathology. Nonspecific lesions; chronic inflammation; granulation tissue; necrosis.

Diagnostic Procedures. *Serology. Biopsy. Cultures.* Rule out tuberculosis, syphilis, Hodgkin, mycosis fungoides, fungus infections, leishmaniasis, leprosy, granuloma venereum and neoplasms of the upper airways, particularly midline malignant reticulosis and certain lymphomas.

Therapy. The treatment of choice is local radiation therapy. Surgery is not useful and actually can worsen the clinical course. Corticosteroids

and cyclophosphamide may be of same effectivenes. Good results reported with trimethoprim and sulfamethoxazole.

Prognosis. High dose radiotherapy to the involved areas results in a high percentage of remissions. The disease should no longer be referred to as lethal.

BIBLIOGRAPHY. McBride P: Case of rapid destruction of the nose and face. J Laryngol 12:64–66, 1897
Stewart JP: Progressive lethal granulomatous ulceration of nose. J Laryngol Otol 48:657–701, 1933
Jaffe ES, Lipford EJ Jr, Margolie JB, et al: Lymphomatoid granulomatosis and angiocentric lymphoma: A spectrum of post-thymic T-cell proliferations. Semin Resp Med 10:167–172, 1989
Rosignoli M, Pezzuto RW, Galli J, et al: Il granuloma centro-facciale e la granulomatosi di Wegener Midline granuloma and Wegener's granulomatosis. Acta Otorhinolaryng Ital (Suppl 38):121–146, 1992

MIEHLKE-PARTSCH

Synonym. Wiedemann variant.

Symptoms and Signs. Observed in neonates. Deformities limited to face and ears; abduction palsy.

Etiology. Thalamidone-induced embryopathy. See Wiedemann.

BIBLIOGRAPHY. Miehlke A, Partsch CH: Ohrmissbildung, Facialis und Abducenslähmung als Syndrom der Thalamidomidschädigung. Arch Ohr Heilk 181:154–164, 1963

MIESCHER I

Synonyms. Acanthosis nigricans—diabetes mellitus (insulin resistant); insulin receptor defect—acanthosis nigricans.

Symptoms and Signs. *Type A (HAIR-AN).* Young females, signs of virilization; accelerated growth. *Type B.* Older females, immunologic disease with circulating antibodies, insulin receptors. Lesions may be present at birth, but usually develop in childhood, seldom after puberty. Pigmentation, dryness, roughness of skin, which assumes a gray, brown, or black color; increased thickness and formation of small papillomatous elevations from velvety to rugose and mammillary. Most frequently involved, unilateral or bilateral axilla, back and sides of neck, groin; less frequently, other flexures, submammary, and umbilical areas. Palms and soles may be thickened. Mucoses rarely show a velvety pattern. Diabetes. Other anomalies have been described in these patients.

Etiology. Autosomal recessive inheritance. Insulin receptor defect.

Pathology. Hyperkeratosis; papillomatosis; acanthosis and pigmentation of variable degree even within single section. Occasionally, horny inclusion cysts.

Diagnostic Procedures. *Blood.* Glycemia (frequent association with lipodystrophic diabetes); insulin in plasma 100 times normal; marked increase in C-peptide. Insulin antibodies. *Biopsy of skin.*

Therapy. Symptomatic.

Prognosis. Slow progression of lesions, which become more severe at puberty and, afterward, may regress or remain static.

BIBLIOGRAPHY. Miescher G: Zwei Faelle von congenitaler familiaerer Akanthosis nigricans, kombieniert mit Diabetes mellitus. Dermatol 32:276–305, 1921
Leme CE, Waichenberg BL, Lerario AC, et al: Acanthosis nigrans, hirsutism, insulin resistance and insulin receptor defect. Clin Endocrinol 17:43–49, 1982
Black MM, Gawkrodger DJ, Seymour CA, et al: Metabolic and nutritional disorders. In Champion RH, Burton JL, Ebling FJG (eds):

Rook/Wilkinson/Ebling Textbook of Dermatology, 5th ed, p 2380. Oxford, Blackwell Scientific, 1992

Flier JS: Syndromes of insulin resistance and mutant insulin. In De Groot LJ (ed): Endocrinology, 3rd ed, pp 1595–1598. Philadelphia, WB Saunders, 1995

MIESCHER II

Synonym. Granulomatous cheilitis. Eponym used to designate the granulomatous cheilitis as a monosymptomatic form of the Melkersson (see).

BIBLIOGRAPHY. Miescher G: Ueber essentielle granulomatöse Makrocheilie (cheilitis granulomatosa). Dermatologica 91:57–85, 1945
Hornstein O: Problems in granulomatous cheilitis (Miescher from an expert testimony viewpoint). Hautarzt 13:302–309, 1962

MIESCHER-LEDER

Synonyms. Miescher III; granuloma disciformis; necrobiosis maculosa.

Symptoms and Signs. Prevalent in women; onset at 50–75 years of age; reported also in adolescents. Plaques, reddish, margined, usually polycyclic shape, center atrophic, edges indurated, present on shins, thighs; abdominal and chest walls may be involved.

Etiology. Today is not considered as an autonomous syndrome but part of the necrobiosis (not diabetic forms). See Granuloma annulare and Oppenheim-Urbach.

BIBLIOGRAPHY. Miescher G, Leder M: Granulomatosis disciformis chronica et progressiva (atypiche tubercolosi). Dermatologica 97:25–34, 1948
Miescher G: Nekrobiosis maculosa. Dermatologica 98:199–204, 1949
Cunliffe WJ: Necrobiotic disorders. In Champion RH, Burton JL, Ebling FJG (eds): Rook/Wilkinson/Ebling Textbook of Dermatology, 5th ed, p 2035. Oxford, Blackwell Scientific, 1992

MIETENS-WEBER

Synonyms. Corneal opacity; nystagmus; elbow contracture; mental retardation; dwarfism; mental retardation of Mietens-Weber.

Symptoms and Signs. *Facies.* Bushy eyebrows; low hairline; ptosis; external ear defects. *Musculoskeletal system.* Muscular defects; digital defects (primarily of hands). Hypertrichosis.

Etiology. Unknown. Autosomal recessive inheritance (?).

Therapy. Keratoplasty.

BIBLIOGRAPHY. Mietens C, Weber H: Syndrome characterized by corneal opacity, nystagmus, flexion contractures of elbows, growth failure and mental retardation. J Pediatr 69:624–629, 1966
Waring GO, Rodriguez MM: Ultrastructural and successful keratoplasty of sclerocornea in Mietens syndrome. Am J Ophthalmol 90:469–475, 1980

MIGRAINE

Synonyms. Classic migraine (with aura); common migraine (without aura); sick headache; hemicrania vera; familial migraine; hemiplegic migraine; abdominal migraine. See Möbius I; Bickerstaff.

Symptoms. Prevalent in women (variable female to male ratio, according to different authors, average 3.5M:7.4F); occasional onset in childhood (10% of patients with migraine have this form); may begin in puberty and cease in menopause; or onset at 40 years of age and termination at 60 years of age. Peak onset between second and third decades.

(Menstrual periods and fluid retention may precipitate attacks.) Premonitory changes in mood and appetite, in classic type aura. Attacks of unilateral throbbing pain (hemicrania), periodic and recurrent. Nervous tension (usually in these patients starting when relaxed). Prodromes include contralateral visual manifestations, occasionally motor and sensory phenomena. Attacks last 4–6 hours, occasionally longer, days. They are partially relieved by darkness and quiet. Anorexia; abdominal colic of variable intensity lasting minutes or days. Vomiting (may relieve pain), diarrhea. Followed occasionally by polyuria.

Signs. Hyperidrosis; pallor or flushing of skin.

Etiology. Personality factors of significant importance in precipitating and establishing condition. Autosomal dominant (70% penetrance) or recessive.

Diagnostic Procedures. *EEG.* May show minimal changes. *Ergotamin test.* Prevention of attack in aureal stage.

Therapy. Once attack is begun, sumatriptan succinate per, or s.c. relieves the pain. Ergotamin in association with caffeine and other compounds taken in prodromal state may abort the attacks. Methysergide for prophylaxis (with care because of risk of retroperitoneal fibrosis, see Ormond). Good results also with propranolol or amytriptyline for prevention.

Prognosis. With age tendency of headache and nausea to decrease in severity leaving only neurologic abnormalities that recur with decreasing frequency (see Symptoms). Attacks may be followed by permanent deficit of visual field.

BIBLIOGRAPHY. Allan W: Inheritance of migraine. Arch Intern Med 42:590–599, 1928
Alvarez WC: Was there sick headache in 3000 B.C.? Gastroenterology 5:524, 1945
Editorial: Classification and diagnostic criteria for headache disorders cranial neuralgia and facial pain. Cephalalgia 8(Suppl 7):1–96, 1988
Diamond S: Migraine headaches. Med Clin No Am 75:545–566, 1991
Editorial: Subcutaneous sumatriptan international study group: Treatment of migraine attacks with sumatriptan. N Engl J Med 325:316–321, 1991

MIGRAINE, MALIGNANT

Synonyms. Malignant migraine; hemiplegic migraine.

Symptoms and Signs. Frequently affecting patients with OXPHOS syndromes (see), especially in M.E.L.A.S. (see). Migraine attacks (undistinguishable from classic form) that may evolve into stroke-like episodes, frequently followed by seizures.

Etiology. See migraine classic. In cases of OXPHOS syndromes, association with mtDNA mutations.

Pathology. See M.E.L.A.S.

Diagnostic Procedures. See migraine classic and M.E.L.A.S

Therapy. See migraine classic and M.E.L.A.S.

Prognosis. Stroke-like episodes may resolve spontaneously or leave permanent reliquates.

BIBLIOGRAPHY. Shoffner JM, Wallace DC: Oxidative phosphorylation diseases. In Scriver CR, Beaudet AL, Sly WS, et al: The Metabolic and Molecular Bases of Inherited Disease, 7th ed. New York, McGraw-Hill, 1995

MIGRATORY OSTEOLYSIS

Synonyms. Transient osteoporosis of hip; regional migratory osteoporosis. See Observation hip.

Symptoms. Prevalent in males; onset in youth and middle age. Intensely painful regional swelling in one of the lower extremities, seldom preceded by trauma. Pain aggravated by weight-bearing and motion. Similar segmental episodes may occur in other areas of opposite leg without an initiating cause.

Signs. Swelling of hip, knee, or foot. Overlying skin is dry; superficial veins are dilated.

Etiology. Unknown. Condition similar to Sudeck (see).

Pathology. Periosteal reaction under edematous areas; increase of synovial fluid; membrane injected and thickened. Microscopically, minimal or absent signs of inflammation.

Diagnostic Procedures. *X-ray.* Normal during first 2–3 weeks, then severe localized osteoporosis.

Therapy. Analgesics.

Prognosis. Self-limited condition. Spontaneous resolution in months with return to normal density of the bone. Possibly recurrence in other areas.

BIBLIOGRAPHY. Curtiss PH, Kincaid WE: Transitory demineralization of the hip in pregnancy: A report of three cases. J Bone Joint Surg (Am) 41:1327–1333, 1959

De Marchi E, Santacroce A, Salarino GB: Su di una peculiare artropatia rarefacente dell'anca. Arch Putti 21:62–75, 1966

Hunder GG, Kelly PJ: Roentgenologic transient osteoporosis of the hip: A clinical syndrome? Ann Intern Med 68:538–552, 1968

Pinals RS: Traumatic arthritis and allied conditions. In Hollander JL, McCarty DJ: Arthritis and Allied Conditions, 8th ed, p 1397. Philadelphia, Lea & Febiger, 1978

MILIAN I

Synonym. Ninth day erythema.

Symptoms. Onset after the injection of arsphenamine, neoarsphenamine, oxophenarine hydrochloride (Mapharsen) or acetylglycarsenobenzene. Abrupt onset of prodromal symptoms between the fifth and 19th days. Malaise; chills; fever; anorexia; vomiting; headache; sore throat; followed after 1 day (average 9 days) by generalized rash, lasting 1–12 days, and followed by desquamation.

Signs. Rash described as macular erythematous, rarely urticarial; generalized lymphadenopathy; conjunctival suffusion. Occasionally, hepatomegaly, jaundice, and splenomegaly.

Etiology. Unknown; not observed since penicillin has been substituted for arsenical compounds in the treatment of syphilis. Reaction to arsenophenamine compounds not related to presence of syphilis.

Pathology. In addition to the skin manifestation, visceral manifestations have been observed; hepatomegaly; splenomegaly; nephritis. Pathology reports are not available, however.

Therapy. Palliative.

Prognosis. Self-limited condition; spontaneous recovery; never fatal. Recurrence not constant when the drugs are administered again.

BIBLIOGRAPHY. Milian G: Arsénobenzol, érythème et rubéole. Paris Med 23:131–135, 1917

Peters EE: The syndrome of Milian's erythema of the ninth day: Report of 54 cases. Am J Syph 25:527–556, 1941

Macaluso S, Magalini SI: Reazioni avverse a farmaci: le vasculiti tossiche. Gior Ital Angiol 14:120–124, 1994

MILIAN II

Synonyms. Atrophia alba; progressive fibrosis telangiectasis; progressive telangiectasis; white atrophy; livedoid vasculitis.

Symptoms and Signs. Prevalent in women. On the foot or ankle, formation of a white plaque with stippled telangiectasia and pigmented edges. Tender petechiae, blistering, and crusting may precede the lesion. Associated usually with venous incompetence. (See Lower leg stasis.) Ulceration follows in 30% of cases.

Etiology. Unknown; defect of circulation (possibly, primary capillaritis).

Pathology. Atrophy of epidermis; scleroderma-like changes; no inflammatory changes. Thrombosis of small vessels; fibrinoid changes. Ulcer necrosis bordered by acanthosis and hyperkeratosis.

Therapy. Rest; compression (with poor results). Steroids accelerate ulcer healing. Low molecular weight dextran, phenformin, ethyl estradiol, stanazol, heparin among the many agents tried.

Prognosis. Ulcer slow to heal. Chronic condition.

BIBLIOGRAPHY. Milian G: Les atrophies cutanées syphilitiques. Bull Soc Fr Dermatol 36:865–871, 1929

Ryan TJ, Burnand K: Diseases of the veins and arteries leg ulcers. In Champion RH, Burton JL, Ebling FJG (eds): Rook/Wilkinson/Ebling Textbook of Dermatology, 5th ed, pp 1985–1986. Oxford, Blackwell Scientific, 1992

MILIARY HEMANGIOMAS, CONGENITAL

Synonyms. Hematoangiomatosis eruptive neonatal; diffuse neonatal hemoangiomatosis.

Symptoms and Signs. Both sexes affected; evident at birth. Two clinical forms: I, benign, and II, malignant. The malignant form is associated with visceral lesion. In the malignant form, large number of hemangiomas scattered over skin, mucosae. Dyspnea; tachycardia; jaundice.

Etiology. Unknown; no evidence of hereditary transmission. Possible relation with Rendu-Osler-Weber syndrome.

Pathology. Hemangiomas on skin, mucosae, and practically all organs (liver; spleen; mesentery; pancreas; trachea; central nervous system). Some invasion and destruction of normal tissue, but no evidence of malignancy.

Diagnostic Procedures. *Biopsy. Angiography.* (If feasible.) *Echography of liver.*

Therapy. Systemic corticosteroids. Hepatic artery ligation, partial lobectomy, transarterial embolization when indicated.

Prognosis. *Benign form.* Favorable outlook. *Malignant form.* Death in early infancy, generally from high output failure.

BIBLIOGRAPHY. von Falkowski A: Ueber eigenartige mesenchymale Hämartome in Leber and Milz neben multiplen eruptiven. Angiomen der Haut bei einem Säugling. Beitz Pathol Anat 57:385–414, 1914

Burman D, Mansell PWA, Warin RP: Miliary hemangiomata in the newborn. Arch Dis Child 42:193–197, 1967

Weismann K, Graham RM: Systemic disease and the skin. In Champion RH, Burton JL, Ebling FJG (eds): Rook/Wilkinson/Ebling Textbook of Dermatology, 5th ed, p 2436. Oxford, Blackwell Scientific, 1992

MILKMAN

Synonyms. Looser-Milkman; Looser zones; osteoporosis; osteomalacia; pseudofractures.

Symptoms. Prevalent in females; onset in middle age. Fatigue; pain in back, legs.

Signs. Tenderness on pressure of affected bones; possibly, limping.

Etiology. Disorder of phosphorus, calcium metabolism; osteomalacia (adult counterpart of rickets). The eponym Milkman syndrome has been used to indicate the radiologic feature of pseudofractures.

Pathology. Ribbon-like zone of calcification. Decalcification along paths of vessels; incomplete fractures; defect filled by active osteoblasts; lack of calcification of matrix.

Diagnostic Procedures. *Blood.* Low serum calcium and phosphorus; high alkaline phosphatase level. *X-ray.* Pseudofractures zone of Looser or Milkman, small fissures in cortex of long bones in symmetric locations; generalized demineralization.

Therapy. Vitamin D.

Prognosis. Chronic condition; occasionally, spontaneous disappearance of manifestations during pregnancy or menopause.

BIBLIOGRAPHY. Looser E: Ueber pathologische Formen von Infraktionen und Callusbildungen bei Rachitis und Osteomalackie und anderen Knochenerkrankungen. Zentralbl Chir 47:1470–1474, 1920
Milkman LA: Pseudofractures (hunger osteopathy; late rickets; osteomalacia). Am J Roentgenol 24:29–37, 1930
Steinback HL, Noetzli M: Roentgen appearance of the skeleton in osteomalacia and rickets. Am J Roentgenol 91:955–972, 1964
Goldring SR, Krane SM, Avioli LV: Disorders of calcification osteomalacia and rickets. In De Groot LJ (ed): Endocrinology, 3rd ed, p 1210. Philadelphia, WB Saunders, 1995

MILLARD-GUBLER

Synonyms. Gubler, abducens—facial hemiplegia alternans; alternating inferior hemiplegia. See Foville.

Symptoms and Signs. Hemiplegia and contralateral internal strabismus, diplopia, and loss of power to rotate eye outward.

Etiology. Vascular lesions; encephalitis; tumors at the base of pons, affecting abducens (VI) and facial (VII) nerves and pyramidal tract.

BIBLIOGRAPHY. Gubler A: De l'hémiplégie alterne envisagée comme signe de lesion de la protubérance annulaire et comme preuve de la décussation des nerfs faciaux. Gaz Hebd Med Paris 3:749–789; 811, 1856
Adams RD, Victor M: Principles of Neurology, 5th ed, p 1173. New York, McGraw-Hill, 1993

MILLER-DIEKER

Synonyms. Lissencephaly I.

Symptoms. From birth. Infantile spasms, hypotonia, inability to swallow. Mental retardation.

Signs. *Head.* Microcephaly, small mandible, hollow temples, dolicocephaly, micrognathia, nostrils anteversion, failure to thrive. *Muscles.* Poor development, poor reflexes, decorticate decerebrate postures. *Lungs.* Frequent infections. *Occasionally.* Hirsutism, corneal clauding, duodenal atresia, fingers anomalies, congenital heart disease, renal anomalies, cryptorchidism, hepatosplenomegaly, jaundice.

Etiology. Unknown. Possibly autosomal recessive inheritance; usually denovo. Deletion of chromosome 17 (p13.3), one X-linked pedigree reported.

Pathology. Microcephaly and thickened cortex with 4 rather than 6 layers (type I). Golgi stain shows many inverted pyramidal cells.

Diagnostic Procedures. X-rays. CT scan. MRI. Ultrasonography. Smooth cortex of brain. See Signs. *Electroencephalography.* Hypsarrhythmia.

Prognosis. Death in early infancy.

BIBLIOGRAPHY. Miller JB: Lissencephaly in 2 siblings. Neurology 13:841–850, 1963
Dieker H, Edward RH, Zurhein GM, et al: The lissencephaly syndrome: The clinical delineation of Birth Defects II. Malformation Syndromes, pp 53–64. New York, N.F. March Dimes 1969
Dobyns WB, van Tuinen P, Ledbetter DH: Clinical diagnosis criteria for Miller-Dieker syndrome. Am J Hum Genet 43:A46, 1988
Ledbetter DH, Ballabio A: Molecular cytogenetics of contiguous gene syndromes: Mechanisms and consequences of gene dosage imbalance. In Scriver CR, Beaudet AL, Sly WS, et al: The Metabolic and Molecular Bases of Inherited Disease, 7th ed, pp 823–824. New York, McGraw-Hill, 1995

MILLER (M.)

Synonyms. Postaxial acrofacial dysostosis. Acrofacial dysostosis postaxial.

Symptoms and Signs. From birth. *Head.* Malar hypoplasia, ectropion of lower lid, micrognathia, cup shaped ears. *Limb.* Postaxial deficiency, bilateral in both hands and feet.

Etiology. Autosomal recessive inheritance.

BIBLIOGRAPHY. Miller M, Fineman R, Smith DW: Postaxial acrofacial dysostosis syndrome. J Pediatr 95:970–975, 1979
Barbuti D, Orazi C, Reale A, et al: Postaxial acrofacial dysostosis or Miller syndrome: A case report. Eur J Pediatr 148:445–446, 1989

MILLES

Synonyms. Jenning-Milles. Sturge-Weber (see) associated with choroid angioma without glaucoma.

BIBLIOGRAPHY. Jenning-Milles W: Nevus of the right temporal and orbital region: Nevus of the choroid and detachment of the retina in the right eye. Trans Ophthalmol Soc UK 4:168–171, 1884
Sahel JA, Albert DM: Phakomatoses and neurocristopathies. In Garner A, Klintworth GK (eds): Pathobiology of Ocular Disease: A Dynamic Approach, 2nd ed, p 1361. New York, Marcel Dekker, 1994

MILLIKAN-SIEKERT

Synonyms. Basilar artery insufficiency; brachial—basilar insufficiency; subclavian steal; vertebral basilary artery.

Symptoms. Numbness; coldness; pain; claudication of arm and hand (left arm more frequently involved; bilateral involvement also possible). Exercise of involved arm precipitates neurologic symptoms: syncopal attacks; facial paresthesia; blindness; headache. Neurologic symptoms may be absent, however.

Signs. Bruit over supraclavicular area; pulse reduction and reduction of blood pressure in ipsilateral arm.

Etiology. Stenosis of proximal part of subclavian artery (congenital atherosclerosis) draining the blood from the vertebral artery to upper extremity resulting in basilar insufficiency.

Pathology. Congenital or acquired (atherosclerosis; thrombosis; extrinsic compression) stenosis of subclavian artery proximal to vertebral artery branch.

Diagnostic Procedure. *Angiography.* Reversed blood flow in vertebral artery.

Therapy. Ligation of vertebral artery close to its origin or (better) end-to-side bypass graft, between common carotid artery and subclavian artery distal to vertebral origin. Antiaggregant and/or anticoagulant therapy.

Prognosis. Symptoms disappear with surgical correction.

BIBLIOGRAPHY. Millikan CH, Siekert RG: Studies in cerebrovascular disease: The syndrome of intermittent insufficiency of the basilar arterial system. Proc Staff Meetings Mayo Clin 30:61–68, 1955
Berger RL, Sidd JJ, Ramaswamy K: Retrograde vertebral-artery flow

produced by correction of subclavian-steal syndrome. N Engl J Med 277:64–69, 1967

Schlant RC, Alexander RW: Hurst's The Heart, 8th ed, p 2176. New York, McGraw-Hill, 1994

MILLS

Obsolete.

Synonym. Ascending progressive spinal paralysis; spinal paralysis progessive ascending.

Symptoms. Paralysis affecting one leg and gradually ascending to involve the arm. The other side is affected later in the same fashion.

Signs. Slowly developing muscular atrophy without fibrillations. Extrapyramidal signs may develop during course of disease.

Etiology. Unknown. Considered by Mills and Spiller a spinal paralysis and by Cossa and colleagues of cerebral origin, due to an abiotrophic process (form of senile paraplegia). The characterization of this very doubtful clinical entity is given by the exclusive involvement of the motor neurons. Many different agents show this clinically selective action.

Pathology. Cortical atrophy; ventricular dilatation.

Diagnostic Procedures. *CSF.* Pleocytosis. *EEG. CT scan. MRI of brain and spine.*

Therapy. Symptomatic.

Prognosis. Very slow progressive evolution lasting decades.

BIBLIOGRAPHY. Mills CK, Spiller WG: On Landry's paralysis, with the report of a case. J Nerv Ment Dis 25:365–391, 1898

Spiller WG, Llongcope WT: Multiple motor neuritis including Landry's paralysis and lead palsy with reports of cases. Med Record 70:81–88, 1906

Cossa P, et al: Revision du syndrome de Mills. Presse Med 60:419–420, 1952

MINAMATA

Named for the bay in Japan near where the condition was first observed.

Synonym. Alkyl-mercury poisoning, mad hatter.

Symptoms. Both sexes affected; onset several weeks or months after ingestion of fish from water contaminated by methyl mercury (industrial waste) or ingestion of animals (hogs) fed with grain treated with methyl mercury fungicide. From very severe to extremely mild. Mouth, tongue, and extremity paresthesia; constriction of visual fields up to blindness; hearing decreases up to complete loss; asthenia; fatigue; inability to concentrate; dysarthria; tremors; apallic syndrome (see Kretshmer) or persistent vegetative state.

Etiology. Chronic alkyl-mercury poisoning. Paresthesias are associated with an estimated total body burden of 40 mg, whereas death occurred at an estimated 200 mg.

Pathology. Degenerative changes in cerebral cortex and cerebellum.

Diagnostic Procedures. *Blood, hair, and tissues.* Presence of mercury. *EEG.* Severe abnormalities. *CT scan.*

Therapy. Withdrawal from exposure. No specific treatment. BAL not useful. Trial with DMPS (2,3-dimercapto-1-propanosulfonic acid).

Prognosis. Poor. Severe residual effects after remission of acute phase. More than 100 fatal cases and 17 babies with cerebral palsy.

BIBLIOGRAPHY. Kurland LT, Faro SN, Siedler HL: Minamata disease. World Neurol 1:370–395, 1960

Takeuchi T, Eto N, Eto K: Neuropathology of childhood cases of methylmercury poisoning (Minamata disease) with prolonged symp-

toms, with particular reference to the decortication syndrome. Neurotoxicology 1:1–20, 1979

De Francisci G, Magalini SI: L'avvelenamento da mercurio. Rec Progr Med 74:438–450, 1983

Matsumoto SC, Okajima T, Inayoshy S, et al: Minamata disease demonstrated by computed tomography. Neuroradiology 30:42–4,6 1988

MINIMAL CHANGE, NEPHROTIC

Synonyms. Steroid-responsive, nephrotic; SRNS.

Symptoms and Signs. In children (20–40 new cases per million) and in adults (two cases per million). Edema, particularly of eyelid and scrotum; ascitis (especially in children). Hypovolemic shock (especially in children) heralded by abdominal pain. Blood hypertension; venous thrombosis; infections.

Etiology. Unknown. Reported in siblings. Autoimmunopathogenesis. Abnormal glomerular permeability.

Pathology. *Kidney.* Light microscopy glomeruli normal. *Immunohistology.* No IgG or complement components are demonstrable in glomeruli, only IgM occasionally demonstrated in mesangeal region. *Electronmicroscopy.* Retraction of epithelial foot processes.

Diagnostic Procedures. *Blood.* Hypoalbuminemia. Hematocrit reduced; hyperviscosity; increase of fibrinogen and fibrin complexes; spontaneous platelet aggregation increase; reduced IgG; LDL increased.

Therapy. Glucocorticoids; alkylating agents; levamisole; cyclosporin A.

Prognosis. Reduced mortality with modern management. Death occurs from hypovolemia, thrombosis, and sepsis.

BIBLIOGRAPHY. Churg J, Habib R, White RHR: Pathology of the nephrotic syndrome in children: A report of the international study of kidney disease in children. Lancet 1:1299–1302, 1970

Neuhaus TJ, Barratt TM: Minimal change disease. In Massry SG, Glassock RJ: Textbook of Nephrology, 3rd ed, pp 710–719. Baltimore, Williams & Wilkins, 1995

MINKOWSKI-CHAUFFARD

Synonyms. Vanlair-Masius; Gaensslen-Erb; alcoholic jaundice; hemolytic icterus, congenital; HS; spherocytosis, hereditary.

Symptoms. Recognized at all ages; both sexes equally affected. Positive family history. At least one of the parents affected (mother, gallbladder disease) and about 50% of siblings. Rarely, sporadic cases. Usually first noticed in childhood or early adolescence, with various degrees of intensity; occasionally so mild as to pass unnoticed. Anorexia; lassitude; delayed puberty. Recurrent acute episodes characterized by fever, tachycardia, abdominal pain, dyspnea, vomiting.

Signs. Persistent slight jaundice; not infrequently, chronic leg ulcer, splenomegaly; occasionally, moderate hepatomegaly and various developmental anomalies may be present.

Etiology. Autosomal dominant inheritance (75% of families) and autosomal recessive (25%). Primary defect of red cell membrane: abnormal spectrin that binds protein 4.1 poorly and interacts weakly with actin. When red blood cells pass through the spleen they are conditioned by the inhospitable environment and become spherocytes that in circulation are more susceptible to destruction by the reticuloendothelial system or during successive passages through the spleen.

Pathology. *Spleen.* Splenomegaly, absence of adhesions, pulp dry, dark, homogeneous, malpighian bodies undistinguished. *Sinus.* Apparently empty (containing red cell stromas); macrophages increased; active erythrophagocytosis. *Liver.* Increased iron content. *Gallbladder.* Bilirubin stones. *Bone marrow.* Hyperplastic erythroid hyperplasia; myeloid metaplasia in bones.

Diagnostic Procedures. *Blood.* Hemoglobin 9–12 g/100 ml; during crisis 3–4 g/100 ml; mean corpuscular volume (MCV) variable (83:5:85); mean corpuscular hemoglobin (MCH) variable; mean corpuscular hemoglobin concentration (MCHC) 37–39 g/100 ml. Mean diameter of red cells reduced; absence of central pallor. Reticulocytes increased. Polychromatophilia; red cell fragility increased. Osmotic fragility (especially incubating variant) increased. Coombs negative. Leukocytes normal. Serum bilirubin (indirect) increased. Serum iron normal or increased. *Urine.* Urobilin increased. *Stool.* Urobilin increased.

Therapy. Splenectomy.

Prognosis. Death possible during crisis. Repeated crises may cause several complications (e.g., cerebral, cardiac, biliary tract). Possibly, spontaneous improvement without recurrence of jaundice.

BIBLIOGRAPHY. Vanlair CF, Masius JB: De la microcythémie. Bull R Acad Med Belg 5:515, 1871

Minkowski O: Ueber eine hereditäre, unter dem Bilde eines chronischen Ikterus mit Urobilinurie: Splenomegalie und Nierensiderosis verlaufende Affection. Verh Dtsch Kongr Inn Med 18:316–319, 1900

Chauffard MA: Pathogenie de l'ictére congenital de l'adulte. Sem Med (Paris) 27:25–29, 1907

Becker PS, Lux SE: Hereditary spherocytosis and hereditary elliptocytosis. In Scriver CR, Beaudet AL, Sly WS, et al: The Metabolic and Molecular Bases of Inherited Disease, 7th ed, pp 3530–3539. New York, McGraw-Hill, 1995

MINOR

Synonyms. Minor-Oppenheim; central hematomyelia; hematorrhachis.

Symptoms and Signs. Onset usually after trauma (e.g., bending, falling); onset sudden, occasionally, delayed. Complete or almost complete paralysis; below lesion vasomotor changes, absence of sphincter control, absence of deep reflexes (according to spinal shock), extensor plantar reflex usually elicited. Sensory changes variable according to extension and location of primitive injury.

Etiology. Direct and indirect injury to spine. Blood dyscrasias, syphilis, tumor, myelitis, angioma, aneurysm, administration of anticoagulants are other possible causes.

Pathology. Bleeding in spinal cavity, without direct spinal cord involvement.

Diagnostic Procedures. *Spinal fluid.* Hemorrhagic. *Myelography.* Not indicated. *CT scan. Selective spinal angiography. MRI.*

Therapy. Microsurgery if needed.

Prognosis. After progression of symptoms for 2–3 days, static period; then improvement up to complete disappearance of symptoms if spinal cord is not involved.

BIBLIOGRAPHY. Minor L: Central haematomyelia. Arch Psychiatr (Berlin) 24:693–729, 1892

Adams RD, Victor M: Principles of Neurology, 5th ed, pp 1096–1097. New York, McGraw-Hill, 1993

MIRHOSSEINI-HOLMES-WALTON

Synonym. Retinopathy, pigmentary; mental retardation. See Cohen (may be the same or allelic to).

Symptoms. Both sexes. Visual impairment caused by pigmentary retinal degeneration, cataract. Mental retardation.

Signs. Microcephaly, hyperextensible joints, scoliosis, arachnodactyly. Occasionally hypogonadism.

Etiology. Autosomal recessive inheritance.

BIBLIOGRAPHY. Mirhosseini SA, Holmes LB, Walton DS: Syndrome of pigmentary retinal degeneration cataract, microcephaly and severe mental retardation. J Med Genet 9:193–196, 1972

Mendez HMM, Paskulin GA, Vallandro C: The syndrome of retinal pigmentary degeneration, microcephaly and severe mental retardation (Mirhosseini-Holmes-Walton syndrome) report of two patients. Am J Med Genet 22:223–228, 1985

MIRIZZI

Synonym. Ductus hepaticus obstruction.

Symptoms and Signs. Those of chronic cholecystitis and hepatocholangitis.

Etiology. Cystic duct stone, shrinkage of gallbladder, and stenosis of hepatic duct.

Pathology. Segmental hepatocholangitis.

Diagnostic Procedures. *Cholangiography.* Timed biliary drainage. Combined cholecystokinin-pancreozymin-secretin test. *Echography.* 99m Tc IDA cholescintigraphy. *CT scan. MRI.* Smooth common hepatic duct stenosis, or short, round filling defect; intrahepatic ducts may be dilated.

Therapy. Surgery or antispastic agent, according to etiology.

Prognosis. Good if stenosis treated.

BIBLIOGRAPHY. Mirizzi PL: Sindrome del conducto hepatico. G Int Chir 8:731–777, 1948

Albot G, Corteville M: De pathologie van de ductus hepaticus. Belg Geneesk 10:452–465, 1954

Hilger DJ, Ver Steeg KR, Beaty PJ: Mirizzi syndrome with common septum: Ultrasound and computed tomography findings. J Ultrasound Med 7:409–411, 1988

Prober A, Cogacov C, Barkai M: A variant of the Mirizzi syndrome. Br J Radiol 61:331–332, 1988

MIRROR PSEUDOTOXEMIA

Synonyms. Toxemic maternal; pseudotoxemic.

Symptoms. Occurs in Rh-negative isoimmunized pregnant patients around 28th or 30th week of pregnancy.

Signs. Increased weight gain; edema refractory to the usual diuretics; mild elevation of blood pressure. These signs and symptoms in an Rh-negative isoimmunized pregnant woman represent an ominous complex and universally predict an immediate intrauterine fetal death or delivery of a baby who cannot survive.

Etiology. Unknown. Possibly disturbance in aldosterone secretion leading to fluid accumulation in the fetus and mother. This increased size of uterine content conceivably could produce anoxia of the decidua and perhaps result in the increased production of the oxytocin and hence symptoms of toxemia.

Pathology. Hydrops fetalis; large placenta.

Diagnostic Procedures. *Urine.* Mild proteinuria.

Therapy. Nothing can be done at that stage to save the baby, except to induce labor. The management is that of Rh-isoimmunized pregnant women, namely repeated amniocentesis if necessary, induction of labor around 34th–36th week if deemed necessary. If earlier, intrauterine blood transfusion and then induction of labor at 34th–36th week. Finally, intramuscular injection in all Rh-negative primigravidas after delivery, of Rho (D antigen) immune globulin (RhoGAM) to immunize against further isoimmunization in susequent pregnancies.

Prognosis. Poor for the baby; good for the mother after termination of pregnancy.

BIBLIOGRAPHY. Jeffcoate TNA, Scott JS: Some observations on the placental factor in pregnancy toxemia. Am J Obstet Gynecol 77:475–489, 1959

Speck G: Eclampsia at the sixteenth week of gestation, with Rh isoimmunization and cystic degeneration of the placenta. Obstet Gynecol 15:70–72, 1960

Nicolay KS, Gainey HL: Pseudotoxemic state associated with severe Rh isoimmunization. Am J Obstet Gynecol 89:41–45, 1964

Morison DH: Anaesthesia and preeclampsia. Can J Anesth 34:415–422, 1987

MITCHELL I

Synonyms. Gerhardt II; Weir Mitchell I; erythermalgia primary.

Symptoms and Signs. Burning distress of extremities; redness; increased skin temperature; often induced by increased environmental temperature during summer months, and at night in bed. Relieved by cooling. Trophic changes rare. Both sexes; onset usually over middle age.

Etiology. Unknown; often preceding for years the onset of a myeloproliferative syndrome. Autosomal dominant inheritance reported in some families.

Pathology. Little known.

Diagnostic Procedures. *Blood.* Studies for typical blood changes of myeloproliferative syndromes. Thrombocythemia reported in several cases. Induction of attack by application of heat.

Therapy. Treatment of underlying condition if present. Aspirin may produce relief for days. Ultraviolet radiation may be beneficial. Avoidance of causes of vasodilation in extremities.

Prognosis. As mentioned. Often an early clue, preceding for years the development of severe (often fatal) conditions.

BIBLIOGRAPHY. Mitchell SW: Clinical lecture on certain painful affections of the feet. Philadelphia, Med Times 3:81–82, 113; 115, 1872

Champion RH: Reactions to cold. In Champion RH, Burton JL, Ebling FJG (eds): Rook/Wilkinson/Ebling Textbook of Dermatology, 5th ed, p 837. Oxford, Blackwell Scientific,1992

MITOCHONDRIAL MYOPATHIES

Synonyms. Megaconial myopathy; pleoconial myopathy. Group that includes, in addition to the reported ones, many other not yet well-defined syndromes that, in some cases, involve also other organs. Abnormal mitochondria are the common feature. In most cases demonstrated abnormalities of OXPHOS (see) owing to mt DNA alterations

BIBLIOGRAPHY. Shy GM, Gonatas NK, Perez M: Two childhood myopathies with abnormal mitochondria. I Megaconial myopathy. II Pleoconial myopathy. Brain 89:133–158, 1966

Shoffner JM, Wallace DC: Oxidative phosphorylation diseases. In Scriver CR, Beaudet AL, Sly WS, et al: The Metabolic and Molecular Bases of Inherited Disease, 7th ed, pp 1555, 1565, 1578. New York, McGraw-Hill, 1995

MITOCHONDRIAL MYOPATHY, BENIGN, INFANTILE

Synonyms. Benign, infantile mitochondrial myopathy; BIMM. See OXPHOS.

Symptoms and Signs. At birth. Weakness, hypotonia, difficulty in feeding, respiratory impairment.

Etiology. Autosomal recessive or new autosomal dominant inheritance. Nuclear DNA mutation with alterations of complex IV. See complex IV and OXPHOS syndromes.

Diagnostic Procedures. *Blood.* Lactic acidosis. *Muscle biopsy. Histochemstry.* abnormal complex IV, that normalizes after first year.

Therapy. See OXPHOS.

Prognosis. Clinical and biochemical improvement during first year of life.

BIBLIOGRAPHY. Di Mauro S, Nicholson JF, Hays AP, et al: Benign infantile mitochondrial myopathy due to reversible cytochrome c oxidase deficiency. Ann Neurol 14:226–234, 1983

Shoffner JM, Wallace DC: Oxidative phosphorylation diseases. In Scriver CR, Beaudet AL, Sly WS, et al: The Metabolic and Molecular Bases of Inherited Disease, 7th ed, pp 1552–1553. New York, McGraw-Hill, 1995

MITOCHONDRIAL MYOPATHY–CARDIOMIOPATHY, BENIGN, INFANTILE

Synonyms. Benign, infantile mitochondrial myopathy—cardiomyopathy; BIMC. See OXPHOS.

Symptoms and Signs. Severe variant of mitochondrial myopathy, infantile, benign (see), involving skeletal and cardiac muscle.

Etiology. See OXPHOS syndromes.

Prognosis. Death shortly after birth or survival and gradual improvement.

BIBLIOGRAPHY. Wikstrom M, Krab K, Saraste M: Proton-translocating cytochrome complexes. Ann Rev Biochem 50:623–655, 1981

Shoffner JM, Wallace DC: Oxidative phosphorylation diseases. In Scriver CR, Beaudet AL, Sly WS, et al: The Metabolic and Molecular Bases of Inherited Disease, 7th ed, p 1554. New York, McGraw-Hill, 1995

MITOCHONDRIAL MYOPATHY, LETHAL, INFANTILE

Synonyms. Lethal infantile mitochondrial myopathy; LIMB. See OXPHOS.

Symptoms and Signs. Normal at birth. Onset at 3 weeks, failure to thrive, weakness, hypotonia. Occasionally progressive external ophthalmoplegia, hepetic dysfunction, de Ton-Fanconi-Debré syndrome, generalized aminoaciduria, etc.

Etiology. Genetics unclear. Autosomal dominant or recessive with variable expressivity. Depletion of mtDNA causing multiple defects of OXPHOS (see complex syndromes): complex I, II, IV, alone or in combinations.

Pathology. Muscle fibers lipid and glycogen accumulation and abnormal mitochondria, absence of paracrystalline inclusions

Diagnostic Procedures. *Blood.* Severe lactic acidosis. *Muscle biopsy.*

Therapy. See OXPHOS.

Prognosis. Death within first year.

BIBLIOGRAPHY. Di Mauro S, Mendell JR, Sahenk Z, et al: Fatal infantile mitochondrial myopathy end renal dysfunction due to cytochrome-c-oxidase deficiency. Neurology 30:795–804, 1980

Shoffner JM, Wallace DC: Oxidative phosphorylation diseases. In Scriver CR, Beaudet AL, Sly WS, et al: The Metabolic and Molecular Bases of Inherited Disease, 7th ed, pp 1553–1554. New York, McGraw-Hill, 1995

MITRAL VALVE ATRESIA

Synonyms. Hypoplastic heart ventricle; hypoplastic left ventricle. (Hypoplasia of aortic tract complex associated with functionally adequate left ventricular chamber not to be considered within this entity.)

Symptoms and Signs. Predominant in male infants. Mild cyanosis; pallor; tachypnea; congestive heart failure; frequently, peripheral pulses absent or weak. Systolic murmur (grade 2⅗) at left sternal border. Second sound loud and single. Failure to thrive. Syncope.

Etiology. Unknown; congenital heart malformation.

Pathology. Hypoplasia of left ventricle associated with a small aortic arch and small ascending and transverse aorta, large pulmonary artery and orifice, and normally related arterial trunks.*

Diagnostic Procedures. *X-ray.* Cardiomegaly; passive congestion increases vascularity of the lungs. *ECG.* Right axis deviation and right ventricular hypertrophy; vectorcardiography: P-wave broad, tall, notched. *Cardiac catheterization.* Elevated left atrial pressure. *Two-dimensional echocardiography with color flow imaging and spectral Doppler interrogation.*

Therapy. Surgery; only palliative to reinforce the interatrial communication left to right and patency of ductus arteriosus right to left. Medical treatment of intercurrent infection and congestive failure.

Prognosis. Very poor; death in early infancy.

BIBLIOGRAPHY. Noonan JA, Nadas AS: The hypoplastic left heart syndrome, an analysis of 101 cases. Pediatr Clin N Am 5:1029–1056, 1958
Gittenberger-de Groot AC, Weuick ACG: Mitral atresia: morphological details. Br Heart J 51:252, 1984
Nugent EW, Plauth WH, Edwards JE, et al: The pathology, pathophysiology recognition and treatment of congenital heart disease. In Schlant RC, Alexander RW, Hurst's The Heart, 8th ed, p 1816. New York, McGraw-Hill, 1994
Perloff JK: The Clinical Recognition of Congenital Heart Disease, 4th ed, p 727. Philadelphia, WB Saunders, 1994

MITRAL VALVE REGURGITATION

Symptoms. Both sexes affected but prevalent in males. Onset at all ages. Initially asymptomatic; then cough, asthenia. Occasionally, dyspnea, palpitation, hemoptysis, angina.

Signs. Strong left-downward displaced apical beat. Holosystolic murmur replacing first apical sound and radiating toward axilla; systolic thrill; second pulmonic sound accentuated; frequently, third sound.

Etiology. Rheumatic infection; subacute bacterial endocarditis; ischemia; trauma; hereditary (see Leopard). Undue restraint upon leaflets or chordae (bacterial endocarditis, myxomatous mitral valve, Loeffler endomyocardiac fibrosis, lupus erythematosus). Calcification mitral ring.

Pathology. Mitral valve insufficiency; left ventricle hypertrophy.

Diagnostic Procedures. *ECG.* Left ventricular predominance. *X-rays. Fluoroscopy. Angiography. Cineangiography. Echocardiography. Cardiac catheterization. Radionuclide studies.*

Therapy. Surgical treatment. Valve prothesis and prevention of bacterial endocarditis. If indicated, medical management of cardiac failure.

Prognosis. From asymptomatic to various degrees of cardiac failure.

BIBLIOGRAPHY. Hope J: Signs of disease of the mitral valve. In A Treatise on the Diseases of the Heart, p 387. London, Churchill, 1939
Gaasch WH, O'Rourke RA, Cohn LH, et al: mitral valve disease. Nugent EW, Plauth WH, Edwards JE, et al: The pathology, pathophysiology recognition and treatment of congenital heart disease. In Schlant RC, Alexander RW: Hurst's The Heart, 8th ed, pp 1491–1502. New York, McGraw-Hill, 1994

MITRAL VALVE STENOSIS

Symptoms. *Congenital form.* Equal distribution in both sexes (possibly, female prevalence); onset before 6 months of age. From asymptomatic to severe acute illness (see the following); seldom syncope; no hemoptysis. *Acquired form.* Onset in childhood, adolescence, seldom later. Palpitation; distress in cardiac area; dyspnea; orthopnea; cough; frequent respiratory infections; hoarseness or aphonia; weakness; abdominal discomfort; hemoptysis; angina; syncope.

Signs. Left displaced apical beat and thrust; presystolic or early diastolic crescendo rumble (with onset of atrial fibrillation the rumble disappears). First sound loud and high pitched; second sound reinforced. Congestion of neck veins; later, edema and pulmonary congestion.

Etiology. Congenital defect (rare); rheumatic infection. Thrombus formation; atrial myxoma; bacterial vegetation and calcification.

Pathology. Narrowing of mitral valve from various morphologic defects.

Diagnostic Procedures. *ECG.* QRS vertical axis; seldom, right deviation; large, broad P-waves. *X-rays.* Left atrium and right ventricle enlarged; displacement of esophagus. *Heart catheterization.* Two-dimensional echocardiography with color flow imaging and spectral Doppler interrogation. Decrease of the E-F slope of the anterior leaflet of mitral valve, abnormal posterior leaflet movement, decreased valve motion, thick echoes around valve (calcification). *Radionuclide studies.*

Therapy. Surgical treatment if indicated. Medical management of cardiac failure and prevention of bacterial endocarditis.

Prognosis. According to degree of lesions. Common complications and causes of death are atrial fibrillation, pulmonary edema, bacterial endocarditis, peripheral and pulmonary embolism, cardiac failure.

BIBLIOGRAPHY. Vienssen SR: Traite Nouveau de la Structure et des Causes du Mouvement Naturel du Coeur, p 101. Toulouse, Guillemette, 1715
Gaasch WH, O'Rourke RA, Cohn LH, et al: mitral valve disease. Nugent EW, Plauth WH, Edwards JE, et al: The pathology, pathophysiology recognition and treatment of congenital heart disease. In Schlant RC, Alexander RW: Hurst's The Heart, 8th ed, pp 1483–1491. New York, McGraw-Hill, 1994
Perloff JK: The Clinical Recognition of Congenital Heart Disease, 4th ed, pp 171–178. Philadelphia. WB Saunders, 1994

MITRAL VALVE STENOSIS–BALL VALVE THROMBUS

Synonyms. Atrial thrombosis massive; thrombosis, atrial, massive.

Symptoms. Occurs in 9–20% of mitral stenosis patients (percentage increasing with age); insidious onset. Dyspnea; disorientation; mental confusion; rarely, syncope.

Signs. Severe pulmonary congestion with intervals of temporary improvement. Occasionally, episodes of acrocyanosis; absence or weakness of pulse; engorgement of neck veins, relieved by sitting up or leaning forward.

Etiology. Rheumatic disease. Large thrombus of left atrium occluding mitral valve. Myxoma or pedunculated sarcoma may produce the same syndrome.

Pathology. See Etiology.

Diagnostic Procedures. *ECG. Angiocardiography.* Interatrial filling defect. Radionuclide studies. *CT scan. Transesophageal echocardigraphy.*

Therapy. Anticoagulants; digitalis ineffective.

Prognosis. Poor.

BIBLIOGRAPHY. Surawicz B, Nierenberg MA: Association of silent mitral

*Blind dimple in floor of left atrium; frequently association with aortic atresia; patent foramen ovale; transposition of great vessels; hypoplasia of left ventricle (see) ventricular septal defects.

stenosis with massive thrombi in the left atrium. New Engl J Med 263:423–431, 1960

MITTELSCHMERZ

Synonym. Graafian follicle cyst.

Symptoms. Sharp abdominal pain, recurrent at periodic intervals. Menstrual irregularity and pelvic discomfort.

Etiology. Follicular ovary cyst; atresia of ovarian follicle.

BIBLIOGRAPHY. Kenigsberg D, Rosenwaks Z, Hogden GD: Ovarian follicular maturation ovulation and ovulation induction. In De Groot: Endocrinology 3rd ed, p 2036. Philadelphia, WB Saunders, 1995

MIXED SCLEROSING BONE DYSPLASIA

Synonyms. Melorheostosis; osteopoikilosis; ostheopathia striata; generalized sclerosis; MSBD.

Symptoms. Asymptomatic.

Signs. Subcutaneous nodules, lymphedema, hemangiomata.

Etiology. Sporadic occurrence.

Diagnostic Procedures. *Blood.* Creatine phosphokinase, alkaline phosphatase, and parathormone: elevated; Calcium and phosphourus: decreased; mild anemia. *X-rays.* Skeleton: combination of melorheostosis, dense linear striation, asymmetric generalized sclerosis. *Bone scans.* In all lesions increased uptake.

BIBLIOGRAPHY. Walker GF: Mixed sclerosing bone dystrophies. J Bone Joint Surg (Br) 46:546–552, 1964
Pescaud-Ged E, Rihovet WA, Pascaud JL, et al: Melorheostosis—osteopoikilosis and linear scleroderma. Ann Radiol 24:643–646, 1981
Pacific R, Murphy WA, Teitelbaum SL: Mixed-sclerosing bone dystrophy. Calcif Tissue Int 38:175–185, 1986

M.N.G.I.E.

Synonyms. Myo-neuro-gastrointestinal disorder and encephalopathy; P.O.L.I.P. (polyneuropathy, ophthalmoplegia, leukoencephalopathy intestinal pseudo-obstruction). See OXPHOS.

Symptoms and Signs. From birth. Progressive external ophthalmoplegia, limb weakness, peripheral neuropathy; gastroenteropathy with chronic diarrhea, intestinal pseudo-obstruction.

Etiology. Defect may be in mitochondrial and inheritance would thus be maternal fenomen, partial deficiency of COX. Autosomal recessive inheritance also possible.

Pathology. Brain leukodystrophy. Muscle ragged red fibers. Peripheral nerves: endoneural fibrons, demyelinization.

Diagnostic Procedures. *Blood.* Lactic acidosis. *MRN.* Leukodystrophy. *Liver and muscle.* Defect of cytochrome-c-oxidase.

Therapy. Parenteral nutrition if necessary. Symptomatic.

Prognosis. Death from cachexia.

BIBLIOGRAPHY. Bardosi A, Creutzfeld W, Di Mauro S, et al: Myo-Neurogastrointestinal encepohalopathy (MNGIE syndrome) owing to the partial deficiency of cytochrome c oxidase. Acta Neuropathol 74:248–258, 1987
Simon LT, Horoupian DS, Dorfman LJ, et al: Polyneuropathy, opthalmoplegia, leukoencephalopathy, and intestinal pseudo-obstruction: POLIP syndrome. Ann Neurol 28:349–360, 1990
Shoffner JM, Wallace DC: Oxidative phosphorylation diseases. In Scriver CR, Beaudet AL, Sly WS, et al: The Metabolic and Molecu-

lar Bases of Inherited Disease, 7th ed, p 1587. New York, McGraw-Hill, 1995

MÖBIUS I

Synonyms. Hemicrania hemiplegic; hemiplegic—ophthalmoplegic migraine; hemiplegic familial migraine; neurologic migraine.

Symptoms. Occurs in young adults. Moderate hemicrania accompanied by extraocular palsy (oculomotor [III] and other oculomotor nerves); frequently followed (after 3–5 days of onset and when pain subsides) by hemiparesis. Recovery usually follows after a few days.

Etiology and Pathology. Unknown. Indirect indications of unilateral cerebral edema owing to vasomotor phenomena; in some cases aneurysm of internal carotid or neoplasia.

Diagnostic Procedures. *X-ray of skull. Angiography. Brain CT scan. MRI. EEG.*

Therapy. Same as for migraine, classic (see). Corticosteroids; diuretics; if aneurysm identified, surgery.

Prognosis. Permanent damage of oculomotor (III) nerve may occur.

BIBLIOGRAPHY. Möbius PJ: Ueber periodische wiederkehrende Oculomotoriuslachennung. Klin Wochenschr 21:604–608, 1884
Frideman AP: The migraine syndrome. Bull NY Acad Med 44:45–62, 1968
Adams RD, Victor M: Principles of Neurology, 5th ed, p 156. New York, McGraw-Hill, 1993

MÖBIUS II

Synonyms. von Graefe II; Graefe II; akinesia algera; arthrogryposis; congenital facial diplegia; nuclear agenesis; oculofacial paralysis; paralysis congenita 6th–12th cranial nerves; MOBS.

Symptoms. Facial paralysis; inability to abduct the eyes beyond midpoint; nutritional difficulty because of tongue and palate atrophy or deformities. Mental deficiency often associated.

Signs. Mask-like expression; open mouth; paralysis of soft palate and muscles of mastication; atrophy of tongue. Also observed: absence of pectoralis muscles, talipes, syndactyly.

Etiology. Possibly, failure of development of facial nerve cells or primary defect of muscles deriving from first two branchial arches or both. Chromosomal abnormalities (short arm of chromosome 1 or long arm of chromosome 13). Congenital myopathies may also cause this syndrome.

Pathology. Studies are few, incomplete, and inadequate to draw any conclusions about real pathology of the condition. Extensive asymmetric changes in brain stem, medulla, and pons. Aplasia, hypoplasia of facial and extraocular muscles. Facial nerves small or absent.

Diagnostic Procedures. *EMG. Biopsy of muscle. X-ray of skull. EEG. CT scan. MRI. Brainstem auditory evoked potentials (BAEP).* Abnormal.

Therapy. Surgery to protect cornea. Surgical correction of associated defects. Pulsatile administration of gonadotropin-realizing hormone for 3 months when indicated.

Prognosis. Recovery in a few weeks or nonprogressive permanent paralysis of face, always bilateral, often asymmetric, and when incomplete, usually sparing lower face and platysma.

BIBLIOGRAPHY. von Graefe A: Graefe-Saemisch Handbuch, vol 6, p 60. Leipzig, Engelmann, 1880
Möbius PJ: Ueber angeborene doppelseitige Abduces-Facialis-Lahmung. Munch Med Wochenschr 35:91–94; 108–111, 1888
Thomas HM: Congenital facial paralysis. J Nerv Ment Dis 25:571–593, 1898
Kumar D: Moebius syndrome. J Med Genet 27:122–126, 1990

MacDermot KD, Winter RM, Taylor D, et al: Oculofacial-bulbar palsy in a mother and son: Review of 26 reports of familial transmission within "Moebius spectrum of defects." J Med Genet 28:18–26, 1991

MOELLER-HUNTER

Synonyms. Hunter (W.); Hunter glossitis; glossitis Moeller; atrophic glossitis.

Symptoms. Occurs as complication in 50% of cases of pernicious anemia. Pain on the tip and side of tongue and partial loss of taste.

Signs. Vivid red patches (beefy red) on edges of tongue or entire dorsum of tongue. Seldom, entire mouth and throat involved.

Etiology. Pernicious anemia (see Addison-Biermer).

Prognosis. With treatment, rapid regression of symptoms and signs; papillae may be regenerated in 1 week.

BIBLIOGRAPHY. Moeller JOL: Klinische Bemerkungen über einige weniger bekannte Krankheiten der Zunge. Dtsch Klin 3:273–275, 1851
Hunter W: Further observation on pernicious anaemia (severe cases). A chronic infective disease: Its relation to infection from the mouth and stomach; suggested serum treatment. Lancet I:221–224, 1900
Lee GR: Megaloblastic and non megaloblastic macrocytic anemias. In Lee GR, Bithell TC, Foerster J, et al (eds): Wintrobe's Clinical Hematology, 9th ed, p 756. Philadelphia, Lea & Febiger, 1993

MOENCKEBERG

Synonyms. Medial arteriosclerosis; medial calcified sclerosis.

Symptoms. Prevalent in males; onset after 50 years of age. Intermittent claudication with pain in foot, calf, thigh, or buttock.

Signs. Palpation of leg vessels reveals nodularity.

Etiology. Unknown. Various factors correlated with arteriosclerotic changes: stress; diet; toxic; nicotine.

Pathology. Larger arteries involved: rings or plaques of calcification of media; tortuosity and elongation. Adventitia respected; endothelium intact, but deformed.

Diagnostic Procedures. *Evaluation of arterial flow. X-ray.* Calcium deposits along arterial tracts.

Therapy. None; or surgical bypass.

Prognosis. That of associated atherosclerotic changes.

BIBLIOGRAPHY. Moenckeberg JG: Ueber die reine Mediaverkalkung der Extremitätenarterien und ihr Verhalten zur Arteriosklerose. Virchows Arch Pathol 171:141–167, 1903
Morris PJ: Periferal arterial disease. In Weatherall DJ, Ledingham JGG, Warrell DA (eds): Oxford Textbook of Medicine, 3rd ed, pp 2362–2375. Oxford, Oxford Med Pub, 1996

MOERSCH-WOLTMANN

Synonyms. Muscular rigidity; progressive spasm; see Stiffman and Kok.

Symptoms. Predominant in men (70%). Prodromal intermittent aching and tightness of body and limb muscles, evolving into a permanent stiffness that affects voluntary mobility. In addition, paroxysmal, painful spasms that are precipitated by physical and emotional stimuli and that may result in bone fractures. Profuse sweating, tachycardia associated with spasms. Sleep suppresses contractions. Sensory system and intellect are not affected.

Signs. Board-like stiffness of muscles. Reflexes normal.

Etiology. Unknown. Postulated: abnormal activity of small gamma motor neurons that induce contraction of muscle spindles, which in turn maintain excitability of lower motoneuron system correlation with hyperthyroidism or hypothalamic dysfunction or both. Familial occurrence reported (autosomal dominant [?], X-linked [?]). Autoimmunity.

Pathology. *Biopsy of muscle.* Normal or various abnormalities; increase in fibers and collagen; degeneration phenomena; sarcolemmal hyperplasia.

Diagnostic Procedures. *Urine.* In 30% of cases, abnormal reducing substance. *Blood.* Increased serum phosphorus during glycogen deposition (insulin administration). *Basal metabolic rate.* Increased. *EMG.* Tonic contraction continuing at rest.

Therapy. Dramatic improvement (produce good remission) with diazepam; cortisol or correction of other hormone specific derangements.

Prognosis. Progressive condition; weight loss and fractures.

BIBLIOGRAPHY. Moersch FP, Woltmann HW: Progressive fluctuating muscular rigidity and spasm ("stiff-man" syndrome): Report of case and some observations in 13 other cases. Proc Staff Meet Mayo Clinic 31:421–427, 1956
Gordon EE, Januszku DM, Kaufman L: A critical survey of stiff-man syndrome. Am J Med 42:582–599, 1967
Layzer RB: Stiff-man syndrome: An autoimmune disease? N Engl J Med 318:1060–1061, 1988
Adams RD, Victor M: Principles of Neurology, 5th ed, pp 1093, 1195, 1273, 1274. New York, McGraw-Hill, 1993

MOHR

Synonyms. Mohr-Claussen; acrocephalosyndactyly IV; orofacial-digital II; OFD II. See Papillon-Leage-Psaume and Majewski (may be the same syndrome).

Symptoms. Both sexes affected equally. Present from birth. Feeding difficulties; mental and physical development retardation; deafness (conductive type). Frequent respiratory infections.

Signs. *Facies.* Broad nasal bridge; hypoplasia alae nasi, pleudocleft (median) of upper lip; irregular teeth; multiple hypertrophic frenula of labia; cleft tongue; narrow arched palate; molar and maxillar hypoplasia. *Limbs.* Short humerus, femur, and tibia; bilateral manual exadactyly and bilateral polysyndactyly of halluces. *Muscle.* Hypotonia. *Hair and skin.* No changes. Mental retardation frequent; various neurologic abnormalities.

Etiology. Unknown. Autosomal recessive inheritance.

Prognosis. Frequently death from respiratory infections in infancy.

BIBLIOGRAPHY. Otto G: Monstrorum sexcentorum descriptio anatomica. SF Hirt Vratislaviae, 1841
Mohr OL: A hereditary sublethal syndrome in man. Avhandl Norske Videnskaps-Akademi Oslo. J Mat Naturwiss Klasse 14:1–3, 1941
Claussen O: Et arvelig syndrom omfattende tugemisdannelse of polydactyly. Nord Med 30:1147–1151, 1946
Anneren G, Arvidson B, Gustavson KH, et al: Oro-facio-digital syndromes I and II: Radiological methods for diagnosis and the clinical variations. Clin Genet 26:178–186, 1984
Anneren G, Gustavson KH, Jozwiak S, et al: Abnormalities of the cerebellum in oro-facio-digital syndrome II (Mohr syndrome). Clin Genet 38:69–73, 1991

MOLLARET

Synonym. Meningitis benign recurrent.

Symptoms and Signs. Observed particularly in infants. Recurrent hyperthermia; cephalalgia; nausea; vomiting; nuchal rigidity; myalgia; Kernig and Brudzinski signs. Occasionally, convulsions.

Etiology. Viral infection suspected (herpes simplex type I [HVS-1]).

Diagnostic Procedures. *Cerebrospinal fluid.* Pleocytosis of mixed type; lymphocytes, neutrophils, and endothelial cells.

Therapy. Symptomatic.

Prognosis. Good. Symptoms recede in 2–3 days but may recur for weeks or months. Apparently, however, a self-limited condition.

BIBLIOGRAPHY. Mollaret P: Méningite endothélio-leucocytaire multirécurrente benigne. Syndrome nouveau ou maladie nouvelle? Presentation de deux malades Bull Soc Méd Paris 60:121–122, 1944; Press Méd 52:210–211; Rev Neurol (Paris) 76:57–76, 1944
Frederiks JAM, Bruyn GW: Mollaret's meningitis. In Vinken PJ, Bruyn GW: Handbook of Clinical Neurology, vol 34, pp 545–552. Amsterdam, North-Holland, 1978
Adams RD, Victor M: Principles of Neurology, 5th ed, p 650. New York, McGraw-Hill, 1993

MOLYBDENUM COFACTOR DEFICIENCY

Synonyms. Xanthine oxidase and sulfite oxidase, combined deficiency.

Symptoms and Signs. Normal birth, moderate neonatal depression, occasionally dysmorphic features of head: large head, full cheeks, upturned nose, esophthalmus, telecanthus, cleft palate, microcephaly, large ears, loose skin, wrinkles of forehead. First–second week: feeding difficulties, characteristic neurological symptoms: tonic/clonic seizures (not responding to therapy), axial hypotonia, peripheral hypertonicity, lens dislocation.

Etiology. Autosomal recessive inheritance. Absence of molybdenum cofactor synthesis that causes absence of sulfite oxidase and xanthema oxidase with consequent neurological damage for either toxic sulfite products or insufficient sulfite or sulfate available for brain development.

Pathology. Cerebral atrophy, microgyria, ventricular enlargement, multicystic focal lesions of white matter spongiosis. Loss of neurons.

Diagnostic Procedures. *Urine.* Detection of sulphite by strip-test. *Tissue samples.* Absence of sulfite oxidase and xanthine dehydrogenase activities. Prenatal diagnosis is possible.

Therapy. None clinically effective to date. Only positive biochemical responses with diet low in sulfur containing amino acids and supplemented with sulfate and molybate.

Prognosis. Poor death at early age or severe mental retardation.

BIBLIOGRAPHY. Duran M, Beemer FA, Van der Heiden C, et al: Combined deficiency of xanthine oxidase and sulphite oxidase: A defect of molybdenum metabolism or transport. J Inherit Metab Dis 1:175–178, 1978
Gray RGF, Green A, Basu SN, et al: Antenatal diagnosis of molybdenum cofactor deficiency. Am J Obstet Gynec 163:1203–1204, 1990
Johnson JL, Wadmans SK: "Molybdenum cofactor deficiency" and isolated sulfite oxidase deficiency. In Scriver CR, Beaudet AL, Sly WS, et al: The Metabolic and Molecular Bases of Inherited Disease, 7th ed, pp 2277–2278. New York, McGraw-Hill, 1995

MONBRUN-BENISTY

Synonym. Ocular stump causalgia.

Symptoms. Occurs 1 month after rupture of the eyeball. Severe refractory pain starting from orbital cavity and extending on the face and the corresponding hemicranium. Congestion and hyperhidrosis of region involved.

Etiology. Sympathetic irritation of resected sympathetic fiber to the eye.

Pathology. Neuroma of resected sympathetic fibers.

Therapy. Cervical ganglion or Gasser ganglion resection; alcoholization of superior branch of trigeminal (V) nerve brings temporary relief.

Prognosis. Ablation of stump ineffectual. Good result with cervical or Gasser ganglion resection.

BIBLIOGRAPHY. Monbrun M, Mme Benisty: C R Soc Neurol Paris, 1916
Barre JA, Klein M: Un cas de syndrome de Monbrun-Benisty (causalgie du moignon oculaire) gueri par Gasserectomie. Rev Otoneuroophthalmol 11:755–758, 1934
Barraco P, Morax S: Chirurgie mutilante du globe. Encycl Méd Chir (Paris, France) Ophtalmologie 213000 A10, 10, 1987

MONDAY FEVER

Synonyms. Byssinosis; cotton mill fever; cotton miller fever. See Allergic alveolitis syndromes.

Symptoms. Occupational disease. Wheezing; dyspnea; cough with mucoid expectoration. Onset on Monday morning when returning to work at place with high concentration of industrial cotton dust.

Signs. Rales; hyperresonance on chest percussion.

Etiology. Hypersensitivity to cotton dust.

Pathology. Emphysema; chronic bronchitis; interstitial fibrosis; small granuloma contains bodies similar to asbestos.

Diagnostic Procedures. *X-ray of chest. Skin test.* Reaction to cotton dust.

Therapy. Avoidance of exposure to cotton dust.

Prognosis. Good if exposure discontinued; otherwise, chronic bronchitis, respiratory failure, or cor pulmonale.

BIBLIOGRAPHY. Chan-Yeung M: Occupational asthma. In Lynch JP, DeRemee RA: Immunological Mediated Pulmonary Diseases, p 360. Philadelphia, Lippincott, 1991

MONDINI

Synonyms. Dysplasia, inner ear; inner ear anomaly; congenital deafness; inner ear anomaly; cochlear malformation.

Symptoms. Both sexes. Onset from birth. Unilateral or bilateral. Deafness, vertigo, ataxia. Frequently found in association with many syndromes: Klippel-Feil, Pendred, Trisomies, Di George, and other undefined associations.

Signs. Usually children are slightly built, have failure to thrive, and also are mute.

Etiology. Malformation of the inner ear that may be associated with other congenital anomalies or occur in isolated form. In some cases may be consequence of teratogenic drugs assumed during pregnancy.

Pathology. *Ear.* Dysplasia consisting of flattened bony cochlear capsule with underdeveloped bony structure in the apical part of cochlea characterized by defects in the interscalar septum, modiolous, and osseous spiral lamina, reduction in numbers of cochlear turns and dilated endolymphatic system.

Diagnostic Procedures. *CT scan.* Reduction in size of cochlea (dwarf cochlea) more than reduction in number of coils. *Caloric test.* Reduced response of affected ear.

Therapy. Correction of perilymphatic fistulas if present.

Prognosis. Loss of auditory and vestibular function may be static or progressive from mild to total.

BIBLIOGRAPHY. Mondini C. Anatomica surdi nati sectio'. De Bononiensi Scientarum et artium institute atque academia commentarii. Banoniae 7:419–431, 1791

Illum P: The Mondini type of cochlear malformation. A survey of the literature. Arch Otolaryngol 96:305–311, 1972

Schuknecht H F: Mondini dysplasia. A clinical and pathological study. JAMA 3–23, 1994

MONDOR

Synonyms. Superficial breast phlebitis; chest wall phlebitis; sclerosing breast periphlebitis; sclerosing breast phlebitis.

Symptoms. Predominant in females; onset in third to sixth decade. No or slight discomfort.

Signs. Usually, unilateral red linear cord from lateral margin of breast, crossing costal margin to abdominal wall, attached to skin, not to deep fascia.

Etiology. Obliterative phlebitis of thoracoepigastric vein. Frequently, history of trauma.

Pathology. Periphlebitis of lateral thoracic or thoracoepigastric vein. Thrombosis; adventitia and media destruction.

Therapy. Topical application of heparinoid compounds.

Prognosis. Usually, all manifestations disappear in a few weeks.

BIBLIOGRAPHY. Mondor H: Tronculite souscutanée subaiguë de la paroi thoracique antérolatérale. Mem Acad Chir (Paris) 65:1271–1278, 1939

Hogan GF: Mondor's disease. Arch Intern Med 113:881–885, 1964

Sabiston DC: Textbook of Surgery, 14th ed, p 1496. Philadelphia, WB Saunders, 1991

Schlant RC, Alexander RW: Hurst's The Heart, 8th ed, p 242. New York, McGraw-Hill, 1994

MONDOR PHLEBITIS, PENIS

Symptoms and Signs. In males 20–40 years old; onset 24–48 h after intercourse: painless, single or grouped doughy purplish, cord-like lesion from or around coronal sulcus. Occasionally extending to dorsal lymphatics, seldom ulcerating.

Etiology and Pathology. Unknown trauma considered, viral and bacterial infections coincidental; early changes affecting veins with occlusion by a neutrophils-clot and granulation tissue on vein walls.

Prognosis. Self-limiting in weeks.

BIBLIOGRAPHY. Findlay GH, Whiting DA: Mondor's phlebitis of penis. Clin Exp Dermatol 2:65–67, 1977

Ive FA: The umbilical, perianal and genital regions. In Champion RH, Burton JL, Ebling FJG (eds): Rook/Wilkinson/Ebling Textbook of Dermatology, 5th ed, p 2818. Oxford, Blackwell Scientific, 1992

MONGE

Synonyms. Mountain sickness chronic; high altitude; polycythemia chronic secondary mountain; seroche.

EMPHYSEMATOUS TYPE

Symptoms. Dyspnea; frequently, bronchitis; laryngitis.

Signs. Cyanosis; globular chest.

ERYTHREMIC TYPE

Symptoms. Fatigue; exertional dyspnea; decrease in mental fitness; headache; epistaxis; gum bleeding; hemoptysis; anorexia; nausea; vomiting; decreased visual acuity; tinnitus; cough. Loss of libido; paresthesia and pain in the extremities. Aphonia, lethargy up to coma.

Signs. Severe cyanosis (increasing with exertion); frequently purpura. Eyelids edematous; bluish scleral injection; thickening of tongue; turgor of hands; clubbing of fingers; hepatosplenomegaly (in 10% of cases).

Etiology. Unknown. Possibly, minimal intrinsic pulmonary disease too mild to give manifestation at low altitude. Similar to Ayerza, differentiated by the fact that the latter condition does not respond to transfer to low altitude.

Pathology. Polycythemia.

Diagnostic Procedures. *Blood.* Erythrocytosis; reticulocytes normal or increased. Leukocytes normal; platelets normal; indirect bilirubin high; increase of blood volume; increased excretion of urobilinogen.

Therapy. Transfer to sea level.

Prognosis. Remission and relapses frequently observed. Complete remission if patient transferred to sea level. Death from hemorrhages, bronchopneumonia; or cardiac disorders late and frequently cause of death.

BIBLIOGRAPHY. Monge C: High altitude disease. Arch Intern Med 59:32–40, 1937

Monge C, Lozano R, Carcelen A: Renal excretion of bicarbonate in high altitude natives and in natives with chronic mountain sickness. J Clin Invest, 43:2303–2309, 1964

Houston CS: Altitude illness. Emerg Med Clin N Am, 2:503–512, 1984

Grover RF, Reeves JT, Rowell LB, et al: The influence of environmental factors on the cardiovascular system. In Schlant RC, Alexander RW: Hurst's The Heart, 8th ed, pp 2117–2122. New York, McGraw-Hill, 1994

MONGOLIAN BLUE SPOTS

Synonym. Dermal melanocytosis.

Symptoms and Signs. Present in 90% of Asian neonates and in 1% of white infants (maximal frequency in those of Mediterreanean areas). Incidence in other nationalities range between these two. Faint, blue-grayish, macular pigmentation, usually a single patch in lumbosacral area that, occasionally, may extend to loins and shoulders.

Etiology. Unknown.

Pathology. Dermal collagen fibers and neurovascular bundles mixed with melanocytes, disposed parallel to skin. Absence of macrophages and no alteration of collagen and elastic fibers.

Prognosis. For some time after birth, pigmentation tends to increase in depth; then, usually, it fades completely in seventh and occasionally, 13th year. Rarely discoloration remains for life.

BIBLIOGRAPHY. El Bahrawy AA: Arch Dermatol Syph 141:171, 1922

MacKie: Melanocytic Naevi and Malignant Melanoma. In Champion RH, Burton JL, Ebling FJG (eds): Rook/Wilkinson/Ebling Textbook of Dermatology, 5th ed, pp 1537–1538. Oxford, Blackwell Scientific, 1992

MONTEGGIA

Synonym. Ulnar fracture—radial head dislocation. See Galeazzi.

Symptoms. More common in children. Pain in forearm.

Signs. Fracture dislocation of forearm with dislocation of radial head proximally. Elbow partially flexed and rotated inward.

Etiology. Blow to forearm.

Diagnostic Procedures. *X-ray of elbow.* Fracture of ulna radial head points through the middle of the capitellum. Four types of this fracture have been described.

Therapy. Most fractures treated by closed methods. If unsuccessful, open reduction is needed.

Prognosis. If not recognized and treated, poor function may result.

BIBLIOGRAPHY. Monteggia GB: Istituzioni Chirurgiche, vol 5. Milan, Pirotta Maspero, 1814
Sabiston DC: Textbook of Surgery, 14th ed, pp 1306–1307. Philadelphia, WB Saunders, 1991

MONTREAL PLATELETS

Synonyms. Giant platelets; MPS. See thrombocytopathia hereditary.

Symptoms and Signs. Both sexes. Healthy subjects with only prolonged bleeding time.

Etiology. Autosomal dominant inheritance.

Diagnostic Procedures. *Blood.* Thrombocytopenia; platelets on smear appear enlarged, spontaneous aggregation of platelets; normal clot retraction and thromboplastin formation, normal. Ristocetin-induced aggregation but low to absent thrombin-induced aggregation.

BIBLIOGRAPHY. Lacombe M, d'Angelo G: Etudes sur une thrombopathie familiale. Nouv Rev Fr Hematol 3:611, 1963
Milton JC, Frojmovic MM: Shape-changing agents produce abnormally large platelets in a hereditary "giant platelet" syndrome (MPS). J Lab Clin Med 93:154–161, 1979

MOORE (E.M.)

Eponym used to indicate a fracture of distal end of radius, dislocation of the ulna, and trapping of styloid process under the annular ligaments.

BIBLIOGRAPHY. Moore EM: A luxation of the ulna not hitherto described, with a plan of reduction and mode of after-treatment; including the management of Colles' fracture. Albany, NY, Weed, 1872
Saito H, Takahaschi Y, Zenzai K: Intra-articular fracture of the distal radius. Treatment and results. In Vastamaeki M: Current Trends in Hand Surgery, pp 131–160. Netherlands, Excerpta Medica, 1995

MOORE-FEDERMAN

Synonym. Dwarfism—stiff joints—ocular abnormalities. See also Leri.

Symptoms and Signs. Both sexes affected; apparently normal at birth; noticed at 3–5 years of age. Joint stiffness. Symptoms slowly progress to produce inability to completely clench hand. Delayed growth: adult reaches 130–150 cm. Hyperopia; asthma; hoarseness; hepatomegaly.

Etiology. Autosomal dominant inheritance.

Diagnostic Procedures. *X-rays.* Diminished height of vertebrae; slightly widened phalangeal metaphyses. *Urine.* No mucopolysaccharides and amino acid excretion.

Prognosis. Good quoad vitam. Dwarfism. Frequent respiratory infections.

BIBLIOGRAPHY. Moore WT, Federman DD: Familial dwarfism and "stiff joints." Report of a kindred. Arch Intern Med 115:398–404, 1969
Winter RM, Patton MA, Challener J, et al: Moore-Federman syndrome and acromicric dysplasia. Are they the same entity? J Med Genet 26:320–325, 1989

MOORE LIGHTNING STREAKS

Synonyms. Flashes.

Symptoms and Signs. In patient with migraine sudden vision of a rapid bright zigzag line rapidly disappearing.

Etiology. Ischemia of nerve cells in the occipital lobe.

Diagnostic Procedures. See migraine.

Prognosis. Benign manifestation.

BIBLIOGRAPHY. Adams RD, Victor M: Principles of Neurology, 5th ed, p 222. New York, McGraw-Hill, 1993

MOORE (M.T.)

Synonyms. Abdominal epilepsy; paroxysmal pain; visceral epilepsy.

Symptoms. Cramps, pain; nausea; strange feeling in the abdomen and chest, followed or not followed by seizures. General pattern of attack remains the same in each patient, although initiating symptoms may vary. Percentages of incidence of paroxysmal symptoms: gastrointestinal (Moore) (65%); cardiorespiratory (50%); genitourinary (5%); rising visceral sensation (17%); generalized convulsions (50%); psychiatric disturbances (46%).

Etiology. Usually, lesions of frontal parasagittal regions, or idiopathic.

Diagnostic Procedures. *EEG. X-ray. CT scan. MRI. Stereoelectroencephalography.* Of skull and organ involved for differential diagnosis and localization of focus.

Therapy. Anticonvulsant drugs.

Prognosis. Good response to treatment. Recovery with possible development of recurrent convulsions in later years.

BIBLIOGRAPHY. Morgagni GB: The Seats and Causes of Diseases Investigated by Anatomy; in Five Books, Containing a Great Variety of Dissection with Remarks, vol I, pp 192–195. Alexander B (trans) London, Millar Cadell, 1769
Moore MT: Paroxysmal abdominal pain: A form of focal symptomatic epilepsy. JAMA 124:561–563, 1944
Mulder DW, Daly D, Bailey AA: Visceral epilepsy. Arch Intern Med 91:481–493, 1954
Dalessio DJ: The nervous system. In Haubrich WS, Schaffner F, Berk JE (eds): Bockus Gastroenterology, 5th ed, pp 3386–3387. Philadelphia, WB Saunders, 1995

MOOREN

Synonyms. Ulcus rodens corneal; serpiginous cornea ulcer; cornea serpiginous ulcer.

Symptoms. No significant race or sex incidence. Primarily affects adults. Ocular pain (in one eye or both eyes) and photophobia that appear simultaneously or at different times in the absence of any known systemic disease.

Signs. Superficial corneal erosion starting as a corneal infiltrate, just inside the limbus and spreading in serpiginous manner. Central margin presents an overhanging lip; the anterior corneal layers are involved. Lesion is progressive and chronic; the cicatricial reaction is minimal. Signs of iritis are frequently present. The perforation of cornea and hypopyon are rarely seen. Conjunctiva and sclera are never affected by the ulcer.

Etiology. Unknown. Allergy and hypersensitivity have been considered (weak evidence for type III hypersensitivity reaction). Other postulated etiologic mechanisms: metabolic disorders; malnutrition; hereditary familial primary changes in trigeminal (V) nerve or sympathetic fibers; trophic disturbances secondary to local disease.

Pathology. Ulceration of cornea undermined at its central edge. Microscopically, scanty inflammatory reaction in the region of the cleft and central lip of ulcer, absence of neovascularization of the cornea. Intracellular edema of basal layer of corneal epithelium. Lip of ulcer covered by thinned epithelium, curled into thick squamous fragments. Bowman membrane absent beneath ulcer. Inflammatory pannus of limbus formed by plasma cells in anterior chamber; eosinophilic material bordering the endothelium and polymorphonuclear cells, filling angle and trabecular meshwork behind ulcer. Iris may be normal or show signs of inflammation.

Diagnostic Procedures. *Tears.* Search for bacteria, viruses, fungi; allergens and immune complexes and corneal antibodies.

Therapy. Analgesic and topical agents for secondary infections; trial with antiallergic or corticosteroid compounds and cytotoxic chemotherapy; removal of conjunctiva adjacent to the ulcerating cornea, combined with resection of the necrotic, ulcerating cornea and application of a tissue adhesive to exclude access of neutrophils to the region.

Prognosis. Chronic progressive disease.

BIBLIOGRAPHY. Nettleship E: Chronic serpiginous ulcer of the cornea (Mooren's ulcer). Trans Ophthalmol Soc UK 22:103–115, 1902
Edwards WC, Reed RE: Mooren's ulcer. Arch Ophthalmol 80:361–364, 1968
Wood TO, Kaufman HE: Mooren's ulcer. Am J Ophthalmol 71:417–427, 1971
Foster CS: Ocular manifestations of immune disease. In Garner A, Klintworth GK (eds): Pathobiology of Ocular Disease: A Dynamic Approach, 2nd ed, pp 166–168. New York, Marcel Dekker, 1994

MOREL-WILDI

Eponym used to indicate nodular formations (of probably dysgenetic origin) of the frontal cortex. Asymptomatic.

BIBLIOGRAPHY. Morel F, Wildi F: Dysgénésie nodulaire disséminée de l'écorce frontale. Rev Neurol (Paris) 87:251–270, 1952

MORGAGNI-ADAMS-STOKES

Synonyms. MAS; Adams-Stokes; Stokes-Adams; Spen; cardiac syncope (arrhythmic); atrioventricular heart block.

Symptoms. Onset usually after 40 years of age. Episodes of sudden weakness, fainting, convulsions regardless of body position or particular time. Syncope, however, occurs more readily when patient is standing or sitting.

Signs. Paleness becoming cyanosis; unconsciousness; clonic jerks; during attacks pulse very slow (usually under 20), or absent (asystole of 4–15 seconds duration); fall of blood pressure; difficult breathing; fixed pupils; incontinence; bilateral Babinski with resumption of heart beats; flushing of the face.

Etiology. Intensity and progression of symptoms and signs depend on degree of bradycardia. Cerebral hypoxia due to atrioventricular block; asystolic fibrillation.

Pathology. Atherosclerotic heart disease findings; congenital or rheumatic heart disease; myocarditis (infections, particularly diphtheria).

Diagnostic Procedures. ECG. Holter. Atrioventricular block, transient or permanent.

Therapy. During attacks and if no pulse, strike a blow over precordium. If ineffective, institute resuscitation procedures (massage; artificial respiration; defibrillation). If ventricular fibrillation etiologic cause, start intravenous injection of isoproterenol in dextrose; epine-

phrine (intramuscular, or intravenous, or intracardiac if needed). Type and severity of attacks or failure of medical management (long-term oral isoproterenol, atropine, epinephrine, corticosteroid therapy, chlorothiazide) indicate the need for implantation of an artificial cardiac pacemaker.

Prognosis. Guarded, depending on pathogenetic factors.

BIBLIOGRAPHY. Morgagni JB: De Sedibus et Causis Morborum. Letter the Ninth: Which Treats of the Epilepsy (description of heart block), 1761
Adams R: Cases of diseases of the heart accompanied with pathological observations. Dublin Hosp Repts 4:353–453, 1827
Stokes W: Memoir on slow pulse. Dublin Q J Med Sc 2:73–85, 1846
Bondoulas H, Lewis RP: Cardiac syncope: Diagnosis, mechanism and management. In Myerburg RJ, Kessler KM, Castellanos A: Recognition clinical assessment and management of conduction disturbances. In Schlant RC, Alexander RW: Hurst's The Heart, 8th ed, pp 748–750. New York, McGraw-Hill, 1994

MORGAGNI HERNIA

Synonyms. Anterior diaphragmatic hernia; hernia Morgagni.

BIBLIOGRAPHY. Morgagni GB: The Seats and Causes of Diseases Investigated by Anatomy; in Five Books, Containing a Great Variety of Dissection with Remarks, liber III Alexander B (trans). London, Millar Cadell, 1769
Sabiston DC: Textbook of Surgery, 14th ed, p 1165. Philadelphia, WB Saunders, 1991

MORGAGNI-STEWART-MOREL

Synonyms. Stewart-Morel; Morgagni-Pende; Morel-Moore; hyperostosis frontalis interna; metabolic craniopathy; including hyperostosis cranialis interna (Manni JJ) and cranial hyperostosis-galactorrhea.

Symptoms. Predominant in women. Symptoms frequently appearing at menopausal time. Subacute and progressive development of frontal headache, often severe; seldom seizures; mental impairment, depression, weakness, fatigue, vertigo. In HCI recurrent facial palsy and signs of other cranial nerve entrapment.

Signs. Obesity and hirsutism. Many cases with hyperostosis without symptoms and vice versa. In some cases intestinal malfunctions and galactorrhea.

Etiology. Unknown. The disorder may be autosomal dominant but X-linked inheritance also possible. May be related to hyperprolactinemia.

Pathology. Hyperostosis of inner table of frontal bone reducing the anterior part of cranial cavity. Frontal cortex sufferance possible.

Diagnostic Procedures. *X-rays. Scintigraphy. CT scan. MRI. Radionucleotide images of brain.* See Pathology. *Blood.* Serum alkaline phosphatases (in 50% of cases) elevated. Hyperprolactinemia in many cases. In some cases hyperglycemia.

Therapy. Symptomatic.

Prognosis. Relatively benign.

BIBLIOGRAPHY. Morgagni GB: De sedibus and causes morborum Lib. 1 De Morbis Capitis. Venezia Typographia Remondiniana, 1761
Moore S: Hyperostosis Cranii (Stewart-Morel syndrome: Metabolic craniopathy, Morgagni's syndrome [Ritvo], le syndrome de Morgagni-Morel). Springfield, IL, Charles C Thomas, 1955
Morel F: L'hyperostose frontale interne. Syndrome de l'hyperostose frontale interne avec adipose et troubles cèrebraux. Paris, Gaston, Doin e Co, 1930
Stewart RM: Localized cranial hyperostosis in the insane. J Neurol Psychopathol (London) 8:321, 1928
Pawlikowski M, Komorowski J: Hyperostosis frontalis, galactorrhea

(hyperprolactinemia and Morgagni-Stewart-Morel syndrome). Lancet 1:474, 1983

Manni JJ, Scaf JJ, Huygen PLM, et al: Hyperostosis cranialis interna: A new hereditary syndrome with cranial nerve entrapment. N Engl J Med 322:450–454, 1990

MORNING GLORY

Synonym. Optic disk central glial anomaly; axial coloboma; papilla "en fleur de liseron"; peripapillary scleral staphyloma; posterior ectasia papillae.

Symptoms. Present from birth. Severe decrease in visual acuity.

Signs. Strabismus. Unilateral enlarged pink optic disk, flower-like with fluffy dot in the center nerve head, inscribed in a ring of altered chorioretinal pigment. At the edge of disk, narrow branches of retinal arteries, presence of exudates, subretinal hemorrhages, and neovascularization. Periphery of retina normal. Possibly abnormality of anterior chamber. Occasionally: retinal detachment, retinoschisis, cataract, cleft lip/palate.

Etiology. Unknown. Trisomy 4q has been reported.

Pathology. Papillae large and excavated, central bouquet of glia hyperplasia; retinal vessels oriented radially from the periphery of the disk. Occasionally: glomerulonephritis.

Diagnostic Procedures. *CT scan. Ultrasonography. MRI.* Colobomatous area, retinal detachment; thickened optic nerve, normal retro-bulbar optic nerve; occasionally: encephalic midline defects, renal dysplasia.

BIBLIOGRAPHY. Handmann M: Erbliche, vermütlich angeborene zentrale Gliöse; Entartung des Sehenerven mit besonderer Beteiligung der Zentralgefaesse. Klin Monatsbl Augenheilkd 83:145–152, 1929

Kindler P: Morning glory syndrome: Unusual congenital optic disk anomaly. Am J Ophthalmol 69:376–384, 1970

Manschot WA: Morning glory syndrome: A histopathologic study. Br J Ophthalmol 74:560–580, 1990

Nucci P, Mets MB, Gabianelli EB: Trisomy 4q with morning glory disk anomaly, Ophthalmic Paediatr Gen 11:143–145, 1990

MORNING SICKNESS

Synonyms. Vomiting in pregnancy. See Hyperhemesis gravidarum.

Symptoms and Signs. In approximately 50% of pregnancies, especially if primiparae.

Etiology. Possibly high estrogen levels.

Pathology. None. May be a sign of Hydatiform mole (see).

Diagnostic Procedures. According to severity of symptoms. If severe. *Blood gas analysis.* Acidosis. *Osmolality.* Dehydration. Assesment of nutritive status.

Therapy. Vitamin B$_6$ potentially useful usually; superfluous: antiemetics, antihistaminics, and antispasmodics.

Prognosis. In majority of cases this syndrome does not imply complications.

BIBLIOGRAPHY. Sahakaian V, Rouse D, Sipes S, et al: Vitamin B$_6$ is effective therapy for nausea and vomiting: A randomized, double blind placebo-controlled study. Obstet Gynecol 78:33–36, 1991

MORPHEA

Synonyms. Addison keloid; Alibert keloid; circumscribed scleroderma. See Scleroderma and Romberg-Wood.

Symptoms. Prevalent in females (3:1); onset usually in second to fourth decades. Migraine; arthralgia; abdominal pain in only 15% of cases; generalized joint pain in 40% of cases.

Signs. Five varieties recognized: (1) Plaques, usually multiple, asymmetric (2–15 cm in diameter), zones of skin induration that in months become smooth, shiny, hairless, nonsweating, and ivory color with purplish edges. Bullae, vesicles, hemorrhages, and telangiectases may develop. Hypoesthesia of zone involved. Trunk, limbs, face, and genital areas may be involved. (2) Guttate lesions, bigger and less numerous lesions, similar to white spot (see). (3) Linear lesions, usually single (occasionally bilateral) lesions of linear shape similar to plaque lesion described. (4) Frontoparietal scleroderma en coupe de sabre. Linear scleroderma affecting frontal or frontoparietal region of face and scalp, associated more or less with minor subcutaneous atrophic changes. (5) Generalized, larger plaques usually appearing first on the trunk, sometimes involving the entire body. Face becomes expressionless; contractures appear.

Etiology. Unknown. Occasionally, onset associated with trauma, pregnancy, menopause, nature of relationship not established.

Pathology. Epidermis normal or atrophic. Dermis edematous, swelling, and degeneration of collagen; moderate perivascular lymphocytic infiltrates. Reduction of elastic tissue. Atrophy of hair, follicle, and sweat glands.

Diagnostic Procedures. *Biopsy of skin. Blood.* Normal; occasionally eosinophilia, hypocomplementaemia; increased sedimentation rate; rarely, anti DNA and ENA antibodies. *X-ray.* Spine abnormality in 47% of patients (especially linear lesions).

Therapy. Penicillamine and pyridoxine per os in early stage; sapazopyrin (enteric coated) to slow down rapidly developing forms; antimalarials useful for inflammation aspects. Infiltration with corticosteroids if indicated. Surgery occasionally used if sclerosis interferes with different functions.

Prognosis. Plaque: spontaneous improvement; 3–5 years duration. Linear: spontaneous improvement; lasts longer. Occasionally, development of systemic sclerosis syndrome. Generalized form: improvement after 3–5 years; severe disability in some cases. Death from other causes.

BIBLIOGRAPHY. Fagge CH: On keloid, sclerosis, morphoea and some allied affections. Guy's Hosp Rep 13:255–328, 1868

Wartenberg R: Progressive facial hemiatrophy. Arch Neurol Psychiatr 54:75–96, 1945

Dawber RPR, Ebling FJG, Wojnarowska FT: Disorders of hair. In Champion RH, Burton JL, Ebling FJG (eds): Rook/Wilkinson/Ebling Textbook of Dermatology, 5th ed, p 2603. Oxford, Blackwell Scientific, 1992

MORQUIO

Synonyms. Brailsford-Morquio; Dale (Morquio type B). Chondrosteodystrophy; eccentro-osteochondrodysplasia; keratan sulfaturia; hereditary osteochondrodystrophy deformans; mucopolysaccharidosis IV; MPS IV A and B.

Symptoms. Both sexes affected; become clinically evident at end of first year of life. Deafness; weak extremities; waddling gait. Absence of mental retardation; subtle or evident symptoms of myelopathy up to quadriplegia.

Signs. Dwarfism (growth stops at 6 years of age); short trunk and neck. *Facies.* Coarse broad mouth; spaced teeth. *Thorax.* Pectus carinatum. Aortic regurgitation in some cases. *Extremities.* Knock-knees; joints very loose and unstable. Absence of hypoplasia of odontoid process, possibly resulting in atlantoaxial subluxation (see).

Etiology. Autosomal recessive inheritance. Two forms are now recognized. Type A owing to absence of N-acetylgalactosamine-6-sulfatase and type B (milder Dale syndrome owing to B-galactosidase deficiency). Both give defective degradation of keratan sulfate.

Pathology. Irregular growth of cartilage and epiphysis and focal aseptic necrosis. Chondrocytes packed with vacuoles.

Diagnostic Procedures. *Urine.* Excretion of keratan sulfate. *X-rays.* Skeletal survey. Platyspondyly; epiphyseal changes; spotty calcification. *Blood.* Reilly bodies in lymphocytes. Prenatal diagnosis now is possible.

Therapy. Orthopedic surgery.

Prognosis. After 6–7 years of age situation becomes stabilized without further growth, however, death usually occurs before 20–30 years of age. Longer survival reported. Myelopathy and pulmonary complications are the leading causes of death.

BIBLIOGRAPHY. Morquio L: Sur une forme de dystrophie osseuse familiale. Bull Soc Pediatr Paris 27:145–152, 1929
Dale T: Unusual forms of familial osteochondrodystrophy. Acta Radiol 12:337–358, 1931
Neufeld EF, Muenzer J: The mucopolysaccharidoses. In Scriver CR, Beaudet AL, Sly WS, et al: The Metabolic and Molecular Bases of Inherited Disease, 7th ed, pp 2476–2477. New York, McGraw-Hill, 1995

MORQUIO-ULLRICH

Terminology proposed by Wiedemann to distinguish these patients from those with classic Morquio.

Symptoms and Signs. Typical symptoms and signs of Morquio, plus one or more features usually associated with Hurler: Hepatosplenomegaly; corneal opacity; deafness; granulation in leukocytes. This eponym is unnecessary since it appears that these extraskeletal manifestations develop in all patients with Morquio syndrome, if they survive to adolescence.

BIBLIOGRAPHY. Wiedemann HR: Ausgedehnte und allgemeine erblich bedingte Bildungs-und Wachstumsfehler des Knockengerüstes. Mschr Kinderheilkd 102:136–140, 1954
Kaplan D, McKusick V, Trebach S, et al: Keratosulfatechondroitin sulfate peptide from normal urine and from urine of patients with Morquio syndrome (mucopolysaccharidosis IV). J Lab Clin Med 71:48–55, 1968

MORRIS

Synonyms. Hairless women; androgen insensitivity; androgen receptor deficiency; AIS, complete form; dihydrotestosterone receptor deficiency; complete androgen resistance; testicular feminization (term to be abandoned). See also Male pseudohermaphroditism, incomplete hereditary type I.

Signs. Individual who appears externally to be a normal, well-developed female in body contour, distribution of body hair, voice, and breast development. *Amenorrhea.* Raised psychologically and socially as a female. Vagina well developed, blind ending; small clitoris, no cervix; absence of uterus; external genitalia female in character, although there may be in some cases an ambiguous phallic enlargement and scant pubic hair. Often inguinal hernias, containing palpable gonad (testis).

Etiology. Unknown. Possibly a sex-linked recessive gene. Inability of end organs to respond to normal circulating levels of testosterone or ectopic testes fail to secrete.

Pathology. Fallopian tubes and uterus are rudimentary or absent. Sometimes testis in the inguinal canal, intra-abdominal or in the labia; with no spermatogenesis, nor wolffian duct structures.

Diagnostic Procedures. *Chromosome studies.* Sexual chromatin ab-

sent; XY pattern. *Blood.* Testosterone level may be similar to those found in normal males. Elevated plasma luteinizing hormone (LH) levels. *Echography.* Absence of uterus and fallopian tubes. Variable location of testis.

Therapy. No attempt to change sex. If vagina inadequate, use of dilators or plastic surgery. Removal of undescended testicles (better at early age) to avoid possible neoplastic transformation. Estrogen administration at time of puberty.

Prognosis. Good psychological adjustment and life, including satisfactory sexual activity, as female possible.

BIBLIOGRAPHY. Dieffenbach H: Familiaerer Hermaphroditismus Inagural Dissertation. Stuttgart, 1912
Goldberg MB, Maxwell AF: Male pseudohermaphroditism proved by surgical exploration and microscopic examination: A case report with speculations concerning pathogenesis. J Clin Endocrinol 8:367–379, 1948
Morris JM: The syndrome of testicular feminization in male pseudohermaphrodites. Am J Obstet Gynecol 65:1192–1211, 1953
Bals-Pratsch M, Schweikert H-U, Nieschlag E: Androgen receptor disorder in three brothers with bifid prepenile scrotum and hypospadia. Acta Endocr 123:271–276, 1990
Forest MG: Diagnosis and treatment of disorders of sexual development. In De Groot LJ (ed): Endocrinology, 3rd ed, pp 1920–1921. Philadelphia, WB Saunders, 1995

MORROW-BROOKE

Synonyms. Brooke epidemic acne; epidemic acne; keratosis follicularis contagiosa; acne venenata includes chloracne.

Symptoms. Outbreak in different world regions; in each episode, it may be prevalent in one sex or age group. Pruritus; general discomfort.

Signs. On the face and ears, but possibly also on limbs and trunk. At onset, erythematous follicular papules, which rapidly change into comedo and follicular cysts that later form large keratinized brown plaques, tending to become confluent.

Etiology. Not clearly established. Strongly suspected toxic nature, especially chlorinated compounds. Acne venenata; DDT, neat cutting oils, crude petroleum, distilled, heavy coal-tar cosmetics, asbestos, topical corticosteroids.

Therapy. Avoid contact with suspected agents. Exfoliative pastes; retinoic acid.

Prognosis. Regression. Little or no scarring. Chloracne may persist for years.

BIBLIOGRAPHY. Morrow PA: Keratosis follicularis associated with fissuring of the tongue and leukoplakia buccalis. J Cutan Dis NY 4:27–65, 1886
Brooke HA: Keratosis follicularis contagiosa. In International Atlas of Rare Skin Diseases, No 7, plate 22, 1892
Rycroft RJG: Occupational dermatoses. In Champion RH, Burton JL, Ebling FJG (eds): Rook/Wilkinson/Ebling Textbook of Dermatology, 5th ed, pp 759–761. Oxford, Blackwell Scientific, 1992

MORT D'AMOUR

Symptom and Sign. Sudden death during sexual intercourse.

Etiology. Increase in blood pressure; arrhythmia; heart ischemia; rupture of cerebral aneurysm.

Therapy. Prophylaxis: a skillful, cooperative partner.

Prognosis. Pleasant death.

BIBLIOGRAPHY. Heggveit HA: La mort d'amour. Am Heart J 69:287–294, 1965

MORTENSEN

Synonyms. Di Guglielmo II; Revol; hemorrhagic thrombocythemia; hyperthrombocytic myelosis. See Myeloproliferative.

Symptoms. Both sexes equally affected; onset in third decade or later. Spontaneous bleeding manifestations of variable severity (e.g., hemoptysis, melena, menorrhagia). Excessive bleeding after minor trauma and at surgery. Thrombotic manifestations may be present in splenic vein and superficial and deep veins of legs.

Signs. Splenomegaly of variable size.

Etiology. Possible autosomal dominant trait. Suggested but not confirmed relationship to 21 chromosome deletion.

Pathology. No characteristic changes in spleen. Seldom, myeloid metaplasia in liver, spleen, or lymph nodes.

Diagnostic Procedures. *Blood.* Usually, anemia; occasionally, moderate erythrocytosis. Leukocytes increased (10,000–30,000, occasionally, over 60,000). Platelets extremely increased (millions); bizarre morphologic changes; various functional abnormalities. In some cases, mild deficiency of clotting factors II, V, and VI. *Bone marrow.* Panhyperplasia with marked increase of megakaryocytes, some showing morphologic abnormalities.

Therapy. According to severity of manifestations from none to busulfan; melphalan, uracil mustard, radioactive phosphorus. Splenectomy usually disastrous. Controversial results with anticoagulants. Encouraging results with aspirin and other platelet antiaggregating agents.

Prognosis. Survival at 5 years in 75%. May progress to myeloproliferative disease, Vaquez.

BIBLIOGRAPHY. Di Guglielmo G: Megacariociti e piastrine negli organi emopoietici e nel sangue circolante. Atti R Acad Chir Napoli 83:19, 1919
Epstein E, Goedel A: Hämorrhagische Thrombocythamie bei vascularer Schrumpfmilz. Virchows Arch 292:233–248, 1934
Mortensen O: Thrombocythemia hemorrhagica. Acta Med Scand 129:547–549, 1948
Revol L: La myélose hyperthrombocytaire (thrombocytémie hémorragique). Sang 21:409–423, 1950
Brière J, Brière JF: Thrombocythèmies, Encicl Med Chir (Paris) Sang Fasc. 13006, R-10 (7–1987)
Bithell TC: Thrombocytosis. In Lee GR, Bithell TC, Foerster J, et al (eds): Wintrobe's Clinical Hematology, 9th ed, pp 1391–1393. Philadelphia, Lea & Febiger, 1993

MORTON (D.)

Synonyms. Morton triad; short first metatarsal syndrome; metatarsus primus brevis varus.

Symptoms. Usually bilateral condition. Excessive foot fatigue; burning pain under metatarsal heads and metatarsophalangeal articulations of second and third metatarsal bones; longitudinal arch pain; radiation of pain to the calf, hamstring, and back muscles; pain typically beginning while walking or after longstanding and is relieved by rest.

Signs. Feet appear nearly normal. Careful inspection may reveal that first metatarsal may be slightly displaced upward and medially, abnormally movable, and covered with soft smooth skin, whereas the heads of second and third metatarsal are prominent and a hard callus is localized under their heads.

Etiology. Congenital malformation of first metatarsal bone. Autosomal dominant trait. Acute symptoms owing to synovitis of second or third metatarsal joints and middle cuneiform; chronic symptoms owing to secondary hypertrophic osteoarthritis.

Diagnostic Procedures. *X-ray.* Short first metatarsal bone and secondary changes.

Therapy. Compensating insoles; metatarsal pad or transverse bar.

Prognosis. In 75% of cases, fast recovery (1 week) with treatment; in 15% minor functional residual impairment; 10% require further treatment.

BIBLIOGRAPHY. Morton DJ: Metatarsus atavicus: The identification of a distinct type of foot disorder. J Bone Joint Surg 9:531–544, 1927
Morton DJ: Foot disorders in general practice. JAMA 109:1112–1119, 1937
Jahss MR: Disorders of the Foot. Philadelphia, WB Saunders, 1982
Klippel JH, Dieppe PA: Rheumatology, p 3.4.11. St Louis, CV Mosby, 1995

MORTON (T.)

Synonyms. Digital neuroma; metatarsalgia.

Symptoms. Predominant in women. Unilateral or, occasionally, bilateral. Recurrent burning pain between third and fourth metatarsal space, radiating to adjacent part of foot. Soreness may persist also when at rest and prevent sleep. Occasionally clicking sound in interspace (Moulder click).

Signs. Foot appears normal. Pain may be elicited by pressure applied between third and fourth metatarsal heads.

Etiology. Compression of digital nerve between metatarsal head and ground; syndrome may also occur with neurofibromas and angioneurofibromas of medial plantar nerve.

Pathology. Swelling not true neuroma of digital nerve affected; initially, simple perineural edema, then fibrosis.

Diagnostic Procedures. *X-ray. Ultrasonography of foot.*

Therapy. Felt pad proximal to head of fourth metatarsal. Injection of procaine and steroid relieves the pain. Once conservative treatment fails surgical excision of interdigital neuroma.

Prognosis. Responds well to conservative or surgical treatment.

BIBLIOGRAPHY. Durlacher L: A Treatise on Corns, Bunions and Diseases of Nails and the General Management of the Feet. London, Simpkin Marshall, 1845
Morton TG: Peculiar and painful affection of the fourth metatarsophalangeal articulation. Am J Med Sci 71:37–45, 1876
Alexander IJ, Johnson KA, Parr JW: Morton's neuroma: A review of recent concepts. Orthopedics 10:103–106, 1987
Reynolds JC: Morton's neuroma interdigital neuroma. In Gould JS: The Foot, p 101, 1991
Klippel JH, Dieppe PA: Rheumatology, pp 5.13.9–10, 5.19.10–11. St Louis, CV Mosby, 1995

MORVAN II

Synonyms. Analgesic paralysis; whitlow.

Symptoms and Signs. Progessive analgesia. Trophic lesions of digits; loss of soft tissue and resorption of phalanges. Muscular atrophy.

Etiology. Different types of lesions of the spinal cord (hereditary, sensory neuropathies; leprosy, Syringomyelia, etc.).

BIBLIOGRAPHY. Morvan AM: De la parésie analgésique à panaris des extrémités supérieures ou paréso-analgésiques des extrémités supérieures Gaz hebd méd. (Paris) 20:580–590, 624, 721, 1883

MORVAN III

Synonyms. Chorea fibrillaris; myoclonus multiplex fibrillaris. See also Chorea.

Symptoms and Signs. Attacks of chorea limited to calves and thighs, seldom involving the trunk.

Etiology. See Chorea.

BIBLIOGRAPHY. Morvan AM: De la chorée fibrillaire. Gaz Hebd Med 27:173–176, 1890

MOSCHCOWITZ

Synonyms. Baehr-Schiffrin; Upshaw factor deficiency; Schulman-Upshaw; hemolytic thrombocytopenic purpura; thrombohemolytic purpura; TTP; microangiopathic hemolytic anemia; hemolytic; uremic.

Symptoms. Prevalent in females; onset from infancy to old age; majority of cases 10–40 years of age. Constant fluctuation of neurologic symptoms: headache; mental changes; paresis; syncope; aphasia; dysarthria; visual changes; coma. Almost constant hemorrhagic manifestations: purpura; retinal hemorrhages; melena; hematemesis; hematuria. Less frequently observed: weakness; myalgia; arthralgia; nausea; vomiting.

Signs. Pallor; petechiae; ecchymosis; jaundice (not constant); moderate adenopathy; hepatomegaly (25%); splenomegaly (20%).

Etiology. Deficiency of a plasma factor (thrombopoietin-like substance). Defect in processing of a very large VIII: vWF multimers after synthesis and secretion by endothelial cells. Autosomal recessive inheritance postulated.

Pathology. Widespread hyaline occlusion (platelets and fibrin) of arterioles and capillaries; absence of inflammatory signs; rarely infarctions.

Diagnostic Procedures. *Blood.* Various degrees of thrombocytopenia; anemia occasionally very severe; reticulocytosis; presence of fragmented and altered cells (burr cells; helmet cells); accelerated red cell breakdown; hyperbilirubinemia. Coombs test negative; marked increase of leukocyte number (leukemoid reaction); azotemia. Biopsy revealing typical pattern (see Pathology). *Bone marrow.* Increased number of immature megakaryocytes and myeloid–erythroid hyperplasia. *Urine.* Proteinuria; hematuria; casts.

Therapy. Steroids and splenectomy of little or no benefit; conflicting reports with heparin. Dextran, aspirin, and dipyridamole reported useful. Excellent results reported with plasma transfusions, whole blood exchange and plasmapheresis, also in terminal cases. Following treatment neurologic manifestations and laboratory data are corrected within few hours

Prognosis. Progressive course; prior treatment with plasmapheresis 80% death in 3 months. Now with energetic treatment 80% of patients survive the initial episode.

BIBLIOGRAPHY. Moschcowitz E: Acute febrile pleiochromic anemia with hyaline thrombosis of terminal arterioles and capillaries: An undescribed disease. Arch Intern Med 36:89–93, 1925
Schulman I, Pierce M, Lukens A, et al: Studies on thrombopoiesis I. A factor in normal human plasma required for platelets production; chronic thrombocytopenia due to its deficiency. Blood 16:943–957, 1960
Upshaw JD: Congenital deficiency of a factor of normal plasma that reverses microangiopathic hemolysis and thrombocytopenia. N Engl J Med 298:1350–1352, 1978
Martin DL, MacDonald KL, White KE, et al: The epidemiology and clinical aspects of the hemolytic uremic syndrome in Minnesota. N Engl J Med 323:1161–1167, 1990
Bithell TC: Thrombotic thrombocytopenic purpura and other forms of nonimmunologic platelet destruction. In Lee GR, Bithell TC,

Foerster J, et al (eds): Wintrobe's Clinical Hematology, 9th ed, pp 1356–1360. Philadelphia, Lea & Febiger, 1993

MOSSE

Synonyms. Liver cirrhosis; polycythemia.

Symptoms and Signs. According to Mosse, polycythemic symptoms and signs appearing first, followed by clinical features of liver cirrhosis including splenomegaly.

Etiology. It is not established if this may be considered a pathologic entity or rather a simple coincidence. However, erythrocytosis is observed in 10% of hepatocellular carcinoma that usually develop in patients with liver cirrhosis.

Pathology. That of polycythemia vera and liver cirrhosis. Splenomegaly. Occlusion of hepatic vein in polycythemia (Budd-Chiari syndrome) frequently observed. Frequent evolution into hepatocellular carcinoma.

Diagnostic Procedures. *Blood.* Polycythemia; liver functions altered; low fibrinogen. *Bone marrow.* Hyperplasia. *Biopsy of liver.* Cirrhosis.

Therapy. That of polycythemia and cirrhosis, if tumor surgery.

Prognosis. Poorer than for simple polycythemia. Tumor death in few months.

BIBLIOGRAPHY. Mosse, M: Ueber Polycythemie mit Uroblinikterus und Milztumor. Dtsch Med Wochenschr 33:2175–2176, 1907
Athens JW, Lee GR: Polycythemia: Erythocytosis. In Lee GR, Bithell TC, Foerster J, et al (eds): Wintrobe's Clinical Hematology, 9th ed, p 1257. Philadelphia, Lea & Febiger, 1993

MOTION SENSITIVITY

Synonyms. Air sickness; kinetosis; motion sickness; naupathia.

Symptoms and Signs. Occurs in persons traveling in automobiles, trains, ships, or airplanes. Pallor; sweating; sialorrhea; nausea; vomiting. Prostration may follow when condition persists.

Etiology. Not clear. Familial aggregation reported. Labyrinth stimulation by motion, plus psychic factors. Visual and olfactory stimuli may play important part.

Therapy. Prophylaxis with many drugs; scopolamine, meclizine (Bonine), dimenhydrinate (Dramamine) given 30 minutes before starting trip. Avoiding the intake of fluid and eating only solid foods. Pure lemon juice taken immediately before trip often prevents vomiting. Nausea may be repelled by lying down with a firm support for the head, closing the eyes, and breathing fresh air. Exhaustion owing to prolonged vomiting cured by fluid replacement.

Prognosis. Symptoms disappear following termination of journey.

BIBLIOGRAPHY. Treisman M: Motion sickness: an evolutionary hypothesis. Science 197:493–495, 1977
Bia FJ, Barry M: Special health considerations for travelers. Med Clin North Am 76:1295, 1992
Weatherall DJ, Ledingham JGG, Warrell DA (eds): Oxford Textbook of Medicine, 3rd ed, pp 322, 1203, 1821. Oxford, Oxford Med Pub, 1996

MOTORCYCLE

Symptoms and Signs. In adolescence or less frequently in adult life. Unusual emotional investment in the motorcycle, accident proneness (frequent incidents) extending to early childhood. Motorcycle becames part of life dreams, and conscious and unconscious fantasies. Fear of physical injuries. Conflict with the father figure (usually competent and highly critical) and identification with mother; passivity and inability to compete; deficient self-image; poor control impulses; fear of involvement with aggressive girls; impotence and intense homosexual concerns.

Etiology. Ego defect deriving from poor father relationship. The motorcycle used to strenghten a fragile ego.

Therapy. Psychotherapy.

Prognosis. Highly prone to accidents.

BIBLIOGRAPHY. Nicoli AN Jr: The motocycle syndrome. Am J Psychiatr 126:1588–1595, 1970
Nicoli AM Jr: The adolescent. In The Harvard Guide to Modern Psychiatry. Cambridge, Belknap Press Harvard Univ Press, 1978

MOTOR-SCOOTER HANDLEBAR

Symptoms and Signs. Occurs usually in young subjects after falling from motor scooter. Evidence of trauma in the groin may or may not be present. Typical history of claudication of one leg developing soon after trauma.

Etiology and Pathology. Compression of external iliac with damage of the intima and reactive proliferation and occlusion of the vessel.

Diagnostic Procedures. Doppler. Femoral and distal arteries of involved leg not palpable. Lumbar aortography. Obstruction of vessel.

Therapy. If recognized early, simple arteriotomy; if recognized later, complicated bypass procedures necessary.

Prognosis. If unrecognized, spontaneous rupture may occur. Good with treatment.

BIBLIOGRAPHY. Deutsch V, Sinkover A, Bank H: The motor-scooter handlebar syndrome. Lancet II:1051–1053, 1968

MOUCHET

Eponym used to indicate the paralysis of the cubital nerve following fracture of external humeral condyle.

BIBLIOGRAPHY. Mouchet A: Paralyses tardives du nerfe cubital à suite de fractures du condyle externe de l'humerus. J Chir (Paris):437–456, 1914

MOULDED BABY

Synonyms. Watson; plagiocephaly; hip dislocation—scoliosis—bat ears—stenomastoid tumor.

Symptoms and Signs. From birth. Both sexes (prevalent females). Plagiocephaly (head moulding); torticollis; unilateral dislocation of hip; scoliotic convexity and sternomastoid tumor all tending to be on the same side and unilateral bat ears on the opposite one.

Etiology. Possibly owing to posture of the fetus into the uterus. No hereditary factors evidenced.

Diagnostic Procedures. *X-rays.* Pelvic obliquity; normal acetabula; with one hip in abduction and the other in adduction.

Therapy. Parents reassurance. Hip streching into abduction in flexion. Do not overtreat (splintage, plaster, immobilization, etc.).

Prognosis. Spontaneous resolution of hip disorder to complete normality before age 2.

BIBLIOGRAPHY. Watson GH: Relation between the side of plagiocephaly, dislocation of hip, scoliosis, bat ears and sternomastoid tumors. Arch Dis Child 46:203–210, 1971
Dunn PM: Congenital postural deformities. Br Med Bull 32:71–76, 1976

Good C, Walker G: The hip in the moulded baby syndrome. J Bone-Joint Surg (Br) 66:491–492, 1984

MOUNIER-KUHN

Synonyms. Bronchiectasis—ethmoid sinusitis; sinusitis—bronchiectasis; tracheobronchomegaly.

Symptoms. Predominant in males; onset in third to fourth decade. Symptoms indistinguishable from those of chronic bronchitis and ethmoiditis: cough; inability to expectorate.

Signs. On chest auscultation, harsh, rasping sounds.

Etiology. Unknown. Familial incidence of congenital malformation of the trachea, that leads to increased compliance of its own and of the bronchial walls.

Pathology. Cartilagineous and membranous parts of trachea and bronchi show thin atrophic muscular and elastic tissue; tracheobronchial collapse and signs of chronic infections.

Diagnostic Procedures. *X-ray of chest.* Increased caliber of trachea and bronchi; in lateral projection (especially) the air columns present corrugated aspect. Diagnosis is made when coronal diameter of trachea (measured 2 cm from projection of aortic arch) exceeds 30 mm. *Bronchoscopy.* Aspect may simulate multiple diverticula.

Therapy. Antibiotics. Fluidification. In some cases, surgery.

Prognosis. Variable. Repeated infections lead to respiratory insufficiency and pulmonary heart.

BIBLIOGRAPHY. Czyhlarz ER: Ueber in Pulsiondivertikel der Trachea mit Bemerkungen ueber das Verhalten der elastischen Fasern an normalen Tracheen und Bronchien Pathologie. Centralblatt Allg Pathol Anat 18:721, 1897
Mounier-Kuhn P: Dilatation de la trachée, constatations radiographiques et broncoscopiques. Lyon Med 150:106–109, 1932
Mounier-Kuhn P: Le syndrome "ethmoidoantrie et bronchiectasis." Clinique. Etiologie, Hypothèse. Pathogéniques. Ann d'Otolaryngol 12:387–404, 1945
Davis PB, Hubbard VS, McCoy K: Familial bronchiectasis. J Pediatr 102:177–185, 1983
Mildenberger P, Schild HH: Tracheobronchomegalie Der Radiologie 28:236– 238, 1988
Weatherall DJ, Ledingham JGG, Warrell DA (eds): Oxford Textbook of Medicine, 3rd ed, p 2724. Oxford, Oxford Med Pub, 1996

MOUNT-REBACK

Synonyms. Choreoathetosis, familial, paroxysmal; paroxysmal dystonic choreoathetosis.

Symptoms and Signs. Both sexes from first infancy choreic attacks lasting only few minutes, few times a day, without loss of consciousness. Hunger, fatigue, and later alcohol, coffee and tobacco are precipitating agents. Attacks may be preceded by aura.

Etiology. Autosomal dominant inheritance.

BIBLIOGRAPHY. Mount LA, Reback S: Familial paroxysmal choreoathetosis: Preliminary report on an hitherto undescribed clinical syndrome. Arch Neurol Psychat 44:841–847, 1940
Muller U, Kupke KG: The genetics of primary torsion dystonia. Hum Gen 84:107–115, 1990

MOYA-MOYA

Synonyms. Kawakita; Leed; Maki; Taveras; progressive arterial intracranial occlusions; intracranial arteries progressive occlusions.

Symptoms and Signs. Most cases in Japanese; a few black and Caucasian patients. Both sexes affected with slight female prevalence; onset from infancy to young adulthood, usually following some nonspecific infectious process or cold.

Paralysis and focal epileptic attacks, alternating between both sides, usually evidence onset of the condition, together with twitching, speech disturbances, unsteady gait, hemianopia, and headache. In some cases (especially in adults), psychiatric manifestations are prominent. These manifestations may be followed by signs of intracranial hemorrhage.

Etiology. Unknown. Considered a nonspecific inflammation owing to autoimmune reaction.

Pathology. Occlusion of distal internal carotid artery, proximal anterior, and middle cerebral arteries, and sometimes basilar and proximal posterior cerebral arteries. Absence of atherosclerotic changes.

Diagnostic Procedures. *X-ray of skull.* Usually normal. *Angiography.* Occlusion usually situated in internal carotid artery at its bifurcation; development of a large network of vessels in basal ganglia and upper brainstem areas from basilar artery and trunk of anterior and middle cerebral arteries. Marked degree of vascularization and visualization of rete mirabile. *CT brain scan. MRI.* Cerebral atrophy. *Spinal tap.* Occasionally, hemorrhagic.

Therapy. The first attempts at treatment were medical, seeking to increase blood flow pharmacologically, either by vasodilatation or reduction of blood viscosity. Today, surgical intervention is increasingly popular, and a variety of operations have been described, including cervical carotid sympathectomy and superior cervical ganglionectomy, intracranial transplantation of omentum or temporalis muscle with an intact vascular supply, direct superficial temporal artery-middle cerebral anastomosis and more recently, encephalo-duro-arterio synangiosis.

Prognosis. Serious progress to complete obstruction of most of major arterial network along base of brain that eventually stops spontaneously. Majority of patients survive with moderate or no disability. Mental retardation in one-third of children.

BIBLIOGRAPHY. Kawakita Y, Abe K, Miyata Y, et al: Spontaneous thrombosis of internal carotid artery in children. Folia Psychiatr Neurol Japn 19:245–255, 1965

Leed NE, Abbott KH: Collateral circulation in cerebrovascular disease in childhood via rete mirabile and perforating branches of anterior choroidal and posterior cerebral arteries. Radiology 85:628–634, 1965

Maki Y, Nakata Y: Autopsy case of hemangiomatous malformation of bilateral internal carotid artery at the base of brain. Brain Nerve (Tokyo) 17:764–766, 1965

Taveras JM: Multiple progressive intracranial arterial occlusion: A syndrome of children and young adults. Am J Roentgenol Rad Ther Nucl Med 106:235–268, 1969

Satoh S, Shibuya H, Matsushima Y, et al: Analysis of the angiographic findings in cases of childhood Moya Moya disease. Neuroradiology 30:111–119, 1988

MOYNAHAN I

Synonyms. Alopecia; epilepsy; oligophrenia; epilepsy—alopecia—oligophrenia.

Symptoms and Signs. Both sexes. At birth alopecia (delay in the growth of hair for two 4 years); seizures; mental retardation. In same cases microcephaly.

Etiology. Possibly autosomal recessive inheritance.

Diagnostic procedures. *EEG.* Unusual patterns.

Prognosis. Hair may grow at 2–4 years of age.

BIBLIOGRAPHY. Moynahan EJ: Familial congenital alopecia, epilepsy, mental retardation with unusual electroencephalograms. Proc Roy Soc Med 55:411–412, 1962

van Haeringen A, Hurst JA, Savidge R, et al: A familial syndrome of microcephaly, sparse hair, mental retardation and seizures. J Med Genet 27:127–129, 1990

MOYNAHAN II

Synonym. XTE. See Rapp-Hodgkin.

Symptoms and Signs. Cleft palate; hypohidrosis; defective enamel; nail anomalies; hair coarse and dry; absence of eyelashes of lower lid; short-lasting skin bullae.

Etiology. Unknown; autosomal dominant inheritance.

BIBLIOGRAPHY. Moynahan EJ: X.T.E. (Xeroderma, talipes, and enamel defect). A new heredo-familial syndrome. Two cases. Homozygous inheritance of a dominant gene. Proc Roy Soc Med 63:447–448, 1970

MSILINI JOINT

Symptoms and Signs. In Southern Africans; female prevalence onset before age 40. In children and adolescents, initial deformities also may be seen. Slowly progressing disability from hip joint and/or knee and/or ankle joint deformities.

Etiology. Unknown.

Diagnostic Procedures. *Blood.* Usually normal; occasionally alkaline phosphatase low and phosphates slightly reduced. *X-ray.* Deformity and medial subluxation of femoral head. Altogether, changes are reminiscent of osteoarthritis.

Prognosis. Slow progression.

BIBLIOGRAPHY. Yach D, Botha JL: Msilini joint disease in 1981 decreased prevalence rates, wider geographical location than before and socioeconomic impact of and endemic ostheoarthrosis in an underdeveloped community in South Africa. Int J Epidemiol 14:276–284, 1985

MUCHA-HABERMANN

Synonyms. Wise; parapsoriasis guttata; parapsoriasis varioliformis; pityriasis lichenoides—varioliformis; varicelliform parapsoriasis; lymphomatoid papulosis.

Symptoms and Signs. Prevalent in men (70%); onset in adolescence and adulthood; seldom in childhood. (In childhood, acute form prevalent; in other ages chronic form more usual). *Acute.* Mild systemic manifestations occasionally may precede by 2 or 3 days; eruptions; fever; malaise; headache; joint swelling; arthralgia. Crops of edematous pinkish papules with central vesiculation and hemorrhagic necrosis evolving to superficial crusting or to scarring ulcerations. Moderate burning, or no symptoms with eruptions. Trunk, thighs, flexor sides of upper arms preferred zones; generalized form involving occasionally also palms and soles. Face and scalp usually spared. *Chronic.* Small lichenoid papules, brownish color, scaling, leaving shining brown surface. Scarring seldom. Leukoderma transitory or (seldom) permanent may follow both acute and chronic forms.

Etiology. Unknown; possibly virus or allergic vasculitis.

Pathology. Variable according to form and stage. Early lymphocyte infiltration; dilated capillaries with endothelial proliferation. Necrotic changes. Chronic similar to resolving eczema or psoriasis.

Diagnostic Procedures. *Blood.* Exclude syphilis. *Biopsy of skin.*

Therapy. No specific treatment. *Acute.* Systemic steroids. *Chronic.* Ultraviolet light, tar preparations; or no treatment. Tetracycline, erythromycin long term, PUVA have been proposed.

Prognosis. *Acute.* New crops stop appearing after a few weeks. Most cases clear in 6 months; others recur for years. *Chronic.* Scaling for 3–4 weeks; then clearing. Recurrence of new manifestations for years.

BIBLIOGRAPHY. Mucha V: Ueber einen der Parakeratosis variegata (Unna) bzw. Pityriasis lichenoides chronica (Neisser-Juliusberg) nahestehenden eigentüflmlichen Fall. Arch Derm Syph 123:586–592, 1916

Habermann R: Ueber die akut verlaufende, nekrotisier ende Unterart der Pityriasis lichenoides (Pityriasis lichenoides et varioliformis acuta). Dermatol Z 45:42–48, 1925

Ryan TJ: Cutaneous vasculitis. In Champion RH, Burton JL, Ebling FJG (eds): Rook/Wilkinson/Ebling Textbook of Dermatology. Oxford, Blackwell Scientific, 5th ed, pp 1957–1958, 1992

MUCKLE-WELLS

Synonym. Amyloidosis—deafness—urticaria—limb pain; deafness—amyloidosis—urticaria—limb pain.

Symptoms and Signs. Both sexes affected; onset in adolescence. Recurrent attacks of urticaria-like rash, with systemic manifestations; paresthesia; limb pain (ague-like bouts); pain; progressive perceptive deafness; premature loss of libido with relative infertility. Associated physical malformation: pes cavus; skin thickening; glaucoma. Nephrotic syndrome appears in middle age: forme fruste with one or more features missing.

Etiology. Unknown. Autosomal dominant inheritance.

Pathology. Kidney small, shriveled; adherent capsules; narrowed cortex; poor corticomedullary demarcation. Temporal bone section shows complete absence of Corti's organ and vestibular sensory epithelium; atrophy of cochlear nerve; amyloidosis.

Diagnostic Procedures. *Blood.* High sedmentation rate; polycythemia. *Urine.* Trace of reducing substances; hyperglycinuria.

Therapy. Symptomatic. Trial with colchicine seems indicated.

Prognosis. Progressive, ending in uremia.

BIBLIOGRAPHY. Muckle TJ, Wells M: Urticaria, deafness and amyloidosis: A new hetero-familial syndrome. Q J Med 31:235–248, 1962

Benson MD, Amyloidosis. In Scriver CR, Beaudet AL, Sly WS, et al: The Metabolic and Molecular Bases of Inherited Disease, 7th ed, p 4180. New York, McGraw-Hill, 1995

MUELLER-KUGELBERG

Synonyms. Myopathy—Cushing; steroid myopathy; corticosteroid myopathy. See Perkoff.

Symptoms and Signs. Insidious onset years after the first manifestations of the endocrine disorder, Cushing syndrome. Weakness of the pelvic girdle and thighs, minor in legs and shoulders.

Etiology. Excessive corticosteroids cause atrophy of muscle fibers.

Pathology. Muscle fiber degeneration and hyalinization. Increased fat content of muscles.

Diagnostic Procedures. *Biopsy of muscle.* See Pathology. *Electromyography.* Decreased duration and voltage; no fibrillation or pronounced irritability.

Therapy. Removal of adrenocortical tumor.

Prognosis. Complete recession of symptoms after tumor excision.

BIBLIOGRAPHY. Mueller R, Kugelberg E: Myopathy in Cushing's syndrome. J Neurol Neurosurg Psychiatr 32:314–320, 1959

Adams RD, Victor M: Principles of Neurology, 5th ed, pp 1235–1236. New York, McGraw-Hill, 1993

MUELLER-WEISS

Synonym. Os naviculare pedis malacia. See Epiphyseal ischemic necrosis.

Symptoms. Pain in the feet enhanced by ambulation, or asymptomatic.

Etiology. Unknown.

Pathology. Symmetric malacia of os naviculare pedis.

BIBLIOGRAPHY. Mueller W: Ueber eine eigenartige doppelseitige Veraenderung des Os naviculare pedis beim Erwachsenen. Dtsch Z Chir 201:84–87, 1927

Weiss K: Ueber die "Malazie" des Os naviculare pedis. Fortschr Roentgenol 45:63–67, 1927

MUENZER-ROSENTHAL

Eponym used to indicate the triad of hallucination, anxiety, catalepsy that may be found in several psychotic disorders.

BIBLIOGRAPHY. Muenzer ET: Zur Frage der symptomatischen Narkolepsie nach Enzephalitis lethargica. Mschr Psychiatr Neurol 63:97–111, 1927

Rosenthal C: Ueber das Auftreten von halluzinatorisch-kataleptischem Angstsydrom, Wachanfaellen und ählichen Storerungen bei Schizophrenen. Mschr Psychiatr Neurol 102:11–38, 1939

MULTICENTRIC RETICULOHISTIOCYTOSIS

Synonyms. Lipoid dermatoarthritis; reticulocytoma cutis.

Symptoms and Signs. Prevalent in females (3:1); all races affected; age of onset from second to tenth decade. Gradual development of nodules in skin, mucosae, subcutaneous tissues, synovia, periostium, and bone, resulting in deforming polyarthritis. In about 25%, nodules and arthritis appear simultaneously; in 60% arthritis precedes the nodules by months or years; seldom, nodules precede arthritis. Other symptoms: weight loss; pruritus; weakness; fever; paresthesias; xanthelasma (40%): hypertension (27%); lymphadenopathy (16%); malignant neoplasms (28%).

Etiology. Unknown. Granulomatous histiocytic reaction to unidentified stimulus; association with malignancies (28%) unknown if genetic or casual: very likely a paraneoplastic process since it improves with the successful treatment of associated neoplasm when this is detected.

Pathology. Nodular lesions: finely vacuolated histiocytes close to small blood vessels; lymphocytes and plasma cells dispersed in the nodules; multinucleated giant cells with small vacuoles and eccentric nuclei with one or two large nucleoli. Vacuoli stained by oil red (partially). Destructive arthritis.

Diagnostic Procedures. *Blood.* Hyperlipemia; all fractions increased; high beta lipoprotein. *Biopsy. X-ray.*

Therapy. Trial with adrenocorticotropic hormone (ACTH) nitrogen mustard, chlorambucil, hydroxychloroquine. Cyclophosphamide seems to bring better results. Surgery.

Prognosis. Disease may become spontaneously inactive after 10 years and nodules become stable or decrease. Patients usually are left crippled by arthritis and with leonine facies.

BIBLIOGRAPHY. Targett JH: Giant cell tumours of the integuments. Trans Pathol Soc (London) 48:230–255, 1897

Parkes-Weber F, Freudenthal W: Nodular non-diabetic cutaneous xanthomatosis with hypercholesterolemia and typical histologic features. Proc Roy Soc Med 30:522–526, 1937

Nunnink JC: Multicentric reticulohistiocytosis and cancer: A case report and review of the literature. Med Pediat Oncol 13:273–279, 1985

Hess CE: Hairy cell leukemia, malignant histiocytosis, and related disorders. In Lee GR, Bithell TC, Foerster J, et al (eds): Wintrobe's Clinical Hematology, 9th ed, p 2192. Philadelphia, Lea & Febiger, 1993

MULTICORE-MINICORE MYOPATHY

Synonyms. See minicore myopathy.

Symptoms and Signs. See Shy-Magee. Arms and legs more affected. Mild facial muscle weakness, external ophthalmoplegia scolions, and seldom cardiomyopathy.

Etiology. Both autosomal dominant and recessive inheritance described.

Pathology. Nonspecific features of congenital myopathies (see Shy-Magee, type I fiber predominance and type I fiber atrophy, multi- and minicores (see Shy-Magee). Z-band streaming. Loss of mitochondria of glycogen and sarcotubular systems.

Diagnostic Procedures. *EMG. Muscle biopsy. Blood enzymes.*

Therapy. None.

Prognosis. Favorable, however, clinical deterioration may occur.

BIBLIOGRAPHY. Engel AG, Gomez MR, Grover RV: Multicore disease—a recognized congenital myopathy associated with multifocal degeneration of muscle fibers. Proc Mayo Clin 46:661–681, 1971
Vanneste JAL, Stam FC: Autosomal dominant multicore disease. J Neurol Neurosurg Psychiatr 45:360–365, 1982
Goebel HH, Lenard HG: Congenital myopathies. In Rowland LP, Di Mauro S (eds): Handbook of Clinical Neurology, vol 18: Myopathies, p 331. Amsterdam, Elsevier, 1992

MULTIFIDUS TRIANGLE

Symptoms. Single or, more frequently, recurrent attacks of sharp, localized pain followed by persistent discomfort below posterior superior iliac spine, often initiated by physical exercise (bending and twisting of lumbar spine).

Signs. Point of localized tenderness; pressure on trigger point increases pain and causes typical radiation.

Etiology and Pathology. Deep liagmentous or myofascial injury, exacerbated by trauma, inflammations. The area involved is referred to as the multifidus triangle (inferior portion of multifidus muscle).

Diagnostic Procedure. *X-ray of spine.*

Therapy. Injection of procaine or corticosteriods at trigger point.

Prognosis. Majority of attacks cured by a single injection at trigger point.

BIBLIOGRAPHY. Livingston WK: Back disabilities due to strain of multifidus muscle: Cases treated by novocain injection. West J Surg 49:259–265, 1941
Bauwens P, Coyer AB: The "multifidus triangle" syndrome as a cause of recurrent low-back pain. Br Med J 2:1306–1307, 1955
Weatherall DJ, Ledingham JGG, Warrell DA (eds): Oxford Textbook of Medicine, 3rd ed, p 3148. Oxford, Oxford Med Pub, 1996

MULTIPLE ENDOCRINE NEOPLASIA II SYNDROMES

Synonyms. Familial chromaffinomatosis; MEN II; multiple neuroma; pheochromocytoma; thyroid medullary carcinoma; including Sipple and William-Pollock. Today the MEN II is subdivided in various subsyndromes:

FMTC: familial medullarythyroid carcinoma without pheochrocytoma; in some cases development of parathyroid hyperplasia or tumors

CLASSICAL MEN IIA (Sipple): medullary thyroid carcinoma and pheochromocytoma both frequently bilateral

MEN IIA: cutaneous lichen amyloidosis

MEN IIB (Williams-Pollock): medullary thyroid carcinoma with pheochromocytoma, multiple mucosal neuromas, intestinal ganglioneuromatosis, marfanoid habitus, muscular weakness, high arched palate, pes cavus, and various other abnormalities.

Symptoms and Signs. Both sexes affected. The symptoms and signs in the subsyndromes depend on the various tumors and their phases of development, the eventual predominance of one of them, and of the associated lesions in different stages of evolution.

Familial medullary thyroid carcinoma only (FMTC): diarrhea may be presenting complaint, from minor to severe; the ectopic ACTH syndrome (see) is frequently associated. Early phase hyperparathyroidism and its typical clinical manifestations seldom are present (considered a variant of MEN IIA).

MEN IIA

See preceding plus symptoms related to presence of pheochromocytoma: clinically detectable in approx 50% of cases (larger percentage show presence of the tumor at autopsy): marked palpitations, tachycardia, and nervousness with lack of hypertension in early phase.

MEN IIB

Etiology. Clinically may be considered a different syndrome, but some overlap exists. As a mechanism for the development of neoplasias it is considered the clonal expansion of C-cells within the various glands affected. Causes leading to hyperplasia are considered to be: point mutations of the RET protooncogene and other events leading to the neoplastic transformation. Autosomal dominant inheritance.

Pathology. Medullary carcinoma of thyroid: group of cells varying in size and shape from small and round, to large ovoid or spindle cells, sometimes palisaded, indistinct cellular outline, scanty cytoplasm. In all cases amyloid is found in various amounts up to the point of dominating the pattern, or to exclude cellular elements. Metastasis to cervical nodes in two thirds of the cases and distant sites in one third. Pheochromocytoma frequently bilateral, seldom malignant.

Diagnostic Procedures. *Radioactive iodine uptake.* Studies for pheochromocytoma (see).

Therapy. Surgery. Chemotherapy.

Prognosis. Patient with medullary carcinoma of thyroid or pheochromocytoma should be followed for development of other lesions or manifestations of the syndrome.

BIBLIOGRAPHY. Eisenberg AA, Wallerstein H: Pheochromocytoma of the suprarenal medulla (paraganglioma): Clinicopathological study. Arch Pathol 14:818–836, 1932
Beer EC, King FM, Prinzmetal M: Pheochromocytoma with demonstration of pressor (adrenalin) substances in the blood preoperatively during hypertensive crises. Ann Surg 106:85–91, 1937
Sipple JH: The association of pheochromocytoma with carcinoma of the thyroid gland. Am J Med 31:163–166, 1961
Williams ED: Medullary carcinoma of the thyroid. In De Groot LJ (ed): Endocrinology, 3rd ed, p 863. Philadelphia, WB Saunders, 1995
Gagel RF: Multiple endocrine neoplasia type 2. In De Groot LJ (ed): Endocrinology, 3rd ed, pp 2835–2836. Philadelphia, WB Saunders, 1995

MULTIPLE ENDOCRINE NEOPLASIA IIB

Synonyms. Williams-Pollock; MEN III; neuromata—mucosal endocrine tumors; mucosal neuroma. See also Wermer and Sipple.

Symptoms and Signs. Both sexes equally affected. May be present at birth or develop later. Fifty percent show complete syndrome of multiple neuromas (lips; tongue; eyelids), bumpy lips, pheochromocytoma, and medullary carcinoma; 7% show neuromas, pheochromocytoma, and medullary carcinoma; the others exhibit variable combinations of the preceding, without the pheochromocytoma. Some patients have diarrhea. Marfanoid habitus in about 50% of patients.

Etiology. Mutation in a gene controlling a papacrine growth factor possibly responsible for this condition; autosomal dominant inheritance demonstrated in some cases. MEN III (IIB) has been separated from the MEN IIA because of low incidence of associated parathyroid disease in these cases.

Pathology. Neuromas: masses of convoluted nerves, enveloped by thick perineurium; absence of capsule; less connective tissue than in von Recklinghausen (see). For features of other neoplasias, see Wermer and Sipple.

Therapy. Surgical excision when indicated and feasible.

Prognosis. Poor.

BIBLIOGRAPHY. Braley AE: Medullated corneal nerves and plexiform neuroma associated with pheocromocytomata. Trans Am Ophthal Soc 52:189–197, 1954

Williams ED, Pollock DJ: Multiple mucosal neuromata with endocine tumors: A syndrome allied to von Reckinghauser's disease. J Pathol Bacteriol 91:71–80, 1966

Fryns JP, Chrzanowska K: Mucosal neuromata syndrome (MEN type IIb [III]). J Med Genet 25:703–706, 1988

Gagel RF: Multiple endocrine neoplasia type 2. In De Groot LJ (ed): Endocrinology, 3rd ed, pp 2835–2836. Philadelphia, WB Saunders, 1995

MULTIPLE ORGAN FAILURE

Synonyms. M.O.F.; post-traumatic septic; hypermetabolism; organ failure complex; gut origin septic states; M.O.D.S. multiple organ dysfunction.

Symptoms and Signs. In patients with sepsis or in prolonged state of shock. Fever (or hypothermia or normothermia), progressive failure of several organs (or dysfunction), i.e., lungs, heart, kidney, liver, pancreas, gastrointestinal tract, brain, bone marrow, clotting system, etc.

Etiology. Exact mechanisms leading to individual organ failure are not known—endotoxin, cellular injury, impaired organ perfusion, neuroumoral and metabolic responses likely play a major role. Stress ulceration, acidosis, diffuse intravascular coagulation are at the same time main complications and contributing factors.

Diagnostic Procedures. *Blood.* Acid-base balance, rheology, hypebilirubinemia, evaluation of metabolic status and kidney function. *Urine.* Oliguria. *X-ray. CT scan. MRI.* Lung (typical pattern). *ECG.* Hemodynamic evaluation.

Therapy. Ventilatory assistance; treatment of infection. Antibiotics and immunotherapy, prevention and treatment of kidney failure, treatment of hemodynamic failure and acidosis, restoration of clotting factors, cytoprotection of gastric mucosa, parentaral alimentation.

Prognosis. Poor. Thirty percent or higher mortality with optimal treatment.

BIBLIOGRAPHY. Burke JF, Pontoppidan H, Welch CE: High output respiratory failure: An important cause of death ascribed to peritonitis or ileus. Ann Surg 158:581–595, 1963

Eiseman B, Beart R, Norton L: Multiple organ failure. Surg Gynecol Obstet 144:323–326, 1977

Taylor RW: Sepsis, sepsis syndrome, and septic schock. In Civetta JM, Taylor RW, Kirby RR (eds): Critical Care, 2nd ed. Philadelphia, JB Lippincott, 1992

Baue AE: What's in a name? An acronym or a response. Am J Surg 165:299–301, 1993

MULTIPLE SCLEROSIS

Synonyms. MS; disseminated sclerosis; insular sclerosis; sclerosis, multiple; sclerose en plaques.

Symptoms. Prevalent in females; onset difficult to identify, usually between 20 and 40 years of age. Increasing risk with increase in latitude. Precipitating factors (?): infection, trauma, and pregnancy. Variable; multiple combinations of symptoms may represent the initial episode; because of their occasional mildness and spontaneous remission they may be forgotten or not associated with the disease. Unilateral blurring of vision; pain of the eye at rest; remission and recurrences typical, eventually resulting in central and paracentral scotoma. Attacks of double vision; trigeminal neuralgia; attacks of vertigo; intentional tremor (usually later manifestation); speech changes (usually later): slurring; long pause; monotony. Spastic paresis (80% of cases) starting with weakness, usually in legs, and "jumping of legs" at night or before falling asleep. Hemiplegia attacks; mild sensory changes; bladder disorders. Mental symptoms: deterioration; depression; hypomania; euphoria (most common symptom). Several variants of MS may occur with specific course and type of clinical findings: Schilder (see), Devic (see), acute multiple sclerosis (acute course with possible death in weeks or months); MS and peripheral neuropathy.

Signs. In eyes; optic disk normal or moderately hyperhemic or abnormal temporal pallor (occasional); pupillary reaction normal; nystagmus. Pathologic reflexes; abdominal reflexes absent. Atrophy of muscles (rare).

Etiology. Unknown. Very likely more than one disease included under this heading. Possibly, toxic viral, allergic, or metabolic factors. Importance of environmental factors not specified yet. Familial cases reported (5% observed in siblings) without definite genetic pattern.

Pathology. Large gray-yellowish areas, consistency soft or firm, scattered throughout neuraxis from optic (II) nerve to conus medullaris, particularly in white matter. Microscopically, plaques of demyelination scattered with no perivascular distribution, and edema. In old lesion, fragmentation and destruction of axons. In recent lesion, axons are intact, microglial reaction, phagocytic cells laden with fat, perivascular round cell infiltration.

Diagnostic Procedures. *Blood. Urine.* Normal. *Cerebrospinal fluid.* Lumbar puncture adverse effect. Occasionally, increased total proteins. IgG index: ratio over 1:7. Moderate pleocytosis. *EEG.* Nonspecific changes in acute stage (90%), in subacute (68%), in remission (33%). *CT scan. MRI.* May reveal asymptomatic plaques.

Therapy. No specific treatment. Symptomatic, physical therapy, good nutrition, and vitamins. Some beneficial effect with ACTH and corticosteroids. Hyperbaric oxygen of some benefit, especially in early stage. Experimentally, azathioprine, cyclophosphamide, and total lymphoid irradiation may improve condition.

Prognosis. Remission and relapses, usually with downhill course, characterize the disease. Years of well-being may follow any episode. Benign form with early arrest and clinically silent forms reported. Average survival 10–20 years from initial episode (except in benign form). In late onset (over 40), faster evolution and shorter length of survival.

BIBLIOGRAPHY. Cruveilhier J: Anatomie pathologique du corps humain, ou descriptions avec figures lithographiées et coloriées, des diverses alterations morbides dont le corps humain est susceptible, vol 2. Paris, Baillière, 1829–1852

Mackay RP, Hirano A: Forms of benign multiple sclerosis: Report of two "clinically silent" cases discovered at autopsy. Arch Neurol 17:588–600, 1967

Mussini JM: Sclérose en plaques. Encyclop Méd Chir Paris Neurol Fasc 17074 B–10 (3–1978)

Adams RD, Victor M: Principles of Neurology, 5th ed, pp 777–790. New York, McGraw-Hill, 1993

MULTIPLE SYNOSTOSIS

Synonyms. Synostosis tarsal—carpal—digital.

Symptoms and Signs. From birth. Both sexes. Carpal and tarsal synostoses (coalition) radial head subluxation; aplasia or hypoplasia of middle phalanges and metacarpophalangeal and metacarpophalangeal synostoses.

Etiology. Autosomal dominant inheritance.

BIBLIOGRAPHY. Pearlman HS, Edkin RE, Warren RF: Familial tarsal and carpal synostosis with radial-head subluxation (Nievergelt's syndrome). J Bone Joint Surg 46A:585–592, 1964
Da-Silva ED, Filho SM, Albuquerque SC: Multiple synostosis syndrome: study of a large Brazilian kindred. Am J Med Genet 18:237–247, 1984

MÜNCHHAUSEN

Synonyms. Baron Münchhausen; fictitious chronic; hospital addiction; hospital hoboes; hysterical malingering; peregrinating problem patient.

Symptoms. Male-to-female ratio, 3:1; age range 19–62 (mean 39). Subject feigns severe illness of dramatic or emergency nature; pathologic lying; aggressive, truculent, and at the same time evasive behavior; departure from hospital against medical advice; history of many hospital admissions and extensive traveling; police record and borderline drug addiction.

Signs. Evidence of many previous surgical procedures; laparotomies; cranial burr holes; evidence of interference with diagnostic procedures and self-mutilation.

Etiology. Psychopathologic entity distinct from vagrancy, self-mutilation, and malingering, but including all features of these conditions; stemming from antisocial personality, neurosis, brain damage, or unknown causes.

Pathology. Resulting from iatrogenic procedures or self-inflicted.

Diagnostic Procedures. Hypnosis may be useful to elucidate repressed affect or memories.

Therapy. No cure reported. Sympathetic attitude toward patient; long-term supervision, psychotherapy, and institutionalization.

Prognosis. Patient may die of iatrogenic procedures, suicide, intercurrent real diseases; or, losing vitality, abandon hospital addiction.

BIBLIOGRAPHY. Asher R: Münchausen's syndrome. Lancet I:339–341, 1951
De Francisci G, Parisi N, Magalini SI: La sindrome di Münchausen. Il Policlinico, sez med 88:292–303, 1981
Schwegler U, Krengel HG, Kuntz HD, et al: Muenhhausen-Syndrom. Med Welt 36:1439–1442, 1985
Weatherall DJ, Ledingham JGG, Warrell DA (eds): Oxford Textbook of Medicine, 3rd ed, pp 4211, 4258. Oxford, Oxford Med Pub, 1996

MURCHISON-PEL-EBSTEIN FEVER

Synonyms. Murchison-Saunderson; Pel-Ebstein fever.

Symptoms. Observed more frequently in children than in adults. Relapsing fever; intermittent periods of normal or subnormal temperature. Cycles of various length, usually 15–28 days, varying from patient to patient, but constant in the same patient. Sweats usually associated with pyrexia. Weakness and fatigue often out of proportion to extent of disease or anemia; weight loss.

Signs. Pulse rate usually slightly higher than expected from temperature. If lymph nodes are present, increase in size during febrile episode observed.

Etiology and Pathology. This syndrome is observed in the majority of cases associated with Hodgkin syndrome (see); occasionally observed also with reticular cell sarcoma, some cases of malignant nephroma, other necrotic tumors, or tuberculosis.

Diagnostic Procedures. *X-ray of chest, abdomen. Skin test.* For tuberculosis. *Biopsy.* Of lymph node.

Therapy. Good remission with chemotherapy (nitrogen mustard or similar agent) or radiation therapy when associated with Hodgkin disease. Cortisone and adrenocorticotropic hormone (ACTH) also control the temperature.

Prognosis. That of the disease responsible.

BIBLIOGRAPHY. Murchison C: Case of "lymphoadenoma" of the lymphatic system, etc. Trans Pathol Soc (London) 21:372–389, 1870
Pel PK: Zur Symptomatologie der sogenannten Pseudo-Leukamie. Berl Klin Wochenschr 22:3–7, 1885
Ebstein W: Das chronische Rückfallsfieber, eine neue Infektionskrankheit. Berl Klin Wochenschr 24:565; 837, 1887

MURRI

Synonyms. Presenile ataxia cerebellaris; parenchymatous cortical cerebellum degeneration; presenile cerebellar ataxia; toxic cerebellar degeneration. See Holmes I.

Symptoms. Prevalent in males; gradual onset in the fourth to seventh decade. Difficulty in walking. Manifestation usually remains localized to legs; occasionally spreads to trunk and arms.

Signs. Hyperreflexia (occasionally); usually, absence of nystagmus.

Etiology. Uncertain; toxic factor (primarily alcohol); heart; stroke; malignancy; chronic gastrointestinal diseases; hereditary familial trait; subacute form reported with Hodgkin. Question of nutritional cause considered.

Pathology. Cerebellar atrophy: loss of Purkinje cells and preservation of basket cells; granular and molecular layer of cerebellum sparse.

Diagnostic Procedures. *EEG. Angiography. Echoencephalography. Brain isotope scan. CSF.* Increase in protein; lymphocytic pleocytosis. *CAT and MRI brain scan.*

Therapy. Symptomatic.

Prognosis. Progressive course 1–15 years. Spontaneous arrest occasionally observed, especially if patient abstains from alcohol. In idiopathic form, subacute or chronic course.

BIBLIOGRAPHY. Murri A: Degeneratione cerebellare da intossicazione endogena. Riv Crit Clin Med 1:593; 609, 1900
Adams RD, Victor M: Principles of Neurology, 5th ed, pp 868–870. New York, McGraw-Hill, 1993

MUSCLE PHOSPHOGLYCERATE KINASE DEFICIENCY

Synonyms. PGK deficiency, glycogenosis type IX.

Symptoms and Signs. Condition in more evident in males. From clinically silent to hemolytic anemia. Usually, seizures; mental retardation. Rarely, myopathy with cramps; intolerance to exercise.

Etiology. X-linked recessive. Locus Xq13. Different nonfunctioning variants of enzyme are known. Defect of anaerobic glycolysis.

Pathology. Muscle: normal.

Diagnostic Procedures. *Urine.* Myoglobinuria. *Blood.* CK increased, signs of hemolytic anemia.

Therapy. Symptomatic.

Prognosis. Death in early age.

BIBLIOGRAPHY. Rosa R, George C, Fardeau M, et al: A new case of phosphoglycerate kinase deficiency. PGK Creteil associated with rhabdomyolysis and lacking hemolytic anemia. Blood 60:84–91, 1982

Guis MS, Karadsheh N, Mentzer WC: Phosphoglycerate kinase San Francisco: A new variant associated with hemolytic anemia but not with neuromuscular manifestations. Am J Hemat 25:175–182, 1987

MUSCLE PHOSPHOGLYCERATE MUTASE DEFICIENCY

Synonyms. Deficiency of M subunits of PGAM, PGAM-M deficiency; glycogenosis, type X.

Symptoms and Signs. Both sexes. In adults, intolerance for exercise, cramps.

Etiology. Isolated defect of PGAM owing to defect of muscle (MM) subunits. Residual activity is owing to brain (BB) subunits. Autosomal recessive. Gene defect probably on chromosome 7.

Pathology. Muscle: normal or patchy glycogen storage therapy.

Diagnostic Procedures. *Urine.* Recurrent myoglobinuria. *Blood.* Ischemic exercise: low rise of venous lactate.

Therapy. Symptomatic.

Prognosis. Stable condition.

BIBLIOGRAPHY. Di Mauro S, Miranda AF, Kahn S, et al: Human muscle phosphoglycerate mutase deficiency: A newly discovered metabolic myopathy. Science 212:1277–1279, 1981

Vita G, Toscano A, Bresolin N, et al: Muscle phosphoglycerate mutase (PGAM) deficiency in the first Caucasian patient. Neurology 40:297, 1990

Chen YT, Burchell A: Glycogen storage diseases. In Scriver CR, Beaudet AL, Sly WS, et al: The Metabolic and Molecular Bases of Inherited Disease, 7th ed, p 936. New York, McGraw-Hill, 1995

MUSCULAR DYSTROPHY, LATE ONSET DISTAL NONAKA TYPE

Synonyms. Nonaka type muscolar dystrophy; myopathy Japanese type, late onset distal; autosomal recessive distal muscular dystrophy; ARDMD.

Symptoms and Signs. In Japanese. Onset in second to third decade. Difficulty in running, tendency to fall, difficulty in toe walking (vs heal walking difficulty in other distal myopathies). After some time or contemporarily mild forearm wasting and weakness. Cranial and respiratory muscles spared.

Etiology. Autosomal recessive inheritance.

Diagnostic Procedures. *Muscle biopsy.* Rimmed vacuoles in type I and II fibers. *Electromicroscopy.* Demonstrates numerous intracytoplasmatic vacuoles with lamellar bodies.

Therapy. None. Corticosteroids guarantee some improvement.

Prognosis. In 15 years patient becomes bedridden.

BIBLIOGRAPHY. Miyoski K, Saijo K, Kuru T, et al: Four cases of distal myopathy in two families. Jpn J Human Genet 12:113, 1967

Nonaka I, Sunohara N, Ishiura S, et al: Familial distal myopathy with rimmed vacuole and lamellar (myeloid) body formation. I Neurol Sci 51:141–155, 1981

Isaacs H, Badenhorst ME, Whistler T: Autosomal recessive myopathy. J Clin Pathol 41:188–194, 1988

Buchman AS, Coehran EJ: Distal myopathies. In Rowland LP, Di Mauro S: Handbook of Clinical Neurology, vol 18, p 197. Elsevier, Amsterdam, 1992

MUSCULAR DYSTROPHY, PROXIMAL, AUTOSOMAL DOMINANT, LATE ONSET TYPE

Synonyms. Muscular dystrophy limb girdl; LGMD1.

Symptoms and Signs. From late second decade, progressive weakness of limb girdle muscles. More frequent and earlier involvement of pelvis femoral muscles than scapulohomeral.

Etiology. Autosomal dominant inheritance. Suggest linkage with Pelger-Huet anomaly (may be caused by a gene defect mapped to 5 q).

Diagnostic Procedures. *EMG.* Not reported. *Blood.* Serum creatinine kinase may be elevated.

Therapy. None.

Prognosis. Good quoad vitam.

BIBLIOGRAPHY. Schneidermann LJ, Sampson WI, Schoene W, et al: Genetic studies of a family with two unusual autosomal dominant conditions: Muscular dystrophy and Pelger-Huet anomaly. Am J Med 46:380–393, 1969

Gilchrist JM, Pericak-Vance M, Silverman L, et al: Clinical and genetic investigations in autosomal dominant limb-girdle muscular dystrophy. Neurology 38:3–9, 1988

MUSCULOAPONEUROTIC FIBROMATOSIS

Synonym. Desmoid tumor.

Symptoms and Signs. Prevalent in women (70%); onset in third to fifth decade, frequently after pregnancy. Tender, firm, subcutaneous mass usually arising from muscular aponeurosis of lower abdominal wall, and progressively spreading.

Etiology. Unknown. Possibly, trauma, endocrine factors. Reported in association with Gardner (see).

Pathology. Gray-white, not encapsulated, consistent mass that invades the muscle. Histologically, fibroblast proliferation and infiltration, areas of mucoid degeneration.

Diagnostic Procedures. *Biopsy. Bioassay.* Could reveal elevated levels of estrogenic and gonadotropic hormones.

Therapy. Wide surgical excision.

Prognosis. Cured by surgery. No metastasis.

BIBLIOGRAPHY. Thorbjarnarson B, Pack GT, et al (eds): Treatment of Cancer and Allied Diseases, vol 8. New York, Hoeber, 1964

Reitamo JJ, Scheinin TM, Hayry P: The desmoid syndrome: New aspects in the cause, pathogenesis and treatment of the desmoid tumor. Am K Surg 151:230–237, 1986

Enzinger FM, Weiss SW (eds): Soft Tissue Tumors, 2nd ed, pp 153–159. St Louis, CV Mosby, 1988

MYASTHENIA, CONGENITAL. EPSILON SUBUNIT MUTATION

Synonyms. AChR deficiency, prolonged open time, low conductance, epsilon subunit mutation.

Symptoms and Signs. In females. From birth. Myasthenic symptoms of different severity, that slowly progress in intensity.

Etiology. Autosomal recessive inheritance hypothesized. May be defect of epsilon subunit of ACh receptor, that causes alterations of ion channel.

Pathology. Muscle: alteration at electron microscopy of end plates.

Diagnostic Procedures. *EMG.* Decremental response. AChR antibodies: negative. *Muscle biopsy.* No immune complexes at neuromuscular function.

Therapy. Nonresponsive to antimyasthenic therapy except for short periods.

Prognosis. Slowly progressive condition.

BIBLIOGRAPHY. Engel AG, Hutchinson D, Nakano S, et al: Congenital myasthenic syndrome attributed to a mutation of the epsilon subunit of the acetylcholine receptor. Neurology 42:307–311, 1992

Engel AG, Hutchinson D, Nakano S, et al: Myasthenic syndromes attributed to mutations affecting the epsilon subunit of the acetycholine receptor. Ann NY Acad Sci 681:496–508, 1993

MYASTHENIA GRAVIS, FAMILIAL INFANTILE

Synonyms. FIM, familial infantile myasthenia.

Symptoms and Signs. In early infancy. Fluctuating ptosis, poor suck and cry, feeding difficulties. Secondary respiratory infections with episodic exacerbation of symptoms by fever, excitement, vomiting. Apneic episodes may cause anoxic brain injury. Between exacerbations patients are normal except after exercise. After 10 years of age exacerbations less frequent, but complaint of weakness. Tendon reflexes normal, muscle normal.

Etiology. Defect in ACh resynthesis and packaging. Autosomal recessive inheritance.

Diagnostic Procedures. *EMG.* Decremental response at 2–H2 stimulation similar to MG (see Erb Goldfflam). Edrophonium test positive. *Muscle biopsy.* No abnormalities, no immune complexes at neuromuscular junction. Only synaptic vescicles are smaller in rested FIM and increase paradoxically in size after stimulation.

Therapy. Modest doses of anticholinesterase drugs. Information as to possible worsening of condition and occurrence of crises. Intrathracheal intubation and assisted ventilatory device if necessary.

Prognosis. Death by apnea possible. Usually good quoad vitam.

BIBLIOGRAPHY. Greer M, Schotland M: Myasthenia gravis in the newborn. Pediatrics 26:101–108, 1960

Mora M, Lambert EH, Engel AG: Synaptic vescicle abnormality in familial infantile myasthenia. Neurology 37:206–214, 1987

Penn AS, Richman DP, Ruff RL (eds): Myasthenia gravis and related disorders: Experimental and clinical aspects. Ann NY Acad Sci 681. 1993

MYASTHENIA GRAVIS, TRANSIENT NEONATAL

Synonyms. Strickroot, neonatal myasthenia gravis; transient neonatal myasthenia gravis.

Symptoms and Signs. After few hours from birth, feeding difficulty, generalized weakness, respiratory difficulty, feeble cry, facial paresis, ptosis.

Etiology. Transplacental transfer of Anti-AChR antibodies from myasthenic mother to child.

Therapy. That of myasthenia (see Erb Goldfam).

Prognosis. Disease lasts 18–47 days.

BIBLIOGRAPHY. Strickroot FL, Schaeffer BL, Bergo HL: Myasthenia gravis occurring in an infant born of a myasthenic mother. JAMA 120:1207–1209, 1942

Trartos SJ, Efthimiadis A, Morel E, et al: Neonatal myasthenia gravis antigenic specificities of antibodies in sera from mothers and their infants. Clin Exp Immunol 80:376–380, 1990

MYASTHENIA, FAMILIAL LIMB–GIRDLE

Synonyms. Familial limb—girdle myasthenias.

Symptoms and Signs. During childhood or teens, weakness of limb-girdle muscles. Ocular and cranial muscle spared. Possible joint contractures, cardiac repolarization defects.

Etiology. Autosomal recessive.

Pathology. Muscle: possible type 1 fiber atrophy. Tubular aggregates.

Diagnostic Procedures. *EMG.* Decremental response

Therapy. Response to anticholinestherase drugs but not prednisone.

Prognosis. Slowly progressive condition.

BIBLIOGRAPHY. McQuillen MP: Familial limb-girdle myasthenia. Brain 89:121–132, 1966

Engel AG: Myasthenia gravis and myasthenic syndromes. In Roland LP, Di Mauro S: Handbook of Clinical Neurology, vol 18: Myopathies, p 391. Amsterdam, Elsevier, 1992

MYELOCEREBELLAR

Synonyms. Ataxia—pancitopenia; pancitopènia—ataxia.

Symptoms and Signs. From early infancy. Cerebellar ataxia and successive development of leukemia with hypoplastic bone marrow and relative symptoms: bleeding, infections, etc.

Etiology. Unknown. Autosomal dominant inheritance.

Pathology. Cerebral atrophy and myelomonocytic leukemia.

Diagnostic Procedures. *Blood. Bone marrow.* Evidence of pancitopenia and myelomonovytic leukemia.

Therapy. Symptomatic.

Prognosis. From early death to survival to adolescence or adulthood with variable degree of manifestations.

BIBLIOGRAPHY. Li FP, Potter NU, Buchanan GR, et al: A family with acute leukemia, hypoplastic anemia and cerebellar ataxia: Association with bone marrow C-monosomy. Am J Med 65:933–940, 1978

Daghistani D, Curless R, Toledano SR, et al: Ataxia-pancytopenia and monosomy 7 syndrome. J Pediatr 115:108–110, 1989

MYELOFIBROSIS

Synonyms. Vaughan; Harrison-Vaughan including Lewis-Szur; osteopathia condensans disseminata-myeloid-megakaryocytic-hepatosplenomegaly; chronic nonleukemic myelosis (see Myeloproliferative syndromes); agnogenic myeloid metaplasia.

Symptoms. Both sexes affected. Onset usually after fifth decade; very rare in childhood. Insidious onset. Weakness; fatigue; weight loss; anorexia; left quadrant or generalized abdominal discomfort. Mild hemorrhagic manifestations.

Signs. Pallor; splenomegaly; frequently hepatomegaly; seldom, moderate lymphadenopathy.

Etiology. Unknown. At the side of idiopathic form myelofibrosis may occur in numerous malignant conditions—leukemias, lymphomas, carcinomas, etc—and nonmalignant conditions—granulomatous, endocrine, collagen diseases, toxic agents, radiation exposure, Paget, etc.

Pathology. Spleen, huge; liver, usually enlarged; myeloid metaplasia is found in spleen, liver, renal capsules, and lymph nodes. Increased bony trabeculae and replacement of marrow space by connective tissue, with few scattered areas of hematopoiesis.

Diagnostic Procedures. *Blood.* Normocytic (seldom macrocytic) anemia of variable degree; seldom, polycythemia, reticulocytosis, polychromatophilia. Occasionally, nucleated red cells. Leukocytes initially normal (40%), elevated (40%, seldom 50,000), decreased (20%); immature cells occasionally found; increased basophils. Leukocyte alkaline phosphatase elevated. Uric acid high; hyperbilirubinemia moderate. Platelet normal or decreased; occasionally, giant platelets or megakaryocyte fragment. *Bone marrow.* Increased bone consistency, usually dry tap. *Biopsy of bone.* Typical feature (see Pathology). *Splenic puncture.* Myeloid hyperplasia. *X-ray of bone.* Typical findings.

Therapy. Symptomatic. Androgens. Busulfan, splenic radiation, or splenectomy only when splenic symptoms, including hemolysis, are overwhelming.

Prognosis. Usually, slow progressive course leading to death after 1–33 years because of infections, hemorrhage, cardiac failure, leukemic conversion, hepatic failure, or thrombosis. A "malignant" form (Lewis-Szur syndrome) has been reported: description of a group of patients who showed findings inconsistent with the possible characterization of a definite syndrome with rapid evolution.

BIBLIOGRAPHY. Heuck, G: Zwei Faelle von Leukämie mit eigent-hünlichen Blut-Resp Knochenmarksbefunde. Virchows Arch Pathol Anat 78:475–496, 1879

Meyer E, Heineke A: Ueber Blutbildung bei schweren Anaemien und Leukaemie. Dtsch Arch Klin Med 88:435–492, 1907

Stephens DJ, Bredek JF: A leukemic myelosis with osteosclerosis. Ann Intern Med 6:1087–1096, 1933

Vaughan JM: Leuco-erythroblastic anaemic. J Pathol Bacteriol 42:541–564, 1936

Vaughan JM, Harrison CV: Leukoerythroblastic anaemia and myelosclerosis. J Pathol Bacteriol 48:339–352, 1939

Lewis SM, Szur L: Malignant myelosclerosis. Br Med J 7:472, 1963

Athens JW: Myelofibrosis. In Lee GR, Bithell TC, Foerster J, et al (eds): Wintrobe's Clinical Hematology, 9th ed, pp 2018–2933. Philadelphia, Lea & Febiger, 1993

MYELOPEROXIDASE DEFICIENCY

Synonyms. MPO. Grignaschi.

Symptoms and Signs. Healthy subjects or presenting disseminated or visceral candidiasis. Diabetes mellitus and defects in chemotaxis are associated in some cases. In this case patients also may present acne follicularis and pustular psoriasis.

Etiology. Lack of peroxidase activity in the azurophilic granules of neutrophils and the primary lysosomes of monocytes. Autosomal recessive inheritance proposed and considered, also the possibility of variable expression of the gene or defects in structural as well as regulatory genes. Gene for MPO is located on chromosome 17 at q22–23. Other causes of this defect include pregnancy, lead poisoning, Hodgkin, sepsis, megaloblastic anemia, ceroid lipofucinosis, leukemias.

Diagnostic Procedures. *Blood.* MPO deficiency in neutrophils and monocytes.

Therapy. No specific therapy. Treat presumed fungal infections earlier.

BIBLIOGRAPHY. Grignaschi VJ, et al: A new cytochemical picture: Spontaneous negativity of the peroxydase oxidase and lipid reactions in the neutrophil progeny and in the monocytes of two siblings. Rev Assc Med Argent 77:218, 1963

Undritz E: Die Alius-Grignaschi-anomalie: Der erblich kostitutionelle peroxydasedefekt der neutrophilen und monocyten. Blut 14:129, 1966

Lehrer RI, Cline MJ: Leukocyte myeloperoxydase deficiency and disseminated candidiasis: The role of myeloperoxydase on resistance to Candida infection. J Clin Invest 48:1478–1488, 1969

Forehand JR, Nauseef WM, Cornutte JT, et al: Inherited disorders of phagocyte killing. In Scriver CR, Beaudet AL, Sly WS, et al: The Metabolic and Molecular Bases of Inherited Disease, 7th ed, pp 4011–4013. New York, McGraw-Hill, 1995

MYELOPROLIFERATIVE SYNDROMES

Included in this category are all the idiopathic persistent (or transitory) intense proliferations in the bone marrow of erythroid, myeloid, megakaryocytic, or fibroblastic types, singly or in various combinations with corresponding changes in peripheral blood. This group includes Vaquez-Osler (see), myelofibrosis (see), chronic myelocytic leukemia, primary thrombocythemia, and intermediate forms, including combinations with multiple myeloma.

BIBLIOGRAPHY. Dameshek W: Some speculations on the myeloproliferative syndromes. Blood 6:372–375, 1951

Lopas H, Josephson AM: Myeloproliferative syndrome: Evaluation of myelosclerosis and chronic myelogenous leukemia to polycythemia vera. Arch Intern Med 114:754–759, 1964

Wintrobe MM (ed): Clinical Hematology, 8th ed. Philadelphia, Lea & Febiger, 1981

MYELOPROLIFERATIVE, TRANSITORY

Synonyms. Transitory myeloproliferative; leukemia, transient.

Symptoms and Signs. In newborn with Down syndrome and seldom in normal infants. Variable symptoms according to degree of leukemoid reaction.

Etiology. Unknown; see Down.

Diagnostic Procedures. *Blood and bone marrow.* Leukemoid reaction.

Therapy. Symptomatic.

Prognosis. Disappearance of hematologic manifestation.

BIBLIOGRAPHY. Seibel NL, Sommer A, Miser J: Transient neonatal leukemoid reactions in mosaic trisomy 21. J Ped 104:251–254, 1984

Niikawa N, Deng H-X, Abe K, et al: Possible mapping of the gene for transient myeloproliferative syndrome at 21 q11.2. Hum Genet 87:561–766, 1991

MYHRE

Synonyms. Growth, mental deficiency.

Symptoms and Signs. Pre- and postnatal growth deficiency (adult, 140 cm). Mental retardation. Early onset deafness (conductive and sensory type). Unusual facies (maxillary hypoplasia, prognathism, short palpebral fissures, small mouth). Muscle hypertrophy; decreased joint mobility; cryptorchidism; cardiac anomalies.

Etiology. Unknown. Possibly autosomal dominant inheritance.

Diagnostic Procedures. *X-rays.* Cranium thickened; ribs broadened; vertebrae large and flattened; iliac wings hypoplastic; long bones short.

BIBLIOGRAPHY. Myhre SA, Ruvalcaba RHA, Graham CB: A new growth deficiency syndrome. Clin Genet 20:1–5, 1981

Saljak MA, Aftimos S, Gluckman PD: A new syndrome of short stature, joint limitation on muscle hypertrophy. Clin Genet 23:441–446, 1983

MYOCLONIC EPILEPSY

Synonyms. Berger. Includes Focal cortical myoclonus. See also Etiology.

Symptoms and Signs. Myoclonic attacks may initiate in any period of life, more frequent in childhood. Irregular twitches of one part of the body (group, single, or part of a muscle). Cerebellar components of variable degrees, dementia (variable component according to single pathologies, see Etiology).

Etiology. Multiple etiologies. Autosomal dominant, recessive, or X-linked inheritance; viral, bacterial infections; degenerative (in old people usually related to ischemia); dysplasic, neoplastic; toxic or metabolic disorders. Includes a vast group of conditions: See Unverrich-Lundburg; Lafora bodies; Baltic myoclonus; Cherry-red spot; Sialidosis I; Heidenhain; Gaucher (late childhood variety); Rasmussen; Subacute sclerosing encephalitis; Alpers; Subacute spongiform encephalopathy; Ramsay-Hunt.

Pathology. Variable according to type of basic disorder

Diagnostic Procedures. *EEG.*

Therapy. Phenytoin, Valproic acid in Balcan myoclonus (see). When indicated cortical resection.

Prognosis. Variable from transient (in case of infections) to stationary or progressive at variable speed (in other forms hereditary or degenerative).

BIBLIOGRAPHY. Berger H: Ueber das Elektrenkephalogramm des Menschen. Siebente Mitteilung. Arch Pschiat Nervenkr 100:301–320, 1933
Kuzniecky R, Berkovic S, Andermann F, et al: Focal cortical myoclonus on Rolandic cortical dysplasia: Clarification by magnetic resonance imaging. Ann Neurol 23:317–325, 1988
Adams RD, Victor M: Principles of Neurology, 5th ed, pp 90–91. New York, McGraw-Hill, 1993

MYOFIBRILLAR LYSIS MYOPATHY

Synonyms. Cancilla; myopathy, lysis type I myofibrills.

Symptoms and Signs. Rare. From birth stable or progessive myopathy.

Etiology. Autosomal recessive inheritance. Failure of protein synthesis.

Pathology. Muscle fibers (type I): large areas devoid of sarcomas, myofilaments, and organelles, replete with fine granular amorphous material of nonglycogen character (lysis of myofibrills).

Diagnostic Procedures. *Muscle biopsy.*

Therapy. None.

Prognosis. Usually progressive condition.

BIBLIOGRAPHY. Cancilla PA, Kalyanaraman K, Verity MA, et al: Familial myopathy with probable lysis of myofibrills in type I fibers. Neurology 21:279–285, 1971

MYOPATHY, CONGENITAL FIBER-TYPE DISPROPORTION

Synonyms. Fiber-type disproportion myopathy; CFTD.

Symptoms and Signs. From asymptomatic to death from respiratory failure. Rarely ophthalmoplegia and ptosis. Floppy infants.

Etiology. Autosomal and recessive inheritance described. May be caused by a defect of maturation of muscle fibers.

Pathology. Muscle: different patterns characterized by difference and size or distribution of type I and type II fibers (selective type I atrophy, for example).

Diagnostic Procedures. Muscle biopsy.

Therapy. Symptomatic.

Prognosis. Varies greatly among different conditions

BIBLIOGRAPHY. Brooke MH, Engel WK: The histographic analysis of human muscle biopsies with regard to fiber types IV children's biopsy. Neurology 19:591–605, 1969
Mizuno Y, Komiya K: A serial muscle biopsy study, in a case of congenital fiber type disproportion associated with progressive respiratory failure. Brain Dev 12:431–436, 1990

MYOPATHY X-LINKED, EXCESSIVE AUTOPHAGY

Synonyms. XMEA; MFAX.

Symptoms and Signs. In Finns. Slowly progressing muscle weakness of legs. Walking not impaired.

Etiology. X-linked inheritance.

Pathology. Muscle: Excessive number of autophagic vacuoles.

Diagnostic Procedures. *Blood.* CK elevated. *Muscle biopsy.*

Therapy. Symptomatic.

Prognosis. Slow progression.

BIBLIOGRAPHY. Kalimo H, Savontaus ML, Lang H, et al: X-linked myopathy: A new hereditary muscle disease. Ann Neurol 23:258–265, 1988
Saviranta P, Lindlof M, Lehesjoki A-E, et al: Linkage studies in a new X-linked myopathy suggesting exclusion of DMD locus and tentative assignment to distal Xq. Am J Hum Genet 42:84–88, 1988

MYOSITIS, LOCALIZED

Symptoms and Signs. Muscle tenderness; enlargement and induration of all or part of a muscle.

Etiology. Inflammatory reaction secondary to injury to muscle fibers and connective sheaths.

Pathology. Inflammatory cells infiltrating regenerated muscle fibers and connective tissue.

Diagnostic Procedures. *Biopsy of muscle.*

Therapy. None specific.

Prognosis. Subsidence of the condition with residual permanent pseudocontraction of the affected muscle.

BIBLIOGRAPHY. Adams RD, Denny-Brown D, Pearson CM: Diseases of the Muscles, 3rd ed, p 367. New York, Harper & Row, 1975
Perry JD: Sports medicine: The clinical spectrum of injury. In Klippel JH, Dieppe PA: Rheumatology, p 5.21.3. St Louis, CV Mosby, 1994

MYOTONIC FLUCTUANS

Synonyms. Familial muscle cramps, Becker type II.

Symptoms and Signs. See Thompsen. Variations in severity in hours or days. No temporal progression like myotonia congenita recessive form. Pain accompanies myotonic contractions.

Etiology. Autosomal dominant.

Diagnostic Procedures. EMG. Classic myotonic pattern.

Therapy. Type I antiarrhythmic: phenitoine, quinine procainamide, mexiletine, and others, but patients often spontaneously discontinue drugs because their severe side effects outweigh their therapeutic advantage.

Prognosis. Good.

BIBLIOGRAPHY. Becker PE: Myotonic Congenita and Syndromes Associated with Myotonia. Stuttgart, Thieme, 1977

Ricker K, Lehmann-Horn F, Moxley R: Myotonia fluctuans. Arch Neurol 47:268–272, 1990

MYOTONIC GENERALIZED

Synonyms. Myotonia congenita; MCR.

Symptoms and Signs. Not manifest at birth, Onset 4–12 years, or later, especially in males. Myotonic contracture first of leg muscles and then of arms and facies. Depression of reflexes. Cold exacerbates condition, but less than in Thomsens. Susceptibility to malignant hyperthermia. Muscular hypertrophy present.

Etiology. Autosomal dominant condition; defect of skeletal chloride channel gene on chromosome 7.

Diagnostic Procedures. *EMG.* Typical myotonic pattern.

Therapy. Type I antiarrhythmic: phenitoine, quinine procainamide, mexiletine, and others, but patients often spontaneously discontinue drugs because their severe side effects outweigh their therapeutic advantage.

Prognosis. Lifelong clumsiness. Worsening in 20–30 years.

BIBLIOGRAPHY. Becker PE: Zur Genetik der Myotonien. In Kuhh E (ed): Progressive Muskeldystrophie, Myotonic, Myathenic, pp 247–255. Berlin: Springer-Verlag, 1966

Kock MC, Steinmeyer K, Lorenz C, et al: The skeletal muscle chloride channel in dominant and recessive human myotonia. Science 257:797–800, 1992

MYOTUBULAR MYOPATHY

Synonym. Centronuclear myopathy; descending ocular myopathy of early childhood.

Symptoms and Signs. Both sexes affected. Onset at birth or in early childhood. Ptosis; symmetric weakness of limbs (in one case, facial diplegia). Symptomatically not distinguishable from progressive external ophthalmoplegia (see) except for limb weakness.

Etiology. Persistence of fetal muscle proteins. In chidlhood; autosomal recessive and dominant inheritance.

Pathology. Called myotubular myopathy from the presenting hypotrophic round muscle fibers (type I) with central nuclei that resemble myotubes. (Similar cells are seen in muscle specimen from fetus at 12–20 weeks gestation.)

Diagnostic Procedures. *Biopsy of muscle.* (See Pathology.) *EMG.* Myopathy pattern. *Blood. Urine.* Not contributory.

Therapy. Symptomatic.

Prognosis. Usually progressive. Improvement reported.

BIBLIOGRAPHY. Spiro AJ, Shy GM, Gonatas NK: Myotubular myopathy. Arch Neurol 14:1–14, 1966

Kinoshita M, Cadman TE: Myotubular myopathy. Arch Neurol 18:265–271, 1968

Pavone L, Mollica F, Grasso A, et al: Familial centronuclear myopathy. Acta Neurol Scand 62:33–40, 1980

Goebel HH, Lenard HG: Congenital myopathies. In Rowland LP, Di Mauro S (eds): Handbook of Clinical Neurology, vol 18: Myopathies, p 331. Amsterdam, Elsevier, 1992

MYOTUBULAR MYOPATHY, X-LINKED

Synonym. Van Wingaarden; myopathy centronuclear; MTM1; MTMX.

Symptoms and Signs. In males. From birth or prenatal diagnosis (hydramnios, decreased fetal movements). Floppy infants. Extraocular facial and neck muscles always affected. Severe respiratory distress up to asphyxia; height over 90th percentile.

Etiology. X-linked inheritance. "Maturation arrest" of muscle fibers with persistence of fetal muscle proteins.

Pathology. Muscle fibers: ultrastructurally appear immature (even after weeks of life) with large nuclei, numerous ribosomes, myofibrils not striated, and large lakes of glycogen.

Diagnostic Procedures. *X-rays. Ultrasonography.* Thin ribs; elevated diaphragm. *Biopsy and culture of muscle fibers.* See Pathology. Unusual ability to proliferate in numerous passages.

Therapy. Symptomatic.

Therapy. Poor. Death in early infancy.

BIBLIOGRAPHY. Van Wjngaarden GK, Fleury P, Bethlem J, et al: Familial "myotubular" myopathy. Neurology 19:901–908, 1969

Oldfors A, Kyllerman M, Wahlstrom J, et al: X-linked myotubular myopathy: Clinical and pathological findings in a family. Clin Genet 36:5–14, 1989

Goebel HH, Lenard HG: Congenital myopathies. In Rowland LP, Di Mauro S (eds): Handbook of Clinical Neurology, vol 18: Myopathies, p 331. Amsterdam, Elsevier, 1992

MYXEDEMA, COMA

Symptoms and Signs. Prevalent in females and in old age. In hypothyroid patients, infections, cardiovascular, or respiratory diseases are usually precipitating cause; other causes; cold anesthesia (it occurs mostly in winter); drugs. Hypothermia, hypotension, seizures, cardiac failure progressing to shock, coma.

Etiology. Inability to cope with stress; adrenal insufficiency.

Pathology. That of hypothyroidism.

Diagnostic Procedures. *Blood.* Sodium and chloride low, hypoglycemia; hypercapnia and respiratory acidosis; T4; TSH, cortisol levels. *Urine.* 17-Ketosteroids low. Usually no time to do studies because emergency treatment required.

Therapy. Triiodothyronine (10–25 mcg or more) by gastric tube or parenterally every 8 hours, or sodium levothyroxinrtisone (100 mg) every 8 hours (Synthyroid, 200–400 mcg intravenously and 100–200 mcg/24 hr). Hydrocortisone. Treat eventual infections. Administer fluids cautiously. Do not warm the patient (only adequate covering). Provide ventilation.

Prognosis. Very poor; high mortality. Fifty percent survival with adequate treatment.

BIBLIOGRAPHY. LeMarquand HS, Hausmann W, Hemsted EH: Myxoedema as a cause of death: Report of two cases. Br Med J 1:704–706, 1953

Catz B, Russell S: Myxedema, shock and coma. Arch Intern Med 108:407–417, 1961

Murkin JM: Anesthesia and hypothyroidism: A review of thyroxine physiology, pharmacology, and anesthetic implications. Anesth Analg 61:371–383, 1982

Utiger RD: Hypothyroidism. In De Groot LJ (ed): Endocrinology, 3rd ed, pp 765–766. Philadelphia, WB Saunders, 1995

MYXEDEMA, JUVENILE

Synonyms. Juvenile hypothyroidism. See also Gul and cryptothyroidism.

Symptoms and Signs. Both sexes affected, onset in adolescence. After a period of normal growth and mental development, variable slowing of growth, from complete to mild delay. Dentition delayed; constipation;

placid behavior (often considered normal and pleasant by parents). Puberty delayed or, occasionally, isosexual maturation may be precocious.

Etiology. Associated with defects in thyroid hormone synthesis (presence of goiter) or exhaustion. Atrophy of small amounts of aberrant thyroid tissue (see Cryptothyroidism) or examples of Hashimoto (see).

Pathology. See Etiology.

Diagnostic Procedures. *Blood.* T4; T3; thyroid antibodies; thyroid-stimulating hormone (TSH) and, eventually, measurements of other pituitary hormones (e.g., gonadotropins, prolactin).[131]I uptake. *X-ray.* Sella turcica normal; bone age and growth delayed.

Therapy. Thyroid hormone by slow, gradual increases up to needed dose.

Prognosis. Optimal response to a well-conducted treatment. Growth resumes; obesity and myxedematous changes revert. Precocious puberty, including galactorrhea, also reverts.

BIBLIOGRAPHY. Utiger RD: Hypothyroidism. In De Groot LJ (ed): Endocrinology, 3rd ed, pp 765–766. Philadelphia, WB Saunders, 1995

MYXEDEMA, MADNESS

Symptoms and Signs. Among the many psychologocal and behavioral manifestations of hypothyroidism (thought and movement slowing, decreased attention, loss of ambition, memory decay, sleep cycle alterations, headache, slow and hesitant speech), seldom there may be associated severe anxiety and agitation (myxedema madness).

Etiology. See Gull.

BIBLIOGRAPHY. Swanson JW, Kelly JJ Jr, MacConahey WM: Neurologic aspects of thyroid dysfunction. Mayo Clin Proc 56:504–512, 1981

MYXEDEMA, NODULAR THYROTOXICOSIS

Synonyms. Pretibial mixedema.

Symptoms and Signs. Occurs in patients with thyrotoxicosis. Appearance of nonpitting, elevated plaques on the skin of lower extremities (seldom upper extremities) after onset of thyrotoxicosis or more frequently after thyroidectomy. Hypertrophic osteoarthropathy may also be associated.

Etiology. Unknown.

Pathology. Thyroid; see Flajani. Typical skin changes for myxedema.

Therapy. None.

Prognosis. Lesion persists despite thyroidectomy or thyroid administration after surgery.

BIBLIOGRAPHY. Sollier P: Maladie de Basedow avec Myxoédeme. Rev Med 11:1000–1013, 1891
Cohen BC, Benua RS, Rawson RW: Localized myxedema involving upper extremity. Arch Intern Med 111:641–645, 1963
McKenzie JM, Zakarija M: Hyperthyroidism. In De Groot LJ (ed): Endocrinology, 3rd ed, Philadelphia, WB Saunders, 1995

MYXEDEMATOUS, CEREBELLAR

Synonyms. Hypothyroidism, cerebellar ataxia; ataxia cerebellaris myxedema; cerebellar ataxia myxedema.

Symptoms and Signs. Occurs in patients with hypothyroidism. Signs of myxedema and cerebellar symptoms (ataxia; incoordination) appearing at the same time or years after onset of myxedema.

Etiology. Thyroid hormone deficiency.

Pathology. That of myxedema.

Diagnostic Procedures. *Blood.* Evaluation of thyroid function. *Echography, scintigraphy.*

Therapy. Thyroid hormone.

Prognosis. Cerebellar symptoms and signs disappear after 2–3 weeks of treatment.

BIBLIOGRAPHY. White EW: Myxedema associated with insanity. Lancet I:974–976, 1884
Jellinek EH, Kelly RE: Cerebellar syndrome in myxoedema. Lancet II:225–227, 1960
Cremer GM, Goldstein NP, Paris J: Myxedema and ataxia. Neurology 19:37–46, 1969
Swanson JW, Kelly JJ Jr, MacConahey WM: Neurologic aspects of thyroid dysfunction. Mayo Clin Proc 56:504–512, 1981

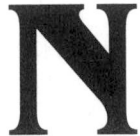

N

NAEGELI

Synonyms. Franceschetti-Jadassohn; Jadassohn-Franceschetti; chromatophore nevus; hyperhidrosis; skin pigmentation; keratosis pilaris; enamel dysplasia; melanophoric nevus.

Symptoms. Both sexes affected with equal frequency. Onset in second or third year of life. Development of reticular pigmentation (in fine network) that becomes generalized, without preliminary inflammatory changes. Usually, keratoderma and hypohidrosis of palms and soles. Temperature regulation may be disturbed by reduction of number of sweat glands. Hair and nails normal. Teeth normal or defective with yellow spotting. Nystagmus, strabismus, and optic atrophy.

Etiology. Unknown; autosomal dominant inheritance (rare).

Diagnostic Procedure. *Biopsy of skin.*

Therapy. Symptomatic.

Prognosis. Progressive condition. Mental and physical development normal.

BIBLIOGRAPHY. Naegeli O: Familiärer Chromatophore-naevus. Schweiz Med Wchnschr 57:48, 1927

Franceschetti A, Jadassohn W: "A propos de l'incontinentia pigmenti" delimitation de deux syndromes différents figurants sous le même terme. Dermatologica 108:1–28, 1954

Sparrow GP, Samman PD, Wells RS: Hyperpigmentation and hypohidrosis (the Naegeli-Franceschetti-Jadassohn syndrome): Report of a family and review of literature. Clin Exp Dermatol 1:127–140, 1976

Bleehen SS, Ebling FJG, Champion RH: Disorders of skin color. In Champion RH, Burton JL, Ebling FJG (eds): Rook/Wilkinson/Ebling Textbook of Dermatology, 5th ed, p 1584. Oxford, Blackwell Scientific, 1992

NAGER-REYNIER

Synonyms. Mandibulofacial dysostosis; preaxial acrofacial dysostosis; acrofacial dysostosis. See Treacher-Collins and Franceschetti-Klein.

Symptoms and Signs. Bilateral hypoplasia of mandibular ascending ramus; aplasia of temporomandibular joint; atresia of external auditory canal, frequently, with cleft palate and without lid anomalies or macrostomia. Thumbs hypoplastic or absent; radius and ulna may be fused or one of the two may be absent.

Etiology. Unknown. Most cases sporadic. Autosomal dominant inheritance suggested. Evidence for cases with recessive form presented as well.

Diagnostic Procedure. *X-rays.* See Signs.

Therapy. Avulsion of abnormally implanted teeth and prostheses.

BIBLIOGRAPHY. Slingenberg B: Missbildungen von Extramitaeten. Virchows Arch (Pathol Anat) 193:1–91, 1908

Nager FR, de Reynier JP: Das Gehoerorgan bei den angeborenen Kopfmissbildung. Pract Otorhinolaryngol (Basel) (Suppl 2) 10:1–128, 1948

Halal F, Herrmann J, Pallister P, et al: Differential diagnosis of Nager acrofacial dysostosis syndrome: report of four patients with Nager syndrome and discussion of other related syndromes. Am J Med Genet 14:209–224, 1983

Aylsworth AS, Lin AE, Friedman PA: Nager acrofacial dysostosis male-

to-male transmission in two families. Am J Med Genet 41:83–88, 1991

NAJJAR

Synonyms. Genital anomaly; mental retardation; cardiomyopathy; cardiogenital.

Symptoms and Signs. From birth. Micropenis; Hypoplastic or bifid scrotal sac; small testes. Mental retardation. Cardiomyopathy.

Etiology. Possibly autosomal recessive inheritance.

BIBLIOGRAPHY. Najjar SS, der Kaloustian VM, Nassif SI: Genital anomaly, mental retardation, and cardiomyopathy: a new syndrome. J Pediatr 83:286–288, 1973

Najjar SS, der Kaloustian VM, Nassif SI: Genital anomaly, mental retardation, and cardiomyopathy: A new syndrome. Clin Genet 26:371–373, 1984

NAKAGAWA

Synonyms. Angioblastoma; tufted angioma; progressive capillary hemangioma

Symptoms and Signs. Rarely congenital, onset usually in early life, seldom in adults. Local pain and localized sweating. Firm, indurated, red-brown or red-blue, centrally depressed, plaque or patch with irregular margins and finger-like projections, usually involving trunk or neck, progressively enlarging for several years.

Etiology. Unknown.

Pathology. Collection of blood vessels in the dermis that appear as oblong tufts (cannonball pattern), resembling glomeruli, absence of cytologic atypia.

Diagnostic Procedures. *Biopsy.*

Therapy. Clobetasol propionate ointment (scarce symptomatic benefit), dye laser, cryosurgery, X-ray, electrocautery and surgical treatment (frequent recurrence).

Prognosis. Benign lesion without malignant transformation.

BIBLIOGRAPHY. Nakagawa K: Case report of angioblastoma of the skin. Jp J Sermatol 59:92–94, 1949

Bernstein EF, Kantor G, Howe N, et al: Tufted angioma of the thigh. J Am Arch Dermatol 31:307–311, 1994

NAKAIZUMI

Synonym. Lewkojeva; amyloid hereditary corneal deposits; corneal dystrophy, gelatinous drop-like; Japanese-type corneal dystrophy, lattice type III.

Symptoms. Most frequent in Japan, where the onset is from 70 to 90 years of age. In other countries earlier onset. Photophobia; excessive lacrimation.

Signs. Raised gelatinous mulberry-like masses over central cornea. Cataract may be associated.

Etiology. Unknown. Possibly autosomal recessive inheritance.

Pathology. Significant amyloid deposition in Bowman layer and epithelium and moderate in anterior stroma.

Therapy. Corneal graft.

BIBLIOGRAPHY. Lewkojewa EF: Ueber einen Fall primaerer Degeneration Amyloidose der Kornea. Klin Monatsbl Augenheilkd 83:117–137, 1930

Mondino BJ, Rabb HF, Sugar J, et al: Primary familial amyloidosis of the cornea. Am J Ophthalmol 92:732–736, 1981

Hida T, Proia AD, Kigasawa K, et al: Histopathological and immunochemical features of lattice corneal dystrophy type III. Am J Ophthalmol 104:249–252, 1987

Gorevic PD, Munoz PC, Gorgone G, et al: Amyloidosis due to a dystrophy type II. N Engl J Med 325:1780–1785, 1991

NAKED STENT

Synonyms. Hemolysis after transjugular intrahepatic portosystemic shunting; post-TIPS hemolytic anemia.

Symptoms and Signs. In approximately 12% of patients submitted to transjugular intrahepatic portosystemic shunting (excellent new technique for treatment of portal hypertension). Onset 10–30 days after implantation: jaundice, anemia, dizziness.

Etiology. Traumatic, naked stent-related hemolysis.

Pathology. Naked, not endothelized, stent wire observed in explanted livers.

Diagnostic Procedures. Hemoglobin decreased; reticulocytosis and schistocytes increased. Bilirubin increased.

Therapy. Removal of stent. Liver transplantation if indicated.

Prognosis. Remission of symptoms after stent removal or liver transplantation. Spontaneous remission reported in some cases.

BIBLIOGRAPHY. Sanyal AJ, Freedman AM, Purdum PP: Progressive encephalopathy and intravascular hemolysis following transjugular intrahepatic porto-caval shunt (TIPPS) (correspondence). Ann Int Med 117:443–444, 1992

Sanyal AJ, Freedman AM, Shiffman ML: Portosystemic encephalopathy after transjugular intrahepatic portosystemic shunt: Results of a prospective controlled study. Hepatology 20:46–55, 1994

Editorial: Hemolysis after transjugular intrahepatic portosystemic shunting: The naked stent syndrome. Hepatology 23:177–181, 1996

NANCE

Synonyms. Deafness, stapes fixation; perilymphatic gusher—deafness; deafness (mixed), perilymphatic gusher.

Symptoms and Signs. In males, progressive mixed hearing loss; vestibular response lacking or strongly reduced. In females, slight hearing loss. Profuse drainage of perilymph and cerebral fluid at surgical mobilization of stapes.

Etiology. X-linked trait.

Pathology. Dilatation of internal auditory meatusi deficient or absent bone between lateral end of meatus and basal turn of cochlea. Communications between subarachnoid space and perilymph in the cochlea (perilymphatic hydrops).

Diagnostic Procedures. *Audiometry.* Vestibular function. *X-rays.* CT scan. *MRI.*

Therapy. Stapes surgery is to be avoided to prevent complications.

BIBLIOGRAPHY. Nance WE, Setleff R, McLeod AC, et al: X-linked mixed deafness with congenital fixation of the stapedial footplate and perilymphatic gusher. Birth Defect Orig Art Ser VII (4):64–69, 1971

Pheps PD, Reardon W, Pembrey M, et al: X-linked deafness, stapes gushers, and distinctive defects of the inner ear. Neuroradiology 33:326–330, 1991

NANCE-HORAN

Synonyms. Brachymetacarpia, cataract, mesiodens; cataract, dental; mesiodens, cataract.

Symptoms and Signs. Both sexes affected. Present from birth. Normal intelligence. *Male.* Supernumerary central incisor (mesiodens); incisors screwdriver-like; cataract, posterior suture microcornea; short fourth metacarpals. *Female.* Heterozygous. Progressive punctate cataracts diastemata; normal vision (usually); incisor teeth with edges narrower than normal (Hutchinson-like).

Etiology. X-linked inheritance. The gene has been mapped to X21.1–p22.3.

Diagnostic Procedure. *Blood.* Serum alkaline phosphatase elevated. *X-rays.* See Signs.

Therapy. Surgery for cataract at early age (difficult to remove).

BIBLIOGRAPHY. Nance WE, Warburg M, Bixler D, et al: Congenital sex-linked cataract, dental anomalies, and brachymetacarpalia. Birth Defects 10:285–291, 1974

Horan MB, Billson FH: X-linked cataract and Hutchinsonian teeth. Aust Paediatr J 10:98–102, 1974

Walpole IR, Hockey A, Nicoll A: The Nance-Horan syndrome. J Med Genet 27:632–634, 1990

NANCE-SWEENEY

Synonyms. Nance dwarfism; Nance-Insley; deafness—chondrodysplasia; chondrodystrophy—sensineural deafness; otospondylomegaepiphyseal dysplasia; O.S.M.E.D.

Symptoms and Signs. Both sexes. Deafness progressing and severe. Rhizomelic micromelia; ear deformities; saddle nose; thin hair; thick leathery skin; soft tissue calcification; cleft palate, occasionally.

Etiology. Autosomal recessive inheritance.

Diagnostic Procedure. *X-ray.* Scoliosis; flattened base of skull; cartilage calcifications; achondroplasia-type deformity of pelvis.

Prognosis. Deafness severe and progressive. Adult height 120 cm.

BIBLIOGRAPHY. Nance WE, Sweeney A: A recessively inherited chondrodystrophy. Birth Defects 6:25–27, 1970

Insley J, Astley R: A bone dysplasia with deafness. Br J Radiol 47:244–251, 1974

Miny P, Lenz W: Autosomal recessive deafness with skeletal dysplasia and facial appearance of Marshall syndrome. Am J Med Genet 21:317–324, 1985

Salinas CF, deBotero D, Isaza C: Bone Dysplasia, Deafness and Cleft Palate Syndrome, p 259. Berlin, 7th Int Cong Hum Genet, 1986

NARCOLEPSY, DIABETOGENIC HYPERINSULINISM

Synonyms. Chronic refractory fatigue; euthyroid hypometabolism; hyperinsulinism—narcolepsy; hypothyroid hypometabolism; metabolic obesity; psychosomatic obesity. See Pickwickian.

Symptoms. Family history of narcolepsy (48%). Irresistible drowsiness with pathologic and inappropriate sleep (100%); cataplexy (50%); usually following sudden emotion; hypnagogic hallucination (56%); sleep paralysis (49%); inability to move on awaking or predormitum. Frequently associated, vascular headache (65%) (see cluster headache syndrome), peripheral neuropathy, especially of lower limbs (34%), spontaneous leg cramps (37%) (see Wittmaak-Ekbon). Angina pectoris and arrhythmias (32%). Psychiatric features; anxiety and depression.

Signs. Obesity (75%); therapeutic response to trial of analeptic agent (100%). Frequently associated; recurrent edema (50%), cafe au lait spots (29%); occipital nevus and white forelock.

Etiology. Hypoglycemia related to feeding habit; narcoleptic hypokinesia; accelerated lipogenesis related to chronic hyperinsulinism; deranged nervous system function.

Pathology. Obesity.

Diagnostic Procedures. *Blood.* Glucose determination with fasting; morning glucose tolerance test; afternoon glucose tolerance test. Insulin and insulin-like activity determination. Electrolytes; cholesterol; uric acid; protein bound iodine. *Urine.* Volume (diurnal and nocturnal collection). *Pulmonary function tests. ECG. EEG. Metabolic rate. Pharmacologic studies.* (1) Methylphenidate hydrochloride; (2) insulin; (3) tolbutamide; (4) liothyronine.

Therapy. Diet (gradual decrease); moderate exercise; analeptics (ritalin). If diabetes, treat; if prediabetic state, institute preventive measures. Avoid needless administration of thyroid; decrease fluid intake; avoid therapeutic fasting.

Prognosis. Good response to treatment; realistic weight reduction and analeptics.

BIBLIOGRAPHY. Roberts HJ: Obesity due to the syndrome of narcolepsy and diabetogenic hyperinsulinism: Clinical and therapeutic observations in 252 patients. J Am Geriatr Soc 15:721–743, 1967
Fugger L, Tisch R, Libau R, et al: The role of human major histocompatibility complex (HLA) genes in disease. In Scriver CR, Beaudet AL, Sly WS, et al: The Metabolic and Molecular Bases of Inherited Disease, 7th ed, p 574. New York, McGraw-Hill, 1995

NARCOLEPTIC TETRAD

Includes narcolepsy, cataplexy, sleep paralaysis, and hypnagogic hallucinosis. See Gelineau.

NASAL DEVELOPMENT DEFECTS

Synonyms. Nasal aplasia; heminasal aplasia; proboscis lateralis; arhinia; arhinogenesis.

Symptoms and Signs. Aplasia of both nasal side or of half the nose that may be found with or without a nasal proboscis and in association with other facial anomalies. The proboscis 2–4 cm in length × 0.5–1 cm wide may be located (rarely in the midline) or attached to an eyelid or laterally to it. Seldom bilateral. Intelligence usually is normal.

Etiology. Unknown. Congenital development defect. In specific association may be inherited.

BIBLIOGRAPHY. Tiefenthal G: Total Aplasia einer Nasenhaelfte. Mschr Ohrenheilkd 44:1071–1075, 1910
Antoniades K, Baraitser M: Proboscis lateralis. A case report. Teratoloy 40:193–197, 1989

NASU

Synonyms. Membranous dystrophy.

Symptoms and Signs. Fat necrosis with cysts; observed in association with many different diseases. Bone fractures, neuropsychiatric conditions, diabetes, myeloma, lupus erythematosus, ischemia, infections.

Etiology. Unknown. Suggested ischemic injury of adipose tissue.

Pathology. Cysts lined by wavy hyaline, acidophilic membranes; inside the cyst membrane convolutes and assume arabesques pattern. Membrane shows periodic acid-Schiff staining and resistance to diastase.

BIBLIOGRAPHY. Nasu T: A lipid metabolic disease "membranous lipodystrophy." Acta Pathol Japan 23:539–558, 1973
Alègre VA, Winkelmann RK, Aliaga A: Lipomembranous changes in chronic panniculitis. J Am Acad Dermatol 19:39–46, 1988

NEGLECT

Synonyms. Attentional neglect; inattention.

Symptoms and Signs. Failure to respond, report, or orient to novel or meaningful stimuli presented to the side opposite a brain lesion. Major behavorial manifestations are hemi-inattention; akinesia; hemispatial neglect. Associated frequently, allesthesia, anognosia, and anosodiaphoria.

Etiology. Attributed to disorders of sensation; abnormalities of body schema; or disorders of attention or perception owing to dysfunction in a corticolimbic reticular formation loop. Hemorrhage most frequent cause.

Pathology. Lesions may be present in the following areas: inferior parietal lobule; dorsolateral frontal lobe; cingulate gyrus; neostriatum; thalamus.

Diagnostic Procedures. *CT scan. MRI.*

Therapy. When the acute phase has passed, adjust the environment so that interaction with people or things may take place on the good side. Training.

Prognosis. Symptoms may diminish, with different evolution in a period of weeks to months or years; frequently incomplete.

BIBLIOGRAPHY. Poppelreuter WL: Die psychischen Schaedigungen durch Kopfschuss. Im Kriege 1914–1916: Die Stoerungen der niederen und hohern Leistungen durch Feletzungendes Oksipitalhirn, 6th ed. Leipzig, L Voss, 1917
Heilman KM, Valenstein E, Watson RT: The neglect syndrome. In Vinken PJ, Bruyn GW (eds): Handbook of Clinical Neurology, pp 153–183. Amsterdam, North-Holland, 1984

NÉKAM

Synonyms. Keratosis lichenoides chronica; porokeratosis striata lichenoides; lichen ruber moniliformis; lichen verucosus et reticularis. Morbus Moniliformis Lichenoides.

Symptoms and Signs. *Face.* Seborrheic dermatitis-like eruption. *Limbs.* Violaceus papular and nodular lesions in linear and reticulate pattern, most marked on hands and feet.

Etiology. Unknown. Unusual variant of lichen planus or distinct entity.

Pathology. Nonspecific. Chronic dermatitis and lichenoid features.

Therapy. Favorable response to photochemotherapy and etetrinate.

BIBLIOGRAPHY. Kaposi M: Lichen Ruber Planus, p 571 Vierteljahr, 1886
Nékam L: Lichen moniliformis. Presse Med 46:1000, 1938
Black MM: Lichen planus and lichenoid disorders. In Champion RH, Burton JL, Ebling FJG (eds): Rook/Wilkinson/Ebling Textbook of Dermatology, 5th ed, p 1696. Oxford, Blackwell Scientific, 1992

NELATON

Synonyms. Acro-osteolysis; mutilating ulcer; acropathy. See Neuropathy, hereditary sensory radicular.

Symptoms and Signs. Onset at puberty. Ulceration of the soles of feet. Occasionally development of "elephant foot."

Etiology. Unknown. See HSAN syndromes. Relationship with other foot ulceration syndromes (see also Morvan; Biemond III). Not yet completely elucidated.

Pathology. Trophic ulceration of foot; osteoporosis and compression of metatarsals and phalanges.

Diagnostic Procedures. *X-ray.* Of feet. *Blood.* Glucose curve. *Doppler.*

Therapy. Symptomatic. Amputation sometimes required.

Prognosis. Successive attacks with intermittent periods of various length. Danger of infections.

BIBLIOGRAPHY. Nélaton A: Affection singulière des os du pied. Gaz Hop 4:13, 1852
Thevenard A: L'acropathie ulcero-mutilante familiale. Rev Neurol (Paris) 74:193–212, 1942
Denny-Brown D: Hereditary sensory neuropathy. J Neurol 14:237–252, 1951

NELSON

See Addisonian syndromes.

Symptoms and Signs. Occurs in patients with adrenal hyperplasia; onset 6 months to 12 years after adrenalectomy. Deep pigmentation of the skin and mucosae, restricted visual fields, and other neurologic signs of pituitary tumor.

Etiology. Chromophobe tumor of the hypophysis developing after removal of hypertrophic adrenal. Excessive secretion of adrenocorticotropic hormone (ACTH) and beta-lipotropin.

Pathology. Chromophobe tumor of the hypophysis.

Diagnostic Procedures. *X-ray of skull. Blood.* Plasma ACTH level. *X-rays.* Sellar enlargement and deformity; pituitary tumor.

Therapy. Radiation of hypophysis or hypophysectomy; Nivazol.

Prognosis. Fair. Pigmentation and other neurologic and metabolic signs may respond to treatment.

BIBLIOGRAPHY. Nelson DH, Meakin JW, Thorn GW: ACTH-producing pituitary tumors following adrenalectomy for Cushing's syndrome. Ann Intern Med 52:560–569, 1960
Kasperlik-Zaluska AA, Nielubowicz J, Wislawski J, et al: Nelson's syndrome: Incidence and prognosis. Clin Endocrinol 19:693–698, 1983
Ball JA, Williams G, Yeo TH, Joplin GF: Effect of nivazol in Nelson's syndrome. Postgraduate Med J 64:220–221, 1988
Sherwood LM: Paraneoplastic endocrine disorders (ectopic hormone syndromes). In De Groot LJ (ed): Endocrinology, 3rd ed, pp 2774–2775. Philadelphia, WB Saunders, 1995

NEMALINE MYOPATHIES

Synonym. Rod body myopathy. See Floppy infant syndromes.

EARLY ONSET TYPE

Symptoms. Onset at birth. Delayed motor development; proximal limb weakness. Respiratory failure.

Signs. Reduced muscle bulk; muscle hypotonia. Reflexes usually absent, normal in some cases. Associated malformations; high palate; pigeon breast; pes cavus; kyphosis or scoliosis.

Etiology. Unknown. Autosomal dominant and possibly recessive inheritance.

Pathology. In muscles, type I fiber predominance. Twenty to fifty percent of fibers affected. Fibers containing variable amount of rods or filamentous formation (that are made up of regular giant lattices of Z-disc occasionally observed within nuclei). Nuclei of affected cell vesicular with prominent nucleoli.

Diagnostic Procedures. *Biopsy.* Of muscle (see Pathology). *Blood.* Creatine index increased, serum glutamic-oxaloacetic transaminase (SGOT) normal. *Urine.* Amino acid excretion normal. *Electromyography.* Decreased duration of potentials.

Therapy. Symptomatic. In cases of GH deficiency, growth hormone (GH) should be used with caution and under strict supervision.

Prognosis. Static weakness; unexplained death reported in some cases.

LATE ONSET TYPE

Symptoms. Both sexes affected. Onset in fourth to sixth decade in reported cases. Occurs in subjects previously well and without developmental abnormalities. Gradual onset of distal leg or pelvic girdle weakness, progressing to affect proximal part and then distal part of all limbs and neck flexors.

Signs. Muscle hypotonia, some wasting. Reflexes usually normal or decreased.

Etiology. Unknown. Nonfamilial (or clinical variant of the preceding). Nonspecific reaction of Z band to various insults.

Pathology. See Early onset type.

Diagnostic Procedures. See Early onset type.

Therapy. Symptomatic.

Prognosis. Progressive course.

BIBLIOGRAPHY. Shy GM, Engel WK, Somers JE, et al: Nemaline myopathy: A new congenital myopathy. Brain 86:793–810, 1963
Heffernan LP, Rewcastle NB, Humphrey JG: The spectrum of rod myopathies. Arch Neurol 18:529–542, 1968
Wallgren-Pettersson C, Kaariainen H, Rapola J, et al: Genetics of congenital nemaline myopathy: A study of 10 families. J Med Genet 27:480–487, 1990
Goebel HH, Lenard HG: Congenital myopathies. In Rowland LP, Di Mauro S (eds): Handbook of Clinical Neurology, vol 18: The Myopathies, p 331. Amsterdam, Elsevier, 1992

NEOCEREBELLAR

Synonym. Posterior cerebellar lobe.

Symptoms and Signs. Both sexes affected. Onset at all ages. Generalized or homolateral hypotonia; pendular reflexes; static tremor; during voluntary movements, disturbance in station, past-pointing, and spontaneous deviation of limbs; gait disturbances (deviation and tendency to fall toward side of lesion); asthenia; delay in starting and stopping muscular contractions; dysmetria; adiadochokinesia; speech disturbances: slow, monotonous, scanning; later, utterance, jerkiness, explosiveness; disturbances in writing.

Etiology and Pathology. Neoplastic vascular, inflammatory, or traumatic lesion of posterior lobe or of lateral part of cerebellum.

Diagnostic Procedures. *Angiography. CT brain scan. MRI. Spinal tap.*

Therapy. Surgery if indicated.

Prognosis. Depends on etiology.

BIBLIOGRAPHY. Holmes G: The symptoms of acute cerebellar injuries due to gunshot injuries. Brain 40:461–535, 1917
Bremer F: Le cervelet. In Roger GH, Benet L: Traite de Physiologie Normale et Pathologique, vol 10, Pt 1–2. Paris, Masson, 1935
Adams RD, Victor M: Principles of Neurology, 5th ed, p 74. New York, McGraw-Hill, 1993

NEONATAL HEPATITIS

Synonyms. Giant cell hepatitis; thick bile hepatitis neonatal.

Symptoms and Signs. Both sexes affected. At birth infant appears normal. In first weeks of life becomes icteric. Hepatomegaly develops. Slow weight gain and thriving. Hemorrhagic tendency may develop. Frequently, splenomegaly.

Etiology. Unknown in 70% of cases. In other cases: infective; genetic (AT deficiency)-metabolic defects; chromosomal abnormalities; toxins; various cholestatic conditions. Familial form. Probably autosomal recessive inheritance, with manifestation extremely variable from very severe to very mild.

Pathology. In liver; multinuclear giant cells, cholestasis, and occasionally fibrosis.

Diagnostic Procedures. *Blood. Urine.* Standard tests of liver function abnormal, but do not distinguish various forms of the syndrome; general evidence of cholestasis. *Biopsy.* Of liver. Pathologic findings are diagnostic.

Therapy. Symptomatic.

Prognosis. Long-term studies still lacking; 6–12 months after recovery, two thirds in good health; in the rest, signs of cirrhosis or death.

BIBLIOGRAPHY. Craig JM, Landing BH: Form of hepatitis in neonatal period simulating biliary atresia. Arch Pathol 54:321–333, 1952
Aagenaes O, Van Der Hagen CB, Refsum S: Hereditary recurrent intrahepatic cholestasis from birth. Arch Dis Child 43:646–657, 1968
Sandor T, Surinya M, Monus Z: Familial occurrence of giant cell hepatitis in infancy. Acta Hepato-Gastroent 23:101–104, 1976
Cox DW: 1-Antitrypsin deficiency. In Scriver CR, Beaudet AL, Sly WS, et al: The Metabolic and Molecular Bases of Inherited Disease, 7th ed, pp 4140–4141. New York, McGraw-Hill, 1995

NEONATAL LUPUS ERYTHEMATOSUS

Synonym. Heart block, congenital; lupus erythematosus, neonatal.

Symptoms and Signs. In newborns of mothers with lupus erythematosus, more frequent in females. Petecchiae, hemorrhages, pneumonitis, splenomegaly, cutaneous lupus lesions second to sixth month of life: macules, papules, plaques; congenital heart block, with associated malformation (transposition of great vessels). Hemolytic anemia.

Etiology. Antibodies present in mother that pass to fetus and determine inflammatory myocarditis (causing endocardial fibroelastosis and atrioventricular block). Possibly antibodies involved are SS-A (Ro) and SS-B (La) (RNA–protein complexes).

Pathology. *Heart.* Replacement of atrial septal musculature by elastic, fibrous, and adipose tissue.

Diagnostic Procedures. *Blood.* Thrombocytopenia; anemia; presence of lupus markers (see SLE); leukopenia.

Therapy. Permanent pacemaker. Plasmapheresis during pregnancy. Surgery.

Prognosis. In some cases progression to adult SLE, in others resolution.

BIBLIOGRAPHY. McCuistion CH, Schoch EP Jr: Possible discoid lupus erythematosus in newborn infants. Arch Derm Syph 70:782–785, 1954
Watson RM, Lane AT, Barnett NK, et al: Neonatal lupus erythematosus: A chemical serological and immunogenetic study with review of the literature. Medicine 63:362–378, 1984
Neonatal lupus syndrome. Editorial. Lancet II:489–490, 1987
Miesher PA (ed): Systemic Lupus Erythematosus. Berlin, Springer, 1995

NEOPLASTIC PORPHYRIA TARDA

Synonym. Porphyria cutanea tarda; hepatic tumor.

Symptoms and Signs. Those of porphyria cutanea tarda (see).

Etiology. Hepatic tumor exhibiting defect of porphyrin metabolism.

Pathology. Benign or malignant primary tumor of the liver, not associated with cirrhosis. Fluorescence limited to tumoral tissue.

Diagnostic Procedures. See Porphyria cutanea tarda.

Therapy. Surgical excision of tumor.

Prognosis. Disappearance of all symptoms of porphyria tarda after removal of neoplastic tissue.

BIBLIOGRAPHY. Kordac V: Frequency of occurrence of hepatocellular carcinoma in patients with porphyria cutanea tarda in long-term follow-up. Neoplasia 19:135–139, 1972
Kappas A, Sassa S, Anderson KE: The porphyrias. In Lee GR, Bithel TC, Foerster J, et al (eds): Wintrobe's Clinical Hematology, 9th ed, pp 1277–1280. Philadelphia, Lea & Febiger, 1993

NEPHRITIS, RADIATION

Synonyms. Radiation nephritis.

Symptoms. Onset 6–12 months after exposure to radiation (proteinuria, elevation of blood pressure may be evident sooner). Anorexia; cephalalgia; nausea; vomiting, dyspnea.

Signs. Generalized edema; pallor; high blood pressure; heart failure.

Etiology. Exposure to 2500 or more rads in a period of 5 weeks.

Pathology. Kidney normal size; occasionally, surrounded by fibrous tissue; glomeruli show thick basement membrane, hyalinization, and swollen cells; tubular atrophy.

Diagnostic Procedures. *Blood.* Anemia; high blood urea nitrogen and creatinine. *Urine.* Proteinuria; reduced glomerular filtration rate.

Therapy. Symptomatic. Kidney transplantation.

Prognosis. Poor. Death within months or years, or evolution into chronic renal disease.

BIBLIOGRAPHY. Luxton RW: Radiation nephritis. Q J Med 22:215, 1953
Luxton R: Radiation nephritis: A long-term study of 54 patients. Lancet 2:1221–1224, 1961
Glassock RJ: Radiation nephritis. In Massry SG, Glassock RJ: Textbook of Nephrology, 3rd ed, pp 981–982. Baltimore, 1995

NEPHROPHTHISIS, FAMILIAL JUVENILE

Synonyms. Fanconi III; medullary cystic kidney. See Polycystic disease.

Symptoms. Reported in children and young adults. Polydipsia and polyuria; night blindness followed by progressive constriction of peripheral fields and, finally, blurred vision.

Signs. In eyes, retinal arterioles narrowed, disk pale, yellow pigment deposit present throughout retina, macular degeneration, no lens opacity. Blood pressure usually normal until late stage of disease.

Etiology. Unknown. Autosomal recessive inheritance.

Pathology. *Kidney.* Contracted; cortex thin. Thickening of Bowman capsule to hyalinization of glomeruli; nephrons coiled; tubular basal membrane thickened; tubules atrophic (areas of hypertrophy may be observed); interstitial fibrosis. *Eyes.* See Signs. In older subject, medullary cysts may be found in the kidney.

Diagnostic Procedures. *Urine.* Normal, low specific gravity, or moderate proteinuria and minimal hematuria; high excretion of K. Cultures negative. Pyelography. Reduction in size of kidney. Creatine tolerance and phenolsulfonphthalein excretion abnormal. *Blood.* Hyperazotemia. *Echography. CT scan.* Medullary areas with mottled aspect of increased density and cystic lucencies. *Electroretinography.* Pattern consistent with retinitis pigmentosa. *Audiography.* Normal.

Therapy. Symptomatic. Hemodialysis. Kidney transplantation.

Prognosis. Usually, death from renal failure before reaching adulthood. Some longer survival reported. Good results without recurrences with transplantation.

BIBLIOGRAPHY. Fanconi G, Hanhart E, von Albertini A, et al: Die familiare juvenile Nephronophthise. Helv Pediat Acta 6:1–49, 1951

Steele BT, Lirenman DS, Beattie GW: Nephrophthisis. Am J Med 68:531–538, 1980

Cohen AH, Hoyer JR: Nephrophthisis: A primary tubular basement membrane defect. Lab Invest 55:564–572, 1986

Chapman AB, Gabow PA: Hereditary and congenital cystic diseases. In Massry SG, Glassock RJ: Textbook of Nephrology, 3rd ed, pp 553–555, 921–922. Baltimore, Williams & Wilkins, 1995

NETHERTON

Synonym. Comèl-Netherton; ichthyosiform erythroderma variant; ichtiosis linearis circumflexa.

Symptoms and Signs. Occurs almost exclusively in females; present from birth or early infancy. Ichthyosiform erythroderma: generalized erythema and dry and fine scaling; in some cases loss of abundant amount of fluid across skin. On trunk and limbs lesions may be associated with polycyclic eruption with horny margin; or remain inconspicuous but always with flexural disposition. Sparse, brittle hair; trichorrhexis invaginata (bamboo deformity). Occasionally atopic manifestations.

Etiology. Autosomal recessive inborn error of metabolism of variable expressivity (?).

Pathology. Acanthosis, thickening of parakeratotic horny layer. In cytoplasm of upper dermis edema with perivascular infiltration of plasmacells and lymphocytes. Malpighian cells; presence of periodic acid-Shiff-positive granules.

Diagnostic Procedures. *Biopsy.* Of skin. *Urine.* In one case reported, aminoaciduria. *Blood.* Hypoglobulinemia.

Therapy. Etretinates. PUVA.

Prognosis. With age (especially at puberty) partial remissions, but little tendency to spontaneous recovery. In some cases severe immunocompromision leading to death.

BIBLIOGRAPHY. Comèl M: Ichtiosis linearis circumflexa. Dermatologica 98:122–136, 1949

Netherton EW: A unique case of trichorrhexis nodosa: Bamboo hairs. Arch Dermatol 78:483–487, 1958

Traupe H: The Ichtioses. Berlin, Springer-Verlag, 1989

NETTLESHIP (E.) I

Synonyms. Urticaria perstans hemorrhagica; urticaria pigmentosa; xanthelasmoidea; mastocytosis. Includes urticaria aquagenic; urticaria localized heat.

Symptoms and Signs. No sex prevalence; onset in infancy and childhood, or later. Solitary lesion or multiple lesions. Tan macules on the skin, which when stroked, produce urticariation (Darier sign), itching. Vesiculation not constantly present (absent in patient with later onset). When present, gradual decline and disappearance in 2 years. Frequently associated with history of hay fever and asthma. Dermatographia in more than half of cases. Generalized flushing; tachycardia; headache; gastrointestinal complaints. Various bone abnormalities may also be associated. Occasionally, hepatosplenomegaly.

Etiology. Unknown. Sporadic cases and congenital inheritance with simple autosomal dominance, with reduced penetrance described or recessive inheritance. In affected family, frequent occurrence in twins. In aquagenic form, caused by contact with water and in localized heat form (limited to area of contact) by exposure to a warm source.

Pathology. On skin biopsy, dense mast cell infiltrates.

Diagnostic Procedures. *Biopsy.* Of skin. *Urine.* Elevated level of histamine in some cases.

Therapy. Excision of lesion only if symptoms acute, attacks of excessive vesiculation and flushing, or occasionally for cosmetic reasons. Calcium lactate gives some symptomatic benefit.

Prognosis. Usually, spontaneous regression of cutaneous lesions in a few years; lightly pigmented asymptomatic macular lesions may persist. In patients with onset after childhood, symptomatic activity persists indefinitely and systemic mast cell involvement may occur. About 30% develop malignant variety.

BIBLIOGRAPHY. Nettleship E: Rare forms of urticaria. Br Med J 2:323–324, 1869

Fowler JF, Parseley WM, Cotter PG: Familial urticaria pigmentosa. Arch Derm 122:80–81, 1986

Anstey A, Lowe DG, Kirby JD, et al: Familial mastocytosis: A clinical immunophenotypic, light and electron microscopic study. Br J Dermatol 125:583–587, 1991

NETTLESHIP-FALLS

Synonyms. Nettleship (E) II; Vogt albinism X-linked ocular albinism; sex-linked nystagmus; albinism ocular sex-linked; OA1.

Symptoms and Signs. Onset from birth. *Males.* Severely affected. Skin normal or mottled with presence of pigmented nevi and freckles. Hair normal to light colored. Eyes normal color range. Nystagmus and photophobia present; moderate to severe vision reduction. Head nodding and tilting (50%). Strabismus (60%). Reproductive system anomalies common. *Females.* Carriers with absent signs or, occasionally, as severely affected as males.

Etiology. X-linked inheritance involvement of several DNA markers in the distal portion of Xp 22.3 locus.

Pathology. Fewer melanocytes than normal and giant melanosomes present in neuroepithelium-derived pigmented epithelia of eye as well as in the skin.

Diagnostic Procedures. Ophthalmoscopy. Transillumination of iris: males show cartwheel; females diaphanous aspect. In males red reflex present; fundal pigment absent; in females mosaic retina ("splashes of mud") present. Incubation of hair bulb. With tyrosine. Pigmentation.

Therapy. Symptomatic.

Prognosis. With age, possibly, darkening of iris and decreased nystagmus.

BIBLIOGRAPHY. Nettleship E: On some hereditary diseases of the eye. Trans Ophthalmol Soc UK 29:57–198, 1908–1909

Bergen AAB, Samanns C, Schuurman EJM, et al: Multipoint linkage analysis in X-linked ocular albinism of the Nettleship-Falls type. Hum Genet 88:162–166, 1991

Klintworth K: Disorders of amino acid metabolism and melanine pigmentation. In Garner A, Klintworth GK (eds): Pathobiology of Ocular Disease: A Dynamic Approach, 2nd ed, p 948. New York, Marcel Dekker, 1994

NEUHAUSER

Synonyms. Del Giudice; megalocornea—mental retardation; MMR; MMMM.

Symptoms and Signs. In children. Hypotonia; seizures; frontal bossing; antimongoloid slant of eyes; epicanthal folds; broad nasal base; megalocornea accompanied occasionally by iris hypoplasia; large fleshy ears and long fingers.

Etiology. Unknown. Autosomal recessive inheritance.

BIBLIOGRAPHY. Neuhauser G, Kaveggia EG, France TD, et al: Syndrome of mental retardation, seizures, hypotonic cerebral palsy and megalocornea, recessively inherited. Z Kinderheilk 120:1–18, 1975

Del Giudice E, Sartorio R, Romano A, et al: Megalocornea and mental retardation syndrome: Two new cases. Am J Med Genet 26:417–420, 1987

Frydman M, Berkenstadt M, Raas-Rothschild A, et al: Megalocornea, macrocephaly, mental and motor retardation (MMMM). Clin Genet 38:149–154, 1990

NEUHAUSER-BERENBERG

Synonyms. Chalasia cardiac sphincter; cardioesophageal relaxation; esophagus chalasia; gastroesophageal reflux.

Symptoms and Signs. Affects both sexes, usually in infancy. Onset a few days after birth. Vomiting occurs following feeding of child and when he or she is positioned horizontally. Excessive regurgitation, failure to thrive, and danger of aspiration.

Etiology. Unknown. Transitory motor disorder of esophagus with lack of closure of gastroesophageal junction after passage of food.

Diagnostic Procedure. *Fluoroscopy.* Retrograde filling of esophagus in inspiration and with increase of intra-abdominal pressure.

Therapy. Keep infant in orthostatic position during and after feeding.

Prognosis. Variable according to severity of form. For 1 hour in mild form, up to 24 hours in severe form. Bethanechol and antacids prior to meals and thickened food may improve situation. If lack of response surgery ater 6 weeks.

BIBLIOGRAPHY. Neuhauser EB, Berenberg W: Cardioesophageal relaxation as a cause of vomiting in infants. Radiology 48:480–483, 1947

Ogorek CP: Gastroesophageal reflux and disese. In Haubrich WS, Schaffner F, Berk JE (eds): Bockus Gastroenterology, 5th ed, vol 2, p 450. Philadelphia, WB Saunders, 1995

NEU-LAXOVA

Synonyms. Microcephaly; growth retardation; flexion deformities.

Symptoms and Signs. Both sexes affected. Intrauterine growth retardation; flexion deformities; overlapping fingers; rocker-bottom feet; protruding heels; toes syndactyly. Marked microcephaly; ocular hypertelorism; exophthalmos; absent eyelids; short neck. Occasionally, tiny nose.

Etiology. Multiple dysplasia, malformation entity. Possibly autosomal recessive inheritance.

Pathology. Brain atrophy; absence corpus callosum.

Prognosis. Early death.

BIBLIOGRAPHY. Neu RL, Kajii T, Gardener LI, et al: A lethal syndrome of microcephaly with multiple congenital anomalies in three siblings. Pediatrico 47:611–612, 1971

Laxova R, Ohdra PT, Timothy JAD: A further example of a lethal autosomal recessive condition in sibs. J Ment Defic Res 16:139–143, 1972

Mueller RE, Winter RM, Naylor CPE: Neu-Laxova syndrome: two further case reports and comments on proposed sub-classification. Am J Med Genet 16:645–649, 1983

Meguid NA, Temtamy SA: Neu-Laxova syndrome in two Egyptian families. Am J Med Genet 41:30–31, 1991

NEUMANN (E.)

Synonyms. Epulis, congenital; neonatal myoblastoma. See Abrikossov myoblastoma.

Symptoms. Both sexes affected; observed in newborns. Pedunculated tumor in the oral mucosa, usually on the margin of tongue, but may be found also anywhere. Smooth nodule 1–3 cm in diameter.

Etiology. Unknown.

Pathology. See Abrikossov.

Therapy. Surgical excision.

Prognosis. No tendency to recur after excision.

BIBLIOGRAPHY. Neumann E: Eine Fall von congenitaler Epulis. Arch Heilk 12:189, 1871

Scully C: The oral cavity. In Champion RH, Burton JL, Ebling FJG (eds): Rook/Wilkinson/Ebling Textbook of Dermatology, 5th ed, p 2706. Oxford, Blackwell Scientific, 1992

NEUMANN (I.)

Synonym. Pemphigus vegetans (Neumann variety).

Symptoms and Signs. Both sexes affected. Onset in young and middle-aged adults. Localized lesions in the mouth and other mucosae (e.g., vagina); may or may not precede skin lesions; usually present in some stage of the disease. *Skin.* Bullae that break and develop into exudative vegetative lesions with small pustules; when drying, hyperkeratosis and fissures occur. Skin in flexure zones most frequently involved.

Etiology. Unknown. It may develop in the recuperation phase of pemphigus vulgaris.

Pathology. Bullae as in pemphigus vulgaris; acantholysis associated with acanthosis; microabscesses with eosinophils.

Therapy. Corticosteroids.

Prognosis. Spontaneous remission reported, but usually fatal without treatment.

BIBLIOGRAPHY. Neumann I: Ueber Pemphigus vegetans (frambosioides). Vrtljschr Dermatol 13:157–178, 1886

Korman NJ: Pemphigus. Semin Dermatol 8:689–700, 1990

Pye RJ: Bullous eruptions. In Champion RH, Burton JL, Ebling FJG (eds): Rook/Wilkinson/Ebling Textbook of Dermatology, 5th ed, p 1636. Oxford, Blackwell Scientific, 1992

NEUMANN (M.A.)

Synonyms. Dementia, familial (Neumann type). Subcortical glyosis.

Symptoms and Signs. See Senile dementia.

Etiology. Sporadic. Autosomal recessive inheritance reported.

Diagnostic Procedures. *Brain biopsy.* Normal level of neurotransmitters; subcortical glyosis. *MRI. EEG. Cerebrospinal fluid.* Normal level of neurotransmitters.

BIBLIOGRAPHY. Neumann MA: Pick's disease. J Neuropath Exp Neurol 8:255–282, 1949
Kronbesserian P, Davons P, Bianco C, et al: Demence familiale de type Neumann (glyose sous corticale). Rev Neurol (Paris) 141:706–712, 1985
Khoubesserian P, Dvous P, Bianco C, et al: Demence familiale de type Neumann (gliose sous corticale). Rev Neurol (Paris) 141:706–712, 1985

NEURITIS MULTIPLEX CUTANEA

Synonym. Wartenberg; multiple sensory neuritis, acquired.

Symptoms. Minimal and unnoticed for a long time. Changes of skin sensitivity from hypoesthesia to anesthesia. Spontaneous pain rare, elicited by slight trauma of the skin; distribution of affected areas is disseminated but never symmetric. Most frequently involved nerves are digital, upper and lower extremity, saphenous, femoral cutaneous, lateralis calcanei.

Signs. Subjecting an involved sensory nerve to brisk "stretching," a brief sharp pain is elicited in the area innervated. Motor nerves never involved. No vasomotor or trophic manifestations; no general or systemic disturbances.

Etiology. Unknown. The syndrome may be an expression of diabetes, carcinoma, malnutrition or abuse of alcohol or drugs.

Pathology. Unknown.

Prognosis. Chronic course with remission and intermission, affecting one sensory nerve or another one remotely located.

BIBLIOGRAPHY. Schlesinger H: Ueber Neuritis multiplex cutanea. Neurol Centralbl 30:1218–1221, 1911
Wartenberg R: Multiple sensory neuritis: A clinical entity. Trans Am Neurol Assoc 71:101–104, 1946
Savin JA: Skin and the nervous system. In Champion RH, Burton JL, Ebling FJG (eds): Rook/Wilkinson/Ebling Textbook of Dermatology, 5th ed, pp 2472–2473. Oxford, Blackwell Scientific, 1992

NEURITIS, PATELLAR PLEXUS

Synonyms. Gonalgia paresthetica (similar condition); neuralgia traumatic prepatellar (similar condition).

Symptoms. Complaint of "electric shock" when well-defined unilateral or bilateral trigger areas of prepatellar or adjacent zones are even lightly touched. Sensation appears, disappears, and recurs without apparent reason.

Etiology. Unknown. Previous minor and forgotten injury. Anatomic accident in misplacement of infrapatellar branch of saphenous or other nerve of prepatellar plexus, vulnerable to mechanical trauma or ischemia produced by movement.

BIBLIOGRAPHY. Wartenberg R: Digitalgia paresthetica and gonyalgia paresthetica. Neurology 4:106–115, 1954
Smillie IS: Injuries of the Knee Joint. Edinburgh, Churchill Livingstone, 1962

NEUROBLASTOMA

Synonyms. Congenital neuroblastoma; sympathicoblastoma, sympathicogonioma. See Hutchinson and Pepper.

Symptoms and Signs. Incidence slightly higher in males. Median age 2 years, with 90% of cases diagnosed before 6 years of age. Seldom symptomatic until tumor reaches a massive size; a hard painless mass in the neck, a localized intrathoracic mass incidentally observed radiographically, a palpable abdominal mass, or bone pain or other metastasis (60–75% present at diagnosis).

Etiology. Unknown. Autosomal dominant or recessive inheritance with variable penetrance or expression suggested.

Pathology. Primary site not always easily identified. Most common areas involved are adrenal, retroperitoneal (other organs), mediastinal. In the least differentiated type, grade III, cell structure small, no evident cytoplasm, presence of rosettes. In grade II, cell separated by fibrillar eosinophilic stroma. In grade I, ganglion cell present.

Diagnostic Procedures. *X-ray. CT scan. MRI. Echography. Bone marrow.* Presence of cancer cells (50%). *Urine.* Increased excretion of dopamine, norepinephrine, vanillylmandelic acid. A variety of biological and genetic markers used to refine risk-directed therapy. Staging according to variable systems based on clinical or laboratory data provide therapeutical and prognostic guidelines.

Therapy. Extended radical surgery within reason (see Prognosis). Radiotherapy; systemic chemotherapy.

Prognosis. According to age at diagnosis, staging at time of intervention and type of treatment, 4-year survival 24–100%. *X-rays.* No recurrence at site of irradiation, but possible metastasis. Spontaneous involution and regression (especially in neonatal stage D), well-documented.

BIBLIOGRAPHY. Dodge HJ, Benner MC: Neuroblastoma of adrenal medullar in siblings. Rocky Mt Med J 42:35–38, 1945
Hecht F, Hecht BK, Northrup JC, et al: Genetics of familial neuroblastoma: Long-range studies. Cancer Genet Cytogenet 7:227–230, 1982
Hayes FA, Smith EI: Neuroblastoma. In Pizzo PA, Poplack DG, Pediatric Oncology, p 607. Philadelphia, JB Lippincott, 1989
Santana VM: Neuroblastoma. In Behrman RE, Kliegman Arvin Nelson: Textbook of Pediatrics, 15th ed, pp 1460–1463. Philadelphia, WB Saunders, 1995

NEUROFIBROMATOSIS SYNDROMES

1. NF I: Von Recklinghausen (see)
2. NF II: Familial acoustical neurinoma
3. NF III: Riccardi (NF III)
4. NF IV: Riccardi (NF IV)

BIBLIOGRAPHY. Riccardi VM, Eichner JE: Neurofibromatosis: Phenotype, Natural History, and Pathogenesis. Baltimore, Johns Hopkins Univ Press, 1986
Mulvihill JJ, Parry DK, Sherman JL: Neurofibromatosis 1 (Recklinghausen disease) and neurofiromatosis 2 (bilateral acoustic neurofibromatosis): An update. Ann Inter Med 113:39–52, 1990

NEUROGENIC BLADDER

Synonyms. Spastic bladder; reflex bladder.

Symptoms. Precipitous micturition; nicturia; leakage around catheters; intolerance of catheter. Throbbing headache; profuse sweating; nasal obstruction; "goose bumps" accompany the spastic contractions.

Signs. Blood hypertension, bradycardia accompany spastic contraction.

Etiology. Spinal cord lesions above the conus medullaris.

Pathology. Tumor; trauma; infections; degenerative changes of spine at level immediately above the conus medullaris. Hydronephrosis may develop.

Diagnostic Procedures. *X-ray.* Of spine. *Myelography. Cystometrography.*

Therapy. Propantheline and oxybutine in cases refractory to pharmacological treatment. Convert spastic to flaccid bladder. (1) Subarachnoid injection of alcohol to abolish hyperreflexia. (2) Cordectomy. (3) Selective rhizotomy of third and fourth sacral roots bilaterally is best procedure since it is not accompanied by extensive damage to nervous structure and by the resulting conus medullaris syndrome.

Prognosis. That of etiology, plus renal complication. Good result with last procedure indicated.

FLACCID BLADDER SYNDROME

Symptoms and Signs. Desire, initiation, and inhibition of micturition are absent. Usually, part of the conus medullaris syndrome.

Etiology and Pathology. Trauma, tumor, vascular lesion, or infection at level of conus medullaris.

Diagnostic Procedures. *X-ray. Spinal tap. Myelogram. Urologic evaluation. Cystometry. Cystoscopy.*

Therapy. Bethanecol or, if feasible, surgery to remove compression of cord. Symptomatic.

Prognosis. Infection of bladder, a common complication.

BIBLIOGRAPHY. Bors E: Neurogenic bladder. Urol Surv 7:177–250, 1957
Adams RD, Victor M: Principles of Neurology, 5th ed, p 475. New York, McGraw-Hill, 1993

NEUROLEPTIC, MALIGNANT

Synonyms. Delay; NMS. (Includes Deuschl familial occurrence).

Symptoms and Signs. In patients treated with neuroleptics. Incidence estimated from 0.02–3.23. Sex-age not meaningful risk factors. Exhaustion, psychomotor activity, dehydration considered risk factors. It occurs in the early phases of treatment. Preceded; not invariably, by insidious neurologic and autonomic signs (obtundation, new-onset catatonia, tachycardia, tachypnea, hypertension, dysarthria, dysphagia, diaphoresis, sialorrhea, incontinence, minor temperature increase, rigidity, myoclonus, tremors). Full syndrome represented by hyperthermia, with profuse sweating (98%) (possible brain or cerebellar damage if not promptly treated) "lead-pipe" rigidity (97%) (associated with myonecrosis). Changes in mental status (97%) up to deliirium, coma, catatonic features; autonomic activation and instability; sinus tachycardia (88%), hypertension (61%); coarse tremor myoclonus, and less frequently other extrapyramidal and bulbar signs. In 31% of cases evidence of pulmonary embolism that may lead to respiratory arrest.

Etiology. Acute reduction of brain dopamine activity. Neuroleptic-induced disruption of regulation in hypothalamus, and basal ganglia that cause failure to compensate for an increasd rate of endogenous metabolic activity and heat production.

Diagnostic Procedures. *Laboratory findings.* None specific. CPK increased (95%) other enzymes may be elevated; leukocytosis; metabolic acidosis or hypoxia; myoglobinuria (67%). *EEG.* Generalized slowing.

Therapy. Discontinuation of drug, fluid balance temperature control monitoring of general conditions. Dopamine antagonist or dantrolene should be considered. Electroshock has also been adopted in refractory cases.

Prognosis. Last 7–10 days in uncomplicated cases. High risk of recurrences on reintroduction according to time elapsed since recovery and dosage used.

BIBLIOGRAPHY. Delay J, Pichot P, Lamperiere T, et al: Un neuroleptique majeur non-phenothiazine et non reserpinique, l'haloperidol, dans le traitment des psychoses. Ann Med Psychol 118:145–152, 1960
Caroff SN, Mann SC: Neuroleptic malignant syndrome. Med Clin N Am 77:185–201, 1993

NEUROPATHY, HEREDITARY, SENSORY, RADICULAR

Synonyms. Hicks-Camp; Denny-Brown; H.S.A.N.I.

Symptoms. Both sexes. Onset 15–35 years of age. Deafness and shooting pains from the feet to the legs initially. No loss of sensation of touch, heat, and cold on the feet.

Signs. Starting with a corn on big toe, development painless, deepening to the bone and extending to other toes. Reduction then disappearance of tendon reflexes. Arms and cranial reflexes normal (except auditory).

Etiology. Unknown. Autosomal dominant trait. Relationship with other foot ulceration syndromes (see Nelaton; Morvan; Biemond III) not yet completely elucidated; restless legs and lancinating pain could be minor presentation of the same condition (?).

Pathology. Marked loss of ganglion cells in sacral and lumbar dorsal root ganglia with, in some cases, clear hyaline bodies (amyloid?).

Diagnostic Procedures. *X-ray.* Electrophysiologic studies of nerve. *Biopsy.* Of nerve and ganglia.

Therapy. Prevention of foot ulcers. Conservative treatment of ulcers preferable to surgery.

Prognosis. Progressive condition leading to severe ulceration and complete deafness.

BIBLIOGRAPHY. Hicks EP, Camp MB: Hereditary perforating ulcer of the foot. Lancet I:319–321, 1922
Denny-Brown D: Hereditary sensory radicular neuropathy. J Neurol Neurosurg Psychiatr 14:237–252, 1951
Danon MJ, Carpenter S: Hereditary sensory neuropathy biopsy: Study of an autosomal dominant variety. Br Med J 2:737–740, 1985
Adams RD, Victor M: Principles of Neurology, 5th ed, p 1148. New York, McGraw-Hill, 1993

NEUROPATHY, SERUM

Symptoms and Signs. Predominant in males; onset 7–10 days after injection of serum (preventive or curative) for conditions such as tetanus, diphtheria. Local pain; swelling of tissues and joints; edema of mucous membranes; hyperthermia. After 2 or 3 days paralysis of one or more spinal nerve territories, usually (mono or bilateral) of shoulder-girdle, but occasionally more extensive involvement. Possibly convulsions, meningeal reaction. Absence of sensory alterations (usually).

Etiology. Complication of injection of foreign proteins.

Pathology. Polyneuritis changes; edema of involved areas.

Diagnostic Procedure. *Electromyography.*

Therapy. During acute stage, antihistaminic drugs. Physical therapy after onset of paralysis.

Prognosis. Variable recovery in 1 to several months. Residual weakness and muscle wasting in 10–20%.

BIBLIOGRAPHY. Garvey JL: Serum neuritis: 20 cases following use of antitetanic serum. Postgrad Med 13:210–213, 1953
Adams RD, Victor M: Principles of Neurology, 5th ed, p 1159. New York, McGraw-Hill, 1993

NEUTROPENIA, IMMUNOGLOBULIN ABNORMALITIES

Synonyms. Immunoglobulinopathia; neutropenia; granulocytopenia; hypogammaglobulinemia; hypogammaglobulinemia; neutropenia.

Symptoms. In early infancy (familial form) or various ages (nonfamilial form). Oral, pharyngeal, respiratory infection.

Signs. Lymphoadenopathy, splenomegaly.

Etiology. Familial forms. Suggested X-linked inheritance. Nonfamilial form: unknown.

Pathology. Pneumonitis without granuloma formation. Lymph node and thymus normal.

Diagnostic Procedures. *Familial form.* Blood: hypogammaglobulinemia. Bone marrow: maturation arrest at myelocyte level. Absence of antibodies againt leukocytes. Skin window: delayed and hypocellular response. *Nonfamilial form.* Blood cyclic or chronic neutropenia. Hypogammaglobulinemia. Bone marrow. Almost complete absence of plasma cells.

Therapy. Gamma globulins.

Prognosis. In many cases good temporay response to chronic gamma globulins administration.

BIBLIOGRAPHY. Good RA, Zak S: Disturbances in gammaglobulin synthesis as "experiments of nature." Pediatrics 18:109, 1956
Loudsdale D, Deodhar SD, Mercer R: Familial granulocytopenia and associated immunoglobulin abnormality. J Pediatr 71:790–801, 1967
Athens JW, Neutropenia. In Lee GR, Bithell TC, Foerster J, et al (eds): Wintrobe's Clinical Hematology, 9th ed, p 1602. Philadelphia, Lea & Febiger, 1993

NEUTROPENIA, NEONATAL

Synonyms. Isoimmune neonatal neutropenia.

Symptoms and Signs. Occurs in newborns. Mild recurrent infections or fulminating infections. Skin infection is the most frequent clinical finding.

Etiology. Passage to the fetus of leukocyte antibodies produced by the mother. The phenomenon of passage of these antibodies is rather frequent, while the effect on neutrophil number and clinical manifestations is very rare.

Diagnostic Procedures. *Blood.* Leukopenia with severe neutropenia, accompanied by monocytosis. No anemia or thrombocytopenia. Maternal blood contains agglutinins against neutrophils. *Bone marrow.* Rich myeloid series, but few or absent mature neutrophils. Severe neutropenia, with a normal total leukocyte count. Monocytosis is frequent, and eosinophilia sometimes is observed.

Therapy. Antibiotics (if infections); corticosteroid or adrenocorticotropic hormone.

Prognosis. Usually excellent; complete spontaneous recovery, except in fulminating cases. (The duration of the neutropenia varies 2–17 weeks.)

BIBLIOGRAPHY. Hitzig WH, Gitzelmann R: Transplacental transfer of leukocyte agglutinins. Vox Sang (NS) 4:445–456, 1959
Athens JW: Neutropenia. In Lee GR, Bithel TC, Foerster J, et al (eds): Wintrobe's Clinical Hematology, 9th ed, p 1603. Philadelphia, Lea & Febiger, 1993

NEVO

Synonyms. See Sotos.

Symptoms and Signs. Features similar to Sotos; accelerated intrauterine growth. At birth generalized edema, muscle hypotonia and contractures, clumsiness, dolichoephaly, malformed ears, large extremities; clinodactyly. Retarded motor and speech development.

Etiology. Autosomal recessive inheritance.

BIBLIOGRAPHY. Nevo S, Zeltzer M Benderly A: Evidence for autosomal recessive inheritance in cerebral gigantism. J Med Genet II:158–165, 1974
Cohen MM Jr: Overgrowth syndromes. In El-Shafie M, Klippel CH (eds): Associated Congenital Malformations, pp 71–104. Baltimore, Williams & Wilkins, 1981

NEVUS FLAMMEUS

Synonyms. Capillary nevus; plane nevus; telangiectatic nevus; Unna nevus; salmon patches; port-wine stain.

Symptoms and Signs. May present three distinct groups of features: (1) Salmon patches. Both sexes affected; present at birth. On the nape, forehead, and eyelids; pinkish patches, with fine telangiectasis. They may disappear within 1 year, or later; 5–7% of those of the nape of neck persist throughout life (Unna nevus). (2) Port-wine nevus. Both sexes affected; present at birth. In any part of the body, more frequent on face and upper trunk (membranes may be involved) patches, pink to bright red of various dimensions (a few millimeters to several centimeters in diameter). (3) Nevus increasing in size. Same characteristics as the preceding, but appearing after a traumatic injury of the part.

Etiology. Unknown. Neurogenic factor related to birth postulated. Autosomal dominant inheritance. Part of many hereditary syndromes.

Pathology. Variable. Ectasia of superficial or deeper vessels associated more or less with connective hypertrophic changes.

Therapy. Several approaches, but all unsatisfactory. Excision and grafting; ionizing radiation; dermabrasion. Cosmetic masking remains the safest and most efficient procedure.

Prognosis. From spontaneous disappearance to permanence.

BIBLIOGRAPHY. Shelly WB, Livingood CS: Familial multiple nevi flammei. Arch Derm Syph 59:343–345, 1949
Merlob P, Reisner SH: Familial nevus flammeus of the forehead and Unna's nevus. Clin Genet 27:165–166, 1985
Atherton DJ: Naevi and other developmental defects. In Champion RH, Burton JL, Ebling FJG (eds): Rook/Wilkinson/Ebling Textbook of Dermatology, 5th ed, pp 483–484. Oxford, Blackwell Scientific, 1992

NEZELOF

Synonyms. Lymphopenia; normoglobulinemia; S.C.I.D.; severe combined immunodeficiency; T-lymphocyte deficiency; thymic alymphoplasia; see Beck-Ibrahim.

Symptoms and Signs. Both sexes affected. Seventy-five percent male; onset in infancy. Virus and fungus infections. Herpes labialis, bronchopulmonary infections leading to emphysema and bronchiectasis.

Etiology. It represents the other end of the spectrum of combined immunodeficiency, which originates from the De Vaal syndrome (see). (See also intermediate form of Glanzmann-Rinikier.) In Nezelof the defect seems to be limited to the thymus system (responsible for cellular immunity). Proper reference is Nezelof in case of presence of oligoclonal or polyclonal immunoglobulins. Autosomal recessive inheritance.

Pathology. Thymic dysplasia residues of thymus can be found in the neck consisting in islands of endodermal cells without lymphoid tissue and Hassall corpuscles. In peripheral lymph nodes, spleen, and other organs lymphocyte depletion and presence of numerous plasma cells.

Diagnostic Procedures. *Blood.* Coombs test positive. Hemolytic anemia; normal granulocytes number; lymphopenia deficiencies of both B- and T-lymphocytes. Normal immunoglobulins; however, antigen stimulation does not produce increase in antibodies. Cases reported with selective deficit of immunoglobulins IgG, IgM, and IgA. Impaired delayed hypersensitivity. Absence of skin reactions to various antigens.

Therapy. Trimethorpim-sulfamethoxazole, immunoglobulin (varicellazoster immune); blood products obtained from cytomelovirus-negative donors and always irradiated before use. Only effective treatment: bone marrow transplantation from istoidentical donor, or from haploididentical after T-cell depletion.

Prognosis. Death by third to fourth year of life primarily from varicella, herpes, adenovirus, and cytomegalovirus infection.

BIBLIOGRAPHY. Nezelof C, Jammet ML, Lortholary P, et al: L'hypoplasie héréditaire du thymus sa place et sa responsabilité dans une observation d'aplasie lymphocytare normoplasmacytaire et normoglobulininémique du nourissau. Arch Fr Pediatr 21:897–920, 1964
Lukens JN: Immune deficiency diseases: inherited and acquired. In Lee GR, Bithel TC, Foerster J, et al (eds): Wintrobe's Clinical Hematology, 9th ed, pp 1683–1684. Philadelphia, Lea & Febiger, 1993

NICOLAU I

Synonyms. Nicolau-Hoigné; accidental embolization; embolia cutis medicamentosa.

Symptoms. Occurs following an intramuscular injection of bismuth (original report), penicillin, tetracyclines. Somnolence; acoustic sensation; occasionally, visual loss; sudden pain in extremities or abdomen; paresis or paralysis; shock.

Signs. Pallor; cyanosis; peripheral edema; tachycardia; motor irritability; arterial hypotension.

Etiology. Accidental injection of drug into artery. Reaction of nonallergic type, but of embolic nature.

Pathology. According to arterial district involved.

Therapy. Symptomatic. Amputation occasionally required when failling attempt of restoring circulation or revascularization.

Prognosis. Variable. Death in severe cases.

BIBLIOGRAPHY. Nicolau S: Dermite livédode et gangrë-neuse de la fesse, consécutive aux injections intramusculaires, dans la syphilis. A propos d'un cas de'embolie artérielle bismuthique. Ann Mal Vénéreol (Paris) 20:321–339, 1925
Hoigné R: Akute Nebenreaktionen auf Penicillin-prä-parate. Acta Med Scand 171:201–208, 1962
Domula M, Weissbac G, Lenk H: Das Nicolau-Syndrom nach Benzathinpenizillin. Ein Überblick an Hand von 5 eigenen Beobachtungen. Kinderärztl Praxis 40:437–448, 1972
Littmann K, Albrecht RM, Richter HJ, et al: Embolia cutis. Dtsch Med Wschr 109:800–805, 1984

NIEDEN

Synonym. Cataract telangiectasia.

Symptoms and Signs. Both sexes affected. Onset from birth. Telangiectasia of face and upper limbs; sparse eyebrows; skin thickened; increased pigmentation of neck; signs of heart enlargement and congenital valvular defects. Bilateral cataract. Glaucoma.

Etiology. Unknown. Familial cases reported.

Pathology. Telangiectasia. Heart enlargement; valvular defects; hypoplasia of aorta. Defect of iris mesenchyma.

Therapy. Heart surgery where indicated.

Prognosis. Variable. Reported cases still alive in their third and fourth decades.

BIBLIOGRAPHY. Nieden A: Cataractbildung bei teleangiectätischer Ausdehnung der Capillaren der ganzen Gesichtshaut. Centbl Prarkt Augenheilkd 11:353–357, 1887
Waardenburg PJ, Franceschetti A, Klein D: Genetics and Ophthalmology, vol 1, p 906. Springfield, IL, Charles C Thomas, 1961

NIELSEN (H.)

Synonym. Congenital dystrophia brevicollis.

Eponym used to indicate a combination of Klippel-Feil (see) and Bonnevie-Ulrich.

BIBLIOGRAPHY. Nielsen H: Dystrophia brevicollis congenita. Hospitalstidende 77:409–431, 1934

NIELSEN-JAKOBS

Synonyms. Agnosia; apraxia; aphasia; anterior cingulate gyri; cingulate gyri.

Symptoms. Apathy; akinesia; mutism; incontinence.

Signs. Open eyes; normal muscle tone; indifference to pain. Babinski sign bilaterally. Increased respiration rate.

Etiology. Bilateral damage to the cingulate gyri.

Prognosis. Severe

BIBLIOGRAPHY. Nielsen JM: Agnosia, Apraxia and Aphasia. New York, Hoeber, 1946
Nielsen J, Jacobs JC: Bilateral lesions of the anterior cingulate giry. Bull LA Neurol Soc 16:231–234, 1951
Brown JW: Frontal lobe syndromes. In Vinken PJ, Bruyn GW (eds): Handbook of Clinical Neurology, vol 45, p 33. Amsterdam, North-Holland, 1984

NIELSEN (J.M.) I

Synonyms. Exhaustive psychosis; neuromuscular exhaustion; disaster; compassion fatigue. See chronic fatigue.

Symptoms. Develops subacutely after severe overexertion during a period of euphoria. Degree of overwork is variable and depends on age and other factors. Feeling of deep exhaustion of entire body, more severe in abused muscles. Headache pain, tenderness, twitching, and then atrophy of muscles involved. Dizziness. Generalized restlessness that prevents sleeping and rest; weight loss.

Signs. In acute stage, muscle flaccidity, absence of deep reflexes. Later, reflexes return to normal.

Etiology. Unknown; metabolic disturbance caused by overwork or trauma.

Pathology. Unknown.

Diagnostic Procedures. *Cerebrospinal fluid.* Normal. *Electromyography. Thyroid function tests.*

Therapy. Symptomatic. Rest, diet.

Prognosis. Very slow; partial recovery of moderate activity. Lack of recovery of previous tone and strength.

BIBLIOGRAPHY. Nielsen JM: Subacute generalized neuromuscular exhaustion syndrome. Bull Los Angeles Neurol Soc 5:128–130, 1940

Nielson JM: Subacute generalized neuromuscular exhaustion syndrome. Report of 3 cases. Calif Med 66:338–340, 1947

Stutman RK, Bliss EL: Postraumatic stress disorder: hypnotizability and imagery. Am J Psychiatr 142:741–743, 1985

Straus SE: Chronic Fatigue Syndrome. New York, Marcel Dekker, 1995

Figley CR (ed): Compassion Fatigue. New York, Brunner-Mazel, 1995

NIEMANN-PICK

Synonyms. Lipid histiocytosis; sphingomyelin lipidosis; sphingomyelin reticuloendotheliosis; sphingomyelin—cholesterol lipidoses.

TYPE I

Lipidosis with sphingomyelinase deficiency and primary sphingomyelin storage.

TYPE IA: ACUTE FORM

Symptoms. Affects both sexes equally. About 40% of patients are Jewish, but all races may be affected. Usually normal at birth; onset at 1–2 months. Failure to thrive; mental retardation; progressing to apathy and dullness.

Signs. Debility and wasting of extremity; abdominal enlargement; hepatosplenomegaly. Cherry red spot in macular region (50%). Skin may show plaques of brown pigmented areas; blue brown discoloration; xanthomas are rare.

Etiology. Deficiency of lysosomal sphingomyelinase (activity less than 5%). Autosomal recessive inheritance. Probably in the different cases and phenotypes of type I (ASC) there is more than one mutation in enzyme form.

Pathology. All organs show infiltration with typical foamy vacuolated cells, containing sphingomyelin-sterol. Organs primarily involved are liver, spleen, lungs, lymph nodes, bone marrow. Brain shows marked degenerative changes.

Diagnostic Procedures. *Blood.* Anemia; vacuolated leukocytes. High cholesterol level. Kampine-Brady-Kanfer test on washed white blood cells shows low level of enzymatic activity for hydrolysis of sphingomyelin and glucocerebrosides. *Bone marrow.* Presence of typical cells. *Biopsy and biochemical studies.* Of tissues.

Therapy. None. However, in some cases, splenectomy, although it does not change the final prognosis.

Prognosis. Death within 5 years.

TYPE IS (CHRONIC NON-NEURONOPATHIC)

Symptoms and Signs. Onset at the same age as the preceding or, more typical, slightly later. Splenomegaly first sign; hepatomegaly later. Respiratory infection. Absence of signs of central nervous system involvement; possibly, high intellectual capacity.

Etiology. See the preceding. Sphingomyelinase activity less than 10%.

Pathology. In spleen, liver, lungs, bone marrow, presence of birefringent foam cells.

Diagnostic Procedures. *Blood.* Anemia; evidence of minor liver function impairment. *Bone marrow.* See Pathology. *X-ray.* Of chest. Diffuse infiltration.

Therapy. Symptomatic.

Prognosis. Poor.

TYPE IC

Symptoms and Signs. Accidental discovery of hepatosplenomegaly and/or foam cells or blue histiocytes in bone marrow. Splenic rupture, bilary cirrhosis, respiratory problems. Sometime described cherry red spot and cerebellar ataxia

Etiology. See the preceding.

Diagnostic Procedures. *Bone marrow.* Foam cells. *Liver and spleen biopsy.* Increase of sphingomyelin.

Prognosis. Good.

TYPE II

Lipidosis with primary defect uncertain and secondary sphingomyelin storage.

TYPE IIA

Acute form includes neonatal hepatitis like forms and cases with psychomotor retardation.

Symptoms and Signs. Appearing between first days of life and 2 years of age. Jaundice and clinical picture of hepatitis. Later in some cases progressive psychomotor retardation with hypertonicity of limbs and loss of coordination.

Etiology. Autosomal recessive inheritance. Enzyme defect is not known but in the pathway of metabolism of glycolipids, sphingomyelins, or cholesterol.

Pathology. Presence of foamy cells in bone marrow and other organs. Droplets are less birifrangent than in type I.

Diagnostic Procedures. See the preceding.

Therapy. Symptomatic.

Prognosis. Progressive failure of mental and motor skills. Death at 5–15 years of age.

TYPE IIS

Subacute form includes type C of Crocker (Chronic neuronopathic), type D (Nova Scotia), juvenile dystonic lipoidosis, neurovisceral storage with vertical supranuclear ophthalmoplegia, juvenile Nieman-Pick disease with blue histiocytes, DAF syndrome (down gaze paresis, ataxia, athetosis, foam cells).

Symptoms and Signs. Normal at birth and for first 2 years (occasionally longer), then loss of speech, ataxia, gran mal seizures, hypertonia, hyperreflexia, moderate hepatosplenomegaly, jaundice.

Etiology. Autosomal recessive inheritance. Basic enzyme defect not known. In type D (Nova Scotia). Common ancestry to a couple born in Nova Scotia, Canada in 1600.

Synonyms. Farber-Crocker.

Symptoms. Limited to population from Nova Scotia; onset in second to fourth year of life. Unsteady gait; lack of coordination; epilepsy (grand and petit mal); mental deterioration.

Signs. Hepatosplenomegaly. Jaundice.

Etiology. See the preceding. Sphingomyelinase normal or slightly reduced.

Pathology. Foamy cells in bone marrow and different organs.

Prognosis. Poor.

BIBLIOGRAPHY. Niemann A: Ein unbekanntes Krankheitbild. Jahrb Kinderh N F 29:1–10, 1914

Pick L: Ueber die lipoidzellige Splenohepatomegalie Typus Niemann-Pick als Stoffwecheslerkrankung. Med Klin 23:1483–1488, 1927

Pick L, Bielschowsky M: Ueber lipoidzellige Splenomegalie (Typus Niemann-Pick) und amaurotische Idiotie. Klin Wochenschr 5:1631, 1927

Schuchman EH, Desnick RJ: Nieman-Pick disease type A and B: Acid sphingomyelinase deficiencies. In Scriver CR, Beaudet AL, Sly WS, et al: The Metabolic and Molecular Bases of Inherited Disease, 7th ed, pp 2602–2604. New York, McGraw-Hill, 1995

NIERHOFF-HUEBNER

Synonym. Endochondral dysostosis.

Symptoms. Onset during first days of life. Convulsion; somnolence; muscular flaccidity.

Signs. From birth, normal body length, micromelia; short neck; microcephaly (occasional); mild cyanosis; jaundice.

Etiology. Considered a variant of Morquio (osteochondrodystrophy). Autosomal recessive inheritance or dominant with incomplete penetrance.

Pathology. Cranial sutures dehiscent. Rib junctures. Rachitic rosary. *Heart.* Ventricle dilatation and myocardial swelling. *Kidney.* Swelling. Leptomeninges. Hemorrhages. Microscopically, bone structure changes, especially of proximal end of femur and distal end of ulna.

Diagnostic Procedures. *Blood.* Hyperazotemia. *X-ray. CT scan. MRI.* Of skeleton. Abnormal calcification of epiphyseal and metaphyseal part of bones and cranial vault. *Cerebrospinal fluid.* Normal. *EEG.* Altered patterns.

Therapy. Symptomatic.

Prognosis. Fatal within a few weeks.

BIBLIOGRAPHY. Nierhoff H, Heubner O: Familiaere systemisierte enchondrale Dysostose bei 3 Geschwistern. Z Kinderh 78:497–521, 1956

NIEVERGELT

Synonyms. Nievergelt-Erb; Nievergelt-Pearlman; mesomelic dyplasia Nievergelt; multiple synostosis syndrome; radioulnar synostosis.

Symptoms. Both sexes affected. Prevalent in males; onset from birth. Dwarfism. Symmetric dysplasia of elbows; luxation of ulna or radial heads; radioulnar synostosis; brachydactyly; flexion of fingers; symmetric dysplasia of lower legs; genu valgum; clubfoot; deformed great toes. Hearing loss.

Etiology. Unknown. Autosomal dominant inheritance.

Diagnostic Procedures. *X-ray.* Of skeleton. Superior radioulnar synostosis; fibula relatively longer; tarsal bone synostosis; epiphyseal line obliquity. *Chromosome studies.* Negative.

Therapy. Orthopedic procedures.

Prognosis. Poor quoad functionem.

BIBLIOGRAPHY. Nievergelt K: Positiver Vaterschafs nachweis auf Grund erblicher Missbildungen der Extremitäten. Arch Klaus Stift Vererbungforsch 19:157–160, 1944
Wiedemann HR, Dibbern H: Niegervelt syndrome. Med Welt 31:374–375, 1980
Taybi H, Lachman R: Radiology of Syndromes and Metabolic Disorders and Skeletal Dysplasia, 3rd ed. St Louis, Mosby-Year Book, 1990

NIGHT EATING

Synonym. Morning anorexia; hyperphagia; insomnia.

Symptoms. Apparently prevalent in women; occurs in obese patients or patients with weight disorders. Nocturnal hyperphagia, insomnia, and anorexia in the morning. Difficulty in losing weight.

Etiology. Unknown. Response to stress in emotionally disturbed individual.

Therapy. Psychotherapy; environmental manipulation; diet; amphetamine and similar medications.

Prognosis. This syndrome influences the result of weight reduction programs.

BIBLIOGRAPHY. Stunkard AJ, Grace WJ, Wolff HG: The nighteating syndrome: A pattern of food intake among certain obese patients. Am J Med 19:78–86, 1955
Field HL, Domanque BB: Eating Disorders Throughout the Life Span. London, Greenwood Press, 1988
Giannini AJ, Slaby AE (eds): The Eating Disorders. Ijmuiden, Netherlands, Springer, 1993

NOACK

Synonyms. Acrocephalopolysyndactyly I; progressive synostosis. Now considered included in Pfeiffer syndrome (see).

BIBLIOGRAPHY. Noack M: Ein Betrag zum Krankheitsbild der Akrozephalosyndaktylie (Apert). Arch Kinderh 160:168–171, 1959
Vanek J, Losan F: Pfeiffer's type of acrocephalosyndactyly in two families. J Med Genet 19:289–292, 1982

NOCTURNAL FREQUENCY IN WOMEN

Synonym. Nocturnal stranguria.

Symptoms. Nocturnal frequency in women with or without disturbance of micturition during the day, with or without menstrual irregularity in the premenopausal group, and vasomotor disturbances or atrophic vaginitis in the menopausal group.

Signs. Majority have fibromyomas.

Etiology. Cardiovascular renal diseases; anatomic defects of urinary tract; genitourinary infections, psychogenic factors. Possibly, hormonal factors.

Diagnostic Procedures. *Urine. Culture.* Frequently negative.

Therapy. Recommended by Greenblatt: Implantation of testosterone pellets.

Prognosis. According to Greenblatt, total or partial relief of symptoms with testosterone. Surgery for fibromyomatas not necessary in many cases to eliminate nocturia.

BIBLIOGRAPHY. Greenblatt RB: Syndrome of nocturnal frequency alleviated by testosterone propionate. J Clin Endocrinol 2:321–324, 1942
Komaroff AI: Urinalysis and urine culture in women with dysuria. Ann Int Med 104:212–218, 1986
Bayley B: Urinary tract infections. In Weatherall DJ, Ledingham JGG, Warrell DA (eds): Oxford Textbook of Medicine, 3rd ed, pp 3205–3214. Oxford, Oxford Med Pub, 1996

NOMA

Synonyms. Cancrum oris; gangrenous stomatitis.

Symptoms and Signs. Usually occurs in children. On oral mucosae, ulcer rapidly extending into a gangrenous greenish black lesion. Possible complications: alveolar bone destruction and sepsis.

Etiology. Fusospirochetal infection in debilitated patient; frequently associated with severe basic conditions (e.g., leukemia; virus infection; lymphomas).

Pathology. Cellulitis and necrosis of affected zone.

Diagnostic Procedures. *Blood.* Leukocytosis. *Culture.* Bacillus fusiformis and many secondary infectious agents.

Therapy. Antibiotics; treatment of the basic condition. Topical clorhexidine. Metronidazole per os (7 day treatment).

Prognosis. Severe. Fundamental control of basic condition for a positive outcome.

BIBLIOGRAPHY. Trible GB, Dick A: Noma. Arch Otolaryngol 16:1–8, 1932
Scully C: The oral cavity. In Champion RH, Burton JL, Ebling FJG (eds): Rook/Wilkinson/Ebling Textbook of Dermatology, 5th ed, p 2698. Oxford, Blackwell Scientific, 1992

NONKETOTIC HYPERGLYCINEMIA

Symptoms and Signs. Onset in first days of life. Listlessness; lack of spontaneous movements; spasticity; seizures; myoclonus; opisthotonos; hiccups; progressive to apnea, if surviving (regaining spontaneous respiration) failure to thrive; severe mental retardation. In a minority of cases symptoms appear later (6 months) and develop progressive spastic diplegia and optic atrophy, intellectual functions are spared and seizures are absent. A transitory form without consequences has been described also.

Etiology. Autosomal recessive inheritance. Defects in the P-, H-, and T-proteins; according to the defect three or four subtypes have been identified. Type NKHI (80% of cases with protein P-defect), and NKH2, NKH3. The gene for P-protein maps to chromosome 9p13.

Diagnostic Procedures. *Blood. CSF. Urine. Glycine.* Markedly elevated. *Cerebrospinal fluid.* Plasma ratio 0.08 diagnostic. *EEG.* Abnormal.

Therapy. None effective. Exchange transfusion life saving, but with temporary effect. Glycine restriction. Sodium benzoate.

Prognosis. Overwhelming illness in early life in the majority of cases. See Symptoms and Signs.

BIBLIOGRAPHY. Gerritsen T, Kaveggia E, Waisman HA: A new type of hyperglycinemia with hypoxaluria. Pediatrics 36:882–891, 1965
Hamosh A, Johnston MV, Valle D: Nonketotic hyperglycinemia. In Scriver CR, Beaudet AL, Sly WS, et al: The Metabolic and Molecular Bases of Inherited Disease, 7th ed, pp 1337–1348. New York, McGraw-Hill, 1995

NONNE

Synonyms. Quincke; Symond; intracranial hypertension benign; meningeal hydrops; hydrops; otitic hydrocephalus; pseudotumor cerebri; serous meningitis. Two types are recognized: Borries and benign hydrocephalus.

BORRIES SYNDROME

Symptoms. Occurs in both sexes; onset at all ages. Headache; nausea; vomiting; listlessness; mild fever; diplopia; blurred vision; occasionally tinnitus. Mental state unchanged; no seizures.

Signs. Bilateral papilledema; all other neurologic signs usually negative (benign abducens [VI] nerve palsy syndrome, possible in children). In some cases, otologic examination reveals perforated tympanic membrane with purulent discharge or discolored, distorted drum (prevalence in right ear); mastoid tenderness. In other cases, no otologic findings.

Etiology. Multiple etiologies; infection of middle ear or head injury.

Pathology. Mastoiditis with obstruction of lateral sinus, most frequently observed on the right side. A localized associated edema of cerebrum adjacent to the focal infection has been postulated.

Diagnostic Procedures. *Blood.* Mild leukocytosis; moderate increase of erythrocyte sedimentation rate. Serology for syphilis negative. *CSF.* Increased pressure. Lack or minimal increase with compression of jugular vein ipsilateral to infected mastoid; normal response contralaterally. Sugar and cells normal. *EEG.* Minimal alterations or normal. *X-ray.* Of mastoid. Clouding air cells and disruption of normal trabecular pattern. Widening of skull sutures observed in some children. *Carotid angiography. CT scan. MRI.*

Therapy. Antibiotic therapy and serial spinal punctures. If this fails, simple mastoidectomy.

Prognosis. Two weeks after mastoidectomy majority of cases cured; if intracranial pressure persists after mastoidectomy, recovery takes up to 6 months. Eventually, 100% recovery with adequate treatment.

BENIGN HYDROCEPHALUS SYNDROME

Symptoms and Signs. Prevalent in women; onset in middle age. Symptoms and signs as earlier with exception of absence of otologic pathology. If pregnant, evidence of progressive ocular signs owing to atrophy of retina.

Etiology. Unknown. Frequently associated with pregnancy, obesity, Addison syndrome, steroid, or other hormone and vitamins A and D imbalances (see Marie-See).

Pathology. None, except increased amount and tension of cerebral fluid.

Diagnostic Procedures. As in the preceding.

Therapy. Repeated spinal tap may relieve all symptoms.

Prognosis. Generally good. Disappearance of symptoms in 2–6 months. In pregnancy, good prognosis for mother and child.

BIBLIOGRAPHY. Quincke H: Die Lumbarpunktion des Hydrocephalus Klin Wochenschr 28:929, 1981
Nonne M: Ueber Falle vom Symptomenkomplex "tumor cerebri" mit Ausgang in Heilung (pseudotumor cerebri). Ueber lethal verlaufene Falle von "pseudotumor cerebri" mit Sektionsbefund. Dtsch Z Nervenheilk 27:169–216, 1904
Mestrezat W: Le liquide cephalo-rachidien normal et pathologique: Valeur clinique de l'examen clinique: Le syndromes humoraux dans le diverses affections. Paris, A Maloin, 1912
Borries GVT: Otogene encephalitis. Soc Danoise d'Oto-laryngology, 2 Feb. 1921; Zschz Ges Neurol Psychiatr 70:93–101, 1921
Symonds CP: Otitic hydrocephalus. Brain 54:55, 1931
Gneer M: Benign intracranial hypertension I. Mastoiditis and lateral sinus obstruction. Neurology 12:472–476, 1962
Nickerson CW, Krik RF: Recurrent pseudotumor cerebri in pregnancy. Report of two cases. Obstet Gynecol 26:811–813, 1965
Adams RD, Victor M: Principles of Neurology, 5th ed, pp 547–549. New York, McGraw-Hill, 1993

NONNE-MILROY-MEIGE

Synonyms. Elephantiasis, congenital; tropholymphedema hereditary; lymphedema, hereditary I (Nonne-Milroy); lymphedema, hereditary II (Meige).

Symptoms. Prevalent in females (70–80%); onset gradual and asymptomatic; three varieties: congenital at birth; precox (Nonne-Milroy), at birth to 35 years of age; tarda (Meige), after 35 years.

Signs. Unilateral or bilateral edema of ankle ascending to the knee and eventually above; initially easily pitting; disappearing with elevation of the leg; seldom on the arms, genitalia, face, and other areas. Skin smooth, firm, and natural color. Later, harder edema, not relieved by elevation with rough, pigmented skin over swollen parts. Persistent pleural effusion; in the variety tarda, possible association with deafness, primary pulmonary hypertension, cerebrovascular malformations, peculiar facial features (puffiness, deep creases, excessive wrinkling, cleft palate).

Etiology. Autosomal dominant inheritance. Cases of secondary lymphedema (malignancy, surgery, roentgen, pressure, filariasis, inflammation) were described by authors together with the hereditary ones. Today the use of eponym is restricted to the hereditary variety.

Pathology. Layer of spongy subcutaneous tissue; replacement of part of adipose tissue by lymphatic spaces. Fibrosis; thickening of blood vessel walls.

Diagnostic Procedures. *Blood.* Hypoproteinemia. *Pleural tap.* Hyperproteinemia.

Therapy. Early stage. Frequent elevation and elastic stockings; massages; skin toilet; penicillin (prophilaxis of erysipelas); surgery (removal of excessive skin).

Prognosis. Chronic course; permanent condition; normal life span. Rarely, lymphosarcoma may arise.

BIBLIOGRAPHY. Nonne M: Vier Fälle von Elephantiasis congenita hereditaria. Arch Pathol Anat (Paris) 125:189–196, 1891
Milroy WF: Undescribed variety of hereditary oedema. New York, Med J 56:505–508, 1892
Meige H: Dystrophie oedematose hereditaire. Presse Med 6:341–343, 1898
Herbert FA, Bowen PA: Hereditary late onset lymphedema with pleural effusion and laryngeal edema. Arch Intern Med 143:913–915, 1983
Ryan TJ, Champion RH: Disorders of lymphatic vessels. In Champion RH, Burton JL, Ebling FJG (eds): Rook/Wilkinson/Ebling Textbook of Dermatology, 5th ed, pp 2019–2022. Oxford, Blackwell Scientific, 1992

NONNENBRUCH

Synonym. Extrarenal oliguria (see Hepatorenal).

Eponym (obsolete) used to indicate all forms of oliguria owing to extrarenal factors: e.g., dehydration, shock.

BIBLIOGRAPHY. Nonnenbruch W: Ueber das entzüdliche dem der Niere und das hepatorenale Syndrom. Dtsch Med Wochenschr 63:7–10, 1937

NOONAN

Synonyms. Female pseudo-Turner; Turner-like; male Turner.

Symptoms. Both sexes affected. Mental retardation (rare in gonadal dysgenesis); stunted growth. Functional fetal gonads: differentiation of male genitalia or complete absence or disappearance; in female, from normal sexual development, to absent development and primary amenorrhea.

Signs. Many different types of congenital anomalies (in most cases minor) none characteristic or obligatory for diagnosis. Generally, shortness of stature (not as severe as in gonadal dysgenesis). In male, cryptorchidism (77%). Pulmonary valvular or arterial stenosis or other congenital heart malformation. (As a general rule, lesions prevalent in right heart as contrasted with gonadal dysgenesis, in which the left lesions predominate.) *Facial anomalies.* Ptosis; hypertelorism; antimongoloid slanting of palpebrae; ear abnormalities; micrognathia; dental anomalies; uvula and, less frequently, palate anomalies. *Chest anomalies.* Pectus carinatum; vertebral anomalies; digital anomalies; dysonychia; hirsutism; occasionally webbing of neck. Some cases have been reported in which the syndrome was associated with multiple cafe au lait spots, compatible in size and number with Von Recklinghausen neurofibromatosis. These features may represent a distinct genetic entity rather than the coincidence of two diseases.

Etiology. Unknown. Usually sporadic; multifactorial inheritance. Male-to-male transmission has been reported, suggesting an autosomal dominant gene with variable expressivity.

Pathology. See Symptoms and Signs. Gonads normal or rudimentary.

Diagnostic Procedures. *Chromosome studies.* Normal karyotypes. X-rays. *Cardiologic studies. Hormone secretion studies. Blood.* Thrombocytopenia and various coagulation defects reported. One family reported with high alkaline phosphatase in all members of family, with or without major or minor manifestations of syndrome.

Therapy. If hormonal deficiency, replacement either in continuous or cyclic fashion. Treatment has to be started early and continued as long as needed. Surgery for heart malformation when feasible.

Prognosis. According to degree, number, and type of anomalies. Relatives of proband are affected much less severely as a general rule.

BIBLIOGRAPHY. Kobilinski O: Ueber eine flughautähnliche Ausbreitung am Halse. Arch Anthropol 14:342–348, 1883
Noonan JA, Ehmke DA: Associated noncardiac malformations in children with congenital heart disease. J Pediatr 63:468–470, 1963
Ranke MB, Heideman P, Knupfer C, et al: Noonan syndrome: Growth and clinical manifestations in 144 cases. Eur J Pediat 148:220–227, 1988
Winters SJ: Clinical disorders of the testis. In De Groot LJ (ed): Endocrinology, 3rd ed, pp 2390–2391. Philadelphia, WB Saunders, 1995

NOONAN-LIKE CHERUBISM; POLYARTICULAR PIGMENTED, VILLONODULAR SYNOVITIS

Symptoms and Signs. *Facies.* Mild hypertelorism, oculomotor defect, low-set ears. Jaw lesions. Cavernous hemangioma of lip and orbit reported. Multiple lentiges; lymphedema. Various heart abnormalities. Villo nodular syndrome involving several joints before age 10.

Etiology. Autosomal dominant inheritance. Contiguous gene syndrome with polyarticular villonodular synovities and other malformations.

Pathology. The jaw lesions debated if fibrous dysplasia? Giant cell granuloma? Cherubism?

BIBLIOGRAPHY. Hoyer PF, Neuman FW: Cherubism-eine osteofibroese. Kiefererkrankung im Kindersalter. Klin Paediatr 194:128–131, 1982
Gorlin RJ, Cohen MM Jr, Levin LS: Syndromes of Head and Neck, p 899. New York, Oxford University Press, 1996

NORMAN-LANDING

Synonyms. Caffey; pseudo-Hurler; neurovisceral lipoidosis familial; neurovisceral pseudo-Hurler lipoidosis; beta-galactosidase deficiency; generalized gangliosidosis (type I); GM1 (type I); infantile GM1.

Symptoms. Both sexes affected. Onset from birth. Mental and motor retardation; startle response to sound; seizures; blindness; deafness; spastic quadriplegia. Poor appetite, feeding difficulties. Recurrent bronchopneumonia.

Signs. Facial and peripheral edema; macrocephaly. Facial abnormalities: coarse features; broad nose; frontal bossing; long philtrum; prominent maxilla; mild macroglossia. Cherry-red macular spot (50%); retinitis pigmentosa. Joint movement limitation; kyphoscoliosis. Hepatosplenomegaly.

Etiology. Autosomal recessive inheritance. Severe deficit of lysosomal enzyme beta-galactosidase. Defect on chromosome 3.

Pathology. Neural lipidosis. Visceral histiocytosis: foamy cells in bone marrow, lymph nodes, liver, spleen, and various visceral organs. Ballooning renal glomeruloepithelial cytoplasm.

Diagnostic Procedures. *Blood.* Vacuolated lymphocytes. Beta-galactosidase assay of leukocytes. *Bone marrow.* Foamy histiocytes. *Urine.* Mucopolysacchariduria. *Beta-galactosidase assay. Biopsy of skin.* Presence of foamy cells. *Fibroblast culture. Beta-galactosidase assay.*

Therapy. Symptomatic.

Prognosis. Death at 6 months to 2 years.

BIBLIOGRAPHY. Caffey J: Gargoylism (Hunter-Hurler disease), dystomatosis multiplex, lipochondrodystrophy; prenatal and neonatal bone lesions and their early postnatal evolution. Bull Hosp Joint Dis 12:38–66, 1951
Norman RM, Tingey AH, Newman CGH, et al: Tay Sachs disease with visceral involvement and its relation to gargoylism. Arch Dis Child 39:634–640, 1964
Landing BH, Silverman FN, Craig JM, et al: Familial neurovisceral lipidosis. Am J Dis Child 108:503–582, 1964
Suzuki Y, Sakuraba H, Oshima A: Galactosidase deficiency (galactosidosis): Gm1 gangliosidosis and Morquio B Disease. In Scriver CR, Beaudet AL Sly WS, et al: The Metabolic and Molecular Bases of Inherited Disease, 7th ed, pp 2785–2791. New York, McGraw-Hill, 1995

NORMAN-ROBERTS

Synonym. Lissencephaly II.

Symptoms and Signs. From birth. Similar to Miller-Dieker. Low, sloped forehead and prominent nasal bridge are the distinguishing features.

Etiology. Autosomal recessive inheritance. Chromosomal normalcy.

BIBLIOGRAPHY. Norman MG, Roberts M, Sirois J, et al: Lissencephaly. Can J Neurol Sci 3:39–46, 1976
Dobyns WB, Stratton RF, Greenberg F: Syndromes with lissencephaly I: Miller-Dieker and Norman-Roberts syndromes and isolated lissencephaly. Ann J Med Genet 18:509–526, 1984

NORRBOTTEN*

Symptoms and Signs. Those of Greither. Extremely severe symptoms that may reach mutilating degree.

Etiology. Autosomal recessive inheritance.

BIBLIOGRAPHY. Gamborg Nielsen P: Two different clinical and genetic forms of hereditary palmoplantar keratoderma in the northernmost county of Sweden. Clin Genet 28:361–366, 1985

NORRIE

Synonyms. Andersen-Warburg; Whitnall-Norman; Episkopi blindness; atrophia bulborum hereditaria; fetal iritis; oligophrenia microphthalmus; bilateral retinal pseudotumor; oculoacoustic dysplasia, congenital.

Symptoms. Only males affected. Present from birth. Multiple recurrent vitreous hemorrhages. Blindness; in some cases, mental retardation (25%) that begins at any age; deafness of different severity developing at ages 9–45 years.

Signs. Presence of a mass behind clear lens; cataract (developing later); corneal opacification; phthisis bulbi, and, occasionally, iris atrophy and synechiae.

Etiology. Sex-linked inheritance, complete penetrance but different expressivity gene defect on Xp 21.

Pathology. Malformation of retinal layers of sensory cells, optic nerves, and tracts. Persistent hyperplastic primary vitreous intraocular hemorrhages. Other organs not studied.

Therapy. Symptomatic.

Prognosis. Blindness; possibly, development of mental retardation and deafness (one third of cases).

*Town in Sweden.

BIBLIOGRAPHY. Clarke E: Pseudo-glioma, in both eyes. Trans Ophthalmol Soc UK 18:136–138, 1898
Norrie G: Causes of blindness in children: Twenty-five years' experience of Danish Institutes for the blind. Acta Ophthalmol (Kopenh) 5:357–386, 1927
Warburg M: Norrie's disease: A congenital progressive oculo-acoustic-cerebral degeneration. Acta Ophthalmol 89(Suppl):1–147, 1966
Collins FA, Murphy DL, Reiss AL, et al: Clinical, biochemical and neuropsychiatric evaluation of a patient with a contiguous gene syndrome due to a microdeletion X p11.3 including Norrie disease locus and monoamineoxidase (MSOA and MAOB) genes. Am J Med Genet 42:127–134, 1992
Klintworth K: Genetically determined disorders affecting the eye. In Garner A, Klintworth GK (eds): Pathobiology of Ocular Disease: A Dynamic Approach, 2nd ed, pp 811–812. New York, Marcel Dekker, 1994

NORUM

Synonyms. Lecithin cholesterol acyltransferase deficiency familial; L.C.A.T. deficiency; serum cholesterol; ester familial deficiency. See also Fish eye.

Symptoms and Signs. Prevalent in Scandinavia. From childhood, corneal opacities that form an arcus lipoides, impairment of vision. Normochromic anemia; progressive renal failure; early atherosclerotic manifestations.

Etiology. Autosomal recessive inheritance. Absence of L.C.A.T. (chromosome 16), which impairs metabolism of HDL and consequently alters lipoprotein pattern.

Diagnostic Procedures. *Cornea.* Grayish dots that cause "misty" appearance. *Blood.* Erythrocytes, altered lipid composition; hemolytic anemia. *Plasma.* High unesterified cholesterol and lecithin and low cholesterol ester and lysolecithin. No pre-beta-lipoprotein band; hypertriglyceridemia. Alteration of composition of VLDL and HDL; LDL2 are abnormally large. *Bone marrow and spleen.* Foam cells (sea blue histiocytes). *Urine.* Proteinuria, hematuria, hyaline casts. *Renal biopsy.* Foam cells.

Therapy. Plasma transfusion, restriction of dietary fat intake. Kidney transplantation (good results).

Prognosis. Increased incidence of myocardial infarction.

BIBLIOGRAPHY. Norum KR, Gjone E: Familial serum cholesterol esterification failure: A new inborn error of metabolism. Biochim Biophys Acta 144:698–700, 1967
Vergani C, Catapano AL, Roma P, et al: A new case of familial LCAT deficiency. Acta Med Scand 214:173–176, 1983
Gotoda T, Yamada N, Murase T, et al: Differential phenotypic expression by three mutant alleles in familial lecithin: Cholesterol acyltransferase deficiency. Lancet 338:778–781, 1991

NOTHNAGEL II

Synonym. Ophthalmoplegia—cerebellar ataxia; cerebellar ataxia; ophthalmoplegia. See Pretectal and Brun.

Symptoms. Unilateral oculomotor palsy (ipsilateral to lesion); ataxia of gait. Poorly coordinated upper extremity movements.

Pathology. Unilateral midbrain lesion (tectum); infarction; neoplasia.

BIBLIOGRAPHY. Nothnagel H: Topische Diagnostik der Gehirnkrankheiten: Eine Klinische Studie, p 220. Berlin, Hirschwald, 1879
Keane JR: The pretectal syndrome: 206 patients. Neurology 40:684–690, 1990
Adams RD, Victor M: Principles of Neurology, 5th ed, p 1173. New York, McGraw-Hill, 1993

NOWAKOWSKI-LENZ

Synonyms. Androgen-resistant (type II); incomplete form of AIS; incomplete, hereditary male pseudohermaphroditism (type II); pseudovaginal perineoscrotal hypospadias; 5-alpha reductase deficiency. See Reifenstein.

Symptoms and Signs. At birth, external female phenotype; bilateral testes and normal virilized wolffian structures terminating in vagina. At puberty, variable degrees of virilization of external genitalia and partial development of secondary sexual characteristics; prostatic tissue not palpable; no gynecomastia; no acne.

Etiology. Deficiency of 5-alpha-reductase; autosomal recessive inheritance. Part of the spectrum of incomplete androgen insensitivity syndromes.

Pathology. See Symptoms and Signs.

Diagnostic Procedures. *Chromosome study.* 46XY. *Hormonal study.* Testosterone normal or elevated; dihydrotestosterone low in adulthood; ratio of urinary 5-beta-reduced to 5-alpha-reduced steroids decreased; reduction in vitro of testosterone to dihydrotestosterone; decreased 5-alpha-reductase activity in tissues.

Therapy. If decision is to raise as female, castration is needed before puberty to prevent virilization. If decision is to raise as male, repair of hypospadias and cryptorchidism.

Prognosis. As female (with early castration), usually successful adjustment; as male, at puberty usually a change in gender role.

BIBLIOGRAPHY. Ferriman DG: Familial hypogonadism. Proc Roy Soc Med 47:439–442, 1954
Nowakowski H, Lenz W: Genetic aspects on male hypogonadism. Rec Proc Horm Res 17:53–95, 1961
Forest MG: Diagnosis and treatment of disorders of sexual development. In De Groot LJ (ed): Endocrinology, 3rd ed, p 1921. Philadelphia, WB Saunders, 1995

NUMB CHIN

Synonyms. Mental neuropathy; MN.

Symptoms and Signs. Numbness of chin and lower lip, possibly associated with pain and swelling.

Etiology. Considered a potentially ominous symptom indicating the presence of metastasis or primary tumor of the lower jaw. Trauma, inflammatory disorders, cyst, or benign tumor seldom responsible for such a clinical manifestation.

Diagnostic Procedures. *X-ray. CT scan. MRI.* Frequently, symptoms may precede the instrumental evidence by a month. *Cerebrospinal fluid.*

Therapy. Surgical, roentgen, ray, or chemical treatment of primary or metastatic lesions.

Prognosis. If neoplasia, ominous.

BIBLIOGRAPHY. Seldin HM, Seldin SD, Rakower W: Metastatic carcinoma of the mandible: Report of cases. J Oral Surg 11:336–340, 1953
Coverley JR, Mohnec AM: Syndrome of numb chin. Arch Intern Med 112:819–821, 1963
Burt RK, Sharfman WH, Karp BI, et al: Mental neuropathy (Numb chin syndrome): A harbinger of tumor progression or relapse. Cancer 70:877–881, 1992

NUTCRACKER

Synonyms. Renal vein compression, renal vein hypertension of; varicosities; renal pelvis and ureter; hematuria essential.

Symptoms and Signs. Both sexes. Essential hematuria, left varicocele. Anemia, abdominal and flank pain.

Etiology. Abnormal branching of superior mesenteric artery from aorta that compresses left renal vein, leading to venous hypertension. Renal pelvis and ureteral venous varicosities ensue that leak into urinary tract.

Diagnostic Procedures. *Phlebography. Venous pressure measurements. Urography. MRI (procedure of choice). Urine.* hematuria. *Blood.* Anemia.

Therapy. Conservative treatment, nephropexy, excision of pelvic varicosities, renal venous bypass, renal decapsulation transposition of left renal vein, interruption of inferior mesenteric artery.

Prognosis. Good with surgery.

BIBLIOGRAPHY. De Schepper A: "Nutcracker" phenomenon of the renal vein causing left renal veni pathology. J Belg Radiol 55:507–511, 1972
Hohenfellner M, Steinbach F, Schultz-Lampel D, et al: The nutcracker syndrome: New aspects of pathophysiology, diagnosis and treatment. J Urol 146:685–688, 1991

NUTRITIONAL AMBLYOPIA

Synonyms. Obal; alcohol amblyopia; deficiency amblyopia; retrobulbar neuropathy; tobacco–alcohol amblyopia.

Symptoms. Occurs in chronic undernourished individuals; onset slow, insidious. Progressive visual loss; dimness for close and far objects; difficulty in reading; photophobia; retrobulbar discomfort.

Signs. Initially, slight redness of temporal margins of optic disks; later pallor; symmetric bilateral central or paracentral scotoma; intact peripheral fields.

Etiology. Chronic malnutrition in vitamin B_{12} deficiency; diabetes mellitus, after isonicotinic acid-hydrazide treatment. The notion that tobacco or cyanide could be responsible has been discarded by logic and by experimental data.

Pathology. Bilateral symmetric loss of myelinated fibers in central part of optic (II) nerve. In severe forms, loss of ganglion cell in the macula.

Diagnostic Procedures. *Blood.* Hypoproteinemia; hypochromic microcytic or macrocytic anemia. Low level of B_{12} (occasional); low transketolase activity. *Urine.* Abnormal excretion of methylmalonic acid.

Therapy. Improved nutrition; vitamin B complex.

Prognosis. Degree of recovery according to degree of damage and time of onset of treatment.

BIBLIOGRAPHY. Obal A: Nutritional amblyopia. Am J Ophthalmol 34:857–865, 1951
Dreyfus PM: Nutritional disorders of obscure etiology. Med Sci 17:44–48, 1966
Giannini AJ, Slaby AE (eds): The Eating Disorders. Ijmuiden, Netherlands, Springer, 1993

NUTRITIONAL RECOVERY

Symptoms and Signs. Occurs in undernourished children when they begin to recover, following the administration of adequate food. The symptoms and signs appear in the following order, increase for 2 weeks, and then slowly decrease and disappear within about 3 months: transient weight loss followed by progressive increase; edema that disappears in approximately 20 days; progressively increasing hepatomegaly, normal consistency, sharp edge, no tenderness, appearing at the 20th day; abdominal distension; moderate congestion of thoracoabdominal venous network; ascites (in 50% of cases) of short duration (1–2 weeks); persistent hypertrichosis of shoulders, thighs, and face (in 50% of cases).

Etiology. Unknown. Complex metabolic disorder. It is supposed that following the removal of fat infiltration, binding of water at the liver level determines intrahepatic-portal hypertension.

Pathology. Liver biopsies show the progressively decreasing fatty infiltrations.

Diagnostic Procedures. *Blood.* Before syndrome; total proteins, albumin, alpha and beta globulins low; gamma globulins high. Two weeks after beginning of syndrome, total protein normal, albumin still low; gamma-globulin rising. After disappearance of edema, same pattern plus correction of alpha-globulin level, hepatic function tests abnormal, with the exception of cephalincholesterol. Increase of eosinophils in blood 60–75 days after onset. *Biopsy.* Of liver (see Pathology).

Prognosis. Disappearance of the syndrome in about 3 months.

BIBLIOGRAPHY. Gomez F, Galvan RR, Munoz JC: Nutritional recovery syndrome. Pediatrics 10:513–526, 1952
Symposium on Nutrition. The Pediatric Clinics of North America, vol 32, no 2. Philadelphia, WB Saunders, 1985
Giannini AJ, Slaby AE (eds): The Eating Disorders. Ijmuiden, Netherlands, Springer, 1993

NYGAARD-BROWN

Obsolete.

Synonyms. Essential thrombophilia. See also Trousseau syndrome.

Symptoms and Signs. Variable manifestations related to venous obstruction involving localized districts.

Etiology. Unknown. Possibly, a paraneoplastic syndrome.

Diagnostic Procedure. *Blood.* Enhanced coagulation.

Therapy. Heparin.

Prognosis. According to basic pathology and district(s) affected. Gangrene is a frequent complication.

BIBLIOGRAPHY. Nygaard KK, Brown GE: Essential thrombophilia. Report of five cases. Arch Intern Med 59:82:106–107, 1937

NYSSEN-VAN BOGAERT

Synonyms. Deafness; opticocochleodentate degeneration; quadriparesis; mental retardation.

Symptoms and Signs. Both sexes. Onset in infancy. Visual loss; hearing loss; quadriparesis; physical and mental retardation.

Etiology. Autosomal recessive inheritance.

Pathology. Marked cachexia, muscular atrophy. Specific systematized lesions involving optic pathways, cochlear pathways, rubrodentate pathways, medial lemnisci, and pyramidal tracts. Brain is small and atrophic.

Diagnostic Procedures. *CSF.* Normal. *EEG.* Dysrhytmia. *CT scan. MRI.*

Therapy. Symptomatic.

Prognosis. Progression of neurologic defects is slow. After infantile onset deterioration into immobilized idiots in 1 year; in some cases, however, the disease may appear arrested and later assume a rapid course.

BIBLIOGRAPHY. Nyssen R, van Bogaert L: La dégénérescence systématisée optico-cochléo-dentelée. Rev Neurol 2:321–345, 1934
Zeman W: Dégénérescence systématisée optico-cochléo-dentelée. In Vinken PJ, Bruyn GW (eds): Handbook of Clinical Neurology, vol 22, pp 535–552. Amsterdam, Elsevier, 1975

NYSTAGMUS COMPENSATION

Symptoms. Onset preceded by nystagmus. Infantile esotropia; abnormal head posture toward the adducted fixing eye, amblyopia. Nystagmus is reduced with fixing eye adduced.

BIBLIOGRAPHY. Von Noorden GK: The nystagmus compensation (blockage) syndrome. Am J Ophthalmol 82:287, 1976
Frank JW: Diagnostic signs in the nystagmus compensation syndrome. J Pediatr Ophthalmol Strabism 16:317–320, 1979

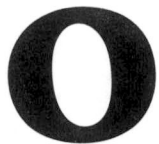

O

OASTHOUSE

Synonyms. Smith-Strang; beery baby; methionine malabsorption.

Symptoms and Signs. Onset in infancy. White hair; severe mental defect; unresponsiveness to stimuli; flaccidity. Recurrent episodes of generalized edema. Distinctive odor of dried malt or hops.

Etiology. Congenital enzymatic block. This condition resembles phenylketonuria but is considered a separate entity because of a different enzymatic block. Defect of utilization of alphaketoacids of essential aminoacids. Autosomal recessive inheritance

Pathology. No specific changes. Unduly soft consistency of all parts of brain; widespread defect of myelinization in cerebrum, brain stem, and cord.

Diagnostic Procedures. *Urine.* Large amounts of alpha-hydroxybutyric and phenylpyruvic acids; ferric chloride test positive.

Therapy. None specific; symptomatic.

Prognosis. Poor. Condition persists until death, which may occur within first year of life.

BIBLIOGRAPHY. Smith AJ, Strang LB: An inborn error of metabolism with the urinary excretion of a hydroxy-butyric acid and phenyl-pyruvic acid. Arch Dis Child 33:109–113, 1958

Cone TE: Diagnosis and treatment: Some diseases, syndromes, and conditions associated with an unusual odor. Pediatrics 41:993–995, 1968

Hooft C, Carton D, Snoeck J, et al: Further investigation in the methionine malabsorption syndrome. Helv Paediatr Acta 23:334–349, 1968

Mudd SH, Levy HL, Skovby F: Disorders of transsulfuration. In Scriver CR, Beaudet AL, Sly WS, et al: The Metabolic and Molecular Bases of Inherited Disease, 7th ed, pp 1283–1284. New York, McGraw-Hill, 1995

O'BRIEN

Synonyms. Actinic granuloma.

Symptoms and Signs. In sunny countries in fair persons over 30 years of age in an area compromised by actinic elastosis (see), appearance of pink papules that slowly organize in an area (0.2–0.5 cm) of annular inflammatory reaction with thickened edge and atrophic center. Usually asymptomatic.

Etiology. Autonomous entity or nonspecific expression of a granulomatous disease occurring on area of skin altered by light exposure.

Pathology. *Skin biopsy.* External zone with actinic elastosis, intermediate zone histocytic and giant cell inflammatory reaction, and central zone (within the annulus) absent or very scarce elastic tissue. Minimal or no lysosome activity in histiocytes of inflamed zone (differential feature with granuloma annulare where abundant activity is present).

Therapy. Sunscreen to prevent further lesions and corticosteroid infiltration in the annular edge.

Prognosis. Fair.

BIBLIOGRAPHY. O'Brien JP: Actinic granuloma: An annular connective tissue disorder affecting sun and heat-damaged (elastotic) skin. Arch Dermatol 111:460–470, 1975

Burton JL: Disorders of connective tissue. In Champion RH, Burton JL,

Ebling FJG (eds): Rook/Wilkinson/Ebling Textbook of Dermatology, 5th ed, p 1788–1789. Oxford, Blackwell Scientific, 1992

OBSERVATION HIP

Synonyms. Transitory coxitis; coxitis serosa seu simplex; acute transient epiphysitis; toxic synovitis; synovitis transient. See Migratory osteolysis of the hip.

Symptoms. Occurs in children. Limp with or without referred pain to the knee, thigh, or groin.

Signs. Slight limitation of passive hip movements.

Etiology. Varied: minor injury; focal infections; allergy; most frequently, idiopathic.

Pathology. Mild osteoarthritis or synovitis.

Diagnostic Procedures. *X-ray.* Normal. *Blood.* Sedimentation rate normal. *Mantoux test.* Positive only in some subjects. *Biopsy.* Of lymph node. Slight hyperplasia; no evidence of tuberculosis.

Therapy. Preventon of weight bearing and observation (hence the name of the syndrome).

Prognosis. Symptoms disappear spontaneously in weeks or months, seldom recur. Sequelae long after the episodes are sometimes observed with radiologic changes in hip joint.

BIBLIOGRAPHY. Lovett RW, Morse JL: A transient or ephemeral form of hip disease with report of cases. Boston Med Surg J 127:161–163, 1892

Hunder GG, Kelly PJ: Roentgenologic transient osteoporosis of the hip: A clinical syndrome? Ann Intern Med 68:539–552, 1968

OCCIPITAL HORN

Synonyms. Ehler-Danlos type IX; Ehlers-Danlos X-linked; cutis laxa.

Symptoms and Signs. Inguinal hernias, complications from bladder and ureteric diverticulae, skin and joint laxity. Chronic diarrhea. Palpable ossified occipital horn. IQ low normal or mildly retarded range.

Etiology. X-linked inheritance (in some part of Xp). May be an allelic mutation of Menkes II (see).

Diagnostic Procedures. *X rays.* Ossified occipital horn, "hammerlike" expansion of lateral end of clavicles, wavy outline of cortex of long bones. *Arteriography.* Arterial tortuosity elongation and stenosis. *Skin culture.* Low lysyl oxidase levels, in cultured fibroblasts, analysis of copper transport. *Blood.* Serum copper reduced. Prenatal diagnosis possible.

Therapy. Symptomatic.

Prognosis. Good. Mild mental retardation.

BIBLIOGRAPHY. Lazoff SG, Rybak JJ, Parker BR, et al: Skeletal dysplasia, occipital horns, intestinal malabsorption and obstructive uropathy: A new hereditary syndrome. Birth Def Orig Art Ser XI:71–74, 1975

Blackston RD, Hirshhorn K, Elsas LJ: Ehlers-Danlos syndrome (EDS), type IX: Biochemical evidence for X-linkage (Abstract). Am J Med Genet 41:A49, 1987

Danks DM: Disorders of copper metabolism. In Scriver CR, Beaudet AL, Sly WS, et al: The Metabolic and Molecular Bases of Inherited Disease, 7th ed, p 2227. New York, McGraw-Hill, 1995

OCCUPATIONAL NOSEBLEEDS

Synonyms. Apple packer; rosaniline nosebleeds.

Symptoms. Mild rhinorrhea and conjunctival irritation. Nosebleeds occurring in people working with tray manufacturing for apple and apple-packing or other industries that use rosaniline dyes.

Signs. Seldom (1%), septal ulcer ringed with blue dust.

Etiology. Mucosal irritation by rosaniline dyes (gentian violet; crystal violet; methyl violet).

Pathology. Hyperemia and hemorrhage of nasal mucosa.

Therapy. Corticosteriods may prevent bleeding and minimize irritation. Ulcer requires cautery or other prolonged treatment.

Prognosis. Nosebleeds stop with cessation of exposure, except when ulcer is present.

BIBLIOGRAPHY. Quinby GE: Epidemic nosebleeds in apple packers. JAMA 197:165–168, 1966
Quinby GE: Gentian violet as a cause of epidemic occupational nosebleeds. Arch Environ Health 16:485–489, 1968

OCHOA

Synonyms. Urofacial.

Symptoms and Signs. Both sexes. Evident when crying, smiling, or grimacing. Constipation (65%). Signs from difficulty in passing urine from neuropathic bladder. Males. Cryptorchidism (100%).

Etiology. Autosomal recessive.

Pathology. Vesical mucosal hypertrophy, trabeculation and diverticula, hydroureter and hydronephrosis.

BIBLIOGRAPHY. Elejade BR: Genetic and diagnostic considerations in three families with abnormalities of facial expression and congenital urinary obstruction: The Ochoa syndrome. Am J Med Genet 3:97–108, 1979
Ochoa B, Gorlin RJ: Urofacial syndrome. Am J Med Genet 27:661–668, 1987

OCKULY-MONTGOMERY

Synonyms. Lichenoid tuberculid; papulonecrotic tuberculid.

Symptoms and Signs. On the limbs, sudden, symmetric eruption of pea-like, brownish lesions, possibly, annular shape and in groups.

Etiology. Unknown. Considered by the authors a tuberculid rash, which, however, is similar to sarcoidosis (see Besnier-Boeck-Schaumann).

Pathology. In upper dermis; well-defined, usually perivascular, tubercle; inconstant causation. Coexistent (occasionally) with glandular or systemic tuberculosis.

Therapy. *Biopsy. Tuberculosis tests. X-ray. Sputum cultures. Mantoux test* (generally negative).

Prognosis. Lesion fades with residual brown discoloration, without scarring.

BIBLIOGRAPHY. Ockuly OE, Montgomery H: Lichenoid tuberculid: Clinical and histopathologic studies. J Invest Dermatol 14:415–426, 1950
Savin JA: Mycobacterial infections. In Champion RH, Burton JL, Ebling FJG (eds): Rook/Wilkinson/Ebling Textbook of Dermatology, 5th ed, p 1052. Oxford, Blackwell Scientific, 1992

OCULO-CEREBELLO-TEGMENTAL

Symptoms and Signs. Both sexes affected. Onset at older ages. Transitory hemiplegia of sudden onset associated with bilateral cerebellar manifestations and paralysis of associated ocular movements.

Etiology and Pathology. Vascular lesion of mesencephalon. Softening of peduncular tegmentum.

BIBLIOGRAPHY. Rodriguez B, Rodriguez BR, Oreggia A: Un nuevo tipo de sindrome peducolar; oftalmoplejia internuclear anterior y sindrome cerebelosobilateral par lesion tegmental. Arch Urug Med 10:353–370, 1945
Fournier A, Ducoulombier H, Coussin J, et al: Oculocerebellar-myoclonic syndrome and neuroblastoma. J Sci Med Lille 90:189–197, 1972
Adams RD, Victor M: Principles of Neurology, 5th ed, pp 225–240. New York, McGraw-Hill, 1993

OCULO-DENTO-DIGITAL DYSPLASIA

Synonyms. Gillespie; Lohman; Weyers III; Mohr; Mohr-Clausen; Meyer; Schwickerath-Weyers; dyscraniopygophalangia; microphthalmos; oculodentoosseus, ODD, acrocephalopoly syndactyly IV, orofacial-digital II, OFDII. See also Hallermann-Streiff, Rieger, Peter, Rutherford, Gorlin-Chandhry-Moss

Symptoms and Signs. Both sexes affected. Present from birth. Two types. Dysplasia oculodentodigitalis. Symptoms and signs less severe than in type II. Dyscraniopygophalangial. Hypertelorism; microphthalmia; microcornea; eccentric pupil; changes in iris structure; remnant of pupillary membrane. Myopia; hyperopia. Thin small nose; anteverted nostrils; hypoplastic teeth (enamelogenesis imperfecta); mandible wide, alveolar ridge. Syndactyly (fourth and fifth fingers; third and fourth toes). Camptodactyly (fifth finger). Hypoplasia of one or more digits. Sparse hair growth. Visceral malformations. Usually mentally normal. Cases with progressive spastic paraparesis reported.

Etiology. Autosomal dominant with variable expressivity. Described autosomal recessive form with more severe ocular effect.

Diagnostic Procedures. *X-ray.* Broad tubular bones. *MRI.* Abnormal white matter diffuse, abnormally high signal intensity in subcortical zones bilaterally (with paraparesis).

Prognosis. *Type I.* Fair. *Type II.* Fatal because of associated visceral malformations.

BIBLIOGRAPHY. Lohmann W: Beitrug zur Kenntnis des reinen Mikrophthalmus. Arch Augenheilkd 86:136–141, 1920
Mohr, OL: A hereditary sublethal syndrome in man. Avhandl Norske Videnskaps-Akademi Oslo. J Mat Naturwiss Klasse 14:1–3, 1941
Claussen O: Et arvelig syndrom omfattende tugemis-dannelse of polydactyly. Nord Med 30:1147–1151, 1946
Meyer-Schwickerath G, Gruterich E, Weyers H: Mikrophthalmus-Syndrome. Klin Monatsbl Augenheilkd 131:18–30, 1957
Patton MA, Lawrence KM: Three cases of oculodentodigital (ODD) syndrome: Development of the facial phenotype. J Med Genet 22:386–389, 1985
Gutmann DH, Zackai EH, McDonald-McGinn DM, et al: Oculodental digital dysplasia syndrome associated with abnormal cerebral white matter. Am J Med Genet 41:18–20, 1991

OCULOMELIC AMYOPLASIA

Synonyms. Arthrogryposis, oculomotor limitation; flectoretinal anomalies. See Arthrogryposis distal type II.

Symptoms and Signs. From birth. Limb contractures; limitation of ocular movement; visual reduction. Absence of stature reduction, short neck, or epicanthal folds.

Etiology. Possibly autosomal dominant inheritance.

Pathology. Replacement of muscle by fibrous bands and fat.

Diagnostic Procedures. Electroretinogram abnormalities.

BIBLIOGRAPHY. Lai MMR, Tettenborn MA, Hall JG, et al: A new form of autosomal dominant arthrogryposis. J Med Genet 28:701–703, 1991

OCULOPHARYNGEAL MUSCULAR DYSTROPHY

Synonyms. Von Graefe; Graefe, OPMD; dysphagia—ptosis—muscular dystrophy.

Symptoms and Signs. Equal sex distribution onset from infancy to fifth decade; insidious onset and slow progression. Progressive ptosis and dysphagia (cardinal symptoms); occasionally associated, weakness of facial, extraocular, and limb-girdle muscles. Dysphagia precedes the ptosis by an interval of 1 month or years. All patients share common ethnic background.

Etiology. Inherited condition of dominant type. Most affected individuals in the United States and Canada descend from a Frenchman who immigrated to Canada in 1634. The European cases descend from different individuals. A variety with predominant distal myopathy has been reported (Satoyoshy) also. A family with a recessive form (possibly a different condition) has been reported as well (Serimgeour). A few sporadic cases have been reported also.

Pathology. *Muscle biopsy.* Isolated or clustered fibers with accumulation of sarcoplasmic matter. *Electronmicroscopy.* Degenerative fiber changes and abnormalities in muscle cell mitochondria. Typical nuclear inclusions and no RRF (ragged red fibers).

Diagnostic Procedures. *Deglutition studies.* Abnormality confined to pharynx, hypopharynx, and upper third of esophagus. *Electromyography.* Consistent with myopathic process.

Therapy. Cricopharyngeal myotomy to improve deglution.

Prognosis. Slow progression (years of ptosis and dysphagia), and wasting of affected muscles.

BIBLIOGRAPHY. Von Graefe AF: Demonstration in der Berlin medizinschen Gesellschaft. Berlin Klin Wochenschr 5:127, 1868
Taylor EW: Progressive vagus glossopharyngeal paralysis and ptosis: Contribution to a group of family diseases. J Nerv Ment Dis 42:129–139, 1915
Kiloh LG, Nevin S: Progressive dystrophy of external ocular muscles (ocular myopathy). Brain 74:115–143, 1951
Knoblanch A, Koppel M: Die okulopharyngeale Muskeldystrophy. Schweiz Med Wochenschr 114:557–561, 1984
De Braekeleer M: Hereditary Disorders in Saguenay-Lac-St Jean (Quebec, Canada). Hum Hered 41:141–146, 1991
Rowland LP: Progressive external ophthalmoplegia and ocular myopathies. In Rowland LP, Di Mauro S (eds): Handbook of Clinical Neurology, vol 18: Myopathies, p 287. Amsterdam, Elsevier, 1992

O'DONNELL-PAPPAS

Synonyms. See Karsch and Neugenbauer.

Symptoms and Signs. Nystagmus and presenile cataract; nystagmus and mild foveal hypoplasia; peripheral corneal pannus.

Etiology. Unknown autosomal dominant.

BIBLIOGRAPHY. O'Donnell FE Jr, Pappas HR: Autosomal dominant foveal hypoplasia and presenile cataracts. Arch Ophthalmol 100:279–281, 1982

ODONTOHYPOPHOSPHATASIA

Synonyms. See acid phosphatase deficiencies.

Symptoms and Signs. Dental disease without other features of hypophosphatasia, adult (see).

BIBLIOGRAPHY. Pimstone B, Eisenberg E, Silverman S: Hypophosphatasia: Genetic and dental studies. Ann Int Med 65:722–729, 1966
Page RC, Baab DA: New look at the etiology and pathogenesis of early periodontitis. J Periodomtol 56:748, 1985
Whyte MP: Hypophosphatasia. In Scriver CR, Beaudet AL, Sly WS, et al: The Metabolic and Molecular Bases of Inherited Disease, pp 4095–4111. New York, McGraw-Hill, 1995

OECKERMAN

Synonyms. Acid-alpha-mannosidase deficiency; alpha-mannosidosis deficiency; mannosidosis. See Mucopolysaccharidosis syndromes (Hurler, Scheie, etc.). Syndrome today is divided into type I with infantile onset and type II with juvenile onset and less severe course.

Symptoms and Signs. Both sexes affected. In first year of life, normal, except for recurrent respiratory infections; then, in succeeding years the following progressive changes and manifestations: delayed early motor and speech development; clumsy movements; coarse facies (less than in MPS I and later than in ML II); low nasal bridge; prominent forehead and mandible; occasionally, macroglossia and wide teeth; lens opacities and vision reduction; frequently, neural deafness. Generalized muscle hypotonia; brisk tendon reflexes; protuberant abdomen.

Etiology. Autosomal recessive inheritance. Lysosomal condition with deficiency of acid-alpha mannosidase. Enzyme defect is mapped to chromosome 19 p13 q13.

Pathology. Lymphocytes: vacuolated. Liver biopsy: vacuolated cells with reticulogranular pattern. Central nervous system: widespread ballooning of cells.

Diagnostic Procedures. *Blood.* Vacuolization of peripheral lymphocytes; presence of dark granules in neutrophils; presence of reduced alpha-mannosidase in serum, leukocytes, tissues, and urine. *X-ray. MRI.* Dysostosis multiplex. Prenatal diagnosis possible.

Therapy. Symptomatic.

Prognosis. Survival to adult age reported.

BIBLIOGRAPHY. Oeckerman PA: A generalized storage disorder resembling Hurler's syndrome. Lancet II:239–241, 1967
Thomas GH, Beaudet AL: Disorders of glycoproteins degradation and structure: mannosidosis, fucosidosis, sialidosis, and aspartylglycosaminuria and carbohydrate-deficient glycoprotein syndrome. In Scriver CR, Beaudet AL, Sly WS, et al: The Metabolic and Molecular Bases of Inherited Disease, 7th ed, pp 2533–2537. New York, McGraw-Hill, 1995

OFUJI

Synonyms. Eosinophilic pustular folliculitis; papulo-erythroderma Ofuji.

Symptoms and Signs. In Japan. Rare in other countries. Formation of itching, circinate or serpiniginous plaques formed by pustules and papules, clearing centrally and peripherally spreading on the face, trunk, and extensor aspect of arms, seldom on palms and soles. Remission and relapses characterize the condition.

Etiology. Unknown.

Pathology. In seborrheic areas of skin usually centered on hair follicles, development of sterile pustules infiltrated with eosinophils, some neutrophils and mononuclear cells. Moderate spongiosis; perivascular dermal infiltrare.

Diagnostic Procedures. *Blood.* In concomitance with exacerbations leucocytosis and eosinophilia.

Therapy. Erratic response to corticosteroids or dapsone, oxyphenbutazone.

Prognosis. Relapses and remission recurrent, slight residual pigmentation.

BIBLIOGRAPHY. Ofuji S, Ogino A, Horio T, et al: Eosinophilic pustular folliculitis in infancy. Ped Dermatol 50:195–203, 1970

Comacho-Martinez F: Eosinophilic pustular folliculitis. J Am Acad Dermatol 17:686–689, 1987

Burton JL: Eczema, lichenification, prurigo and erythroderma. In Champion RH, Burton JL, Ebling FJG (eds): Rook/Wilkinson/Ebling Textbook of Dermatology, 5th ed, p 588. Oxford, Blackwell Scientific, 1992

OGILVIE

Synonyms. Colonic pseudo-obstruction, acute; pseudo-obstruction of colon; colonic false obstruction; intestinal pseudo-obstruction; ileus of colon.

Symptoms and Signs. In old age. Both sexes. Variable pathologic conditions have been associated: neurologic, cardiovascular, pulmonary, renal, intra-abdominal process, retroperitoneal, after surgery, after trauma, drugs. Abdominal distention (100%), hyperactive or high-pitched bowel sounds (88%), abdominal tenderness, nausea, vomiting, fever, constipation, and diarrhea. Perforation, 14.8%.

Etiology. Unknown. Imbalance between sympathetic and parasympathetic innervation hypothesized.

Pathology. Distended colon, with possible cecal perforation.

Diagnostic Procedures. *X-ray.* Plain film of abdomen. Signs of intestinal obstruction without fluid level. *Barium enema.* No signs of mechanical obstruction. *Blood.* Mild imbalance of electrolytes.

Therapy. Conservative. Nasogastric aspiration, colonic decompression. Correction of electrolyte imbalance. Antibiotics, metronidazole. Treatment of underlying condition. Reported that epidural anesthesia may resolve condition. Surgery. Colonoscopic decompression and, if the case warrants, perforation.

Prognosis. It resolves completely in 3–6 days with adequate therapy. Medical mortality rate 25–30%; 46% in perforated cases.

BIBLIOGRAPHY. Ogilvie H: Large intestine colic due to sympathetic deprivation: New clinical syndrome. Br Med J 2:671–673, 1948

MacFarlane JA, Kay SK: Ogilvie's syndrome of false colonic obstruction: Is it a new clinical entity? Br Med J 2:1267–1269, 1949

Nanni G, Garbini A, Luchetti P, et al: Olgivie's syndrome (acute colonic pseudo-obstruction): Review of literature and report of 4 additional cases. Dis Colon Rectum 25:157–177, 1982

Vanek VW, AP-Salti M: Acute pseudo-obstruction of the colon (Ogilvie's syndrome): An analysis of 400 cases. Dis Colon Rectum 29:203–210, 1986

Manten HD: Pseudo-obstruction. In Haubrich WS, Schaffner F, Berk JE (eds): Bockus Gastroenterology, 5th ed, vol 2, pp 1261–1263. Philadelphia, WB Saunders, 1995

OGUCHI

Synonyms. Night blindness stationary; nyctalopia (misnomer) hemeralopia (correct term). See also Uyemura.

Symptoms. Majority of cases observed in Japan; reported also in Caucasians and blacks. Both sexes affected; manifest at early age. Stable nyctalopia in dimmed illumination; reduced dark adaptation fields and night visual acuity. With light, normal visual acuity.

Signs. Unusual color of fundus, from grayish-white to yellow, extending throughout entire fundus or in small section(s); Mizno phenomenon (after 2–3 hours in the dark the fundus assumes a normal reddish appearance).

Etiology. Unknown. Autosomal recessive inheritance.

Pathology. Indirect evidence of thinning or defect in the pigmented epithelium of fundus. Cones longer and anatomically modified.

Diagnostic Procedures. *Ophthalmoscopy.* Evidence of Mizno phenomenon using eye patches. *Electroretinography.* Absence of B-waves. *Fluorescent angiography.*

Therapy. None. Vitamin A may be tried.

Prognosis. Static Hemeralopia.

BIBLIOGRAPHY. Oguchi C: Ueber einen Fall Von eigenartiger. Hemeralopie Nippon Ganka Gakkai Zasshi 11:123, 1907

Oguchi C: Ueber die eigenartiger Hemeralopie mit diffuser weissgränlicher Verfarhung des Augenhintergrundes. Graefe Arch Ophthalmol 81:109–117, 1912

Bird AC, Jay B, Hussain AA, et al: Retinal photoreceptor disorders. In Garner A, Klintworth GK (eds): Pathobiology of Ocular Disease: A Dynamic Approach, 2nd ed, p 1225. New York, Marcel Dekker, 1994

O.H.A.H.A.

Synonyms.
Ophthalmoplegia—hypotonia—ataxia—hypoacusia—athetosis.

Symptoms and Signs. Both sexes. Onset: After learning to speak sudden deafness; ophthalmoplegia (only convergence persists) and latter (10–18 months of age) ataxia and athetosis of variable severity. Tendency to keep the mouth open. Mental development normal, but impression of stupidity because of mentioned handicaps.

Etiology. Autosomal recessive inheritance. Possibly a polyneuropathy.

Diagnostic Procedures. Ear: loss of caloric response.

BIBLIOGRAPHY. Kallio A-K, Jauhiainen J: A new syndrome of ophthalmoplegia hypoacusis, ataxia, hypotonia and athetosis (OHAHA). Adv Audiol 3:84–90, 1985

McKusick VA: Mendelian Inheritance in Man, X ed, vol 2, p 1604. Baltimore, University Press, 1992

OKIHIRO

Synonyms. Duane with radial defect; DR; acrorenal—ocular; radial ray defect; see Duane.

Symptoms and Signs. Both sexes. Variable ocular defects: Duane's syndrome (see); coloboma, ptosis. Variable degrees of hypoplasia of thumb, polydactyly, and reduction of mobility of interphalangeal joints. Variable renal anomalies: kidney malrotation, crossed renal ectopia, urinary tract anomalies. Also associated: Klippel-Feil (see), Goldenhar's (see), Wildervanck, cleft palate, spinal meningocele, deafness, etc.

Etiology. Autosomal dominant inheritance of the radial defect

Diagnostic Procedures. *X-rays of skeleton. Urography. Dermatoglyphic pattern. Abnormalities.*

BIBLIOGRAPHY. Okihiro MM, Tasaki T, Nakano KK, et al: Duane syndrome and congenital upper limb anomalies. Arch Neurol 34:174–179, 1977

Halal F, Homsy M, Perrault G: Acro-renal-ocular syndrome: Autosomal dominant thumb hypoplasia, renal ectopia, and eye defect. Am J Med Genet 17:753–762, 1984

McDermot KD, Winter RM: Radial ray defect and Duane anomaly: Report of a family with autosomal dominant transmission. Am J Med Genet 27:313–319, 1987

OLDFIELD

Obsolete.

Synonyms. Colonic poliposis; carcinoma; sebaceous cysts. See Gardner.

Symptoms and Signs. It has been presented as a possible variant of Gardner syndrome where the colonic polyposis is associated with sebaceous cysts or sebocystomatosis.

Etiology. Question about the origin of "retention versus neoformation" is discussed. No reason to retain this eponym.

Pathology. Cysts containing cheesy material.

Diagnostic Procedures. *X-ray. Barium enema. Coloscopy. CT scan. MRI. Cyst biopsy.*

Therapy. Surgery.

BIBLIOGRAPHY. Ingram JT, Oldfield MC: Hereditary sebaceous cysts. Br Med J i:960–963, 1937
Oldfield MC: The association of familial poliposis of the colon with multiple sebaceous cysts. Br J Surg 41:534–541, 1954
Kenny PJ, O'Neill J: Familial intestinal polyposis associated with further abnormalities of growth. Austr NZ J Surg 28:145–150, 1958

OLD SERGEANT

Synonym. Neurotic battle behavior.

Symptoms. Occurs in well-motivated, previously efficient soldiers without neurotic factors in previous history, who are able to handle responsibility (60% noncommissioned officers) have leadership quality, strong self-esteem; onset after a long period of combat, without rest. Abnormal tremulousness; first into foxhole, last to leave shelter; decreased effectiveness in battle to complete incapacitation; inability to make quick decisions and assume responsibility. No complaints and seldom on sick call. Symptoms disappear once patient is removed from environment, but quickly return if re-exposed, despite willingness to perform. Strong sense of discipline and devotion to unit (squad, company) in which he or she is serving. Frequently, dyspepsia.

BIBLIOGRAPHY. Sobel R: "Old sergeant" syndrome. Psychiatry 10:315–321, 1947
Belenky G: Contemporary Studies in Combat Psychiatry. London, Greenwood Press, 1987

OLIVER

Synonym. Postaxial polydactyly; mental retardation.

Symptoms and Signs. Two girls and one boy with said combination reported.

Etiology. Autosomal recessive inheritance.

BIBLIOGRAPHY. Oliver CP: Recessive polydactylism associated with mental deficiency. J Hered 31:365–367, 1940

OLIVER-MCFARLANE

Synonyms. Gray; trichomegaly; mental retardation; dwarfism; retina pigmentary degeneration.

Symptoms and Signs. Normal development in first few months of life. Bilateral destruction of tear canals. Slow dentition; poor vision (pigmentary degeneration of retina); heterochromia; hypertrichosis of eyebrows and eyelashes; alopecia (developing at 4–5 years of age), dwarfism; normal mentality, or retardation.

Etiology. Unknown. Form of ectodermal dysplasia. Usually sporadic. Partial trisomy of chromosome 13 suggested.

Pathology. See Signs. Biopsy of scalp skin shows degenerated hair follicles with patchy lymphocytic infiltration.

Diagnostic Procedures. *Blood.* Normal. *Spinal fluid.* Normal. *Chromosome study.* Normal.

Therapy. Growth hormone.

Prognosis. Normal mental development; partially sighted. Hormone treatment benefits growth.

BIBLIOGRAPHY. Gray H: Trichomegaly or movie lashes. Stanford Med Bull 2:157–158, 1944
Oliver GL, McFarlane DC: Congenital trichomegaly with associated pigmentary degeneration of the retina, dwarfism, and mental retardation. Arch Ophthalmol 74:169–171, 1965
Delleman JW, Van Walbeek K: The syndrome of trichomegaly, tapetoretinal degeneration and growth disturbances. Ophthalmologica 171:313–315, 1975
Sampson JR, Tolmie JL, Cant JS: Oliver-McFarlane syndrome: A 25-year follow-up. Am J Med Genet 34:199–201, 1989

OLIVOPONTOCEREBELLAR ATROPHY III

Synonyms. OPCA III; OPCA; retinal degeneration; Froment.

Symptoms and Signs. Both sexes. Onset in middle age, occasionally in adolescence or in severe cases in infancy. Progressive loss of vision and ataxia.

Etiology. Autosomal dominant inheritance.

Pathology. Retinal degeneration (various patterns, mainly macular). Cerebellar degenerative changes.

Prognosis. Variable period of survival according to severity. Variable in different families.

BIBLIOGRAPHY. Froment J, Bonnet P, Colrat A: Heredo-degenerations retinienne et spino-cerebeleuse; variantes ophthalmoscopiques et neurologique presentees par trois generations successive. J Med Lyon, 153–163, 1937
Konigsmark BW, Weiner LP: The olivopontocerebellar atrophy: A review. Medicine 49:227–241, 1970
Cooles P, Michaud R, Best PV: A dominantly inherited progressive disease in a black family characterized by cerebellar and retinal degeneration, external ophthalmoplegia, and abnormal mitochondria. J Neurol Sci 87:275–288, 1988

OLIVOPONTOCEREBELLAR ATROPHY V

Synonyms. OPCA V; Carter-Sukavaiana.

Symptoms and Signs. Prevalent in males. Cerebellar signs followed at later age by rigidity and progressive mental deterioration up to dementia.

Etiology. Autosomal dominant inheritance.

Pathology. Cerebellar and substantia nigra degeneration up to atrophy. Cortical evidence of degenerative process.

BIBLIOGRAPHY. Chandler JH, Bebin J: Hereditary cerebellar ataxia: Olivopontocerebellar type. Neurology 6:187–195, 1956
Carter HR, Sukavajana C: Familial cerebello-olivary degeneration with late development of rigidity and dementia. Neurology 6:876–884, 1956
Konigsmark BW, Lipton HL: Dominant olivopontocerebellar atrophy

with dementia and extrapyramidal signs: Report of a family through three generations. Birth Defects Orig Art Ser VII (1):178–191, 1971

OLIVOPONTOCEREBELLAR ATROPHY, X-LINKED

Synonyms. Cerebellar ataxia.

Symptoms and Signs. In males. Onset in infancy (or adolescence). Nystagmus, ataxia, dysarthria, orthopedic problems, normal or slighty impaired mental development; absence of pyramidal signs: normal strength, reflexes, and sensations.

Etiology. X-linked inheritance.

Diagnostic Procedures. *CT scan. MRI. Other neuroimaging techniques.*

Therapy. Symptomatic.

Prognosis. Does not seem to affect life span. Death from intercurrent diseases.

BIBLIOGRAPHY. Brandberg F, Kasuistische Beitrage zur gleichgeschlectlichen Vererburg. Arch Rass-u Ges Biol 7:290–305, 1910
Turner EV, Roberts E: A family with a sex linked hereditary ataxia. J New Ment Dis 87:74–80, 1938
Lutz R, Bodensteiner J, Schefer B, et al: X-linked olivopontocerebellar atrophy. Clin Genet 35:417–422, 1989

OLIVOPONTOCEREBELLAR DEGENERATION SYNDROMES

1. Menzel (see)
2. Fincler-Winkler (see)
3. Froment (see)
4. Shut-Haymaker (see)
5. Olivopontocerebellar degeneration, V (see)
6. Olivopontocerebellar degeneration, X-linked (see)
7. Dejerine-Thomas (see)

BIBLIOGRAPHY. Adams RD, Victor M: Principles of Neurology, 5th ed, p 991. New York, McGraw-Hill, 1993

OLLIER

Synonyms. Unilateral chondromatosis; endochondromatosis multiple; osteochondromatosis Ollier. See Maffucci.

Symptoms. Onset usually in infancy, present at all ages. Various functional disturbances of hands, feet, femora, fibulas, and pelvis (in that order), usually unilateral. Occasionally, pathologic fractures and vision impairment.

Signs. Deformity of mentioned bones; occasionally, abnormally short distal end of ulna. Ophthalmoplegia. Absence of hemangiomas (present instead in Maffucci).

Etiology. Unknown. Sporadic. Few instances of familial occurrence (Autosomal dominant type with reduced penetrance).

Pathology. Epiphyseal plates fail to undergo normal bone replacement and become incorporated in mature bone. Expansion of enchondromas with resulting deformities of bones. Occasionally association with granulose tumor of ovary, parasellar chondrosarcoma or astrocytoma.

Diagnostic Procedures. *X-ray.* Of skeleton. Radiolucent patches or fragmented, explosion-like pattern in metaphysis. *Biopsy.* Of bone.

Therapy. Orthopedic correction of deformities and pathologic fractures.

Prognosis. Severe disease may result in crippling and invalidism. Enchondroma sometimes develops into chondrosarcoma (10%). Growth of enchondroma may stop after puberty and calcification take place; some-

times it continues to grow throughout life. Tendency in some cases (30%) to become malignant chondrosarcomas.

BIBLIOGRAPHY. Ollier L: De la dyschondroplasie. Bull Soc Chir Lyon 3:22, 1899
Ollier M: Sur une nouvelle affection: La dyschondroplasie. Rev Chir Paris, 21:396–398, 1900
Vaz RM, Turner C: Ollier disease (enchondromatosis) associated with ovarian juvenile granulosa cell tumor and precocius pseudopuberty. J Pediatr 108:945–947, 1986
Rimoin DL, Lachman RS: Genetic disorders of the osseous skeleton. In Beithon P (ed): McKusick's Heritable Disorders of Connective Tissue, 5th ed, p 670. St Louis, CV Mosby, 1993

OLMSTED

Synonyms. Palmo-plantar—perioral keratoderma.

Symptoms and Signs. Well-defined palms amd plants keratoderma; deformity in flexion of fingers, leading to spontaneous amputation; periorificial erythema; warty hyperkeratosis. Occasionally: total alopecia; nail and tooth anomalies; joint laxity.

Therapy. See palmo-plantar keratoderma syndromes.

BIBLIOGRAPHY. Olmsted HC: Keratoderma palmaris et plantaris congenitalis: Report of a case showing associated lesions of unusual location. Am J Dis Child 33:757–764, 1927
Atherton DJ, Sutton C, Jones BM: Mutilating palmoplantar keratoderma with periorificial keratotic plaques (Olmsted's syndrome). Br J Dermatol 122:245–252, 1990

OMENN

Synonyms. Immunodeficiency, combined reticuloendotheliosis-eosinophilia; Rethiculoendotheliosis, familial combined immunodeficiency. See Sezary; erythroderma, and cutaneous T-cell lymphomas.

Symptoms and Signs. In infancy. Erythematous scaly rash, evolving into diffuse erythroderma. Hepato-spleno-adenomegaly. Diarrhea. Recurrent infections. Failure to thrive.

Etiology. Autosomal recessive inheritance.

Pathology. Skin: perivascular dense lymphohistiocytic-eosinophilic infiltration; lymph nodes: massive histiocytes; lymphocytes; eosinophil infiltration.

Diagnostic Procedures. *Blood.* Lymphocytosis, eosinophilia. Immunoglobulin decreased; IgE markedly increased. Lymphocytes as well as histiocytes are activated T-cells.

Therapy. Bone marrow transplantation.

Prognosis. Poor. Frequent termination in lymphoma.

BIBLIOGRAPHY. Omenn GS: Familial reticuloendotheliosis with eosinophilia. N Engl J Med 273:427–432, 1965
Glover MT, Atherton DJ, Levinsky RJ: Syndrome of erythroderma, failure to thrive and diarrhea in infancy: A manifestation of immunodeficiency. Pediatrics 81:66–72, 1988
Atherton DJ: The neonate. In Champion RH, Burton JL, Ebling FJG (eds): Rook/Wilkinson/Ebling Textbook of Dermatology, 5th ed, pp 426–427. Oxford, Blackwell Scientific, 1992

OMOHYOID

Symptoms. May occur when patient is in state of well-being; more frequent in subjects suffering from cramps in other areas. Onset usually following the act of yawning and swallowing at the same time as turning the head. Immediate excruciating pain in side of neck extending from the hyoid region to the omolateral scapula. Pain eases after a few minutes, but does not disappear. Inability to swallow saliva. Voice alteration and slurring of speech.

Signs. Pain spontaneous and on pressure over omohyoid muscle. Throat and larynx normal.

Etiology. Acute spasm or cramps of omohyoid muscle.

Therapy. Parenteral analgesic if pain lasts more than 1 hour. In cases of refractory pain or repeated attacks, division of central tendon of affected muscle.

Prognosis. Usually a moderate residual discomfort for 1 or 2 days. According to author, personal condition disappeared after a few years.

BIBLIOGRAPHY. Zuchary RB, Young A, Hammond JDS: The omohyoid syndrome. Lancet II:104–105, 1969

ONCOGENIC HYPOPHOSPHATEMIC OSTEOMALACIA

Synonyms. OHO.

Symptoms and Signs. Insidious onset, usually in adulthood. Fatigability; bone pain; skeletal deformities. When in children, also growth retardation.

Etiology. Humoral factors from small mesenchymal tumors (hemangiopericytoma; odontogenic tumor; fibroma; angiosarcoma; angiofibroma; myoma; oat-cell carcinoma; osteoblasmoma, etc.). Clinical pattern very similar to Hypophosphatemia, X-linked (see).

Pathology. Osteomalacia.

Diagnostic Procedures. *Blood.* P/GFR reduced; hypophosphatemia, low plasma 1,25(OH)2D. Calcium normal. *X-ray.* Rickets.

Therapy. Surgical removal of tumor. If tumor not found: combined phosphate and 1,25(OH)2D.

Prognosis. All signs revert as soon as tumor is removed.

BIBLIOGRAPHY. MacGuire MH, Merenda JT, Etzkorn JR, et al: Oncogenic osteomalacia: A case report. Clin Orthop 244:305, 1989
Rasmussen H, Tenenhouse HS: Mendelian Hypophosphatemias. In Scriver CR, Beaudet AL, Sly WS, et al: The Metabolic and Molecular Bases of Inherited Disease, 7th ed, pp 3737–3738. New York, McGraw-Hill, 1995

ONDINE CURSE

Synonyms. Primary alveolar hypoventilation; idiopathic hypoventilation, nonobese; congenital central hypoventilation; forgotten respiration; CCHS. See Pickwickian.

Symptoms and Signs. Most cases reported have presented the syndrome within a few hours of birth. In 50% of patients prior history of central nervous system disease. Patient breathes relatively normally during the day but presents long periods of apnea during the night. Even death may occur during sleep. Possibly, various symptoms of hypothalamic dysfunction present.

Etiology. Diagnosis by exclusion. Rule out central nervous system disease, upper airway obstruction, neuromuscular disorders. It appears to result from a defect in the brain stem control and possibly a deficient transmission chemoreceptor.

Diagnostic Procedures. *Pulmonary function tests.* With patient awake, gas exchange normal or almost normal; during sleep, respiratory failure. *X-ray. CT scan.* Normal lung findings and diaphragm movement. Of skull: normal, neurocristopathy as associated lesion. *ECG.* Absence of right cardiac hypertrophy. *Blood.* Absence of polycythemia.

Therapy. Various drugs have been tried, with variable results. The most

beneficial include doxapram and almitrine. The mainstay of treatment is tracheostomy with mechanical ventilation during the night. Phrenic nerve pacing (bilateral) has been used both in adults and children.

Prognosis. Children can grow up with mechanical ventilation. There is a definite risk of death owing to respiratory infection, cor pulmonale, or autonomic disturbances with cardiorespiratory failure or cardiac arrest.

BIBLIOGRAPHY. Giraudoux J: "Ondine." In Four Plays, vol 1, p 253. New York, Hill & Wang, 1958
Severinghaus JW, Michell RA: Ondine's curse: Failure of respiratory center automaticity while awake. Clin Res 10:122, 1962
Fishman LS, Samson JH, Sperling DR: Primary alveolar hypoventilation syndrome (Ondine's curse). Am J Dis Child 110:155–161, 1965
Weatherall DJ, Ledingham JGG, Warrell DA (eds): Oxford Textbook of Medicine, 3rd ed, pp 2670, 2916, 3888. Oxford, Oxford Med Pub, 1996

ONYALAI

Synonym. Werlhof variant.

Symptoms and Signs. Occurs in Bantu tribes in Africa. Only males affected. Onset at any age, mostly in adulthood. Hemorrhagic bullae in mouth and other mucosal cavities.

Etiology. Unknown. Variant of idiopathic thrombocytopenic purpura.

Diagnostic Procedures. *Blood.* Thrombocytopenia.

BIBLIOGRAPHY. Strongway WE, Strongway AK: Ascorbic acid deficiency in the African disease onyalay. Arch Intern Med 83:372–376, 1949
Lewis SM, Lurie A: Onyalai: A clinical and laboratory survey. J Trop Hyg 96:281–285, 1958
Bithell TC: Thrombocytopenia caused by immunologic platelet destruction: Idiopathic thrombocytopenic purpura (ITP), drug-induced thrombocytopenia, and miscellaneous forms. In Lee GR, Bithell TC, Foerster J, et al (eds): Wintrobe's Clinical Hematology, 9th ed, p 1342. Philadelphia, Lea & Febiger, 1993

OPALSKI

Synonyms. Cervicomedullary; vertebrospinal artery, posterior.

Symptoms and Signs. Crossed hemianesthesia to pain and temperature and uncrossed hemiplegia.

Etiology and Pathology. Extended area of ischemia in the medulla and dorsal to the olive (as in Wallenberg, see), extending below the medulla involving the crossed pyramidal tract in an area of gliosis. Type of lesion stretching out longitudinally, with upper part affecting medulla and lower part the high cervical cord (in contrast with brain stem syndromes extending transversally).

BIBLIOGRAPHY. Opalski A Un nouveau syndrome sous-bulbaire. Syndrome partiel de l'artère vertébro spinale postérieur. Paris Med 36:214–220, 1946
Rondot P: Syndromes of central motor disorder. In Vinken PJ, Bruyn GW: Handbook of Clinical Neurology, vol 1, p 189. Amsterdam, Elsevier, 1969

OPHTHALMIA, SYMPATHETIC

Synonym. Sympathetic uveitis.

Symptoms. Occurs 3–8 weeks after injury to one eye. Development in contralateral eye, photophobia, pain, lacrimation, and vision impairment.

Signs. Tenderness; uveitis white drusen-like spots (Dalen-Fuchs nodules), vitreous cell; subretinal edema; papillitis.

Etiology. Penetrating injury to one eye that causes sympathetic reaction in the other eye through reflex mechanism. Uveal pigment possible offending agent. Immunopathogenesis of condition still fundamentally obscure.

Pathology. Changes in uninjured eye: granulomatosis; inflammation; nodular accumulation of lymphocytes in uveal tract, followed by epithelioid cell infiltration.

Diagnostic Procedures. *Ophthalmoscopy.* Uveitis; retinal edema up to detachment. *Blood.* Antiuveal antibodies reported in high percentage of cases.

Therapy. Rapid intervention, up to removal of injured eye before changes in the contralateral one became established.

Prognosis. Without treatment, chronic course, marked tendency to relapse, and possibly progression leading to blindness.

BIBLIOGRAPHY. Pusey B: Cytotoxins and sympathetic ophthalmia. Arch Ophthalmol 32:334–338, 1903

Foster CS: Ocular manifestations of immune disease. In Garner A, Klintworth GK (eds): Pathobiology of Ocular Disease: A Dynamic Approach, 2nd ed, pp 172–174. New York, Marcel Dekker, 1994

OPITZ-FRIAS

Synonyms. Opitz-Christian; Opitz-G; Christian-Opitz; G; B.B.B.; dysphagia—hypospadias—hypertelorism—esophageal abnormality; telecanthus-associated abnormalities; hypertelorism—hypospadias.

Symptoms. Males affected (in female carriers, partial expression). Present from birth. Swallowing problems with recurrent aspiration. Stridulous breathing; nonconstant wheezing; hoarse cry.

Signs. Hypertelorism. Palpebral fissures slanted; nasal bridge flat; mild to severe micrognathia. Occasionally, short frenulum of tongue, bifid scrotum, imperforate anus, prominent parietal-occipital areas. Females have normal genitalia.

Etiology. Unknown. Considered autosomal dominant, sex-limited or sex-linked.

Diagnostic Procedures. *Cinefluorography* of swallowing.

Therapy. If repeated aspirations, gastrostomy or jejunostomy considered.

Prognosis. Persistence of respiratory problems; bronchiectasis. Intelligence development normal; mild mental retardation in one family.

BIBLIOGRAPHY. Opitz JM, Frias JL, Gutenberger JE, et al: The G syndrome of multiple congenital anomalies. Birth Defects 5:95–103, 1969

Opitz JM, Summit RL, Smith DW: The BBB syndrome: Familial telecanthus with associated congenital anomalies. Birth Defects Orig Art Ser V (2):86–94, 1969

Silva EO: The hypertelorism-hypospadias syndrome. Clin Genet 23:30–34, 1983

Opitz JM: "G" syndrome (hypertelorism with esophageal abnormalities and hypospadia or hypospadia-dysphagia, or Opitz-Frias or Opitz G syndrome. Perspective in 1987 and bibliography (editorial). Am J Med Genet 28:275–285, 1987

OPITZ-KAVEGGIA

Synonyms. FG (initials represent patient surname); Keller.

Symptoms and Signs. In males. Congenital macrocephaly; striking facies; imperforate or displaced anus; hypotonia; joint contractures; heart defects. Mental retardation; seizures, occasionally sensineural deafness, short stature. Striking personalities.

Etiology. X-linked inheritance, incompletely recessive.

Pathology. Partial agenesis of corpus callosum; variable gastrointestinal and heart malformations.

Prognosis. From death in first days of life to adulthood with short stature, muscle hypotonia, constipation, and variable degrees of mental retardation.

BIBLIOGRAPHY. Opitz JM, Kaveggia EF: The FG syndrome: An X-linked recessive syndrome of multiple congenital anomalies and mental retardation. Z Kinderheilk 117:1–18, 1974

Keller MA, Jones KL, Nyhan WL, et al: A new syndrome of mental deficiency with craniofacial, limb and anal abnormalities. J Pediatr 88:589–591, 1976

Thompson EM, Baraitser M, Lindenbaum RH, et al: The FG syndrome: 7 new cases. Clin Genet 27:582–594, 1985

OPPENHEIM

Synonyms. Amyotonia congenita; myotonia congenita; hypotonia benign congenital; muscle hypoplasia congenital benign.

Hypotonia represents a symptom of various conditions. The old syndrome, representing a too-heterogeneous group, has been subdivided into Nording-Hoffman; infantile muscular atrophy; myopathies (Shy-Magee; nemaline mitochondrial; myotubular), and undifferentiated forms of hypotonia and muscle underdevelopment (see Walton, Krabbe, and Floppy infant). Tendency to use the eponym to indicate generically primary nonprogressive myopathies and differentiate them from forms secondary to central nervous system pathology.

BIBLIOGRAPHY. Oppenheim H: Textbook of Nervous Disease. New York, GE Steckert, 1911

Adams RD, Denny-Brown D, Pearson CM: Diseases of the Muscle, 3rd ed, p 256. New York, Harper & Row, 1975

Goebel HH, Lenard HG: Congenital myopathies. In Rowland LP, Di Mauro S (eds): Handbook of Clinical Neurology, vol 18: Myopathies, p 331. Amsterdam, Elsevier, 1992

OPPENHEIMER (A.)

Synonyms. Spondylitis ossificans ligamentosa I; physiologic vertebral ligamentous calcification. See Forestier.

Symptoms. Occurs in patients over 50 years of age. Mild or no symptoms in the back, but decreased mobility of spinal column. No symptoms or evidence suggestive of rheumatoid arthritis.

Etiology. Limitation of spinal motion; degenerative changes followed by calcification of longitudinal vertebral ligaments.

Diagnostic Procedures. *X-ray.* One or multiple interspaces involved; thoracic region most frequently affected with calcification of ligament and a tortuous appearance. Vertebrae normal density; apophyseal, and costovertebral joints normal. *Blood.* Normal; normal sedimentation rate.

Therapy. Physical therapy. Patients should be instructed to sleep supine on a firm bed without a pillow and to practice postural and deep-breathing exercises regularly. Indomethacin can be used for the control of pain. Surgical treatment to correct some spine and hip deformities can be of value in selected cases.

Prognosis. Good.

BIBLIOGRAPHY. Oppenheimer A: Calcification and ossification of vertebral ligaments (spondylitis ossificans ligamentosa) roentgen study of pathogenesis and clinical significance. Radiology 38:160–173, 1942

Smith CF, Pugh DG, Polley HE: Physiologic vertebral ligamentous calcification: An aging process. Am J Roentgenol 74:1049–1058, 1955

Bjelle A: Age and rheumatic diseases. In Klippel JH, Dieppe PA: Rheumatology, p 1.15.4. St Louis, CV Mosby, 1994

OPPENHEIM-SCHOLZ-MOREL

Synonyms. Dyshoric angiopathia.

Symptoms and Signs. Post-mortem diagnosis except one case. No particular symptomatology. Visual gnosias.

Etiology and Pathology. Alteration of arteriolar and precapillary permeability (dyshoria) with transudation of plasmatic substances (amyloid material?) through endothelium and diffusion in the brain parenchyma producing discrete lesions, especially occipital area. Suggested autosomal recessive inheritance.

BIBLIOGRAPHY. Morel F: Petite contribution à l'étude d'une angiopathie apparentemant dysphoric and topistique. Monatschr Psychiat Neurol 120:352–357, 1950

Costantinidis J: Dyshoric angiopathia (Oppenheimer-Scholz-Morel). In Vinken PJ, Bruyn GW: Handbook of Clinical Neurology, vol 42, pp 728–729. Amsterdam, Elsevier, 1981

OPPENHEIM-URBACH

Synonyms. Urbach; extracellular cholesterosis; dermatitis atrophicans maculosa lipoides diabetica, necrobiosis diabeticorum; necrobiosis lipoidica.

Symptoms and Signs. Rare. Prevalent in females. Seventy-five percent of patients have diabetes. Onset at all ages. *Variety I.* Purple red plaque with yellow-brown center and nodules developing rapidly on extremities and dorsa of hands and feet. Ears, tongue, and chest may also be involved. *Variety II.* Purplish macular lesions interspersed with yellowish nodules and papules. Liver and spleen may be enlarged in both forms.

Etiology. Two-thirds to three-fourths of patients have diabetes mellitus; association not clear (only 0.3% of diabetic patients present the syndrome). Deposition of glycoprotein in small vessel walls may underlie the development of the condition as well as other forms of microangiopathies.

Pathology. Granulomatous reaction and fat deposit to necrobiotic and inflammatory localized changes with minimal evidence of vascular changes (except for lesion of the legs).

Diagnostic Procedures. *Biopsy of skin. Blood.* Glucose (in etiology); in many cases increase of alpha-2-macroglobulin.

Therapy. Treat when diabetes; extensive ulceration: excision and grafting. Proposed: aspirin and dipyridamole and perilesion infiltration with heparin or steroids.

Prognosis. Chronic, possibly incapacitating, but relatively benign course. Possibly, spontaneous remission after years.

BIBLIOGRAPHY. Oppenheim M: Eine noch nicht beschrieben Hauterkrankung bei Diabetes mellitus (Dermatitis atrophicans lipoides diabetica). Wien Klin Wchnschr 45:314–315, 1932

Urbach E: Beiträge zu einer physiologischen und pathologischen Chemie der Haut; eine neue diabetische Stoffwechseldermatose: Nekrobiosis lipoidica diabeticorum. Arch Derm Syph 166:273–285, 1932

Cunliffe WJ: Necrobiotic disorders. In Champion RH, Burton JL, Ebling FJG (eds): Rook/Wilkinson/Ebling Textbook of Dermatology, 5th ed, pp 2033–2038. Oxford, Blackwell Scientific, 1992

OPSISMODYSPLASIA

Symptoms. Both sexes. At birth. Hypotonia respiratory infections. Neurologic symptoms in case of subluxation of C1 vertebra.

Signs. Short stature, short hands and fingers, facial abnormalities, short nose and depressed nasal bridge; short rhizomelic limbs; narrow thorax.

Etiology. Generalized delay of endochondrial ossification. Suggested autosomal recessive inheritance.

Pathology. Chondro-osseous tissue shows large and widened hypertrophic area and wide connective tissue septa around hypertrophic cells.

Diagnostic Procedures. *X-rays. Echography. CT scan.* Severe hypoplasia of vertebrae, base of skull and long bones epiphyses ossification.

Therapy. Prevention of subluxation of C1; Symptomatic.

Prognosis. Death in the first few years of life.

BIBLIOGRAPHY. Maroteaux P, Stanescu V, Stanescu R: Four recently described osteochondrodysplasias. In Papadatos CJ, Bartsocas CS (eds): Skeletal Dysplasias. New York, Alan R Liss, 1982

Maroteaux P, Stanescu V, Stanescu R, et al: Opsismodysplasia: A new type of chondrodysplasia with predominant involvement of the bones of the hands and the vertebrae. Am J Med Genet 19:171–182, 1984

ORBITAL APEX

Synonyms. Déjean; Rollet; orbital apex-sphenoidal; orbital superior fissure; sensorimotor ophthalmoplegia. It belongs to a group of syndromes with extremely similar clinical characteristics. In particular it is difficult to distinguish it from Rochon-Davigneau since these syndromes share many symptoms, but in the latter blindness is absent. See also Tolosa-Hunt.

Symptoms. Sudden onset, sometimes following recent respiratory infection, trauma. Impairment or loss of vision (owing to optic nerve involvement); diplopia. Severe pain in retro-orbital and temporoparietal areas (area of ophthalmic branch of trigeminal nerve plus involvement of III, IV, and VI nerve); especially in case of trauma associated damage to the internal carotid artery, cerebrospinal fluid rhinorrhea, posttraumatic diabetes insipidus.

Signs. Little or no displacement of bulb, from limited movement in various directions, to complete ophthalmoplegia. Bulb fixed in straight ahead position caused by the paralysis of third, fourth, and sixth cranial nerves. Anesthesia of upper eyelid and forehead. Pupil dilated and fixed.

Etiology and Pathology. Infection, cysts, aneurysm, neoplasm, or trauma of sinuses (primarily frontal and ethmoidal) affecting the sphenoid fissure. Low-grade, nonspecific inflammation of cavernous sinuses.

Diagnostic Procedures. *X-ray. Angiography. CT scan. MRI.* Patterns according to etiology. *Blood.* In some cases, elevation of leukocytes and sedimentation rate. *CSF.* Highly variable; sugar normal or depressed; protein and cell normal or slightly elevated.

Therapy. Antibiotics or surgery. Heparin in cases with thrombosis. Corticosteroids for granulomatous lesions.

Prognosis. Depends on etiology. Much improved by use of antibiotics; some cases of nonspecific infection respond to corticosteroids.

BIBLIOGRAPHY. Hirschfeld L: Epanchemant de sang dans de sinus caverneux du cote gauche diagnostique pendant la vie. C R Soc Biol 138, 1858

Déjean C: Les syndromes paralytiques du sommet de l'orbite. Arch Ophthalmol 44:657–690, 1927

Zachariades N, Vairaktaris E, Papavassiliou D, et al: Orbital apex syndrome. Int J Oral Maxillofac Surg 16:352–354, 1987

Postma MP, Seldomridge GW, Vines FS: Superior orbital fissure syndrome and bilateral internal carotid pseudoaneurysms. J Oral-Maxillofac-Surg 48:503–508, 1990

Unger JM, Gentry LR, Grossman JE: Sphenoid fractures: Prevalence, sites and significance. Radiology 175:175–180, 1990

ORBITAL MYOSITIS

Synonyms. Orbital pseudotumor; ocular myositis; euthyroid Graves. See progressive external ophthalmoplegia.

Symptoms and Signs. In adults (but also in children) preceded by manifestations of nonspecific virus-like symptoms, unilateral or bilateral edema, and congestion of periorbital soft tissues and conjunctiva. Proptosis. Prominent local pain enhanced by movement of eyes. Diplopia. Sometimes ortbital hemorrhage and ecchymosis of eyelid. Attack usually stops within few days spontaneously or following therapy (scc). Sometimes chronic ophthalmoplegia.

Etiology. May be part of Flajani (see) proceeding hyperthyroidism or viral-induced reaction of eye muscles.

Pathology. *Muscle biopsy.* Inflammatory cells infiltrating between muscles, perivascular degeneration, and fibrosis.

Diagnostic Procedures. *CT scan. MRI.* To establish differential diagnosis with tumors or Flajani. Study of thyroid hormones: negative.

Therapy. Steroids (prednisone 50–80 mg day for 7–10 days, followed by tapering).

Prognosis. Relapses are possible. Fibrosis may limit passive mobility of eyes.

BIBLIOGRAPHY. Gleason JE: Idiopathic myositis involving the extraocular muscles. Ophthalmic Rec 12:471–478, 1903
Keane JR: Alternating proptosis: A case report of acute orbital myositis definied by the computerized tomographic scan. Arch Neurol 34:642–643, 1977
Rowland LP: Progressive external ophthlmoplegia and ocular myopathies. In Rowland LP, Di Mauro S (eds): Handbook of Clinical Neurology, vol 18: Myopathies, p 287. Amsterdam, Elsevier, 1992

ORGANIC HYPERINSULINISM

Synonym. Hyperinsulinism, endogenous. See Harris and hypoglycemic, neonatal.

Symptoms and Signs. Those of acute and chronic hypoglycemia, sometimes with irreversible brain damage. Whipple triad: (1) history of attack of hunger, weakness, sweating, and paresthesias coming during the fasting state; (2) blood glucose level of 40 mg/100 ml during the attacks; (3) immediate recovery with administration of glucose. Sudden hunger; weakness; headache; faintness; vertigo; sweating; paresthesias (on the face); tremors; palpitation. Central nervous system changes: diplopia; ataxia; aphasia; paralysis; convulsion; coma.

Etiology and Pathology. Adenoma of islets of Langerhans (beta cells), multiple, small, a few malignant with functional metastasis. Familial (usually), associated often with adenoma of parathyroids and pituitary. Hypertrophy or hyperplasia of pancreas in children; age; insulin resistance; malnutrition.

Differential Diagnosis. Other causes of hypoglycemia: *Organic.* (1) Hypopituitarism; (2) hypoadrenocorticism; (3) chronic passive congestion of the liver; (4) tumors of different types (e.g., mesodermal; hepatomas; adrenal); (5) central nervous system lesions. *Functional.* (1) Functional hypoglycemia; (2) alimentary hypoglycemia; (3) early diabetes; (4) alcohol abuse; (5) lactation; intense muscular exertion; (6) renal glycosuria. *Factitious hepatic enzyme defects.* (1) Glycogen storage diseases; (2) hereditary fructose imbalance; (3) hereditary galactosemia. *Therapeutic.* Overdosage in treatment of diabetes. Idiopathic in infancy. (1) Newborn of diabetic mother; (2) leucine sensitivity; (3) leucine insensitivity (a) absence of alpha cells, (b) poor epinephrine secretion.

Diagnostic Procedures. (1) Prolonged fasting; no food for 72 hours; only water. Only mild exercises. If patient has islet cell adenoma there is a reduction of blood glucose of 30%. (2) Five-hour glucose tolerance test: 1 g injected intravenously. If adenoma, in 30 minutes the glucose falls 50–80% and remains low for several hours. If functional, glucose falls but then rises to normal level in 1–2 hours. (3) Tolbutamide tolerance test. (4) Assay of insulin (excessive rise after tolbutamide) may be of great value. More important the longer hypoglycemia persists. (5) Leucine tolerance test. (6) Liver function test: fructose-galactose

tolerance test, glucagon and epinephrine tolerance test. (7) Angiography. Selective celiac and superior mesenteric artery studies.

Therapy. Surgery; blood glucose monitoring and glucose infusion with the aid of closed loop artificial pancreas; glucagon; diazoxide (300–600 mg daily orally) with concomitant thiazide diuretic. (Verapamil can be used in patients unable to tolerate diazoxide.) For islet cell carcinomas, streptozocin has been tried with success, without kidney toxicity.

Prognosis. Complete remission with adequate therapy. *Complications:* Retinal cerebrovascular hemorrhage; coronary insufficiency; central nervous system irreversible damage (fast drop; muscle atrophy; pyramidal signs); after surgery, transient or permanent diabetes; pancreatic insufficiency; gastric ulcerations.

BIBLIOGRAPHY. Flier JS: Syndromes of insulin resistance and mutant insulin. In De Groot LJ (ed): Endocrinology, 3rd ed, p 1594. Philadelphia, WB Saunders, 1995

ORKEL

Synonyms. Multiple epiphyseal dysplasia tarda (type IV), MEDT (type IV); see Fairbank.

Symptoms and Signs. Both sexes affected; normal at birth. At age of 4 or 5 ambulation problems; ankle and foot deformities; hip joint abnormally wide; bowlegs. At age 15, evidence of paraparesis; hyperactive leg reflexes; dorsal Babinski sign; ankle clonus; visual trouble (retinitis pigmentosa).

Etiology. Autosomal recessive inheritance (?); of uncertain classification. Chromosome 19q12.

Diagnostic Procedures. *X-ray.* See Symptoms and Signs. *Blood. Urine.* Normal. *Ophthalmoscopy.* Retinal (retinitis pigmentosa) and vascular abnormalities.

Therapy. Orthopedic and surgical.

Prognosis. Difficulty in walking in spite of therapy. Progression of vision impairment.

BIBLIOGRAPHY. Watt JK: Multiple epiphysial dysplasia: Report of four cases. Br J Surg 39:533–535, 1952
Bailey JA: Disproportionate Short Stature: Diagnosis and Management, p 429. Philadelphia, WB Saunders, 1973
Beighton P: McKusick's Heritable Disorders of Connective Tissue, 5th ed, pp 622–625. St Louis, CV Mosby, 1993

ORMOND

Synonyms. Gerota fascitis; periureteral fibrosis; periureteritis plastica; retroperitoneal fibrosis; retroperitoneal idiopathic fibrosis.

Symptoms. More frequent in males; average age at onset 46 years for males, 32 years for females. Pain in the back, of variable intensity, usually progressing and radiating in pattern of ureteral colic, or abdominal pain without specific localization. Pain usually persisting for 1 month. Frequently associated: vomiting; nausea; anorexia; malaise; fatigue; weight loss, constipation or diarrhea. Seldom associated: ADH-resistant diabetes insipidus syndromes (see) with nicturia; oliguria; backache; edema; headache; dysuria; thirst.

Signs. Not contributory. Moderate blood pressure elevation; seldom, fever. A mass may be palpated and tenderness elicited in the costal vertebral angle.

Etiology. Unknown. Possibly a fasciculitis of collagen disease; multiple etiologies possible. See Sclerosing lipogranulomatosis syndromes. Methysergide and ergotamine can occasionally cause this syndrome.

Pathology. Periureteral fibrosis; fibrous band that locally constricts ureter, sometimes iliac vessel or aorta as well. Microscopically, chronic inflammatory reaction with prevalent lymphocytes and fibroblastic proliferation. Pyelonephritis frequently observed. Fibrous band occluding bile duct also occasionally present (suggesting systemic disease).

Diagnostic Procedures. *Blood.* Anemia (constant); high blood urea nitrogen, high sedimentation rate. *Retrograde pyelography. CT scan. Ultrasonography. Biopsy.* Multiple deep biopsies to rule out neoplastic disease.

Therapy. Surgery, nephrectomy, or nephrostomy with ureterolysis, and subsequent operation of other side to free the ureter. Antibiotics.

Prognosis. Good with therapy; diabetes insipidus-like syndrome disappears as a result of treatment of local condition. Pyelonephritis may persist. In patients with unilateral involvement, involvement of other side occurs in about 25% of cases. Surgical treatment for relief of ureteral obstruction from the fibrous encasement. Steroid therapy of questionable value.

BIBLIOGRAPHY. Oberling C: Retroperitoneal xanthogranuloma. Am J Cancer 23:477–489, 1935

Ormond JK: Bilateral ureteral obstruction due to envelopment and compression by an inflammatory retroperitoneal process. J Urol 59:1072–1079, 1948

Morad N, Strongwater SL, Eypper S, Woda BA: Idiopathic retroperitoneal and mediastinal fibrosis mimicking connective tissue disease. AM J Med 82:363–366, 1987

Weatherall DJ, Ledingham JGG, Warrell DA (eds): Oxford Textbook of Medicine, 3rd ed, pp 3244–3246. Oxford, Oxford Med Pub, 1996

ORO-FACIAL-DIGITAL III

Synonyms. OFD III; "see-saw winking."

Symptoms. From birth. Both sexes. Mental retardation.

Signs. Eye abnormalities (in some cases "see-saw winking"); hypertelorism; hamartomatous tongue; teeth abnormalities; uvula bifida; hexadactyly of hands and feet; pectus excavatum; kyphosis; spasticity.

Etiology. Possibly autosomal recessive inheritance.

BIBLIOGRAPHY. Ford FR: Diseases of the Nervous System in Infancy, Childhood, and Adolescence, p 811. Springfield IL, Charles C Thomas, 1960

Sugarman GI, Katakia M, Menkes JH: See-saw winking in a familial oro-facial-digital syndrome. Clin Genet 248–254, 1971

OROTIC ACIDURIA I and II

Synonyms. Orotidylic pyrophosphorylase and orotidylic decarboxylase deficiency; orotate phosphorybosyltransferase and OMP decarboxylase deficiency; uridine monophosphate synthase deficiency; UMP synthase deficiency; megaloblastic orotic anemia.

Symptoms. Prevalent in males. No abnormalities at birth. During first year, failure to thrive. Apathy; some degree of mental retardation, lassitude; repeated infections. Possible urinary obstruction from orotic acid in high concentration.

Signs. Pallor; muscle hypotonia; no neurologic defects.

Etiology. In form I reduced activity in both orotate-phosphoribose-transferase (OPRT) and orotidine 5-phosphate-decarboxylase (ODC); In form II only one enzyme defective (orotidine-5-phosphate decarboxylase). Autosomal recessive inheritance. Several other causes of orotic aciduria have been found: urea cycle defects, nutritional and liver damage, lysinuric protein intolerance, formiminotransferase/cyclodeaminase deficiency. PP-ribose P-synthetase deficiency, other purine metabolic defects, pregnancy, administration of several drugs, etc.

Diagnostic Procedures. *Blood.* Megaloblastic anemia with marked anisopoikilocytosis (not responding to B_{12}, folic acid). Hypochromic circulating red cell (that do not respond to iron or pyridoxine administration) good response to uridylic and cytidylic acids. Leukogenic normal platelets. *Urine.* Excessive excretion of orotic acid. *Bone marrow.* Atypical megaloblastic changes.

Therapy. Yeast nucleotides (poorly tolerated: gastrointestinal symptoms). Uridylic acid and cytidilic acid; glucocorticoids.

Prognosis. Good remission with yeast nucleotides. Good remission with treatment.

BIBLIOGRAPHY. Huguley CM Jr, Bain JA, Rivers SL, et al: Refractory megaloblastic anemia associated with excretion of orotic acid. Blood 1:615–634, 1959

Bensen JT, Nelson LH, Pettenati MJ, et al: First report of management and outcome of pregnancies associated with hereditary orotic aciduria. Am J Med Genet 41:426–431, 1991

Webster DR, Becroft DMO, Suttle DP: Hereditary orotic aciduria and other disorders of pyrimidine metabolism. In Scriver CR, Beaudet AL, Sly WS, et al: The Metabolic and Molecular Bases of Inherited Disease, 7th ed, pp 1809–1823. New York, McGraw-Hill, 1995

ORTHOSTATIC SYNCOPE

Synonyms. Hypotension orthostatic; hyperadrenergic orthostatic hypotension.

Symptoms. More frequent in tall, asthenic subjects with poor muscle structure. In the morning hours, enhanced by heat, humidity, heavy meals, and exercise and when assuming upright posture. Lightheadedness, blurred vision, weakness, and unsteadiness; may reach loss of consciousness.

Signs. Progressive hypotension over seconds or minutes, tachycardia, pallor, cold extremities, and sweating.

Etiology. May be classified into three categories: (1) venous pooling and/or blood volume depletion (anemia, hemorrhage, gastrointestinal fluid loss, prolonged fever, dialysis, intense sweating, diabetes insipidus); (2) pharmacological agents (antihypertensive, diuretics, nitrates, vasodilatotors, antidepressants, tranquilizers, and other central nervous system agents); (3) neurogenic (neuropathies, spinal cord diseases, intracranial tumors, Parkinson, CNS atherosclerosis, etc.). Deficiency of autonomic functions.

Pathology. According to etiology.

Diagnostic Procedures. Evaluation of possible general causes (see Etiology) for autonomic imbalances differential diagnosis (see Bradbury-Eggleston and Shy-Drager syndromes).

Therapy. See Bradbury-Eggleston.

Prognosis. Variable according to basic condition. Single episodes tend to be overcome spontaneously.

BIBLIOGRAPHY. Schatz IJ: Orthostatic hypotension. Arch Intern Med 144, 773–777; 1037–1041, 1984

Lewis RP, Budoulas H, Schaal SF, et al: Diagnosis and management of syncope. In Schlant RC, Alexander RW: Hurst's The Heart, 8th ed. New York, McGraw-Hill, 1994

ORTNER

Synonym. Cardiovocal.

Symptoms. Hoarseness plus symptoms of cardiovascular conditions: aortic arch lesions; mitral stenosis; congenital cardiac defects; hypertensive heart disease; coronary artery disease.

Signs. Faulty movements or palsy of left vocal cord.

Etiology and Pathology. Left laryngeal nerve injury by compression between aorta and dilated pulmonary artery.

Diagnostic Procedures. Those for cardiac disease.

Differential Diagnosis. In infancy, vocal cord paralysis has usually been associated with central nervous system lesions, especially meningocele with Arnold-Chiari malformation. Increased intracranial pressure can compress the vagus nerves at the foramen magnum, causing bilateral vocal cord paralysis. Birth trauma could cause either bilateral or unilateral paralysis. If the traction on the left recurrent laryngeal nerve is relieved in infancy, full recovery of vocal cord function is to be expected.

Therapy. That of cardiac disease.

Prognosis. Depends on etiology.

BIBLIOGRAPHY. Ortner N: Recurrenslähmung bei Mitralstenose. Wien Klin Wochenschr 10:753–755, 1897
Stocker HH, Enterline HT: "Cardiovocal syndrome": Laryngeal paralysis in intrinsic heart disease. Am Heart J 56:51–59, 1958
Condon LM, Katkov H, Singh A, et al: Cardiovocal syndrome in infancy. Pediatrics 76:22–25, 1985

ORZECHOWSKI

Synonyms. Truncular ataxia—opsoclonia; ataxia truncular opsoclonia; encephalitis; opsoclonia; tremulousness.

Symptoms. Follows a benign upper respiratory infection. (1) Opsoclonia: involuntary oscillations of eyes in horizontal and vertical directions, persisting with closed eyes. Sometimes associated with blinking, lacking the rhythmicity and regularity of nystagmus. (2) Incapacitating postural tremulousness of the body. (3) Fever and various symptoms and signs of encephalitis.

Etiology. Unknown; very likely viral.

Pathology. Unknown.

Diagnostic Procedures. *Spinal tap.* Pleocytosis, or normal. Viral isolation studies should be performed on cerebrospinal fluid, stool, and pharyngeal secretion.

Therapy. Tetracycline (?). Supportive and symptomatic.

Prognosis. Alarming and incapacitating for a few weeks. Spontaneous resolution without sequelae.

BIBLIOGRAPHY. Orzechowski K: De l'ataxie dysmetrique des yeux: Remarques sur l'ataxie des yeux dite myoclonique (opsoclonie, opsochorie). J Psychol Neurol 35:1–18, 1927
Winkler GF, Baringer JR, Sweeney VP: An acute syndrome of ocular oscillations and truncal ataxia. Trans Am Neurol Assoc 91:96–99, 1966
Cogan DG: Opsoclonus, body tremulousness and benign encephalitis. Arch Ophthalmol 79:545–551, 1968
Carp RI, Loeve A, Wisniewski H (eds): Slow infections of the central nervous system Proc NY Acad Sci 94:34, June, 1993

OSEBOLD-REMONDINI

Synonyms. Brachydactyly type A6; brachymesophalangy mesomelic short limbs; carpal and tarsal abnormalities.

Symptoms and Signs. From birth. Hypoplasia or absence of middle phalanges of all digits (hands and feet). Radial deviation of index fingers. Mesomelic shortening of limbs. Decreased distal joint motion; numbness, dysestesia. Normal intelligence.

Etiology. Autosomal dominant inheritance.

Pathology. Bone: nonspecific disarray of columnization. PAS-positive cytoplasmic inclusions.

Diagnostic Procedures. *X-ray wrist.* Hamate and capitate bones fused; delayed coalescence of bipartite calcanei.

Prognosis. Good. Patient will only reach a short stature.

BIBLIOGRAPHY. Osebold WR, Remondini DS, Lester EL, et al: An autosomal dominant syndrome of short stature with mesomelic shortness of limbs, abnormal carpal and tarsal bones, hypoplastic middle phalanges and bipartite calcanei. Am J Med Genet 22:791–809, 1985
Sheffield LJ, Mayne VM, Danks DM: Osebolt-Remondini syndrome vs chondrodysplasia punctata. Am J Med Genet 28:507, 1987

OSGOOD-SCHLATTER

Synonyms. Schlatter; tibial tubercle osteochondrosis. See Epiphyseal ischemic necrosis.

Symptoms. More common in males. Onset in early adolescence. Pain in the medial area of knee, aggravated by active extension.

Signs. Swelling over tibial tubercle; tenderness on palpation.

Etiology. Epiphyseal ischemic necrosis trauma (see).

Diagnostic Procedures. *X-rays.* Fragmentation of tibial tubercle.

Therapy. Conservative treatment: restriction of activities, cast immobilization for 3–6 weeks. Surgery seldom indicated; if symptoms persist, bone pegs may be inserted into tibial tuberosity.

Prognosis. Conservative treatment frequently successful with spontaneous recovery in a few weeks.

BIBLIOGRAPHY. Osgood RB: Lesions of the tibial tubercle occurring during adolescence. Boston Med Surg J 148:114–117, 1903
Schlatter C: Verletzungen des schnabelförmigen Forsatzes der oberen Tibiaepiphyse. Beitr Klin Chir 38:874–887, 1903
Kujala UM, Kvist M, Heinonen O: Osgood-Schlatter's disease in adolescent athletes: Retrospective study of incidence and duration. Am J Sports Med 13:236–241, 1985
Beighton P: Other heritable and generalized disorders of connective tissue. In Beithon P (ed): McKusick's Heritable Disorders of Connective Tissue, 5th ed, pp 547–548. St Louis, CV Mosby, 1993

OSLER (W.) II

Synonym. Ball-valve gallstone.

Symptoms. Recurrent episodes of colic pain, with typical radiation to back; possibly jaundice.

Etiology. Presence of mobile gallstone in Vater diverticulum periodically obstructing the bile outflow.

Diagnostic Procedures. Cholecystography.

Therapy. Surgery. Lithotripsy; contact dissolution therapy; percutaneous cholecystolithotomy; antispastic medication.

Prognosis. Fair.

BIBLIOGRAPHY. Osler W: The ball-valve gallstone in the common duct. Lancet I:1319–1323, 1897
Malet PF, Rosenberg DJ: Cholelithiasis; gallstone pathogenesis, natural history, biliary pain and nonsurgical therapy. In Haubrich WS, Schaffner F, Berk JE (eds): Bockus Gastroenterology, 5th ed, vol 2, pp 2702–2703. Philadelphia, WB Saunders, 1995

OSMOTIC DEMYELINATION

Synonyms. Hyponatremia rapid correction.

Symptoms and Signs. In patient with severe hyponatremia 3–4 days after effectuation of a rapid correction (<115 mmol/L). Seizures and coma.

Pathology. Central pontine and extrapontine myelinolysis.

Prognosis. High risk of death.

BIBLIOGRAPHY. Sterns RH. Riggs J. Schochet SS: Osmotic demyelination syndrome following correction of hyponatremia. N Engl J Med 314:1535–1542, 1986

Verbalis JG, Martinez AJ: Determinants of brain myelinolysis following correction of chronic hyponatremia in rats. In Jard S, Jamison R (eds): Vasopressin, pp 539–547. Montrouge, France, J. Libbey, 1991

OSTEOARTHRITIS, HYPERTROPHIC, GENERALIZED

Synonyms. Kellgren-Moore. See also Forestier and Oppenheimer (A). Possibly same conditions.

Symptoms. Prevalent in women; onset in middle age. Acute inflammatory phase usually precedes articular symptoms; pain and functional limitation, usually milder than anatomic changes suggest.

Signs. Predilected sites are interphalangeal and carpometacarpal joints of hands; other articulations usually are involved successively.

Etiology. Unknown. Hereditary. Two groups recognized: One has more severe symptoms (associated with Heberden nodes, see); the second is occasionally associated with inflammatory polyarthritis (negative rheumatoid arthritis test).

Pathology. Narrowing of joint spaces; osteophytes.

Diagnostic Procedures. *X-ray.* Facets, arches, and spinous processes of column enlarged ("kissing spines"); molten-wax osteophytes. *Blood.* Sedimentation rate.

Therapy. Physical therapy. Calcium; vitamin D; testosterone derivates; anti-inflammatory agents.

Prognosis. Variable rate of progression toward incapacitation.

BIBLIOGRAPHY. Kellgren JH, Moore R: Some concepts of rheumatic disease. Br Med J 1:1152–1157, 1952

Khan MA: Ankylosing spondylitis clinical features. In Klippel JH, Dieppe PA: Rheumatology, pp 3.25.1–3.25.10. St Louis, CV Mosby, 1994

OSTEOGENESIS IMPERFECTA

Synonyms. Adair-Dighton; Dighton-Adair; Ekman-Lobstein; Eddowes; Hoeve-Dekleyn; Lobstein; Porak-Durante; Spurway; van der Hoeve; Vrolick; blue sclerae—brittle bones—deafness; fragilitas ossiumosteopsathyrosis; OIC; OIT. Four clinical varieties are distinguished.

OI TYPE I

Synonyms. OI tarda; OI with blue sclerae.

Symptoms and Signs. All races affected; time of onset variable. Blue sclerae may be only manifestation. Fractures may or may not occur at a later age, usually from minor traumas. Decrease in fracture incidence after puberty; incidence may increase again after menopause. Short legs (bowing or sequela of fractures); round back; conical thorax; joint hypermobility.

Etiology. Autosomal dominant inheritance. Metabolic defect of collagen causing extreme fragility of bones.

Pathology. Thin cortical layer and trabeculae; normal periosteum and epiphyseal cartilage; metaphysis shows calcified cartilage, which tends to fracture. Normal osteoblasts. Bone fragmentation; fractures and healing, usually with hypertrophic callus.

Diagnostic Procedures. *X-ray.* Thin cortices; long bones have slender shaft widening at epiphyses. *Blood.* Normal calcium; phosphorus alkaline phosphatase may be increased. Coagulation studies: occasionally abnormalities.

Therapy. Calcitonin. Surgical correction of deformities.

OI TYPE IA AND B

Synonyms. OI imperfecta; opalescent teeth; dentinogenesis imperfecta; osteogenesis imperfecta.

Symptoms and Signs. Same as the preceding. Some patients may lack blue sclerae. Opalescent teeth (type IA) or normal teeth (type IB).

Etiology. Autosomal dominant inheritance.

Prognosis. Type IA more severe growth impairment owing to greater occurrence of fractures. Type IB milder.

OI TYPE II

Synonym. OI congenital—perinatal, lethal form.

Symptoms and Signs. All races, both sexes affected. Present from birth (stillborn or short survival). Caput membranaceum (cranium soft and membraneous); extremities short and clumsy; pelvic, spinal, scapular abnormalities; cleft palate; micrognathia; flat face; flail chest; severe respiratory troubles. Fracture liability. Blue sclerae (ocular hallmark of the condition). Embryotoxon and hyperopia are frequent. Cornea may be thinned, leading to keratoconus and megalocornea. Skin thin and translucent; subcutaneous hemorrhages. Deafness. Teeth abnormal: color, amber or bluish.

Etiology. Autosomal dominant. Metabolic defect of collagen: point mutation of amino acids involved in sulfide bonds. Forms with autosomal recessive inheritance have been called Vrolik syndrome.

Prognosis. Death at birth or early age.

OI TYPE III

Synonyms. OI progressively deforming; normal sclerae.

Symptoms and Signs. Sclerae bluish color at birth that normalizes with growth. Progressive deformity of limbs in childhood and of spine in adolescence. Dentinogenesis imperfecta.

Etiology. Autosomal recessive inheritance. Metabolic defect of collagen: altered collagen glycosylation.

Prognosis. Progressive deformity.

OI TYPE IV

See Beighton.

BIBLIOGRAPHY. Ekman OJ: Dissertation Medica. Descriptionem et Casus Aliquot Osteomalaciae Sistens. Uppsala, Sweden, 1788

Lobstein J: De la Fragilité des Os ou l'osteopsathyrose, traite de l'anatomie pathologique. Paris 2:204–212, 1883

Vrolick W: Tabulae ad Illustrandan Embryogenesis Hominis et Mammalium. Tam Naturalem quam Abnormen. Lipsiae, Weigel, 1854

Spurway J: Hereditary tendency to fracture. Br Med J 2:844, 1896

van Der Hoeve J, Kleyn A: Blaue Sclera, Knochenbruchigkeit und Schwerhorigkeit. Arch Ophthalmol 95:81–93, 1918

Patterson CR, McAllion S, Miller R: Heterogeneity of osteogenesis imperfecta type I. J Med Genet 20:203–205, 1983

Cetta G, Ramirez F, Tsipouras P: Third Intern Conf Osteogenesis Imperfecta, New York. Ann NY Acad Sci 543. 1988

Byers PH: Disorders of collagen biosynthesis and structure. In Scriver CR, Beaudet AL, Sly WS, et al: The Metabolic and Molecular Bases of Inherited Disease, 7th ed, pp 4039–4051. New York, McGraw-Hill, 1995

OSTEOGENESIS IMPERFECTA, MICROCEPHALY, CATARACTS

Synonym. Buyse-Bull. See Oosteogenesis imperfecta.

Symptoms and Signs. Both sexes (three sibs). Stillborn or afterbirth. Microcephaly, bilateral cataract, prenatal bone fractures. Blue sclerae.

Etiology. Autosomal dominant inheritance.

Pathology. Short and bowed long bones. Soft calvaria, small and smooth cortex.

BIBLIOGRAPHY. Buyse M, Bull MJ: A syndrome of osteogenesis imperfecta microcephaly and cataracts. Birth Defects Orig Ser 14:6 B:95–98, 1978

OSTEOGLOPHONIC DWARFISM

Synonym. Craniofacial dysostosis; fibrous metaphyseal defects.

Symptoms and Signs. Both sexes. Facies distorted; depression of nasal bridge; frontal bossing; prognathism; craniostenosis; rhizomelic dwarfism; occasionally lumbar lordosis.

Etiology. Autosomal dominant inheritance.

Pathology. Biopsy of lytic lesion. Benign, whorled, fibrous tissue.

Diagnostic Procedures. *X-ray.* Of skeleton. Typical Rx appearance of unusual spondyloepimetaphyseal dysplasia; symmetrical lucent metaphysis defects (osteoglophonic = hollowed out). *Blood.* In some cases reported hypophosphatasia (see).

BIBLIOGRAPHY. Fairbank T: An Atlas of General Affections of the Skeleton, pp 181–183. Baltimore, Williams & Wilkins, 1951
Kelley RI, Borns PF, Nichlas D, et al: Osteoglophonic dwarfism in two generations. J Med Genet 20:436–440, 1983
Beighton P: Osteoglophonic dysplasia. J Med Genet 26:572–576, 1989

OSTEOMESOPYKNOSIS

Synonym. Axial osteosclerosis.

Symptoms and Signs. In adolescents and young adults. Pelvic pain; low back pain; thigh pain; sterility.

Etiology. Autosomal dominant trait.

Pathology. Localized increased density of bones. The lesions are localized to the spine, the pelvis, and the heads of femora. "Ovarian sclerosis" and infertility in one proband.

Diagnostic Procedures. *X-rays. CT scan. MRI.* Of the pelvis, the spine, and the femora. Increased radiodensity with patchy sclerotic lesions.

Therapy. Symptomatic.

Prognosis. Unknown.

BIBLIOGRAPHY. Simon D, Cazalis P, Dryll A, et al: Une osteosclerose axiale de transmission dominante autosomatique: Nouvelle entite? Rev Rheum 46:375–382, 1979
Maroteaux P: L'osteomesopycnose: Une nouvelle affection condensante de transmission dominante autosomique. Arch Fr Pediatr 37:153–157, 1980
Proschek R, Labelle H, Bard C, et al: Osteomesopiknosis. J Bone Joint Surg (Am) 67:652–653, 1985

OSTEOPATHIA STRIATA, CRANIAL STENOSIS

Synonyms. Cranial stenosis; striated bones; hyperostosis generalisata with striations. See Voorhoeve.

Symptoms. Both sexes. Possible prenatal diagnosis. Asymptomatic in 50% of cases. Vague recurrent pains, hearing dificulties, up to deafness; facial nerve palsy. Occasionally mental retardation, premature cataracts, respiratory infections.

Signs. From mild cranial enlargement to macrocephaly, facial abnormalities (with Pierre Robin syndrome). Occasionally scoliosis; spondylolisthesis.

Etiology. Unknown. Autosomal dominant trait.

Diagnostic Procedures. *X-rays.* Typical bone striation (see Voorhoeve) and craniostenosis. *Ultrasound examination.* For prenatal diagnosis.

BIBLIOGRAPHY. Fairbank T: An Atlas of General Affections of the Skeleton, Baltimore, Williams & Wilkins, 1951
Kornreich L, Grunebaum M, Ziv N, et al: Osteopathia striata, cranial sclerosis with cleft palate and facial nerve palsy. Eur J Pediatr 147:101–103, 1988

OSTEOPATHIA STRIATA, PIGMENTARY DERMOPATHY

Synonyms. See Voorhoeve.

Symptoms and Signs. In females. From birth. Macular, hyperpigmented dermopathy including white forelock.

Etiology. Unknown. Consistent with X-linked inheritance.

Diagnostic Procedures. *X-rays.* Typical osteopathia striata (see Voorhoeve).

BIBLIOGRAPHY. Whyte MP, Murphy WA: Osteopathia striata associated with familial dermopathy and white forelock: Evidence for postnatal development of osteopathia striata. Ann J Genet 5:227–234, 1980

OSTEOPOROSIS, PSEUDOGLIOMA

Symptoms and Signs. Appears to be more frequent in Mediterranean area. Those of osteogenesis imperfecta (see) plus bilateral retinoblastoma manifesting after a few weeks of life. Muscular hypotonia; ligaments laxity. Intelligence normal in most cases. Occasionally, congenital heart disease.

Etiology. Autosomal recessive inheritance.

Pathology. Retinal pseudoglioma.

Therapy. Eye enucleation after irradiation. Calcitonin.

BIBLIOGRAPHY. Bianchine JW, Murdoch JL: Juvenile osteoporosis in a boy with bilateral enucleation of the eyes for pseudoglioma. Birth Defects Orig Art Ser V (4):225–226, 1969
Somer H, Palotie A, Somer M, et al: Osteoporosis-pseudoglioma syndrome: Clinical, morphological and biochemical studies. J Med Genet 25:543–549, 1988

OSTERTAG

Synonyms. Amyloid nephropathy hereditary; Amyloidosis familial visceral; amyloidosis VIII; German amyloidosis.

Symptoms and Signs. Both sexes affected; age of onset variable. Arterial hypertension; marked hepatosplenomegaly; hematuria; pitting edema (clinical impression of nephritis or nephrosis).

Etiology. Unknown. Possibly, autosomal dominant inheritance.

Pathology. Widespread amyloidosis, most striking in the kidneys.

Diagnostic Procedures. *Blood. Urine.* Evidence of nephropathy. *Biopsy.* Congo red test.

Therapy. Hemodialysis. Kidney transplantation.

Prognosis. That of chronic renal failure.

BIBLIOGRAPHY. Ostertag B: Demonstration einer eigenartigen familiaren paramyloidose. Zbl Path 56:253–254, 1932
Ostertag B: Familiäre Amyloid-Erkrankung. Z Menschl Vererb Konstit-Lehre 30:105–115, 1950
Libbey CA, Talbert ML: A 43-year-old woman with hepatic failure after renal transplantation because of amyloidosis. N Engl J Med 317:1520–1531, 1987

OSUNTOKUN

Synonyms. Pain indifference; deafness; deafness—analgesia congenita.

Symptoms and Signs. Brother and half sister with different father. Analgesia congenital (see Biemond I) and deafness.

Etiology. Unknown.

BIBLIOGRAPHY. Osuntokun BO, Odeku EL, Luzzatto L: Congenital pain asymbolia and auditory imperception. J Neurosurg Psychiatr 31:291–296, 1968

OTA

Synonyms. Nevus fuscoceruleus—ophthalmomaxillaris; oculodermal melanocytosis.

Symptoms. Frequent in Japanese, rarer in Caucasians and blacks; onset in childhood. Asymptomatic.

Signs. Bluish pigmented spots in the periorbital area and of sclera; may extend to include cheeks, forehead, scalp, nose, and ears (seldom, the trunk). Not always unilateral.

Etiology. Unknown.

Pathology. See Mongolian spot. Area affected usually that of first and second division of trigeminal (V) nerve.

Diagnostic Procedures. *Biopsy.*

Therapy. Cosmetics. Carbon dioxide snow may lighten the pigmentation.

Prognosis. Lesions may become confluent in some areas; they usually become darker with time and persist in adult life.

BIBLIOGRAPHY. Ota M: Nevus, fusco-coeruleus ophthalmomaxillaris. Tokyo Med J 63:143–145, 1939
Grossniklaus HE, Green WR: Uveal tumors. In Garner A, Klintworth GK (eds): Pathobiology of Ocular Disease: A Dynamic Approach, 2nd ed, p 1425. New York, Marcel Dekker, 1994

OTHELLO

Synonyms. Erotic jealousy; psychotic jealousy; sexual jealousy; paranoia, conjugal.

Symptoms. Both sexes may be affected. Apparently prevalent in men; sudden onset. Minor symptoms of a few months of suspicion. Onset usually in fourth decade. Delusion of infidelity of sexual partner; accusation on the basis of a particular episode that allegedly proves the fact, misinterpretation, and distortion of past episodes. Meticulous and obsessive search for proof. Continuous repeated interrogations to obtain confession. Increased sexual activity; if rejected, interpreted as proof of infidelity, avoids partner to seek certain proof. Irritability, tension, and depression distracting from proper performance of job. Frequently explosion of violence, particularly against spouse.

Etiology. Unknown. Pure form is a special variety of paranoia. It may be a feature of maniac depressive psychosis, epilepsy, alcoholism.

Therapy and Prognosis. If part of psychosis, follows evolution of basic condition. If pure form, long lasting, often persisting, and resistant to therapy.

BIBLIOGRAPHY. Todd J, Dewhurst K: Othello syndrome: A study in psychopathology of sexual jealousy. J Nerv Ment Dis 122:367–374, 1955
Kaplan HI, Sadock BJ: Comprehensive Textbook of Psychiatry, 6th ed, p 169. Baltimore, Williams & Wilkins, 1995

OTTO-CHROBAK

Synonyms. Otto pelvis; sunken acetabulum; acetabular protrusion; arthrokatadysis.

Symptoms. Onset in pubertal period or later. Progressive and frequently bilateral loss of hip joint movement without pain.

Signs. Deformity on hip flexion and abduction.

Etiology. Unknown. Degenerative condition. Usually, congenital defect and familial occurrence.

Diagnostic Procedures. *X-ray.* Acetabulum assumes a spherical form, completely surounding the femoral head; thinning of acetabulum floor, which appears displaced medially and bulges into pelvis.

Therapy. None for basic defect. Orthopedic treatment of secondary osteoarthropathy.

Prognosis. Osteoarthropathic changes during adult life.

BIBLIOGRAPHY. Sokoowsky A, Kopera Z: Przypadek pierwotnego wgobiemia panewki stawn biodrowego (protrusio acetabuli primaria Otto-Chrobak) viekn modocianym. Post Reum Warszava 3:140–145, 1957
Richardson EG. Miscellaneous non traumatic disorders. In Crenshaw AH (ed): Campbell's Operative Orthopedics, 7th ed, pp 1060, 1361, 1363. St Louis, CV Mosby, 1987

OUCH-OUCH

Synonyms. Itai-itai byo, cadmium intoxication.

Symptoms and Signs. Endemic in the Jinzu river basin of the Toyama prefecture in Japan. Typical patients: middle age postmenopausal, multiparous woman with lombar pains, leg myalgia, duck-like gait. Pressure on bone elicits pain.

Etiology. Cadmium contamination of soil and water.

Pathology. Osteomalacia. Kidney: contracted tubular atrophy and dilation eosinophilic casts, interstitial fibrosis normal glomeruli.

Diagnostic Procedures. *X-ray.* Pseudofractures and typical osteomalacia findings. *Urine.* Proteinuria and glycosuria, aminoaciduria, decreased tubular reabsorption of phosphorus, low phenolsulfonphtalein excretion, decreased urine concentration ability.

Therapy. Chelating agents: meso-2,3-dimercaptosuccinic acid.

Prognosis. Progressive condition, seldom renal failure.

BIBLIOGRAPHY. Mason HJ, Davison AG, Wright AL, et al: Relations between liver cadmium, cumulative exposure, and renal function in cadmium alloy workers. Br J Ind Med 45:793–802, 1988

OUDTSHOORN* SKIN

Synonym. Keratolytic winter erythema.

Symptoms and Signs. In South Afrikaaners. Onset from infancy to early adulthood. Manifest in cold weather. Intermittent and recurrent

---

*Name of South Africa province.

redness with centrifugal peeling of palms and soles. In severe cases extension to all body.

Etiology. Unknown. Autosomal dominant inheritance.

Prognosis. Tendency to subside after age 30.

BIBLIOGRAPHY. Findley GH, Nurse GT, Heyl T, et al: Keratolytic winter erythema of "Oudtshoon skin": A newly recognized inherited dermatosis prevalent in South Africa. S Afric Med J 52:871–874, 1977

OVARIAN FAILURE, PREMATURE

Synonyms. Premature menopause; premature familial ovarian failure included, resistant ovary syndrome included.

Symptoms and Signs. Onset of menopause before 40 years of age.

Etiology. Various causes may determine the syndrome: (1) idiopathic; (2) antiovarian or antireceptor antibodies; (3) viral infections (mumps) (4) cytotoxic drugs; (5) radiation; (6) familial cases owing to partial deletion of long arm of X chromosome (Xq 26–27).

Diagnostic Procedures. *Blood.* High gonadotropin levels. Genetic analysis and chromosome mapping (DNA hybridization techniques).

Therapy. Replacement therapy with cyclical estrogen and progesteron.

Prognosis. Usually final cessation of reproduction.

BIBLIOGRAPHY. Board JA, Redwine FO, Moncure CW, et al: Identification of differing etiologies of clinically diagnosed premature menopause. Am J Obstet Gynecol 134:936–944, 1979
Krauss CM, Nurant Turksoy R, Atkins L, et al: Familial premature ovarian failure due to an interstitial deletion of the long arm of the X chromosome. N Engl J Med 317:125–131, 1987
Baird DT: Amenorrhea, anovulation, and dysfunctional uterine bleeding. In De Groot LJ (ed): Endocrinology, 3rd ed, p 2064. Philadelphia, WB Saunders, 1995

OVARIAN HYPERSTIMULATION

Synonym. Meigs secondary; OHSS.

Symptoms. Occurs in patients who undergoes ovulation induction for treating amenorrhea and infertility. Weight gain (good indicator of severity of syndrome). Nausea, abdominal pain and distension; acute abdominal crisis (paralytic ileus); tachycardia; oliguria; hematuria; chest pain; dyspnea; increased blood pressure. Occasionally venous thrombosis.

Signs. Ascites; marked ovarian enlargement (very gentle examination for risk of rupture—vaginal examination contraindicated); hydrothorax; ascites.

Etiology. Grossly exaggerated angiogenic response to the administration of human menopausal gonadotropins, clomiphene; human chorionic gonadotropins; follicle stimulating hormone or luteinizing hormone.

Pathology. Ovarian enlargement, necrosis. Ascites; hydrothorax; in some cases; intra-abdominal hemorrhages.

Diagnostic Procedures. *Blood. Urine.* Monitoring of serum estradiol. *Electrolytes.* Hyponatremia, hyperkalemia, and acidosis. Nonprotein nitrogen; increased coagulation. *ECG. X-ray. CT scan. Ultrasound.*

Therapy. Discontinuation of administration of drug; rest; fluid (crystalloid and colloids—do not overinfuse) therapy; potassium exchange resin, mannitol or aspiration of thoracic fluids and in some cases interruption of pregnancy may be necessary. If surgery necessary, wedge resection indicated rather than castration, except in uncontrollable hemorrhage.

Prognosis. Generally good. Cases of death reported.

BIBLIOGRAPHY. Vandiest L, DeBast A: Syndrome adbominal aigü par dégénérescence kystique massive et totale des ovaires due a l'administration des gonadotrophines. Brux Med 38:1636–1642, 1958
Neuwirth RS, Turksoy RN, Vande Wiele RL: Acute Meig's syndrome secondary to ovarian stimulation with human menopausal gonadotropins. Am J Obstet Gynecol 91:977–981, 1965
Editorial: Ovarian hyperstimulation syndrome. Lancet 338:1111–1112, 1991

OVARIAN HYPERTHECOSIS

Symptoms and Signs. Amenorrhea; infertility; hirsutism; virilism occasionally noted.

Etiology. Unknown. Regarded as one form of Stein-Leventhal (see) (severe form).

Pathology. Endometrial hyperplasia. Ovaries are enlarged and firm with nests of theca-lutein cells in stroma and hyperthecosis. Differential diagnosis: Stein-Leventhal syndrome; differentiation possible only on the basis of the microscopic findings. Adrenal tumor and masculinizing ovarian tumor.

Diagnostic Procedures. *Blood.* Levels of androgen higher in Stein-Leventhal.

Therapy. Wedge resection of ovaries; clomiphene citrate.

Prognosis. Good.

BIBLIOGRAPHY. Givens JR, Niser WL, Coleman SA, et al: Familial ovarian hyperthecosis: A study of two families. Am J Obstet Gynec 110:959–972, 1971
Scully RE: Ovarian tumors with endocrine manifestations. In De Groot LJ (ed): Endocrinology, 3rd ed, p 2124. Philadelphia, WB Saunders, 1995

OVARIAN VEIN

Existence discussed.

Synonyms. Included, postpartum thrombophlebitis of ovarian vein.

Symptoms and Signs. Onset in second or third decade. Rarely observed in nulliparous women; primarily occurring or beginning during pregnancy. Periodic pain in the flank on the right side and right lower quadrant, which appears several days before onset of menstruation and disappears after 1 or 2 days of menstruation. Infection of urinary tract and administration of progesterone aggravate the symptoms.

Etiology. Related to hydronephrosis and pyelonephritis of pregnancy; extension of this condition. May result from repeated frequent pregnancies, use of oral contraceptives, and increased vascularity from gynecologic disorders, causing incompetence of ovarian vein valves. May also be caused by thrombophlebitis (postpartum) of the ovarian vein (1/600 deliveries); which case, however, represents a more serious condition because of the possible extension to the vena cava; this specific condition has been attributed to coagulation defects during pregnancy.

Pathology. Right ovarian vein is larger than the left one, and dilatation and incompetence of valves occur during pregnancy and may persist in multiparas. Connective tissue sheath is thickened with adherence of vein and ureter, where the iliac vessels are crossed. The wall of the vein is thick, its muscle hypertrophic.

Diagnostic Procedures. *Excretory urography.* Right side abnormalities; mild to moderate calicectasis; pyelectasis; ureterectasis; upper portion of ureter dilated; tortuous middle portion lateral deviation; junction of middle pelvic portion medial deviation. *Cystoscopy.* Negative. Right retrograde urography. Normal pelvic ureter; poor filling at iliac vessels crossing; in the middle portion, minor deformities; in the proximal portion, irregular extrinsic deformities. *Pelvic phlebography.* Evidence of closeness of right ovarian vein and ureter. *Echography. CT scan. MRI.*

Therapy. Prolonged medical treatment for urinary tract infection. In case of failure with persistence of infection and signs of progressive obstructive changes, excision of ovarian vein and arteriolysis (excision of vein does not prevent pregnancy).

Prognosis. Good. If medical treatment fails, surgery succeeds in 75% of cases. In case of postpartum phlebitis of ovarian vein potentially lethal from pulmonary embolism.

BIBLIOGRAPHY. Clark JC: The right ovarian vein syndrome. In Emmitt JL: Clinical Urography, 2nd ed, pp 1227–1236. Philadelphia, WB Saunders, 1964

Dykhuizen RF, Roberts JA: The ovarian vein syndrome. Surg Gynecol Obstet 130:443–452, 1970

Melnick RG, Bromwit DM: Bilateral ovarian vein syndrome. AM J Roentegenol Radim Ther Nucl Med 113:503, 1971

Dure-Smith P: Ovarian vein syndrome: It is a myth? Urology 13:355, 1979

Baran GW, Frisch KM: Duplex Doppler evaluation of puerperal ovarian vein thrombosis. AJR 149:321, 1987

OVERLAP

Synonym. Sharp; mixed connective tissue disease, MCTD.

Symptoms and Signs. Prevalent in females; onset in adolescence or early adulthood (median age of onset 10 years). Presenting symptoms tenosynovitis, and polyarthritis, then symptoms and signs of scleroderma (see Morvan) combined with those of lupus erythematosus systemic (SLE, see). Observed in about 10% of patients with scleroderma. Other overlapping conditions are mitral valve prolapse; SLE and rheumatoid arthritis; scleroderma and Sjogren (see); scleroderma and Hashimoto (see); and scleroderma and hypoglobulinemic syndromes.

Etiology. Autoimmune conditions. A phenotype continuum autosomal dominant in some cases. Controversial entity.

Diagnostic Procedures. *Blood.* Extractable nuclear antigen (ENA) that contains ribonucleoproteins and is associated with a speckled pattern of antinuclear antibodies (ANA). *X-ray. Bones:* Osteoporosis, joint derangement (narrowing, erosion, ankylosis, subluxation necrosis), penciling of phalangeal tips. *Intestine:* Esophageal dysfunction, gastric reflux. *Lungs:* Pleural thickening, ilar adenopathy.

Therapy. Corticosteroid and nonsteroidal anti-inflammatory agents.

Prognosis. Usually good. Six years after onset, mortality 6%. Majority of patients develop scleroderma.

BIBLIOGRAPHY. Bianchi FA, Bistue AR, Wendt VE, et al: Analysis of 27 cases of progressive systemic sclerosis and a review of literature. J Chron Dis 19:953–977, 1966

Sharp GC, Irvin WS, Tan EM, et al: Mixed connective tissue disease: An apparently distinct rheumatic disease syndrome associateed with specific antibody to an extractable nuclear antigen (ENA). Am J Med 52:148–159, 1972

Allen RC, St Cyr C, Maddison PJ, et al: Overlap connective tissue syndromes. Arch Dis Childhood 61:284–288, 1986

Glesby MJ, Pyeritz RE: Association of mitral valve prolapse and systemic abnormalities of connective tissue: A phenotypic continuum. JAMA 262:523–528, 1989

Maddison PJ: Mixed connective tissue disease, overlap syndromes, and eosinophilic fasciitis. Ann Rheum Dis 50:887–893, 1991

OVERSUPPRESSION

Synonyms. Contraceptive amenorrhea; anovulation following oral contraceptive; postcontraceptive anovulation. Postpill amenorrhea.

Symptoms and Signs. Amenorrhea of 3 months or longer, or marked irregularity of menstrual cycles, and infertility following discontinuation of oral contraceptive therapy, sometimes with galactorrhea.

Etiology. Suspected dysfunction of hypothalamic centers concerned with gonadotropin release.

Diagnostic Procedures. Determination of follicle-stimulating hormone (FSH), luteinizing hormone (LH), and estrogen levels, and prolactin level (if elevated, a pituitary prolactinoma may be present).

Therapy. Usually, recovery without treatment. Bromocriptine (Parlodel) if elevated level of prolactin; otherwise clomiphene (Clomid).

Prognosis. Good response to treatment.

BIBLIOGRAPHY. Whitelow MJ, Nola VF, Kalman CF: Irregular menses, amenorrhea, and infertility following synthetic progestational agents. JAMA 195:780–782, 1966

Horowitz BJ, Solomkin M, Edelstein SW: The oversuppression syndrome. Obstet Gynecol 31:387–389, 1968

Mishell DR: Contraception. In De Groot LJ (ed): Endocrinology, 3rd ed, pp 2144–2155. Philadelphia, WB Saunders, 1995

OWREN

Synonyms. Factor V deficiency; labile factor deficiency; parahemophilia; proaccelerin deficiency. See Prothrombin deficiency syndromes.

Symptoms and Signs. Both sexes; great variability in time of onset and severity. Symptoms similar to those of hemophilia with the exception of the lack of hemarthrosis. Menorrhagia usually serious problem. Postpartum bleeding a few days after delivery. In heterozygous relatives, only epistaxis or minor manifestations.

Etiology. Absence of proaccelerin in the plasma. Autosomal recessive inheritance; autosomal dominant inheritance also suggested. Also acquired form.

Diagnostic Procedures. *Prothrombin time.* Prolonged; corrected by fresh plasma deprived of vitamin K-dependent clotting factors; not corrected by proaccelerin-poor plasma (stored or oxalated). Thromboplastin generation usually abnormal. Other coagulation tests. May be abnormal.

Therapy. Fresh plasma or fresh frozen plasma. Vitamin K ineffective.

Prognosis. Good, but death from bleeding may occur.

BIBLIOGRAPHY. Owren PA: The coagulation of blood: Investigations of a new clotting factor. Acta Med Scand (Suppl 194) 128:1–327, 1947

Friedman IA, Quick AJ, Higgins F, et al: Hereditary labile factor (factor V) deficiency. JAMA 175:370–374, 1961

Bithell TC: Hereditary coagulation disorders. In Lee GR, Bithel TC, Foerster J, et al (eds): Wintrobe's Clinical Hematology, 9th ed, p 1443. Philadelphia, Lea & Febiger, 1993

5-OXOPROLINASE DEFICIENCY

Synonyms. Oxoprolinuria owing to oxoprolinase deficiency.

Symptoms and Signs. Starting in infancy vomiting, diarrhea, abdominal pain, kidney colics, absence of neurologica symptoms and hemolysis.

Etiology. Autosomal recessive inheritance. Deficiency of oxoprolinase.

Diagnostic Procedures. *Urine.* Excessive excretion of 5-oxo-L-proline. *Blood.* Glutathione synthetase activities of erythrocytes, leukocytes, and cultured skin fibroblasts normal. Cultured skin fibroblasts show low level of 5-oxoprolinase. *X-rays.* Urinary stones (oxalate and carbonate).

BIBLIOGRAPHY. Larsson A, Mattsson B, Wauters EAK, et al: 5-Oxoprolinuria due to hereditary 5-oxoprolinase deficieny in two brothers: A new inborn error on gamma-glutamyl cycle. Acta Paediat Scand 70:301–308, 1981

Meister A, Larsson A: Glutathione synthetase deficiency and other disorders of the glutamyl cycle. In Scriver CR, Beaudet AL, Sly WS, et al: The Metabolic and Molecular Bases of Inherited Disease, pp 1472–1473. New York, McGraw-Hill, 1995

5-OXOPROLINURIA

Synonyms. Jellum; pyroglutamic aciduria, glutathione synthetase deficiency.

Symptoms and Signs. From childhood: mental retardation, epileptic seizures, spasticity, cerebellar lesion; IQ 60; hemolysis.

Etiology. Autosomal recessive. Deficiency glutamylcysteine synthetase that mediates glutathione synthesis.

Diagnostic Procedures. *Urine.* Elevated amount of 5-oxoproline. *Blood.* Metabolic acidosis, hemolysis; red cells contain none or less than 2% of glutathione synthetase; neutropenia.

Therapy. Still experimental with inhibitors of glutamyl transpeptidase; vitamin E increases red cell survival and ameliorates neutropenia.

Prognosis. Mental retardation in some cases. Otherwise good.

BIBLIOGRAPHY. Jellum E, Kluge T, Borresen HC, et al: Pyroglutamic aciduria: A new inborn error of metabolism. Scand J Clin Lab Invest 26:327–335, 1970
Robertson PL, Buchanan DN, Muenzer J: 5-Oxoprolinuria in an adolescent with chronic metabolic acidosis, mental retardation and psychosis. J Pediat 118:92–95, 1991
Tanaka KR, Paglia DE: Pyruvate kinase and other enzymopathies of the erythrocyte. In Scriver CR, Beaudet AL, Sly WS, et al: The Metabolic and Molecular Bases of Inherited Disease, 7th ed, p 3499. New York, McGraw-Hill, 1995

OXPHOS SYNDROMES

Synonyms. Oxydative phosphorylation.

Large group that includes an high number of syndromes subdivided according to clinical and biochemical criteria that do not provide completely satisfactory definitions since seldom individuals exhibit complete phenotype. Classification of the historical individual syndromes according to molecular genetic criteria into four genetic subgroups has proved to be more useful.

CLASS I MUTATIONS: DISORDERS OF THE NUCLEAR OXPHOS GENES

Mitochondrial myopathy, benign, infantile (see)
Mitochondrial myopathy, lethal infantile (see)
Mitochondrial myopathy-cardiomyopathy, benign, infantile (see)
Barth (see)
Kearns-Sayre (see) and
Ophthalmoplegia chronic progressive external (see)
    (a) autosomal dominant
    (b) autosomal recessive
Myoglobinuria, exertional, inherited (see Rhabdomyolysis exertional)
Leight (see)
Mitochondrial myopathy (see)

CLASS II MUTATIONS: mtDNA POINT MUTATIONS

Leber (optic neuropathy) (see) and clinical variants or associations
MERRF (see)
MELAS (see)
Hypertrophic cardiomyopathy-myopathy
    (a) infantile
    (b) adult

Mytochondrial myopathy (see)
Pigmentary retinopathy-neurodegeneration
Leight (see)
Alzheimer (see)
Parkinson (see)
Maternal inherited sensorineural deafness (see)

CLASS III mtDNA DELATIONS AND DUPLICATIONS

Kearns-Sayre (see) due to mt DNA delation
Ophthalmoplegia chronic, progressive external due to mt DNA delation
Kearns-Sayre (see) due to mt DNA duplication
Ophthalmoplegia chronic, progressive external owing to mtDNA duplication
Pearson (see)
Diabetes mellitus–deafness (see)
Malignant migraine (see)

CLASS IV DISORDERS OF UNKNOWN INHERITANCE

Alpers (see)
Lethal infantile cardiomyopathy
Dystonia, idiopathic, mitochondrial myopathy (see Ziehen-Oppenheim)
M.N.G.I.E. (see)
Ernster-Luft (see)

Etiology. Derangements of *oxydative phosphorylation*; metabolic process, mediated by 5-tintramitochondrial different enzyme complexes (see complex syndromes), and whose assembly and maintenance requires coordinated regulation of nuclear DNA and mitochondrial DNA (mtDNA) genes.

Therapy. Attempts for metabolic management of this eterogeneous group of conditions have been made, and occasional positive therapeutic effects (however, of difficult assessment) reported. Drugs used include coenzyme Q10, phylloquinone, menadione, succinate, ascorbate, and riboflavin.

BIBLIOGRAPHY. Ernster L, Ikkos D, Luft R: Enzymic activities of human skeletal muscle mitochondria: A tool in clinical metabolic research. Nature 184:1851–1854, 1959
Luft R, Ikkos D, Palmieri G, et al: A case of severe hypermetabolism of nonthyroid origin with a defect in the maintenance of mitochondrial respiratory control. J Clin Invest 41:1776–1804, 1962
Shoffner JM, Wallace DC: Oxidative phosphorylation diseases. In Scriver CR, Beaudet AL, Sly WS, et al: The Metabolic and Molecular Bases of Inherited Disease, pp 1535–1609. New York, McGraw-Hill, 1995

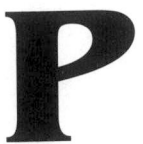

P

PACEMAKER

Symptoms and Signs. In one fifth of patients with well-functioning pacemakers. Dizzy spells, syncope, breathlessness, impaired exercise capacity, postural hypotension. Palpable liver pulsations and common waves in jugular venous pulse.

Etiology. Atrial contraction stimulated by pacemaker occurring during ventricular systole. Atria contract against closed valves producing raised pressure and reduced cardiac output and blood pressure. Occurs when retrograde AV conduction is intact.

Diagnostic Procedure. *Ventricular pacing. Observation of symptoms and signs.*

Therapy. Dual-chamber pacing or reprogramming ventricular pacemaker. Antiarrhythmics: flecainide and dysopyramide.

Prognosis. Good with therapy.

BIBLIOGRAPHY. Alicardi C, Fonad FM, Tarazi RC, et al: Three cases of hypotension and syncope with ventricular pacing: Possible role of atrial reflexes. Am J Cardiol 42:136–142, 1978
Kenny RA, Sutton R: Pacemaker syndrome. Br J Med 293:902–903, 1986
Mond HG: Permanent cardiac pacemakers: Techniques of implantation, testing and surveillance. In Schlant RC, Alexander RW, et al: Hurst's The Heart, 8th ed, pp 437–439. New York, McGraw-Hill, 1994

PACEMAKER-TWIDDLER

Caused by repeated turning of implanted pulse generator under the skin in case of lead retraction from endocardium.

BIBLIOGRAPHY. Mond HG: The Cardiac Pacemaker: Function and Malfunction. New York, Grune and Stratton, 1983
Mond HG: Permanent cardiac pacemakers: Techniques of implantation, testing and surveillance. In Schlant RC, Alexander RW, et al: Hurst's The Heart, 8th ed, pp 437–438. New York, McGraw-Hill, 1994

PACHYDERMOPERIOSTOSIS, SECONDARY

Synonyms. Simond (A); Brugsch; Leva. See also Touraine-Solente-Golé (primary condition).

Symptoms. Reported in many races. Prevalent in males aged 30–70; in females milder symptoms, onset after puberty. Low working capacity.

Signs. Face and scalp skin thickens and folds (expression of despair); increased sebaceous secretion. Hand and foot skin thickens but does not fold and presents hyperhidrosis. Bones of limbs, fingers, and toes thicken, determing cylindrical deformation of fingers and clubbing of toes. Hands and feet remain small (main differential sign). Joint effusions. Occasionally; decrease of facial and pubic hair, gynecomastia.

Etiology. Autosomal dominant inheritance of variable expressivity (sex-influenced) and/or recessive. Usually induced by pulmonary disease, bronchial, bronchiectasis, lung abscess, pleural mesotelioma, seldom by stomach esophagus, or thymus carcinoma, adenocarcinoma.

Pathology. *Skin.* Hypertrophy of connective tissue of epidermis and appendages. *Bones.* Proliferative periostitis with irregular periosteal ossification. Ligaments, tendons, and membranes may ossify.

Diagnostic Procedures. *Blood.* Hyponatremia. *X-rays.* Of skeleton. (See Pathology.) *Endocrine studies.* Normal.

Therapy. Symptomatic. Treatment of primary disease.

Prognosis. Normal life expectancy. Irreversible condition, which, once started, progresses for 5–10 years and then stabilizes. Treatment of primary disease induces regression of skin changes.

BIBLIOGRAPHY. Fredreich N: Hyperostose des gesammten Skelettes. Arch Pathol Anat 43:83–87, 1868
Leva J: Ueber familiare Ackromegalia. Med Klin 11:1266–1268, 1915
Simond's A: Familiare Trommelschlaegelbildung und Knochenhypertrophy. Dtsch Z Nezvenheilk 59:301–321, 1918
Brugsch T: Akromikrie oder Dystrophia osteogenitalis. Med Klin 23:81–82, 1927
Matucci-Cerinic M, Cinti S, Morroni M, et al: Pachydermoperiostosis (primary hypertrophic osteoarthropathy): Report of a case with evidence of endothelial and connective tissue involvement. Ann Rheum Dis 48:240–246, 1989
Harper J: Genetics and genodermatoses. In Champion RH, Burton JL, Ebling FJG (eds): Rook/Wilkinson/Ebling Textbook of Dermatology, 5th ed, pp 362–364. Oxford, Blackwell Scientific, 1992

PACKARD-WECHSEL

Rare eponym used to designate chronic adrenal insufficiency of adult type. See Addisonian syndromes.

PADDED DASH

Synonyms. Larynx–trachea trauma; tracheolaryngeal trauma.

Symptoms. Occurs in passengers involved in car accidents. Seat belt may increase chance of occurrence of this type of lesion. Respiratory distress caused by obstruction of airway; aspiration of saliva, fluid, or solid into airway; hoarseness; pain on swallowing. Neck may appear normal. Presence of subcutaneous emphysema; free cartilage in severe injury. Multiple lacerations of forehead and midface frequently encountered.

Etiology. During crash, forehead strikes windshield, causing hyperextension of neck and exposing anterior neck to trauma from collision with dashboard and injuring laryngotracheal structures.

Pathology. In female (because of longer neck) lesion more frequently supraglottic; in men subglottic. Hematomas; fracture of cartilage; mucosal lacerations.

Diagnostic Procedures. *Laryngoscopy. X-ray.*

Therapy. Maintainance of respiratory exchange (positive-pressure breathing equipment) until tracheostomy may be performed. Conservative treatment in some cases. Surgical exploration, however, frequently indicated.

Prognosis. Asphyxia is cause of death if early treatment not instituted.

BIBLIOGRAPHY. Butler RM, Moser FH: The padded dash syndrome: Blunt trauma to the larynx and trachea. Laryngoscope 78:1172–1182, 1968
Delany HN, Berlin AW: Multiple injuries. In Tinker J, Rapin M (eds): Care of the Critically Ill Patient, p 611. Berlin, Springer-Verlag, 1983

PAGE

Synonyms. Hypertensive diencephalic; mental sweating.

Symptoms. Prevalent in young or middle-aged women, occasionally in men. Onset without any cause or brought on by embarrassment and excitement. Periodic appearance of blotchy flushes covered by small beads of perspiration in the face, upper chest, and seldom, abdomen. Extremities during attack are cold, pale, and show a dusky mottled hue. Watery lacrimation without emotional causes or changes. Headache, tachycardia, and abdominal hyperperistalsis. Emotional polyuria; deep sighing respiration.

Signs. Lability of blood pressure; elevation during attacks. Occasionally presence of low-grade fever.

Etiology. Unknown. Hypothalamic disturbance. A similar syndrome is observed in some patients with tumor compressing hypothalamus (see Penfield).

Pathology. Vascular disease secondary to hypertension minimal in these cases.

Diagnostic Procedure. Injection of 0.25 mg of histamine base intradermally precipitates the attack.

Therapy. Sedatives: reserpine. Topical: ionophoresis. Medical: atropine-like drugs, probanthine, sedatives, tranquilizers, psychiatric treatment. Sympathectomy (in refractory cases).

Prognosis. Relatively benign course with usual minimal complications of essential hypertension (vascular, renal). After sympathectomy the manifestation of syndrome disappears, and may not further be induced by the injection of histamine, but may relapse after few years.

BIBLIOGRAPHY. Page IH: A syndrome simulating diencephalic stimulation occurring in patients with essential hypertension. Am J Med Sci 190:9–14, 1935

Schroeder HA, Goldman ML: Test for the presence of the "hypertensive diencephalic syndrome" using histamine. Am J Med 6:162–167, 1949

Last CG, Hersen M (eds): Handbook of Anxiety Disorders. Elmsford, NY: Pergamon, 1988

PAGET I

Symptoms. Occurs in women 50–60 years of age (breast), in elderly men and women (extramammary), or in men (scrotum). Burning sensation, itching, soreness of the affected area (nipple or apocrine gland areas of genital, perigenital, and axillary areas); scratching lesions.

Signs. In nipple, fissured areola, ulceration, oozing, hyperemia; retraction. Other areas: in acute stage moist erythema; then eczema-like lesion; then denudation and crusting.

Etiology. Unknown. Relationship to or, possibly, extension of carcinoma of mammary duct or ducts of apocrine sweat gland; manifestation of internal malignancy.

Pathology. *Breast.* Intraductal proliferation; paste-like plugs of material; invasion by typical Paget's cells. *Other areas.* Invasion by Paget's cells of skin and apocrine glands.

Diagnostic Procedure. *Biopsy.*

Therapy. Surgery advised in all conditions.

Prognosis. Slow progression. Treatment helpful.

BIBLIOGRAPHY. Paget J: On diseases of the mammary areola preceding cancer of the mammary gland. St Bartholomew Hosp Rep 10:87–89, 1874

Helwig EB, Graham FN: Anogenital (extramammary Paget's disease). Cancer 16:387–404, 1963

Lagios MD, Westdahl PR, Rose MR, et al: Paget's disease of the nipple: Alternative management in cases without or with minimal extent of underlying breast carcinoma. Cancer 54:545–551, 1984

Bulens P, Vanujtsel L, Rijnders A: Breast conservative treatment of Paget's disease. Radiother Oncol 17:305–309, 1990

PAGET II

Synonyms. Pozzi hyperphosphatasemia congenital; hyperostosis corticalis deformans; osteitis deformans.

Symptoms. More frequent in men, but more severe in women; insidious onset after 40 years of age. Frequently asymptomatic. Headache; deep, dull, constant pain in one knee; deafness; waddling gait.

Signs. Enlarged cranial vault; bowing deformities of bones subjected to greater stress (arms, legs); flattening of vertebrae; broadening of pelvis; shortening of stature; kyphosis.

Etiology. Unknown. Possibly, hereditary condition of autosomal dominant type; slow virus infection has been proposed as well (possibly via goat milk).

Pathology. Increased circulation in bones affected, with reabsorption of bone and replacement with osteoid matrix, and fibrotic changes, disorganization of trabeculae. Frequent presence of inclusions in the osteoclasts nuclei of the stacked rows or complex filaments arranged in paracrystalline fashion (paramyxovirus?). Frequently, development of osteogenic sarcoma.

Diagnostic Procedures. *Blood.* Hyperphosphatemia and marked increase of alkaline phosphatase; hypercalcemia; hypercalciuria. *X-ray. CT scan. MRI.* See Pathology. Typical mosaic pattern. *Urine.* Elevated excretion of hydroxyproline peptides. Calcium exchange, marked increase.

Therapy. High calcium phosphate intake. Anabolic steroids; corticosteroids (if cardiac failure or hypercalcemia). With immobilized patients, low calcium and phosphate diet, increased fluids, edetate (EDTA), corticosteroids, or sodium phytate for hypercalcemia, sodium etidronate (5 mg/kg/day), calcitonin.

Prognosis. Progressive condition. Complications: cardiac failure, renal calculi, fractures, osteogenic sarcoma.

BIBLIOGRAPHY. Paget J: On a form of chronic inflammation of bones (osteitis deformans). Med Chir Trans (London) 60:37–63, 1877

Singer FR: Paget's Disease of Bone. New York, Plenum, 1977

Harvey L, Gray T, Beneton MNC, et al: Ultrastructural features of the osteoclasts from Paget's disease of the bone in relation to a viral etiology. J Clin Pathol 35:771–779, 1982

Posen S: Paget's disease: Current concepts. Austr NZJ Surg 62:17–23, 1992

PAGET ABSCESS

Eponym used to indicate an abscess recurrence at the same site after apparent cure.

BIBLIOGRAPHY. Paget J: On residual abscesses. St Bartholomew Hosp Rep 5:73–79, 1869

PAGET, JUVENILE

Synonyms. Osteoectasia, hyperphosphatasia; hyperphosphatasemia, osteoectasia; hyperostosis corticalis deformans juvenilis; familial, osteoectasia.

Symptoms and Signs. Both sexes affected. Bluish sclerae, becoming evident during first year of life. Occasionally, deafness (nerve compression); growth deficiency. Enlarging of head; broadening and then bowing of diaphyses. Pectus carinatum; kyphoscoliosis; teeth caries. Occasionally, fractures. Usually, normal intelligence.

Etiology. Unknown. Possibly autosomal recessive inheritance.

Diagnostic Procedures. *X-ray.* Severe osteoporosis of flat and long bones (see Symptoms and Signs). *Blood.* Serum alkaline and acid phosphatase, leucine aminopeptidase, hydroxyproline, uric acid elevated. *Urine.* Leucine-amino acid peptidase and uric acid elevation.

Therapy. Orthopedic measures of some value; calcitonin.

Prognosis. Fair.

BIBLIOGRAPHY. Bakin H, Eiger MS: Fragile bones and macrocranium. J Pediatr 49:558–564, 1956
Iancu TC, Almagor G, Friedman E, et al: Chronic familial hyperphosphatasemia. Radiology 129:669–676, 1978
Wu RK, Trumble TE, Ruwe PA: Familial incidence of Paget's disease and secondary osteogenic sarcoma: A report of three cases from a single family. Clin Orthop Related Res 265:306–309, 1991

PAGET-SCHRÖTTER

Synonyms. Schrötter; von Schroetter; axillary vein traumatic thrombosis; effort thrombosis; thrombosis intermittent; venous claudication, intermittent.

Symptoms. Occurs in active healthy males; onset usually at 18–40 years of age. Symptoms occur after vigorous work, or occasionally after minimal effort or no exercise. Onset gradual or very rapid. Right arm most often affected. Swelling of all arm from fingers to shoulder girdle and lower part of neck, with dull pain in the joints (particularly intense in the axilla); pain sometimes absent. Absence of systemic manifestations.

Signs. Arm swelling; cyanosis diffuse or mottled; superficial veins prominent; occasionally, hard cord-like mass palpated in the axilla.

Etiology. Idiopathic obstruction of axillary or subclavian vein (not secondary to aneurysm of aorta, cardiac failure, or breast neoplasia). Probably, compressions of vein between muscles and first rib or clavicle. A recent cause of subclavian and axillary vein thrombosis is represented by the introduction of total parenteral nutrition and subclavian cannulas for hemodialysis.

Pathology. In most cases, no signs of thrombus formation. Compression of vein by muscle of phrenic nerve demonstrated.

Diagnostic Procedures. *Blood gas.* Venous pressure; oxygen saturation, and circulation time show stasis. *X-ray.* Normal. *Blood.* Normal.

Therapy. In most cases, conservative. Various surgical procedures to remove obstruction. Anticoagulant helpful. Paravertebral cervical sympathetic block also valuable.

Prognosis. Usually, spontaneous, partial or total recovery in a few days or weeks. Symptoms usually recur.

BIBLIOGRAPHY. Paget J: Clinical Lectures and Essays, p 292. London, 1875
von Schrötter L: Erkrankunger der Gefasse. In Nothnagels Handbuch der Pathologie und Therapie. Wein, 1884; Holder (Nothnagel), 1884
Kieny R, Fontaine R, Suhler A, et al: Thirty-four cases of so-called "exertion" thrombophlebitis of upper extremity (Paget-Schrötter syndrome). J Cardiovasc Surg 13:181–185, 1964
Bithel TC: Thrombosis and antithrombotic therapy. In Lee GR, Bithell TC, Foerster J, et al (eds): Wintrobe's Clinical Hematology, 9th ed, pp 1520–1521. Philadelphia, Lea & Febiger, 1993

PAGON II

Synonym. Anemia sideroblastic; ataxia spinocerebellar; ataxia-anemia, sideroblastic.

Symptoms and Signs. In males. Anemia from birth; ataxia becomes evident by age 1 year, accompanied by clonus, positive Babinski sign.

Etiology. X-linked recessive inheritance.

Pathology. Moderate parenchymal iron storage in tissue.

Diagnostic Procedures. *Blood. Bone marrow.* Hyperchromic microcytic anemia; ring sideroblasts; raised free erythrocyte protoporphyrin levels.

Therapy. None specific.

Prognosis. Nonprogressive neurologic findings.

BIBLIOGRAPHY. Pagon RA, Bird TD, Detter JC, et al: Hereditary sideroblastic anemia and ataxia an X-linked recessive disorder. J Med Genet 22:267–273, 1985
Raskind WH, Wijsman E, Pagon RA, et al: X-linked sideroblastic anemia and ataxia: Linkage to phosphoglycerate kinase at X q13. Am J Hum Genet 48:335–341, 1991

PAINE

Synonym. Microcephaly; spastic diplegia. See Seemanova.

Symptoms. Occurs only in males. Onset from birth. Poor swallowing, requiring gavage feeding. Retarded physical and mental development; seizures (like myoclonic jerks progressing into opisthotonic fits); lack of interest in environment.

Signs. Microcephaly; below third percentile in weight and height; limbs spastic and hyperreflexic. In eye, normal light reflex; early optic atrophy.

Etiology. Unknown. Sex-linked inheritance.

Pathology. Microcephaly; cerebellar hypoplasia. Decreased number of cells in the cerebrum, no gliosis; small interior pontine. Olives only rudimentary. Marked underdevelopment of cerebellar nuclei. Spinal cord normal.

Diagnostic Procedures. *Blood. CSF.* Amino acid ratio reverted (marked increase of cerebrospinal fluid amino acid). *Urine.* Mild aminoaciduria. *X-ray.* Of skull. *CT scan. MRI. EEG.*

Therapy. Orthopedic surgery. Dextroamphetamine; anticonvulsants.

Prognosis. Poor. Death usually within first year. Frequently pulmonary complications.

BIBLIOGRAPHY. Paine RS: Evaluation of familial biochemically determined mental retardation in children, with special reference to amino aciduria. N Engl J Med 262:658–665, 1960
Oka E, Mandarini M: Paine's syndrome in two siblings. Dev Med Child Neurol 10:259, 1968
Opitz JM, Sutherland GR: International workshop on the fragile X and X-linked mental retardation. Am J Med Genet 17:5–94, 1984

PAINE-EFRON

Synonym. Ataxia telangiectasia II. Including Ataxia—telangiectasia—pigmentation; early death.

Symptoms. Onset in late childhood or adulthood. Pain on the back and thighs; then slowly progressing ataxia. No sinopulmonary symptoms (see Louis-Bar). Greater sensory deficit than in Louis-Bar.

Signs. Diffuse telangiectasia (late onset); darkly pigmented nevi.

Etiology. Unknown. Dominant pattern of inheritance. Possibly, spinocerebellar degeneration of a type not classifiable because of lack of adequate histologic reports.

Pathology. Unknown.

Diagnostic Procedures. *Urine.* Absence of urinary substance reported in Louis-Bar (see). *Blood. Cerebrospinal fluid.* Normal.

Prognosis. Much slower evolution in adult life and slight incapacitation. In Ataxia Telangiectasia, pigmentation, early death (second year of life).

BIBLIOGRAPHY. Paine RS, Efron ML: Atypical variants of "ataxia-telangiectasia syndrome." Dev Med Child Neurol 5:14–23, 1963
Tadjoedin MK, Fraser FC: Heredity of ataxiatelangiectasia (Louis-Bar syndrome). Am J Dis Child 110:64–68, 1965
Tsukahara M, Masuda M, Ohshiro K, et al: Ataxia telangiectasia with generalized skin pigmentation and early death. Eur J Pediatr 145:121–124, 1986
Champion RH: Disorder of blood vessels. In Champion RH, Burton JL, Ebling FJG (eds): Rook/Wilkinson/Ebling Textbook of Dermatology, 5th ed, pp 1847–1848. Oxford, Blackwell Scientific, 1992

PAINFUL HEEL

Synonym. Heel pain, idiopathic.

Symptoms. In patients 40–70 years of age, male, active. Pain beneath the anteriolateral prominence of calcaneal tuberosity usually unilateral; pain worse in the morning and after resting, decreases after walking, when tired in the evening, pain may reappear.

Signs. Normally arched foot. Localized tenderness at the inferomedial aspect of calcaneal tuberosity. Swelling and edema may be present.

Etiology. Still unknown. Differential diagnosis includes rheumatoid arthritis, ankylosing spondylitis, Reiter's, osteoarthritis, etc. Possibly related to degenerative process in the calcaneal heel pad of elastic adipose tissue.

Diagnostic Procedure. *X-ray.* Calcaneal spur in 50% of cases (of uncertain significance).

Therapy. Surgery useless. Shoe insert, nonsteroidal anti-inflammatory agents and local corticosteroid injection.

Prognosis. Symptoms last weeks, months, or years. Good response to conservative treatment.

BIBLIOGRAPHY. Still WF: Painful heel. Practitioner 108:345, 1922
Richardson EG: The foot in adolescents and adults. In Crenshaw AH (ed): Campbell's Operative Orthopedics, 7th ed, pp 933–936. St Louis, CV Mosby, 1987

PALANT

Synonym. Cleft palate—face unusual—mental retardation—limb abnormality.

Symptoms. Occurs in females; clinical features present from birth. Normal birth weight. Feeding difficulties; mental, motor, and developmental milestone retardation.

Signs. Short stature; midline cleft palate. *Facies.* Almond-shaped; deep-set eyes; narrow palpebral fissure; mongoloid slant; epicanthal folds; bulbous nose; low hair line. *Limbs.* Bilateral camptodactyly of fourth and fifth fingers; broad distal phalanges of toes; syndactyly of second and third toes; valgus deformity of feet.

Etiology. Unknown. Possibly, autosomal recessive inheritance.

Diagnostic Procedures. *X-ray.* Of skeleton. *Dermatolglyphic pattern.* Normal.

Therapy. Institutionalization.

Prognosis. Good quoad vitam. Severly retarded mental and motor development.

BIBLIOGRAPHY. Palant DI, Feingold M, Berkman MD: Unusual faces, cleft palate, mental retardation, and limb abnormalities in siblings: A new syndrome. J Pediatr 78:686–689, 1971

PALATAL MYOCLONUS

Synonyms. Palatal nystagmus.

Symptoms and Signs. Continuous rhythmic contraction of the uvula and soft palate, with audible click, frequently associated and synchronous with contraction of pharynx, larynx, tongue, floor of the mouth, neck, and diaphragm. Nodding of the head. Seldom, tremor of the hand associated. Ocular movements may also be associated. Frequency of contraction 100–180/min. It may persist during sleep and anesthesia.

Etiology and Pathology. Vascular, neoplastic, traumatic lesion causing denervation of one or a combination of the following structures: nucleus ambiguous, dorsolateral reticular formation, central tegmental tract, olivary nucleus, dentatum.

Diagnostic Procedures. *Spinal tap. EEG. Angiography. Electro-oculogram. CT brain scan. MRI.*

Therapy. Symptomatic. Clonazepam, valproate, tetrabenazine. Barbital decreases frequency, but does not suppress myoclonus.

Prognosis. Depends on nature and extension of lesion.

BIBLIOGRAPHY. Kupper: Ueber klonische Kraempfe der Schingmuskulatur Arch Ohrenheilk 1:296–297 1873
Spencer HR: Pharyngeal and laryngeal "nystagmus" Lancet 2:702–704, 1886
Gallet J: Le nystagmus du voile le syndrome myoclonique de la calotte protubërantielle (thesis). Paris, 1927
Guillain G, Mollaret P: Deux cas de myoclones synchrones et ryhtmées vélo-pharingo-laryngo-oculo diaphragmatiques. Les problèm anatomique et physio-pathologique de ce syndrome. Rev Neurol 2:545–546, 1931
Adams RD, Victor M: Principles of Neurology, 5th ed, p 98. New York, McGraw-Hill, 1993

PALEOCEREBELLAR

Synonym. Cerebellar anterior lobe.

Symptoms. Disturbed postural reflexes; increased extensor tone; tremor; incoordinate, awkward, ataxic movements. Stiff-legged gait.

Signs. Hypotonia or flaccidity of affected muscles.

Etiology. Neoplastic or degenerative lesions of anterior lobe of cerebellum.

Pathology. According to etiology.

Diagnostic Procedures. According to etiology.

Therapy. According to etiology.

Prognosis. Depends on etiology.

BIBLIOGRAPHY. Bailey P: Reflections aroused by an unusual tumor of the cerebellum. J Mt Sinai Hosp 9:299–310, 1942
Adams RD, Victor H: Principles of Neurology, 5th ed, p 74. New York, McGraw-Hill, 1993

PALLISTER-HALL

Synonym. Hall-Pallister; hypothalamic hamartoblastoma; hypopituarism—imperforate anus—postaxial polydactyly. See Smith-Lemli-Opitz.

Symptoms and Signs. Both sexes. Neonatal. Nonconsanguineous parents. Imperforate anus, postaxial polydactyly; in some cases laryngeal cleft, multiple buccal frenula, microphallus, signs of retarded intrauterine growth and signs of cardiac and/or kidney and lung defects.

Etiology. Unknown. Teratogen suspected. Autosomal dominant inheritance postulated. Chromosomal location 3p25.3.

Pathology. Hypothalamic hamartoblastoma on the inferior surface of the cerebrum extending from optic chiasma to interpenducular fossa. (Absence of anterior pituitary in all patients). Histology: cells resembling primitive undifferentiated germinal cells.

Diagnostic Procedures. *X-rays. CT scan. MRI.* See Signs and Pathology.

Therapy. Symptomatic.

Prognosis. Neonatal lethality.

BIBLIOGRAPHY. Hall JG, Pallister PD, Clarren SK et al: Congenital hypothalamic hamartoblastoma, hypopituarism, imperforate anus, and postaxial polydactyly: A new syndrome? Am J Genet 7:47–74, 1980
Iafolla K, Franklin JD, Spiegel PK, et al: Case report and delination of the congenital hypothalamic hamartoblastoma syndrome (Pallister-Hall sundrome). Am J Med Genet 33:489–499, 1989

PALLISTER-KILLIAN

Synonym. Pallister-Teschler Nicola-Killian; Teschler Nicola-Killian. Mosaic tetrasomy 12p; Isochromosome 12p.

Symptoms and Signs. From birth. Mental retardation. Head: prominent forehead, sparse hair and brows; hypertelorism; epicanthal folds; flat nose; macrostomia and -glossia; high palate; abnormal ears. Hypotonia. Occasionally: macrosomia; pigmentary dysplasia, lymphedema; optic hypoplasia, cataracts.

Etiology. Isochrome 12p mosaicism.

Diagnostic Procedures. Culture of lymphocytes and fibroblasts: isochrome present in fibroblasts, absent in lymphs. *X-rays. CT scan. MRI. Sonography. Bone and visceral abnormalities.*

Prognosis. Reach adulthood.

BIBLIOGRAPHY. Teschler-Nicola M, Killian W: Case report 72: Mental retardation, unusual facial appearance, abnormal hair. Syndrome Ident 7:6, 1981
Killian W, Zonana S, Schroer RJ: Case report 102: Abnormal hair, craniofacial dysmorphism and severe mental retardation: A new syndrome. J Clin Dysmorphol 1:6–13, 1983
Lin AE, Clemens M, Garder KL, et al: Case of Pallisteer-Killian syndrome with imperforate anus (letter). Am J Med Genet 31:705–707, 1988

PALLISTER-ULNAR MAMMARY

Synonym. Ulnar, mammary. See Schinzel.

Symptoms and Signs. Both sexes. Absence of body odor and axillary sweating; absence of breast tissue and hypoplasia of nipples and areolas. Postaxial polydactyly or unilateral oligodactyly and abdominal development of ulnar rays. Abnormal development of teeth, palate, vertebral column.

Etiology. Unknown. Autosomal dominant inheritance.

Pathology. See Symptoms and Signs. Plus occasionally absence of kidney.

BIBLIOGRAPHY. Pallister PD, Herrmann J, Opitz JM: A pleiotropic dominant mutation affecting skeletal, sexual and apocrine-mammary development. Birth Defects XII (5):247–254, 1976
Gonzales CH, Herrmann J, Opitz JM: Mother and son affected with ulnar-mammary syndrome of Pallister. Eur J Pediatr 123:225–235, 1976

PALSY, SIXTH NERVE, BENIGN

Synonyms. Benign abducens (VI) nerve paralysis; benign VI nerve palsy.

Symptoms. Occurs in children of any age. Painless paralysis of the abducens (VI) nerve developing 7–21 days after upper respiratory disease. Alertness; no ataxia.

Signs. No papilledema, enlarged head, or other neurologic signs except the paralysis of abducens (VI) nerve.

Etiology. Two mechanisms possible: otitis media and complication or neuritis as part of systemic viral infection. Syndrome to be differentiated from other forms of paralysis expressing presence of tumor, hydrocephalus, meningitis.

Pathology. Not known except in a case in which otitis present.

Diagnostic Procedures. *Blood.* Frequently present, relative lymphocytosis. *Cerebrospinal fluid.* Normal (seldom, transient lymphocytosis). *MRI.* Defer complicated diagnostic studies (arteriography) until lack of regression of the palsy is established.

Therapy. Symptomatic.

Prognosis. Usually, palsy begins to improve within 3–6 weeks, and clears completely within 10 weeks.

BIBLIOGRAPHY. Symond CP: Comment on a paper by Purdom Martin J, et al: Venous thrombosis in central nervous system. Proc R Soc Med 37:383–392, 1944
Knox DL, Clark DB, Schuster FF: Benign VI nerve palsies in children. Pediatrics 40:560–564, 1967
Nelson L: Disorders of the eye. In Behrman RE, Kliegman Arvin Nelson: Textbook of Pediatrics, 15th ed, p 1774. Philadelphia, WB Saunders, 1995

PANCOAST

Synonyms. Ciuffini; Hare; Tobias; apico-ostovertebral; superior pulmonary sulcus.

Symptoms. Severe shoulder pain; paresthesias, paresis, or weakness of one arm.

Signs. Muscle atrophy of shoulder, arm, and hand involved. Signs of apical mass. Mild enophthalmos, ptosis, miosis (Horner).

Etiology. Tumor of pulmonary apex (in less than 5% of cases).

Pathology. Bronchogenic carcinoma or any other tumor in this location. Erosion first of ribs and eventually vertebral involvement.

Diagnostic Procedures. *X-ray.* Of chest. *Bronchoscopy. Cytology.* Of expectorate. *CT scan.* Of chest.

Therapy. Surgery if feasible; chemotherapy; roentgen therapy.

Prognosis. Poor; death usually within 1 year.

BIBLIOGRAPHY. Hare ES: Tumor involving certain nerves. London Med Gaz 23:16–18, 1838
Pancoast HK: Importance of careful roentgen-ray investigations of apical chest tumors. JAMA 83:1407–1411, 1924
Pancoast HK: Superior pulmonary sulcus tumor; tumor characterized by pain, Horner's syndrome, destruction of bone, and atrophy of hand muscles. JAMA 99:1391–1396, 1932
Fraser RS, Paré JAP, Fraser RG, Paré PD: Synopsis of Disease of the Chest, 2nd ed. Philadelphia, WB Saunders, 1994

PANCREATIC PSEUDOCYSTS

Symptoms. Occurs following (sometimes) severe abdominal trauma. One or more attacks of acute pancreatitis, or history of gallbladder disease. Pain mild to severe, usually at epigastrium, right to left quadrant. Nausea and vomiting suggesting paralytic ileus or pyloric obstruction. Loss of weight.

Signs. Abdominal mass smooth, 10–15 cm in diameter in the epigastrium or either lateral upper quadrant. Moderate tenderness; fever; occasionally, paralytic ileus and, less frequently, left side hydrothorax or jaundice or both.

Etiology. Abdominal trauma, or following one or more attacks of acute pancreatitis.

Pathology. Fluid-containing, abnormal sac not lined with epithelium; in the pancreas, usually in the lesser peritoneal sac.

Diagnostic Procedures. *X-ray.* Plain film; contrast medium in stomach, duodenum. *Abdominal CT scan. MRI. Ultrasound.* Chest. Intravenous cholangiography. *Blood.* Serum amylase usually increased (twice normal value). Leukocytosis in about half of cases.

Therapy. Surgery: drainage by cystogastrostomy when feasible.

Prognosis. If untreated, eventually becomes infected, hemorrhagic; develops fistula or produces duodenal or common biliary tract obstruction. Very seldom resolves spontaneously. Cured by cystogastrostomy. Optimal results also obtained by tube drainage; however, recurrences are possible. Once treated, symptoms disappear; patient regains his weight.

BIBLIOGRAPHY. Gussenbayer C: Zur operativen Behandlung der Pankreas-Cysten. Arch Klin Cir 29:358–364, 1883
Goulet RJ, Goodhan J, Schaffer R, et al: Multiple pancreatic pseudocyst disease. Ann Surg 199:6–13, 1984
Freeny PC: Imaging and guided biopsy. In Haubrich WS, Schaffner F, Berk JE (eds): Bockus Gastroenterology, 5th ed, pp 2871–2874. Philadelphia, WB Saunders, 1995

PANCREATOMETAPHYSEAL

Synonym. Metaphyseal pancreatic dysplasia.

Symptoms. Onset shortly after birth. Steatorrhea. Diabetes mellitus develops in childhood or early adolescence. Sometimes associated with Shwachman (see).

Signs. Coxa vara.

Etiology. Unknown. Autosomal recessive inheritance (?).

Diagnostic Procedures. *X-ray.* Of skeleton. Metaphyseal dysostosis. *Pancreatic fluid.* Reduction of pancreatic enzymes. *Blood.* Hyperglycemia and diabetic features. *Biopsy.* Of intestinal mucosa normal.

Therapy. Symptomatic. Administration of pancreatic enzymes, insulin.

BIBLIOGRAPHY. Theodorou SD, Adams J: An unusual case of metaphysial dysplasia. J Bone Joint Surg (Br) 45:364–369, 1963
Giedion A, Prader A, Hadorn B, et al: Metaphysäre Dysostose und angeborene Pankreasinsuffizienz. Fortschr Roentgenstr 108:51–57, 1968

PANIC ATTACK

Symptoms and Signs. Many peripheral manifestations of sudden, massive autonomic nervous system discharge, with fear of dying, of going crazy, or of "doing something uncontrolled during an attack." The attacks occur suddenly, without warning, and for little apparent reason.

Etiology. Predisposition to this disorder may be transmitted as an autosomal dominant trait. Possibly by common environmental disturbances. The syndrome, however, may be considered not as related to a true psychologic problem, but likely to be an organic illness.

Pathology. In patients with the disorder the incidence of mitral valve prolapse has been estimated to be as high as 30–50%. Recent studies oppose any direct relation, however, between panic attacks and mitral valve prolapse.

Diagnostic Procedures. High catecholamine concentrations and elevated lactate levels have been found in affected subjects.

Therapy. One of these drugs can be prescribed (to avoid failure ade-

quate dosage and duration of treatment are fundamental) imipramine hydrochloride phenelzine sulfate; alprazolam; fluoxetine, sertraline usually associated with psychotherapeutical approach.

Prognosis. Relapse rate over 70%. Prolonged treatment is needed. Interruption every 12 months to test need for further medication.

BIBLIOGRAPHY. Sheehan DV: Current perspectives in the treatment of panic and phobic disorders. Drugs Ther 179–190, 1982
Sheehan DV: Panic attacks and phobias. N Engl J Med 307:156–159, 1982
Van Winter J, Stickler GB: Panic attack syndrome. J Pediatr 105:661–665, 1984
Sheehan DV, Raj BA: Panic attacks and the cardiovascular system. In Schlant RC, Alexander RW, et al: Hurst's The Heart, 8th ed, pp 2099–2107. New York, McGraw-Hill, 1994

PANNER II

Synonyms. Capitellum humeri epiphyseal necrosis; Haas; capitellum humeri osteochondrosis; "little league elbow." See Epiphyseal ischemic necrosis.

Symptoms and Signs. Pain in the shoulder aggravated by active movement; swelling and redness over capitellum humeri.

Etiology. See Epiphyseal ischemic necrosis.

BIBLIOGRAPHY. Panner HJ: An affection of the capitellum humeri resembling Calve-Perthes disease of the hip. Acta Radiol (Stockh) 8:617, 1927
Canale ST: Osteochondrosis or epiphysitis? In Crenshaw AH (ed): Campbell's Operative Orthopedics, 7th ed, p 991. St Louis, CV Mosby, 1987

PAPILLARY MUSCLE

Synonym. Papillary muscle dysfunction.

Symptoms. Occurs usually in patients over 40. No specific symptoms. Possibly, symptoms of disease responsible for papillary muscle dysfunction (e.g., angina; congestive failure).

Signs. Apical systolic murmur: delayed in onset; "diamond shaped" with midsystolic accentuation, to moderately loud; "blowing" in quality; best heard at apex radiating at axilla, seldom associated with thrill. If papillary muscle dysfunction associated with left ventricular dilatation and congestive failure, murmur of decrescent quality. Murmur may be a fixed feature (in healing of fibrotic lesions) or transient (in evolving lesions). Absence of late systolic clicks.

Etiology and Pathology. 1. Circulatory insufficiency: angina; infarction of papillary muscle; systemic circulatory disturbances. 2. Left ventricular dilatation: generalized; localized. 3. Nonischemic atrophy of papillary muscle. 4. Defective development. 5. Endocardial diseases. 6. Heart muscle diseases. 7. Functional disturbances of papillary muscle. 8. Rupture.

Diagnostic Procedures. *ECG. Type 1:* Moderate depression of junction J; concavity-upward or slight convexity-downward deformity of ST-T interval. *Type II:* Slight to moderate depression of junction J; prominent convexity-upward deformity of ST interval and terminal inversion of T. *Type III:* Marked depression of junction J; slight convexity, upward deformity of the initial ST interval. *Phonocardiography.* See Signs. *Two-dimensional echocardiography.*

Therapy. That of determining condition and associated manifestations (e.g., congestive failure, angina). Mitral valve replacement if severe mitral regurgitation is present and if left ventricular contractility is preserved.

Prognosis. Depends on etiology.

BIBLIOGRAPHY. Burch GE, DePasquale NP, Phillips JH: Clinical manifestations of papillary muscle dysfunction. Arch Intern Med 112:112–117, 1963

Burch GE, DePasquale NP, Phillips JH: The syndrome of papillary muscle dysfunction. Am Heart J 75:399–415, 1968

Roberts R, Morris D, Pratt CM: Pathophysiology recognition and treatment of acute myocardial infarction and its complications. In Schlant RC, Alexander RW, et al: Hurst's The Heart, 8th ed, p 1150–1151. New York, McGraw-Hill, 1994

PAPILLON-LEFÉVRE

Synonyms. Palmoplantar hyperkeratosis; periodontitis—keratosis, palmoplantaris; periodontopathia; see keratoderma palmoplantar syndromes.

Symptoms and Signs. Appears within first 4 years of life. Hyperkeratosis of palms and soles, usually diffuse type, seldom punctate type, generally not severe, similar to those of Meleda syndrome (see). In some cases, lesion more severe in winter and receding or disappearing during summer. Fetid hyperhidrosis, especially of feet. At the same time of appearance of hyperkeratosis, gingivae become red and swollen and bleed. Bad breath and destruction of periodontal ligament begins and periodontal pockets with pus form. Teeth become mobile and are lost. Period in which the patient is edentulous follows, then the process is repeated with the permanent teeth. In more severe type, complete edentia by 6–10 years of age.

Etiology. Unknown. Autosomal recessive pattern of inheritance.

Pathology. Hyperkeratosis of palms and soles; acanthosis without parakeratosis; gingival pattern similar to ordinary periodontoclasia. Teeth grossly normal with some resorption of cementum and dentin. Calcification of dura mater (third component of syndrome).

Diagnostic Procedures. *X-ray. CT scan. MRI.* Occasionally, ectopic calcification in the tentorium and choroid. Destruction of periodontal structures. *Blood.* In some cases, polycythemia and glucose curve elevated.

Therapy. Vitamin A; etretinate, antibiotics; oral hygiene.

Prognosis. Loss of teeth; dentures well tolerated.

BIBLIOGRAPHY. Papillon MM, Lefèvre P: Deux cas de kératodermie palmaire et plantaire symétrique familiale (maladie de Meleda) chez le frère et la soeur; coexistence dans les deux cas d'alterations dentaires graves. Bull Soc Fr Dermatol Syph 31:82–87, 1924

Cheung HS, Landow RK, Bauer M: Increased collagen synthesis by gingival fibroblasts derived from a Papillon–Lefèvre patient. J Dent Res 61:378–381, 1982

Nazzaro V, Blanchet–Bardon C, Mimoz C et al: Papillon–Lefèvre syndrome. Ultrastructural study and successful treatment with Acitretin. Arch Dermatol 12:533–539, 1988

Gelmetti C, Nazzaro V, Cerri D, et al: Long-term preservation of permanent teeth in a patient with Papillon-Lefèvre syndrome treated with etretinate. Pediatr Dermatol 6:222–225, 1989

PAPILLON-LÉGE AND PSAUME

Synonyms. Orofacial digital dysostosis I; facial orodigital I; Gorlin; linguofacial dysplasia I, OFD, Psaume orofacial digital I. (The original description may include also the OFD II, see.)

Symptoms. Limited to females; lethal in males. (Reported in males; one of the males who had chromosomal study done showed a 47 XXY pattern. See Klinefelter.) Mental retardation and trembling (not constant).

Signs. Constant features: cleft or defect of hard palate; hypertrophic frenulum; cleft of tongue with two or more lobules. Inconstant features: soft palate or uvular cleft; syndactyly; clinodactyly; bradydactyly; hypoplastic nasal cartilages, seborrheic changes; dystopia canthum; pseudocleft of upper lip; alopecia; missing mandibular lateral incisors. A variety of central nervous system malformations.

Etiology. Unknown. Possibly, X-linked dominant mutant condition with variable penetrance.

Diagnostic Procedures. *Blood. Urine.* Normal. *Chromosome study.* No consistent chromosomal abnormality detectable. *X-ray.* Typical findings.

Therapy. Plastic surgery.

Prognosis. Poor.

BIBLIOGRAPHY. Duplouy MS: Communication. Bull Mem Soc Nat Chir Paris 9:456, 1883

Papillon-Léage M, Psaume J: Une malformation héréditaire de la muqueuse buccale, brides et freins anormaux: Generalities. Rev Stomatol 55:209–227, 1954

Gorlin SJ, Anderson VE, Scott CR: Hypertrophied frenuli, oligophrenia, familial trembling and anomalies of hand: Report of four cases in one family and a forme fruste in an other. N Engl J Med 264:486–489, 1961

Gorlin RJ, Psaume J: Orodigitofacial dysostosis: A new syndrome. A study of 22 cases. J Pediatr 61:520–530, 1962

Majewski F, Lenz W, Pfeiffer RA, et al: Das oro-faciodigitale Syndrom. Symptome und Prognose. Z Kinderheilkd 112:89–112, 1972

Goodship J, Platt J, Smith R, et al: A male with type I orofaciodigital syndrome. J Med Genet 28:691–694, 1991

PARANA HARD SKIN

Synonym. See Stiff skin.

Symptoms and Signs. Onset 2–3 months of age. The same as that of stiff skin plus growth retardation.

Etiology. Probably autosomal recessive inheritance.

Prognosis. Malignant course (if compared with stiff skin).

BIBLIOGRAPHY. Cat I, Rodriguez-Magdalena NI, Parolin-Marinoni L, et al: Parana hard-skin syndrome: Study of seven families. Lancet I:215–216, 1974

PARAPLEGIA, PAINFUL

See Putti-Chavany.

Symptoms. Extremely severe pain caused by vertebral root compression (typical specific irradiation) followed by paraplegia, cachexia.

Signs. Pain on compression of specific point of vertebral column. Signs of paraplegia.

Etiology and Pathology. Osteogenic or osteolytic lesions of vertebrae. Multiple myeloma; metastasis of prostate, lung, breast, kidney, or colon malignancy.

Diagnostic Procedures. *X-ray.* Of spine, skeleton. *CT scan. MRI. Blood.* Search for primary anemia, hyperproteinemia (myeloma). *Biopsy.* Of bone marrow.

Therapy. *Myeloma.* Cyclophosphamide; melphalan, testosterone. *Prostate.* Castration; estrogens. *Breast.* Radiation; oophorectomy.

Prognosis. Sometimes dramatic improvement with treatment.

BIBLIOGRAPHY. Vick NA: Grinker's Neurology, 7th ed. Springfield, IL, Charles C Thomas, 1976

Klippel JH, Dieppe PA: Rheumatology, p 4.7.3. St Louis, CV Mosby, 1994

PARAPLEGIC PHANTOM

See Phantom limb.

Symptoms. Occurs in patients with paraplegia and complete cord injury. Phantom phenomena or painful phantom limb of the paraplegic extremity. Phenomena of shortening, telescoping, and decreasing size of phantom, observed in phantom limb syndrome in amputee, are not noted in paraplegic patient with analogous syndrome. In many paraplegic patients, dissociation between position of phantom and actual position of paralyzed limb is eventually noticed within a few days or weeks.

Signs. Paraplegia.

Etiology and Pathology. Different type of cord lesion.

Diagnostic Procedures. See Phantom limb.

Therapy. See Phantom limb.

Prognosis. See Phantom limb.

BIBLIOGRAPHY. Bors E: Phantom limbs of patients with spinal cord injury. Arch Neurol Psychiatr 66:610–631, 1951
Weiss AA: The phantom limb. Ann Intern Med 44:668–677, 1956
Stannard CF: Phantom limb pain. Br J Hosp Med 50:583–587, 1993

PARASPASM, BILATERAL

See Ziehen-Oppenheim.

Symptoms. Gradually increasing intermittent attacks of contractions of all facial muscles and muscles of tongue and neck. Contractions enhanced by emotions, until attacks become almost continuous.

Signs. The patient may sometimes stop the attack temporarily with special maneuvers.

Etiology. Unknown. Extrapyramidal lesions; possibly, part of dystonia lenticularis syndrome (localized form). May occasionally be of psychogenic origin.

Therapy. Phenytoin or carbamazepine (inconstant effect). Quinine sulfate (better result). Diazepam.

BIBLIOGRAPHY. Zeman W, Kaelbling R, Pasamanick B: Idiopathic dystonia musculorum deformans. II. The formes frustes. Neurology 10:1068–1075, 1960
Adams RD, Victor M: Principles of Neurology, 5th ed, pp 1271–1274. New York, McGraw-Hill, 1993

PARASTREMMATIC DYSPLASIA

Synonym. Twisted.

Symptoms. Both sexes. Deformities recognized in first 6–12 month of life. Delay in walking, abnormal gait. Full manifestation by 10 years. Normal intelligence.

Signs. *Legs.* Symmetric, bizarre deformities owing to contracture of major joints: bowing, genu valga, twisted thighs. *Spine.* Kyphoscoliosis. *Neck.* Short.

Etiology. Autosomal dominant inheritance.

Diagnostic Procedures. *Urine.* Absence of mucopolysacchariduria. *X-rays. Bone density.* Decreased. Deformities of cranial vault and long bones; "flocky" aspect in enchondrial areas and calcific stippling of meta-epi and apophysis.

BIBLIOGRAPHY. Rask MR: Morquio-Brailsford osteochondrodystrophy and osteogenesis imperfect: Report of a patient with both conditions. J Bone Joint Surg 45:561–570, 1963

Langer O Jr, Petersen D, Spranger JW: An unusual bone dysplasia: Parastremmatic dwarfism. Am J Roentegen 110:550–560, 1970
Ayura-Gottwald ML, Morla BE: Parastremmatic dwarfism. Bol Med Hosp Infant Mex 39:748–752, 1982

PARENTI-FRACCARO

Synonyms. Fraccaro; Houston-Harris; achondrogenesis I achondrogenesis IA (Houston-Harris); achondrogenesis IB (Fraccaro); lethal chondrogenesis.

Symptoms and Signs. In type IA. Male to female ratio, 15:7; in type IB excess of females. Stillbirth (50%) or neonatal death. Polyhydramnios frequent. Short limbs; dwarfism. Trunk as wide as it is long; wide pelvis. Occasionally congenital heart conditions; cryptorchidism, hernias, urogenital malformations; auditory canal atresia; corneal clouding; cleft palate.

Etiology. Autosomal recessive inheritance.

Pathology. *Type IA:* Cartilaginous matrix normal but for hypervascularity; resting zone is hypercellular. Chondrocytes (with cytoplasmic inclusion bodies) in enlarged lacunae. Bone: hypercellular with persistence of calcified cartilage into metaphysisa. *Type IB:* Ring around chondrocytes. Endochondal ossification severely disorganized. Lack of matrix between resting cartilage cells.

Diagnostic Procedures. *X-ray. Ultrasound* (for prenatal diagnosis). Normal or enlarged skull; normal base; short horizontal ribs; absent sternum ossification; vertebral, sacral, iliac, and pubic anomalies; marked metaphyseal widening and spurs; micromelia. Type IA is distinguished from type IB by the presence of short, cupped flared ribs with multiple fractures.

BIBLIOGRAPHY. Donath J, Vogl A: Untersuchungen ueber den chondrodysteophischen Zwergunchs das Verholten der Wirbelsaule beim chondrodystrophischen Zwerg. Wein Arch Inn Med 10:1–44, 1925
Parenti GC: La anosteogenesi (una varietà della osteogenesi imperfetta). Pathologica 28:447–462, 1936
Fraccaro M: Contributo allo studio delle malattie del mesenchima osteopoietico; l'acondrogenesi. Folia Hered Pathol 1:190–208, 1952
Houston CS, Awen CF, Kent HP: Fatal neonatal dwarfism. J Can Assoc Radiol 23:45–61, 1972
Borochowitz Z, Lachman R, Adomian GE, et al: Achondrogenesis type I: Delineation of further heterogeneity and identification of two distinct subgroups. J Pediatr 112:23–31, 1988

PARINAUD, OCULOGLANDULAR

Synonyms. Cat-scratch; oculoglandular; conjunctiva adenitis, Parinaud.

Symptoms. Both sexes affected. More frequent in children. Tenderness at site of scratch. Irregular fever.

Signs. Granular or ulcerative conjunctivitis; anterior cervical lymphadenopathy; parotid gland swelling.

Etiology. Cat-scratch fever; tularemia; leptotrichosis; tuberculosis; lymphogranuloma venereum; coccidioidomycosis; sporotrichosis; syphilis, sarcoidosis; listeriosis.

Pathology. Conjunctivitis with granulomatous reaction; aspecific lymphadenopathy.

Diagnostic Procedures. *Cultures.* For viruses, mycobacteria, bacteria, and fungi. *Skin test. Kveim test. Fungi.* For tuberculosis, cat-scratch fever. Complement fixation. *Biopsy of conjunctiva.*

Therapy. According to etiology.

Prognosis. Spontaneous recovery (in 1 week or 1 month). Specific treatment speeds recovery.

BIBLIOGRAPHY. Parinaud H, Galezowski X: Conjonctivite infectieuse transmise par les animaux. Ann Ocul 101:252–253, 1889

Müller F: Die differential diagnose des konjunktivoglandulären Syndrome von Parinaud. Dtsch Med Wochenschr 80:152–154, 1955

Margeleth AM: Cat-scratch disease update. Am J Dis Child 138:711–713, 1984

Martin X, Uffer S, Galloud C: Ophthalmia nodosa and the oculoglandular syndrome of Parinaud. Br J Ophthalmol 70:536–542, 1986

Highet AS, Hay RJ, Roberts SOB: Bacterial infections. In Champion RH, Burton JL, Ebling FJG (eds): Rook/Wilkinson/Ebling Textbook of Dermatology, 5th ed, p 1018. Oxford, Blackwell Scientific, 1992

PARKER (N.)

Synonyms. Whispering dysphonia.

Symptoms and Signs. Both sexes. From infancy. Described in Australian kindred. Voice in normal condition comes as a faint whisper. In emotional conditions, after alcohol intake or during sleep normal voice and even shouting is possible. Ailment may progress to almost total aphonia.

Etiology. Unknown. Inherit as autosomal dominant. Distinct disorder in the Dystonic cluster.

Prognosis. In cases remain as an isolated feature, but more frequently in time becomes complicated with symptoms of dystonia musculorum deformans (see Huntington) or isolated dystonic symptoms: tics, torticollis, etc.

BIBLIOGRAPHY. Parker N: Hereditary whispering dysphonia. J Neurol Neurosurg Psychiat 48:218–224, 1985

PARKER (R.W.)

Synonyms. Abercrombie; Smith; adrenal medullary neuroblastoma; gangliosympathicoblastoma; malignant hypernephroma; neuroblastoma; sympathicoblastoma. See also Hutchinson (R.) and Pepper.

Symptoms. Both sexes affected. Present from birth or early infancy or onset in childhood (under age 10 years). Abdominal and back pain. Anorexia; debilitation; diarrhea; or constipation.

Signs. Jaundice (occasionally). Abdominal mass that crosses the midline. Possible association with various congenital malformations: spina bifida; hydrocephalus; polydactyly; aorta coarctation; visceral malformations.

Etiology. Autosomal recessive inheritance. Chromosomal aberration reported.

Pathology. Typically, retroperitoneal neoplasm, usually of adrenal medulla or adjacent sympathetic chain or, less frequently, on ganglia of other areas. Gray or purplish tumor. Microscopically, dense uniform cells, occasionally producing rosettes. *Liver.* Frequently, metastases that may replace the normal tissue almost completely (Pepper). *Long bones.* Typial "onion skin" layering. *Flat bones.* Vertical periosteal spines (Hutchinson).

Diagnostic Procedures. *Bone marrow.* Frequently, presence of typical cells and rosettes. *X-ray. CT scan. MRI.* Typical bone changes. *Biopsy.* See Pathology. *Urine.* Nonconstant increase of catecholamines and vanillylmandelic acid.

Therapy. Roentgen treatment; chemotherapy.

Prognosis. Rapid evolution: death in weeks or months. Spontaneous regression in 3% of cases.

BIBLIOGRAPHY. Parker RW: Diffuse (?) sarcoma of the liver, probably congenital. Trans Pathol Soc London 31:290–293, 1880

Abercrombie J: Multiple sarcomata of the cranial bones. Trans Pathol Soc London 31:216–223, 1880

Smith J: Case of adrenal neuroblastoma. Lancet 2:1214–1215, 1932

Hecht F, Hecht BK, Northrup JC, et al: Genetics of familial neuroblastoma: Long-range studies. Cancer Genet Cytogenet 7:227–230, 1982

Lack EE (ed): Pathology of the Adrenal Glands, p 212. New York, Churchill Livingstone, 1990

PARKINSON

Synonyms. Amyostatic; paralysis agitans; nonencephalitic parkinsonism. See Willige-Hunt.

Symptoms and Signs. Both sexes affected; gradual and insidious onset 50–65 years of age. Tremors at rest, mostly in upper limbs, particularly in the hands (pill-rolling movements); disappear when initiating movements and during sleep. Usually monolateral at onset, then generalized. Muscle rigidity; slowing of voluntary movements initially, then generalized stiffness, fatigue, mild muscle pain, progressing to generalized stiffness. Face mask-like; no wrinkling (youthful aspect); no expression; infrequent winking; pupil reaction prompt; drooling; slow swallowing. Semiflexed posture of head, hand, arm, and trunk; difficulty in straightening. Movements (active or passive) interrupted by cogwheel jerks. Handwriting: small letters; akathisia. Gait: steps short and shuffling; because of postural defect (stooping) the patient has to take a short run to keep his balance while moving; no arm swinging. Voice: monotonous; low pitched.

Etiology. Five etiologic categories: postencephalitic toxic, genetic (mendelenian forms of the disease have been proposed). Autosomal dominant, recessive, and X-linked; idiopathic and simply symptomatic.

Pathology. Degenerative changes mostly in globus pallidus and substantia nigra.

Diagnostic Procedures. *EEG. MRI. Neurophysiological imaging. Serology.*

Therapy. *Medical.* Belladonna; trihexyphenidyl, orphenadrine; levodopa; association of levodopa and decarboxylase inhibitor; benzatropine; ethopropazine; amantadine; bromocriptine; experimental deprenile (β-monoamine-oxidase inhibitor); domperidone (to reduce collateral effects of bromocriptine); pergolide mesylate; lisuride; terguride; ciladopa; L-leucyl-glycinamide. *Surgical.* Transplantation of adrenal medullary tissue or fetal mesencephalic tissue to striatum or caudate nucleus. For the tremor in case of failure of medical treatment. Stereotassic talamotomia or pallidotomia or electric stimulation of ventral intermediate nucleus.

Prognosis. Progressive course; symptomatic relief of some manifestations by medical or surgical treatment.

BIBLIOGRAPHY. Parkinson J: An Essay on the Shaking Palsy. London, Sherwood Neeley-Jones, 1817

Current concepts and controversies in Parkinson's disease. Can J Neurol Sci 11(Suppl), 1984

Koller WC, Paulson G, Therapy of Parkinson's Disease, 2nd ed. New York, Marcel Dekker, 1995

PARROT I

Synonyms. Bednar-Parrot; Parrot pseudoparalysis; Parrot syphilitic osteochondritis; Wegner.

Symptoms. Onset most commonly in first 3 weeks of life, seldom after 3 months. Upper extremities affected more frequently than lower. Pseudoparalysis; periarticular swelling.

Etiology. Congenital syphilis.

Pathology. Complete epiphyseal separation of long bones or fractures. Gelatiniform changes in bone and cartilage forming yellowish fluid.

Diagnostic Procedures. *X-ray.* Widening of joint space; irregular epiphyseal lines; periosteal thickening; bone decalcification.

Prognosis. Adequate, prompt antibiotic treatment brings complete recovery. Deformity if growing line severely affected.

BIBLIOGRAPHY. Wegner G: Ueber hederitäre knochensyphilis bei jungen kindern. Arch Pathol Anat (Berlin) 50:305–322, 1870
Parrot JM: Sur une pseudo-paralysie causée par une altération du système osseux chez les nouveau-nés atteints de syphilis héréditaire. Arch Physiol Norm Pathol Paris 4:319–333; 470–490; 612–623, 1871–1872
McCord JR: Osteochondritis in the stillborn. Am J Obstet Gynecol 42:667–676, 1941
Mascola L, Pelosi R, Blount JH, et al: Congenital syphilis revisited. Am J Dis Child 139:579–580, 1985
Avery GB, Fletcher MA, McDonald MC: Neonatology, 4th ed. Philadelphia, JB Lippincott, 1994

PARROT II

Synonyms. Athrepsia; inanition; infantile atrophy; marasmus.

Symptoms and Signs. Occurs in infants. Failure to thrive; weight loss; emaciation; edema; skin dry and subcutaneous fat loss. Abdomen flat or distended; muscles hypotonic and atrophic; hypothermia; pulse slow; basal metabolic rate decreased. Fretfulness and then listlessness; constipation or diarrhea.

Etiology. Inadequate calorie intake caused by insufficient supply, improper feeding habits, metabolic abnormalities, or congenital malformations. Disturbed parent–child relations.

Diagnostic Procedures. *Blood.* Hypochromic anemia; hypoproteinemia T3, T4, and thyroid-stimulating hormone (TSH). *X-ray.*

Therapy. Dietary correction and correction of specific anatomic or functional defects. Usually there is a slow response to dietary therapy during the first 4 weeks.

Prognosis. Usually poor.

BIBLIOGRAPHY. Parrot JM: L'Athrepsie. Paris, Masson, 1877
Giannini AJ, Slaby AE: The Eating Disorders. Ijmuiden, Netherlands, Springer, 1993

PARRY-ROMBERG

Synonyms. Romberg; hemifacial atrophy; progressive facial hemiatrophy; progressive laminar aplasia; trophoneurosis facialis progressiva. See Scleroderma ("en coupe de sabre").

Symptoms and Signs. Both sexes affected; onset in first two decades, but possible also later. At early stage on paramedian area of face, hair of skull and face affected by alopecia, blanching, often preceding other symptoms. Atrophy of fat and subcutaneous tissue. The process may be bilateral in 5–10% of cases. Extension of the process homolaterally; occasionally occurs involving trunk, extremities, and visceral organs. Cerebral manifestation homolateral to lesion frequently occurs, especially jacksonian type epilepsy and migraine. Sympathetic manifestations also may be present.

Etiology. Unknown. Distinguishing between hemiatrophy and secondary localized scleroderma impossible.

Pathology. Atrophic and secondary inflammatory changes of fat and subcutaneous tissue; skin usually spared except occasionally at later stages. Various degenerative brain lesions; calcification may be found.

Diagnostic Procedures. *Biopsy. EEG. X-rays. CT scan. MRI.* Bone atrophy at same sites of soft tissues athophy; intracranial calcifications. *Blood.* Antinuclear antibodies.

Therapy. Plastic surgery. Symptomatic for neurologic manifestations.

Prognosis. The process usually progresses for number of years, but may become arrested at any stage and then become stable for the rest of life.

BIBLIOGRAPHY. Parry CH: Collections from Unpublished Papers, p 178. London, Underwood, 1825
Romberg MH: Trophoneurosen. In his Klinische Ergebnise, pp 75–81. Berlin, Förstner, 1846
Dilley JJ, Perry HO: Bilateral linear scleroderma en coupe de sabre. Arch Dermatol 97:688–689, 1968
Miller MT, Sloane H, Goldberg MF: Progressive hemifacial atrophy (Parry-Romberg disease). J Pediatr Ophthalmol Strabismus 24:27–36, 1987

PARSONAGE-TURNER

Obsolete.

Eponym once used to indicate many forms of cryptogenic neurologic amyotrophy of the shoulder and cervical plexus. Today different mononeuropathies are described as syndromes and cervical plexus neuropathies are indicated by their etiology.

Synonyms. Neurologic amyotrophy; shoulder girdle, Feinberg, Tinel, Kiloh-Nevin II (see), brachial neuritis, acute brachial neuritis, cryptogenic neuropathy of brachial plexus.

Symptoms and Signs. Sharp pain across the shoulder and proximal part of arm, followed by atrophic paralysis of some muscles of shoulder girdle.

Etiology. Infection or minor surgery with involvement of branches of cervical plexus.

BIBLIOGRAPHY. Parsonage MJ, Turner JWA: Neuralgic amyotrophy, the shoulder-girdle syndrome. Lancet 1:973–978, 1948

PARTINGTON

Synonyms. Russell-Silver, X-recessive.

Symptoms and Signs. Both sexes (severe expression in male, mild in female). Prenatal growth retardation. Asthma. Triangular, face, and café-au-lait spots (different from classic ones) developing on trunk and limbs and sparing the face.

Etiology. IX-linked phenotype.

Prognosis. Facial and skin changes, starting at 1 year of age, are then progressive. Final height in both sexes 160–168.

BIBLIOGRAPHY. Partington MW: X-linked Russell-Silver syndrome. Proc Greenwood Genet Center 4:139, 1985
Partington MW: X-linked Russell-Silver. Short stature with pigmented evidence for heterogeneity of the Russel-Silver syndrome. Clin Genet 29:151–156, 1986

PASCHEFF I

Obsolete.

Synonyms. Conjuntivitis necrotic, infective.

Symptoms and Signs. Conjunctivitis with foci of suppuration and necrosis. Regional lymphoadenopathy.

Etiology. Infection with Microbacillus polymorphicum necroticans.

BIBLIOGRAPHY. Pascheff C: Ueber eine besondere Form von Bindehaut-

Entzuendung (Conjunctivitis necroticans infectiosa). Klin Mbl Augenh 57:517–529, 1916

PASCHEFF II

Synonyms. Trachomatous folliculoma.

Symptoms and Signs. Tumors formed by confluent trachoma follicles in the conjunctiva.

Etiology. C. trachomatis serovars A, B, Ba, and C.

Pathology. Lymphoblastic centers in follicles.

BIBLIOGRAPHY. Pascheff C: Researches on the trachoma: Its etiology and unification of conception. Am J Ophthal 15:690–708, 1932
Treharne JD, Darougar S: Chlamydial infections. In Garner A, Klintworth JK: Pathobiology of Ocular Disease, pp 263–273. New York, Marcel Dekker, 1994

PASINI

Synonyms. Albopapuloid epidermolysis bullosa; epidermolysis bullosa Pasini.

Symptoms and Signs. Both sexes affected; onset seldom in infancy, usually in late childhood or adulthood. Small, firm, white perifollicular papules appearing on the trunk, especially lumbosacral region, slowly enlarging to 15 mm. Features of hyperplastic epidermolysis bullosa.

Etiology. Unknown. Autosomal dominant inheritance. Deranged glycosaminoglycan metabolism.

Pathology. Connective tissue hyperplasia.

Diagnostic Procedures. *Biopsy of skin.*

Therapy. Treatment symptomatic. In season protection of skin from trauma and anhidrotic agents; when blisterings became infected: antibiotics and for severe forms corticosteroids. Phenitoin reported as useful to inhibit collagenase activity.

Prognosis. Healing with scar, frequently of keloid type, or leaving atrophic macula.

BIBLIOGRAPHY. Pasini A: Distrofia cutanea bollosa–atrofizzante ed albopapuloide. G Ital Dermatol Sifil 69:558–564, 1928
Pye RJ: Bullous eruptions. In Champion RH, Burton JL, Ebling FJG (eds): Rook/Wilkinson/Ebling Textbook of Dermatology, 5th ed, p 1626. Oxford, Blackwell Scientific, 1992

PASINI-PIERINI

Synonyms. Atrophoderma progressivum; atrophic morphea variant.

Symptoms. Affects more females than males. May begin in infancy or old age, but usually appears in adolescence and early adult life.

Signs. Slight depression below level of normal skin. Lesions are distributed primarily on back of trunk and shoulders, less on the abdomen, seldom on the limbs. They have different shapes (round or oval) colors (violet, brown), and dimensions (2 cm in diameter or larger). They may become confluent and form patches.

Etiology. Unknown. No genetic basis. See Morphea (may represent one of its variants). Some authors maintain that there may exist two forms of such condition: (1) variant of morphea; (2) stable lesion, possibly congenital.

Pathology. Moderate changes at the lesion sites. At onset edema in lower dermis, and clamping of elastic tissue. Later, reduction of dermal thickness.

Therapy. Symptomatic.

Prognosis. Lesions extend very slowly for 10 years, then stabilize. Eventually, sclerodermatous and other changes are possible.

BIBLIOGRAPHY. Pasini A: Atrofodermia idiopatica progressiva (studio clinico ed istologico). G Ital Mal Venereol 64:785–809, 1923
Pierini LE, Vivoli D: Atrofodermia idiopatica progressiva (Pasini). G Ital Dermatol 77:403–409, 1936
Burton JL: Disorders of connective tissue. In Champion RH, Burton JL, Ebling FJG (eds): Rook/Wilkinson/Ebling Textbook of Dermatology, 5th ed, pp 1779–1780. Oxford, Blackwell Scientific, 1992

PASSWELL

Synonym. Ichthyosis—mental retardation—dwarfism—renal changes.

Symptoms and Signs. Both sexes. From birth. Ichthyosis, mental and physical growth retardation; altered renal functions.

Etiology. Unknown. Autosomal recessive inheritance.

BIBLIOGRAPHY. Passwell JH, Goodman RM, Zprkowski M, et al: Congenital ichthyosis, mental retardation, dwarfism, and renal impairment: A new syndrome. Clin Genet 8:59–65, 1975

PATAU

Synonyms. Bartholin-Patau; D1 trisomy; trisomy 13–15.

Symptoms. Present from birth. Least frequent of live-born autosomal trisomies. Recurrent respiratory infections with episodes of cyanosis and apnea. Severe mental retardation. A few cases with motor seizures.

Signs. Constellation of severe malformations. Arhinencephalia; microphthalmia; coloboma of iris; cleft palate and lip; polydactyly; digit fixed in flexion; cardiac and renal defects. All patients are virtually totally deaf. Diffuse capillary hemangiomas. Cyclopia in 55% of cases.

Etiology. Congenital condition resulting from the presence of an extra chromosome of the 13–15 group (D). In some cases: translocation chromosome or isochromosome for long arm of a group D chromosome. Mosaicism for trisomy D has been described.

Pathology. Arhinencephalia with absent olfactory bulbs; fusion of frontal poles; occasionally, agenesis of corpus callosum and defect of cerebellum; double alveolar ridges of upper jaw; cleft palate and lips. *Heart.* Cardiomegaly; ventricular septal defect; patent ductus arteriosus and foramen ovale; other congenital defects. *Kidney.* Bilateral hydronephrosis. *Other organs.* Various abnormalities.

Diagnostic Procedures. *Chromosome study.* Dermatoglyphic pattern. Transverse palmar crease on one or both hands. Bilateral arch fibular S patterns on the feet (typical findings for this condition). *Blood.* Increased amount of hemoglobin F, Bart and Gower, peduncular projections of leukocytes.

Therapy. Symptomatic.

Prognosis. Frequently, stillbirth. Death in infancy from cardiac or other malformations; 70% die within first 3 months of life; survival to childhood extremely rare. Because of the high infant mortality, surgical or orthopedic corrective procedures should be withheld in early infancy to await the outcome of the first few months. Furthermore, because of the severe brain defect, some authorities believe that no medical means should be used to prolong the life of infants with this syndrome.

BIBLIOGRAPHY. Patau K, Smith DW, Therman E, et al: Multiple congenital anomalies caused by an extra autosome. Lancet 1:790–793, 1960
Valentine GH: The Chromosome Disorders. Philadelphia, JB Lippincott, 1966
Hodes ME, Cole J, Palmer CG, et al: Clinical Experience with Trisomies, 18 and 13. J Med Genet 15:48–60, 1978
Avery GB, Fletcher MA, McDonald MC: Neonatology, 4th ed. Philadelphia, JB Lippincott, 1994

PATELLA APLASIA

Symptoms and Signs. Rare. Both sexes. Aplasia or hypoplasia of patella.

Etiology. Autosomal dominant inheritance (?).

BIBLIOGRAPHY. Bernhang AM, Levine SA: Familial absence of patella. J Bone Joint Surg 55A:1088–1090, 1973
Braun HS: Familial aplasia or hypoplasia of the patella. Clin Genet 13:350–352, 1978
Fulckerson JP, Hungerford DS: Imaging the patello femoral joint. In Disorders of the Patello Femoral Joint. Baltimore, Williams & Wilkins, 1990
Graham GP, Fairclough JA: The knee. In Klippel JH, Dieppe PA: Rheumatology, p 5.12.8. St Louis, CV Mosby, 1995

PATELLO-FEMORAL EXCESSIVE LATERAL PRESSURE

Synonyms. ELPS; patellofemoral pain; patellar compression.

Symptoms and Signs. After traumatic or distortion of knee pain, poorly localized, that increases with exercise and weight bearing especially during clumbing stairs, squatting. Sometimes edema or blockage of knee. Strabismus of patellae, sometimes various knee, baionette deformities. During deambulation pronation may be present.

Etiology. Disorders of patellofemoral alignment with increase of Q angle and excessive tension of external alar ligament excessive tension of external (retinaculum latterale) exacerbated by trauma.

Pathology. External alar ligament may be thick, short and harder than normal. Chondromalacia of articular surfaces is a secondary phenomenon.

Diagnostic Procedures. *Radiography.* Few signs. Sulcus angle may be more open and congruence angle may be smaller. *Bone.* Alteration may be present.

Therapy. *Conservative.* Rest, limitation of movement, exercises for quadriceps muscle, NSAIDs, McConnel rehabilitation program. *Surgical.* Lateral release artroscopic or surgical.

Prognosis. Good with therapy.

BIBLIOGRAPHY. Ficat P, Ficat C, Bailleux A: Syndrome d'hyperpression externe de la rotule (SHPE): Son intérete pour la connaisance del l'arthrose. Rev Chir Orthop 61:39, 1975
Fulckerson JP, Hungerford DS: Imaging the patello femoral joint. In Disorders of the Patello Femoral Joint, p 42. Baltimore, Williams & Wilkins, 1990
Insall JN, Windsor RE, Scott WN, et al (ed): Surgery of the Knee, p 330. New York, Churchill Livingstone, 1993
Graham GP, Fairclough JA: The Knee. In Klippel JH, Dieppe PA: Rheumatology, pp 5.12.8–5.12.9. St Louis, CV Mosby, 1995

PATIN

Synonyms. Guy-Patin; Muenchmeyer; fibrodysplasia ossificans progressiva; fibrosis ossificans progressiva; FOP; interstitial ossifying myositis; myositis ossificans progressiva (misnomer, see Calcinosis universalis); stone man.

Symptoms. Both sexes affected. Prevalent in males (according to various authors 4:1, 3:1, 3:2, or 2:1); onset usually before 10 years of age. Pain and tenderness during contraction of some muscles (which in time become generalized).

Signs. Localized swelling first in neck region, then in the back and, finally, in the limbs; initially, lumps may appear and disappear several times; stiffness of muscles; synostoses of various joints. Frequently associated with microdactyly of little fingers, valgus deviation of great toes,

development of exostoses. Progressive rigidity of thorax with respiratory and cardiac insufficiency. Tendency to ecchymosis. Tongue, heart, larynx, diaphragm, and sphincters not affected.

Etiology. Autosomal dominant inheritance; 90% of cases represent fresh mutation.

Pathology. Biopsy of initial lesions shows extensive proliferation of interstitial cellular connective tissue with very moderate inflammatory changes; formation of reticular fibers and collagen, which retracts and compresses muscle fibers; finally, the muscle fibers fragment and degenerate. The whole process is followed by osteoid formation, which extends peripherally like normal bone (muscle fibers may remain within bone tissue).

Therapy. Symptomatic. Diphosphonate (apparently useful).

Prognosis. Progressive disability and incapacitation. Possibly, arrest of ossifying process. Long survival possible. Death from intercurrent conditions.

BIBLIOGRAPHY. Muenchmeyer E: Ueber Myositis ossificans progressive. Z Ration Med 34:1, 1869
Helferich H: Ein Fall von sogenamter Myositis ossificans progressiva. Aerztl Intelligenz-Blatl 26:485, 1874
Connor JM, Evans DAP: Fibrodysplasia ossificans progressiva: The clinical features and natural history of 34 patients. J Bone Joint Surg 64:76–83, 1982
Connor JM: Soft Tissue Ossification. New York, Springer-Verlag, 1983
Bruni L, Giammaria Tozzi MC, et al: Fibrodysplasia ossificans progressiva: An 11-year-old boy treated with diphosphonate. Acta Ped Scand 79:994–998, 1990

PATTERSON-DAVID

Synonyms. Pseudoleprechaunism. See Danohue.

Symptom and Signs. Both sexes. From birth. Normal birth weight. Large hands, feet, nose and ears. Cutis laxa and generalized bronzed hyperpigmentation. Hirsutism, mental retardation, seizures, generalized skeletal and joint disorders; cushingoid features, premature menarche.

Etiology. Unknown.

Pathology. *Adrenals.* Enlarged (zona fasciculata). *Bones.* Endochondrial calcification, retarded skeletal maturation.

Diagnostic Procedures. *Blood.* Hyperglycemia insulin-resistant, hyperinsulinemia; absence of insulin antibodies, hyperdehydroepiandrosterone and androstenedione.

Therapy. Symptomatic.

Therapy. Survival beyond infancy.

BIBLIOGRAPHY. Patterson JH, Nafkins WL: Leprechaunism in a male infant. J Pediatr 60:730–739, 1962
Patterson JH: Presentation of a patient with leprechaunism. Birth Defects 5:117–121, 1969
David TJ, Webb BW, Gordon IRS: The Patterson syndrome: Leprechaunism and pseudoleprechaunism. J Med Genet 18:294–298, 1981
Gorlin RJ, Cohen MM, Levin LS: Syndromes of Head and Neck, 3rd ed, p 822. New York, Oxford University Press, 1990

PAUTRIER ABSCESS

Symptoms and Signs. Observed in mycosis fungoides (see) and other lymphomas.

Pathology. Intradermal cellular infiltration with foci of reticular cells and eosinophils.

BIBLIOGRAPHY. Weatherall DJ, Ledingham JGG, Warrell DA (eds):

Oxford Textbook of Medicine, 3rd ed, p 3797. Oxford, Oxford Med Pub, 1996

PAUTRIER-WORINGER

Synonyms. Dermatopathic lymphadenopathy; hypomelanotic reticulosis exfoliative.

Symptom. Severe pruritus (not constant).

Signs. Various generalized dermatoses: Exfoliative dermatitis of different etiologies; different types of neurodermatitis; prurigo; seborrheic dermatitis; lichen planus; pemphigus; psoriasis. Lymphadenopathy.

Etiology. Observed in the early stage of mycosis fungoides or with other primary dermopathies. To be differentiated from similar malignant processes, e.g., Hodgkin.

Pathology. *Skin.* That of various dermatoses. *Lymph nodes.* Histopathologic pattern of granulomatous hyperplasia with respect to normal architecture (exceptionally, may be altered); marked degree of hyperplasia of reticular cells, especially in the paracortical area. Varying deposits of melanin and lipid within macrophages. Eosinophilic, polymorphonuclear, and plasma cell infiltration.

Diagnostic Procedures. *Biopsy.* Of lymph node and skin.

Therapy. That of specific dermatosis. Infiltration with half-strength triamcinolone.

Prognosis. Lymph node hyperplasia may regresses according to nature of dermatosis and efficacy of treatment.

BIBLIOGRAPHY. Pautrier LM, Woringer F: Note preliminaire sur un tableau histologique particulier de lésions ganglionnaires accompagnant des eruptions dermatologiques généralisées, prurigineuses, des types cliniques différents. Bull Soc Fr Dermatol Syph 39:947–955, 1932
Pautrier LM, Woringer F: Contribution á l'étude de l'histo-physiologie cutanée; á propos d'un aspect histopathologique nouveau du ganglion lymphatique; la réticulose lipo-maelanique accompagnant certaines dermatoses généralisées; les échanges entre la peau et le ganglion. Ann Dermatol Syph 8:257–273, 1937
Schnyder UW, Schirrer CG: So-called "lipomelanotic reticulosis" of Pautrier-Woringer. Arch Dermatol Syph 70:155–165, 1954
Isaacson PG, Norton AJ: Extranodal Lymphomas, p 152. Edinburgh, Churchill Livingstone, 1994

PAVOR NOCTURNUS

Synonym. Nightmare.

Symptoms. Observed especially in children. Sleep disturbance resulting in moaning, agitation, and difficulty in waking rapidly, or the child awakens abruptly in a state of intense fright, screaming. Possible association with sleepwalking. Usually in the morning there is no memory of the dream.

Signs. Tachycardia, tachypnea.

Etiology. Unknown. In association with frightening dreams.

Diagnostic Procedures. *Electroencephalography.* For differential diagnosis with epilepsy. *EEG.* During the episode shows a waking type of mixed frequency of alpha pattern.

Therapy. None, or psychiatric consultation. Diazepam prevents episode (do not use for protracted periods).

Prognosis. When not expressing major psychotic disturbances, excellent.

BIBLIOGRAPHY. Sheehan DV, Raj BA: Panic attacks and the cardiovascular system. In Schlant RC, Alexander RW, et al: Hurst's The Heart, 8th ed. New York, McGraw-Hill, 1994

PAVY

Synonyms. Cyclic albuminuria; functional proteinuria; asymptomatic proteinuria; transient proteinuria, postural proteinuria; orthostatic proteinuria.

Symptoms and Signs. Asymptomatic. Finding usually discovered accidentally on routine analysis.

Etiology. Unknown. Diagnosis by exclusion after ruling out all possible systemic and local disorders. May represent an after effect of subclinical glomerulonephritis.

Diagnostic Procedures. *Urine.* Proteinuria usually less than 2 g/day. Careful analysis to search for other possible findings. *Blood.* Electrophoresis; creatinine clearance.

Therapy. None. Followup for possible identification of basic pathologic process.

Prognosis. Good. Sometime subsides spontaneously after months or years.

BIBLIOGRAPHY. Pavy FW: Cyclic albuminuria (albuminuria in the apparently healthy). Lancet 2:707–708, 1885
Opas LM, Lieberman E: Fluid and electrolyte disorders in infants and children. In Massry SG, Glassock RJ: Textbook of Nephrology, 3rd ed, pp 530–535. Baltimore, Williams & Wilkins, 1995

PAYR

Synonyms. Splenic flexure. See Irritable bowel and gas syndromes.

Symptoms. Occurs in about 20% of patients with irritable colon, usually postprandially. The abdominal pain is present in the left upper quadrant, radiation pain may be manifested in precordial area, left thoracic or shoulder areas, neck and arm, or pain and pressure in the rectum. Systemic manifestations may also occur; tachycardia; dyspnea.

Signs. Abdominal distention (occasional) on palpation of spastic colon.

Etiology. See Irritable colon. Spasm or intrinsic or extrinsic compression of colon resulting in gas accumulation in splenic flexure.

Diagnostic Procedure. *X-ray.* Gas accumulation and distention localized in the splenic flexure.

Therapy. See Irritable bowel or treat organic obstruction if present.

Prognosis. Depends on etiology.

BIBLIOGRAPHY. Payr E: Ueber eine eigentümliche, durch abnorm starke Klickunge und Adhäsionen bedinge gucartige Stenose der Flexura lienalis und hepatice coli. Verh Dtsch Keng Inn Med 27:276–305, 1910
Lasser RB, Bond JH, Levitt MD: The role of intestinal gas in functional abdominal pain. N Engl J Med 293:524–526, 1975
Eastwood MH, Eastwood J, Ford MJ: The irritable bowel syndrome: A disease or a response? (Discussion paper). J Roy Soc Med 80:219–221, 1987

PEARSON

Synonym. Marrow—pancreas.

Symptoms and Signs. Both sexes. In infancy. Severe refractory anemia (transfusion dependency); malabsorption or other signs of pancreatic exocrine insufficiency. When patients grow they develop Kearns-Sayre (see).

Etiology. Unknown. Possibility of autosomal inheritance.

Pathology. *Pancreas.* Fibrosis. *Spleen.* Aplasia.

Diagnostic Procedures. *Blood.* Sideroblastic anemia. *Bone marrow.*

Normal cellularity, sideroblastic anemia with vacuolization of marrow precursors. *Hepatosplenicpancreatic echography.*

Therapy. Blood transfusions.

Prognosis. Death in early infancy; if survival, hematologic improvement and possible development of Kearns-Sayre.

BIBLIOGRAPHY. Pearson HA, Lobel JS, Kocoshis SA, et al: A new syndrome of refractory sideroblastic anemia with vacuolization of marrow precursors and exocrine pancreatic dysfunction. J Pediatr 95:976–984, 1979

Roting A, Cormier V, Blanche S, et al: Pearson's marrow-pancreas syndrome: A multisystem mitochondrial disorder in infancy. J Clin Invest 86:1601–1608, 1990

McShane MA, Hamman SR, Sweeny M, et al: Pearson syndrome and mitochondrial encephalopathy in a patient with deletion of mtDNA. AM J Hum Genet 48:39–42, 1991

PECTUS EXCAVATUM

Synonyms. Hollow chest; cobbler chest; funnel chest.

Symptoms and Signs. Usually asymptomatic. Deformity of sternum.

Etiology. Autosomal dominant inheritance reported. Observed in Marfan and other congenital syndromes (leopard, Marden-Walker, otopalatodigital). Occupational deformity (cobblers).

Therapy. Surgery to correct defect.

Prognosis. May lead to respiratory insufficiency. Good result with surgery when indicated.

BIBLIOGRAPHY. Peiper A: Ueber die Erblichkeit der Trichterburst. Klin Wschz 1:1647, 1922

Sugiura Y: A family with funnel chest in three generations. Jap J Hum Genet 22:287–289, 1977

Leung AKC, Hoo JJ: Familial congenital funnel chest. Am J Med Genet 26:887–890, 1987

Sabiston DC: Textbook of Surgery, 14th ed, pp 1761–1763. Philadelphia, WB Saunders, 1991

PEL

Synonyms. Ciliary tabetic neuralgia; neuralgic ciliary tabetic; ophthalmic crisis. See Duchenne.

Symptoms and Signs. One of the many possible crises occurring in tabes dorsalis: neuralgic paroxysmal pains affecting the eyes and the ophthalmic area(s).

Etiology. Syphilis (see Duchenne).

Therapy. Specific therapy of little value.

Prognosis. That of tabes.

BIBLIOGRAPHY. Pel PK: Augenkrisen bei Tabes dorsalis (Crisen ophthalmiques). Berl Klin Wochenschr 25:25–27, 1898

Greenwood RJ: Neurosyphilis. In Weatherall DJ, Ledingham JGG, Warrell DA (eds): Oxford Textbook of Medicine, 3rd ed, p 4085. Oxford, Oxford Med Pub, 1996

PELGER-HUET

Synonym. Granulocyte anomaly of Pelger.

Symptoms and Signs. Found chiefly in Germany and Holland (1:1000); in United States (1:10,000). No symptoms. In spite of abnormal leukocytes, resistance to infections is not lowered. Occasionally, other congenital or familial anomalies are associated.

Etiology. Unknown. Autosomal dominant transmission with partial carrier of the trait reported. Some type of leukocyte anomaly may be observed in different conditions: pelgeroid anomalies reported in cases of leukemia, Fanconi anemia syndrome, and following treatment with myelotoxic agents.

Pathology. None.

Diagnostic Procedures. *Blood.* Neutrophils with eccentric and frequently fragmented nuclei with coarse chromatin. Normal cytoplasmic maturation. Condensation of chromatin in lymphocytes, monocytes, and even in megakaryocytes and erythroblasts. *Bone marrow.* Some anomaly observed.

Therapy. None.

Prognosis. Benign condition.

BIBLIOGRAPHY. Pelger K: Demonstratie van een paar zeldzaam voorkomende typen van bloedlichaampjes en bespreking der patiënten. Ned Tijdschr Geneeskd 72:1178, 1928

Huët GJ: Over een familiare anomalie der leucocyten. Mschr Kindergeneesk 1:173–181, 1932; (abstr) Ned Tijdschr Geneeskd 75:5965–5969, 1931

Aznar J, Vaya A: Homozygous form of Pelger–Huet leukocyte anomaly in men. Acta Haematol 66:59–62, 1981

Fishbein JD, Falletta JM: Pelger-Huet anomaly in an infant with multiple congenital anomalies. Am J Hemat 38:240–242, 1991

PELIZAEUS-MERZBACHER (INFANTILE TYPE)

Synonyms. Spielmeyer type PMD; aplasia axialis extracorticalis congenita; brain sclerosis diffuse familial; sudanophilic leukodystrophy. See Schilder; Krabbe; Scholz.

Symptoms. Almost exclusively in males (a few cases reported in females, see Etiology); onset in early childhood except in severe forms (within first 3 months of life). Aimless, wandering eye movements, usually not rhythmic, "eye waggers." Failure to develop normal head control, "head nodders" head and eye movements may later disappear. General lag of development; slow growth and weight gain. Further evolution: spasticity of all extremities, subnormal mental development, and frequently, optic atrophy.

Signs. Head size low-normal or microcephaly; height below third percentile. Sensory system usually well preserved.

Etiology. X-linked inheritance. A certain amount of confusion exists in classification of this syndrome since different criteria have been used in the various reports. When clinical and genetic criteria were used: only male patients (exceptionally, female in Lyon theory) in whom the disease develops in infancy and who have a history of sex-recessive type of genetic inheritance have been (correctly) included. If only pathologic criteria were used, a vast heterogenous group of different clinical entities have been designated with this eponym.

Pathology. Widespread demyelinization in centrum semiovale, cerebellum, and part of brain stem; axis cylinder preserved; throughout white matter, diffuse gliosis and small amounts of perivascular sudanophilic lipid (perinuclear or in fat granules cell). The presence of "myelin islands" in demyelinated areas ("tiger" or "leopard" skin) is considered by many authors the characteristic pathologic finding, and on the basis of its presence the diagnosis of Pelizaeus-Merzbacher made; this diagnosis includes Lowenberg-Hill (dominant inheritance occurring in adult) and other syndromes with this pathologic finding (see Norman-Landing). On the basis of presence or absence of myelin islands, the clinical Pelizaeus-Merzbacher syndrome has also been subdivided in Pelizaeus-Merzbacher type (present) and Seitelberg type (absent).

Diagnostic Procedures. *CSF.* Normal. *X-ray. CT scan. MRI.* Neuroimages normal in first stages then diffuse atrophy (nonspecific). Osteoporosis; kyphoscoliosis (to be interpreted as secondary and not as genetic associated defects). *EEG.*

Therapy. Symptomatic.

Prognosis. In many cases, death in early childhood. Course chronic. Some patients may live to be 60 years old.

BIBLIOGRAPHY. Pelizaeus F: Über eine eigenthumliche Form spastischer Lähmung mit Cerebraler Scheinungen auf hereditärer Grundlage (Multiple Sklerose). Arch Psychiatr Nervenkr 16:698–710, 1885
Merzbacher L: Eine eigenartige familiärhereditare Erkrankungsform (Alpasia axialis extracorticalis congenita). Z Ges Neurol Psychiatr 3:1–138, 1910
Spielmeyer W: Der anatomische Befund bei einem zweiten Fall von Pelizaeus–Merzbacherscher Krankheit. Zentralbl Ges Neurol Psychiatr 32:203, 1923
Norman RM, Tingey AH, Harvey PW, et al: Pelizaeus-Merzbacher disease: A form of sudanophil leukodystrophy. J Neurol Neurosurg Psychiatr 29:521–529, 1966
Cassidy SB, Sheehan NC, Farrell DF, et al: Connatal Pelizaeus-Merzbacher disease: An autosomal recessive form. Pediat Neurol 3:300–305, 1987
Zoghbi HY, Ballabio A: Pelizaeus-Merzbacher disease. In Scriver CR, Beaudet AL, Sly WS, et al: The Metabolic and Molecular Bases of Inherited Disease, 7th ed, pp 4581–4585. New York, McGraw-Hill, 1995

PELLEGRINI-STIEDA

Synonyms. Koehler-Stieda; Stieda-Pellegrini; knee, medial collateral ligament calcification; perarticular knee calcification.

Symptom. Stiffness and pain in and above knee.

Signs. Swelling (not constant).

Etiology. Controversial.

Pathology. Periosteal proliferation or osseous metaplasia of ligament; detached fractured bone fragments from medial femoral condyle; calcified epiperiosteal or soft tissue hematoma; bursa or tendon calcification.

Diagnostic Procedure. *X-ray.*

Therapy. Conservative: physical therapy; roentgen therapy. Surgery: last resort.

Prognosis. Good. Many patients recover spontaneously.

BIBLIOGRAPHY. Pellegrini A: Ossificazione traumatica del legamento collaterale tibiale dell' articolazione del ginocchio sinistro. Clin Mod Firenze 11:433–439, 1905
Graham GP, Fairclough JA: The knee. In Klippel JH, Dieppe PA: Rheumatology, p 5.12.6. St Louis, CV Mosby, 1995

PELLIZZI

Synonyms. Macrogenitosomia precox; pineal; pubertas precox; quadrigeminal plate. See 21- and 11β-Hydroxylase deficiency.

Symptoms and Signs. Onset in childhood. Accelerated increase in height, weight, musculature, and development of sexual characteristics; frequently associated with pineal tumor neurologic syndrome (see).

Etiology. Unknown. Usually associated with destructive tumors of pineal gland. Suppression of an hypothetical pineal hormone that inhibits gonadal development or indirect stimulation of gonadotropin secretion by pressure on the hypothalamus and pituitary. Possible role of pineal through secretion of melatonin as means of timing puberty.

Pathology. Gliomas, teratomas, or necrotic and anaplastic pinealoma.

Diagnostic Procedures. *X-ray of skull. MRI. CT scan.* Occasionally, calcification of pineal gland. *Hormone study.* Gonadotropin determination.

Therapy. Surgery. Radiation therapy.

Prognosis. Depends on etiology and result of surgery.

BIBLIOGRAPHY. Heubner O: Fall von Tumor der Glandula pinealis mit ergenthümlichen Washsthumanomalien. Ver Ges Dtsch Naturf Aerzte, 1898; Leipzig, 1899
Pellizzi GB: La sindrome epifisaria "macrogenitosomia precoce," Riv Ital Neuropatol (Catania) 3:193–207; 250, 1910–1911
Rao YTR, Medini E, Haselow RE, et al: Pineal and ectopic pineal tumors: The role of radiation therapy. Cancer 48:708–713, 1981
Cohen AR, Wilson JA, Sadeghi-Nejad A: Gonadotrophin-secreting pineal teratoma causing precocious puberty. Neurosurgery 28:597–602, 1991

PELVIS-SHOULDER

Synonyms. Scapoloiliac dysostosis.

Symptoms and Signs. Severe hypoplasia of scapulas, pelvis and clavicles. Associated malformations: eye (ectopic pupil); ribs; and spine (bifida).

Etiology. Unknown autosomal dominant inheritance.

BIBLIOGRAPHY. Kosenow W, Niederle J, Sinios A: Becken-Schulter-Dysplasia. Fortschr Roentgenstr 113:39–48, 1970
Moroteaux P: Nomenclature internationale des maladies osseouses constitutionelles. Ann Radiol 13:455–464, 1970
Thomas PS, Reid M, McCurdy AM: Pelvis-Shoulder dysplasia. Pediatr Radiol 5:219–233, 1977

PEMPHIGUS VULGARIS

Symptoms and Signs. Both sexes affected, common in Jews; onset in middle age (40–60 years of age). At first localized lesion in the mouth, bullae, and painful erosion of mouth; other mucosae may also be involved. Eventual appearance of skin lesion: bullae; crusting; erosion; easy bleeding; no tendency to heal; no itching. Any part of skin involved, zones of friction and face more often involved. Eventual healing; no scar; hyperpigmentation.

Etiology. Unknown. Possibly familial condition (autosomal dominant), virus or autoimmune reaction (?).

Pathology. Suprabasal acantholysis, with intraepithelial splitting and bullae.

Therapy. Corticosteroids. Immunosuppressive agents: cyclosporine; azathioprine; cyclophosphamide; methotrexate. Gold sodium thiomalate. Plasma exchange.

Prognosis. Death within 2 years if not treated. Forty percent mortality with treatment.

BIBLIOGRAPHY. Voelter WW, Newell GB, Schwartz SL, et al: Familial occurrence of pemfigus foliaceus. Arch Dermatol 108:93–94, 1973
Alijotas J, Pedragosa R, Bosch J, et al: Prolonged remission after cyclosporine therapy in pemphigus vulgaris: Report of two siblings. J Am Acad Dermatol 23:701–703, 1990
Pye RJ: Bullous eruptions. In Champion RH, Burton JL, Ebling FJG (eds): Rook/Wilkinson/Ebling Textbook of Dermatology, 5th ed, pp 1638–1642. Oxford, Blackwell Scientific, 1992

PENA-SHOKEIR I

Synonyms. Arthrogryposis multiplex congenita; pulmonary hypoplasia; akinesia, fetal sequence; fetal akinesia sequence. See Bowen.

Symptoms and Signs. Both sexes. From birth. Joint contractures, diffuse muscle athrophy, campodactyly, facial anomalies. Respiratory difficulties. Heart arrhythmias.

Etiology. Most cases sporadic or autosomal recessive inheritance. Primary motor neuropathy. Deformation sequence by fetal akinesia (?).

Pathology. Muscle atrophy and substitution by fibers and fat; spinal cord reduction of anterior horn cells; lungs muscle hypoplasia; adrenal hypoplasia.

Diagnostic Procedures. *X-ray. Sonography.* (Prenatal diagnosis) hydramnios, ankyloses; lung hypoplasia.

Prognosis. Repeated respiratory infections cause of death, usually, within first days of life.

BIBLIOGRAPHY. Pena SDJ, Shokeir MHK: Syndrome of campodactyly, multiple ankyloses, facial anomalies and pulmonary hypoplasia: A lethal condition. J Pediatr 85:373–375, 1974
Katzenstein M, Goodman RM: Pre- and postnatal findings in Pena-Shokeir I syndrome: Case report and a review of literature. J Craniofac Genet Dev Biol 8:111–126, 1988
Perlman JM, Burns DK, Twinckler DM, et al: Fetal hypokinesia syndrome in the monochorionic pair of a triplet pregnancy secondary to severe disruptive cerebral injury. Pediatrics 94:521–52,3 1995

PENA-SHOKEIR II

Synonyms. Cerebro-oculo-facio-skeletal; COFS. See also Cockayne, Hallermann-Streiff, Seckel, and Bowen (P.).

Symptoms. Onset from birth. Vomiting, regurgitation. Failure to thrive.

Signs. *Head.* Microcephaly; micrognathia; prominent nasal root; large ears, microphthalmia; blepharophimosis; cataract. *Extremities.* Contractures of elbow and knee; camptodactyly; single palmar crease; clenched fists; longitudinal groove on feet; rocker-bottom feet; coxa valga. *Trunk.* Kyphosis; scoliosis; widely spaced nipples. Muscle hypotonia.

Etiology. Autosomal recessive inheritance. Considered as a different degree of clinical expression of the Bowen's (P.) (or Pena-Shokeir I).

Pathology. See Signs. Generalized cerebral subcortical gliosis.

Diagnostic Procedures. *X-ray.* Osteoporosis; intracranial calcifications; vertical tali and displacement of second metatarsal bone. *Blood. Urine.* Normal.

Therapy. Orthopedic.

Prognosis. Repeated respiratory infections cause of death, usually, within first 3 years.

BIBLIOGRAPHY. Pena SDJ, Shokeir MKH: Autosomal recessive cerebro-oculo-facio skeletal (COFS) syndrome. Clin Genet 5:285–293, 1974
Silego MC, Davi G, Bianco R, et al: The NEW-COPFS (cerebro-oculo-facio-skeletal) syndrome: Report of case. Clin Genet 25:201–204, 1984
Gershoni-Baruch R, Ludatscher RM, Lichting C, et al: Cerebro-oculo-facio-skeletal syndrome: Further delineation. Am J Med Genet 41:74–77, 1991

PENDRED

Synonym. Familial goiter—deaf mutism.

Symptoms. Affects both sexes equally. Various degrees of bilateral sensineural deafness from birth or developing in childhood (perceptive in type; in some cases associated with defective vestibular function); more complete loss in high, than in low tones. Goiters dating from middle childhood that may be of any degree of severity, from just detectable to goitrous cretinism. Usually, normal physical and mental development.

Signs. Size of thyroid from just detectable to 200 g. In children, diffuse enlargement; in adults, more clearly nodular.

Etiology. In majority of cases autosomal recessive inherited defect. The deafness and goiter are independent expressions of same gene defect.

Pathology. Not well known. Mondini defect (malformation of the cochlea).

Diagnostic Procedures. *Audiography.* Sensorineural loss. *Blood. Urine.* Normal except mild glucose intolerance protein-bound iodine (PBI) butanol-extractable iodine (BEI), total and free thyroxine low or normal; antithyroid antibodies absent. Low to absent T4; accumulation and turnover of radioiodine. Perchlorate test (method described to recognize the type of thyroid defect found in this syndrome); rapid discharge of radioiodine from thyroid after administration of perchlorate or sulphocyanide (SCN). *Biopsy.* Hyperplasia; low iodine content; absent or abnormal peroxidase activity.

Therapy. No specific treatment in cases of large goiter or borderline hyperthyroidism thyroxine. If partial thyroidectomy, thyroxine or thyroid extract may prevent regrowth of thyroid.

Prognosis. No treatment may correct deafness. Goiter usually recurs (in absence of treatment) after partial thyroidectomy.

BIBLIOGRAPHY. Pendred V: Deaf-mutism and goiter. Lancet 2:532, 1896
Thould AK, Scowen EF: Genetic studies of the syndrome of congenital deafness and simple goiter. Ann Hum Genet 27:283–293, 1964
Friis J, Johnsen T, Felotta Rasmussen U: Thyroid function in patients with Pendred's syndrome. J Endocrinol Invest 11:97–101, 1988
DeGroot LJ: Congenital defects in thyroid hormone formation and action. In De Groot LJ (ed): Endocrinology, 3rd ed, pp 876–877. Philadelphia, WB Saunders, 1995

PENFIELD

Synonym. Autonomic diencephalic epilepsy.

Symptoms and Signs. Prevalent in males; onset at 6 or 7 years of age. Seizures accompanied by vegetative manifestations: congestion of face; sialorrhea; perspiration; tears; exophthalmos; tachycardia; polypnea; restlessness; logorrhea. The attacks are of different duration and terminate with a short period of obnubilation.

Signs. Proptosis; excessive lacrimation; pupillary abnormalities; tachycardia; blood pressure elevated. Possibility of intermittent hydrocephalus.

Etiology. Hypothalamic dysfunction and epileptic stimulus from lesions located on the floor of third ventricle.

Pathology. One case reported of third ventricle tumor.

Diagnostic Procedures. *Electroencephalography. CT scan. MRI.*

Therapy. Phenobarbital; carbamazepine; primidone. Surgery.

Prognosis. Depends on etiology.

BIBLIOGRAPHY. Penfield W: Diencephalic autonomic epilepsy. Arch Neurol Psychiatr 22:358–374, 1929
Kohler MC: L'association "comitialité, croissance excessive et puberte précoce, arriération mentale," une forme particulière de séquelles d'encéphalopathies ou d'encéphalite infantile. J Med (Lyon) 48:1437–1503, 1967
Adams RD, Victor M: Principles of Neurology, 3rd ed, p 453. New York, McGraw-Hill, 1993

PEPPER

See Parker.

Symptoms and Signs. Those of Parker (see) plus those consequent to liver metastasis.

BIBLIOGRAPHY. Pepper W: A study of congenital sarcoma of the liver and suprarenal with report of a case. Am J Med Sci 121:287–299, 1901

PERHEENTUPA

Synonyms. Mulibrey (muscle—liver, brain—eye) dwarfism; pericardial constriction—growth failure; growth failure—pericardial constriction.

Symptoms. Prevalent in Finns. Low birth weight. Progressive growth failure and delayed puberal development with oligomenorrhea; quiet voice. Amblyopia. Neoplasms are common.

Signs. At birth, asphyxia or cyanosis. Median adult height 135 cm for females, 145 cm for males. Dwarfism with thin limbs; fibrous dysplasia of tibia. *Skin.* Nevus flammeus (see). *Muscle.* Hypotonia. *Facies.* Triangular, bulging forehead; low nasal bridge; alternating esotropic-exotropic strabismus. *Fundus oculi.* Yellowish retinal spots; hypoplasia of chorion capillaries. *Neck.* Prominent veins. *Chest.* Pulmonary congestion; cardiac enlargement; evidence of pericarditis and health failure. *Abdomen.* Ascites; hepatomegaly.

Etiology. Unknown. Autosomal recessive inheritance.

Pathology. See Signs. Myocardial and pericardium fibrosis.

Diagnostic Procedures. *ECG.* Evidence of myocardial hypertrophy and failure. *X-ray. MRI. CT scan of chest.* Pericardial calcium deposit. Of head. Log shallow, J-shaped sella turcica; large cerebral ventricles and cisterns. *Electroretinography.* Normal.

Therapy. Surgery for pericardial constriction.

Prognosis. According to cardiac involvement. Mortality high at all ages. Many patients reach adulthood and may lead a productive life.

BIBLIOGRAPHY. Perheentupa J, Autio S, Leirti S, et al: Mulibrey nanism: Dwarfism with muscle, liver, brain and eye involvement. Acta Paediatr Scand 59:74, 1970
Raitta C, Perheentupa J: Mulibrey nanism: An inherited dysmorphic syndrome with characteristic ocular findings. Acta Ophthalmol (Suppl 123) 52:162–171, 1974
Perheentupa J: The Finnish disease heritage: A personal look. Acta Paed 84:1094–1099, 1995

PERHEENTUPA-VISAKORPI

Synonyms. Protein intolerance defective transport of basic amino acids; dibasic aminoaciduria II.

Symptoms and Signs. Prevalent in Finns. From birth feeding difficulties, vomiting, diarrhea, lethargy, convulsions, hyperammonemic coma. Mental retardation, hepatosplenomegaly, short stature, osteoporosis, lens opacities. Skin hyperelastic, joint hyperextensible, hair brittle.

Etiology. Autosomal recessive inheritance. Defect of intestinal and renal transport of dibasic amino acids. Alteration of the mechanism by which amino nitrogen is transferred to the urea-synthesizing system.

Pathology. *Liver biopsy.* Minimal fatty degeneration. Osteopenia.

Diagnostic Procedures. *Blood.* Hyperammonemia, transaminase elevation; low dibasic amino acid levels, glutamine and alanine increased. *Urine.* Excretion of dibasic amino acids increased. Diagnosis is based on dibasic aminoaciduria without cystinuria. *X-rays.* Marked skeletal fragility.

Therapy. Low protein diet.

Prognosis. Reduced life expectancy.

BIBLIOGRAPHY. Perheentupa J, Visakorpi JK: Protein intolerance with deficient transport of basic amino acids. Lancet 2:813–816, 1965
Carpenter TO, Levy HL, Holtrop ME, et al: Lysinuric protein intoler-

ance presenting as childhood osteoporosis: Clinical and skeletal response to citrulline therapy. N Engl J Med 312:290–294, 1985
Perheentupa J: The Finnish disease heritage: A personal look. Acta Paed 84:1094–1099, 1995

PERINEAL

Symptoms and Signs. Periodic intense perineal itching localized on raphe, accompanied by local sweating; usually worse after prolonged driving, sitting, or fatigue.

Etiology. Unknown. No clear organic basis.

Therapy. Sedatives. Topical corticosteroids.

Prognosis. Period of remission or relapse not always correlated with treatment or alleged pathogenetic factors.

BIBLIOGRAPHY. Champion RH, Burton JL, Ebling FJG (eds): Rook/Wilkinson/Ebling Textbook of Dermatology, 5th ed, p 2801. Oxford, Blackwell Scientific, 1992

PERIODIC ARTHRALGIA

Synonym. Bone pain, periodic.

Symptoms and Signs. Episodic pain located in the shafts of the long bones. It is reminiscent of the pain of sickle cell anemia.

Etiology. Unknown. No instance of male-to-male transmission has been noted; 33 persons in seven generations were considered affected.

Diagnostic Procedures. *X-ray.* For ruling out other diseases.

Therapy. Symptomatic.

Prognosis. Good.

BIBLIOGRAPHY. Reimann HA, Angelides AP: Periodic arthralgia in 23 members of five generations of a family. JAMA 146:713–716, 1951
McKusick V: Mendelian Inheritance in Man. Baltimore, Johns Hopkins University Press, 1992

PERIODIC HYPOTHERMIA

Synonyms. Cyclic hypothermia; hypothermia, recurrent.

Symptoms and Signs. Episodic attacks of icy coldness (rectal temperature below 30°C) with sweating, vasodilatation, vomiting, and bradycardia. Occasionally signs of diabetes insipidus, and signs related to growth hormone deficiency.

Etiology. Possible hypothalamus alteration. In several cases corpus callosum agenesis (see).

BIBLIOGRAPHY. Mooradian AD, Morley GK, McGeachie R, et al: Spontaneous periodic hypothermia. Neurology 34:79–82, 1984

PERIODIC PARALYSIS, III (TYPE A)

Synonym. Normokalemic periodic paralysis; normohyperkalemic periodic paralysis; adynamia episodica.

Symptoms. Onset in early infancy. Stable symmetric proximal weakness (floppy babies); episodes of quadriparesis lasting 2–3 weeks. Trunk ataxia and tremor may be present. Characteristic craving for salt, intense thirst, and stomach pains at onset of attacks, which begin usually in the morning after awaking.

Signs. Muscle hypotonia; no fasciculation or fibrillation; no sensory disturbances; tendon reflexes hypoactive; good coordination taking into consideration degree of hypotonia.

Etiology. Autosomal dominant inheritance autonomy of the condition challenged. Considered the same of hyperkalemic form (see).

Pathology. Muscle biopsy shows two types of fibers: one staining lighter with hematoxylin and eosin (normal); one staining darker, containing small vacuoles that do not stain and are diffuse in the intermyofibrillar areas. Granular material is also contained in the same areas in a lesser number of dark fibers. Cytochemistry shows increased and enlarged mitochondria in 20–40% of muscle cells. Fatty infiltrates in muscle cells.

Diagnostic Procedures. *Blood. Urine.* Normal. *Electromyography.* Myopathic pattern. *Biopsy of muscle.* See Pathology.

Therapy. Sodium chloride, potassium salts do not improve or precipitate attacks.

Prognosis. Improvement between attacks as years pass.

BIBLIOGRAPHY. Poskanzer DC, Kerr DNS: A third type of periodic paralysis with normokalemia and favorable response to sodium chloride. Am J Med 31:328–342, 1961
Shy GM, Gonatas NK, Perez MC: Two childhood myopathies with abnormal mitochondria. I. Megaconial myopathy. II. Pleoconial myopathy. Brain 89:133–158, 1966
Spiro AJ, Prineas JW, Moore CL: A new mitochondrial myopathy in a patient with salt craving. Arch Neurol 22:259–269, 1970
Harper PS: Myotonic dystrophy and other autosomal muscular dystrophies. In Scriver CR, Beaudet AL, Sly WS, et al: The Metabolic and Molecular Bases of Inherited Disease, 7th ed, p 4242. New York, McGraw-Hill, 1995
Walton J, Karpati G, Hilton-Jones D: Disorders of Voluntary Muscle, p 657. Edinburgh, Churchill Livingstone, 1994

PERIODIC SIALADENOSIS

Synonyms. Recurring salivary adenitis; sialorrhea periodic; sialoadenitis chronica.

Symptoms. Sudden, recurrent episodes of discomfort on parotid, submaxillary, or submandibular glands; saliva formation increased or decreased. Cephalalgia; vomiting; diarrhea; occasionally, pain in the abdomen, thorax, or extremities.

Signs. Swelling of involved glands. In some cases, dermographia, urticaria.

Etiology. Unknown. Neurovascular (?); allergic (?); infective (?).

Pathology. Salivary gland edema; after repeated episodes, possibly, signs of chronic inflammation and aspecific eosinophil and monocyte infiltration.

Diagnostic Procedures. *Blood.* Leukocytes normal. *Sedimentation rate.* Normal. *Sialography.* Normal.

Therapy. Corticosteroids. Proposed subtotal paratidectomy.

Prognosis. Episode may last hours or days. Recurrence typical.

BIBLIOGRAPHY. Isacsson G, Ahlner B, Lundquist PG: Chronic sialoadenitis of the submandibular gland. A retrospective study of 108 cases. Arch Otorhinolaryngol 232:91–100, 1981
Schultz PW, Woods JE: Subtotal parotidectomy in the treatment of chronic sialadenitis. Ann Plast Surg 11:459–461, 1983
Brook I: Diagnosis and management of parotitis. Arch Otolaryngol Head Neck Surg 118:469–471, 1992

PERISYLVIAN, DEVELOPMENTAL

Synonyms. Congenital bilateral perisylvian. See Foix-Chavany-Marie.

Symptoms and Signs. Both sexes, prevalent in females. From birth. Oropharyngoglossal dysfunction (100%); moderate to severe dysarthria

(100%); delayed milestone (85%); epilepsy (atypical absence and atonic seizures) (85%); mental retardation (85%); arthrogryposis multiplex (50%); other limbs malformations (50%); infantile spasms (50%).

Etiology. Unknown. Disturbance of cerebral embryogenesis. Genetic with unknown mode of transmission.

Pathology. Bilateral perisylvian cortical dysplasia compatible with polymicrogyria and incomplete opercula formation.

Diagnostic Procedures. *CT scan. MRI. Cerebral angiography.* Symmetrical bilateral sylvian and rolandic macrogyria, extending into parietal regions; cortex is smooth and thick (lesion limited to sylvianrolandic region). *EEG.* Variable abnormalities, nonepileptiform, epileptiform, and ictal.

Therapy. Symptomatic. Corpus callosotomy.

Prognosis. Good for survival. Callosotomy causes improved behavior and cessation of drop attacks.

BIBLIOGRAPHY. Woster-Drpought C: Speech disorders of children of school age. Press 230:419–426, 1953
Kuzniecky R, Andermann F, Guerrini R, et al: Congenital bilateral perisylvian syndrome: Study of 31 patients. Lancet 3421:608–612, 1993
Kuzniecky R, Andermann F, Guerrini R, et al: The epileptic spectrum in the congenital bilateral perisylvian syndrome. Neurology 44:379–385, 1994

PERKOFF

Synonyms. Slocumb; poststeroid myopathy; Cushing-therapeutic myopathy; steroid myopathy; steroid pseudorheumatism. See Mueller-Kugelberg.

Symptoms and Signs. Both sexes affected; onset at all ages. Following prolonged administration of corticosteroids, muscle weakness, mostly of the thighs; moderate muscle atrophy; mild tendon hyporeflexia. Association with other feature of Cushing syndrome (see). Weakness is relieved by short periods of sleep.

Etiology. Corticosteroid administration.

Pathology. Moderate muscle fiber vacuolization.

Diagnostic Procedures. *Urine.* Excretion of large amount of creatine (200–1000 mg/day), reduced creatinine (1 g/day). *Blood.* See Cushing.

Therapy. Cessation of corticosteroid administration.

Prognosis. Prompt restoration of muscle power after discontinuation of steroids.

BIBLIOGRAPHY. Perkoff GT, Silber R, Tyler FH, et al: Myopathy due to the administration of therapeutic amounts of 17-hydroxycorticosteroids. Am J Med 26:981–988, 1959
Slocumb CH: Rheumatoid arthritis. In Brown J, Pearson GM (eds): Clinical Use of Adrenal Steroids, pp 30–43. New York, McGraw-Hill, 1962
Adams RD, Victor M: Principles of Neurology, 5th ed, pp 1235–1236. New York, McGraw-Hill, 1993

PERLMAN

Synonyms. Liban-Kozenitzki; renal hamartomas; nephroblastomatosis; fetal gigantism; nephroblastomatosis; fetal ascites; macrosomia; Willms tumor.

Symptoms and Signs. Both sexes. At birth. Large body size; unusual facies; ascites; polyhydramnios; visceromegaly; cryptorchidism

Etiology. Unknown. Possibly autosomal recessive inheritance.

Pathology. Bilateral renal hamartomas with or without nephroblastomatosis. Pancreas; hypertrophy of Langerhans islets. Described also atrophy of corpus callosum.

Diagnostic Procedures. *Blood.* Hyperinsulinism. *X-rays. Echography.*

Therapy. None attempted. Correction of hyperinsulinism could improve survival chances.

Prognosis. All patients died as infants.

BIBLIOGRAPHY. Liban E, Kozenitzky IL: Metanephric hamartomas and nephroblastomatosis in siblings. Cancer 25:885–888, 1970

Perlman M, Goldberg GM, Bar-Ziv J, et al: Renal hamartomas and nephroblastomatosis with fetal gigantism: A familial syndrome. J Pediatr 83:414–418, 1973

Greenberg F, Coperland Gresik MV, et al: Expanding the spectrum of the Perlman syndrome. Am J Med Genet 29:773–776, 1988

Hamel BCJ, Mannens M, Bokkerink JPM: Perlman syndrome: Report of a case and result of molecular studies. Am J Med Genet 45:A48, 1989

PERNIO

Synonyms. Chilblain, acute; dermatitis hiemalis; perniosis, erythema pernis; erythrocyanosis; lupus pernio. See Immersion foot.

Symptoms and Signs. Acute chilblain. More frequent in children and women. Usually bilateral and symmetric lesions. Dermatitis, bluish red; slight edema. Itching and burning worsened by warm temperature, affecting fingers, toes, and legs (parts exposed to cold). Acute stage usually lasting 1 week; brownish pigmentation may appear and persist for months after lesion heals. Occasionally, hemorrhagic reaction, ulceration, and infection may appear as complications. Chronic chilblain. Repeated acute episodes result in chronic lesions with residual fibrosis and atrophy of skin and subcutaneous tissues. During warm season, lesions may disappear completely.

Etiology. Reaction of peripheral blood vessels to cold (slow-freeze variety).

Pathology. Angiitis; necrosis of panniculus adiposus; chronic inflammatory reaction of subcutaneous tissues. In long-standing lesions, hyperpigmentation and iron deposits.

Therapy. Avoidance of exposure to cold. In chronic severe form, production of fever may clear the lesions quickly. Nifedipine in severe cases may help. Ultraviolet radiation weekly (three doses) at onset of winter. Thyroxin in presence of proved hypothyroidism. Antipruritic local application. In severe form not responding to conservative treatment, sympathectomy.

Pathology. *Acute.* Benign, self-limited. *Chronic.* Avoiding exposure to cold prevents recurrences.

BIBLIOGRAPHY. Miller W: De Pernionibus. Jence, 1680

Champion RH: Reactions to cold. In Champion RH, Burton JL, Ebling FJG (eds): Rook/Wilkinson/Ebling Textbook of Dermatology, 5th ed, pp 835–836. Oxford, Blackwell Scientific, 1992

PERONEAL COMPARTMENT

Synonyms. Peroneal muscles, ischemic necrosis; march gangrene; shin splint.

Symptoms. Follows continuous and prolonged exertion; rapid onset. Leg tired and aching; then swelling and severe pain. Elevation and heat treatment do not relieve the pain.

Signs. Loss of dorsiflexion and inversion; any motion produces pain. Firm consistency of anterolateral portion of leg. Pulses of dorsalis pedis and posterior tibial arteries not palpable.

Etiology. Severe exertion determining diminished blood flow to muscles.

Pathology. Muscle ischemic necrosis of various degrees from massive necrosis to spotty muscle necrosis; no evidence of thrombosis of vessels.

Diagnostic Procedures. *X-ray.* Of leg (to rule out bone trauma). *Blood.* Myoglobulinemia; serum enzymes. *Urine.* Myoglobinuria.

Therapy. Extensive fasciotomy.

Prognosis. Fasciotomy helpful up to 6–9 days after onset. If condition allowed to progress, both anterior tibial (because of secondary compression) and peroneal compartments become impaired, and inversion and clubfoot result.

BIBLIOGRAPHY. Blandy JP, Fuller R: March gangrene: Ischemic myositis of the leg muscles from exercise. J Bone Joint Surg 39B:679, 1957

Reszel PA, Janes JM, Spittell JA Jr: Ischemic necrosis of the peroneal musculature: A lateral compartment syndrome; report of a case. Proc Staff Meet Mayo Clinic 38:130–136, 1963

Lunceford EM Jr: The peroneal compartment syndrome. South Med J 58:621–623, 1965

Slocum DB: The shin splint syndrome. Am J Surg 114:875–881, 1967

Adams RD, Victor M: Principles of Neurology, 5th ed, pp 1164–1165. New York, McGraw-Hill, 1993

PERRAULT

Synonym. Ovarian dysgenesis—deafness; gonadal dysgenesis XX type-deafness; deafness—ovarian dysgenesis.

Symptoms and Signs. *In females.* Bilateral neural-sensory deafness and symptoms of Turner (see). *In males (of same family).* Facultative deafness and normal sexual development.

Etiology. XX dysgenesis; demonstrated a 46 XX karyotype.

BIBLIOGRAPHY. Perrault M, Klotz B, Houset E: Deux cas de syndrome de Turner avec surdi-mutism dans une meme fratrie. Bull Neur Soc Med Hosp (Paris) 16:79–84, 1951

McCarthy DJ, Opitz JM: Perrault's syndrome in sisters. Am J Med Genet 22:629–631, 1985

Forest MG: Diagnosis and teatment of disorders of sexual development. In DeGroot LJ (ed): Endocrinology, 3rd ed, p 1908. Philadelphia, WB Saunders, 1995

PERRY

Synonyms. Parkinsonism; alveolar hypoplasia; mental depression.

Symptoms and Signs. Both sexes. Onset late in V decade. Mental depression (not responsive to pharmacological or electroconvulsive treatment); insomnia, fatigue, weight loss. Parkinson symptoms follow later. Respiratory failure terminal event.

Etiology. Unknown. Autosomal dominant inheritance.

Pathology. Substancia nigra: marked neuronal loss and reactive gliosis. Neurochemical studies. Basal ganglia: depletion of dopamine and also serotonin in substantia nigra.

Diagnostic Procedures. See Parkinson. C.S.F. and blood: taurine decreased and low level (in C.S.F.) of homovalinic acid, GABA and 5-hydroxy indolacetic acid.

Therapy. See Parkinson. Aggressive management for episodes of respiratory failure.

Prognosis. Death occurs 4–6 years from onset of symptoms because of respiratory failure.

BIBLIOGRAPHY. Perry TL, Bratty PJA, et al: Hereditary mental depression and parkinsonism with taurine deficiency. Arch Neurol 32:108–113, 1975

Perry TL, Wright JM, Berry K, et al: Dominantly inherited apathy, central hypoventilation and parkinsonism's syndrome. Clinical, biochemical and neuropathological studies of 2 new cases. Neurology 40:1882–1887, 1990

PERSISTENT HYPERPLASTIC PRIMARY VITREOUS

Synonym. PHPV; persistent tunica vasculosa lentis; pseudophakia fibrosa.

Symptoms and Signs. Usually unilateral, in full term infants of both sexes and all races. Leukoria, rarely presenting signs: nystagmus or squint. Affected eye: usually microphthalmic.

Etiology. Idiopathic persistence and proliferation of normally transient vasculature of primary vitreous, in particular tunica vasculosa lentis leading to formation of retrolental mass with subsequent visual loss. No hereditary influence. It is common in trisomy 13 (see).

Pathology. *Eye.* Opacity induced by a funnel shaped mass of fibro vascular tissue occupyng the retrolental space and site of Cloquet canal. Tissue is vascular and may show evidence of repeated hemorrhages. Iris abnormalities may be associated.

Diagnostic Procedures. Fundoscopy.

Therapy. Surgery: (1) aspiration of all lens material; and (2) creation of clear pupillary space by excision of part of retrolental membrane.

Prognosis. Untreated cases proceed to phthisis bulbi. Vitrectomy has improved outcome. Visual acuity remains poor, but enucleation is not necessary.

BIBLIOGRAPHY. Reese AB: Persistent hyperplastic primary vitreous. Am J Ophthalmol 40:317, 1955

Stark WJ, et al: Persistent hyperplastic primary vitreous: surgical treatment. Ophthalmology 90:452–457, 1983

Torczynski E: Developmental anomalies of the eye. In Garner A, Klintworth GK (eds): Pathobiology of Ocular Disease A Dynamic Approach, 2nd ed, p 1315. New York, Marcel Dekker, 1994

PERSISTENT MUELLERIAN DUCT

Synonyms. PDMS; hernia uteri inguinalis.

Symptoms and Signs. Rare. Normal male virilization, Undescended testes, sometimes located in the same inguinal canal. Testes and hernia (containing uterus and tubes) are palpable; in other cases accidental discovery of the presence of a uterus and fallopian tubes in addition to normal Wolffian structures during surgical interventions.

Etiology. Failure to produce Muellerian-inhibiting hormone, in other cases resitance of the tissue to the action of the hormone. Disorder often familial, either X-linked or sex-limited autosomal inheritance.

Pathology. See Symptoms and Signs.

Diagnostic Procedure. *Echography.*

Therapy. Surgical repair of cryptorchidism.

Prognosis. If spermatogenesis, stored fertility is possible.

BIBLIOGRAPHY. Nilson O: Hernia uteri inguinalis. Acta Chir Scand 83:231–249, 1939

Forest MG: Diagnosis and treatment of disorders of sexual development. In Degroot LJ (ed): Endocrinology, 3rd ed, pp 1921–1922. Philadelphia, WB Saunders, 1995

PETER

To be considered a morphologic entity but not a specific causal entity. See also Ruthenfurd, Gorlin-Chaudhry-Mass, Rieger, and Fraser.

Symptoms and Signs. Visual impairment owing to incomplete separation of lens vesicle, central corneal opacity, synechiae residues of pupillary membrane.

Etiology. Major error in the embryonic development of the eye. Possibly, autosomal recessive inheritance

Therapy. Corneal transplant.

Pathology. Defect of corneogenic mesoderm.

BIBLIOGRAPHY. Peter A: Ueber angeborene Defekbildung der descemetschen Membran. Klin Monatsbl Augenhkeilkd 44:27–40, 105–119, 1906

Stone D, et al: Congenital central corneal Leukoma (Peter's anomaly). Am J Ophthalmol 81:173, 1976

Kivlin JD, Fineman RM, Crandall AS, et al: Peter's anomaly as a consequence of a nongenetic syndromes. Arch Ophthalmol 104:61–64, 1986

Garner A, Klintworth GK (eds): Pathobiology of Ocular Disease: A Dynamic Approach, 2nd ed. New York, Marcel Dekker, 1994

PETER PAN

Symptoms and Signs. Pale soft skin, finely textured lack of hair and a high-pitched voice observed in some syndromes, i.e., Loren-Levi, craniopharyngioma, etc.

BIBLIOGRAPHY. Vinken PJ, Bruyn GW: Handbook of Clinical Neurology, vol 18, p 545. Amsterdam, North-Holland, 1975

PETGES-CLÉJAT

Obsolete.

Synonyms. Poikiloderma atrophicans vasculare; poikilodermatomyositis; Petges-Jacobi; Jacobi. Poikiloderma-mycosis fungoides stage I A (see Etiology).

Symptoms. Usually occurs in young adults. Muscular weakness.

Signs. Areas of skin with pigmented poikiloderma; telangiectasis, atrophy, and calcinosis may also be observed. Muscular wasting.

Etiology. Once excluded lupus erythematodes, dermatomyositis, and drug eruption this condition is better termed poikilodermatous mycosis fungoides (MFT1, or stage I A). Practically the poikiloderma atrophicans vasculare includes MF-associated poikiloderma and forms of poikiloderma non-MF associated.

BIBLIOGRAPHY. Petges G, Cléjat C: Sclérose atrophique de la peau et myosite généralisée. Arch Dermatol Syph 7:550–568, 1906

Guy W, Grauer RC, Jacob FM: Poikilodermatomyositis. Arch Dermatol Syph 40:867–878, 1939

PETIT

Eponym used to indicate mydriasis, increased intraocular pressure, and alterations of retina vessels owing to an irritation of sympathetic nervous system. See Bernard and Horner.

BIBLIOGRAPHY. Petit F: Mémoire dans laquel il est Dé-montré que les Nerfs Intercosteaus Fournissent des Rameaux qui Portens des esprits dans les Yeux. Hist Acad Sci Paris 1–18, 1727

PETIT HERNIA

Symptoms and Signs. Hernia in Petit triangle (lombar region).

BIBLIOGRAPHY. Petit JL: Traité des maladies chirurgicals, et des opérations qui leur conviennent, vol 2, pp 256–268. Paris, Didot 1774
Sabiston DC: Textbook of Surgery, 14th ed, p 1. Philadelphia, WB Saunders, 1991

PETIT MAL

Synonyms. Lennox triad; epilepsia minor; pyknoepilepsy.

Symptoms. Condition starts in childhood; often so mild that no attention is paid to it. Loss of consciousness with or without minimal muscle spasms; loss of contact with environment; usually after a few seconds the patient resumes his activity. No sequelae.

Signs. Eyes look ahead without seeing; small spastic contractions of eyelids, face, or arm occasionally present. Lennox triad: petit mal; akinetic seizures; myoclonic jerks.

Etiology. Unknown. It is felt that this syndrome may represent an hereditary and probably a metabolically determined form of epilepsy.

Diagnostic Procedure. *EEG.*

Therapy. Trimethadione; paramethadione; phensuximide; ethosuximide.

Prognosis. This type of attack tends to decrease or disappear with age; it may be followed in older age by the development of the grand mal syndrome.

BIBLIOGRAPHY. See Epileptic syndromes.
Matthes A, Weber H: Klinische und electroenzephalographische Familienunter-suchungen bei Pyknolepsien. Dsch Med Wochenschr 93:429–435, 1968
Scheuer ML, Pedley TA: The evaluation and treatment of seizures. N Engl J Med 323:1468–1474, 1990

PETZETAKIS-TAKOS

Synonyms. Trophopenic keratitis; keratoconjunctivitis trophica.

Symptoms and Signs. Superficial keratitis (presence of multiple phlyctenules on cornea); palpebral edema; cornea hyperesthesia; photophobia; blepharospasm; decreased iridic reflexes; xerophthalmia; impaired vision; lymph node hypertrophy.

Etiology. Malnutrition (especially vitamin A deficiency); lack of hygiene.

Pathology. Break in corneal epithelium; scars; hypertrophy of preauricular lymph nodes.

Therapy. Diet; antibiotics. Hygienic measures. Control of convulsions and general supportive measures.

Prognosis. Fair with adequate treatment.

BIBLIOGRAPHY. Petzetakis M: Le troubles oculaires pendant la trophopénie (maladie aedémateuse) et l'épidémie de la pellagre. (1941–1944). La keratopathie superficielle trophopenique (Kératopathie épithéliale). Presse Med 58:1082–1084, 1950
Klintworth GK: Vitamin deficiencies and excesses. In Garner A, Klintworth GK (eds): Pathobiology of Ocular Disease: A Dynamic Approach, 2nd ed, p 1152. New York, Marcel Dekker, 1994

PEUTZ-JEGHERS

Synonyms. Hutchinson-Weber-Peutz; Jeghers; Peutz-Touraine; cutaneous pigmentation, intestinal polyposis; lentigiopolypose, digestive; melanoplakia, intestinal polyposis; intestinal polyposis II.

Symptoms. Both sexes, all ethnic groups affected. Symptoms begin in adolescence. Recurrent severe abdominal pain, relieved by vigorous abdominal manipulation; unusual borborygmus; later, occasionally, massive intestinal hemorrhage.

Signs. From birth "black freckles": melanotic pigmentation 2–5 mm in diameter sometimes coalescing on the lips, oral mucosa, cheek, nose, fingers, palms, toes, forearm, or abdominal area. Mucosa pigmentation permanent; cutaneous lesion may appear and fade at puberty or afterward.

Etiology. Congenital autosomal dominant condition.

Pathology. Multiple adenomatous polyps growing in crops in ileum, jejunum, and less frequently, stomach and colon.

Diagnostic Procedures. *X-ray.* Of intestine. Multiple polyps. *Blood.* Anemia. *Stool.* Occult blood.

Therapy. Gastrointestinal tract roentgenograms every 2 years from puberty to full maturity. Uncomplicated polyps removed by excision; if intussusception with necrosis, extensive resection.

Prognosis. If all polyps removed when full adult life reached, no additional polyps develop. If not removed, they may grow and complications arise (hemorrhage; intussusception). Possibly, malignant transformation of gastric and duodenal polyps at early age. Frequent association with tumor development at other sites: breast, ovary, thyroid, pancreas, etc.

BIBLIOGRAPHY. Hutchinson J: Pigmentation of the lips and mouth. Arch Surg London 7:290, 1896
Peutz JLA: Over een zeer merkwaardige, gecombineerde familiairie polyposis van de slimjmvliezen van den tractus intestinalis met die van de neuskeelholte en gepaard met eigenaardige pigemntaties van huiden slijmvliezen. Ned Maandschr Geneesk 10:134–146, 1921
Jeghers H, McKusick VA, Katz KH: Generalized intestinal polyposis and melanin spots of the oral mucosa, lips and digits: Syndrome of clinical significance. N Engl J Med 241:993–1005; 1031–1036, 1949
Spigelman AD, Murday V, Phillips RKS: Cancer and the Peutz-Jeghers syndrome. Gut 30:1588–1590, 1989
Haubrich WS, Schaffner F, Berk JE (eds): Bockus Gastroenterology, 5th ed, pp 1738–1739. Philadelphia, WB Saunders, 1995

PEYRONIE

Synonyms. Buren; van Buren; corpora cavernosa plastic induration; penile fibrosis; induratio penis plastica; penis plastic induration.

Symptoms. Onset in middle-aged or elderly males. Pain and curvature of penis; ability to achieve erection distal to process; interference with coitus.

Signs. Palpation of irregular lump along dorsum of penis.

Etiology. Unknown; frequent association with Dupuytren contracture (see). Induced by adrenergic blockers (propanolol, practolol). Possibility of familial transmission (autosomal dominant male, limited). Reported chromosomal alterations.

Pathology. Pearly gray fibrous area in cavernous sheaths extending linearly or in separate bodies; flat plaques. Microscopically, keloid-like lesion, absence of inflammatory changes, occasionally calcified lesions.

Diagnostic Procedures. *Serology.* Rule out syphilis. *Biopsy.* Rule out malignancy. *Echography.* To evaluate extent and evolution.

Therapy. Reassurance about benign nature of process. Alpha-tocopherol has been used with some benefit. X-rays, diathermy, massage, electrolysis occasionally helpful. A variety of surgical correction proposed.

Prognosis. Chronic condition; poor response to all types of therapeutic approach. Surgical removal of lesion followed by recurrences.

BIBLIOGRAPHY. de la Peyronie F: Sur quelques obstacles qui s'opposent à l'éjaculation naturelle de la semence. Mem Acad Chir Paris 1:425, 1743

Bias WB, Nybery LM Jr, Hochberg MC, et al: Peyronie disease: A newly recognized autosomal dominant trait. Am J Genet 12:227–235, 1982

Guerneri S, Stioui S, Mantovani F, et al: Multiple clonal chromosome abnormalities in Peyronie disease. Cancer Genet Cytogenet 52:181–185, 1991

PFEIFFER (E.)

Synonyms. Acute epidemic infective adenitis; glandular fever; Drüsenfieber. See Infectious mononucleosis. Infectious mononucleosis-like syndrome.

Symptoms. Both sexes affected. Onset usually in childhood. Highly contagious.

Signs. Mild throat inflammation; adenopathy limited to cervical nodes; absence of splenomegaly (except in prolonged cases).

Etiology. Unknown. Several viruses and toxoplasma have been reported. Condition separated from infectious monocytosis (mononucleosis) on clinical and epidemiologic grounds by Hoagland, particularly cytomegalovirus.

Therapy. General supportive measures; for serious infections caused by toxoplasma, sulfadiazine with pyrimethamine.

Prognosis. Much shorter duration than infectious monocytosis.

BIBLIOGRAPHY. Pfeiffer E: Drüsenfieber. Jahrb Kinderheilkd 29:257–264, 1889

Hoagland RJ: Infectious Mononucleosis. NY, Grune & Stratton, 1967

Magnussen CR, Chessin LN: Infectious mononucleosis and mononucleosis-like syndromes. In Reese RE, Gordon DR (eds): A Practical Approach to Infectious Diseases, p 463. Boston, Little, Brown, 1986

Foerster J: Infectious mononucleosis. In Lee GR, Bithell TC, Foerster J, et al (eds): Wintrobe's Clinical Hematology, 9th ed, pp 1850–1851. Philadelphia, Lea & Febiger, 1993

PFEIFFER-PALM-TELLER

Synonym. PPT.

Symptoms and Signs. Brother and sister. Unique amimic facies, ears cup-shaped, narrow palpebral fissure with epicanthal folds, enamel hypoplasia, short stature, progressive joint stiffness, congenital aortic stenosis.

Etiology. Unknown. Possibly autosomal recessive inheritance.

BIBLIOGRAPHY. Pfeiffer RA, Palm D, Teller W: A syndrome of short stature, amimic facies, enamel hypoplasia, slowly progressing stiffness of joint and high-pitched voice in two siblings. J Pediatr 91:955–957, 1977

PFEIFFER (R.A.)

Synonyms. Acrocephalosyndactyly IV; ACS IV; see Noack (possibly same condition).

Symptoms and Signs. Present from birth. *Head.* Brachycephaly; high forehead; hypertelorism; antimongoloid palpebrae; small nose; narrow maxilla; gothic palate. *Hands and feet.* Syndactyly (second and third digits); broad thumbs (pointing outward); broad short great toes. Normal intelligence. Occasionally, elbow synostosis; choanal atresia.

Etiology. Autosomal dominant inheritance.

Pathology. Craniosynostosis; phalangeal malformations and fusion with adjacent bones.

Therapy. None usually required or according to degree of craniosynostosis.

Prognosis. With age facies tends to improve. Normal mental development.

BIBLIOGRAPHY. Pfeiffer RA: Dominante erbliche Akrocephalosyndactylie. Z Kinderheilkd 90:301–320, 1964

Naveh Y, Freidman A: Pfeiffer's syndrome. Report of a family and review of literature. J Med Genet 13:272–280, 1976

Stone P, Trevenen CL, Mitchell I, et al: Congenital tracheal stenosis in Pfeiffer syndrome. Clin Genet 38:145–148, 1990

PHALANGEAL MICROGEODIC

Synonyms. Microgeotic phalangeal.

Symptons and Signs. Both sexes. Mostly from Japan (age 18 months to 2 years). One European report (age 6.5 years). Swelling, redness, heat, and moderate pain in the fingers usually in winter.

Etiology. Unknown.

Diagnostic Procedures. *X-rays.* Small lacunae in bones of affected fingers; mild widening of phalanges.

Therapy. None.

Prognosis. Regression within few months.

BIBLIOGRAPHY. Maroteaux P: Cinq observations d'une affection microgéodique des phalanges du nourisson d'étiologie inconnue. Ann Radiol (Paris) 13:229–239, 1970

Kaibara N, Masuda S, Katsuki I, et al: Phalangeal microgeodic syndrome in childhood. Report of seven cases and review of the literature. Eur J Pediatr 136:41–46, 1981

Inace Miura: Microgeotic disease affecting the hands and feet of children. J Pediat Orthop 11:53–63, 1991

Hoeffel: Microgeodic phalangeal syndrome in an infant: Commentary. Pediatr Radiol 22:80–81, 1992

PHANTOM LIMB

Synonyms. Limb phantom. Includes telescoping (see Prognosis).

Signs. Amputee. Occurs following amputations: 20% of patients no phantom; 67% phantom phenomena; 13% painful phantom. Eighty-five percent of the last groups combined present the syndrome immediately, 7% in less than a month, and remainder within 1 year. "Natural" phantom or phantom phenomena: sensation that amputated part is still present, aligned with the stump and moving with it. Painful phantom limb: phantom pains felt in missing limb from vague unpleasant feeling to crushing pain. Patient may feel missing finger and toes curled up and that they cannot be unclenched.

Etiology. *Organic.* Neuroma of cut nerve or other irritative mechanism in the stump. *Psychogenic.*

Pathology. Scar of stump; neuroma.

Diagnostic Procedures. *X-ray.* Of stump and spine and joints involved indirectly by amputations.

Therapy. Intrathecal fentanyl. Excision (not satisfactory because neuroma reforms). Infiltration of the area of stump (under light anesthesia) with hydrocortisone; elastic stump sock to be worn day and night; postural correction for muscular imbalance. Reamputation to improve vascularity and mobility. Psychotherapy with sedatives or tranquilizers; electroconvulsive therapy. Cordotomy; tractotomy; ablation of postcentral cortex.

Prognosis. "Natural" phantom tingling sensation becomes weaker and usually disappears within 2 or 3 years, sometimes persisting longer. In some cases telescoping phenomenon "gradual reduction of the sensation of persisting limb as from a retraction of a telescope." Best results in painful phantom limb when treatment started early and when local causes of irritation promptly found and removed. Central pain much more difficult to treat.

BIBLIOGRAPHY. Paré A: La manière de traicter les playes faictes tat par hacquebutes que par flèche: et les accidentz d'icelles, côme fractures et caries d'os, gangrene et mortification; avec les pourtraictz des instrumentz necessaires pour leur curation. Et la méthode de curer les combustions principalement faictes par la pouldre à canon, 2nd ed. Paris, Ieau de Brie, on Arnoul l'Angelier, 1552
Mitchell SW: Phantom limbs. Lippincott's Mag 8:563–569, 1871
Gillis L: The management of the painful amputation stump, and a new theory for the phantom phenomena. Br J Surg 51:87–95, 1964
Jacobson L, Chabal C, Brody MC: Relief of persistent postamputation stump and phantom limb pain with intrathecal fentanyl. Pain 37:317–322, 1989
Stannard CF: Phantom limb pain. BR J Hosp Med 50:583–587, 1993

PHENYLKETONURIA II

Synonyms. Dihydropterine reductase deficiency; DHPR deficiency; PKU atypical; quinoid dihydropterine reductase deficiency.

Symptoms and Signs. Both sexes. Onset in neonatal period. Progressive neurological signs (basal ganglia) different from those of classical PKU and that do not respond to low phenylalanine diet.

Etiology. Autosomal recessive inheritance. Possibly a disorder of biopterin metabolism due to a defect of the dihydropterine reductase. Several alleles identified.

Pathology. Basal ganglia and subcortical calcifications.

Diagnostic Procedures. *Blood.* Increased serum phenylalanine. *Urine.* Phenylketonuria. Cultured fibroblasts from liver, brain. Absence of dihydropterine reductase.

Therapy. Intravenous tetrahydropterine. Oral therapy no effect.

Prognosis. Manifestations less severe than in Folling.

BIBLIOGRAPHY. Smith I, Clayton BE, and Wolff OH: New variant of phenylketonuria with progressive neurological illness unresponsive to phenylalanine restriction. Lancet I, 1108–1111, 1975
Scriver CR, Kaufman S, Woo SLC: The hyperphenylalaninemias. In Scriver CR, Beaudet AL, Sly WS, et al: The Metabolic and Molecular Bases of Inherited Disease, 6th ed, pp 495–546. New York, McGraw-Hill, 1989

PHENYLKETONURIA III

Synonyms. Dihydrobiopterin synthetase deficiency; biopterin deficiency; phosphate eliminating enzyme, deficiency of; PEE deficiency; tetrahydropterin deficiency. Phenylketonuria VI.

Symptoms and Signs. From early infancy. Hypotonia and delayed motor development.

Etiology. Autosomal recessive inheritance. Defect in biopterin synthesis postulated.

Diagnostic Procedures. *Blood. Urine.* Biopterin and biopterin-like compounds low. Serum biopterin does not increase with phenylalanine load (as it does in normals and PKU).

Therapy. Dietary control of phenylalanine does not ameliorate situation. Treatment with oral tetrahydropterine restores adequate phenylalanine hydrolase activity and improves CNS function.

Prognosis. Fair with treatment.

BIBLIOGRAPHY. Kaufman S, Holtzman NA, Milstien S, et al: Phenylketonuria due to a deficiency of dihydroperidine reductase. N Engl J Med 293:785, 1975
Rey F, Harpey JP, Leeming RJ, et al: Les hyperphenylalaninemies avec activite normale de la phenylalanine-hydroxylase: les deficit en tetrahydropterine et le deficit en dihydropteridine reductase. Arc Franc Pediat 34:109–120, 1977
Niederweiser A, Shintaku H, Leimbacher W, et al: "Peripheral" tetrahydrobiopterin deficiency with hyperphenylalaninemia due to incomplete 6–pyruvoyl tetrahydropterine synthetase deficiency or eterozygosity. Eur J Pediat 146:228–232, 1987
Scriver CR, Kaufman S, Eisensmith RC, et al: The hyperphenylalaninemias. In Scriver CR, Beaudet AL, Sly WS, et al: The Metabolic and Molecular Bases of Inherited Disease, 7th ed, pp 1046–1051. New York, McGraw-Hill, 1995

PHEOCHROMOCYTOMA

Synonyms. Chromaffinoma; paroxysmal hypertension; medullary paraganglioma. See also Multiple endocrine neoplasia III, Wermer, and Sipple; von Recklinghauser.

Symptoms. Equal incidence in both sexes. Onset from childhood to old age (highest incidence between third and fourth decades). Headache, frequently paroxysmal and associated with palpitations or tachycardia, tachypnea, tremor, sweating, nausea, and emesis. Postural hypotension; weakness and fatigue; chest pain. Seldom: paroxysmal flashing and/or psychic changes.

Signs. Paroxysmal hypertension; weight loss; pallor; decreased GI motility; possibly, neurocutaneous lesions.

Etiology. Autosomal dominant inheritance. It may be associated with many syndromes: von Hippel-Lindau; Von Reckinghausen; MEN II and III; etc

Pathology. Tumor arising from chromaffin cells of paraganglia from the neck through posterior mediastinum, along the aorta to the pelvis. In 19% of cases, multiple; adrenal most frequent site; in 10% of cases, malignant.

Diagnostic Procedures. *Urine. Plasma.* Fasting hyperglycemia. Catecholamines and metabolites increased. *Provocative tests.* Tyramine, glucagon, histamine, or phentolamine (depressor test). Intravenous pyelography, angiography, iodoscan, venography, vena cava catheterization, and venous sampling. *CT scan. MRI.* Localization of tumor.

Therapy. Surgery preceded by and integrated with medical control. Medical therapy: (for inoperable cases only) alpha- and beta-adrenergic blocking agents. Alpha-methylparatyrosine.

Prognosis. Good with surgery. Fair with medical treatment.

BIBLIOGRAPHY. Fraenkel F: Ein Fall von deppelseitigem, voelling latent verlaufenen nebennieren Tumor und gleichzeitiger Nephritis mit veraenderungen am Circulationsapparat und Retinitis. Virchows Arch (A) 103:244–263, 1886
Masson P, Martin J: Paraganglioma surrenal, étude d'un cas humain de tumeurs malignes de la medullo-surrenale. Bull Assoc Fr Cancer 12:135–141, 1923
Mayo C: Paroxysmal hypertension with tumour of retroperitoneal nerve: Report of a case. JAMA 89:1047–1050, 1927
Khosla S, Patel VM, Hay ID, et al: Loss of heterozygosity suggests multiple genetic alterations in pheochromocytomas and medullary thyroid carcinomas. J Clin Invest 87:1691–1699, 1991
Bravo EL: Diagnosis of pheochromocytoma: Reflections on a controversy. Hypertension 17:742–744, 1991
Keiser HR: Pheochromacytoma and related tumors. In De Groot LJ (ed): Endocrinology, 3rd ed, pp 1853–1877. Philadelphia, WB Saunders, 1995

PHLEBECTASIA OF JEJUNUM, ORAL CAVITY, AND SCROTUM

Symptoms. Peptic ulcer symptoms and occasionally symptoms of gastrointestinal bleeding.

Signs. Caviar spot of the tongue; angiokeratoma (spot) of Fordyce of the scrotum; melena.

Etiology. Unknown.

Pathology. *Stomach.* Chronic gastritis; pyloric hypertrophy; duodenal ulcer. *Jejunum.* Thin-walled vessels within submucosa and in the serosa. In some cases, cecum also mildly involved. Phlebectasis of tongue and scrotum.

Diagnostic Procedures. *X-ray.* Of gastrointestinal tract. *Stool.* Gastric analysis. Search for occult blood.

Therapy. Treatment of ulcer; if blood loss, exploratory laparotomy and measures to correct bleeding.

Prognosis. Depends on extent of intestinal tract lesions and bleeding.

BIBLIOGRAPHY. Rappaport I, Schiffman MA: Multiple phlebectasia involving jejunum, oral cavity, and scrotum. JAMA 185:437–440, 1963
Miller DA, Akers WA: Multiple phlebectasia of the jejunum, oral cavity, and scrotum. Arch Intern Med 121:180–182, 1968
Young AE: Combined vascular malformations. In Mulliken JB, Young AE (ed): Vascular Birthmarks. Philadelphia, WB Saunders, 1988

PHLEBOARTERIECTASIS DIFFUSE

Symptoms and Signs. In a part or in the whole limb congenital ectatic of entire arterial and venous system with or without bone hypertrophy.

Etiology. Unknown. Syndrome autonomy contested.

Diagnostic Procedures. Arterio and phlebography.

Therapy. Surgery.

BIBLIOGRAPHY. Malan E, Puglionisi A: Congenital angiodysplasas of the extremities. J Cardiovasc Surg 5:87–130, 1964
Young AE: Combined vascular malformations. In Mulliken JB, Young AE (eds): Vascular Birthmarks, pp 246–274. Philadelphia, WB Saunders, 1988

PHLEBODYNIA

Synonym. Vein pain.

Symptoms. Prevalent in adult females; occurs in epidemic form in community. Severe pain along superficial and deep veins and legs. Mild constitutional symptoms: malaise, headache, and minimal fever.

Signs. Tenderness over affected extremities; no redness or that over course of vein; sensation of turgor of the vein along its course (thickened wall or thrombus?). Homans sign; moderate swelling on one leg or both.

Etiology. Unknown. The possibility of mass hysteria considered.

Pathology. Biopsy of vein shows no gross abnormality. Absence of thrombus; possibly, moderate edema of wall.

Diagnostic Procedures. All negative.

Therapy. No response to conventional method of phlebitis treatment.

Prognosis. Prolonged course; tendency to recur.

BIBLIOGRAPHY. Pearson JS: "Phlebodynia" a new epidemic (?) disease. Circulation 7:370–372, 1953
Brosius GR, Calvert MD, Chin TDY: Epidemic phlebodynia. Arch Intern Med 108:442–447, 1961

Nachbur H, Ris HB: Thrombectomy in acute deep vein thrombosis: Long-term follow-up. In Bergen JJ, Yao JST (eds): Venous Disorders. Philadelphia, WB Saunders, 1991

PHLEGMASIA ALBA DOLENS

Synonyms. Femoral thrombophlebitis; milk leg; postpartum thrombophlebitis.

Symptoms. Postpartum, postsurgical complication. Legs painful.

Signs. Pale, edematous, cool extremity.

Etiology. Thrombosis of deep veins of legs; extension of thrombosis into uterine veins accompanied by arterial spasm and diminished pulse.

Diagnostic Procedures. *Phlebography. Ultrasound. Plethysmography. Fluximetry.* Radioactive fibrinogen. Venous pressure measurement. *Blood.* Coagulation studies. Fibrin products identification.

Pathology. New and pre-existing thrombosis of veins, inflammation of vein walls.

Therapy. Antibiotic; heparin intravenous injection.

Prognosis. Fair with treatment. Possibly, not frequently, pulmonary embolism.

BIBLIOGRAPHY. Barnes RW: Current status of noninvasive tests in the diagnosis of venous disease. Surg Clin North Am 62:489–500, June, 1982
Nachbur H, Ris HB: Thrombectomy in acute deep vein. In Schaub RG, Simmonds CA, Koets MM, et al: Early events in the formation of the venous thrombus following local trauma and stasis. Lab Invest 51:218–221, 1984
Nachbur H, Ris HB: Thrombectomy in acute deep vein thrombosis: Long-term follow-up. In Bergen JJ, Yao JST (eds): Venous Disorders. Philadelphia, WB Saunders, 1991

PHLEGMASIA CERULEA DOLENS

Synonyms. Blue of Gregoire; Gregoire blue; ileofemoral thrombophlebitis; venous phlebitis—gangrene; thrombophlebitis cerulea dolens.

Symptoms. Usually, sudden pain in all toes; occasionally, gradual following recurrent episodes of vein thrombosis; always severe. In some cases progression from phlegmasia alba dolens to cerulea form.

Signs. Clear line of demarcation between involved area and viable tissue; swelling and cyanosis; increase in temperature of discolored parts. Peripheral pulses always palpable, stronger and fuller than unaffected side in early stage till obliterated by progressive edema. In some cases sheathlike appearance involving all sole of foot.

Etiology. Syndrome observed frequently in association with malignancy, or it may be idiopathic. Cessation of blood flow through capillary bed determined by venous thrombosis and edema.

Pathology. Venous thrombosis; edema; gangrene; patency of arterial system.

Diagnostic Procedures. *Blood.* Anemia, high blood urea nitrogen (BUN). Arteriovenous pressure gradient decreased. Phlebography. *Ultrasound.* Plethysmography. Fluximetry. Radioactive fibrinogen venous pressure measurements. *Blood.* Coagulation studies. Fibrin products identification.

Therapy. Antibiotics. Continuous intravenous heparin. Thrombectomy. After demarcation of gangrenous tissue, amputation.

Prognosis. Final loss of tissue less than anticipated. High mortality and morbidity associated with this syndrome.

BIBLIOGRAPHY. Hueter C: Fall von Gangrän in Folge von Venenobliteration. Virchows Arch (Pathol Anat) 17:482–488, 1859

Loewenthal J, May J: Phelgmasia caerulea dolens. Br J Surg 52:584–587, 1965

Bertelsen S, Anker W: Phelgmasia caerulea dolens: Pathophysiology, clinical features, treatment and prognosis. Acta Chir Scand 134:107–112, 1968

Nachbur H, Ris HB: Thrombectomy in acute deep vein thrombosis: Long-term follow-up. In Bergen JJ, Yao JST (eds): Venous Disorders. Philadelphia, WB Saunders, 1991

PHOBIC

See Panic attacks.

Symptoms and Signs. Onset at all ages; both sexes affected (women more than men). Exaggerated and pathologic dread of some precise situation, object, or stimulus, promoting complex maneuvers to avoid it. For example: *Acrophobia.* Dread of high places. *Agoraphobia.* Dread of open places. *Hydrophobia.* Dread of water. *Xenophobia.* Dread of strangers.

Etiology. Usually, resulting from negative experiences during learning stage, or inculcated by parents or teachers. Psychoanalytic role in emphasizing some phobic forms (of higher symbolic value).

Therapy. Psychotherapy.

Prognosis. For phobic reaction in children, good prognosis; in adults, it is more resistant to treatment and seldom spontaneously regresses.

BIBLIOGRAPHY. Westphal (1871)

Barlow DH: Anxiety and Its Disorders: The Nature and Treatment of Anxiety and Panic. New York, Guilford, 1988

Kaplan HI, Sadock BJ: Comprehensive Textbook of Psychiatry, 6th ed, pp 1848, 1205, 1206. Baltimore, Williams & Wilkins, 1995

PHOBIC POSTURAL VERTIGO

Synonyms. Vertigo, phobic postural.

Symptoms and Signs. In both sexes at all ages. Attacks occurring at irregular intervals, sometimes several times a day after typical perceptual stimuli (bridge, staircases, empty rooms, driving a car) or social situation (department store, restaurant, meeting, etc.). Anticipatory anxiety then vertigo, subjective postural unbalance sometimes menancing sensation of impending death, psychomotor restlessness with escape reaction, desire to flee, rigid grasp on arms of chair.

Etiology. In obsessive personalities after periods of stress physical excertion, illness, operation, pregnancy.

Diagnostic Procedures. All exams of vestibular function negative. Psychiatric evaluation: positive.

Therapy. Behavioral therapy good results.

Prognosis. Attacks may recur.

BIBLIOGRAPHY. Brandt T: Vertigo: Its multisensory syndromes. London, Springer-Verlag, 1991

PHOSPHORUS DEPLETION

Symptoms and Signs. Occurs in patients receiving prolonged treatment with nonabsorbable antacids, such as magnesium–aluminum hydroxides, in peptic ulcer therapy, prophylaxis of kidney stones, and others. Weakness, anorexia, and malaise. In severe form, bone pain and joint stiffness; occasionally, intentional tremor.

Etiology. Depletion of phosphorus following the prolonged administration of antacids.

Pathology. Osteomalacia.

Diagnostic Procedures. *Urine.* Hypophosphaturia; hypercalciuria. *Blood.* Hypophosphatemia. Increased calcium gastrointestinal absorption. *X-ray.* Osteomalacia.

Therapy. Adequate dietary phosphorus.

Prognosis. Excellent once adequate amount of phosphorus is given. Severe phosphorus depletion, induced in animals, brings debilitation followed by death.

BIBLIOGRAPHY. Bloom WB, Flinchum D: Osteomalacia with pseudofractures caused by ingestion of aluminum hydroxide. JAMA 174:1327–1330, 1960

Lotz M, Zisman E, Bartter FC: Evidence for a phosphorus-depletion syndrome in man. N Engl J Med 278:409–415, 1968

Knochel JP: The clinical status of hypophosphatemia: An update. N Engl J Med 313:447–449, 1985

Feldman KW, Marcuse EK, Springer DA: Nutritional rickets. Am Fam Phys 42:1311–1318, 1990

Coe FL, Favus MJ: Disorders of Bone and Mineral Metabolism. New York, Raven Press, 1993

PHOTOPHTHALMIA

Synonyms. Desert blindness; electric ophthalmia; snow blindness; ultraviolet keratopathy; keratopathy actinic; actinic keratopathy, acute.

Symptoms. Onset 4–5 hours after exposure. Severe ocular burning pain; itching; smarting of lids; photophobia; lacrimation; blepharospasm; seeing halos around lights.

Signs. Myosis; congestion and swelling of conjunctiva; edema; ulceration of cornea; mucopurulent secretion.

Etiology. Lesion from ultraviolet rays, snow reflection, welding arc, or strong lights.

Pathology. Inflammatory change; eosinophils in secretion.

Therapy. Prevention through use of colored lenses and general anesthetic.

Prognosis. Decrease in vision may result. Usually self-limited. Healing occurs in 12 hours.

BIBLIOGRAPHY. Newell FW: Ophthalmology, Principles and Concepts. St Louis, CV Mosby, 1965

Klintworth GK: Proteins in ocular disease. In Garner A, Klintworth GK (eds): Pathobiology of Ocular Disease: A Dynamic Approach, 2nd ed, pp 1013–1014. New York, Marcel Dekker, 1994

PIBLOKTO

Synonym. Arctic hysteria.

Symptoms. Occurs in eskimos, predominantly in women. Sudden attack of screaming, tearing away clothing, and running wildly. Attacks lasts 1–2 hours. Afterward, complete recovery and amnesia.

Etiology. Hysterical state of dissociation.

BIBLIOGRAPHY. Brill AA: Piblokto or hysteria among Peary's Eskimos. J Nerv Ment Dis 40:514–520, 1913

Willis JS, Martins M: Mental Health in North. Ottawa, Canada, Dept Nat Health Welfare, 1962

Kaplan HI, Sadock BJ: Comprehensive Textbook of Psychiatry, 6th ed, pp 1056–1067. Baltimore, Williams & Wilkins, 1995

PICK (A.)

Synonyms. Arnold Pick; aphasia—agnosia—apraxia; circumscribed brain atrophy; presenile dementia (see Alzheimer); lobar sclerosis.

Symptoms and Signs. Both sexes affected. Onset usually in fifth or sixth decade. Progressive dementia; focal symptoms and signs according to anatomic sites of involvement; temporal and frontal lobes most frequently involved. Anamnestic aphasia. Overall symptomatology very similar to Alzheimer.

Etiology. Unknown. Autosomal dominant inheritance reported.

Pathology. Localized atrophy of temporal lobes; frontal and parietal lobes less involved; basal ganglia normal or shrunken. Cell loss in areas involved; abundant glial proliferation; argentophilic bodies in cell cytoplasm. Absence of senile plaques and intracellular fibrillary degeneration. Blood vessel not involved.

Diagnostic Procedures. *EEG.* Diffuse changes. *CT brain scan. Electroencephalographic brain mapping. Cerebral atrophy. Cerebrospinal fluid.* Normal; occasionally, increase in protein.

Therapy. Symptomatic. Institutional care.

Prognosis. Death in a few years.

BIBLIOGRAPHY. Pick A: Apperzeptive Blindheit der Senilen. Arb Dtsch Psychiatr Klin In Prag 43, 1908
Pick A, Thiele R: Aphasia: Handbuch der Normalen und Pathologischen Physiologie. Berlin, Springer, 1931
Morris JC (ed): Handbook of Dementing Illnesses. New York, Marcel Dekker, 1993

PICK (F.)

Synonyms. Friedel Pick; Hutinel-Pick; constrictive pericarditis; liver pseudocirrhosis; mediastinopericarditis; pericarditis; liver pseudocirrhosis.

Symptoms. Occurs in patients with previous history of chest infection. Dyspnea; weakness; precordial discomfort; anorexia.

Signs. Cervical venous distention: ankle edema; heart normal or slightly enlarged; paradoxic pulse; protodiastolic gallop rhythm, or no significant murmur; hepatomegaly; ascites. Blood pressure usually low.

Etiology. Tuberculosis, various bacterial or viral, radiotherapy, neoplastic infections, or idiopathic, causing obliteration of pericardial cavity. Modern classification distinguishes the following forms: chronic calcific constrictive pericarditis; subacute constrictive pericarditis (rheumatoid arthritis, Hemophilus influenzae infections); postoperative constricting pericarditis; occult constrictive pericarditis; effusive constricting pericarditis (combined tamponade and constrictive lesion).

Pathology. Obliteration, fibrosis, and calcification of pericardial space; chronic inflammatory reaction.

Diagnostic Procedures. *Blood. Urine.* Normal. Low serum albumin; sodium sulfobromophthalein retention usually elevated. Increase of peripheral venous pressure. Circulation time elevated. *X-ray. Echography.* Occasionally, calcification of pericardium; diminished cardiac pulsation on fluoroscopy; pulmonary and pleural pathology frequent. *ECG.* Flattening or inversion of T-waves, elevated RT segment, and possibly elevated ST segment in leads I and II; later, inverted T-wave and diminution of QRS. *Cardiac catheterization.* Signs of constrictive pericarditis.

Therapy. Surgical. Decortication of heart; antitubercular treatment (when indicated).

Prognosis. From complete recovery after surgery to no improvement and death from cardiopulmonary insufficiency according to degree of pulmonary, cardiac, and hepatic involvement.

BIBLIOGRAPHY. Lower R: Tractatus de Corde, pp 104–107. Amstelodami, Apud Danielem Elzevirium, 1669
Pick F: Ueber chronische, unter den Bild der Lebercirrhose verlaufende Pericarditis (pericarditische Pseudolebercirrhose) nebst Bemer-

kungen über die Zuckergussleber (Curschmann). Klin Med 29:385–410, 1896
Shabetai R: Diseases of percardium. In Schlant RC, Alexander RW, et al: Hurst's The Heart, 8th ed, pp 1662–1665. New York, McGraw-Hill, 1994

PICK (L.)

Synonym. Cachectic retinitis; retinitis cachectic.

Symptoms. Decreased visual acuity; reduced field of vision; distortion of shapes of objects.

Signs. Diffuse clouding of retina; peripapillary whitish-gray macula; small hemorrhagic areas; distention of vessels.

Etiology. Cachexia; secondary anemia to carcinoma or severe, chronic, intestinal hemorrhages, or chronic infection conditions.

Pathology. Retinal elements showing fatty degeneration, edema, leukocyte exudates; swelling of nervous fibers; thickening and, occasionally obliteration of vessel walls.

Therapy. Treatment of basic condition.

Prognosis. Poor.

BIBLIOGRAPHY. Pick L: Netzhautveraenderungen bei chronischen Anaemien. Klin Monatsbl Augenheilkd 39:177–192, 1901
Garner A, Sarks S, Sarks JP: Degenerative and related disorders of the retina and choroid. In Garner A, Klintworth GK (eds): Pathobiology of Ocular Disease: A Dynamic Approach, 2nd ed. New York, Marcel Dekker, 1994

PICKWICKIAN

Synonyms. Cardiopulmonary obesity; obesity—hypoventilation. See Narcolepsy, diabetogenic ("functional") hyperinsulinism.

Symptoms. Occurs in about 10% of obese adults; rare in obese children. Somnolence; bulimia. Headache; dyspnea; drowsiness. In children, mental retardation may develop.

Signs. Obesity; limited respiratory chest excursion; cyanosis; nocturnal Cheyne-Stokes respiration; right ventricular failure. Retinal hemorrhages and papilledema.

Etiology. Obesity imposing excessive work load on respiration. Chronic hypoxemia; relative hyperinsulinism may be present. It may be considered as part of the narcolepsy or diabetogenic hyperinsulinism syndromes, where the cardiorespiratory symptoms are present as prominent feature. Role of genetic factors debated.

Pathology. Generalized obesity; excessive fat under diaphragm. Ascites and edema when right ventricular failure develops. Signs of pulmonary hypertension and right heart hypertrophy.

Diagnostic Procedures. *Blood.* Polycythemia; hypoxemia. *Pulmonary function tests.* Alveolar hypoventilation; carbon dioxide retention; total and vital capacity decreased; reduction of expiratory reserve volume. *ECG.* Right axis deviation; changes suggesting ischemia of anterior wall.

Therapy. Diet; analeptic agent; treatment of right ventricular failure. Physical activity.

Prognosis. Fatal if unrecognized; reversible if treated.

BIBLIOGRAPHY. Elliot J: Complete Collection of the Medical and Philosophical Works of John Fothergill. London, 1781
Wadd W: Cursory remarks on corpulence, obesity, considered as a disease: With a critical examination of ancient and modern opinions relative to its causes and cure, containing a reference to the most remarkable cases that have occurred in this country, 3rd ed. London, 1819

Burwell CS, Robin ED, Whaley RD, et al: Extreme obesity associated with alveolar hypoventilation: A Pickwickian syndrome. Am J Med 21:811–818, 1956

Sugarman HY, Baron PL, Fairman RP, et al: Hemodynamic dysfunction in obesity hypoventilation syndrome and the effects of treatment with surgically induced weight loss. Ann Surg 207:609–613, 1988

Newman JH, Ross JC: Chronic cor pulmonale. In Schlant RC, Alexander RW: Hurst's The Heart, 8th ed, pp 1898–1899. New York, McGraw-Hill, 1994

P.I.E.

Synonym. Pulmonary infiltrate eosinophilia. The acronym P.I.E. is used to indicate all eosinophilic lung diseases, which has led to confusion because eosinophilia may not be a constant feature of these conditions.

PIERRE ROBIN

Synonyms. Robin; cleft palate—glossoptosis—micrognathia; glossoptosis—micrognathia—cleft palate. See First arch syndromes.

Symptoms. Difficulty in breathing; difficulty in feeding.

Signs. Micrognathia; cleft palate; glossoptosis; ocular abnormalities; cyanosis; sternum retraction evidence of malnutrition.

Etiology. See First arch syndrome. Autosomal recessive inheritance.

Pathology. See Signs.

Diagnostic Procedures. *X-ray.* Chromosome studies. Normal pattern.

Therapy. Orthostatic nursing (feeding while neonate lying on the abdomen with chest elevated by small pillow). Prevent tongue from slipping backward. False palate of acrylic material.

Prognosis. Usually, infant outgrows feeding and breathing difficulties in weeks or months. There is a significant risk of major airway embarrassment in this disorder, even if the infant seems initially well. Early management of infants with this anomaly should, therefore, be undertaken at centers where skilled airway support is available.

BIBLIOGRAPHY. Sahukowsky WP: Zur Aetologie des Stridor inspiratorisu congenitalis. Jahrb Kinderheilkd NF 73:459–474, 1911.

Robin P: La glossoptose: Son diagnostic, ses consequences, son traitement. J Med Paris 43:235–237, 1923

Sheffield LJ, Reiss JA, Strohm K, et al: A genetic follow up study of 64 patients with Pierre Robin complex. Am J Med Genet 28:25–36, 1987

PIETRANTONI

Eponym used to indicate areas of neuralgia or anesthesia on the face or oral cavity, reported by patients affected by still undetected paranasal tumors.

BIBLIOGRAPHY. Pietrantoni L: Zone nevralgiche e zone di anestesia della regione facciale e della cavità orale come sintomi precoci di alcune forme di tumori maligni delle cavità paranasali. Arch Ital Otol 59:105–108, 1948

PIGEON BREEDER I

Synonyms. Bird breeder lung; bird fancier; pneumonitis of pigeon breeder. See Allergic alveolitis syndromes.

Symptoms. Occurs in individuals who take care of pigeons; onset 4–6 hours after exposure. Malaise; fever; chills; dyspnea; cough; arthralgia.

Signs. Diffuse crepitant rales in both sides of chest.

Etiology. Hypersensitivity reaction to pigeons.

Pathology. Interstitial pneumonitis.

Diagnostic Procedures. *Blood.* Eosinophilia (not a prominent, constant feature). Presence of specific precipitating antibodies. *X-ray.* Of chest. Diffuse coarsening of bronchovascular markings; fine nodulation and reticulation.

Therapy. Corticosteroids.

Prognosis. If contact with birds avoided, symptoms disappear spontaneously in 12–24 hours, pulmonary signs in several days. Repeated, prolonged exposure results in chronic lung disease.

BIBLIOGRAPHY. Reed CE, Sosman A, Barbee RA: Pigeon breeder's lung: A newly observed interstitial pulmonary disease. JAMA 193:261–265, 1965

Unger JD, Fink JN, Unger GF: Pigeon breeder's disease. Radiology 90:683–687, 1968

Fraser RS, Paré JAP, Fraser RG, Paré PD: Synopsis of Diseases of the Chest, 2nd ed. Philadelphia, WB Saunders, 1994

PIGMENTARY GLAUCOMA

Synonym. Pigmentary ocular dispersion—glaucoma; including pigmentary dispersion syndrome (without glaucoma).

Symptoms and Signs. Males affected more frequently than females (4:1). Onset in fourth and fifth decades. Myopia (70%); glaucomatous field changes (39%). Iris translucency (65%); insert anteriorly into the scleral spur (75%); pigment in the posterior trabecular mesh; pigment on equatorial edge of lens capsule.

Etiology. Unknown. Polygenic inheritance. Pigment not cause of glaucoma, but possibly secondary to atrophy of iris epithelium.

Diagnostic Procedures. *Tonometry and tonography.* Ocular hypertension. Typical sign: Krukenberg spindle (which is a deposition of uveal melanin pigment on the posterior surface of cornea).

Therapy. That of glaucoma.

Prognosis. Progressive condition.

BIBLIOGRAPHY. Sugar HS: Pigmentary glaucoma—A 25-year review. Am J Ophthalmol 62:499–507, 1966

Lichter RP: Pigmentary glaucoma: Current concepts. Trans Am Acad Ophthalmol Otolaryngol 78:309, 1974

Maida JW, Spaeth GL: Pigmentary ocular dispersion syndrome. Presented at the 27th Wills Annual Conference, Philadelphia, Jan 30, 1975

Joseph J, Grierson J: Anterior segment changes in glaucoma. In Garner A, Klintworth GK (eds): Pathobiology of Ocular Disease: A Dynamic Approach, 2nd ed, pp 450, 453–453. New York, Marcel Dekker, 1994

PILI ANNULATI

Synonyms. Hair ringed: ringed hair; thrix annulata.

Symptoms. Present at birth or developing in first 2 years of life. Asymptomatic.

Signs. Alternate light and dark bands of scalp hair (occasionally also axillary). Normal or increased hair fragility; hairs breaking at 15–20 cm lengths. Possible association with other congenital defects.

Etiology. Unknown; 50% sporadic cases; 50% hereditary usually autosomal dominant (recessive type possible in some cases).

Pathology. On microscopic examination affected hairs show alternating normally pigmented bands and lighter ones.

Diagnostic Procedures. On transmitted light, light hairs appear black (see Pathology).

Therapy. None.

Prognosis. Permanent condition that does not increase with age.

BIBLIOGRAPHY. Snell GD, Foley F: Inheritance of ringed hair. J Hered 23:155–157, 1932
Degos R: Dermatologie. Paris, Flammarion, 1953
Dawber RPR, Ebling FJG, Wojnarowska FT: Disorders of hair. In Champion RH, Burton JL, Ebling FJG (eds): Rook/Wilkinson/Ebling Textbook of Dermatology, 5th ed, pp 2614–2615. Oxford, Blackwell Scientific, 1992

PILLAY-HORTH

Synonym. Ophthalmomandibulomelic dysplasia; OMM.

Symptoms and Signs. Both sexes affected. Corneal opacities; temporomandibular fusion; obtuse mandibular angle, short forearms.

Etiology. Autosomal dominant inheritance.

Diagnostic Procedures. *X-ray.* Aplasia of lateral condyle head of radius and lower third of ulna; dislocation of radiohumeral and proximal radioulnar joints.

BIBLIOGRAPHY. Pillay VK, Orth MC: Ophthalmo-mandibulomelic dysplasia. An hereditary syndrome. J Bone Joint Surg (Am) 46:858–862, 1964

PINCER NAIL

Symptoms. Severe pain in involved fingers.

Signs. Excessive transverse curvature of nail plate; loss of soft tissue of involved fingers.

Etiology. Unknown.

Diagnostic Procedures. *X-ray.* Of finger. Resorption of phalanx of involved fingers.

Therapy. Surgical avulsion of dystrophic nails.

BIBLIOGRAPHY. Samman PD: The Nails in Disease, p 79. London, Heinemann, 1965
Cornelius CE, Shelley WB: Pincer nail syndrome. Arch Surg 96:321–322, 1968
Wernick J, Gibbs RC: Pedal biomechanics and toenail disease. In Scher RK, Daniel CR (eds): Nails: Therapy, Diagnosis, Surgery, pp 244–249. Philadelphia, WB Saunders, 1990

PINEAL-GONADAL

See Pellizzi and pineal tumor.

Symptoms and Signs. Occurs in young males (hypogonadism and pineal tumor never reported in female). Delayed or absent development of primary and secondary sexual characteristics, associated with pineal tumor neurologic syndrome (see).

Etiology. Unknown. Increased secretion of a hypothetical pineal hormone that inhibits gonadal development.

Pathogenesis. Adenoma or functioning pinealoma.

Diagnostic Procedures. *X-ray. CT scan. MRI.* Of skull. Gonadotropin secretion evaluation.

Therapy. Surgery; substitutional therapy.

Prognosis. Depends on benign or malignant etiology.

BIBLIOGRAPHY. Kitay JI: Pineal lesions and precocious puberty: A review. J Clin Endocrinol 14:622–625, 1954
Cohen AR, Wilson JA, Sadeghi-Nejad A: Gonadotrophin-secreting pineal teratoma causing precocious puberty. Neurosurgery 28:597–602, 1991

PINEAL TUMOR, NEUROLOGIC

Symptoms. Occurs most often in young males. Weakness; headache; vomiting; diplopia; deafness; incoordination; polydipsia; polyphagia; convulsions; mental changes.

Signs. Lack of pupillary reaction; paresis of oculomotor muscle, nystagmus; papilledema; facial paralysis; tremor; ataxia; Romberg sign; hypertonia; tendon hyperreflexia; Babinski sign. Pretectal syndrome (see) most characteristic localizing sign.

Etiology. Unknown. Neoplasia of pineal gland.

Pathology. Gliomas and teratomas (invasion mass, necrosis, and hemorrhage). Cystic hydrops of pineal (lined by glial cells). Pinealoma (composed of pineal parenchymal cells reproducing the mosaic pattern seen in the developing organ). Adenomas and metastasis very rare.

Diagnostic Procedures. *X-ray. CT brain scan. MRI.* Sometimes gland calcified. *Biopsy.* Under steroscopic needle technique.

Therapy. Surgery.

Prognosis. Depends on etiology and result of surgery.

BIBLIOGRAPHY. Kearne JR: The pretectal syndrome: 206 patients. Neurology 40:684–690, 1990
Adams RD, Victor M: Principles of Neurology, 5th ed, pp 578–579. New York, McGraw-Hill, 1993

PINGELAPESE BLINDNESS

Synonyms. Color blindness, myopia; achromatopsia, myopia.

Symptoms and Signs. Affects 4–10% of Pingelapese people. Both sexes. Horizontal pendular nystagmus, photophobia, amaurosis, color blindness, gradually developing cataracts.

Etiology. Autosomal recessive.

Prognosis. Nonprogressive disorder.

BIBLIOGRAPHY. Brodie JA, Hussels I, Brink E, et al: Hereditary blindness among Pingelapese people of Eastern Caroline Island. Lancet I:1253–1257, 1970

PINKUS (F.)

Synonym. Lichen nitidus.

Symptoms. Both sexes affected. Onset usually in childhood and young adulthood. Usually, asymptomatic.

Signs. Eruption of discrete (occasionally grouped) pinhead size, pink or red papules on abdomen, genitalia, forearms, chest, buttocks, seldom on palms and soles. Mucosae rarely affected. Coincidence with lichen planus frequent. Association with Chron (see) reported.

Etiology. Unknown. Possibly related to lichen planus.

Pathology. Papules are formed by a dense circumscribed, infiltrated margin located under the epidermis and formed by lymphocytes, histiocytes, and rarely Langhans cells.

Diagnostic Procedures. *Biopsy.* Of skin. Differential diagnosis with lichen planus, lichen scrofulosum, keratosis pilaris.

Therapy. No treatment required for majority of cases, or topical steroids, PUVA, or astemizole.

Prognosis. Course unpredictable. Finally, recovery without scars.

BIBLIOGRAPHY. Pinkus F: Uber eine neue knoechnfoernige Hauteruption: Lichen nitidus. Arch Dermatol Syph (Berlin) 85:11–36, 1907
Black MM: Lichen planus and lichenoid disorders. In Champion RH, Burton JL, Ebling FJG (eds): Rook/Wilkinson/Ebling Textbook of Dermatology, 5th ed, pp 1696–1698. Oxford, Blackwell Scientific, 1992

PINKUS (H.)

Synonym. Fibroepithelial tumor. This eponym indicates a confusing condition including benign and malignant conditions of the fibromatosis group.

Symptoms and Signs. Appearance and slow growth of a sessile, firm, pink tumor with domed surface, on the abdomen or loins. Associated frequently with seborrheic keratosis or basal cell carcinoma or both.

Etiology. Unknown. Possibly, correlation with X-ray exposure, or arsenic treatment.

Pathology. Tumor formed by fibrotic, cellular, enlarged dermal papillae, enclosed in a nest of small dark cells.

Therapy. Local excision.

Prognosis. Treatment curative.

BIBLIOGRAPHY. Pinkus H: Premalignant fibroepithelial tumors of skin. Arch Dermatol Syph 67:598–615, 1953
MacKie RM: Epidermal skin tumors. In Champion RH, Burton JL, Ebling FJG (eds): Rook/Wilkinson/Ebling Textbook of Dermatology, 5th ed, pp 1496–1497. Oxford, Blackwell Scientific, 1992

PINKUS (H.) II

Synonym. Eccrine poroma.

Symptoms. Both sexes equally affected. Onset in middle age or later. Asymptomatic.

Signs. Usually on the sole, less frequently on palm, and elsewhere on the body, solitary tumor, flat (sole), sessile, or pedunculated, with smooth surface or slightly keratotic; occasionally vascular or ulcerated. Diameter varying from several millimeters to several centimeters.

Etiology. Benign and seldom malignant tumor from eccrine sweat duct epithelium, juxta epidermal localization. Clinically same manifestation of hidroacanthoma simplex (intraepidermal) and dermal duct tumor (intradermal).

Pathology. Cells are small malpighian cells and rich in glycogen. Histochemical reaction of tumor cells similar to those of sudoriparous glands.

Therapy. Surgical excision. Curettage and diathermy sometimes adequate.

Prognosis. Cured by removal.

BIBLIOGRAPHY. Pinkus H, et al: Eccrine poroma. Tumours exhibiting features of the epidermal sweat duct unit. Arch Dermatol 74:511–521, 1956
MacKie RM: Tumors of the skin appendages. In Champion RH, Burton JL, Ebling FJG (eds): Rook/Wilkinson/Ebling Textbook of Dermatology, 5th ed, pp 1516–1517. Oxford, Blackwell Scientific, 1992

PINKUS (H.) III

Synonyms. Alopecia mucinosa; follicular mucinosis.

Symptoms. Both sexes affected. Onset in two age groups: (1) children over 5 and adults under 30; (2) older subjects. *Group 1.* Asymptomatic or paucisymptomatic. *Group 2.* Irritative skin changes and pruritus.

Signs. *Group 1.* On the face, scalp, neck or shoulders, eruption of single or multiple papules or erythematous plaques, with fine scaling, raised follicles, and hair loss. *Group 2.* More numerous lesions with variable aspects: papules, plaques, and nodules; some ulcerated and some developing jelly consistency. Various signs of skin or systemic reticulosis may appear at various times after onset.

Etiology. Unknown. Virus infection (?); nonspecific reaction (?).

Pathology. Edema and mucinous degeneration of sebaceous glands and hair root sheaths. Variable degree of inflammatory changes.

Diagnostic Procedures. *Biopsy.* In Group 2 search for evidence of local or systemic reticulosis.

Therapy. None effective. Superficial radiotherapy; and topical and intralesional steroids, systemic steroids (porpruritic variety), and dapsone may be tried.

Prognosis. *Group 1.* Few, self-limiting lesions, and eventual recovery. *Group 2.* Extensive, polymorphic, persistent lesions with frequent association with malignant reticulosis (20%).

BIBLIOGRAPHY. Pinkus H: Alopecia mucinosa. Inflammatory plaques with alopecia characterized by roots sheath mucinosis. Arch Dermatol 76:419–426, 1957
Tappeiner J: Zuer Problem der Symtomatischen Mucinosis follicularis. Arch Klin Exp Dermatol 227:937–948, 1966
Black MM, Gawkrodger DJ, Seymour CA, et al: Metabolic and nutritional disorders. In Champion RH, Burton JL, Ebling FJG (eds): Rook/Wilkinson/Ebling Textbook of Dermatology, 5th ed, pp 2331–2333. Oxford, Blackwell Scientific, 1992

PINSKI

BIBLIOGRAPHY. Pinsky L, DiGeorge A, Harley R, et al: Microphthalmos, corneal opacity, mental retardation, and spastic-cerebral palsy: An oculocerebral syndrome. J Pediat (St Louis) 67:387–398, 1965

PIRINGER-KUCHINKA

Obsolete.

Synonyms. Lymphadenitis subacuta; lymphadenitis nuchalis and cervicalis.

Eponym used to indicate lymphadenopathy of cervical and nuchal stations (lymphadenitis nuchalis and cervicalis) owing to chronic and subacute infection (e.g., toxoplasmosis).

BIBLIOGRAPHY. Piringer-Kuchinka A: Eigerartiger mikroskopischer Befund an exzidierten Lymphknoten. Verh Dtsch Ges Pathol 36:352–362, 1952

PITT

Synonyms. Pitt-Rogers-Danks; mental retardation—unusual facies—growth retardation (intrauterine).

Symptoms and Signs. Both sexes. From birth. Intrauterine growth retardation. *Facies.* Short upper lip; slanting, prominent eyes; telecanthus large mouth; microcephaly and mental retardation from mild to severe; hyperactive behavior.

Etiology. Possibly autosomal recessive inheritance.

BIBLIOGRAPHY. Pitt DB, Rogers JD, Danks DM: Mental retardation, unusual face and intrauterine growth retardation: A new recessive syndrome? Am J Med Genet 19:307–313, 1984

Donnai D: A further patient with Pitt-Rogers-Danks syndrome of mental retardation, unusual face and intrauterine growth retardation. AmJ Med Genet 24:29–32, 1986

Oortuys JWE, Bleeker-Wagemaker EM: A girl with the Pitt-Rogers-Danks syndrome. Am J Med Genet 32:140–141, 1989

PITT-WILLIAMS

Synonym. Brachydactyly (B + E types).

Symptoms and Signs. Hypoplasia of distal phalanges of ulnar side of hand and shortening of one or several metacarpals. Absence of dwarfism.

Etiology. Autosomal dominant inheritance.

BIBLIOGRAPHY. Pitt P, Williams I: A new brachydactyly syndrome with similarities to Julia Bell type B and E. J Med Genet 22:202–204, 1985

PITUITARY APOPLEXY

Symptoms and Signs. Acute onset. Headache, ophthalmoplegia, amaurosis bilateral, drowsiness or coma.

Etiology. Infarction of a pituitary adenoma.

Diagnostic Procedures. *CSF.* Protein, leukocytes increased; possible presence of red cells. *CT brain scan.* Infarction of the tumor, enlarged sella.

Therapy. Dexamethazone (6–12 mg every 6 hours) and if no improvement transnasal decompression.

Prognosis. Life-threatening situation. Good result with immediate diagnosis and treatment.

BIBLIOGRAPHY. Brougham M, Henser AP, Adams RD: Acute degenerative changes in adenomas of the pituitary body with special reference to pituitary apoplexy. J Neurosurg 7:421–439, 1950
Cooperman D, Maeazkey WB: Pituitary apoplexy. Heart Lung 7:450–454, 1978
Adams RD, Victor M: Principles of Neurology, 5th ed, p 586. New York, McGraw-Hill, 1993

PITUITARY-HYPOTHYROIDISM, FAMILIAL

This group of syndromes includes six syndromes, which are schematically reported. *Isolated TSH deficiency.* Manifested as congenital hypothyroidism. Autosomal recessive. *Thyrotropin, impaired biologic activity.* Partially defective TSH (activity decreased, concentration proportionally increased). *Panhypopituitarism.* With congenital (not sticking) hypothyroidism and associated defects of FSH, HGH, LH, and ACTH—two forms are known—autosomal recessive and X-linked. *Pituitary agenesis.* Only congenital hypothyroidism. Autosomal recessive. *Panhypopituitarism with absent sella turcica.* Congenital hypothyroidism with associated defects of HGH, FSH, LH, ACTH. Autosomal recessive. *Panhypopituitarism with enlarged sella turcica.* Congenital hypothyroidism. Associated deficiency of GH.

BIBLIOGRAPHY. Dumont JE, Refetoff S: Thyroid disorders. In Scriver CR, Beaudet AL, Sly WS, et al: The Metabolic and Molecular Bases of Inherited Disease, 7th ed, pp 2907–2908. New York, McGraw-Hill, 1995

PIULACHS-HEDERICH

See Gas syndromes. Eponym used to indicate a sudden abdominal colic caused by a sudden idiopathic colic gas distention.

BIBLIOGRAPHY. Piulachs P, Hederich H: La "dilatation aguda del colon" complication del dolicomegacolon. Acta Med Hisp 5:131–135, 1947

PIUSSAN

Synonyms. Stiff thumb—brachydactyly (A1)—mental retardation. See Lewis (C.S.).

Symptoms and Signs. In females. Stiff thumbs associated with brachydactyly type A1 and mental retardation.

Etiology. Possibly dominant inheritance (mutation).

BIBLIOGRAPHY. Piussan C, Lenaerts C, Mathieu M, et al: Dominance reguliere d'une ankilose des pouces avec retard mental se transmettant sur trois generations. J Genet Hum 31:107–114, 1983
Barber C, Carpenter NJ, Say B: Bilateral ankylosed thumbs and mental retardation. Am J Med Genet 36:367, 1990

PLACENTAL HEMANGIOMAS

Synonyms. Chorioangiofibromal; fibroangioma; hemangioblastoma; reticulohemangioendothelioma.

Symptoms and Signs. Hemangiomas of the placenta; associated hydramnios in 33% of cases, without fetal anomalies or maternal abnormalities. Often associated with premature labor, premature rupture of membranes, an increased incidence of antepartum and postpartum hemorrhage, and, rarely, dystocia.

Etiology. Not known.

Pathology. Placental hemangiomas vary in size from 2 mm to 22 cm; produce an elevation of the fetal surface. They vary in color from yellow-gray to deep blue-red color and are firm in consistency. Microscopically, hemangioma consists of embryonic cellular tissue with numerous small blood vessels supported by a loose network of chorionic stromal cells. These tumors are well demarcated from the surrounding placental tissue.

Therapy. No special treatment is necessary. The treatment is governed by obstetric conditions.

Prognosis. Good for the newborn, unless causing prematurity.

BIBLIOGRAPHY. Clarke J: Account of a tumor found in the substance of the human placenta. Philos Trans 88:361–368, 1798
Asadourian LA, Taylor HB: Clinical significance of placental hemangiomas. Obstet Gynecol 31:551–555, 1968
Benirschke K, Kaufmann P: Pathology of Human Placenta, 3rd ed. New York, Springer, 1990

PLACENTAL INSUFFICIENCY

Synonyms. Prolonged gestation II; placental dysfunctional II; postmaturity small baby.

Symptoms and Signs. Retardation of uterine growth at about the 30th week of pregnancy; decrease in fetal movements; delivery of an "immature" baby despite the fact that the baby is full-term. Very often intrauterine fetal death.

Etiology. Unknown. Possibly, inability of placenta to transfer, synthesize, transport nutritional and chemical elements necessary for growth of the fetus.

Pathology. A decreased vascular supply and increased fibrosis of the placental tissue; small placenta (200 g).

Diagnostic Procedures. *Urine.* Decrease in urinary estriol excretion; increase of atropine transfer time. *Ultrasonography.*

Therapy. Increased vigilance and active intervention for termination of pregnancy, either vaginally or by cesarean section if and when fetal distress becomes apparent.

Prognosis. Guarded because etiology is unknown. Recurrence of condition is high (40%).

BIBLIOGRAPHY. Rumbolz WL, Edwards MC, McCoogan LS: The small full term infant, placental insufficiency. West J Surg 69:53–60, 1961

Benirschke K, Kaufmann P: Pathology of Human Placenta, 3rd ed. New York, Springer, 1990

PLACENTA PREVIA

Symptoms and Signs. Occurs in 1:100–1:200 deliveries; more frequent in multiparas and in Caucasian patients. Painless hemorrhage during the third trimester of pregnancy. Hemorrhage may come at any time, without warning and even when the patient is asleep. Usually this bleeding is not accompanied by symptoms and signs of pre-eclampsia. Vaginal examination under sterile conditions and double setup reveals the presence of placenta in lower segment of the uterus, partially or totally covering the internal os of the cervix.

Etiology. Little is known about the etiology. It has been suggested that defective vascularization of the decidua, as the result of inflammatory or atrophic processes, may be a contributing factor.

Pathology. According to the degree with which placenta covers the internal os: (1) total or central placenta previa; (2) partial placenta previa; (3) marginal placenta previa.

Diagnostic Procedures. *Ultrasound. MRI.*

Therapy. The uterus should be emptied by the most conservative method as soon as the placenta previa is diagnosed. Such patients should always be hospitalized and be kept under constant observation. Phlebotomy performed for autologous blood banking. *Before labor.* When the fetus is viable and the pregnancy more than 36th week, rupture of the membranes may permit the presenting part to compress the placenta and stop bleeding. If the bleeding does not stop and in case of total placenta previa, cesarean section. If the fetus is not viable, a policy of conservation is taken: complete bed rest; hospitalization; observation. If the fetus is dead, Willett forceps attached to fetal scalp used to obtain additional pressure against the placenta. *During labor.* Depends on variety of previa, dilatation and effacement of cervix, general condition of patient. If dilatation is almost complete, with marginal placenta previa and condition of the patient is good, rupture of membranes and forceps delivery. Under all other circumstances, cesarean section. *Management of third stage.* Beware of alarming postpartum hemorrhage. If bleeding is profuse, Crede method of expression of placenta. If not successful, manual removal of placenta.

Prognosis. Threatened maternal morbidity and mortality. Increased perinatal mortality.

BIBLIOGRAPHY. Hibbard LT: Placenta praevia. Am J Obstet Gynecol 104:172–176, 1969

Gorodeski IG, Neri A, Haimovich L, Bahari CM: Placenta previa: The ultrasonographic localization and its influence on the mode of delivery. J Reprod Med 27:655–657, 1982

Powell MC, Buckley J, Price H, Worthington BS, Symonds EM: Magnetic resonance imaging and placenta previa. Am J Obstet Gynecol 154:565–569, 1986

Benirschke K, Kaufmann P: Pathology of Human Placenta, 3rd ed. New York, Springer, 1990

PLAGIOCEPHALY, FACIAL ASYMMETRY—DENTAL ARTICULATION DERANGEMENT

Synonym. Facial malformation—skull base asymmetry. See Bencze.

Symptoms and Signs. Malformations of vault and base of skull and disturbances of dental articulation. Mandibular compensation may sometimes reduce disturbances of articulation or various degrees of malocclusion may result, associated with various degree of plagiocephaly. Severity of one feature not always correlated with the others.

Etiology. Congenital malformation. Hereditary transmission considered. Torticollis (uncorrected) may be the cause of the progressive plagiocephaly and consequent other symptoms.

Pathology. Not specific.

Diagnostic Procedure. *X-ray.*

Therapy. Adequate data not yet available for an evaluation. If torticollis, helmet treatment.

Prognosis. Tendency toward self-correction of the dental articulation disturbances.

BIBLIOGRAPHY. Korkhaus G: L'influence de l'hérédité et du milieu sur l'architecture du crane facial. Rev Belge Sci Dent 385–403, 1952

Delaire J, Billet J, Ferré JC, et al: Malformations faciales et asymétrie de la base du crane. Rev Stomatol 66:379–396, 1965

Clarren SK: Plagiocephaly and torticollis: Etiology natural history and helmet treatment. J Pediatr 98:92–95, 1981

PLOTT

Synonyms. Laryngeal abductor paralysis; vocal cord dysfunction familial (see Gerhardt).

Symptoms and Signs. From birth. Impairment of phonation or severe inspiratory dyspnea. Psychomotor retardation.

Etiology. X-linked inheritance.

Pathology. Brain damage secondary to respiratory difficulties. Dysgenesis of nucleus ambiguous considered.

BIBLIOGRAPHY. Plott D: Congenital laryngeal abductor paralysis due to nucleus ambiguous dysgenesis in three brothers. N Engl J Med 271:593–597, 1964

Opitz JM, Kaveggia EG, Durkin-Stamm MV, et al: Diagnostic-genetic studies in severe mental retardation. Birth Defects XIV(6B):1–38, 1978

PLUMMER

Synonyms. Toxic nodular goiter; adenoma toxic.

Symptoms. Prevalent in females; onset after 40 years of age. The same symptoms as Flajani, but, typically, slower rate of appearance, in the majority of cases asymptomatic. Usually, predominance of cardiac symptoms and absence of ophthalmopathy, pretibial myxedema, and acropathy.

Signs. Adenomatous thyromegaly (weight usually three times the normal) precedes the symptoms. Single node usually hot, palpable; multinodular. Compression of neck structures rare. Other findings similar to those of the Flajani syndrome.

Etiology. Unknown. Benign neoplasm.

Pathology. Minimal to gross asymmetry of thyroid. Section: variegated surface showing normal tissue with areas of gelatinous aspect. Hyperplastic nodules not encapsulated, occasionally cystic with interposed fibrous scars.

Diagnostic Procedures. Thyroidal ^{123}I normal in 50% of cases; T4 slightly elevated (frequently is the only laboratory finding) thyreoglobulin antibodies negative. *Scintigraphy.* Cold and hot areas. *Ultrasonography. MRI. CT scan.* Nodularity. *Fine-needle aspiration.* Benign lesion. *Histological workup.* Multinodularity or multiple foci of replicating follicular cells.

Therapy. Surveillance mandatory. Radioiodine: treatment of choice in elderly patients or to diminish volume of large euthyroid multinodular goiters. If surgery necessary, make the patient euthyroid first with antithyroid drugs (not all agree on this policy).

Prognosis. Thyrotoxicosis (not obligatory late complication) since possible standstill, spontaneous regression, involution, and degeneration.

BIBLIOGRAPHY. Plummer HS: The clinical and pathological relationship of simple and exophthalmic goiter. Am J Med Sci 146:790–795, 1913
Studer H, Gerber H, Multinodular goiter. In De Groot LJ (ed): Endocrinology, 3rd ed, pp 777–779. Philadelphia, WB Saunders, 1995

PLUMMER-VINSON

Synonyms. Kelly-Paterson; Paterson; Paterson-Brown-Kelly; postcricoid web; Waldenström-Kjellberg; sideropenic dysphagia.

Symptoms. Occurs most often in middle-aged women, rarely in men. Pain and burning sensation behind larynx when swallowing solid food, or sensation of food stuck in the larynx. Fatigue.

Signs. Pallor of skin and mucosae (not constant). Other signs of sideropenic anemia (in hair, nails).

Etiology. An association between sideropenia and one or more webs of mucosa at the juncture between the hypopharynx and the esophagus.

Pathology. Webs of mucosa in the lumen of the esophagus that can narrow the lumen itself. Biopsy of these lesions shows chronic inflammation.

Diagnostic Procedures. *Blood.* Hypochromic anemia (not consistently present); sideropenia (constant). *Stool.* Occult blood. *X-ray.* Thick barium and very short exposures in upper part of esophagus, below cricoid cartilage, shows thin defect of opacity.

Therapy. Repletion of iron stores; rupture the webs or dilate the stenosis by means of bouginage.

Prognosis. Good with therapy. In untreated patients, the dysphagia can interfere with nutrition. Carcinoma in situ is a rare complication.

BIBLIOGRAPHY. Plummer HS: Diffuse dilation of the esophagus without anatomic stenosis (cardiospasm). A report of ninety-one cases. JAMA 58:2013–2015, 1912
Vinson PP: A case of cardiospasm with dilation and angulation of the esophagus. Med Clin North Am 3:623–627, 1919
Kelly AB: Spasm of the entrance of the esophagus. Br J Laryngol Rhinol Otol 34:285–289, 1919
Paterson DR: A clinical type of dysphagia. Br J Laryngol Rhinol Otol 24:289–291, 1919
Lee GR: Iron deficiency and iron-deficiency anemia. In Lee GR, Bithell TC, Foerster J, et al (eds): Wintrobe's Clinical Hematology, 9th ed, pp 813–814. Philadelphia, Lea & Febiger, 1993

PNEUMATIC HAMMER

Synonym. Vibration; hypotenar hammer; hand—arm—vibration; HAVS.

Symptoms. Occurs in individuals exposed to the percussion of vibrating tools. Carpal tunnel syndrome-like symptoms (see). Exposure to cold induces a typical Raynaud phenomenon (see). First affecting only the hand that has been nearer to the end of tool, then all fingers. When attack is severe, complete sensory loss over the fingers may be experienced.

Signs. During attacks, color changes in the fingers; between attacks, normal fingers. No trophic changes.

Etiology. Unknown. Possibly, alteration of the digital vessels (distal ulnar artery or superficial volar arch), so that spasm follows exposure to cold.

Pathology. Some degree of thickening of intima of digital arteries and arterioles. Lesion often located distally to the carpal tunnel.

Diagnostic Procedures. Rule out other causes of Raynaud phenomenon (see). Angiography.

Therapy. Relief from attack by rubbing hands and then immersing them in warm water. Alcohol injection. If intolerable pain, change of activity; if change impossible, sympathectomy or surgical decompression may be considered after careful neurophysiologic assessment.

Prognosis. Relatively benign course; change of occupation may cure the condition.

BIBLIOGRAPHY. President's Monthly Report. The Stonecutter's J 32:5, 1917
Rosen S: von Ein Fall von Thrombose in der Arteria ulnaris nach Einwirchung von Stumpfer Gewalt. Acta Chir Scand 73:500, 1934
Vayssairat M, Defure C, Cormier JM, et al: Hypotenar hammer syndrome: Seventeen cases with long term follow-up. J Vas Surg 5:838–843, 1987
Lundborg G, Dahlin LB: Vibration-induced hand problems. In Vastamaeki M: Current Trends in Hand Surgery, pp 563–571. Netherlands, Excerpta Medica, 1995

PNEUMONIA, LYMPHOID INTERSTITIAL

Synonyms. LIP; plasma cell interstitial pneumonia; PIP.

Symptoms. Both sexes affected. Onset at all ages. Cough; dyspnea.

Signs. Cyanosis and clubbing in 50% of cases.

Etiology. Unknown.

Pathology. Lung infiltrate formed by a mixture of small lymphocytes, plasma cells, and a few large mononuclear elements; in some cases, prevalence of plasma cells (it could represent a variant of this condition). Relative absence of pleural infiltration, involvement of lymph nodes and extrapulmonary tissues.

Diagnostic Procedures. *Blood.* Occasionally, monoclonal gammopathy (IgM and less frequently, IgG). *X-ray.* No specific findings.

Therapy. Trial with corticosteroids.

Prognosis. Progressive condition leading to pulmonary fibrosis.

BIBLIOGRAPHY. Carrington CB, Liebow AA: Lymphocytic interstitial pneumonia. Am J Pathol 48:36A, 1966
Fraser RS, Paré JAP, Fraser RG, Paré PD: Synopsis of Disease of the Chest, 2nd ed. Philadelphia, WB Saunders, 1994

POLAND

Synonym. Pectoralis muscle deficiency—syndactyly.

Symptoms. Incidence 10% of patients with syndactyly. No history. Patient cannot draw arm of affected side across the chest.

Signs. Syndactyly associated with ipsilateral absence of sternal head of pectoralis major. If in a female, asymmetry of breasts; patchy absence of axillary hair; absence of the nipple on affected side.

Etiology. Unknown. Sporadic or occasionally in successive generations autosomal dominant inheritance. Interruption of embryonic blood supply in the succlavian arteries.

Pathology. Absence of pectoralis major; syndactyly.

Diagnostic Procedures. *X-ray.* Of hand and chest. *CT scan. MRI.* To identify possible associated anomalies.

Therapy. Surgical correction of syndactyly in late childhood. Correction with latissimus muscle transposition.

Prognosis. Surgical correction of syndactyly usually brings good results.

BIBLIOGRAPHY. Poland A: Deficiency of the pectoral muscles. Guy Hosp Rep 6:191–193, 1841

Ireland DCR, Tekajama N, Flatt AE: Poland's syndrome: A review of forty-three cases. J Bone Joint Surg 58:52–58, 1976

Der Kaloustian VM, Hoyme HE, Hogg H, et al: Possible common pathogenetic mechanisms for Poland sequence and Adam-Oliver syndrome. Am J Med Genet 38:69–73, 1991

POLAND-MOEBIUS

Combination of the two syndromes (see Poland and Mobius) that is considered to represent a specific genetic malformation with autosomal dominant inheritance.

BIBLIOGRAPHY. Gadot N, Biedner B, Torok G: Moebius syndrome and Poland anomaly case report and review of the literature. J Paediatr Ophthalmol 16:374–376, 1979

Stevenson RE: The Poland-Moebius syndrome. Proc Greenwood Genet Center 1:26–28, 1982

POLLITT

Synonyms. Trichothiodystrophy-neurocutaneous; trichorrhexis nodosa. See Sabouraud.

Symptoms. Both sexes. From birth. Delayed mental and physical retardation. Spastic diplegia.

Signs. Microcephaly; head titubation, jerky eye movements; length and weight below normal. Facies unusual (receding chin, large ears, stubby eyebrows). Trichorrhexis nodosa (hair progressively thinning, brittle, beaded, easily breakable and falling), ichthyosis and eczema, hypoplastic nails. Absent deep tendon reflexes.

Etiology. Possibly autosomal recessive inheritance.

Pathology. *Brain.* Abnormal cortical cell layering.

Diagnostic Procedures. *Hair.* Cystine content 50% normal. *EEG. CT scan. MRI.*

BIBLIOGRAPHY. Pollitt RJ, Jenner FA, Davies M: Sibs with mental and physical retardation and trichorrhexis nodosa with abnormal amino acid composition of the hair. Arch Dis Child 43:211–216, 1968

Gummer CL, Dawber RPR: Trichothiodystrophy: an ultrastructural study of the hair follicle. Br J Dermatol 113:273–280, 1985

Dawber RPR, Ebling FJG, Wojnarowska FT: Disorders of hair. In Champion RH, Burton JL, Ebling FJG (eds): Rook/Wilkinson/Ebling Textbook of Dermatology, 5th ed, pp 2613–2614. Oxford, Blackwell Scientific, 1992

POLYARTERITIS NODOSA CUTANEA

Synonyms. Sneddon-Champion; livedo nodules.

Symptoms and Signs. Prevalent (i.e., described) in male. Onset at all ages (2 months to 69 years). Monosymptomatic: chronic eruption of numerous small (0.5–2 cm), firm, hard, pink, painful nodules on (but not exclusively) the legs; or polysymptomatic: associated with livedo reticularis, myalgia (50%), ulcerations, gangrenous complications, polyneuritis, or arthralgia (50%).

Etiology. Unknown. Cutaneous vasculitis. Allergy (?); autoimmune disorder (?); toxic (?).

Pathology. Necrotizing arteritis at junction of dermis and subcutis; infiltration of vascular walls and fibrinoid necrosis. No inflammatory reaction (in synthesis presence of changes similar to Kussmaul [see], but less intense).

Diagnostic Procedures. *Blood. Normal.* Increase of sedimentation rate; moderate leukocytosis. *Biopsy of skin.* (See Pathology.)

Therapy. Corticosteroids.

Prognosis. Benign. Attacks last a month and may relapse for years; however, no visceral complications have been observed.

BIBLIOGRAPHY. Lyell A, Church R: Cutaneous manifestations of polyarteritis nodosa. Br J Dermatol 66:335–363, 1954

Isolement d'une forme cutanée, pure benigne de periarterite nodeuse (PAN). Instantanés médicaux N.5. Encyclopédie Médico-Chirurgicale, 1979

Champion RH: Reactions to cold. In Champion RH, Burton JL, Ebling FJG (eds): Rook/Wilkinson/Ebling Textbook of Dermatology, 5th ed, p 840. Oxford, Blackwell Scientific, 1992

POLYARTHRITIS, EPIDEMIC, TROPICAL, ACUTE

Symptoms and Signs. Epidemic, seasonal (fall) occurrence of mild fever, cutaneous rash (rubella-like), polyarthritis, lymphadenopathy.

Etiology. Unknown. Infection from mosquito bite virus (?).

Diagnostic Procedures. *Blood.* Agglutination and culture tests negative.

Therapy. Symptomatic.

Prognosis. Self-limited condition lasting 10–20 days; recovery without sequelae.

BIBLIOGRAPHY. Halliday JH, Horan JP: Epidemic of polyarthritis in northern territory. Med J Aust 2:293–295, 1943

Schmidt FR: Unusual features and special types of infectious arthritis. In Hollander JL, McCarty DJ: Arthritis and Allied Conditions, 8th ed, p 1269. Philadelphia, Lea & Febiger, 1972

Klippel JH, Dieppe PA: Rheumatology, p 2.1.6. St Louis, CV Mosby, 1994

POLYCYSTIC

Synonyms. Hepatic cystic; renal cystic. See Caroli. Clinically two varieties are recognized: (1) prevalent renal cystic syndrome, (a) infantile type and (b) adult type; (2) hepatic cystic syndrome, (a) infantile, adolescent type and (b) adult type.

PREVALENT RENAL CYSTIC SYNDROME

INFANTILE TYPE

Symptoms. Nausea; vomiting; dehydration.

Signs. Abdominal distention; palpation of bilateral renal masses (except in small cyst variety). Symptoms and signs may also be observed due to the presence of cysts in other organs (brain, lung, liver, pancreas) but are usually clinically subordinate to kidney pathology.

Etiology. Unknown. May be autosomal recessive. The pathogenetic hypothesis: (1) failure of union of the ureteric bud with convoluted tubules (metanephric; metanephroblastemic); (2) tubules canalization failure; (3) persistence of various generations of "nephrons."

Pathology. Kidney size may be normal or increased and asymmetric. Cysts of various sizes; cystic fluid watery, yellow, bloody, always totally isolated. Degenerative changes of parenchyma, owing to compression, calculi, secondary infections.

Diagnostic Procedures. *Urine.* Albumin; hematuria; epithelial cells.

Blood. Hyperchloremic acidosis. *X-ray.* Intravenous pyelography. *Renal scan with radioactive isotopes.*

Therapy. Medical treatment of infection, renal insufficiency, hypertension. Kidney transplantation.

Prognosis. Excellent results with kidney transplantation.

ADULT TYPE

Symptoms. May be asymptomatic for several decades. Lumbar pains; palpable mass; hypertension; bladder symptoms of dysuria; hematuria; painful or painless. Weakness; abdominal enlargement.

Signs. Hypertension; palpable kidneys.

Etiology. Unknown. Hereditary dominant (in large family, affects 50% of membranes).

Pathology. See Infantile type. Adult cyst may communicate and sometimes contain urinous fluid.

Diagnostic Procedures. See Infantile type.

Therapy. See Infantile type.

Prognosis. Seldom, does not interfere with normal life; usually, progressive symptomatology (e.g., hypertension, uremia infections). Death usually in the middle of sixth decade. Kidney transplantation gives normal life expectancy.

HEPATIC CYSTIC SYNDROME

See Caroli.

INFANTILE, ADOLESCENT TYPE

Symptoms. Both sexes equally affected. Bleeding from esophageal varices is presenting manifestation.

Signs. Splenomegaly.

Etiology. Unknown. Variant of polycystic disease. Other cysts usually present (including kidney) are clinically subordinate. Autosomal dominant.

Pathology. *Liver.* Connective tissue proliferation in periportal spaces; ductules more or less ectasic; lobular architecture preserved; hepatic cell normal. *Kidney.* From minimal microcystic dilatation of tubules in the cortex to macroscopic cysts in cortex and medulla.

Diagnostic Procedures. *Blood.* Normal or slight elevation of bilirubin; elevation of alkeline phosphatase; serum glutamic-oxaloacetic transaminase (SGOT); serum glutamic-pyruvic transaminase (SGPT); moderate decrease of prothrombin. Normal sodium sulfobromophthalein (Bromsulfalein) excretion. *Biopsy.* Of liver. See Pathology. *Urography.* From normal to polycystic pattern. Increase of portal pressure.

Therapy. Portacaval shunt well supported. Liver transplantation attempted.

Prognosis. Fair with treatment.

ADULT TYPE

Symptoms. Dyspepsia; abdominal pain; hemorrhages from esophageal varices.

Signs. Massive hepatomegaly; splenomegaly.

Etiology. See Infantile, adolescent type.

Pathology. See Infantile, adolescent type.

Diagnostic Procedures. See Infantile, adolescent type.

Therapy. See Infantile, adolescent type.

Prognosis. See Infantile, adolescent type.

BIBLIOGRAPHY. Poinso R, Mouges H, Payan H: La maladie kystique du foi. Expansion Scientifique Francaise, 1954

Wilcox RG, Isselbacker KJ: Chronic liver disease in young people. Am J Med 30:185–195, 1961
Clermont RJ, Maillard JN, Benhamon JP, et al: Fibrose hepatique congenitale. Can Med Assoc J 97:1272–1278, 1967
Parfrey PS, Bear JC, Morgan J, et al: The diagnosis and prognosis of autosomal dominant polycystic kidney disease. N Engl J Med 323:1085–1090, 1990
Ravine D, Walker RG, Gibson RN, et al: Treatable complications in undiagnosed cases of autosomal dominant polycystic kidney disease. Lancet 337:127–129, 1991
Weatherall DJ, Ledingham JGG, Warrell DA (eds): Oxford Textbook of Medicine, 3rd ed, pp 3202–3204. Oxford, Oxford Med Pub, 1996

POLYFIBROMATOSIS

Synonyms. See Dupuytren contracture.

Symptoms and Signs. Association of Dupuytren contracture (see) with other fibromatoses: knuckle pads; keloid scarring; Duplay (see), Peyronie (see); myofibromatosis (see).

Etiology. Genetically determined syndromes.

POLYGLANDULAR FAILURE, TYPE I APS

Synonyms. Autoimmune polyglandular I. Familial endocrinopathy-candidiasis. Endocrine deficiency multiple; multiple endocrine; MEN candidiasis endocrinopathy; MEDAC; multiple endocrine deficiency; autoimmune candidiasis; PGA1. See Beck-Ibrahim.

Symptoms and Signs. Both sexes affected. Onset after first year of life. Chronic mucocutaneous candidiasis (usually restricted to skin, nails, oral and perianal mucosa, with remission or progressive course and severe involvement of gastroenteric tract and diarrhea or hemorrhages). associated with symptoms of one of this endocrinopathies: hypoparathyroidism (developing before age 10 years: seizures, carpopedal spasms, laryngospasms, etc.); hypoadrenocorticalism (developing at 10–30 years of age); gonadal insufficiency (more frequent in females: arrest after normal menarche or mestrual irregularities). Associated in addition typical atrophic gastritis (at 15–16 years 15% of cases); teeth and nails abnormal development; keratopathy; tympanic membrane sclerosis; vitiligo; alopecia totalis or partialis; hepatomegaly (10% of cases) Sjoegren; rarely other endocrinopathies (thyroiditis, hypophysitis).

Etiology. Autosomal recessive inheritance. Defective immunoregulation binding together the chronic mucocutaneous candidiasis, the selective IgA deficiencies, and the cluster of autoimmune conditions.

Pathology. Extremely variable according to the manifestations of the syndrome.

Diagnostic Procedures. *Blood.* Hypocalcemia; IgA absent; IgE elevated; polyclonal hypergammaglobulinemia. Search for biochemical changes caused by various endocrine gland deficiencies and tests of hormone deficiency corrections. Humoral immunity studies. With search of specific antibodies to endocrine glands. Histocompatibility profile. Other for differential diagnosis enumeration of T- and B-lymphocytes; lymphocyte stimulation and suppressor T-cell activity. *X-ray.* Absence of rickets; osteomalacia (in hypoparathyroidism form). Nonspecific findings.

Therapy. Symptomatic correction of specific hormone deficiencies or of various condition clusters, and antimycotic agents.

Prognosis. Only temporary benefit from various therapeutic interventions.

BIBLIOGRAPHY. Thorpe ES Jr, Handley HE: Chronic tetany and chronic mycelial stomatitis in a child aged four and one half years. Am J Dis Child 38:328–338, 1929
Sutphin A, Albright F, McCune DJ: Five cases (three in siblings) of

idiopathic hypoparathyroidism associated with moniliasis. J Clin Endocrinol 3:625–634, 1943

Ahonen P: Autoimmune polyendocrino pathycandidosis ectodermal dystrophy (ECED): Autosomal recessive inheritance. Clin Genet 27:535–542, 1985

Muir A, Schatz DA, MacLaren NK: Polyglandular failure syndromes. In De Groot LJ (ed): Endocrinology, 3rd ed, p 3019. Philadelphia, WB Saunders, 1995

POLYGLUCOSAN BODY DISEASE, ADULT FORM

Synonyms. Branching enzyme deficiency, APBD. See Andersen.

Symptoms and Signs. Rare. Observed in Ashkenazi Jews and French Canadians. Onset in the fifth to sixth decade. Upper and lower motor neurone signs, glove stocking sensory loss, sphincter problems, neurogenic bladder, and dementia.

Etiology. Defect of branching enzyme (type glycogenosis type IV) activity limited to single organs. Accumulation of polyglucosan bodies.

Pathology. Nerves. Profusion of microscopic bodies resembling corpora amylacea or Lafora bodies (see) in neurons and astrocytes.

Diagnostic Procedures. *Nerve biopsy. MRI.* Extensive white matter abnormalities. Polymorphonucleates: brancher enzyme 15% of normal.

Therapy. Symptomatic.

Prognosis. Evolution to dementia.

BIBLIOGRAPHY. Robitaille Y, Carpenter S, Karpati G, et al: A distinct form of adult polyglucosan body disease and massive involvement of central and peripheral neuronal processes and astrocytes: a reports of four cases and a review of occurrence of polyglucosan bodies in other conditions such as Lafora's disease and normal aging. Brain 103:315–336, 1980

Lossos A, Barash V, Soffer D, et al: Hereditary branching enzyme dysfunction in adult polyglucosan body disease: A possible metabolic cause in two patients. Ann Neurol 30:655–662, 1991

Bruno C, Servidei S, Shanske S, et al: Glycogen branching enzyme in adult polyglycosan body disease. Ann Neurol 33:88–93, 1993

POLYMER FUME FEVER

Symptoms. Occurs several hours after exposure to fumes of heated polymer. Severe cold symptoms; rigor; shaking of limbs; headache; sore throat.

Signs. None or mild reddening of throat.

Etiology. Inhalation of fumes of pyrolysis of polytetrafluoroethylene (Teflon-fluon). Particles contaminating cigarettes of people smoking when handling these chemicals may be responsible.

Therapy. None. Avoidance of exposure to fumes and smoking when handling these chemicals.

Prognosis. Symptoms disappear spontaneously within a few hours.

BIBLIOGRAPHY. Harris DK: Polymer-fume fever. Lancet 2:1008–1011, 1951

Barnes R, Jones AT: Polymer-fume fever. Med J Aust 2:60–61, 1967

Clayton GD, Clayton FE: Patty's Industrial Hygiene and Toxicology, 4th ed, vol 2, part E, p 3700. New York, John Wiley Sons, 1994

POLYMYALGIA RHEUMATICA

Synonyms. Barber (HS); Bargantum; Bruce; Forestier-Certonciny; anarthritic rheumatoid; anarthritic; myalgic syndrome of aged; pseudopolyarthrite rhizomelique; senile arthritis.

Symptoms. Affects mostly elderly persons; seldom before age 50 onset acute or insidious. Pain and stiffness of the shoulder and hip girdle; occasionally, severe and incapacitating. Fatigue, anorexia, weight loss, and fever. Horton syndrome frequently associated.

Signs. Muscular stiffness and tenderness; absence of joint deformity.

Etiology. Unknown. The diagnosis is based mostly on negative criteria (absence of a definitive alternative diagnosis and exclusion of definitive and probable rheumatoid arthritis, see Diagnostic Procedures).

Pathology. No specific changes in muscle biopsy. Possible association of arteritis (see Horton syndrome).

Diagnostic Procedures. *Blood.* High sedimentation rate; absence of rheumatoid factor and LE cells. *Biopsy.* Of skin, muscle, mucosa. Normal.

Therapy. Good response to corticosteroids and other anti-inflamatory agents

Prognosis. Duration of symptoms 6 months to 6 years. Complete recovery; possibility of recurrence or evolution into Horton.

BIBLIOGRAPHY. Bruce W: College of GP Research Newsletter (9:157); Br Med J 2:811, 1888

Forestier J, Certonciny A: Pseudopolyarthrite rhizomelique. Rev Rheum (Paris) 20:854–862, 1953

Barber HS: Myalgic syndrome with constitutional effects. Polymyalgia rheumatica. Ann Rheum Dis 16:230–237, 1957

How J, Hirst PJ, Bewsher PD, et al: Familial polymyalgia rheumatica. Scot Med J 26:59–61, 1981

Hellmann DB: Immunopathogenesis, diagnosis and treatment of giant cell arteritis, temporal arteritis, polymyalgia rheumatica and takayasu's arteritis. Curr Opin Rheumatol 5:25–32, 1993

POLYMYOSITIS SYNDROMES

Synonym. Idiopathic polymyositis. See Wagner-Unverricht.

Symptoms. Male to female ratio, 1:2. Common to all groups: symmetric muscle weakness (more frequently affecting proximal muscle), shoulder girdle (first group to be affected); tenderness; occasionally, increased consistency; occasionally, progression to fibrotic contractures. Frequently, associated are the Raynaud phenomenon and dysphagia. (See dermatomyositis, same condition.)

Signs. Tendon reflex may be lost when severely affected. Clinically subdivided in the following subgroups: *Group 1.* A. Acute. More frequent in young people (1–20 years). B. Subacute. I: in childhood; chronic; II: early adult life; chronic; III: "late life" muscular dystrophy. *Group 2.* Polymyositis dominant feature; associated connective tissue diseases minor clinical role. *Group 3.* Polymyositis minor feature, associated connective tissues diseases major role. *Group 4.* Polymyositis associated with carcinoma.

However, it appears as best defined as inflammatory myopathy of subacute onset (weeks or months), steady progression in adults who do not present (1) rash, (2) involvement of eyes and facial muscles, (3) family history of neuromuscolar disease, (4) endocrinopathy, (5) exposure to myotoxic drugs (cholesterol lowering agents) or toxins, (6) neurogenic diseases, dystrophies, biochemical muscle disease, or inclusion body myositis (see).

Etiology. Unknown. Systemic disorder when skin manifestations are associated is designated dermatomyositis (see Wegner-Unverricht). In some cases, *Borrelia burgdorferi* or *legionella pneumophila* may be the cause. Pathogenesis is mediated by cytotoxic T-cells that attack muscle fibers expressing MHC-I antigens.

Pathology. Common feature of the polymyositis is acute or subacute degeneration of muscle fibers with variable inflammatory changes. Endomycosial infiltrates mostly within fascicles.

Diagnostic Procedures. *Biopsy.* Of muscle. *Electromyography. Blood.* LE test; rheumatoid test; sedimentation rate; blood enzymes.

Therapy. Adrenal corticoids. Treatment of associated conditions when present.

Prognosis. Very variable. A few cases of acute form have resulted in death. Usually, chronic course with or without muscle atrophy or contractures. When associated with carcinoma, excision of tumor may be followed by disappearance of myositic symptoms.

BIBLIOGRAPHY. Wagner E: Fall einer seltnen Muskelkrankheit. Arch Heilkunde 4:282–283, 1863

Sigurgeirsson B, Lindelof B, Edhag O: Risk of cancer in patients with dermatomyositis or polymyositis: A population-based study. N Engl J Med 326:363–367, 1992

Dalakas MC: Inflammatory myopathies. In Rowland LP, Di Mauro S (eds): Handbook of Clinical Neurology, vol 18: Myopathies, p 369. Amsterdam, Elsevier, 1992

POLYNEUROPATHY, FAMILIAL, RECURRENT

Synonyms. Neuropathy, hereditary; pressure palsies tomaculous neuropathy; bulbs digger palsy; see Jacob (J.C.) (different condition).

Symptoms. Both sexes. Male more severely affected, onset at ages 15–20 years. After kneeling or exercising pressure in other areas of the body, attacks of pain, weakness or transient palsies of selected groups of muscles (peroneal or arms and hands) sometimes, muscle-wasting after repeated attacks. In addition to peroneal and brachial; lower cranial nerves may be affected also.

Etiology. Unknown. Autosomal dominant inheritance trait.

Pathology. In the myelin sheath (of both sensory and motor nerves), sausage-shaped swelling (tomaculous).

Diagnostic Procedures. *Electromyography.* Electric conduction velocity abnormalities. *Sural nerve biopsy.*

Therapy. Corticosteroids.

Prognosis. Attacks usually remit gradually leaving weakness and muscle atrophy.

BIBLIOGRAPHY. De Jong JGY: Over families met Hereditaire disposite tot het optreten van neuritiden, gecorreleard met migraine. Psychiat Neurol Bl 50:60–76, 1947

Davies DM: Recurrent peripheral nerve palsies in a family. Lancet II:266–268, 1954

Fewings JD, Mukherjee TM, Blumbergs PC, et al: Tomaculous neuropathy: Hereditary predisposition to pressure palsies. Aust NZJ Med 15:598–603, 1985

Barisic N, Skarpa D, Jusic A, et al: Steroid responsive familial neuropathy with liability to pressure palsy. Neuropediatrics 21:191–192, 1990

POLYPOSIS COLI, JUVENILE

Synonyms. Juvenile polyposis coli; retention polyposis; solitary polyps rectum—colon; familial discrete polyposis, juvenile familial polyposis coli, including polyposis intestinal IV (Wolff).

Symptoms and Signs. Slightly prevalent in young boys. Blood from anus or stool streaking; diarrhea (occasionally); constipation (rare).

Etiology. Unknown. Autosomal dominant trait. Affected member of a family always shows this type of polyposis and never intestinal polyposis familial (see).

Pathology. Single or several polyps of colon. Prominent stroma; abundant vascular tissue; mononuclear infiltration; frequent eosinophils. Proliferation mucous glands and cysts with mucus.

Diagnostic Procedures. Sigmoidoscopy. Barium enema.

Therapy. Complete local excision; endoscopic excision.

Prognosis. Excellent. Malignant potentiality of such polyps is low; however, there are several reports of older relatives over 40 years of age who had colonic cancer. Removal of polyps cures the condition.

BIBLIOGRAPHY. Woolf CM, Richards RC, Gardner EJ: Occasional discrete polyps of colon and rectum showing inherited tendency in kindred. Cancer 8:403–408, 1955

Rozen P, Baratz M: Familial juvenile colonic polyposis with associated colon cancer. Cancer 49:1500–1503, 1982

Walpole IR, Cullity G: Juvenile polyposis: a case with early presentation and death attributable to adenocarcinoma of the pancreas. Am J Med Genet 32:1–8, 1989

Haubrich WS, Schaffner F, Berk JE (eds): Bockus Gastroenterology, 5th ed, p 1739. Philadelphia, WB Saunders, 1995

POLYSPLENIA

Symptoms and Signs. Prevalent in females. Signs related to (possibly) associated lung and cardiac malformations (especially left isomerism) and caudal deficiency (seven cases reported; distinct entity [?]).

Etiology. Unknown. Suggested identity of this syndrome with Ivemark (see). Family occurrence reported with possible autosomal recessive inheritance.

Pathology. Accessory spleens vary from two to six or more. Associated bilateral, bilobed (left) lungs with symmetric bilateral left bronchi; bilateral morphologic left atria; bilateral superior vena cava with atrial and ventricular defects.

Diagnostic Procedures. *Blood.* Occasionally, presence of Howell-Jolly and Heinz bodies. *CT scan.*

Therapy. Correction of associated cardiac defect when indicated.

Prognosis. Variable.

BIBLIOGRAPHY. Moller JH, Nekib A, Anderson RC, et al: Congenital cardiac disease associated with polysplenia. Circulation 36:789–799, 1967

Rose V, Izukawa I, Moes CAF, et al: Syndromes of asplenia and polysplenia. A review of cardiac and non cardiac malformations in 60 cases with special reference to diagnosis and prognosis. Br Heart J 37:840–852, 1975

Rodriguez JI, Palacios J, Omenaca F, et al: Polyasplenia, caudal deficiency and agenesis of corpus callosum. Am J Med Genet 38:99–102, 1991

Perloff JK: The Clinical Recognition of Congenital Heart Disease, 4th ed, 45–47. Philadelphia, WB Saunders, 1994

POMPE

Synonyms. Cori type II glycogenosis; acid maltase deficiency; AMD; alpha-1,4-glucosidase deficiency; GAA deficiency; glycogenosis (type II); cardiomegalia glycogenica diffusa. Four clinical varieties are recognizable according to the degree of involvement of different organs, although overlapping of symptoms and signs occurs:

1. Cardiomegalic variety
2. Generalized variety
3. Muscular variety
4. Late infantile acid maltase deficiency variety.

Another classification recognizes these varieties:

(1) Infantile onset
(2) Juvenile onset
(3) Adult onset

(4) Lysosomal glycogen disease without alpha-glucosidase deficiency (see).

Both classifications present a certain degree of ambiguity for the overlapping, presence or absence of specific clinical features

CARDIOMEGALIC, GENERALIZED, AND MUSCULAR VARIETIES

Symptoms. Both sexes affected. Clinical onset in first month of life. Vomiting; anorexia; drooling; profound weakness; failure to thrive. Severe mental retardation (may be present); repeated respiratory infections. Later, dyspnea.

Signs. Severe muscle hypotonia (however firm and even hypertrophic); macroglossia (common); cardiomegaly (of various degrees). Apical systolic murmur present; hepatosplenomegaly. Various neurologic defects (generalized variety). Later, cyanosis.

Etiology. Autosomal recessive inheritance. Absent activity of lysosomal hydrolase acid alpha-1,4-glucosidase. Structural gene for acid alpha-glucosidase localized to chromosome 17q23.

Pathology. Generalized glycogen accumulation in heart, muscles, central and peripheral nervous systems, reticuloendothelial system, kidney, liver, adrenal glands.

Diagnostic Procedures. *Blood.* Normal. Leukocytes reveal massive glycogen deposits, absence of alpha-1,4-glucosidase activity. *Blood.* Sugar, glucose, and galactose tolerance; glucagon and epinephrine response normal. *X-ray.* Globular heart enlargement. *ECG.* Shortened PR intervals and large QRS complexes. *EMG.* Pseudomyotonic discharges and irritability. *Biopsy.* Of muscle. Enzymes studies.

Therapy. Trial with vitamin A (to increase lysis of lysosomes).

Prognosis. Death within 1 year usually owing to cardiocirculatory failure.

LATE INFANTILE ACID MALTASE DEFICIENCY SYNDROME

Symptoms and Signs. Clinical onset later than preceding forms. Weakness of hip muscles; Gower signs. Contraction of Achilles tendons; muscles firm and rubbery; anal sphincter may be patulous; defective bladder contraction; aneurysms and vacuolar degeneration of cerebral arteries. Mental retardation or normal development.

Etiology. See the preceding. Markedly reduced activity of enzyme activity.

Pathology. Muscle fibers vacuolated (glycogen deposits); liver glycogen concentration normal; no gross cardiac abnormalities. Glycogen deposit in anterior horn cells of sacral cord.

Diagnostic Procedures. *Biopsy.* Of muscle and liver. Lack of acid maltase. *EMG. Blood.* Leukocytes; absence of alpha-1,4-glucosidase activity.

Therapy. Trial with vitamin A. Epinephrine injections over long period.

Prognosis. This variant allows survival beyond infancy.

BIBLIOGRAPHY. Pompe JC: Over idiopatischehypertrophie von het hart. Ned Tidjdschr Geneeskd 76:304–305, 1932
Roth CJ, Williams HE: The muscular variant of Pompe's disease. J Pediatr 71:567–573, 1967
Swaiman KF, Kennedy WR, Sauls HS: Late infantile acid maltase deficiency. Arch Neurol 18:642–648, 1968
Kretzschamar HA, Wagner H, Hubner G: Aneurysm and vacuolar degeneration of cerebral arteries in late onset acid maltase deficiency. J Neurol Sci 98:169–183, 1990
Hirschhorn R: Glycogen storage disease type II acid-glucosidase (acid maltase) deficiency. In Scriver CR, Beaudet AL, Sly WS, et al: The Metabolic and Molecular Bases of Inherited Disease, 7th ed, pp 2443–2464. New York, McGraw-Hill, 1995

POMPHOLYX

Synonyms. Cheiropompholyx; dyshidrosis.

Symptoms. Both sexes affected; onset after 10 years of age; maximal incidence at 20–40 years. Intense itching, usually limited to palms or soles bilaterally or unilaterally. Attacks are precipitated by such factors as warm weather, stress.

Signs. Sudden appearance of crops of vesicles, which may become confluent in bullae. After repeated attacks, dystrophic nail changes.

Etiology. Form of hyperhidrosis or dyshidrosis; emotional stress is frequently the precipitating factor. In some cases, fungus infection has been proven; in other cases, focal infection, food allergies have been suspected.

Pathology. Eczema-like changes.

Diagnostic Procedures. Evaluation of possible etiologic factors.

Therapy. Soaking in normal saline opens larger bullae; if infection, antibiotics. Mild sedatives helpful.

Prognosis. Recurrent condition, every 2–3 weeks for months or years, or only in warm weather. Recovery or irregular attacks if sporadic.

BIBLIOGRAPHY. Simons RDGP: Eczema of the Hand, 2nd ed. Basel, Karger, 1966
Burton JL: Eczema, lichenification, prurigo and erytroderma. In Champion RH, Burton JL, Ebling FJG (eds): Rook/Wilkinson/Ebling Textbook of Dermatology, 5th ed, pp 559–562. Oxford, Blackwell Scientific, 1992

PONCET

Synonyms. Polyarthritis, aseptic.

Symptoms and Signs. In children and adults. Joint pain and swelling in patients with tubercolosis. Any joint may be affected: knee, ankles and elbows (more frequently).

Etiology. "Allergic mechanism" in tubercolosis. (A mycobacterial heat shock protein-HSP 60 may cross react with cartilage and induce T-cell reactivity in HLA-DR4 + individuals).

Pathology. Aseptic polyarthritis. Tubercolosis elsewhere.

Diagnostic Procedures. *Culture of synovial fluid.* Negative. *X-rays.* Unremarkable.

Therapy. Treatment of tubercolosis.

Prognosis. Resolution of all manifestations with tbc treatment.

BIBLIOGRAPHY. Poncet A: De la polyarthrite tuberculeuse déformante ou pseudorheumatisme chronique tuberculeux Congrès Francaise de Chirurgie 1:732–739, 1897
Isaac AJ, Sturrock RD: Poncet's disease—fact or fiction? A reappraisal of tuberculous rheumatism. Tubercle 55:135–142, 1974
Khoury MI: Does reactive arthritis to tubercolosis (Poncet's disease) exist? J Rheumatol 16:1162–1163, 1989
Winfield JB, Jarjour WN: Heat shock proteins and arthritis. Bull Rheum Dis 41:4–5, 1992

POPLITEAL ARTERY ENTRAPMENT

Synonyms. Pretibial. See Peroneal compartment and anterior tibial compartment syndromes.

Symptoms. Rare. Prevalent in young males; onset at an average of 24–26 years of age. Intermittent unilateral claudication; pain relieved by standing still or sitting; paresthesias when sitting with sharply flexed knee. Absence of signs of generalized atherosclerosis. During crisis, absence of dorsalis pedis pulse, weakness of the posterior tibial pulse. Feet, skin, throphic conditions good. Various types of congenital anomalies may be associated.

Etiology. Entrapment of popliteal artery in relation to medial head of gastrocnemius muscle, generally because of congenital anomaly.

Pathology. Artery loops medially to the medial head of gastrocnemius, instead of passing between lateral and medial heads. Medial head of muscle may be attached in anomalous fashion to the femur. Intermittent compression causes thrombosis and sclerosis or aneurysm of popliteal artery. Early arteriosclerotic muscle changes.

Diagnostic Procedures. *Blood.* Normal. *ECG.* Normal. *Arteriography.* Medial deviation of popliteal artery and, possibly, collateral circulation. *Doppler.* Normal tracing on inferior third of leg when foot is forced in plantar hyperextension.

Therapy. Surgical correction to bypass or reconstruct vessel and remove cause of compression.

Prognosis. Good with proper treatment.

BIBLIOGRAPHY. Stuart TPA: Note on a variation in the course of popliteal artery. J Anat 13:162–165, 1879
Turner GR, Gosney WG, Ellingson W, et al: Popliteal artery entrapment syndrome. JAMA 208:692–693, 1969
Klooster NJ, Kitslaar P, Janevski BK: Popliteal artery entrapment syndrome Fortschr Roentgenst 148:624–626, 1988
Dawson DM, Hallett M, Millender LH: Entrapment Neuropathies, 2nd ed. Boston, Little, Brown, 1990

POPLITEAL PTERYGIUM

Synonyms. PPS; Cleft palate—popliteal web-lip pit—genital; faciogenitopopliteal; "quadruple." See Bartsocas-Papas.

Symptoms and Signs. Present at birth. Intrafamilial variability of manifestations. Normal intelligence. Usually, bilateral pterygium or skin web that extends from heel to ischial tuberosity, limiting extension, abduction, and rotation of legs. Syndactyly of toes and fingers; bony malformations of legs. Club feet; toenail dysplasia. Orofacial cleft lip-palate; lip pits; oral webbing (syngnathia) that impedes mouth opening; fused eyelids. Genital-perineal anomalies. Cryptorchidism; cleft scrotum; inguinal hernia; absence of labia majora.

Etiology. Unknown. Autosomal dominant inheritance with incomplete penetrance and variable expressivity.

Pathology. Pterygium formed by a hard nonelastic subcutaneous cord. Sciatic nerve is free within pterygium covered by a fibromuscular septum. Absence of muscle groups or abnormal insertions. See Symptoms and Signs.

Diagnostic Procedures. *X-ray. Chromosome studies.* Pattern normal.

Therapy. Surgical correction.

Prognosis. Depends on type and extension of lesions.

BIBLIOGRAPHY. Trélat V: Sur un vice conformation trés-rare de la lévre inférieure. J Med Chir Prat 40:442–445, 1869
Gorlin RJ, Sedano HO, Cervenka J: Popliteal pterygium syndrome. Pediatrics 41:503–509, 1968
Hunter A: The popliteal pterygium syndrome: Report of a new family and review of the literature. Am J Med Genet 36:196–208, 1990

POROENCEPHALY

Synonyms. Familial poroencephaly; hemiplegia infantile, poroencephaly.

Symptoms and Signs. Both sexes. From birth. Possible prenatal diagnosis. Hemiplegia, seizures.

Etiology. Autosomal dominant with variable expression and low penetrance. X linked inheritance also reported.

Pathology. Two types. (1) Unilateral cavitation or CSF-filled cyst in brain (resulting from trauma or vascular lesions). (2) Symmetric and bilateral (primary defect in morphogenesis).

Diagnostic Procedures. *X-rays. CT scan. MRI. Ultrasonography.* Ventricular dilatation prominent frontal horns: poroencephaly.

Therapy. Symptomatic.

Prognosis. Poor quoad valitudinem.

BIBLIOGRAPHY. Haar L, Dyken P: Hereditary nonprogressive athetotic hemiplegia: A new syndrome. Neurology 27:849–854, 1977
Zanana J, Adornato BT, Glass ST, et al: Familial poroencephaly and congenital hemiplegia. J Pediatr 109:671–674, 1986
Sensi A, Cerruti S, Calzolari E, et al: Familial poroencephaly. Clin Genet 38:396–397, 1990
Adams RD, Victor M: Principles of Neurology, 5th ed, p 1013. New York, McGraw-Hill, 1993

POROT-FILIU

Synonyms. Epilepsy—iris heterochromia—deafness.

Symptoms and Signs. Rare combination. Both sexes. Congenital deafness (nonconstant), heterochromia or bicolor iris, epilepsy (nonconstant), no neurologic abnormalities, from normal mental development to mental retardation.

Etiology. Unknown.

Diagnostic Procedures. *EEG.* May show generalized abnormalities also in cases without epilepsy.

BIBLIOGRAPHY. Porot M, Filiu M: Un syndrome curieux surdi-mutité, hétérochromie irienne et comitialité. Presse Med 46:1709, 1959
Vinken PJ, Bruyn GW: Handbook of Clinical Neurology, vol 42, p 688. Amsterdam, North-Holland, 1981

PORPHYRIA CUTANEA TARDA

Synonyms. Acquired hepatic porphyria (misnomer); constitutional porphyria (misnomer); symptomatic porphyria (misnomer); latent porphyria; porphyria hepatica III: PCT.

Symptoms and Signs. Highest incidence in Bantu population. Both sexes affected (diagnosed more frequently in men); onset usually at 40–60 years of age, seldom in childhood. Insidious onset. Increased facial pigmentation; intermittent excretion of brown urine; increased skin fragility (in light-exposed areas). Spontaneous eruption of vesicular and then ulcerative lesions on face, neck, extremities, slowly healing and with residual scarring. Hypertricosis of forehead, malar areas, and extremities. Variable sensory neuropathy. Absence of motor disorders; dysreflexia; muscle wasting.

Etiology. Reduced hepatic uroporphyrinogen decarboxylase (URO) activity a common defect in all members of affected families. Considered in recent past an acquired condition, secondary to liver (alcoholic estrogens) injury. Today considered autosomal dominant inheritance, with clinical expression secondary to liver injury. Occurrence in patients on hemodialysis due to insufficient removal of porphyrins.

Pathology. *Liver.* Evidence of hepatic siderosis; cirrhosis; high concentration of porphyrins; increased liver iron. *Skin.* Scarring from repeated lesions.

Diagnostic Procedures. *Urine.* Color pink or brown; pink fluorescence after acidification; high excretion of uroporphyrin (mostly isomer type I). *Stool.* Variable excretion of porphyrin.

Therapy. Serial phlebotomy; desferrioxamine. Avoidance of ethanol or other responsible agents intake.

Prognosis. Spontaneous remission possible (especially after alcohol abstinence). Prognosis good, but, following therapy, remission is temporary. Final outcome not related to porphyria but to cirrhosis and other coexisting pathology.

BIBLIOGRAPHY. Waldenström J: Studien ueber Porphiria. Acta Med Scand (Suppl) 82:1–254, 1937

Kushner JP, Barbuto AJ, Lee GR: An inherited enzymatic defect in porphyria cutanea tarda. Decreased uroporphyrinogen decarboxylase activity. J Clin Invest 56:661–667, 1976

Malina L, Lim CK: Manifestation of familial porphyria cutanea tarda after childbirth. Br J Dermatol 118:243–245, 1988

Lee GR: Porphyria. In Lee GR, Bithell TC, Foerster J, et al (eds): Wintrobe's Clinical Hematology, 9th ed, pp 1277–1280. Philadelphia, Lea & Febiger, 1993

PORTER

Synonym. Pericarditis, idiopathic benign.

Symptoms. Observed at all ages; prevalent in young adult males. Upper respiratory infection precedes, by 1 or 2 weeks, the acute onset of the syndrome. Acute pain in the chest, radiating widely, especially to neck and shoulders; more acute during deep respiration, cough, and sometimes swallowing. Recumbency increases the pain, sitting up decreases it. Cough; dyspnea; fever.

Signs. Pericardial rub; enlarged heart area. Frequently, pleurisy with effusion and pneumonitis are associated.

Etiology. Relationship with virus infection (Coxsackie B) proved only in a certain number of cases. Autoimmune reaction also considered a possible mechanism. In some cases, gout has been observed and considered in the etiology.

Pathology. Pericardial effusion with straw-colored or hemorrhagic fluid.

Diagnostic Procedures. *Blood.* Moderate leukocytosis; increased sedimentation rate. *Electrocardiography.* No destructive changes; sometimes simulates acute myocardial infarction. *Pericardiocentesis. X-ray of chest. Echocardiography.*

Therapy. Analgesic and rest often adequate. In severe cases, rapid response to corticosteroids. Pericardiocentesis seldom necessary.

Prognosis. Benign. Cardiac tamponade, however, may occur and subside spontaneously in a few weeks. Multiple recurrences frequent, especially when corticosteroids are withheld.

BIBLIOGRAPHY. Hodges RM: Idiopathic pericarditis. Boston Med Surg J 51:140–141, 1854

Porter WB, Clark O, Porter RR: Nonspecific benign pericarditis. JAMA 144:749–753, 1950

Shabetai R: Diseases of percardium. In Schlant RC, Alexander RW, et al: Hurst's The Heart, 8th ed. New York, McGraw-Hill, 1994

POSTABORTIVE METRORRHAGIA

Synonym. Metrorrhagia, functional, postabortive.

Symptoms. Vaginal bleeding occurring in the reproductive period of women after either a clinical or unsuspected abortion.

Signs. Signs of early pregnancy (i.e., enlarged uterus, soft cervix) and blood clot in vagina.

Etiology. Due to the persistence of chorionic villi with a variable degree of viability, most often identified by histologic examination. The slowly regressing corpus luteum maintains an estrogen-progesterone imbalance leading to hyperestrinism and disturbance of menstrual rhythm.

Pathology. *Ovaries.* (Findings are not consistent.) Small with degenerative corpora lutea; normal size with cystic or degenerative corpora lutea; enlarged with cystic corpora lutea; normal or enlarged with multiple atretic follicles. Endometrium: hyperplasia.

Diagnostic Procedures. Estimation of gonadotropin in urine and blood is not helpful and is negative in the conventional concentration (2000–100,000 IU/liter). It is possible that minute amounts are present, and are detectable only by special techniques.

Therapy. Curettage is curative.

Prognosis. Good after curettage.

BIBLIOGRAPHY. Aschoff L: Tratado de Anatomia Pathologica, vol 11, p 927. Barcelona, Labor, 1934

Cunningham FG, MacDonald PC, Gant NF, et al (eds): Williams Obstetrics, p 847. Englewood Cliffs, NJ, Prentice-Hall, 1993

POSTCARDIOTOMY, DIPHASIC

This syndrome, occurring after heart surgery, runs a diphasic course. A first phase a few days after surgery characterized by fever and unusual lesions of the mouth (nonulcerative, small, painful induration) disappearing in 2 weeks. A second phase occurs after 3–6 weeks with hepatosplenomegaly, pleural and pericardial friction rubs with a benign course but long lasting (months). This syndrome seems to represent a combination of the postperfusion syndrome (see), and the postpericardiotomy syndrome (see).

BIBLIOGRAPHY. Kahn DR, Ertel PY, Murphy WH, et al: Pathogenesis of the postcardiotomy syndrome. J Thorac Cardiovasc Surg 54:682–687, 1968

Weatherall DJ, Ledingham JGG, Warrell DA (eds): Oxford Textbook of Medicine, 3rd ed, p 2475. Oxford, Oxford Med Pub, 1996

POSTCHOLECYSTECTOMY

Synonyms. Recurrent biliary tract; cholecystectomized painful tomorrow.

Symptoms. Recurrence of same symptoms present before operation, or postoperative occurrence of symptoms such as colicky pain, bloating, nausea, vomiting.

Signs. Pain on palpation of right upper quadrant; sometimes, jaundice.

Etiology and Pathology. Mechanisms of much different natures cause this syndrome. They may be classified in three groups. (1) Unrelated to surgery: (a) erroneous diagnosis for previous operation (symptoms of extrabiliary origin); (b) concomitant pathology (liver, pancreas, neoplasia, stenosis of Oddi sphincter, stenosing choledochitis, cholangitis). (2) Postoperative sequelae: (a) common duct injury or calculi; (b) intrahepatic calculi; (c) cystic duct or gallbladder remnant; (d) adhesion; (e) removal of functioning gallbladder. (3) Functional biliary disorders.

Diagnostic Procedures. *X-ray. CT scan. MRI. Sonography. Scintigraphy. Fine needle cholangiography. Endoscopic retrograde cholepancreotography. Liver and pancreatic function studies.*

Therapy. According to etiology.

Prognosis. Variable according to diagnosis and further treatment.

BIBLIOGRAPHY. Meyers SG, Sandweiss DJ, Saltzstein HC: End results after gallbladder operations. Am J Dig Dis 5:667–674, 1938

Thomas E: Papillitis and the postcholecystectomy syndrome. J Natl Med Assoc 84:238–240, 1992

Burton F R: Postcholecystectomy syndrome: How to determine if the sphincter of Oddi is the cause. Postgrad Med 91:255–258, 1992

Weatherall DJ, Ledingham JGG, Warrell DA (eds): Oxford Textbook of Medicine, 3rd ed, p 2051. Oxford, Oxford Med Pub, 1996

POSTCOARCTATION

Symptoms. Occurs following surgery for resection of coarcted aorta segment. On second postoperative day, anorexia, increased temperature. On fourth day, abdominal pain, vomiting.

Signs. From eighth day, signs of mild peritoneal irritation. Exploration shows petechiae diffused over small bowel. Delayed hypertension (lasting 10 days).

Etiology. Removal of obstructing stenosis subjects vascular bed below coarctation to increased pulse pressure, and greater constant distention of arteries. Vasospasm and ischemia of bowel.

Pathology. Disruption and fragmentation of internal elastic lamina; intimal damage; necrotizing thrombosis; inflammatory reaction.

Therapy. Symptomatic. Prevention of syndrome by control of diastolic blood pressure (sodium nitroprusside, propanolol, reserpine) and insertion of nasogastric tube for decompression of gastrointestinal tract for 48 hours. Antibiotic prophylaxis to prevent risk of infective endocarditis

Prognosis. Guarded. Death from necrotizing mesenteric arteritis or other unrelated postoperative causes.

BIBLIOGRAPHY. Sealy WC: Indication for surgical treatment of coarctation of the aorta. Surg Gynecol Obstet 97:301, 1953.
Mays ET, Sergeant CK: Postcoarctectomy syndrome. Arch Surg 91:58–66, 1965
Kawauchi M, Tada Y, Asano K, et al: Angiographic demonstration of mesenteric arterial changes in postcoarctactectomy syndrome. Surgery 98:602–604, 1985
Bobby JJ, Emami JM, Farmer RTD, et al: Operative survival and 40 year follow up of surgical repair of aortic coarctation. Br Heart J 65:271–276, 1991

POSTDYSENTERIC

Symptoms. Occurs in patients who have recovered from acute dysenteric infections. Recurrence of episodes of abdominal pain and diarrhea.

Signs. Pain and tenderness predominant in lower right abdominal quadrant (in postamebic syndrome) on left side (in postbacillary syndrome).

Etiology. Loss of resistance of bowel to irritation and psychogenic influences are postulated after ruling out residual or recurrent infection.

Pathology. Atrophic changes and ulceration sometimes observed.

Diagnostic Procedures. *Stool.* Function and culture studies. *X-ray.* Of bowel. *Gastric analysis.*

Therapy. Symptomatic.

Prognosis. Symptoms may gradually disappear or persist for many years.

BIBLIOGRAPHY. Fierst SM, Werner A: Postdysenteric syndrome. Gastroenterology 27:281–291, 1954
Weatherall DJ, Ledingham JGG, Warrell DA (eds): Oxford Textbook of Medicine, 3rd ed, p 828. Oxford, Oxford Med Pub, 1996

POSTERIOR FOSSA COMPRESSION

Symptoms and Signs. Patient collapses, respiration stops, heart continues to beat vigorously, cyanosis develops, and heart eventually stops. Artificial respiration restores the heartbeat.

Etiology and Pathology. Increased tension into posterior fossa: hemorrhage from fracture of the base of skull, tumor, or abscess. Greater vulnerability of respiratory center than of cardioinhibitory center.

Therapy. Artifical respiration and prompt surgical relief of posterior fossa hypertension.

Prognosis. Lack of prompt surgical intervention is followed by death. Surgical intervention relieves the condition and offers the possibility of dealing with its determining cause.

BIBLIOGRAPHY. Rogers L: The posterior fossa compression syndrome. Br Med J 2:100–101, 1933

POSTGASTRECTOMY DUMPING SYNDROMES

Synonyms. Postcibal; postcibal hypoglycemia; dumping.

EARLY POSTPRANDIAL DUMPING SYNDROME

Symptoms and Signs. Onset immediately after a meal or within 20–30 minutes. Occurs in 20–30% of gastrectomized patients; in 75% of total patients with dumping. Some patients have symptoms with every meal; some only with heavy meal or with only a single meal during the day. Excessive fullness; crampy abdominal pain; sometimes nausea and vomiting. Borborygmi and sudden diarrhea. Vasomotor symptoms: weakness; palpitation; pallor; sweating; sometimes, syncope; patients with severe symptoms may limit food intake and became malnourished (see Lambling).

Etiology. In gastrectomized patient, rapid filling of jejunum with undigested, hyperosmotic food solution. Inappropriate gut hormone release responsible for vasomotor and GI symptoms.

Diagnostic Procedures. *Blood.* Hyperglycemia coinciding with onset of symptoms; somewhat later, slight potassium and phosphorus fall in the plasma. *X-rays.* Upper GI contrast study to exclude stomal obstruction, or afferent loop syndrome (see). *Endoscopy.* Gastric empting studies with radionuclides. *ECG.* Changes.

Therapy. Individualized according to severity of symptoms. Dietary planning (small feeding; low-carbohydrate, fat-rich diet). Recumbent position after eating or surgical reintervention. Octreotide 50 g s.c. 2–3 times a day before meal. Surgery includes stomal revision, conversion of Billroth II in Billroth anastomosis, pyloric reconstruction, jejunal interposition, Roux-en-Y conversion.

Prognosis. Good in majority of cases.

LATE DUMPING SYNDROME

Symptoms. Occurs in gastrectomized patients (25% of total patients with dumping 2–3 hours after a meal. Prevalence of vasomotor symptoms. Symptoms of hypoglycemia (see Hypoglycemic syndromes).

Etiology. Hypoglycemia following a sharp rise of postprandial blood sugar and exaggerated pancreas response.

Therapy. Symptoms relieved by food. Dietary planning or surgical reintervention.

Prognosis. Good.

BIBLIOGRAPHY. Denecheau D: Les suites médicales éloignées de la gastroenterostomie au cours de l'ulcère de l'estomac et de ses complications. Thèses de Paris, 1907; Semaine Méd 27:316–322, 1907
Hertz AF: The cause and treatment of certain unfavorable after-effects of gastroenterostomy. Ann Surg 58:466, 1913
Carvajal SH, Mulvihill SJ: Postgastrectomy symdromes: dumping and diarrhea in postsurgical syndromes. Gastroenter Clin N Am 23:261–274, 1994

POSTGONOCOCCAL URETHRITIS

Synonym. PGU.

Symptoms and Signs. Occurs usually within 20 days of treatment with penicillin and probenecid for gonorrheal urethritis, with no possibility of sexual reinfection. Recurrence of urethral exudate or pyuria. Syndrome seldom occurs in patient whose gonorrhea was treated with tetracycline.

Etiology. Associated to a significant degree with mycoplasma infection of the urethra.

Pathology. Mild urethritis.

Diagnostic Procedures. Smear and cultures of urethral exudate.

Therapy. Tetracycline.

Prognosis. Cured by tetracycline.

BIBLIOGRAPHY. Shepard MC, Alexander CE Jr, Lunceford CD, et al: Possible role of T-strain mycoplasma in nongonococcal urethritis: A sixth venereal disease? JAMA 188:729–735, 1964
Weatherall DJ, Ledingham JGG, Warrell DA (eds): Oxford Textbook of Medicine, 3rd ed, pp 544–550. Oxford, Oxford Med Pub, 1996

POSTHEPATITIS

Obsolete.

Synonyms. Prolonged hepatitis; convalescent hepatitis.

With new classificaton of different types of hepatitis and their identified variable natural histories (chronicization and persistence of viruses, etc.) the generic term of post-hepatitis cannot any longer be considered an individual clinical syndrome.

BIBLIOGRAPHY. Caravati CM: Posthepatitis syndrome. South Med J 37:251–257, 1944
Weissberg JI, Andres LL, Smith CI, et al: Survival in chronic hepatitis B: An analysis of 379 patients. Ann Intern Med 101:613–616, 1984
Nishioka K, Suzuki H, Mishiro S: Viral Hepatitis and Liver Disease. Ijmuiden, Netherlands, Springer-Verlag, 1994

POSTHERPETIC

Synonym. Neuralgia postherpetica.

Symptoms and Signs. Occurs in patients (especially elderly ones) after herpes zoster infections. Paresthesia; itching; pain of area affected; spontaneous or following change in temperature.

Etiology. Degenerative changes and incomplete regeneration of nerves.

Therapy. Carbamazepine (Tegretol), amitriptyline and perphenazine, useful. Analgesics (poor results). Topical applications of acetyl salicilic acid (700–1550 mg) or indomethacyn (100–150) in ethyl ether/chlorophorm (20–30 ml) applied 3–5 times a day. Acyclovir (400–800 mg/day). With the topical application obtained very encouraging results. Interruption of pain fibers.

BIBLIOGRAPHY. Von Bokay J: Ueber den etiologischen Zusamenhang der varicellen-mit gewissen Fallen von Herpes Zoster. Wien klin Wchnschr 22:1323–1326, 1909
Bell WE: Orofacial Pains Classification: Diagnosis Management. Chicago, Year Book Med Publ, 1985
Olen J (chairman): Classification and diagnostic criteria for headache disorders cranial neuralgia and facial pain. Cephalalgia 8(Suppl 7), 1988
Weatherall DJ, Ledingham JGG, Warrell DA (eds): Oxford Textbook of Medicine, 3rd ed, pp 350, 3945, 4023. Oxford, Oxford Med Pub, 1996

POSTHYPOXIC SYNDROMES

To severe hypoxia a combination or overlapping of the following syndromes may result:

1. Persistent coma or stupor
2. Dementia
3. Visual agnosia
4. Parkinsonism with mental deterioration
5. Choreoathetosis
6. Cerebellar ataxia
7. Epilepsy
8. Impairment of memory and of recent facts acquisition

BIBLIOGRAPHY. Adams RD, Victor M: Principles of Neurology, 5th ed, p 880. New York, McGraw-Hill, 1993
Weatherall DJ, Ledingham JGG, Warrell DA (eds): Oxford Textbook of Medicine, 3rd ed, pp 4237–4238. Oxford, Oxford Med Pub, 1996

POSTIRRADIATION VASCULAR INSUFFICIENCY

Synonym. Radiation vascular insufficiency.

Symptoms and Signs. Occurs following (remotely), radiation therapy, especially after treatment of acromegaly by radiation of pituitary. Symptoms of vascular obstruction with hemiparesis and other signs of reduced or arrested circulation in area involved.

Etiology. Radiation vascular changes. See also Radiation, acute.

Pathology. Not specific; changes of vessels involved; segmental lesions; thickening and fibrosis of vessel wall with marked endothelial proliferation.

Diagnostic Procedure. Arteriography.

Therapy. Anticoagulant.

Prognosis. Guarded.

BIBLIOGRAPHY. Darmondy WR, Thomas LM, Gurdjian ES: Postirradiation vascular insufficiency syndrome. Neurology 17:1190–1192, 1967

POSTOBSTRUCTIVE DIURESIS

Synonym. Water-losing nephritis.

Symptoms and Signs. Occurs 24 or more hours after removal of obstruction from urinary tract. Generally mild and physiologic diuresis, resulting from the correction of the established imbalances; in several cases, however, a "pathologic" diuresis occurs and may last for weeks or longer, causing dehydration, electrolyte imbalance, and hypotension. In the initial phase, hemorrhages from the bladder walls are frequently seen.

Etiology. Defect of sodium reabsorption, causing a solute diuresis; defect in water reabsorption; cellular lack of response to vasopressin.

Diagnostic Procedures. *Blood.* Electrolytes; osmolarity; hematocrit. *Urine.* Volume; electrolytes; osmolarity. *Body weight.* Loss.

Therapy. Fluid and electrolyte balance.

Prognosis. Usually, spontaneous resolution; in some cases, it may be a life threatening event and last weeks or longer.

BIBLIOGRAPHY. Howard SS: Postobstructive diuresis: A misunderstood phenomenon. J Urol 110:537–745, 1973
Klahr S: Obstructive nephropathy. In Massry SG, Glassock RJ: Textbook of Nephrology, 3rd ed, pp 530–535. Baltimore, Williams & Wilkins, 1995

POSTPARTUM BLUES

Synonyms. Postpartum dysphoria; milk fever; milk blues; postpartum psychosis; puerperium depression (20% of parturients); third day blues.

Symptoms. Brief crying episodes, without obvious precipitating factors, not associated with feeling of depression. Usually starting the third day postpartum and ending at the tenth day. Fatigue; increased irritability; sleep disturbances; restlessness; feeling of estrangement from the husband and undue concern for the baby. In other cases the baby is rejected as not belonging.

Etiology. Unknown. Stressful psychological factors; endocrine factors. Altered target organ function (failure of alpha adrenoceptor capacity to fall after delivery). In some cases pregnancy and delivery may precipitate a pre-existing manic depressive condition or prepsychotic schizoid personality.

Therapy. Seldom requires treatment. It has been reported that administration of estrogen for suppression of lactation prevents postpartum depression. In few cases severe form may require electroconvulsive treatment.

Prognosis. Relatively benign self-limited condition: 2 in 1000 women develop psychosis after delivery. Instances of infanticide have been reported.

BIBLIOGRAPHY. Marcè LV: Traite de la follie des femmes enceintes, de nouvelles accouchèes des nourices. Paris, Ballière, 1858
Savage G: Observation on the insanity of pregnancy and childbirth. Guy's Hosp Rep 20:83–117, 1875
Yalom ID, Lunde DT, Moos RH, et al: "Post-partum blues" syndrome; A description and related variables. Arch Gen Psychiatr 18:16–17, 1968
Swyer GIM: Postpartum mental disturbances and hormone changes. Br Med J 290:1232–1233, 1985
Cunningham FG, MacDonald PC, Gant NF, et al (eds): Williams Obstetrics, pp 469–470, 649. Englewood Cliffs, NJ, Prentice-Hall, 1993

POSTPERFUSION

Synonym. Postcardiotomy lymphocytic splenomegaly.

Symptoms. Occurs in young patients operated on for cardiac disease, using cardiopulmonary bypass technique; onset 2–4 weeks after surgery. Fever; absence of chest pain and of definite malaise.

Signs. Splenomegaly (70%); exudative transient pharyngitis (5%); shotty lymphadenopathy (20%); hepatomegaly (30%). Anemia and increased bilirubin in some cases. Maculopapular rash.

Etiology. Unknown. Possibly, infective viral nature because of apparently seasonal distribution. Leukocyte graft-versus-host reaction (?). Probably owing to the Epstein-Barr virus or to the cytomegalovirus from transfused blood.

Pathology. Scanty information; in spleen, decreased follicular pattern. Small follicular germinal centers. Congestion of the pulp. Presence of large mononuclear cells. Irregular structures within the nuclei of these cells (inclusion bodies [?]). Bone marrow hyperplasia; liver passive congestion.

Diagnostic Procedures. *Blood.* Cultures (repeated) negative; lymphocytosis (60%) with atypical cells (virocytes). Serum glutamic-oxaloacetic transaminase (SGOT), serum glutamic-pyruvic transaminase (SGPT), and lactic dehydrogenase (LDH) and mild and transient elevation. *Hepatic function tests.* Abnormal. *Heterophil antibodies.* Moderate elevation or negative.

Therapy. Corticosteroids.

Prognosis. Benign course and spontaneous resolution in 1–4 weeks.

BIBLIOGRAPHY. Kreel I, Zaroff LI, Canter JW, et al: A syndrome following total body perfusion. Surg Gynecol Obstet 111:317–321, 1961
Reyman TA: Postperfusion syndrome. Am Heart J 72:116–123, 1966
Dipak D: Cellular biochemical and molecular aspects of reperfusion injury Proc NY Acad Sci N9420, 1994
Weatherall DJ, Ledingham JGG, Warrell DA (eds): Oxford Textbook of Medicine, 3rd ed, p 2445. Oxford, Oxford Med Pub, 1996

POSTPERFUSION LUNG

Synonyms. Pump lung; postperfusion pulmonary vasculitis.

Symptoms. Occurs in patients operated on for cardiac disease using cardiopulmonary bypass technique; onset immediately after operation (different from postperfusion syndrome, see). Fever; dyspnea.

Signs. Cyanosis; hypotension; signs of pulmonary edema.

Etiology.

1. Arterial mean pressure decreased during bypass.
2. Anoxia.
3. Reaction to denaturation or destruction of blood elements resulting from turbulence in pumping system.
4. Reaction to protein or protein-like materials remaining in heart–lung machine from previous perfusion.

Pathology. Lung dark red, congested; zones of collapse and parenchymal hemorrhages; blood in the bronchi. Intravascular polymorphonuclear leukocytosis. In other organs, diffuse hyperemia.

Diagnostic Procedures. *X-ray.* Of chest. Diffuse clouding of pulmonary fields. *Blood. Electrolytes.*

Therapy. Antibiotic. Corticosteroids. Symptomatic.

Prognosis. Guarded.

BIBLIOGRAPHY. Dodrill FD: The Effects of Total Body Perfusion upon the Lungs, Extracorporeal Circulation, p 327. Springfield, IL, Charles C Thomas, 1958
Neville WE, Kontaxis A, Gavin T, et al: Postperfusion vasculitis. Arch Surg 86:126–137, 1963
Dipak D: Cellular biochemical and molecular aspects of reperfusion injury. Proc NY Acad Sci N9420, 1994

POSTPERICARDIOTOMY

Synonyms. Postcardiotomy; postcommissurotomy. See Dressler.

Symptoms. Postcardiac operative complication appearing several weeks or months after surgical intervention. Patient usually presents slight constitutional disturbance. Pleuropericardial pain, sometimes sharp, radiated to epigastrium, shoulders, and back; aggravated by change of posture and inspiration. Fever; cough (occasional); muscle and joint pain (occasional).

Signs. Pericardial friction rub; features of pleural (unilateral or bilateral) and pericardial effusion. Signs of congestive heart failure, pulmonary infarction, or thrombosis; peripheral veins are absent.

Etiology. Unknown. Possibly, a response to surgical trauma. Following incision of pericardium. Release of autogenous antigen and hypersensitivity reaction (?).

Diagnostic Procedures. *X-ray.* Of chest. *Electrocardiography. Blood.* High sedimentation rate; leukocytosis with absolute neutrophilia; occasionally, eosinophilia; occasionally, anemia.

Therapy. Responds to corticosteroids, not to salicylates.

Prognosis. Benign condition, subsiding spontaneously in a few days or weeks. Frequently recurs.

BIBLIOGRAPHY. Soloff LA, Zatuchni J, Janton OH, et al: Reactivation of rheumatic fever following mitral commissurotomy. Circulation 8:481–493, 1953
Engle MA, Zabriskie JB, Senterpt LB, et al: Viral illness and the postpericardiotomy syndrome: A prospective study in children. Circulation 62:1151–1158, 1980
Khan AM: The postcardiac injury syndromes. Clin Cardiol 15:67–72, 1992
Velander M, Grip L, Mogensen L: The postcardiac injury syndrome

following percutaneous transluminal coronary angioplasty. Clin Cardiol 16:353–354, 1993

Weatherall DJ, Ledingham JGG, Warrell DA (eds): Oxford Textbook of Medicine, 3rd ed, p 2445. Oxford, Oxford Med Pub, 1996

POSTPHLEBITIC

Synonyms. Postphlebitic leg; postthrombotic; venous ulcer; chronic venous insufficiency; ulcus varicosum. See Lower leg stasis.

Symptoms and Signs. Sequelae appearing with 3–10 years of episodes of venous thrombosis; affecting mostly females in middle age. Affecting lower extremities, bilaterally in 25% of cases. Swelling, edema, pain on walking, discoloration, sometimes varicose veins, and ulceration.

Etiology. Venous hypertension owing to postphlebitic incompetence of communicating veins.

Pathology. *Skin.* Epidermis: low degree of intercellular edema with few lymphocytes and granulocytes. Upper dermis: marked edema of connective tissue; swelling of collagen; fragmentation of elastic fibers; dense inflammatory infiltration (lymphocytes and plasma cells). *Blood vessels.* Thickened and dilated. The incompetent veins present uniform thinning of one-half of vein wall and fibrosclerotic thickening of other half.

Diagnostic Procedures. *Serial phlebography. Doppler Trendelenburg test. Perthes test. Determination of venous pressure. Ultrasonography.*

Therapy. Sympathectomy (only with cyanosis, causalgia); ligatures of popliteal veins; superficial femoral veins; valved venous transplants; grafting of internal saphenous vein.

Prognosis. All surgical measures only palliative, but of considerable benefit when specifically indicated.

BIBLIOGRAPHY. Blalock A: Oxygen content of blood in patients with varicose veins. Arch Surg 19:898–905, 1929

Sabiston DC: Textbook of Surgery, 14th ed, pp 1497–1499. Philadelphia, WB Saunders, 1991

Weatherall DJ, Ledingham JGG, Warrell DA (eds): Oxford Textbook of Medicine, 3rd ed, pp 3664–3665. Oxford, Oxford Med Pub, 1996

POSTPHLEBITIC NEUROSIS

Symptoms. Misconception in patient of harboring "clots" that may become free and menace life. Refusal to leave the bed or bear weight or conduct a normal life. Alleged extreme pain and tenderness of the legs.

Etiology. Frequently, iatrogenic. Basic apprehensiveness.

Therapy. Convince patient that danger of embolism has disappeared with recovery.

Prognosis. Frequent conversion to other type of health apprehension.

BIBLIOGRAPHY. Hurst JW: The Heart, 6th ed, p 1887. New York, McGraw-Hill, 1986

POSTPOLIO

Synonyms. Late post-poliomyelitis muscular atrophy. PPMA; progressive post-poliomyelitis muscular atrophy.

Symptoms and Signs. It manifests 15–30 years after recovery from poliomyelitis. Muscle weakness (affecting mostly muscles that had fully or partly recovered fom paralysis), loss of stamina, and occasionally unexplained pains; or new muscle weakness and atrophy. Gastrointestinal problems, difficulties in sleeping and breathing and emotional distress may also occur. For the diagnosis four criteria have been indicated: (1) History of acute polio in childhood or adolescence; (2) partial recovery of motor function and maintanace for at least 15 years; (3) residual asymmetric muscle atrophy in at least one limb, with weak or

missing reflexes and normal sensation; (4) normal functioning of the sphincter muscle.

Etiology. Unknown. Usually no evidence for poliovirus persistence. Immunopathological mechanisms may play a role; or an undetected persistence of virus (or of fragmentary genetic sequences) in the anterior horn cells. Attrition of nerve cells (ongoing denervation and reinnervation stressing the nerve cells) considered among the possible causes.

Diagnostic Procedures. *Cerebrospinal fluid.* Presence of oligoclonal bands, however poliovirus antibodies could not be detected. *Electromyography.* The motor units generate giant potentials even in muscles that appear clinically normal.

BIBLIOGRAPHY. Dalakas MC, Sever JL, Madden DL, et al: Late post-poliomyelitis muscular atrophy: Clinical virologic, and immunologic studies. Rev Infect Dis 6(Suppl2):S562–S567, 1984

Melchers W, deVisser M, Jongen P, et al: The post polio syndrome: No evidence for poliovirus persistence Ann Neurol 32:728–732, 1992

Dalakas MC, Bartfeld H, Kurland G: The post-polio syndrome: Advances in the pathogenesis and treatment. Ann NY Acad Sci 753, 1995

Rodriguez AA, Agre JC, Harmon RL, et al: Electromyographic and neuromuscular variables in post-polio subjects. Arch Phys Med Rehabil 76:989–993, 1995

POSTURAL

Symptoms. Functional type prevalent in children; structural type present at all ages. Only fatigue and backache (in functional type) or significant back pain (in structural type).

Signs. Increase of cervical lordosis; dorsal spine rounded and motion decreased. Exaggerated lordotic lumbar curve; abdominal muscles relaxed and overstretched; pelvis tilted anteriorly and hip flexors shortened. Increase of lumbosacral angle. When patient bends forward, lumbar curve is not properly obliterated.

Etiology. Functional or structural: frequently, pregnancy and obesity determining or accelerating factors.

Diagnostic Procedures. *X-ray.* Spinous processes and facets in contact with each other; secondary degenerative bone changes.

Therapy. Corrective exercises to increase strength of back and abdominal muscles. Weight loss when obesity. Supporting belt or other orthopedic devices to correct curvature of spine.

Prognosis. Persistence of syndrome leads to vertebral column sprain or, when associated with obesity, to emphysema and cardiorespiratory failure.

BIBLIOGRAPHY. Kerr WJ, Lagen JB: The postural syndrome related to obesity leading to postural emphysema and cardiorespiratory failure. Ann Intern Med 10:569–595, 1936

Kuhns JG: Posture and Its Relationship to Orthopedic Disabilities. Ann Arbor, Edward Brothers, 1942

Klippel JH, Dieppe PA: Rheumatology, pp 5.3.1, 5.3.4. St Louis, CV Mosby, 1994

POSTVACCINIAL SYNDROMES

Synonym. Smallpox vaccination complication.

Symptoms.

1. *Accidental infection.* The accidental implantation of vaccinia virus in the eye, mouth, or other parts of the body in the absence of eczema or other pre-existing skin disorder.

2. *Generalized vaccinia.* The generalized spread of vaccinial lesions in the absence of eczema or other pre-existing skin lesion.

3. *Eczema vaccinia.* The generalized spread of vaccinial lesions or local

implantation of vaccinia in a person who has eczema or a past history of eczema. This person may be the patient who was vaccinated or a contact of someone recently vaccinated.

4. *Vaccinia necrosum* (progressive vaccinia). Spreading necrosis at the site of vaccination with or without metastatic necrotic lesions occurring elsewhere on the body.

5. *Encephalitis.* Postvaccinial central nervous system involvement including (separately or in combination) the following symptoms: meningeal signs; ataxia; muscular weakness; paralysis; lethargy; coma or convulsions.

6. *Other.* Vaccinial lesions complicating skin conditions other than eczema in addition to miscellaneous complications not listed above, such as generalized urticarial reactions, bullous erythema multiforme, and secondary bacterial infections.

BIBLIOGRAPHY. Rosen E: A postvaccinial syndrome. Am J Ophthalmol 31:1443–1453, 1948

Neff JM, Lane JM, Pert JH, et al: Complications of smallpox vaccination. 1. National survey in the United States, 1963. N Engl J Med 276:125–132, 1967

Neff JM, Levine RH, Lane JM, et al: Complications of smallpox vaccination in the United States, 1963. II. Results obtained by four statewide surveys. Pediatrics 39:916–923, 1967

Weatherall DJ, Ledingham JGG, Warrell DA (eds): Oxford Textbook of Medicine, 3rd ed, p 368. Oxford, Oxford Med Pub, 1996

POTATO NOSE

Synonym. Nose potato shaped.

Symptoms and Signs. Both sexes. Typical shape of nose. Lack of hypertelorism. Developmental field defect. Autosomal dominant inheritance. Same category of bifid nose (autosomal recessive trait also reported).

BIBLIOGRAPHY. Benjamins CE, Stibbe FH: Sur un cas extraordinaire de difformite congenitale de la pyramide nasale. Acta Otolaryngol 11:274–284, 1927

Toriello HV, Higgins JV, Wallen A, et al: Familial occurrence of a developmental defect of the medial nasal processes. Am J Med Genet 21:131–135, 1985

POTT I

Synonym. Dupuytren fracture.

Symptoms and Signs. Pain; swelling; tenderness in affected foot, which results in shortening it.

Etiology. Direct or indirect trauma.

Diagnostic Procedures. *X-ray.* Transverse fracture of medial malleolus, ankle diastasis; fibula bent inward; both distal fragments displaced laterally.

BIBLIOGRAPHY. Pott P: Some Few General Remarks of Fractures and Dislocations, pp 57–64. London, Howes, 1769

Dupuytren G: Sur la fracture de l'extremité inferieure du peroné, les luxations e les accidents qui en sont la suite. Ann Med Chir Paris 1:2–212, 1819

POTT II

Synonym. Gangrene senilis. Eponym used to indicate the "mortification of toes and feet" due to arterial obstruction. See Mönckeberg.

BIBLIOGRAPHY. Pott P: Chirurgical Observation Relative to the Cataract, the Polypus of the Nose, the Cancer of the Scrotum, the Different Kinds of Ruptures, and the Mortification of the Toes and Feet. London, Howes, 1775

POTT III

Synonyms. David; spine tuberculosis; tuberculous spondylitis. Pott paraplegia.

Symptoms. Occurs in both sexes; onset at all ages. Clinically subdivided in three types: (1) Pott's without paraplegia; (2) paraplegia of early onset, initially during the florid phase of spinal disease (first 2 years); (3) paraplegia of late onset, even after many years, after the disease has become quiescent (also in absence of signs of relapse). Onset gradual. Changes in gait; pain and weakness in the back; abdominal pain, occasionally of buttocks and knee; weight loss; rigidity and upright position of spine; muscular spasm of area involved, followed by acute curvature with backward convexity; reduction of spine length; paralysis.

Etiology. Mycobacterium tuberculosis.

Pathology. Tubercular (caseous) lesion of vertebral bodies and intervertebral disks. Collapse producing angulation. Cold abscess formation localized or extended along anatomic path.

Diagnostic Procedures. *X-ray.* Of spine. See Pathology and Signs. Of thorax. Presence of specific lesions in the lungs. *Blood.* Anemia; increased sedimentation rate. *Stool.* Presence of M. tuberculosis.

Therapy. Specific: streptomycin, amino salicylic acid (PAS); neomycin; rifampin. Ethionamide, and surgical and orthopedic treatment.

Prognosis. According to time of onset of treatment.

BIBLIOGRAPHY. Pott P: Remarks on that Kind of Palsy of the Lower Limbs Which Is Frequently Found to Accompany a Curvature of the Spine and Is Supposed to be Caused by it, Together with a Method of Cure. London, Johnson, 1779

David JP: Dissertation sur les Effets du Mouvement et du Repos dans les Maladies Chirurgicales. Paris, 1779

Strausbaigh LJ: Vertebral osteomyelitis. In Jaauregui LE (ed): Diagnosis and Management of Bone Infection. New York, 1995

Weatherall DJ, Ledingham JGG, Warrell DA (eds): Oxford Textbook of Medicine, 3rd ed, pp 2999–3000. Oxford, Oxford Med Pub, 1996

POTTER

Synonyms. Bilateral kidney agenesis; dysplasia renofacialis; facial-renal dysplasia; oligohydramnios tetrad; renofacial dysplasia; urogenital dysplasia, BRA; HRA.

Symptoms and Signs. Newborn: Potter face: low-set and malformed ears, long epicanthal folds, flattened nose bridge, small mandible. (Note: This finding is found in many renal disorders that interfere with the formation of amniotic fluid and in other instances of prolonged leakage of amniotic fluid); symptoms and signs related to renal agenesis and pulmonary hypoplasia. Oligohydramnios and amnion nodosum. Associated skeletal malformations, including hand and foot clubbing.

Etiology. Autosomal dominant. Potter facies is caused by compression of face resulting from oligohydramnios. This syndrome does not show chromosomal abnormalities, although some syndromes, such as 18 trisomy syndrome, present a very similar clinical pattern.

Pathology. Renal agenesis or malformation; typical facial alterations.

Diagnostic Procedures. *Chromosome studies. CT scan. Digital subtraction angiography. MRI. Ultrasonography.*

Therapy. Symptomatic. Surgery including kidney transplant.

Prognosis. Live-born survival variable according to time and types of possible interventions.

BIBLIOGRAPHY. Potter EL: Bilateral renal agenesis. J Pediatr 29:68–76, 1946

Passarge E, Sutherland JM: Potter's syndrome. Am J Dis Child 109:80–84, 1965

Bankier A, De Campo M, Newell R, et al: A pedigree study of perinatally lethal renal disease. J Med Genet 22:104–111, 1985

Morse R P, Rawnsley E, Crowe HC, et al: Bilateral renal agenesis in three consecutive siblings. Prenatal Diag 7:573–579, 1987

POUTEAU

Eponym used to indicate a variant of the Colles fracture (see).

BIBLIOGRAPHY. Pouteau C: Oeuvres Posthumes de M Pouteau, vol 2, p 251. Paris, Pierres, 1783

PRADER-WILLI

Synonyms. Labhart-Willi; Prader-Labhart-Willi-Fanconi; Willi-Prader; PWS; cryptorchidism—dwarfism—obesity—hypomentia—hypotonia; hypomentia—hypogonadism—obesity; HHHO; H3O.

Symptoms. Frequency 1:25,000. Occurs most often in males, born after normal pregnancy and delivery (prolonged gestation reported by some authors). Weight at birth slightly below normal. *First phase.* At birth hypotonia or atonia, sleepy, convulsions (very seldom) feeding difficulty (tube feeding frequently required). *Second phase.* After about 6 months hypotonia decreases, feeding difficulty disappears to be replaced by hyperphagia and development of obesity. Slow height growth, mental retardation; walking after 2 years of age; speech development poor; emotional disturbances. Frequently observed: polydipsia, polyuria.

Signs. Blue eyes and blond hair frequently observed. Normal size of hands and feet during first year. First 6 months areflexia, poor or absent response to painful stimuli, Moro reflex absent. After 6 months, reflexes active. Obesity; short stature; acromicria; small penis; bilateral or unilateral cryptorchidism; lack of development of secondary sexual characteristic. In female, delayed or absent development of pubertal changes. Other abnormalities occasionally observed; strabismus; micrognathia; abnormal ears; hand and finger abnormalities; teeth defects.

Etiology. Unknown. Hypothalamic disturbance suggested. Sporadic; in some cases autosomal recessive inheritance suggested (lack of evidence). Small interstitial delation of proximal 15q unbalanced translocation has been reported in a great percentage of patients.

Pathology. *Biopsy.* Of testicle. Normal. *Of brain, spinal cord and muscle.* Normal.

Diagnostic Procedures. *X-ray.* Delayed maturation of bones. *Blood.* Hyperglycemia; acetonemia (usually developing after 10th year of life). All tests usually within normal limits, including studies of endocrine functions. *Electromyography.* Normal. *Electroencephalography.* Slow waves; spiky activity; absent sleep spindles.

Therapy. Symptomatic. Diabetic manifestation responds readily to antidiabetic agents. Amphetamine controls hyperphagia. Testosterone replacement. Clomiphene citrate to stimulate rise in luteinizing hormone and sexual development. Low calorie intake. Vagotomy might be worthy of trial for the correction of obesity.

Prognosis. No adequate information. Death from vascular complications if diabetes reported. Possibly increased risk of leukemia.

BIBLIOGRAPHY. Prader A, Labhart A, Willi H: Ein Syndrom von Adipositas, Kleinwuchs, Kryptorchidismus, und Oligophrenia nach myatonieartigem Zustand im Neugeborenenalter. Schweiz Med Wochenschr 86:1260–1261, 1956

Zellweger H, Schneider HJ: Syndrome of hypotonia, hypomentia, hypogonadism, obesity (HHHO) or Prader-Willi syndrome. Am J Dis Child 115:588–598, 1968

Greenswag LR: Adults with Prader-Willy syndrome: A survey of 232 cases. Dev Med child Neurol 29:145–152, 1987

Butler MG: Prader-Willi syndrome: Current understanding of cause and diagnosis. Am J Med Genet 35:319–332, 1990

Robinson WP, Bottani A, Yagang X, et al: Molecular, cytogenetic and clinical investigations of Prader-Willi syndrome patients. Am J Med Genet 49:1219–1234, 1991

Weatherall DJ, Ledingham JGG, Warrell DA (eds): Oxford Textbook of Medicine, 3rd ed, p 4110. Oxford, Oxford Med Pub, 1996

PRASAD (A.S.)

Synonyms. Sarrovy; anemia; hepatosplenomegaly—dwarfism; dwarfism—geophagia; iron deficiency; pica.

Symptoms. Prevalent almost exclusively in males in Iran and Turkey. Geophagia for several years; retarded growth; low-grade fever. In the United States, the geophagia is sometimes observed among black women, especially when pregnant with consequent iron deficiecy anemia.

Signs. Pallor; apparent age not corresponding with chronologic age; lack of development of primary and secondary sexual characteristics; hepatosplenomegaly.

Etiology. Not clearly understood. Among possible mechanisms; alimentation deficient in animal proteins; predominant wheat diet (rich in phosphates interfering with iron absorption) relative deficiency of vitamin C. Pica (ingestion of earth, or clay, laundry starch, and ice) has been reconognized as cause of iron deficiency. Zinc deficiency possibly responsible for hypogonadism. Geophagia interfering with iron absorption. Zinc deficiency (as first proposed) apparently not related to hypochromic anemia. In effect the opposite has been observed where zinc ingestion for prolonged period caused anemia because of secondary copper deficiency.

Pathology. *Biopsy.* Of liver. Normal or moderate fat infiltration. Of testes. Lack of development.

Diagnostic Procedures. *Blood.* Severe hypochromic anemia; liver tests normal; high alkaline phosphatase; low serum iron and zinc; rapid disappearance of zinc after its injection. *X-ray.* Bone age inferior to chronologic age. *Gastric analysis.* Gastric achylia in all patients. *Iron absorption test.* Normal.

Therapy. Oral iron and copper administration; adequate diet.

Prognosis. With iron and diet, anemia and lack of development are corrected and hepatosplenomegaly regresses.

BIBLIOGRAPHY. Prasad AS, Halsted JA, Nadimi M: Syndrome of iron deficiency anemia, hepatosplenomegaly, hypogonadism, dwarfism, and geophagia. Am J Med 31:532–546, 1961

Lee GR: Iron deficiency and iron-deficiency anemia. In Lee GR, Bithel TC, Foerster J, et al (eds): Wintrobe's Clinical Hematology, 9th ed, p 815. Philadelphia, Lea & Febiger, 1993

PRECHTL-STEMMER

Synonyms. Choreiform in children; choreatiform hyperactivity, hyperkinetic. See cocktail party.

Symptoms and Signs. Part of hyperactivity in children syndrome. Normal intelligence, little sleep, wriggling, restlessness, continuous exploratory activity.

Etiology. See Cocktail party.

Therapy. Prednisone (1–2 mg/kg/day) or Haloperidol (0.02–0.1 mg/kg/day) in two divided doses. Do not use phenobarbital (paradoxical effect).

Prognosis. From good response to treatment to remedial education or institutionalization.

BIBLIOGRAPHY. Prechtl HFR, Stemmer CJ: The choreatiform syndrome in children. Dev Med Child Neurol 4:119–127, 1962

Adams RD, Victor M: Principles of Neurology, 5th ed, pp 520–521. New York, McGraw-Hill, 1993

PREINFARCTION

Synonyms. Angina decubitus; angina intermedia; preinfarctional angina; coronary failure; acute coronary insufficiency; coronary intermediate; ischemic heart; impending myocardial infarction; prethrombotic; progressive angina. Unstable angina.

Symptoms. Occurs most often in males, in executive-managerial class. Evidence of pre-existing disease such as hypertension, diabetes, obesity, and past symptoms suggestive of cardiovascular disease in good percentage of cases. Presenting symptoms: chest pain, angina-like, infarction-like, or ill-defined, usually substernal, parasternal, precordial, or anomalously located and radiating to arm, epigastrium, jaw, or back. Shortness of breath; palpitation; fatigue; paresthesia; vomiting; gastrointestinal flatulence. (1) Prolonged attack at rest (in succession or progressively increasing); (2) intensification (with change of pattern) of pain in established angina pectoris; (3) anginal pain at rest after a pain-free period (in cases of old myocardial infarction).

Signs. Usually none except for arrhythmia or gravitational edema.

Etiology. Forerunner of attack of myocardial infarction. Incomplete artherosclerotic obstruction and spasm of coronary arteries. Includes several clinical variants where the patient has been found susceptible to myocardial infarction (symptoms may even be absent). Some patients thus classified may even have had small myocardial infarctions. Angina decubitus is the variety where the pain attacks occur at rest.

Diagnostic Procedures. *Blood.* Leukocytes, sedimentation rate, SGOT normal or show moderate elevation. *X-ray.* Heart size normal. *Electrocardiography.* Myocardial ischemic pattern almost constantly present (95%), RS-T segments downward displacement; T-wave abnormalities. *Coronary angiography.*

Therapy. Rest as for myocardial damage. Monitoring for arrhythmias until crisis over. Pain relievers; prevention and management of anxiety; heparin and antiarrhythmic (not routinely but as needed) plus (as indicated) other drugs used in the treatment of classic angina (see Heberden.) Bypass surgery or angioplasty when surgery not possible and other therapies fail. Methimazole or radioactive iodine (to reduce metabolism) may be tried. Educational before and after resuming activity.

Prognosis. In 50% of cases, development of myocardial infarction. Occasionally, death. Recovery after a variable number of attacks with restoration of normal electrocardiographic pattern.

BIBLIOGRAPHY. Sampson JJ, Eliaser M: The diagnosis of impending acute coronary artery occlusion. Am Heart J 13:675–686, 1937

Feil H: Preliminary pain in coronary thrombosis. Am J Med Sci 193:42–48, 1937

Sherman TC, Litvack F, Grundfest W, et al: Coronary angioscopy in patients with unstable angina pectoris. N Engl J Med 351:913–919, 1986

Cowley MJ, Di Sciascio G, Rehr RB, Vetrovec GW: Angiographic observations and clinical relevance of coronary thrombus in unstable angina pectoris. Am J Cardiol 63:108E–113E, 1989

Thèroux P, Waters D: Diagnosis and management of patients with unstable angina. In Schlant RC, Alexander RW, et al: Hurst's The Heart, 8th ed, pp 1083–1106. New York, McGraw-Hill, 1994

PREISER

Synonym. Scaphoid bone necrosis. See Epiphyseal ischemic necrosis.

Symptoms. Pain and mobility reduction of the wrist.

Etiology. Trauma of the wrist causing avascular necrosis of scaphoid bone.

BIBLIOGRAPHY. Preiser G: Zur Frage der typischen traumatischen Ernaetrungsstoerungen der kurken Hand und Fuss-wurzelknochen. Fortsch Geb Roentgenol 17:360–362, 1911

PREMENSTRUAL

Symptoms. Exaggerated manifestation of normal premenstrual phenomena. It may be considered to occur in about 80% of women. Symptoms begin about 10 days before menstrual period and stop abruptly within 24 hours of menstruation. They begin to recur in a similar fashion on the next cycle. Symptoms of different intensity may be subdivided by systems. Central nervous system. Emotional instability; onset of psychotic manifestations; cyclic headache; nymphomania; visual disturbances. Genital area and breast. Lower abdominal heaviness; distention; low back pain or pain in the legs; anorectal symptoms of pressure and pruritus; mastalgia and swelling of breasts. Nongenital manifestations. Nausea; vomiting; constipation; diarrhea; asthma; rhinorrhea; epistaxis; periocular pigmentation; cyclic localized acneiform eruption; greasy or dry scalp and hair.

Etiology. Not completely assessed; predisposing constitutional factors; evidence of water-salts metabolism involvement; relative excess of estrogen or deficiency of progesterone; overcompensating secretion of aldosterone or antidiuretic hormone (or both) and other causes and mechanisms proposed.

Therapy. Sedative such as phenobarbital, benzodiezepines. Diuretic such as hydrochlorothiazide. Hormonal: medroxyprogesterone starting 5–10 days before cycle. Prostaglandin synthetase inhibitors. Psychotherapy according to intensity of symptoms.

Prognosis. Influenced favorably by treatment.

BIBLIOGRAPHY. Frank FT: Hormonal causes of premenstrual tension. Arch Neurol Psychiatr 26:1053–1057, 1931

Spiegel A: Temporary insanity and premenstrual syndrome: Medical testimony in an 1865 murder trial. New York State J Med 88:482–492, 1988

Rapkin AJ (ed): Premenstrual syndrome. Clin Obstet Gynecol 35:585–586, 1992

Rubinow DR: The premenstrual syndrome: New views. JAMA 268:1908–1912, 1992

PRETECTAL I

Synonyms. Koerber-Salus-Elschnig; Parinaud; Nothnagel; sylvian aqueduct; nystagmus retractorius; sylvian; superior colliculus; divergence paralysis; subthalamus; supranuclear. See Benedikt and Weber-Gubler, pineal.

Symptoms. Headaches; hemiparesis; nausea; vomiting, ataxia; dizziness; vertigo; lethargy; confusion; nystagmus; hemitremor possible.

Signs. Nystagmus (upbeat, downbeat, other); vertical nystagmus (best demonstrated by asking patient to attempt upward gaze or by using target moving downward), convergence-retraction eye movements, paralysis of convergence, disjunctive eye position, skew deviation, upper lid retraction, lid flutter, and lid nystagmus on optokinetic testing. Pupils normal in size (8%), poor reaction to light and near vision, papilledema. Extraocular palsies. Babinski sign; systemic hypertension.

Etiology. Hydrocephalus, neoplasia (pineal, thalamic, midbrain/third ventricle metastasis), vascular lesion (thalamic hemorrhage, primary pretectal, infarction), infection (encephalitis, ventriculitis, abscessbacterial, tubercular, toxoplasma, AIDS, etc.) trauma, arterovenous malformations, Wernicke, Bassen-Kornzweig, hydrocephalus.

Pathology. Lesions of mentioned nature adjacent to periductal gray matter of aqueduct of Sylvius, causing compression or direct invasion of the pretectal region, hydrocephalus in 80% of cases.

Diagnostic Procedures. *X-ray. Isotope brain scan. Angiography. CT scan. MRI. Biopsy of tumor by a CT-guided stereoscopic needle technique.*

Therapy. According to etiology.

Prognosis. Poor, according to etiology.

BIBLIOGRAPHY. Parinaud H: Paralisie des mouvements associés des yeux. Arch Neurol 5:145–172, 1883

Koerber HL: Ueber drei Fälle von Retraktionsbewegung des Bulbus. Ophthalmol Klin 7:65–67, 1903

Salus R: Ueber erworbene Retractionsbewegungen der Augen. Arch Kinderheilkd 47:61–76, 1910

Elschnig A: Nystagmus Retractorius: Ein cerebrales Herd-Symptom. Med Klin 1:8–11, 1913

Pierrot-Descilligny CH, Chain F, et al: Parinaud's syndrome. Electrooculographic and anatomical analyses of six vascular cases with deductions about vertical gaze organization in the premotor structures. Brain 105:667–696, 1982

Keane JR: The pretectal syndrome: 206 patients. Neurol 40:684–690, 1990

PRETIBIAL FEVER

Synonym. Fort Bragg fever.

Symptoms. Sporadic occurrence in North Carolina and Georgia. Sudden onset. Malaise; mild general aching headache; photophobia mild, not persistent; respiratory symptoms; chills; spiking fever (two or more peaks a day) subsiding within 4–8 days.

Signs. On fourth day of illness, patchy erythematous rash usually limited to anterior part of both legs. Usually lasting 2 or a few more days and leaving residual pigmentation for 2 weeks. Splenomegaly; relative bradycardia.

Etiology. Leptospira autumnalis, L. pomona also observed in association with similar syndrome of pretibial as well as generalized rash.

Diagnostic Procedures. *Blood.* Initially leukopenia and then moderate leukocytosis, with moderate relative lymphocytosis; complement fixation for Leptospira. Microscopic agglutination and culture studies.

Therapy. Doxycycline 200 mg orally the first day, then 100 mg per day for 4 days. Prophylaxis by tetracyclines or penicillin given in first 4 days of disease.

Prognosis. Course of 5–10 days and complete recovery.

BIBLIOGRAPHY. Bowdoin CD: A new disease entity (?). J Med Assoc Ga 31:437–438, 1942

Daniels WB, Grennan HA: Pretibial fever. JAMA 122:361–365, 1943

Weatherall DJ, Ledingham JGG, Warrell DA (eds): Oxford Textbook of Medicine, 3rd ed, pp 698–703. Oxford, Oxford Med Pub, 1996

PRIEST-ALEXANDER

Synonyms. Verner-Morrison; water diarrhea—hypokalemia—pancreatic adenoma, WDHA; VIPoma; pancreatic cholera.

Symptoms. May occur as part of MEN I or may coexist with bronchogenic carcinoma. Onset from second to sixth decades, predominant in fifth decade. Flushing. Diarrhea of variable severity and duration, initially intermittent then usually progressive. In acute stages, watery diarrhea (up to 3 L, with 20 L also reported), abdominal pain, nausea, and vomiting. In quiescent state, mushy stools and weight loss. Generalized weakness progressing to paralysis and then to stupor. Duration of symptoms from months to years. Spontaneous remission during pregnancy.

Signs. Weight loss; hypotonia; Blood hypotension sigmoidoscopy negative.

Etiology. Islet cell adenoma in the majority of cases but other tumor may give the same manifestations (ganglioneuroblastoma, pheochromocytoma, neuroblastoma, bronchogenic carcinoma). In a few cases more than one endocrine adenoma observed (thyroid; parathyroid). Production of a vasoactive intestinal peptide (VIP) that stimulates intestinal fluid and electrolyte secretion, decreases acid secretion, relaxes smooth muscle, and keeps stool moist.

Pathology. Islet cell adenoma. In 50% cases metastasis to the liver at time of diagnosis. Secondary effects of chronic severe diarrhea (e.g., weight loss). VIP secretion tumors usually originate in the pancreas (84%) but may also originate in other organs (16%), especially along the sympathetic chain.

Diagnostic Procedures. *Blood.* Hypokalemic alkalosis (metabolic acidosis); glucose intolerance (in 20–50% of cases); hypercalcemia, hypomagnesemia, plasma VIP (by radioimmunoassay) and peptide-histidine-methionine levels. *Stool.* Cultures negative. Alkaline, isotonic, loss of potassium and bicarbonate. *X-ray.* Absence of peptic ulceration and gastric hypersecretion. *CT scans. MRI. Ultrasound.* Most useful identifying techniques.

Therapy. Surgical removal of tumor. Oral glucose-electrolyte solutions. Pharmacologic agents to control diarrhea: prednisone. Trials with alpha adrenergic agonists; norepinephrine; indomethacin; lithium carbonate; somatostatin; phenothiazine; propanolol. Somatostatin analogue octreotide to control diarrhea. Chemotherapy streptozocin and 5-fluorouracil (good palliation), interferon also useful.

Prognosis. Cessation of all symptoms with removal of tumor. Occasional recurrence when metastases are present. Death from dehydration and shock.

BIBLIOGRAPHY. Moldawer MP, Nardi GL, Raker JW: Concomitance of multiple adenomas of the parathyroids and pancreatic islets with tumor of the pituitary: a syndrome with familial incidence. Am J Med Sci 228:190–206, 1954

Priest WM, Alexander MK: Islet cell tumor of the pancreas with peptic ulceration diarrhea and hypokalemia. Lancet 2:1145–1147, 1957

Verner JV, Morrison AB: Islet cell tumor and a syndrome of refractory watery diarrhea and hypokalemia. Am J Med 25:374–380, 1958

Krejs GJ: Vipoma syndrome. Am J Med (Suppl 5B):37–47, 1987

Flier JS: Syndromes of insulin resistance and mutant insulin. In De Groot LJ (ed): Endocrinology, 3rd ed, p 1599. Philadelphia, WB Saunders, 1995

PRIEUR-GRISCELLI

Symptoms. Infantile multisystem inflammatory disease; IMID, CINCA.

Symptoms. At birth or during early infancy. Pain at joints; fever; convulsions (occasionally); feeding problems, visual troubles, deafness, growth and mental retardation.

Signs. Rash (evanescent); arthritic changes; adenopathy; persistence of open fountanellae; head enlargement; hepato-splenomegaly; protruding eyeballs.

Etiology. Unknown.

Diagnostic Procedures. *Blood.* Anemia, leukocytosis, elevated sedimentation rate, and of IgG. *Spinal fluid.* Pleocytosis. *X rays.* Osteoporosis, swelling ends of long bones; moderate joint effusion and contracture, macrocrania, frontal bossing.

Therapy. Symptomatic.

Prognosis. Poor.

BIBLIOGRAPHY. Prieur AM, Griscelli C: Arthropathy with rash, chronic meningitis, eye lesions and mental retardation. J Pediatr 99:79–83, 1981

Lampert F: Infantile multisystem inflammatory disease: Another case of a new syndrome. Eur J Pediatr 144:593–596, 1986

Prieur AM, Griscelli C, Lampert F: A Chronic, infantile, neurological, cutaneous and articular (CINCA) syndrome. A specific entity analyzed in 30 patients. Scand J Rheumatol (Suppl) 66:57–68, 1987

PRIEUR-TRENEL

Eponym used to designate the association of cataract and Sabouraud syndrome (see).

BIBLIOGRAPHY. Prieur M, Trénel M: Monilethrix et cataracte précoce. Bull Soc Ophthalmol Fr 42:794–799, 1930

PRINGLE-BOURNEVILLE

Signs. Subungual and periungual warty fibromas in patient affected by Bourneville syndrome (see).

BIBLIOGRAPHY. Pringle JJ: A case of congenital adenoma seboreum. Br J Dermatol 2:1–14, 1890

PRINZMETAL II

Synonym. Angina pectoris variant.

Symptoms. Precordial angina attacks with the following characteristics:

1. Onset at rest or during normal activity; not induced by strain or emotions.
2. Occurs at the same time each day.
3. During each single attack, time of waxing of pain equal to time of waning (in regular angina waxing time longer than waning one).
4. Intensity and duration of attack greater than that of regular angina.
5. Nitroglycerine protects from crisis and arrests one in progress.

Signs. None.

Etiology and Pathology. Anatomic-pathologic studies have shown the single narrowing of a major coronary branch, in contrast with that found in classic angina, where several minor arteries are involved. Consequently, in this type of angina there is only one single area of ischemia, whereas in classical angina several small areas are involved.

Diagnostic Procedures. *Electrocardiography.* Between attacks, normal; during attack, ST elevation in determinated derivations; increase of R voltage in some derivations; ventricular arrythmias (50%) during pain acme; in rare cases where ECG is abnormal between attacks, it may paradoxically revert to normal during crisis. Effort test does not cause attack or ECG modifications; in rare cases it may induce ST depression. *X-ray.* Of chest. Normal. *Cineangiocardiography.* See Etiology.

Therapy. Does not differ from that of classic angina; anticoagulants useful. Surgical revascularizion particularly indicated.

Prognosis. The ischemic area of the Prinzmetal angina frequently (33%) becomes site of myocardial infarction (and the angina pain disappears). In remaining patients, variable outcome; spontaneous resolution to progressive aggravation. Prognosis is always more severe than in the classic angina.

BIBLIOGRAPHY. Prinzmetal M, Ekmek A, Keimamer R, et al: Variant form of angina pectoris. JAMA 174:1794–1800, 1960
Polese A, De Cesare N, Bartorelli A, Fabbiocchi F, Loaldi A, Montorsi P, Guazzi MD: Different vasomotor action of nifedipine on dynamic coronary obstructions and therapeutic response in effort and Prinzmetal angina. Am J Med Sci 297:73–79, 1989
Thèroux P, Waters D: Diagnosis of patients with unstable angina. In Schlant RC, Alexander RW: Hurst's The Heart, 8th ed, pp 1097–1102. New York, McGraw-Hill, 1994

PRION-RELATED PROTEIN SYNDROMES

Includes (1) Kuru (see); (2) Creutzfeldt-Jakob (see); (3) Gerstmann-Straussler (see); and (4) fatal familial insomnia (see).

Etiology. Disease or diseases both genetic (mutations in the prion protein [PrP] that is encoded by a chromosomal gene), and infectious (sporadicaly transmitted). Prions (protein infectious agent) represent a new class of infectious (?) agent, lacking nucleic acid and replicating with a virus-like strategy; or normal proteins (acute phase reactant) formed in response to other unidentified infections; perhaps these agents absolve important biologic functions in cell membranes.

BIBLIOGRAPHY. Prusiner SB: Prion diseases. In Scriver CR, Beaudet AL, Sly WS, et al: The Metabolic and Molecular Bases of Inherited Disease, pp 4511–4546. New York, McGraw-Hill, 1995
Weatherall DJ, Ledingham JGG, Warrell DA (eds): Oxford Textbook of Medicine, 3rd ed, pp 3977–3981. Oxford, Oxford Med Pub, 1996

PROFICHET

Synonyms. Calcinosis circumscripta; calcinosis cutis; hypodermolithiasis. Including calcinosis of scrotum. See also calcinosis universalis.

Symptoms. Most commonly reported in elderly females; onset insidious. Calcareous deposits, primarily affecting extremities. Usually, lesion not painful; stiffness and aching of joints; coldness of extremities.

Signs. Symmetric hard nodular or plaque formations over pressure points or joints. Skin overlying lesions is dry, red, and hardened. Calcinosis of scrotum and penis reported.

Etiology. Unknown. Possible association with variable conditions: collagen diseases; trauma; neoplasma. Some authors refuse to consider this form an entity and believe it is a part of the calcinosis universalis syndrome.

Pathology. Chalky material in subcutaneous fat associated with collagenous bundles.

Diagnostic Procedures. *X-ray.* To evidence nodules. *Blood.* Hypercalcemia and hyperphosphoremia. *Biopsy.* Calcium phosphate and carbonate deposits.

Therapy. None or surgical removal. Medical treatment usually useless. Cellulose phosphate plus low calcium diet could be considered.

Prognosis. Spontaneous recession possible. Variable degree of incapacitation.

BIBLIOGRAPHY. Hollander: Le diabète phospatique. Thése de Paris. 1877
Profichet GC: Sur une Variété de Concretion Phosphatique Subcutanée (Pierre de la Peau). Paris, 1890
Reines S: Petrificatio cutis circumscripta. Arch Dermatol Syph (Wein) 88:267–289, 1907
Black MM, Gawkrodger DJ, Seymour CA, et al: Metabolic and nutritional disorders. In Champion RH, Burton JL, Ebling FJG (eds): Rook/Wilkinson/Ebling Textbook of Dermatology, 5th ed, p 2369. Oxford, Blackwell Scientific, 1992

PROGRESSIVE EXTERNAL OPHTHALMOPLEGIA

Difficult definition of syndrome because of frequent association with other clinical entities defined as different syndromes. See OXPHOS syndromes.

Synonyms. Opthalmoplegia progressive external, ophthalmoplegia plus; nuclear ophthalmoplegia; PEO; ocular myopathy. See other syndrome reported in the table. PEO is defined in purely clinical terms as presenting the following characteristics.

1. progressive ptosis and immobility of eyes

2. bilateral
3. muscles affected have multiple innervation
4. sparing of pupil
5. gradual progression (years)
6. no remission or exacerbations
7. absence of specific disorders (i.e., thyreopathy, myasthenia, myotonic muscular dystrophy, etc.)

Symptoms and Signs. Age of onset constant in the family members, ptosis with thin or atrophic lids. Limb weakness may be associated.

Etiology. Unknown. May be owing to neurological disease of supranuclear connections or neurons of oculomotor nuclei, diseases of cranial nerves, neuromuscular junction or muscle. Presently it has been demonstrated that many cases share. "Ragged red fibers" with alterations of mitochondrial DNA or other mitochondrial abnormalities. See OXPHOS syndromes.

Diagnostic Procedures. *Muscle biopsy. Brain CT scan, MRI, EEG, CSF, EMG.*

BIBLIOGRAPHY. Von Graef A: Verhandlungen aerztlicher. Gesellschaften. Berl Klin Wochenschr 5:125–127, 1868
Beaumont WM: Notes of a case of progressive nuclear ophthalmoplegia. Brain 13:386–387, 1890
Drachman DA: Ophthalmoplegia plus: a classification of the disorders associated with progressive external ophthalmoplegia. Hand Clin Neurol 22:203–216, 1976
Rowland LP: Progressive external ophthalmoplegia and ocular myopathies. In Rowland LP, Di Mauro S (eds): Handbook of Clinical Neurology, vol 18, Myopathies, p 287. Amsterdam, Elsevier, 1992

Ophthalmoplegia and ptosis (no other manifestations)

Ophthalmoplegia alone

Ptosis alone (different age of onset, etiology autosomal dominant or recessive, maternal mitochondrial DNA deletion present or absent)

OCULAR MYOPATHIES

Ocular and other cranial nerves
Oculopharyngeal muscular dystrophy (autosomal dominant) (see)
Oculopharyngeal myopathy sporadic

Ocular and proximal limb muscles

Ocular and distal limb muscles

Myotonic muscular dystrophy (see)

Myotubular or centronuclear myopathy (see)

Ophthalmoplegia, glycogen storage and abnormal mitochondria

Opthalmopathy of Flajani disease

Orbital myositis (see)

Congenital myopathic ptosis or ophthalmoplegia
Anomalous insertion of ocular muscles
Ocular muscle fibrosis with or without limb weakness

Ptosis of aging

Disorders of neuromuscular function
Erb-Goldflam (see)
Curare sensitive ocular myopathy (today in discussion)
Possibly neural ophthalmoplegias (nuclear and supranuclear)
Moebius (see)
Ophthalmoplegia with myelopathy or encephalopathy of later onset, with mental retardation, optic atrophy and other abnormalities
Hereditary ataxias
Hereditary spastic paraplegia
Hereditary multisystem disease, including Joseph (see)
Dystonia muscolorum deformans (see Ziehen-Oppenheim)
Bassen-Kornzweigg (see)
Progressive supranuclear bulbar palsy (see Steele-Richardson-Olszewiski)

Ophthalmoplegia with motor neuron disease
Werdnig-Offmann (see)

Kugelberg-Welander (see)
Aran-Duchenne (see)
Kearns-Sayre (see)
M.E.L.A.S. (see)
M.E.R.R.F. (see)
M.N.G.I.E. (see) (ophthalmoplegia with peripheral neuropathy in myo-neuro-gastrointestinal encephalopathy)
O.S.P.O.M. (ophthalmoplegia, sensorimotor peripheral neuropathy intestinal pseudo-obstruction and mitochondrial myopathy)

*From Rowland LP (Modified) Progressive external ophthalmoplegia. In Vinken GW Bryn (eds): Handbook of Clin Neurol, vol 22, pp 177–202. Amsterdam, 1975

PROLIDASE DEFICIENCY

Synonyms. Lathyritic. See also lathyrism.

Symptoms and Signs. From birth. Mental retardation. Characteristic features: prominent skull sutures, ptosis eyelids, ocular proptosis, splenomegaly, chronic dermatitis, leg ulcers, recurrent respiratory infections, obesity from early age. Joint laxity, waddling gait, protuberant abdomen, osteoporosis, mild mental retardation.

Etiology. Autosomal recessive. Deficiency of prolidase which metabolizes proline (collagen).

Diagnostic Procedures. *Urine.* Imidodipeptiduria.

Therapy. Administration of L-proline does not benefit dermatological signs. Trials for enzyme replacement.

Prognosis. According to level of deficiency, from poor quoad vitam to minor manifestations.

BIBLIOGRAPHY. Goodman SI, Solomons CC, Muschenheim F, et al: A syndrome resembling lathyrism associated with imidopeptiduria. Am J Med 45:152, 1968
Milligan A, Graham-Brown RAC, Burns DA, et al: Prolidase deficiency: A case report and literature review. Br J Dermatol 121:405–409, 1989
Endo F, Tanoue A, Kitano A, et al: Biochemical basis of prolidase deficency: Polypeptide acid RNA phenotypes and the relation to clinical phenotypes. J Clin Invest 85:162–169, 1990

PRONATOR TERES

Synonyms. Anterior interosseous nerve; median nerve.

Symptoms. Two clinical patterns according to level of nerve compression (see Etiology).

1. Median nerve: sensory and motor changes in area of nerve distribution.
2. Interosseous nerve: no sensory loss, weakness limited to pronator quadratus, flexor pollicis, flexor digitorum to II and III fingers.

Etiology. Trauma or fibrous band compressing median nerve before it gives off the anterior interosseous nerve or of the interosseous nerve at the elbow as it passes between the two heads of pronator teres muscle.

Therapy. Decompression surgery, sometimes required

Prognosis. Variable

BIBLIOGRAPHY. Dawson DM, Hallett M, Millender LH: Entrapment Neuropathies. Boston, Little, Brown, 1983
Seror P: Le syndrome du nerf interosseux antérier: charactéristiques èlectromyographiques (2 cas) et revue de la littérature (62 cas): Rev EEG Neurophysiol Clin 16:153–163, 1986

PROPERDIN DEFICIENCIES

Symptoms and Signs. The most frequent manifestation is fulminate meningococcemia and meningococcal meningitis. Systemic lupus erythematosus and discoid lupus also are seen.

Etiology. X-linked inheritance. Gene for properdin maps to X p11.23–21.1. Three varieties of the condition recognized marked reduction (1%); reduction to 10% of normal; normal level but dysfunctional.

BIBLIOGRAPHY. Ross SC, Densen P: Complement deficiency states and infection: Epidemiology, pathogenesis and conseqences of Naisserial infections in an immune deficiency. Medicine (Baltimore) 63:243, 1984

Winkelstein JA, Sullivan KE, Colten HR: Genetically determined disorders of the complement system. In Scriver CR, Beaudet AL, Sly WS, et al: The Metabolic and Molecular Bases of Inherited Disease, 7th ed, p 3928. New York, McGraw-Hill, 1995

PROPIONIC ACIDEMIAS

Synonyms. Glycinemia ketotic I, glycinemia ketotic II, hyperglycinemia; ketoacidosis; leukopenia I and II; PPC I and II.

Symptoms and Signs. The clinical picture is that of the ketotic hyperglycinemia syndrome (see) but the metabolic defects can be various.

1. Propionyl CoA carboxylase deficiency (beta-methylcrotonyl glycinuria II) I and II.
2. Multiple carboxylase deficiency.

BIBLIOGRAPHY. Weatherall DJ, Ledingham JGG, Warrell DA (eds): Oxford Textbook of Medicine, 3rd ed, pp 137–1372. Oxford, Oxford Med Pub, 1996

PROTEUS

Synonyms. Elephant man; gigantism (partial) of hands and feet; nevi; hemihypertrophy; macrocephaly. See Klippel-Trenaunay-Weber, Ollier, and Maffucci.

Symptoms and Signs. No sex predilection. Birth weight increased growth velocity leading to partial gigantism of hands and feet; gyriform hyperplasia of hands and feet, mocassin-type plantar hyperplasia, hemihypertrophy, subcutaneous tumors (lipomas), macrocephaly, or other skull anomalies. Nevi. Visceral manifestations from abdominal and pelvic lipomatosis. Moderate mental deficiency (55%); convulsion in some cases.

Etiology. Unknown. Perhaps genetic. Autosomal dominant (?).

Diagnostic Procedures. *CT scan. MRI. Sonography.* Macrocrania; exostoses; cranial hyperostosis; cerebral atrophy; overgrowth of adipose tissue in the hands and feet; vertebrae, ribs and scapulae anomalies; intraabdominal lipomas and lymphangiomas.

Prognosis. Final height normal.

BIBLIOGRAPHY. Wieland E: Zur Pathologie der dystrophischen Form des angeborenen partiellen Riesenwuchses. Jahrb Kinderheilk 65:519–594, 1907

Cohen MM Jr: Understanding Proteus syndrome, unmasking the elephant man and stemming elephant fever. Neurofibromatosis 1:260–280, 1988

Samlaska CP, Levin SW, James WD, et al: Proteus syndrome. Arch Dermatol 125:1109–1114, 1989

Atherton DJ: Naevi and other developmental defects. In Champion RH, Burton JL, Ebling FJG (eds): Rook/Wilkinson/Ebling Textbook of Dermatology, 5th ed, pp 491–492. Oxford, Blackwell Scientific, 1992

PROTHROMBIN DEFICIENCY SYNDROMES

CONGENITAL

Synonyms. Factor II deficiency, hypoprothrombinemia. Including constitutional dysthrombinemia.

Symptoms and Signs. Both sexes affected; present usually from infancy (latest onset at 13 year). Mild hemorrhagic manifestations.

Etiology. Autosomal recessive inheritance. Two variants are recognized: (1) cross-reacting material (CRM) positive (rare) constitutional dysprothrombinemia (2) CRM-negative (more common).

Pathology. Effects and sequelae of hemorrhagic diathesis.

Diagnostic Procedures. *Form 1. Blood.* Immunoelectrophoresis normal amount of antigenically competent prothrombin, which does not yield normal amount of thrombin. Prothrombin time about 10% of normal. *Form 2. Blood.* One-stage prothrombin time normal or almost normal. Two-stage reveals true hypothrombinemia.

Therapy. No specific treatment available. Vitamin K has no effect. Plasma transfusion has some effect on bleeding.

Prognosis. Poor. Death from bleeding at different ages. See also Owren and Hemophilia, classic.

ACQUIRED HYPOPROTHROMBINEMIA SYNDROMES

Symptoms and Signs. Hemorrhagic manifestation.

Etiology.

1. Vitamin K deficiency (deficiency of prothrombin; Factor VII, X, occasionally also IX)
2. Hepatocellular diseases (deficiency of prothrombin, Factor V, VII, X, occasionally IX)
3. Dicumarol medication (deficiency of prothrombin, Factor VII; slower fall also of IX and X).
4. Hemorrhagic, neonatal (see)

Diagnostic Procedures. See Etiology.

Therapy. Vitamin K; fresh plasma.

Prognosis. Depends on etiology.

BIBLIOGRAPHY. Josso F, Prou–Wartelle O, Soulier JP: Étude d'un Cas D'Hypoprothrombinemie congenitale. Nouv Rev Fr Hematol 2:647–672, 1962

Bithell TC: Hereditary coagulation disorders. In Lee GR, Bithel TC, Foerster J, et al (eds): Wintrobe's Clinical Hematology, 9th ed, pp 1442–1443, 1501. Philadelphia, Lea & Febiger, 1993

High KA, Roberts HR: Molecular Basis of Thrombosis and Hemostasis. New York, Marcel Dekker, 1995

PRUNE BELLY

Synonyms. Obrinsky; Eagle-Barett; abdominal muscle deficiency; abdominal muscles absence, urinary tract, cryptorchidism.

Symptoms. Almost exclusively in males, where the full syndrome is seen. Inability to move from lying to sitting position without the help of the arms. Frequent respiratory infections (unable to cough effectively). Frequently, urinary obstruction and infections. An association with pulmonic stenosis, mental retardation, and deafness has been reported as well.

Signs. Absence of abdominal muscles in lower and medial region of abdomen. Lower ribs flared outward; testicles retained; kidney palpable. Possibly, association of other congenital defects: lower extremities deformities; gastrointestinal anomalies; cardiac abnormalities.

Etiology. Unknown. Possibly sex-linked recessive trait. Chromosomal pattern normal in subject studied. Recent studies indicate that the urogenital anomalies can be attributed to a functional urethral obstruction that in turn is the result of prostatic hypoplasia. Prostatic maldevelopment causes weakness of the prostatic wall with resultant sacculation of the prostatic urethra.

Pathology. *Abdomen.* Abdominal wall formed by skin, superficial fascia, and peritoneum, bilateral cryptorchidism. (The abdominal muscle hypoplasia is a nonspecific lesion, resulting from fetal abdominal distention secondary to early bladder distention.) Absence of inguinal canal and gubernaculum. *Urinary tract.* Lower urinary obstruction (in some cases). Dysplastic kidney, sometimes cystic; dilatation and elongation of ureters; enlargement of bladder.

Diagnostic Procedures. *Cystography. Blood.* Blood urea nitrogen (BUN) determination. The syndrome can be diagnosed prenatally by means of ultrasonography.

Therapy. Abdominal belt; orchiopexy (if feasible). Urinary tract surgery to allow micturition when indicated. Fetal therapy in utero: drainage of the distended urinary tract.

Prognosis. About 20% stillborn; 50% die within 2 years. Record of occasional patients who reach old age (70 years).

BIBLIOGRAPHY. Fröhlich F: Der Mangel der Muskeln, insbesondere der Seitenbauchmuskelnn. Wurzburg, Dissert, 1839.
Parker RW: Case of an infant in whom some of the abdominal muscles were absent. Trans Clin Soc (London) 28:201–203, 1895
Osler W: Congenital absence of abdominal muscle with destended and hypertrophied urinary bladder. Bull Johns Hopkins Hosp 12:331–333, 1901
Greskovich FJ, Myberg LM Jr: The prune belly syndrome: A review of its etiology, defects, treatment and prognosis. J Urol 140:707–713, 1988
Burton JL: Disorders of connective tissue. In Champion RH, Burton JL, Ebling FJG (eds): Rook/Wilkinson/Ebling Textbook of Dermatology, 5th ed, p 1782. Oxford, Blackwell Scientific, 1992

PRURITUS GRAVIDARUM

Synonyms. Pregnancy pruritus (including early onset pruritus pregnancy or Besnier pruritus gestationis).

Symptoms and Signs. Besnier pruritus gestationis. One of three hundred pregnancies, onset about 25th week of pregnancy. Itching, absence of urticated lesions on the extensor aspect of limbs and shoulders; groups of crusted papules. Pregnancy pruritus. Onset in the third month increasing during all pregnancy. Localized in the abdominal region, may become generalized.

Etiology. Bound to cholestasis owing to estrogen increases.

Diagnostic Procedures. Liver function tests.

Therapy. Choleretics. Antihistamines.

Prognosis. When severe sign of increased occurrence of cholelithiasis.

BIBLIOGRAPHY. Besnier E: Premiére note et observations préliminaires pour servir d'ntroduction l'étude des prurigos diathésiques (dermatites multiformes prurigineuses choniques exacerbantes et paroxystiques, du type du prurigo de Hebra). Ann Derm Syph Paris 3:634–648, 1892
Weatherall DJ, Ledingham JGG, Warrell DA (eds): Oxford Textbook of Medicine, 3rd ed, p 1804. Oxford, Oxford Med Pub, 1996

PSEUDOACANTHOSIS NIGRICANS

See Acanthosis nigricans syndromes.

Symptoms and Signs. Affects both sexes equally; onset in adulthood (25–60 years of age). Frequent association with obesity and dark complexion. Patches of pigmentation and thickening present in any body fold, inner and upper thighs.

Etiology. Unknown. Not to be confused with acanthosis nigricans. Association with obesity and moderate extension of lesion are the differential diagnostic elements.

Diagnostic Procedures. None.

Therapy. Hypocaloric diet.

Prognosis. Regression and thickening with weight loss; pigmentation reduces or may persist.

BIBLIOGRAPHY. Ollendorff-Curth H: Pseudo-acanthosis nigricans. Ann Dermatol Syph 78:417–429, 1951
Griffiths WAD, Leigh IM, Marks R: Disorders of keratinization. In Champion RH, Burton JL, Ebling FJG (eds): Rook/Wilkinson/Ebling Textbook of Dermatology, 5th ed, pp 1384–1386. Oxford, Blackwell Scientific, 1992

PSEUDOACHONDROPLASIA

Synonym. Spondyloepiphyseal dysplasia.

Symptoms. Both sexes affected. Short stature becoming evident during adolescence. Short trunk variety. Precocious osteoarthrosis of hips, occasionally also of knees and shoulders. Absence of clinical abnormality of face and skull.

Etiology. Unknown. Autosomal dominant and recessive inheritances. Still debated, abnormal synthesis or processing of cartilage protein core. Four types, two autosomal dominant (I and III) and two recessive (II and IV) types have been classified.

Pathology. Fragmentation of epiphyseal ossification centers.

Diagnostic Procedures. *X-ray.* Of skull. Absence of lesion. In children, fragmentation of epiphyseal ossification center. Spinal change characteristic in adult. Lumbar vertebrae formed by eburnated bone in central and posterior parts of superior and inferior plates. Osteoarthrosis. In the two dominant forms X-ray changes more severe.

Pathology. In type III: cytoplasmic metachromasia of fibroblasts and specific ultramicroscopic alteration in the chondrocytes.

Therapy. Symptomatic.

Prognosis. Final height 130–150 cm.

BIBLIOGRAPHY. Maroteaux P, Lamy M: Les formes pseudo-achondroplastiques des dysplasies spondyloépiphysaires. Presse Méd 67:383–386, 1959
Stanescu V, Maroteaux P, Stanescu R: The biochemical defect of pseudoachondroplasia. Eur J Pediatr 138:221–225, 1982
Hall JG, Dorst JP, Rotta J, et al: Gonadal mosaicism in pseudoachondroplasia. Am J Med Genet 28:143–151, 1987
Weatherall DJ, Ledingham JGG, Warrell DA (eds): Oxford Textbook of Medicine, 3rd ed, p 3089. Oxford, Oxford Med Pub, 1996

PSEUDOARTHROGRYPOSIS

Synonyms. Siwon; elbow—knee congenital rigidity; ankylosis elbow knee.

Symptoms and Signs. From birth. Females. Rigidity of elbows and knees.

Etiology. Autosomal dominant.

Pathology. Ankylosis and proximal fusion of tibia and fibula or humerus, radius, and ulna.

BIBLIOGRAPHY. Siwon P: Kongenital, hereditaere, doppelseitige Ankylosen der Ellenbogengelenke. Dtsch Z Chir 209:338–349, 1928
Pasina A, Wildervank LS: Hereditary occurrence of congenital rigidity

of elbows and knees (congenital multiple arthrogryposis). Arch Chir Neurol 8:43–56, 1956

PSEUDOBULBAR PALSY

Synonyms. Limbic system; includes Lhermitte-Cornil. See Foix-Chavany-Marie.

Symptoms. Occurs in patients over 40 years of age. Dysarthria (but not dysphasia); temporary complete aphonia; dysphagia; disorder of gait; disturbed reflex; emotional reactions; spontaneous crying and laughing that cannot be controlled. Neurogenic bladder (see); intelligence affected or not.

Signs. Paresis of voluntary motion; exaggeration of automatic and reflex movements. Facial expression may be similar to that in parkinsonism; voice nasal without intonation; volume low; whispering; drooling of saliva.

Etiology. Arteriosclerosis with multiple areas of softening. Syphilis, infections, trauma, and degenerative diseases may also be responsible.

Pathology. Softening in any place where supranuclear fibers pass through: cortical; subcortical; corona radiata; internal capsula zones. Supranuclear fibers must be destroyed on both sides to produce this syndrome. Vascular lesions.

Diagnostic Procedures. None specific. *EEG. CT scan. MRI. Angiography. Blood.* Cholesterol may be elevated.

Therapy. None specific. Antibiotic for frequent pulmonary complications.

Prognosis. Remission of this syndrome rare, especially after emotional component becomes manifested. Rehabilitation of patient extremely difficult. Death from pulmonary complications or inanition.

BIBLIOGRAPHY. Magnus A: Fall von Aufhebung des Willenseinflusses auf einige Hirnnerven. Arch Anat Physiol Wissensch Med 258:567, 1837
Lhermitte J Cornil L Syndrome stié à debut apoplectique et à expression choréo-athéthosique et pseudobulbaire. Rev Neurol 38:419–421 1922
Adams RD, Victor M: Principles of Neurology, 5th ed, pp 448–449. New York, McGraw-Hill, 1993
Weatherall DJ, Ledingham JGG, Warrell DA (eds): Oxford Textbook of Medicine, 3rd ed, p 4122. Oxford, Oxford Med Pub, 1996

PSEUDOCHROMHIDROSIS

See Chromhidrosis.

Symptoms and Signs. Similar to those of chromhidrosis.

Etiology. Differing from chromhidrosis in that the sweat changes color after having reached the skin, from the activity of chromogenic bacteria, especially Corynebacterium, usually located in hairy areas.

Therapy. Hygiene and topical antibacterial agents.

Prognosis. Condition disappears with adequate treatment.

BIBLIOGRAPHY. Hurley HJ, Shelley WB: The Human Apocrine Gland in Health and Disease. Springfield, IL, Charles C Thomas, 1960
Champion RH: Disorders of sweat glands. In Champion RH, Burton JL, Ebling FJG (eds): Rook/Wilkinson/Ebling Textbook of Dermatology, 5th ed, p 1761. Oxford, Blackwell Scientific, 1992

PSEUDO-CUSHING

Symptoms. Seen especially in young subjects. Overeating.

Signs. Truncal obesity; purple striae on abdomen and thighs.

Etiology. Among the many possible causes: psychological maladjustment; constitutional factors; strenuous exercise; renal failure; hypoglycemia; hypercortisolism secondary to alcoholism (chronic and withdrawal).

Pathology. Obesity.

Diagnostic Procedures. *Urine.* Increased secretion of cortisol (greater than normal, less than in Cushing). Increased excretion of hydrocortisone metabolites. Plasma cortisol level in low-normal range. Adrenocorticotropic hormone (ACTH) test, metyrapone test, and adrenal suppression tests (Decadron) normal (see Cushing).

Therapy. Treatment of obesity; diet; psychotherapy.

Prognosis. Weight loss, disappearance of striae, and return to normal adrenal function with treatment.

BIBLIOGRAPHY. Nieman L, Cutler GB Jr: Cushing's syndrome. In De Groot LJ (ed): Endocrinology, 3rd ed, p 1746. Philadelphia, WB Saunders, 1995
Weatherall DJ, Ledingham JGG, Warrell DA (eds): Oxford Textbook of Medicine, 3rd ed, p 1643. Oxford, Oxford Med Pub, 1996

PSEUDOCYESIS

Synonyms. Fantasized pregnancy; false pregnancy.

Symptoms. Occurs usually in later fertile period. Amenorrhea; morning sickness; appetite variation; breast sensitivity; constipation; impression of fetal movements.

Signs. Abdominal enlargement, which disappears after anesthesia; cervix firm; uterus normal size.

Etiology. Delusion of pregnancy. Psychogenic mechanisms.

Diagnostic Procedures. *Pregnancy test.* Negative.

Therapy. Psychiatric.

Prognosis. Possible conversion to other delusional states.

BIBLIOGRAPHY. Cunningham, MacDonald, Gant, et al (eds): Williams Obstetrics, pp 23, 31. Englewood Cliffs, NJ, Prentice-Hall, 1993
Kaplan HI, Sadock BJ: Comprehensive Textbook of Psychiatry, 6th ed, p 1702. Baltimore, Williams & Wilkins, 1995

PSEUDODIASTROPHIC DWARFISM

Synonyms. Dwarfim pseudodyastropic. See Diastrophic dysplasia.

Symptoms. In early infancy unexplained hyperthermia and contractures.

Signs. Short at birth, blue gray sclera, hypertelorism, flat nasal bridge, malformed ears; cleft palate; elbow dislocation; interphalangeal dislocation; club feet; scoliosis.

Etiology. Autosomal recessive inheritance.

Pathology. No modification of chondro-osseous morphology (differing from diastrophic dysplasia).

Therapy. Orthopedic correction and surgery.

Prognosis. Often fatal in first year. Clubfoot responds better to physical and surgical therapy than the diastrophic form.

BIBLIOGRAPHY. Burgio GR, Belloni C, Beluffi G: Nanisme pseudodiastrophique: etude de deux soeurs nouveau-nees. Arch Franc Pediatr 31:681–696, 1974
Eteson DJ, Beluffi G, Burgio GR, et al: Pseudodiastrophic dysplasia: A distinct newborn skeletal dysplasia. J Pediatr 109:635–641, 1986
Canky-Klain N, Stanescu V, Bebler P, et al: Pseudodiastophic dysplasia evolution with age and management: Report of two new cases and review of literature. Ann Genetic 33:129–136, 1990

PSEUDOGOUT

Synonyms. Chondrocalcinosis; calcium gout; crystal synovitis; synovitis crystal.

Symptoms. Occurs most often in females over 40. Articular symptoms from mild arthralgias to acute arthritis mimicking gout attack (lasting from 21 hour to 50 days). Joints most frequently affected: knees, hands, and feet; 20% polyarthralgias.

Sign. Mild or acute inflammation of joints involved.

Etiology. Metabolic defect; precipitation of crystal of calcium pyrophosphate in synovial fluid cartilage and periarticular structures.

Pathology. Possibly, genetically determined or subacute inflammation owing to the presence of calcium crystals.

Diagnostic Procedures. *Synovial fluid aspiration* (diagnostic). Intracellular and extracellular. Calcium crystal in some cases. *Blood.* Hyperuricemia and diabetes findings or alteration of glucose tolerance curve. Sedimentation rate usually elevated. Serum calcium and phosphorus normal in majority of patients. Serum alkaline phosphatase normal. *X-ray.* Articular calcification as a thin line paralleling contour of bone or granular deposit in fibrochondrial structures; degenerative changes of joints.

Therapy. Colchicine gives good to fair response; aspirin, corticosteroid good to fair. Aspiration of synovial fluid also may give relief from symptoms.

Prognosis. Relatively benign condition; articular degeneration develops, but not as severe as in rheumatoid arthritis.

BIBLIOGRAPHY. McCarty DJ, Kohn NN, Faires JS: Significance of calcium phosphate crystals in the synovial fluid arthritic patients: The "pseudogout syndrome." I. Clinical aspects. Ann Intern Med 56:711–737, 1962

Moskowitz RW, Katz D: Chondrocalcinosis and chondrocalsynovitis (pseudogout syndrome). Am J Med 43:322–334, 1967

Riestra JL, Sanchez A, Rodriguez-Valverde V, Castillo E, Calderon J: Roentgenographic features of the arthropathy associated with CPPD crystal deposition disease. A comparative study with primary osteoarthritis. J Rheumatol 12:1154–1158, 1985

McCarty DJ (ed): Crystalline Deposition Diseases. Rheum Dis Clin N America (14):2. Philadelphia, WB Saunders, 1988

Weatherall DJ, Ledingham JGG, Warrell DA (eds): Oxford Textbook of Medicine, 3rd ed, pp 2988–2990. Oxford, Oxford Med Pub, 1996

PSEUDO-GRAEFE

Synonym. Fuchs sign.

Symptoms and Signs. While the eye may be adducted and lid elevated, no movement up or down occurs when the vertical recti contract together.

Etiology and Pathology. Trauma or tumor at the base of skull. Regenerating fibers growing to wrong muscles, or spreading of a localized stimulation to an injured third nucleus so that when one tries to move the eye in one direction, impulses also flow into all other muscles innervated by oculomotor (III) nerve.

Diagnostic Procedures. *X-ray. CT scan. MRI. Angiography. CSF. EEG.*

Therapy and Procedures. According to etiology.

BIBLIOGRAPHY. Bender MB: Nerve supply to orbicularis muscle and physiology of movement of upper eyelid, with particular reference to the Pseudo-Graefe phenomenon. Arch Ophthalmol 15:21–30, 1936

Walsh FB, King AB: Ocular signs of intracranial saccular aneurysms. Arch Ophthalmol 27:1–33, 1942

Anderson JR: Ocular vertical deviations. Br J Ophthalmol (Suppl) 12:7–99, 1947

Adams RD, Victor M: Principles of Neurology, 5th ed, p 233. New York, McGraw-Hill, 1993

PSEUDOHERMAPHRODITISM, MALE, DEFICIENCY OF 17–20 DESMOLASE TESTIS

Synonyms. 17–20 lyase deficiency. See also Pseudohermaphroditism male—gynecomastia.

Symptoms and Signs. At birth: females, normal internal and external genitalia; at puberty, lack of pubertal development and infertility. Males, variable phenotypes from complete female external genitalia, through severe hypospadiats to normal male phenotype. No hypertension.

Etiology. Possibly X-linked (or autosomal recessive [?]); deficiency of 17–20 desmolase of testis. Association with 18q deletion.

Diagnostic Procedures. Cortisol and metabolites: normal; increased progesterone, 17-hydroxyprogesterone and variably, pregnelone, 17-hydroxypregnenolone, and pregnenolone sulfate. Normal or low DHEA, and 4-androstenodione. Testosterone and DHEA do not increase following ACTH stimulation.

Therapy and Procedures. Surgical repair of external genitalia and sex steroid substitution at age of expected puberty.

BIBLIOGRAPHY. Zachmann M, Hamilton W, Vollmin JA et al: Testicular 17–20 desmolase deficiency causing male pseudohermaphroditism. Acta Endocrinol (Suppl) 155:65–80, 1971

Forest MG: Diagnosis and treatment of disorders of sexual development. In De Groot LJ (ed): Endocrinology, 3rd ed, p 1917. Philadelphia, WB Saunders, 1995

PSEUDOHERMAPHRODITISM, MALE, GYNECOMASTIA

Synonyms. 17-Hydroxysteroid deficiency, 17-ketosteroid reductase deficiency testis, 17-KSR deficiency, 17-β-HSD deficiency.

Symptoms and Signs. At birth. External genitalia female type with or without moderate ambiguity. Testis palpable in inguinal canal or labial folds. Diagnosis usually at puberty or adult age because of development of male body habitus and secondary sexual characteristics. Gynecomastia not always present.

Etiology. Autosomal recessive inheritance. 17-Ketosteroid reductase deficiency limited to the testis.

Diagnostic Procedures. *Blood.* Accumulation of 4-androstenedione, whereas testosterone is normal or low. LH elevated FSH normal or low; ACTH and gluco- and mineralo-corticoids are normal; 17-hydroxyprogesterone is increased; DHEA occasionally is mildly increased while 5-androstenediol is decreased.

Therapy. Diagnosis before puberty: removal of abnormal testis.

Prognosis. According to therapy. Female habitus appears as the best choice.

BIBLIOGRAPHY. Neher R, Kahnt FW: Gonadal steroid biosynthesis in vitro in four cases of testicular feminization. In Vermeulen A, Exley D (eds): Androgens in Normal and Pathological Conditions, p 132. Amsterdam, Excerpta Med, 1966

de Peretti E, Saez J, Bertrand J: Familial male pseudohermaphroditism (MHP) due to 17–Ketosteroid reductase defect: in vitro study and testicular incubation. Amsterdam, Excerpta Med, p 205, 1970

Saez JM, De Peretti E, Morera AM, et al: Familial male pseudohermaphroditism with gynecomastia due to a testicular 17–ketosteroid reductase defect I: Studies in vivo. J Clin Endocrinol 32:604–610, 1971

Balducci M, Toscano V, Wright F, et al: Familial male pseudohermaphroditism with gynecomastia due to 17-beta-hydroxysteroid dehydrogenase deficiency: A report of three cases. Clin Endocrinol 23:439–444, 1985

Forest MG: Diagnosis and treatment of disorders of sexual development. In De Groot LJ (ed): Endocrinology, 3rd ed, pp 1917–1918. Philadelphia, WB Saunders, 1995

PSEUDOHERMAPHRODITISM, MALE, INCOMPLETE HEREDITARY (TYPE I)

Synonym. Androgen resistance (type I); incomplete androgen insensitivity.

Symptoms. Clinically includes a variety of subsyndromes (previously considered autonomous entities): from the extreme feminine end of the spectrum with Lub through Gilber-Dreyfus and Reifenstein to the other extreme of the Rosewaters, which presents an almost complete male phenotype. Each form will present its own relative psychological problems and different needs of role adjustment.

Signs. From phenotypic female with pseudovagina (Lub) to normal sterile male (common hypospadias). Normal body hair; scanty or absent beard.

Etiology. X-linked inheritance (or autosomal recessive [?]). See Seabright-Bantam.

Pathology. See individual syndromes. Normal gonads; incomplete spermatogenesis. Wolffian ducts vary in development; absence of ducts derivatives.

Diagnostic Procedures. *Chromatin studies.* Male sex chromatin 46XY karyotype. *Blood.* Testosterone production normal or increased. Estrogen production greater than in normal men. Gonadotropin levels elevated.

Therapy. See individual syndromes. Resistance to androgenic and anabolic effects of testosterone.

Prognosis. Good quoad vitam. See individual syndromes.

BIBLIOGRAPHY. Griffin JE, Wilson JD: The androgen resistance syndromes: 5-α-reductase deficiency, testicular feminization and related disorders. In Scriver CR, Beaudet AL, Sly WS, et al: The Metabolic and Molecular Bases of Inherited Disease, 6th ed, p 1932. New York, McGraw-Hill, 1989

Forest MG: Diagnosis and treatment of disorders of sexual development. In De Groot LJ (ed): Endocrinology, 3rd ed, p 1921. Philadelphia, WB Saunders, 1995

PSEUDO-HIRSCHSPRUNG

Synonyms. Colonic inertia; acquired functional megacolon; idiopathic megacolon; psychogenic megacolon; sluggish colon.

Symptoms and Signs. Occurs in children. Symptoms and signs of partial intestinal obstruction.

Etiology. Unknown.

Pathology. No signs of gross mechanical obstruction or disease that may cause secondary symptomatic megacolon. Histologically, intramural plexes are normal, and there is no evidence of degenerative changes.

Diagnostic Procedures. *Barium enema.* Proximal megacolon with undilated distal segment. *Biopsy of intestinal mucosa.* Normal.

Therapy. Rectosigmoidectomy. Cases treated with temporary colostomy recovered after closure of colostomy.

Prognosis. Excellent with treatment.

BIBLIOGRAPHY. Bill AH Jr, Creighton SA, Stevenson JK: The selection of infants and children for the surgical treatment of Hirschsprung's disease. Surg Gynecol Obstet 104:151–156, 1957

Ehrenpreis T: Pseudo-Hirschsprung's disease. Arch Dis Child 40:177–179, 1965

Watier A, Feldman P, Martelli H, et al: Hirschsprung's disease. In Haubrich WS, Schaffner F, Berk JE (eds): Bockus Gastroenterology, 5th ed, vol 2, pp 1611–1612. Philadelphia, WB Saunders, 1995

PSEUDO-HURLER POLYDYSTROPHY

Synonyms. ML III; mucolipidosis III.

Symptoms and Signs. Both sexes affected. Onset usually at 2–4 years of age. Hands and shoulder stiffness, progressing to clawhand deformity (at 6–8 years of age) and striking dwarfism. Carpal tunnel syndrome (see). Coarse facies. Fine peripheral corneal clouding (progressive). Cardiac murmurs. Mild mental retardation (in 50%). Occasionally inguinal hernia; acne. Clinical picture is similar to Maroteaux-Lamy of intermediate severity.

Etiology. Autosomal recessive inheritance. Multiple enzyme defects apparently confined to connective tissue. Defect allelic to the one for Leroy I cell disease (see). Defect of phosphorylation of hydrolases, which does not enable them to enter lysosomes and thus become active. Many mucopolysaccharides are not metabolized.

Pathology. Histologic changes similar to those of Leroy I cell syndrome (see); inclusions not as prominent in I cells.

Diagnostic Procedures. *Fibroblast culture.* See Pathology. *Urine.* Absent or moderate mucopolysacchariduria. *Blood.* Increased lysosomal enzymes value. Amniotic fuid: prenatal diagnosis. *X-ray.* Lesions more severe in males. Dysostosis multiplex; particularly striking changes in the hip.

Therapy. Orthopedic.

Prognosis. Adulthood reached with severe dysostosis.

BIBLIOGRAPHY. Maroteaux P, Lamy M: La pseudopolydystrophie de Hurler's. Presse Med 74:2889–2892, 1966

Kornfeld S, Sly WS: I cell disease and pseudo-Hurler polydystrophy: Disorders of lysosomal enzyme phosphorylation and localization. In Scriver CR, Beaudet AL, Sly WS, et al: The Metabolic and Molecular Bases of Inherited Disease, 7th ed, pp 2497–2498. New York, McGraw-Hill, 1995

Weatherall DJ, Ledingham JGG, Warrell DA (eds): Oxford Textbook of Medicine, 3rd ed, pp 1434–1435, 3985. Oxford, Oxford Med Pub, 1996

PSEUDOHYPOALDOSTERONISM I

Synonym. Cheek-Perry; salt-wasting. See low salt.

Symptoms. Reported in Caucasians, Arabs, Asians, Indians, Mexican-Americans, Persian Jews, and one Afro-American. Prevalent in males. Onset from 5 days to 7 months of age. Variable severity of manifestations. Vomiting; anorexia; failure to gain weight; cyanotic attacks when exposed to elevated temperature.

Signs. Poor weight gain; dehydration.

Etiology. Insensitivity of the renal tubules to action of aldosterone. It may overlap with the Thorn syndrome and Inappropriate antidiuretic hormone syndrome. Evidence for various genetic defects. In a group of cases observed target organ unresponsiveness to mineralocorticoids and severe clinical course, in others unresponsiveness appears limited mainly to the kidney and the clinical expression is mild or absent (see Gordon). Type I can be differentiated from other similar conditions from its mineralocorticoid insensitivity, adequate steroid production, altered Na/K ratio in biological fluids, renal salt wasting (hyponatremia), renal K retention and tubular acidosis.

Pathology. Unknown. In some cases, renal biopsy showed 25% of small glomeruli and glomerulosclerosis of varying degrees, no major tubular changes.

Diagnostic Procedures. *Blood.* Hyponatremia; hyperkalemia. *Urine.* Normal 17-ketosteroids; high aldosterone level. Good response to adrenocorticotropic hormone (ACTH) with increased excretion of aldosterone. *Kidney biopsy.*

Therapy. Unresponsive to desoxycorticosterone (DOCA), fludrocortisone, and aldosterone; aggravated by spironolactone. Responds optimally to vigorous replacement of sodium and intravascular volume.

Prognosis. Death (8%) caused by salt depletion and hyperkaliemia. Good response and height and weight gain with salt administration, which, in the majority of cases, may be discontinued after infancy in spite of the persistence of excess of aldosterone

BIBLIOGRAPHY. Cheek DB, Perry JW: A salt wasting syndrome in infancy. Arch Dis Child 33:252–256, 1958
Royer P, Bonnette J, Mathieu H, et al: Pseudo-hypoaldosteronism. Ann Pediatr 10:596–605, 1963
Kuhnle U, Nielsen MD, Tietze HU, et al: Pseudohypoaldosteronism in eight families: Different forms of inheritance are evidence for various genetic defects. J Clin Endocr Metab 70:638–641, 1990
Hanukoglu A: Type I pseudohypoaldosteronism includes two clinically and genetically distinct entities with either renal or multiple target organ defects. J Clin Endocr Metab 73:936–944, 1991
Melby JC, Azar ST: Hypoaldosteronism and mineralocorticoid resistance. In De Groot LJ (ed): Endocrinology, 3rd ed, pp 1804–1808. Philadelphia, WB Saunders, 1995

PSEUDOHYPOALDOSTERONISM II

Synonyms. Gordon (RD).

Symptoms and Signs. Late childhood or adulthood: blood hypertension.

Etiology. Unknown. Enhanced chloride reabsorption at distal nephron, no salt wasting.

Diagnostic Procedures. *Blood.* Hyperkalemia, acidosis, aldosterone levels normal or slightly reduced.

Therapy. Thiazide diuretics very effective. Scarce effect of furosemide.

Prognosis. Good.

BIBLIOGRAPHY. Gordon RD, Hodsman GP: The syndrome of hypertension and hyperkalemia without renal failure. Long term correction by thiazide diuretic. Scott Med J 31:43, 1986
DuBose TD, Alpern RJ: Renal tubular acidosis. In Scriver CR, Beaudet AL, Sly WS, et al: The Metabolic and Molecular Bases of Inherited Disease, 7th ed, pp 3679–3681. New York, McGraw-Hill, 1995

PSEUDOHYPOPHOSPHATASIA

Synonyms. Scriver. See acid phosphatase deficiencies.

Symptoms and Signs. Extremely rare form with all the classic features of infantile hypophosphatasia (see) with normal or increased serum alkaline phosphatase.

BIBLIOGRAPHY. Scriver CR, Cameron D: Pseudohypophosphatasia. N Engl J Med 281:604–606, 1969
Moore CA, Wappner RS, Coburn SP, et al: Pseudohypophosphatasia: Clinical, radiographic, and biochemical characterization of a second case. Am J Hum Genet 47:A-68, 1990
Whyte MP: Hypophosphatasia. In Scriver CR, Beaudet AL, Sly WS, et al: The Metabolic and Molecular Bases of Inherited Disease, pp 4095–4111. New York, McGraw-Hill, 1995

PSEUDOLIPOMATOSIS, SYMMETRICAL

Synonyms. Symmetrical pseudolipomatosis; see Dercum.

Symptoms and Signs. See adenolipomatosis symmetric.

Etiology. Probably a form of myxedema with cervico-clavicolar localization.

PSEUDOLYMPHOMA

Synonym. Anticonvulsant hypersensitivity drug sensitivity; AHS; Dilantin hypersensitivity.

Symptoms. Estimated frequency between 1 in 1000 and 1 in 10,000. Onset 1 week to 2 years after exposure to one of the drugs (phenytoin, carbamazepine, and phenobarbital). Fever, malaise, and arthralgia.

Signs. Polymorphic skin eruption; generalized lymphadenopathy; hepatosplenomegaly; joint swelling.

Etiology. Sensitivity to anticonvulsant. Diphenylhydantoin (Dilantin) and mephenytoin (Mesantoin) are most common offenders.

Pathology. Lymph node biopsy shows complete loss of normal architecture and replacement of germinal center by reticuloendothelial cells of monstrous size. Skin biopsy normal or myocosis fungoides-like pattern of infiltration with eosinophils. In liver, moderate or minimal fat metamorphosis; eosinophilic infiltration. In bone marrow, marked eosinophilic hyperplasia.

Diagnostic Procedures. *Blood.* Mild anemia, leukopenia, or leukocytosis; eosinophilia. Serum glutamic-oxaloacetic acid (SGOT), lactic dehydrogenase, alkaline phosphatase high. *X-ray of chest.* Normal. *Lupus erythematosus (LE) test.* Negative.

Therapy. Discontinuation of anticonvulsant drug.

Prognosis. Good if drug is suspended (cure in 7–14 days) and substituted. Cross-sensitization possible. If condition not identified, death may result.

BIBLIOGRAPHY. Coope R, Burrows RGR: Treatment of epilepsy with sodium diphenyl hydantoinate. Lancet 1:490–492, 1940
Schreiber MM, McGregor JG: Pseudolymphoma syndrome. A sensitivity to anticonvulsant drugs. Arch Dermatol 97:297–300, 1968
Vittorio CC, Muglia JJ: Anticonvulsant hypersensitivity syndrome. Arch Int Med 155:2285–2290, 1995

PSEUDO-MEIGS

Term given by Meigs. Same as true Meigs syndrome, except that in the pseudo-Meigs syndrome the tumor may be in the ovary, tubes, uterus, or round ligament. After removal of the tumor, ascites and hydrothorax do not necessarily disappear as in the case of true Meigs syndrome.

Therapy. Removal of the tumor.

Prognosis. Depends on nature of tumor and or its metastasis.

BIBLIOGRAPHY. Meigs JV: Pelvic tumors other than fibromas of the ovary with ascites and hydrothorax. Obstet Gynecol 3:471–486, 1954
Brenner WE, Scott RB: Meigs-like syndrome secondary to Krukenberg's tumor. Obstet Gynecol 31:40–44, 1968

PSEUDOMEMBRANOUS ENTEROCOLITIS

Synonyms. Hemorrhagic enterocolitis; ischemic enterocolitis; necrotizing colitis; postoperative enterocolitis; staphylococcal enterocolitis; toxic pseudomembranous intestinal inflammation; uremic colitis, including Janbon.

Symptoms and Signs. Both sexes affected. Usually a severe underlying disease of extremely variable nature. Abrupt onset (usually after 2 days from beginning of antibiotics up to 3 weeks after their discontinuation). Nausea; vomiting; abdominal cramps and distention; watery, occasionally hemorrhagic, diarrhea; shock. Absence of abdominal tenderness and frequently also of bowel sounds. Frequently, same symptoms as in paralytic ileus.

Etiology. Antibiotics and metronidazole the most frequent causative agents (Janbon syndrome) of the enhanced development of Clostridium difficile (a normal resident of the intestine).

Pathology. Multiple isolated or confluent white yellowish plaques, slightly elevated, from 1–3 mm to 20 mm in diameter, covering superficial ulceration. Remaining mucosa edematous and hyperemic. Histologically, pseudomembranes are composed of fibrin, mucus, desquamated cells, and leukocytes.

Diagnostic Procedures. *Sigmoidoscopy.* See Pathology. *X-ray.* Plain film reveals edema and distortion of haustra. *Blood.* Leukocytosis. *Stools.* Culture of C. difficile and detection of C. difficile cytotoxin.

Therapy. Cessation of antibiotic therapy. Fluid-electrolyte balance. Albumin or blood replacement or both. Vancomycin (500 mg × 4/day × 7–10 days), orally metronidazole (1.5–2 g/day p os), avoid antidiarrheals. Surgery for perforation or toxic dilatation.

Prognosis. Overall mortality 15%.

BIBLIOGRAPHY. Janbon M: Le syndrome choleriforme de la terramycine. Montpellier Med 41:300–311, 1952
LaHatte LJ, Tedesco FJ, Schuman BM: Antibiotic-associated injury to the gut. In Haubrich WS, Schaffner F, Berk JE (eds): Bockus Gastroenterology, 5th ed, vol 2, pp 1657–1671. Philadelphia, WB Saunders, 1995

PSEUDO-OBSTRUCTION, INTESTINAL, CHILDHOOD

Synonym. Chronic idiopathic intestinal pseudo obstruction (CIIP); functional intestinal obstruction; hereditary hollow visceral myopathy; familial visceral myopathy; familial megaduodenum (see also megaduodenum); megacysts intestinal hypoperistalsis (see).

Symptoms and Signs. Rare onset in utero (fetal abdominal distension, material polyhydramnios). At birth (22%), first month (43%), first year (65%). Abdominal distension, constipation, vomiting, diarrhea; failure to thrive; seizures; temperature instability; dysphagia; urological abnormalities.

Etiology. Disorder of nerves and ganglia: hyper and hypoganglionosis. Diseases of smooth muscle coats various hereditary pattern described in different families.

Diagnostic Procedures. *Plain film of abdomen.* Rx esophagus, stomach, small intestinal with barium reveals: gastroesophageal reflux, dilatation of small bowel, delayed gastric emptyng; megaduodenum. *Esophageal manometry intestinal studies. Exploration laparotomy. Biopsy.* With silver stain. According to etiology.

Therapy. Diet, total parenteral nutrition, nasogastric suction, surgery for intractable pain or massive diarrhea. Antibiotics, metoclopramide, bethanechol not effective. Cisapride seldom useful.

Prognosis. Severe in preterm infants, surgery often necessary. Most children die in 2 years. Milder forms may live to old middle age before correct diagnosis is made.

BIBLIOGRAPHY. Anuras S, Shaw A, Christensen J: The familial syndromes of intestinal pseudo-obstruction. Am J Hum Genet 33:584–591, 1981
Schuffler MD: Chronic intestinal pseudo obstruction syndromes. Med Clin North Am 65:1331–58, 1981
Vargas JH, Ament ME: Chronic intestinal pseudo-obstruction syndrome (CIPS) in pediatrics results of a North American survey. Clin Res 35:210, 1987

Milla PJ: Disorders of gastrointestinal motility in childhood. Chichester, Wiley & Sons, 1988
Manten HD: Pseudoobstruction. In Haubrich WS, Schaffner F, Berk JE (eds): Bockus Gastroenterology, 5th ed, pp 1260–1261. Philadelphia, WB Saunders, 1995

PSEUDOPANCREATIC CHOLERA

Synonym. Diarrhea, secretory, chronic, idiopathic; secretory diarrhea, chronic, idiopathic.

Symptoms and Signs. In patients with or without intestinal resections. Symptoms and signs like those of Verner-Morrison (see).

Etiology. Unknown or endocrine tumor or elevated plasma level secretagogue.

Diagnostic Procedures. Same as Verner-Morrison. *Blood research for VIP.* Negative.

Therapy. Somatostatin.

Prognosis. Good with therapy.

BIBLIOGRAPHY. Read NW, Read MG, Krejs GJ, et al: A report of five patients with large volume secretory diarrhea, but no evidence of endocrine tumor or laxative abuse. Dig Dis Sci 27:193–201, 1982
Ammon HV: Diarrhea. In Haubrich WS, Schaffner F, Berk JE (eds): Bockus Gastroenterology, 5th ed, pp 89–91. Philadelphia, WB Saunders, 1995

PSEUDOPELADE

Symptoms and Signs. Sex and age incidence according to etiology. Idiopathic cases usually occur in females in third to fifth decades. Onset insidious. Formation of small, round, bald areas, smooth, soft, without signs of inflammation (moderate erythema may be present), enlarging and confluent. Vertex most frequently affected.

Etiology. Lupus erythematosus; lichen planus; scleroderma; keratosis pilaris; idiopathic.

Pathology. Lymphocytic infiltrate around hair follicle; bulb spared; followed by atrophy of hair follicles and sebaceous glands. Sweat glands spared.

Diagnostic Procedures. *Biopsy.* (In early stage.) Diagnosis of associated disorder. *Direct immunofluorescence.*

Therapy. Lesion irreversible. Treatment of underlying condition prevents spreading. Autograph from other areas of scalp.

BIBLIOGRAPHY. Degos R, Rabut R, Duperrat B, et al: L'état pseudo-peladique, réflexions à propos de cent cas d'alopécies cicatricielles en aires, d'appearance primitive du type pseudopelade. Ann Dermatol Syph 81:5–26, 1954
Dawber RPR, Ebling FJG, Wojnarowska FT: Disorders of hair. In Champion RH, Burton JL, Ebling FJG (eds): Rook/Wilkinson/Ebling Textbook of Dermatology, 5th ed, pp 2599–2600. Oxford, Blackwell Scientific, 1992

PSEUDOPHAKIC BULLOUS KERATOPATHY

Symptoms and Signs. After intraocular lens implantations decreased vision and corneal decompensation manifested by vascularization and scarring, keratitis, ulcers, descematocele, and melting and perforation.

Etiology. Reaction to IOL after cataract surgery. (1) Mechanical (iris supposed IOL sometimes dislocate anteriorly causing endothelial chaffing). (2) Sublineal, chronic, smoldering inflammation usually at loop fixation sites. Oxidative free radicals formed by inflammatory cells could be toxic to endothelial cells.

Pathology. Bullous separation of epithelium in cornea from underlying stroma.

Therapy. Corneal transplantation or penetrating keratoplasty or exchange of offending IOL.

Prognosis. Good with therapy.

BIBLIOGRAPHY. Apple DL, Rabb MF: Ocular Pathology, 4th ed, p 153. St Louis, CV Mosby, 1991
Morris DA: Ocular trauma. In Garner A, Klintworth GK (eds): Pathobiology of Ocular Disease: A Dynamic Approach, 2nd ed, pp 418–419. New York, Marcel Dekker, 1994

PSEUDO-PSEUDOHYPOPARATHYROIDISM

Synonym. Albright II.

Symptoms and Signs. All those of Martin-Albright (see) except there are normal calcium and phosphate values and lack of related symptomatology.

Etiology. Unknown. Probably inherited as X-linked disorder. Coexistence of pseudohypoparathyroidism (PHP) and pseudopseudohypoparathyroidism in the same families indicates that anatomy and lack of hormonal response, although related, are not interdependent. Same deficiency in Gs (ubiquitous protein required for cAMP production), as expressed in PHP syndrome.

Diagnostic Procedures. *Blood. Urine.* Normal. *X-ray.* Calcification seen in PHP not seen in this form.

BIBLIOGRAPHY. Albright F, Forbes AP, Henneman PH: Pseudopseudohypoparathyroidism. Trans Assoc Am Phys 65:337–350, 1952
Levine MA, Spiegel AM: Pseudopseudohypoparathyroidism. In De Groot LJ (ed): Endocrinology, 3rd ed, pp 1140–1142. Philadelphia, WB Saunders, 1995

PSEUDOSYRINGOMYELIC

Synonyms. See Morvan.

Symptoms and Signs. Disproportionate involvement of pain and temperature fibers in several peripheral nerves: seldom may affect cranium and arms, sparing trunk and legs.

Etiology. Observed in Tangier (see) and amyloid neuropathies.

BIBLIOGRAPHY. Adams RD, Victor M: Principles of Neurology, 5th ed, New York, McGraw-Hill, 1993

PSEUDO-VITAMIN D-DEFICIENCY RICKETS

Synonyms. Prader; vitamin D-dependent rickets; rickets, autosomal recessive; pseudodeficiency rickets; autosomal recessive vitamin D deficiency (ARVDD); vitamin D-dependent rickets, VDDR. Classified in type I and type II.

TYPE I

Symptoms and Signs. The same as in ordinary rickets owing to vitamin D deficiency. Both sexes affected; onset in first 6–9 months of life. Growth deficiency; hypotonia; skeletal changes typical of rickets; seizures (hypocalcemia); occasionally fractures. Teeth enamel hypoplasia.

Etiology. Autosomal recessive. Characterized by organ resistance owing to a genetic defect of 25-hydroxylcholecalciferol 1-α-hydroxylase, that converts 25-(OH) to 1, 25-(OH2) D.

Diagnostic Procedures. *Blood.* Hypocalcemia, serum 1,25-(OH2) D low. PTH high. Plasma phosphate normal or low.

Therapy. Vitamin D in daily doses or 1, 25-(OH2) D3.

Prognosis. Good with therapy.

TYPE II

Symptoms and Signs. Same as the preceding. Frequent association with alopecia totalis.

Pathology. Probably autosomal recessive. Abnormal function of target organs: intestinal mucosa and bone.

Diagnostic Procedures. *Blood.* Hypocalcemia, hypophosphatemia, high PTH; 1,25-(OH2) D level high.

Therapy. Resistance to treatment with vitamin D at high doses because of end-organ refractoriness. Patients without alopecia are more responsive to pharmacologic doses than patients with alopecia.

BIBLIOGRAPHY. Prader A, Illig R, Hirerli E: Eine besondere Form der primaeren Vitamin D resistenten Rachitis mit Hypocalcaemie und autosomal-dominantem Erbgana: die hereditaere Pseudo-Mangelrachitis. Helv Paediatr Acta 16:456–458, 1961
Rosen JF, Fluschman AR, Finberg L, et al: Rickets with alopecia: An inborn error of vitamin D metabolism. J Paediatr 94:729, 1979
De Braekeleer M: Hereditary disorders. In Saguenay-Lac-St-Jean (Quebec, Canada) Human Hered 41:141–146, 1991
Demay MB: Hereditary defects in vitamin D metabolism and vitamin D receptor defects. In De Groot LJ (ed): Endocrinology, 3rd ed, pp 1173–1178. Philadelphia, WB Saunders, 1995

PSEUDO-WILLEBRAND

Synonyms. Platelet Willebrand, Willebrand-Jurgens.

Symptoms and Signs. In Puerto Ricans. Those of von Willebrands (see).

Etiology. X-linked or autosomal dominant inheritance. Platelets remove factor VIII at abnormal rate because of augmented glycoprotein I b.

Diagnostic Procedures. *Blood.* Diminished platelets; large in size. Increased ristocetin-induced platelet aggregation, decreased plasma FV III VWF.

Therapy. Fresh blood transfusions.

Prognosis. Good. See von Willebrand.

BIBLIOGRAPHY. Miller JL, Castella A: Platelet type von Willebrand's disease: Characterization of a new bleeding disorder. Blood 60:790–794, 1982
Weiss HJ, Meyer D, Rabinowitz R, et al: Pseudo von Willebrand's disease: An intrinsic platelet defect with aggregation by unmodified human factor VIII, von Willebrand factor and enhanced absorption of its high molecular weight multimers. N Engl J Med 306:326–333, 1982
Bithell TC: Hereditary coagulation disorders. In Lee GR, Bithel TC, Foerster J, et al (eds): Wintrobe's Clinical Hematology, 9th ed, pp 1436–1437. Philadelphia, Lea & Febiger, 1993

PSEUDO-ZOLLINGER-ELLISON

Synonyms. Antral G-cell hyperfunction; includes retained antrum.

Symptoms and Signs. Rare: After surgery for gastric ulcer (antrectomy and Billroth II reconstruction). Recurrence of pain and ulcer.

Etiology. Obstruction of gastric outlet or retained antrum, that causes hyperplasia of G-cells and hypergastrinemia and hypersecretion of acid in absence of islet cell tumors.

Pathology. Hyperplasia of G-cells.

Diagnostic Procedures. *Endoscopy. Blood.* Determination of serum gastrin level, calcium, aspirin level (for possible surreptious use).

Therapy. *Medical.* Anti-H2 antagonists, aspirin use and smoking discontinuation. *Surgical.* If after 3 months ulcer has not healed, reintervention: resection of a cuff of antral tissue at the end of the afferent limb.

Prognosis. Good with therapy.

BIBLIOGRAPHY. Friesen SR, Tonita T: Pseudo-Zollinger-Ellison syndrome: hypergastrinemia, hyperchloridria, without tumor. Ann Surg. 194:481–493, 1981
Thirlby RC: Postoperative recurrent ulcer in postsurgical syndromes. Gastroenterol Clin N Am 23:295–311, 1994

PSOAS MYOSITIS–FIBROSIS

Symptoms. Onset insidious or sudden. Unilateral or bilateral pain in lower quadrants of abdomen, dull and aching, lasting from days to years with periodic exacerbations and remissions. Pain is enhanced by activity and is partly relieved by rest. Fibrositis of different muscles frequently associated (see Fibrositis). Anxiety manifestations.

Signs. Tenderness over psoas muscle. Contraction or stretching of muscles reproduces symptoms. When bilateral, pain stronger on one side.

Etiology. Unknown. Trauma, postural defects, acute infections, pregnancy may be the exciting factor.

Pathology. See Fibrositis.

Diagnostic Procedures. Rule out abdominal, urinary tract, gynecologic, and vertebral pathology conditions. *Blood. Leukocytosis. X-ray.*

Therapy. See Treatment of Fibrositis. Diagnosis is important to prevent useless surgery. Treatment of anxiety manifestation: psychotherapy and tranquilizers.

Prognosis. Generally good response to treatment. See Prognosis in Fibrositis.

BIBLIOGRAPHY. Greene JA: The syndrome of psoas myositis and fibrositis: Its manifestations and its significance in the differential diagnosis of lower abdominal pain. Ann Intern Med 23:30–34, 1945
Weatherall DJ, Ledingham JGG, Warrell DA (eds): Oxford Textbook of Medicine, 3rd ed, p 4157. Oxford, Oxford Med Pub, 1996

PSYCHOGENIC CHEST PAIN

Synonyms. Cardiac psychosis; chest discomfort. See Anterior chest wall syndromes.

Symptoms. Gradual onset of a vague distress, usually related to a very limited area (apex of heart, nipple [finger tip sign]), or extensive area covering left anterior and lateral chest. May or may not be associated with arm symptoms. Headache, weakness, fatigability in the morning that disappear with activity or distraction are often associated. Description of type of pain extremely variable. No relation with activity, posture, or meals.

Signs. Psychologic support.

Etiology. Anxiety reaction often precipitated by death or illness of relative or friend or other psychologic deep-seated derangements. Sometimes iatrogenic. Sometime chest discomfort bound to depression, self-gain motivations, or could be a real cardiac psychosis (with obsessive idea).

Therapy. Psychotherapy according to intensity and functional manifestation of the condition.

Diagnostic Procedures. Rule out cardiogenic origin. In borderline cases a coronary arteriogram may be needed.

Prognosis. Good response to psychotherapy. Frequent conversion to other psychosomatic conditions.

BIBLIOGRAPHY. Senay E, Offenkrantz WC: A case study of psychosomatic symptoms. Consultant 9:42–47, 1969
Eliot RS, Morales-Ballejo HM: The heart, emotional stress and psychiatric disorders. In Schlant RC, Alexander RW: Hurst's The Heart, 8th ed, p 2090. New York, McGraw-Hill, 1994
Weatherall DJ, Ledingham JGG, Warrell DA (eds): Oxford Textbook of Medicine, 3rd ed, pp 2168–2169. Oxford, Oxford Med Pub, 1996

PSYCHOGENIC POLYDIPSIA

Synonym. Compulsive water drinker; polydipsea psychogenic.

Symptoms. Occurs usually in women (80%); age at onset 8–60, most often 35–60 years. Onset sudden or vague, usually associated with menopause, delusional illness, stress of various kinds. Neurotic trait common in childhood; frequent history of sleep walking. No stable and satisfactory sex life; stormy and dramatic medical history for psychological and organic illness. Excessive fluid intake fluctuating irregularly by the hour or day; polyuria. Periods of remission and relapses lasting months.

Signs. Few physical signs. In some, scars from multiple operations; generally, obesity; fluctuation of blood pressure.

Etiology. Psychotic compulsion associated with other psychotic manifestations, from severe to minor neurotic behavior.

Pathology. Unknown.

Diagnostic Procedures. *Blood.* Plasma osmolality significantly lower than normal. *Urine.* Ability to concentrate urine varies considerably and in most patients is impaired. Vasopressin makes the patient sick, without affecting polydipsia.

Therapy. Continuous narcosis or electroconvulsive therapy.

Prognosis. Spontaneous remissions and relapses. Transient improvement with therapy.

BIBLIOGRAPHY. Bralow ED, de Wardener HE: Compulsive water drinking. QJ Med 28:235–258, 1959
Weatherall DJ, Ledingham JGG, Warrell DA (eds): Oxford Textbook of Medicine, 3rd ed, p 3121. Oxford, Oxford Med Pub, 1996

PSYCHOMOTOR ATTACKS

Synonym. Psychomotor convulsion; epilepsy psychomotor; precursive epilepsy, psychomotor equivalent; temporal lobe epilepsy. Complex partial seizures. See Grand mal and Petit mal.

Symptoms. Onset at any age. Change in consciousness with alteration of thoughts and feelings. Motor activity partially correlated. Aura of hallucinogenic type may precede the attack. Patient acts and talks as if partially conscious; his behavior is erratic and he may commit strange acts, sometimes violent. Occasionally, he may fall asleep after the attack and have partial amnesia of events. These patients also may have a deep alteration of their personality between attacks: paranoid; homicidal tendency; various types of psychoses.

Etiology. Idiopathic or cerebral lesion (temporal) and frontal or amygdaloid-hippocampal.

Diagnostic Procedure. *EEG.*

Therapy. Diphenylhydantoin; primidone; phenobarbital. Surgical removal of temporal lobe lesion.

Prognosis. Poor for emotional and psychic stability.

BIBLIOGRAPHY. Falconer MA, Serafetinides EA, Corsellis JAN: Etiology and pathogenesis of temporal lobe epilepsy. Arch Neurol 10:233–248, 1964

Adams RD, Victor M: Principles of Neurology, 5th ed, pp 237, 282–283. New York, McGraw-Hill, 1993

PSYCHOPHONASTHENIA

Synonym. Conversion aphonia/dysphonia; includes relapsing aphonia. See Functional voice syndromes.

Symptoms. Male to female ratio, 1/10. Frequently starting in late adolescence or following some crisis in private or professional life; no history of prior laryngitis. Occurs in a person, usually cultured (singer, minister, lawyer), intelligent, but with strong, withdrawn personality, who is timid and highly sensitive. Sensitivity of the throat; choking sensation when attempting to speak, paresthesias of head and neck; dryness or excessive secretion of mouth. Cracking of the voice and, when speaking for some time, aching of vocal cords. The dysfunction is stable thus differing from other functional syndromes.

Signs. Occasionally, accompanying signs may be tachycardia, palpitation, and sweating.

Etiology. Neurotic manifestation deriving from feeling of inadequacy. To be differentiated from other forms of phonasthenia or where local pathology exists.

Diagnostic Procedures. *Laryngoscopy.* Voice frequency, waveform. *Spectrographic analysis, laryngeal airway resistance measurement.*

Therapy. Psychotherapy.

Prognosis. Good with treatment. Relapse or other neurotic manifestations may appear.

BIBLIOGRAPHY. Greene JS: Psychophonasthenia syndrome. Ann Otol Rhinol Laryngol 50:1177–1184, 1941

Koufman JA, Blalock PD: Functional voice disorders. In Otolaryngol Clin N Amer 24:1059–1073, 1991

PTEROGOPALATINE FOSSA

Synonym. Behr; Foix-Jefferson; sphenomaxillary fossa; see orbital apex.

Symptoms. More or less continuous, severe pain in the upper jaw (mistaken for toothache) in the region of upper back molar teeth; disturbed sensitivity on the cheek and infraorbital foramen. Distribution second branch of trigeminal (V) nerve. Later, extension of pain to lower jaw. Homolateral deafness (middle ear type). Later, palate paralysis and anesthesia and paralysis of pterygoid muscles (deviation of jaw on opening the mouth); homolateral blindness.

Signs. On posterior rhinoscopy, fullness of lateral wall of nasopharynx. Fullness of temporal fossa visible externally (late). Unilateral or bilateral enlargment of cervical and retropharyngeal glands. Later, antral lavage may show bleeding.

Etiology. More frequently, metastatic lesion in the pterygopalatine fossa; less frequently, primary lesions spreading from lateral wall of posterior part of nose or from sinus of Morgagni. In the latter case, Trotter syndrome is included; this syndrome may precede, follow, or occur in combination.

Pathology. Neoplastic, metastatic, or primary lesion in the pterygopalatine fossa, successively invading antrum, pterygoid lamina, eustachian tube, alveolus, temporal fossa, optic (II) nerve, interior of orbit. Metastasis in lymph node, liver, and skeleton.

Diagnostic Procedures. *X-ray. CT scan. MRI.* Involvement of foramen. Foramen ovale normal at first. *Biopsy.*

Therapy. Deep X-ray; radium implantation; chemotherapy.

Prognosis. Poor; treatment only palliative.

BIBLIOGRAPHY. Asherson N: Trotter's syndrome and associated lesions. J Laryngol Otol 65:349–366, 1951

Adams RD, Victor M: Principles of Neurology, 5th ed, p 1172. New York, McGraw-Hill, 1993

P.U.G.H.

Synonyms. Pseudouveitis, glaucoma, hyphema. See U.G.H.

Symptoms and Signs. Pseudouveitis, glaucoma, and hyphema (UGH syndrome) plus neovascular membrane over iris and occlusion of central retinal veins.

Etiology. Unknown. Trauma possible cause unrelated to presence of intraocular lens.

BIBLIOGRAPHY. Pallin SL: Condition mimicking UGH syndrome unrelated to presence of IOL. Ophthal Times, Aug, 1983, p 50

Morris DA: Ocular trauma. In Garner A, Klintworth GK (eds): Pathobiology of Ocular Disease: A Dynamic Approach, 2nd ed, p 389. New York, Marcel Dekker, 1994

PULMONARY ARTERIES STENOSIS

Synonyms. Pure pulmonary arteries stenosis; supravalvular pulmonic stenosis.

Symptoms. Age at onset from infancy to adulthood. Usually, asymptomatic for a long time; sooner or later fatigue, exertional dyspnea, occasionally chest pain, or syncope on effort.

Signs. High-pitched ejection type of systolic murmur ending before second sound. Maximal on second left interspace. Administration of amyl nitrate intensifies murmur. Palpable thrill in area of maximal intensity of sound. Increased split of second sound. Occasionally, hemoptysis.

Etiology. Unknown. Congenital cardiac anomaly. Familial association with autosomal dominant pattern in some cases. This syndrome may also be simulated by external compression of pulmonic artery. Occasionally, rubella infection in the mother (see Gregg).

Pathology. Pulmonic stenosis at level of infundibulum, valve, or main pulmonary artery.

Diagnostic Procedures. *X-ray.* Early, normal size of heart; later; right ventricular enlargement. Pulmonary fields clear. *Angiocardiography.* Moderate or absent dilatation of pulmonary trunk, poststenotic dilatation of intrapulmonary vessels. *Electrocardiography. Cardiac catheterization. Pressures. Oxymetry. Two-dimensional echography* with color flow imaging and spectral Doppler interrogation.

Therapy. Surgical enlargement of stenotic passage. Balloon angioplasty, pericardial or synthetic patch angioplasty.

Prognosis. Surgical mortality below 10%, with mild or moderate stenosis; usually, no sign of deterioration. In severe stenosis, progressive deterioration. Median age of death from pure pulmonic stenosis 20 years. Half do not reach adult life; but survival beyond 70 years in some cases reported.

BIBLIOGRAPHY. Oppenheimer EH: Partial atresia of main branches of pulmonary artery occurring in infancy and accompanied by calcification of pulmonary artery and aorta. Bull Johns Hopkins Hosp 63:261–277, 1838

Currens JH, Kinney TD, White PD: Pulmonary stenosis with intact interventricular septum. Am Heart J 30:491–510, 1945

Lock JE, Castaneda-Zuniga WR, Fuhrman BP, et al: Balloon dilatation angioplasty of hypoplastic and stenotic pulmonary arteries. Circulation 67:962–967, 1983

Perloff JK The Clinical Recognition of Congenital Heart Disease, 4th ed, pp 198–229. Philadelphia, WB Saunders, 1994

PULMONARY ARTERIOVENOUS FISTULA

Synonyms. Pulmonary arteriovenous aneurysm; arteriovenous varix; lung hemangioma. See Rendu-Osler-Weber.

Symptoms. Occurs usually in young adults of both sexes; may be observed in infancy and childhood. Symptoms depend on size of shunt: from asymptomatic to exertional dyspnea, chest pain, dizziness, syncopal or epileptiform seizures, Morgagni-Adams-Stokes syndrome, hemoptysis.

Signs. Cyanosis; clubbing of fingers and toes. Continuous murmur may be heard over affected lung; heart enlarged (but not as much as in acquired arteriovenous fistula). Hemangiomas of skin and mucosae frequently associated.

Etiology. Unknown. Inherited familial condition in cases where Rendu-Osler-Weber is present.

Pathology. Single or multiple arteriovenous fistulas in the lung, more common in right lower lobe.

Diagnostic Procedures. *Blood.* Polycythemia. *X-ray.* Pulmonary density. *Fluoroscopy.* Pulsating or nonpulsating masses. *Tomography.* *CT scan.* *MRI.* Spherical lesion attached to a vessel. *Angiocardiography.* *Two-dimensional echography* with color flow imaging and spectral Doppler interrogation.

Therapy. Resection of aneurysm; lobectomy or pneumonectomy; bilateral resection reported.

Prognosis. Cure obtained by resection of fistula(s).

BIBLIOGRAPHY. Churton T: Leeds and West-Riding Medico-Chirurgical Society: Multiple aneurysm of pulmonary artery. Br Med J 1:1223, 1897

Smith HL, Horton BT: Arteriovenous fistula of lung associated with polycythemia vera: Report of case in which diagnosis was made clinically. Am Heart J 18:589–592, 1939

Mattila S, Meurala H, Jarvinen A, et al: Pulmonary arteriovenous fistulas. Scand J Thorac Cardiovasc Surg 16:165–168, 1982

Perloff JK: The Clinical Recognition of Congenital Heart Disease, 4th ed, pp 714–726. Philadelphia, WB Saunders, 1994

PULMONARY ARTERY COMPRESSION, ASCENDING AORTA ANEURYSM

Symptoms and Signs. Occurs in syphilitic patients. Aortic incompetence; right ventricular hypertrophy; single second sound.

Etiology. Syphilitic aneurysm of ascending aorta compressing pulmonary artery.

Diagnostic Procedures. *X-ray.* Enlargement of heart; marked enlargement of pulmonary artery with clear lung fields (one lung more oligemic than the other); calcification of the aneurysm. *ECG.* Right axis deviation; vertical position; biventricular hypertrophy. *Catheterization.* Right ventricle displaced to the left; failure to push the tip on compressed pulmonary artery. *Angiocardiography.* Demonstration of compression and absence of valvular stenosis. *Aortogram.* *Blood.* Serology positive. *Two-dimensional echocardiography* with color flow imaging and spectral Doppler interrogation.

Therapy. Penicillin; surgery to correct aneurysm.

Prognosis. Progressive disease leading to death. Good results with surgery.

BIBLIOGRAPHY. Pearson JR, Nichol ES: The syndrome of compression of the pulmonary artery by a syphilitic aortic aneurysm resulting in chronic cor pulmonale, with a report of a case. Ann Intern Med 34:483–492, 1951

Kulkarni TP, Gandhi MJ, Datey KK: The syndrome of compression of the pulmonary artery by an aneurysm of the ascending aorta. Am Heart J 65:678–682, 1963

DeBakey ME, Noon GP: Aneurysm of the thoracic aorta. Mod Concepts Cardiovasc Dis 44:53–58, 1975

Linsay J Jr, DeBakey ME, Beall AC: Diagnosis and treatment of diseases of the aorta. In Schlant RC, Alexander RW: Hurst's The Heart, 8th ed, pp 2167–2169. New York, McGraw-Hill, 1994

PULMONARY CYSTIC LYMPHANGIECTASIS

Synonyms. CPCL; pulmonary lymphangiectasia.

Symptoms. Onset at birth (some stillborn) or in first day of life. Cyanosis and respiratory distress. Conditions associated with pulmonary hypertension, particularly when the pulmonary venous pressure chronically exceeds 30 mmHg.

Signs. Numerous rales in both lungs; heart sounds normal; associated pleural effusion in some cases. Lymphedema of other organs also occasionally seen. Occasionally, associated with congenital cretinism or congenital heart disease (one-third of cases).

Etiology. Autosomal recessive inheritance.

Pathology. Lungs larger than normal; pale firm, numerous small cysts with tense walls, transparent and glistening, containing clear colorless serous fluid. Localized lung atelectasis. Cyst wall lined with flat endothelium. No signs of inflammation in connective tissue. No connection between air passage and cysts.

Diagnostic Procedures. *X-ray.* Of lung. *Respiratory function tests.*

Therapy. Symptomatic.

Prognosis. Poor. Death in early infancy.

BIBLIOGRAPHY. Virkow R: Gesammelte Abhandlungen zur Wissenschaflichen Medicin. Frankfurt, 1851

Felman AH, Rathigan RM, Pierson KK: Pulmonary lymphangiectasia: Observation in 17 patients and proposed classification. Am J Roentgenol 116:548–553, 1972

Scott-Emnakpor AB, Warren ST, et al: Familial occurrence of congenital pulmonary lymphangiectasis: Genetic implication. Am J Dis Child 135:532–534, 1981

Avery GB, Fletcher MA, McDonald MC: Neonatology, 4th ed. Philadelphia, JB Lippincott, 1994

PULMONARY EOSINOPHILIC GRANULOMA

Synonyms. Primary pulmonary histiocytosis X; eosinophilic granuloma pulmonary; see histiocytosis syndromes; Carrington; Churg-Strauss; Hinson-Pepys.

Symptoms and Signs. In adults. Male predominance; more frequent in Caucasians. From asymptomatic to: fatigue, fever, weight loss, nonproductive cough, dyspnea, chest pain, pneumothorax, osteolytic rib lesions, hemoptysis, pleural effusion. May affect extrapulmonary organs (see other histocytosis X syndromes).

Etiology. Unknown. May be an hypersensitivity disease to tobacco smoke that starts by accumulation of Langerhans cells.

Pathology. *Lung biopsy.* Subpleural nodules (2–10 mm) and small cysts. Accumulation of H-X cells (with Birbeck granules) (with progression of disease: fibrosis). BAL: Langerhans cells are 2–20% of effector cells. They are positive for OKT6 monoclonal antibody, S-100 protein, HLADR.

Diagnostic Procedures. *Chest X-ray.* *CT scan.* Diffuse bilateral peripheral cysts and nodules. Later on: reticulonodular pattern. *Open lung biopsy.* See Pathology.

Therapy. Corticosteroids, Vinca alkaloids; refrain from smoking.

Prognosis. Spontaneous remission is possible.

BIBLIOGRAPHY. Farinacci C, Jeffrey H, et al: Eosinophic granuloma of the lung: Report of two cases. U.S. Armed Forces Med L 2:1085, 1951
Prakash UBS: Pulmonary eosinophilic granuloma. In Lynch JP, De Remee RA: Immunologically Mediated Pulmonary Diseases, p 432. Philadelphia, Lippincott, 1991

PULMONARY STENOSIS–PATENT FORAMEN OVALE OR OSTIUM SECUNDUM DEFECT

Synonyms. Fallot trilogy (with reversed shunt).

Symptoms. Cyanosis especially on exertion may appear shortly after birth, but more frequently occurs later; occasionally, after puberty or in adult life; eventually becoming persistent. Squatting posture occasionally; inadequate weight gain; frequent pulmonary infections; fatigue; exertional dyspnea.

Signs. Clubbing of fingers and toes; high-pitched ejection murmur (briefer and earlier than that observed in pure pulmonic stenosis, see); second sound single. Administration of amyl nitrate decreases murmur.

Etiology. Unknown. Congenital heart malformation.

Pathology. Pulmonary stenosis with patent foramen ovale.

Diagnostic Procedures. *X-ray.* Of chest. *Angiocardiography. ECG. Cardiac catheterization. Pressure. Oximetry. Two-dimensional echocardiography with color flow imaging and spectral Doppler interrogation. Frank vectocardiogram.*

Therapy. Surgery.

Prognosis. Mortality from surgery 10%. Right-sided heart failure appears in third or fourth decade and is main cause of death. Occasionally subacute bacterial endocarditis (SBE) and cerebral abscesses causes of death.

BIBLIOGRAPHY. Morgagni JB: Seats and Causes of Diseases. London, Millar Cader in the Stand: and Johnson Paine in Pater-Noster Row, 1769
Perloff JK: The Clinical Recognition of Congenital Heart Disease, 4th ed, pp 381–395. Philadelphia, WB Saunders, 1994

PULMONARY SUBVALVULAR STENOSIS

Synonyms. Infundibular pulmonary stenosis; subinfundibular pulmonary stenosis; double-chambered right ventricle; two-chambered right ventricle.

Symptoms and Signs. Rare as isolated defect. Both sexes affected; present from birth. Same characteristics as pulmonary valve stenosis with the following differentiating signs: right ventricular impulse does not reach third left interspace; murmur and thrill maximal in fourth interspace; ejection sound absent.

Etiology. Congenital sporadic malformation. Hypertrophy of infundibular muscle may be responsible for stenosis.

Pathology. Infundibular stenosis more frequent than subinfundibular. Absence of poststenotic dilatation. Infundibulum may be dilated. Defect usually associated with ventricular septal defect, pure form seldom seen.

Diagnostic Procedures. *X-ray.* Absence of dilatation of pulmonary trunk; right aortic arch; local indentation at ostium of infundibulum. *ECG. Angiocardiography. Echocardiography. Cardiac catheterization. Right ventricular angiography.*

Therapy. Surgical valvotomy in cardiopulmonary bypass.

Prognosis. Good with surgery.

BIBLIOGRAPHY. Keith A: Malformations of the heart, Lancet 2:359, 1909
Perloff JK: The Clinical Recognition of Congenital Heart Disease, 4th ed, pp 198–199. Philadelphia, WB Saunders, 1994

Schlant RC, Alexander RW: Hurst's The Heart, 8th ed, p 1842. New York, McGraw-Hill, 1994

PULMONARY TRUNK IDIOPATHIC DILATATION

Symptoms. Absent.

Signs. Characteristic auscultatory and phonocardiographic findings: split apical first sound; first component of equal or greater intensity than second component; systolic click ushers in a systolic ejection murmur louder in pulmonary area. Second sound widely split. A short diastolic murmur may be present in the second intercostal space.

Etiology. Unknown. (A forme fruste of Marfan must be excluded). Criteria for diagnosis of this rare form are (1) simple dilatation of pulmonary artery or its main branches; (2) occasionally, association of hypoplasia of aorta; (3) absence of heart congenital anomalies, lung diseases, rheumatism, and syphilis.

Pathology. In some cases cystic medial necrosis of wall of pulmonary artery may be found. Medial degeneration can be severe enough to result in aneurysm, rupture, or dissection that is found in the main pulmonary arteries.

Diagnostic Procedures. *ECG.* Normal. *X-ray.* Dilatation of pulmonary artery. (Exclude presence of straight back syndrome [see] that may lead to an erroneous diagnosis). *Phonocardiography. Cardiac catheterization.* Normal right ventricular systolic pressure and systolic pressure difference across pulmonic valve of 15 mmHg or less during stress (diagnostic). *Two-dimensional echography with color flow imaging and spectral Doppler interrogation.*

Therapy. None or symptomatic according to evolution.

Prognosis. Benign; however, it may be aggravated by pulmonary regurgitation or may progress to aneurysm formation.

BIBLIOGRAPHY. Wessler H, Jackes L: Clinical Roentgenology of Disease of the Chest, pp 26–29. Troy, NY, Southworth, 1923
Ramsey HW, De la Torre A, Linhart JW, et al: Idiopathic dilatation of the pulmonary artery. Am J Cardiol 20:324–330, 1967
Perloff JK: The Clinical Recognition of Congenital Heart Disease, 4th ed, pp 230–235. Philadelphia, WB Saunders, 1994

PULMONARY VALVE ATRESIA, INTACT VENTRICULAR SEPTUM

TYPE I

Symptoms and Signs. Cyanosis from birth; distress and acute illness from first days of life. On heart auscultation, soft systolic murmur, maximal intensity mid-left sternal border, or high frequency and located in lower left sternal border. Diastolic murmur absent; quiet, single second sound. Hepatomegaly; seldom, liver pulsation.

Etiology. Unknown.

Pathology. Pulmonary valvular atresia with intact ventricular septum, small volume, thick-walled right ventricle, and hypoplastic tricuspid orifice (Type I).

Diagnostic Procedures. *X-ray.* Transverse heart configuration with moderate enlargement; concavity in main pulmonary segment; decreased vascularity. *ECG catheterization. Angiocardiography. Two-dimensional echocardiography with color flow imaging and spectral Doppler interrogation.*

Therapy. Surgery.

Prognosis. Death from first day to 15 months; when operated, from 2 days to 5 years. High mortality at surgery.

TYPE II

Symptoms and Signs. Impossible to differentiate from Ebstein (see) on clinical data. Only difference, more severe respiratory distress.

Etiology. Unknown.

Pathology. Pulmonary valvular atresia with intact ventricular septum, normal-sized or dilated right ventricle, and tricuspid orifice regurgitation (Type II).

Diagnostic Procedures. *X-ray. ECG. Cardiac catheterization. Angiocardiography. Two-dimensional echocardiography* with color flow imaging and spectral Doppler interrogation. Allow differentiation between this syndrome and the Ebstein syndrome.

Therapy. Differential diagnosis important because emergency pulmonary valvotomy may benefit this condition while surgery is contraindicated in Ebstein.

Prognosis. Poor.

BIBLIOGRAPHY. Peacock TB: On malformation of the human heart. London. J Churchill and Sons, 1858
Freedom RM, Wilson G, Trusler GA, et al: Pulmonary atresia and intact ventricular septum. Scand J Thorac Cardiovasc Surg 17:26–36, 1983
Perloff JK: The Clinical Recognition of Congenital Heart Disease, 4th ed, pp 598–613. Philadelphia, WB Saunders, 1994

PULMONARY VALVE DYSPLASIA

Synonyms. See Pulmonary valve stenosis and Noonan.

Symptoms and Signs. Abnormal facies, hypertelorism, ptosis, low-set ears, and mental retardation. Growth retardation. No ejection sound or pulmonic component of second sound. Is especially common in patients with Noonan syndrome.

Etiology. Congenital hereditary disorder.

Pathology. Pulmonary valve characterized by three distinct cusps, absence of commissural fusion, and annular hypoplasia. Cusps contain myxomatous tissue.

Diagnostic Procedures. *X-ray.* See Pulmonary valve stenosis, plus absence of poststenotic dilatation. *ECG. Two-dimensional echocardiogram with color flow imaging and spectral Doppler interrogation. Cardiac catheterization. Vectocardiogram.*

Therapy. Surgical valvotomy.

Prognosis. Fair with surgery.

BIBLIOGRAPHY. Koretzky ED, Moller JH, Korus ME, et al: Congenital pulmonary stenosis resulting from dysplasia of the valve. Circulation 40:43–53, 1969
Linde LM, Turner SW, Sparkes RS: Pulmonary valve dysplasia: A cardiological syndrome. Br Heart J 35:301–304, 1973
Nugent EW, Plauth WH, Edwards JE, et al: The pathology, pathophysiology recognition and treatment of congenital heart disease. In Schlant RC, Alexander RW: Hurst's The Heart, 8th ed, p 1797. New York, McGraw-Hill, 1994
Perloff JK: The Clinical Recognition of Congenital Heart Disease, 4th ed, p 203. Philadelphia, WB Saunders, 1994

PULMONARY VALVE INSUFFICIENCY

Symptoms. Characteristically absent or nonspecific; mild exertional dyspnea. Hyperdynamic right ventricular impulse.

Signs. Diastolic murmur of low frequency, heard best at pulmonary area or a little lower along left sternal border, increasing in intensity during inspiration. Short systolic ejection murmur may also be present.

Etiology. Congenital valve defect, or idiopathic dilatation of pulmonary artery.

Diagnostic Procedures. *ECG.* Normal or right ventricular hypertrophy. *Phonocardiography and intracardiac phonocardiography. Cardiac catheterization (diagnostic). X-ray of chest. Two-dimensional echocardiography with color flow imaging and spectral Doppler interrogation. Angiocardiography.*

Therapy. None specific. Antibiotic prophylaxis during dental procedures and conditions leading to bacteremia.

Prognosis. Patients asymptomatic. They may reach adulthood free of limitation. Increased incidence of bacterial endocarditis.

BIBLIOGRAPHY. Kezdi P, Priest WS, Smith JM: Pulmonic regurgitation. Q Bull Northwest Univ Med School 29:368–373, 1955
Criscitiello MG, Harvey WP: Clinical recognition of congenital pulmonary valve insufficiency. Am J Cardiol 20:765–772, 1967
Rackley CE, Wallace RB, Edwards JE, et al: Tricuspid and pulmonary valve disease. In Schlant RC, Alexander RW: Hurst's The Heart, 8th ed. New York, McGraw-Hill, 1994
Perloff JK: The Clinical Recognition of Congenital Heart Disease, 4th ed, pp 236–246. Philadelphia, WB Saunders, 1994

PULMONARY VALVE STENOSIS

Synonym. Valvular pulmonic stenosis.

Symptoms and Signs. Both sexes equally affected. Present from birth. Diagnosis usually suspected, however, during first year of life. Frequent malformation. From asymptomatic to fatigue, dyspnea with exertion (according to degree of obstruction), squatting, seldom syncope. Prominent midsystolic murmur and thrill maximal in second left interspace; pulmonic ejection sound. History of unimpaired growth; acyanosis; occasionally, high colored cheeks. Hepatomegaly.

Etiology. Congenital defect. Rarely, acquired (e.g., rheumatic fever, bacterial endocarditis). Familial cases reported.

Pathology. Heart conical or dome-shaped structure with a narrow outlet. Poststenotic dilatation of pulmonary trunk and left pulmonary artery dilatation. In adults calcification. In case of dome-shaped stenosis with patent foramen ovale or atrial septal defect, the term trilogy of Fallot is applied.

Diagnostic Procedures. *ECG.* Right atrial and ventricular hypertrophy. *X-ray.* Normal or reduced pulmonary arteries. *Blood.* Hematocrit elevated; normal oxygen saturation. *Two-dimensional ultrasonography with color flow imaging and spectral Doppler interrogation. Vector cardiography. Cardiac catheterization.*

Therapy. Surgical correction. Valvotomy.

Prognosis. According to degree of stenosis. Generally, survival into adulthood (death at average age 26 years).

BIBLIOGRAPHY. Edwards JE: Pulmonary stenosis with intact ventricular septum. In Gould SE: Pathology of the Heart, 2nd ed. Springfield, IL, Charles C Thomas, 1960
Nugent EW, Plauth WH, Edwards JE, et al: The pathology, pathophysiology, recognition and treatment of congenital heart disease. In Schlant RC, Alexander RW: Hurst's The Heart, 8th ed, pp 1797–1800. New York, McGraw-Hill, 1994
Perloff JK: The Clinical Recognition of Congenital Heart Disease, 4th ed, pp 198–229. Philadelphia, WB Saunders, 1994

PULMONARY VEIN STENOSIS

Synonyms. Congenital pulmonary vein stenosis. See Pulmonary vein stenosis; patent foramen ovale. The obstruction in the venules and small veins is designated as pulmonary veno-occlusive disease.

Symptoms and Signs. Uncomplicated vein stenosis rare. Both sexes affected; present from birth. Dyspnea; tachypnea; failure to thrive. Repeated respiratory infections. Hemoptysis.

Etiology. Congenital malformation.

Pathology. Two varieties recognized: (1) narrowing near junction with left atrium (extrapulmonary); (2) narrowing at various distances in extrapulmonary or intrapulmonary sections. Usually, several veins involved.

Diagnostic Procedures. *X-ray.* Symmetric or asymmetric pulmonary congestion; absence of left atrial enlargement. *Cardiomegaly* (right atrium and ventricle). *ECG.* Sinus rhythm; right atrial enlargement and right axis deviation. P-waves, left atrial absent; occasionally, normal. *Cardiac catheterization and two-dimensional echocardiography with color flow imaging and spectral Doppler interrogation.* To exclude mitral stenosis and cor triatriatum. Stenosis of individual pulmonary veins (first variety).

Therapy. Medical management of congestive heart failure. Surgical management: discrete stenosis of pulmonary veins has seldom been relieved by operation or balloon dilatation.

Prognosis. Death ranges from 5 months to 10 years. Pulmonary veno-occlusion disease (second variety) average survival from onset: 20 months.

BIBLIOGRAPHY. Nakib A, Moller JH, Kanjuh VI, et al: Anomalies of the pulmonary vein. Am J Cardiol 20:77–90, 1967

Driscoll DJ, Hesslein PS, Mullins CE: Congenital stenosis of individual pulmonary veins: Clinical spectrum and unsuccessful treatment by transvenous balloon dilatation. Am J Cardiol 49:1767–1773, 1982

Nugent EW, Plauth WH, Edwards JE, et al: The pathology, pathophysiology, recognition and treatment of congenital heart disease. In Schlant RC, Alexander RW: Hurst's The Heart, 8th ed. New York, McGraw-Hill, 1994

Perloff JK: The Clinical Recognition of Congenital Heart Disease, 4th ed, pp 185–186. Philadelphia, WB Saunders, 1994

PULMONARY VENOUS ANOMALOUS DRAINAGE, MITRAL STENOSIS

Symptoms and Signs. Clinical impression of interatrial septal defect and tight mitral stenosis.

Etiology. Congenital defect.

Pathology. Pulmonary vein entering superior vena cava or right atrium determining a left-to-right shunt. Mitral stenosis; absence of interatrial septal defect.

Diagnostic Procedures. *ECG.* Right ventricular hypertrophy. *X-ray.* Of chest. Enlargement of right ventricle; hypoplastic aorta. *Cardiac catheterization.* Pulmonary wedge pressure elevated; large left-to-right shunt; high oxygen saturation in right atrium. *Echocardiogram. Cardiac catheterization:* findings of high or low pulmonary wedge pressure in different parts of lungs may represent additonal evidence for the presence of the partial anomalous venous drainage.

Therapy. Surgical correction of mitral stenosis and resection of pulmonary lobe if correction of left-to-right shunt not otherwise possible.

Prognosis. Good with surgery. Decrease of subjective and objective symptoms.

BIBLIOGRAPHY. Hughes CW, Rumore PC: Anomalous pulmonary veins Arch Pathol 37:364–366, 1944

Wassermil M, Hoffman MS: Partial anomalous pulmonary venous drainage associated with mitral stenosis with an intact atrial septum. Am J Cardiol 10:894–899, 1962

Nugent EW, Plauth WH, Edwards JE, et al: The pathology, pathophysiology, recognition and treatment of congenital heart disease. In Schlant RC, Alexander RW: Hurst's The Heart, 8th ed. New York, McGraw-Hill, 1994

PULMONARY VENOUS ANOMALOUS DRAINAGE TO HEPATIC VEIN

Synonym. Anomalous pulmonary venous drainage to hepatic vein.

Symptoms. Both sexes affected. Present from birth. Dyspnea.

Signs. Cyanosis; edema; second pulmonic sound accentuated; absence of murmurs; pulsating hepatomegaly.

Etiology. Congenital defect.

Pathology. Pulmonary veins united entering the hepatic vein. Left atrium and ventricle very small; right atrium and ventricle enlarged. Marked pulmonary congestion.

Diagnostic Procedures. *ECG.* Right axis deviation; right ventricle hypertrophy. Peaked, high P-waves. *Angiocardiography.* Shows dye below diaphragm. *Two-dimensional echocardiography with color flow imaging and spectral Doppler interrogation.*

Therapy. Symptomatic. Early surgical correction.

Prognosis. Fatal. Congestive failure in first month of life.

BIBLIOGRAPHY. Perloff JK: The Clinical Recognition of Congenital Heart Disease, 2nd ed, p 284. Philadelphia, WB Saunders, 1978

Nugent EW, Plauth WH, Edwards JE, et al: The pathology, pathophysiology, recognition and treatment of congenital heart disease. In Schlant RC, Alexander RW: Hurst's The Heart, 8th ed. New York, McGraw-Hill, 1994

PULMONARY VENOUS ANOMALOUS DRAINAGE TO RIGHT ATRIUM

Synonyms. Taussig-Snellen-Alberts; anomalous pulmonary venous drainage; anomalous pulmonary venous connection (Taussig-Snellen-Alberts); partial anomalous pulmonary venous connection.

Symptoms. Both sexes affected; present from birth. Dyspnea; asthenia; easy fatigability; recurrent respiratory infections.

Signs. Cyanosis absent; skin semitranslucent; occasionally, deformity of left side of thorax; tachypnea; distended veins of neck; pulsating hepatomegaly; right atrium and ventricle enlarged; accentuation of second pulmonary sound; precordial systolic and midsystolic apical murmurs; arrhythmias.

Etiology. Congenital defect.

Pathology. Right pulmonary veins join the left atrium close to the rim of ostium secundum defect; or one or more pulmonary veins enter the right atrium or a systemic vein (anomalous connection). Atrial septal defect of patency of foramen ovale frequently associated. Right lung preferentially involved (10:1).

Diagnostic Procedures. *ECG.* Right axis deviation; right ventricle hypertrophy; P-waves elevated. *Cardiac catheterization.* Oxygen saturation of right auricle greater than superior vena cava. Pulmonary artery increased pressure. *Cineangiography. Echocardiography. Cardiac catheterization.*

Therapy. Surgical correction. Early surgical correction when large pulmonary blood flow, congestive failure, or pulmonary arterial hypertension is present.

Prognosis. Possibly, cardiac failure. Survival into adulthood.

BIBLIOGRAPHY. Snellen HA, Alberts FH: The clinical diagnosis of anomalous pulmonary venous drainage. Circulation 8:801–816, 1952

Taussig HB: Congenital Malformation of the Heart. Cambridge, The Commonwealth Fund, Harvard University Press, 1960

Lucas RV Jr: Anomalous venous connections, pulmonary and systemic. In Adams FH, Emmanonillides GC (eds): Mass Heart Diseases in

Infants, Children and Adolescents, p 458. Baltimore, Williams & Wilkins, 1983

Nugent EW, Plauth WH, Edwards JE, et al: The pathology, pathophysiology, recognition and treatment of congenital heart disease. In Schlant RC, Alexander RW: Hurst's The Heart, 8th ed. New York, McGraw-Hill, 1994

PULPOSUS

Synonyms. Traumatic discopathy; herniated disk; intervertebral disk protrusion; herniated nucleus pulposus.

Symptoms and Signs. Both sexes affected. Onset in vigorous subjects of middle age. Minimal form. Asymptomatic or minor symptoms (see the following) subsiding with bed rest (diagnosed by myelography). Classical form. History of backache. Initial episode usually follows a minor traumatic injury (following a snap); progressive increase of pain and then distal radiation. Backache that subsides, whereas the full sciatica syndrome (see Cotugno) develops with all its sensorial and eventually motor features.

Etiology. Single trauma or more frequently minor trauma or strain acting on already partly degenerated annulus, which causes a prolapse of nucleus pulposus and of degenerated annulus toward the weakest point (left or right of posterior midline). According to the degree of protrusion and extrusion of the nucleus, various clinical patterns are elicited.

Pathology. Most frequent sites of herniation are L4–L5, L5–S1, less frequently L3–L4; more rarely other locations.

Diagnostic Procedures. *X-ray.* In various projections and positions. *CT scan. MRI.*

Therapy. Bed rest; analgesics; anti-inflammatory agents; vitamin B_{12}. Operative treatment with or without vertebral fusion.

Prognosis. Attacks usually subside in 2–3 weeks with treatment or may assume subchronic or chronic evolution.

BIBLIOGRAPHY. Mixter WJ, Barr JS: Rupture of intervertebral disc with involvement of spinal canal. N Engl J Med 211:210–215, 1934

Weinstein J, Stratt KF, Lehman T, et al: Lumbar disc herniation: A comparison of the results of chemonucleolysis and open discectomy after ten years. J Bone Joint Surg (Am) 68A:43–54, 1986

Nyström B: Experience of microsurgical compared with conventional techniques in lumbar disc operations. Acta Neurol Scand 76:129–141, 1987

Adams RD, Victor M: Principles of Neurology, 5th ed, pp 179–181. New York, McGraw-Hill, 1993

PUPILLOTONIC PSEUDOTABES

Synonyms. Argyll Robertson with mydriasis; Ross; myotonic pupil; pupillotonia; iridoplegia interna. If combined with altered deep tendon reflexes: Adie; Holmes IV; Holmes-Adie; Markus; Reys; Holmes; Saengers; Weill.

Symptoms. Relatively sudden impairment of vision, with blurring, difficulty in reading, and headache. More frequent in females in the second and third decades.

Signs. Dilatation of affected pupil (80% unilateral); absent or delayed light accommodation and less severely involved convergence accommodation response. The pupil may occasionally after contracting slowly become smaller than the normal one. Diminution or absence of tendon reflexes may be present. Tonic pupil dilates with atropine. Differential diagnosis with Argyll Robertson pupil (see Argyll Robertson).

Etiology. Unknown. Occasionally, in association with post-traumatic conditions or infective diseases; autosomal dominant inheritance also reported.

Pathology. Partial degeneration of postganglionic fibers to the sphincter muscles from ciliary ganglion.

Diagnostic Procedures. Methacholine test. Solution (2.5%) instilled into conjunctival sac gives rapid constriction of miotic pupil; pupil reacts normally to epinephrine and cocaine.

Therapy. Trial with parenteral administration of mecholyl.

Prognosis. Once developed, the syndrome remains; benign condition. The pupil tends to become smaller with increasing years.

BIBLIOGRAPHY. Mylius NI: Ueber familiares Vorkommen der Pupillotonic. Klin Monatsbl Augenheilkd 101:598–599, 1938

Lowenstein O, Loewenfeld IE: Pupillotonic pseudotabes (syndrome of Markus-Weill and Reys-Holmes-Adie): A critical review of the literature. Surv Ophthalmol 10:129–185, 1965

Richwien R: Pathophysiology of tonic pupil and other stages of iridoplegia along with observation on the iridoplegia-areflexia syndrome (Weill-Reys-Holmes-Adie syndrome). Adv Ophthalmol 25:166–187, 1972

Agbeja AM, Dutton GM: Adie's syndrome as a cause of amblyopia. J Pediatr Ophthalmol Strabismus 24:176–177, 1987

Weatherall DJ, Ledingham JGG, Warrell DA (eds): Oxford Textbook of Medicine, 3rd ed, pp 3877, 4085. Oxford, Oxford Med Pub, 1996

PURE GONADAL DYSGENESIS 46 XX

Synonyms. Savage; gonadal dysgenesis, pure (XX); pure ovary failure (XX).

Symptom. Normal growth. Amenorrhea.

Signs. Sexual infantilism, marked variability of clinical expression up to good breast development; normal axillary and pubic hair; lack of signs of Turner and normal female internal and external genitalia. Occasionally mild virilization (clitoral enlargement, hirsutism) may be observed.

Etiology. Sporadic or autosomal inheritance. Ovarian tissue resistant to follicle-stimulating hormone (FSH). Stimulation (see Seabright-Bantam) or failure of normal ovarian development owing to environmental factors or imperceptible deletion of part of long arm of one X chromosome.

Pathology. Ovary resembling "fat" streak; presence of numerous primordial follicles; none showing development beyond antrum stage; stromal cell hyperplastic in some areas and luteinized in others.

Diagnostic Procedures. *Urine.* Total gonadotropins elevated both FSH and luteinizing hormone (LH), estrogen 5–10 ug/24 h, pregnanediol 1 mg/24 h. Chromosome study. Normal pattern. (46 XX sex chromatin positive). *Ultrasonography. MRI.* Absence of normal ovary.

Therapy. Estrogen replacement and withdrawal to induce bleeding. Trial with clomiphene citrate 100 mg daily, which does not change FSH or LH values. Human chorionic gonadotropin, 10,000 IU after previous treatment has been completed; however, results in an increased evidence of estrogenic activity.

BIBLIOGRAPHY. Solivar AR: The syndrome of pure gonadal dysgenesis. Am J Med 38:615–619, 1965

Jones GS, Ruehsen-DeMoraes M: Communication to AMA, San Francisco Meeting, 1968

Aleem FA: Familial 46XX gonadal dysgenesis. Fertil Streil 35:317–320, 1981

Forest MG: Diagnosis and treatment of disorders of sexual development. In De Groot LJ (ed): Endocrinology, 3rd ed, pp 1907–1908. Philadelphia, WB Saunders, 1995

PURE RED CELL APLASIA

Synonym. Erythrocytic hypoplasia.

Cluster of syndromes, including erythrocytic anemias acquired, acute and chronic (see) and Blackfan-Diamond (see).

BIBLIOGRAPHY. Krantz SB: Annotation: Pure red cell aplasia. Br J Haematol 25:11, 1973; N Engl J Med 291:345, 1974
Williams DM: Pancytopenia, aplastic anemia, and pure red cell aplasia. In Lee GR, Bithel TC, Foerster J, et al (eds): Wintrobe's Clinical Hematology, 9th ed, pp 911–943. Philadelphia, Lea & Febiger, 1993

PURE RED CELL APLASIA–THYMOMA

Synonyms. Erythrocytic hypoplasia—thymoma. Thymoma—erythrocytic hypoplasia.

Symptoms. Average age of onset 60 years (range 20–78 years). Prevalent in females (4:1). In patients with thymoma, the aregenerative anemia association is present in 5–10% of cases. In adult patients with a regenerative anemia, thymoma is present in 50% of cases. Fatigue; weakness; shortness of breath; hemorrhagic manifestations in some cases progressive. Symptoms of myasthenia gravis may be associated.

Signs. Pallor; no lymphadenopathy or splenomegaly. Retrosternal dullness when tumor sufficiently enlarged.

Etiology. Unknown. Possibly autoimmune disorder.

Pathology. Thymomas, almost always benign. Usually, spindle cell or spindle cell-lymphocytic varieties; less frequently lymphoepithelioma, lymphocytic, fibrous, and cystic.

Diagnostic Procedures. *Blood.* Hemoglobin level usually below 6 g; normocytic-normochromic type. Reticulocytes low or absent. Thrombocytopenia (10%), pancytopenia (10%), neutropenia and anemia (8%); hypogammaglobulinemia (10%); hypergammaglobulinemia (8%). *Bone marrow.* Marked hypoplasia of erythroid series; lymphocytosis.

Therapy. Chest X-rays; thymectomy; corticosteroids; testosterone.

Prognosis. Thymectomy induces remission of symptoms, permanent or temporary, in about 25% of cases. Steroids may induce remission; more effective after thymectomy. Some cases may respond to testosterone. All cases of complete cure belong to the pure red cell type.

BIBLIOGRAPHY. Matras A, Priesel A: Ueber einige Gewächse des Thymus. Beitr Pathol Anat 80:270–306, 1928
Rogers GH, Manaligod JR, Blazek WV: Thymoma associated with pancytopenia and hypogammaglobulinemia: Report of a case and review of the literature. Am J Med 44:154–164, 1968
Kranz SR, Kao V: Studies on red cell aplasia. II. Report of a second patient with an antibody to erythroblast nuclei and a remission after immunosuppressive therapy. Blood 34:1–13, 1969
Williams DM: Pancytopenia, aplastic anemia, and pure red cell aplasia. In Lee GR, Bithel TC, Foerster J, et al (eds): Wintrobe's Clinical Hematology, 9th ed, pp 911–943. Philadelphia, Lea & Febiger, 1993

PURETIC

Synonyms. Mucopolysaccharidosis variant; hyalinosis systemic.

Symptoms. Painful contractures of joints, developing at 3 months of age. Usually death in infancy or stunted growth. Recurrent suppurative infection of skin, eyes, nose, ears.

Signs. Skull and face deformed. Multiple subcutaneous nodules at joints (elbow, shoulder, knees); osteolysis of terminal phalanges.

Etiology. Unknown. Considered a variant of mucopolysaccharidosis. Possibly autosomal recessive inheritance. Considered the same as juvenile hyalinefibromatosis.

BIBLIOGRAPHY. Murray J: On three peculiar cases of molluscum fibrosum in one family. Med Chir Trans London 56:235–238, 1873

Puretic S, Puretic B, Fiser-Herman M, Adamcic M: A unique form of mesenchymal dysplasia. Br J Dermatol 74:8–19, 1962
Ishikawa H, Hori Y: Systematisierte Hyalinose in Zusammenhang mit Epidermolysis bullosa polydystrophica und Hyalinosis cutis et mucosae. Arch Klin Exp Dermatol 218:30–51, 1964
Gorlin RJ, Cohen MM Jr, Levin LS: Syndromes of Head and Neck, pp 849–850. New York, Oxford Press, 1990
Bedford CD, Sills JA, Sommelet-Olive D, et al: Juvenile Hyaline fibromatosis a report of two severe cases. J Pediatr 119:404–410, 1991

PURINE NUCLEOSIDE PHOSPHORYLASE DEFICIENCY

Synonyms. PNP deficiency, NP deficiency, purine nucleoside: orthophosphate ribosyl transferase deficiency.

Symptoms and Signs. From birth defect of cellular immunity. Symptoms may be delayed for several years. Infections of skin, lung, ears, and urinary tract. Candida and virus infections. Anemia. Increased susceptibility to vaccinations. Spastic tetraparesis.

Etiology. Autosomal recessive inheritance. Deficiency of PNP of various degrees leads to altered function of T cells. Gene mapped to chromosome 14.

Diagnostic Procedures. Tests for cellular immunity. *Blood.* Anemia: Both T-cells and B-cells normal at birth, followed by a gradual decrease in T-cell immunity, whereas B-cell function remains normal. Polynucleates BC activity: low or absent. Hypouricemia. High level of inosine and guanosine levels. *Urine.* Hypouricosuria, excessive amounts of purines.

Therapy. Attempted correction of immune deficiency with bone marrow, embryonal thymus transplants, and thymosine (clinically ineffective), PNP.

Prognosis. Fatal in some cases for infections and blood transfusions. In some patients who survive, vaccination may be fatal. Lymphoma development is a possibility.

BIBLIOGRAPHY. Giblett ER, Ammann AJ, Wara DW, et al: Nucleoside phosphorylase deficiency in a child with severely defective T-cell immunity and normal B-cell immunity. Lancet 1:1010–1013, 1975
Rijksen G, Kuis W, Wadman SK, et al: A new case of purine nucleoside phosphorylase deficiency enzymologic, clinical and immunologic characteristics. Ped Res 21:137–141, 1987
Lukens JN: Immune deficiency diseases: Inherited and acquired. In Lee GR, Bithel TC, Foerster J, et al (eds): Wintrobe's Clinical Hematology, 9th ed, p 1685. Philadelphia, Lea & Febiger, 1993

PURPLE PEOPLE

Synonym. Chlorpromazine toxicity, chronic.

Symptoms. Both sexes affected (previously thought to occur only in women). Occurs in psychiatric patients on long-term, high doses of chlorpromazine. Peculiar purplish-gray pigmentation of sun-exposed skin areas, progressing to permanent blue-black or purplish-gray metallic color. In some patients, corneal and lens opacities may also develop.

Etiology. Deposition in the skin of a chlorpromazine metabolite that reacts with sunlight. Ultraviolet light with wavelengths above 320 nm seems to be primarily responsible for the effects.

Therapy. Special window glass to reduce ultraviolet light in institutions where this treatment is conducted.

BIBLIOGRAPHY. Greiner AC, Berry K: Skin pigmentation and corneal and lens opacities with prolonged chlorpromazine therapy. Can Med Assoc J 90:663–665, 1964
AHFS Q5: Drug Information, p 1510. Bethesda, MD, 1995
Weatherall DJ, Ledingham JGG, Warrell DA (eds): Oxford Textbook of Medicine, 3rd ed, p 4252. Oxford, Oxford Med Pub, 1996

PURPURA, MECHANICAL

Synonym. Orthostatic purpura (included).

Symptoms and Signs. Localized cutaneous hemorrhagic manifestations: petechiae and ecchymoses. In the mechanical form, localization prevalent on head, neck, and upper extremities; in orthostatic form, on lower extremities.

Etiology. Miopragia of capillaries and small arteries.

Diagnostic Procedures. *Blood.* Frequently associated, mild thrombocytopenia.

Therapy. Vitamin C; rutin; sodium carbazochrome sulfonans.

Prognosis. Benign persistent condition.

BIBLIOGRAPHY. Bithell TC: Bleeding disorders caused by vascular abnormalities. In Lee GR, Bithel TC, Foerster J, et al (eds): Wintrobe's Clinical Hematology, 9th ed. Philadelphia, Lea & Febiger, 1993

PURPURA, PSYCHOGENIC

Synonyms. Psychosomatic; bleeding stigmata hysteric purpura.

Symptoms and Signs. Occurs in subjects with strong emotional involvement or other psychotic manifestations; most often in females. Occurrence of hematomas or bleeding in connection with certain complex psychic experiences. Spontaneous reproduction of wounds and bodily suffering of Christ, of battle wounds of Mohammed, or unrelated to religious experiences; repeated spontaneous bleeding in old healed scars associated with strong emotional experiences when memory of the experience is elicited, or symbolic of repressed sexual or aggressive feelings. Menstruation equivalent in various parts of the body (axilla, nose) or bloody hand.

Etiology. Unknown. Opinions divided about the pathogenesis of these manifestations, from supernatural origin, hysteric conversion phenomena and self-induced.

Pathology. Ecchymosis or blood oozing through apparently normal skin.

Diagnostic Procedures. Psychoanalysis reproduces symptomatology by reproduction of stimulating psychic conditions. Rule out self-induction by protection or observation. Rule out Werlof (see). Coagulation studies.

Therapy. Psychotherapy.

Prognosis. Recurrence of the phenomena. Difficult treatment. Possible conversion to other types of hysterical manifestations.

BIBLIOGRAPHY. Hyde JH: A contribution to the study of bleeding stigmata. J Cutan Dis 15:557, 1897
Agle DF, Ratnoff OD: Purpura as a psychosomatic entity. Arch Intern Med 109:685–694, 1962
Bithell TC: Bleeding disorders caused by vascular abnormalities. In Lee GR, Bithel TC, Foerster J, et al (eds): Wintrobe's Clinical Hematology, 9th ed. Philadelphia, Lea & Febiger, 1993

PURPURA SIMPLEX, HEREDITARY

Symptoms and Signs. Females almost exclusively affected. Spontaneous ecchymoses; positive tourniquet test. Rheumatic fever, rheumatoid arthritis, and ptosis frequently associated.

Etiology. Autosomal dominant trait.

Therapy. None. Deficit of only esthetic significance.

BIBLIOGRAPHY. Davis E: Hereditary familial purpura simplex. Lancet 1:145–146, 1941
Bithell TC: Bleeding disorders caused by vascular abnormalities. In Lee

GR, Bithel TC, Foerster J, et al (eds): Wintrobe's Clinical Hematology, 9th ed. Philadelphia, Lea & Febiger, 1993

PURPURA SIMPLEX, SPORADIC

See Purpura, psychogenic.

Symptoms and Signs. Prevalent in females. Mild purpura; small ecchymoses in the legs. Exacerbation during menstrual periods.

Etiology. Unknown.

Diagnostic Procedures. Diagnosis by exclusion. *Blood.* Normal platelets; normal clotting factors; tourniquet test occasionally shows abnormality.

BIBLIOGRAPHY. Bithell TC: Bleeding disorders caused by vascular abnormalities. In Lee GR, Bithel TC, Foerster J, et al (eds): Wintrobe's Clinical Hematology, 9th ed. Philadelphia, Lea & Febiger, 1993

PURTSCHER

Symptoms. Duane retinopathy; Valsalva retinopathy, traumatic, retinal; angiopathy; fat embolism; lymphorrhagia, traumatic.

Symptoms. Occurs following trauma of different degrees. Transient visual impairment.

Signs. Retinal and preretinal hemorrhages, exudates, edema, venous congestion; papilledema.

Etiology. Sudden rise in blood pressure; head and chest congestion. Fat embolism to be considered.

Pathology. Possibly, partial retinal vein obstruction. See Signs.

Therapy. Antiedema treatment.

Prognosis. Usually good.

BIBLIOGRAPHY. Purtscher O: Angiopathie retinae traumatica. Lymphorrhagien des Augengrundes. Albrecht Von Graefes Arch Ophthalmol 82:341–371, 1912
Hoare GW: Traumatic retinal angiopathy resulting from chest compression by safety belt. Br J Ophthalmol 54:667–674, 1970
Morris DA: Ocular trauma. In Garner A, Klintworth GK (eds): Pathobiology of Ocular Disease: A Dynamic Approach, 2nd ed, p 407. New York, Marcel Dekker, 1994

PUTSCHAR-MANION

Synonyms. Splenogonadal fusion, limb defects, micrognathia.

Symptoms. In male (only one female reported). Ectromelia, micrognathia, numerous unerupted teeth, crowding of upper incisors, V-shaped palate (no cleft).

Etiology. Autosomal dominant inheritance.

Pathology. See Signs. Fusion of spleen and gonads.

Prognosis. Death in infancy.

BIBLIOGRAPHY. Putschar WGJ, Manion WC: Splenic-gonadal fusion. Am J Pathol 32:15–35, 1956
Pauli RM, Greenlaw A: Limb deficiency and splenogonadal fusion. Am J Med Genet 13:81–90, 1982

PUTTI-CHAVANY

Synonyms. Paralyzing sciatica; sciatica paralysant.

Symptoms and Signs. Unilateral sciatica (see Cotugno) associated with paralysis of the foot.

Etiology. See Cotugno.

Prognosis. Rapid resolution of painful episode followed by onset of sensory troubles.

BIBLIOGRAPHY. Putti V: Lomboartrite e Sciatica Vertebrale. Bologna, 1936.

Chavany JA: Petite histoire de la sciatique paralysant. Prog Med 86:427–435, 1958

Weatherall DJ, Ledingham JGG, Warrell DA (eds): Oxford Textbook of Medicine, 3rd ed, pp 2992, 3906, 4097. Oxford, Oxford Med Pub, 1996

PYCNODYSOSTOSIS

Synonyms. Maroteaux-Lami II; Toulouse-Lautrec; pyknodysostosis.

Symptoms and Signs. Both sexes affected; evident from early infancy. Dwarfism; easy fractures of bones; partial agenesis of terminal digits of hands and feet; persistent opening of cranial fontanelles; occipital bossing; parrot-like nose; micrognathism; scoliosis (Toulouse-Lautrec seems to have suffered from this syndrome). Occasionally, mental retardation. Two-thirds of patients had fractures, especially of lower extremities; poor dentition and frequent caries.

Etiology. Unknown. Autosomal recessive inheritance.

Pathology. Osteopetrosis.

Diagnostic Procedures. *Blood.* Normal; no anemia. *X-ray.* Skull dolichocephaly; opening of fontanelles. Bone dense; absence of diploë; absence of frontal sinuses. In other bones, diffuse osteopetrosis.

Therapy. Special dental care; orthopedic provision for fractures.

Prognosis. Good; no anemia, blindness, or other complication as observed in similar syndromes (e.g., Albers-Schönberg). There may be, however, progressive loss of distal phalanges; persistence of open fontanelles.

BIBLIOGRAPHY. Montanari U: Acondroplasia e disostosi cleidocranica digitale. Chir Organi Mov 7:379–391, 1923

Collado-Otero F: Una forma mas de distrofia osea. Acta Pediatr Esp 14:1–27, 1956

Maroteaux P, Lamy M: La pycnodysostose. Presse Med 70:999–1002, 1962

Maroteaux P, Lamy M: The malady of Toulouse-Lautrec. JAMA 191:715–717, 1965

Sedano HD, Gorlin RJ, Anderson VE: Pycnodysostosis: clinical and genetic considerations. Am J Dis Child 116:70–77, 1968

Mills KLG, Johnston AW: Pycnodysostosis. J Med Genet 25:550–553, 1988

PYLE

Synonyms. Bakwin-Krida; metaphyseal dysplasia; leontiasis ossea. See Craniometaphyseal dysplasia.

Symptoms. Both sexes affected. Often asymptomatic. Onset in early infancy. Progressing headache; vomiting; irritability. Late motor development; vacuous expression; blindness; deafness; facial muscle paralysis, joint pain.

Signs. Large head; nasal bridge broad and flat; hypertelorism; open mouth; scoliosis, limitation of elbow extension, genu valgum (early onset).

Etiology. Unknown. Autosomal recessive inheritance.

Pathology. Cranium enlarged and heavier; bone ivory-like; diploë eliminated; paranasal sinuses obliterated; suture lines indistinct; reduction of foramina. Microscopically, compact bone, dilated Haversian canals, no osteoclasts. Long bones (femur in particular) flask-shaped in metaphyseal region; decreased density.

Diagnostic Procedures. *Blood.* Normal; calcium, phosphorus, alkaline phosphatase normal. *X-ray.* Of skull and long bones.

Therapy. Surgical decompression of nerves at foramina (surgery at multiple stages).

Prognosis. Poor; death from bone encroachment in area of foramen magnum.

BIBLIOGRAPHY. Smith GE, Jones FW: The archeologic survey of Nubia, report for 1907–1908. Rep Remains Cairo 2:289, 1910

Pyle E: A case of unusual bone development. J Bone Joint Surg 13:874–876, 1931

Vohra V: Pyle's disease: familal metaphyseal dysplasia: A case report. Australas Radiol 31:75–78, 1987

Rimoin DL, Lachman RS: Genetic disorders of the osseous skeleton. In Beithon P (ed): McKusick's Heritable Disorders of Connective Tissue, 5th ed, pp 663–664. St Louis, CV Mosby, 1993

Klippel JH, Dieppe PA: Rheumatology, p 7.45.5. St Louis, CV Mosby, 1995

PYODERMA GANGRENOSUM

Synonyms. Brocq phagedena geometricum; Meleney undermining burrowing ulcer; phagedena geometricum; Cullen postoperative serpiginosus ulceration; burrowing phagedenic ulcer.

Symptoms. Both sexes equally affected; onset generally in adult life, seldom in childhood. It occurs frequently in association with ulcerative colitis, rheumatoid arthritis, chronic infections, malnutrition.

Signs. Extremely variable manifestations owing to the pyoderma gangrenosum and associated condition. On the lower limbs or trunk, usually at the site of insect bite, needle puncture or trauma, appearance of single or multiple tender nodules, which evolve in pustules and then, breaking down, form ulcers slowly enlarging to 10 cm or more. Ulcers assume various shapes (round, oval, serpiginous) and present a bluish reddish edge, central, and necrotic base.

Etiology. Unknown. Various aspecific germs isolated, but not considered responsible. (Defective immune response?)

Pathology. No specific changes.

Diagnostic Procedures. *Biopsy and culture.* To exclude other diagnosis. *Blood.* In several cases, hypoproteinemia or presence of paraglobulins; assessment of nutritive status; rheumatoid factor. *X-ray.* Of intestine. To search for ulcerative colitis.

Therapy. In cases without demonstrable underlying diseases, trials with antibiotics, gamma globulins, corticosteroids (of relative benefit).

Prognosis. Extremely variable. Ulcers may last for weeks or years; successive crops recur at variable intervals. Usually, in previously healthy subjects, course with slower progression and faster recovery and general health not affected; with associated condition, the course follows the evolution of the basic pathology.

BIBLIOGRAPHY. Brocq JL: Nouvelle contribution à l'étude du phagédénisme géométrique. Ann Dermatol Syph 5:6:1–39, 1916

Goldgraber MB, Korsner JB: Gangrenous skin lesion associated with chronic ulcerative colitis: A case study. Gastroenterology 39:94–103, 1960

Ryan TJ: Cutaneous vasculitis. In Champion RH, Burton JL, Ebling FJG (eds): Rook/Wilkinson/Ebling Textbook of Dermatology, 5th ed, pp 1922–1927. Oxford, Blackwell Scientific, 1992

PYODERMA VEGETANS

Synonyms. Dermatitis vegetans, including: genitocrural dermatitis and intertrigo. See also Hallopeau II.

Symptoms and Signs. Both sexes affected. Onset at all ages. Several clinical variants, but the general characteristics are shared by all forms. Occurs in subjects with normal skin and good health, or in malnutrition and chronic alcoholism, but most frequently in individuals with preexisting eczema or infective dermatitis. Generally, in flexures and genitalia, appearance of small pustules and granulomatous reaction that form foul-smelling, moist plaques; in other variants, formation of red crusted plaques, surrounded by vesiculopustules; if mucosae (oral cavity) involved, term pyostomatitis is used.

Etiology. Unknown. Nonspecific skin reaction.

Pathology. Nonspecific chronic granulomatous reaction and pseudo-epitheliomatous hyperplasia. Abscess may contain many eosinophils.

Diagnostic Procedures. *Biopsy. Blood. Urine. Stool.* In cases of associated or underlying pathology, evidence of ulcerative colitis, hepatopathies, malnutrition.

Therapy. That of underlying conditions. Moist compresses. Antibiotics (systemic or topical) unpredictable response.

Prognosis. Chronic condition. Possibly, spontaneous remission with residual scars. If cure of identified underlying condition achieved, fast recovery.

BIBLIOGRAPHY. Nanta A, Bazex A: Formes cliniques des pyodermites végétantes. Ann Dermatol Syph 8:609–623, 1937
Melezer N: Zur Kenntnis der chronishcen vegetierenden Pyodermien. Minerva Dermatol 34:308–313, 1959
Highet AS, Hay RJ, Roberts SOB: Bacterial infections. In Champion RH, Burton JL, Ebling FJG (eds): Rook/Wilkinson/Ebling Textbook of Dermatology, 5th ed, pp 1021–1022. Oxford, Blackwell Scientific, 1992

PYRAMIDAL DECUSSATION

Synonyms. Hemiplegia cruciata; ventromedial.

Symptoms. Paralysis of one upper extremity and contralateral paralysis of lower extremity. Face is spared.

Signs. Spasticity; increase in tone of affected muscles; hyperreflexia; ankle clonus; Babinski sign; absent abdominal reflexes on side of involved leg.

Etiology. Usually, trauma and causes other than softening. Seldom, softening.

Pathology. Lesion (see Etiology) in lower part of medulla at specific point distal to decussation of arm fibers, and proximal to decussation of leg fibers.

Diagnostic Procedures. *Spinal tap. Angiography, serology.*

Therapy. Symptomatic.

Prognosis. Depends on etiology.

BIBLIOGRAPHY. Chavany JA, Taptas JN, Haggenmueller D: Les faux syndromes alternes d'origine hémisphérique; l'hemiplegia cruciata par lésions corticales bilatérales. Presse Med 60:1126–1128, 1952
Adams RD, Victor M: Principles of Neurology, 5th ed, pp 42, 56. New York, McGraw-Hill, 1993

PYRIDOXINE CEREBRAL DEFICIENCY

Synonym. Hunt (AD).

Symptoms. Occurs in newborn with a traumatic birth; onset a few hours after delivery. (Seizure activity may have begun even in utero.) Repeated and intractable convulsions; shrill cries. Mental retardation.

Signs. Convulsions preceded by faint pallor and rolling of the eyes.

Etiology. Autosomal recessive inheritance. Possibly high intake of pyridoxine during pregnancy. Enzymatic abnormality of central nervous system in which there is a continuing high requirement for pyridoxine in excess of normal dietary intake owing to a disorder of GABA synthesis.

Pathology. *Brain.* Edema; neural degeneration (hypoxic type). *Adrenal cortex.* Areas of degeneration. *Liver.* Fatty degeneration; local congestion.

Diagnostic Procedures. *EEG.* Marked dysrhythmia and slow wave activity (findings present when signs of incipient convulsion are present). After injection of pyridoxine, significant decrease of slow wave activity. *Tryptophan loading and xanthurenic acid excretion test.* Normal.

Therapy. Pyridoxine hydrochloride will dramatically stop the convulsions and continuous treatment for life prevents their recurrence.

Prognosis. Death without treatment. With treatment, control of seizures, but mental retardation persists.

BIBLIOGRAPHY. Hunt AD, Stokes J Jr, McCrory WW, et al: Pyridoxine dependency: Report of a case of intractable convulsions in an infant controlled by pyridoxine. Pediatrics 13:140–145, 1954
Frimpter GW: Pyridoxine (B6) dependency syndromes. Ann Intern Med 68:1131–1132, 1968
Goutierez F, Aicardi J: A typical presentation of pyridoxine-dependent seizures: a treatable cause for intractable epilepsy in infants. Ann Neurol 17:117–120, 1985
Scriver CR, Gibson KM: Disorders of aminoacids in free and peptide-linked forms. In Scriver CR, Beaudet AL, Sly WS, et al: The Metabolic and Molecular Bases of Inherited Disease, 7th ed, pp 1359–1360. New York, McGraw-Hill, 1995

PYRIFORMIS

Symptoms. Occurs in patients with history of trauma to the sacroiliac or gluteal region (sometimes forgotten because of long gap in time between trauma and onset of symptoms). Pain in zone of sacroiliac joint; greater sciatic notch and pyriformis muscle; radiating in the leg and causing difficulty in walking. Acute reexacerbation of chronic pain by stooping or lifting weight.

Signs. Palpable, sausage-shaped mass over pyriformis (during attack of pain), and tenderness, Lasègue sign; gluteal atrophy according to duration of condition.

Etiology. Lesion of pyriformis muscle affecting sciatic nerve in cases where close relation between this muscle and nerve exist.

Pathology. Adhesion between pyriformis and sciatic nerve.

Diagnostic Procedures. *X-ray.* To rule out other pathologic conditions of lumbar, sacral, and hip articulation areas.

Therapy. Sectioning of pyriformis muscle and separation of sciatic nerve from any attachment to the muscle.

Prognosis. Excellent result with treatment indicated. Immediate and permanent relief of syndrome. Section of muscle does not interfere with any movement of hip joint and does not cause disability.

BIBLIOGRAPHY. Yoemans W: The relation of arthritis of the sacroiliac joint to sciatica. Lancet 2:1119–1122, 1928
Robinson DR: Pyriformis syndrome in relation to sciatic pain. Am J Surg 73:355–358, 1947

PYRUVATE CARBOXYLASE DEFICIENCY

Synonyms. PC deficiency. See Leigh.

Symptoms and Signs. Rare, both sexes. Three different clinical presentations. In the first one (group A) (18 cases) onset is soon after birth with chronic lactic acidemia and delayed neurologic development and seizures. Normal lactate/pyruvate ratio, ammonia, citrulline and lysine, elevated alanine, and proline. The second one (group B) (9 cases) presents early lactico-acidosis, hepatomegaly, with elevated levels of ammonia, citrulline, proline, lysine, and elevated lactate/pyruvate ratio (5×). In the third one (group C) (1 case) onset 14 months acute metabolic acidosis, normal blood ammonia and citruline, elevated alanine, lysine, and proline.

Etiology. Autosomal recessive inheritance. Deficiency of pyruvate carboxylate.

Pathology. Autopsy: reduction of white matter, hepatic fibrosis.

Diagnostic Procedures. *Blood.* Lactic acidosis, elevated pyruvate levels, intermittent hypoglycemia, and ketosis.

Therapy. Reported benefits with thiamine and lipoic acid.

Prognosis. In group A death in early infancy; two cases survived to 5 years with mental retardation. In group B all dead within 3 months. In group C 7 years survival with normal development.

BIBLIOGRAPHY. Delvin E, Neal JL, Scriver CR: Pyruvate carboxylase: Two forms of human liver. Pediatr Res 6:392, 1972

Atkin BM, Buist NRM, Utter MF, et al: Pyruvate carboxylase deficiency and lactic acidosis in a retarded child without Leigh's disease. Pediatr Res 13:109–120, 1979

Robinson BH, Oci J, Sherwood WG, et al: The molecular basis for two different clinical presentations of classical pyruvate carboxylase deficiency. Am J Hum Genet 36:283–294, 1984

Robinson BH: Lactic acidemia. In Scriver CR, Beaudet AL, Sly WS, et al: The Metabolic and Molecular Bases of Inherited Disease, 7th ed, p 1491. New York, McGraw-Hill, 1995

PYRUVATE KINASE DEFICIENCY, HEMOLYTIC ANEMIA

Synonym. Dacie anemia (type); PK1 deficiency. High red cell ATP; ATP-pyruvate phosphotransferase.

Symptoms. Both sexes equally affected. Onset in infancy or early childhood, seldom in adulthood. Weakness; fatigue. Exacerbation of symptoms with intercurrent diseases or surgery.

Signs. All signs may appear from very mild to very severe. Jaundice; pallor; splenomegaly; hepatomegaly (rare); chronic leg ulcers (rare); prominent frontal bosses (in severe cases). Cholelithiasis at relatively early age.

Etiology. Specific erythrocyte deficiency of pyruvate kinase. Autosomal recessive inheritance with variable penetrance.

Pathology. In bone marrow, normoblastic hyperplasia, increased hemosiderin. Spleen enlarged; no specific changes; hyperplasia of reticulum; ischemia of red pulp. Absence of extramedullary hyperplasia. Cholelithiasis.

Diagnostic Procedures. *Blood.* Anemia; relative macrocytosis; reticulocytosis; variable number of nucleated red cells. Leukocytes and platelets normal; moderate hyperbilirubinemia; serum haptoglobulin absent or decreased. Osmotic fragility normal. Incubated fragility test: various abnormalities. Autohemolysis test positive; not corrected by addition of glucose and adenosine. Coombs test negative; Heinz bodies absent. Ferrokinetic study (59Fe): rapid plasma clearance. Survival time of cells shortened. *Stool.* Fecal urobilinogen increased.

Therapy. Splenectomy. Hyperbilirubinemia in newborn may require blood exchange tranfusion. Avoid use of salycilates.

Prognosis. Extremely variable, from fulminating cases to long survival with minimal manifestations. Splenectomy beneficial in most cases.

BIBLIOGRAPHY. Dacie JV, Mollison PL, Richardson N, et al: A typical congenital haemolytic anaemia. QJ Med 22:79–98, 1953

Brewer GJ: A new inherited abnormality of human herithrocyte-elevated erythrocyte adenosine triphosphate. Biochem Biophys Res Commun 18:430–434, 1965

Zurcher C, Loos JA, Prins HK, et al: Hereditary high ATP content of human herithrocytes. Folia Haemat 83:366–376, 1965

Beutler E, Forman L, Rios-Larrain E: Elevated pyruvate kinase activity in patients with hemolytic anemia due to pyruvate kinase deficiency. Am J Med 83:899–904, 1987

Tanaka KR, Paglia DE: Pyruvate kinase and other enzymopathies of the erythrocyte. In Scriver CR, Beaudet AL, Sly WS, et al: The Metabolic and Molecular Bases of Inherited Disease, p 3492. New York, McGraw-Hill, 1995

QI-GONG

Synonyms. Chi-gong; vital energy exercise.

Symptoms and Signs. In Chinese communities in mainlands or emigrated. Practice of special exercises aiming to improve physical, mental, and spiritual health by reduction of stagnation of Qi (vital energy) circulation. According to people who practice these exercises in addition to positive results (reduction of stress and of various physical and psychological symptoms) it may induce transient or permanent psychotic symptoms (hallucinations, delusions, etc.).

Etiology. Psychotic disorder culture bound. Locally included in diagnostic system for mental disorders.

BIBLIOGRAPHY. Lin K-M: Cultural influences on the diagnosis of psychotic and organic disorders. In Mezzich JE, Kleinman A Fabrega H, et al: Culture and Psychiatric Diagnosis. Washington, American Psychiatry Press, 1995

QUADRICEPS MYOPATHY

Synonyms. Quadriceps amyotrophy. Contraversial definition that probably includes different clinical entities.

Symptoms and Signs. Usually in adult male. Atrophy of quadriceps of leg occasionally brachioradialis; knee jerks. Females may present milder manifestations.

Etiology. Polymyositis; or genetically inherited myopathy X-linked type.

Diagnostic Procedures. *Blood.* Increased creatinine kinase. *Muscle biopsy.* Evidence of muscular atrophy. *EMG.* Muscle or neurologic pattern.

Therapy. None.

Prognosis. Good quoad vitam.

BIBLIOGRAPHY. Bramwell E: Observations on myopathy. Proc R Soc Med 16:1–12, 1922
Espir MLE, Matthews WB: Hereditary quadriceps myopathy. J Neurol Neurosurg Psychiatr 36:1041–1045, 1973
Serratrice G, Pou-Serradel A, Pellisier JF, et al: Chronic neurogenic quadriceps amyotrophy. J Neurol 232:150–153, 1985
Walton J, Karpati G, Hilton-Jones D: Disorders of Voluntary Muscle, p 580. Edinburgh, Churchill Livingstone, 1994

QUADRILATERAL SPACE

Symptoms. In young adults. Following forward flexion, abduction of arms: intermittent paresthesia. Humerus rotation aggravates symptoms.

Etiology. Compression of posterior humeral circumflex artery and axillary nerve in quadrilateral space.

Therapy. Surgery.

BIBLIOGRAPHY. Cahill BR, Palmer RE: Quadrilateral space syndrome. J Hand Surg 8:65–69, 1983
Cormier PJ: Quadrilateral space syndrome: A rare cause of shoulder pain. Radiology 167:797–798, 1988

QUARELLI

Eponym used to indicate Parkinson syndrome (see) that follows chronic intoxication with carbon disulfide.

BIBLIOGRAPHY. Quarelli G: Del tremore parkinsonsimile dell'intossicazione cronica da disolfuro di carbonio. Med Lavoro 21:58–64, 1930

QUEYRAT

Synonyms. Queyrat erythroplasia. See also Bowen. Erythroplasia Queyrat.

Symptoms. It is not observed in circumcised males. Painless thickening of external genitalia, usually on penis, less frequently on vulva, and described also in mouth and tongue.

Signs. Slightly raised, intense red, glistening plaque with sharply outlined edge; later, scaling.

Etiology. Unknown. Intraepithelial carcinoma, not associated with internal cancer (Bowen).

Pathology. Cutaneous surface of stratum corneum stripped and covered by parakeratosis. Epidermis thick with interpapillary ridges extending into dermis, which is edematous and inflamed. Acanthosis with variety of abnormal cells; increased mitosis.

Diagnostic Procedures. *Biopsy and bacteriologic exams* (in case of doubt).

Therapy. Topical application of anti-irritating agents (colchicine analogues); if tendency to invasion, surgical excision. Thiocalciran cream; 5-fluorouracil cream; radium mold.

Prognosis. Lesion usually tends to remain unlimited; in some cases, diffusion and possibility of metastasis.

BIBLIOGRAPHY. Queyrat A: Erythroplasie du gland. Bull Soc Fr Dermatol Syph 22:378–382, 1911
Ive FA: The umbilical perianal and genital regions. In Champion RH, Burton JL, Ebling FJG (eds): Rook/Wilkinson/Ebling Textbook of Dermatology, 5th ed, pp 2822–2823. Oxford, Blackwell Scientific, 1992

QUIE-HILL

Synonyms. See Hyperimmunoglobulin E and Job.

Symptoms and Signs. Allergic rhinitis. Recurrent foruncolosis. Abscesses and eczema-like dermatoses.

Diagnostic Procedures. *Blood.* Immunoglobulin E, slight elevation.

BIBLIOGRAPHY. Moore EC, Cohen F: Skin manifestations if immunodeficiency. In Stone J (ed): Dermatologic Immunology and Allergy, pp 297–331. St Louis, CV Mosby, 1985

QUINCKE I

Synonyms. Bannister; Milton-Quincke; angioderma; circumscribed edema; giant urticaria; wandering edema; angioedema-urticaria; including urticaria chronic.

Symptoms. Male to female ratio, 1:2. In 50% of cases associated with urticaria (intensely itchy, worse at night). Nausea; vomiting; cephalalgia; diarrhea; severe respiratory distress according to areas involved. Polyuria, in some cases, at termination of attacks.

Signs. Rapid onset of single or multiple, nonpitting, tense, pink or red, surrounded by a red flare swellings or wheals, from dime to palm size, usually lasting less than 24 hours, then fading with no trace. Any part of body may be affected; most frequently involved areas: lips, eyelids, genitalia. Tongue and larynx may be involved.

Etiology. Idiopathic. Allergy to various agents; possibly, emotional factors are involved.

Pathology. Capillary stasis in subcutaneous tissue, without evidence of vascular damage. Affected skin contains increased mast cells.

Diagnostic Procedure. *Allergy tests. Blood* IgE total and specific. Evidence of thyroid disease in high number of cases. Wheal formation in response to autologous serum.

Therapy. Antihistamines. Epinephrine and related drugs; corticosteroids. Endotracheal intubation if larynx involved. Trials of specific desensitization if allergy proven.

Prognosis. Attacks usually last 1–2 hours, but may persist for 2–3 days (average 12 hours) before spontaneous or therapeutic remission. Chronic form defined by daily recurrences for at least 6 weeks. Recurrent attacks. Life-threatening in case of laryngeal involvement. Prognosis for life usually not as serious as in angioneurotic edema, hereditary (see).

BIBLIOGRAPHY. Quincke HI: Über akutes umbeschrie-benes Hautderm. Mhefte Prakt Dermatol 1:129–131, 1882

Bannister HM: Acute angioneurotic edema. J Nerv Ment Dis 21:627–631, 1894

Milton JL: On giant urticaria. Edinburgh Med J 22:513–526, 1976

Champion RH: Urticaria. In Champion RH, Burton JL, Ebling FJG (eds): Rook/Wilkinson/Ebling Textbook of Dermatology, 5th ed, pp 1877–1879. Oxford, Blackwell Scientific, 1992

Graves MW: Chronic urticaria. N Engl J Med 332:1867–1772, 1995

QUINSY

Term derived from Greek κψναγχηε, which means a bad sore throat.

Synonym. Peritonsillar abscess.

Symptoms. Malaise; chills; pain radiating from one side of throat to ear and neck; dysphagia; dysphonia; malodorous breath; trismus; drooling; stiff neck; hyperthermia.

Signs. Tonsillitis; edema and displacement prevalent in one side; tongue coated; difficulty in inspecting pharynx.

Etiology. Tonsillitis initially owing to streptococcal infection, then to Gram-negative microorganisms.

Pathology. Abscess into tonsil and extending into surrounding neck tissue.

Diagnostic Procedures. *Blood.* Leukocytosis. *Throat culture.* Mixed flora, usually of Gram-negative type.

Therapy. Antibiotics. After fluctuation, drainage of abscess.

Prognosis. Much improved by antibiotics and surgery.

BIBLIOGRAPHY. Harley EH: Quinsy tonsilectomy as the treatment of choice for peritonsillar abscess. Ear Nose Throat J 67:84–87, 1988

Weatherall DJ, Ledingham JGG, Warrell DA (eds): Oxford Textbook of Medicine, 3rd ed, p 572. Oxford, Oxford Med Pub, 1996

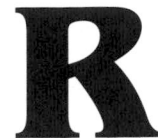

RABENHORST

Synonyms. Cardio—acro—facial. See Cayler.

Symptoms and Signs. From birth. Narrow face, micrognathia, high and narrow nose, prominent septum; microstomia; attached earlobe; ventricular septal defect and pulmonary stenosis; minor hand and foot malformations.

Etiology. Unknown.

BIBLIOGRAPHY. Gosse FR: The Rabenhorst syndrome. Z Kinderheilk 117:109–114, 1974

RABE-SALOMON

Synonyms. Salomon l; afibrinogenemia congenital; fibrinogenopenia congenital; congenital hypofibrinogenemia. See Dysfibrinogenemia and Hypofibrinogenemia.

Symptoms. Occurs in both sexes; manifestations from birth. Bleeding from umbilical cord usually profuse. After trauma or surgery, severe bleeding. Episodes of ecchymosis, hematomas, epistaxis, hemopthysis, hematuria, hemorrhage in central nervous system, alternated with long periods of freedom from hemorrhages. Menses may be normal.

Signs. Very rarely, hemarthroses; seldom, permanent damage to tissue after hemorrhage; pseudocyst in the bone may occur.

Etiology. Failure to synthetize fibrinogen. Autosomal recessive inheritance. Mutation in one or another of the three fibrinogen genes (alpha, beta, or gamma).

Diagnostic Procedures. *Blood.* Anemia at time of hemorrhages; blood does not clot spontaneously or after addition of thrombin. Absence of fibrinogen (traces may be revealed with immunologic method). All other coagulation factors normal (slight depression of proaccelerin seldom observed). Bleeding time prolonged. Tourniquet test normal. Sedimentation rate nonexistent (after 24-hour red cells still floating). Fibrinogen antibodies (appearing after repeated transfusions).

Therapy. Bleeding treated by injection of fibrinogen. Infusion of cryoprecipitate.

Prognosis. Patients may reach adulthood; death from bleeding into vital area or severe blood loss. Possible thrombosis of pulmonary district.

BIBLIOGRAPHY. Rabe F, Salomon E: Ueber Faserstoffmangel im Blute bei einem Falle von Haemophilie. Dtsch Ark Klin Med 132:240–244, 1920
Mammen EF: Congenital abnormalities of the fibrogen molecule. Semin Tromb Hemost 1:184, 1974
Lord ST: Fibrinogen. In High KA Roberts HR (eds): Molecular Basis of Thrombosis and Hemostasis. New York, Marcel Dekker, 1995

RABSON-MENDENHALL

Symptoms and Signs. In infancy. Thick, rapidly growing hair, abnormal teeth and nails, acanthosis nigricans (see). Frequently accelerated growth, enlarged phallus, precocious pseudopuberty.

Etiology. Unknown. Mutation in the insulin receptor gene.

Pathology. Pineal gland and adrenal cortex hyperplasia.

Diagnostic Procedures. *Blood.* Hyperglycemia (developing in childhood) with insulin resistance; severe ketoacidosis (observed but not typical).

Therapy. Symptomatic.

BIBLIOGRAPHY. Mendenhall EN: Tumor of the pineal body with high insulin resistance. J Ind Med Assoc 43:32–36, 1950
Rabson SM, Mendenhall EN: Familial hypertrophy of the pineal body, hyperplasia of adrenal cortex and diabetes mellitus: Report of 3 cases. Am J Clin Pathol 26:283–290, 1956
Flier JS: Syndromes of insulin resistance and mutant insulin. In De Groot LJ (ed): Endocrinology, 3rd ed, p 1599. Philadelphia, WB Saunders, 1995

RACINE

Synonyms. Premenstrual salivary; premenstrual sialorrhea.

Symptoms and Signs. Tumefaction of one or more salivary glands, beginning 4–5 days prior to menstrual cycle and disappearing at its onset.

Etiology. Unknown. Part of the premenstrual syndrome (see).

Pathology. Interstitial edema and temporary dilatation of excretory canals of salivary glands.

Therapy. See Premenstrual.

BIBLIOGRAPHY. Racine W: Le syndrome salivaire prémenstruel. Schweiz Med Wchschr 69:1204–1207, 1939
Gooren LJG, Money J: Normal and abnormal sexual behavior. In De Groot LJ (ed): Endocrinology, 3rd ed, p 1985. Philadelphia, WB Saunders, 1995

RADIATION, ACUTE

Synonyms. Radiation injuries; accidental radiation.

Symptoms and Signs. Sequential stages of the radiation syndrome as well as the characteristic forms of the syndrome (cerebral, gastrointestinal, hematopoietic) develop according to the amount of radiation received, and to a lesser extent, to individual susceptibility. "Typical" radiation-induced syndrome evolves after whole body doses of 2 or more Sv (200 rem) according to the following pattern:

1. *Prodromal stage.* Within 2 hours of exposure, anorexia, nausea, malaise, listlessness, fatigue. Progressing to prostration and culminating at about 8 hours, and then subsiding rapidly. Or second day nausea and (occasionally) vomiting, but marked improvement of general situation.

2. *Latent stage.* Third day, asymptomatic and able to return to normal activity about the 20th day. Epilation starts at second week if dose greater than 3 Sv (300 rem).

3. *Bone marrow depression stage.* Anemia; leukopenia; thrombocytopenia. Abrupt malaise; fatigue; exertional dyspnea; frank hemorrhages; purpura; stomatitis; fever. This stage culminates at the 30th day.

4. *Recovery phase.* After having survived the crisis, progressive recovery and subsidence of symptoms within another 30 days.

5. *Convalescence.* Starting approximately at the 60th day and complete by 90th day.

Etiology. Exposure to penetrating X-ray, gamma, or neutron radiation.

See table for relation between dose and effect. Depending on dose received, three main clinical forms result:

1. *Hematopoietic form* (1 Sv). Already described in stage 3; death may result within 2 months.

2. *Gastrointestinal form* (5 Sv). Prodromal: nausea within a few minutes, vomiting, diarrhea. Latent: asymptomatic up to sixth day. Third stage: hematologic changes plus nausea, vomiting, diarrhea, paralytic ileus, circulatory collapse, death. *Pathology.* Small intestine distended; congestion of wall; mucosa edematous, hemorrhagic; erosion of epithelial lining, and ulceration with superimposed infection. Bone marrow and lymphatic system aplasia.

3. *Cerebral form* (20 Sv). Prodromal: weakness, drowsiness within 1 hour progressing to apathy, lethargy. Within 3 hours, seizures, ataxic movements. If surviving this phase, prostration and death in 2–3 days. *Pathology.* Brain edema; pyknosis of granule cell layer of cerebellum.

Diagnostic Procedures. *Blood.* Leukopenia; anemia; thrombocytopenia; chromosomal aberrations (dyantrics, rings).

Therapy. Prodromal stage. Psychological reassurance.

Dose (Sv)	Clinical Effect
<0.5	Asymptomatic or trivial effects (moderate bone marrow depression).
0.5–1	Trivial and transitory clinical manifestations.
1.0–1.5	30% of patients: prodromal phase and bone marrow depression phase. Ambulatory; no major medical problem.
1.5–2.0	80% show typical four stages of radiation syndrome. Hospitalization required from third stage on. Generally good prognosis, recovery to normal life.
2–4	Typical acute radiation syndrome; serious manifestation requiring hospitalization and intensive care. Recovery, possibly to normal life, depending on prompt and adequate treatment.
4–6	Typical picture of acute radiation syndrome or fulminating course: up to 5 Sv, hematopoietic changes determine clinical effects and outcome (see); up to 6 Sv, gastrointestinal form of acute radiation syndrome (see).
10–20	Fulminating course, cerebral form of acute radiation syndrome

If necessary, sedation. Hematopoietic form. Antibiotic as soon as signs of infection appear. (*Caution:* bone marrow depression.) Transfusion of blood or separated platelets (or both) and leukocytes. Injection of compatible bone marrow (on well-defined conditions). *Gastrointestinal form.* Parenteral nutrition; fluid and electrolyte balance. Antibiotics; aseptic environment; blood transfusion. *Cerebral form.* Heavy sedation to prevent seizures.

Prognosis. See Therapy.

BIBLIOGRAPHY. Gerstner HB: Acute radiation syndrome in man: Military and civil defense aspects. US Armed Forces Med J 9:313–354, 1958
Upton AC: Radiation Injury. The University of Chicago Press, 1969
Milory NC: Management of irradiated and contaminated casualty victims. Emerg Med Clin North Am 2:667–686, 1984
American Medical Assoc: A Guide to the Hospital Management of Injuries Arising from Exposure to or Involving Ionizing Radiation. Chicago, AMA, 1985
Strambi E: Accidental radiation injuries, whole-body radiation syndrome. In Manni C, Magalini SI (eds): Emergency and Disaster Medicine, pp 355–360. Berlin, Springer-Verlag, 1985
Tubiana M, Dutreix J, Wambersie A: Radiobiologie. Hermann, Paris, 1986
Weatherall DJ, Ledingham JGG, Warrell DA: Oxford Textbook of Medicine, pp 1218–1219. Oxford, Oxford Med Pub, 1996

RADIATION ARTHROPATHY

Symptoms and Signs. Occurs after radiation exposure. Asymptomatic for years; then pain and swelling and erythema of tender areas.

Etiology. Roentgen radiation.

Pathology. Degenerative changes of cartilage. Chondrocalcinosis; ankylosis; rheumatoid-like changes; osteochondritis.

Diagnostic Procedures. *X-ray.* Narrowing of articular spaces; periarticular osteoporosis; marginal bone formation.

Therapy. None.

Prognosis. Variable evolution with final ankylosing of degeneration changes.

BIBLIOGRAPHY. Kolar J, Urabe CR, Chyba J: Arthropathies after irradiation. J Bone Joint Surg (Am) 49:1157–1166, 1967

RADIATION FIBROMATOSIS

Synonyms. Postradiation pseudosarcoma. See Pinkus (H.) I.

Symptoms and Signs. Onset usually 5 years after radiotherapy (from 16 months to 27 years). Firm small nodule developing at the radiation site.

Etiology. Exaggerated response to previous radiation.

Pathology. Histology varies greatly: Poorly differentiated fibroblastic lesions with bizarre mitotic figures, giant nuclei, to orderly interlacing bundles of spindle cells of connective tissue.

Therapy. Excision.

Prognosis. Benign; lack of recurrence after excision. No metastasis.

BIBLIOGRAPHY. Schultz F, ed. The X-ray Treatment of Skin Diseases, pp 135–151. London, Rebman, 1912
Samitz MH: Pseudosarcoma, pseudomalignant neoplasm as a consequence of radiodermatitis. Arch Dermatol 96:283–285, 1967
Schneider AB, Shore-Freedman E, Ryo UV, et al: Radiation induced tumors of the head and neck following childhood irradiation: Prospective study. Medicine 64:1–15, 1984
Dawber RPR, Ebling FJG, Wojnarowska FT: Disorders of hair. In Champion RH, Burton JL, Ebling FJG (eds): Rook/Wilkinson/Ebling Textbook of Dermatology, 5th ed, p. 2607. Oxford, Blackwell Scientific, 1992

RADIATION HEPATITIS

Synonym. Liver radiation

Symptoms and Signs. Onset usually 4 weeks after radiation of liver area. Mimics Budd-Chiari (see). Jaundice; ascites; painful hepatomegaly.

Etiology. Radiation.

Pathology. Intrahepatic venules damaged with resulting congestion of liver. Minimal histologic changes in the parenchyma.

Diagnostic Procedures. Demonstration of patency of hepatic vein. *Biopsy.* Of liver. *Angiography. Liver scan. Blood.* Liver function tests. Alkaline phosphatase high.

Prognosis. Variable according to amount of radiation. Acute venous congestion may result in death.

BIBLIOGRAPHY. Ingold JA, Reed GB, Kaplan HS, et al: Radiation hepatitis. Am J Roentgenol 93:200–208, 1965
Lansing AM, Davis WM, Brizel HE: Radiation hepatitis. Arch Surg 96:878–882, 1968

RADIATION MYELOPATHY

Symptoms and Signs. Several months after radiation therapy: (1) transitory purely sensory, subjective symptoms; (2) acute onset of paraplegia or quadriplegia; and (3) progressive myelopathy; atrophy of irradiated cord segments.

Etiology. X-ray radiation. Vascular damage plays an important role, and neurologic damage appears secondary.

BIBLIOGRAPHY. Alajouanine TH, Ullmann M: Ramollisement médulaire au-dessus d'une tumeur extra-durale métastatique par compression des vaisseaux radiculaires correspondants. Rev Neur 69:169–175, 1938

Lazorthes G: Pathology classification and clinical aspects of vascular diseases of the spinal cord. In Vinken PJ, Bruyn GW: Handbook of Clinical Neurology, vol 12, p 501. Amsterdam, North-Holland, 1972

RADIATION NEPHRITIS

Synonyms. Irradiation nephritis, nephritis radiation.

Symptoms and Signs. Rare today because of better protective techniques. Onset after 6–12 months from exposure; shorter period of latency in children. Blood hypertension; symptoms and signs of anemia.

Etiology. Radiation of renal areas.

Diagnostic Procedures. *Urine.* Proteinuria. *Blood.* Evidence of progressive renal insufficiency.

Therapy. Responds to nephrectomy when one kidney is protected or to renal transplantation.

Prognosis. According to evolution benign or malignant hypertension and treatment.

BIBLIOGRAPHY. Hartman FW, Bolliger A, Doub HP: Experimental nephritis produced by irradiation. Am J Med Sci 172:487–500, 1926

Luxton RW: Radiation nephritis: A long term study of 54 patients. Lancet 2:1221, 1961

Weatherall DJ, Ledingham JGG, Warrell DA: Oxford Textbook of Medicine, p 3231. Oxford, Oxford Med Pub, 1996

RADIATION PNEUMONITIS

Synonym. Irradiation pneumonia.

Symptoms. Insidious onset 1–6 months after completion of roentgen therapy. Dry nonproductive cough; asthenia; fever; exertional dyspnea. Inability to inhale at full lung capacity; seldom, hemopthysis.

Signs. Tachycardia; crepitation at inspiration; signs of consolidation; seldom, friction rubs.

Etiology. From doses of 20 Gy, possibility of radiation pneumonitis; dose of 50–60 Gy (in 5–6 weeks) always causes the syndrome.

Pathology. Initially, electron microscopy shows loss of type II alveolar cells and surfactant depletion; then pulmonary hypertension develops from obliteration of vascular bed. Effects from superimposed infections and heart failure are difficult to separate from primary X-ray effects. The acute pneumonic reaction is characterized by exudation and desquamation of cells into alveolar space, vascular lesions, and deposit of connective tissue and lymphocytes into septa. The late or fibrotic stage is characterized by replacement of normal tissue by fibrous tissue.

Diagnostic Procedures. *X-ray.* Consolidation of lung parenchyma, patchy or confluent; volume loss; in rare cases, hyperlucent lung (see Burke). Pulmonary function tests.

Therapy. Symptomatic. Prednisolone or mustine hydrochloride.

Prognosis. Acute pneumonia may last 1 month and regress completely or evolve into pulmonary fibrosis and chronic respiratory insufficiency. Radiation therapy may be responsible for successive development of carcinomas.

BIBLIOGRAPHY. Gross NJ: Pulmonary effects of radiation therapy. Ann Intern Med 86:81–92, 1977

Roberts CM, Foulchene E, Zaunders JJ, et al: Radiation pneumonitis: A possible lymphocyte-mediated hypersensitivity reaction. Ann Int Med 119:1050–1051, 1993

RAEDER

Synonyms. Hornes incomplete; paratrigeminal paralysis; oculopupillary paratrigeminal paralysis. See Horton and orbital apex.

Symptoms. Reported almost exclusively in males. Unilateral, deep, severe pain concentrated around the eyes, sometimes self-limited, with complete recovery. Other times, continuous with exacerbations or relapsing after free periods. Occasionally with various combinations of parasellar nerve involvements: optic (II), oculomotor (III), trochlear (IV), abducens (VI).

Signs. Ptosis and myosis (sometimes not easily noticeable). Absence of facial sweating (differentiates this syndrome from Horner's); conjunctival injection and lacrimation (usually present).

Etiology. Neoplastic, traumatic, inflammatory, vascular, or idiopathic lesion that damages the oculosympathetic fibers distally to the bifurcation of the external carotid artery (in this way sparing the sweating fibers).

Pathology. Tumor; abscess; aneurysms. When parasellar involvement (Raeder paratrigeminal syndrome group I lesion in anterior part of middle cranial fossa), some causes with various localization in group II (without parasellar nerves involvement), such as abscessed tooth, internal carotid aneurysms.

Diagnostic Procedures. *X-ray.* Of skull and neck. *Arteriography.*

Prognosis. According to etiology.

BIBLIOGRAPHY. Raeder JG: Paratrigeminal paralysis of oculopupillary sympathetic. Brain 47:149–158, 1924

Law WR, Nelson ER: Internal carotid aneurysm as a cause of Raeder's paratrigeminal syndrome. Neurology 18:43–46, 1968

Brandel JP, Chapon F, Viader F, et al: Syndrome de Raeder du a une dissection carotidienne. Press Med 16:541, 1987

Weatherall DJ, Ledingham JGG, Warrell DA: Oxford Textbook of Medicine, p 3877. Oxford, Oxford Med Pub, 1996

RAMBAN-HASHARON

Symptoms and Signs. In males. Cranio-facial dysmorphism; microcephaly; central hypotonia; seizures; mental development retardation; recurrent respiratory infections.

Etiology. Autosomal recessive inheritance. Possibility of glycosylation defect. Patients fail to incorporate fucose into cell-surface carbohydrates, thus lack carbohydrate ligands for selection family of adhesion molecules.

Diagnostic Procedures. *Blood.* Remarkable neutrophilia, with defects of random and directed migration and decreased homotypic aggregation, opsonophagocytic and bacterial activity is normal; absence of red-blood cell H antigen (manifest Bombay (hh) phenotype). *X-ray. MRI. Cortical atrophy.*

BIBLIOGRAPHY. Frydman M, Etzioni A Eidlitz-Markus T, et al: Rambam-Hasharon syndrome of psychomotor retardation, short stature defective neutrophil motility and Bombay phenotype. Am J Med Genet 44:297–302, 1992

RAMON

Synonyms. Cherubism; gingival fibromatosis; epilepsy; mental deficiency; hypertrichosis.

Symptoms and Signs. Both sexes. Seizures. Mental deficiency becomes evident in first years; gengival fibromatosis by second year; seizures by fourth year. Evident after fourth year: cherubism (maxillary fibrous dysplasia) and stunted growth. Hypertrichosis (50%), juvenile rheumatoid arthritis (may be a component of the syndrome).

Etiology. Unknown. Autosomal recessive inheritance. Some of the same features are induced by phenytoin administration.

Pathology. Gengival biopsy. Perivascular pattern of collagen fibers that compress blood vessels.

BIBLIOGRAPHY. Ramon Y, Berman W, Bubis JJ: Gingival fibromatosis combined with cherubism. Oral Surg 24:436–448, 1967
Pina-Neto JM, Moreno AFC, Silva LR, et al: Cherubism, gingival fibromatosis, epilepsy and mental deficiency (Ramon syndrome) with juvenile rheumatoid arthritis. Am J Med Genet 25:433–441, 1986

RAMOS-ARROYO

Synonyms. Corneal hypoesthesia; retinal abnormality; deafness; unusual facies; ductus arteriosus; mental retardation.

Symptoms. Both sexes. Hypoesthetic corneas, visual disturbances, sensineural deafness. Mental retardation.

Signs. *Unusual facies.* Hypertelorism, flat profile, frontal bossing, depressed nasal bridge, midface hypoplasia.

Etiology. Unknown. Possible autosomal dominant inheritance.

Pathology. *Eye.* Lack of pericapillary choriocapillaritis and retinal pigment epithelium. Persistent ductus arteriosus.

Therapy. Surgery for patent ductus.

Prognosis. Good quoad vitam.

BIBLIOGRAPHY. Ramos-Arroyo MA, Clark GG, Saksena SS, et al: Congenital corneal anesthesia, with retinal abnormalities, deafness, unusual facies, persistent ductus arteriosus and mental retardation: A new syndrome? Am J Med Genet 26:349–354, 1987

RAPADILINO

Synonyms. Radial aplasia (RA); patellar aplasia/hypoplasia and cleft/high palate (PA); diarrhea and dislocated joints (DI); little size and limb malformations (LI); long slender nose and normal intelligence (NO).

Symptoms. Both sexes. All families originate from Finland. Diarrhea in infancy. Normal intelligence.

Signs. Main signs radial and patellar aplasia. Additional feature: joint dislocation. *Face.* Long nose, small chin, unusual ears, cleft or high arched palate. Small stature.

Etiology. Sporadic and autosomal recessive inheritance.

BIBLIOGRAPHY. Kaariainen H, Ryoppy S, Norio R: RAPADILINO syndrome with radial and patellar aplasia/hypoplasia as main manifestation. Am J Med Genet 33:346–351, 1989

RAPE TRAUMA

Symptoms and Signs. Begin with the physical assault; however, weeks may elapse between the assault and the emergence of reaction. *Phase 1.* Disorganization (acute). *Phase 2.* Reorganization (long-term process).

Etiology. Distress of psychological trauma, compounded by added medical and legal stresses.

BIBLIOGRAPHY. Burgess A, Hofmstrom L: Rape trauma syndrome. Am J Psychiatr 131:981–986, 1974
Ochberg F (ed): Post-traumatic therapy and victims of violence. New York, Brunner/Mazel, 1988
Prentky RA, Vernon L: Human sexual aggression: Current perspectives. NY Acad Sci 528, 1988
Kaplan HI, Sadock BJ: Comprehensive Textbook of Psychiatry, 6th ed, pp 1733–1736. Baltimore, Williams & Wilkins, 1995
Weatherall DJ, Ledingham JGG, Warrell DA: Oxford Textbook of Medicine, pp 4313, 4314, 4257. Oxford, Oxford Med Pub, 1996

RAPIDLY PROGRESSING NEPHRITIS

Synonyms. Nephritis, rapidly progressing. This condition includes three types of disease: See Idiopathic diffuse crescenting glomerulonephritis types I, II, and III.

Symptoms. Extracapillary proliferative glomerulonephritis; rapidly progressing nephritis.

Symptoms. Prevalent in males. Onset in adolescence and young adulthood (in women at any age). Onset seldom acute, usually insidious. Anorexia; diarrhea; smoky urine; oliguria (more severe than in acute nephritic syndrome).

Signs. *Blood.* Hypertension (less severe than in acute nephritis).

Etiology. Usually idiopathic. In 30% of cases preceding streptococcal infection. This syndrome may be associated also with other conditions, e.g., Goodpasture; infective endocarditis; Schönlein-Henoch; vasculitis; lupus erythematosus.

Pathology. See Idiopathic diffuse crescenting glomerulonephritis.

Therapy. Anticoagulants; adrenocorticosteroids. Chronic dialysis. Kidney transplantation. Plasmapheresis may be helpful.

Prognosis. See specific diseases.

BIBLIOGRAPHY. Oredugba O, Mazumdar DC, Meyer JS, et al: Pulse methylprednisolone therapy in idiopathic rapidly progressive glomerulonephritis. Ann Intern Med 92:504–506, 1980
Weatherall DJ, Ledingham JGG, Warrell DA: Oxford Textbook of Medicine, pp 3162–3167. Oxford, Oxford Med Pub, 1996

RAPP-HODGKIN

Synonyms. Ectodermal hypohidrotic dysplasia; anhidrotic ectodermal dysplasia. See also Christ-Siemens.

Symptoms and Signs. Both sexes affected. Recognized in early infancy. Hyperthermia (episodes); hypohidrosis; variable growth deficiency. Low nasal bridge; narrow nose; hypoplastic maxilla; small mouth; cleft lip, palate, uvula. Thin skin; sparse fine hair (pili canaliculi); small dysplastic nails; hypodontia; conical teeth. Hypospadias. Purulent conjunctivitis and otitis media.

Etiology. Autosomal dominant inheritance. Of doubtful autonomy; appears to be a mild variant of Christ-Siemens (see).

Pathology. See Symptoms and Signs. Sweat pores present but reduced in number. Hairs show canal-like depression along length of axis.

BIBLIOGRAPHY. Rapp RS, Hodgkin WE: Anhidrotic ectodermal dysplasia. Autosomal dominant inheritance with palate and lip anomalies. J Med Genet 5:269–272, 1968

Stasiowska B, Sartoris S, Goitre M, et al: Rapp-Hodgkin ectodermal dysplasia syndrome. Arch Dis Child 56:793–795, 1981

Breslau-Siderius EJ, Laveijsen APM, Otten FWA, et al: The Rapp-Hodgkin syndrome. Am J Med Genet 38:107–110, 1991

RAPUNZEL

Synonyms. Bezoar; phytobezoar; trichobezoar.

Symptoms. Dragging or fullness in upper abdominal quadrant; epigastric pain (70%); nausea and vomiting (64%).

Signs. Mass palpable in epigastric region of phytobezoar (54%) and of trichobezoar (88%). Signs of peritonitis (7–10%).

Etiology. Food or ingurgitated matter that has formed a compact body, occasionally assuming the aspect of long strands of twisted hair extending from the bezoar through the intestine.

Diagnostic Procedures. *X-ray.* Direct demonstration of the presence of foreign body. *Gastroscopy.* Best diagnostic tool. *Endoscopic biopsy. Blood.* Hypochromia; microcytic anemia; slight white blood cell elevation.

Therapy. Enzymatic approach (papain every 3 hours); endoscopic fragmentation; surgery.

Prognosis. Spontaneous resolution may occur. Good with treatment.

BIBLIOGRAPHY. Vaugh EE Jr, Sawyers JL, Scott HW Jr: The Rapunzel syndrome: An unusual complication of intestinal bezoar. Surgery 63:339–343, 1968

Clearfield HR: Trauma, bezoar, and other foreign bodies. In Haubrich WS, Schaffner F, Berk JE (eds): Bockus Gastroenterology, 5th ed, pp 836–838. Philadelphia, WB Saunders, 1995

RAVENNA

Synonyms. Achondroplasia tarda; atypical achondroplasia; hypochondroplasia; Leri hypochondroplasia.

Symptoms and Signs. Both sexes affected. Evident at birth or within third year. At birth, height 47.7 cm and weight 2.9 kg. Characteristic sign; a block just short of full extension of elbow. Head larger than rest of body. Shortened limbs; leg bowing less frequent than in achondroplasia. Mild motor delay; unusual mental retardation; behavioral problems common. Slow growth eventually determining a mild disproportionate dwarfism (with short limbs); final height 127–152.4 cm; joint relaxation; small but normal hands and feet.

Etiology. Autosomal dominant inheritance with complete penetrance. This syndrome probably is caused by an allele of achondroplasia (see).

Pathology. See Diagnostic Procedures.

Diagnostic Procedures. *X-ray.* Normal bones of skull, hands, and feet. Long bone short and larger, with exaggerated physiologic bowing. Femoral neck length shortened; greater trochanters prominent. Knee epiphyses squared aspect. Fibulas longer, causing mild varus ankle. Vertebral canal narrowed. Sacrum hypoplastic. *Blood. Urine.* Normal.

Therapy. Minor orthopedic correction for feet, knees. Physical therapy. Cesarean section for pregnancy.

Prognosis. Adults report myofascial pain, bursitis, lumbosacral strain. No neurologic alteration. IQ reduced to 50–80 points.

BIBLIOGRAPHY. Ravenna F: Achondroplasia et chondrohypoplasie: Contribution clinique. Nouv Iconogr Salpetriere 26:157–184, 1913

Leri A, Linossier M: Hypochondroplasia hereditaire. Bull Méd Soc Med Hop (Paris), 48:1780–1787, 1924

Sillence DO, Horton WA, Rinoin DL: Morphologic studies in the skeletal dysplasias: A review. Am J Pathol 96:813–870, 1979

Rimoin DL: Genetic disorders of the osseous system. In Beithon P: McKusick's Heritable Disorders of Connective Tissue, 5th ed, p 578. St Louis, CV Mosby, 1993

RAY

Synonym. Amorality. Eponym used to indicate a lack of moral sense and of relative restraints to comply with socially accepted moral rules, and the consequent antisocial activity related to the violation of established rules. Antisocial behavior is found in several psychiatric disorders, and this eponym is of only historical value.

BIBLIOGRAPHY. Ray I: A Treatise on the Medical Jurisprudence of Insanity. London, Hendersonn, 1837

Staller RJ: Does sexual perversion exist? Johns Hopkins Med J 134:43–57, 1974

Kaplan HI, Sadock BJ: Comprehensive Textbook of Psychiatry, 4th ed, pp 959, 2047. Baltimore, Williams & Wilkins, 1985

RAYMOND-CÉSTAN

Synonyms. Céstan; Foville, superior type. Raymond-Foville, dissociation of lateral gaze; pontine.

Symptoms and Signs. Unilateral abducens paralysis; paralysis of lateral conjugate gaze; contralateral hemiplegia; anesthesia of face, extremities, and trunk.

Etiology. Hemorrhage; thrombosis tumor with nuclear lesion involving pyramidal tract. The postlongitudinal bundle and the medial lemniscus also may be involved.

BIBLIOGRAPHY. Raymond F, Céstan R: Trois observations de paralysie des mouvements associés des globes oculaires. Rev Neurol (Paris) 9:70–77, 1901

Adams RD, Victor M: Principles of Neurology, 5th ed, p 1173. New York, McGraw-Hill, 1993

RAYNAUD

Synonyms. Symmetric gangrene; symmetric asphyxia. See also Raynaud phenomenon.

Symptoms. Prevalent in females (5:1); usually begins in first or second decade. Reported in five children in whom no clinical, hematologic, or immunologic evidence of a collagen disorder was found. As a rule, cold is the precipitating factor for onset of symptoms. Emotional stress also may be a precipitating factor. Episodes of color change in fingers beginning and increasing gradually; occasionally, dramatic onset of intense manifestation (dead finger phenomenon). Usually after exposure of the fingers to cold, pallor, cyanosis, and rubor appear, followed by pain and paresthesia. Initially only the tips of one or two fingers are involved. With time, the phenomenon extends to involve all fingers and rest of the hand. Bilaterality (diagnostic criterion). Absence of systemic manifestation.

Signs. Transient changes in color of fingers; cold and slight swelling during attacks. Sclerodermatous changes of the skin after repeated attacks and occasionally minor gangrenous changes.

Etiology. Unknown. Functional vasospastic condition. Raynaud syndrome (idiopathic) has to be differentiated from Raynaud phenomenon syndrome (see) and from thromboangiitis obliterans, arteriosclerosis obliterans, Mitchell syndrome I, and scleroderma. Described cases with autosomal dominant phenotype.

Pathology. In advanced stages, thickening of intima of digital arteries. When trophic lesion, obstructed arteries and area of necrosis eventually develop.

Diagnostic Procedures. Rule out conditions associated with Raynaud phenomenon (see).

Therapy. Protection of extremities from cold and injuries. Moving to a warmer climate is sometimes indicated. Mild Raynaud disease, when associated with menopausal symptoms or menstrual periods, may benefit from estrogen administration. Tolazoline hydrochloride, phenoxybenzamine hydrochloride, Hydergine. Local application of glyceryl trinitrate and reserpine may be used with moderate success in mild form, but usually results are disappointing. In the reported children, oral phenoxybenzamine proved useful for maintenance treatment, whereas during acute attacks infusions of prostacyclin, nitroprusside, and ketanserin were used. Sympathectomy when attacks frequent and severe.

Prognosis. Normal life span. Several patients present a nonprogressive course with periodic exacerbations. Results of sympathectomy are fairly good in idiopathic Raynaud (60%), but are disappointing in secondary Raynaud phenomenon. (Importance of correct diagnosis before major treatment considered.)

BIBLIOGRAPHY. Raynaud AGM: De L'asphyxie Local et de la Gangrène Symaetrique des Extrémités, pp 6–9. Paris, Rignoux, 1862

Fries JF: Clinical significance of Raynaud's phenomenon. Med Digest June 15–20, 1967

Burns EC, Dunger DB, Dillon MJ: Raynaud's disease. Arch Dis Child 60:537, 1985

Champion RH: Reactions to cold. In Champion RH, Burton JL, Ebling FJG (eds): Rook/Wilkinson/Ebling Textbook of Dermatology, 5th ed, pp 842–843. Oxford, Blackwell Scientific, 1992

Weatherall DJ, Ledingham JGG, Warrell DA: Oxford Textbook of Medicine, pp 2365, 2374. Oxford, Oxford Med Pub, 1990

RAYNAUD PHENOMENON

Episode of constriction of small arteries or arterioles (or both) of extremities, with change in color of the skin, pallor, cyanosis. This phenomenon is observed in several clinical entities:

1. *Raynaud syndrome*

2. *Post-traumatic conditions*
   Frostbite
   Pneumatic hammer syndrome
   After injury or surgery
   Typists' and pianists' vasospastic phenomenon

3. *Neurogenic conditions*
   Carpal tunnel syndrome
   Diseases of nervous system
   Shoulder-girdle compression syndromes

4. *Occlusive arterial diseases*
   Arteriosclerosis obliterans
   Embolism
   Thromboangiitis obliterans
   Thrombosis

5. *Intoxications*
   Ergot
   Heavy metals

6. *Miscellaneous conditions*
   Cold hemoagglutination
   Dermatomyositis
   Lupus erythematosus
   Marchiafava-Micheli syndrome
   Rheumatoid arthritis
   Scleroderma syndromes
   Waldenström syndrome I

BIBLIOGRAPHY. Raynaud AGM: De l'asphyxie Locale et de la Gangrene Symètrique des Extrémitiés. Paris, Rignoux, 1862

Coffman JD: Raynaud's Phenomenon. New York, Oxford, 1989

Weatherall DJ, Ledingham JGG, Warrell DA: Oxford Textbook of Medicine, p 3028. Oxford, Oxford Med Pub, 1990

REAVEN

Synonyms. Insulin resistance; X (not to be confused with the other X-syndrome, the Microvascular angina, so denominated by cardiologists); C.H.A.O.S. (coronary artery disease, hypertension, adult onset diabetes, obesity, stroke); deadly quartet (upper body obesity, glucose intolerance, hypertriglyceridemia, hypertension); G.H.O. (glucose intolerance, hypertension, obesity). See Rabson-Mendenhall.

Symptoms and Signs. The possible clustering of risk factors for coronary artery disease–high blood pressure and associated insulin resistance are indicated with this eponym; where there are interacting hyperinsulinemia, impaired glucose tolerance, or non-insulin-dependent diabetes mellitus, increased plasma triglyceride concentration, and decreased HDL-cholesterol concentration.

Etiology. Suggested that resistance to insulin-stimulated glucose uptake is involved in the etiology of non-insulin-dependent diabetes mellitus, hypertension, and coronary artery disease.

BIBLIOGRAPHY. Reaven GM: Role of insulin resistance in human disease. Diabetes 37:1595–1607, 1988

Davidson MB: Clinical implications of insulin resistance syndromes. Am J Med 99:420–426, 1995

REBEITZ-KOLODNY-RICHARDSON

Synonyms. R.K.R.; achromasia neural—corticodentatonigral degeneration.

Symptoms. Occurs in late middle age. Clumsiness and slowness of movement of left limbs (presenting symptoms), then widespread. Severe impairment in control of muscular movements, postural abnormalities, involuntary muscular activity. Moderate muscular weakness. Mental faculties relatively spared. Tremor constant but not too severe. Finally, severe contractures, dysphagia, and speech impairment.

Signs. Paralysis of ocular muscles; exaggeration of myotonic reflexes and increased resistance to passive stretching of affected muscles. Babinski sign.

Etiology. Unknown. Possibly, metabolic failure at cellular level. Richardson-Steele-Oslzewski syndrome (see) bears some similarity with this syndrome, but pathologically the two syndromes appear different. Some clinical aspects of this syndrome are also shared with Pick (see), Alzheimer (see), Huntington (see), Parkinson (see), and, most of all, with Jakob-Creutzfeldt (see). So many clearly different features of each of these syndromes from the present one, however, allow this to be considered as a separate clinical entity.

Pathology. Alterations limited to brain: convolutional atrophy, especially parietal and frontal; lateral and third ventricles enlarged. No vascular alterations. Nerve cells in anterior cortex disappear. Astrocytic gliosis; slight microglial activity; signs of inflammation absent. Some of remaining nerve cells show swelling of cell body, displacement of nucleus, achromasia, hyaline cytoplasm, and vacuolization. Substantia nigra also shows loss of pigmented cells; corpus of Louys, dentate, and roof nuclei of cerebellum also loss of cells. Cerebellar cortex unaffected.

Diagnostic Procedures. *CSF. Normal. EEG.* Unspecific slow and sharp waves activity. *CT brain scan. MRI. Cerebral atrophy.*

Therapy. Symptomatic.

Prognosis. Years of slowly progressing incapacity. Death within 6–8 years of onset.

BIBLIOGRAPHY. Rebeitz JJ, Kolodny H, Richardson EP: Corticodentatonigral degeneration with achromasia. Arch Neurol 18:20–33, 1968

Adams RD, Victor M: Principles of Neurology, 5th ed, p 974. New York, McGraw-Hill, 1993

RECLUS II

Synonyms. Cooper; ligneous phlegmon.

Symptoms and Signs. Abscess on the neck that causes a woody induration of subcutaneous connective tissue; pain; fever; general malaise.

Etiology. Infective.

Pathology. Suppuration with secondary fibrosis of subcutaneous tissue.

Therapy. Surgery and antibiotics.

Prognosis. According to the adequacy of treatment.

BIBLIOGRAPHY. Reclus P: Phlégmon ligneux du cou. Rev Chir (Paris) 16:522–531, 1896

RECTAL ULCER

Synonyms. Solitary rectal ulcer.

Symptoms and Signs. Long history of defecation disorders; rectal bleeding.

Etiology. Disthrophic reaction to chronic injury.

Pathology. Benign mucosal lesion in the distal anterior wall of rectum.

Diagnostic Procedures. *Rectoscopy.* Granulation of rectal mucosa, rectal stricture, thick rectal folds. *Barium enema; defecography.* Rectocele, prolapse, abnormal perineal descent.

Therapy. Surgical.

BIBLIOGRAPHY. Madigan MR, Morson BC: Solitary ulcer of the rectum. Gut 10:871–881, 1969
Goei R, Baeten C, Arends JW: Solitary rectal ulcer syndrome: Findings at barium enema study and defecography. Radiology 168:303–306, 1988

RECTUS MUSCLE

Synonym. Rectus muscle hematoma.

Symptoms. Occurs in late middle life; more frequent in women than in men. Sudden, severe pain on either side of midline, always below the level of umbilicus; moderate increase in temperature, prostration; vomiting; hyperpnea; shock. In some cases, slow development of a mass without acute symptoms.

Signs. Very tender mass at site of pain, remaining fixed; ecchymotic discoloration; tachycardia. If patient partially sits up, the mass cannot be moved laterally. No tenderness elicited in tissues surrounding the mass. Localized tonic contraction; absence of generalized rigidity.

Etiology. Sudden muscular contraction (cough; sneeze; vomiting; movement); associated frequently with infections or other conditions (pregnancy; intoxication) that result in weakening and atrophy of muscle. Degeneration of blood vessels; blood dyscrasia. In many spontaneous cases no causes can be found.

Pathology. Vascular hyaline degeneration; muscle granulation; and hyaline degeneration suggesting degenerative process prior to rupture. Hematoma formed by blood extravasated among degenerated fibers, or may be completely separated.

Diagnostic Procedures. See Signs. *Needle aspiration. Laboratory. Noncontributory. X-ray and/or xerography of abdominal wall. Surgical exploration.*

Prognosis. Good, depending on underlying or concurrent disease.

Mortality 4–5%; in pregnancy, maternal mortality 12% and fetal mortality 25–50%.

BIBLIOGRAPHY. Payne RL: Spontaneous rupture of the superior and inferior epigastric arteries within the rectus abdominal sheath. Ann Surg 108:757–768, 1938
Jones TW, Merendino KA: The deep epigastric artery: Rectus muscle syndrome. Am J Surg 103:159–169, 1962

RED DIAPER

Synonym. Serratia marcescens gastrointestinal.

Symptoms. None.

Signs. Diaper turns red 24–36 hours after soiling.

Etiology. Serratia marcescens established as predominant gastrointestinal bacterial species.

Pathology. None.

Diagnostic Procedures. *Stool.* Culture.

Therapy. Sulfasalazine, gentamycin, and revision of diet.

Prognosis. Serratia marcescens is overgrown by usual bacterial intestinal flora as soon as change in diet is begun and sulfa treatment given.

BIBLIOGRAPHY. Waisman H, Stone WH: The presence of Serratia marcescens as the predominating organism in the intestinal tract of the newborn: The occurrence of the "red diaper syndrome." Pediatrics 21:8–12, 1958

RED-EYED SHUNT

Synonym. Carotid cavernous fistula.

Symptoms. Ocular pain; diplopia; noise in the head.

Signs. Red eye, proptosis, evident episcleral vessels, exophthalmos, limited eye motion.

Etiology. Carotid-cavernous fistula.

Diagnostic Procedures. *Sonography.* Dilatation of superior ophthalmic vein. Increased intraocular pressure.

Therapy. Surgical.

Prognosis. Good with treatment.

BIBLIOGRAPHY. The diagnosis and prognosis of atypical carotid-cavernous fistula (red eyed shunt syndrome). Am J Ophthal 93:424–436, 1982

REDLICH

Obsolete.

Synonym. Flatau; Munch-Patersen. Abortive disseminated encephalomyelitis; cerebrospinal meningitis, epidemic; encephalomyelitis funicularis infectiosa. Could be considered as a variant of von Economo encephalitis (see).

BIBLIOGRAPHY. Redlich E: Ueber abortive Formen der Encephalomyelitis disseminata. Dtsch Med Wochenschr 55:562–563, 1929

RED MAN

Synonym. Rifampicin toxicity, including Red-neck.

Symptoms and Signs. Orange and red "glowing" discoloration of the skin, facial or periorbital edema, pruritus of the head, vomiting.

Etiology. It is a toxic reaction and/or allergic among children inadvertently given excessive doses of rifampicin for chemoprophylaxis of Haemophilus influenzae disease (20–200 times normal dose) or suicidal attempt in adults. Described also after vancomycin administration (Redneck).

Diagnostic Procedures. *Serum*. Transient liver enzymes alteration.

Therapy. Symptomatic. Prevention: Attention to detail in calculating the dose to be given and in the preparation and administration of the drug. Corticosteroids.

Prognosis. Rapid remission.

BIBLIOGRAPHY. Newton RW, Forrest ARW: Rifampicin overdosage. "The red man syndrome." Scot Med J 20:55–56, 1975
Bolan G, Laurie RE, Broome CV: Red man syndrome: Inadvertent administration of an excessive dose of rifampin. Pediatrics 77:633–635, 1986
Levi M, Koren G, Dupuis L, et al: Vancomycin-induced red man syndrome. Pediatrics 86:572–580, 1990
AHFS 95: Drug Information, p 398. HFS Bethesda, 1995

REDUCING BODY MYOPATHY

Synonyms. Granular body myopathy; myopathy, reducing body.

Symptoms and Signs. The cases have been grouped only because of similar istophatological findings. Wide variability of symptoms and signs, shared with various congenital myopathies.

Etiology. Unknown. Reported in sisters.

Pathology. Muscle biopsy: Fibers with inclusions that without enzymatic activity are positive in menandione-linked alpha-glycerophosphate dehydrogenase (MAG) preparation. Two proteins have been identified inside reducing bodies.

Diagnostic Procedures. *Muscle biopsy*. EMG.

Therapy. Symptomatic.

Prognosis. Good quoad vitam.

BIBLIOGRAPHY. Brooke MH, Neville HE: Reducing body myopathy. Neurology 22:829–840, 1972
Huebner G, Pongrate D: Granular Koerper-Myopathie (reducing body myopathy?) Beitrag zur Feinstuktur und Klassifierung. Virkows Arch A (Pathol Anat) 392:97–104, 1981
Goebel HH, Lenard HG: Congenital myopathies. In Rowland LP, Di Mauro S (eds): Handbook of Clinical Neurology, vol 18: The Myopathies, p 331. Amsterdam, Elsevier, 1992

REDUNDANT CAROTID ARTERY

Synonyms. Carotid artery, redundant; kinking carotid artery; intermittent carotid obstruction. See Carotid system ischemia.

Symptoms. Vertigo or transient hemiparesis or episodes of blindness of one eye, when turning the head to one side. Return of vision or disappearance of paresis when turning the head to the midline.

Etiology and Pathology. Tortuosity of carotid artery. Turning of the head produces artery obstruction through kinking of the vessel. Possibly, congenital malformation of carotid artery or acquired arterial dilatation and tortuosity.

Diagnostic Procedures. Arteriography. Doppler.

Therapy. Surgical resection of tortuous vessel with end-to-end anastomosis.

Prognosis. Treatment will usually completely relieve the symptoms.

BIBLIOGRAPHY. Riser M, Geraud J, Ducoudray J, et al: Dolicho-carotide

interne avec syndrome vertigineux. Rev Neurol (Paris) 85:145–147, 1951
Kellogg DR, Smith LL: Recurrent monocular blindness due to a redundant carotid artery. Arch Surg 95:908–910, 1967
Adams RD, Victor M: Principles of Neurology, 5th ed, p 676. New York, McGraw-Hill, 1993

REED

Synonyms. Tietz-Reed; see Woolf; Ziprkowski-Margolis and Albinism oculocutaneous.

Symptoms and Signs. Both sexes affected. Profound deafness and piebaldness (large white forelock and symmetric white spots on arms, legs, and abdomen). Albinism does not affect the eyes (blue iris). Affected subjects tan normally.

Etiology. Autosomal dominant inheritance.

BIBLIOGRAPHY. Tietz WA: Syndrome of deaf-mutism associated with albinism showing autosomal dominant inheritance. Am J Med Genet 15:259–264, 1963
Reed WB, Stone VM, Boder E, et al: Pigmentary disorders in association with congenital deafness. Arch Dermatol 95:176–186, 1967

REESE-BLODI

Synonyms. Reese retinal dysplasia; Krause-Reese; retinal dysplasia Reese.

Symptoms and Signs. Variable owing to malformation of the retina and persistence of primary vitreus. Visceral malformations may be associated.

Etiology. Possibily autosomal recessive inheritance syndrome. It is a characteristic eye change in the Bartolin-Patau (see). It must be differentiated from microphthalmos, anophthalmos, and Norrie (see).

Diagnostic Procedures. Chromosomal studies.

BIBLIOGRAPHY. Yudkin AM: Congenital bilateral microphthalmos accompanied by other malformations of the body. Am J Ophthal II:128–131, 1928
Krause AC: Congenital encephalo-ophthalmic dysplasia. Arch Ophthal 36:387–444, 1946
Reese AB, Blodi FC: Retinal dysplasia. Am J Ophthal 33:23–32, 1950
Matthes A, Stenzel K: Familiaere, encephalo-retinale Dysplasia (Krause-Reesem syndrom) mit myoklonischastatischem Petit Mal. Z Kinderheilk 103:81–89, 1968
Torczynski E: Developmental anomalies of the eye. In Garner A, Klintworth GK (eds): Pathobiology of Ocular Disease: A Dynamic Approach, 2nd ed, p 1316. New York, Marcel Dekker, 1994

REESE-ELLSWORTH

Synonym. Anterior chamber cleavage; iridogoniodysgenesis. See also Axenfeld and Rieger. The three syndromes must be grouped under Axenfeld or Axenfeld-Rieger eponym.

Symptoms. Both sexes affected. Present at birth (80% bilaterally). Decreased visual acuity according to anatomic lesions of cornea. Mental retardation.

Signs. Adhesion between iris and cornea. Mesenchymal tissue in chamber angle. Shallow anterior chamber. Iris coloboma and hypoplasia; corneal opacities of variable density; sclerocornea; anterior pole cataract. Cleft palate, syndactyly, craniofacial dysostosis, myotonic dystrophy may be present.

Etiology. Abnormalities of embryologic development of anterior chamber because of failure of normal migration of mesodermal cells or failure of their differentiation. Virus (rubella) is one of the most frequent agents responsible.

Diagnostic Procedures. Increased intraocular pressure. Remains of hyaloid artery in retina.

Therapy. Surgery according to lesions.

Prognosis. Variable.

BIBLIOGRAPHY. Reese AB, Ellsworth RM: The anterior chamber cleavage syndrome. Arch Ophthalmol 75:307–318, 1966

Holmark J, Jensen OA: Anterior chamber cleavage syndrome: A typical case of Peter's anomaly with primary aphakia. Acta Ophthalmol 50:877–886, 1972

Torczynski E: Developmental anomalies of the eye. In Garner A, Klintworth GK (eds): Pathobiology of ocular disease: A dynamic approach, 2nd ed, p 1397. New York, Marcel Dekker, 1994

REFETOFF

Synonym. Thyroid hormone resistance—deaf mutism—goiter—euthyroidism. See Seabright-Bantam syndrome.

Symptoms and Signs. Both sexes. From infancy: recurrent goiter; deafmutism. No history to suggest thyrotoxicosis or hypothyroidism; other physical signs negative. Growth, development, and intelligence: normal.

Etiology. Possibility of both autosomal dominant and recessive inheritance owing to different mutation in the same gene. Particular resistance of peripheral tissue to the action of thyroid-stimulating hormone (TSH), pituitary also partially resistant to thyroid hormone suppressive action.

Pathology. Thyroid: follicles of unequal size, lined by flat to cuboidal cells with round-oval nuclei; abundant colloid in areas of epithelium projecting into lumen. No lymphocytic infiltration.

Diagnostic Procedures. *Blood.* Markedly elevated serum total and free T3 and T4 levels; normal or elevated serum TSH. Defective function of receptor could be identified (in some cases) in studies of lymphocytes and fibroblasts. *X-ray.* Skeleton survey: stippled epiphyses.

Therapy. No evidence that treatment with thyroid hormone is useful. Thionamides, radioactive iodine or surgery could induce subclinical hypothyroidism.

Prognosis. Except for goiter no other manifestations affect life or functions.

BIBLIOGRAPHY. Refetoff S, DeWind LT, DeGroot LJ: Familial syndrome combining deaf-mutism, stippled epiphyses, goiter and abnormally high. PBI: Possible target organ refractoriness to thyroid hormone. J Clin Endocrinol 27:279–294, 1967

Takeda K, Balzano S, Sakurai AQ, et al: Screening of nineteen unrelated families with generalized resistance to thyroid hormone for known point mutations in the thyroid hormone receptor beta gene and the detection of a new mutation. J Clin Invest 87:496–502, 1991

De Groot LJ: Congenital defects in thyroid hormone formation and action. In De Groot LJ (ed): Endocrinology, 3rd ed, p 881. Philadelphia, WB Saunders, 1995

REFLEX EPILEPSIES

Symptoms. Seizures following a specific external photic stimulus (example: television watching); particular sounds; music; some particular movement; somatosensory; reading. See Sensory seizures syndromes.

BIBLIOGRAPHY. Hall M: Synopsis of Cerebral and Spinal Seizures of Inorganic Origin and of Paroxysmal Form as a Class and of Their Pathology as Involved in the Structures and Action of the Neck, 2nd ed. London, Mallett, 1851

Hishikawa Y, Yamamoto J, Furuya E, et al: Photosensitive epilepsy: Relationships between the visual evoked responses and the epileptiform discharges induced by intermittent photic stimulation. Electroencephalogr Clin Neurophysiol 23:320–334, 1967

Weatherall DJ, Ledingham JGG, Warrell DA: Oxford Textbook of Medicine, p 3918. Oxford, Oxford Med Pub, 1990

REFSUM

Synonyms. Refsum-Thiebaut; ataxia hereditaria—hemeralopia polyneuritiformis; hemeralopia heredoataxia polyneuritiformis; heredopathia atactica polyneuritiformis; phytanic acid storage.

Symptoms. Children develop the condition between 4 and 7 years of age, in some persons, however, as late as fifth decade. Progressive nerve deafness; concentric constriction of visual fields; night blindness; chronic polyneuropathy; involving motor and sensory nerves; cerebellar ataxia; loss of sense of smell. Dramatic exacerbation following febrile episodes, surgery, pregnancy; gradual partial recovery at the end of precipitating episodes.

Signs. Ichthyosis; atypical retinitis pigmentosa; pupillary abnormalities. Reported also, epiphyseal dysplasia, pes cavus, long metacarpal and metatarsal bones, signs of cardiomyopathy.

Etiology. Autosomal recessive inheritance. Defect of alpha-oxidation of phytanic acid of exogenous (plant) origin that accumulates principally in the nervous system, altering the myelin sheath.

Pathology. Nerves enlarged; accumulation of exudate between nerve bundles and beneath perineurium. Increased amount of fibrous tissue periaxon and thickening of perineural sheath (secondary changes).

Diagnostic Procedures. *Blood.* Increased content of phytanic acid. hypocholesterolemia. *CT scan. MRI. CSF.* Increased protein without pleocytosis. *EEG.* Frequent changes, nonspecific.

Therapy. Diet free of chlorophyll, phytol, and phytanic acid. Repeated cycles of plasmapheresis may be useful.

Prognosis. Spontaneously progressing; terminating with death after several years. Improvement reported with treatment. Early treatment may prevent or minimize symptoms.

BIBLIOGRAPHY. Refsum S: Heredo-ataxia hemeralopia polyneuritiformis-et tidligere ikke beskrevet familiaert syndrom? en fozel Obig moddelelse. Nord Med 28:2682–2685, 1945

Steinberg D: Refsum disease. In Scriver CR, Beaudet AL, Sly WS, et al: The Metabolic and Molecular Bases of Inherited Disease, 7th ed, pp 2351–2369. New York, McGraw-Hill, 1995

Weatherall DJ, Ledingham JGG, Warrell DA: Oxford Textbook of Medicine, p 1437. Oxford, Oxford Med Pub, 1990

REICHEL

Synonyms. Henderson-Jones; synovial chondromatosis; tenosynovial periarticular chondrometaplasia; synovial osteochondromatosis.

Symptoms. More common in males; onset in youth or middle age. Asymptomatic, or pain, swelling, and motion limitation of affected joint (in order of frequency: knee; hip; elbow; shoulder). Rarely, polyarticular.

Signs. Often. Presence of loose bodies in joint and increased synovial fluid.

Etiology. Unknown.

Pathology. Cartilage nodules originating from synovia and loose bodies in cavity. Histologically, metaplastic transformation of synovial tissue. Occasionally, it calcifies (osteochondromatosis).

Diagnostic Procedures. *X-ray.* Typical pattern in case of calcification; otherwise negative.

Therapy. None, or surgery.

Prognosis. Benign condition; very rarely, malignant evolution.

BIBLIOGRAPHY. Reichel P: Chondromatose der Kniegelenkkapsel. Arch Klin Chir 6:717–724, 1900
Klippel JH, Dieppe PA: Rheumatology, pp 3.39.3–3.39.4. St Louis, CV Mosby, 1994

REICHERT

Synonyms. Jacobson nerve neuralgia; geniculate ganglion neuralgia; tympanic plexus neuralgia. See Hunt I and Weisenburg.

Symptoms. Paroxysm of stabbing pain in external auditory meatus, associated with other pains in the face and postauricular zone. It may be differentiated from Weisenburg by the fact that it is not induced by eating, swallowing, or talking, and no increase in salivation is observed.

Etiology and Pathology. Neoplastic, herpes infection, inflammatory irritation of the tympanic branch of the glossopharyngeal (IX) nerve (Jacobson nerve).

Therapy. Intracranial division of the glossopharyngeal (IX) nerve.

Prognosis. Cured by division of the glossopharyngeal (IX) nerve. After section of this nerve, unilateral loss of sensation of soft palate-pharyngeal wall from eustachian tube to epiglottis and posterior third of tongue.

BIBLIOGRAPHY. Reichert FL: Tympanic plexus neuralgia. True tic douloureux of the ear or so-called geniculate ganglion neuralgia: Cure effected by intracranial section of the glossopharyngeal nerve. JAMA 100:1744–1746, 1933
Reichert FL: Neuralgias of the glossopharyngeal nerve with particular reference to the sensory, gustatory and secretory functions of the nerve. Arch Neurol Psychiatr 32:1030–1037, 1934
In Champion RH, Burton JL, Ebling FJG (eds): Rook/Wilkinson/Ebling Textbook of Dermatology, 5th ed, pp 842–843. Oxford, Blackwell Scientific, 1992
Weatherall DJ, Ledingham JGG, Warrell DA: Oxford Textbook of Medicine, pp 4023–4024. Oxford, Oxford Med Pub, 1990

REIFENSTEIN

Synonyms. Gynecomastia—hypospadias; androgen insensitivity partial. See Male pseudohermaphroditism, incomplete hereditary (type I).

Symptoms and Signs. Occurs in males. Developing at puberal age. Gynecomastia; small penis; normal testes; high-pitched voice; sparse beard; small prostate; female pelvic development; female fat distribution. Some men in the family may be infertile but phenotypically normal.

Etiology. Unknown. Sex-linked recessive inheritance. Increase of estriol level.

Pathology. Gynecomastia compatible with estrogen stimulation. Testes normal size; biopsy shows decreased Leydig cell. Spermatozoal maturation onset with normal number of primary and secondary spermatocytes, few or no spermatids or sperm.

Diagnostic Procedures. *Blood.* Normal 17-ketosteroids; plasma concentration of testosterone and luteinizing hormones high; low gonadotropins; receptor deficiency in cultured fibroblasts. *Sperm.* Oligo or azoospermia. *Chromosome studies.* Normal karyotype.

Therapy. Resistance to androgenic and anabolic effects of testosterone.

Prognosis. Good quoad vitam; poor quoad functionem.

BIBLIOGRAPHY. Reifenstein EC Jr: Hereditary familial hypogonadism. Recent Prog Horm Res 3:224, 1948
Schweikert HU, Weissbach L, Stangeberg C, et al Clinical and endocrinological characterization of two subjects with Reifenstein syn-

drome associated with qualitative abnormalities of the androgen receptor. Horm Res 25:72–75, 1987
Forest MG: Diagnosis and treatment of disorders of sexual development. In De Groot LJ (ed): Endocrinology, 3rd ed, p 1921. Philadelphia, WB Saunders, 1995

REIMANN

Synonyms. Hyperviscosity; purpura hyperglobulinemia; rheologic.

Symptoms. Visual troubles; epistaxis and mucosal bleeding; vertigo; deafness; weakness; fatigability; anorexia; dyspnea; syncope and convulsions.

Signs. Eyes dilated; sausage-shaped veins; retinal hemorrhage; nystagmus. Peripheral edema; decreased pulse pressure.

Etiology. Increase in blood viscosity above a certain threshold level. Increase in viscosity due to the presence of abnormal amount of macroglobulins (M component) or other dysproteinemias (molecules with asymmetric configurations, aggregates of IgG M components that affect blood viscosity).

Pathology. That of primary Waldenström II (macroglobulinemia) syndrome (see) or secondary macroglobulinemia owing to lymphomas, reticulum cell sarcoma, tumors, multiple myeloma. Diffuse mucosal bleeding; retinopathy.

Diagnostic Procedures. *Blood.* Anemia; white blood cells normal or increased lymphocytes; thrombocytes normal. Viscosity determination; protein electrophoresis. *SIA test,* and other indirect and direct studies for quantitative and qualitative determination of pathologic proteins. *Biopsy of bone marrow and lymph node. EEG.* Aspecific changes.

Therapy. The specific symptoms owing to hyperviscosity may be well controlled by plasmapheresis. To be repeated as symptoms return or once individual threshold established every time this is approached. Treatment with support. Treatment of basic disorders: penicillamine; corticosteroids; chemotherapy for lymphomas.

Prognosis. Symptomatic relief. Natural progress of the basic condition.

BIBLIOGRAPHY. Reimann HA: Hyperproteinemia as cause of autonomous agglutination: Observations in a case of myeloma. JAMA 99:1411–1414, 1932
Fulton JE, Hurley HJ, Kennedy R: Purpura hyperglobulinemia. Arch Dermatol 97:446–449, 1968
Andrews JC, Hoover LA, Lee RS, et al: Vertigo in the hyperviscosity syndrome. Otolaryngol Head Neck Surg 98:114–149, 1988
Foerster J: Plasma cell dyscrasias: General considerations. In Lee GR, Bithell TC, Foerster J, et al (eds): Wintrobe's Clinical Hematology, 9th ed, pp 2208–2210. Philadelphia, Lea & Febiger, 1993

REIMANN-ANGELIDES

Synonyms. Bone pain, periodic; periodic arthralgia.

Symptoms and Signs. Both sexes. From infancy episodes of pain localized in the shafts of long bones.

Etiology. Unknown. Autosomal dominant inheritance. Sporadic cases in the experience of the author (SIM), in which episodes disappear after adolescence.

Pathology. Unknown.

Prognosis. In congenital form persistence for life.

BIBLIOGRAPHY. Reimann HA, Angelides AP: Periodic arthralgia in 23 members of five generations of a family. JAMA 146:713–716, 1951
Thompson BH, Merritt AD: Dominantly inherited period of bone pain. Birth Defects 10:245–248, 1974

Klippel JH, Dieppe PA: Rheumatology, p 7.4.2. St Louis, CV Mosby, 1994

REINHARDT-PFEIFFER

Synonyms. Clyde mesomelic dwarfism; ulna—fibula hypoplasia. See Langer; brachymelia and Nievergelt.

Symptoms and Signs. At birth, short forearms and ulnar deviation of hands. Height remaining below zero percentile. Cutaneous dimple.

Etiology. Suggestive of autosomal dominant inheritance.

Diagnostic Procedures. *X-rays. Ulna.* Distal hypoplasia. *Radii.* Flat and curved, proximal dislocation. *Tibie.* Short. *Fibulae.* Hypoplastic and curved skeletal architecture of hands and humeri relatively normal.

Therapy. Night splints for correction of hand deviation.

BIBLIOGRAPHY. Pfeiffer RA: Beitrag zur erblichen Verkuerzung von Ulna und Fibula. In Weidemann HR (ed): Dysostosen, Stuttgart, G Fisher, Verlag, 1966
Reinhardt K, Pfeiffer RA: Ulno-fibula dysplasie-Eine autosomal-dominant vererbte Mikromesomelie aehnlich dem Nievergeltsyndrom. Fortschr Roentenschtr 107:379–391, 1967
Rimoin DL, Lachman RS: Genetic disorders of the osseous skeleton. In Beithon P (ed): McKusick's Heritable Disorders of Connective Tissue, 5th ed, p 636. St Louis, CV Mosby, 1993

REINKE EDEMA

Synonyms. Vocal process polypoid degeneration.

Symptoms and Signs. Female predominance; long-term smoking, may be associated with hypothyroidism, reflux or drugs. Long-standing stable vocal dysfunction with some fluctuation, vocal fatigue, changes of voice quality. Laryngoscopy fusiform submucosal edema (polypoid degeneration).

Etiology. Vocal abuse chronic irritating factors (smoke, allergens, drugs, etc.).

Diagnostic Procedures. *Laryngoscopy.* Frequency (pitch) analysis; waveform analysis; spectrography; laryngeal airway resistance.

Therapy. Voice rest and therapy; refrain from smoking; anti-inflammatory agents.

Prognosis. High percentage of good response to treatment. In rare cases malignant degeneration.

BIBLIOGRAPHY. Reinke F: Untersuchungen ueber das menschliche Stimmband. Fortsch Med 13:469–478, 1895
Koufman JA, Blalock PD: Functional voice disorders. Otolaryngol Clin N Am 24:1059–1073, 1991

REINSTEIN-CHALFIN

Synonyms. Retinitis pigmentosa central inverse, central inverse retinitis pigmentosa—deafness; deafness—retinitis pigmentosa inversa.

Symptoms. Both sexes in Askenazi family. Early loss of central vision, preference for dim illumination.

Signs. Retinitis pigmentosa with predominant pigmention around disc and macula, sensorineural deafness, hypogenitalism.

Etiology. Autosomal recessive inheritance.

Prognosis. Deafness progresses slowly in second and third decades.

BIBLIOGRAPHY. Reinstein NM, Chalfin AI: "Inverse retinitis pigmentosa deafness and hypogenitalism." Am J Ophthal 72:332–341, 1971
Garner A, Sarks S, Sarks JP: Degenerative and related disorders of the retina and choroid. In Garner A, Klintworth GK (eds): Pathobiology of Ocular Disease: A Dynamic Approach, 2nd ed. New York, Marcel Dekker, 1994

REIS-BUECKLERS

Synonyms. Corneal dystrophy (Reis-Buecklers) ring dystrophy. See Groenouw type I (may be same condition); including Grayson-Wilbrandt.

Symptoms. Onset variable, age 8–20 years. Increased severity after 40 years of age. Infrequent episodes of eye pain, reduction of vision. Frequent strabismus. In Grayson-Wilbrandt variety: variable effect on vision, normal corneal sensitivity.

Signs. Corneal changes: dusty opacity and mottled scarring with peripheral condensation ring separated from limbs by a strip of normal cornea. In Grayson-Wilbrandt variety same pattern or small, macular, gray raised opacity.

Etiology. Autosomal dominant.

Pathology. Bowman membrane erosive lesions with secondary involvement of epithelium. Ultrastructural examination shows swollen mitochondria, large vacuoles, swelling and disruption of the endoplasmic reticulum of epithelial cell, especially of the basal ones. Bowman membrane replaced by clusters of disoriented collagen fibrils and electron dense fibrils.

Therapy. Corneal transplant when needed.

Prognosis. Progressive vision reduction; in some cases vision has minimal reduction or is not affected.

BIBLIOGRAPHY. Buecklers M: Ueber eine weitere familiaere Hornhautdystrophie (Reis). Klin Monatsbl Augenheilkd 114:386–397, 1949
Grayson M, Wilbrandt H: Dystrophy of anterior limiting membrane of the cornea (Reis-Buecklers type). Am J Ophthalmol 61:345–349, 1966
Moller HU: Granular corneal dystrophy Groenouw type I (Grl) and Reis-Bucklers' corneal dystrophy (R-B): One entity? Acta Ophthalmol 67:678–684, 1989
Moller HU: Granular corneal dystrophy Groenouw type I: Clinical and genetic aspects. Acta Ophthalmol 69(Suppl 198):1–40, 1991
Rodrigues MM, Rajagopalan S, Jones KA: Anterior and posterior corneal dystrophy. In Garner A, Klintworth GK (eds): Pathobiology of Ocular Disease: A Dynamic Approach, 2nd ed, pp 1190–1193. New York, Marcel Dekker, 1994

REITER

Synonyms. Fiessinger-Leroy-Reiter; Ruhr; Waelsch. Blennorrheal idiopathic arthritis; arthritis urethritica; venereal arthritis; conjunctivourethrosynovial; polyarthritis enterica; urethro—oculo—articular.

Symptoms and Signs. Prevalent in males; onset between second and fourth decades. *Urethritis.* May pass unnoticed or severe painful micturition; hematuria; purulent discharge. Usually first manifestation of the triad. In enteric form, usually mild. *Balanitis circinata.* Develops later. *Conjunctivitis.* In over 50% of cases; usually follows after 10 days from onset of urethritis. Intensity varies from simple congestion to purulent discharge. Iritis and keratitis seldom occur concomitantly. *Arthritis.* Most constant element of the triad. Symmetrical; involving mostly knees, ankle, metatarsal and midtarsal joints, seldom wrists. Swelling; skin pale and warm; arthralgia; mild fever.

Some cases present diarrhea as first symptom. Other elements of the triad follow, isolated or at the same time, after 2 or 3 weeks or much later (years), usually in a mild fashion. Skin lesions: keratoderma, limited or generalized; oral muscosal lesions may also occur as part of the syndrome, occurring concomitantly with the arthritis or later onset.

Etiology. Numerous agents are suspected of being responsible for this syndrome: pleuropneumonialike organisms (PPLO), Chlamydia, Shigella flexneri (for the enteric form). Autoimmune condition.

Pathology. Dermatologic lesions similar to pustular psoriasis, hyperparakeratosis, spongiform pustules. Synovial changes aspecific, later similar to rheumatoid arthritis lesions.

Diagnostic Procedures. *Culture and serology.* To rule out venereal diseases and possibly to identify agent (usually sterile culture). *X-ray of joints.* Early cortical erosion; new bone formation and articular destruction, followed by osteoporosis. *Blood.* Sedimentation rate increased during acute stage. HLA-B27 positive in 80% of white patients and in 30% of blacks.

Therapy. Symptomatic. Antibiotics ineffective, most effective nonsteroidal anti-inflammatory drugs; gold. Induced hyperthermia (pyrotherapy) (prolonged remission).

Prognosis. Symptoms may remit spontaneously. Conjunctivitis usually lasts 5–10 days, occasionally 1 month. Recurrences usually unilateral. Arthritis lasts for months. Recurrences frequent and lead to ankylosis. Complications include myocarditis, pericarditis, pleurisy, aortic valve lesions, heart block, pulmonary infiltration, glaucoma, and thrombophlebitis.

BIBLIOGRAPHY. Brodie BC: Pathological and Surgical Observations on Diseases of Joint, 2nd ed, p 54. London, Longman, 1818

Reiter H: Ueber eine bisher unerkannte Spirochäteninfektion (Spirochaetosis arthritica). Dtsch Med Wochenschr 42:1535–1536, 1916

Fiessinger N, Leroy E: Sur une Syndrome caractérisé par l'inflammation simultanée de toutes les muqueses externes coexistant avec une éruption vesiculeuse des quatre membres, non doloreuse et non recidivante Paris Méd 25:54 1917

Deer T, Rosencrance JC, Chillag SA: Cardiac conduction manifestations of Reiter's syndrome. South Med J 84:799–800, 1991

Weatherall DJ, Ledingham JGG, Warrell DA: Oxford Textbook of Medicine, Oxford Med Pub, pp 2970–2972, 1996

REJCHMAN

Synonyms. Gastrosuccorrhea; hypertrophic—hypersecretory gastropathy.

Symptoms and Signs. Those of gastritis with acid regurgitation.

Etiology. Unknown.

Pathology. Florid gastric mucosa presenting mammillary or cobblestone surface between folds, associated with large parietal cell mass and otherwise normal histologic findings.

Diagnostic Procedures. Gastric endoscopy and biopsy.

Therapy. Antacids; cimetidine, omeprazol.

Prognosis. Good.

BIBLIOGRAPHY. Rejchman M: Przpadek chorobowo wzmozonego wydzielania sokn zaladkowego. Gaz Lek Warszawa 2:516–522, 1882

Stempien SJ, Daradi AE, Reingold MM, et al: Hypertrophic hypersecretory gastropathy. Am J Dig Dis 9:471–493, 1964

Silvis SE, Blackwood WM, Vennes J: The selection of gastric hypersecretory patients by blind gastroscopy film review. Gastrointest Endosc 19:116–119, 1972

Golberg RI, Calleja GA: Protein losing gastroenteropathy. In Haubrich WS, Schaffner F, Berk JE (eds): Bockus Gastroenterology, 5th ed, p 1083. Philadelphia, WB Saunders, 1995

RELAPSING POLYCHONDRITIS

Synonyms. Jaksch Wartenhorst; Meyenburg-Altherz-Vehlinger; von Meyenberg II. Chondromalacic arthritis; cartilagineous-arthritic deafness; systemic chondromalacia; perichondritis; diffuse perichondritis;

chronic atrophic polychondritis; rheumatic perichondritis; granulomatous arteritis-polyarthritis.

Symptoms. Both sexes equally affected. Onset usually in middle life (but reported at all ages). Onset acute. Recurrent episodes of malaise, fever, occasionally polyarthritic pains; occasionally, dyspnea, visual trouble, changes of pitch of voice; hearing impairment; vertigo.

Signs. After subsidence of inflammatory phase, various cartilage changes take place at various involved sites. *Ears* (88%). Pinnas thickened, deformed; perceptive deafness (48%). Labyrinthine vertigo (25%). *Nose* (82%). Cartilage atrophy; saddle deformity with dropping and softening of the tip. *Joints* (78%). In hands and feet, multiple articular dislocation. Big joints (synovial) usually spared, but all cartilages may be involved (symphysis pubis; manubrium sterni; vertebrae). *Chondrocostal cartilage* (47%). Softening with sternum retraction in deep inspiration. *Larynx and trachea* (70%). Flatness in anteroposterior direction. *Eye.* Episcleritis and conjunctivitis (47%); iritis (27%). *Heart.* Signs of aortic valve insufficiency (14%).

Etiology. Unknown. Lysosomal labilizing factor of esogenous or exogenous toxic nature implied. Immunologic reactions considered. Familial occurrence has been reported (autosomal dominant).

Pathology. Dissolution and lysis of cartilage; loss of basophilia; acidophilic coloration of the matrix. Lymphocyte and plasma cell infiltration in perichondral tissue plus fibroblastic granulation.

Diagnostic Procedures. *Blood.* During attacks, increased sedimentation rate; anemia; low titer of rheumatoid factor, HLA-DR4 antigen present. *CT scan. MRI. X-ray.* Of joints. Moderate destruction. Of heart. Enlargement (if aortic insufficiency). Of chest (tomography). Tracheal stenosis.

Therapy. Corticosteroids suppress acute inflammatory reactions; if respiratory involvement, long-term treatment. Azathioprine; cyclophosphamide (early management).

Prognosis. Average life span from onset 7 years (range 10 months to 10 years). Death from airway stenosis, respiratory complications, and cardiovascular insufficiency.

BIBLIOGRAPHY. Jaksch R, Wartenhorst R: Polychondropathia. Wien Arch Inn Med 6:93–100, 1923

von Meyenburg H: Ueber Chondromalacia. Schweiz Med Wochenschr 66:1239–1240, 1936

Altherz F: Ueber einen Fall von systematisierter Chondromalacie. Virchows Arch Pathol 297:445–479, 1936

Michet CJ Jr, McKenna CH, Luthra HS, et al: Relapsing polychondritis: Survival and predictive role of early disease manifestations. Ann Int Med 104:74–78, 1986

Stewart SS, Ashigava T, Dudley A, et al: Cerebral vasculitis in relapsing polychondritis. Neurology. 38:150–152, 1988

Weatherall DJ, Ledingham JGG, Warrell DA: Oxford Textbook of Medicine, pp 3015–3016. Oxford, Oxford Med Pub, 1996

RENAL GLYCINURIA

Synonym. Iminoglycinuria type II.

Several conditions may affect glycine transport through the kidney, traits that must be distinguished from prerenal hyperglycinuria.

1. Renal hyperglycinuria and nephrolithiasis (DeVries)
2. Renal hyperglycinuria, autosomal dominant (Käser); type B renal diabetes and glucoglycinuria
3. Hypophosphatemic rickets and glucoglycinuria X-linked (Scriver); type A diabetes

BIBLIOGRAPHY. DeVries A, Kochwa S, Lazebuik J, et al: Glycinuria: A hereditary disorder associated with nephrolithiasis. Am J Med 23:408–414, 1957

Käser H, Cottier P, Antener J: Glucoglycinuria: A new familial syndrome. J Pediatr 61:386–394, 1962

Scriver CR, Goldbloom RB, Ray CC: Hypophosphatemic rickets with renal hyperglycinuria, renal glucosuria and glycyloprolinuria: A syndrome with evidence for renal tubular secretion of phosphorus. Pediatrics 34:357–371, 1964

Chesney RW: Iminoglicinuria. In Scriver CR, Beaudet AL, Sly WS, et al: The Metabolic and Molecular Bases of Inherited Disease, 7th ed, pp 3650–3651. New York, McGraw-Hill, 1995

RENAL TUBULAR ACIDOSIS, TYPE I

Synonyms. Persistent primary renal tubular acidosis; distal renal tubular acidosis; RIA 1; classic renal tubular acidosis; hyperchloremic renal tubular acidosis; renal tubular acidosis "gradient" defect; San Francisco, Oklahoma, Atlanta, Philadelphia; see Lightwood-Albright.

Symptoms. Predominant in females (70%) owing to strong association with autoimmune disease. Onset from second year of life to early adulthood. Exertional dyspnea, anorexia; lethargy; failure to thrive; bone pain and pathologic fractures, rickets; nephrocalcinosis; uretheral colics; polyuria; flaccid paralysis; mild fever.

Signs. Stunted growth. *Blood.* Hypertension; cardiac arrhythmias.

Etiology. Can be primary in hereditary or sporadic form and secondary to autoimmune disorders, nephrocalcinosis, drug- or toxin-induced nephropathy, renal diseases, genetically transmitted systemic diseases and hepatic cirrhosis. Different genetic forms of hereditary RIA 1 have been described: *San Francisco syndrome:* Prevalent characteristics from birth are hypercalcinuria and hypocitraturia with relevant metabolic acidosis. *Philadelphia syndrome:* May be an incomplete form of San Francisco in which nephrocalcinosis may not be present until adulthood and only then can cause metabolic acidosis. *Atlanta syndrome:* Prevalent manifestation is hypercalcinuria accompanied or not by nephrocalcinosis and impairment of renal function. *Oklahoma syndrome:* Hypercalcinuria is primary defect, that only over time damages the tubule, impairs acidification, and causes nephrocalcinosis.

Pathology. Osteomalacia; nephrocalcinosis; renal stones; pyelonephritis.

Diagnostic Procedures. *Blood.* Acidosis, hyperchloremia, hyponatremia, hypokalemia; hypocalcemia, hypophosphatemia, elevated alkaline phosphate, decreased ammonia and titrable acid, increased excretion of potassium, calcium, and phosphorus. *X-ray.* Osteomalacia, nephrocalcinosis; kidney stones.

Therapy. Sodium and potassium bicarbonate and citrate in daily doses of 1–3 mEq/kg. Zinc therapy also might be effective. Therapy must be continued for life.

Prognosis. Good with therapy. Tendency to permanent condition with progression of the disease and its complications partially controlled and prevented by treatment.

BIBLIOGRAPHY. Lightwood R: Calcific infarction of the kidney in infants. Communication Proc Br Paediatr Soc Arch Dis Child 10:205–206, 1935

Albright F: Metabolic studies and therapy in a case of nephrocalcinosis with rickets and dwarfism. Bull Johns Hopkins Hosp 66:7–33, 1940

Du Bose TD Jr, Alpern RJ: Renal tubular acidosis. In Scriver CR, Beaudet AL, Sly WS, et al: The Metabolic and Molecular Bases of Inherited Disease, 7th ed, pp 3655–3689. New York, McGraw-Hill, 1995

RENAL TUBULAR ACIDOSIS, TYPE II

Synonyms. Soriano (J.R.); RIA 2; proximal renal tubular acidosis bicarbonate wasting type renal tubular acidosis, Fanconi (see). RIA 2 occurs almost always as a feature of Fanconi syndrome. See Lightwood-Albright.

Symptoms and Signs. In the congenital form most (or all) cases are males. As an isolated defect: growth retardation. Also reported: mental retardation, nystagmus, cataract, corneal opacities, glaucoma, teeth defects. Tubular dysfunction similar to that of Fanconi's syndrome.

Etiology. Primary form possibly X-linked recessive inheritance or sporadic. Inability to reabsorb bicarbonate in the proximal tubules. Caused also by: congenital malabsorption causing vitamin D deficiency, hypocalcemia, secondary hyperparathyroidism, hypophosphatemia. Observed also as feature of several genetically transmitted diseases: cystinosis, Lowe; Wilson; etc., or nongenetic condition: nephrosis, renal transplant, renal vein thrombosis; amyloidosis, etc.

Diagnostic Procedures. *Urine.* pH down to 5 during acidosis. *Blood.* Hyperchloremic acidosis; opokaliemia; red cells with increased osmotic resistance; failure of bicarbonate administration to correct acidosis; bicarbonate titration curve grossly impaired. *X-ray.* Seldom nephrocalcinosis.

Therapy. Vitamin D; correction of hyperparathyroidism; bicarbonate and potassium.

Prognosis. In congenital form: transitory condition, with growth retardation or in secondary forms persisting condition and evolving according to specific renal defects and basic condition.

BIBLIOGRAPHY. Worthey HG, Good RA: The de Toni-Fanconi syndrome with cystinosis. Am J Dis Child 95:653, 1958

Lamy M, Freza J, Rey J, et al: Etude metabolique du syndrome de Lowe. Rev Eur Etud Clin Biol 7:271, 1962

Soriano JB, Boichis H, Stark H, et al: Proximal renal acidosis: A defect in bicarbonate reabsorption with normal urine acidification. Ped Res 1:81–98, 1967

Du Bose TD Jr, Alpern RJ: Renal tubular acidosis. In Scriver CR, Beaudet AL, Sly WS, et al: The Metabolic and Molecular Bases of Inherited Disease, 7th ed, pp 3655–3689. New York, McGraw-Hill, 1995

RENAL TUBULAR ACIDOSIS, TYPE III

Synonyms. RTA 3; bicarbonate wasting—distal RTA.

Designation of this type of RTA has been abanoned.

Symptoms and Signs. Children with distal acidification defect and renal bicarbonate wasting are now considered to suffer from classical distral RTA (see Type I).

BIBLIOGRAPHY. Alpern RJ: Renal tubular acidosis. In Scriver CV, Beaudet AL, Sly WS, et al: The Metabolic and Molecular Bases of Inherited Disease, 7th ed, p 3677. New York, McGraw-Hill, 1995

RENAL TUBULAR ACIDOSIS, TYPE IV

Synonyms. RTA 4; hyperkalemic distal renal tubular acidosis; hyporeninemic hypoaldosteronism; SHH; hypoaldosteronism isolated, secondary.

Symptoms and Signs. More frequent in males; occurs during and after late middle age (average, 68 years old). Symptoms related to diabetes mellitus in 50% of cases, chronic renal insufficiency in 80% of cases, and those of hyperkalemia and underlying condition determining renal insufficiency.

Etiology. Aldosterone deficiency, diabetic nephropathy pseudohypoaldosteronism, other causes of renal insufficiency. Among possible mechanisms: hyporeninemia from damaged juxtaglomerular apparatus, sympathetic insufficiency, abnormal prostaglandin production, and altered conversion of prorenin.

Diagnostic Procedures. *Blood. Urine.* Hyperkalemia; decreased fractional excretion of K in relation to GFR and reduced response to kaliuretic stimuli including Na bicarbonate, Na sulfate, diuretics, and K chloride IV. *Urine.* Low pH; low K$^+$.

Therapy. None specific. Therapy from none to different approaches according to etiology and clinical status of patient, restriction of dietary potassium, resins, loop diuretics; fluorocortisone (with caution).

Prognosis. That of underlying condition.

BIBLIOGRAPHY. Du Bose TD Jr, Alpern RJ: Renal tubular acidosis. In Scriver CR, Beaudet AL, Sly WS, et al: The Metabolic and Molecular Bases of Inherited Disease, 7th ed, pp 3655–3689. New York, McGraw-Hill, 1995
Melby JC, Azar ST: Hypoaldosteronism and mineralocorticoid resistance. In Groot LJ (ed): Endocrinology, 3rd ed, pp 1805–1806. Philadelphia, WB Saunders, 1995

RENDU-OSLER-WEBER

Synonyms. Babington; Goldstein; Osler-Rendu-Weber; ORW; hemorrhagic telangiectasia hereditaria; angiomatosis, hemorrhagic familial; telangiectasia, hemorrhagic hereditaria.

Symptoms. both sexes equally affected. Occasional patients may be constantly asymptomatic. Repeated epistaxis often beginning in childhood. Occult or frank gastrointestinal bleeding (melena; hematemesis) manifest in middle or later life. Hemophysis also occurs at various ages. In older age group, weakness, pallor, and dyspnea are the presenting symptoms.

Signs. During second or third decade, circumscribed punctiform lesions in the skin and mucous membranes; bluish reddish capillary and venous telangiectasis and spider angiomas may appear. If pulmonary aneurysm syndrome, clubbing, cyanosis, polycythemia, and other typical signs.

Etiology. Unknown. Autosomal dominant hereditary transmission of high penetrance.

Pathology. No complete agreement. Dilated capillaries and venules without muscular or elastic layer; new formation of vessels; congenital anomalies with weak capillary endothelium; lesion of mesenchymal tissue in which capillaries are imbedded.

Diagnostic Procedures. *Blood.* Coagulation studies negative, except when in association with (1) other coagulation defects as in Minot-von Willebrand syndrome or (2) hypochromic anemia. *Biopsy of lesions. Angiography. High-resolution helical computed tomography. MRI.*

Therapy. Treatment of bleeding and correction of anemia (iron). Caustic agents, photocoagulation; electrocautery, laser, embolotherapy, septal dermoplasty; X-ray treatment of lesions that may be easily reached, ligation of arterial supply. Recurrences frequent and occasionally more severe. Administration of ethynyl estradiol has been reported to give good results. Danazol also reported as beneficial. If pulmonary aneurysm, surgery may cure the manifestations. Future gene replacement.

Prognosis. The severity of this syndrome is extremely variable; 4% mortality for severe uncontrollable bleeding has been reported. Some members of affected family found to have the condition only when carefully interrogated and examined.

BIBLIOGRAPHY. Sutton HG: Epistaxis as an indication of impaired nutrition, and of degeneration of the vascular system. Med Mirror 1:769–781, 1864
Rendu M: Epistaxis répétées chez un sujet porteur de petits angiomes cutanés et muquex. Bull Mem Soc Méd Hôp Paris 13:731–733, 1896
Osler W: On a family form of recurring epistaxis, associated with multiple telangiectases of the skin and mucous membranes. Bull Johns Hopkins Hosp 12:333–337, 1901
Weber FP: Haemorrhagic telangiectasia of the Osler-type "telangiectatic dysplasia" and isolated case, with discussion on multiple pulsating stellate telangiectases and other striking haemangiectatic conditions. Br J Dermatol 48:182–193, 1936

Guttmacher AE, Marchuk DA, White RI Jr: Hereditary hemorrhagic telangiectasia. N Engl J Med 333:918–924, 1994

RENON-DELILLE

Obsolete.

Synonym. Acromegaly, thyroid—ovarian deficiency. See Launois.

Symptoms and Signs. Hypotension; tachycardia; hyperhidrosis; intolerance to heat; insomnia; oliguria; acromegaly.

Etiology. Unknown. See Multiple endocrine deficiency.

BIBLIOGRAPHY. Rénon L, Delille A: Insuffisance thyro-ovarienne et hyperactivité hypophysaire (troubles acromégaliques). Amélioration par l'opothérapie Thyro-ovarienne; Augmentation de l'acromégalie par la médication hypophysaire. Bull Mem Soc Med Hôp Paris 25:973–979, 1908

RESIDUAL OVARY

Symptoms. Occurs in patients who have had hysterectomy and salvage of one or both ovaries. Continuous or intermittent pelvic pain and tenderness; occasionally dyspareunia.

Signs. Persistent pelvic mass usually larger than 5 cm.

Etiology. Continued or attempted ovarian function.

Pathology. Ovary cystic, atretic, hemorrhagic follicles, corpora lutea, perioophoritis. Occasionally, endometriosis and neoplasia.

Therapy. When indicated, exogenous hormone treatment. If this treatment does not relieve symptoms, consider correction of adhesions and, as last resort, oophorectomy.

Prognosis. Neoplasia and malignant degeneration present in 8% of residual ovaries indicate the necessity of a definite diagnosis and adequate surgical procedure.

BIBLIOGRAPHY. Grogan RH: Reappraisal of residual ovaries. Am J Obstet Gynecol 97:124–129, 1967

RESPIRATORY DISTRESS SYNDROME

Synonym. Hyaline membrane disease.

Symptoms. (Over one half of infants have difficulty in initiating normal respiration.) Expiratory grunting or whining, sternal and intercostal retractions, nasal flaring, cyanosis.

Signs. Auscultation: diminished air entry.

Etiology. The disease is owing to the absence, deficiency, or alteration of the pulmonary surfactant. Alteration or absence of surfactant results in decreased compliance and reduced alveolar ventilation. Right-to-left shunt, because of large lung areas not perfused.

Pathology. *Gross.* The lung is collapsed, firm, dark red, and liver-like. *Microscopic.* Alveolar collapse, overdistention of the dilated alveolar ducts, pink-staining membrane on alveolar ducts. *Electron microscopy.* Damage of alveolar epithelial cells, swelling of capillary endothelial cells.

Diagnostic Procedures. *X-ray.* Reticulogranular, ground-glass appearance with air bronchograms. *Blood gas analysis.* Hypoxemia, often hypercarbia, metabolic acidosis.

Therapy. Neutral thermal environment, oxygen administration, assisted ventilation, continuous positive airways pressure (CPAP), no oral feeding, continuous monitoring of respiration, ECG, and temperature. In cases that need mechanical ventilation with more than 60% of O$_2$ instillation into airway through an endotracheal tube of a preparation of swine or ox pulmonary surfactant or a synthetic preparation of phospholipids and emulsifying agents. Trial with TSH.

Prognosis. Poor. Intensive care may completely reverse the outcome.

BIBLIOGRAPHY. Strang LB, MacLeishm MH: Ventilatory failure and right to left shunt in newborn infants with respiratory distress. Pediatrics 98:17–27, 1961

Klaus M: Respiratory function and pulmonary disease of the newborn. In Barnett H (ed): Pediatrics, 15th ed, pp 1255–1261. New York, Appleton-Century-Crofts, 1972

Farrel P, Avery M: Hyaline membrane disease. Am Rev Resp Dis 111:657–688, 1975

Charon A, Taeusch W, Fitzgibbon C, et al: Factors associated with surfactant treatment response in infants with severe respiratory distress syndrome. Pediatrics 83:348–354, 1989

Collaborative European Multicentre Study Group, Eur J Pediatr, 152:372, 1992

RETINAL CONE DEGENERATION

Synonyms. Includes a number of genetic disorders that cannot be clearly distinguished one from another; usually subdivided according to inheritance and aspects of the fundus (see individual syndromes).

Symptoms and Signs. Progressive loss of vision. Photophobia, defective color vision. Rarely, loss of side vision and night blindness.

BIBLIOGRAPHY. Krill AE, Deutman AF, Fishman M: The cone degeneration. Doc Ophthalmol 35:1–80, 1973

Bird AC, Jay B, Hussain AA, et al: Retinal photoreceptor disorders. In Garner A, Klintworth GK (eds): Pathobiology of Ocular Disease: A Dynamic Approach, 2nd ed, p 1217. New York, Marcel Dekker, 1994

RETINAL CONE DEGENERATION, AUTOSOMAL DOMINANT

Symptoms and Signs. Progressive loss of vision. Photophobia, defective color vision. Rarely, loss of side vision and night blindness.

Etiology. Autosomal dominant.

Diagnostic Procedures. *Fundus.* Macular lesion with bull's eye appearance (edema). *Electroretinography.* Distinctive findings.

BIBLIOGRAPHY. Davis CT, Hollenhorst RW: Hereditary degeneration of the macula, occurring in five generations. Am J Ophthalmol 39:637–643, 1955

Krill AE, Deutman AF, Fishman M: The cone degeneration. Doc Ophthalmol 35:1–80, 1973

Bird AC, Jay B, Hussain AA, et al: Retinal photoreceptor disorders. In Garner A, Klintworth GK (eds): Pathobiology of Ocular Disease: A Dynamic Approach, 2 ed, p 1217. New York, Marcel Dekker, 1994

RETINAL DISINSERTION, CONGENITAL

Synonyms. See Walker-Warburg.

Symptoms and Signs. Blindness from birth associated with other ocular abnormalities: unilateral microphthalmos; central anterior and posterior central cataracts; colobomas of lens: temporal retina paving stone-like degeneration.

Etiology. Congenital factors.

BIBLIOGRAPHY. Gonin J Pathogénie et anatomie pathologique des décollementes rétiniens. Bull Soc Ophthalmol 33:1–18, 1920

Boniuk M, Hittner HM: Congenital retinal disinsertion syndrome. Trans Am Acad Ophthalmol Otolaryngol 79:827–834, 1975

Torczynski E: Developmental anomalies of the eye. In Garner A, Klint-

worth GK (eds): Pathobiology of Ocular Disease: A Dynamic Approach, 2nd ed, p 1322. New York, Marcel Dekker, 1994

RETINAL NECROSIS, ACUTE

Synonyms. Includes panuveitis; retinal arteritis; necrotizing retinitis.

Symptoms and Signs. Anterior uveitis, vitreous opacity, cement-like retinal exudates. CNS can be involved.

Etiology. Viral infection (herpes simplex virus type 1 and varicella zoster virus).

Diagnostic Procedures. Slit-lamp examination. *Blood.* Serological methods. Neuroimaging to assess neurological involvement.

Pathology. Uveitis, vasculitis, vitritis, and necrosis of retina. Periarteritis, peripheral exudates, and necrosis.

Therapy. Large doses of steroid and antiherpes agents (acyclovir).

Prognosis. Retinal detachment possible.

BIBLIOGRAPHY. Culbertson W, Blumenkranz M, Haines H, et al: The acute retinal necrosis syndrome. Ophthalmology 89:1317–1325, 1982

Hayreh SS: So-called "acute retinal necrosis syndrome": An acute panuveitis syndrome. Dev Ophthalmol 10:40–77, 1985

Matsno T, Makayama T, Koyama T, et al: Mild type acute retinal necrosis: Syndrome involving both eyes of three-year interval. Jpn J Ophthalmol 31:455–460, 1987

Easty DL, Willams C: Viral and rickettsial disease. In Garner A, Klintworth GK (eds): Pathobiology of Ocular Disease: A Dynamic Approach, 2nd ed, pp 236–245. New York, Marcel Dekker, 1994

RETINAL PIGMENT EPITHELIUM HYPERTROPHY

Synonyms. Congenital hypertrophy, retinal pigment epithelium; CHRPE. See Gardner syndrome.

Symptoms and Signs. Retinal lesions, "pigmented scar," unilateral, solitary of 1 or 2 disc diameters. In the center chorioretinal atrophy, and at periphery hyperpigmentation surrounded by depigmentation. Frequently found in patients affected by Gardner syndrome and may represent a valuable clue for the presence of the latter.

Etiology. Autosomal dominant inheritance. Possibly identical genetic lesion of Gardner.

BIBLIOGRAPHY. Blair NT, Trempe CL: Hypertrophy of the retinal pigment epithelium associated with Gardner syndrome. Am J Ophthalmol 90:661–667, 1980

Bull MJ, Ellis FD, Sato S, et al: Hypertrophy of retinal pigment epithelium in Gardner syndrome. Proc Greenwood Genet Ctr 4:136, 1985

McCartney E, Alison CE: Intraocular epithelial tumors and cysts. In Garner A, Klintworth GK (eds): Pathobiology of Ocular Disease: A Dynamic Approach, 2nd ed, pp 1415–1416. New York, Marcel Dekker, 1994

RETINA: POSTPOLE COLLOIDAL DEGENERATION

1. Hutchinson. Guttate choroiditis
2. Wagnes. "Malattia levantinese"
3. Doyne. Honeycombed degeneration (typical)
4. Holthose-Batten. Honeycombed degeneration

RETINITIS PIGMENTOSA–DEAFNESS– MENTAL RETARDATION-HYPOGONADISM

Synonyms. Deafness—mental retardation—retinitis—hypogonadism.

Symptoms and Signs. Both sexes. From birth. Retinitis pigmentosa (see), deafness, mental retardation. Hypogonadism: in males, gynecomastia small testis, subvirilization; in females, oligomenorrhea. Nystagmus, acanthosis nigra, multiple keloids.

Etiology. Autosomal recessive inheritance.

Diagnostic Procedures. *Blood.* Hyperinsulinism, altered glucose metabolism.

BIBLIOGRAPHY. Edwards JA, Sethi PK, Scoma AJ, et al: A new familial syndrome characterized by pigmentary retinopathy, hypogonadism, mental retardation, nerve deafness and glucose intolerance. Am J Med 60:23–32, 1976

RETINO-HEPATO-ENDOCRINOLOGIC

Synonyms. R.H.E.

Symptoms and Signs. Total color blindness (progressive). Evidence of degenerative liver disease and various endocrine dysfunctions: hypothyroidism, diabetes type II, infertility or repeated aborption. Hearing defects.

Etiology. Autosomal recessive inheritance.

Diagnostic Procedures. *Blood.* Increase of creatine phosphokinase. *Fundus oculi.* Attenuated retinal vessels, pallor of the disc, generalized atrophy without pigmentation. Scotopic function normal; phototopic function lost.

BIBLIOGRAPHY. Hansen E, Froyshov-Larsen I, Berg K: A familial syndrome of progressive cone dystrophy, degenerative liver disease, endocrine dysfunction and hearing defects I: Ophthalmological Findings. Acta Ophthal 54:129–144, 1976
Berg K, Froyshov-Larsen I, Hansen E: Familial syndrome of progressive dystrophy, degenerative liver disease and endocrine dysfunction III: Genetic studies. Clin Genet 13:190–200, 1978

RETINOSCHISIS

Synonyms. Blessing-Iwanoff; Iwanoff; Sorby macular dystrophy; retinal cystoid degeneration. Including ablatio falciformis congenita.

Symptoms. Sex predominance according to inheritance type. Visual handicap mild up to age 40–50 years, then sudden impairment of vision.

Signs. Retinal cystic degeneration, splitting, detachment, and finally atrophy.

Etiology. Unknown. X-linked and autosomal dominant and recessive families reported.

Pathology. Cystic degeneration mainly of deep nerve layer of retina, all layers involved, cystic areas coalesce with adjacent areas splitting in two layers, detachment and atrophy with sclerosis of choroid.

Diagnostic Procedures. *Ophthalmoscopy.* On retinal periphery small translucent areas or branching channels. *Electroretinogram.* From normal to various abnormalities.

Prognosis. Variable according to evolution.

BIBLIOGRAPHY. Forsius HR, Erikson AW: Retinoschisis X-chromosomalis. In Erikson AW, Forsing HR, Nevaullinna HR, et al (eds): Population Structure and Genetic Disorders, p 673. New York, Academic Press, 1900
Mann I, McRae A: Congenital vascular veils in the vitreous. Br J Ophthalmol 22:1–10, 1938
Wave H: Ablatio falciformis congenita (retinal fold). Br J Ophthalmol 22:456–470, 1938
Alitalo T, Kruse TA, de la Chapelle A: Refined localization of the gene causing X-linked-juvenile retinoschisis. Genomics 9:505–510, 1991
Torczynski E: Developmental anomalies of the eye. In Garner A, Klint-

worth GK (eds): Pathobiology of Ocular Disease: A Dynamic Approach, 2nd ed, pp 1317–1318. New York, Marcel Dekker, 1994

RETIREMENT

Symptoms. Affecting people before or after retirement from jobs or careers (especially military personnel who retire at an early age). Irritability; loss of interest; lack of energy; increased alcohol intake; somatic complaints without physical basis (gastrointestinal tract, cardiovascular system).

Etiology. Psychic maladjustment to a changed status, resulting in depression-anxiety complex.

Therapy. Opportunity for activity that will provide new ambitions and goals.

BIBLIOGRAPHY. Figley CR, McCubbin H (eds): Stress and the Family, vol I: Coping with Normative Transitions. New York, Brunner/Mazel, 1983

RETT

Synonyms. Cerebroatrophic hyperammonemia; hyperammonemia cerebroatrophic; autism—dementia—ataxia; loss of purposeful use of hand.

Symptoms and Signs. Occurs in females. After normal initial development up to 7–18 months combination of psychic deterioration that in a year and a half leads to: severe dementia, autism, loss of finalized use of hands, truncal ataxia, and lack of progression of head growth (acquired microcephaly). Situation remains stable for decades except for insidious appearance of the additional symptoms: seizures, spastic paraparesis, vasomotor disturbances of legs.

Etiology. X-linked inheritance with lethality for males. No chromosomal abnormality is found. Other hypotheses have been advanced: metabolic interference.

Diagnostic Procedures. *Blood.* Mild hyperammonemia. *EEG.* Multifocal epileptiform discharges. *Cerebral CT scan. MRI.* Cerebral atrophy.

BIBLIOGRAPHY. Rett A: Ueber ein cerebral-atrophisches. Syndrom bei Hyperammonaemie. Monatsschr Kinderheilkd 116:310–311, 1968
Moeschler JB, Charnan C, Berg S, et al: Rett syndrome: Natural history and management. Pediatics 82:1–10, 1988
Editorial: The Rett syndrome diagnostic criteria work group: Diagnostic criteria for Rett syndrome. Ann Neurol 23:425–428, 1988
Akesson HO, Hagberg B, Wahlstrom J, et al: Rett syndrome: A search for gene source. Am J Med Genet 42:104–108, 1992

REYE (R.K.D.) II

Synonyms. Reye-Johnson hepatic encephalopathy; liver degeneration—encephalopathy; encephalopathy—fatty hepatomegaly.

Symptoms. Both sexes affected. Onset from 6 months to 10 years. Upper respiratory infection (50%); seldom gastrointestinal involvement. Onset 3–21 days after recovery from infection. Progressive vomiting, frequently hemorrhagic; dyspnea; fever; hypotonia; coma; convulsions.

Signs. Some patients have characteristic posture: flexion of elbows, hands clenched, legs extended; dilated pupils; abnormal reflexes; fluctuating liver enlargement. Seldom, rash.

Etiology. Probably owing to aspirin or salicylate use during viral illness. Possibly, hepatoxic substance or virus: influenzae B (mostly), A, echo virus, reovirus, rubella, rubeola, herpes simplex, Epstein-Barr.

Pathology. *Liver.* Hepatomegaly; fatty degeneration; focal necrosis; mild inflammation; inclusion bodies in some cases. *Kidney.* Fat changes.

Brain. Edema; nonspecific, noninflammatory changes. *Lung.* Occasionally, pneumonia.

Diagnostic Procedures. *Blood.* Leukocytosis with neutrophilia; hypoglycemia (in 50% of cases); hyperammonemia; metabolic acidosis; high serum glutamic-oxaloacetic transaminase (SGOT); serum glutamic-pyruvic transaminase (SGPT); and blood urea nitrogen (BUN). *CSF.* Increased pressure, acellular; marked hypoglycorrhachia (50%). *Urine.* Ketonuria; aminoaciduria. *EEG.* Diffuse arrhythmic delta activity progressing in cases to silence (cerebral death).

Therapy. Intensive care based on fluid restriction, dexamethasone, neomycin, vitamin K, dextrose (25%). Integrated with endotracheal intubation, mechanical ventilation, hypothermia, and, if intracanial pressure increased, mannitol. Exchange transfusions have been used with success.

Prognosis. Greatly improved by intensive treatment; mortality about 5–10%. Some spontaneously recover without sequelae.

BIBLIOGRAPHY. Brain WR, Hunter D: Acute meningoencephalomyelitis of childhood: Report of six cases. Lancet 1:221–227, 1929

Reye RDK, Morgan G, Baral J: Encephalopathy and fatty degeneration of the viscera. A disease entity in childhood. Lancet 2:749–752, 1963

Hansen JR, McCray PB, Bale JF, Corbett AJ, Flanders DJ: Reye syndrome associated with aspirin therapy for systemic lupus erythematosus. Pediatrics 76:202–205, 1985

Banett MJ, Hurwitz ES, Schonberger LB, Rogers M: Changing epidemiology of Reye's syndrome in the United States. Pediatrics 77:598–602, 1986

Weatherall DJ, Ledingham JGG, Warrell DA: Oxford Textbook of Medicine, pp 2025–2026, 4072–4073. Oxford, Oxford Med Pub, 1996

RHABDOMYOLYSIS, EXERTIONAL

Synonym. March hemoglobinuria, including Myoglobinuria, exertional, inherited. See OXPHOS; MacArdle, anterior tibial, and peroneal compartment.

Symptoms and Signs. Onset at all ages. More frequently occurring in young men just enrolled in the military service or in athletic clubs; extremely rare in females. The attacks follow stressing calisthenics executed without previous gradual preparation. Severe myalgia of stressed muscles (tender, crampy, and swelling), lasting from a few days to 1 month, or original capacity for exercise returns in 1 to several months. The subjects notice emission of dark brown urine 24–38 hours after the exercise and preceded by malaise and oliguria.

A familial form is characterized by recurrent episodes of rabdomyolysis after strenuous excercise, heavy alcohol ingestion, or fasting and the symptoms: weakness, fatigability, muscle pain, and myoglobinuria. No other manifestation of OXPHOS disease.

Etiology. Rhabdomyolysis following strenuous exercise, particularly when to the point of exhaustion. Sporadic or familial (autosomal recessive?). Different pathogenetic mechanisms postulated.

Attack onset in some cases seems related to muscle glycogen depletion caused by alteration of muscle lipid metabolism including carnitine palmitoyl transferase deficiency, in others to derangements of OXPHOS owing to mtDNA deletions.

Pathology. Muscular inflammatory changes; coagulation necrosis of muscle fibers.

Diagnostic Procedures. *Urine.* Myoglobinuria; proteinuria. *Blood.* Creatine phosphokinase (CPK) aldolase, serum glutamic-oxaloacetic transaminase (SGOT), lactic dehydrogenase increased; blood urea nitrogen (BUN) may increase. *EMG.*

Therapy. Rest; prevention through gradual exercise, especially with subject in sedentary occupation, wearing appropriate shoes and eventually change running style. Possibility of kidney damage and anuria to be considered, and eventually treated. In familial form avoid prolonged

fasting, treat infections promptly, avoid physical stress. See also OXPHOS syndromes.

Prognosis. Good. No physical impairment left after complete disappearance of symptoms.

BIBLIOGRAPHY. De Langen CD: Myoglobin and myoglobinuria. Acta Med Scand 124:213–226, 1946

Hed R: Myoglobinuria Arch Intern Med 92:825–832, 19

Christensen TE, Saxtrup O, Hansen TI, et al: Familial myoglobinuria: A study of muscle and kidney pathophysiology in three brothers. Dan Med Bull 30:112–115, 1983

Arcangeli A, Cavaliere F, Carducci P, Proietti R, Magalini SI: Acute rhabdomyolysis during heroin abuse. Italian J Med 2:23, 1986

Ziskind A: Jet-ski rhabdomyolysis. JAMA 225:1879–80, 1986

Shoffner JM, Wallace DC: Oxidative phosphorylation diseases. In Scriver CR, Beaudet AL, Sly WS, et al: The Metabolic and Molecular Bases of Inherited Disease, 7th ed, p 1555. New York, McGraw-Hill, 1995

RHIZOMELIC CHONDRODYSPLASIA PUNCTATA

Synonyms. Koala bear recessive; chondrodystrophia calcificans punctata; stippled epiphyses; chondrodystrophia calcificans; chondrodysplasia epiphysealis punctata. See also Conradi-Huenermann.

Symptoms and Signs. Both sexes affected. Present from birth. Marked irritability (relieved by analgesics); thermoregulatory instability; feeding difficulties; recurrent otitis and airway infections; Rhizomelic dwarfism; joint contractures. *Head.* Flat facies; low nasal bridge; nonconstant upward palpebral slanting; microcephaly. Cataracts (72%) seldom optical atrophy. *Skin.* Ichthyosiform dermatosis with alopecia (28%); mental deficiency. Spastic tetraplegia and seizures in patients who survive.

Etiology. Autosomal recessive inheritance. Peroxisomal disorder without abnormal bile acid synthesis.

Pathology. Altered enchondrial bone formation; lack of columnar arrangement; formation of cancellous bone in necrotic areas.

Diagnostic Procedures. *X-ray.* Present only in early infancy: Punctate epiphyseal ossification centers stippling. Later: symmetric short humeri and femora; metaphyseal splaying and cupping; vertical clefting of vertebrae on lateral projection; trapezoid dysplasia of ileum.

Therapy. Symptomatic.

Prognosis. Poor; death by 2 years of age. Rarely longer survival.

BIBLIOGRAPHY. Putschar WGJ: Chondrodystrophia calcificans congenita (dysplasia epiphysialis punctata). Bull Hosp Jt Dis Orthop Inst 11:514–527, 1951

Spranger JW, Opitz JM, Bidder U: Heterogeneity of chondrodysplasia punctata. Hum Genet II:190–212, 1971

Wardinsky TD, Pagon RA, Powell BR, et al: Rhizomelic chondrodysplasia punctata and survival beyond one year: A review of the literature and five case reports. Clin Genet 38:84–93, 1990

Poll-The BT, Maroteaux P, Narcy C, et al: A new type of chondrodysplasia punctata associated with peroxisomal dysfunction. J Inherit Metab Dis 14:361–363, 1991

Weatherall DJ, Ledingham JGG, Warrell DA: Oxford Textbook of Medicine, p 1441. Oxford, Oxford Med Pub, 1996

RICCARDI (NF III)

Synonym. Neurofibromatosis, mixed; palmocutaneous neurofibromas included.

Symptoms and Signs. Those of von Recklinghausen (NF I) (freckling and cutaneous neurofibromas are pale, scarcer, and relatively larger) and familial acoustic neuromas (NF II) (bilateral acoustic neuroma, meningiomas and spinal neurofibromas giving symptoms in the second or early third decade and developing rapidly); absence of optical gliomas.

Etiology. Autosomal dominant inheritance.

Prognosis. A rapid and usually fatal course (from tumors in CNS).

BIBLIOGRAPHY. Riccardi VM, Eichner JE: Neurofibromatosis: Phenotype, Natural History and Pathogenesis. Baltimore, Johns Hopkins Univ Press, 1986

RICCARDI (NF IV)

Synonyms. Neurofibromatosis, variant forms. Neurofibromatosis, atypical.

Symptoms and Signs. Heterogeneous groups of cases that do not present sufficient clinical features to be included in NF I, NF II, NF III.

Etiology. Unknown.

Prognosis. Different evolution and requiring different genetic counseling from other groups.

BIBLIOGRAPHY. Riccardi VM, Eichner JE: Neurofibromatosis: Phenotype, Natural History and Pathogenesis, Baltimore, Johns Hopkins Univ Press, 1986

RICHARD-RUNDLE

Synonyms. Sylvester (PE); ketoaciduria—mental deficiency; ataxia—deafness—retardation, ketoaciduria.

Symptoms and Signs. From infancy. Underdevelopment of sexual characteristics; ataxia; deafness; mental retardation; peripheral muscle wasting.

Etiology. Unknown. Autosomal recessive inheritance.

Diagnostic Procedures. *Urine.* Ketoaciduria.

Prognosis. No risk to life.

BIBLIOGRAPHY. Koennecke W: Friedreichsche Ataxia und Taubstummheit. Z Neurol Psychiat 53:161–165, 1920
Richard BW, Rundle AT: A familial hormonal disorder associated with mental deficiency, deafmutism and ataxia. J Ment Def Res 3:33–55, 1959
Sylvester PE: Spinocerebellar regeneration hormone disorder, hypogonadism, deafmutism and mental deficiency. J Ment Def Res 16:203–214, 1972
Konigsmark BVW: Hereditary diseases of the nervous system with hearing loss. In Vinken PJ, Bruyn GW (eds): Handbook of Clinical Neurology, vol 22, pp 499–526. Amsterdam, North-Holland, 1975

RICHARDSON-STEELE-OSLZEWSKI

Synonyms. Steele-Richardson-Oslzewski; dementia—nuchal dystonia; supranuclear palsy; progressive supranuclear palsy.

Symptoms and Signs. Occurs mostly in males. Onset during sixth decade. Insidious, vague changes in personality; visual, speech alteration; unsteady gait; altered facies: deeply lined; spastic with jaw and facial jerks. Dementia with changes in personality appear early but remain usually mild. Constant pseudo-ophthalmoplegia affecting chiefly vertical gaze; pseudobulbar palsy; dysarthria; dystonic rigidity of neck and upper trunk and various inconstant cerebellar and pyramidal symptoms and signs. No forced laughter and crying. No parkinsonian tremor; tendon hyperreflexia; Babinski (inconstant).

Etiology. Unknown. Possibly, degenerative conditions or virus infections. To be differentiated from paralysis agitans, cerebellar degenera-

tion, Creutzfeldt-Jakob; presenile dementia syndromes, Parkinson. It may clinically overlap (to some extent) with Lhermitte, Cruetzfeldt-Jakob, Hirano parkinsonism-dementia, and corticodental degenerative with neuronal achromasia. Differences in clinical manifestations or anatomic-pathologic changes, however, do not permit unifying all these syndromes under a single label at the present time.

Pathology. Neurofibrillary tangles (Hirano globose type); granulovacuolar degeneration; occasionally torpedoes on the axons of Purkinje cells. Loss of nerve cells in basal ganglia, brain stem, cerebellum. Fibrillary gliosis in all areas with loss of nerve cells and fibrillary tangles. Demyelinization in various tracts; saccules in substantia nigra and subthalamic nucleus; perivascular cuffing.

Diagnostic Procedures. *CSF.* Normal. *EEG. X-ray.* Of skull. *CT scan. MRI.*

Therapy. L-dopa and anticholinesterase drugs, bromocriptine give temporary benefit.

Prognosis. Steady progressive course leading to death in 5–7 years.

BIBLIOGRAPHY. Chavany JA, von Bogaert L, Godlewski S: Sur un syndrome de rigidité à prédominance axiale avec perturbation des automatismes oculo-palpébraux d'origine encéphalitique. Presse Med 59:958–962, 1951
Richardson JC, Steele J, Oslezwski J: Supranuclear opthalmoplegia, pseudobulbar palsy, nuclear dystonia and dementia. Trans Am Neurol Assoc 88:25–30, 1963
LeChevalier B, Viader F: La paralysie supranucleaire progressive (maladie de Steele-Richarson-Olzewski) vingt et un ans apres. La Press Med 19:1879–1881, 1990
Morris JC: Handbook of Dementing Illnesses. New York, Marcel Dekker, 1993

RICHNER-HANHART

Synonym. Tyrosinemia type II; oculocutaneous tyrosinemia; tyrosine aminotransferase deficiency; TAT deficiency; keratosis palmaris—corneal dystrophy.

Symptoms. Affects closely inbred families from Italy (approximately 50%), Australia, Canada, Switzerland, and United States. Both sexes equally affected. From birth: lacrimation, photophobia redness; painful nonpruritic lesions of palms and soles that blister and become hyperkeratotic. Mental retardation, self-mutilating behavior.

Signs. Corneal herpetiform erosions, dendritic ulcers corneal and conjunctival plaques, nystagmus, glaucoma.

Etiology. Autosomal recessive inheritance. Deficiency of hepatic tyrosine aminotransferase (TAT) and formation of tyrosine crystaline inclusions.

Pathology. *Biopsy.* Of skin: the plantar hypercheratotic lesion shows simple hypercheratosis and some aberrant keratinocytes with multipe nuclei. *Ultrastructural examination.* In affected keratinocytes, aggregation of tonofilaments and intracytoplasmatic needle-shaped inclusions (tyrosine crystals).

Diagnostic Procedures. *Blood.* Tyrosinemia. *Urine.* Tyrosiluria and tyrosine metabolites over normal levels.

Therapy. Low tyrosine, low phenylalanine diet. Control of maternal plasma tyrosine during pregnancy, in TAT deficient patients.

Prognosis. Good with early diet. If not treated, mental retardation.

BIBLIOGRAPHY. Richner H: Hornhaul affection bei Keratoma palmare et plantare hereditarium. Klin Monatsbl Augenheilkd 100:580–588, 1938
Hanhart E: Neue Sondeformen von Keratosis palmoplantaris, u.a. eine regelmass g-dominanten mit systematisierten, Lipomen, ferner 2

einfach-rezessive mit Schwachsinn und Z.T. mit Hornhautveranderungen des Auges (Ektadermal syndrome). Dermatologica 94:286–308, 1947

Shimizu N, Ito M, Ito K, et al: Richner-Hanhart syndrome: Electron microscopic study of the skin lesions. Arch Dermatol 126:1342–1346, 1990

Mitchell GA, Lambert M, Tanguay RM: Hypertyrosinemia. In Scriver CR, Beaudet AL, Sly WS, et al: The Metabolic and Molecular Bases of Inherited Disease, 7th ed, pp 1082–1083. New York, McGraw-Hill, 1995

RICHTER

Synonyms. Reticulum cell sarcoma; diffuse histiocytic lymphoma.

Symptoms and Signs. In patients with pre-existing and persisting evidence of chronic lymphocytic leukemia, development of a solid cell lymphoma. Weight loss, fever, generalized lymphoadenopathy, and symptoms related to kidney, lung, and/or gastrointestinal tract.

Etiology. Unknown. Clonal transformation of CLL cells into histiocytic lymphoma cells or development of an independent B-cell malignancy.

Pathology. Pielomorphic large cell lymphoma.

Diagnostic Procedures. *X-ray. CT scan. MRI.* Development of localized lymphoadenopathy *Blood.* Anemia, lymphocytes typical changes of leukemia, dysglobulinemia. *Lymph node biopsy.* (See Pathology.)

Therapy. Chemotherapy and X-ray treatment similar to those used in Hodgkin (see).

Prognosis. Median survival of less than months from presentation.

BIBLIOGRAPHY. Richter MN: Generalized reticular cell sarcoma of lymph nodes associated with lymphatic leukemia. Am J Pathol 4:285, 1928

Catovsky D: Chronic lymphocytic leukemia and other leukemias of mature B- and T-cells. In Weatherall DJ, Ledingham JGG, Warrell DA: Oxford Textbook of Medicine, p 3422. Oxford, Oxford Med Pub, 1996

RICHTER HERNIA

Symptoms and Signs. Hernia with partial protrusion of intestinal lumen.

BIBLIOGRAPHY. Richter AG: Abhandlung von den Bruechen, pp 596–597. Goettingen, Dietrich, 1785

Sabiston DC: Textbook of Surgery, 14th ed, p 1. Philadelphia, WB Saunders, 1991

RIDDOCH

Synonym. Visual disorientation II. See Head-Holmes.

Symptoms and Signs. Patient not aware of defect. Visual disorientation in homonymous half field with preservation of stereoscopic vision and visual attention. Ability to fix gaze on an object and to maintain it on contralateral side, but less so on affected side. Pupillary and convergence reflexes normal. Visual acuity normal or slightly reduced.

Etiology and Pathology. Unilateral lesion of parietal lobe (neoplastic; traumatic; infective).

Diagnostic Procedures. *CT brain scan. MRI. Angiography.*

Therapy. Surgery or according to etiology.

Prognosis. Depends on etiology. After removal of cause, symptoms recede.

BIBLIOGRAPHY. Riddoch G: Dissociation of visual perceptions due to occipital injuries, with especial reference to appreciation of movement. Brain 40:15–57, 1917

Riddoch G: Visual disorientation in homonymous half fields. Brain 58:376–382, 1935

Adams RD, Victor M: Principles of Neurology, 5th ed, p 403. New York, McGraw-Hill, 1993

RIDLEY

Eponym used to indicate dyspnea in heart failure.

BIBLIOGRAPHY. Ridley H: Observationes quaedam medico-praticae et physiologicae; inter quas aliquanto fusius agitur, de asthmate et hydrophobia. Quarum etiam decem ultimis subjiciuntur administrationes totidem corporum morbis quorum tituli observationibus iis praesigunture affectorum anatomicae, cum particulari, et non ante observata, de cordis in embryone vasorum structura, et sanguinis juxta eam circuitu, dissertatione, pp 224. Lugduni Batavorum, G Langerak et LT Lucht, 1738

Hope J: A Treatise on Diseases of the Heart and Great Vessels. London, 1833

Osler W: Lectures on Angina Pectoris and Allied States, p 81. New York, Appleton, 1897

Cohn JN, Sonnenblick EH: Diagnosis and therapy of heart failure. In Schlant RC, Alexander RW: Hurst's The Heart, 8th ed, pp 561–562. New York, McGraw-Hill, 1994

RIEDEL

Synonyms. Ligneous thyroiditis; struma Riedel; fibrous thyroiditis, chronic; woody thyroiditis; sclerosing thyroiditis.

Symptoms. Female to male ratio, 2–4:1. Onset most frequently 30–70 years of age. Onset insidious; occasionally, asymptomatic. Dyspnea; dysphagia; hoarseness; aphonia. Later (and not seldom) signs of hypothyroidism (see Gull). In some cases association with extracervical fibrosclerosis (approximately 30%).

Signs. Thyroid normal size or enlarged, usually symmetrical or unilateral, and of hard consistency.

Etiology. Unknown. No explanation for the typical fibroblastic proliferation. Sporadic. Apparently no genetic predisposition.

Pathology. Thyroid tissue replaced by dense fibrotic tissue, where scattered follicular cells and acini remain; the fibrotic tissue is adherent to trachea and muscle.

Diagnostic Procedures. *Thyroid tests.* Usually normal; thyroid antibodies (in 45%); later T4 concentration and ^{131}I uptake may be depressed. *Blood.* Normal sedimentation rate and white blood cell count. *Biopsy.* See Pathology.

Therapy. Surgery usually only to relieve obstruction. Medical treatment if hypothyroidism.

Prognosis. Process may remain stable for years or progress slowly and produce hypothyroidism that may stabilize or regress. In some case evolution into Hashimoto (see).

BIBLIOGRAPHY. Riedel BM: Die chronische zur Bildung eisenharter Tumoren fuehrende Entzuendung der Schilddruese. Verh Dtsch Ges Chir 25:101–105, 1896

Hamburger J: The various presentations of thyroiditis: Diagnostic considerations. Ann Intern Med 104:219–224, 1986

Volpé R: Subacute and sclerosing thyroiditis. In De Groot LJ (ed): Endocrinology, 3rd ed, pp 747–748. Philadelphia, WB Saunders, 1995

RIEGER

Synonyms. Axenfeld posterior embryotoxon-juvenile glaucoma; dysgenesis mesodermalis cornae et iridis; iris dysplasia—hypodontia—myotonic dystrophy—iris dysplasia—hypertelorism—psychomotor retardation; iridogoniodysgesis; somatic anomalies.

Symptoms. Juvenile glaucoma beginning in childhood with great oscillation in tension; frequently associated with neurologic manifestations.

Signs. Various anterior segment disturbances: dyscoria; pseudopolycoria; corectopia; iridostasis; iris dehiscences; prominence of iris sphincter; aplasia of the mesodermal leaf of the iris; ectropion uveae; corneal opacification; anterior polar cataract; ectopia lentis. Frequently associated, microphthalmos, strabismus, ptosis palpebralis, and hemangioma conjunctivalis. Extraocular associated manifestations: absence of or irregular teeth; hypertelorism; partial absence of facial bones; myotonic dystrophy, and umbilical hernia.

Etiology. Unknown. Hereditary autosomal dominant condition. Chromosomal aberrations (4, 6, 9, 13, 18, 21) have been reported in association with this syndrome.

Pathology. Elevated intraocular pressure. Embryotoxon (prominent anterior border ring of Schwalbe), associated with anterior segment disturbances (see Signs).

Diagnostic Procedures. *Gonioscopy. X-rays.*

Therapy. Limboscleral trephination; miotics.

Prognosis. With trephination; ocular tension usually becomes regulated and visual deterioration does not progress.

BIBLIOGRAPHY. Brailey WA: Double microphthalmos with defective development of iris, teeth and anus. Glaucoma at an early age. Trans Ophthalmol Soc UK 10:139, 1890
Axenfeld T: Embriotoxon corneal posterius. Berl Dtsch Ophthalmol Ges 42:301, 1920
Rieger H: Beiträge zur Kenntnis seltener Missbildungen der Iris: Über Hypoplasie des Irisvorderblattes mit Verlagerung und Entrundung der Pupille. Albrecht Von Graefes Arch Ophthalmol 133:602–635, 1935
Friedman JM: Umbilical dysmorphology: The importance of contemplating the belly button. Clin Genet 28:343–347, 1985
Pedersen OO, Rushood A, Olsen EG: Anterior mesenchymal dysgenesis of the eye. Acta Ophthalmol (Copenh) 67:470–476, 1989

RIEHL

Synonyms. Jute spinner melanosis; melanosis Riehl; reticulated pigmented poikiloderma; tar melanosis; war melanosis. See Civatte.

Symptoms. More frequent in women. Onset at any age. Mild constitutional (unexplained) symptoms.

Signs. Brownish gray pigmentation of the face, more intense in forehead and temples, occasionally extension to neck and scalp, chest, seldom, hands, and forearms.

Etiology. Unknown. Tar derivatives, cosmetic, nutritional factors suspected.

Pathology. Degenerative changes of basal layer; perivascular dermal infiltrates; melanin free in dermis and in melanophores. Horny plugs in follicles.

Therapy. Symptomatic.

Prognosis. Chronic condition, slowly fading.

BIBLIOGRAPHY. Riehl G: Ueber eine eigenartige Melanose Vorläufige Mitterung. Wien Klin Wochenschr 30:780–781, 1917

Civatte A: Poikiloderma réticulée du visage et du cou. Ann Dermatol Syph 4:605–609, 1923
Bleehen SS, Ebling FJG, Champlon RH: Disorders of skin color. In Champion RH, Burton JL, Ebling FJG (eds): Rook/Wilkinson/Ebling Textbook of Dermatology, 5th ed, p 1597. Oxford, Blackwell Scientific, 1992

RIETTI-GREPPI-MICHELI

Obsolete.

Synonym. Microelliptopoikilocytic anemia. See also Thalassemia syndromes. Clinical classification used prior to the discovery of the characteristic physiochemical behavior of hemoglobins. This eponym indicated the presence of hypochromic iron-resistant anemia, hemolytic jaundice, and decreased osmotic fragility.

BIBLIOGRAPHY. Rietti F: Sugli itteri emolitici primitivi. Atti Acc Sci Med Nat Ferrarae, 1925
Greppi E: Ittero emolitico familiare con aumento della resistenza dei globuli. Minerva Med (Pt 2) 8:1–11, 1928
Micheli F: Le splenomegalic emolitiche. Att 35th Congr Soc Ital Med Int, 1929

RIGA-FEDE

Synonyms. Cardarelli diphtheroid subglossitis; Fede; cachectic aphthae; subglossitis diphtheroides; sublingual fibrogranuloma.

Symptoms. Sublingual pain arising in children affected by whooping cough or diphtheria.

Signs. Small sublingual ulcerated tumor.

BIBLIOGRAPHY. Riga A: Di una Malattia Della Prima Infanzia, Probabilmente non Trattata, di Movimenti Patologici. Napoli, 1881
Fede F: Della produzione sottolinguale, malattia di Riga. I Congr Pediatr Ital Napoli, pp 251–260, 1890–1891
Scully C: The oral cavity. In Champion RH, Burton JL, Ebling FJG (eds): Rook/Wilkinson/Ebling Textbook of Dermatology, 5th ed, p 2709. Oxford, Blackwell Scientific, 1992

RIGHT RECTUS

Synonyms. Right rectus muscle; pseudoappendiceal.

Symptoms. Severe pain localized from onset to right lower quadrant. Nausea but no vomiting (absence of crampiform generalized abdominal pain).

Signs. Marked tenderness, spasticity over McBurney's point. No rebound tenderness. Persistence of tenderness when rectus muscle tenses (patient raising neck or trying to sit without the help of hands). Signs of rheumatic fever may be present.

Etiology and Pathology. Rheumatic myositis; strain of right rectus muscle.

Diagnostic Procedures. *Blood.* In rheumatic fever, elevated sedimentation rate, moderate leukocytosis, normal differential antistreptolysine titer. *ECG.* In rheumatic fever. In strain, normal blood findings. *Echography. Xerography.*

Therapy. That of rheumatic fever. Topical infection with procaine.

Prognosis. According to etiology.

BIBLIOGRAPHY. Geptill P: Differential diagnosis of abdominal manifestations of acute rheumatic fever from acute appendicitis. Ann Surg 99:650–660, 1934

Babbage ED, McLaughlin CW Jr, Fruin RL: Strain of right rectus muscle simulating acute appendicitis. War Med 5:280–282, 1944

Reitman N: Abdominal manifestations of rheumatic fever: Description of a right rectus syndrome. Ann Intern Med 22:671–687, 1945

Steinheber FV: Medical conditions mimicking the acute surgical abdomen. Med Clin North Am 57:1559–1567, 1974

Haubrich WS: Abdominal pain. In Haubrich WS, Schaffner F, Berk JE (eds): Bockus Gastroenterology, 5th ed, pp 27–28. Philadelphia, WB Saunders, 1995

RILEY-DAY

Synonyms. Familial dysautonomia; hereditary sensory autosomal neuropathy III; HSAN III.

Symptoms. Almost completely confined to Ashkenazic Jews. Condition often manifested in first days of life. Defective lacrimation; corneal hypoalgesia; relative insensitivity to pain; defective taste sensation; defective swallowing; orthostatic hypotension; paroxysmal hypertension; attacks of unexplained pyrexia; poor muscular coordination and dysarthria; emotional lability; cyclic vomiting; frequent pulmonary infections. Failure to thrive.

Signs. Frequent ulceration of cornea (50%); absence of vallate and fungiform papillae of tongue (pathognomonic); kyphoscoliosis; neuropathic joints (may also be observed). Areflexia; Romberg sign.

Etiology. Partial or complete absence of plasma dopamine-beta-hydroxylase activity; hereditary condition (autosomal recessive inheritance).

Pathology. Nonconstant findings: hypoplasia and cytologic changes of autonomic ganglia; cytologic alterations in hypothalamus and brain stem.

Diagnostic Procedures. Characteristic response to certain drugs: absence of flushing to histamine injection and exaggerated response to methacholine and norepinephrine; potentiated miosis following instillation of methacholine into conjunctival sac. *X-ray.* Of bones and joints; scoliosis. *EEG.* Epileptic patterns. *Urine.* Elevated ratio of homovanillic acid to vanillylmandelic acid.

Therapy. No satisfactory treatment available. Tarsorrhaphy. Anesthesia high risk.

Prognosis. Poor. Aspiration pneumonia, hyperpyrexia, nephrosclerosis as causes of death.

BIBLIOGRAPHY. Riley CM, Day RL, Greeley DM, et al: Central autonomic dysfunction with defective lacrimation. I. Report of five cases. Pediatrics 3:468–478, 1949

Axelrod FB, Kania I, Fish I, et al: Progressive sensory loss in familial dysautonomia. Pediatrics 67:517–522, 1981

Kaplan M, Schiffmann R, Shapira Y: Diagnosis of familial dysautonomia in the neonatal period. Acta Paediatr Scand 74:131–132, 1985

Weatherall DJ, Ledingham JGG, Warrell DA: Oxford Textbook of Medicine, p 4104. Oxford, Oxford Med Pub, 1996

RILEY-SHWACHMAN

Symptoms. Described in two children. Anorexia; cachexia; asthenia.

Signs. Characteristic ambulation with stiff legs, wide base, and calcaneal limp. Deep reflexes increased; ankle clonus.

Etiology. Unknown.

Diagnostic Procedures. *X-ray.* Generalized osteoporosis and increased density at the base of the skull.

BIBLIOGRAPHY. Riley CM, Shwachman H: Unusual osseous disease with

neurologic changes: Report of two cases. Am J Dis Child 66:150–154, 1943

RIMMED VACUOLE MYOPATHY

Synonyms. Myopathy with ringed vacuoles including granulovacuolar myopathy.

Symptoms and Signs. Similar to those of Cylindrical spiral myopathy (see). Onset in childhood or later, progressive muscle weakness, especially of legs.

Etiology. Probably autosomal dominant inheritance.

Pathology. Muscle: Rimmed or autophagic vacuoles located closely to cell surface, demarcated by a fine granular rim in light microscopic sections.

Diagnostic Procedures. *Muscle biopsy. EMG.*

Therapy. Symptomatic.

Prognosis. Slowly progressive condition. In some cases fatal outcome.

BIBLIOGRAPHY. Argov Z, Yarom R: Rimmed vacuole myopathy sparing the quadricipis: A unique disorder in Iranian Jews. J Eur Sci 64:33–43, 1984

Goebel HH, Lenard HG: Congenital myopathies. In Handbook of Clinical Neurology, 18: Rowland LP, Di Mauro S (eds): The Myopathies, p 331. Amsterdam, Elsevier, 1992

RIMOIN-McALISTER

Synonyms. Metaphyseal dysplasia (type A-V); dysostosis metaphyseal (type A-V).

Symptoms and Signs. Occurs in males. Present from birth. Recurrent ear infections. Conductive hearing loss; mental retardation; short limb dwarfism.

Etiology. Autosomal recessive inheritance.

Diagnostic Procedures. *X-ray.* Widening, shortening, and irregularity of metaphyses of long bones of upper and lower extremities.

BIBLIOGRAPHY. Rimoin DL, McAlister WH: Metaphyseal dysostosis, conductive hearing loss and mental retardation: A recessive inherited syndrome. Birth Defects 7:116–122, 1971

RING CHROMOSOME r (2)

Symptoms and Signs. Mild to severe intrauterine and severe postnatal growth deficit, microcephaly, and not typical dysmorphisms and visceral defects.

Etiology. Ring r(2) chromosome including two mosaics.

BIBLIOGRAPHY. Sutherland GR, Carter RF: 46, XX/46, xx, r(2)(p25q37) mosaicism clinical and cytogenetic studies. Ann Genet (Paris) 21:164–167, 1978

Schinzel A: Catalogue of Unbalanced Chromosome Aberrations in Man, pp 106–107. Berlin, de Gruyer, 1984

RING D2 CHROMOSOME

Symptoms and Signs. Aplasia of thumbs; mental and physical retardation; trigonocephaly. Other similarities in common among patients with this syndrome are microcephaly, ptosis of eyelids, epicanthal folds, malrotation of ears, micrognathia, hypoplastic nipple, widely spaced first and second toes.

Etiology. Chromosomal deletion associated with ring D2 chromosome. Clinical differences associated with variable degrees of chromosomal loss or differences in genetic background. Lack of thumbs is a common feature.

Diagnostic Procedure. *Chromosome study.*

BIBLIOGRAPHY. Bain AD, Gauld IK: Multiple congenital abnormalities associated with ring chromosome. Lancet 2:304–305, 1963

Sparkes RS, Carrel RE, Wright SW: Absent thumbs with a ring D2 chromosome: A new deletion syndrome. Am J Hum Genet 19:644–659, 1967

RING DERMOID

Symptoms and Signs. Usually bilateral amblyopia, astigmatism (irregular cornea), strabismus, dermoid choristoma, conjunctival plaque of keratinization and hairs growing from tumor mass.

Etiology. Unknown. Autosomal dominant.

Pathology. Tan firm nodule(s) in lower temporal quadrant of corneoscleral limbus, coverd by keratinized statified squamous epithelium and containing adipose tissue, collagen hair follicles, sweat and sebaceous glands and occasionally cartilage.

BIBLIOGRAPHY. Henkind P: Bilateral corneal dermoids. Am J Ophthalmol 76:972–977, 1973

Mattos J: Ring dermoid syndrome. Arch Ophthalmol 98:1059–1061, 1980

Torczynski E: Developmental anomalies of the eye. In Garner A, Klintworth GK (eds): Pathobiology of Ocular Disease: A Dynamic Approach, 2nd ed, pp 1303–1304. New York, Marcel Dekker, 1994

RITSCHER-SCHINZEL

Synonyms. Dandy-Walker-like; atrioventricular septal defect: craniocerebellocardiac; 3C.

Symptoms and Signs. From birth. Macrocephaly, hypertelorism, downslanting palpebrae, depressed nasal bridge, narrow palate low set ears. Mild mental retardation. Signs of heart malformations (atrioseptal defect).

Etiology. Unknown. Possibly autosomal recessive inheritance.

Pathology. Atrioseptal malformation. Dandy-Walker malformation (see) with communicating hydrocephalus (in one case) cerebellar variable malformations.

Diagnostic Procedures. See Pathology. *Blood. Low immunoglobulin level.*

Therapy. Symptomatic. Heart surgery.

Prognosis. Poor.

BIBLIOGRAPHY. Ritscher D, Schinzel A, Bolthauser E, et al: Dandy-Walker (like) malformation, atrioventricular septal defect and a similar pattern of minor anomalies in 2 sisters: A new syndrome? Am J Med Genet 26:481–491, 1987

Verloes A, Dresse MF, Javanovic M, et al: 3C syndrome: Third occurrence of cranio-cerebellar-cardiac dysplasia (Ritscher-Schinzel syndrome). Clin Genet 35:205–208, 1989

RITTER

Synonyms. Lyell; exfoliative neonatal dermatitis; keratolysis neonatorum; staphylococcal-scalded skin; SSS. Including TEN (toxic epidemic necrolysis).

Symptoms. Occurs in infants around seventh day of life or in childhood. Male to female ratio, 4:1. Irritability; pain.

Signs. Erythema spreading all over the body, followed by desquamation of epidermis in large sheets. Nikolsky sign. Red, weeping areas result from desquamation. In the few adults recorded, usually renal failure and immunologic incompetence.

Etiology. Unknown. Association with staphylococcal infection (hemolytic, coagulase positive). Identical with Lyell syndrome.

Pathology. Epidermal necrosis; lack of involvement of corium.

Diagnostic Procedure. *Culture.* To identify bacteria.

Therapy. Antibiotics; cortisone. General supportive treatment.

Prognosis. Healing of the skin quite complete 10 days after onset of desquamation in more than two thirds of cases. Fatality in the remaining cases with high fever, severe toxicity, and shock. (TEN form toxic epidermal necrolysis.)

BIBLIOGRAPHY. Ritter von Rittershain G: Dermatitis erysipelatosa, Gangraena, Enkephalitis. Oesterr Jb Paediatr Wien 1:23–24, 1870

Ritter von Rittershain G: Die exfoliative Dermatitis jungerer Sauglinge. Ztsahr Kinderheilk 2:3–23, 1878

Lyell A: The staphylococcal-scaled skin syndrome in historical perspective: Emergence of dermopathic strains of Staphylococcus aureus and discovery of the epidermolytic toxin. A review of events up to 1970. J Am Acad Dermatol 9:285–294, 1983

Blanc MF, Jarnier M: Staphylococcies exfoliantes (SSSS) de l'adulte. Ann Dermatol Venerol 113:833–843, 1986

Pye RJ: Bullous eruptions. In Champion RH, Burton JL, Ebling FJG (eds): Rook/Wilkinson/Ebling Textbook of Dermatology, 5th ed, pp 1665–1667. Oxford, Blackwell Scientific, 1992

ROBERTS

Synonyms. Appelt-Gerken-Lenz; cleft lip-palate-tetraphocomelia; facial hemangioma—hypomelia—hypotrichosis; pseudothalidomide; SC.

Symptoms and Signs. Present from birth. At birth, length 40 cm, weight 1.5–2 kg; microbrachycephaly; hypertelorism; shallow orbit; prominent eyes, cataracts, corneal opacity, coloboma; midfacial capillary hemangiomas; thin nares; malformed ears; cleft lip, occasionally left palate; micrognathia. Sparse, silver blond hair. Hypomelia (of all degrees from phocomelia to minor and variable alterations); cryptorchidism. In the few survivors, severe mental defect. Occasionally, hydrocephalus, cardiac and renal defects.

Etiology. Autosomal recessive inheritance.

Diagnostic Procedures. *Blood.* Possible thrombocytopenia. *X-rays. CT scan. Sonography.* See Signs.

Therapy. Not advisable in cases of severe defects in midfacial and severe limbs defects.

Prognosis. Frequently, stillbirth or early death. Survivors show severe growth defects and mental deficiency.

BIBLIOGRAPHY. Krueger R: Die Phocomelic und ihre Uebergaenga (case 87), p 92. Berlin, A Hirschwald, 1906

Roberts JB: A child with double cleft of lip and palate, protrusion of the intermaxillary portion of the upper jaw and imperfect development of bones of the four extremities. Ann Surg 70:252–254; 1919

Grundy HO, Burlbaw J, Walton S, Dannar C: Roberts syndrome: Antenatal ultrasound: A case report. J Perinat Med 16:71–75, 1988

ROBERTSON-KIHARA

Synonyms. Juxtaglomerular apparatus tumor.

Symptoms and Signs. Those of secondary aldosteronism (see).

Etiology. Unknown. Neoplastic production of renin and secondary aldosteronism.

Pathology. Juxtaglomerular apparatus, benign tumor.

Diagnostic Procedures. *Blood.* Plasma renin and aldosterone increase hypokalemia. *Renal arteriogram. CT scan. MRI.* Demonstration of tumor.

Therapy. See hyperaldosteronism.

Prognosis. Fair.

BIBLIOGRAPHY. Robertson PW, Klidjian A, Harding LK, et al: Hypertension due to a renin secreting tumor. Am J Med 43:963–976, 1967
Samsom SC, Giebisch GH: Control of potassium excretion. In Massry SG, Glassock RJ: Textbook of Nephrology, 3rd ed, p 318. Baltimore, Williams & Wilkins, 1995

ROBINOW

Synonyms. Covesdem; Robinow-Silverman-Smith; achondroplasia-like dwarfism; acral dysostosis—facial—genital abnormalities; achondroplastic dwarfism; mesomelic dwarfism; fetal face—mesomelic dwarfism.

Symptoms and Signs. Both sexes affected, especially females. Marked variability, especially in females. Present from birth. Mild shortness. *Head.* Macrocephaly; frontal bossing; hypertelorism; small upturned nose; small mouth; micrognathia; crowded teeth. *Extremities.* Brachymelia; brachydactyly. *Genitalia.* Penis or clitoris and labia majora hypoplasia. *Cryptorchidism.* Other associated anomalies: facial nevus (23%), rudimentary uvula (18%), cleft palate (9%), scoliosis (50%), mental retardation (5–27%), umbilical hernia (20%).

Etiology. Autosomal dominant or recessive (Covesdem) inheritance.

Diagnostic Procedures. *Blood.* Thrombocytopenia. *Urine.* Normal. *Chromosome study.* Normal. *X-ray.* Of skeleton. Does not confirm clinical impression of achondroplastic changes; multiple rib anomalies (40%), hemivertebrae (70%), urinary system anomalies (29%).

Pathology. See Signs; hemivertebrae.

Therapy. Question of sex rearing because penile hypoplasia.

Prognosis. Usually, normal mental performance.

BIBLIOGRAPHY. Robinow M, Silverman FN, Smith HD: A newly recognized dwarfing syndrome. Am J Dis Child 117:649–651, 1969
Butler MG, Wadlington WB: Robinow syndrome: Report of two patients and review of literature. Clin Genet 31:77–85, 1987
Israel H, Johnson GF: Craniofacial pattern similiarities and additional orofacial findings in siblings with the Robinow syndrome. J Craniofacial Genet Dev Biol 8.63–73, 1988
Rimoin DL: Genetic disorders of the osseous system. In Beithon P: McKusick's Heritable Disorders of Connective Tissue, 5th ed, pp 636, 637, 719. St Louis, CV Mosby, 1993

ROBINOW-SORAUF

Synonyms. Craniosynostosis—bifid hallux; acrocephalosyndactyly RS.

Symptoms and Signs. Facies equal to Saethre-Chotzen (see), plus bilaterally broad toes (duplication of distal phalanx).

Etiology. Autosomal dominant.

BIBLIOGRAPHY. Robinow M, Sorauf TJ: Acrocephalopolysyndactyly (type Noack) in a large kindred. Birth Defects XI (5):99–106, 1975
Young ID, Harper PS: An unusual form of acrocephalosyndactyly. J Med Genet 19:286–288, 1982

ROBINSON (A.R.)

Synonym. Hidrocystoma.

Symptoms. Prevalent in females. Onset in middle age. Occurs in persons exposed to heat (e.g., cooks). Lesion of cheeks and eyelids of cystic aspect, which progressively enlarges with repeated heat exposure.

Etiology. Unknown.

Pathology. Dilated and convoluted sweat ducts, containing amorphous debris, not connected with surface.

Therapy. Excision. Avoidance of exposure to heat.

Prognosis. Benign.

BIBLIOGRAPHY. Robinson AR: Hidrocystoma. J Cutan Dis 11:293–303, 1893
MacKie RM: Tumors of the skin appendages. In Burton JL, Cunlife WJ: Subcutaneous fat. In Champion RH, Burton JL, Ebling FJG (eds): Rook/Wilkinson/Ebling Textbook of Dermatology, 5th ed, p 1517. Oxford, Blackwell Scientific, 1992

ROBINSON (E.M.)

Synonyms. Dysmenorrhea; unilateral genital atresia.

Symptoms. Occurs in patients 12–27 years of age. Dysmenorrhea setting in shortly after menarche, increasing in severity with subsequent menstruations. Concomitant symptoms; nausea; vomiting; constipation or diarrhea; dysuria.

Signs. Unilateral pelvic tumor.

Etiology. Incomplete fusion of müllerian ducts or faulty adaptation of the müllerian ducts resulting in atresia of one side and therefore accumulation of the menstruation flow on that side with each menstruation.

Pathology. Pelvic cystic mass filled with blood occupying either the left or right lower quadrant. The mass on section represents one side of the ovary, tube, uterine cavity, and cervix.

Therapy. Early surgical removal of mass and surgical correction of the defect.

Prognosis. Good.

BIBLIOGRAPHY. Robinson EM: Supernumerary uterus in a girl eighteen years old: Removal; recovery. Ala Med J 23:152–154, 1910–1911
Merckel GC, Sucoff MC, Sender B: The syndrome of dysmenorrhea and unilateral gynatresia in a double uterus: Report of a case and review of literature. Am J Obstet Gynecol 80:70–75, 1960
Schulman LP, Elias S: Developmental anomalies of the female reproductive tract: Pathogenesis and nosology. Adolesc Pediatr Gynecol 1:203–238, 1988

ROBINSON (G.C.)

Synonyms. Deafness; nail dystrophy; ectodermal dysplasia.

Symptoms and Signs. Nonconstant presence of all features: partial anodontia; peg-shaped teeth; hypoplasia and dystrophy of nails (altered dermatoglyphics); mental retardation; seizures; moderate deafness (sensorineural type); less frequently, syndactyly, polydactyly.

Etiology. Autosomal dominant inheritance (Robinson) and autosomal recessive (D.O.O.R.).

Diagnostic Procedures. *Sweat test.* Increase of sweat electrolytes. *Skin biopsy. Plasma. Urine.* Increase of organic 2-oxoglutarate.

BIBLIOGRAPHY. Robinson GC, Miller JR, Bensimon JR, Bensimon JR:

Familial ectodermal dysplasia with sensorineural deafness and other anomalies. Paediatrics 30:797–802, 1962

Feinmessers M, Zelig S: Congenital deafness associated with onyco-dystrophy. Arch Otolaryngol 74:507–508, 1961; 90:474–477, 1969

Qazy QH, Nangia BS: Abnormal distal phalanges and nails, deafness, mental retardation and seizures disorder: A new familial syndrome. J Pediat 104:391–394, 1984

Harper J: Genetics and genodermatoses. In Champion RH, Burton JL, Ebling FJG (eds): Rook/Wilkinson/Ebling Textbook of Dermatology, 5th ed, p 346. Oxford, Blackwell Scientific, 1992

ROCHON-DAVIGNEAU

Synonyms. Superior orbital fissure; orbital fissure superior. Includes: Behr (pterygopalatine fossa) and Dejan (orbital fossa). See Rollet and Jacod.

Symptoms and Signs. Ophthalmoplegia (involvement of third, fourth, and sixth cranial nerves); sensory changes in the trigeminal ophthalmic area: ptosis, high proptosis, dilatation and fixation of pupil; anaesthesia of upper high lid and forehead. No blindness. Seldom areas of V/I and V/II contemporaneous involvement.

Etiology and Pathology. (1) Fracture of the zygomatic area; (2) Infections in retrobulbar space, cavernous sinus and/or CNS; (3) Neoplasia from the nose extending through orbital floor (Dejan) or pterygopalatine fossa (Behr); (4) Hematoma.

Diagnostic Procedures. *X-ray. Angiography.* Patterns according to etiology. *Blood.* In some cases, elevation of leukocytes and sedimentation rate. *Cerebrospinal fluid.* Highly variable; sugar normal or depressed; protein and cell normal or slightly elevated.

Therapy. Antibiotics or surgery. Heparin in cases with thrombosis.

Prognosis. Depends on etiology. Much improved by use of antibiotics; some cases of nonspecific infection respond to corticosteroids.

BIBLIOGRAPHY. Rochon-Duvigneaud A: Quelques cas de paralysie de tous les nerfs orbitaires (ophtalmoplegie totale avec amaurose et anesthésie dans le domaine de l'ophtalmique d'origine syphilitique). Arch Ophthalmol 16:746–760, 1896

Zachariades M, Vairaktaris E, Papavassiliou D, et al: The superior orbital fissure syndrome. J Maxillofac Surg 13:125–128, 1985

Gorlin RJ, Cohen MM, Levin LS: Syndromes of the Head and Neck, p 602. New York, Oxford University Press, 1990

ROENHELD

Synonyms. Postprandial cardiogastric; postprandial gastrocardiac; hysteric tympanism.

Symptoms. Following a meal, atypical chest pain lasting several hours, palpitations.

Etiology. Unknown.

Diagnostic Procedures. *ECG.* Normal before meal; 30 minutes after feeding; sinus tachycardia, linear ST depression, flat T-waves; 2–3 hours after meal, normal. In cases with heart block, bradycardia after meal.

Therapy. In many cases atropine, domperidone, and other anticholinergic agents prevent manifestations.

BIBLIOGRAPHY. Roenheld L: Der gastrocardiale Symptomenkomplex, eine besondere Form sogenannter Herzneurose. Z Phys Diat Ther 16:339–349, 1912

Gilbert NC, Fenn GK, LeRoy GV: The effect of distention of abdominal viscera. JAMA 115:1962–1967, 1940

Utsu F, Enescu V, Boszormenyi E, et al: Postprandial syndrome. New Physician 15:102–103, 1966

O'Rourke RA: Chest pain. In Schlant RC, Alexander RW: Hurst's The Heart, 8th ed, p 464. New York, McGraw-Hill, 1994

ROGER

Synonym. Small septal ventricular heart defect. Two types of this defect are recognized:

WITH MILD PULMONIC STENOSIS

Symptoms. Asymptomatic; absence of cyanosis.

Signs. Murmur of ventricular septal defect.

Diagnostic Procedures. *ECG.* Mild right ventricular hypertrophy. *X-ray.* Normal.

Therapy. None.

Prognosis. Good.

WITH SEVERE PULMONIC STENOSIS

Symptoms and Signs. See Pulmonary subvalvular stenosis (infundibular with intact ventricular septum).

BIBLIOGRAPHY. Roger H: Reserches cliniques sur le communication congénitale des deux coeurs, par inocclusion des septum interventriculare. Bull Acad Med 8:1074–1094, 1879

Nugent EW, Plauth WH, Edwards JE, et al: The pathology, pathophysiology recognition and treatment of congenital heart disease. In Schlant RC, Alexander RW: Hurst's The Heart, 8th ed, pp. 1768–1773. New York, McGraw-Hill, 1994

ROGERS (L.E.)

Synonyms. Megaloblastic anemia; thiamine responsive diabetes mellitus; sensory neural deafness; thiamine responsive anemia.

Symptoms and Signs. Both sexes. Megaloblastic anemia responding to thiamine therapy. Sensory neural deafness; situs viscerum inversus. Hepatosplenomegaly: generalized subedema, hoarseness, cardiac and neurologic disturbances. Those of diabetes.

Etiology. Autosomal recessive. Reduced α-ketoglutarate dehydrogenase activity.

Diagnostic Procedures. *Blood.* Megaloblastic anemia; hyperglycemia. *Bone marrow.* Megaloblastic erythropoiesis and many ringed sideroblasts. *ECG.* Variable patterns. *X-rays.* Situs inversus viscerum reported.

Therapy. Thiamine corrects anemia but not diabetes.

Prognosis. Fair with treatment. Relapses with discontinuation of thiamine.

BIBLIOGRAPHY. Rogers LE, Poster FW, Sidbury JB Jr: Thiamine-responsive megaloblastic anemia. J Pediat 74:494–504, 1969

Duran M, Wadman SK: Thiamine-responsive inborn errors of metabolism. J Inherit Metab Dis 8 (Suppl 1):70–75, 1985

Saudubray JM, Charpentier C: Clinical phenotypes: Diagnosis/algorithms. In Scriver CR, Beaudet AL, Sly WS, et al: The Metabolic and Molecular Bases of Inherited Disease, 7th ed, pp 382, 384, 392. New York, McGraw-Hill, 1995

ROKITANSKY-VAN BOGAERT

Synonyms. Hamartomatous meningeal melanosis; melanoblastic hyperplasia; melanosis neurocutaneous; neurocutaneous melanosis.

Symptoms. Both sexes affected. Onset in fetal life. Variable neurologic symptoms from normalcy to severe mental deficiency and other neurologic deficits.

Signs. Numerous pigmented skin nevi; frequent typical feature is "bathing trunk" nevus, involving skin of lower abdomen, buttocks, and upper parts of legs.

Etiology. Congenital dysplasia of neural crest. Autosomal recessive inheritance.

Pathology. *Skin.* Typical appearance of pigmented dermal nevi. *Central nervous system.* Dura-pia-arachnoid or brain, cerebellum (almost entirely confined to gray matter) pigmented cells; pigment-laden macrophages; melanophoric cells.

Diagnostic Procedures. *X-rays. CT scan. MRI.* Hydrocephalus; calcifications in suprasellar cistern, silvian fissure, occipital lobe; spinal cord distorsion syringomyelia.

Therapy. Symptomatic.

Prognosis. Variable; stillbirth or death in early childhood. Survival up to adulthood possible. Possibility of malignant transformation of lesions to be considered.

BIBLIOGRAPHY. Rokitansky J: Ein ausgezeichneter Fall von Pigmentmal mit ausgebreiteter Pigmentierung der inneren Hirn- und Rückemarkshäute. Allg Wien Met Ztg 6:113, 1861
Van Bogaert L: La melanose neurocutanée diffuse heredofamiliale. Bull Acad R Med Belg (6th series) 13:397, 1948
Zuniga S, Casheras J, Benveniste S: Rhabdomyosarcoma arising in a congenital giant nevus associated with neurocutaneous melanosis in a neonate. J Pediat Surg 22:1036, 1038, 1987

ROLANDO FRACTURE

Symptoms and Signs. Comminuted intra-articular fracture of proximal end of metacarpal.

BIBLIOGRAPHY. Sabiston DC: Textbook of Surgery, 14th ed, p 1. Philadelphia, WB Saunders, 1991

ROLLAND-DEBUQUOIS

Synonyms. Dissegmental dysplasia; R-D. See Silverman-Handmaker and Kniest-like, lethal.

Symptoms and Signs. Neonatal distress. Short limbed chondrodysplasia (Kniest-like) presenting same features that the Silverman-Handmaker (see).

Etiology. Autosomal recessive inheritance.

Pathology. Chondro-osseous tissue with patches of broad collagen fibers.

Diagnostic Procedures. *X-rays.* Radiologic changes similar but less severe than those observed in Silverman-Handmaker.

Prognosis. Lethal disorder, many survive past infancy.

BIBLIOGRAPHY. Rolland JC, Langier J, Grenier B, et al: Nanisme chondrodystrophique et division palatine chez un nouveaue-ne. Ann Pediatr 19:139–142, 1972
Alek KA, Grix A, Clericuzio C, et al: Dyssegmental dysplasia: Clinical, radiographic and morphologic evidence of heterogeneity. Am J Med Genet 27:295–312, 1987

ROMANO-WARD

Synonyms. Ward-Romano; long QT; LQT; QT syndrome; ventricular fibrillation, prolonged QT interval. See also Jervell-Lange-Nielsen.

Symptoms and Signs. Include all those present in Jervel's and Lange-Nielsen with and without deafness.

Etiology. Unknown. Possibly, congential subnormal activity of right stellate ganglion combined with reflex overactivity of left stellate ganglion. Autosomal dominant inheritance reported.

Diagnostic Procedures. See Jervell-Lange-Nielson.

Therapy. Quinidine or procainamide. Proposed therapy with beta-blocking agents. Automatic implantable defibrillator.

Prognosis. Repeated automatic attacks of dysrhythmias, syncope, and sudden death after psychologic or physical stress.

BIBLIOGRAPHY. Locati E, Moss AJ, Schwartz PJ, et al: The long QT syndrome. Am J Cardiol 3:516, 1948
Romano C, Gemma G, Pongiglione R: Aritmie cardiache rare dell'età pediatrica. II. Accessi sincopali per fibrillazione ventricolare parossistica. Clin Pediatr 45:656–683, 1963
Ward OC: A new familial cardiac syndrome in children. J Irish Med Assoc 54:103–106, 1964
Bhandari AK, Scheinman M: The long QT syndrome. Mod Concepts Cardiovasc Dis 54:45–50, 1985
Schlant RC, Alexander RW: Hurst's The Heart, 8th ed, pp 937, 1725, 1731, 1745. New York, McGraw-Hill, 1994

ROMBERG-WOOD

Synonym. Primary pulmonary hypertension.

Symptoms. Female to male ratio, 5:1 (in childhood equal incidence). Onset usually 12–40 years of age; but ranging from early infancy to eighth decade. Effort syncope; angina pectoris; dyspnea; asthenia; fatigue (in otherwise healthy young women) after exertion, cold exposure, or excitement, or spontaneously. Raynaud phenomenon (see) occasionally associated.

Signs. In infants asthenia and cough may lead to malnutrition and failure to thrive. Occasionally, mild acrocyanosis. Pulse small; large vein (cervical) pulsation. Palpation of right ventricular systolic impulse and of main pulmonary artery: presystolic distention of right ventricle. Auscultation; loud pulmonic component of second sound with ejection sound; right-sided fourth sound. Hepatomegaly.

Etiology. Idiopathic instrinsic obstructive disease of small arteries and arterioles of pulmonary bed. Multiple causes, mostly unknown, but resulting in vicious cycle (pulmonary hypertension begets pulmonary hypertension). Both autosomal dominant and recessive inheritance reported. Angiitis or Marfan associated in some cases.

Pathology. Histology: in small arteries and arterioles, medial hypertrophy, intima proliferation, fibrous vascular occlusion, secondary dilatation (angiomatoid lesions), necrotic and thrombotic changes.

Diagnostic Procedures. *ECG.* Initially, normal sinus rhythm; later, atrial flutter or fibrillation and various degrees of systolic overload of right atrium; up to frank right axis deviation. *X-ray.* Variable from mild to extreme enlargement of pulmonary trunk and branches; lung fields clear. *Fluoroscopy.* Pulsation of pulmonary arteries. *Catheterization.* Pulmonary arterial hypertension; without left-to-right or right-to-left shunt; normal pulmonary wedge pressure.

Therapy. No satisfactory therapy. Long-term anticoagulants. Symptomatic.

Prognosis. Variable according to course. Death in 4–5 years from onset of symptoms. Reported a persistent familial neonatal form with death in a few days.

BIBLIOGRAPHY. Romberg E: Ueber Sklerose der Lungernarterie. Dtsch Arch Klin Med 48:197–206, 1891–1892
Wood P: Pulmonary hypertension. Mod Concepts Cardiovasc Dis 28:513–518, 1959

Loyd JE, Primm RK, Newman JH: Familial primary pulmonary hypertension: Clinical patterns. Am Rev Respir Dis 129:194–197, 1984

Fishman AP: Pulmonary Hypertension. In Schlant RC, Alexander RW: Hurst's The Heart, 8th ed, pp 1857–1874. New York, McGraw-Hill, 1994

Weatherall DJ, Ledingham JGG, Warrell DA: Oxford Textbook of Medicine, pp 2511–2513. Oxford, Oxford Med Pub, 1996

RONCHESE

Synonyms. Pili torti, twisted hair.

Symptoms and Signs. In females, from infancy. Shafts of hair, flat and twisted at regular intervals through 180 degrees, dry, coarse, lusterless, and fragile. Occasionally hypoplastic tooth enamel.

Etiology. Unknown. Autosomal recessive inheritance. This condition is observed also in Menkes syndrome (see).

Prognosis. Usually hair becomes normal at puberty.

BIBLIOGRAPHY. Ronchese F: Twisted hairs (pili torti). Arch Dermatol Syph 26:98–109, 1932

Schutz J: Pili moniliformis Arch Dermatol Syphilol 53:69–73, 1946

Gedda L., Cavalieri R: Rilievi genetici della distrofia congenita dei capelli. Proc Sec Intern Cong Hum Genet Roma Sept 6/12/61, 2:1070–1077, 1963

Dawber RPR, Ebling FJG, Wojnarowska FT: Disorders of hair. In Champion RH, Burton JL, Ebling FJG (eds): Rook/Wilkinson/Ebling Textbook of Dermatology, 5th ed, pp 2609–2610. Oxford, Blackwell Scientific, 1992

ROQUES

Eponym used to indicate the combination of effects of pulmonary and cardiac sclerosis observed in old patients with cor pulmonale secondary to chronic respiratory insufficiency.

BIBLIOGRAPHY. Roques R: Les scléroses parallélles du coeur et du poumon. Sem Hop Paris 25:721–724, 1949

ROSACEA

Synonyms. Acne rosacea (misleading name); couperose.

Symptoms. In adolescence, more common in males; in adulthood, male to female ratio, 1:3; onset usually 30–40 years of age. Variable according to different variants of the syndrome: heat and congestion in areas involved; soreness and irritability of eye (ocular rosacea). Recurrence of symptoms in the spring or following stress or fatigue.

Signs. Progressive. Initially intermittent flushing, becoming a permanent erythema on the cheeks, chin, forehead; associated with papules and pustules and telangiectasis. In some cases, thickening of skin of affected areas, and association of edema of the eyelids.

Etiology. Unknown. Gastrointestinal, nutritional, psychological, endocrine, and infective factors, seborrheic status and vasomotor reactivity considered.

Pathology. Initially, vasodilatation; then, edema of dermal vessels, ectasia with lymphocytic infiltration followed by formation of epithelial cell foci.

Therapy. Psychological treatment; rest; sedation. If sunlight aggravates the symptoms, antimalarial drugs. Tetracycline per os or topical when per os contraindicated (pregnancy). Metronidazole per os or topical (1%). Corticosteroid may make rosacea worse (use of bland type for short period may be helpful).

Prognosis. Unpredictable. Recurrence of minor manifestations in spring for years (10 or more) then thickening of lesions without further remission. Many cases may subside spontaneously in a shorter period. In adolescent males the milder form lasts 4–5 years.

BIBLIOGRAPHY. Kissmeyer A: Sur la kératite et autres affections oculaires de la couperose. Ann Dermatol Syph 5:22–48, 1934

Pendelesco C, Valdeman J: La kératite rosacée. Arch Ophthalmol 2:1080–1087, 1938

Miescher G: Rosacea und rosacea: Ähnliche Tuberkulide. Dermatologice 88:150–170, 1943

Marks R: Rosacea, flushing and perioral dermatitis. In Champion RH, Burton JL, Ebling FJG (eds): Rook/Wilkinson/Ebling Textbook of Dermatology, 5th ed, pp 1851–1858. Oxford, Blackwell Scientific, 1992

ROSAI-DORFMAN

Synonyms. Sinus histiocytosis; massive lymphadenopathy; SHML.

Symptoms and Signs. All races. Male to female ratio, 1.8:1; from birth to seventh decade (median, 20.6 years). Lymphoadenopathy (100%): cervical most frequent (84%); all other stations may be involved with minor frequency. Extranodal disease (present in 43% of cases): skin, nasal cavities, paranasal sinuses, soft tissue bones, eyelid, orbit, salivary glands, CNS. At onset unusual hepatosplenomegaly. Fever (27%). Pallor (anemia 66%). Various rheumatic manifestations.

Etiology. Unknown.

Pathology. *Lymph node.* Proliferation of histocytes with round, eight staining nuclei and apparently benign nucleoli, vacuolated on sinuses and occasionally in interfollicular areas. Others hyperplastic germinal center with thick fibrous capsulae and areas of necrosis. Hysticocytes show, characteristically lymphocytophagocytosis (normal, viable lymphocytes, less frequently, neutrophils and plasma cells inside vacuolated histiocytes).

Diagnostic Procedures. *Blood.* Anemia, neutrophilia elevated sedimentation rate, polyclonal gammopathy. *Frozen tissue.* Immunophenotic profile 5–100 protein (100%). HAM 56 (100%), alfa, -antitripsin and alfa1-chymotrypsin (95%). Lysozyme (85%). CD1A (Leu6) negative. *X-rays.* Possible lytic areas.

Therapy. Surgery, radiotherapy, prednisone, chemotherapy (prednisone + vinca alkaloids + alkylating agents, apparently best combination).

Prognosis. Course protracted. Few cases with complete remission reported. With treatment, course is protracted and in most cases patient recovers.

BIBLIOGRAPHY. Rosai J, Dorfman RF: Sinus histiocytosis with massive lymphoadenopathy: A newly recognized benign clinopathologic entity. Arch Pathol Lab Med 87:63, 1969

Fourcar E, Rosai J, Dorfman R: Sinus histiocytosis with massive lymphadenopathy (Rosai-Dorfman disease): Review of the entity. Semin Diagn Pathol 7:19–73, 1990

Weatherall DJ, Ledingham JGG, Warrell DA: Oxford Textbook of Medicine, p 3609. Oxford, Oxford Med Pub, 1996

ROSEMBERG-LOHR

Synonyms. Metaphyseal—sella turcica dysplasia; Rosemberg; ulnar–metaphyseal dysplasia.

Symptoms and Signs. Wrist pain. Thickening of the wrists.

Etiology. Autosomal dominant inheritance.

Diagnostic Procedures. *X-rays. CT scan.* Metaphyseal irregularities; wide epiphyseal plate and metaphyses. Dorsum sella: thickened. Vertebrae: wedged, and plate sclerosis; coxa valga.

BIBLIOGRAPHY. Rosemberg E, Lahr H: A new hereditary bone dysplasia with characteristic bowing and thickening of the distal ulna. Eur J Pediatr 145:40–45, 1986

ROSENBERG-BARTHOLOMEW

Synonyms. Hyperuricemia; ataxia; deafness.

Symptoms and Signs. In females, full expression: ataxia and deafness. In males, less severely affected.

Etiology. Possibly consistent with autosomal recessive or X-linked inheritance.

Diagnostic Procedures. *Blood.* Hyperuricemia. Alteration related to renal impairment. Red cell: hypoxanthine-guanine phosphoribosyl transferase normal.

BIBLIOGRAPHY. Rosenberg AL, Bartholomew BA: Hyperuricemia neurologic deficits: A family study abstracted. Arthritis Rheum 17:837, 1968
Rosenberg AL, Bergstrom L, Troost BT, et al: Hyperuricemia and neurologic deficits: A family study. N Engl J Med 282:992–997, 1970

ROSENBERG-CHUTORIAN

Synonym. Optic atrophy—polyneuropathy—deafness; deafness—polyneuropathy—optic atrophy.

Symptoms and Signs. Males. Distal muscular atrophy (type Charcot-Marie-Tooth, see), progressive optic atrophy and hearing loss.

Etiology. Unknown. Suggested X-linked semidominant inheritance.

BIBLIOGRAPHY. Rosenberg RN, Chutorian A: Familial opticoacoustic nerve degeneration and polyneuropathy. Neurology 17:827–832, 1967
Konigsmark BM, Gorlin RJ: Genetic and Metabolic Deafness. Philadelphia, WB Saunders, 1976

ROSENBLOOM-ZEICHEN

Synonyms. Limited joint mobility, diabetes; cheiroarthropathia diabetica; periarticular joint contraction, diabetes.

Symptoms and Signs. Reported in 50% of postadolescent patients with diabetes mellitus of 5 years duration. Painless and not disabling. Limited joint mobility, beginning typically on fifth finger. Moving radially, involving interphalangeal, metacarpophalangeal and large joints. Growth failure. Association with thick waxy skin, decreased pulmonary function, retinopathy, nephropathy, and neuropathies independently from duration of diabetes.

Etiology. Diabetes mellitus. Age more important than duration of diabetes.

Diagnostic Procedures. *X-rays.* Periarticular thickening. *Blood.* Hyperglycemia.

Therapy. That of diabetes.

Prognosis. Growth failure not related to diabetic control.

BIBLIOGRAPHY. Rosenbloom AL, Frias JL: Diabetes mellitus, short stature and joint stiffness: a new syndrome. Clin Res 22:92A, 1974
Benedetti A, Noaaco C: Cheiroarthropathy of juvenile diabetes. Acta Diabetol Lat 13:94, 1975
Rosenbloom AL: Limited joint mobility in insulin dependent childhood diabetes. Eur J Pediatr 149:380–388, 1990

ROSEN-CASTLEMAN-LIEBOW

Synonyms. Alveolar proteinosis; lung alveolar proteinosis; pulmonary alveolar proteinosis; PAP; pulmonary phospholipidosis—lipoproteinosis; phospholipoproteinosis.

Symptoms. Onset at all ages. Most often in adult males. Majority of patients chronically exposed to sawdust, fumes, or other irritating substances. Onset insidious. In half of cases, prodromal febrile illness considered pneumonia. Progressive dyspnea; productive cough; sputum thick, chunky, and yellow-whitish, seldom red streaked. Fever usually absent. Fatigability, chest pain, and weight loss.

Signs. Few; pulmonary rales (rare); finger clubbing (rare); cyanosis (terminally).

Etiology. Defective clearence of intra-alveolar material owing to a dysfunction of type II alveolar pmneumocytes. Reported associated with hematologic malignancies; lymphoma; infection (bacterial, fungal, viral). Possible familial occurrence (autosomal dominant [?]).

Pathology. Beneath pleura, multiple yellow-grayish nodules firm on palpation, size from a few millimeters to 2 cm, areas of consolidation; marked increase in weight. Microscopically, alveoli filled by PAS-positive proteinaceous material, rich in lipid; aveolar cell ghosts. Alveolar septa and interstitial tissue and capillaries normal. Interstitial fibrosis may occur in some cases.

Diagnostic Procedures. *X-ray.* Fine, diffuse, perihilar, radiating nodular or reticular pattern of increased density. Calcification does not occur; lymph nodes not enlarged. *Blood.* Moderate tendency to polycythemia. Leukocytes normal or moderate neutrophilia; LDH elevated. *Sputum.* Culture negative. *Skin test.* Negative. *Open lung biopsy.* See Pathology.

Therapy. Antibiotics for superimposed infections. Ambroxol; lung lavage useful. Corticosteroid ineffective.

Prognosis. Chronic course. Cases of spontaneous recovery in 5 months to 5 years. Clinical remission with persistence of radiographic features frequent. Progressive dyspnea, cyanosis, and death after chronic course in 25% of cases.

BIBLIOGRAPHY. Rosen SH, Castleman B, Liebow AA: Pulmonary alveolar proteinosis. N Engl J Med 258:1123–1142, 1958
Hoffman RM, Rogers RM: Pulmonary alveolar proteinosis. In Lynch JP, Remee RA: Immunologically Mediated Pulmonary Diseases, p 449. Philadelphia, Lippincott, 1991
Weatherall DJ, Ledingham JGG, Warrell DA: Oxford Textbook of Medicine, pp 2833–2835. Oxford, Oxford Med Pub, 1996

ROSENTHAL (C.)

Synonyms. Sleep paralysis; night palsy; sensory paroxysm. See pavor nocturnus. (No to be confused with sleep palsies, see Saturday night paralysis.)

Symptoms. Occurs at moment of falling asleep or awaking. Anxiety usually accompanied by hypnagogic hallucinations. Inability to talk or shout, and moaning, being half asleep and half awake with a dim awareness of environment. Attacks last 1 or 2 minutes, but subjectively seem to last a long time. May be interrupted by a sudden movement or by somebody touching the patient. Some differences from pavor nocturnus (see).

Signs. None.

Etiology. Unknown. Related to narcolepsy (see Gelineau), cataplexy, hypnagogic paralysis, and hallucinations with which it constitutes a clinical tetrad of no special clinical significance.

Therapy. None specific.

Prognosis. Variable. Some people may experience the attack only once or twice in life; some have repeated attacks for life.

BIBLIOGRAPHY. Mitchell SW: On some of the disorders of sleep. Virginia Med Monthly 2:769–781, Feb 1876

Rosenthal C: Ueber das verzoegerte psychomotorische Erwachen, seine Entspehung und seine nosologische Bedentung. Arch Psychiatr 81:159–171, 1927

Wilson SAK: The narcolepsies. Brain 51:63–109, 1928

Schneck JM, Fuseli H: Nightmare and sleep paralysis. JAMA 207:725–726, 1969

Adams RD, Victor M: Principles of Neurology, 5th ed, p 345. New York, McGraw-Hill, 1993

ROSENTHAL-KLOEPFER

Synonyms. Acromegaloid changes; cutis verticis gyrata; corneal leukoma. See Cutis verticis gyrata; Sotos and Touraine-Solente-Gole syndromes.

Symptoms and Signs. Both sexes affected. Onset in early childhood. Visual troubles owing to corneal leukomas; acromegaloid development; horn-like projection of lateral supraorbital ridges. From fourth decade hyperplasia and furrowing of skin of face and scalp. Normal mental development.

Etiology. Unknown. Autosomal dominant inheritance.

Therapy. Symptomatic.

Prognosis. Good quoad vitam.

BIBLIOGRAPHY. Rosenthal JW, Kloepfer HW: An acromegaloid cutis verticis gyrata, corneal leukoma syndrome. A new medical entity. Arch Ophthalmol 68:722–726, 1962

Gardner-Medwin D: Cerebral gigantism. Dev Med Child Neurol 11:796–797, 1969

ROSENTHAL (R.L.)

Synonyms. Factor XI deficiency; hemophilia C; plasma thromboplastin antecedent deficiency; PTA deficiency.

Symptoms. Both sexes affected. Common in European Jews and Japanese. Clinical manifestation similar to hemophilia but milder. Rarely, spontaneous bleeding, purpura, or hemarthrosis. Usually, manifestation secondary to trauma or surgery. Important feature is bleeding, occasionally occurring 2–3 days after surgery. Severe form exists.

Etiology. Congenital deficiency of Factor XI. Incompletely recessive autosomal inheritance; major manifestation in homozygous, minor in heterozygous individuals.

Diagnostic Procedures. *Blood.* Normal bleeding time; slightly prolonged clotting time; increased partial thromboplastin time, corrected by normal absorbed plasma or aged serum; abnormal thromboplastin generation test when all reagents are from patient; abnormal prothrombin consumption test; normal one-stage prothrombin time.

Therapy. Plasma; stored plasma effective.

Prognosis. Variable according to severity of form. Surgical or postsurgical bleeding most threatening feature.

BIBLIOGRAPHY. Rosenthal RL, Dreskin OHN: New hemophilia-like disease caused by deficiency of a third plasma thromboplastin factor. Proc Soc Exp Biol Med 82:171–174, 1953

Muir WA, Ratnoff OD: The prevalence of plasma thromboplastin antecedent (PTA, factor X1 deficiency). Blood 44:569, 1974

Fujikawa K, Chung DW: Factor XI. In High KA, Roberts HR (eds): Molecular Basis of Thrombosis and Hemostasis. New York, Marcell Dekker, 1995

ROSEWATER

Synonym. Familial gynecomastia. See male pseudohermaphroditism,

incomplete hereditary (type I); gynecomastia familial. See Reifenstein (same condition or variant of).

Symptoms and Signs. Gynecomastia; sterility. External genitalia normal.

Etiology. X-linked inheritance. Resistance to androgen action. Gwinup denies this interpretation because of the rapid masculinization apparently obtained by testosterone admistration (200 mg monthly).

Pathology. Normal internal genital system.

Diagnostic Procedures. *Blood.* Testosterone level increased; estrogens (for men) increased. Gonadotropins increased.

BIBLIOGRAPHY. Rosewater S, Gwinup G, Hamwi G: Familial gynecomastia. Ann Intern Med 63:377–385, 1965

Gwinup G: Incomplete male pseudohermaphroditism. N Engl J Med 308. 1974

Griffin JE, McPhaul MJ, Russell DW, et al: The androgen resistence syndromes: 5-reductase deficiency, testicular feminization, and related disorders. In Scriver CR, Beaudet AL, Sly WS, et al: The Metabolic and Molecular Bases of Inherited Disease, 7th ed, p 2981. New York, McGraw-Hill, 1995

ROSS

Synonyms. Holmes-Adie; segmental hypohidrosis; progressive selective sudomotor denervation.

Symptoms and Signs. Time of onset of pupillotonia, hypoactive deep tendon reflexes, and hypohidrosis is variable. Localized (patchy) progressive hyperhidrosis to anhidrosis, following a dermatomal pattern; no vasoconstriction or alteration of blood flow.

Etiology. Unknown. The coexistence of hypohidrosis and Holmes-Adie syndrome appears not to be a chance association.

Pathology. Unknown. Skin biopsy of affected areas normal. Selective, degenerative changes of sympathetic pathways.

Diagnostic Procedures. *Sweat test.* Localized hypohidrosis (quinizarin compound test, pilocarpine test). Tests indicated for pupillotonic-pseudotabes (see).

Therapy. None.

Prognosis. Usually progressive hypohidrosis.

BIBLIOGRAPHY. Ross AT: Progressive selective sudomotor denervation: A case with coexisting Adie's syndrome. Neurology 8:809–817, 1959

Lucy DD, Van Allen MW, Thompson HS: Holmes-Adie syndrome with segmental hypohidrosis. Neurology 17:763–769, 1967

Heath PD, Moss C, Cartlidge NEF: Ross syndrome and skin changes. Neurology 32:1041–1042, 1982

ROSSELLI-GULIENETTI

Synonyms. Walker-Clodius; Zlotogora-Ogur (considered different entity only by some AA); EEC; ectrodactyly—ectodermal dysplasia—clefting; lobster claw deformity; nasolacrimal obstruction. See also Aase-Smith; Gross-Groh-Weppl; Holt-Oram, Robert.

Symptoms. Both sexes affected. Onset from birth. Photophobia.

Signs. *Facies.* Hypertelorism; constant epiphora; mucopurulent conjunctival discharge; cleft palate and lips. Partial anodontia, microdontia severe cheratitis, choanal atresia. *Extremities.* Deformities of hands: syndactyly; absence of second metacarpal of index and middle finger; and rudimentary third metacarpal of same digits; and feet: absence of first and fifth metacarpal and occasionally of the toe; mild nail dysplasia. *Hair.* Sparse, thin, light colored. Occasionally: deafness; ear malformation; renal anomalies.

Etiology. Autosomal dominant inheritance.

Diagnostic Procedures. *X-rays. CT scan. MRI. Sonography:* See Signs. *Blood.* Growth hormone level deficiency.

Therapy. Surgery. Trial with corticosteroids and antibiotics.

Prognosis. Good quoad vitam.

BIBLIOGRAPHY. Cockaine EA: Cleft palate-lip, hare-lip, dacruocystitis, and cleft hand and foot. Biometrika 28:60–63, 1936

Rosselli D, Giulienetti R: Ectodermal dysplasia. Br J Plas Surg 14:190–204, 1961

Walker JC, Clodius L: The syndrome of cleft lip, cleft palate and lobster claw deformities of hand and feet. Plast Reconstr Surg 32:627–636, 1963

Zlotogora J, Zilberman Y, Tenenbaum A, et al: Cleft lip and palate, pili torti, malformed ears, partial syndactyly of fingers and toes and mental retardation: A new syndrome? JMed Genet 24:291–293, 1987

Christodoulow J, McDongall PN, Scheffield LJ: Choanal atresia as feature of ectrodactyly-ectodermal dysplasia-clefting (EEC) syndrome. J Med Genet 26:586–589, 1989

Rodini ESO, Richieri Costa A: Autosomal recessive ectodermal dysplasia, cleft lip palate, mental retardation and syndactyly: The Zlotogora-Ogur syndrome. Am Med Genet 36:473–476, 1990

ROSTAN

Synonyms. Cardiac asthma; paroxysmal dyspnea. Eponym used to indicate dyspneic attacks generally occurring during the night in patients with congestive heart failure.

BIBLIOGRAPHY. Rostan LL: Mémoire sur cette question, l'asthme des veillards est-il une affection nerveuse? Nouv J Med Chir Pharm 3:3–30, 1818

ROTENSTEIN

Synonym. Arteritis familial granulomatous polyarthritis-uveitis. See Job.

Symptoms and Signs. Both sexes, fever, erythematous rash, hypertension, uveitis. Large vessel nodules; hand, knee, and ankles warm and red, pericardial and pleural effusion, seizures.

Etiology. Autosomal dominant.

Pathology. Systemic noncaseating granulomatous lesions. Periarticular osteoporosis.

Diagnostic Procedures. *Arteriography.* Stenosis and poststenotic dilatations. *Skin. Liver biopsy.* See Pathology.

Therapy. Prednisone, cyclophosphamide.

Prognosis. Improvement with prolonged treatment. Fatal outcome at various ages.

BIBLIOGRAPHY. Rotenstein D, Gibbas DL, Majmudar B, et al: Familial granulomatous arteritis with polyarthritis of juvenile onset. N Engl J Med 306:86–90, 1982

ROTH-BIELSCHOWSKY

Synonym. Pseudo-ophthalmoplegia.

Symptoms and Signs. Complete paralysis of all conjugate movements of eyes in one or more directions, except those under labyrinthine control. Vertical movements are relatively or preferentially affected. Stimulation of one labyrinth induces reflex deviation of eyes to side opposite that of paralysis; stimulation of other labyrinth induces deviation of eyes to side of paralysis.

Etiology and Pathology. Lesion of basal ganglia or tectum.

Therapy. According to etiology.

Prognosis. Depends on etiology.

BIBLIOGRAPHY. Roth W: Demonstration von kranken mit Ophthalmoplegie. Neurol Centralbl 20:921, 1901

Bielschowsky A: Das klinische Bild der assozierten Blicklähmung und seine Bedeutung für die topischen Diagnostik. MMW 50:1666–1670, 1903

Cogan DG, Adams RD: Type of paralysis of conjugate gaze (ocular motor apraxia). Arch Ophthalmol 50:434–442, 1953

Adams RD, Victor M: Principles of Neurology, 5th ed, pp 229–230. New York, McGraw-Hill, 1993

ROTHMANN-MAKAI

Synonyms. Makai; lipogranulomatosis subcutanea.

Symptoms and Signs. Both sexes affected. Prevalent in children. Appearance (usually symmetric) of nodules or plaques, slightly tender, firm, elastic consistency in subcutaneous tissue (up to 10 or 15 cm in diameter) on the trunk, occasionally on limbs and face as well. Area most affected front of thighs. No systemic symptoms.

Etiology. Unknown. Possibly trauma or vascular damage.

Pathology. At onset, vasodilatation; fat cell necrosis, infiltration with neutrophils. Intermediate: histiocytes with foamy cytoplasm. Terminal: fibrosis with lobular atrophy.

Diagnostic Procedures. Biopsy.

Therapy. None.

Prognosis. Slowly evolving condition; duration 6 months to 1 year; seldom longer (years).

BIBLIOGRAPHY. Rothmann M: Ueber Entzündung und Atrophie des subcutanen Fettgewebes. Virchows Arch (Pathol Anat Physiol) 136:159–169, 1894

Makai E: Über Lipogranulomatosis subcutanea. Klin Wochenschr 7:2343–2346, 1928

Niemi KM, Forström L, Hannuksela M, et al: Nodules on the legs: A clinical, histological and immunohistological study of 82 patients representing different types of nodular panniculitis. Acta Dermatol Venerol 57:145, 1977

Burton JL, Cunlife WJ: Subcutaneous fat. In Champion RH, Burton JL, Ebling FJG (eds): Rook/Wilkinson/Ebling Textbook of Dermatology, 5th ed, p 2144. Oxford, Blackwell Scientific, 1992

ROTHMUND-THOMSON

Synonyms. Bloch-Stauffer; Thomson-Rothmund; cataract—telangiectasia—pigmentation; poikiloderma atrophicans—cataract juvenilis. See Werner.

Symptoms and Signs. Prevalent in females (16:5); appearing 3–6 months after birth. Cutaneous changes: telangiectasia; brownish pigmentation; atrophy of skin; lesions appearing on the face, ears, buttocks, extremities. At 4–6 years of age, development of bilateral cataracts (50%); occasionally later and in some cases do not develop (see Thomson). Mental and physical development normal or deficient. In some cases, sexual retardation (1:4).

Etiology. Unknown. Recessive hereditary familial trait.

Pathology. *Skin.* Thin and pliable; no ulceration. Distended veins form a characteristic netlike arrangement around atrophic scaling areas. Brownish pigmented spots in the vicinity of telangiectasia. No inflammatory reaction or homogenization of subcutaneous tissue. Other organs and tissues. Normal. In some cases, hypogenitalism (25%) and bone defect (1:3).

Diagnostic Procedures. *Biopsy.* Of skin. *Blood.* Low vitamin A.

Therapy. Cataract extraction.

Prognosis. Progressive in first years of life, then tends to remain static. Average life span, even to old age. Possibly, carcinomatous changes of skin.

BIBLIOGRAPHY. Rothmund A: Über Cataracten in Verbindung mit einer eigenthümlichen Hautdegeneration. Albrecht Von Graefes Arch Ophthalmol 14:159–182, 1868
Thomson MS: Poikiloderma congenitale. Br J Dermatol 48:221–234, 1936
Silver HK: Rothmund-Thomson syndrome: An oculocutaneous disorder. Am J Dis Child 111:182–190, 1966
Dechenne C, Chantraine JM, Davin JC: A Rothmund-Thomson case with hypertension. Clin Genet 24:266–272, 1983
Klintworth GK: Genetic disorders affecting the eye. In Garner A, Klintworth GK (eds): Pathobiology of Ocular Disease: A Dynamic Approach, 2nd ed, p 813. New York, Marcel Dekker, 1994

ROTHMUND-WERNER

Cases in which features of Rothmund and Werner syndromes overlap.

BIBLIOGRAPHY. Thannhauser SJ: Werner's syndrome (progeria of the adult) and Rothmund's syndrome: Two types of closely related heredofamilial atrophic dermatosis with juvenile cataracts and endocrine features. Ann Intern Med 23:559–626, 1945
Merz EH, Tausk K, Dukes E: Mesoecto-dermal dysplasia and its variants. Am J Ophthalmol 55:488–504, 1963

ROTOR

Synonym. Hyperbilirubinemia idiopathic.

Symptoms and Signs. Both sexes affected. Onset shortly after birth or in childhood. Mild fluctuating jaundice. Attacks of intermittent epigastric discomfort and occasionally abdominal pain, fever, and hepatomegaly.

Etiology. Autosomal recessive inheritance. Organic anion transport defect with reduced biliary excretion of coproporphyrins.

Pathology. *Liver.* Normal histology.

Diagnostic Procedures. *Blood.* No evidence of hemolysis. Serum bilirubin (conjugated) slight to moderate increase. Sulfobromophthalein in serum sample taken at 45 minutes shows a marked elevation (in Dubin-Johnson the same elevation has been seen at 90–120 min). *Urine.* Bilirubinuria. Increased total urinary coproporphyrin; absent increase of fraction III. *Cholangiography.* Normal.

Therapy. None.

Prognosis. Good.

BIBLIOGRAPHY. Rotor AB, Manahan L, Florentin A: Familial nonhemolytic jaundice with direct van den Bergh reaction. Acta Med Philippina 5:37–49, 1948
Chawdhury JR, Wolkoff AW, Chawdhury NR, et al: Hereditary jaundice and disorders of bilirubin metabolism. In Scriver CR, Beaudet AL, Sly WS, et al: The Metabolic and Molecular Bases of Inherited Disease, 7th ed, p 2190. New York, McGraw-Hill, 1995

ROUSSET

Synonym. Anodontia—monilethrix. See Sabouraud.

Symptoms and Signs. Association of various tooth abnormalities (pointed; development limited to few permanent teeth; absence of permanent dentition) and monilethrix.

Etiology. Unknown. Monilethrix could have autosomal or recessive inheritance and is one feature of many syndromes: Menkes'; argininosuccinicaciduria; Pollit; hair-brain; Netherton.

BIBLIOGRAPHY. Strandberg J: A contribution to our knowledge of aplasia moniliformis. Acta Dermatol Venereol 3:650–655, 1922
Rousset J: Génodermatose difficilement classable (trichorrhexis nodosa) predominant chez lan quatre générations. Bull Soc Fr Dermatol Syph 59:298–300, 1952
Gorlin RJ, Pindborg JJ: Syndromes of the Head and Neck. New York, McGraw-Hill, 1964

ROUSSY-CORNIL

Synonyms. Hypertrophic neuropathy sporadic; interstitial hypertrophic neuritis; polyradiculoneuropathy.

Symptoms. Onset in second to third decade or later. Wide distribution of lancinating pains (not constant); peripheral weakness; fasciculation; disturbed vision; ataxia.

Signs. Nerves are occasionally palpable and tender when touched; peripheral atrophy; tendon reflexes disminished or abolished; myosis; sluggish pupils; scoliosis.

Etiology. Unknown. Regarded as form of von Recklinghausen neurofibromatosis, associated with cerebellar diseases. (To be differentiated from Charcot-Marie-Tooth, leprosy, polyneuritis, amyloid, and collagen diseases.) Its autonomous entity doubted by some authors. It may be considered also as the adult type of Dejerine-Sottas.

Pathology. Uniform nerve trunk thickening; hypertrophy of Schwann sheaths (onion-like laminated structure). Secondary lesions: thickening of spinal roots; degeneration of posterior columns.

Diagnostic Procedures. Laboratory. Normal (occasionally increase in protein in cerebrospinal fluid). Biopsy of sensory nerve.

Therapy. None. General care and splinting of weak muscles. Corticosteroids.

Prognosis. Progressive. Occasionally remissions and exacerbations.

BIBLIOGRAPHY. Roussy G, Cornil L: Névrite hypertrophique progressive non-familial de l'adulte. Ann Med 6:296–305, 1919
Dyck PJ, Lambert EH: Lower motor and primary sensory neuron diseases with peroneal muscular atrophy. Arch Neurol 18:603–618, 1968
Adams RD, Victor M: Principles of Neurology, 5th ed, pp 1149–1150. New York, McGraw-Hill, 1993

ROUSSY-LÉVY

Synonym. Symonds-Show; ataxia hereditary; muscular atrophy.

Symptoms. Onset early in childhood. Variable manifestations with constant patterns within affected family. Difficulty in walking, clumsiness, and tremor of hands, mental deficiency.

Signs. Muscular wasting of legs and hands. Ataxia; bilateral pes cavus; tendon areflexia; kyphoscoliosis. Sensory changes and cerebellar signs minimal or absent.

Etiology. Unknown. Confuse entity considered form of hypertrophic neuriti, fortuitous association of Charcot-Marie-Tooth and essential tremor, peroneal muscular atrophy, Dejerine-Sottas and forms of spinocerebellar degeneration. Autosomal dominant inheritance.

Pathology. Degeneration of spinal cord radicular areas and posterior roots (see Friedreich ataxia, Pathology).

Diagnostic Procedures. *Electromyography. CT scan. MRI.*

Therapy. Symptomatic. Orthopedic, physical therapy, avoid alcohol and fatigue.

Prognosis. Slowly progressive. Death from intercurrent diseases, spontaneous remission observed.

BIBLIOGRAPHY. Roussy G, Lévy G: Sept cas d'une maladie familiale particuliére: troubles de la marche, pieds bots et aréfléxia tendineuse généralisée, avec accessoirement, légère maladresse des mains. Rev Neurol (Paris) 33:427–450, 1926
Symonds CP, Show ME: Familial claw-foot with absent tendon jerks: A forme fruste of the Charcot-Marie-Tooth disease. Brain 49:387–403, 1926
Rombold GR, Riley HA: The abortive type of Friedreich's disease. Arch Neurol Psychiatr 16:301–302, 1926
Yudell A, Dyck PJ, Lambert EA: A kinship with Roussy-Levy syndrome. Arch Neurol 13:432–440, 1965
Weatherall DJ, Ledingham JGG, Warrell DA: Oxford Textbook of Medicine, p 4103. Oxford, Oxford Med Pub, 1996

ROUX

Synonyms. Roux limb; Roux stasis gastric atony postgastrectomy, devagotomized Roux limb; gastroparesis chronica.

Symptoms and Signs. In patients who have undergone a Roux-en-Y procedure for reconstruction after partial gastrectomy with vagotomy because of alkaline gasritis (see bile reflux). Symptoms occur either postopertively or months or years after operation. More frequent in women. Nausea and vomiting of solid food (38%), epigastric pain and fullness (46%), gastroparesis (26%), weight loss (32%)

Etiology. The vagotomy of the Roux limb is the cause of gastric atony and delayed empting.

Diagnostic Procedures. Gastric empting studies: delayed empting. Endoscopy.

Therapy. *Medical.* Prokinetic drugs (metoclopramide, bethanechol, domperidone, lisapride); adequate nutritional support; intermittent or chronic gastric decompression via nasogastric tube or gastrectomy, avoid narcotics for pain. *Surgical.* Removal of dysfunctional gastric remnant: total gastrectomy; with Roux-en-Y reconstruction, gastrojejunostomy (Billroth II-type anastomosis) with diverting Braun enteroenterostomy duodenal switch operation, Tanner Roux 19 modification; exclusion jejunoduodenostomy.

Prognosis. Medical therapy: success 50%; surgical therapy: optimal result.

BIBLIOGRAPHY. Gustavson S, Ilstul D, Morrison P, et al: The Roux stasis syndrome after gastrectomy. Am J Surg 155:490–494, 1988
Vogel SB, Haking MP: Etiology and treatment of the Roux syndrome. Prob Gen Surg 10:308–320, 1993
Schirmer BD: Gastric atony and the Roux syndrome in Postsurgical syndromes. Gastroenterol Clin N Am 23:327–343, 1994

ROWELL

Synonym. Multiform-like erythema; lupus erythematosus.

Symptoms and Signs. Without precipitating factors, episodic development of annular multiform-like erythema lesions on the face, mouth, neck, and chest, in patients affected by lupus erythematosus, discoid (see) or lupus erythematosus, systemic (see). Initially, lesions are papular, than ringform and, finally, bullous and necrotic.

Etiology. Unknown. See Lupus erythematosus.

Diagnostic Procedures. *Blood.* Typical serologic abnormalities. Speckled type of antinuclear factor associated with precipitine antibody to saline extract of human tissues and rheumatoid factor. Homogeneous type of antinuclear antibody may be present.

Therapy. That of lupus erythematosus.

Prognosis. Episodes last few days up to over 1 month. According to intensity, various degrees of scarring.

BIBLIOGRAPHY. Rowell NR, Beck JS, Anderson JR: Lupus erythematosus and erythema multiform-like lesions. A syndrome with characteristic immunological abnormalities. Arch Dermatol 88:176–180, 1963
Miesher PA (ed): Systemic Lupus Erythematosus. Berlin, Springer, 1995

ROWLAND PAYNE

Synonyms. Horner ipsilateral vocal cord; phrenic nerve palsies.

Symptoms. In women with metastatic breast tumor 6–42 months after first recurrence after chemo- or roentgen therapy. Scarce: pain and weakness in the shoulder, change in voice.

Signs. Horner syndrome (see) plus ipsilateral vocal cord and phrenic nerve palsies. Nonconstant motor involvement in cervical distribution. Lymphoadenopathy of ipsilateral supraclavicular fossa.

Etiology. Metastatic lesion from breast cancer. Possibility that other malignancies (lung) can elicit same manifestations.

Pathology. Neoplastic infiltration at the level of sixth cervical vertebra.

Diagnostic Procedures. *CT brain scan. MRI.*

Therapy. That of breast cancer.

Prognosis. Preterminal syndrome. All patients died within 6 months from onset.

BIBLIOGRAPHY. Rowland Payne CME: Newly recognized syndrome in the neck: Horner's syndrome with ispilateral vocal cord and phrenic nerve palsies. J R Soc Med 74:814–818, 1981
Vaghadia H, Splitte M: Medical letter. J R Soc Med 76:7, 1983

ROWLEY-ROSENBERG

Synonyms. Busbi syndrome (family name); renal aminoaciduria—growth retardation—cor pulmonale—dwarfism; renal aminoaciduria—cor pulmonale—growth retardation; pulmonary hypertension—aminoaciduria.

Symptoms. Rate of growth begins to slow at 1 year of age, in spite of apparently normal nutritional intake; slow motor development; waddling gait; frequent respiratory infections; normal mental development.

Signs. Growth retardation; reduced muscle and adipose tissue. Signs of recurrent pulmonary infections of various degrees (e.g., pneumonia; bronchitis); right ventricular hypertrophy.

Etiology. Unknown. Familial recessive disorders; renal etiology for aminoaciduria; several factors in the growth disturbance. Aminoaciduria without other signs of the condition may exist in other members of the family.

Pathology. Poor muscular development; diffuse changes; fatty infiltration; loss of cross striation; foci of flocculation suggestive of nonspecific primary myopathic lesion. Subcutaneous fat practically absent. Left lung weight below average. Cardiomegaly with marked right ventricular hyperplasia (absence of congenital defects); kidney normal.

Diagnostic Procedures. *Blood.* Increase of free fatty acids; normal amino acid level; PCO_2 elevated, SO_2 decreased. *Urine.* Aminoaciduria: increased excretion of alpha-amino nitrogen (serine, threonine, histidine, lysine, tyrosine primarily). *ECG.* Right ventricular hypertrophy. *X-ray.* Minimal osteoporosis.

Therapy. Symptomatic.

Prognosis. Death of patient with full syndrome before 12 years of age. Simple aminoaciduria results in a normal life.

BIBLIOGRAPHY. Rowley PT, Mueller PS, Watkin DM, et al: Familial growth retardation, renal aminoaciduria, and cor pulmonale. Am J Med 31:187–204, 1961

Rosenberg LE, Mueller PS, Watkin DM: Familial growth retardation, renal aminoaciduria, and cor pulmonale. Am J Med 31:205–214, 1961

Fraser RG, Paré JAP: Diagnosis of Diseases of the Chest, 2nd ed, p 1765. Philadelphia, WB Saunders, 1977

ROYER

Eponym to indicate the association of diabetes mellitus and Prader-Willi syndrome (see).

BIBLIOGRAPHY. Royer P: Le diabéte sucré dans la syndrome de Willi-Prader. J Ann Diabetol Hôtel Dieu 4:91–99, 1963

ROYER-WILSON

Eponym used to indicate ventricular septal defect and absent pulmonary valve. See Kurtz-Sprague-White.

BIBLIOGRAPHY. Royer BF, Wilson JD: Incomplete heterotaxy with unusual heart malformations: A case report. Arch Pediatr 25:881–896, 1908

ROZYCKI

Synonyms. Deafness; vitiligo; achalasia.

Symptoms and Signs. Both sexes. Congenital deafness, dwarfism, vitiligo, muscle wasting and achalasia.

Etiology. Autosomal recessive inheritance (?)

BIBLIOGRAPHY. Rozychi DL, Ruben RJ, Rapin I, et al: Autosomal recessive deafness associated with short stature, vitiligo, muscle wasting and achalasia. Arch Otorynolaryng 93:194–197, 1971

Konigsmark BM, Gorlin RJ: Genetic and Metabolic Deafness. Philadelphia, WB Saunders, 1976

RUBINSTEIN-TAYBI

Synonyms. Broad digits; broad thumb; great toe.

Symptoms. Psychomotor retardation; history of respiratory infections. Mental deficiency (IQ 17–86).

Signs. Facial features: (variable) high arched eyebrows; down- and medially-slanting palpebral fissures (with or without epicanthic folds); ptosis; exophthalmos; strabismus; broad nose bridge; prolonged nasal septum; maxillary hypoplasia; anomalies of size, shape, and position of ears; high-arched palate. Broad thumbs and great toes; changes of dermatoglyphic pattern-low ridge count, extra triradius on tip of thumb, characteristic pattern of thenar area, ulnar loop at base of hypothenar area and in allucal area lateral displacement of E. triradius with or without triradius. Dwarfism; cryptorchidism; nevus flammeus (see). Keloid scars easily form.

Etiology. Most cases sporadic. Possibly polygenic or multifactorial inheritance or autosomal dominant inheritance. 16p13.3 site of the syndrome.

Pathology. See Signs.

Diagnostic Procedures. *EEG.* Abnormal. *X-ray.* Skeletal age retarded; large foramen magnum; low acetabular angle.

Therapy. Symptomatic.

Prognosis. Good quoad vitam except when associated with defect such as congenital cardiac anomalies. Ability to walk with typically abnormal gait; poor speech development.

BIBLIOGRAPHY. Rubinstein JH, Taybi H: Broad thumbs and toes and facial abnormalities: A possible mental retardation syndrome. Am J Dis Child 105:588–608, 1963

Gillies DRN, Roussounis SH: Rubinstein-Taybi syndrome: Further evidence of a genetic aetiology. Dev Med Child Neurol 27:751–755, 1985

Breuning MH, Dauwerse HG, Fugazza G, et al: Rubinstein-Taybi syndrome caused by submicroscopic deletions within 16p13.3. Am J Hum Genet 52:249–254, 1993

Weatherall DJ, Ledingham JGG, Warrell DA: Oxford Textbook of Medicine, p 4110. Oxford, Oxford Med Pub, 1996

RUBROTHALAMIC

Synonyms. Thalamoperforate; thalamic anterolateral.

Symptoms and Signs. In adult and senior subjects. Involuntary movements (resting or intentional tremor, choreoathetotic movements); thalamic hand; and sometime gaze paralysis; no pain or definable disorders of deep sensation.

Etiology and Pathology. Vascular lesion in the anterothalamic area.

BIBLIOGRAPHY. Martin JJ: Thalamic syndromes. In Vinken PJ, Bruyn GW: Handbook of Clinical Neurology, vol 2, p 485. Amsterdam, North-Holland, 1969

RUD

Synonyms. Dwarfism—ichthyosiform erythroderma—mental deficiency. Ichthyosis—neurologic disorder—hypogonadism.

Symptoms and Signs. Both sexes affected (male to female ratio, 2:1). Onset in infancy. Erythroderma ichthyosiform; dwarfism; mental deficiency; hypogonadism; epilepsy; chronic anemia; muscular atrophy; arachnodactyly.

Etiology. Unknown. Not yet completely established clinical entity. Possibly, X-linked recessive.

Pathology. In brain, immature nerve cells; beta cells show chronic chromatolysis; increased oligodendroglia in frontal cortex; binucleated cells in cortex and basal ganglia.

Diagnostic Procedures. *Blood.* Anemia, megaloblastic type. *Biopsy of skin.*

Therapy. Symptomatic.

Prognosis. Poor.

BIBLIOGRAPHY. Rud E: Et Tilfaelde af Infantilisms med Tetani, Epilepsy, Polyneuritis, Ichthiosis og Anaemia of Pernicios type. Hospitalstidende 70:525–538, 1927

York-More ME, Rundle AT: Rud's syndrome. J Ment Def Res 6:108–118, 1962

Wisniewski K, Lewis AR, Shanske AL: X-linked inheritance of the Rud syndrome. Am J Hum Genet 37:A83, 1985

RUDIMENTARY TESTES

Synonyms. Wilkins-Bergada; Leydig cell deficiency; microgenitosomia; normal male chromosome; primary testicular hypoplasia.

Symptoms and Signs. From birth, only males, small gonads either in the scrotum or inguinal channel, small penis and hypospadias. Not associated other anomalies.

Etiology. Probably familial with X-linked inheritance. The syndrome is part of congenitally hypoplastic testis that range from pure XY gonadal dysgenesis to congenital anorchia.

Pathology. Testes: small with differentiated tubules interstitial fibrosis. Internal genitalia in some cases, persistence of structures with vagina and uterus.

Diagnostic Procedures. *LHRH test.* Normal. Testosterone production: low. In postpuberal age: gonadotropins high. Karyotype: 46 XY.

Therapy. Sex assignment according to external genitalia.

Prognosis. Good quoad vitam. Sex assignment may be difficult. No fertility.

BIBLIOGRAPHY. Wilkins L: The Diagnosis and Treatment of Endocrine Disorders in Childhood and Adolescence, pp 276–277. Springfield, IL, Charles C Thomas Publisher, 1965

Bergada C, Cleveland WW, Jones HW, et al: Variants of embryonic testicular dysgenesis: Bilateral anorchia and the syndrome of rudimentary testes. Acta Endocrinol 40:521–536, 1962

Acquafredda A, Vassal J, Job JC: Rudimentary testes syndrome revisited. J Paediatr 80:209–214, 1987

RUEDIGER

Synonym. See hand-foot-uterus.

Symptoms and Signs. A brother and a sister described. Present from birth. *Facies.* Coarse; clefting of soft palate. *Extremities.* Flexion contracture of hands; thick palmar creases; small fingers and nails, arches in all fingers. Ureteral stenosis; retarded growth. The girl had bicornuate uterus and cystic ovaries, the boy small penis and large inguinal hernia.

Etiology. Possibly, autosomal recessive inheritance.

Prognosis. Death within first year of life.

BIBLIOGRAPHY. Ruediger RA, Schimdt W, Loose DA, et al: Severe developmental failure with coarse facial features, distal limb hypoplasia, thickened palmar creases, bifid uvula, and urethral stenosis: A previously undescribed familial disorder with lethal outcome: J Pediatr 79:977–981, 1971

RUFOUS ALBINISM

Symptoms and Signs. In black inhabitants of New Guinea. Mahogany skin and red hair. Irides reddish brown. Mild nystagmus and photophobia.

Etiology. Autosomal recessive inheritance.

Diagnostic Procedures. Hairbulbs test. Accumulation of tyrosine.

Therapy. None.

Prognosis. Stable condition.

BIBLIOGRAPHY. Pearson K, Nettleship E, Usher CH: A monograph on albinism in man: Drapers Company Research Tumors. Biometric Series 6, 8, 9; parts 1, 2, 4. London, Dulan, 1911–1913

Harvey RG: The "red skins" of Lufa sub-district. Further observations on the distinctive skin pigmentation of some New Guinea indigenes. Hum Biol Oceania 1:103, 1971

RUKAVINAS

Synonyms. Amyloid neuropathy (type II); Indiana type amyloidosis neuropathy; Maryland type amyloidosis neuropathy; amyloidosis serine 84.

Symptoms. Both sexes affected. Onset in third and fourth decades. Symptoms of peripheral neuropathy most severely affecting upper limbs. Same symptoms as in carpal tunnel syndrome (see). Gastrointestinal symptoms are minor (if compared with above form).

Signs. Impairment of sensation in the distribution of median nerve; little motor involvement. Scleroderma-like changes in skin of hands and arms. Vitreous opacities in eyes leading to blindness.

Etiology. Unknown. Autosomal dominant inheritance.

Pathology. Diffuse parenchymal infiltration with amyloid substance.

Diagnostic Procedures. *Blood.* Serum electrophoresis shows unusual peak in alpha-2–globulin area; reduced retinol binding protein. *Congo red test. EVG. Biopsy of rectum and nerve.*

Therapy. Symptomatic. Carpal tunnel decompression.

Prognosis. Extremely slow progression, usually leading normal life. Death 14–40 years after onset of symptoms. Cardiomyopathy cause of death.

BIBLIOGRAPHY. Falls HF, Jackson J, Carey JH, et al: Ocular manifestations of hereditary primary systemic amyloidosis. AMA Arch Ophthalmol 54:660–664, 1955

Rukavinas JB, Block WD, Jackson CE, et al: Primary systemic amyloidosis: A review and an experimental genetic and clinical study of 29 cases with particular emphasis on the familial form. Medicine 35:239–334, 1956

Benson MD, Duwler FE: Prealbumin and retinol binding protein serum concentration in the Indiana type hereditary amyloidosis. Arthritis Rheum 26:1493–1498, 1983

Benson MD: Amyloidosis. In Scriver CR, Beaudet AL, Sly WS, et al: The Metabolic and Molecular Bases of Inherited Disease, 7th ed, pp 4161–4163. New York, McGraw-Hill, 1995

RUMINATION

IN INFANTS

Symptoms. Ingested food is regularly regurgitated and rechewed and partially reswallowed. Associated with failure to thrive, marasmus.

Etiology. Attributed to psychological causes. Abnormal mother–infant relationship, with immaturity of the mother and attempted autogratification of the infant (?). Considered also a conditioned response.

Therapy. In severe form, hospitalization and care of psychic aspect. In the past, conditioning therapy even by electroshock.

Prognosis. Good if habit broken, otherwise may even lead to death.

IN ADULTS

Symptoms. Onset 15–30 minutes after a meal, for about 1 hour, regurgitation of food, one mouthful at a time, chewing and reswallowing it, without effort, involuntarily. The practice is not associated with nausea, pyrosis, or abdominal pain. Rumination stops when food regurgitated becomes acid. In some cases, the practice may be stopped voluntarily.

Etiology. Unknown. Attributed to psychogenetic mechanism.

Diagnostic Procedures. Rule out hiatal hernia.

Therapy. None. Psychological counseling.

Prognosis. Embarassing, nondebilitating habit.

BIBLIOGRAPHY. Wivship DH, Zboralske FF, Weber WN, et al: Esophagus in rumination. Am J Physiol 207:1189–1194, 1964

Amarnath RP, Abell TL, Malagelada JR: The rumination syndrome in adults. Ann Int Med 105:513–518, 1986

Achord JL: Nausea and vomiting. In Haubrich WS, Schaffner F, Berk JE (eds): Bockus Gastroenterology, 5th ed, vol 2, pp 41, 44. Philadelphia, WB Saunders, 1995

RUMMO

Eponym used to indicate cardioptosis.

BIBLIOGRAPHY. Rummo G: Sulla cardioptosis, primo abbozzo anatomo-clinico. Arch Med Int 1:161–183, 1898

RUNEBERG

Eponym to indicate a particular form of Addison-Biermer disease (see), where the course is characterized by spontaneous complete remissions followed by progressively more severe relapses.

BIBLIOGRAPHY. Runeberg JW: Zur Kenntnis der sogenannten progressiven perniciösen Anämie. Dtsch Arch Klin Med 28:499–520, 1880–1881

RUNNER ANEMIA

Synonyms. Jogger anemia.

Symptoms and Signs. In 56% of joggers and especially in long distance runners. Iron-deficiency anemia.

Etiology. Unknown. Considered gastrointestinal bleeding from transient ischemia during exercise, hematuria (see march hemoglobinuria, mild hemolysis).

Diagnostic Procedures. *Urine. Fecies.* Hemoglobin present. *Blood.* hemoglobinemia.

BIBLIOGRAPHY. Dufaux B, et al: Serum ferritin, transferrin, haptoglobin and iron in middle and long-distance runners, elite rowers and professional racing cyclists. Int J Sports Med 2:43–46, 1981
Lee GR: Iron deficiency and iron-deficiency anemia. In Lee GR, Bithel TC, Foerster J, et al: Wintrobe's Clinical Hematology, p 817. Philadelphia, Lea & Febiger, 1993

RUNNER KNEE

Synonyms. Iliotibial band friction.

Symptoms and Signs. In runners, especially in subjects with genu varum and planus feet. Pain over lateral epicondyle of femur during run and tenderness on palpation of areas.

Etiology. Friction between iliotibial band and femur or bursitis.

Therapy. Rest or injection with corticosteroids.

BIBLIOGRAPHY. Renne JW: The iliotibial band syndrome. J Bone Joint Surg 57:1010–1011, 1975
Graham GP, Fairclough JA: The knee. In Klippel JH, Dieppe PA: Rheumatology, p 15.12.6. St Louis, CV Mosby, 1995

RUSSELL

Synonym. Diencephalic infantilis.

Symptoms. Both sexes affected. Onset at 3 months to 2 years. Good to increased appetite; apparent well-being; euphoria; hyperkinesia; vomiting.

Signs. Pallor of skin, not of mucosae; emaciation. Blindness or severe visual loss; homonymous hemianopia; nystagmus present in 50% of cases. The autonomic disturbance consists of excessive sweating, easy flushing of the skin, tachycardia, and vomiting. No other physical signs.

Etiology and Pathology. "Silent" neoplasm of hypothalamic region and floor of third ventricle or adjacent structures causing compression of hypothalamus. The tumor can be astrocytoma, glioma, or craniopharyngioma.

Diagnostic Procedures. *Blood.* Paradoxically, normal values; increase in eosinophils sometimes observed; hypoglycemia (occasional). *CSF.* Protein elevation (not constant). *X-ray. CAT. MRI.* Of skull. Erosion

under anterior clinoid processes. Radiographic appearance of extremity: normal fat lines more completely obliterated than in severe emaciation or starvation. *Isotope brain scan. Echoencephalography.*

Therapy. Cobalt irradiation; condition usually not amenable to surgery because of location.

Prognosis. Severe; 2- to 4-year remission with irradiation treatment and fatal outcome.

BIBLIOGRAPHY. Goebel F "Hypophysaere Kachexie" beim Kleinkind ohne Zwergwuchs bei inactiver. Hypophyse Z Kinderheilk 53:575, 1932
Russell A: A diencephalic syndrome of emaciation in infancy and childhood. Arch Dis Child 26:274, 1951
Carradori R, Miele A, Ricci C: Su di un caso di craniofaringioma con sindrome diencefalica cachetizzante (Sindrome di Russell). Aggiornamento Pediatrico 37:117–119, 1986

RUSSELL III

Synonyms. Hyperammonemia (type II); OCT: ornithine carbamyl transferase deficiency.

Symptoms and Signs. Both sexes affected. Difference of severity: very severe in males, milder in females. *Male.* Normal at birth; within few hours or 1–2 days, lethargy, poor feeding, dyspnea, ataxia, convulsions, hyperthermia, rapid progression to coma and respiratory failure. *Female.* Onset in early infancy. Variable symptoms from dislike of protein food, to recurrent vomiting, with or without screaming, headache, confusion, ataxia, dyslalia, progressing or not progressing to coma, and seizures.

Recurrent hepatomegaly during attacks. Patients with minor symptoms are mentally normal; those with intermediate or severe symptoms have variable degrees of mental retardation. Pattern of recurrent episodes is similar to that of migraine.

Etiology. Sex-linked dominant inheritance. Ornithine carbamyl transferase (OCT) deficiency.

Pathology. Minimal and nonspecific changes.

Diagnostic Procedures. *Blood.* Postprandial blood hyperammonemia: elevation directly correlated to degree of enzyme deficiency and clinical manifestations (from simple increase in postprandial period to constant extreme elevation). Serum glutamic-oxaloacetic transaminase (SGOT) and serum glutamic-pyruvic transaminase (SGPT) increased, plasma amino acids normal; pyrimidine metabolites increased (also increased urinary excretion). *Enzyme studies.* Deficiency of OCT in liver biopsy.

Therapy. Reduction of protein from diet.

Prognosis. *Males.* Death in neonatal period. *Females.* Death at later age or survival, generally, with mental and physical retardation.

BIBLIOGRAPHY. Russell A, Levin B, Oberhalzer VG, et al: Hyperammoniemia: A new instance of an inborn enzymatic defect of the biosynthesis of urea. Lancet 2:699–700, 1962
Walser M: Urea cycle disorders and other hereditary hyperammoniemic syndromes. In Brusilow SW, Horwich AL: Urea cycle enzymes. In Scriver CR, Beaudet AL, Sly WS, et al: The Metabolic and Molecular Bases of Inherited Disease, 7th ed, pp 1187–1188. New York, McGraw-Hill, 1995

RUSSELL-SILVER

Synonyms. Silver; asymmetry—dwarfism. See Partington.

Symptoms and Signs. No sex preponderance. Small size for gestational age. Significant congenital asymmetry (78%) from marked hemihypertrophy to limited asymmetry involving skull, spine, extremity. Shortness of stature (93%); pattern of growth parallel to normal but below the third percentile. Usually, small at birth; variation in sexual development (34%): precocious sexual development; dissociation between physical evidence of maturation and epiphyseal development. Other occasional manifestations: cafe au lait areas of skin; short and incurved fifth fingers; downturning of mouth; triangular shape of face; syndactyly of toes; mental retardation; renal anomaly; hypospadias.

Etiology. Unknown. May arise from different causes; sporadic, autosomal dominant in one family. Six cases of this syndrome with growth hormone deficiency have been reported, three of which had additional pituitary abnormalities.

Diagnostic Procedures. *Blood.* Elevated gonadotropins, evidence of estrogenic stimulation in desquamated cells; tendency toward fasting hypoglycemia (from 10 months to 3 years); investigation for pituitary abnormalities. *X-ray.* In some cases, dissociation between epiphyseal age and physical evidence of sexual development.

Therapy. Symptomatic. High replacement doses of growth hormone may be required to overcome deficiency.

Prognosis. Tendency toward improvement in growth and appearance in childhood and adolescence; 10% association with Wilms tumor (see Wilms tumor-hemihypertrophy).

BIBLIOGRAPHY. Silver HK, Kiyasu W, George J, et al: Syndrome of congenital hemihypertrophy, shortness of stature, and elevated urinary gonadotropins. Pediatrics 12:368–376, 1953

Russell A: A syndrome of "intrauterine" dwarfism recognizable at birth with craniofacial dysostosis disproportionately short arms and other anomalies (5 examples). Proc R Soc Med 47:1040–1044, 1954

Davis PSW, Davies PS, Valley R, et al: Adolescent growth and puberty progression in the Silver-Russell syndrome. Arch Dis Child 63:130–135, 1988

Adams RD, Victor M: Principles of Neurology, 5th ed, p 1018. New York, McGraw-Hill, 1993

RUST

Synonyms. Malum suboccipitale; suboccipital vertebral.

Symptoms and Signs. Pain in suboccipital area, which the patient tries to reduce by keeping the head in flexed position. Trigeminal neuralgia; hypoglossal and vagus paralysis; tongue atrophy; cardiac arrhythmias. Localized swelling or suboccipital region.

Etiology. Variable: traumatic, rheumatic, neoplastic, infective (e.g., tuberculosis, syphilis).

Therapy. According to etiology.

BIBLIOGRAPHY. Rust JN: Aufsaetze und Abhändlungen aus dem Gebiete der Medizin. Chirurgie und Staatsarzneikunde, vol 1, p 196. Berlin, Enslin, 1834

RUTHERFURD

Synonyms. Oculodental; corneal dystrophy; gum hypertrophy; gingival hypertrophy; corneal dystrophy. See also Gorlin-Chaudhry-Moss, Peter, Reger, and Meyer-Schwickerath-Weger.

Symptoms. Both sexes affected. Present from birth. Iris anomalies; oligodontia; microdontia; hypoplastic enamel; gum hypertrophy; mental retardation.

Etiology. Autosomal dominant inheritance.

BIBLIOGRAPHY. Rutherfurd ME: Three generations of inherited dental defects. Br Med J 2:9–11, 1931

Houston IB, Shotts N: Rutherfurd's syndrome. A familial oculo-dental disorder: A clinical and electrophysiologic study. Acta Paediatr Scand 55:233–238, 1966

RUTLAND

Synonym. Ciliary disorientatation.

Symptoms and Signs. Pulmonary problems from first week of life.

Etiology. Suggested autosomal recessive inheritance.

Diagnostic Procedures. Quantitative methods for measuring "ciliary orientation": random orientation observed (as compared to parallel observed in normal subjects as well as in patients with recurrent respiratory tract infections).

Therapy. Symptomatic.

Prognosis. Unknown. Suggestion that the patients might be fertile since disorientation of sperm tails will not have effect on fertility.

BIBLIOGRAPHY. Rutland J, DeIongh RV: Random ciliary orientation: a cause of respiratory tract disease. N Engl J Med 323:1681–1684, 1990

RUVALCABA

Synonym. Hunter; Sugio-Kajii; brachymetapody; hypogenitalism; retardation; trichorhinophalangeal III.

Symptoms. Very rare. Occurs in males. Present from birth. Mental and physical retardation; visual disturbances; intestinal disorders.

Signs. Head microcephaly. *Face.* Antimongoloid slant; narrow beaked nose, micrognathia with crowded teeth, low set ears, white forelock. *Thorax.* Pectus carinatum, kyphoscoliosis. *Abdomen.* Inguinal hernias. *Limbs.* Limited motion of the elbow, short metacarpal and metatarsal. *Skin.* Hypoplastic, hyperchromic areas on glans and penile shaft, large areolae.

Etiology. Autosomal dominant inheritance.

Pathology. See signs. lipid storage myopathy; hematomatous intestinal polyps.

Diagnostic Procedures. *X-rays.* See Signs. Chomosomal studies.

BIBLIOGRAPHY. Ruvalcaba RH, Reichert A, Smith DW: A new familial syndrome with osseous dysplasia and mental deficiency. J Pediatr 79:450–455, 1971

Hunter A: Ruvalcaba syndrome. Am J Med Genet 21:785–786, 1985

Niikawa N, Kamei T: The Sugio-Kajii syndrome. Proposed Trichorhinophalangeal syndrome type III (letter). Am J Med Genet 24:759–760, 1986

Bieler MG, Wilson WG, Kelly TE: Apparent Ruvalcaba syndrome with genitourinary abnormalities. Am J Med Genet 33:314–317, 1989

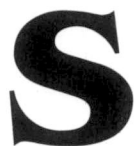

SABIN-FELDMAN

Synonyms. Cerebral damage; chorioretinopathy; pseudotoxoplasmosis; microcephaly; chorioretinopathy.

Symptoms and Signs. Onset in early infancy. Variable neurologic symptoms, related to extensive destruction of cerebral tissue. Hydrocephalus; chorioretinopathy and degenerative changes of small retinal vessels.

Etiology. Unknown. The clinical pattern is identical to that caused by toxoplasmosis, but this agent was not identified in these patients. Familial cases with a similar syndrome, also defined, pseudotoxoplasmosis (microcephaly and chorioretinopathy), reported with both autosomal dominant and recessive inheritance.

Diagnostic Procedures. *Blood.* No toxoplasma antibodies. *X-ray.* Of brain. Scattered calcifications.

Therapy. Symptomatic.

Prognosis. Fatal.

BIBLIOGRAPHY. Sabin AB, Feldman HA: Chorioretinopathy associated with other evidence of cerebral damage in childhood: A syndrome of unknown etiology separable from congenital toxoplasmosis. J Pediatr St Louis 35:296–309, 1949
Parke JT, Riccardi VM, Lewis RH, et al: A syndrome of microcephaly and retinal pigmentary abnormalities without mental retardation in a family with coincidental autosomal dominant hyperreflexia. Am J Med Genet 17:585–594, 1984
McKusick VA: Mendelian Inheritance in Man, 10th ed. Baltimore, Johns Hopkins Univ Press, 1992

SABOURAUD

Synonyms. Beaded hair; monilethrix. See Pollitt.

Symptoms. Both sexes affected. Onset usually in first 2 months, but later onset up to adult life also reported. No clinical features except higher incidence of cataracts and related visual impairment.

Signs. Hair normal at birth, progressively thinning up to second month, when there is complete loss. In the entire scalp or selected zones (e.g., nape, occipital), from small follicular, horny papules, development of brittle, beaded hairs easily breakable before they reach 1–2 cm in length. Other hairy regions may also be affected, with resulting areas of alopecia.

Etiology. Unknown. Autosomal dominant inheritance. Families with recessive inheritance also described but not proven. A metabolic disorder (enzyme defect) suggested.

Pathology. *Hair.* Beading, elliptical nodes 1 mm apart, separated by constricted zone lacking medulla. *Follicles.* Horny plugging; otherwise normal.

Diagnostic Procedures. *Urine.* Arginoaminic aciduria not found consistently.

Therapy. Symptomatic.

Prognosis. Variable. Increasing severity through childhood; improvement in summer; persistence or regression in adult life.

BIBLIOGRAPHY. Sabouraud R: Sur les cheveux moniliformes (trichorhexies et monilethrix). Ann Dermatol Syph 3:781–793, 1892

Renwick JH, Izatt MM: Linkage data on moniletrix. Cytoget Cell Genet 47:108, 1988
Dawber RPR, Ebling FJG, Wojnarowska FT: Disorders of hair. In Champion RH, Burton JL, Ebling FJG (eds): Rook/Wilkinson/Ebling Textbook of Dermatology, 5th ed, pp 2607–2609. Oxford, Blackwell Scientific, 1992

SACCHAROPINURIA

Synonyms. Carson; saccharopine dehydrogenase deficiency; AASS deficiency. See Hyperlysinemia.

Symptoms and Signs. Mental retardation in some cases; short stature, no seizures, spastic diplegia.

Etiology. Autosomal recessive inheritance supposed. Disease caused by mutation of a single locus that codes for aminoadipic semialdehyde synthetase (AASS) causing altered lysine degradation. May be considered a variation of hyperlysinemia.

Diagnostic Procedures. *Urine.* Excretion of large quantity of lysine, citrulline, histidine, and saccharopine. *Blood.* Serum saccharopine and homocitrulline, present in small quantity. Lysine four to five times higher than normal, and similar increase for the citrulline. *Cerebrospinal fluid.* High concentration of saccharopine. *EEG.* Abnormalities.

Therapy. Symptomatic; diet.

Prognosis. Good quoad vitam. Neurologic abnormalities.

BIBLIOGRAPHY. Carson NAJ, Scally BB, Neill DW, et al: Saccharopinuria: A new inborn error of lysine metabolism. Nature 218:679, 1968
Sim Ell O, Johansson T, Aula P: Enzyme defect in saccharopinuria. J Pediatr 82:54–57, 1973
Cox RP, Markovitz PJ, Chuang DT: Familial hyperlysinemia-multiple enzyme deficiency associated with the bifunctional aminoadipic semialehyde synthase. Trans Am Clin Chim Assoc 97:69–81, 1985
Cox RP, Dancis J: Errors of lysine metabolism. In Scriver CR, Beaudet AL, Sly WS, et al: The Metabolic and Molecular Bases of Inherited Disease, 7th ed, p 1237. New York, McGraw-Hill, 1995

SACHSALBER

Synonyms. Hemihypertrophy, facial; neurofibromatosis—buphtalmos.

Symptoms and Signs. Both sexes. Facial hemihypertrophy, more frequently on left side. Unilateral exophtalmos with decreased vision. Symptoms and signs of neurofibromatosis (see) frequently affecting homolateral eyelid. Possibly associated signs of status dysraphicus (see Bremer). Glaucoma is a frequent complication.

Etiology. Unknown.

Pathology. True hemihypertrophy of both skull and integuments. See von Recklinghausen. *X-ray.* Enlargement of hemiskull, especially of orbita optic canal and other foramens.

Diagnostic Procedure. *Biopsy.* Of skin lesion.

BIBLIOGRAPHY. Sachsalber A: Ueber das Rankenneurom der orbita mit sekundaeren buphtalmos. Beitr Augenheilk 27:1–43, 1897
Kramer W: Klippel-Trenaunay syndrome. In Vinken PJ, Bruyn GW (eds): Handbook of Clinical Neurology, vol 14, p 398. Amsterdam, North-Holland, 1972

SACK-BARABAS

Synonyms. Ehler-Danlos IV type; polyaneurysmatic. See Ehler Danlos.

Symptoms and Signs. Early appearance: aneurysm in skin, bowel, uterus, and major blood vessels. Bruises, recurrent abdominal pain and eventual intestinal perforation, uterine rupture in pregnancy.

Etiology. Autosomal recessive or dominant. Altered synthesis of type III collagen.

Diagnostic Procedures. *Microscopy.* Alteration of elastic lamina of vessels, absence of myofilaments in smooth muscle cells. *Derma.* Scarce elastin. *Urine.* Increased excretion of hydroxyproline. *Blood.* Sometimes anti-smooth muscle antibodies.

Therapy. Surgery.

Prognosis. Poor because of complications.

BIBLIOGRAPHY. Sack G: Status Dysvascularis, ein Fall von besonderer Zerreisslichkeit der Blutgefässe. Dtsch Arch Klin Med 178:663–669, 1936

Barabas AP: Vascular complications in the Ehler-Danlos syndrome. J Cardiovasc Surg 13:160–167, 1972

Stella A, Gessaroli M, Cifiello BI, et al: Sack-Barabas (Ehler-Danlos IV type) (Clinical and histopathologic ultrastructural correlations). Vasc Surg 20:67–73, 1986

Byard RW, Keeley FW, Smith CR: Type IV Elher-Danlos syndrome presenting as sudden infant death. Am J Clin Pathol 93:579–582, 1990

Weatherall DJ, Ledingham JGG, Warrell DA: Oxford Textbook of Medicine, p 3084. Oxford, Oxford Med Pub, 1996

SAETHRE-CHOTZEN

Synonyms. Chotzen; acrocephalosyndactyly III; ACS III; SCS, acrocephaly; skull asymmetry; mild syndactyly. Including: auralcephalosyndactyly, and Robinow-Sorauf (all three possible different expressions of same gene).

Symptoms. Both sexes affected. Present from birth. Mild to moderate mental retardation; convulsions; multiple respiratory infections.

Signs. Short stature (primary or secondary [?]). *Head.* Flat occiput; prognathism; hypertelorism; deviated nasal septum; ear deformity; strabismus. Defective teeth (primary or secondary [?]). *Limbs.* Partial syndactyly of second and third or fourth and fifth fingers and toes; radioulnar synostoses; simian palmar creases. *Cryptorchidism.* Heart murmur (cardiac anomaly [?]). Forme fruste possible in relatives.

Etiology. Unknown. Autosomal dominant transmission, with variable expressions suggested.

Pathology. See Signs. Also, renal anomalies.

Diagnostic Procedures. *Blood.* Normal; absence of amino acid abnormalities. *X-ray.* Of skeleton. *Chromosome studies.* Apparently normal.

Therapy. Craniosynostosis.

Prognosis. Permanent condition. Facial appearance tends to improve during childhood.

BIBLIOGRAPHY. Saethre H: Ein Beitrag zum Turmschä-del problem. (Pathogenese, Erblichkeit und Symptomatologie). Dtsch Z Nervenheilk 117–119; 533–555, 1931

Chotzen F: Eine eigenartige familiäre Entwicklungsstörung (Akrocephalosyndaktlylie, Dystostosis craniofacialis und Hypertelorismus). Mschr Kinderheilkd 55:97–122, 1932

Legius E, Fryns JP, Van den Berghe H: Auralcephalosyndactyly: A new craniosynostosis syndrome or a variant of the Saethe-Chotzen syndrome? J Med Genet 26:522–524, 1989

Niemann-Seyde SC, Eber SW, Zoll B: Saethe-Chotzen syndrome (ACS III) in four generations. Clin Genet 40:271–276, 1991

ST. HELENIAN CELLULITIS

Synonym. Helenia.

Symptoms. Cases observed on St. Helena Island. Female to male ratio, 3:1. Intense burning pain in legs, accompanied by headache, rigor and sometimes by pulmonary edema.

Signs. After 24 hours, unilateral leg lesion, accompanied by redness from calf to ankle; development of small blisters, which may coalesce in large blisters or burst.

Etiology. Unknown. Probably infective.

Diagnostic Procedures. *Blood.* Neutrophilic leukocytes increased.

Therapy. None.

Prognosis. The lesions dry, scab, and resolve in 6 weeks. Brown discoloration may remain. The episodes may recur.

BIBLIOGRAPHY. Shine IB: St. Helenia's cellulitis. Br J Dermatol 76:357–361, 1964

Rook A, Wilkinson DS, Ebling FJG, et al: Textbook of Dermatology, 4th ed, p 751. Oxford, Blackwell Scientific, 1986

ST. LOUIS*

Synonyms. St. Louis encephalitis.

Symptoms. Onset in late summer and early fall; occurs in infancy and later. Occurs in different locations but especially along the Mississippi river. From asymptomatic to severe. Prodromal: lassitude; malaise; cephalalgia; sore throat. Or acute onset. Severe cephalalgia; hyperthermia; stiff neck; mental confusion, delirium; transitory blurring of vision.

Signs. Increase in deep reflexes; absence of abdominal reflexes; Kernig sign. Cranial nerves may be involved; ocular signs rare.

Etiology. Arbovirus transmitted by Culex mosquito vector.

Pathology. Cerebral edema; diffuse hemorrhages in all central nervous system areas. Focal lymphocyte infiltration of meninges; neuronal degeneration; glial proliferation.

Diagnostic Procedures. *Blood.* Leukocytosis; presence of neutralizing antibodies. *Cerebrospinal fluid.* Leukocytes, proteins, and pressure increased.

Therapy. Symptomatic. Sedation.

Prognosis. Mortality 20%; prolonged period of convalescence and possible sequelae.

BIBLIOGRAPHY. Weatherall DJ, Ledingham JGG, Warrell DA: Oxford Textbook of Medicine, p 416. Oxford, Oxford Med Pub, 1996

SAINT SYNDROMES

1. *St. Agatha.* Mastopathic inflammatory
2. *St. Aignan* or Agnan. Favus ringworm; tinea
3. *St. Arman.* Pellagra
4. *St. Anthony.* Eponym applied to several different conditions:
   A. *St. Anthony dance.* Chorea (see), also called *St. Vitus* dance.
   B. *St. Anthony fire.* Ergotism (epidemic gangrene and psychotic alterations).
   C. *St. Anthony fire.* Erysipelas

---

*Term refers to "first" epidemic observed in St. Louis in July, 1933; actually observed previously in Paris in 1932.

D. *St. Anthony fire*. Herpes zoster
5. *St. Apollonia*. Toothache
6. *St. Avertin*. Epilepsy (see)
7. *St. Avidus*. Deafness
8. *St. Blasius*. Quinsy (see) (or Blaize)
9. *St. Dymphna*. Mental derangements
10. *St. Erasmus*. Colic pain
11. *St. Fiacre* or *Flacre*. Hemorrhoids
12. *St. Francis*. Erysipelas
13. *St. Gervasius*. Juvenile or adult rheumatic pains
14. *St. Gete*. Carcinoma
15. *St. Giles*. Leprosy
16. *St. Gothard*. Ancylostomiasis
17. *St. Guy dance*. Chorea
18. *St. Hubers*. Rabies
19. *St. Ignatius*. Pellagra
20. *St. Louis*. Encephalitis (see)
21. *St. Kilda*. Colds, infection
22. *St. Main*. Scabies
23. *St. Martin*. Alcoholism
24. *St. Mathurin*. Idiocy
25. *St. Modestus*. Chorea (see)
26. *St. Roch* or *Roche*. Plague
27. *St. Sebastian*. Plague
28. *St. Valentine*. Epilepsy (see)
29. *St. Vitus dance*. Chorea (see)
30. *St. Zachary*. Mutism

SAINT TRIAD

Synonyms. Hiatus hernia; gall stones; diverticulosis.

Symptoms. Occurs in both sexes. Prevalent in females; onset in middle to late life. (1) Those of Bochdalek diaphragmatic hernia: vague, intermittent abdominal pain; bloating; regurgitation or chest pain or both; dyspnea and cardiovascular symptoms or those of acute intestinal obstruction. (2) Those of cholelithiasis: right upper abdominal pain with typical back irradiation; vomiting; nausea; fatty food intolerance. (3) Those of diverticulosis: abdominal pain in various areas; constipation or diarrhea.

Etiology. Unknown.

BIBLIOGRAPHY. Hueller CJB: Hiatus hernia diverticulosis coli and gallstones. Saint's triad. South Afr Med J 22:376, 1948
Palmer ED: Saint's triad (hiatus hernia, gallstones, and diverticulosis coli): The problem of properly directing surgical therapy. Am J Dig Dis 22:314–315, 1955
Small LD: Cholelithiasis. In Bockus HL: Gastroenterology, 3rd ed, vol 3, p 774. Philadelphia, WB Saunders, 1976

SAKATI-NYHAN-TISDALE

Synonyms. Acrocephalopolysyndactyly III, ACPS; ACPS—leg hypoplasia.

Symptoms and Signs. One case reported in a boy of 8 years. Multiple abnormalities noted at birth: craniosynostosis with acrocephaly; brachydactyly; polydactylysyndactyly of toes; bowed femora; hypoplastic tibias; posterior displacement of fibulas on the femora; congenital heart disease; inguinal hernia; areas of alopecia and cutaneous atrophy of scalp; lineal submental scars resembling clefts. In the first year, difficult breathing, with frequent respiratory infections, attacks of cyanosis. Development slow, eventually with help, patient partially overcame difficulty of ambulation, learned to walk with special crutches at 5 years of age. Intelligence normal despite signs of increased intracranial pressure.

Etiology. Possibly, single gene mutation. Not to be excluded the action of teratogen. It shares elements with Apert (see), Laurence-Moon-Bartet-Biedl (see) and other acrocephalosyndactyly syndromes (see).

Pathology. See Symptoms and Signs.

Diagnostic Procedures. *X-rays*. Described bone anomalies; signs of increased intracranial pressure. Epiphyseal center frequently missing. Generalized osteoporosis. *ECG*. Left axis deviation; incomplete right bundle branch block. *Urine*. Amino acid normal. *Cytology*. Normal. *Dermatoglyphic pattern*. Altered.

Therapy. None. Physical therapy.

Prognosis. Fair quoad vitam.

BIBLIOGRAPHY. Sakati N, Nyhan WL, Tisdale WK: A new case with acrocephalopolysyndactyly, cardiac disease, and distinctive defects of the ear skin and lower limbs. J Pediatr 79:104–109, 1971

SALAMON

Synonyms. Woolly hair hypotrichosis, everted lower lip, outstanding ears. See Woolly hair.

Symptoms and Signs. See Synonyms.

Etiology. Possibly autosomal recessive inheritance.

BIBLIOGRAPHY. Salamon T: Ueber eine Familie mit recessiver Kraushaarigkeit, Hypotrichose und anderen Anomalien. Haut Arzt 14:540–544, 1963
Salamon T, Cubela V, Bogdanovic B, et al: Ueber ein Geschwisterpaar mit einer eigenartigen ektodermalen dysplasie. Arch Klin Exper Dermatol 230:60–68, 1967

SALDINO-MAINZLER

Synonyms. Acrodysplasia; retinitis pigmentosa; nephropathy; cone-shaped epiphyses; nephropathy; retinitis pigmentosa.

Symptoms. Rare. In childhood. Polypsia, polyuria, visual deficit; cerebellar ataxia; short stature, hands and feet.

Signs. Elevated blood pressure; short middle phalanges of digits; retinitis pigmentosa; liver fibrotic; pigmented midline nevi.

Etiology. Autosomal recessive inheritance.

Pathology. *Kidney*. Diffuse tubular atrophy; fibrosis. *Eye*. Tapetoretinal degeneration.

Diagnostic Procedures. *X-rays*. Cone-shaped epiphyses of hand (especially middle phalanges) and feet; flattened capital femoral epiphyses. *Excretory urography*. Small kidneys, poor concentration of contrast medium. *Blood*. Evidence of renal failure.

Therapy. Symptomatic.

Prognosis. Poor.

BIBLIOGRAPHY. Saldino RM, Mainzler F: Cone-shaped epiphyses (CSE) in siblings with hereditary renal disease and retinitis pigmentosa. Radiology 98:39–45, 1971
Ellis DS, Heckenlivery SR, Martin CL, et al: Leber's congenital amaurosis associated with familial juvenile nephropthisis and cone-shaped epiphyses of the hands (Saldino-Mainzler syndrome). Am J Ophthalmol 97:233–239, 1984
Rimoin DL, Lachman RS: Genetic disorders of the osseous skeleton. In Beithon P (ed): McKusick's Heritable Disorders of Connective Tissue, 5th ed, pp 642–643. St Louis, CV Mosby, 1993

SALDINO-NOONAN

Synonym. Le Marec; chondoroectodermal dysplasia (lethal type). SRP-1; short rib-polydactyly I.

Symptoms and Signs. Female sex preponderance (9/13). Hydrop at birth; head dolichocephaly, micrognathia. *Thorax.* Short and narrow. *Abdomen.* Protuberant. *Limbs.* Micromelia; polydactyly, brachydactyly. *Occasionally.* Genital, cardiovascular, gastrointestinal, lung, and renal anomalies.

Etiology. Autosomal recessive inheritance.

Pathology. *Bones.* Altered or absent zone of proliferation, loss of columnization.

Diagnostic Procedures. *X-rays. Ultrasonography.* (Prenatal diagnosis). Dolichocephaly, poor mineralization on frontal bones, mantibular hypoplasia, short ribs, small scapulae and iliac bones, vertebrae misshapen and squared, tubular bones short and misshapen.

Prognosis. Death in perinatal period.

BIBLIOGRAPHY. Saldino RM, Noonan CD: Severe thoracic dystrophy with striking micromelia, abnormal osseous development, including the spine and multiple visceral abnormalities. Am J Roentgenol 114:257–263, 1972
Sillence D: Perinatally lethal short rib-polydactyly syndrome. Pediatr Radiol 17:474–480, 1987
Rimoin DL, Lachman RS: Genetic disorders of the osseous skeleton. In Beithon P (ed): McKusick's Heritable Disorders of Connective Tissue, 5th ed, pp 587–589. St Louis, CV Mosby, 1993

SALLA*

Synonyms. Finish type sialuria. See Sialic acid storage and Sialidoses.

Symptoms and Signs. Both sexes. Onset at 12–18 months. Mental retardation. Ataxia, athetosis, rigidity, spasticity, impaired speech. Growth retardation (50%) exotropia (50%).

Etiology. Form of sialuria (allelic form [?]). Defect in transmembrane transport in the lysome causing lysosomal storage of free fatty acids. Autosomal recessive inheritance.

Pathology. Lysosomal inclusions in peripheral lymphocytes and various tissues

Diagnostic Procedures. *Blood.* Vacuolated lymphocytes (4–15%). *Urine.* Excretion of sialic acid. *EEG.* Progressive diminution of amplitude. *X-rays.* Thick calvarium (50%).

Prognosis. Normal life span.

BIBLIOGRAPHY. Aula P, Antio S, Raivio KO, et al: "Salla disease," a new lysosomal storage disorder. Arch Neurol 36:88–94, 1979
Renlund M, Aula P: Prenatal detection of Salla disease based upon increased free sialic acid in amniocytes. Am J Med Genet 28:377–384, 1987
Whitley CB: The mucopolysaccharidoses. In Beithon P (ed) McKusick's Heritable Disorders of Connective Tissue, 5th ed, p 472. St Louis, CV Mosby, 1993

SALLERAS-ORTIZ

BIBLIOGRAPHY. Salleras A, Ortiz de Zarate JC: Recessive sex-linked inheritance of external ophthalmoplegia and myopia coincident with other dysplasias. Br J Opthalmol 34:662–667, 1950

---

*Geographic area in Finland.

SALPINGITIS ISTMICA NODOSA

Synonyms. Chiari; SIN; tubular diverticulosis; adenomyohyperplasia; adenomyosis; endosalpingiosis.

Symptoms and Signs. In women in the reproductive age (average 26–30) rare in premenarche or postmenopause. High incidence in blacks of North America or Jamaica. Usually no symptoms or signs. Discovered in infertility testing, after ectopic pregnancy, or miscarriages.

Etiology. Unknown. Probaby acquired inflammatory infectious condition.

Pathology. One or both tubes misplaced, nodular hyperplasia and hypertrophy of muscularis that surrounds pseudo gland-like structures lined by tubular epithelium.

Diagnostic Procedures. *Istero-salpingography.* Single or multiple diverticula of the tube. *Laparoscopy.* Nodular fungiform enlargement of the tube.

Therapy. In advanced cases tubo-cornual anastomosis may be indicated.

Prognosis. Progressive condition that may evolve toward tubal lumen obliteration causing infertility, ectopic pregnancy, miscarriage. Better pregnancy outcome with surgery.

BIBLIOGRAPHY. Chiari H: Zur pathologischen Anatomie des Eleiter catarrhs Z Heilkunde 8:457–473, 1887
Creasy JF, Clark RL, Cuttino JT, et al: Salpingitis istmica nodosa: Radiological and clinical correlates. Radiology 154:597–600, 1985
MacComb PF, Rowe TC: Salpingitis istmica nodosa: Evidence it is a progressive disease. Ferti Steril 51:542–545, 1989

SALZMANN

Synonym. Nodular cornea dystrophy.

Symptoms. Both sexes affected. More common in females. Onset at any age in persons with corneal disease. Vision impairment; ocular pain.

Signs. Yellow-white superficial nodular masses on the cornea.

Etiology. Complication of phlyctenular keratitis or trachoma.

Pathology. Nodular dystrophy of cornea with progressive vascularization and degeneration of epithelium and Bowman membrane. Because of alternating thickening and thinning of epithelium, pannus formation and hyaline thickening of superficial stroma by deposition of nodular collagen.

Therapy. Lamellar keratoplasty.

Prognosis. Slow progression.

BIBLIOGRAPHY. Salzmann M: Ueber eine eigentümliche Form von Hornhautentzündung. Mitt Verein Aertze Steiermark 53:194–198, 1916
Vannas A, Hogan MJ, Wood I: Salzmann's nodular degeneration of the cornea. Am J Ophthalmol 79:211–219, 1975
Klintworth GK: Proteins in ocular disease. In Garner A, Klintworth GK (eds): Pathobiology of Ocular Disease: A Dynamic Approach, 2nd ed, pp 1007–1014. New York, Marcel Dekker, 1994

SANCHEZ-CORONA

Synonyms. Spinocerebellar ataxia; dysmorphism. See Friedreich ataxia.

Symptoms and Signs. Both sexes (one family reported). *Hair.* Abundant, rough; mild palpebral ptosis; thick lips with down-curved angles. Dysarthria, ataxia, psychomotor development delayed; scoliosis; foot deformity.

Etiology. Autosomal recessive inheritance probable.

BIBLIOGRAPHY. Sanchez-Corona J, Garcia-Cruz D, Gonzales-Angulo A, et al: A distinct dysmorphic syndrome with spinocerebellar ataxia and probable autosomal recessive inheritance. Hum Genet 69:243–245, 1985

SANDERS

Synonyms. Epidemic keratoconjunctivitis; macular keratitis; shipyard keratoconjunctivitis; keratoconjunctivitis epidemica.

Symptoms. Both sexes affected. Onset at all ages. High incidence in factories, shipyards, and eye clinics. Malaise; cephalalgia; pain in the affected eyes; photophobia; lacrimation; no increase in temperature.

Signs. Unilateral preauricular adenopathy.

Etiology. Virus infections, possibly by adenovirus 8–11.

Pathology. Edema and hyperemia of conjunctiva; hypertrophy of affected lymph nodes.

Diagnostic Procedures. *Smear of tears.* Mononuclear cells. *Electromicroscopy.* Viral particles.

Therapy. Antibiotics.

Prognosis. Spontaneous remission. Possible complications: keratosis and persistent visual impairment.

BIBLIOGRAPHY. Sanders M: Epidemic keratoconjunctivitis ("shipyard conjunctivitis"). I. Isolation of a virus. Arch Ophthalmol 28:581–586, 1942

Adenovirus keratoconjiunctivitis (editorial). Br J Ophthalmol 61:73, 1977

Lund OE, Stephani FH: Corneal histology after epidemic keratoconjunctivitis. Arch Ophthalmol 96:2085–2088, 1978

Easty DL, Williams C: Viral and rickettsial disease. In Garner A, Klintworth GK (eds): Pathobiology of Ocular Disease: A Dynamic Approach, 2nd ed, pp 245–247. New York, Marcel Dekker, 1994

SANDHOFF

Synonyms. Jatzkewitz-Pilz; gangliosidosis II; GM-2; hexosaminidases A and B deficiency.

Symptoms. Onset at 6 months of age. Motor weakness; startle reaction to sound; early blindness; progressive mental and motor deterioration. Frequent respiratory infections.

Signs. Macrocephaly; doll-like facies; macroglossia; cherry red spots in macula. Signs of heart involvement (pansystolic murmur, cardiomegaly, etc.) usually precede those from nervous system.

Etiology. Autosomal recessive inheritance. Enzyme defect (deficiency of hexosaminidase A and B). Same or allelic form defects of hexosaminidases have been found with juvenile and adult onset and generally milder symptomatology.

Pathology. Brain cortex, cerebellar, spinal, and autonomic neuronal lipoidosis; cytoplasm of neurons ballooned and enlarged with nucleus displacement. Accumulation of osmiophylic cytoplasmic bodies. Secondary demyelinization. Gliosis. Presence of vacuolated histiocytes in viscera, with possible preeminence of Henle renal loop localization.

Diagnostic Procedures. *Body tissues and fluids.* Activity of hexosaminidase A and B deficiency. *Blood.* Hexosaminidase assay of serum (lymphocytes vacuolization scarce). *Bone marrow.* Rarely, foamy histiocytes. *Biopsy.* Not necessary.

Therapy. No specific therapy. Enzyme replacement therapy hazardous.

Prognosis. Death by 3 years of age from respiratory infections.

BIBLIOGRAPHY. Sandhoff K, Harzer K: Total hexosaminidase deficiency in Tay-Sachs disease (variant O). In Hero HG, Van Hoff F (eds): Lysosomes and Storage Diseases, p 345. New York, Academic, 1973

Banerjee P, Siciliano L, Oliveri D, et al: Molecular basis of an adult form of betahexosaminidase B deficiency with motor neuron disease. Biochem Biophys Res Commun 181:108–115, 1991

Gravel RA, Clarke JTR, Kaback MM: The G_{m2} gangliosidoses. In Scriver CR, Beaudet AL, Sly WS, et al: The Metabolic and Molecular Bases of Inherited Disease, 7th ed, pp 2848–2849. New York, McGraw-Hill, 1995

SANDIFER

Synonym. Hiatus hernia; torticollis.

Symptoms. Prevalent in males. Onset in infancy. Epigastric pain; vomiting. In infancy; asthenia.

Signs. Pallor. Head rotation with neck stretching, which is enhanced during eating or reading. Strabismus. Malnutrition.

Etiology. Unknown. All manifestations seem correlated to the presence of the hiatus hernia.

Diagnostic Procedures. *Blood.* Iron deficiency anemia. *X-ray.* Of stomach. Hiatus hernia.

Therapy. Surgical correction of hernia.

Prognosis. Anemia, torticollis, strabismus, malnutrition disappear with treatment of hernia.

BIBLIOGRAPHY. Sutcliffe J: Torsion spasms and abnormal posture in children with hiatus hernia: Sandifer's syndrome. Prog Pediatr Radiol 2:190–197, 1969

Nanayakkara CS, Patton FY: Sandifer syndrome: An overlooked diagnosis? Dev Med Child Neurol 27:816–819, 1985

SANDMANN-ANDRA

Symptoms and Signs. From birth. Both sexes. Hypohidrosis reduction of number of teeth.

Etiology. Autosomal dominant inheritance.

BIBLIOGRAPHY. Sandmann H, Andra A: Beitrag zum Krankheitsbild der ektodermalen. Dysplasie Z Kinderheilk 82:238–255, 1959

SANDOZ

Synonyms. Pulmonary fibrosis, familial.

Symptoms and Signs. Occurs in younger age than idiopathic pulmonary fibrosis (see) but has an identical course.

Etiology. Autosomic dominant inheritance with variable penetrance. Possible association with immunoglobulin haplotype Gm1 and chromosome 14.

Pathology. See idiopathic pulmonary fibrosis.

Diagnostic Procedures. See idiopathic pulmonary fibrosis.

Therapy. See idiopathic pulmonary fibrosis.

Prognosis. See idiopathic fibrosis.

BIBLIOGRAPHY. Sandoz E: Uber zwei Falle von fetaler Bronchektasie. Beitr Pathol Anat 41:495–516, 1907

Murphy A, O'Sullivan BJ: Familial fibrosing alveolitis. Ir J Med Sci 150:204–209, 1981

Bitterman PB, Rennard SI, Keogh BA, et al: Familial idiopathic pulmonary fibrosis. Evidence of lung inflammation in unaffected family members. N Engl J Med 314:1343–1347, 1986

Weatherall DJ, Ledingham JGG, Warrell DA: Oxford Textbook of Medicine, pp 2786–2794. Oxford, Oxford Med Pub, 1996

SANFILIPPO

Synonyms. Sanfilippo-Good (types A, B, C, D); heparinuria; mucopolysaccharidosis III, MPS III; polydystrophic oligophrenia.

Symptoms. Both sexes affected. Severe mental retardation, becoming fully evident at school age. Minor somatic changes in facial features and joints. Good body strength.

Signs. Dwarfism and stiff joints (less severe than in other mucopolysaccharidoses); moderate hepatosplenomegaly. Absence of corneal opacification. Generalized hirsutism.

Etiology. Autosomal recessive inheritance. Four forms of enzymatic defect in degradation of heparan N-sulfate have been distinguished.

Type A: heparan N-sulfatase
Type B: α-N-acetylglucosaminidase
Type C: specific N-acetyl transferase
Type D: α-N-acetylglucosamine-6-sulfatase

These different enzymopathies share the same clinical picture, with type A presenting the most severe symptoms (earlier onset, more rapid progression, and earlier death).

Pathology. Presence of metachromatic inclusion positive for mucopolysaccharide and acid phosphatase in cells of all types. Heparan sulfate found in brain.

Diagnostic Procedures. *Urine.* Excretion of heparan sulfate only; in some cases, absence of this finding. *Enzymes assay.* In fibroblasts and other cells or serum. *X-rays.* Mild dysostosis multiplex. Prenatal diagnosis is now possible.

Therapy. None. Institutionalization required in most cases.

Prognosis. Death in second decade in majority of cases.

BIBLIOGRAPHY. Sanfilippo SJ, Podosin R, Langer LO Jr, et al: Mental retardation associated with acid mucopolysacchariduria (heparin sulfate type). J Pediatr 63:837–838, 1963
Neufeld EF, Muenzer J: The Mucopolysacchridoses. In Scriver CR, Beaudet AL, Sly WS, et al: The Metabolic and Molecular Bases of Inherited Disease, 7th ed, 2474–2476. New York, McGraw-Hill, 1995

SANGUE DORMIDO

Synonyms. Sleeping blood.

Symptoms and Signs. In people from Cape Verde. Pain, tremor, numbness, paralysis, convulsions, blindness, infections, stroke, and miscarrige.

Etiology. A miscellaneous group of organic and psychotic origin, culturally grouped together by Islanders and immigrants in Europe or United States.

BIBLIOGRAPHY. Kaplan HI, Sadock BJ: Comprehensive Textbook of Psychiatry, 6th ed, p 1053. Baltimore, Williams & Wilkins, 1995

SANTAVUORI-HALTIA

Synonyms. Finnish type ceroid lipofuscinosis; neuronal ceroid-lipofuscinosis, infantilis, Finnish; INCL. See ceroid lipofuscinosis.

Symptoms and Signs. Both sexes affected. Onset at 8–18 months. Mental development arrested; hypotonia; ataxia; seizures; early visual impairment. Blind by age 2. *Fundus.* Oculi hypopigmentation, atrophy; discoloration of macula with yellow-gray areas. *Liver and spleen.* Not enlarged and no bone abnormalities. Later stage, severe dementia muscle wasting. A late infantile and a juvenile form described CLN1 gene appears located at 1p32.

Etiology. Autosomal recessive inheritance. Disturbance of linoleic acid metabolism.

Pathology. Deposits of autoflourescent lipopigments in all tissues, predominant in the brain. *Brain.* Small, loss of nerve cells and status spongiosus; various sizes and structures of lipopigment deposits (lamellar, granular, "fingerprint" aspect), with acid phosphatase activity. *Retina.* Loss of cones and rods; degeneration of epithelial cells; lipoid pigment accumulation.

Diagnostic Procedures. *ERG.* Waveforms lost when retina compromised. *EEG.* High voltage; triphasic waves; later only delta waves. *CT scan. MR imaging.* Lateral ventricles slighly dilated. *Electromicroscopy.* Of eccrine glands of skin. No enzyme deficiency has been yet demonstrated. *Bone marrow and other tissue biopsy.* Presence of lipopigments. *Urine.* Presence of lipopigments in sediment. *Blood.* Lipopigments in lymphocytes; azurophilic hypergranulation in neutrophils and lymphocyte vacuolization (only in homozygotes).

Prognosis. Within 3 years, total incapacitation. Death in 10–15 years.

BIBLIOGRAPHY. Santavuori P, Haltia M, Rapola J, et al: Infantile type of so-called neuronal ceroid-lipofuscinosis: A clinical study of 15 patients. J Neurol Sci 18:257–267, 1973
Jarvela I, Santavuori P, Vesa J, et al: Assignment of the infantile form of neural ceroid lipofuscinosis (INCL, CLN1) to the short arm of chromosome 1. Cytogenet Cell Genet 58:1856–1857, 1991
Weatherall DJ, Ledingham JGG, Warrell DA: Oxford Textbook of Medicine, p 3985. Oxford, Oxford Med Pub, 1996

S.A.P.H.O.

Synonyms. Andrews bactérides-arthrites pseudoseptiques. Synovitis—acne—pustolosis—hyperostosis—oateomyelitis; acne-associated spondyloarthropathy; see Tietze.

Symptoms and Signs. Acne conglobata; acne fulminans; hidradenitis suppurativa; palmo-plantar pustolosis; sterno-costo-clavicular hyperotosis; chronic recurrent osteomyelitis and spondyloarthropathy. Skin lesions may occur before simultaneously or even 20 years after onset of bone or joints symptomatology.

Etiology. Unknown. Possibly weak association with HLA-B27.

Diagnostic Procedures. *Blood.* Seronegativity. *X-ray.* Asymmetric oligoarthritis; sacroiliitis syndesmophytes; enthesopathies; anterior chest lesions.

Therapy. Anti-inflammatory agents.

Prognosis. Course generally prolonged and unpredictable. Peripheral articular synovitis short duration, bone lesions long duration (up to over 20 years) with bouts of pain and recurrent inflammation. Occasionally monocyclic course.

BIBLIOGRAPHY. Kato T, Kambara A, Hoshi E: Case of bilateral clavicular osteomyelitis with palmar and plantar pustulosis. Seiki Geka 19:590–593, 1968
Khan MA, Chamot A-M: Sapho syndrome. Rheum Dis N Am 18:225–245, 1992
Khan MA: Ankylosing sponditis: Clinical features. In Klippel JH, Dieppe PA: Rheumatology, p 3.25.8. St Louis, CV Mosby, 1995

SARCOID MYOPATHY

See Besnier-Boeck-Schaumann.

Symptoms. Onset most often in middle and old age. Muscular pain; weakness of legs or, less frequently, of arms.

Signs. Muscle wasting or firm enlargement of muscles with nodules; contractures.

Etiology. Unknown. See Besnier-Boeck-Schaumann.

Pathology. On muscle biopsy, appearance of changes described in sarcoidosis: interstitial infiltration with giant cells; epithelioid cells and lymphocytes; palisade-like and reticular collagen fiber network, replacing tissue; muscle fiber degeneration with floccular necrosis.

Diagnostic Procedures. *Blood.* Intermittent monocytosis and eosinophilia; leukopenia and increased calcium; hyperproteinemia; increased alkaline phosphatases. Kveim test (60% positive).

Therapy. Corticosteroids.

Prognosis. Good response to treatment.

BIBLIOGRAPHY. Licharew A: Demonstration. Dermatol Centralbl 11:253–254, 1908
Talbot PS: Sarcoid myopathy. Br Med J 4:465–466, 1967
Weatherall DJ, Ledingham JGG, Warrell DA: Oxford Textbook of Medicine, p 4156. Oxford, Oxford Med Pub, 1996

SARCOPLASMIC BODY MYOPATHY

Synonyms. Edstroem; myopathy sarcoplasmic body; hereditary distal neuropathy, late onset. See Gowers-Welander (possibly same condition) and Gober (Cytoplasic-spheroid body complex group).

Symptoms and Signs. Same as in Gowers-Welander (see) but with cardiomyopathy.

Etiology. Autosomal dominant inheritance.

Pathology. *Muscle biopsy.* Sarcoplasmic bodiies, filamentous bodies, and intermediate filaments of desmin.

Diagnostic Procedures. See Gowers-Welander.

Therapy. None.

Prognosis. Slowly progressive

BIBLIOGRAPHY. Edstroem L, Thornell LE, Eriksson A: A new type of hereditary distal myopathy with characteristic sarcoplasmic bodies and intermediate (skeleton filaments). J Neurol Sci 47:171–190, 1980
Goebel HH, Lenard HG: Congenital myopathies. In Handbook of Clinical Neurology 18: Rowland LP, Di Mauro S (eds): The Myopathies, p 331. Amsterdam, Elsevier, 1992

SATURDAY NIGHT PALSIES

Synonym. Alcoholic neuropathy.

Symptoms. Occurs in heavy drinkers. Discovered when awaking after alcohol intoxication and having fallen asleep or "passed out" in various positions with arm abducted, resting over edge of a chair or with head over arm. Most frequently, paralysis of muscle innervated by radial nerve (extension of elbow, wrist, fingers); also peripheral nerve of lower extremities affected; especially peroneal nerve.

Etiology. Compression neuritis. Frequently, pre-existing alcoholic neuritis.

Therapy. Abstention from alcohol. Thiamine; vitamin B$_{12}$; pyridoxine; diet rich in carbohydrates and protein. Physical therapy.

BIBLIOGRAPHY. Mayer RF: Recent studies in man and animal of peripheral nerve and muscle dysfunction associated with chronic alcoholism. Ann NY Acad Sci 215:370–372, 1973
Weatherall DJ, Ledingham JGG, Warrell DA: Oxford Textbook of Medicine, p 4094. Oxford, Oxford Med Pub, 1996

SAUNDERS-SUTTON

Synonym. Delirium tremens.

Symptoms. Occurs in chronic alcoholic patients; onset associated with alcohol withdrawal or intercurrent trauma or infection. Irritability; food aversion; insomnia; constant confabulation; hallucinations of terrifying objects or animals; generalized tremor and seizures (occasional).

Signs. Perspiration; coated tongue; tachycardia.

Etiology. In chronic alcoholic condition, dehydration associated with any condition is usually the precipitating cause.

Pathology. *Brain edema.* Swelling and granular degeneration of ganglion cells. Perivascular hemorrhages.

Diagnostic Procedures. *Body fluid.* Presence of alcohol. *Blood.* Leukocytosis. *Urine.* Albuminuria.

Therapy. Prevent self-injury (physical restraints). Drugs for sedation: clomethiazol; diazepam; chlordiazepoxide; beta-blockers. High-caloric intake; thiamine and multivitamins containing folic acid. Maintenance of fluid and electrolyte balance (hypomagnesemia and hypoglycemia are frequent).

Prognosis. Easy collapse and death from exhaustion; heart failure; pneumonia. After period of rest, treatment, and long period of sleep, gradual improvement.

BIBLIOGRAPHY. Sutton T: Tracts on Delirium Tremens, on Peritonitis and on Some Other Internal Inflammatory Affections on the Gout. London, Underwood, 1813
Adams RD, Victor M: Principles of Neurology, 5th ed, pp 912–913. New York, McGraw-Hill, 1993
Weatherall DJ, Ledingham JGG, Warrell DA: Oxford Textbook of Medicine, pp 1251, 2084, 2093, 4259, 4290. Oxford, Oxford Med Pub, 1996

SCAPULOCOSTAL

Synonym. Postural drag paradox.

Symptoms. Occurs in middle-aged individuals; insidious onset. Deep shoulder pain with different patterns of irradiation: neck, occiput, chest, or combinations.

Signs. Trigger point at or under medial angle of scapula at posterior thoracic wall.

Etiology and Pathology. Traumatic or nontraumatic factors (arthritis, bursitis, myositis).

Diagnostic Procedures. *X-ray.* Of shoulder, cervical spine. *ECG.* To rule out cardiopathy.

Therapy. Physical therapy: massage, exercises. Injection of procaine or hydrocortisone at the trigger point. Firm digital pressure of trigger point often followed by mitigation of acute symptoms.

Prognosis. Spontaneous remission 70%.

BIBLIOGRAPHY. Michele AA: Scapulocostal syndrome: Its mechanism and diagnosis. NY J Med 55:2485–2493, 1955
Klippel JH, Dieppe PA: Rheumatology, p 5.8.2. St Louis, CV Mosby, 1995

SCAPULOILIOPERONEAL ATROPHY, CARDIOMYOPATHY

Synonyms. Emery-Dreifuss muscular dytrophy M.D. (with early contractures and cardiomyopathy); Hauptmann-Thannhauser muscular dystrophy, FSH. See scapulo-peroneal syndromes; Charcot-Marie-Tooth and Kungelberg-Welander.

Symptoms and Signs. Both sexes. Onset myopathy 17–42 years of age, cardiac signs later. Muscle contractures, neck stiffness slowly progressing; weakness of humeral and peroneal muscles, pelvic involvement, tendon areflexia.

Etiology. Unknown. Autosomal dominant inheritance. There are both myopathic and neurogenic dominant forms.

Pathology. *Muscle.* Inflammatory changes, perivascular cuffing.

Diagnostic Procedures. *EEG.* Motor nerve conduction velocity, borderline or normal values.

Therapy. Orthopedic; heart transplant.

Prognosis. Progressive condition.

BIBLIOGRAPHY. Hauptmann A, Thannhauser SJ: Muscular shortening and dystrophy: A heredofamilar disease. Arch Neurol Psychiatr 46:654–664, 1941

Davidenkow S: Scapuloperoneal amyotrophy. Arch Neurol Psychiatr 41:694–701, 1939

Jennekens FGI, Busch HFM, van Hemel NM, et al: Inflammatory myopathy in scapulo-ilio-peroneal atrophy with cardiomyopathy: A study of two families. Brain 98:709–722, 1975

Emery AEH: Emery-Dreifuss syndrome. J Med Genet 26:637–641, 1989

Stevenson WG, Perloff JK, Weiss JN, et al: Facioscapulohumeral muscular dystrophy: Evidence for selective, genetic electrophysiologic cardiac involvement. J Am Coll Cardiol 15:292–299, 1990

SCAPULO-PERONEAL MUSCULAR DYSTROPHY

Synonyms. See Erb III.

Symptoms and Signs. Onset median 20 years of age. Seldom younger or older (to 40). In the majority of cases muscles of shoulder and face first affected and dropfoot follows after years. Seldom onset with weakness of anterior tibial muscles and then years later upper girdle involvement. Scapula alata is prominent. Asymmetric involvement of muscles frequent. Absence of fasciculation and sensory disturbance and pes equino varus.

Etiology. Sporadic cases or autosomal dominant inheritance. Considered a variant of Erb III (see).

Diagnostic Procedures. *EMG. Biopsy.* Evidence of muscular dystrophy. *Blood.* Serum enzymes slightly and nonconstantly elevated.

Therapy. Physiotherapy.

Prognosis. Course slow and benign.

BIBLIOGRAPHY. Gowers WR: A lecture on myopathy and distal form. Br Med J 2:89–92, 1902

Kaeser HE: Scapulo-peroneal syndrome. In Vinken PJ, Bruyn GW (eds): Handbook of Clinical Neurology, vol 22, pp 58–59. Amsterdam, Elsevier, 1985

SCAPULO-PERONEAL MUSCULAR DYSTROPHY, SPINAL; RECESSIVE TYPE

Synonyms. Includes Brossard.

Symptoms and Signs. Nonhomogeneous group with inconstant scapulo-peroneal distribution of muscle involvement. Onset at birth or within first year (in Brossard cases, 14 and 22 years). Onset contemporary or dissociated of lower leg and shoulder girdle muscle involvement. Foot deformities frequent.

Etiology. Autosomal recessive inheritance.

BIBLIOGRAPHY. Brossard J: Etude clinique sur une forme héréditaire d'atrophie musculaire progressive débutant par les membres inférieurs (type fémoral avec griffe des orteils), p 174. Paris, Steinheil, 1886

Kaeser HE: Scapulo-peroneal syndrome. In Vinken PJ, Bruyn GW (eds): Handbook of Clinical Neurology, vol 22, pp 62–63. Amsterdam, Elsevier, 1985

SCAPULO-PERONEAL SYNDROMES

A. Scapulo-peroneal muscular dystrophy (see)
B. Dawidenkow (see)
C. Kaeser (see)
D. Emery-Dreifuss (see)
E. Scapulo-peroneal spinal recessive type (see)
F. Scapuloileoperoneal atrophy, cardiomyopathy

See also Erb III.

SCARRING FOLLICULAR KERATOSIS

Synonyms. According to minor differences or stages of the same process various syndromes have been differentiated; many intermediate forms exist as well. The three main entities are Keratosis pilaris atrophicans (see), Honeycomb atrophy (see), Keratosis pilaris decalvans (see).

Etiology. Sporadic or autosomal dominant, recessive or sex-linked defects.

SCASSELLATI-SFORZOLINI

Synonym. Vertical bilateral retraction. See Duane and A and V syndromes.

Symptoms and Signs. Unilateral or bilateral partial or almost complete loss of upward gaze; some limitation of downward gaze; retraction upon depression and pseudoptosis. A exotropia or V exotropia can be found. Associated congenital anomalies include unilateral partial ptosis, facial asymmetry, and anomalies of the optic (II) nerve heads.

Etiology. Unknown. Congenital inherited condition.

Pathology. Unknown.

Diagnostic Procedures. *Electromyography.*

BIBLIOGRAPHY. Scassellati-Sforzolini G: Una sindrome molto rara: Difetto congenito monolaterale della elevazione con retrazione del globo. Riv Otoneurooft 33:431–439, 1958

Khodadoutst AA, von Noorden GK: Bilateral vertical retraction syndrome: A family study. Arch Ophthalmol 78:606–612, 1967

SCHACHTER

Synonyms. Nevo-osteo-oligophrenic.

BIBLIOGRAPHY. Karczewska K: Nevo-osteo-oligofrenic syndrome of infants. Pediatr Pol 41:1187–1192, 1966

SCHAEFER-SOERENSEN

Synonyms. Bagolini; Schaffer II; plagiocephaly—superior oblique deficiency; ocular torticollis.

Symptoms and Signs. Prevalent in females. Combination of plagiocephaly (unilateral coronal sutures stenosis), strabismus (particularly dissociation of conjugate movements), and torticollis.

Etiology. Various intrauterine influences on developing cranial sutures. Possible pathogenetic mechanism proposed for strabismus: palsy or motor imbalance caused by shortened length of superior oblique muscle and variation of its mechanical effect on rotation of eyeball because of enlarged angle.

Diagnostic Procedures. *X-ray of skull. Bielchowsky head-tilt test.*

Therapy. Resection of inferior oblique muscle.

Prognosis. According to severity: good for torticollis and binocular function in less severe cases.

BIBLIOGRAPHY. Archer DB, Gordon DS, Maguire CJF, et al: Ophthalmic aspects of craniosynostosis. Trans Ophthalmol Soc UK 94:172–196, 1974
Schaefer WD, Sorensen N: Motilitatsstorungen bei Koronarnaht-Synostosen. Meeting of Berufsverband Augenarzte. Wiesbaden, Germany, 1979
Bagolini B, Campos EC: Plagiocephaly causing superior oblique deficiency and ocular torticollis: A new clinical entity. Arch Ophthalmol 100:1093–1096, 1982
Bagolini B: Personal communication, 1995

SCHÄFFER I

Synonym. Schaffer I; keratosis palmoplantaris variant.

Symptoms and Signs. Disseminated follicular keratosis of skin; leukokeratosis of oral mucosa; small foci of alopecia; dysonychia; congenital cataracts; microcephaly; mental retardation; hypogenitalism and dwarfism.

Etiology. Unknown. Autosomal dominant inheritance.

BIBLIOGRAPHY. Schäfer E: Zur Lehre von den congenitalen Dyskeratosen. Arch Dermatol Syph 148:425–432, 1925
Silver HK: Rothmund-Thompson syndrome: An oculocutaneous disorder. Am J Dis Child 111:182–190, 1966

SCHAMBERG

Synonyms. Loewenthal; purpuric pigmentary dermatosis; pigmentary progressive dermatosis.

Symptoms and Signs. Occurs more often in males; onset at any age. Irregular plaques, orange brownish with "cayenne pepper" spots, within and at edges of lesions, erupting most frequently on the legs, occasionally other parts of the body. Occasionally, slight pruritus. No systemic symptoms.

Etiology. Unknown. Stasis may play a role. Autosomal dominant trait.

Pathology. Slight changes in epidermis; hemosiderin deposits.

Therapy. None.

Prognosis. Chronic recurrences; years duration.

BIBLIOGRAPHY. Schamberg JF: A peculiar progressive pigmentary disease of the skin. Br J Dermatol 13:1–5, 1901
Loewenthal LJA: Itching purpura. Br J Dermatol 66:95, 1954
Champion RH: Purpura. In Champion RH, Burton JL, Ebling FJG (eds): Rook/Wilkinson/Ebling Textbook of Dermatology, 5th ed, pp 1888–1889. Oxford, Blackwell Scientific, 1992

SCHANZ II

Synonym. Spinal insufficiency.

Symptoms. Moving from erect to a prone position causes a feeling of fatigue and lumbar pain.

Etiology. Lumbar spine pathology of different etiologies: rheumatic, inflammatory, neoplastic, muscle weakness, congenital or acquired.

BIBLIOGRAPHY. Schanz A: Eine typische Erkrankung der Wirbelsaeule (insufficientia vertebrale). Klin Wochenschr 44:989–992, 1907

SCHATZKI

Synonyms. Esophagogastric ring; lower esophageal ring.

Symptoms. Both sexes affected; onset after 50 years of age. Asymptomatic or episodes of substernal pain, dysphagia on swallowing solid food, and pyrosis.

Signs. Diameter of lower esophageal ring normal or reduced.

Etiology. Unknown. Motor disorder of lower esophageal ring or anatomic malformation, associated frequently with diaphragmatic hernia.

Pathology. Mucosal strands of connective muscular tissue 4 or 5 cm above diaphragm at the gastroesophageal area.

Diagnostic Procedures. *Fluoroscopy.* With barium swallow. *Esophageal manometry.*

Therapy. Repair of an associated hernia insufficient to control dysphagia. Bougienage or excision of the ring followed by treatment of esophagitis.

BIBLIOGRAPHY. Schatzki R, Gary JE: Dysphagia due to a diaphragm-like localized narrowing in lower esophagus ("lower esophageal ring"). Am J Roentgenol 70:911–922, 1953
Blanchon P, Dupuis J, Babok D: L'anneau de Schatzki. Atlas Radiol Clin 47:1–4, 1968
Wilkins EW Jr: The lower esophageal ring: How unique? (editorial). Ann Thorac Surg 37:101–102, 1984
Lichtenstein GR: Esophageal rings, webs, and diverticula. In Haubrich WS, Schaffner F, Berk JE (eds): Bockus Gastroenterology, 5th ed, vol 2, pp 518–533. Philadelphia, WB Saunders, 1995

SCHEIBE

Synonyms. Nadol-Burges; Cochleo—saccular malformation, cataracts.

Symptoms and Signs. Postnatal sensorneural deafness, congenital or slowly progressing. Later (third to fourth decade) development of cataracts. Ataxia and staggering gait (suggesting drunkeness) and vertigo eventually appear. Occasionally patient may complain of diverticula of small bowel. Cases in which hearing loss is noticed about 30 years later are described also.

Etiology. Sporadic and autosomal dominant inheritance. May be a feature of Rubella syndrome (see).

Pathology. Inner ear changes are limited to cochlea and saccule bilaterally. Cochleo-saccular dysplasia in congenital deafness and cochleo-saccular degeneration in postnatal degeneration.

Therapy. Symptomatic.

Prognosis. According to type. Progression of symptoms to ataxia and blindness occurs in degenerative types.

BIBLIOGRAPHY. Scheibe A: A Case of deafmutism with auditory atrophy and anomalies of development in the membranous labyrinth of both ears. Arch Otol 21:12–22, 1892
Nadol JB, Burges B: Cochleosaccular degeneration of the inner ear and progressive cataracts inherited as an autosomal dominant trait. Laryngoscope 92:1028–1037, 1982
Bandt T: Vertigo: Its Multisensorial Syndromes. London, Springer-Verlag, 1991

SCHEIE

Synonyms. Spat-Hurler; Hurler, late; alpha-L-iduronidase deficiency;

mucopolysaccharidosis V (formerly); MPSV (formerly); MPS IS; mucopolysaccharidosis IS.

Symptoms. Both sexes affected. Visual impairment; normal intelligence; cases with psychosis reported.

Signs. Stiff joints; claw hand; carpal tunnel syndrome; facies characteristically "broad mouthed." Clouding of cornea, uniform in early stage, later becoming densest peripherally. Retinitis pigmentosa. Stature normal or low-normal range; excessive body hair; aortic valve regurgitation.

Etiology. Autosomal recessive inheritance. Alpha-L-iduronidase deficiency.

Pathology. Same alterations as in Hurler (see). Cortical neuron normal (different from Hurler).

Diagnostic Procedures. Same as in Hurler. Differential diagnosis on clinical basis only. Prenatal diagnosis possible.

Therapy. Surgery for correction of carpal tunnel, glaucoma; aortic valve prothesis.

Prognosis. Good quoad vitam; normal intelligence and stature.

BIBLIOGRAPHY. Scheie HG, Hambrick GW Jr, Barness LA: A newly recognized forme fruste of Hurler's disease (gargoylism). Am J Ophthalmol 53:753–769, 1962

Madhava Rao B, Gupta SK, Abraham KA, et al: Rare multivalvular involvement in a family of Scheie syndrome. Indian J Pediatr 55:317–322, 1988

Klintworth GK: Disorders of glycosaminoglycans (mucopolysaccharides) and proteoglycans. In Garner A, Klintworth GK (eds): Pathobiology of Ocular Disease: A Dynamic Approach, 2nd ed, pp 862–863. New York, Marcel Dekker, 1994

Neufeld EF, Muenzer J: The mucopolysaccharidoses. In Scriver CR, Beaudet AL, Sly WS, et al: The Metabolic and Molecular Bases of Inherited Disease, 7th ed, pp 2472–2473. New York, McGraw-Hill, 1995

SCHEUERMANN

Synonyms. Kyphosis dorsalis juvenilis; epiphyseal osteochondritis; vertebral osteochondrosis; osteochondrosis spinal.

Symptoms. Both sexes affected. Early manifestation from 12 years of age. Backache.

Signs. Kyphosis originating in late childhood in which there is a rigid arcuate backward curvature (round shoulders). In many cases, however, absence of kyphosis and presence of flat thoracic area (with loss of lordosis in lumbar tract) and the localized scoliosis (thoracic or lumbar) are the only clinical signs.

Etiology. Growth disorder: transition from cartilage to bone irregular and patchy, usually sporadic. Families with autosomal dominant inheritance.

Pathology. Osteochondrosis of affected vertebral bodies.

Diagnostic Procedures. *X-ray. CT scan. MRI.* Of spine. Increased anteroposterior diameter of vertebral bodies (wedge-shaped); disk spaces reduced; kyphosis; Schmorl nodes.

Therapy. *Orthopedic.* To correct deformity, relieve or reduce pain, prevent an increase in the kyphotic angle and relative complications. *Medical.* Early surgical treatment advocated.

Prognosis. Early manifestations mild, but have serious effects on future capacity for sports and physical activities.

BIBLIOGRAPHY. Scheuermann H: Kyphosis dorsalis juvenilis. Über geshkrift. Laeger 82:385–393, 1920

Murray PM, Weinstein SL, Spratt KF: The natural history and long term follow-up of Scheuermann's kyphosis. J Bone Joint Surg (Am) 75A:236–248, 1993

Ferreira-Alves A, Resina J, Palma-Rodrigues R: Scheuermann's kyphosis. J Bone Joint Surg 77B (Am):943–950, 1995

SCHILDER

Synonyms. Heubner-Schilder; myelinoclastic diffuse sclerosis, sudanophilic leukodystrophy, encephalitis periaxialis diffusa (incorrect eponym). The Crome-Zapella seems to represent an ulterior variant in the confused group of leukodystrophies.

Symptoms. Very rare. Both sexes. Two major phenotypes identified. *Type I* (German type). Onset in infancy. Normal development in first months of life then headache, cerebral blindness, central deafness, mental changes, myoclonic seizures, dullness, apathy progressing to stupor. Bilateral or monolateral spastic weakness progressing to paralysis. Multiple neurologic symptoms (motor and sensorial according to areas involved). *Type II* (Japanese type). Milder intellectual impairment in adults.

Signs. *In Type I. Eyes.* Nystagmus; extranuclear palsy (occasional); hemianopia; papilledema (15–20%). Seldom, bronzing of skin or jaundice. *Type II.* Angiokeratoma corporis diffusum in one case.

Etiology. Autosomal recessive inheritance. In some past classification only sporadic type indicated with this eponym. Deficient activity of alpha-N-acetylgalactosaminidase (former alpha-galactosidase B). In the past, this disease was considered a variant of multiple sclerosis (Charcot) and this eponym was (improperly) used to indicate a heterogeneous group of conditions, probably including cases of adrenoleukodystrophy, Dawson disease, and other disorders with diffuse cerebral damage.

Pathology. Cerebral edema. Disseminated plaques may be present with extensive involvement of white matter. Affects centrum semiovale: perivascular lymphocytes infiltration, astrocytes proliferation; some enormous and multinucleated; vacuolated cells containing oil red O-positive material, osmophilic bodies.

Diagnostic Procedures. *Spinal tap.* Increased pressure, slight pleocytosis, high immunoglobin G content with oligoclonal bands. *Blood. Urine.* Rule out adrenoleukodystrophy by analysis of long-chain fatty acids of plasma cholesterol esters. *CT scan. MRI.* Hypodense lesions with contrast enhancement in brain stem cerebellum, and cortex. *EEG.* Diffuse dysfunction with multifocal irritative features. *Brain stem.* Auditory, somato-sensory, and visual evoked potential, low amplitude, and/or delayed responses.

Therapy. Corticosteroids.

Prognosis. Variable according to types.

BIBLIOGRAPHY. Schilder P: Zu Kenntnis der sogenannten diffusen Sklerose. Ueber Encephalitis periaxialis diffusa. Z Ges Neurol Psychiatr (Berlin) Leipzig 10:1–60, 1912

Crome L, Zapella M: Schilder's disease (sudanophilic leukodystrophy) in five male members of one family. J Eur Neurosurg Psychiatr 26:431–438, 1963

Poser CM, Goutieres F, Carpentier M, Aicardi J: Schilder's myelinoclastic diffuse sclerosis. Pediatrics 77:107–112, 1986

Klintworth GK: Ocular involvement in disorders of the nervous system. In Garner A, Klintworth GK (eds): Pathobiology of Ocular Disease: A Dynamic Approach, 2nd ed, p 1717. New York, Marcel Dekker, 1994

Desnick RJ, Wang AM: N-Acetylgalactosaminidase deficiency: Schindler disease. In Scriver CR, Beaudet AL, Sly WS, et al: The Metabolic and Molecular Bases of Inherited Disease, 7th ed, pp 2509–2527. New York, McGraw-Hill, 1995

SCHILDER-FOIX

Synonym. Centrilobar symmetric sclerosis. See Schilder.

Eponym used to indicate variable neurologic manifestations related to sclerosis of white matter; nonprogressive lesions possibly caused by anoxic encephalopathy. See Pelizaeus-Merzbacher, Scholtz, Krabbe.

BIBLIOGRAPHY. Schilder P: Zur Frage der Enzephalitis periaxialis diffusa (sogenannte diffuse Sklerose). Z Ges Neurol 15:359, 1913
Foix C, Marie J: La sclérose cérébrale centrolobulaire à tendence symetrique: Ses rapports avec l'encephalite periaxiale diffuse. Encephale 22:81, 1927

SCHINZEL I

Synonyms. Atrichia; somatic mental retardation; skeletal anomalies.

Symptoms and Signs. Almost complete alopecia; nail dysplasia, hyperkeratosis of skin (legs) small hands and feet; syndactyly. Short stature, microcephaly, mental retardation.

Etiology. Unknown.

Diagnostic Procedures. *X-rays.* Fusion of vertebral bodies; of talusnavicular, of lunate-triquetral, of IV–V metacarpals; hip dislocation.

BIBLIOGRAPHY. Damste TJ, Prakken JR: Atrichia with papular lesions: a variant of ectodermal dysplasia. Dermatologica 108:114–121, 1954
Schinzel A: A case of multiple skeletal anomalies, ectodermal dysplasia and severe growth and mental retardation. Helv Paediatr Acta 35:243–251, 1980

SCHINZEL II

Synonyms. See Ulnar-mammary. Pallister (possibly identical condition in Pallister; mostly female subjects).

Symptoms and Signs. Mostly male. Congenital. Ulnar finger and fibular toe ray defects. Delayed growth and onset of puberty, hypogenitalism, hypoplasia of nipples and apocrine glands (lack or reduced sweating). Occasionally, various intestinal stenoses: subglottic, pyloric, anal. Signs of ventricular septal defect. Short stature, obesity.

Etiology. Unknown. Autosomal dominant inheritance.

BIBLIOGRAPHY. Schinzel A: Ulnar-mammary syndrome. J Med Genet 24:778–781, 1987
McKusick VA: Mendelian Inheritance in Man, 10th ed, p 1003. Baltimore, Johns Hopkins Univ Press, 1992

SCHINZEL-GIEDION

Symptoms. Mental retardation; seizures.

Signs. *Facies.* Coarse, frontal bossing; midface retraction; ocular hypertelorism. Nose, short, upturned; choanal stenosis. Ears, low set. Teeth, delayed eruption. Neck, short with redundant skin. Hypertrichosis; hypoplastic nipples; hypoplastic dermal ridges; hyperconvex nails. Genitourinary anomalies. Skeletal anomalies

Etiology. Possible autosomal recessive inheritance.

BIBLIOGRAPHY. Schinzel A, Giedion A: A syndrome of middle face retraction, multiple skull anomalies, club feet, and cardiac and renal malformations in sibs. Am J Med Genet 1:362–375, 1978
Hall BD: Schinzel-Giedion syndrome: Report of the fifth case. David W Smith workshop on malformations and morphogenesis. Madrid, Spain 23–29, May 1989

SCHIRMER

Synonyms. Sturge Weber variant.

Symptoms and Signs. Bisymptomatic form of Sturge Weber ocular and cutaneous: precocius glaucoma and buphthalmos.

BIBLIOGRAPHY. Schirmer RS: Ein Fall von Teleangiektasie Albrecht v. Graefes Arch Ophth 7:119–121, 1860
Alexander GL: Sturge Weber syndrome. In Vinken PJ, Bruyn GW (eds): Handbook of Clinical Neurology, vol 22, p 227. Amsterdam, North-Holland, 1975

SCHMID (B.J.)

Synonym. Spondylometaphyseal dysplasia (type C-III).

Symptoms and Signs. Both sexes affected. Onset of clinical manifestations in early infancy. Abnormalities of sternum and ribs; altered gait. Later becoming more evident; short neck; prognathism; kyphoscoliosis; genu valgum.

Etiology. Unknown. Karyotypic alterations of chromosomes questionable.

Pathology. Normal structure of bone; proliferation of connective and osteoid tissue with increased osteoblasts in medullary space.

Diagnostic Procedures. *Blood. Urine.* Normal. *X-rays.* Of spine, hips, and metaphyses of long bones. Dorsolumbar kyphosis; acetabular "blowout"; delayed ossification metaphyseal defects of ossification; major vertical streaks in upper extremities.

Therapy. Corrective osteotomy. Trials with vitamin D.

Prognosis. Poor quoad functionem.

BIBLIOGRAPHY. Schmid BJ, Becak W, Becak ML, et al: Metaphyseal dysostosis: Review of literature, study of a case with cytogenetic analysis. J Pediatr 63:106–112, 1963
Rimoin DL, Lachman RS: Genetic Disorders of the Osseous Skeleton. In Beithon P(ed): McKusick's Heritable Disorders of Connective Tissue, 5th ed, pp 620–621. St Louis, CV Mosby, 1993

SCHMID (F.)

Synonyms. Chondrodystrophia adolescentium sui tarda; dysostosis enchondralis metaphysaria; metaphyseal chondrodysplasia Schmid; M CH D Schmid; metaphyseal dysostosis (type BI).

Symptoms and Signs. Both sexes affected. Onset in early childhood. Clinically, no characteristic features: retarded growth with bow legs and short diaphyses. Leg pains in childhood. No face and skull involvement. Trunk may be normal or short. Metaphysis less affected than in Jansen. Hands and feet not involved or minimally involved. Women affected have children with little difficulty.

Etiology. Possibly autosomal dominant inheritance. Families with possible autosomal recessive form also reported.

Pathology. Cartilage hypoplasia. Biopsy. Rough-surfaced endoplasmic reticulum cisternae of chondrocytes from accumulation of a protein (?). Normal osteoid.

Diagnostic Procedures. *X-ray.* Changes described. Vertebrae may show same features as in Jansen syndrome. Epiphyses close prematurely.

Therapy. High doses of vitamin D have been tried, with doubtful success. Orthopedic measures limited to major deformities.

Prognosis. Metaphyseal lesions appear healed in adults. Sequelae of coxa vara and shortening of bones. Osteoarthritic manifestations minimal or absent.

BIBLIOGRAPHY. Schmid F: Beitrag zur Dysostosis enchondralis metaphysaria. Monatsschr Kinderheilkd 97:393–397, 1949
Lachman RS, Rimoin DL, Spranger J: Metaphyseal chondrodysplasia Schmid type: Clinical and radiographic delineation with review of the literature. Pediatr Radiol 18:93–102, 1988
Rimoin DL, Lachman RS: Genetic disorders of the osseous skeleton. In

Beithon P (ed): McKusick's Heritable Disorders of Connective Tissue, 5th ed, pp 630–631. St Louis, CV Mosby, 1993

SCHMIDT (A.)

Synonym. Vagoaccessory.

Symptoms. Stiff neck; inability to turn the head; speech disorders, swallowing disorders.

Signs. Unilateral and ipsilateral paralysis of soft palate, vocal cords, sternocleidomastoid and trapezius muscles (partial or total).

Etiology and Pathology. Most frequently, vascular lesion affecting cranial nerves within medulla oblongata or at their point of exit from skull. Neoplasm and infections less frequently.

Diagnostic Procedures. *X-ray. Angiography. Spinal tap. Serology.* For syphilis.

Therapy. According to etiology.

Prognosis. Guarded. According to etiology.

BIBLIOGRAPHY. Schmidt A: Doppelseitige Accessormslähmung bei Syringomyelie. Dtsch Med Wochenschr 18:606–608, 1892
Adams RD, Victor M: Principles of Neurology, 5th ed, pp 1180–1181. New York, McGraw-Hill, 1993

SCHMIDT (M.B.)

Synonyms. Thyroid—adrenocortical—pancreatic insufficiency; polyglandular autoimmune II, multiple endocrine deficiency (APS II); M.E.N.A.P.S. II; multiple endocrine deficiency, autoimmune II; polyglandular failure type II APS; diabetes mellitus—Addison—myxedema.

Symptoms and Signs. More frequent than type I. Onset at all ages (more frequently in the third, fourth decade; seldom before or after); predominantly in females (3–4 times). Manifestations of chronic lymphocytic thyroiditis or Flajani Syndrome (see) may precede or follow the manifestations of Addison syndrome. Very often coexists with insulin-dependent diabetes mellitus; their onset may precede or follow thyroid or subrenal involvement. Possible anemia (pernicious). Alopecia or vitiligo (less frequent occurrence than in type I).

Etiology. Unknown. An autoimmune mechanism postulated with common antibodies against thyroid and adrenal and possibly pancreas. Possibly autosomal dominant inheritance.

Pathology. *Adrenal.* Changes consistent with slowly progressive necrosis of cortex, with lymphocytic plasma cells and macrophage infiltration. *Thyroid.* Extensive lymphocytic infiltration; fewer plasma cells than in adrenals; mild fibrosis; no frank necrosis of epithelium. Generalized changes: those observed in Addison and hypothyroidism.

Diagnostic Procedures. *Humoral immunity studies.* With search of specific antibodies to endocrine glands. Histocompatibility profile. Other for differential diagnosis. enumeration of T- and B-lymphocytes; lymphocyte stimulation and suppressor T-cell activity. *Blood. Urine.* Search for biochemical changes owing to various endocrine gland deficiencies and tests of hormone deficiency corrections.

Therapy. Symptomatic correction of specific hormone deficiencies or of various condition clusters.

Prognosis. Variable according to degree of involvement and treatment. Usually only temporary benefit from various therapeutic interventions.

BIBLIOGRAPHY. Schmidt MB: Eine biglanduläre Erkrankung (Nebennieren und Schilddrüsse) bei Morbus Addisonii. Verh Dtsch Pathol Ges 21:212–221, 1926
Carpenter CC, Solomon N, Silverberg SG, et al: Schmidt's syndrome (thyroid and adrenal insufficiency): A review of the literature and a report of fifteen new cases including ten instances of co-existent diabetes mellitus. Medicine 43:153–180, 1964
Meyerson J, Lechuga-Gomez EE, Bigazzi PE, et al: Polyglandular autoimmune syndrome: Current concepts. Canad Med Assoc J 138:605–612, 1988
Muir A, Schatz DA, MacLaren NK: Polyglandular failure syndromes. In De Groot LJ (ed): Endocrinology, 3rd ed, p 3019. Philadelphia, WB Saunders, 1995

SCHMITT-WIESER

Synonym. Clay shoveler.

Symptoms and Signs. Occurs following overstraining in shoveling or performing similar activity. Lesion of spinous process of first thoracic vertebra and displacement of apophysis.

Prognosis. Spontaneous repair within a few months.

BIBLIOGRAPHY. Schmitt HG, Wieser P: Die Schipperkrankenkheit bei Jugendlichen. Arch Klin Chir (Berl) 268:333–340, 1961

SCHNECKENBECKEN* DYSPLASIA

Synonym. Cochlea—pelvis dysplasia; snail—pelvis dysplasia.

Symptoms and Signs. Very rare. Born from consanguineous parents. Polyhydramnios; lethal edema. *Head.* Large. *Face.* Flat. *Palate.* Cleft. *Neck.* Short.

Etiology. Autosomal recessive inheritance.

Pathology. *Bones.* Increased cellular density, typical resting cartilage, normal chondrocytes with central nucleus, hypervascularization.

Diagnostic Procedures. *X-rays.* Diagnostic snail-shaped ilia. Dumbbell short long bones: wide fibula; round vertebra; short splayed ribs and clavicles; scapulae hypoplastic; brachydactyly. *Ultrasound imaging.* Intrauterine diagnosis.

Prognosis. Lethal in the newborn period.

BIBLIOGRAPHY. Borochowitz Z, Jones KL, Silbey R, et al: A distinct lethal neonatal chondrodyplasia with snail-like pelvis "Schneckenbecken" dysplasia. Am J Med Genet 25:47–59, 1986
Knowles S, Winter R, Rimoin D: A new category of lethal short-limbed dwarfism. Am J Med Genet 25:41–46, 1986
Camera G, Scarano G, Tronci A, et al: "Snail-like pelvis" chondrodysplasia: A further case report. Am J Med Genet 40:513–514, 1991
Rimoin DL, Lachman RS: Genetic disorders of the osseous skeleton. In Beithon P (ed): McKusick's Heritable Disorders of Connective Tissue, 5th ed, pp 582–583. St Louis, CV Mosby, 1993

SCHNEIDER

Synonym. Central cervical spinal cord injury; central cord.

Symptoms. Weakness prevalent in upper extremities up to paresis and paralysis; sensory loss of variable degree; radicular pain.

Signs. Paralysis of fingers and arms, and paresis of upper part of legs; feet spared.

Etiology. Arthritis; trauma causing compression of cervical cord between osteophytes and ligamentum flavum; associated with vascular insufficiency because of compression of vertebral artery on hyperextension of cervical spine.

---

*Name given to indicate the iliac wing configuration.

Diagnostic Procedures. *X-ray.* Of spine. Fractures or osteoarthritic changes. *CSF.* Abnormal proteins.

Therapy. Orthopedic measures for spine stabilization. Corticosteroids to reduce edema.

Prognosis. Variable.

BIBLIOGRAPHY. Schneider HC: Trauma to the spine and spinal cord. In Kahn EA, Basset RC, Scheined RC, et al: Correlative Neurosurgery. Springfield, IL, Charles C Thomas, 1955
Merriam WF, Taylor TR, Ruff SJ, et al: A reappraisal of acute traumatic central cord syndrome. J Bone Joint Surg (Br) 68:708–713, 1986
Adams RD, Victor M: Principles of Neurology, 5th ed, p 1080. New York, McGraw-Hill, 1993

SCHNITZLER

Synonyms. Macroglobulinemia—urticaria; urticaria—macroglobulinemia.

Symptoms and Signs. Urticaria on trunk and limbs, sparing face palms and soles atypical, persistent (years) not always itchty; each lesion lasts from a few hours to a few days; eruptions accompanied by fever, pain on legs (with hyperostosis); hepato-, spleno-, and adeno-megaly may occur. General status good.

Etiology. Unknown. An IgM monoclonal gammopathy (with deposit in the skin) considered as a possible cause.

Pathology. Biopsy of lesion: perivascular infiltration in superficial dermis with lymphocytes, histiocytes, eosinophils and numerous polymorphonuceares with leucocytoclasis. Vessel wall swelled, with mild fibrinoid necrosis. Direct immunofluorescence negative.

Diagnostic Procedures. *Biopsy.* See Pathology. *Blood.* High sedimentation rate; hyperfibrinogenemia; hyperleukocytosis; throbocytosis; elevated globulins; immunoelectrophoresis. *Serum.* Monoclonal IgM-k, IgA, and IgG normal. Serum complement and c1 inhibitor normal.

Therapy. Antihistamines, dapsone, colchicine no effect. Nonsteroidal anti-inflammatory agents effective for control of bone pain. High dosage corticosteroids: transitory effect on urticaria.

Prognosis. Benign for a long term follow-up in one case development (after 20 years from onset) of lymphoplasmacytic lymphoma. Other cases died because of opportunistic infections.

BIBLIOGRAPHY. Schnitzler L, Schubert B, Boasson M, et al: Urticaire chronique, lésions osseuses, macroglobulinémie IgM: Maladie de Waldenstroem? 2e présentation. Bull Soc Fr Dermatol Syph 81:363, 1974
Janier M, Bonvalet D, Blanc MF, et al: Chronic urticaria and macroglobulinemia (Schnitzler's syndrome): Report of two cases. J Am Acad Dermatol 20:206–211, 1989

SCHNYDER

Synonyms. Crystalline corneal dystrophy; corneal–crystalline dystrophy.

Symptoms. Both sexes affected. Onset early in life. Moderate decrease of visual acuity.

Signs. Arcus juvenilis appearing early in life as oval or annular cloudy opacification of central part of cornea with clear periphery. Progressive extension of opacity toward periphery, but never reaching the limbus.

Etiology. Unknown. Autosomal dominant inheritance.

Pathology. Normal epithelium; small needle-like crystal of cholesterol in the area located in anterior portion of stroma posterior to Bowman membrane.

Diagnostic Procedures. *Slit-lamp examination. Biopsy.* Of cornea.

Blood. Hyperlipemia (particularly hypercholesterolemia and type III dysbetalipoproteinemia).

Therapy. Full thickness keratoplasty.

Prognosis. After keratoplasty graft remains clear for at least 15 months. Hyperlipemia accentuates the relapses.

BIBLIOGRAPHY. Van Went JM, Wibaut F: Hereditary anomaly in cornea. Ned Tijdschr Geneeskd 1:2996–2997, 1924
Schnyder W: Mitteilung ueber einen neuen Typus von familiaerer Hornhauterkrankung. Schweiz Med Wochenschr 10:559, 1929
Schnyder W: Scheibenförmige Kristalleinlagerungen in der Hornhautmitte las Erbleiden (degeneratio cristallinea corneal hereditaria). Klin Monatsbl Augenheilkd 103:494–502, 1939
Bron AJ, Williams HP, Carruthers ME: Hereditary crystalline stromal dystrophy of Schnyder. I. Clinical features of family with hyperlypoproteinemia. Br J Ophthalmol 56:383–399, 1972
Winder AF: Disorders of lipid and lipoprotein metabolism. In Garner A, Klintworth GK (eds): Pathobiology of Ocular Disease: A Dynamic Approach, 2nd ed, p 1112. New York, Marcel Dekker, 1994

SCHOEPF

Synonym. Hypotrichosis—oligodontia—palmoplantar keratosis. Could be included into the Papillon-Lefevre syndrome (see).

Symptoms and Signs. Hypospadias; oligodontia. At puberty, palmoplantar hyperkeratosis. At 25 years of age, hair loss; at 50 years of age, rosacea; at 60, cysts of both eyelids. Occasionally, photophobia, basal cell carcinoma, eccrine poroma.

Etiology. Debated autosomal recessive inheritance.

BIBLIOGRAPHY. Schoepf E, Schulz HJ, Passage E: Syndrome of cystic eyelids, palmoplantar keratosis; hypospadias and hypotrichosis as a possible autosomal recessive trait. Birth Defects 7:219–221, 1971
Nordin H: Familiar occurrence of eccrine tumors in a family with ectodermal dysplasia. Acta Derm Venereolog (Stockh) 68:523–530, 1988
Gorlin RJ, Cohen MM Jr, Levin LS: Syndromes of Head and Neck, pp 870–871. New York, Oxford, 1990

SCHÖNENBERG

Synonym. Cardiopathy—dwarfism.

Symptoms and Signs. Present from birth. Symptoms and signs of various types of congenital cardiac defects. Blepharophimosis; epicanthal folds; pseudoptosis of eyelids. Proportionate dwarfism.

Etiology. Unknown. Consanguinity of parents and familial occurrence reported.

BIBLIOGRAPHY. Schönenberg H: Über ein neues Kombinationsbild multipler Abartungen (Minderwuchs, Vitium cordis, beiderseitige congenitale Ptose). Ann Pediatr 182:229–240, 1954
François J: L'heredité en ophthalmologie. Bull Soc Belge Ophthal 94–300, 1958
Buffoni L, Chiossi FM: Presentatione di un caso di' una rara sindrome malformativa—la sindrome di Schönenberg. Minerva Pediatr 23:1549–1554, 1971

SCHÖNLEIN

This eponym is sometimes used in place of the term Schönlein-Henoch syndrome (see) when the rheumatoid pain and cutaneous lesions are predominant.

SCHÖNLEIN-HENOCH

Synonyms. Henoch-Schönlein; anaphylactoid purpura; hemorrhagic capillary toxicosis; peliosis rheumatica.

Symptoms and Signs. Most often seen in childhood and young adulthood, seldom later in life; prevalent in males. Onset variable: headache; anorexia; fever (moderate and irregular); abdominal pains or pain on the joint (cutaneous manifestation) may each be first complaint. Abdominal pain (35–60% of patients) have colicky character and come frequently at night; occasionally, vomiting, diarrhea, and melena or severe constipation accompany the colic. No abdominal rigidity. Rheumatoid pains affecting all joints, most frequently legs; periarticular effusion frequent. Cutaneous mainfestations may present different types of lesions: purpura; urticaria wheals; angioneurotic edema; diffuse erythema; necrotic ulcer, most frequently affecting legs, seldom oral mucosa. Nervous system and special sense organs may be affected: paresis; convulsions; optic atrophy; ophthalmitis. Hematuria, progressive renal failure.

Etiology. Allergic reaction to bacteria, food, drugs. A case is reported in which the syndrome, in a 9-year-old girl, was associated with selective IgA deficiency.

Pathology. *In skin.* Perivascular inflammation, necrotizing arteriolitis (in severe cases), plasma and cells pericapillary extravasation. Gastrointestinal mucosae may show some of the lesions described. *Kidney biopsy.* Light microscopy mesangial proliferative glomerulonephritis. *Electron microscopy.* Electron dense deposits. Immunofluorescence: granular deposits of IgA, IgG and IgM. *Skin biopsy immunofluorescence.* Deposits of IgA C3 and C5.

Diagnostic Procedures. *Blood.* Normal platelet number or only very moderate decrease. *X-rays.* Of gastrointestinal tract. May initially reveal "spiking" of bowel outline and later "thumb-print" or rigid effacement of mucosa; these changes disappear with recovery.

Therapy. Symptomatic; bed rest; removal of cause if identified. Corticosteroids and adrenocorticotrophic hormone (ACTH) less effective than expected.

Prognosis. Generally good. Edema of glottis the main life-threatening feature. Intestinal intussusception not a rare complication.

BIBLIOGRAPHY. Schönlein JL: Allgemeine und specielle Pathologie und Therapie. Nach dessen Vorlesungen niedergeschrieben und hrsg. von einigen seiner Zuhörer. 3 aufl, Herisou, Lit-Comp 1837
Henoch E: Über eine eigenthumliche Form von Purpura. Klin Wochenschr 11:641–643, 1874
Martini A, Ravelli A, Notarangelo RD, et al: Henoch-Schönlein syndrome and selective IgA deficiency. Arch Dis Child 60:160, 1985
Bithell TC: Bleeding disorders caused by vascular abnormalities. In Lee GR, Bithell TC, Foerster J, et al (eds): Wintrobe's Clinical Hematology, 9th ed, pp 1377–1379. Philadelphia, Lea & Febiger, 1993

SCHPRINTZEN-GOLDBERG

Synonyms. Golberg-Schprintzen; Montefiore; marfanoid—craniostenosis.

Symptoms and Signs. From birth. Obstructive apnea. Craniosynostosis, ocular hypertelorism, and proptosis; strabismus, downslanting of palpebral lids; maxillar hypoplasia; micrognathia; low-set ears. Normal intelligence. Arachnodactyly, campodactyly; talipes equinovarus; umbilical and inguinal hernias.

Etiology. Unknown. Sporadic.

Diagnostic Procedures. Normal chromosomal pattern.

BIBLIOGRAPHY. Schprintzen RJ, Goldberg RB: A recurrent pattern syndrome of craniosynostosis associated with arachnodactyly and abdominal hernias. J Craniofac Genet Dev Biol 2:65–74, 1982

Cohen MM Jr: Craniosynostosis: Diagnosis, Evaluation and Management. New York, Raven Press, 1986

SCHROEDER I (H.A.)

Synonym. Acute "Lowsalt." See Hyponatremic syndromes.

Symptoms and Signs. Occurs in patients treated intensively for congestive heart failure. Rapid physical and mental deterioration. Further unresponsiveness to diuretics; thirst; anorexia; nausea; prostration; calf cramps; tendency to syncope in the erect position; narrowing of pulse pressure (rise of diastolic level); oliguria and finally renal failure.

Etiology. Acute dehydration as hyponatremia or as hypochloremia developing after iatrogenic profuse diuresis. (Not to be confused with hyponatremia, chronic dilution [see] and reminded that hyponatremia is common "per se" in severe congestive failure and its development is correlated with increased activity of the renin-angiotensin system.)

Diagnostic Procedures. *Blood.* Predominant decrease of chloride or depression of sodium as well as chloride; BUN increased.

Therapy. In the acute form with dehydration, oral administration of water and salt. Parenteral administration only in emergency or with inability to take fluid by mouth.

Prognosis. Guarded.

BIBLIOGRAPHY. Schroeder HA: Renal failure associated with low extracellular sodium chloride: The low salt syndrome. JAMA 141:117–124, 1949
Vogl A: The low-salt syndromes in congestive heart failure. Am J Cardiol 3:192–198, 1959
Ehrlich EN, Friedman AL, Shenken Y: Hormonal regulation of electrolyte and water metabolism. In De Groot LJ (ed): Endocrinology, 3rd ed, p 1704. Philadelphia, WB Saunders, 1995

SCHROEDER II (H.A.)

Synonyms. Endocrine hypertensive. Including maternal obesity syndrome.

Symptoms. Prevalent in females; seldom in males; relatively sudden onset of obesity, occurring at menarche, menopause, after multiple pregnancies or gynecologic operations. Headache; menstrual irregularity; aversion to salty food and high fluid intake. Tendency to easy bruising and ecchymosis.

Signs. Obesity of central type with pale striae on thighs; mild hirsutism. *Blood.* Hypertension occurring after the weight gain; fundus oculi changes. In no instance should the preceding signs and symptoms be confused with those of Cushing syndrome.

Etiology. The pathogenesis and etiology of this syndrome are obscure. A hereditary factor may predispose to this variety of hypertension. See Cohen syndrome.

Pathology. Left ventricular hypertrophy; slight to moderate arteriolar nephrosclerosis; polyps or myomas of uterus; adenomas or focal hyperplasia of the adrenal cortex.

Diagnostic Procedures. *Blood.* Mild polycythemia; abnormal carbohydrate metabolism; several abnormally low concentrations of sodium and chlorides. Differential diagnosis: (1) The maternal obesity syndrome, characterized by the rapid gain in weight observed in women during pregnancy or after childbirth. (2) Large baby diabetic syndrome. (3) Cushing syndrome.

Therapy. The hypertension responds favorably to severe restriction of dietary salt, and lesions in the ocular fundi may regress.

Prognosis. Good.

BIBLIOGRAPHY. Schroeder HA, Davies DF, Clark HE: A syndrome of

hypertension, obesity. Menstrual irregularities and evidence of adrenal cortical hyperfunction. J Lab Clin Med 34:1746, 1949
Schroeder HA, Davies DF: Studies on "essential" hypertension. V. An endocrine hypertensive syndrome. Ann Intern Med 40:516–539, 1954
Bray GA: The syndromes of obesity: An endocrine approach. In De Groot LJ (ed): Endocrinology, 3rd ed, pp 2625–2662. Philadelphia, WB Saunders, 1995

SCHROEDER (C.H.)

Synonyms. Luxation congenital hereditary; humeroradial synostosis. See Larsen and Pfeiffer.

Symptoms and Signs. Bizarre pinnas; bilateral radial luxation; radiohumeral ankylosis; bilateral hip, shoulder, and knee dislocation: camptodactyly.

Etiology. Unknown. Either dominant or recessive autosomal inheritance.

BIBLIOGRAPHY. Schroeder CH: Familiaere kongenitale Luxationem. Z Orthop Chir 57:500–596, 1932
Kentel J, Kindermann J, Mockel H: Eine wahrscheinlich autosomal recessiv vererbte Skeletmissbildung mit Humeroradialsynostose. Humangenetik 9:43–53, 1970
Hunter AGW, Cox DW, Rudd NL: The genetics of an associated clinical findings in humero-radial synostosis. Clin Genet 9:470–478, 1976

SCHROETTER

Synonyms. Von Schroetter; diaphragmatic chorea; laryngeal chorea.

Symptoms. Nonpainful tics that cause utterance of a peculiar cry.

BIBLIOGRAPHY. von Schroetter L: Uber "Chorea laryngis." Allg Wien Med Ztg 24:67–68, 1879

SCHULTZ (W.)

Synonyms. Agranulocytosis acute; agranulocytic angina; granulocytopenia acute; pernicious leukopenia; neutropenia, malignant.

Symptoms. More frequent in adults and in females (3:1); onset in middle age. Acute onset. Prostration; chills; fever. Ulceration of mucous membranes, principally of mouth and throat.

Etiology. Hematopoietic disorders: aleukemic leukemia; therapeutical and chemical agents as hematopoietic depressants; ionizing radiation; idiopathic.

Pathology. Gangrenous ulceration of mucosae.

Diagnostic Procedures. *Blood.* Extreme leukopenia (1000); almost complete absence of neutrophil leukocytes. The few present show toxic granulation and nuclear and cytoplasmatic changes. Usually no anemia and thrombocytopenia. *Bone marrow.* May be hypoplastic, normal, or hyperplastic. When hypoplastic, only immature myeloid elements present.

Therapy. Find, if possible, the offending agent and avoid exposure of the patients to it; smears and cultures to identify the organism causing infection, and then administration of the most suitable antibiotics, general care of the patient, with particular emphasis on oral hygiene; neutrophil transfusion. Adrenocorticosteroids and ACTH are not indicated.

Prognosis. Continuously improving with the constant development of potent antibiotics, and with the progress in general intensive care.

BIBLIOGRAPHY. Brown PK, Ophuls WA: A fatal case of acute primary infectious pharyngitis. Am Med 3:649–651, 1902

Tuerk W: Septische Erkrankungen bei verkuemmerung des Granulocytensystems. Wien Klin Wochenschr 20:157, 1907
Schultz W: Über eigenartige Halserkrankungen. Dtsch Med Wochenschr 48:1495–1496, 1922
Athens JW: Neutropenia. In Lee GR, Bithel TC, Foerster J, et al (eds): Wintrobe's Clinical Hematology, 9th ed, pp 1594–1600. Philadelphia, Lea & Febiger, 1993

SCHUTZ-HAYMAKER

Synonym. Olivopontocerebellar atrophy IV.

Symptoms and Signs. Both sexes. Adult onset. High variability of symptomatology: spinocerebellar ataxia to spastic paraplegia, involvement of cranial nerves (IX, X, XII).

Etiology. Autosomal dominant inheritance. Deficiency of glutamic dehydrogenase in some patients.

Pathology. High variability of data. Changes in inferior olivary nucleus and cerebellum with different degree of pontine involvement, loss of anterior motor cells of spinal cord in the spinocerebellar tracts and posterior funiculus.

BIBLIOGRAPHY. Schutz JW: Hereditary ataxia: Clinical study through six generations. Arch Neurol Psychiatr 63:535–568, 1950
Schutz JW, Haymaker W: Hereditary ataxia: Pathologic study of 5 cases of common ancestry. J Neuropathol Clin Neurol 1:183–213, 1951
Plaitakis A, Nicklas WJ, Dresnick RJ: Glutamate dehydrogenase deficiency in the patients with spinocerebellar syndrome. Ann Neurol 7:297–303, 1980
Auburger G, Orozco Diaz G, Capote RF, et al: Autosomal dominant ataxia: Evidence for locus heterogeneity from a Cuban founder: effect population. Am J Hum Genet 46:1163–1177, 1990

SCHWARTZ-BARTTER

Synonyms. Bartter-Schwartz; ADH; inappropriate antidiuretic hormone; cerebral hyponatremia; salt-wasting cerebral.

Symptoms. Headache; confusion; disorientation; hostility and other mental aberrations without motor or sensory defects.

Signs. Normal reflexes; no dehydration; no edema; no signs of renal, hepatic, or cardiac disease.

Etiology. Syndrome associated with carcinoma of lung or following head trauma, brain tumor, cerebral vascular disease, encephalitis, tuberculosis, meningitis. This syndrome is the result of electrolyte imbalance, namely hyponatremia owing to inappropriate secretion by neoplastic tissues of antidiuretic hormone (ADH) or other chemical substances that have ADH-like effect on renal collecting tubule.

Diagnostic Procedures. *Blood.* Hyponatremia, moderate or severe. Normal blood urea nitrogen (BUN). *Urine.* Hypertonic; increased sodium and chloride excretion. Poor response of hyponatremia to hypertonic saline infusion. *X-ray. CT scan. MRI.* Demonstration of malignancy, infection, trauma. *CSF. EEG.* Possibly, different types of abnormalities.

Therapy. Restriction of fluid intake. In severe hyponatremia: furosemide diuresis plus electrolyte replacement; demeclocycline to correct antidiuresis.

Prognosis. Depends on association with malignant or benign etiology. Water restriction sufficient in inducing remission of symptoms. Recurrence with increase of fluid intake.

BIBLIOGRAPHY. Leaf A, Bartter FC, Santos RF, et al: Evidence in man that urinary electrolyte loss induced by pitressin is function of water retention. J Clin Invest 32:868–878, 1953
Schwartz WB, Bennett W, Curelop S, et al: A syndrome of renal sodium

loss and hyponatremia probably resulting from inappropriate secretion of antidiuretic hormone. Am J Med 23:259–542, 1957

Lipscomb HS, Retiene WK, Matsen F, et al: The syndrome of inappropriate secretion of antidiuretic hormone. Cancer Res 28:378–383, 1968

Ehrlich EN, Friedman AL, Shenken Y: Hormonal regulation of electrolyte and water metabolism. In De Groot LJ (ed): Endocrinology, 3rd ed. Philadelphia, WB Saunders, 1995

SCHWARTZ-JAMPEL-ABERFELD

Synonyms. Aberfeld; blepharophimosis, myopathy, dwarfism osteochondromuscular dystrophy. SJA; myotonic myopathy, dwarfism, chondrodystrophy, oculofacial abnormalities; chondrodystrophic myotonia.

Symptoms. Onset within first month of life. Myotonia; contractures.

Signs. Short stature; hypoplastic facial bones; micrognathia. Eyes upward slanting; blepharophimosis; exotropia; myopia; microcornea; low-set auricles; hypertrichosis; arachnodactyly; hypoplastic larynx; abnormal epiglottis; short neck; pectus carinatum; kyphoscoliosis; abnormal acetabulum. Muscles are hypertrophic and stiff.

Etiology. Postulated membrane defect with inability to maintain proper gradient of Na and K. Autosomal recessive inheritance, possibility of heterozygote manifestation in some cases (?). Autosomal dominant inheritance suggested as well.

Pathology. Muscle biopsy shows diffuse atrophy with replacement of muscle fibers by adipose and connective tissue. Skeletal lesions similar to that of Morquio (see).

Diagnostic Procedures. *Blood. Serum enzymes. Urine. Amino acids. Chromosome studies.* Pattern normal. *X-ray.* Osteoporosis. *Electromyography.* Pattern differs from that of myotonia congenita because of relative little waxing and waning of amplitude and frequency. Electrical activity does not disappear during sleep. Abnormalities found also on relative of patients.

Therapy. Type I antiarrhytmic agents: phenytoine, quinine, procainamide, mexiletine, and others; however, patients spontaneously, often discontinue drugs because of their severe collateral effects versus their beneficial effects.

BIBLIOGRAPHY. Pinto LM, de Spuza JS: Un caso de "doenca muscular" de difficil classificacao. Rev Port Pediatr Pueric 6:1, 1961

Schwartz O, Jampel RS: Congenital blepharophimosis associated with a unique generalized myopathy. Arch Ophthalmol 68:52–57, 1962

Aberfeld DS, Hinterbuchner LP, Schneider M: Myotonia, dwarfism, diffuse bone disease and unusual ocular and facial abnormalities (a new syndrome). Brain 88:313–322, 1965

Pascuzzi RM, Gratianne R, Azzarelli B, et al: Schwartz-Jampel syndrome with dominant inheritance Muscle Nerve 13:1152–1163, 1990

Spaans F, Theunissen P, Reekers AD, et al: Schwartz-Jampel syndrome: I. Clinical electromyographic and histologic studies. Muscle Nerve 13:516–527, 1990

SCHWARZ-LELEK

Synonym. Frontal bossing-genu varum. See Pyle.

Symptoms and Signs. Two cases reported. Onset from birth. Frontal bossing; genu varum.

Etiology. Unknown. Autosomal recessive inheritance (?).

Diagnostic Procedures. *X-ray.* Of head. Hyperostosis and sclerosis, more marked in frontal, occipital, maxillary, and mandibular areas. Paranasal sinuses obliterated. Of clavicles, ribs, humeri, hands. Hyperostosis (see Pyle). Of femur. Bowing; radiolucency of metaphyseal area. *Blood.* Alkaline phosphatases elevated.

BIBLIOGRAPHY. Schwarz E: Craniometaphyseal dysplasia. Am J Roentgenol 94:461–466, 1960

Lelek I: Camurati–Engelmannische Erkrangungen. Fortschr Roentgenst 94:702–712, 1961

Gorlin RJ, Spranger JW, Koszalka MF: Genetic craniotubular bone dysplasia and hyperostose: A critical analysis. Birth Defects V (4):79–95, 1969

Gorlin RJ, Cohen MM Jr, Levin LS: Syndromes of Head and Neck, pp 231–232. New York, Oxford, 1990

SCHWENINGER-BUZZI

Obsolete.

Synonym. Identified today with anetoderma (see), in which there are no preceding inflammatory lesions. Different from Jadassohn-Pellizari type (see), where lesions are preceded instead by erythema or urticaria.

BIBLIOGRAPHY. Schweninger E, Buzzi S: Multiple benigne geschwulstartige Bildundgen der Haut. Internat. Atlas seltener Hautkrankht. Heft V. Hamburg und Leipzig, Voss, 1891

Korting GW, Cabré J, Holzmann H: Zur Kenntnis der Kollagenveränderungen bei der Anetodermie von Typus Schweninger-Buzzi. Arch Klin Exp Dermatol 218:274–297, 1964

Burton JL: Disorders of connective tissue. In Champion RH, Burton JL, Ebling FJG (eds): Rook/Wilkinson/Ebling Textbook of Dermatology, 5th ed, p 1773. Oxford, Blackwell Scientific, 1992

SCIMITAR

Synonyms. Hypogenetic lung; turkish sabre; scimitar vein.

Symptoms. Prevalent in females. Twenty-five percent of cases are diagnosed in early infancy; they suffer from recurrent respiratory infections. Can be completely asymptomatic or paucisymptomatic. Fatigue; dyspnea; history of pneumonia; cough, chest pain; wheezing. Seldom, growth failure.

Signs. Right displacement of heart; infrequently, decreased size and motion of right chest; rales; loud cardiac murmurs over the sternum or on either side of it. Occasionally, physical examination normal.

Etiology. Congenital malformation (see Pathology). Some familial cases reported.

Pathology. Anomalous venous drainage through abnormal pulmonary vein of the right lung that joins the inferior vena cava. Right pulmonary artery frequently hypoplastic. Lung lobation or bronchial distribution frequently abnormal. Diverticula and cysts of bronchi. Small right lung; heart displacement to the right. Diaphragmatic defects and congenital heart defect may also be associated.

Diagnostic Procedures. *X-ray.* Displacement of heart to the right; abnormal venous trunk "scimitar sign" lying parallel to right heart border distally, broader and curving medially and anteriorly. *Fluoroscopy.* Absence of pulsation. Opacity of right lung. *Tomography. Bronchoscopy. Bronchography. Angiocardiography. Catheterization. Pulmonary function tests. Two dimensional echocardiography with color flow imaging and spectral Doppler interrogation.*

Therapy. Physiologically corrective operations: connection of anomalous vein to right atrium, plus creation of atrial septal defect, or direct transplantation to left atrium, or, if a branch leading to left atrium is present, simple ligation between the branch and the inferior vena cava. Pneumonectomy or lobectomy in some cases with severe pulmonary disease.

Prognosis. Condition frequently occurs without serious symptoms and with good prognosis. Association with pulmonary and cardiac malformations makes the prognosis guarded.

BIBLIOGRAPHY. Cooper G: Case of malformation of the thoracic viscera:

Consisting of imperfect development of right lung and transposition of the heart. Lond Med Gaz 18:600–602, 1836

Chassinat R: Observations d'anomalies anatomiques remarquables de l'appareil circulatoire, avec hépatocéle congéniale, symptom particulier. Arch Gen, Med 11:80–91, 1836

Oakley D, Naik D, Verel D, Rajan S: Scimitar vein syndrome: Report of nine new cases. Am Heart J 107:596–598, 1984

Schlant RC, Alexander RW: Hurst's The Heart, 8th ed, p 1777. New York, McGraw-Hill, 1994

SCLERODERMA

Synonyms. Acrosclerosis; hidebound skin; progressive systemic sclerosis; PSS.

Symptoms and Signs. Predominantly in females (4:1). Onset usually in fourth decade in females; later in males. Raynaud phenomenon (see) usually presenting symptoms; less frequently, hand swelling or joint swelling; ulceration of fingers or legs. Weight loss; dyspnea; gastroesophageal reflux; diarrhea or constipation; abdominal pain. *Skin changes.* Face and hands usually involved; lesion spreading to forearm, chest. Typical faces: smooth, shiny forehead; skin thickened; lines cancelled; nose becoming small; radial furrows around the mouth; mouth opening reduced; hardening of skin prevents depression of eyelids. Telangiectases. *Hand.* Swelling initially; bulbous appearance, then atrophy; painful ulcer; gangrene; retraction holding the hand in semiflexion. *Feet.* Similar but usually less severe changes. Calcinosis localized or generalized. *Gastrointestinal.* Esophageal reflux; dysphagia; colicky abdominal pains; malabsorption (see). *Respiratory.* Dyspnea; dry or productive cough; cyanosis; recurrent pneumothorax. *Cardiac.* Arrhythmia; cardiomegaly. *Muscular weakness. Joint.* Arthralgia; rheumatoid arthritis, typical changes.

Etiology. Unknown. Collagen disorder, autoimmunity. Rare instances of familial occurrence reported. Trigger for condition unknown virus as external trigger proposed in genetically predisposed subject.

Pathology. Sclerotic changes in skin, lungs, heart, submucosa, muscularis of gastrointestinal tract, and skeletal muscles. Vascular intimal proliferation; occlusive thrombosis; hyalinization; perivascular infiltration with lymphocytes.

Diagnostic Procedures. *Biopsy.* Of skin and muscle. *Blood.* Increased sedimentation rate (50%); and globulin level (50%); false-positive serology (5%); cold agglutinins (25%); rheumatoid factor test positive (30%); antinuclear antibodies (78%). *Urine.* Proteinuria (moderate); may develop Epstein syndrome (see). *X-ray.* Of bones and joints. Lesion equal to rheumatoid arthritis. Of gastrointestinal tract. Esophageal dilatation; abnormal peristalsis strictures; stomach seldom affected; duodenum may have ulceration; jejunum and ileum seldom involved; colon frequently involved; wide-mouthed diverticula; appearance of ulcerative colitis. Of chest. Diffuse reticular infiltration, usually in lower two-thirds; cystic changes; pleurisy; pneumonia (frequent). *ECG.* Usually abnormal. Kidney and pulmonary function tests.

Therapy. Corticosteriods (as symptomatic); low molecular weight dextran intravenously. (No consistent benefit.) Prostaglandin E1, prostacyclin, reserpine, guanethidine ketanserin, nifedipine, prazosin to decrease Raynaud phenomenon intensity and frequency. D penicillamine: to decrease skin thickness and rate of further visceral involvement. Azathioprine: useful in 30% of cases. Symptomatic treatment: minoxidil, captopril, hemodialysis. Hyperbaric O_2.

Prognosis. Variable, from death in 1–2 years, to many years after onset. Men have poorer prognosis than women. Carcinoma of lungs develops frequently in cases with pulmonary involvement; malignant hypertension, carcinoma, or perforation of gastrointestinal tract.

BIBLIOGRAPHY. Curzio C: Discussioni anatomo-pratiche di un raro e stravagante morbo cutaneo in una giovane donna felicemente curato in questo gŕande ospedale degli Incurabili. Napoli G di Simone, 1753

Gintrac E: Note sur la sclerodermie. Rev Med Chir (Paris) 2:263–267, 1847

Le Roy EC: The pathogenesis of systemic sclerosis. Clin Exper Rheumatol 7:135–137, 1989

Rowell NR, Goodfield MJD: The connective tissue diseases. In Champion RH, Burton JL, Ebling FJG (eds): Rook/Wilkinson/Ebling Textbook of Dermatology, 5th ed, pp 2233–2235. Oxford, Blackwell Scientific, 1992

SCLEROSTEOSIS

Synonyms. Hansen; cortical hyperostosis—syndactyly. See van Buchem.

Symptoms and Signs. In Afrikaaners of Dutch extraction. From early infancy progressive. Headaches; deafness (childhood), blindness (adulthood) anosmia, facial asthesia, strabismus and exophthalmos; overgrowth progressing to moderate gigantism; prominent asymmetric (occasional) mandible; syndactyly, second to third finger; nail dysplasia.

Etiology. Autosomal recessive. Possibly a modification of same gene causing van Buchem.

Diagnostic Procedures. *X-ray skeletal studies.*

Therapy. Skull decompression.

Prognosis. Progression of bone thickening leads to occlusion of multiple cranial foramina. Intracranial pressure if not relieved may be fatal.

BIBLIOGRAPHY. Mirsch IS: Generalized osteitis fibrosa. Radiology 13:44–84, 1929

Hansen HG: Sklerosteose. In Opitz J, Smith F (eds): Handbook der Kinderheilkunde, vol 6, pp 351–355. Berlin, Springer, 1967

Beighton P, Barnard A, Hamersma H, et al: The syndromic status of sclerosteosis and van Buchem disease. Clin Genet 25:175–181, 1984

Weatherall DJ, Ledingham JGG, Warrell DA: Oxford Textbook of Medicine, pp 3089–3090. Oxford, Oxford Med Pub, 1996

SCLEROTYLOSIS

Synonyms. Mennecier; scleroatrophic—keratotic dermatosis limbs.

Symptoms and Signs. Present at birth. Both sexes. Atrophic fibrinosis of skin of limbs, nail hypoplasia, tylosis palms and soles. Frequently associated cancer of skin and bowel.

Etiology. Autosomal dominant trait.

BIBLIOGRAPHY. Mennecier M: Individualisation d'une nouvelle entite: la genodermatose sclero-atrophiante et keratodermique des extremities frequentement degenerative. Etude clinique et genetique (possibilite de linkage avec le system MNSS). M.D. Thesis Univ de Lille, 1967

Fisher S: La genodermatose scleroatrophiante et keratodermique des extremites (au sujet de trois nouveaux cas familieux). Ann Dermatol Venerol 105:1079–1082, 1978

SCOE

Symptoms and Signs. Palmoplantar keratoderma. Short stature, facial dysmorphism, hypodontia.

Etiology. Autosomal dominant.

BIBLIOGRAPHY. Scoe WK: A new syndrome. Pediatr Deut 11:145–150, 1989

SCOTOMA, HOMONYMOUS HEMIANOPTIC

Symptoms. Sudden onset of difficulty in reading and fixing objects located close to the central field of the affected eye. No reduced visual acuity; homonymous scotoma that excludes the macula; maintenance of peripheral field in such a manner that unaffected part of the field lies between periphery and scotoma.

Signs. Normal ophthalmologic findings.

Etiology. Unknown. Possibly, a vascular accident, embolus, toxic condition, infection (?).

Pathology. Unknown. Possible lesion of lateral geniculate bodies or above that point.

Therapy. Symptomatic. Thrombolytic anticoagulants.

Prognosis. Good for visual acuity. The patient accommodates for the presence of the blind spot in his field of vision.

BIBLIOGRAPHY. Wilbrand H: Ueber die makulärhemianopische Lesestörung und die von Monakowsche Projektion der Makula auf die Sehsphäre. Klin Monatsbl Augenheilkd 45:1–39, 1907
Allen T, Carman H: Homonymous hemianoptic paracentral scotoma. Arch Ophthalmol 20:846–849, 1938
Adams RD, Victor M: Principles of Neurology, 5th ed, pp 219–220. New York, McGraw-Hill, 1993

SCOTT

Synonym. Craniodigital—mental retardation. See Saethre-Chotzen

Symptoms and Signs. Present from birth. Brachycephaly; pointed nose; micrognathia; long lashes; prominent and arched eyebrows; hirsutism; cutaneous syndactyly of second, third, and fourth fingers. Mental and somatic retardation.

Etiology. X-linked recessive inheritance (?).

BIBLIOGRAPHY. Scott CR, Bryant JL, Graham CB: A new craniodigital syndrome with mental retardation. J Pediatr 78:658–663, 1971
Lorenz P, Hinkel GH, Hoffmann C, et al: The craniodigital syndrome of Scott Report of a second family. Am J Med Genet 37:224–226, 1990

SEA-BLUE HISTIOCYTE

Synonyms. Sawitsky; Silverstein; bleu histiocyte.

Symptoms. Both sexes affected. Onset from infancy to old age, usually in subjects under 40. Asymptomatic or increased bleeding tendency.

Signs. Marked splenomegaly; mild purpura; occasionally, liver cirrhosis.

Etiology. Autosomal recessive inheritance (?). Dominant variant reported (Lewis type, from family name considered now a form of Niemann-Pick, see). Secondary form associated with several conditions: idiopathic thrombocytopenic purpura; thalassemia; chronic myeloid leukemia; Vaquez disease; Besnier-Boeck-Schaumann; Wolman; various lipoidoses.

Pathology. In bone marrow, diffuse infiltration by a distinct histiocyte ($20–60\mu$ in diameter), single eccentric nucleolus; cytoplasm granules staining (Giemsa or Wright) sea-blue. Granules are stainable with Sudan black B; para-aminosalicylic acid (PAS) and acid-fast staining. Spleen similarly infiltrated. Other organs occasionally infiltrated.

Diagnostic Procedures. *Bone marrow.* See Pathology. *X-rays.* Lung infiltration in 30% of patients.

Therapy. Corticosteroids tried.

Prognosis. Usually benign and uncomplicated course; possibility, however, of extension of infiltration and involvement of various organs and fatality. The younger the age of onset, the poorer the prognosis.

BIBLIOGRAPHY. Silverstein MN, Young DG, ReMine WH, et al: Splenomegaly with rare morphologically distinct histiocyte: A syndrome. Arch Intern Med 114:251–257, 1964

Lee RE: Histiocytic disease of bone marrow. Hematol Oncol Clin No Am 2:657–667, 1988
Viana MB, Giugliani R, Leite VHR, et al: Very low levels of high density lipoprotein cholesterol in four sibs of a family with non-neuropathic Niemann-Pick disease and blue sea histiocytosis. J Med Genet 27:449–504, 1990

SEABRIGHT-BANTAM SYNDROMES

Used restrictively as eponym for pseudohypothyroidism, or, more correctly to indicate a failure of a tissue to respond to a specific endocrine stimulation. In the Seabright-Bantam rooster, the tail feathers have the appearance of female plumage, and represent a failure of an organ to respond to a specific stimulation, in this case androgenic hormone. This lack of response of a target organ to hormonic stimulation is observed in many syndromes.

1. In pseudohypothyroidism, the failure of response of the biochemical changes to the administration of parathyroid hormone
2. ADH-resistant diabetes insipidus (see)
3. De Morsier II
4. Dwarfism (Seabright-Bantam type) (see)
5. Savage (see)
6. Goldberg-Maxwell (see)
7. Pseudohypohermaphroditism, male, incomplete hereditary (see)
8. Thyroidal insensitivity to TSH
9. Rosewater (see)
10. Nowakowski-Lenz (see)
11. Reifenstein (see)
12. Laron

BIBLIOGRAPHY. Albright F, Burnett, CH, Smith PH, et al: Pseudo-hypoparathyroidism. Example of "Seabright-Bantam syndrome": Report of 3 cases. Endocrinology 30:922–932, 1942

SEASONAL AFFECTIVE DISORDER

Synonyms. SAD; winter depression; summer depression.

Symptoms and Signs. Both sexes. Changes in mood that go from normal (?) rhythms in mood and behavior present in general population to the morbid (?) extreme of the spectrum of such changes. The winter SAD is characterized by oversleep, gain in weight, and depression; the summer SAD by lost sleep and weight and decreased appetite. Both groups reported decreased energy, desire of socialization, and sadness.

Etiology. The pathologization of a normal rhythmic pattern related to changes in the physical environment (known for centuries) seems to me as excessive, and created to satisfy the need of a medical diagnosis for a psychologic reaction by emotionally labile individuals. Attempts also have been made to establish possible genetic trait and establish pattern of inheritance.

Therapy. Enhanced environmental lighting (with some success in winter type).

BIBLIOGRAPHY. Castiglione A: A history of Medicine. New York, Alfred A Knopff, 1941
Madden PAF, Heath AC, Rosenthal NE, et al: Seasonal changes in mood and behavior: The role of genetic factors. Arch Gen Psychiatr 53:47–55, 1996

SEAT BELTS

Not a clinical entity. Under this heading are included all injuries resulting directly from wearing the belt during a car accident. Many types of abdominal injuries, as well as injury in the chest, heart contusion, vascular and lung injuries, caused by shoulder belts. "Chance" fractures of vertebrae have been reported.

BIBLIOGRAPHY. Chance GA: Note on type of flexion fracture of the spine. Br J Radiol 21:452, 1948

LeMire JR, Earley DE, Hawley C: Intra-abdominal injuries caused by automobile seat belts. JAMA 201:735–737, 1957

Doersch KB, Dozier WE: The seat belt syndrome, the seat belt sign, intestinal and mesenteric injuries. Am J Surg 116:831–833, 1968

Taylor GA, Eggli KD: Lap-belt injuries of the lombar spine in children: A pitfall in CT diagnosis. AJR 150:1355–1358, 1988

SECKEL

Synonyms. Virchow-Seckel; bird-headed dwarfism; nanocephaly; microcephalic primordial dwarfism.

Symptoms. Both sexes affected. Present at birth. Low birth weight; failure to grow; mental retardation; sweet disposition. Recently a case has been described in which all the features of the syndrome were present, but not the dwarfism. This could be an incomplete form of the syndrome or a variant.

Signs. Dwarfism; small head; prominent beaked nose, strabismus; sparse hair. Different congenital malformations: dislocation of hip; clubfoot; absent thumb; cloaca-like malformation of genitourinary tract and rectum.

Etiology. Unknown. Autosomal recessive inheritance.

Pathology. See Signs. Small brain with primitive convolutional pattern; ectopic and small kidney; deformed liver.

Diagnostic Procedures. *Chromosome studies. Virus studies. Cytomegalic. X-ray. CT scan. MRI. Sonography. Biochemical studies. Blood. Urinary excretions.* Reported case with pancytopenia.

Therapy. Symptomatic.

Prognosis. Good quoad vitam. Patient may survive to advanced age, but with moderate to severe mental retardation.

BIBLIOGRAPHY. Mann TP, Russel A: Study of microcephalic midget of extreme type. Proc R Soc Med 52:1024–1029, 1959

Seckel HPG: Bird-headed Dwarfs: Studies in Developmental Anthropology Including Human Proportions. Springfield, IL, Charles C Thomas, 1960

Majewski F, Goecke T: Studies of microcephalic primordial dwarfism I: Approach to a delineation of the Seckel Syndrome. Am J Med Genet 12:7–21, 1982

Thompson E, Dembry M: Seckel syndrome: An overdiagnosed syndrome. J Med Genet 22:192–201, 1985

Gorlin RJ, Cohen MM Jr, Levin LS: Syndromes of Head and Neck, pp 313–315. New York, Oxford, 1990

SECRETAN

Symptoms and Signs. Post-traumatic, marked restriction of digital flexion (except the thumb), or edema of dorsal metacarpal region and base of fingers. If trauma on the foot, posttraumatic edema of the dorsum of foot.

Etiology. Overload and dilatation of lymphatics caused by constricting band, tourniquet on wrist, base of finger, above the knee.

Pathology. Edema of dorsum of hand or foot.

Therapy. Psychiatric advice, if no response to conservative measures, closed lymphangioplasty.

Prognosis. Treatment prevents permanent deformity and achieves excellent cosmetic and functional results. Possible conversion to other neurotic manifestation.

BIBLIOGRAPHY. Secretan H: Oedeme dur et hyperplasie traumatique du metacarpe dorsal. Rev Med Suisse Rom 21:409–416, 1901

Grobmyer AJ III, Bruner JM, Dragstedt LR II: Closed lymphangioplasty in Secretan's disease. Arch Surg 97:81–83, 1968

Ryan TJ, Burnand K: Diseases of the veins and arteries leg ulcers. In Champion RH, Burton JL, Ebling FJG (eds): Rook/Wilkinson/Ebling Textbook of Dermatology, 5th ed, pp 1982–1984. Oxford, Blackwell Scientific, 1992

SEDLACKOVA

Synonyms. Shprintzen; velo-cardio-facial; VCF; VCF. See Di George (significant overlap demonstrated).

Symptoms. From birth. Both sexes. Hypotonia in infancy. Conductive hearing caused by chronic otitis media loss (75%), learning disability (100%) intellectual impairment.

Signs. Shorter stature (30%); microsomy (30–40% of patients); microcephaly (40%); long facies; retracted mandible; cleft of secondary palate and velopharyngeal insufficiency; prominent nose; narrow palpebral fissures; abundant hair (50%); minor auricular deformities; slender and hypotonic limbs; ventricular septal defect (70%); right aortic arch (45%); tetralogy of Fallot (see) (15%); aberrant left subclavian artery (15%); adenoids (85%); tonsils (50%); slender hands and digits (63%).

Etiology. Generally sporadic. Reported also, autosomal dominant (X-linked dominance not excluded). Deletion within long arm of chromosome 22(22q11) (in 10–15% of patients).

Diagnostic Procedures. *Blood.* Hypocalcemia (100% of cases). *X-ray. CT scan.* Absent thymus (10%), platibasia (75%), scoliosis.

Therapy. Correction of cleft and cardiosurgery.

Prognosis. Reduced learning ability and intellectual skills. Depends on cardiac anomalies.

BIBLIOGRAPHY. Sedlackova E: The syndrome of the congenital shortened velum: The dual innervation of the soft palate. Folia Phonat 19:441–443 1967

Shprintzen RJ, Goldberg RB, Lewin ML, et al: A new syndrome involving cleft palate, cardiac anomalies, typical facies, and learning disabilities: Velo-cardio-facial syndrome. Cleft Palate J 15:56–59, 1978

Lipson AH, Yuille D, Angel M, et al: Velocardiofacial (Shprintzen) syndrome: An important syndrome for the dysmorphologist to recognize. J Med Genet 28:596–604, 1991

Motzkin B, Marion R, Goldberg R, et al: Variable phenotypes in velo-cardiofacial syndrome with chromosomal deletion. J Pediatr 123:406–410, 1993

S.E.D. TARDA-LIKE GROUP

Synonyms. Spondyloepiphyseal dysplasis late onset; late onset spondylodysplasias. See Jacobsen.

Symptoms and Signs. Includes a group of conditions clinically similar to Jacobsen, but different in etiology (autosomal recessive or dominant) and radiographic findings.

BIBLIOGRAPHY. Rimoin DL, Lachman RS: Genetic disorders of the osseous skeleton. In Beithon P (ed): McKusick's Heritable Disorders of Connective Tissue, 5th ed, p 615. St Louis, CV Mosby, 1993

SEELIMUELLER

Synonym. Syphilitic neuralgia. It is a sign rather than a syndrome: Pain elicited by pressure on cranial areas associated with diffused neuralgic pains.

Etiology. Syphilis.

BIBLIOGRAPHY. Seelimueller OLG: Ueber syphilitische Neuralgien. Dtsch Med Wochenschr 9:624–625, 1883

SEEMANOVA

Synonyms. See Paine syndrome.

Symptoms and Signs. Similar to those of Paine (see) except for: absence of abdominal reflexes; normality of level of amino acid in cerebrospinal fluid, absence of hypoplasia of cerebellum, pons, and inferior olive.

Etiology. X-linked inheritance. Debated if same condition as that described by Paine.

BIBLIOGRAPHY. Seemanova E, Lesny I, Hyanek J, et al: X-chromosomal recessive microcephaly with epilepsy spastic tetraplegia and absent abdominal reflex. New variety of "Paine syndrome?" Humangenetik 20:113–117, 1973
Opitz JM, Sutherland GR: International workshop on the fragile X and X-linked mental retardation. Am J Med Genet 17:5–94, 1984

SEGAWA

Synonyms. Dystonia progressive, diurnal variation; dystonia; parkinsonism, diurnal variations.

Symptoms and Signs. Appears (insidiously) between 1 and 9 years of age. Postural and motor disturbances with marked diurnal variations. Minor in the morning and aggravated in the late evening; relieved by sleep. Initially they are affecting one limb and within 5 years from onset, progressivelly extending to all four. Rarely torsion of trunk. Absent: rigidity, resting tremors, changes of sensory, pyramidal, or cerebellar origin, and intellectual developmental disorders.

Etiology. Unknown. Autosomal dominat inheritance.

Therapy. L-dopa produces remarkable improvement.

Prognosis. Moderate progression in adulthood.

BIBLIOGRAPHY. Yamamura Y, Sobue I, Audo K, et al: Paralysis agitans of early onset with marked diurnal fluctuation of symptoms. Neurology 23:239–244, 1973
Segawa M, Hoseka A, Miyagawa F, et al: Hereditary progressive dystonia with marked diurnal fluctuation. Adv Neurol 14:215–233, 1976
Nygard TG, Duvoisin RC: Hereditary dystonia: Parkinsonism syndrome of juvenile onset. Neurology 36:1424–1428, 1986
Ellenberg JH, Koller WC, Langston JW: Etiology of Parkinson's Disease. New York, Marcel Dekker, 1995

SEIDLMAYER

Synonyms. Postinfection purpura; purpura postinfectiva.

Symptoms and Signs. Occurs especially in children after episodes of infections, which may have been mild or ignored. Appearance of a purpuric eruption characterized by coin-like elevations.

Etiology. Direct vascular damage or allergic mechanism.

BIBLIOGRAPHY. Seidlmayer H: Die fruehinfantile, postinfektiose Kokarden-Purpura. Z Kinderheilkd 61:217–255, 1939
Bithell TC: Bleeding disorders caused by vascular abnormalities. In Lee GR, Bithel TC, Foerster J, et al (eds): Wintrobe's Clinical Hematology, 9th ed, p 1379. Philadelphia, Lea & Febiger, 1993

SEITELBERGER

Synonym. Prenatal neuroaxonal dystrophy. See Pelizaeus-Merzbacher; Hallervorden-Spatz.

Symptoms and Signs. Both sexes affected. Normal at birth; normal development up to second year of life. Then difficulty in standing and walking; progressive deterioration of neurologic function; speech; incontinence during sleep; nystagmus; strabismus; blindness; seizures; tendon hyporeflexia or areflexia; or initially pathologic reflexes, flexion, and deformities.

Etiology. Unknown. Still undetermined metabolic disorder. Usually sporadic. Familial tendency suspected (autosomal recessive inheritance), but not proved. Relationship with Hallenvorden-Spatz (adult) is postulated.

Pathology. Widespread lesions in central nervous system with the appearance of eosinophilic round or oval structures (Schollen or spheroids) mostly in the gray matter; swelling of axons and dendrites; degeneration of nerve cells; accumulation of fat granules in parts of basal ganglia; cerebellar atrophy with sclerosis; degeneration of optic pathway; degeneration of tracts of spinal cord.

Diagnostic Procedures. *Urine.* Creatine increased; creatinine decreased. Possible diabetes insipidus. *Blood.* Thyroid-stimulating hormone decreased. *CT brain scan. MRI.* Acoustical and visual evoked potentials. *EEG brain mapping. Electromyography. CSF. Biopsy of muscle and skin. Ultrastructural exams.*

Prognosis. Poor. Death from complications within months or a few years of onset.

BIBLIOGRAPHY. Seitelberger F: Eine unbekannte Form von infantiler lipoidspeicher Krankheit des Geshirns. In Proc 1st Inter Cong Neuropath (Rome Sept 8–13, 1952) vol. 3, p 323. Turin, Rosenberg-Sellier, 1952
Nagashima K, Suzuki I, Ichikawa E, et al: Infantile neuroaxonal dystrophy: Perinatal onset with symptoms of diencephalic syndrome. Neurology 35:735–738, 1985
Ozmen M, Caliskan M, Goebel HH, et al: Infantile neuroxanal dystrophy: Diagnosis by skin biopsy. Brain Dev 13:256–259, 1991
Adams RD, Victor M: Principles of Neurology, 5th ed, pp 822–823. New York, McGraw-Hill, 1993

SELIGMAN

Synonyms. Alpha-heavy chain; alpha HCD.

Symptoms and Signs. Both sexes affected. Onset in childhood and adolescence. Severe malnutrition; diarrhea; failure to thrive or weight loss; asthenia; respiratory complications; bleeding. Digital clubbing. Affects individuals in poor hygienic environment.

Etiology. Unknown. Probably a true intestinal sarcoma with Sternberg-like cells. Infective disease hypothesized.

Pathology. Infiltration of lamina propria of intestine, visceral lymph nodes, respiratory tract by plasma cells, lymphocytes, reticular cells; occasionally, bone marrow also infiltrated. Peripheral lymph nodes are not involved.

Diagnostic Procedures. *Blood.* Hypocalcemia; rise in alkaline phosphatase. *Electrophoresis.* Increased alpha-2 beta fractions. Immunoelectrophoresis reaction with anti-alpha sera. Immunofluorescent study. Anemia. *Bone marrow.* Usually normal. *Biopsy.* Of small bowel. Typical infiltration. *Lymphography, barium enema.* Hypertrophic folds and pseudopolyposis of duodenal and jejunal mucosa.

Therapy. Patients without evidence of immunoblastic changes: first treatment antibiotic alone (tetracycline or ampicillin and metronidazole). If no improvement in 3 months: combination chemotherapy, nitrogen mustard, vincristine, prednisone, and procarbazide (MOPP), or cyclophosphamide, adriamicin, vincristine, and prednisone (CHOP). Continue antibiotics in any cases. Total abdominal irradiation and prednisone.

Prognosis. Encouraging results with treatments adequate to the clinical and histological evaluation.

BIBLIOGRAPHY. Seligman M, Davon F, Hurer D: Alpha chain disease: A new immunoglobulin abnormality. Science 162:1396–1397, 1968
Foerster J: Heavy chain diseases. In Lee GR, Bithell TC, Foerster J, et al (eds): Wintrobe's Clinical Hematology, 9th ed, pp 2261–2266. Philadelphia, Lea & Febiger, 1993

SELYE

Synonyms. Adaptation; GAS; stress, general adaptation. Eponym in use to indicate the sum of all reactions that follow prolonged stress (independent from its nature of physical or psychologic origin). The typical pathologic findings are represented by adrenal cortical hyperplasia, thymic and lymphatic involution, and gastrointestinal erosion or ulcers.

BIBLIOGRAPHY. Selye H: The Physiology and Pathology of Exposure to Stress: A Treatise Based on the Concepts of the General-Adaptation Syndrome and the Disease of Adaptation. Montreal, 1950
Selye H: The Stress of Life. New York, McGraw-Hill, 1956
Chrousos GP, Cizza G, Kvernansky R, et al: Stress mechanisms and clinical implications. NY Acad Sci 771. 1995

SEMINAL VULVITIS

Symptoms and Signs. Vulvar edema; itching and erythema after intercourse, occasionally followed by generalized urticaria.

Etiology. In atopic subjects with allergy to human seminal plasma or other antigens transmitted that way. A case of interest, attacks after the partner had eaten walnuts.

BIBLIOGRAPHY. Mathias CG, Frick OL, Caldwell TM, et al: Immediate hypersensitivity to seminal fluid and atopic dermatitis. Arch Dermatol 116:209–212, 1980

SENEAR-USHER

Synonyms. Ormsby; pemphigus erythematosus.

Symptoms and Signs. Bullae appearing in normal skin of trunk and limbs, which, after breaking, result in crusted lesions similar to seborrheic dermatitis. Lesion on the face; erythematous scaling and crusts; butterfly distribution on malar areas; transient mucosal involvement possible.

Etiology. Unknown. Possibly autoimmune, viral infection, but not proved. In most cases it is suggested the combination of lupus erythematosus (LE) and pemphigus; in some cases observed combination with Erb-Goldflam.

Pathology. Acantholysis; dark-staining cells (acantholytic), but smaller than cells of pemphigus vulgaris (pyknotic acantholytic cells).

Diagnostic Procedures. *Biopsy of skin. LE test. Antinuclear antibodies.*

Therapy. Corticosteroids. Immunosuppressive agents (azathioprine, cyclophosphamide, methotrexate). Gold sodium thiomalate.

Prognosis. Better than in pemphigus vulgaris. Localized lesions may continue for years before becoming generalized, bullous reactions recurrent at different times. Patient reported by Senear and Usher was alive and well at the age of 78.

BIBLIOGRAPHY. Senear F, Usher B: An unusual type of pemphigus; combining features of lupus erythematosus. Arch Dermatol Syph 13:761–781, 1926
Pye RJ: Bullous eruptions. In Champion RH, Burton JL, Ebling FJG (eds): Rook/Wilkinson/Ebling Textbook of Dermatology, 5th ed, pp 1643–1644. Oxford, Blackwell Scientific, 1992

SENILE DEMENTIA

Synonyms. Diffuse brain atrophy; senile psychosis; see Alzheimer; Pick (A.); brain-bone-fat.

Symptoms. Occurs in both sexes. Onset over 60 years of age. Insidious onset. Deficit of immediate memory, and interest focused on the past. Power of concentration decreased; change in behavior and paranoid tendency; depression. Lack of interest and disregard for personal appearance; occasionally, hallucination, delirium (see Brain syndrome, chronic). Focal symptoms may be present.

Signs. Decreased reflexes; sluggish pupil, loss of vibratory sensibility.

Etiology. Unknown. Considered genetically different from arteriosclerotic dementia. Autosomal dominant gene with low penetrance. Today considered same as Alzheimer presenile dementia (see), although in some families this diagnosis has been ruled out by cerebral biopsy.

Pathology. Shrinking of brain; thickening of meninges. Alteration of cortex; dilatation of ventricles; shrinking of basal ganglia; alteration of nerve cells.

Diagnostic Procedures. *EEG. CT scan. MRI. Arteriography. Leukocyte culture and chromosomal count.* Loss of chromosomal material. Increased loss of chromosomes, mainly X chromosomes in female patients. *CSF.* Normal.

Therapy. Symptomatic.

Prognosis. Poor. Death after chronic progression of mental and focal symptomatology.

BIBLIOGRAPHY. Larsson T, Sjögren T, Jacobson G: "Senile dementia," a clinical, sociomedical and genetic study. Acta Psychiatr Scand (Suppl 167) 39:1–259, 1963
Mesulman MM: Dementia: Its definition, differential diagnosis and subtypes. JAMA 253:2559–2561, 1985
Morris JC (ed): Handbook of Dementing Illnesses. New York, Marcel Dekker, 1993
Weatherall DJ, Ledingham JGG, Warrell DA: Oxford Textbook of Medicine, p 3973. Oxford, Oxford Med Pub, 1996

SENIOR-LOKEN

Synonyms. Letterer-Senior-Loken; nephropathy, tapetal, retinal degeneration; oculorenal retinal degeneration; tubulointerstitial nephropathy, retinal degeneration.

Symptoms. Both sexes affected. Onset in early childhood. Thirst; polyuria; mental retardation. Visual loss progressing to complete blindness.

Signs. Tapetoretinal degeneration of eyes. Arterial hypertension (late development).

Etiology. Unknown. Familial condition, possibly induced by pleotropic gene with variable expression.

Pathology. *Kidneys.* Tubulointerstitial nephropathy. *Eyes.* Tapetoretinal degeneration similar to Leber type (see).

Diagnostic Procedures. *Urine.* Minimal hematuria and albuminuria. *Blood.* Anemia, blood urea nitrogen (BUN), and creatinine increased.

Therapy. Symptomatic. Diet, dialysis.

Prognosis. Poor. Death before adulthood.

BIBLIOGRAPHY. Senior B, Friedmann AI, Brando JL: Juvenile familial nephropathy with tapetoretinal degeneration: A new oculorenal dystrophy. Am J Ophthalmol 52:625–633, 1961

Schuman JS, Lieberman KV, Friedman AH, et al: Senior-Loken syndrome (familial renal retinal dystrophy) and Coat's disease. Am J Ophthalmol 100:822–827, 1985

Weatherall DJ, Ledingham JGG, Warrell DA: Oxford Textbook of Medicine, p 3205. Oxford, Oxford Med Pub, 1996

SENSENBRENNER

Synonym. Levin I; cranioectodermal dysplasia.

Symptoms and Signs. Both sexes affected. Dolichocephaly; frontal bossing; hypertelorism; antimongoloid slant; epicanthal fold; full cheeks; elevated lower lip; slow-growing fine hair teeth small and spaced; multiple frenula. Short and thin thorax; short limbs; abnormal distal phalanges; fifth finger clinodactyly. Normal intellectual development. Occasionally sagital suture synostosis.

Etiology. Autosomal recessive inheritance (?).

Diagnostic Procedures. *X-ray.* Of long bones. Flattening epiphyses. Of hands. Bones short.

BIBLIOGRAPHY. Sensenbrenner JA, Dorst JP, Owens RP: New syndrome of skeletal, dental and hair anomalies. Birth Defects 11:372–379, 1975

Levin LS, Perrin JCS, Ose L, et al: A hereditable syndrome of craniostenosis, short thin hair, dental abnormalities and short limbs: Cranioectodermal dysplasia. J Pediatr 90:55–61, 1977

Young ID: Cranioectodermal Dysplasia (Sensenbrenner's syndrome). J Med Genet 26:393–396, 1989

Lang GD, Young ID: Cranioectodermal dysplasia in sibs. J Med Genet 28:6, 1991

SENSORY SEIZURES SYNDROMES

Synonym. Seizures sensory; epileptic sensory. See grand mal, petit mal, vestibular epilepsy.

Several types of this form of epilepsy are known:

1. Auditory
2. Vertiginous: "vestibulogenic epilepsy." Must be differentiated from vestibular epilepsy (see).
3. Visual
4. Olfactory (uncinate seizures)
5. Gustatory
6. Cutaneous

Symptoms. According to the form the patient experiences, hallucination of different senses, usually of unpleasant nature. Movement of mouth and lips occurs sometimes, followed by major seizure. Memory may be disturbed.

Etiology. Lesions of different cerebral centers or idiopathic. In uncinate seizures, lesions are usually found.

Diagnostic Procedures. *EEG. X-ray.* Of skull. *Angiography. CT scan. MRI.* Auditory, sensorial, visual evoked potential.

Therapy. See grand mal.

BIBLIOGRAPHY. Gowers WR: The Borderlands of Epilepsy. London, Churchill, 1907

Brandt T: Vertigo: Its Multisensory Syndromes, p 95. London, Springer-Verlag, 1991

SEPTO-OPTIC DYSPLASIA

Synonyms. De Morsier II; dwarfism, septo–optic dysplasia. See also Lorain-Levi and Gilford-Burnier.

Symptoms. Visual impairment. Partial to complete amblyopia. Symptoms related to partial or complete panhypopituitarism and diabetes insipidus and less commonly thyroid dysfunctions. Anosmia. Usually, normal intelligence.

Signs. Growth deficiency and other signs related to pituitary deficiencies. Cleft palate, ear deformities, syndactyly, hypertelorism, micropenis. Pendular nystagmus.

Etiology. Unknown. Usually sporadic.

Pathology. Association of optic (II) nerve and pellucid septumor corpus callosum hypoplasia.

Diagnostic Procedures. *Funduscopic evaluation.* Hypoplasia of optic disk. *Pituitary function test. Hormone studies.*

Therapy. Pituitary single hormone deficiency replacement.

Prognosis. Fair with therapy. In severe cases, poor.

BIBLIOGRAPHY. De Morsier G: Etudes sur les dysraphies crânioencéphaliques; agénésie du septum lucidum avec malformation du tractus optique. La dysplasie septo-optique. Schweiz Arch Neurol Psychiatr 77:267–292, 1956

Blethen SL, Weldon VV: Hypopituitarism and septo-optic dysplasia in first cousins. Am J Med Genet 21:123–129, 1985

Hanna CE, Mandel H, La Franchi SH: Puberty in the syndrome of septo-optic dysplasia. AJDC 143:186–189, 1989

Weatherall DJ, Ledingham JGG, Warrell DA: Oxford Textbook of Medicine, p 4113. Oxford, Oxford Med Pub, 1996

SERUM SICKNESS

Synonym. Inoculation reaction.

Symptoms. Onset 7–15 hours (or up to 2 weeks) after exposure (injection) to a foreign antigen (heterologous protein) for prophylaxis of infections (e.g., rabies, diphtheria, Clostridium, snake venom) or administration of certain drugs (e.g., penicillin; sulfa compounds). Fever; myalgia; arthralgia. Rare complication: laryngeal edema.

Signs. Arthritis; urticaria; lymphadenopathy; splenomegaly.

Etiology. Antigen excess causing the formation of soluble antigen-antibody complexes, which, diffusing into tissues and activating the complement, cause the inflammatory response.

Diagnostic Procedures. *Blood.* Increased sedimentation rate; leukocytosis; occasionally, eosinophilia. Hemoagglutinating antibodies level rises and complement level decreases. *Urine.* Hematuria; proteinuria; synovial fluid. Leukocytosis (20,000), mostly polynucleated.

Therapy. Epinephrine; antihistamines; salicylates; in severe form, corticosteroids.

Prognosis. Good. Self-limited condition; no residual.

BIBLIOGRAPHY. Patterson R, Anderson J: Allergic reactions to drugs and biologic agents. JAMA 248:2637–2645, 1982

Weatherall DJ, Ledingham JGG, Warrell DA: Oxford Textbook of Medicine, p 164. Oxford, Oxford Med Pub, 1996

SETLEIS

Synonyms. Forceps marks, unusual face; temporal forceps marks, unusual face; facial ectodermal dysplasia.

Symptoms and Signs. Present from birth. Bitemporal aplasia of skin (forceps mark-like scarring); vertical groove below lip; polystichia of upper eyelids; lower eyelid astichia and absence of meibomian glands; widow's peak; wrinkling of skin around eyes; rubbery consistency of nose and chin; flattening of thenar and hypothenar areas. In one family reported imperforate anus.

Etiology. Possibly, autosomal recessive.

Prognosis. Normal growth and development

BIBLIOGRAPHY. Setleis H, Kramer B, Valcarcel M, et al: Congenital ectodermal dysplasia of the face. Pediatrics 32:540–548, 1963
Rudolph RI, Schwartz W, Leyden JJ: Bitemporal aplasia cutis congenita. Arch Dermatol 110:615–618, 1974
Clark RD, Golabi M, Lacassie Y, et al: Expanded phenotype and ethnicity in Setleis syndrome. Am J Med Genet 34:354–357, 1989

SEVER

Synonyms. Calcaneous apophysitis; osteochondrosis os calcis.

Symptoms and Signs. Occurs in children. Pain and tenderness over posterior part of heel.

Etiology. See Epiphyseal ischemic necrosis.

BIBLIOGRAPHY. Gordon BL: Current Medical Information and Terminology, 4th ed. Chicago, American Medical Association, 1971

SEXUAL IMPOTENCE, LOW BACK INJURY

Symptoms. Occurs in male patients with back injuries. Development of impotence (complete or partial). This group of patients, when compared with potent counterpart, presents double amount of subjective physical complaints, requests for hospitalization, surgical procedures.

Etiology. Unknown. Psychological factors partially involved. History reveals that patient was an only child or youngest child in a family of many siblings, came from unstable home, or suffered parental loss or separation.

BIBLIOGRAPHY. LaBan MM, Burk RD, Johnson EW: Sexual impotence in men having low-back syndrome. Arch Phys Med 47:715–723, 1966
Weatherall DJ, Ledingham JGG, Warrell DA: Oxford Textbook of Medicine, pp 3901, 4224. Oxford, Oxford Med Pub, 1996

SEZARY-BOUVRAIN

Synonyms. Erythrodermia with Sezary cells.

Symptoms and Signs. In adult (younger than in Chronic lymphatic leukemia) sudden appearance of recurring eczematous, erythematous lesions similar to lesions observed in the Alibert-Bazin syndrome (see). Lesion may be dry and scaly, but frequently it is associated with edema localized or diffuse to the entire surrounding area. Occasionally: pigmentation (10–20%), palmoplantar keratoderma, alopecia, nail disorders, adenomegaly (66% of cases), hepatomegaly (rare), splenomegaly (exceptional).

Etiology. Unknown. The syndrome may be located between the Alibert-Bazin and the lymphoid leukemia (T-lymphocytes type). A retrovirus isolated in one case of hairy cell leukemia.

Pathology. *Skin biopsy.* Band of infiltration by macrophages, lymphocytes, and typical Sezary cells (two types have been identified—the large and the small). The first, 12–20 μ in diameter with basophilic cytoplasm, irregular, frequently multilobulated nucleus without nucleoli. The second, 8–10 μ in diameter with less irregular nucleus.

Diagnostic Procedures. *Blood.* Moderate leukocytosis 10–99% of lymphocytes are Sezary cells. *Bone marrow.* For a long time respected by neoplastic cells. Moderate presence of Sezary cells (number not related to circulating cells).

Prognosis. Subacute or chronic evolution, with good general conditions. Between 2 and 10 years from onset, death from complications (infections, heart, kidney failure, conversion into malignant lymphoma). The small type variety has a more favorable outcome.

BIBLIOGRAPHY. Sezary A, Bouvrain Y: Erythrodermie avec presence de cellules monstrueuses dans le derme et le sang circulant. Bull Soc Fr Dermatol Syphylogr 45:254–260, 1938
Guilhon JJ, Meynadier J, Clot J: Le syndrome de Sezary. Conceptions actuelles. Nouv Presse Med 7:29–34, 1979
Flaudrin G, Daniel MJ: Sezary syndrome cytochemistry and ultrastructure. In Polliack A (ed): Human Leukemia, pp 327–330. Boston, Grune & Stratton, 1984
Foerster J: Chronic lymphocytic leukemia. In Lee GR, Bithell TC, Foerster J, et al (eds): Wintrobe's Clinical Hematology, 9th ed, p 2041. Philadelphia, Lea & Febiger, 1993

SHABBIR

Synonyms. Laryngo–onycho–cutaneous.

Symptoms and Signs. In Pakistan. Hoarseness, nail dystrophy, chronic skin ulceration, present mainly on the face.

Etiology. Autosomal recessive inheritance.

BIBLIOGRAPHY. Shabbir G, Hassan M, Kazmi A: Laryngo-onicho-cutaneous syndrome: A study of 22 cases: A new syndrome. Biomedica 2:15–25, 1986

SHAKEN BABY

Synonyms. Retinal hemorrhage; subdural hemorrhage. See Battered child.

Symptoms and Signs. Usually in small children (less than 1 year, often less than 6 months). Seizures, failure to thrive, vomiting, lethargy or drowsiness, hypothermia, bradycardia, hyper or hypotension, respiratory irregularities, coma.

Etiology. Violent shaking by caretaker.

Diagnostic Procedures. *CT scan.* Subdural hemorrhage. *Fundus.* Retinal hemorrhages in different stages.

Therapy. Isolation of baby and therapy of specific complication.

Prognosis. Compromise of visual acuity. Neurological damage, coma, or death. If therapy is sufficiently prompt, good quoad vitam.

BIBLIOGRAPHY. Spaide RF, Swengel RM, Scharre DW, et al: Shaken baby syndrome. Am Fam Phys 41:1145–1152, 1990
Morris DA: Ocular trauma. In Garner A, Klintworth GK (eds): Pathobiology of Ocular Disease: A Dynamic Approach, 2nd ed, pp 406–407. New York, Marcel Dekker, 1994

SHATTOCK

Synonyms. Pseudotubercoloma silicoticum, silicotic granuloma.

Symptoms and Signs. Granuloma of skin or mucosa.

Etiology and Pathology. Foreign body reaction to silica particles.

BIBLIOGRAPHY. Shattock SG: Pseudotubercoloma of the lip. Proc Roy Soc Med 10 (sect Path) 6–17, 1916–1917

SHAVER

Synonyms. Bauxite pneumoconiosis; aluminum oxide Shaver-Ridell; non-nodular silicosis.

Symptoms. Onset gradual. Nonproductive cough; expectoration, dyspnea; anorexia; asthenia; retrosternal pain.

Signs. Cyanosis; pulmonary rales.

Etiology. Inhalation of aluminum oxide, silicone dioxide fumes produced by melting of bauxite.

Pathology. In lungs, nonnodular fibrosis; emphysematous bullous areas. Intra-alveolar fibrosis; bronchiolectasis; typical particles (double refracting).

Diagnostic Procedures. *X-ray.* Reticulation of lungs; fine spotting. Lymph node enlargement. In advanced cases cystic shadows. *Pulmonary function tests.* Decrease in diffusing capacity.

Therapy. Symptomatic

Prognosis. Progression with rapid aggravation of symptoms.

BIBLIOGRAPHY. Shaver CG, Ridell AR: Lung changes associated with manufacture of alumina abrasives. J Indust Hyg 29:145–157, 1947
Weatherall DJ, Ledingham JGG, Warrell DA: Oxford Textbook of Medicine, p 2847. Oxford, Oxford Med Pub, 1996

SHEEHAN

Synonyms. Reye-Sheehan; Simmonds-Sheehan; postpartum; panhypopituitarism; postpartum hypopituitarism. See Simmonds and Pituitary apoplexy.

Symptoms. Onset postpartum. Acute initial shock; failure of lactation; asthenia; hypoglycemic crisis; amenorrhea or menstrual irregularity.

Signs. Pallor out of proportion to anemia; loss of pubic and axillary hair; dryness of skin; atrophy of vaginal mucosa; return phase of tendon reflexes slow.

Etiology. Spasm of infundibular arteries, which are drained by hypophyseal portal vessels. If spasm persists for several hours, most of tissue in the anterior lobe necrotizes; when blood starts to flow, stasis or thrombosis occurs in the stalk and adenohypophysis.

Pathology. Pituitary thrombosis, necrosis, and scar formation; secondary atrophy of thyroid, adrenal cortex, and ovaries.

Diagnostic Procedures. *Basal metabolic rate.* Low. *Blood.* High cholesterol; low protein-bound iodide. *Urine.* Low excretion of corticosteroids, estrogen, and pituitary gonadotropins.

Therapy. Replacement therapy.

Prognosis. Remarkable improvement with replacement therapy.

BIBLIOGRAPHY. Simmonds M: Ueber Hypophysisschwund mit tödlichem Ausgang. Dtsch Med Wochenschr 40:322–323, 1914
Sheehan HL: Post-partum necrosis of the anterior pituitary. J Pathol Bacteriol 45:189–214, 1937
Lakhdar AA, McLaren EH, Davda NS, McKay EJ, Rubin PC: Pituitary failure from Sheehan's syndrome in the puerperium: Two case reports. Br J Obstet Gynaecol 94:998–999, 1987
Baird DT: Amenorrhea, anovulation, and dysfunctional uterine bleeding. In De Groot LJ (ed): Endocrinology, 3rd ed, p 2069. Philadelphia, WB Saunders, 1995

SHEFFIELD

Synonym. Chondrodystrophy punctata, mild type; brachytelephalangic chondrodysplasia punctata.

Symptoms and Signs. From birth. Male to female ratio, 2:1. Failure to thrive. Moderate growth disturbance. Abnormal facies; flattened tip and depressed bridge of nose. Moderate mental retardation; hypoplasia of distal phalanges.

Etiology. Possibly X-linked recessive phenotype (deletion of Xp?).

Diagnostic Procedures. *X-rays.* Epiphyseal stippling disappearing after 3 years of age. Phalangeal anomalies important for diagnosis at later age.

Prognosis. Good quoad vitam.

BIBLIOGRAPHY. Sheffield LJ, Danks DM, Mayne V, et al: Chodrodystrophia punctata: 23 cases of a mild and relatively common variety. J Pediatr 89:916–923, 1976
Maroteaux P: Brachytelephalangic chrondrodysplasia punctata: A possible X linked recessive form. Hum Genet 82:167–170, 1989
Royce PM, Steinmann B (eds): Connective Tissue and Its Heritable Disorders: Molecular, Genetic and Medical Aspects. New York, Wiley-Liss, 1993

SHELL NAIL

Signs. Atrophy of nail bed; atrophic bony changes. Mirror image of clubbing, where there is proliferation of soft tissue and periostitis, with new bone formation and bulging of nail.

Etiology. Unknown. This type of lesion has been found associated with bronchiectasis.

BIBLIOGRAPHY. Cornelius CE III, Shelley WB: Shell nail syndrome associated with bronchiectasis. Arch Dermatol 96:694–695, 1967
Barak R, Dawber RPR (eds): Diseases of the Nail and Their Management. Oxford, Blackwell Scientific Publications, 1994

SHENKUI

Synonyms. Schen-k'uei.

Symptoms and Signs. In Chinese. Anxiety, or panic (fear for life threatening) and somatic complains (without evidentiable physical causes): dizziness, backache, fatigability, insomnia, sexual dysfunctions (impotence, premature ejaculation).

Etiology. Locally attributed to excessive semen loss (loss of vital essence) from frequent intercourse, masturbation, night emissions, or passage of white torbit urine (alleged semen loss).

BIBLIOGRAPHY. Lin K-M: Cultural influences on the diagnosis of psychotic and organic disorders. In Mezzich JE, Kleinman A, Fabrega H, et al: Culture and Psychiatric Diagnosis. Washington, American Psychiatry Press, 1995

SHEPHERD

Synonym. Astragaloid (talar) fracture. Eponym used to indicate a fracture of the astragalus with separation of the external margin.

BIBLIOGRAPHY. Shepherd FJ: A hitherto undescribed fracture of the astragalus. J Anat Physiol (Lond) 17:79–81, 1882

SHIN SPLINT

Synonyms. Charley horse; quadriceps femoris contusion.

Symptoms. Occurs in athletes (with absence of direct injuries). Pain and discomfort in the leg gradually increasing from repetitive running on a hard surface or forcible, excessive use of foot flexors. Usual sites of pain in lower half of postmedial border of tibia, tibial compartment, interosseous membranes. At first, pain is relieved by rest, then becomes continuous and incapacitating to the point of forcing discontinuation of sport.

Signs. Tenderness over area involved; moderate swelling. Anterior tibial pulse good.

Etiology and Pathology. Sterile mechanical inflammation of muscle-tendon determined by overexertion of leg muscles. Minimal tears of periosteum, interosseous membrane, muscle, or muscle-tendon junction. To be differentiated from fractures and ischemic disorders, fascial hernias.

Diagnostic Procedures. *X-ray. Electromyography.* Normal.

Therapy. Rest. Athletes try to prevent it by ingesting NaCl. Quinine sulfate (300 mg tid) or diphenhydramine hydrochloride (50 mg) may prevent it in subjects prone to cramps.

Prognosis. Ten to twenty-four days' duration.

BIBLIOGRAPHY. Rachun A, Allman FL, Blazina ME, et al: Standard Nomenclature of Athletic Injuries. Chicago, American Medical Association, 1966
Slocum DB: The shin splint syndrome: Medical aspects and differential diagnosis. Am J Surg 114:875–881, 1967
Klippel JH, Dieppe PA: Rheumatology, p 5.21.9. St Louis, CV Mosby, 1994

SHONE

Synonyms. Parachute mitral valve. Heart congenital malformation complex including the following:

1. Parachute mitral valve (chorda tendineae of both leaflets inserted into single left ventricular papillary muscle obstructing valve flow)
2. Supravalvular stenosing ring
3. Subvalvular aortic stenosis
4. Coarctation of aorta. In individual patients, each of the malformations mentioned may be missing from the complex.

Symptoms and Signs. Those of mitral valve stenosis (see) or regurgitation if chordae are elongated and not fused. Not all four obstructive lesions are necessarily significant or even present, and other anomalies may coexist.

BIBLIOGRAPHY. Shone JD, Sellers RD, Anderson RC, et al: The development complex of "parachute mitral valve" supraventricular ring of left atrium, subaortic stenosis and coarctation of aorta. Am J Cardiol 11:714–725, 1963
Perloff JK: The Clinical Recognition of Congenital Heart Disease, 4th ed, p 173. Philadelphia, WB Saunders, 1994

SHORT

Synonyms. Laslett-Short; tachycardia-bradycardia.

Symptoms. Affects females in higher (but not significant) percentage. Onset usually after sixth decade (average 68 years). Syncope (55%); palpitations (12%); vertigo (6%); ingravescent angina (12%); other symptoms caused by ingravescent congestive cardiac insufficiency (15%).

Signs. Not diagnostic. Out of crisis, heart frequency at 60 beats; asystole after tachycardia episodes; also, episodes of isolated bradycardia and tachycardia.

Etiology. Sick sinus node abnormally susceptible to suppressive influence of ectopic atrial activity. Coronaropathy; hypertension; cardiopathies (e.g., rheumatic, congenital, idiopathic).

Diagnostic Procedures. *ECG.* Prolonged registration to document episodes (usually 6–12 hours adequate). Reported to be of diagnostic value, but discussed: massage of carotid sinus or injection of atropine

during ECG registration to evidentiate sinus malfunction; atrial stimulation with evaluation of recovery time.

Therapy. Responds poorly to pharmacologic treatments: digitalis plus propanolol; quinidine plus propanolol; diuretics; antihypertensive agents. Permanent artificial pacemaker usually required.

Prognosis. Chronic, progressive; uncomfortable condition. Good results with pacemaker.

BIBLIOGRAPHY. Laslett EE: Syncopal attacks associated with prolonged arrest of whole heart. Q J Med 2:347, 1909
Short DS: The syndrome of alternating bradycardia and tachycardia. Br Heart J 16:208–214, 1954
Stein B, Roberts R: Syncope, presyncope, palpitations, and sudden death. In Schlant RC, Alexander RW: Hurst's The Heart, 8th ed, pp 475–479. New York, McGraw-Hill, 1994

S-H-O-R-T

Synonyms. S (short stature), H (hypersensibility of joints), H (hernia) O (ocular depression), R (Rieger anomaly), T (teething delay); lipodystrophy, unusual facies, short stature, Rieger anomaly.

Symptoms. Both sexes. Prevalent in males. Poor weight gain and frequent illness; normal intelligence; speech and dental eruption delayed.

Signs. Lipoatrophy of face and limbs (buttocks); eyes deep set and Rieger anomaly (see); alae nasi outstanding hypoplastic; nasal bridge wide; stature reduced; joints hyperextendable; inguinal hernia. Occasionally: hypospadias; hypotrichosis.

Etiology. Autosomal recessive inheritance. Cases with possible dominance reported.

Diagnostic Procedures. *Blood.* Diabetes (becomes manifest at later age).

Prognosis. Patient remains short and lipoatrophic. Normal survival.

BIBLIOGRAPHY. Gorlin RJ: Rieger anomaly and growth retardation (the S-H-O-R-T syndrome). Birth Defects 11:46–48, 1975
Sensenbrenner JA, Hisserles JE, Levin LS: A low birthweight syndrome; Rieger's syndrome. Birth Defects 11:423–426, 1975
Lipson A, Cowell C, Gorlin RJ: The SHORT syndrome: Further delineation and natural history. J Med Genet 26:473–475, 1989

SHORT BOWEL

Synonym. Small intestinal insufficiency.

Symptoms and Signs. Occurs in patients in whom a long portion of the intestine has been removed. A spectrum of deficiency patterns. Overall result of malabsorption consisting of weight loss, muscle wasting weakness, lassitude, diarrhea, pallor.

Etiology. Lack of adequate absorbing surface causes selective deficiencies resulting from removal of specialized areas of the intestine. This syndrome appears and persists when more than half of small bowel is removed. Removal of two thirds usually is compatible with life, but severe deficiencies occur and survival is not certain. Permanence of 3–4 feet is the minimal length for reasonable health.

Diagnostic Procedures. *Blood.* Anemia; glucose tolerance test; low protein; low cholesterol; electrolytes studies. *Stool.* Steatorrhea and undigested product.

Therapy. *Supportive.* Diet high in calories and supplying all essential elements; low in residue. Integrated with or substituted by parenteral administration. Anemia treated with vitamin B_{12}, folic acid, and iron according to type. Drugs to prolong transit time (codeine paregoric). *Surgical.* Reversal of a segment of small intestine to slow transit; vagotomy.

Prognosis. When this syndrome is present after surgery, it has to be kept in mind that spontaneous recovery usually occurs because of improvement of absorption and eventual increase of transit time through remaining tract. As pointed out before, pathologic manifestations are directly related to extent of intestine removed, from minor transient symptoms to a severe progressive pathology and death.

BIBLIOGRAPHY. Colcock BP, Braasch JW: Surgery of Small Intestine in the Adult. Philadelphia, WB Saunders, 1968

Weser E, Urban E: Short bowel syndrome. In Haubrich WS, Schaffner F, Berk JE (eds): Bockus Gastroenterology, 5th ed, vol 2, pp 1063–1071. Philadelphia, WB Saunders, 1995

SHOULDER MUSCULOTENDINOUS CUFF

Symptoms. History of trauma to the shoulder; sensation of "snap"; sudden pain, frequently followed by a pain-free period and then recurrence. Disability; inability to raise arm or initiate abduction. Chronic symptoms; soreness of shoulder; impaired mobility; night discomfort.

Signs. Local discoloration; tenderness over shoulder; crepitation.

Etiology. Trauma of periarticular soft tissue of the shoulder; "aging" tissues.

Pathology. Rupture of supraspinatus and other shoulder tendons; degenerative, inflammatory changes.

Diagnostic Procedures. *X-ray.* Negative.

Therapy. Conservative measures when possible, and surgical measures when indicated by evidence of tear or rupture of tendons.

Prognosis. Depends on etiology and degree of lesions.

BIBLIOGRAPHY. Klippel JH, Dieppe PA: Rheumatology, p 5.8.5. St Louis, CV Mosby, 1995

Weatherall DJ, Ledingham JGG, Warrell DA: Oxford Textbook of Medicine, p 2995. Oxford, Oxford Med Pub, 1996

SHRINKING LUNG

Symptoms and Signs. In lupus erythematous systemic (see). Dyspnea.

Etiology. Diaphragmatic defect causing reduction of transdiaphragmatic pressure and reduced expansion of lungs.

Diagnostic Procedures. *Chest radiogram.* Small clear lungs.

Therapy. Beta-adrenergic drugs.

Prognosis. Dyspnea stable in time. Consequences from evolution of the basic disease.

BIBLIOGRAPHY. Rubin LA, Urowitz MB: Shrinking lung syndrome in SLE: A clinical pathological study. Rheumatology 10:973–976, 1983

SHULMAN

Synonyms. Posttransfusion purpura; purpura post-transfusion.

Symptoms and Signs. Rare reaction reported only in middle-aged females after repeated blood transfusions. Onset about 1 week after blood transfusion. Severe purpura.

Etiology. Possibly, formation of a cross-reacting antibody that destroys patient platelets.

Diagnostic Procedures. *Blood.* Severe thrombocytopenia; presence of platelet isoantibody in plasma. Platelet agglutination test; inhibition of clot retraction; complement fixation test.

Therapy. Adrenocorticotropic hormone (ACTH); prednisone; exchange transfusion in extremely severe cases.

Prognosis. Thombocytopenia persists for 24 hours to 44 days, except if exchange transfusion is done. Antibody titer also falls in weeks. After

recovering, injection of platelets has no untoward effect and antibodies are not recalled.

BIBLIOGRAPHY. Van Loghem JJ, Dorfmeijer H, Van der Hart M: Serological and genetical studies on platelet antigen (Zw.) Vox Sang 4:161–169, 1959

Shulman NR, Aster RH, Leitner A, et al: Immunoreactions involving platelets. V. Posttransfusion purpura due to a complement fixing antibody against a genetically controlled platelet antigen. A proposed mechanism for thrombocytopenia and its relevance in "autoimmunity." J Clin Invest 40:1597–1620, 1961

Bithell TC: Thrombocytopenia caused by immunologic platelet destruction: Idiopathic thrombocytopenic purpura (ITP), drug-induced thrombocytopenia, and miscellaneous forms. In Lee GR, Bithell TC, Foerster J, et al (eds): Wintrobe's Clinical Hematology, 9th ed, p 1345. Philadelphia, Lea & Febiger, 1993

SHULMAN II

Synonyms. Eosinophilic fascitis; fascitis eosinophilica.

Symptoms and Signs. Subcutaneous. Indurations of limbs: bilateral and symmetric.

Etiology. Unknown.

Pathology. Typical eosinophilic infiltration of muscular fascias.

Diagnostic Procedures. *Blood.* Eosinophilia. *Biopsy.* Of fascia, see.

Therapy. Corticosteroids.

BIBLIOGRAPHY. Shulman LE: Diffuse fascitis with eosinophilia. A new syndrome. Trans Assoc Phys 88:70–86, 1975

Contant G, Bletry O: Pathologie de l'eosinophile. Aspects cliniques prognostiques et therapeutiques. Ed Tech Encycl Med Chir (Paris France) Hématologie 13,009a10 1993 12 pp

Weatherall DJ, Ledingham JGG, Warrell DA: Oxford Textbook of Medicine, pp 3039, 3791. Oxford, Oxford Med Pub, 1996

SHUNT-HAYMAKER

Synonyms. Olivofrontocerebellar degeneration IV.

Symptoms and Signs. Both sexes. From infancy. Clinical manifestation variable from the classic ones of spinocerebellar ataxia to spastic paraplegia and involvement of cranial nerves (IX, X, XII).

Etiology. Autosomal dominant inheritance. Finding of linkage to makers on 6p.

Pathology. Major lesions in inferior olivary nucleus and cerebellum with variable pontine involvement and loss of anterior motor horn cells in spinocerebellar tracts and funiculus.

Diagnostic Procedures. *CT scan. MRI. Neuroimaging techniques.*

Therapy. Symptomatic.

Prognosis. Death from intercurring diseases.

BIBLIOGRAPHY. Shunt JW: Hereditary ataxia: Clinical study through six generations. Arch Neurol Psychiatr 65:535–568, 1950

Shunt JW, Haymaker W: Hereditary ataxia: Pathologic study of 5 cases of common ancestry. J Neuropath Clin Neurol 1:183–213, 1951

Auburger G, Orozco-Diaz G, Capote RF, et al: Autosomal dominant ataxia: Genetic evidence for locus heterogeneity from Cuban founder-effect population. Am J Human Genet 46:1163–1177, 1990

SHWACHMAN

Synonyms. Burke (V); Shwachman-Bodian; Shwachman-Diamond; metaphyseal chondrodysplasia (type B IV); neutropenia-pancreatic insufficiency; pancreatic insufficiency-bone marrow dysfunction; lipomatosis of pancreas, congenital.

Symptoms and Signs. Onset at 2–10 months of age. In childhood, may be asymptomatic, or one or both features of the syndrome: (1) malabsorption, steatorrhea; (2) recurrent infections. Bleeding tendency. Absence of chronic respiratory diseases.

Etiology. Unknown. A familial incidence observed, but not an adequate number of cases to establish mode of inheritance; autosomal recessive inheritance presumed.

Pathology. Small intestine biopsy shows mild inflammatory changes. *Pancreas.* Hypoplasia of exocrine tissue (replaced by fat) with normal islets. *Bone marrow.* Myeloid series hypoplasia; occasionally, megakaryocyte deficiency. Bone marrow findings may drastically change according to cyclic phase of proliferation and depression of myeloid series. *Bone.* Metaphyseal chondrodysplasia; focal lack of mineralization in epiphyses.

Diagnostic Procedures. *Blood.* Neutropenia; hypochromic anemia in some cases; thrombocytopenia (occasionally). *Stool.* Steatorrhea; decrease of serum pancreatic enzymes (lipase, amylase, trypsine). *Fat balance study. X-ray. CT scan.* In some cases, metaphyseal dysostosis. *Sweat studies.*

Therapy. Pancreatic enzymes; antibiotic for infections.

Prognosis. Steatorrhea decreases as patient grows older; however, pancreatic exocrine secretion remains low. Tendency to hematologic malignancies.

BIBLIOGRAPHY. Shwachman H, Diamond LK, Oski FA, et al: Pancreatic insufficiency and bone marrow dysfunction: A new clinical entity. J Pediatr 63:835–843, 1963

Shwachman H, Diamond LK, Oski FA, et al: The syndrome of pancreatic insufficiency and bone marrow dysfunction. J Pediatr 65:645–663, 1964

Dossetor JFN, Spratt HC, Rolles CJ, et al: Immunoreactive trypsin in Shwachman's syndrome. Arch Dis Child 64:395–406, 1989

D'Angio CT, Lloid JK: Nephrocalcinosis in Shwachman's syndrome. Arch Dis Child 64:614–615, 1989

Weatherall DJ, Ledingham JGG, Warrell DA: Oxford Textbook of Medicine, pp 2039, 3559. Oxford, Oxford Med Pub, 1996

SHY-DRAGER

Synonyms. Orthostatic hypotension, neurologic; orthostatic hypotension variant; Shy-McGee-Drager; multiple system atrophy, MSA.

Symptoms. Occurs in adults. Onset gradual. Orthostatic hypotension; impotence; general or localized anhidrosis; loss of sphincter control; visual troubles; rigidity; tremor; adiadochokinesis; fasciculations; muscle wasting leading to severe invalidism. Occasionally, dysphagia. Central nervous system manifestations may be identical to those of Parkinson (see).

Signs. Iris atrophy; external ophthalmoparesis; hyperactive muscle stretch reflexes; pathologic reflexes.

Etiology. Unknown. Progressive degenerative process of nervous system. Inflammatory nature cannot be completely excluded. A slowly evolving familial form of this condition has been reported. The autonomic defect appears to be located centrally or partially in the afferent pathways controlling reflex adjustment to postural changes.

Pathology. Nonspecific. Bilateral symmetric neuronal loss and demyelinization of basal ganglia, cerebellar system, corticospinal motor system, and autonomic nervous system.

Diagnostic Procedures. *Blood.* Electrolyte alterations. In recumbent position normal plasma level of norepinephrine; failure of the level to be modified by change in position or exercise. Low level of dopamine beta-hydroxylase. Significant vasoconstrictor response to intra-arterial tyramine, and normal response to norepinephrine. *Urine.* Increased excre-

tion of deaminated metabolites of norepinephrine. Injection of acetyl methylcholine; absence of any change. *EMG. EEG.*

Therapy. Administration of 9-fluorohydrocortisone and salt may correct the orthostatic hypotension, but the neurologic symptoms continue to progress. Mechanical measures; volume expanders; pharmacologic agents (sympathomimetics, vasoconstrictors, β-receptor blockers, α2-receptor agonists, prostaglandin synthesis inhibitors, antiserotoninergics, MAO inhibitors, vasopressin). Atrial tachypacing (100 rate).

Prognosis. Progressive. General debilitation leading to fatal complications.

BIBLIOGRAPHY. Shy GM, Drager GA: A neurological syndrome associated with orthostatic hypotension. Arch Neurol 2:511–527, 1960

Lee S, Chen CN: Clinical diversity of the Shy-Drager syndrome: A case in Hong Kong. J R Soc Med 82:225–226, 1989

Lewis RP, Budoulas H, Schaal SF, et al: Diagnosis and management of syncope. In Schlant RC, Alexander RW: Hurst's The Heart, 8th ed, p 931. New York, McGraw-Hill, 1994

Cryer PE: Orthostatic postural hypotension. In De Groot LJ (ed): Endocrinology, 3rd ed, p 2937. Philadelphia, WB Saunders, 1995

SHY-GONATAS

Synonyms. Oculopharyngeal—muscular dystrophy. See also Hunter and Refsum.

Symptoms. Onset in middle age. High variability among families where any one of the symptoms may be dominating. Pharyngeal symptoms. Weight loss up to starvation. Weakness of proximal section of extremities; ataxia (cerebellar); double vision and decreased acuity; especially in night vision; dementia.

Signs. Gargoylism; reflexes absent; cardiac arrhythmias; proptosis; hypertelorism; keratopathy.

Etiology. Unknown. Metabolic defect in myelinization. Autosomal dominant trait (recessive inheritance also reported). Membrane abnormalities suggested. According to Gonatas, anatomic-pathologic findings distinguish the form from gargoylism.

Pathology. Accumulation of lipids and mitochondrial inclusion bodies in muscles. Extensive demyelinization and pathologic cytosomes (zebra bodies) in Schwann cells and axons. In liver cells, inclusion bodies. In cornea, ulcers. Retinal pigmentary degeneration.

Diagnostic Procedures. *Electromyography.* Suggests myopathy. *Blood.* Normal enzymes.

Therapy. None specific. If pharyngeal symptoms prevent feeding, artificial alimentation; if cardiologic, pacing may be required.

Prognosis. Progressive condition to starvation and motor incapacitation.

BIBLIOGRAPHY. Shy GM, Silberberg DH, Appel SM, et al: A generalized disorder of the nervous system, skeletal muscle and heart resembling Refsum's disease and Hurler's syndrome. I. Clinical, pathologic, and biochemical characteristics. Am J Med 42:163–169, 1967

Gonatas NK: A generalized disorder of the nervous system, skeletal muscle and heart resembling Refsum's disease and Hurler's syndrome. II. Ultrastructure. Am J Med 42:169–178, 1967

Pauzner R, Blatt I, Mouallem M, et al: Mitochondrial abnormalities in oculopharyngeal muscular dystrophy. Muscle Nerve 14:947–952, 1991

SHY-MAGEE

Synonyms. Central core; CCD; muscle core; nonprogressive congenital myopathy. See Floppy infant syndromes.

Symptoms. Both sexes affected. Onset in first year of life or later; cases reported of onset in adult life. Proximal muscular weakness and cramps following exercise; delayed physical development in walking, climbing (some patients take 5 years to start to walk). Normal mental development. Association with malignant hyperthermia syndrome reported in some families. Clinical varieties include mild, moderate, and severe forms.

Signs. Symmetric hypotonia of proximal muscles, greater in lower extremities than upper. No fasciculation or myotonia. Minor wasting; tendon flexes normal or diminished.

Etiology. Unknown. Autosomal, dominant inheritance, with variable penetrance or expression. CCD gene mapped to proximal 19q13.1

Pathology. *Muscle.* Densely packed core of altered striated myofibrils on the center of muscle fiber. Partial disorganization of normal striation and irregular Z disk in the core. Occasionally, floccular changes in isolated muscle fibers.

Diagnostic Procedures. *Biopsy.* Of muscle. See Pathology. Biochemical studies of muscle metabolism. *Blood.* Creatine index increased. Serum glutamic-oxalacetic transaminase (SGOT) normal. *Urine.* Creatinine greatly increased. EMG. Decreased duration of action potential.

Therapy. Symptomatic.

Prognosis. Defect remains without progression.

BIBLIOGRAPHY. Shy GM, Magee KR: A new congenital non-progressing myopathy. Brain 79:610–621, 1956
Gamstrop I: Non-dystrophic myogenic myopathies with onset in infancy or childhood: A review of some characteristic syndromes. Acta Pediatr Scand 71:881–886, 1982
Kausch K, Leheman-Horn F, Janka M, et al: Evidence for linkage of the central core disease locus to the proximal long arm of human chromosome 19. Genomics 10:756–769, 1991
Goebel HH, Lenard HG: Congenital myopathies. In Rowland LP, Di Mauro S (eds): Handbook of Clinical Neurology, vol 18: Myopathies, p 331. Amsterdam, Elsevier, 1992

SIALIDOSIS I AND II

Synonyms. Cherry red spot, myoclonus; myoclonus, cherry red spot; Mucolipidosis I, ML I; neuraminidase deficiency; glycoprotein neuraminidase deficiency. See Goldberg.

Symptoms and Signs. *Type I.* More frequent in Italians. From second decade. Myoclonus; decreased vision; night blindness; painful neuropathy (see Fabry); tendon hyperreflexia; nystagmus; ataxia; grand mal. Cherry red spot in macula. *Type II.* Dysmorphic type, divided into juvenile and infantile forms. *Juvenile form.* In Japanese from second decade: coarse facies, dysostosis multiplex, myoclonus, same ocular symptoms of type I. Angiokeratoma and glucosidosis. Vacuolated lymphocytes. *Infantile form.* Normal at birth, then development of mucopolysaccharidosis phenotype. Abnormal renal function. Congenital form with hydrops fetalis and ascites reported in family groups. Another classification recognizes five forms: (1) primary N D without dysmorphism (congenital); (2) primary N D with dysmorphism (congenital); (3) primary N D with dysmorphism (childhood); (4) combined neuraminidase/beta-galactosidase deficiency (infantile); (5) combined neuraminidase/beta-galactosidase deficiency (juvenile).

Etiology. Autosomal recessive inheritance. Defect of α-neuraminidase. Enzyme defect on pter-q23 region of chromosome 10. Possible role of serotonin in the pathogenesis of myoclonus.

Pathology. Vacuolation in Kupffer cell, of minor degree in hepatocytes; vacuolation in nerve; fibroblasts; myoenteric plexus neurons; brain cells; neuronal lipoidosis.

Diagnostic Procedures. *Urine.* High sialic acid containing oligosaccharides. *Blood.* Vacuolated lymphocytes (except in type I). *Biopsies.* Of liver and nerve. See Pathology. *Direct measurement of sialidase activity in fresh tissue samples.* Prenatal diagnosis possible.

Therapy. Hydroxytryptophan; anticonvulsive therapy.

Prognosis. Death in second decade for infantile form. Later (fourth to fifth) for other forms.

BIBLIOGRAPHY. Terry K, Linker A: Distinction among four forms of Hurler's syndrome. Proc Soc Exp Biol Med 115:394–402, 1964
Lowden JA, O'Brien JS: Sialidosis: A review of human neuraminidase deficiency. Am J Hum Genet 31:1–18, 1979
Young ID, Young EP, Mossmamn J, et al: Neuraminidase deficiency case report and review of the phenotype. J Med Genet 24:283–290, 1987
Thomas GH, Blaudet AL: Disorders of glycoprotein degradation and structure: Mannosidosis, -mannosidosis, sialidosis aspartylglycosamininuria and carbohydrate-deficient glycoprotein syndrome. In Scriver CR, Beaudet AL, Sly WS, et al: The Metabolic and Molecular Bases of Inherited Disease, 7th ed, pp 2542–2545. New York, McGraw-Hill, 1995

SIALURIA

Synonyms. See Salla, ISSD, and Sialidoses (different entities).

Symptoms and Signs. From birth. Coarse facies. Hepatosplenomegaly. Normal growth and development.

Etiology. Possibly autosomal recessive inheritance. Feedback inhibition of an enzyme of sialic acid synthesis.

Diagnostic Procedures. *Urine.* Massive excretion of free sialic acid. Different from sialidoses because of normal or increased level of neuraminodase activity.

BIBLIOGRAPHY. Montrenil J, Biserte G, Strecker G, et al: Description d'un nouveau type de meliturie: la sialurie. Clin Chim Acta 21:61–68, 1968
Sappala R, Tietze F, Krasnewich D, et al: Sialic acid metabolism in sialuria fibroblasts. J Biol Chem 266:7456–7461, 1991
Gahl WA, Schneider JA, Aula PP: Lysosomal transport disorders: Cystinosis and sialic acid storage disorders. In Scriver CR, Beaudet AL, Sly WS, et al: The Metabolic and Molecular Bases of Inherited Disease, 7th ed, pp 3785–3789. New York, McGraw-Hill, 1995

SICCA

Synonym. Sjögren group E, A, B. See Alacrima. Association of keratoconjunctivitis sicca and xerostomia without an associated collagen disease (see Sjögren's).

BIBLIOGRAPHY. Deutsch HJ: Sjögren's syndrome and pseudolymphoma. Ann Otol 76:1074–1084, 1967
Hakin KN, Lightman S: The eye in systemic disorders. In Garner A, Klintworth GK (eds): Pathobiology of Ocular Disease: A Dynamic Approach, 2nd ed, pp 191–193. New York, Marcel Dekker, 1994

SICCARDI

Symptoms and Signs. Described in one Italian boy. Recurrent infections, skin slate-gray pigmentation, silver-colored hair; lymphoadenopathy, hepatosplenomegaly.

Etiology. Unknown. Parents related that the father was completely healthy, but showed defect of neutrophil bactericidal activity.

Diagnostic Procedures. *Blood.* Thrombocytopenia. Neutrophil defect of bactericidal activity.

Therapy. Symptomatic.

Prognosis. Patient died at 4 years of age from cerebral hemorrhage.

BIBLIOGRAPHY. Siccardi AG, Bianchi E, Calligari A, et al: A new familial defect in neutrophilbactericidal activity. Helv Paediatr Acta 33:401–412, 1978

SICK BUILDING

Symptoms and Signs. In workers in a so-called "sick building," where igigenic conditions (ventilation, humidity, dust), are deficient. Variable skin complaints: dryness, itching. Symptoms reported in epidemic form are more pronounced than actual lesions. The face is frequently affected. Some patients complain of respiratory symptoms up to frank asthmatic attacks.

Etiology. Combination of environmental factors and suggestion.

Pathology. In several patients, rosacea and mild dermatological lesions.

Therapy. Bonification of environment.

Prognosis. Symptoms disappear with bettering of working conditions.

BIBLIOGRAPHY. Berg M: Facial skin complaints and work at visual display units: Epidemiolgical clinical and histopathological studies. Acta Derm Venereol 69:(Suppl 150) 6–9, 1989
Tucker WG: Sources of indoor air contaminants: Characterizing emissions and health impacts. NY Acad Sci 641. 1992
Weatherall DJ, Ledingham JGG, Warrell DA: Oxford Textbook of Medicine, pp 1231, 1232. Oxford, Oxford Med Pub, 1996

SICK EUGONADAL

Symptoms and Signs. Observed in a number of nonendocrine conditions (acute or chronic diseases, as well as in severe dietary weight loss or anorexia nervosa [see] or exessive excercise). Oligo or amenorrhea and other signs of hypogonadism.

Etiology. Deranged hormonal metabolism in liver and kidney or from altered peripheral aromatization of estrogens in the decreased quantities of adipose tissue.

Diagnostic Procedures. *Blood.* Hormonal levels decreased; gonadotrophin secretion.

Therapy. Treatment of basic pathological condition and hormonal substitution.

BIBLIOGRAPHY. Weatherall DJ, Ledingham JGG, Warrell DA: Oxford Textbook of Medicine, p 1718. Oxford, Oxford Med Pub, 1996

SICK EUTHYROID

Synonyms. Sick cell.

Symptoms and Signs. In patients with severe pathological conditions (liver, kidney, heart, severe burn, major surgery, etc.). Those of hypothyroidism.

Etiology. Unclear.

Diagnostic Procedures. *Blood.* Low T3 (because of decreased conversion from T4) elevated reverse T3 (because of reduced clearance). Normal basal or depressed TSH

Therapy. Treatment with thyroid hormones does not affect the outcome.

Prognosis. Poor. Bound to general condition evolution.

BIBLIOGRAPHY. Docter R, Krenning EP, DeJong M, et al: The sick euthyroid syndrome: Changes in thyroid hormone serum parameters and hormone metabolism. Clin Endocr 39:499–510, 1993

SICKLE CHEST

Symptoms and Signs. Complication of sickle cell disease (see Herrick). Chest pain, fever, leukocytosis.

Etiology. Intravascular sickling in lung that causes alveolar necrosis. Infection usually is secondary.

Diagnostic Procedures. *Blood.* Sickle cell anemia. *Angiography.* Occlusion of distal pulmonary vessels. *Pulmonary artery pressure.* Increased.

Therapy. Exchange transfusion: artificial ventilation with positive pressure or prepulmonary oxygenation with extracorporeal membrane.

Prognosis. High mortality in spite of good intensive treatment.

BIBLIOGRAPHY. Davies SC, Luce PJ, Riordan PJ, et al: Acute chest syndrome in sickle cell disease. Lancet I:36–38, 1984
Gillett DS, Gunning KEJ, Sawicka EH, et al: Life-threatening sickle chest syndrome treated with extracorporeal membrane oxygenation. Br J Med 294:81–82, 1987
Weatherall DJ, Clegg JB, Higgs DR, et al: The hemoglobinopathies. In Scriver CR, Beaudet AL, Sly WS, et al: The Metabolic and Molecular Bases of Inherited Disease, 7th ed, p 3435. New York, McGraw-Hill, 1995

SICK LIBRARY

Symptoms and Signs. Manifestations of allergic reactions (sneezing, coughing, etc.).

Etiology. Allergy to molds, bacteria, dust, and other organic compounds deriving from aged books.

Diagnostic Procedures. *Skin.* Allergy tests. *Blood.* Immunoglobulin E level, RAST.

Therapy. Prophylaxis with cromoglycate nasal spray, or inhalation and eye drops, or specific desensitization. An interesting measure to protect books from damage from insects and relative formation of organic debris is that adopted by the University Library in Coimbra (Portugal), where bats have nested behind the book shelves and during the night perform the task. This measure seems to have been effectively functioning now for centuries.

Prognosis. According to treatment and frequency of library frequentation.

BIBLIOGRAPHY. Brook SJ, Brook I: Are public library books contaminated by bacteria? J Clin Epidemiol 47:1171–1174, 1994
Leon FS: Bacteri no! Fungi yes! J Clin Epidemiol 48:1183–1184, 1995
Hay RJ: Sick library syndrome. Lancet 346:1573–1574, 1995

SICK SINUS

See Short.

Symptoms. Symptoms of periodic mild cerebral artery insufficiency. Slight changes in personality; irritability; fleeting memory losses; sleep alterations. Fatigue; weakness; mild digestive troubles; modest periodic oliguria. In more severe form, speech slurring, paresis, judgment alterations.

Signs. Persistent, severe, sudden sinus bradycardia; cessation of sinus rhythm for short intervals with other rhythms supervening; long periods of sinus arrest resulting in cardiac arrest; bouts of ventricular rhythm following chronic atrial fibrillation with slow ventricular rate. Failure to resume sinus rhythm after cardioversion.

Etiology. Considered an inadequate descriptive term since it includes any form of sinus nodal depression. It is applied as synonym of Short syndrome. It implies disease of the atrioventricular (AV) junction. The pathogenetic mechanism is represented by transient pressure injury of the sinus, from catheter or destruction of nodal tissue by ischemic, sclerotic, or inflammatory process. Symptoms are caused by hypoperfusion of brain, kidney, and heart.

Pathology. Lesion of sinoatrial node. Other features of pre-existing cardiac pathology.

Diagnostic Procedures. *ECG.*

Therapy. Electrical pacing. Isoproterenol not practical. Atropine may not be effective.

Prognosis. Fair with electrical pacing.

BIBLIOGRAPHY. Ferrer MI: The sick sinus syndrome in atrial disease. JAMA 206:645–646, 1968

Myerburg RJ, Kessler KM, Castellanos A: Recognition, clinical assessment and management of conduction disturbances. In Garner A, Klintworth GK (eds): Pathobiology of Ocular Disease: A Dynamic Approach, 2nd ed, p 748. New York, Marcel Dekker, 1994

Weatherall DJ, Ledingham JGG, Warrell DA: Oxford Textbook of Medicine, p 2266. Oxford, Oxford Med Pub, 1996

SIDEROBLASTIC ANEMIA, HEREDITARY

Synonyms. Rundless-Falls; pyridoxine-responsive anemia; iron loading, hereditary, anemia. See Pearson.

Symptoms. Occurs most often in males. In females, carrier status with minor manifestations. In a minority, anemia is congenital or discovered during childhood. In the majority, discovered from 12–87 years. Weakness, tiredness, occasionally, leg pain and paresthesias of feet. Symptoms associated with pyridoxine deficiency, such as mental retardation, convulsions, peripheral neuropathy, glossitis, dermatitis lacking in these patients.

Signs. Pallor, hepatomegaly, and splenomegaly. Occasionally, pretibial edema and skin pigmentation.

Etiology. X-linkage inheritance (see Rudles-Falls). Cases reported also with autosomal and more rarely recessive inheritance The enzyme defect may involve δ-aminolevulinic acid synthetase among many other possible mechanisms considered.

Pathology. See Diagnostic Procedures.

Diagnostic Procedures. *Blood.* Anemia from mild to severe; hypochromia; microcytosis frequent; normocytosis and macrocytosis less frequently observed. Marked anisopoikilocytosis. Hemoglobin electrophoresis normal. Reticulocytes low, siderocytes frequently increased, rate of destruction of erythrocytes moderately increased. Coombs test negative. Osmotic fragility, increased resistance to hypotonic saline. White blood cell number normal or decreased, in some cases increased; platelets normal or occasionally thrombocytopenia or thrombocytosis; Serum iron increased; iron-binding capacity saturated; associated hypolipemia and hypocholesterolemia. *Bone marrow.* Marked normoblastic hyperplasia; reduction of myeloerythroid ratio. Evolution to myelofibrosis possible. Increased iron-staining granules in the erythroblasts and reticuloendothelial cells. Tryptophan load-xanthurenic acid excretion test. Increased excretion in many cases.

Therapy. Pyridoxine (100–200 mg/day): Good response for the anemia in one third of patients; complete remission seldom occurs. Crude liver extract or androgen or both enhance the therapeutic effect of pyridoxine in some cases. Splenectomy (abandoned because of thromboembolic complications and possible fatal outcome). Iron depletion program when indicated.

Prognosis. Optimal or suboptimal response of the anemia and defective tryptophan metabolism. No consistent changes in associated leukocyte abnormalities. In rare cases, thrombotic episodes coincident with pyridoxine response. Relapses usually recurring with discontinuation of treatment. In some cases, spontaneous temporary remission after a period of treatment. Death occurs from overwhelming infections or hemochromatosis with liver insufficiency or both.

BIBLIOGRAPHY. Cooley TB: A severe type of hereditary anemia with elliptocytosis interesting sequence of splenectomy. Am J Med Sci 209:561–568, 1945

Rundles RW, Falls HF: Hereditary (sex linked) anemia. Am J Med Sci 211:641–658, 1946

Pasanen AVO, Eklof M, Tenhumen R: Coproporphyrinogen oxidase activity and porphyrin concentrations in peripheral red blood cells in hereditary sideroblastic anaemia. Scand J Haematol 34:235–237, 1985

Bottomley SS: Sideroblastic anemias. In Lee GR, Bithell TC, Foerster J, et al (eds): Wintrobe's Clinical Hematology, 9th ed, pp 856–858. Philadelphia, Lea & Febiger, 1993

SIEGRIST

Synonyms. Siegrist-Hutchinson; pigmented choroidal vessels.

Symptoms and Signs. Prevalent in females. Onset in advanced age. Decreasing vision; exophthalmos; granular pigmented areas in the choroid that follows the path of the larger choroidal vessels. *Blood.* Hypertension.

Etiology. Unknown.

Pathology. Changes of choroid and other manifestations related to arteriosclerotic changes.

Diagnostic Procedures. *Urine.* Albuminuria.

Therapy. None.

Prognosis. The occurrence of these choroidal changes indicate an unfavorable prognosis.

BIBLIOGRAPHY. Siegrist A: Zur Kenntnis der Arteriosclerose der Augengefässe. IX Cong Internat D'Opht d'Utrecht pp 131–139, 1900

Garner A: Vascular diseases. In Garner A, Klintworth GK (eds): Pathobiology of Ocular Disease: A Dynamic Approach, 2nd ed, p 1641. New York, Marcel Dekker, 1994

SILFVERSKIÖLD

Obsolete.

Synonyms. Grudzinski; Morquio variant; extremity osteochondrodystrophy. Possibly a variant of Morquio syndrome.

BIBLIOGRAPHY. Silfverskiöld N: A forme fruste of chondrodystrophia, with changes simulating several of the known local malacias. Acta Radiol 4:44–57, 1925

Helweg-Larsen HF, Morch ET: Hereditary of osteochondrodystrophy: Silfverskiöld and Morquio syndromes. Nord Med 30:377–882, 1946

SILLENCE

Synonym. Brachydactyly—symphalangism.

Symptoms and Signs. Brachydactyly, distal symphalangism (chess pawn); scoliosis; pes equinus; normal stature.

Etiology. Autosomal dominant inheritance.

BIBLIOGRAPHY. Sillence DO: Brachydactyly, distal symphalangism, scoliosis, tall stature, and club feet: A new syndrome. J Med Genet 15:208–211, 1978

SILO-FILLER DISEASE

Synonym. Bronchiolitis obliterans (see). Allergic alveolitis (see).

Symptoms. In subjects who enter silos from the time of filling until 6 weeks thereafter. For diagnosis, consider temporal relationship between exposure and development of the syndrome. Irritation from fumes prompting to leave the silo within few minutes, or sudden unconsciousness. After a latency of hours: fever, cough, myalgias, and progressive dyspnea.

Signs. Acute respiratory distress, cyanosis, coarse rales and sibils, collapse (if not promptly assisted).

Etiology. Generally limited to silo-gas or NO₂ related effect and hypoxia owing to anaerobic fermentation.

Pathology. *Lungs.* Heavy full of frothy white fluid and its consolidation in all lobes; exudation of neutrophils in alveolar spaces, alveolar walls infiltrated by lymphocytes, necrotizing bronchiolitis.

Diagnostic Procedures. *X-rays.* Chest: pulmonary edema, bilateral patchy infiltrates. Respiratory and cardiovascular monitoring. *Blood gasses.* Acid base balance.

Therapy. Early respiratory assistance with high concentration of O₂. High dosage of corticosteroids.

Prognosis. Death in untreated patients. If assisted, good. Possible complication or evolution into bronchiolitis obliterans (see) (most often reversible); late bronchiolitis obliterans with scarring and chronic airway obstruction (rare) in the latter case lung transplantation is indicated.

BIBLIOGRAPHY. Elper GR: Silo-filler's disease: A new perspective. Mayo Clin Proc 64:368–370, 1989

Weatherall DJ, Ledingham JGG, Warrell DA: Oxford Textbook of Medicine, pp 2815, 2847. Oxford, Oxford Med Pub, 1996

SILVERMAN-HANDMAKER

Synonym. Dyssegmental dysplasia S-H; anisospondylic camptomicromelic dwarfism. See Kniest-like, lethal and Rolland-Desbuquois.

Symptoms and Signs. Hispanic background. Stillborn or live only hours. Hydrocephalus, cleft palate, orbital hypoplasia, flat face, narrow chest; reduced joint mobility. Occasionally: hirsutism, ear abnormalities, evidence of congenital heart disease and genitourinary abnormalities.

Etiology. Autosomal dominant inheritance.

Pathology. Hydrocephaly and occipital exencephalocele, polymicrogyria; cerebellar hypoplasia. Enchondrial ossification disturbed; lack of columnization; ballooning of cartilage cells; mucoid degeneration; accumulation of mucopolysaccharides, no increase in collagen fibers.

Diagnostic Procedures. *X-ray. Ultrasound.* Typical spine changes: coronal cleft and oversized vertebral sagittal clefting. Short trunk, narrow thorax; severe symmetric shortening of tubular bones (somewhat folded on themselves).

Prognosis. Stillborn or death within 48 hours.

BIBLIOGRAPHY. Simmonds M. Untersuchungen von Missbildungen mit. Hilfe des Roentgenverfahrensr (case 2). Fortschz Geb Roentgenstr 4:197–211, 1900–1901

Silverman FN: Forms of dysostotic dwarfism of uncertain classification. Am Radiol 12, 1005–1008, 1969

Handmaker SD, Robinson LD, Campbell J, et al: Dissegmental dwarfism: A new syndrome of lethal dwarfism. Birth Defects Orig Art 12:79–80, 1977

Aleck Ka, Grix A, Clericuzio C, et al: Dyssegmental dysplasia: Clinical, radiographic and morphologic evidence of heterogeneity. Am J Med Genet 27:295–312, 1987

Rimoin DL, Lachman RS: Genetic disorders of the osseous skeleton. In Beithon P (ed): RS McKusick's Heritable Disorders of Connective Tissue, 5th ed, pp 601–603. St Louis, CV Mosby, 1993

SILVESTRINI-CORDA

Synonym. Endocrine deficiency—hepatic cirrhosis. See Sick euthyroid and Sick eugonadal.

Symptoms. Occurs in patients with liver cirrhosis. Anorexia; asthenia;

loss of libido; impotence; menstrual disorders (menorrhagia; amenorrhea; postmenopausal bleeding.)

Signs. Gynecomastia (Silvestrini); testicular atrophy (Corda). Loss of axillary hair; vascular arterial "spider" plus all signs of liver cirrhosis (e.g., liver enlarged at onset, reduced and nodular, later ascites).

Etiology. Secondary endocrinologic changes caused by failure of liver to metabolize different hormones.

Pathology. That of liver cirrhosis; gynecomastia; atrophy of testicular germinal epithelium; prostatic nodular hyperplasia. Decrease of lipid content of adrenals.

Diagnostic Procedures. *Blood.* Typical changes of liver cirrhosis. *Urine.* Increased excretion of estrogen and decrease of 17-ketosteroids and androgen.

Therapy and Prognosis. That of liver cirrhosis.

BIBLIOGRAPHY. Corda L, Sulla CD: Reviviscenza della mammella maschile nella cirrosi epatica. Minerva Med 5:1067–1069, 1925

Silvestrini R: La reviviscenza mammaria nell'uomo affetto da cirrosi del Laennec. Riforma Med 42:701–704, 1926

Lloyd CW, Williams RH: Endocrine changes associated with Laennec's cirrhosis of the liver. Am J Med 4:315–330, 1948

Wisgerhof M: Adrenal glands and gonads: The steroid hormones. In Haubrich WS, Schaffner F, Berk JE (eds): Bockus Gastroenterology, 5th ed, pp 3473–3474. Philadelphia, WB Saunders, 1995

SILVESTRONI-BIANCO

Synonyms. Microdrepanocytosis; sickle cell-thalassemia; Hb-S-beta Thalassemia.

Symptoms. Variable pattern including features of Herrick and thalassemia syndromes. From mild anemia to severe anemia; abdominal crisis; splenomegaly.

Etiology. Combination of two pathologic genes usually inherited one from each parent, seldom both from same parent.

Diagnostic Procedures. *Blood.* Findings of sickling and thalassemia. Hemoglobin electrophoresis usually shows 60–80% of hemoglobin S, 20% of hemoglobin F, and balance hemoglobin A; hemoglobin A2 usually increased.

Prognosis. Variable according to biochemical defect. Death in infancy or childhood, or survival into adulthood.

BIBLIOGRAPHY. Silvestroni E, Bianco I: Prime osservazioni di resistenze globulari aumentate in soggetti sani e rapporto fra questi soggetti e i malati di cosidetto ittero emolitico con resistenze globulari aumentate. Bull Atti Acc Med Romana 49:1–16, 1943

Silvestroni E, Bianco I: Una nuova entita nosologica: la malattia microdrepanocitica Haematologica. 1–34, 1946

Silvestroni E, Bianco I: Genetic aspects of sickle cell anemia and microdrepanocytic disease. Blood 7:429–435, 1952

Lukens JN: The thalassemias and related disorders: Quantitative disorders of hemoglobin synthesis. In Lee GR, Bithel TC, Foerster J, et al (eds): Wintrobe's Clinical Hematology, 9th ed, p 1126. Philadelphia, Lea & Febiger, 1993

SIMELL-TAKKI

Synonyms. Jacobsohn; gyrate atrophy of choroid and retina; retinitis pigmentosa, atypical, hyperornithinemia, Finnish type.

Symptoms and Signs. Both sexes. Prevalent in Finnish people. From childhood, progressive loss of vision, blindness reached in fourth decade. Posterior subcapsular cataracts. Sometimes associated anomalies of body hair.

Etiology. Autosomal recessive. Chromosome 10 defect in ornithine-[A5]d-aminotransferase that causes accumulation of ornithine, which inhibits creatine synthesis. Apparently, hyperornithinemia is toxic to the eye.

Diagnostic Procedures. In childhood: demarcated circular areas of chorioretinal degeneration which enlarge and coalesce in adult life. *Electroretinography.* Reduced conduction with progression of disease. *Muscle biopsy.* Abnormalities of muscle fibers (type II). *Body fluids.* Elevation of ornithine level. Level of ornithine aminotransferase in transformed lymphocytes in obligate heterozygous carriers is approximately 50% of normal value.

Therapy. Exogenous creatine and pyridoxine. Pyridoxal phosphate give some results (in responsive subjects).

Prognosis. Progressive condition.

BIBLIOGRAPHY. Jacobsohn E: Ein Fall von Retinitis pigmentosa atypica. Klin Monatsbl Augenheilkd 26:206, 1888

Simell O, Takki K: Raised plasma ornithine and gyrate atrophy of the choroid and retina. Lancet 1:1031, 1973

Kennaway NG, Weleber RG, Buist NRM: Gyrate atrophy of the choroid and retina, with hyperornithinemia: Biochemical and histological studies and response to vitamin B6. Am J Hum Genet 32:529–541, 1980

Klintworth GH: Disorders of aminoacid metabolism and melanin pigmentation. In Garner A, Klintworth GK (eds): Pathobiology of Ocular Disease: A Dynamic Approach, 2nd ed, pp 957–960. New York, Marcel Dekker, 1994

SIMMONDS

Synonyms. Glinski-Simmonds; hypopituitarism; panhypopituitarism; postpuberal panhypopituitarism. See Sheehan.

Symptoms. Prevalent in females. Onset in postpuberal period. Asthenia; prolonged inanition to emaciation. Loss of libido and potency.

Signs. Weight loss; atrophy of all body tissues; loss of body hair; atrophic skin gives the appearance of premature aging. Atrophy of genital organs. Sensitivity to cold; bradycardia. Low blood pressure may reach shock level with patient in upright position. Psychic changes.

Etiology. Lesion and hypofunction or atrophy (or both) of anterior pituitary gland (idiopathic; tumor; infections; X-rays; surgery).

Pathology. *Pituitary.* See Etiology. *Thyroid adrenal, gonads.* Secondary atrophy.

Diagnostic Procedures. *Blood.* Thyroid-stimulating hormone (TSH) and adrenocorticotropic hormone (ACTH) level. Anemia of various degrees according to degree of hypofunction. *Basic metabolic rate* low. *Urine.* Low 17-ketosteroids, 11-oxysteroids, and gonadotropins.

Therapy. ACTH, gonadotropins, thyroid, and other deficient hormones.

Prognosis. Dramatic improvement with treatment.

BIBLIOGRAPHY. Simmonds M: Ueber Hypophysisschwund mit tödlichem Ausgang. Dtsch Med Wochenschr 40:322–323, 1914

Hickstein DD, Chaundler WF, Marshall JC: The spectrum of pituitary adenoma. West J Med 144:433–436, 1986

Kasa-Vubu JZ, Kelch RP: Precocious and delayed puberty: Diagnosis and treatment. In De Groot LJ (ed): Endocrinology, 3rd ed, pp 1960–1961. Philadelphia, WB Saunders, 1995

SIMPSON

Synonym. Hysterical abdominal bloating.

Symptoms. Occurs in women or occasionally men (see Couvade). Abdominal swelling; pseudocyesis.

Signs. Depression of diaphragm and lordosis of spine.

Etiology. Unknown. Delusion of pregnancy a symptom of many psychotic states.

Diagnostic Procedures. Under anesthesia abdominal swelling disappears, and returns as soon as patient awakes.

BIBLIOGRAPHY. Simpson J: Clinical Lectures on Diseases of Women, p 363. Edinburgh, Black, 1872

Enock MD, Trethouan WH, Barker JC: Some Uncommon Psychotic Syndromes. Baltimore, Williams & Wilkins, 1967

SIMPSON-GOLABI-BEHMEL

Synonyms. Golabi-Rosen; bulldog; dysplasia—gigantism.

Symptoms and Signs. In males. Partial manifestations in female carrier. At birth: overgrowth that continues. *Head.* Large; prominent skull sutures; coarse facies; hypertelorism; broad nose; wide mouth; macroglossia; spotty palatal and perioral pigmentation; mental deficiency. *Limbs.* Hands: large and square, broad hypoplastic nails. Thumbs: postaxial hexadactyly, foot deformity, broad halluces. *Skeleton.* Mild scoliosis and pectus excavatum. *Skin.* Thickened and brown nipples.

Etiology. X-linked inheritance.

Diagnostic Procedures. *X-rays.* Skeletal vertebral segmentation defects. *Bone.* Age advanced. *Kidney.* Large, lobulate, cystic, hydronephosis. *Gut.* Malrotation, pyloric ring. *Blood.* Occasional polycythemia. *ECG.* Conduction defects.

Prognosis. When patients reach adulthood (heigh above average) they lose some of the clumsiness and general typical features become less evident.

BIBLIOGRAPHY. Simpson JL, Landey S, New M, et al: A previously unrecognized X-linked syndrome of dysmorphia. Birth Defects. Orig Art Ser 11:18–24, 1975

Golabi M, Rosen L: A new X-linked mental retardation: Overgrowth syndrome. Am J Med Genet 17:345–358, 1984

Behmel A, Ploechl E, Rosenkranz W: A new X-linked dysplasia gigantism syndrome: Follow up in the first family and report on a second Austrian family. Am J Med Genet 30:275–285, 1988

SIMPSON (S.L.)

Obsolete.

Synonym. Adipose gynandrism. Adipose gynism (equivalent syndrome in female). See Pseudo-Cushing.

Symptoms and Signs. Onset in preadolescence. Tendency toward obesity and delayed sexual maturation. Some morphologic features suggest female habitus (owing to fat distribution and delayed sexual development). Patient somewhat taller than average.

Etiology. Unknown. Genetic factor: endocrine changes possibly secondary to obesity. One of the many shades of the hypogenitalism group of syndromes.

Diagnostic Procedures. See Pseudo-Cushing.

Therapy. Diet.

Prognosis. Good. Eventually, normal development and fertility.

BIBLIOGRAPHY. Simpson SL: Clinical and pathological aspects of adrenal glands. Proc R Soc Med 27:383–387, 1934

Simpson SL: Adrenal hyperfunction and function. Bull NY Acad Med 27:723–742, 1951

Rosenfield RL, Cara JF: Somatic growth and maturation. In De Groot LJ (ed): Endocrinology, 3rd ed, pp 2549–2589. Philadelphia, WB Saunders, 1995

SINDING-LARSEN-JOHANSSON

Synonyms. Sinding-Larsen; patellar chondropathy; osteochondritis patellae; chondromalacia patellae; including jumper knee. See Osgood-Schalatter.

Symptoms and Signs. Prevalent in boys in early teenage years. Pain and tenderness over inferior pole of patella. Limping; pain on flexion and slight swelling at area of tenderness.

Etiology. Traction apophysitis, related to overuse. Inflammation of a secondary or accessory center of calcification of patella (accessory center present in 3% of cases, in most cases remaining asymptomatic). Trauma or vascular disturbance considered important factor in initiating the osteochondritic process. Occasionally, autosomal dominant inheritance (male-to-male transmission).

Pathology. Synovial thickening; effusion; cartilage gray or yellow, fissured and flaking; loose bodies.

Diagnostic Procedure. *X-ray.* Fragmentation of patella.

Therapy. Rest; reassurance; immobilization seldom required. Testosterone to accelerate ossification.

Prognosis. Mild course. Recovery. It may persist into adolescence (see Jumper knee).

BIBLIOGRAPHY. Sinding-Larsen CMF: A hitherto unknown affection of the patella in children. Acta Radiol 1:171–173, 1921
Johansson S: En foerut icke beskriven sjnkdom i patella. Hygiea 84:161–166, 1922
Lopez R, Lewis H: Larsen-Johansson disease: Osteochondritis of the accessory ossification center of the patella. Clin Pediatr 7:697–700, 1968
Fulckerson JP, Hungerford DS: Imaging the patella femoral joint. In Disorders of the Patella Femoral Joint. Baltimore, Williams & Wilkins, 1990
Graham GP, Fairclough JA: The knee. In Klippel JH, Dieppe PA: Rheumatology, p 5.12.8. St Louis, CV Mosby, 1995

SINGLE ATRIUM

Synomyms. Common atrium; cor triloculare biventriculare.

Symptoms. Both sexes affected. Present from early age. Effort dyspnea; frequent respiratory infections; constant or transitory crying on exercise; cardiac failure (in severe form).

Signs. Physical appearance can be normal. In mild form: moderate cynosis after exercise or crying, red cheeks, and digital redness. In severe form: physical underdevelopment. Frequently associated with Ellis-van Creveld (see) and asplenia (see Ivemark) and polysplenia (see). On auscultation, pulse and precordial movements are those characterizing the large atrial septal defect.

Etiology. Congenital malformation.

Pathology. Complete absence of atrial septum; right and left sides of the common cavity have the respective characteristics of the right and left atrium.

Diagnostic Procedures. *ECG.* Tendency for leftward deviation of P-wave axis; QRS similar to those observed in endocardial cushion defect. Volume overload of right ventricle. *X-ray.* Size of right atrium unimpressive. *Two-dimensional echography with color flow imaging and spectral Doppler interrogation.*

Therapy. Surgical correction. Heart transplantation.

Prognosis. Extremely variable according to type and intensity of left-

to-right shunts or right-to-left shunts and pulmonary vascular resistance.

BIBLIOGRAPHY. Cunningham GJ: Trilocular heart with bilateral aneurysmal dilatation of pulmonary arteries. J Pathol Bacteriol 60:379–386, 1948
Nugent EW, Plauth WH, Edwards JE, et al: The pathology, pathophysiology, recognition and treatment of congenital heart disease. In Schlant RC, Alexander RW: Hurst's The Heart, 8th ed, p 1779. New York, McGraw-Hill, 1994
Perloff JK: The Clinical Recognition of Congenital Heart Disease, 4th ed, pp 328–333. Philadelphia, WB Saunders, 1994

SINGLETON-MERTEN

Synonyms. Aortic arch calcification; osteoporosis; toothbuds hypoplasia.

Symptoms and Signs. Occurs in both sexes. Failure of some teeth eruption; reduction in number; widening of hand bones; cardiomegaly; muscular weakness and poor physical development. Occasionally psoriatic skin manifestation.

Etiology. Sporadic.

Diagnostic Procedures. *X-ray.* Cardiomegaly; calcification of aortic arch; osteoporosis of cranial vault and long bones.

Prognosis. In two cases, death from ventricular fibrillation.

BIBLIOGRAPHY. Singleton EB, Merten DF: An unusual syndrome of widened medullary cavities of the metacarpals and phalanges, aortic calcification and abnormal dentition. Pediatr Radiol 2:2–4, 1973
Gay B Jr, Kuhn JP: A syndrome of widened medullary cavities of bone, aortic calcification, abnormal dentition and muscular weakness (The Singleton-Merten syndrome). Radiology 118:389–395, 1976

SINGLE VENTRICLE

Synonyms. Cor triloculare biatriatum. Common ventricle; univentricular heart. See Holmes.

Symptoms. Male to female ratio, 2–4:1. Present from birth. Frailty; orthopnea.

Signs. Moderate or absent cyanosis; edema; left sternal edge; holosystolic murmur of low pitch; blurred mid-diastolic or late diastolic murmur; accentuated second pulmonic sound. Cardiomegaly.

Etiology. Congenital malformation.

Pathology. Single ventricle with anatomic features of left ventricle; associated with two atria; two separated atrioventricular A-V valves enter the single ventricle, occasionally, joined to form a single valve. Possibly, stenosis or narrowing of pulmonary trunk.

Diagnostic Procedures. *Blood.* Polycythemia. *X-ray.* Cardiomegaly with globular shape. *Angiocardiography. ECG. Two-dimensional echocardiography with color flow imaging and spectral Doppler interrogation. Cardiac catheterization.*

Therapy. Medical management for congestive heart failure and anoxic periods; bacterial endocarditis prevention. Palliative surgery frequently needed.

Prognosis. Sixty percent of patients require hospital admission within first month of life.

BIBLIOGRAPHY. Chemineau, 1699, quoted by Perloff (see)
Peacock TB: On Malformations of the Human Heart. London, John Chercill, 1858
Perloff JK: The Clinical Recognition of Congenital Heart Disease, 4th ed, pp 635–657. Philadelphia, WB Saunders, 1994
Nugent EW, Plauth WH, Edwards JE, et al: The pathology, pathophysi-

ology recognition and treatment of congenital heart disease. In Schlant RC, Alexander RW: Hurst's The Heart, 8th ed, pp 1816–1817. New York, McGraw-Hill, 1994

SINOVIAL SHELF

Synonyms. Plica, medial shelf; patellar (medio) plica.

Symptoms and Signs. Usually adolescent girls with femors patellar dysplasia or condromalacia. Anterior knee pain (90%), swelling knee that gives away. Usually pain is referred to the medial femoral condyle. Symptoms are exacerbated by movement and may be associated with congenital malalignment. A thickened band may be palpated over femoral condile.

Etiology. Abnormal or hypertrophic plica in the knee (suprapatellar, medial, infrapatellar) that causes inflammation and pain.

Pathology. Plica may present hemorrhages or partial laceration.

Diagnostic Procedures. Arthroscopy diagnostic.

Therapy. *Medical.* Rest, anti-inflammatory drugs. *Surgical.* Arthroscopic resection of plica.

Prognosis. Good with treatment.

BIBLIOGRAPHY. Hughston JC, Stone M, Andrews JR: The suprapatellar plica: Its role in internal derangement of the knee. J Bone Joint Surg (Am) 55:1318–1324, 1973
Broukhim B, Fox JM, Blazine ME, et al: The synovial shelf syndrome. Clin Orthop 142:135–138, 1979
Fulckerson JP, Hungerford DS: Imaging the patello femoral joint. In Disorders of the Patello Femoral Joint. Baltimore, Williams & Wilkins, 1990
Insall JN, Windsor RE, Scott WN, et al (eds): Surgery of the Knee. New York, Churchill Livingstone, 1993

SIX S SIGN

Synonyms. Sunbed Suntan Sacro-Scapular Sparing Sign.

Symptoms and Signs. Usually women aged 18–35 years, using sunbeds with a transparent surface that allows the simultaneous irradiation of anterior and posterior aspects of the body. Total body tanning except for the presence of a palm-sized macule of untanned skin overlying the sacrum and two smaller symmetrical areas overlying the scapulae.

Etiology. Pressure and oxygen-deprivation that prevent UVA light effect on tanning.

Therapy. Advise patients on risk of long-term sunbed abuse.

BIBLIOGRAPHY. Payne CMER: The sunbed suntan sacroscapular sparing sign. Dermatology 190:172, 1995

SJAASTAD-DALE

Synonym. Hemicrania chronic, paroxysmal.

Symptoms and Signs. Those of cluster headache (see). Unilateral pains of temporo-orbital are paroxysmal of short duration (20–30 min). Different from cluster headache; episodes occur many times each day, for years.

Etiology. Unknown. See Migraine, classic.

Therapy. Different from cluster headache; attacks are stopped dramatically by indomethacin.

BIBLIOGRAPHY. Sjaastad O, Dale I: A new clinical headache entity: Chronic paroxysmal hemicrania. Acta Neurol Scand 54:140–156, 1976

Nappi G, Savoldi F: Headache: Diagnostic system and taxonomic criteria. London, J Libbey Eurotext, 1985
Cady RK, Fox AW: Treating the Headache Patient. New York, Marcel Dekker, 1994

SJÖGREN I

Synonyms. Gougerot-Sjögren; Gougerot-Houwer-Sjögren; dacryosialoadenopathia atrophicans; keratoconjunctivitis sicca—xerostomia; secreto-inhibitor—xerodermatostenosis. KCS; SS.

Symptoms and Signs. Prevalent in females (80–90%). Onset in middle age (36% before menopause; 64% at or after menopause). In male patients, average age at onset 47 years. Insidious onset. Diminution or cessation of lacrimation (keratoconjunctivitis sicca KCS) (A); of salivary gland secretion (xerostomia) (B); pharyngitis; laryngitis; rhinitis sicca; swelling of parotid gland (50% initial symptoms). Polyarthritis (C). Combinations of AB, AC, BC diagnostic. When associated with autoimmune rheumatic disease defined as secondary SS. Other possible association: excessive dental cavities; tracheobronchitis; vaginitis; achlorhydria; Raynaud phenomenon; purpura; arteritis; focal myositis; neuropathy; alopecia; splenomegaly; hepatomegaly.

Etiology. Unknown. Possible factors; endocrine; infectious; allergic; autoimmune; congenital or familial (autosomal or recessive); associated with collagen disorders 30–60% in patients with rheumatoid arthritis and 20–70% with scleroderma.

Pathology. In parotid gland, lymphocytic infiltration with recognizable architecture of gland, not folliculoid pattern, proliferation of myoepithelial cells, atrophy of some acini (pattern similar to Mikulicz pattern, see). Alacrimal keratoconjunctivitis with lymphocytic infiltration. In submandibular, tracheal, esophageal, vaginal, subepithelial mucous glands, similar pattern with parotid gland. In kidney (occasional), chronic interstitial nephritis. Focal myositis (occasional); focal peripheral arteritis (occasional).

Diagnostic Procedures. Labial salivary gland biopsy. Initially focal periductal lymphocytic infiltration that eventually replaces normal ducts and acini; in major salivary glands presence of myoepithelial islands surrounded by lymphocytes. *Schirmer test.* Measure of extent to which a thin paper strip inserted into conjunctival sac is moistened. *Sialography. Blood.* Leukopenia; eosinophilia; thrombocytopenia; hyperglobulinemia; cephalin flocculation; thymol turbidity; rheumatoid factor (in 70%); tissue antibodies; antibodies against cytoplasmic antigens SS-A (or Ro) and SS-B (or La); RANA antigen and antibodies against salivary ducts increased sedimentation rate.

Therapy. Corticosteroids; adrenocorticotropic hormone (ACTH); occlusion of the puncta by electrocautery may alleviate keratoconjunctivitis. Topical fibronectin.

Prognosis. Chronic disease, only partially responsive to treatment. Usually, mild form for years, then some patients may develop lymphoma or reticular cell sarcoma or simple generalized adenopathy (pseudolymphoma). Other cases complicated by various collagen diseases.

BIBLIOGRAPHY. von Graefes AF: Demonstration in der Berliner Medizinischen Gesellschaft. Klin Wochenschr 5:127, 1868
Sjögren H: Zur Kenntnis der Keratoconjunctivitis sicca (Keratitis filiformis bei Hypofunktion der Tramendrüsen). Acta Ophth (Suppl II) 1–151, 1933
Sjögren H: A new conception of kerato-conjunctivitis sicca. Hamilton JB (trans), Sidney, Australasian Medical, 1943
Hakin KN, Lightman S: The eye in systemic immune disorders. In Garner A, Klintworth GK (eds): Pathobiology of Ocular Disease: A Dynamic Approach, 2nd ed, pp 191–193. New York, Marcel Dekker, 1994
Weatherall DJ, Ledingham JGG, Warrell DA: Oxford Textbook of Medicine, pp 3036–3038. Oxford, Oxford Med Pub, 1996

SJÖREN-LARSSON

Synonyms. Spastic diplegia; ichthyosis; oligophrenia; ichthyosiform erythroderma. See Ichthyosis syndromes and Rud.

Symptoms. No sex predilection. Consanguinity between parents; high incidence in siblings. Neurologic disorders seldom diagnosed at birth, usually within first year. Stiff awkward movement of legs, then in the arms (spastic diplegia). Severe mental deficiency (idiocy or imbecility). No patients reported with low or normal intelligence.

Signs. Usually evident at birth. Scalp hair normal or thin and brittle; moderate hyperkeratosis face and scalp; slightly scaling ichthyosis of trunk, back, neck, and extremities (more marked in flexural areas). Erythema of various degrees; moderate hyperkeratosis of palms and soles, but no keratoderma. Dysplasia of tooth enamel may be present. Macular lesions and recurrent corneal ulceration may be observed. Deep hyperreflexia for the legs; ankle clonus; Babinski sign; minor or no hyperreflexia for the arms. Short stature.

Etiology. Fatty alcohol oxidoreductase deficiency causes accumulation of long-chain fatty alcohol; autosomal recessive inheritance.

Pathology. On skin biopsy, hyperkeratosis and acanthosis; stratum granulosum diminished or absent. No reported autopsy studies.

Diagnostic Procedures. *Biopsy.* Of skin (see Pathology). *CT scan. MRI.* Hydrocephalus; sclerotic cortical atrophy; no intracerebral calcifications. *EEG.* Slow paroxysmal activity.

Therapy. Symptomatic, corneal graft to save sight when there are corneal ulcerations. Proposed diet of medium-chain triglycerides.

Prognosis. Spastic diplegia usually remains stationary after 5 years of life.

BIBLIOGRAPHY. Pardo-Castello V, Faz H: Ichthyosis: Little's disease. Arch Dermatol 26:915, 1932

Sjögren T, Larsson T: Oligophrenia in combination with congenital ichthyosis and spastic disorders: A clinical and genetic study. Acta Psychiatr Neurol Scand 32 (Suppl 113):1–112, 1957

Jagell S, Linden S: Ichthyosis in the Sjögren-Larsson syndrome. Clin Genet 21:243–252, 1982

Weatherall DJ, Ledingham JGG, Warrell DA: Oxford Textbook of Medicine, p 3985. Oxford, Oxford Med Pub, 1996

SKIN PEELING

Synonyms. Skin shedding, keratolysis exfoliativa, congenita deciduous skin; peeling skin.

Symptoms and Signs. Rare 20 cases circa reported. Continuous or periodic seasonal shedding of extensive areas of body skin (statum corneum) hyperkeratosis of palms and soles (usualy spared of massive peeling), nail spared (but in one case); easily pluckable anagen hairs (in one case). Short stature (in two cases). General good health.

Etiology. Sporadic or possibly autosomal recessive inheritance.

Pathology. Massive desquamation of thick layer of stratum corneum.

Diagnostic Procedures. *Blood. Urine.* Usually normal findings. In two cases aminoaciduria, decreased plasma tryptophan levels (in the cases with short stature).

Therapy. Symptomatic bland oil application.

Prognosis. Continuous or recurrent manifestation.

BIBLIOGRAPHY. Stone RM: Keratolysis or "skin shedding." JAMA 35:557, 1900

Fox H: Skin shedding (keratolysis exfoliativa congenita): Report of a case. Arch Dermatol 3:202, 1921

Tolat SN, Gharpuray MB: Skin peeling syndrome. Cutis 53:255–257, 1994

SLEEP APNEA

Symptoms and Signs. All ages. Three varieties of syndromes identified.

1. *Predominant obstructive type.* Frequently overweight, short and fat neck. Average age 46 years; daytime fatigue, deficit in learning, memory, and vocabulary.
2. *Predominantly central sleep apnea.* Usually normal or under weight; average age 63 years; no daytime fatigue. Apneic events lead to cardiac arrhythmias and to arousal.
3. *Mixed type.* Features of type 1 and 2. Frequently hypertension. Type 1 subjects awake: normal pulmonary function; subject sleeping: apneic events, frequently accompanied by cardiac arrhythmias and hemodynamic changes.

Etiology. Multifactorial.

Diagnostic Procedures. *Type I.* Sleep-induced airway obstruction or upper airway apnea. *Type II.* Decreased diaphragmatic activity during sleep. During sleep various techniques noninvasive or invasive (in severe forms) to document number and predominant type of apneic events. *ECG.* 24-hour monitoring. Progressive sinus bradycardia during episodes, followed by abrupt reversal and sinus acceleration at termination; may occur also atrioventricular blocks, prolonged sinus pause, ventricular tachycardia, atrial fibrillation. *Systemic and pulmonary arterial pressure:* rise during episodes.

Therapy. Weight loss; atropine sulfate and oxygen (in severe cases use compressed positive airway pressure. C-pap), blunt the marked sinus variations. Propanolol no obvious effect.

Prognosis. Life-threatening arrhythmias and sudden death during sleep possible. It seems, however, that the prevalence of serious arrhythmias and conduction defects during sleep in patients with this syndrome is lower than reported.

BIBLIOGRAPHY. Bond WC, Ebey J Jr, Welf S: Rhythm heart rate variability (sinus arrhythmias) related to stages of sleep. Cond Reflex 8:98–107, 1973

Tilkian AG, Guilleminault C, Schroeder KL, et al: Sleep induced apnea syndrome: Prevalence of cardiac arrhythmias and their reversal after tracheostomy. Am J Med 63:348–358, 1977

Miller WP: Cardiac arrhythmias and conduction disturbances in the sleep apnea syndrome. Prevalence and significance. Am J Med 73:317–321, 1982

Weatherall DJ, Ledingham JGG, Warrell DA: Oxford Textbook of Medicine, pp 2909, 2916–2918. Oxford, Oxford Med Pub, 1996

SLIM DISEASE

Symptoms and Signs. Fever, itching maculopapular, general malaise, prolonged diarrhea, occasional respiratory symptoms. Maculopapular rash, oral candidiasis; extreme wasting and weight loss. Lymphadenopathy and Kaposi sarcoma are not as common in slim disease as found among western homosexual patients with AIDS. Kaposi sarcoma is commoner among slim disease patients than among western hemophiliacs infected with AIDS virus.

Etiology. HTLV-III infection, transmitted by heterosexual contact, homosexual contact, insect vectors such as mosquitos, bed bugs or lice, and injections.

Diagnostic Procedures. HTLV-III serum. ELISA assay.

Therapy. Antibiotics. Symptomatic treatment.

Prognosis. Not known (a very new disease).

BIBLIOGRAPHY. Serwadda D, Mugerwa R, Sewan-Kambo N, et al: Slim disease: A new disease in Uganda and its association with HTLV-III infection. Lancet 2:849–852, 1985

Weatherall DJ, Ledingham JGG, Warrell DA: Oxford Textbook of Medicine, pp 485, 487, 4078. Oxford, Oxford Med Pub, 1996

SLIT VENTRICLE

Symptoms and Signs. *Acute form.* Symptoms of increased intracranial pressure; symptoms of cerebral edema; decrease of the consciousness level. *Subacute form.* Increased tendency to convulsions; headache; ataxia; balance disturbances; changed sleeping patterns and drowsiness; nausea. *Chronic form.* Recurrent and postural symptoms, as in the subacute form.

Etiology. Overdrainage of cerebrospinal fluid (CSF) in patients with hydrocephalus who had a ventriculoatrial or ventriculoperitoneal shunt.

Pathology. *Acute form.* Subdural effusion and epidural hemorrhage. *Subacute and chronic forms.* Collapsed ventricles, ventricular catheter closed by the ventricular wall, no CSF drained through the shunt. The chronically collapsed ventricle loses its flexibility and does not reinflate easily.

Diagnostic Procedures. *CT scan.* Acute and subacute form: collapsed ventricles, periventricular lucency, subarachnoid accumulation of CSF; chronic form: recurrent, total, or partial collapse of ventricles. *EEG.* Increased abnormalities.

Therapy. Replacement of the valve with a high resistance one; use of an antisiphon device; full neurosurgical evaluation.

BIBLIOGRAPHY. Hide-Brown MD, Rekate HL, Nulsen FE: Re-expansion of previously collapsed ventricles: The slit ventricle syndrome. J Neurosurg. 56:536–539, 1981
Epstein F, Lapras C, Wisoff JH: Slit ventricle syndrome: etiology and treatment. Pediatr Neurosci 14:5–10, 1988
Adams RD, Victor M: Principles of Neurology, 5th ed, p 547. New York, McGraw-Hill, 1993

SLOW CHANNEL

Synonyms. See myasthenic syndromes.

Symptoms and Signs. Onset may vary. Progression is gradual and intermittent. Severe involvement with weakness and fatigability of cervical, scapular, and finger extensor muscles. Moderate weakness of eyelid elevators, occasionally diplopia. Legs usually are spared, whereas trunk and arm muscles may be affected. Tendon reflexes usually normal.

Etiology. Autosomal dominant gene with high penetrance and variable expressivity. Also sporadic cases. Mutation of AChR subunit that hinders closure of AChR ion channel.

Pathology. *Muscle.* Predominance of type I fibers with variations in size and increase of connective tissue. *Electron microscopy.* Functional fields degeneration with electron dense debris.

Diagnostic Procedures. *Muscle biopsy.* EMG. Single nerve stimuli evoke repetitive compound muscle action potentials. Decremental response at 2–3 Hz stimulation; decay of MEEP and EPP is prolonged. *AChR antibody test.* Negative. AChE inibitors ineffective.

Therapy. Until now flunarizine has proven ineffective.

Prognosis. Slowly progressive condition.

BIBLIOGRAPHY. Engel AG, Lambert EH, Mulder DM, et al: A newly recognized congenital myasthenic syndrome attributed to a prolonged open time of the acetylcholine-induced ion channel. Ann Neurol 11:553–569, 1982
Engel AG, Walls TJ, Nagel A, et al: Newly recognized congenital myasthenic syndromes. I. Congenital paucity of synaptic vesicles and reduced quantal release. II. High conductance fast channel syndrome. III. Abnormal acetylcholine receptor (AChR) interaction with ace-

tylcholine. IV. AChR deficiency and short channel open time. Prog Brain Res 84, 125–137, 1990

SLUDER

Synonyms. Lower facial neuralgia; sphenopalatine neuralgia; sphenopalatine ganglion neuralgia. See also Ethmoidal anterior nerve and Charlin.

Symptoms. Episodic recurrences of vague head pains, in nose and orbit (maxillary division of fifth cranial nerve) and occasionally in other parts of face. Also, shoulder and neck pains, never extending over the ear. Associated congestion of nose and eye; lacrimation. Attacks last minutes, hours, or days.

Etiology. Sphenopalatine ganglion irritation. Little reason to believe that such condition exists (Grinker) as an autonomous entity; variant of cluster headache.

Therapy. Injection of the ganglion with alcohol or application of cocaine over the ganglion reported effective by some authors. Others were not successful with this treatment.

BIBLIOGRAPHY. Sluder G: The role of sphenopalatine (Meckel's) ganglion in nasal headaches. NY Med J 87:989–990, 1908
Olen J (Chairman): Classification and diagnostic criteria for headache disorders cranial neuralgia and facial pain. Cephalalgia 8 (Suppl 7), 1988
Camaioni D, Camaioni A, Sabato AF, et al: La sindrome di Sluder edi Charlin. Contributo clinico. Agopuntura e tecniche di terapia antalgica, Vol VI, N. I, p17–20, 1989

SLY

Synonyms. Mucopolysaccharidosis VII; MPS VII; beta-glucuronidase deficiency.

Symptoms. Both sexes affected. Onset in early infancy or later (milder form with onset after 4 years of life). Repeated respiratory infections. Visual impairment; mental and physical retardation (not constant).

Signs. From delayed growth to normal stature. *Facies.* Coarse. Gross corneal clouding (not constant); other occasional findings are hepatosplenomegaly, umbilical, or inguinal hernias, anterior chest deformities, vertebral column deformities, extremity deformities (e.g., clubfoot, genu valgum, metatarsus adductus).

Etiology. Deficiency of beta-glucuronidase responsible for block of degradation of heparan sulfate. Autosomal recessive inheritance. Several alleles postulated as responsible for different phenotypes. Gene encoding-glucuronidase is localized on chromosome 7q21.1–q22.

Diagnostic Procedures. Test for glucuronidase. In fibroblast leukocytes and serum. *Blood.* Inclusion bodies in leukocytes. Prenatal diagnosis is now possible.

Therapy. Allogeneic bone marrow transplantation. Attempts with enzyme and gene replacement are presently under development.

Prognosis. Variable; periods of survival not yet assessed.

BIBLIOGRAPHY. Sly WS, Quinton BA, McAlister WN, et al: Beta-glucuronidase deficiency. Report of clinical, radiological and biochemical features of a new mucopolysaccharidosis. J Pediatr 82:249–257, 1973
Neufeld EF, Muenzer J: The mucopolysaccharidoses. In Scriver CR, Beaudet AL, Sly WS, et al: The Metabolic and Molecular Bases of Inherited Disease, 7th ed, p 2478. New York, McGraw-Hill, 1995

SMALL

Synonyms. Coat disease; deafness; muscular dystrophy mental retardation.

Symptoms and Signs. Both sexes. From birth. Visual impairment, neural deafness, immobile facies, muscular weakness, accentuated spinal curvature, mental retardation.

Etiology. Unknown. Autosomal recessive trait.

Pathology. Fundus oculi: vessels tortuosity, telangiectases, retinal detachment. Type of muscular defect not identified.

Diagnostic Procedures. Fundus oculi. Tortuosity of retinal vessels, exudative retinitis.

Prognosis. Muscle disease progresses from childhood.

BIBLIOGRAPHY. Small RG: Coat's disease and muscular dystrophy. Trans Am Acad Ophthalmol Otolaryngol 72:225–231, 1968

SMALL CUFF

Synonym. Nonhypertension.

Symptoms and Signs. When a small cuff is used to determine arterial pressure, gross error may result in the auscultatory systolic and diastolic values. Erroneous diagnosis may result with unnecessary anxiety and possibly therapeutic mismanagement. To determine the blood pressure in infants and children where this situation may more easily arise, the use of cuffs of different sizes is suggested. In newborn; 2.5 cm cuff; in infants (2 weeks to 1 year), 5.0 cm cuff; in children (1–13 years), 9.0 cm cuff. The same concept applies to extremely obese patients where a larger cuff has to be used instead of the regular one.

BIBLIOGRAPHY. Robinow M, Hamilton WF, Woodbury RA, et al: Accuracy of clinical determination of blood pressure in children with values under normal and abnormal conditions. Am J Dis Child 58:102–118, 1939
Hansen RL, Stickler GB: The "nonhypertension" or "small-cuff" syndrome. Clin Pediatr 5:579–580, 1966
O'Rourke RA: Physical examination of the arteries and veins (including blood pressure determination). In Hurst JW: The Heart, 6th ed, p 139. New York, McGraw-Hill, 1986

SMITH-LEMLI-OPITZ

Synonyms. Cerebrohepatorenal. SLO, RSH (initials of three families).

Symptoms. Onset in fetal life. (Feeble fetal activity; at birth short stature.) Prevalent in males. Growth retardation; failure to thrive; mental retardation; vomiting in infancy.

Signs. Several combinations of the following features: short stature; moderate muscle hypertonicity or, more rarely, hypotonicity; microcephaly. Epicanthal folds; ptosis of eyelids; strabismus; broad nose; upturned nares; micrognathia; arched palate; posterior palatal cleft. Ear auricles low set, abnormal shape; small external canal. Hypospadias; cryptorchidism. Hands with horizontal upper palmar creases; dermal pattern 10/10 whorls; distal palmer axial triradius; short third fingers; short thumb and toes; cutaneous syndactyly of second and third toes; metatarsus adductus.

Etiology. Unknown. Autosomal recessive inheritance.

Pathology. See Signs. Small brain, kidneys; duplication of pelvis; cortical renal cysts; congenital pyloric stenosis in some cases. Hepatomegaly; intrahepatic biliary dysgenesis. Congenital heart diseases may be associated.

Diagnostic Procedures. *EEG. X-ray. Chromosome studies.*

Therapy. Symptomatic.

Prognosis. Death from complications at early age. Survival to adulthood reported.

BIBLIOGRAPHY. Smith DW, Lemli L, Opitz JM: Newly recognized syndrome of multiple congenital anomalies. J Pediatr 64:210–217, 1964
Fine RN, Gwin JL, Young EF: Smith-Lemli-Opitz syndrome, radiologic and postmortem findings. Am J Dis Child 115:483–488, 1968
Opitz JM, Penchaszadeh VB, Holt MC, et al: Smith-Lemli-Opitz (RSM) syndrome bibliography. AM J Med Genet 28:745–750, 1987
Lachman MF, Wright Y, Whiteman DAH, et al: Brief clinical report: A 46, XY Phenotypic female wuth Smith-Lemli-Opitz syndrome. Clin Genet 39:136–141, 1991
Weatherall DJ, Ledingham JGG, Warrell DA: Oxford Textbook of Medicine, pp 130, 4111, 4121. Oxford, Oxford Med Pub, 1996

SMITH-McCORT

Synonyms. Osteochondrodystrophy, Eponym suggested for a case of Dyggve-Melchior-Clausen (see), with normal intelligence.

BIBLIOGRAPHY. Smith R, McCort J: Osteochondrodystrophy (Morquio-Brailsford Type). Cal Med 88:55–59, 1958
Kaufman RL: Mental retardation with dwarfism (Dyggve-Melchior-Clausen syndrome). In Vinken PJ, Bruyn GW: Handbook of Clinical Neurology, vol 43, p 266. Amsterdam, North-Holland, 1982

SMITH (R.W.)

Synonym. Reversed Colles fracture.

Symptoms. Pain in the wrist following fall on dorsum of flexed hand.

Signs. Tenderness. Spade handle deformity.

Pathology. Nonarticular fracture of distal radius with dorsal angulation and volar displacement.

Therapy. Open reduction seldom indicated except in young adult.

BIBLIOGRAPHY. Smith RW: Fractures of the Bones of the Fore-arm in the Vicinity of the Wrist Joint in His: A Treatise on Fracture in the Vicinity of Joint and on Certain Forms of Accidental and Congenital Dislocations, pp 129–175. Dublin, Hodges Smith, 1847
Saito H, Takahashi Y, Zenzai K: Intra-articular fracture of the distal radius: Treatment and results. In Vastamaeki M: Current Trends in Hand Surgery. Netherlands, Excerpta Medica, 1995

SMOKER RESPIRATORY

Synonym. Tabagism.

Symptoms. Occurs in smokers of all ages. Chronic condition with exacerbation after increase in smoking. Chronic pharyngitis; hoarseness; cough and expectoration; wheezing relieved by expectoration. Occasionally, dyspnea, chest constriction, and pain may be observed.

Signs. Those of chronic pharyngitis and bronchitis.

Etiology. Tobacco smoke.

Pathology. Chronic bronchitis and inflammatory changes and edema of pharynx and larynx.

Diagnostic Procedures. *X-ray.* Of chest.

Therapy. Eliminate cause (stop smoking). Antibiotics in acute stage.

Prognosis. Excellent if smoking is stopped.

BIBLIOGRAPHY. Fogg AH: Queries and minor notes: Allergy to tobacco smoke. JAMA 144:810–811, 1950
Waldbott GL: Smoker's respiratory syndrome: A clinical entity. JAMA 151:1398–1400, 1953
Hunninghake GW, Crystal RG: Cigarette smoking and lung destruction. Am J Respir Dis 128:833–838, 1983

Weatherall DJ, Ledingham JGG, Warrell DA: Oxford Textbook of Medicine, pp 2674–2675. Oxford, Oxford Med Pub, 1996

SNEDDON

Synonyms. Livedo reticularis, systemic involvement. Includes anti-cardiolipin (possibly same condition).

Symptoms and Signs. Predominantly affects young females with onset after menarche. Those of livedo reticularis (see), associated with arterial disease involving cerebral, ocular, coronary, renal and peripheral arteries. Frequent Raynaud phenomenon (see).

Etiology. Sporadic in some cases autosomal dominant inheritance observed. Female reproductive hormones, antiphospholipid antibodies vasculitis have been hypothesized as possible etiologic factors.

Pathology. Intimal proliferation involving small and medium-sized cutaneous arteries, leading to considerable reduction of vascular lumen, similar changes may be observed also in other organs.

Diagnostic Procedures. See livedo reticularis. Only some cases shows the presence of anticardiolipin or lupus anticoagulant.

Therapy. Low-dose aspirin and dipyridamole. Corticosteroids and immunosuppressive drugs not effective.

Prognosis. Poor. Death caused by thrombosis.

BIBLIOGRAPHY. Sneddon IB: Cerebro-vascular lesions and livedo reticularis. Br J De4rmatol 77:180–185, 1965
Burton JL: Cutaneous polyarteritis nodosa, porcellain white scars and cerebral thromboses. Lancet I:1263–1264, 1988
Al Meshari K, Al Eisa A, Akthar M: Sneddon's syndrome: A systemic arterio-occlusive disorder. Am J Kid Dis 26:368–372, 1995
Weatherall DJ, Ledingham JGG, Warrell DA: Oxford Textbook of Medicine, pp 3020, 3724. Oxford, Oxford Med Pub, 1996

SNEDDON-WILKINSON

Synonyms. Duhring-Sneddon-Wilkinson; subcorneal pustular dermatosis.

Symptoms and Signs. Predominantly in women (4:1). Onset after 40 years of age. Seldom in children. Eruption of pustules in the groin, axillae, submammary areas, flexor surfaces of limbs, occasionally palms and soles. Face and mucosae spared. Erythema around pustules at onset. Pustules are usually oval, flaccid, turbid. They dry in a few days, leaving superficial crusts. Their grouping produces a serpiginous outline.

Etiology. Unknown. Possibly a variant of Stevens-Johnson. Reported in association with IgA and IgG gammopathy pyoderma gangrenosum and ulcerative colitis.

Pathology. Subcorneal pustule, covered by thin keratin layer; base formed by granular tissue or prickle cells layer. In the fluid, many neutrophils and red cells, scanty eosinophils. Mild acanthosis; questionable acantholysis; no bacteria.

Diagnostic Procedures. *Biopsy.*

Therapy. Dapsone 100 mg a day. If gammopathy found vitamin A acid, and corticosteroid topically.

Prognosis. Benign condition of several years duration. Possible myeloma appearance in older patients.

BIBLIOGRAPHY. Sneddon IB, Wilkinson DS: Subcorneal postular dermatosis. Br J Dermatol 68:385–394, 1956
Sneddon IB, Wilkinson DS: Dermatose pustuleuse sous-cornée. Bull Soc Fr Dermatol Syph 64:226–233, 1957
Pye RJ: Bullous eruptions. In Champion RH, Burton JL, Ebling FJG (eds): Rook/Wilkinson/Ebling Textbook of Dermatology, 5th ed, pp 1669–1670. Oxford, Blackwell Scientific, 1992

SOEMMERING

Synonyms. Ring cataract Soemmering; post cataract surgery.

Symptoms and Signs. After cataract surgery or spontaneous or traumatic loss of internal content of lens. Proliferation of new fibers that form an opaque doughnut-shaped lens.

Etiology. See Symptoms and Signs.

Pathology. Anterior and posterior part of lens capsule apposed and new lens fibers appear on the equatorial region of lens.

BIBLIOGRAPHY. Soemmering W: Beobachtungen ueber die organischen Veraenderungen im Auge nach Staaroperationen. Frankfurt, 1828
Klintword GK, Garner A: The causes types and morphology of cataracts. In Garner A, Klintworth GK (eds): Pathobiology of Ocular Disease: A Dynamic Approach, 2nd ed, p 519. New York, Marcel Dekker, 1994

SOLAR ELASTOSIS AND KERATOSIS SYNDROMES

Synonyms. Actinodermatosis; lucite, chronic; keratosis, includes acrokeratoelastosis; Dubreuilh; Jodassohn cutis rhomboidalis nuchal; Milian citron skin; Path.

Symptoms. Both sexes. Occurring usually at late age (fourth decade) in people subjected to prolonged exposure to the sun.

Signs. May be different and combinations have been designed by various eponyms:

1. *Acrokeratoelastosis.* Small, warty papules, yellowish or pinkish, in narrow bands; occasionally, telangiectasic at the border or palmodorsal skin of hand, from tip of thumb to radial side of index finger.
2. *Debreuilh.* Yellow plaques, more or less marginated on face or neck.
3. *Favre-Racouchot.* (see).
4. *Jadassohn cutis rhomboidalis nuchal.* Skin of back of neck thickened by yellowish infiltration subdivided by furrows in a network-like pattern; occasionally lesion extends to the sides and upper chest.
5. *Milian citron skin.* Yellowish thickening and wrinkling of the skin.
6. *Path.* Multiple keratotic lesions of the skin with pattern similar to squamous carcinomas; spontaneously disappear.

Etiology. Sun exposure; trauma; possibly, genetic factors also involved.

Pathology. Elastotic degeneration of collagen into amorphous elastotic mass with blood vessels becoming sparse and tortuous.

Therapy. Sunscreens for susceptible persons.

BIBLIOGRAPHY. Debreuilh MW: De la melanose circonscrite precancereuse. Ann Dermatol Syph (Paris) 3:129–151, 205–230, 1912
Milian G, Manson M: Erytheme polymorphe photobiotrophique avec localization préternale. Bull Soc Fr Dermatol 39:651–652, 1932
Path DD: Tumor-like keratosis: Report of a case. Arch Dermatol 39:228–238, 1936
Burton JL: Disorders of connective tissue. In Champion RH, Burton JL, Ebling FJG (eds): Rook/Wilkinson/Ebling Textbook of Dermatology, 5th ed, p 1787. Oxford, Blackwell Scientific, 1992

SOLITARY HUNTER

Synonyms. Lonely hunter; monosomatic hypochondrial psychosis pain-prone; psychogenic pain. See Women who fall syndrome.

Symptoms. Average age at onset 28 years. Intractable pain, not organic, with evidence of psychogenic nature; solitary hunting; conflict over the expression of aggression and depression; tendency to drive fast cars; accident proneness; unrealistic ambitions and problems with work.

Etiology. Patients with this syndrome do not belong to any definite psychiatric category. Character disorders with problems of impulse, control, and conversion symptoms. Hunting and solitude may be considered defense against murderous impulses. Pain as atonement for guilt feeling. Different clinical syndromes (masochism, pain proneness, phantom limb pain, primary atypical facial neuralgia, late-onset schizophrenia, involutionary psychotic reaction, and some painful post-traumatic states) belong (with others) to this entity (psychogenic pain).

Therapy. Difficult. Positive approach and showing that pains are real; cautious referral to psychiatrist. Some results reported with pimozide, haloperidole, trycyclic antidepressants, monoaminooxidase inhibitor traylcypromine, and selective serotonin re-uptake inhibitors. Hospitalization may be necessary.

Prognosis. Progressively unable to perform work, and progressive depression.

BIBLIOGRAPHY. Engel GL: "Psychogenic" pain and the pain-prone patient. Am J Med 26:899–918, 1959
Tinling DC, Klein RF: Psychogenic pain and aggression: The syndrome of solitary hunter. Psychosom Med 28:738–748, 1966
Sedler MJ: The Psychiatric Clinics of North America: Delusional Disorders, p 384. Philadelphia, WB Saunders, 1995

SOLITARY RECTAL ULCER

Synonyms. SRUS; Hamartomatous malformation, congenital; colitis cystica profunda localized.

Symptoms and Signs. In fourth–fifth decade. Male to female ratio 1:2. Rectal bleeding (95%), staining of stool (60%), mucous discharge (50%), rectal prolapse (50–80%), especially in anterior rectal wall, constipation (40%), diarrhea (20%), tenesmus (40%).

Etiology. Probably not single etiology. Rectal prolapse or intussusception, high intrarectal pressure, pudendal nerve neuropathy.

Pathology. Fibrous obliteration of lamina propria, extension of muscle fibers into lamina propria in localized colitis cystica prufonda (LCCP) also mucus-filled cysts.

Diagnostic Procedures. *Sigmoidoscopy.* Presence of mucosal ulcerations and erosion in the rectum. In 30–50% of patients no ulcer is present, only erythema and granulation. In LCCP (possibly an early stage of SRUS) mucus-filled cysts are observed in submucosa of colon.

Therapy. Conservative therapy unsuccessful. Sucralfate enemas; surgery; local excision of affected areas; abdominal rectopexy, in some cases diverting colectomy.

Prognosis. Fair with therapy. Recurrences possible.

BIBLIOGRAPHY. Cruveilheir J: Ulcere chronique due to rectum In Anatomie pathologique du corps humaine. Maladie due rectum V2 Libre 25 Paris, Balliere, 1829
Madigan MR: Solitary ulcer of the rectum. Proc R Soc Med 57:403, 1964
Maxson CS, Klein HD, Rubin W: Atypical forms of inflammatory bowel disease. Med Clin N Amer 78:1259–1273, 1994

SOLUTE LOADING-HYPERTONICITY

Synonym. Water loss, solute excess.

Symptoms and Signs. The same as in pure water depletion syndrome, with two exceptions: (1) Patient gains, instead of loses, weight. (2) Patient is polyuric with low specific gravity urine instead of oliguric.

Etiology and Pathology. Nasogastric feeding with inadequate water. Bleeding ulcer patient treated with milk and alkali, without adequate water. Infants fed with too-concentrated milk. Diabetic with polyuria or when overtreated with unnecessary electrolyte replacement and insulin.

Diagnostic Procedures. *Urine.* Polyuria with low specific gravity.

Therapy. The same as in pure water depletion syndrome (see) plus the correction of iatrogenic causes.

Prognosis. If condition not recognized and treated early, death occurs.

BIBLIOGRAPHY. Goldberger E: A Primer of Water, Electrolyte, and Acid-base Syndromes, 3rd ed. Philadelphia, Lea & Febiger, 1965
Garcia-Perez A, Burg MB: Role of organic osmolytes in adaptation of renal cells to high osmolality. J Memb Biol 119:1–13, 1991
Senkfor SI, Anger MS, Berl T: Control of water excretion. In Massry SG, Glassock RJ: Textbook of Nephrology, 3rd ed, pp 288–292. Baltimore, Williams & Wilkins, 1995

SOMATOSTATINOMA

Symptoms and Signs. Rare (1/40 million). Malabsorption and steatorrhea. Weight loss. Frequently associated with von Recklinghausen type I (see). Symptoms related to diabetes (90%) present in patient with pancreatic tumor. In case of duodenal tumor, cholestatic jaundice.

Etiology. Tumor producing somatostatin (tetradecapeptide) substance with neurocrine or paracrine activity: suppression of secretion of growth hormone, of thyrotropin, and inhibition of numerous intestinal endocrine and exocrine functions (all intestinal hormones release). It is produced by the D-cells of pancreas and gut and found in ganglia and nerve cells of intestine. Also may be associated with other endocrine tumor of gastroenteropancreatic axis.

Pathology. Two main types: Pancreatic (large). Duodenal (small and well-localized). The presence of elevated somatostatin in the tumor may be evidenced by immunohistochemical staining. Frequently metastatic at time of discovery.

Diagnostic Procedures. *Blood.* Evidence of mild diabetes mellitus (nonketotic except for rare exceptions). Seldom hypoglycemia. Somatostatic levels increased (RIA methodology). Differential rate of release of S14 and S28 account for different clinical manifestations. *Ultrasound. Endoscopy.* For tumor localization. *X-ray.* Cholelithiasis and gallbladder reduced contractility. *Gastric juice.* Hypochlorhydria, decreased gastrin release. *Stool.* Steatorrhea, evidence of exocrine pancreatic secretion.

Therapy. Surgery with tumor debulking, followed by chemotherapy or palliation with chemotherapy or hepatic embolization.

BIBLIOGRAPHY. Larson LI, Holst JJ, Kuhl C, et al: Pancreatic somatostatinoma: Clinical features and physiological implications. Lancet 1:666–668, 1977
Harris GJ, Tio F, Cruz AB: Somastatinoma: A case report and review of the literature. J Surg Oncol 36:8–16, 1987
Ohtsuki Y, Sonobe H, Mizobuchi T, et al: Duodenal carcinoid (Somastatinoma) combined with von Recklinghasen's disease: A case report and review of the literature. Acta Pathol Jpn 39:141–146, 1989

SORIANO (M.)

Synonym. Periostitis deformans. See Leri-Joanny.

Symptoms and Signs. Both sexes affected. Recurrent pains in areas of bone where the formation of pseudotumoral masses occurs. The attack may recur several times. During more severe episodes anorexia and general debilitation may be associated.

Etiology. Unknown.

Pathology. Hyperplastic osteogenic osteoperiostitis.

Diagnostic Procedures. *X-ray.* Of bones.

Therapy. Analgesics.

Prognosis. In 2–12 months, regression of the masses. Each individual attack is less severe than the previous one.

BIBLIOGRAPHY. Soriano M: Periostitis deformans. Ann Rheum Dis 11:154–161, 1952

SORSBY I

Synonyms. Macular hereditary coloboma. Coloboma of macula-brachydactyly B; apical dystrophy; coloboma of macula. See also Laurence-Moon and Biemond.

Symptoms. Both sexes affected. Onset from birth. Reduced visual acuity.

Signs. *Hands and feet.* Dystrophy; rudimentary or absent nails of index fingers; bifurcation of distal phalanges of thumbs; absence of big toes; hallux valgus. *Face.* Cleft palate. *Eye.* Hyperopia; nystagmus; bilateral macular colobomas with variable pigmentation and sharp borderline.

Etiology. Autosomal dominant inheritance.

Pathology. See Signs. Kidney aplasia. Chondrocytes surrounded by densely packed staining material.

Therapy. Symptomatic.

Prognosis. Poor.

BIBLIOGRAPHY. Sorsby A: Congenital coloboma of the macula; together with an account of the familial occurrence of bilateral macular coloboma in association with apical dystrophy of hands and feet. Br J Ophthalmol 19:65–90, 1935
Smith RD, Fineman RM, Sillence DO, et al: Congenital macular colobomas and short-limb skeletal dysplasia. Am J Med Genet 5:365–371, 1980
Torczynski E: Developmental anomalies of the eye. In Garner A, Klintworth GK (eds): Pathobiology of Ocular Disease: A Dynamic Approach, 2nd ed, pp 1295–1300. New York, Marcel Dekker, 1994

SORSBY II

Synonym. Fundus dystrophy, pseudoinflammatory. See Best (can be identical syndrome).

Symptoms and Signs. Both sexes affected. Onset in third and fourth decades of life, occasionally in fifth decade. Visual trouble with clouding of central vision, first in one eye and then in the other. Fundus shows hemorrhages and exudates on central areas, with scar and pigmentary deposits; eventually, evolution into choroid atrophy with disappearance of vessels.

Etiology. Unknown. Autosomal dominant inheritance. Retina metabolic needs of vitamin A and other factors suggested

Pathology. Before reduction of vision may be seen fine drusen or confluent deposit of yellow subretinal material. Later atrophy of outer retina or growth of subretinal new vessels

Diagnostic Procedures. *Electrophysiological studies.* Reduced light rise on electroculography; *angiography.*

BIBLIOGRAPHY. Sorsby A, et al: A fundus dystrophy with unusual features (late onset and dominant inheritance of a central retinal lesion showing oedema, haemorrhage and exudates developing into generalized choroidal atrophy with massive pigment proliferation). Br J Ophthalmol 33:67–100, 1949
Kalmus H, Seedburgh D: Probable common origin of a hereditary fundus dystrophy (Sorsby's familial) pseudoinflammatory macular dystrophy in an English and Australian family. J Med Genet 13:271–276, 1976
Thompson EM, Baraitser M: Sorsby syndrome: A report on further generations of the original family. J Med Genet 25:313–321, 1988
Bird AC, Jay B, Hussain AA, et al: Retinal photoreceptor disorders. In Garner A, Klintworth GK (eds): Pathobiology of Ocular Disease: A Dynamic Approach, 2nd ed, pp 1220–1221. New York, Marcel Dekker, 1994

SOTOS

Synonym. Cerebral gigantism in childhood.

Symptoms and Signs. Both sexes. Birth weight and length greater than normal; accelerated growth during the first 4–5 years of life; then growth seems to approach normal, remaining, however, two standard deviations above mean for chronologic age. Macrocrania, dolichocephaly; prognathism; hypertelorism; antimongoloid obliquity of palpebral fissures; characterizing facies; high-arched palate; mental retardation; clumsiness or ataxia. Occasionally, obesity, convulsions, abnormal dermatoglyphic pattern.

Etiology. Unknown. Possibly, pathogenic mechanism operating in uterus or impaired function of hypothalamic-pituitary axis. Failure of growth hormone to rise following hypoglycemia. Possibly, variant of Lawrence-Seip and Russell syndromes. The three forms are parts of the same spectrum. Most cases sporadic; autosomal dominant inheritance reported. The autosomal dominant gene may be located either at 3p21 or 6p21.

Pathology. See Signs.

Diagnostic Procedures. *CT brain scan. MRI.* Dilated ventricular system (mainly lateral and third). *Chromosome studies.* Normal. *Blood.* Oral glucose tolerance test abnormal in some cases; fasting plasma growth hormone levels normal. GH levels and GH dynamics normal. Increase of 17-ketosteroids; high level of valine, isoleucine, and leucine; normal OHCS. *EEG.* No specific changes.

Therapy. Symptomatic. Supportive counseling.

Prognosis. Generally, good health after childhood. Only a few achieve an excessive adult height. Problem of social adjustment owing to aggressiveness.

BIBLIOGRAPHY. Sotos JF, Dodge PR, Muirhead D, et al: Cerebral gigantism in childhood, a syndrome of excessively rapid growth with acromegalic features and a nonprogressive neurologic disorder. N Engl J Med 271:109–116, 1964
Bale AE, Drum MA, Parry DM, et al: Familial Sotos syndrome (cerebral gigantism): Craniocephalic and psychological characteristics. Am J Med Genet 20:613–624, 1985
Cole TRP, Hughes HE: Sotos syndrome. J Med Genet 27:571–576, 1990
Weatherall DJ, Ledingham JGG, Warrell DA: Oxford Textbook of Medicine, pp 1700, 4111. Oxford, Oxford Med Pub, 1996

SPAET-DAMESHEK

Synonym. Chronic hypoplastic neutropenia; neutropenia, chronic hypoplastic.

Symptoms. Onset at 14–67 years of age. Repeated severe, prolonged infections of the skin, mouth, throat, ears, paranasal sinuses, and lungs.

Signs. No characteristics except for scar of previous infections. Finger clubbing absent. Splenomegaly of moderate degree.

Etiology. Unknown. Bone marrow selective (neutrophil) hypoplasia. Reported familial occurrence with both autosomal dominant and recessive type (see Gaensslen).

Diagnostic Procedures. *Blood.* Total leukocyte count usually normal. Severe neutropenia; almost constant monocytosis. Only occasionally, moderate anemia, and thrombocytopenia. No hyperglobulinemia *Bone marrow.* Marked selective granulocytic hypoplasia. Other series normal.

Therapy. Antibiotics. This neutropenia is not affected by splenectomy, corticosteroids, adrenocorticotropic hormone (ACTH), and immunosuppressive agents.

Prognosis. Good. Extremely chronic condition, very lengthy course.

BIBLIOGRAPHY. Hattersley PG: Chronic neutropenia. Report of case not cured by splenectomy. Blood 2:227–234, 1947

Spaet TH, Dameshek W: Chronic hypoplastic neutropenia. Am J Med 13:35–45, 1952

Athens JW: Neutropenia. In Lee GR, Bithel TC, Foerster J, et al (eds): Wintrobe's Clinical Hematology, 9th ed, p 1605. Philadelphia, Lea & Febiger, 1993

SPAHR

Synonyms. Metaphyseal dysplasia (type A-1); metaphyseal dysostosis (type A-1).

Symptoms and Signs. Marked bowing of legs.

Etiology. Possibly autosomal recessive inheritance.

Therapy. If needed, osteotomy.

BIBLIOGRAPHY. Spahr A, Spahr-Hartmann I: Dysostose metaphisaire familiale étude de 4 cas dans une fratrie. Helv Paediat Acta 16:836–849, 1961

Bailey JA: Disproportionate Short Stature: Diagnosis and Management, p 273. Philadelphia, WB Saunders, 1973

SPANLANG-TAPPEINER

Synonyms. Alopecia; hyperhidrosis; corneal dystrophy; keratosis palmoplantaris; corneal dystrophy.

Symptoms and Signs. Both sexes affected. Onset at 5–20 years. Alopecia partial, total, or localized; nail dystrophy; hyperkeratosis of palms and soles. Teeth normal, visual impairment because of tongue-shaped corneal opacities.

Etiology. Unknown. Autosomal dominant inheritance.

BIBLIOGRAPHY. Unna PG: Über das Keratoma Palmare et Plantare Heretitatium. Vjschr Dermatol 15:231, 1883

Spanlang H: Beiträge zur Klinik und Pathologie seltener Hornhauterkrankungen (Dystrophia adiposa corneal, Dystker atosis corneae congenital). Z Augenheilk 62:21–41, 1927

Stevanovic DV: Alopecia congenita: The incomplete dominant form of inheritance with varying expressivity. Acta Genet 9:127–132, 1959

SPASMODIC DYSPHONIA

Synonyms. Includes Adductor spasmodic dysphonia. See Voice functional disorders syndromes.

Symptoms and Signs. Family history of dystonia may be present (23%). It may be associated with other dystonias (19%) such as Meige, blepharospasm, torticollis, etc. Symptoms may vary among patients. Under stress usually worsening of symptoms. Onset according to patients related to a possible upper respiratory infection (no data support the statement) and/or to a stressful event. Strained, strangled quality of the voice, that initially may be intermittent and then become constant, even if a fluctuation of severity persists. A compensatory mechanism induces the patient to whisper or speak during inspiration to facilitate communication. Vocal folds adduct or close too tightly during phonation (Adductor spasmodic dysphonia) or present intermittent spastic contraction.

Etiology. It falls in the group of movement disorders (focal dystonias); disorders of alteration of central motor processing.

Diagnostic Procedures. *Laryngoscopy.* Laryngeal electromyography.

Therapy. No effective treatment found. Under study botulin toxic injection, anterior laryngoplasty, implantable stimulator.

Prognosis. Complete recovery of function not possible.

BIBLIOGRAPHY. Traube L: Spastisch Form der Nervosen Hiserkeit Gerammelte. Beitr Pathol Physiol 2:677, 1971

Miller RH, Woodson GE: Treatment options in spasmodic dysphonia. Otolaryngologic Clin N Am 24:1227–1237, 1991

SPASMODIC LAUGHTER

Synonyms. Forced laughter; homeric laughter; sham mirth. See also Gelolepsy.

Symptoms. Uncontrollable laughter without the emotion of pleasure (mirthless): spontaneous or following different slight stimulations that normally arouse no emotional response, such as pointing the finger or a normal sound.

Etiology. It must be considered a symptom more than a syndrome. It is observed in the following conditions: multiple sclerosis; pseudobulbar palsy; epilepsy; intracranial hemorrhages; after premotor lobotomy. May be caused by release of paleothalamus from phylogenetically younger thalamic structures, suprasegmental, frontal cerebral cortex. Observed also in Kuru (see).

Pathology. Severe diffuse organic brain lesions. See Etiology.

Prognosis. Poor. Bad omen symptoms.

BIBLIOGRAPHY. Homer: Iliad and Odyssey: "an unextinguished laughter shakes the skies."

Martin JP: Fits of laughter (sham mirth) in organic cerebral disease. Brain 73:453–464, 1950

Poeck K: Pathologic laughter and cryng. In Vinken PJ, Bruyn GW (eds): Handbook of Clinical Neurology, vol 45, pp 219–225. Amsterdam, North-Holland, 1984

SPASMODIC TORTICOLLIS

Synonym. Wry neck.

Symptoms. Both sexes affected. The head is suddenly intermittently pulled and turned to one side. Slight movement at first gradually increasing in intensity. Emotions and stress make them more severe. Movements cease during sleep. With time muscle may become permanently contracted and the head deviated to one side. With special maneuver the patient may decrease or stop movements. See also Torticollis.

Signs. Contraction and hypertrophy of muscles involved (especially sternocleidomastoid, posterior, and lateral muscles of neck, upper part of trapezii). Familial cases reported. Difficult distintiction from Ziehen-Oppenheim forms with autosomal dominant and recessive inheritance described

Etiology. Unknown. As localized dystonia part of the dystonic lenticular syndrome; as sequela of chronic encephalitis.

Therapy. Psychotherapy does not help. Supporting padded collar of some help. Section of intraspinal portion of spinal accessory nerves and upper three or four anterior roots of spinal cord gives good results. Periodic injection of botulinum neurotoxin type A into affected muscles.

Prognosis. Usually progressing; 10% show involvement of other muscles of body; may become static or spontaneously regress.

BIBLIOGRAPHY. Poppen JL, Martinez-Niochet A: Spasmodic torticollis. Clin No Am 31:883–890, 1951

Thompson F, McManus S, Colville J: Familial congenital muscular torticollis: Case report and review of literature. Clin Orthop Rel Res 202:193–196, 1986

Denislic M, Pirtosek Z, Vodusek DB, et al: Botulinum toxin in the treatment of neurological disorders. In Soput D, Zorec R: Toxin and exocytosis. Ann NY Acad Sci 710:76–87, 1994

SPASMUS NUTANS

Symptoms. Both sexes affected. Onset at 6–18 months; never after third year. Aggravated by cold weather. Rhythmic movements of the head in the upright position associated with rapid, horizontal bilateral nystagmus. Attempt at gaze fixation intensifies manifestations. During sleep, it disappears.

Etiology. Unknown. It seldom may betray the presence of chiasmal or third ventricle tumor.

Prognosis. Spontaneous disappearance by the age of 3 or 4 years. In this period remission and relapses possible. No residue.

BIBLIOGRAPHY. Adams RD, Victor M: Principles of Neurology, 5th ed, p 238. New York, McGraw-Hill, 1993

SPIEGHEL

Synonyms. Spiegelian hernia, hernia Spieghel.

Symptoms and Signs. Pain of hernia site, usually above level of the inferior epigastric vessels level on the linea semilunaris. Pain is enhanced by increase in intra-abdominal pressure. The mass is made more evident with patient standing and straining, and may disappear with gurgling sound on pressure, thus allowing the palpation of the orifice. Occasionally the mass is not evident.

Etiology. Acquired condition.

Diagnostic Procedures. *Ultrasound. CT scan. MRI.*

Therapy. Aponeurotic repair of the orifice.

Prognosis. High incidence of incarceration. Good with repair.

BIBLIOGRAPHY. Spieghel A: Opera quae extore omnia, p 103. Amsterdam, John Bloew, 1645
Spangen L: Spieghelian hernia. Surg Clin No Am 64:351–366, 1984

SPIEGLER-FENDT

Synonyms. Bäfverstedt, Kaposi-Spiegler; lymphadenosis, benigna cutis; miliary lymphocytoma.

Symptoms and Signs. Prevalent in females (3:1). Onset at any age (more frequently second and third decades). *Variety 1.* Circumscribed lymphocytoma cutis. No systemic symptoms, except secondary to lesion displacing genitourinary structures. One or several purple yellowish, rubbery, elevated nodules, usually appearing on the face (60%), earlobes, and tip of nose. Nipple, scrotum, vagina less frequently affected. Regional lymph nodes seldom enlarged; no splenomegaly. *Variety 2.* Miliary eruption of several bluish nodules on face, trunk, and limbs. Itching especially in summer months. No lymph node or spleen enlargement.

Etiology. Benign hyperplasia of reticuloendothelial tissue of the skin. Trauma, insect bite, photosensitivity among precipitating causes.

Pathology. Lymphocyte infiltration of dermis separated from epidermis by normal connective tissue. Occasionally assuming a follicular pattern. Eosinophil accumulation at the periphery (occasional).

Diagnostic Procedures. *Biopsy. Blood.* Normal.

Therapy. Radiotherapy (effects not substantiated). Topical steroids for miliary lesions.

Prognosis. Good response to treatment. Circumscribed form may disappear spontaneously. Generalized form may persist for life or regress and relapse, without affecting general health or life expectancy.

BIBLIOGRAPHY. Spiegler E: Ueber die sogenannte Sarkomatosis cutis. Arch Dermatol Syph 27:163–174, 1894
Fendt H: Beiträge zur Kenntnis der sogenannten sarcoiden Geswülste der Haut. Arch Dermatol Syph 53:213–242, 1900
Höfer W: Lymphadenosis benigna cutis. Arch Klin Exp Dermatol 203:23–40, 1956
Burton JL: Disorders of connective tissue. In Champion RH, Burton JL, Ebling FJG (eds): Rook/Wilkinson/Ebling Textbook of Dermatology, 5th ed, pp 2101–2103. Oxford, Blackwell Scientific, 1992

SPIELMEYER-VOGT

Synonyms. Vogt-Spielmeyer, Batten; ceroid lipofuscinosis, juvenilis; neuronal ceroid—lipofuscinosis, juvenilis. See also Ceroid lipofuscinosis.

Symptoms and Signs. Both sexes affected. Onset at 3–8 years. Mental development arrest; hypotonia; ataxia; polymyoclonia, seizures; extrapyramidal signs; visual impairment up to blindness. Fundus oculi hypopigmentation, atrophy; discoloration of macula with yellow-gray areas. Liver and spleen not enlarged and no bone abnormalities. Later stage, severe dementia, muscle wasting.

Etiology. Autosomal recessive inheritance. Disturbance of linoleic acid metabolism.

Pathology. Deposits of autoflourescent lipopigments in all tissues, predominant in the brain. *Brain.* Small, loss of nerve cells and status spongiosus; various sizes and structures of lipopigment deposits (lamellar, granular, "fingerprint" aspect), with acid phosphatase activity. *Retina.* Loss of cones and rods; degeneration of epithelial cells; lipoid pigment accumulation.

Diagnostic Procedures. *ERG.* Waveforms lost when retina compromised. *EEG.* High voltage; triphasic waves; later only delta waves. *CT scan. MRI.* Lateral ventricles slighly dilated. *Electromicroscopy.* Of eccrine glands of skin. No enzyme deficiency has been yet demonstrated. *Bone marrow and other tissue biopsy.* Presence of lipopigments. *Urine.* Presence of lipopigments in sediment. *Blood.* Lipopigments in lymphocytes; azurophilic hypergranulation in neutrophils and lymphocyte vacuolization (only in homozygotes).

Prognosis. Within 3 years, total incapacitation. Death in 10–15 years.

BIBLIOGRAPHY. Batten FE: Cerebral degeneration with symmetrical changes in the maculae in two members of a family. Trans Opthalmol Soc UK 23:386–390, 1902
Vogt H: Ueber familiäre amaurotische Idiotie und verwandte Krankheitsbilder. Mschr Psychiat 18:161–171, 310–357, 1905
Spielmeyer W: Klinische und anatomische Untersuchungen über einen besonderen Fall von amaurotischer Idiotie. Nissle Beitr Nerv Geistes Krh, Berlin 1908
Gardiner M, Sandford A, Deadman M, et al: Batten disease (Spielmeyer-Vogt disease): Juvenile onset (neuronal ceroid-lipofuscinosis) gene (CLN3) maps to human chromosome 16. Genomics 8:387–390, 1990
Weatherall DJ, Ledingham JGG, Warrell DA: Oxford Textbook of Medicine, p 3985. Oxford, Oxford Med Pub, 1996

SPILLER

Obsolete.

Synonyms. Charcot-Joffroy; epidural ascending paralysis; hypertrophic spinal meningitis. See also Erb-Charcot.

Symptoms and Signs. Severe pain in the neck, back of the head, upper shoulder, chest, and arms; enhanced by movement of the neck. Atrophy and fasciculation of muscles of those regions develop in weeks or months. Hyporeflexia or areflexia of tendons of arms and hands first; later weakness and spasticity of legs and sensory loss below level of lesions. Vasomotor and atrophic changes, and sphincter insufficiency may develop.

Etiology. Nonspecific etiology; syphilis in some cases.

Pathology. Granulomatous infiltration of dura mater usually of the cervical region, sometimes of thoracic region. Roots of cervical cord constricted and inflamed.

Diagnostic Procedures. *Lumbar puncture.* Complete, partial, or no block of spinal subarachnoid space. *CT scan, MRI, electromyography.*

Therapy. Extirpation of dura mater from posterior portion of affected part.

Prognosis. Dramatic improvement if treatment is not delayed.

BIBLIOGRAPHY. Charcot JM, Joffroy A: Deux cas d'atrophie musculaire progressive avec lésions de la substance grise et des faisceaux antéro-latéraux de la moelle épinière. Arch Physiol 2:354–367, 1869

Spiller WG: Epidural ascending spinal paralysis. Rev Neurol Psychiatr 9:494–498, 1911

Vick NA: Grinker's Neurology, 7th ed. Springfield, IL, Charles C Thomas, 1976

SPINAL ANTERIOR

Synonyms. Anterior spinal; anterior myelopathy; cornual anterior.

Symptoms. Motor disturbance caused by muscular atrophy and paralysis of different muscles of extremities or trunk or both, in combination or affecting single muscles; urinary disturbances if bladder is affected.

Signs. Fasciculation and finally after weeks or months, paralysis and atrophy of single (occasional) or group of muscles, loss of reflexes, sensorium intact or temporarily mildly affected. Electric reaction of degeneration can be demonstrated in denervated muscles. Trophic changes of the overlying skin, which appears cyanotic and cold.

Etiology. Degenerative lesions of nervous tissue selectively involving anterior cornua of spinal cord. Progressive muscular atrophy; poliomyelitis; amyotrophic lateral sclerosis; syphilis.

Pathology. Varies according to etiology. Initial hyperemia of pia vessels and affected gray matter; later edema and yellow-gray color and softening of gray matter. Microscopically, degenerative and necrotic changes.

Diagnostic Procedures. Findings vary according to etiology. *Blood.* Leukocytosis in poliomyelitis. *Cerebrospinal fluid.* Various changes according to stages.

Therapy. Depends on etiology.

Prognosis. Depends on etiology.

BIBLIOGRAPHY. Adams RD, Victor M: Principles of Neurology, 5th ed, p 1105. New York, McGraw-Hill, 1993

Weatherall DJ, Ledingham JGG, Warrell DA: Oxford Textbook of Medicine, p 3856. Oxford, Oxford Med Pub, 1996

SPINAL CHRONIC ARACHNOIDITIS

Synonyms. Hypertrophic cervical pachymeningitis; arachnoiditis spinal; meningitis circumscripta spinalis.

Symptoms and Signs. Insidious onset. Pain, weakness, sensorimotor loss (paralysis, paresthesias) involving lower extremities asymmetrically, then ascending. Prominent fasciculation.

Etiology. It follows one of the chronic infective processes; or occasionally, after intrathecal injection. A family with autosomal inheritance of this syndrome reported (analogy with Peyronie and Dupuytren proposed).

Pathology. Fibrous tissue proliferation in delimitated areas or diffused with chronic type of inflammatory reactions. Interference with cerebrospinal fluid flow.

Diagnostic Procedures. *Blood.* Leukocytosis. *Cerebrospinal fluid.* Partial or complete spinal block; xanthochromia or Froin syndrome (see); increased proteins. *CT scan. MRI.* May reveal single or multiple locations of process.

Therapy. No effective medical or surgical treatment. Corticosteriods not beneficial.

Prognosis. Progressive condition.

BIBLIOGRAPHY. Winkelman NW, Eckel JL: Focal lesions of the spinal cord due to vascular disease. JAMA 99:1919–1926, 1932

Duke RJ, Hashimoto SA: Familial spinal arachnoiditis: A new entity. Arch Neurol 30:300–303, 1974

Weatherall DJ, Ledingham JGG, Warrell DA: Oxford Textbook of Medicine, p 3894. Oxford, Oxford Med Pub, 1996

SPINAL CORD INJURY, PROGRESSIVE CONFUSIONAL

Symptoms. Occurs in patients with fracture of cervical vertebrae and in nontraumatic injury of spinal cord. Mental symptoms: loss of memory; hallucination; delirium.

Signs. Those of spinal cord lesion. In some patients, circulation appears to fail before respiration (opposite to posterior fossa compression, see); slight cyanosis.

Etiology. Unknown. Previously considered a result of cerebral contusion. Interruption of vasomotor pathways and sensory tracts in nontraumatic cases.

Pathology. Traumatic or pathologic fractures of vertebrae, hematomyelia, or sarcoma and other pathology of spinal cord. Atelectasis of lungs.

Diagnostic Procedures. *X-ray. CT scan. MRI. Spinal tap (?).*

Therapy. Symptomatic. Corticosteroids, naloxone. If compression, surgery.

Prognosis. All patients who developed this syndrome died shortly thereafter.

BIBLIOGRAPHY. Putnam T: The progressive confusional syndrome following injuries to cervical portion of the spinal cord. Science 86:542–543, 1937

SPINAL SHOCK

Synonyms. Marshall-Hall, Riddock; including "autonomic dysreflexia."

Symptoms and Signs. All ages. After spinal cord injury. Clinically divided in two stages: *Areflexia.* The symptomatology present in this stage is of variable degree from fully manifested or minimal. All neural elements below the lesion fail. Tetraplegia (if lesion at C4–C5 segments); paraplegia (if lesion at thoracic level); accompanied by bladder (overflow incontinence) and bowel paralytic ileus, atonic paralysis, gastric atony; sensory loss, muscular flaccidity; loss of reflexes, loss of autonomic activity (sweating, vasomotor, tone, etc.). Skin pale and dry, decubital ulcerations; depression of genital reflexes. *Hyperreflexic activity.* After a few weeks reflexes return and become gradually stronger and finally exaggerated up to flexor spasms "mass reflex" elicited by stimulation, variety of paresthesias or dull pain. Above lesion successively may develop the "autonomic dysreflexia" syndrome: episodic response to specific stimuli (i.e., distended bladder) or exaggerated sweating, flushing, headache, blood hypertension, bradycardia.

Etiology. Spinal trauma.

Pathology. Functional (edema) or anatomic interruption of corticospinal tracts.

Therapy. Usually symptomatic and conservative. Avoid movement, especially flexion and traction (surgical fixation may be adopted in a second stage) or early decompression may be adopted. Spinal cord cooling. In acute phase: corticosteroids, naloxone; endogenous opiate antagonists, bladder catheterization, enemas. In chronic phase: physiotherapy according to evaluation.

Prognosis. Complete areflexia duration varies from hours to permanent. In the majority minimal activity returns within 1–6 weeks. Paresis and hyperreflexic activity duration extremely variable according to intensity of trauma and treatment.

BIBLIOGRAPHY. Marshall Hall M: Synopsis of the Diastaltic Nervous System. London, J Mallett, 1850

Riddock G: The reflex functions of the completely divided spinal cord in men, compared with less severe lesions. Brain 40:264, 1917

Guttman L: Spinal Cord Injuries: Comprehensive Management and Research. Oxford, Blackwell Scientific, 1976

Mathias CJ, Frankel H: The cardiovascular system in tetraplegia and paraplegia. In Vinken PJ, Bruyn GW, Klawans GL: Handbook of Clinical Neurology, vol 61, p437–440. Amsterdam, North-Holland, 1992

Weatherall DJ, Ledingham JGG, Warrell DA: Oxford Textbook of Medicine, p 3896. Oxford, Oxford Med Pub, 1996

SPIRA

Synonym. Fluoride toxicity.

Symptoms and Signs. Onset in late childhood to early adulthood. Mottling or brown discoloration of teeth. Nausea; anorexia; vomiting; constipation. In older patients, possibly, stiffness, rheumatalgia. Osteosclerotic changes in the skeleton and rarely central nervous system involvement.

Etiology. Fluoride chronic intoxication from water, food, dust (in cryolite mines), or dusts and vapors (industry and agriculture).

Pathology. Hypoplasia of dental enamel and defective bone calcification.

Therapy. None specific. Cessation of exposure or consumption.

Prognosis. Rheumatalgia and stiffness may regress. Teeth lesions remain.

BIBLIOGRAPHY. Spira D: Br Med Rev 5:61, 1928

Dean HT: Chronic endemic fluorosis. JAMA 107:1269–1273, 1936

Hodge HC, Smith FA: Biological effects of inorganic fluorides. In Simons SH (ed): Fluorine Chemistry, vol 4. New York, Academic Press, 1965

Ellenhorn MJ, Barceloux DG: Medical Toxicology, pp 533–534. New York, Elsevier, 1988

SPITZER-WEINSTAIN

Synonyms. Renal tubular potassium secretion defect.

Symptoms and Signs. In children. Short stature. Occasionally weakness, hypertension, and associated hypoplasia of upper incisors, urinary tract infections, and renal colics.

Etiology. Unknown. Decreased secretion of potassium, and secondary impairment of proximal tubule bicarbonate reabsorption.

Diagnostic Procedures. *Urine.* Normal. *Blood.* Hyperkalemia, metabolic acidosis; no reduction of GFR

Therapy. Chlorothizide corrects both acidosis and hyperkalemia. Bi-carbonate, if persistent acidosis; sodium restriction sometimes is sufficient to correct all derangements.

Prognosis. Good.

BIBLIOGRAPHY. Spitzer A, Edelmann CM Jr, Goldberg LD, et al: Short stature hyperkalemia and acidosis: a defect in renal transport of potassium. Kidney Int 3:251–257, 1973

Weinstein SF, Allan DME, Mendoza SA: Hyperkalemia, acidosis, and short stature associated with a defect in renal potassium excretion. J Pediat 85:355–358, 1974

Dubose TD, Alpern RJ: Renal tubular acidosis. In Scriver CR, Beaudet AL, Sly WS, et al: The Metabolic and Molecular Bases of Inherited Disease, 7th ed, pp 3679–3681. New York, McGraw-Hill, 1995

SPLIT NOTOCHORD

Synonyms. Caudal dysplasia. Includes the malformation reported in the past as posterior enteric sinus, posterior enteric cyst, posterior spina bifida, diastematomyelia or diplomyelia, anterior spina bifida, prevertebral enteric cyst, rachischisis. See also Meckel-Gruber, Mermaid and membraneous aplasia cutis.

Symptoms. Variable according to nature and extent of malformation.

Signs. Posterior enteric cysts or sinuses; small protrusion of distal end of the intestine dorsal to the split vertebrae. Split spine without herniation of alimentary canal observed.

Etiology. Unknown. Autosomal dominant inheritance reported.

Pathology. See Synonyms and Signs.

Diagnostic Procedures. *X-ray.*

Therapy. Surgery when feasible.

Prognosis. Several of the manifestations of this syndrome compatible with life, but syndrome often fatal.

BIBLIOGRAPHY. Meckel JR: Beschreibung zweier durch sehrähnliche Bildungsabweichung entstellter Geschwister. Dtsch Arch Phys 7:99–172, 1822

Gruber GB: Zur Frage der neurenterischen Offnung bei Früchten mit vollkommener Wirbelspaltung. Z Anat Entwicklungsgesch 80:433–453, 1926

Denes J, Gonti J, Leb J: Dorsal herniation of gut: A rare manifestation of the split notochord syndrome. J Pediatr Surg 2:359–363, 1967

Welch JP, Alterman K: The syndrome of caudal dysplasia: A review, including etiologic considerations and evidence of heterogeneity. Pediatr Pathol 2:313–327, 1984

Jones KL: Smith's Recognizable Patterns of Human Malformations, p 72. Philadelphia, WB Saunders, 1988

SPO.NA.STRI.ME.

Synonyms. Spondylar—nasal alteration—striated metaphyses.

Symptoms and Signs. Prevalent in females. Normal intelligence. *Face.* Asian look, midface hypoplasia, saddle nose, frontal bossing, large head. *Limbs.* Short; dwarfism. Kyphoscoliosis, lumbar lordosis.

Etiology. Autosmal recessive inheritance.

Pathology. *Bone.* Pseudocystic transformation; defect in collagen synthesis and proteoglycans.

Diagnostic Procedures. *X-rays.* Striation in methaphyses; osteoporosis; codfish vertebrae.

BIBLIOGRAPHY. Fanconi CI, Giedion A, Prader A: The SPONASTRIME dysplasia: familial short-limb dwarfism with saddle nose, spinal alterations and metaphyseal striation. Helv Paediat Acta 38:267–280, 1983

Lachman RS, Stoss M, Spranger S: Sponastrime dysplasia: A radiologic-pathologic correlation. Pediatr Radiol 19:417–424, 1989

SPONDILODYSPLASTIC GROUP, PERINATALLY LETHAL

Synonyms. Lethal platyspondylic dwarfism, thanatophoric variants; platyspondyly-perinatal lethality. Includes Torrance, San Diego, and Luton varieties; see thanatophoric.

Symptoms and Signs. Several entities. Three well-defined—Torrance, San Diego, and Lutton, plus a number of less defined ones. Characterized by perinatal mortality and severe platospondyly, large head, short neck, coarse facies, small chest, large abdomen, very short limbs.

Etiology. Sporadic.

Pathology. *Torrance.* Hypercellular resting cartilage with large chondrocytes and normal growth plate. *San Diego.* Testing cartilage normal, large round chondrocytes, normal column formation. *Luton.* Hypercellular cartilage, normal large cells, focal degenerating chondrocytes, and focal disorganization.

Diagnostic Procedures. *X-ray.* Decreased calcification of cranial base, short ribs, vertebral bodies ossified and very small, hypoplastic ilia ischia and pubic bones, relatively straight long bones widened, with cupped or rounded methaphyses.

Prognosis. Perinatal mortality.

BIBLIOGRAPHY. Rimoin DL, Lachman RS: Genetic disorders of the osseous skeleton. In Beithon P (ed): McKusick's Heritable Disorders of Connective Tissue, 5th ed, p 580. St Louis, CV Mosby, 1993

SPONDYLOENCHONDRO DYSPLASIA

Synonyms. Shorr; enchondromatosis-spondylometaphyseal dysplasia. See Ollier; Spranger.

Symptoms and Signs. In males. Short stature; rhizomelia, genu valgum, enlarged chest (antero-posterior), with kyphosis; lombar lordosis; large joints.

Etiology. Probably autosomal recessive inheritance.

Diagnostic Procedures. *X-rays.* Long and flat bones: enchondromatous changes; (hand and feet spared); platyspondyly with endplate irregularity.

BIBLIOGRAPHY. Shorr S, Legum C, Ochshorn M: Spondyloenchondrodysplasia: Enchondromatosis with severe platyspondyly in two brothers. Radiology 118:113–139, 1976
Menger H, Kruse K, Spranger J: Spondyloenchondro dysplasia. J Med Genet 26:93–99, 1989
Horton WA, Hecht JT: The chondrodysplasias. In Royce PM, Steinmann B (eds): Connective Tissue and Its Heritable Disorders: Molecular, Genetic and Medical Aspects. New York, Wiley-Liss, 1993

SPONDYLOEPIMETAPHYSEAL DYSPLASIA, HYPOTRICHOSIS

Symptoms and Signs. Both sexes. From infancy. Mild rhizomelic short stature, hypotrichosis.

Etiology. Autosomal dominant inheritance.

Diagnostic Procedures. *X-rays.* Metaphyseal flaring and irregularities; delayed and irregular epiphyseal calcification. Changes greatest in proximal femurs. Development of lytic areas with age.

BIBLIOGRAPHY. White MP, Petersen DJ, McAlister WH: Hypotrichosis

with spondyloepimetaphyseal dysplasia in three generations: A new autosomal dominant syndrome. Am J Med Genet 45(Suppl):A68, 1989
White MP, Petersen DJ, McAlister WH: Hypotrichosis with spondyloepimetaphyseal dysplasia in three generations a new autosomal dominant syndrome. AM J Med Genet 36:288–291, 1990

SPONDYLOEPIPHYSEAL DYSPLASIA, CONGENITAL

Synonyms. Spranger-Wiedemann; SED congenita. See MacDermot.

Symptoms and Signs. Both sexes. From birth. Main characterizing signs—affection of vertebrae and juxtatruncal epiphyses (short stature). Occasionally associated: cleft palate, myopia, sensineural deafness, hypoplasia of abdominal muscles, hernias, mental retardation.

Etiology. Autosomal dominant inheritance or sporadic. Probably result of mutation in the COL2A1 gene. Defect of type II collagen. It fits into a continuous spectrum of several clinical syndromes.

Pathology. Demonstration of PAS-positive cypoplasmic inclusion in chondrocytes after diastase digestion.

Diagnostic Procedures. *X-rays.* Flattening of vertebrae, lack of ossification in proximal tibial epiphyses and other flat or long bones.

BIBLIOGRAPHY. Spranger JW, Wiedemann HR: Dysplasia spondyloepiphysaria congenita. Helv Paediat Acta 21:598–611, 1966
Anderson IJ, Goldberg RB, Marion RW, et al: Spondyloepiphyseal dysplasia congenita: Genetic linkage to type II collagen (COL2A1). Am J Med Genet 46:896–901, 1990

SPONDYLOEPIPHYSEAL DYSPLASIA TARDA, AUTOSOMAL DOMINANT

Synonyms. See Jacobsen.

Symptoms and Signs. Onset ranging 2–20 years. Stiff gait precedes pain; eventually pain and stiffness in the back, knees, shoulders, and elbows.

Etiology. Autosomal dominant inheritance. Probably includes several phenotypes.

Diagnostic Procedures. *X-rays.* Platyspondily; in childhood irregularity of femoral head; in adulthood degenerative changes therein with moderate changes of hands, joints.

Prognosis. Final height ranging from 140–150 cm. In adulthood generalized osteoarthropathy.

BIBLIOGRAPHY. Moldauer M, Hanelin J, Bauer W: Familial precocious degenerative arthritis and a natural history of osteochondrodystrophy. In Blumenthal HT (ed): Medical and Clinical Aspects of Aging, pp 226–233. New York, Columbia University Press, 1962
Anderson IJ, Tsipouras P, Scher C, et al: Spondyloepiphyseal dysplasia, mild autosomal dominant type is not due to primary defects of type II collagen. Am J Med Genet 37:272–276, 1990

SPONDYLOEPYPHYSEAL DYSPLASIA TARDA, PROGRESSIVE ARTHROPATHY

Synonyms. Progressive pseudorheumatoid dysplasia; pseudorheumatoid dyslasia, progressive. See SED tarda-like group and Jacobsen.

Symptoms. Both sexes. Onset at 3–8 years. Morning stiffness, difficulty on walking, easy fatigability, muscular weakness, joint stiffness (first on the hips).

Signs. Swelling of finger joints and contractures at larger joints, occasionally kyphoscoliosis.

Etiology. Autosomal recessive inheritance.

Pathology. Abnormal addensation of chondrocytes, pycnotic nuclei, defective column formation.

Diagnostic Procedures. *Blood.* Normal sedimentation rate, absence of rheumatoid factor. *X-ray.* Narrowing of all articular spaces and absence of rheumatoid characteristics. Various alterations of hands, hip, spine, joints, and epiphysis of long bones. Platyspondyly, anterior end-plate erosion.

Therapy. Symptomatic.

Prognosis. Progessive condition.

BIBLIOGRAPHY. Wynne-Davis R, Hall C, Anselm BM: Spondylo-epiphyseal dysplasia tarda with progressive arthropathy: A "new" disorder of autosomal recessive inheritance. J Bone Joint Surg 64 (B):442–445, 1982
Rimoin DL, Lachman RS: Genetic disorders of the osseous skeleton. In Beithon P (ed): McKusick's Heritable Disorders of Connective Tissue, 5th ed, p 615. St Louis, CV Mosby, 1993

SPONTANEOUS OSTEONECROSIS OF THE KNEE

Synonyms. Avascular subcondral necrosis of knee; painful knee of the elderly; knee spontaneous osteonecrosis.

Symptoms and Signs. Classically in elderly subjects. Sudden knee pain. Sometimes secondary arthrosis.

Etiology. Unknown. Maybe vascular component or corticosteroid therapy. Differs from Koenig I because of site of lesion.

Pathology. Osteonecrosis of medial condyle of femur, rarely loose bodies.

Diagnostic Procedures. *X-ray.* Radiotransparent areas of medial condyle of femur. *Bone scan.* Hyperactivity long before radiologic evidence.

Therapy. Noninteventional. Reduction of load, anti-inflammatory drugs, physiotherapy. Rarely surgery.

Prognosis. Resolution in 6 months.

BIBLIOGRAPHY. Ahlbaeck S, Bauer GCH, Bohne WN: Spontaneous osteonecrosis of the knee. Arthritis Rheum 11:705, 1968
Aichroth P: Osteocondritis dissecans of the knee. In Insall JN, Windsor RE, Scott WN, et al: Surgery of the Knee. New York, Churchill Livingstone, 1993

SPOTTED LEG

Synonyms. Diabetic shin spots.

Symptoms and Signs. Occurs in diabetic patients; onset at a mean age of 50–60 years. Most patients show evidence of neuropathy or retinopathy or both. A few or many bilateral, asymmetric, round or oval, circumscribed, shallow lesions covered by atrophic, shiny, pigmented skin. Lesions not painful, not ulcerated. Distributed over anterior, lateral, and medial aspects of legs below the knees. Patient aware of lesions; no recollection of trauma; usually ignores them and does not call the physician attention to them. Associated neuropathy of hypoesthesia type and diminished or absent reflexes.

Etiology. Manifestation of vascular disease in diabetes; possibly, trauma, a factor in the development of lesions.

Pathology. Atrophy of epidermis; slight fibrosis; separation of collagen fibers of dermis; pigmentation owing to hemosiderin and increased evidence of melanin (because of atrophy). Abnormal capillaries with thick walls and obliteration of lumen.

Therapy. Diabetes treatment. Surgery with distal revascularization gives good results.

Prognosis. That of diabetes and its complications.

BIBLIOGRAPHY. Melin H: An atrophic circumscribed skin lesion in the lower extremities of diabetics. Acta Med Scand 176 (Suppl 423):1–75, 1964
Murphy RA: Skin lesions in diabetic patients: the "spotted leg" syndrome. Lahey Clin Found Bull 14:10–14, 1965
Black MM, Gawkrodger DJ, Seymour CA, et al: Metabolic and nutritional disorders. In Champion RH, Burton JL, Ebling FJG (eds): Rook/Wilkinson/Ebling Textbook of Dermatology, 5th ed, p 2378. Oxford, Blackwell Scientific, 1992

SPRANGER

Synonyms. Geleophysic dwarfism; mucopolysaccharidoses variant.

Symptoms. Present from birth. Unusual, pleasant, and happy face (geophysic). Behavior intelligence and development normal.

Signs. Dwarfism; lean habitus Dysostosis: multiflex-like alteration primarily involving the hands and feet. Frequently evidence of cardiac valvulopathies. Hepatomegaly, splenomegaly.

Etiology. Unknown. Autosomal recessive inheritance. Possibly, a variant of mucopolysaccharidosis.

Pathology. Heart valves. Striking abnormalities. Focal accumulation of mucopolysaccharides in the liver, cardiovascular system cartilage, trachea.

Diagnostic Procedures. *Urine.* Mucopolysaccharides normal excretion. *X-rays.* Hands and feet tubular bones short and plump. *Skin biopsy.* Lysosomal storage vacuoles.

Therapy. Symptomatic. Heart valve prothesis.

Prognosis. Poor. Death usually in infancy.

BIBLIOGRAPHY. Vanace PW, Friedman S, Wagner BM: Mitral stenosis in an atypical case of gargoylism: A case report with pathologic and histochemical studies of the cardiac tissues. Circulation 21:80–98, 1960
Spranger JW, Filbert EF, Tuffli GA, et al: Geleophysic dwarfism: A "focal" mucopolysaccharidosis? Lancet 2:97–98, 1960
Shohat M, Grubert HE, Pagon RA, et al: Geleophysic dysplasia: A storage disorder affecting the skin, bone, liver, heart, and trachea. J Pediatr 117:227–232, 1990

SPRENGEL

Synonyms. High scapula congenita; shoulder elevation.

Symptoms and Signs. One scapula (seldom both) short in vertical axis and wider in transverse and closer to the midline than the other one. Retracted during movement, except when fixed to thoracic spine or ribs. Because of this malformation, the shoulder on affected side is elevated and advanced. Scoliosis frequently is present, and torticollis may occasionally be associated. Abduction of shoulder beyond 90 degrees is impossible.

Etiology. Unknown. Autosomal dominant inheritance.

Pathology. Bands of connective tissue or bony bridge between scapula and ribs or spine. Trapezius or serratus magnus muscle may be replaced by connective tissue.

Diagnostic Procedures. *X-ray.*

Therapy. None, or attempted orthopedic correction.

Prognosis. Nonprogressive condition.

BIBLIOGRAPHY. Sprengel: Die angeborene Verschiebung des Schulterblattes nach oben. Arch Klin Chir Berl 42:545–549, 1891

Hodgson SV, Chin DC: Dominant transmission of Sprengel's shoulder and cleft palate. J Med Genet 18:263–265, 1981

SPRUE, TROPICAL

Synonyms. Aphthae tropical; Ceylon sore mouth; Cochin China diarrhea; tropical diarrhea; Hill diarrhea.

Symptoms. More common in certain tropical and subtropical regions, affecting particularly recently immigrated Caucasians. Onset usually insidious. Explosive diarrhea with foul smelling, bulky, pale, greasy, frothy stools during day and night. Weight loss; nausea; vomiting; anorexia; paresthesia; pain in the mouth and anal region; disinterest in self and surroundings.

Signs. Pallor; cheilosis; stomatitis; aphthae; glossitis with smooth, beefy red tongue; teeth partially or totally absent; bleeding manifestations; moderate to severe wasting; premature aging; hair dry. Heart frequently small; hypotension; abdomen protuberant (especially on standing). Liver smooth, soft, easily palpable, but not enlarged. Neurologic examination in some cases: Lichtheim syndrome (see).

Etiology. Unknown. Possibly, specific infectious agent not yet clearly identified. It could be the alpha-Prototheca partoricensis in zygote form.

Pathology. External and internal wasting with disappearance of fat deposits, viscera reduced in size and weight. Intestinal villi shortened and thick; tendency to fuse together; blunted edematous free margins. Infiltration of mucosa with inflammatory cells, especially eosinophils.

Diagnostic Procedures. *Blood.* Macrocytic anemia; leukopenia; moderate or severe thrombocytopenia; occasionally, hypoprothrombinemia; hypocholesterolemia; hypoproteinemia; hyperbilirubinemia. *Serum.* Iron normal; liver function usually normal. *Bone marrow.* Megaloblastosis; giant metamyelocytes. *Gastric fluid.* Anacidity. Cytologic changes similar to those of pernicious anemia. *Stool.* See Symptoms. Increase in fatty acids. Vitamin A tolerance curve, flat curve, D-xylose test generally depressed. *X-ray.* Sprue pattern. *Biopsy.* Of small intestine. See Pathology.

Therapy. Folic acid (15 mg/day); vitamin supplement; antibiotics. Diet complete and compatible with diet to which the patient was previously accustomed. Vitamin B_{12} (parenteral). Treatment of symptomatic complications or other coexisting conditions (e.g., parasistosis).

Prognosis. Excellent recovery following treatment; maintenance treatment necessary. Most sprue patients remain lean. Without treatment, poor prognosis.

BIBLIOGRAPHY. Ketelaer V: Commentarius medicus, de aphthis nostratibus, seu Belgarum sprouw. Ludg Bat, 1672
Hillary W, Severini A: Observations on the Changes of the Air, and the Concomitant Epidemical Diseases in the Island of Barbados, 2nd ed, p 103. London, Hawkes, Clarke, and Collins, 1766
Bartholomew C, William: Hillary and sprue in the Caribbean 230 years later. Gut 30:17–21, 1989
Garrido JA, Sheehy TW: Tropical sprue. In Haubrich WS, Schaffner F, Berk JE (eds): Bockus Gastroenterology, 5th ed, vol 2, pp 1049–1062. Philadelphia, WB Saunders, 1995

SRB

Synonym. Costosternal malformation.

Symptoms and Signs. Present from birth. Neuralgic pains of scapulohumeral girdle. Aplasia and synostosis of first two ribs; horniform protrusion of manubrium; secondary atrophy of muscles supplied by first two thoracic nerves; local venous congestion.

Etiology. Unknown.

Diagnostic Procedures. *X-ray.* See Symptoms and Signs.

Therapy. Surgical decompression of nerves and blood vessels.

BIBLIOGRAPHY. Srb J: Ueber Missbildung en der ersten Rippe. Med Jahrb Wien 5:75, 1862–1865
Wenz W, Geipert G: Röntgenologie und Klinik der erbschen rippensternum anomalie. Radiologie 7:53–58, 1967

STANESCU

Synonyms. Osteochondrosis; osteopetrosis; craniofacial dysostosis; diaphyseal hyperplasia; osteosclerosis dominant type. See also Maroteaux-Lamy II.

Symptoms. Present from birth. Both sexes affected. Slow growth. Normal intelligence and normal fertility.

Signs. Small stature (short limbs especially, upper arms and hands). Brachycephaly; depression at frontoparietal sutures; exophthalmos; narrow maxilla; small mandible; crowded teeth. Possible: exostoses; fractures.

Etiology. Autosomal dominant inheritance.

Pathology. Osteopetrosis.

Diagnostic Procedures. *X-ray.* Bone tends to become denser with age and to show thick cortex. Diaphyseal hyperplasia. Thin skull. Occasionally, sacralization S1.

Therapy. None.

Prognosis. Good quoad vitam.

BIBLIOGRAPHY. Stanescu V, Maximilian C, Poenaru S, et al: Syndrome héréditaire dominant, réussissant une dyostose cranio-faciale de type particulier, une insuffisance de croissance d'aspect chondrodystrophique et un épaississement massif de la corticale des os longs. Rev Fr Endocrinol Clin 4:219–231, 1963
Dipierri JE, Guzman JD: A second family with autosomal dominant osteosclerosis typical Stanescu. Am J Med Genet 18:13–18, 1984
Rimoin DL, Lachman RS: Genetic disorders of the osseous skeleton. In Beithon P (ed): McKusick's Heritable Disorders of Connective Tissue, 5th ed, p 657. St Louis, CV Mosby, 1993

STAPHYLOCOCCAL SCALDED SKIN

Synonyms. SSSS; Lyell; Fuchs-Lyell (drug reaction variety); Fuchs-Salzmann-Terrier; Debré-Lamy-Lyell; dermatitis medicamentosa; toxic epidermolysis; epidermolysis necroticans combustiformis; bullous erythroderma epidermolysis; toxic epidermal necrolysis; scalded skin.

All the synonyms have been used to indicate a generalized erythema-inflammation-necrosis of epidermis following a bullous phase. Today two different syndromes have been classified: the Ritter (see) that represents the proper Staphylococcal scalded syndrome and the Toxic epidermal necrolysis.

BIBLIOGRAPHY. Fuchs E: Ueber Knoechenfoermige Hornhautruebung. debrecht Von Graefes. Arch Ophthalmol 53:423–435, 1902
Fuchs E: Ueber Knochenförnige Horhauttrübungen. Arch Ophthalmol 89:337–349, 1915
Debré R, Lamy M, Lamotte M: Un cas d'erythrodermie avec epidermolyse chez un enfant de 12 ans. Bull Soc Pediatr 37:231–238, 1939
Lyell A: Toxic epidermal necrolysis: Eruption resembling scalding of the skin. Br J Dermatol 68:355–361, 1956
Pye RJ: Bullous eruptions. In Champion RH, Burton JL, Ebling FJG (eds): Rook/Wilkinson/Ebling Textbook of Dermatology, 5th ed, pp 1665–1667. Oxford, Blackwell Scientific, 1992

STARGARDT

Synonyms. Macular degeneration, juvenile; Stargardt type; fundus flavimaculatus—atrophic macular dystrophy. See Franceschetti.

Symptoms. Onset at 6–20 years of age. Gradual bilateral decrease of vision (previously reported as normal).

Signs. Initially, no ophthalmologic changes. Later, disappearance of foveal reflex (first signs) and then changes in the pigmented epithelium (grayish-yellow spots); fovea granulated, covered by a snail slime-like material; perifoveal flecks beneath vessels; later, horizontal oval area of atrophy of pigment "beaten bronze atrophy," surrounded by flecks, which progressively enlarges with its halo of flecks without, however, reaching the periphery. Disk and vessels are spared. In 50% of cases association with fundus flavimaculatus (see Franceschetti). In same families association with nephrolithiasis, interstitial nephritis or Pierre Marie syndrome.

Etiology. Primary defect is in the pigment epithelium or in neuroepithelium. Autosomal recessive inheritance; possibly, dominant in some families. It has been suggested that Stargardt syndrome be used only to refer to the atrophic form with flecks and not to include in it all forms of juvenile macular dystrophies.

Pathology. Disappearance of visual elements in the macular and perimacular areas. The substance accumulated seems to be of mucopolysaccharide nature.

Diagnostic Procedures. *Fluorescein angiography and photography. Retinal function studies. Fundoscopy.* Mottled pigmentary spots accumulation in the macula.

Therapy. None.

Prognosis. Slowly evolving condition.

BIBLIOGRAPHY. Stargardt K: Ueber familiäre, progressive Degeneration in der Maculagegende des Auges. Albrecht von Graefes Arch Klin Ophthalmol 71:540–550, 1909
Smith BF, Smith JB, Low J: Stargardt's disease: The evolution of a diagnosis. J Pediatr Ophthalmol Strabismus 24:259–262, 1987
Bither PP, Berns LA: Stargardt's disease: A review of the literature. J Am Ophthalmol Assoc 59:106–111, 1988
Montyjarvi M, Tuppurainen K: Stargardt's disease: Family studies. Doc Ophthalmol 79:79–89, 1992

STARTLE EPILEPSY

Synonyms. Epileptic startle.

Symptoms and Signs. Audiogenic violent starts, characterized by limb and trunk flexion (and desynchronization of EEG activity). With time starts blend into more prolonged (1–30 seconds) tonic spasms, and occasionally may be followed by bilateral symmetrical or focal seizure

Etiology and Pathology. Most frequently in perinatal encephalopathy (see) or Tay-Sachs (see).

BIBLIOGRAPHY. Gastaut H, Tassinari CA: Triggering mechanisms in epilepsy: The electroclinical point of view. Epilepsia 7:85–138, 1966
Hallett M, Marsden CD, Fahn S: Myoclonus. In Vinken PJ, Bruyn GW: Handbook of Clinical Neurology, vol 49, pp 620–621. Amsterdam, North-Holland, 1986

STATUS DYSRAPHICUS

Association of Morvan with external congenital malformations such as cervical rib syndrome, Klippel-Feil, and Arnold-Chiari.

STATUS EPILEPTICUS

Synonyms. Epilptic status.

Symptom. Successive seizures without regaining consciousness between attacks.

Signs. Exhaustion; stupor; coma; tachycardia; dyspnea. If patient recovers, hemiplegia may follow.

Etiology. Complication of epilepsy, grand mal or petit mal, usually following withdrawal of medication or change in therapy.

Therapy. Support vital functions. Phenytoin, intravenous infusion without exceeding 50 mg/minute (loading dose 15–18 mg/kg). Diazepam, 5–10 mg intravenously for a rapid stop of the seizures while waiting for the phenytoin to have effect. In very severe cases: sodium thiopental 0.5–1 mg/kg.

Prognosis. Severe. Death if situation is not brought under control.

BIBLIOGRAPHY. Adams RD, Victor M: Principles of Neurology, 5th ed, pp 273–297. New York, McGraw-Hill, 1993

STEAKHOUSE

Synonyms. Lower esophageal ring; café coronary. See Schatzki.

Symptoms. Intermittent, complete esophageal obstruction often during rapid eating, commonly at steak dinner. The symptoms may arise also when a person aspirates food, sometimes by eating peanut butter, bubble gum, honey. The victim clutches the chest, becomes cyanotic and may die.

Signs. Endoscopy frequently does not show any esophageal stricture.

Etiology. Passive fibrous stricture at the esophagogastric junction uniformly with hiatus herniation.

Pathology. Shell consisting of connective tissue without inflammation and overgrowth of muscularis mucosae, esophageal mucosa on upper, and gastric mucosa on the lower surface.

Diagnostic Procedures. *X-ray.* Of esophagus. Smooth, sharp, concentric narrowing of the distal part of esophagus, not easily seen at routine fluoroscopy. Seen when esophagus is fully distended by thick barium.

Therapy. Change of eating habit. A blow over the back to produce expulsion of bolus of food, manual removal of obstructing bolus (in case of meat) or the "bear clutch" maneuver over the abdomen with repeated quick thrusts until food is expelled. Bougienage and pneumatic dilatation or endoscopic punch biopsy; direct surgical approach for severe cases and repair of hiatus hernia.

Prognosis. Good. Dilatation usually adequate; surgery in more severe cases prevents recurrences.

BIBLIOGRAPHY. Ingelfinger FJ, Kramer P: Dysphagia produced by contractile ring in lower esophagus. Gastroenterology 23:419–430, 1953
Schatzki R, Gary JE: Dysphagia due to diaphragm-like localized narrowing in the lower esophagus ("Lower esophageal ring"). Am J Roentgenol 70:911–922, 1953
Atlas DH: Cafe coronary from peanut butter. N Engl J Med 296:399, 1977

STEATOCYSTOMA MULTIPLEX

Synonyms. Multiple atheromas; sebaceous cystis, multiple.

Symptoms. Both sexes equally affected. Onset in adolescence or adult life. Asymptomatic.

Signs. Smooth, yellowish swellings on the skin. Diameter 1 or 2 mm to 2 cm, distributed on proximal parts of limbs and presternal region. Absence of punctum on lesions; some inflammation and suppuration.

Etiology. Autosomal dominant inheritance.

Pathology. Dermoid cysts formed by keratinizing epithelium with oily content, some containing hair.

Therapy. Excision when feasible, mostly for cosmetic reasons.

Prognosis. Benign; permanent condition. One case of malignant transformation reported.

BIBLIOGRAPHY. Mount LB: Steatocystoma multiplex. Arch Dermatol Syph 36:31–39, 1937

Hodes ME, Norins AL: Pachonychia congenita and steatocytoma multiplex. Clin Genet 11:359–364, 1977

Cuccia-Belvedere M, Brazzelli V, Martinetti M, et al: Familial steatocystoma multiplex HLA Gm, Km genotyping and chromosomal analysis in two unrelated families. Clin Genet 36:136–140, 1989

STEEL

Synonyms. Puerto Rican; Hips; radial heads dislocation; carpal coalition, short stature. See Hip, congenital dislocation; Larsen; Beals; Fairbank.

Symptoms and Signs. Both sexes. In Puerto Rican children of Hispanic descent. Bilateral Trendelenburg gait. Bilateral dislocation of the hip (100%), dislocated radial heads (72%), short stature (87%), carpal coalition (85%), and other variable and inconstant musculoskeletal anomalies, scoliosis (65%), anomaly of cervical spine (13%), talipes cavus bilaterally (35%).

Etiology. Suggested autosomal dominant inheritance. Blood. Urine. Normal.

Diagnostic Procedures. X-ray. Skeletal survey.

Therapy. Closed reduction and adductor tenotomy and or other orthopedic surgical interventions according to need.

Prognosis. Dismal possibility to maintain reduction of dislocated hips; however, even when the hip remains out of the socket the functional result may be considered satisfactory.

BIBLIOGRAPHY. Steel HH: The Puerto Rican syndrome. Read at the Annual Meeting of Shrine Surgeons San Francisco, Oct 10, 1973

Steel HH, Piston RW, Clancy M, et al: A syndrome of dislocated hips and radial heads, carpal coalition, and short stature in Puerto Rican children. J Bone Joint Surg 75A:259–264, 1993

STEIDELE

Synonyms. Steidele complex; aortic arch atresia; aortic arch interruption.

Symptoms. According to different combinations of associated defects.

1. *Aortic arch atresia, patent ductus arteriosus, and ventricular septal defect.* Prevalent in males. May appear normal at birth; then cardiac failure and death within first month of life, seldom later. Clinical recognition difficult. Cyanosis mild or inconspicuous.
2. *Aortic arch atresia without supracardiac or intracardiac shunts.* Seldom, congestive heart failure in infancy. In postadolescence or early adulthood, dyspnea, cephalalgia, epistaxis, leg fatigue, and soreness on walking.

Signs. Usually no difference between upper and lower arterial pulses in type 1. Marked difference in type 2.

Etiology. Congenital malformation.

Pathology. Complete anatomic interruption of aortic arch. A patent ductus arteriosus virtually always present. A ventricular septal defect is frequently present. Other malformations may coexist.

Diagnostic Procedures. *ECG.* Right ventricular hypertrophy with high peaked P-waves. In older patients without shunts, also left ventricular hyperplasia. *Two-dimensional echocardiography. Cardiac catheterization. X-ray.* Cardiomegaly; pulmonary venous congestion; in type without shunt, rib notching possible.

Therapy. Prevention of bacterial endocarditis. Medical management. Palliative surgery attempted in type 1. In type 2 surgical correction when indicated.

Prognosis. In type 1 death within first month; a few may reach early adulthood. In type 2 survival into third decade.

BIBLIOGRAPHY. Steidele RJ: Sammlg. Verschiedener in der chirurg. prakt. Lehrshule Germachten Beobb 2:114, 1777–1778

Van Mierop LHS, Kutsche LM: Embryology of Heart. In Schlant RC, Alexander RW: Hurst's The Heart, 8th ed, p 1722. New York, McGraw-Hill, 1994

Perloff JK: The Clinical Recognition of Congenital Heart Disease, 4th ed, p 156. Philadelphia, WB Saunders, 1994

STEINBACK-BROWN

Synonyms. Acrodysplasia IV; epiphyseal dysplasia; diastrophic dwarfism variant (?); epiphyseal dysostosis.

Symptoms and Signs. Normal height; acromelic shortening.

Etiology. Unknown.

Diagnostic Procedures. X-ray. Axial skeletal changes. Malsegmentation of hands and feet.

BIBLIOGRAPHY. Steinback HI, Brown RA: Epiphyseal dysostosis. Am J Roentgenol 105:860–869, 1969

Bailey JA: Disproportionate Short Stature: Diagnosis and Management, p 197. Philadelphia, WB Saunders, 1973

STEINBROCKER

Synonyms. Coronary scapular; shoulder–hand; sympathetic reflex dystrophy. See Sudeck.

Symptoms and Signs. Affects both sexes, slight predominance of females; onset after 50 years of age (90%). Gradual stiffness, discomfort, weakness in shoulder and hand. Sudden severe pain and stiffness, swelling, hyperesthesia of hand. Three stages. (1) Lasting 3–6 months; complete hand and shoulder involvement. (2) Lasting 3–6 months; partial or total resolution of swelling and vasospasm or vasodilatation. Early trophic changes and contractures, and muscle atrophy. (3) Varying duration (in some cases years); atrophic and dystrophic changes; contractures of fingers; "frozen" shoulder; residual pain infrequent.

Etiology. Reflex dystrophy secondary to internal lesions; postmyocardial infarction (20%); cervical disk or intraforaminal spurs (20%); post-traumatic (10%); posthemiplegic (6%); miscellaneous causes (Herpes zoster, vasculitis, tumor, arthritis) (10%), or idiopathic (25%).

Pathology. *Shoulder tissue.* Inflammatory aspecific changes similar to those seen in capsulitis, periarthritis. *Skin of finger.* Edema; fat depletion, small hemorrhages (see Sudeck).

Diagnostic Procedures. *X-ray RA test. Sedimentation rate.* To rule out rheumatoid arthritis. *ECG. X-ray.* Of chest, cervical spine, and shoulder.

Therapy. Treatment of underlying condition: analgesic; physical therapy; exercise; corticosteroids; stellate ganglionic blocks; sympathectomy.

Prognosis. Variable and unpredictable; lack of correlation with extent and nature of etiology. Residual contractures observed frequently.

BIBLIOGRAPHY. Steinbrocker O: Painful homolateral disability of the shoulder and hand, with swelling and atrophy of the hand. Ann Rheum Dis 6:80–84, 1947

Schlant RC, Alexander RW: Hurst's The Heart, 8th ed, p 209. New York, McGraw-Hill, 1994

STEINDLER

Eponym used for sacralgia. See Fibrositis.

BIBLIOGRAPHY. Steindler AV, Luck JV: Differential diagnosis of pain low in the back: Allocation of the source of pain by procaine hydrochloride method. JAMA 110:106–113, 1938

STEINERT

Synonyms. Batten-Gibb; Curshmann-Batten-Steinert; myotonic dystrophy; myotonia atrophica.

Symptoms. Marked ethnic distribution of the disease (frequent incidence) in Canadian Quebec area. Appears slightly more frequently in male 20–30 years of age. Weakness; myotonia (inability to relax the grasp properly due to abnormal, delayed relaxation of skeletal muscles); motions slow and inefficient. Loss of libido; impotence, oligomenorrhea to amenorrhea. Frequent pulmonary infection. Development of myotonic dystrophy personality: whining dependency. Anticipation. Earlier occurrence of symptoms in second generation.

Signs. Atrophy of muscles (facial, sternocleidomastoideus, quadriceps femoris, distal forearm, and hand). Frontal alopecia; myotic pupils that react sluggishly to light and accommodation; ptosis; cataracts. Percussion of a muscle stimulates contraction of many fibers determining a prolonged localized contraction of the muscle. Tendon reflexes diminished or absent; cardiac conduction defects with arrhythmias. Early frontal balding

Etiology. Autosomal dominant inheritance. Gene defect lies in segment q13.32cM of chromosome 19.DM is owing to a 50 or more CTG reapeat instead of 5 CTG repeat that occurs in normal subjects. The greater the expression of CTG repeat the more severe is the disease manifestation. Maybe this defect is the cause of alteration of function of chloride channel.

Pathology. Atrophy of muscle fibers, replaced by fat and connective tissue interposed with normal and hypertrophic fibers. Brain: cerebral atrophy, specific thalamic inclusions described, neurofibrillary changes. Atrophy of testis (80%) or ovary.

Diagnostic Procedures. *Blood. Urine. CSF.* Normal. *EMG.* Characteristic pattern. *ECG.* Reveals abnormality. *Pulmonary function studies. Endocrine studies.* Increased insulin resistance. *X-ray.* Of skull. *CT scan. MRI.* Radiologic image abnormalities (60%). With DNA probes (Southern blotting, PCR techniques) possibility of prenatal and presymptomatic diagnosis.

Therapy. Pregnant women require particular assistance (abortion, failed labor, retained placenta, etc.). Cataracts corrected surgically. Symptomatic for orthopedic problems. Pacemaker for conduction defects. Nasal ventilation for sleep apnea. Methylphenidate for hypersomnia. Careful management in anesthesia. Therapeutical trials include testosterone growth hormone administration and exercise training.

Prognosis. Slowly progressive. Patient may reach old age.

BIBLIOGRAPHY. Steinert H: Myopathologische Beitrage: Ueber das klinische und anatomische Bild des Muskelschwunds der Myotoniker. D Ptsch Z Nervenheilk 37:58–104, 1909
Batten FE, Gibbs HP: Myotonia atrophica. Brain 32:187–205, 1909
Curshmann H: Ueber familiaere atrophische Myotonia. Dtsch Z Nervenheilk 45:161–202, 1912
Moxley RT III: Myotonic muscular dystrophy. In Rowland LP, Di Mauro S (eds): Handbook of Clinical Neurology, vol 18: Myopathies, p 209. Amsterdam, Elsevier, 1992

STEINER-VOERNER

Synonyms. Angiomatosis miliaris; miliary angiomatosis.

Symptoms. Prevalent in females. Onset at all ages, especially in adolescence. In patients with vasomotor and thermal lability. Frequently concurrent with eruptions (see Signs); cephalalgia; vertigo; nausea; vomiting; diarrhea; tachycardia; anhidrosis; polyuria; various visual impairments; fever.

Signs. Appearance of small diffuse angiomas on cutaneous and mucosal areas.

Etiology. It represents one of the forms of miliaria according to recent classification: crystallina (sudamina); rubra (prickly heat); profunda (mamillaria) owing to epidermal injury in susceptible individuals, where because of sweat the skin flora produces a toxin that damages luminal sweat cells and causes obstruction of the sweat glands by a PAS-positive material.

Therapy. Sedatives. Antiserotonin compounds.

BIBLIOGRAPHY. Steiner L, Voerner H. Angiomatosis miliaris. Eine idiopathische Gefaesserkrankung. Dtsch Arch Klin Med 96:105–116, 1909
Champion RH: Disorders of sweat glands. In Champion RH, Burton JL, Ebling FJG (eds): Rook/Wilkinson/Ebling Textbook of Dermatology, 5th ed, pp 1758–1759. Oxford, Blackwell Scientific, 1992

STEIN-LEVENTHAL

Synonyms. Polycystic bilateral ovarian; persistent anovulation. See Ovarian hyperthecosis.

Symptoms. Onset after puberty or in late teenage years. Menstruation normal at onset and for some time; then progressive oligomenorrhea and finally amenorrhea. Sometimes, primary amenorrhea and menorrhagic episodes. Sterility. Minor voice change.

Signs. Obesity (40%), hypertrichosis (70%), and sometimes virilism (20%). In familial form, males abnormally hairy.

Etiology. Still not quite settled, but numerous researchers think it might be an abnormality in the steroidogenesis of ovarian hormone: A block in the conversion of androstenedione to estrogen, because of enzymatic deficiencies concerned with aromatization of androstenedione into estrogens. If primary abnormality resides in hypothalamus or pituitary still not clear. Autosomal dominant inheritance reported in some families.

Pathology. Ovaries are usually enlarged and often described as "oyster-like." Numerous cystic follicles underneath a thickened ovarian capsule; hyperplastic fibrosis of cortical stroma; hypertrophy and hyperplasia of endometrium. Hyperplasia of theca cells in atretic follicles, sparse primordial and developing follicles stromal hyperplasia.

Diagnostic Procedures. *Blood. Urine.* Slight elevation of 17-ketosteroids in urine; slight elevation of plasma androstenedione or testosterone level, slight elevation of luteinizing hormone levels. Estradiol and follicle-stimulating hormone low. *X-ray. Gynecography. Culdoscopy. Exploratory laparotomy.*

Therapy. Weight reduction. Induction of ovulation is the key to success. Trial with cortisone for a minimum of 6 months. If pregnancy is desired, induction of ovulation with clomiphene. Wedge resection of both ovaries; should be last method. If patient does not desire pregnancy medroxyprogesterone 10 mg/d for the first 10 days of each month. Spironolactone for the treatment of hirsutism or in severe cases hysterectomy and bilateral oophorectomy and estrogen replacement (better epilation and electrolysis).

Prognosis. Good with medical or surgical treatment. Eighty percent cured with wedge resection in well-selected patients; however, recurrences are common.

BIBLIOGRAPHY. Stein IF, Leventhal ML: Amenorrhea associated with bilateral polycystic ovaries. Am J Obstet Gynecol 29:181–191, 1935
Stein IF: The Stein-Leventhal syndrome: A curable form of sterility. N Engl J Med 259:420–423, 1958
Schwartz M, Gindoff PR, Jewelewicz R: Polycystic ovary syndrome: An enigma awaiting solution. Bull NY Acad Med 63:134–155, 1987

Goldzieher JW, Young RW: Selected aspects of polycystic ovarian disease. Endocrinol Metab Clin No Am 1:141–171, 1992

STEVENS-JOHNSON

Synonyms. Baader; Fissinger-Rendu; Klauder; Neumann II. Erythema multiforme exudativum; respiratory mucosa; mucocutaneocular. See Erythema multiforme and Lyell.

Symptoms. Affects all ages, greatest incidence in first and third decades; moderate prevalence in men. Occurs (1) in individuals in good general health, without exogenous factors evident (17%); (2) in individuals presenting vague symptomatology of headache, upper respiratory or urinary tract infections (prodromata?) and where some drugs (see Etiology) have been given (50%); (3) in individuals to whom drugs were given for symptoms not suggesting prodromata of Stevens-Johnson syndrome. Malaise; mild pruritus; burning sensation; arthralgia; myalgia; fever.

Signs. Vesiculobullous lesions of skin (target or bulls-eye lesion) inacral localization and bullae evolving into painful ulcerations in two or more mucous membrane sites (oral cavity; genitourinary tract; conjunctiva). Nikolsky signs negative. Tracheobronchial mucosa and conjunctiva involvement

Etiology. Unknown. Only some cases of unequivocal correlation with drug administration. Viral infections (most cases follow outbreaks of herpes simplex infection) allergic mechanism suspected. Drugs most frequently involved: sulfonamides; penicillin; phenolsulfophthalein; sedatives; also many other unrelated drugs.

Pathology. Hyperkeratosis; acanthosis; vesicles with eosinophils, fibrin precipitate, lymphocytes and neutrophils. Lymphocyte perivascular infiltrate in dermis.

Diagnostic Procedures. Cytology and culture of bullae aspirate. *X-ray.* Of chest. Frequently, finding of pneumonitis. *Blood.* Sedimentation rate, white blood cells increased. *Skin biopsy.* Keratinocyte necrosis perivascular lymphocytic infiltration.

Therapy. Bed rest; liquid diet; gargles; calamine lotion; bacitracin ointment for skin; corticosteroid eye drops. Corticosteroids in moderate doses in severe cases stopped if no prompt response. Acyclovir oral effective in preventing herpes complications.

Prognosis. Approximately 10-day course with severe manifestations; 15–30 days for healing lesions. Usual recovery; possible recurrence. In some cases, persistent corneal lesions, loss of vision. Fatal in some cases.

BIBLIOGRAPHY. Stevens AM, Johnson FC: A new eruptive fever associated with stomatitis and ophthalmia: Report of two cases in children. Am J Dis Child 24:526–533, 1922
Bianchine JR, Macaraeg PVJ, Lasagna L, et al: Drugs as etiologic factors in the Stevens-Johnson syndrome. Am J Med 44:390–405, 1968
Savill JS, Barrie S, Ghosh S, et al: Fatal Stevens-Johnson syndrome following urography with iopamidol in systemic lupus erythematosus. Postgrad Med J 64:392–394, 1988
Bastuji-Garin S, Rzany B, Stern RS: Clinical classification of cases of toxic epidermal necrolysis, Stevens-Johnson syndrome, and erythema multiforme. Arch Dermatol 129:92–96, 1993

STEWART-BERGSTROM

Synonyms. Arthrogrypoticlike hands; sensorineural deafness; deafness; sensorineural—arthrogrypotic-like hands.

Symptoms. Both sexes. Onset early after birth. Hand abnormalities (arthrogrypotic-like), and minor abnormalities of feet. Sensorineural deafness with external ear canal, tympanic membranes normal.

Etiology. Autosomal dominant inheritance with complete penetrance and variable expressivity.

Diagnostic Procedures. *Blood.* Normal. *X-ray.* Hand abnormalities and occasional minor alterations of acetabulum. Palmar dermatoglyphics. Similar to those observed in arthrogryposis. *Audiography.*

Therapy. Orthopedic correction.

Prognosis. Nonprogressive condition.

BIBLIOGRAPHY. Stewart JM, Bergstrom L: Familial hand abnormality and sensorineural deafness. A new syndrome. J Pediatr 78:102–110, 1971
Akbarnia BA, Bowen JR, Doegherty J: Familial arthrogrypotic hand abnormality and sensorineural deafness. Am J Dis Child 113:403–405, 1979

STEWART-HOLMES

See Jackson cerebellar fits.

Symptoms. Attacks last 2–3 minutes. Jerking movements of one arm (unilateral); irregular in sequence and distribution; occasionally affecting the contralateral arm to a slighter degree; frequently associated with vertigo. Other signs of cerebellar lesion may be observed.

Etiology and Pathology. Lesion in cerebellum; traumatic; vascular; neoplastic.

Diagnostic Procedures. *EEG. Angiography. CT brain scan.*

Therapy. Surgery if indicated.

Prognosis. According to nature of lesion.

BIBLIOGRAPHY. Stewart TG, Holmes G: Symptomatology of cerebellar tumours: A study of forty cases. Brain 27:522–591, 1904
Dow RS, Moruzzi G: The Physiology and Pathology of the Cerebellum. Minneapolis, University of Minnesota Press, 1958
Adams RD, Victor M: Principles of Neurology, 5th ed, pp 79–80. New York, McGraw-Hill, 1993

STEWART-TREVES

Synonyms. Lymphangiosarcoma of extemities; postmastectomy lymphangiosarcoma.

Symptoms and Signs. Occurs in patients with chronic lymphedematous extremity; majority of cases in women with breast cancer after mastectomy. Reported in cases (male and female) of groin dissection and radiation for cancer, and in cases of congenital lymphedema without evidence of previous malignancy. Appearance on edematous extremity of a mass, usually dark, slightly tender, enlarging.

Etiology. Alteration in lymphatic circulation, owing to surgery or irradiation or idiopathic, causing neoplastic changes of vascular cells.

Pathology. Lymphangiosarcoma. In postmastectomy cases, the sarcomatous nature of tumor has been challenged by some authors, and considered instead as retrograde metastasis from carcinoma.

Diagnostic Procedures. *Biopsy.*

Therapy. Amputation. External radiotherapy. Intra-arterial 90y in ceramic microspheres.

Prognosis. Generally poor. Frequent widespread metastasis.

BIBLIOGRAPHY. Stewart FW, Treves N: Lymphangiosarcoma in postmastectomy lymphedema. Report of 6 cases of elephantiasis chirurgica. Cancer 1:64–81, 1948
Haltberg BM: Angiosarcokomas in chronically lymphedematous extremities: Two cases of Stewart-Treves syndrome. Am J Dermatol 9:406–412, 1987
MacKie RM: Soft tissue tumors. In Champion RH, Burton JL, Ebling

FJG (eds): Rook/Wilkinson/Ebling Textbook of Dermatology, 5th ed, p 2092. Oxford, Blackwell Scientific, 1992

STIFF HEART

Synonyms. Restrictive cardiac; restrictive hemodynamic including diastolic compliance, acute changes. See also Pick (F.).

Symptoms. Exertional dyspnea; finally orthopnea; occasionally, pain in the chest.

Signs. Elevation of systemic venous pressure; pulsus paradoxus; Kussmaul sign may be present; heart sound faint or normal; additional diastolic sounds (strong evidence for the condition); hepatomegaly; ascites and edemas. Episodes may occur with or without angina pectoris.

Etiology and Pathology. Chronic constrictive pericarditis (tuberculosis, trauma, radiation, rheumatoid arthritis, mycosis, idiopathic). Primary and secondary myocardiopathies (myocardial fibrosis, subendocardial fibroelastosis). Loeffler subendocardial fibroelastosis, amyloidosis, hemochromatosis, and in diastolic compliance acute changes by abnormalities of intracellular uptake of calcium by sarcoplasmic reticulum.

Diagnostic Procedures. *ECG.* Normal or some abnormalities. *X-ray.* Helpful in differential diagnosis. *Two-dimensional echocardiography with color imaging and spectral Doppler interrogation. Cardiac catheterization.* Diagnostic. Other tests. As needed, according to etiology and symptoms.

Therapy. Not specific. According to etiology and symptoms. Digitalization of little benefit.

Prognosis. Chronic evolution; results according to etiology.

BIBLIOGRAPHY. Shabetai R, Fowler NO, Fenton JC: Restrictive cardiac disease, pericarditis and the myocardiopathies. Am Heart J 69:271–280, 1965
Kilpatrick TR, Horack HM, Moore CB: "Stiff heart" syndrome: An uncommon cause of heart failure. Med Clin No Am 51:959–966, 1967
Schlant RC, Sonnenblick EH: Pathophysiology of Heart Failure (p 521), and Shabetai R: Diseases of pericardium (p 1647). In Schlant RC, Alexander RW, et al: Hurst's The Heart, 8th ed. New York, McGraw-Hill, 1994

STIFF-MAN

Synonyms. Ambiguous eponym since it is used to indicate the Moersch-Woltman (see) original desciption, the Grund (see) the fasciculation-weakness (see) the neuromyotonia (observed after lesions of peripheral nerve with stiffness, fasciculation, myokymia, delayed relaxation, and occasionally muscle hypertrophy).

BIBLIOGRAPHY. Weatherall DJ, Ledingham JGG, Warrell DA: Oxford Textbook of Medicine, p 4159. Oxford, Oxford Med Pub, 1996

STIFF SKIN

Synonym. Mucopolysaccharidosis variant.

Symptoms. Rare. Both sexes affected. Congenital or noticed in early childhood. Limited mobility of various joints.

Signs. Localized areas of stony-hard skin involving primarily buttocks and upper thighs. Lordotic stance.

Etiology. Unknown. Probably, autosomal dominant inheritance. Could belong, as a variant, in mucopolysaccharidosis group.

Pathology. Epidermis unremarkable; in the upper dermis interstitial ground substance granular and eosinophilic; abnormal amount of hyaluronidase-digestible acid mucopolysaccharide; appendages are normal.

Diagnostic Procedures. *Biopsy.* Of skin. See Pathology. *Blood.* Normal. *Urine.* Normal. No increased excretion of mucopolysaccharides. *X-ray.* Of skeleton. Normal.

Therapy. None.

Prognosis. Stable condition.

BIBLIOGRAPHY. Pichler E: Hereditaere Kontrakturen mit sclerodermie-artigen Hantveraenderungen. Z Kinderheilkd 104:349–361, 1968
Esterly NB, McKusick NA: Stiff skin syndrome. Pediatrics 47:360–369, 1971
Stevenson RE, Lucas TL Jr, Martin JB Jr: Symmetrical lipomatosis associated with stiff-skin and systemic manifestations in four generations. Proc Greenwood Genet Ctr 3:56–64, 1984
Burton JL: Disorders of connective tissue. In Champion RH, Burton JL, Ebling FJG (eds): Rook/Wilkinson/Ebling Textbook of Dermatology, 5th ed, p 1810. Oxford, Blackwell Scientific, 1992

STILL

Synonyms. Chauffard-Ramon; Chauffard-Still; Dreier; juvenile rheumatoid arthritis; acute polyarthritis. Eponym also used for subacute and chronic juvenile rheumatoid arthritis.

Symptoms and Signs. More frequent in females; onset before puberty (never before 6 months of age), or in adults. High spiking fever antedating arthritis for months; skin rash (erythema morbillifom salmon colored); nonconstant pneumonitis; pericarditis; iridocyclitis; failure to thrive; lymphadenopathy; hepatomegaly; splenomegaly. Eventually monoarticular or polyarticular arthritis becomes evident.

Etiology. Unknown. Possibility of genetic origin not assessed. Relation with collagen and autoimmune diseases.

Pathology. Nonspecific synovitis in joint with granulation tissue, erosion of cartilage, fibrosis, bony ankylosis. Nonspecific lymph node hyperplasia. Myocarditis.

Diagnostic Procedures. *Blood.* Leukocytosis (50%); moderate anemia; high sedimentation rate. Lupus erythematosus test negative. Test for rheumatoid arthritis positive (20%). *X-ray.* Of joints. Demineralization; erosions; reduction of joint space. *Synovial biopsy.*

Therapy. Corticosteroids; naproxen, diclofenac, tolmetin, aspirin; chloroquine.

Prognosis. Persistent activity for 2 or 3 years. Pain disappearing 10 years after onset. Possible ankylosis and failure to grow or transient and reversible lesions.

BIBLIOGRAPHY. Cornil V: Mémoire sur les coïncidences pathologiques du rhumatisme articulaire chroniques. C R Soc Biol 1 (2):3–25, 1864–1865
Still GF: On a form of chronic joint disease in children. Proc R Med Chir Soc (Lond) 9:10–15, 1896
Pouchot J, Sampalis J, Beaudet F: Adult Still's disease: Manifestations, disease course and an outcome in 62 patients. Medicine 70:118–136, 1991
Weatherall DJ, Ledingham JGG, Warrell DA: Oxford Textbook of Medicine, pp 2973–2974. Oxford, Oxford Med Pub, 1996

STILLER

Synonyms. Asthenia universalis congenita; morbus asthenicus.

Symptoms. Asthenia; gastric atonia; pallor. Tall and skinny individual; scarce subcutaneous tissue; splanchnoptosis.

Etiology. Unknown.

Prognosis. In the past, this habitus was associated with a high incidence of tubercular diseases.

BIBLIOGRAPHY. Stiller B: Die asthenische Konstitutionskrankheit (Asthenia universalis congenita. Morbus asthenicus). Stuttgart, Enke, 1907

STIMMLER

Synonyms. Alaninuria—microcephaly—dwarfism—diabetes mellitus.

Symptoms and Signs. At birth. Female. Microcephaly, small teeth, low weight. Then physical (dwarfism) and mental retardation.

Etiology. Autosomal recessive inheritance.

Diagnostic Procedures. *Blood.* Alanine, pyruvate, lactate increased. *Urine.* Alanine excretion increased.

BIBLIOGRAPHY. Stimmler L, Jensen N, Toseland P: Alaninuria associated with microcephaly, dwarfism, enamel hypoplasia, and diabetes mellitus in two sisters. Arch Dis Child 45:682–685, 1970
Scriver CR, Gibson KM: Disorders of aminoacids in free and peptide-linked forms. In Scriver CR, Beaudet AL, Sly WS, et al: The Metabolic and Molecular Bases of Inherited Disease, 7th ed, p 1351. New York, McGraw-Hill, 1995

STOKVIS-TALMA

Synonyms. Autotoxic cyanosis; enterogenous cyanosis; idiopathic methemoglobinemia; van den Bergh. Eponym obsolete; no longer considered an entity. The symptoms today are attributed to ingestion of a product that produces methemoglobinemia. The possibility persists, however, that bacterial overgrowth in the intestine may damage the red cells' metabolism and make them more sensitive to the action of ingested products, with oxidant properties (e.g., analgesics, antipyretics).

BIBLIOGRAPHY. Stokvis BJ: Kihdrage tot de casuistick der autotoxiche enterogene Cyanosen (Methaemoglobinaemia [?]) et Enteritis parassitaria. Med Tschr Geneesk 36:678–693, 1902
Talma S: Intraglobulare Methaemoglobinaemia beim Menschen. Berl Klin Wochenschr 39:865–867, 1902
Lukens JN: Methemoglobinemia and other disorders accompanied by cyanosis. In Lee GR, Bithell TC, Foerster J, et al (eds): Wintrobe's Clinical Hematology, 9th ed, p 1263. Philadelphia, Lea & Febiger, 1993

STOMATOCYTOSIS

Synonym. Hydrocytosis.

Symptoms and Signs. A peculiar morphologic feature of red cells that are uni-concave, with a slit-like area of central pallor. These erythrocytes show shorter survival and increased osmotic fragility resulting in hemolytic anemia.

Etiology. Stomatocytes are found in more than one type of congenital hemolytic anemia both on autosomal and recessive inheritance. Defect also is caused by a potassium-sodium disorder, higher Na, and lower K content in red cells. A cold-sensitive variety also has been described.

Therapy. Splenectomy may be beneficial in severe forms.

BIBLIOGRAPHY. Lock SP, Smith R, Hardisty RM: Stomatocytosis: A hereditary red cell anomaly associated with haemolytic anaemia. Br J Haemat 7:303–314, 1961
Eber SW, Lande WM, Iarocci TA, et al: Hereditary stomatocytosis: consistent association with an integral membrane protein deficiency. Br J Haematol 72:452–455, 1989
Huppi PS, Ott P, Amato M, et al: Congenital haemolytic anaemia in a low birth weight infant due to congenital stomatocytosis. Eur J Haemat 47:1–9, 1991
Lukens JN: Hereditary spherocytosis and other hemolytic anemias associated with abnormalities of the red cell membrane and the cyto-

skeleton. In Lee GR, Bithell TC, Foerster J, et al (eds): Wintrobe's Clinical Hematology, 9th ed, pp 977–979. Philadelphia, Lea & Febiger, 1993

STONE HEART

Synonym. Ischemic contracture of heart.

Symptoms. Occurs in both sexes. Onset at any age in people with acquired severe heart disease (class III or IV) after cardiac surgery. Sudden development of myocardial failure owing to a small spastic heart, stopped in systole, where not even vigorous manual massage succeeds in producing an adequate stroke volume. The contracted state is irreversible.

Etiology. Unknown. State of rigor of the ischemic myocardium failing to relax, attributed to loss of myocardial energy stores, leading to depletion of adenosine triphosphate (ATP) in the region occupied by the myofilaments.

Pathology. *Heart.* Hypertrophy of concentric type; presence of fibrosis; small left ventricular chamber.

Therapy. Attempt to prevent by ensuring continued oxygen supply to myocardium during surgery, perfusion with low-calcium solutions, maintaining a relative condition of acidosis, and administration of ATP and potassium. The best management in preventing stone heart is the reduction of aortic clamping time; a corrected myocardial protection with cardioplegic solution during clamping time and finally, after declamping, adequate coronary reperfusion.

Prognosis. Once developed, the condition presently appears irreversible.

BIBLIOGRAPHY. Cooley DA, Reul GJ, Wukasch DC: Ischemic contraction of the heart: "Stone heart." Am J Cardiovasc 29:575–577, 1972
Katz AM, Tada M: The "stone heart": A challenge to the biochemist. Am J Cardiol 29:578–580, 1972
Lell WA: Myocardial protection during cardiopulmonary by-pass. In Kaplan JA (ed): Cardiac Anesthesia, p 1031. Philadelphia, WB Saunders, 1993
Vinten-Johansen J, Hammon JW: Myocardial protection during cardiac surgery. In Gravlee GP, Davis RP, Utley JR (eds): Cardiopulmonary Bypass, p 115. Baltimore, Williams & Wilkins, 1993

STOOKEY

Obsolete.

Synonyms. Cervical cord compression, extradural chondromas. See Cervical spondylotic myelopathy.

Etiology. The alleged chondromas were recognized as soft disk herniation or bony osteophytes.

BIBLIOGRAPHY. Stookey B: Compression of spinal cord due to ventral extradural cervical chondromas: Diagnosis and surgical treatment. Arch Neurol Psychiatr 20:275–291, 1928

STORAGE POOL

Synonyms. Dense granules defects; platelet storage pool. See also Hermansky-Pudlak and Chediak-Higashi.

Symptoms and Signs. Mild to moderate bleeding.

Etiology. Deficiency in total platelet. ADP, Autosomal dominant inheritance.

Diagnostic Procedures. *Blood.* Abnormalities in platelet aggregation patterns. Absence of second wave of aggregation in response to ADP and epinephrine and absent in response to collagen. Decreased level of platelet serotonin and decreased ADP/ATP ratio.

Therapy. DDAVP, platelet transfusion for severe bleeding episodes.

Prognosis. Fair.

BIBLIOGRAPHY. Caen JP, Sultan Y, Larriccu MJ: A new familial platelet disease. Lancet II:203–204, 1968
Newman PJ, Poncz M: Inherited disorders of platelets. In Scriver CR, Beaudet AL, Sly WS, et al: The Metabolic and Molecular Bases of Inherited Disease, 7th ed, p 3348. New York, McGraw-Hill, 1995

STORM

Synonyms. Werner-like; calcific cardiac valvular degeneration; premature aging.

Symptoms and Signs. Both sexes. Early progressive signs of cardiopathy. In adolescence loss of eyebrows thinning and graying of hair; wrinkling. Frequently polyarthropathy. Occasionally malabsorption. Absence of cataracts and sclerodermatous changes.

Etiology. Autosomal dominant inheritance.

Pathology. *Heart.* Calcification in the mitral and aortic valves, with mitral prolapse and myxedematous degeneration. See also signs for other organs.

Diagnostic Procedures. *X-rays. Heart.* Calcified anuli in both valve with serate stenosis. *Joints.* Polyarthropathy.

BIBLIOGRAPHY. Weisman HF, Gaither NS, Moore J, et al: The Storm syndrome: A new, pleiotropic, autosomal dominant disorder affecting connective tissue. Am J Med Genet 45:A67, 1989

STORMORKEN

Synonyms. Thrombocytopathy—asplenia—miosis.

Symptoms. From early infancy. Asthenia, cephalea, dyslexia, easy bleeding.

Signs. Ichthyosis, miosis.

Etiology. Unknown. Familial occurrence (autosomal dominant?).

Diagnostic Procedures. *CT scan.* Absence of spleen. *Blood.* Red cells with Howell-Jolly bodies. Platelets in normal number.

BIBLIOGRAPHY. Stormorken H, Sjaastad O, Langslet A, et al: A new syndrome: Thrombocytopathy, muscle fatigue, asplenia, miosis, migraine, dyslexia, and ichthyosis. Clin Genet 28:367–374, 1985

STRACHAN

Synonyms. Howes-Pallister-Landor; Strachan-Scott; ariboflavinosis—amblyopia—painful neuropathy—orogenital dermatitis.

Symptoms. Amblyopia; paresthesias of feet, hands, trunk, and occasionally face. Dizziness; deafness; hoarseness; spasticity; ataxia.

Signs. Reflex loss; genital dermatitis; corneal degeneration; glossitis; stomatitis. Features of chronic malnutrition.

Etiology. Chronic malnutrition.

Pathology. Bilateral symmetric loss of myelinated fibers in central part of optic nerves. Loss of ganglion cells in the macula (in severe form).

Diagnostic Procedures. *Blood.* Hypoproteinemia; hypochromic, microcytic, or macrocytic anemia; reduced level of B_2 and B_{12} (occasional); low transketolase activity. *Urine.* Abnormal excretion of methylmalonic acid.

Therapy. Oral or parenteral B vitamin group; improved nutrition.

Prognosis. Degree of recovery according to degree of amblyopia and time of onset of treatment.

BIBLIOGRAPHY. Strachan H: On a form of multiple neuritis prevalent in the West Indies. Practitioner (Lond) 59:477–484, 1897
Adams RD, Victor M: Principles of Neurology, 5th ed, p 864. New York, McGraw-Hill, 1993
Weatherall DJ, Ledingham JGG, Warrell DA: Oxford Textbook of Medicine, p 4100. Oxford, Oxford Med Pub, 1996

STRAEUSSLER

Synonyms. Spinocerebellar ataxia; dementia; plaque-like deposits.

Symptoms and Signs. Onset in adults. Sensory ataxia, cerebellar syndrome followed by dementia, pseudobulbar signs and distal spinal muscular atrophy.

Pathology. Cerebral cortex, basal ganglia, and particularly cerebellum: characteristic senile plaque-like deposits. Glyosis in parts of cerebral hemispheres, external pallidum, thalamus, sustantia nigra, red and dentate nucleus. Loss of spinal anterior horn cells and glyosis.

Diagnostic Procedures. Autosomal dominant inheritance. Disorder similar to Kuru (see).

Therapy. Symptomatic.

Prognosis. Leading to death in 2–7 years after a progressive course.

BIBLIOGRAPHY. Seitelberger F: Einegartige familiaer-hereditaere Krankait des Zentralnervensystems in einer niederoesterreichischer. Sippe Wien Klin Wschr 74:687–692, 1962
Crémieux A, Recordier M, Boudouresques J, et al: Dégénérescence spino-cérébelleuse familiale et maladie d'Alzheimer Etude anatomo-clinique d'un cas. Rev Neurol 109:45–54, 1963

STRAIGHT BACK

Synonym. Back straight.

Symptoms. Delusion of heart disease (because of faulty diagnosis) affecting activities and employment of the patient. In some cases, dyspnea.

Signs. Loss of kyphotic curve of upper dorsal spine (flattened palm of examiner's hand on the area does not have normal deviation of fingers). Heart auscultation: harsh, late systolic murmur, ejection type from grade IV to grade I at the base. Increased pulmonic closure sounds.

Etiology and Pathology. Congenital abnormality of upper dorsal spine that decreases anteroposterior diameter of chest and causes spurious heart enlargement and mechanical murmurs. In some cases, pulmonary obstruction with elevation of pulmonary arterial pressure.

Diagnostic Procedures. *Echocardiography. X-ray.* Of chest, frontal and lateral view. Anterior concavity of vertebral column in upper dorsal region absent, with compression of heart against the sternum and kinking of great vessels. *Fluoroscopy. ECG.* Normal.

Therapy. None. If dyspnea and signs of pulmonary hypertension, surgery to correct chest cage deformity.

Prognosis. Benign condition; correct diagnosis avoids iatrogenic heart disease.

BIBLIOGRAPHY. Ravlings MS: The "straight back" syndrome: A new cause of pseudoheart disease. Am J Cardiol 5:333–338, 1960
Leinbach RC, Harthorne JW, Dinsmore RE: Straight back syndrome with pulmonary venous obstruction. Am Cardiol 21:588–592, 1968
Schlant RC, Alexander RW: Hurst's The Heart, 8th ed, pp 225, 290, 364. New York, McGraw-Hill, 1994
Weatherall DJ, Ledingham JGG, Warrell DA: Oxford Textbook of Medicine, p 2874. Oxford, Oxford Med Pub, 1996

STRANSKY-REGALA

Obsolete.

Synonym. Chronic congenital hemolytic anemia. Eponym used to indicate a variety (?) of congenital chronic hemolytic anemias occurring in the Philippines; splenectomy controlled the hemolytic component but not the anemia.

BIBLIOGRAPHY. Stransky E, Regala A: New type of familial congenital chronic hemolytic anemia. Am J Dis Child 71:492–505, 1946

STRAUSS-CHURG-ZAK

Synonyms. Churg-Strauss; allergic granulomatosis—angiitis.

Symptoms and Signs. Prevalent in women. Asthmatic attacks; recurrent eruptions on trunk and limbs of erythema multiform-like; hemorrhagic and nodular lesions in the skin. Peripheral neuropathies, Raynaud phenomenon, pericarditis or myocarditis, less frequently intestinal complications and mild kidney function impairment.

Etiology. Unknown. Related to vasculitis syndrome and collagen diseases. Differing from periarteritis nodosa (see Kussmaul-Maier) because of lung involvement and peculiar granulomatous skin lesions.

Pathology. Endothelial necrosis; edema; fibrinoid necrosis of collagen; granulomas with prevalence of eosinophils, histiocytes, giant cells.

Diagnostic Procedures. *Blood.* Anemia; eosinophilia; high sedimentation rate. *Biopsy.* Of skin. *X-rays.* Chest frequent pleuropulmonary and/or cardiac anomalies.

Therapy. Corticosteroids. Cyclophosphamide.

Prognosis. Very poor. The condition evolves through remissions and relapses always preceded by intense eosinophilia.

BIBLIOGRAPHY. Strauss L, Churg J, Zak FG: Cutaneous lesions of allergic granulomatosis: Histopathologic study. J Invest Dermatol 17:349–359, 1951
Lenham JG, Elkan KB, Pusey CD, et al: Systemic vasculitis with asthma and eosinophilia: A clinical approach to Churg-Strauss syndrome. Medicine 63:65–81, 1984
Leavitt RV, Fauci AF: Pulmonary vasculitis. Am Rev Resp Dis 134:149–166, 1986
Hass C, Geneau C, Odinot JM, et al: L'angeite allergique avec granulomatose: syndrome de Churg et Strauss Etude retrospective de 16 observations. Ann Med Int 142:335–342, 1991

STRAW PETER

Synonyms. Struwwelpeter; cerebral dysfunction infantilis; hyperkinetic; hypokinetic; minimal brain dysfunction; slovenly Peter; see Prechtel-Stemmer and cocktail party.

Symptoms. Estimated to affect 5–20% of general school population. In preschool age, manifested as clumsiness (general coordination deficits); abnormal activity level (hyperkinetic, restless, fidgety, disorganized thought processes, or hypokinetic); impulsivity; emotional lability. At school, excessive distractibility, specific learning disability (reading, spelling, arithmetic, abstract concepts), perceptual motor deficits (poor drawing, printing).

Signs. Transient strabismus, poor coordination of fingers, impaired auditory or visual (or both) perceptual systems; motor awkwardness.

Etiology. *Variable.* Prechtel-Stemmer syndrome (see). From psychosociologic environmental factors to minimal brain dysfunction; genetic predisposition.

Pathology. Nonspecific.

Diagnostic Procedures. Multidisciplinary approach. *EEG.* Borderline or minimal abnormalities observed. *Otologic, ophthalmologic, psychological, psychiatric, and educational evaluations.*

Therapy. Home management: routinized and scheduled program, decrease in environmental stimulation. School management: close cooperation between doctors and teachers; special tutorial education, if needed. Medication to reduce hyperactivity and increase attention: Captodiamine hydrochloride, thioridazine hydrochloride, and amphetamines.

Prognosis. Usually symptoms subside by puberty. Mild degree of mental retardation; epilepsy, other disabilities may become evident.

BIBLIOGRAPHY. Clements SD, Peter JE: Minimal brain dysfunctions in school-age child. Arch Gen Psychiatr 6:185–197, 1962
Pincus JH, Glaser GH: The syndrome of "minimal brain damage" in childhood. N Engl J Med 275:27–35, 1966
Hoffmann H: "Struwwelpeter" (quoted by ed). JAMA 202:28–29, 1967
de la Cruz FF, Fox BH, Roberts RH (eds): Minimal brain dysfunction. Ann NY Acad Sci 205:1–396, 1973
Adams RD, Victor M: Principles of Neurology, 5th ed, p 520. New York, McGraw-Hill, 1993

STREPTOCOCCAL, TOXIC SHOCK-LIKE

Synonyms. Toxic, steptococcal shock-like; necrotizing fascitis; gangrene, acute hemolytic streptococcal; streptococcal fascitis/myositis; gas infection; invasive group A streptococcal infection.

Symptoms and Signs. Occasionally epidemic, often sporadic. In all ages in normal or immunocompromised patients. From small contaminated wounds or surgical incisions rapidly developing fasciitis or myositis. In 12–48 hours: diarrhea, vomiting, shock, signs of renal failure, and multiorgan failure. Erythema darkens to purple and presents blisters or bullae. In a less severe case, on tenth day formation of line of demarcation and rupture of skin that reveals extensive area of necrotic tissue.

Etiology. Invasive infection by streptococcus Group A but hemolytic stains that cause this type of infection usually are M1, or M3, T1 and produce A, B, or C exotoxins.

Pathology. Extensive fascial and muscular necrosis. Foci of bacterial necrosis may be present also in different visceral organs.

Diagnostic Procedures. *Culture of necrotic tissue; hemoculture.* Streptococal presence.

Therapy. Antibiotics, intensive therapy for shock; extensive surgical debridement; amputation

Prognosis. Death in 40–60% of cases.

BIBLIOGRAPHY. Pfanner W: Zur Kenntnis und Behandlung des nekrotisierenden Erysipels. Dtsch Ztschr Chir 144:108, 1918
Meleney GL: Hemolytic sterptococcus gangrene. Arch Surg 9:317–364, 1924
Cone LA, Voodard DR, Schlievert PM, et al: Clinical and bacteriological observations of a toxic-shock-like syndrome due to streptococcus pyogenes. N Eng J Med 317:146–149, 1987
Stevens DL: Invasive group A streptococcus infections. Clin Infec Dis 14:2–13, 1992
Weatherall DJ, Ledingham JGG, Warrell DA: Oxford Textbook of Medicine, p 502. Oxford, Oxford Med Pub, 1996

STRESS FRACTURE OF FIBULA

Synonym. Fibular fatigue fracture. See Shin splint.

Symptoms. Common in athletes and in children. Abrupt onset; severe pain above and behind lateral side of ankle. Insidious onset (more frequent); gradually increasing pain during or following activity. Frequently limp. Running or climbing stairs causes severe pain.

Signs. Tenderness above lateral ankle and occasionally swellings that become bone-hard with time.

Etiology. Fracture of fibula usually at tibiofibular joint owing to excessive stress during sports activity.

Pathology. Fracture of fibula; formation of callus (see also Stress fracture of tibia).

Diagnostic Procedures. *X-ray.* Fracture seldom seen at onset except with special studies (macrograph). Typical appearance may not be seen before 4 weeks.

Therapy. Rest from sport; adhesive elastic strapping.

Prognosis. With treatment, usually cure in about 6 weeks; then gradual return to sport activity. Without treatment, the entire sport season may be lost.

BIBLIOGRAPHY. Burrows HJ: Fatigue fractures of fibula. J Bone Joint Surg (Br) 30:266–279, 1948
Devas MB, Sweetnam R: Stress fractures of the fibula: A review of 50 cases in athletes. J Bone Joint Surg (Br) 38:818–829, 1956
Slocum DB: The shin splint syndrome: Medical aspects and differential diagnosis. Am J Surg 114:875–881, 1967
Perry JD: Sports medicine: The clinical spectrum of injury. In Klippel JH, Dieppe PA: Rheumatology, pp 5.21.9–5.21.10. St Louis, CV Mosby, 1995

STRESS FRACTURE OF TIBIA

Synonym. Periostitis tibiae ab excercitio.

Symptoms. Occurs in athletes (runners); insidious onset of dull pain in the shin at the end of a run. It increases over the days or months until it prevents continuation of sport activities. At beginning pain is relieved by rest; later pain remains after activity. Abrupt onset also observed, although less frequently.

Signs. Tenderness and swelling over tibia (lower third). Absence of inflammatory reaction. Good tibial pulse.

Etiology. Repeated stress fractures of cortex at first, then spreading to the bone. To be differentiated from shin splint syndrome and other overuse syndromes.

Pathology. At onset localized osteoclastic reabsorption, then linear fracture, then periosteal and endosteal callus.

Diagnostic Procedures. *X-ray.* Changes appear usually late, 3–4 weeks after onset.

Therapy. Rest from sport; adhesive strapping.

Prognosis. Complete recovery after 3–4 months.

BIBLIOGRAPHY. Aleman O: Tumors of foot from long marches. Tidskr Militar Hälsovard 54:191–208, 1929
Devas MB: Stress fractures of the tibia in athletes or "shin soreness." J Bone Joint Surg (Br) 40:227–239, 1958
Slocum DB: The shin splint syndrome: medical aspects and differential diagnosis. Am J Surg 114:875–881, 1967
Perry JD: Sports medicine. The clinical spectrum of injury. In Klippel JH, Dieppe PA: Rheumatology, pp 5.21.9–5.21.10. St Louis, CV Mosby, 1995

STRING

Symptoms and Signs. Appears as a complication of cerclage suture used to oppose choroid and retina and retinal detachment. Onset between 4th and 19th postoperative day. Intense pain in the eye; edema of eyelids; proptosis of the globe; chemosis of conjunctiva; uveitis; ocular hypertension. Cornea remains clear; anterior chamber is very deep; iris is fixed and assumes green color.

Etiology and Pathology. Complication of cerclage operation. Suture causing vascular obstruction; configuration of eye predisposing factor.

Therapy. Responds slowly to steroids. Application of diathermy in conjunction with cerclage suture may prevent the occurrence of the syndrome.

Prognosis. Persists for weeks, ultimately resolves; secondary changes persist and result in complete detachment of retina.

BIBLIOGRAPHY. Mason N: The "string syndrome": Seen as a complication of Arruga's cerclage suture. Br J Ophthalmol 48:70–74, 1964
Pauh H: Differential Diagnosis of Eye Disease. Philadelphia, WB Saunders, 1978

STROKE SYNDROMES

Three types or stages clinically distinguished.

1. Transient ischemic attacks
2. Stroke in evolution
3. Completed stroke

STROKE IN EVOLUTIONS

Synonym. Progressive stroke.

Symptoms. Sudden onset of relentless progression of symptoms. Sensorial alterations from stupor to coma.

Signs. Breathing irregular (Cheyne-Stokes or other anomalies). Focal signs of lesions; flaccidity; hemiplegia. This stage is the cerebral shock.

COMPLETE STROKE

Symptoms. Partial or total recovery of consciousness; lessening of paralysis; flaccidity converted to spasticity.

Etiology. Cerebrovascular accident: hemorrhagic or thrombotic.

Pathology. Focal injury of brain and peripheral or general edema.

Diagnostic Procedures. *Cerebrospinal fluid.* Increased pressure. Red cells in some cases. *EEG.* Focal signs. *Angiography. CT scan.* Evidence of area of lesion.

Therapy. General supportive measures. Antiedema treatment. Consideration and evaluation of neurosurgical intervention. Antibiotics.

Prognosis. Variable from deepening of coma and death, to recovery and partial to almost complete remission of symptoms.

BIBLIOGRAPHY. Adams RD, Victor M: Principles of Neurology, 5th ed, pp 670–672. New York, McGraw-Hill, 1993

STRONG

Synonyms. Right-sided aortic arch; mental deficiency; facial dysmorphism; aortic arch anomaly; peculiar facies; mental retardation. See Rubinstein-Taybi, Russell-Silver, and Floppy infant.

Symptoms and Signs. Evident from birth. Both sexes affected. Low birth weight; mental retardation; microcephaly; hypotonia; hyperactive patellar reflexes. *Facies.* Asymmetric, triangular. Nose, prominent; septal deviation. Antimongoloid slant. Large ears; rotated posteriorly. Broad forehead. Small, downturned mouth. Teeth abnormalities. *Hands.* Syndactyly. *Heart.* Significant murmur.

Etiology. Unknown. Genetic mutation, followed by dominant inheritance without apparent sex linkage.

Pathology. See Signs. Fourth and sixth aortic arch abnormalities.

Diagnostic Procedures. *X-ray.* Of chest, with barium swallow. Right-sided aortic arch and esophageal indentation. Bone age normal. Asymmetry of facial bones; deviation of nasal septum; slight hypertelorism. *ECG.* Normal. *Psychometric evaluation.* Mental retardation or subnormality. *Karyotype study.* Normal. *Urine. Amino acid chromatogram.* Normal.

Therapy. Symptomatic.

Prognosis. Good quoad vitam. A few patients may grow normally, complete schooling, and hold skilled jobs; however, majority fail to be promoted a grade at least once.

BIBLIOGRAPHY. Strong WB: Familial syndrome of right-sided aortic arch, mental deficiency and facial dysmorphism. J Pediatr 73:882–888, 1968

STRUDWICK*

Synonyms. Murdock-Walker; Lowsky-Zychowicz; Sutcliffe; SEMD-Strudwick; spondylometaphyseal dysplasia (type C-V); spondylometaphyseal dysostosis (type C-IV); spondyloepimetaphyseal dysplasia; dappled metaphysis; KO2; metaphyseal dysostosis (type B-II).

Symptoms and Signs. Both sexes affected. Present from birth. Short trunk and extremities. Normal weight. Nose broad and flat. Eye problems. Sternum prominent. Breathing short and impaired (rib retraction), hyperpneic. Moderate hepatosplenomegaly; protuberant abdomen. Delayed growth and motor milestones. Joint laxity; elbows do not extend fully; coxa vara; knock-knee; scoliosis and lordosis. Other possible malformations: cleft palate; hemangiomas; hernias; foot malformations.

Etiology. Autosomal recessive trait.

Diagnostic Procedures. *Blood. Urine.* Normal. *X-rays.* Metaphyseal irregularities; "paint brush" and radiologic hyperlucency. "Dappling" alternated zones of osteosclerosis and osteopenia maximal in the ulna and fibula.

Therapy. Control of respiratory infections. Surgical correction of cleft palate, hernias, and significant sternum deformities, and nonsurgical orthopedic measures to correct various defects.

Prognosis. Fair quoad vitam. Increased mortality in early age. Poor for function; frequently, episodic polyarthritis in later life. Severe scoliosis and cord compression in early adulthood.

BIBLIOGRAPHY. Kozolowsky K, Zichowicz C: Metaphyseal dystosis of mixed type in a female child. Am J Roentgen 88:443–449, 1962
Murdock JL, Walker BA: A new form of spondylometaphyseal dysplasia. Birth Defects 5:368–370, 1969
Kousseff BG, Nichols P: Autosomal recessive spondylometaepiphyseal dysplasia type Strudwick. Am J Med Genet 17:547–550, 1984

STRUEMPELL-LORRAIN

Synonyms. Spastic infantile paralysis; spastic familial paraplegia. See Kugelberg-Welander and Behr I.

Symptoms. Prevalent in males; onset in early life. Lower extremities hypertonicity and weakness, followed by involvement of upper limbs, dysarthria, and dysphagia.

Signs. Clumsy ambulation; pes cavus (frequent); exaggerated deep reflexes; Babinski sign; decreased or abolished abdominal reflexes; sphincters slightly affected (later).

Etiology. Autosomal (usually) recessive inheritance or sex-linked.

Could be considered a variant of Friedreich ataxia (see) and some heredoataxias with cerebellar atrophy.

Pathology. Degeneration of corticospinal and spinocerebellar tracts of cord, greatest in lumbar and thoracic segments. Possibly, agyria.

Diagnostic Procedures. *CSF.* Normal. *EMG. Blood.* Creatine phosphokinase (CPK). Normal or slightly elevated.

Therapy. None. Orthopedic measures.

Prognosis. Slowly progressive in years; finally, confines patient to bed. Death from intervening conditions.

BIBLIOGRAPHY. Struempell A: Beitraege zur Pathologie des Rueckenmarks. Arch Psychiatr 10:676–717, 1880
Lorrain M: Contribution a l'étude de la paraplégie spasmodique familiale (thesis). Paris, 1898
Strupell A: Die Primaere Seitenstangsklerose (spastische Spinalparalyse). Dtsch Z Nervenheilk 27:291–339, 1904
Scheltens P, Bruyn RPM, Hazenberg GJ: A Dutch family with autosomal dominant pure spastic paraparesis (Struempell's disease). Acta Neurol Scand 82:169–173, 1990
Adams RD, Victor M: Principles of Neurology, 5th ed, p 1098. New York, McGraw-Hill, 1993

STRUMA OVARY

Synonym. Ovary-thyroid tumor.

Symptoms. Onset usually from 30–50 years of age. Sensation of abdominal pressure and fullness. In 10% of patients, variable combinations of symptoms of hyperthyroidism (see Flajani).

Signs. Movable mass in adnexal area; occasionally, bilateral masses.

Etiology. Unknown.

Pathology. Benign teratoma, nodular surface, small cystic spaces. Typical thyroid follicle.

Diagnostic Procedures. *X-ray. Echography. CT scan. Abdominal scan. Blood.* See Flajani.

Therapy. Oophorectomy and same procedures used for carcinoma of thyroid gland.

Prognosis. Hyperthyroidism signs disappear after surgery.

BIBLIOGRAPHY. Kempers RD, Dockerty MB, Hoffman DL, et al: Struma ovarii ascites, hyperthyroid and asymptomatic syndromes. Ann Intern Med 72:883–893, 1970
Scully RE: Ovarian tumors with endocrine manifestations. In De Groot (ed): Endocrinology, 3rd ed, pp 2121–2122. Philadelphia, WB Saunders, 1995
Weatherall DJ, Ledingham JGG, Warrell DA: Oxford Textbook of Medicine, p 1717. Oxford, Oxford Med Pub, 1996

STRÜMPELL-LEICHTENSTERN

Synonyms. Weston Hurst; leukoencephalitis, acute hemorrhagic; encephalomyeliyis, acute, hemorrhagic. Includes hemorrhagic necrotizing encephalomyelitis.

Symptoms. Both sexes affected. Onset at all ages, prevalent in children. Onset rapid or apoplectiform (necrotizing). Prodromata of cephalalgia and fever. Convulsions; mental dullness; delirium; coma.

Signs. Focal manifestations; tachypnea; neck rigidity; myoclonus; aphasia; optic atrophy; ataxia.

Etiology. Multiple: viral; postvaccinal; drug-induced; hypersensitive mechanisms.

Pathology. In brain, scattered hemorrhagic foci usually in white matter

---

*Name of prototype patient.

(intranuclear inclusion bodies in some cases). In necrotizing variety, liquefaction of white matter.

Diagnostic Procedures. *Blood.* Usually, leukocytosis and high sedimentation rate. *CSF.* Normal or lymphocytic pleocytosis and a few scattered red cells. *Angiography. CT scan, MRI.* May suggest presence of occupying lesion. *EEG.*

Therapy. Symptomatic. Trial with antibiotics; corticosteroids.

Prognosis. Usually fatal. The few recoveries will show severe residuals. In necrotizing form, death may supervene in 24 hours.

BIBLIOGRAPHY. von Strümpell A: Ueber primaere acute Encephalitis. Dtsch Arch Klin Med 47:53–74, 1890

Leichtenstern O: Ueber primaere acute haemorrhägische Encephalitis. Dtsch Med Wochenschr 18:39–40, 1892

Hurst EW: Acute haemorrhagic leukoencephalitis: Previously undefined entity. Med J Australia 2:1–6, 1941

Adams RD, Victor M: Principles of Neurology, 5th ed, pp 794–796. New York, McGraw-Hill, 1993

STRYKER-HALBEISEN

Obsolete.

Synonym. Erythroderma; macrocytic anemia.

Symptoms. Weakness; fatigue; intense pruritus.

Signs. Late feature: patchy, scaly, vesicular erythroderma on face, neck, and upper chest.

Etiology. There are no absolute cutaneous markers of pernicious anemia except a frequent association with vitiligo (10 times more frequent occurrence than in normal population).

Diagnostic Procedures. *Blood.* Macrocytic anemia.

Therapy. Pyridoxine and other B complex vitamins; crude liver extract.

Prognosis. Skin lesions and blood changes corrected by treatment.

BIBLIOGRAPHY. Stryker GV, Halbeisen WA: Determination of macrocytic anemia as an aid in diagnosis of certain deficiency dermatoses. Arch Dermatol Syph 51:116–123, 1945

Rook A, Wilkinson DS, Ebling FJG, et al: Textbook of Dermatology, 4th ed, p 2365. Oxford, Blackwell Scientific Publications, 1986

STUART-PROWER* FACTOR DEFICIENCY

Synonym. Factor X deficiency. See Prothrombin deficiency syndromes.

Symptoms and Signs. Same manifestations as factor VII deficiency (see). Childhood bleeding from mild to severe resembling hemophilia. Thromboembolism.

Etiology. Autosomal recessive. An abnormal factor X (Factor X Friuli) also reported. Acquired form described (amyloidosis).

Diagnostic Procedures. *Blood.* Prolonged prothrombin time and partial thromboplastin time. Different from factor VII deficiency because thromboplastin generation and viper venom (Stypven) time abnormal. Immunodiffusion techniques and antibody neutralization show two variants of this defect: (cross-reacting material) CRM positive and CRM negative.

Therapy. Blood, plasma, plasma concentrate. Trial with progestational agents. In acquired cases splenectomy.

Prognosis. Good, but death from hemorrhage may occur.

*Names of first described patients.

BIBLIOGRAPHY. Telfler TP: A new coagulation defect. Br J Haematol 2:308–316, 1956

Denson KWE, Lurie A, De Cataldo F, et al: The factor X defect: Recognition of abnormal forms of factor X. Br J Haematol 18:317, 1970

Watzke HH, Wallmark A, Hamaguchi N, et al: Factor X (Santo Domingo) evidence that the severe clinical phenotype arises from a mutation blocking secretion. J Clin Invest 88:1685–1689, 1991

Bithell TC: Hereditary coagulation disorders. In Lee GR, Bithell TC, Foerster J, et al (eds): Wintrobe's Clinical Hematology, 9th ed, pp 1444, 1500–1501. Philadelphia, Lea & Febiger, 1993

STUB THUMB

Synonyms. Brachydactyly type D, potter thumbs, murder thumb. brachymegalodactylism.

Symptoms and Signs. Both sexes. Unilateral 25% or bilateral 75%. Both sexes. Short and large terminal phalanx of digits.

Etiology. Autosomal dominant with variable penetrance.

BIBLIOGRAPHY. Breitenbecher JK: Hereditary shortness of thumbs. J Hered 14:15–21, 1923

Gray E, Hurt BK: Inheritance of brachydactyly type D. J Hered 75:297–299, 1984

STUEHMER

Synonyms. Balanitis xerotica obliterans; penis kraurosis.

Symptoms. Usually young adult men. Pain during erection. Pruritus.

Signs. May present different aspects: ivory white patches on the penis; hemorrhagic periurethral bullae; parchment-like membrane covering glans; with progression, shrinkage and atrophy of penis, with meatal narrowing and fissuring of prepuce. Regional lymphadenopathy.

Etiology. May be an advanced stage of several conditions; for example lichen sclerosus, chronic balanitis.

Pathology. Atrophic epidermis; collagen homogenization; infiltration under collagen by lymphocytes and histiocytes.

Therapy. Corticosteroid ointments; intralesional corticosteroid injections; circumcision; dorsal slit; urethral dilatation.

Prognosis. Evolving form toward atrophy of penis. Occasionally, malignant transformation.

BIBLIOGRAPHY. Stuehmer A: Pigmentnaevi und ihre Behandlung. Medizinische 735–739, May 30, 1953

Rook A, Wilkinson DS, Ebling FJG, et al: Textbook of Dermatology, 4th ed, pp 2272, 2273, 2813, 2814. Oxford, Blackwell Scientific, 1986

STURGE-WEBER

Synonyms. Dimitri hemoangiomatosis; Jahnke (variant without glaucoma); Kalisher; Krabbe II: Lawford (variant with glaucoma, without increased ocular pressure); Parkes Weber; Weber-Dimitri; encephalofacial angiomatosis; encephalotrigeminal angiomatosis; meningocutaneous; neurooculocutaneous; phacomatosis; vascular encephalotrigeminal. See Klippel-Trenaunay-Weber.

Symptoms. Usually promising start, even intellectual precocity, before onset of mental retardation and epileptic seizures. Convulsions are of focal type and on the contralateral side of facial nevus. Seldom hemorrhage from angiomas.

Signs. Unilateral facial nevus (port wine) along area of distribution of trigeminal (V) nerve. Atrophy or spasticity on contralateral side of nevus. Increase or decrease of intraocular tension. Glaucoma, enophthalmos, exophthalmos, optic atrophy, and vascular malformation frequently observed. Limb hypertrophy. Obesity (not constant).

Etiology. Congenital; dysplasia of embryonic vascular system occurring during sixth week of embryonic life, affecting vessels between those surrounding the brain wall and those of membranous skull and integument. No evidence of heredity clearly confirmed.

Pathology. Hemangioma of face and brain. Mesodermal defect of capillary or cavernous blood vessels; arteriovenous aneurysm.

Diagnostic Procedures. *X-ray. CT scan. MRI.* Evidence of intracerebral calcifications same side as nevus (becoming detectable at age 2). *EEG.* Gross dysrhythmia.

Therapy. Cerebral lobectomy has to be considered in infancy before epilepsy occurs. In cases with hemiparesis, promising results with hemispherectomy. Symptomatic treatment of epilepsy when surgery not feasible. Alternative forms of treatment include injection of sclerosing solution, radiation therapy or radium implant, carbon dioxide snow, electrodissection, or insertion of steel wire electrodes.

Prognosis. Mental retardation and hemiparesis eventually develop if surgery does not prevent them.

BIBLIOGRAPHY. Sturge WA: A case of partial epilepsy, apparently due to a lesion of one of the vaso-motor centers of the brain. Trans Clin Soc Lond 12:162–167, 1879; Br Med J 1:704, 1879

Weber FP: Right-sides, hemi-hypotrophy resulting from right-sided congenital spastic hemiplegia with a morbid condition of the left side of the brain revealed by radiogram. J Neurol Psychopathol (Lond) 37:301–311, 1922

Dimitri V: Tumor cerebral congénito (angioma cavernosum). Rev Assoc Med Argent 36:63, 1923

Sahel JA, Albert DM: Phakomatoses and Neurocristopathies. In Garner A, Klintworth GK (eds): Pathobiology of Ocular Disease: A Dynamic Approach, 2nd ed, pp 1361–1363. New York, Marcel Dekker, 1994

SUBDURAL HEMATOMA SYNDROMES

ACUTE

Synonym. Hemorrhagic internal pachymeningitis.

Symptoms. Onset immediately after trauma. Unconsciousness; coma.

Signs. Dilated pupil on one side; loss of corneal reflexes; fundic venous congestion; progressive weakness of contralateral arm and leg.

Etiology. Trauma.

Pathology. Laceration of veins crossing to superior longitudinal sinus.

Diagnostic Procedures. *Angiography. CT scan. MRI.*

Therapy. Immediate operation.

Prognosis. Poor. High mortality.

SUBACUTE

Symptoms. Appears 1 week or longer after trauma. Headache; irritability; neck stiffness; hemiplegia and aphasia.

Signs. Hemiplegia; Babinski sign; changes in pulse and respiration; strabismus.

Pathology. Laceration of brain or veins crossing superior longitudinal sinus (or both). Hematoma with membranous capsule containing hemorrhagic fluid and clots.

Diagnostic Procedures. *X-ray. Angiography. CT scan. MRI.*

Therapy. Surgical evacuation.

Prognosis. Mortality 25%.

CHRONIC

Symptoms. Occurs in infants and in adults, especially in alcoholics. Onset weeks or months after severe or mild trauma of the head. Gradual progression. Severe unremitting headache. Some patients present convulsions as first symptoms. Irritability; inattention; lethargy; finally stupor. Hemiplegia (usually contralateral, occasionally ipsilateral). Hemianopsia (seldom). Sensory changes not frequent.

Signs. Frequently absent; papilledema (in only 20% of cases). Dilated fixed pupil; external ophthalmoplegia.

Etiology. Trauma.

Pathology. Not true hematomas but hemorrhagic cysts. Small bleeding cysts in which disintegration increases the osmotic pressure and attracts fluid so that the volume of the cyst progressively enlarges. Content of cyst chocolate-colored fluid.

Diagnostic Procedures. *Spinal tap.* Frequently, normal pressure and chemistry. Fluid clear or slightly xanthochromic; normal cell count; protein slightly increased. *X-ray. CT scan. MRI.* Often negative (shift of Pineal body). *EEG.*

Therapy. Removal of fluid through trephine opening or, if needed, removal of capsule and clotted content.

Prognosis. According to time of removal. In some cases, spontaneous regression. If symptomatic, surgery indicated.

IN INFANTS

Symptoms. Onset during first 6 months of life. Vomiting; failure to eat; irritability; convulsions; stupor.

Signs. Low-grade fever; bulging of fontanelles and head enlargement; distention of scalp veins; retinal hemorrhages; seldom papilledema.

Etiology. Trauma or clotting defect.

Pathology. Accumulation of blood and fluid.

Diagnostic Procedures. Puncture of subdural space through lateral angle of anterior fontanelle or coronal suture.

Therapy. According to need: (1) daily tapping and drainage of 10 ml of fluid; (2) bilateral holes and evacuation of hematoma; (3) craniotomy with excision of membrane and evacuation of clot.

Prognosis. Fair. Good response to treatment.

BIBLIOGRAPHY. Adams RD, Victor M: Principles of Neurology, 5th ed, pp 762–764. New York, McGraw-Hill, 1993

SUBDURAL HYGROMA

Symptoms and Signs. Similar to those of subdural hematoma. In order of frequency: headache, nervousness and irritability; stupor; loss of memory and confusion; hemiparesis or hemiplegia; dizziness.

Etiology. Cranial trauma (tearing of arachnoid). Subdural effusion secondary to infections. Rupture of arachnoid at basal cistern in communicating hydrocephalus.

Pathology. Collection of clear or yellowish fluid in subdural space, with high concentration of protein.

Diagnostic Procedures. See Subdural hematoma syndromes.

Therapy. See Subdural hematoma syndromes.

Prognosis. See Subdural hematoma syndromes.

BIBLIOGRAPHY. Naffziger HC: Subdural fluid accumulation following head injury. JAMA 82:1751–1752, 1924

Wycis HT: Subdural hygroma: Report of seven cases. J Neurosurg 2:340–357, 1945

Adams RD, Victor M: Principles of Neurology, 5th ed. New York, McGraw-Hill, 1993

SUBMERSION

Synonyms. Near drowning.

Symptoms. Occurs in individuals who have been near drowning. Tachypnea; mild fever; restlessness; vertigo; confusion and occasionally nausea; vomiting; shock.

Signs. Cyanosis, signs of pulmonary congestion and edema, and abdominal distention.

Etiology. Unknown. Possibly related to asphyxia and effect of stress.

Pathology. No evidence of aspiration of water into the lung. Lung congestion and edema.

Diagnostic Procedures. *Blood.* White blood cells increased.

Therapy. Rest; symptomatic.

Prognosis. Good. Transitory condition.

BIBLIOGRAPHY. Saline M, Baum GL: The submersion syndrome. Ann Intern Med 41:1134–1138, 1954
Conn AW, Modell JH: Current neurological considerations in near-drowning. Can Anaesth Soc J 27:197–198, 1980
Civetta JM, Taylor RW, Kirby RR (eds): Critical Care, 2nd ed. Philadelphia, Lippincott, 1992

SUCROSE-DEXTRINOSE DEFICIENCY

Synonyms. Sucrose-isomaltose malabsorption, disaccharide intolerance I, sucrose-isomaltose deficiency.

Symptoms and Signs. Early childhood. Symptoms of alactasia (see) evoked by table sugar or sweetened foods. Association of renal calculi (oxalate) possible.

Etiology. Autosomal recessive.

Diagnostic Procedures. *Small intestine biopsy.* Low activity of sucrose and isomaltose. *Oral sucrose tolerance test.* Oral administration of a test dose (1–2 mg/kg) of lactose, glucose, or galactose and of maltose produces a normal rise of blood sugar concentration. Ingestion of sucrose is followed by explosive diarrhea. *Stool.* pH is low.

Therapy. Suspension of sucrose from diet. Enzyme of fungal origin may be tried. Sucrose-free diet is provided by milk, meat, fish, fowl, eggs, animal fat, glucose, vegetables, and cheese.

Prognosis. Good with therapy.

BIBLIOGRAPHY. Moore D, Lichtman S, Durie P, et al: Primary sucrose-iso-maltase deficiency: Importance of clinical judgment. Lancet II:164–165, 1985
Semenza G, Auricchio S: Small intestinal disaccharidases. In Scriver CR, Beaudet AL, Sly WS, et al: The Metabolic and Molecular Bases of Inherited Disease, 7th ed, pp 4467–4468. New York, McGraw-Hill, 1995

SUDDEN DEATH, ADULT

Synonyms. See Mort d'amour; voodoo death.

Symptoms and Signs. In subjects of all ages in apparent good health. Clinically unexplainable sudden death.

Etiology. Pathologic findings retrospectively will indicate the previously unidentified causes as: congenital cardiac malformations, infective-immune, thrombolytic, atherosclerotic, or other degenerative processes.

Therapy. Early. Attempt to resuscitate.

BIBLIOGRAPHY. Lancisi GM: De subitaines mortibus. Buegni Roma 1707 Translation: White PD, Boursey AV, St John's University Press, New York, 1971
Stein B, Roberts R: Syncope, presyncope, palpitations, and sudden death. In Schlant RC, Alexander RW: Hurst's The Heart, 8th ed. New York, McGraw-Hill, 1994

SUDDEN INFANT DEATH

Synonyms. SIDS; crib death; cot death.

Symptoms. Distinctive age distribution. Almost never occurs before 2 weeks or after 8 months of age. Higher incidence among nonwhite and poor families and in lower-weight-range babies. Seasonal: highest incidence late autumn, winter, and spring. It occurs almost exclusively during sleep. Babies who are completely healthy and normal occasionally, except for history of minor respiratory symptoms for 1–2 weeks, are discovered dead in the morning, lying in a characteristic abdominal position, with face to side.

Etiology. Unknown. Parathyroid insufficiency theory rejected; thymo-lymphaticus habitus theory rejected; suffocation excluded. Death may result from the combination of many interrelated factors in which possibly virus infections, low birth weight, and laryngospasm seem to play a role. To be differentiated from other forms of unexpected death, where etiologic findings may be identified. Inherited forms reported.

Pathology. Petechial hemorrhages (93%) appearing only in the thoracic contents. Pulmonary edema; heart dilated, containing fluid blood. Urinary bladder empty; redness of pharynx and minor inflammatory changes of airway.

Diagnostic Procedures. *Autopsy.* Cannot explain death or presence of described findings.

Prognosis. Sudden death syndrome represents 10% of deaths occurring in first year of life. Prophylaxis unknown.

BIBLIOGRAPHY. Beckwith JB, Bergman AB: The sudden death syndrome of infancy. Hosp Pract 2:44–52, 1967
Proceedings of the first Australian Rotary Health Research Fund Conference on "cot death." Aust Paediatr J 22:Suppl 1, 1986
Nelson EAS, Taylor BJ, Weatherall IL: Sleeping position and infant bedding may predispose to hyperthermia and the sudden infant death syndrome. Lancet 1:199–200, 1989
Hunt CE: Sudden infant death. In Behrman, Kliegman, Arvin: Nelson Textbook of Pediatrics, 15th ed, pp 1991–1999. Philadelphia, WB Saunders, 1995

SUDECK

Synonyms. Kienboeck; Sudeck-Leriche; post-traumatic atrophy; post-traumatic bone atrophy; post-traumatic sympathetic dystrophy; post-traumatic osteoporosis; peripheral trophoneurosis; post-traumatic osteoporosis; reflex dystrophy. See Mitchell I and Causalgia.

Symptoms and Signs. Prevalent in old people and in women. Those of Steinbrocker (see). Typical bone changes, however, are not always associated with trauma.

Etiology. Unknown (see Steinbrocker syndrome).

Pathology. Patchy osteoporosis, especially around joints.

Diagnostic Procedures. *X-ray.* Radionucleotide uptake study, thermography: typical pattern of localized osteoporosis initiating after 1–2 months from onset of symptoms.

Therapy. See Steinbrocker.

Prognosis. Osteoporosis sometimes remains after the patient has recovered from other symptoms of Steinbrocker syndrome.

BIBLIOGRAPHY. Sudeck P: Ueber die acute enzündliche Knockenatrophie. Arch Klin Chir 62:147–156, 1900

Sudeck P: Ueber die acute enzündliche Knochenatrophie. Verh Dtsch Ges Chir 29:673–682, 1900

Schwartzman RJ, McLellan T: Reflex sympathetic dystrophy: A review. Arch Neurol 44:555–561, 1987

Klippel JH, Dieppe PA: Rheumatology, p 7.38.1. St Louis, CV Mosby, 1994

Weatherall DJ, Ledingham JGG, Warrell DA: Oxford Textbook of Medicine, pp 3096–3097. Oxford, Oxford Med Pub, 1996

SUGARMAN I

Synonyms. Oral–facial–digital III; seesaw winking–oral–facial–digital; postaxial digital polydactyly.

Symptoms and Signs. In two females. Mental retardation. Facies in one case continuous alternating winking and numerous malformations. Both cases. *Tongue.* Lobulated, hamartomatous. *Teeth.* Anomalus, malocclusion. *Uvula.* Bifid. *Palate.* Normal. *Limbs.* Postaxial hexadactyly of hands and feet. Pectus excavatum; short sternum; kyphosis.

Etiology. Possibly autosomal recessive inheritance.

BIBLIOGRAPHY. Sugarman GI, Katakia M, Menkes J: See-saw winking in a familial oral-facial-digital syndrome. Clin Genet 2:248–254, 1971

SUGARMAN II

Synonym. Brachydactyly; major proximal phalanges shortening.

Symptoms and Signs. Short fingers with no motility at proximal interphalangeal joints. Hallux more proximal and dorsal than usual.

Etiology. Possibly autosomal recessive inheritance or dominant with reduced penetrance.

Diagnostic Procedures. *Rx hand.* Double first metacarpal bilaterally.

Therapy. Amputation of big toe.

BIBLIOGRAPHY. Sugarman GI, Hager D, Kulik WJ: A new syndrome of brachydactyly of hands and feet with duplication of the first toes. Birth Defects 5:1–8, 1974

Fujimoto A, Smolensky LS, Wilson MG: Brachydactyly with major involvement of proximal phalanges. Clin Genet 21:107–111, 1982

SULZBERGER-GARBE

Synonyms. Savill; exudative discoid lichenoid dermatosis; lichenoid chronic dermatosis; polymorphic prurigo.

Symptoms. Prevalent in men (especially Jews); abrupt onset in fourth to sixth decade. Cyclothymic or neurotic personalities. Severe pruritus, nocturnal and paroxysmal, localized on genitals, under breast, around the mouth or extremities, often following a local infection.

Signs. Ephemeral exudative lesions; follicular papules and urticaria-like lesions. Lichenification, crusting and serous discharge may develop. Penile and scrotal lesions almost pathognomonic.

Etiology. Unknown. Emotional disturbances and secondary reaction to rubbing and scratching the lesion. Infectious eczematoid dermatitis has been described under this term.

Pathology. Similar to seborrheic dermatitis with greater crusting and lichenification. Cocci in corneal layer of epidermis not constantly found.

Diagnostic Procedures. *Biopsy.* Of skin. *Psychiatric evaluation. Blood.* Eosinophilia.

Therapy. If infection, treat topically; psychiatric treatment; antipruritics; anesthetics and combinations. Systemic steroids (temporary effect). Azathioprine (rapid response reported).

Prognosis. Control of superimposed infection and psychotherapy may give good results. Usually, chronic and difficult to control. Relapses frequent; spontaneous remissions occasional, usually after months or years.

BIBLIOGRAPHY. Savill T: On an epidemic skin disease. Br Med J 2:1197–1202, 1891

Sulzberger MB, Garbe W: Nine cases of a distinctive exudative discoid and lichenoid chronic dermatosis. Arch Dermatol Syph 36:247–278, 1937

Burton JL: Eczema, lichenification, prurigo and erythroderma. In Champion RH, Burton JL, Ebling FJG (eds): Rook/Wilkinson/Ebling Textbook of Dermatology, 5th ed, p 568. Oxford, Blackwell Scientific, 1992

SUMMERSKILL-WALSHE

Synonyms. Tygstrup; cholestasis, benign, recurrent, intrahepatic; BRIC; intrahepatic cholestasis benign.

Symptoms. Prevalent in males. Steatorrhea with malabsorption and weight loss: first episode usually before 20 years of age; number of attacks very variable. Duration 2 weeks to 18 months. Fatigue; nervous tension; anorexia; occasionally, nausea and vomiting; pain in upper right abdominal quadrant (50%); bleeding tendency.

Signs. Jaundice; occasionally, abdominal tenderness; liver enlargement; easy bruising; pruritus.

Etiology. Benign intrahepatic disorder; cholestasis resulting from defect of excretion of conjugated bilirubin from liver cells and canaliculi. Possibility of recessive genetic condition with poor penetrance. Features to distinguish it from cholestasis, intrahepatic hereditary recurrences are not clear, except for milder course and later age of onset.

Pathology. Liver biopsy during jaundice: bile stasis in the canaliculi; round cell infiltration in portal tracts. No changes indicating extrahepatic obstruction; no irreversible change of hepatic architecture. In asymptomatic periods: no changes. Electromicroscopic studies during attack: numerous vescicles containing low-medium density material present in many cells. Following recovery they disappear.

Diagnostic Procedures. *Blood.* Increase of conjugated bilirubin; high alkaline phosphatase; normal protein and electrophoretic pattern; colloidal lability tests normal; prothrombin time prolonged in some cases. Abnormal findings reverting to normal during remission. *Urine.* Urobilin present. *Stool. Steatorrhea. X-ray.* Of gallbladder. Good visualization.

Therapy. None specific. Correction of malabsorption (vitamins). Steroids and phenobarbital may reduce bilirubin level without affecting course of disease; cholestyramine relieves some symptoms (pruritus).

Prognosis. Good, with recurrence of condition.

BIBLIOGRAPHY. Summerskill WHJ, Walshe JM: Benign recurrent intrahepatic "obstructive" jaundice. Lancet 2:686–690, 1959

Tygstrup N: Intermittent possibly familial intrahepatic cholestatic jaundice. Lancet 1:1171–1172, 1960

Chowdhury JR, Wolkoff AW, Arias IM: Hereditary jaundice and bilirubin metabolism. In Scriver CR, Beaudet AL, Sly WS, et al: The Metabolic and Molecular Bases of Inherited Disease, 6th ed, p 1367. New York, McGraw-Hill, 1989

SUMMITT

Synonyms. Summitt acrocephalosyndactyly; craniosynostosis; syndactyly; obesity. See Carpenter (of which both Summitt and Goodman are considerd variants).

Symptoms and Signs. Present from birth. *Head.* Acrocephaly; occipital irregularity; epicanthal folds; strabismus; narrow palate; delayed teeth eruption. *Extremities.* Syndactyly from mild to severe; genu valgum and coxa valga (occasional). *Trunk.* Obesity; moderate gynecomastia. Normal mental development.

Etiology. Autosomal recessive inheritance (?).

BIBLIOGRAPHY. Summitt RL: Recessive acrocephalosyndactyly with normal intelligence. Birth Defects 5:35–38, 1969

Sells CJ, Hanson JW, Hall JG: The Summitt syndrome: Observation of a third case. Am J Med Genet 3:27–33, 1979

Cohen DM, Green JG, Miller J, et al: Acrocephalopolysyndactyly type II Carpenter syndrome: Clinical spectrum and an attempt at unification with Goodman and Summitt syndromes. Am J Med Genet 28:311–324, 1987

SUNRISE-SUNSET

Synonyms. Sunset-Sunrise; East-West; Movement intraocular lens. See also Windshield wiper.

Symptoms and Signs. After implantation of IOL after cataract extraction. Defect of vision.

Etiology. Displacement of IOL; zonalur rupture.

Diagnostic Procedures. *Ophthalmoscopy.* Displacement as rising or setting sun of IOL.

Therapy. Replacement of IOL.

BIBLIOGRAPHY. Apple DJ, Rabb MF: Ocular Pathology, 4th ed, p 146. St Louis, CV Mosby, 1991

SUPERIOR LONGITUDINAL SINUS THROMBOSIS

Symptoms. More frequent in children. Headache; nausea; vomiting; general prostration; aplasia, urinary incontinence (in bilateral cases); convulsions. Occasionally, symptoms of spastic paraplegia.

Signs. Scalp edema; distention of veins near fontanelles. Homonymous hemianopsia or quadrantanopia, paralysis of conjugate gaze.

Etiology. Infective or aseptic thrombosis of superior longitudinal sinus (less frequent than in lateral sinus, see); extension of infection or reaction from paranasal sinuses; skull infection; brain abscess or because of extension from other cerebral venous sinuses.

Pathology. See Etiology. Frequent intracranial hemorrhagic complications.

Diagnostic Procedures. Difficult diagnosis. *X-ray.* Direct injection of radiopaque dye into longitudinal sinus. *CT scan. MRI.*

Therapy. Antibiotics. Surgery.

Prognosis. Frequently fatal or severe residual neurologic manifestations; in some cases, complete recovery.

BIBLIOGRAPHY. Vick NA: Grinker's Neurology, 7th ed. Springfield, IL, Charles C Thomas, 1976

Adams RD, Victor M: Principles of Neurology, 5th ed, pp 547, 611–612. New York, McGraw-Hill, 1993

SUPERIOR RIM SYNDROME

Synonym. Coloboma of temporal inferior and nasal rims.

Symptoms and Signs. Scotoma of the involved areas.

Etiology. Autosomal dominant inheritance or associated with congenital toxoplasmosis, varicella, syphilis.

Diagnostic Procedures. *Slit lamp microscopy.* Intact superior optic disc rim with extensive coloboma of temporal, inferior, and nasal rims.

Prognosis. Good.

BIBLIOGRAPHY. Apple DJ, Rabb MF: Ocular Pathology. 4th ed, p 20. St Louis, CV Mosby, 1991

SUPINE HYPOTENSIVE

Synonym. Inferior vena cava.

Symptoms. Occurs in last month of pregnancy in 3–11%. Sudden fall of systolic blood pressure; circulatory collapse; retching and nausea when assuming supine position.

Signs. Tachycardia; fall of arterial pressure over 30 mm Hg. A few patients presenting this syndrome have premature separation of placenta because of sudden increase in venous pressure when lying down causing compression of vena cava.

Etiology and Pathology. Compression of inferior vena cava by flaccid full-term pregnant uterus, thus reducing venous return to heart and decreasing cardiac output.

Therapy. Lying down on left lateral position. If drop of pressure occurs on delivery table, tilting the right pelvis to the left.

Prognosis. Good. Spontaneously corrected after termination of pregnancy.

BIBLIOGRAPHY. Runge H: Venous pressure during pregnancy, delivery, and puerperium. Arch Gynäkol 122:142–157, 1924

Robbins RA, Estrara T, Russell C: Supine hypotensive syndrome and abruptio placenta. Am J Obstet Gynecol 80:1207–1208, 1960

McAnulty JH, Metcalfe J, Ueland K: Heart disease and pregnancy. In Schlant RC, Alexander RW: Hurst's The Heart, 8th ed, p 2043. New York, McGraw-Hill, 1994

Weatherall DJ, Ledingham JGG, Warrell DA: Oxford Textbook of Medicine, pp 1726, 1735. Oxford, Oxford Med Pub, 1996

SURVIVOR

Synonyms. Concentration camp II; postconcentration camp.

Symptoms. Occurs in victims who survived concentration camp or physical and mental distress owing to persecution (hiding and striving for survival). Chronic state of tension; vigilance; irritability; depression; unrest and fear; sleep disturbances; nightmares. Headache; fatigue; excessive sweating. Avoidance of company and, in severe cases, complete withdrawal. Feeling of guilt (especially if only survivor of family) because of survival. Memory defects; parapraxia.

Etiology. Persistence of after effect of psychological trauma.

Therapy. Psychotherapy. Group therapy in some cases indicated.

Prognosis. Difficult therapy.

BIBLIOGRAPHY. Niederland WG: Psychiatric disorders among persecution victims. A contribution to the understanding of concentration camp pathology and its after-effects. J Nerv Ment Dis 139:458–474, 1964

McCann IL, Pearlman LA: Psychological Trauma and the Adult Survivor. New York, Brunner/Mazel, 1990

SUSPENDED HEART

Synonym. Vasoregulatory asthenia.

Symptoms. Onset at all ages. No sex preference. Chest pain or palpitation or both.

Signs. Usually, asthenic habitus; no evidence of cardiovascular disease.

Etiology. Alteration of position of heart so that it appears elongated and vertical or disturbance of the autonomic nervous system with hyperdynamic circulation.

Diagnostic Procedures. *ECG.* Depression of the ST segment in leads III and IIIR (during deep inspiration); lesser depression in II and CR7; not changed by change to upright position. *X-ray.* Anterior view: apparently normally located heart. During deep inspiration left cardiophrenic junction moves toward the middle. Right oblique view: during inspiration, heart and diaphragm separated widely. Left oblique view: during inspiration, gap between heart and diaphragm.

Therapy. Symptomatic.

Prognosis. Excellent. This syndrome represents only an innocuous electrocardiographic variation. Its importance is owing to the fact that an ST depression (in absence of digitalization) usually indicates the presence of a myocardial infarction.

BIBLIOGRAPHY. Evans W, Lloyd-Thomas HG: The syndrome of the suspended heart. Br Heart J 19:153–158, 1957
Stein B, Roberts R: Syncope, presyncope, palpitations, and sudden death. In Schlant RC, Alexander RW: Hurst's The Heart, 8th ed. New York, McGraw-Hill, 1994

SUSTO

Synonyms. Fright; soul loss; espanto; pasmo; tripa ida; chibih.

Symptoms and Signs. In Mexico, Central and South America and some Latinos in United States; but also present in many parts of the world. After a frightening event, delusion that the soul has left the body, and left sickness and unhappiness. Deep social discomfort; loss of appetite; sleep disturbances; intense dreaming activity; loss of motivation for all kind of activities; low self-consideration and feeling of dirtiness. Muscle ache and pains; headache digestive troubles and diarrhea.

Etiology. Major depressive disorder, postraumatic stress.

Therapy. Ritual approaches according to cultural backgrounds; psychotherapy.

BIBLIOGRAPHY. Lin K-M: Cultural influences on the diagnosis of psychotic and organic disorders. In Mezzich JE, Kleinman A, Fabrega H, et al: Culture and Psychiatric Diagnosis. Washington, American Psychiatry Press, 1995

SUTTON I

Synonyms. Halo leukoderma; leukoderma acquisitum centrifugum; halo nevus.

Symptoms. Both sexes affected. Onset in young adulthood (range 4–45 years). Asymptomatic.

Signs. Halo of hypomelanosis (0.5–1.0 cm) developing around a cutaneous nevus (benign or malignant). The phenomenon is observed usually with lesion on the trunk; less frequently on the head; seldom on the extremities. The central nevus tends to disappear slowly. In 30% of patients development of vitiligo.

Etiology. Unknown. Part of process of involution of melanotic nevi; genetic defect in melanogensis. Familial occurrence (autosomal recessive reported).

Pathology. The histology of central lesions shows the substitution of the melanocytes by lymphocytes and reticular cells.

Diagnostic Procedures. Biopsy of central lesion (if clinical doubt especially in older people).

Therapy. Reassurance and sunscreen in young, especially if multiple lesions; if clinical doubt arises, surgery.

Prognosis. Good in most instances.

BIBLIOGRAPHY. Sutton R: An unusual variety of vitiligo (leucoderma acquisitum centrifugum). J Cutan Dis 34:797–800, 1916
MacKie RM: Melanocytic Naevi and Malignant Melanoma. In Champion RH, Burton JL, Ebling FJG (eds): Rook/Wilkinson/Ebling Textbook of Dermatology, 5th ed, pp 1535–1536. Oxford, Blackwell Scientific, 1992

SUTTON II

Synonym. Periadenitis, mucosa, necrotica, recurrens; ulcer of Sutton. See Zahorsky and Behçet.

Symptoms and Signs. Onset in childhood or adolescence. Painful nodular lesions in the mucosa of mouth, frequently affecting the tongue also. Occasionally, vagina may be involved. After 3 or 4 days, detachment of necrotic plug and ulceration.

Etiology. Unknown. Variant of aphthosis.

Pathology. See Zahorsky.

Therapy. See Zahorsky.

Prognosis. Chronic recurrent lesions.

BIBLIOGRAPHY. Sutton RL Jr: Recurrent scarring painful aphthae. Amelioration with sulfathiazole in two cases. JAMA 117:175–176, 1941
Ive FA: The umbilical perianal and genital regions. In Champion RH, Burton JL, Ebling FJG (eds): Rook/Wilkinson/Ebling Textbook of Dermatology, 5th ed, p 2848. Oxford, Blackwell Scientific, 1992

SWAN I

Synonyms. Blindspot; squint; monofixation.

Symptoms and Signs. Periodic diplopia; concomitant compensating esotropia of 12–18 degrees. No other clinical findings.

Etiology. Physiological mechanism to project the image of nondeviating eye onto blindspot of the deviating one, thus allowing its plotting as a central scotoma for the latter. There is criticism against considering such as mechanism a syndrome.

Therapy. Optical correction suggested.

Prognosis. Of no significant clinical importance.

BIBLIOGRAPHY. Swan KC: The blind spot syndrome. Arch Ophthalmol 40:371–388, 1940
Verhaeff FC: The so-called blindspot syndrome. Am J Ophthalmol 40:802–808, 1955
Bolet RV: Development of monofixation syndrome in congenital atropia. J Pediatr Ophthalmol Strabismus 18:49–51, 1981

SWAN II

Synonym. Congenital epiblepharon; inferior oblique insufficiency.

Symptoms and Signs. Observed in infants. (1) Epiblepharon, bilateral or unilateral; little irritation of cornea or occasionally keratitis. (2) Little or no eye deviation except in the field of action of the affected inferior oblique muscle (involved only unilaterally). Lack of contraction of the antagonists.

Etiology. Unknown. Rare combination: 4:5000 cases examined at the University of Oregon Medical School.

Therapy. Control the inversion of the lash line, possibly by nonsurgical means. Antibiotic for infections.

Prognosis. Patient learns to avoid rotation of his eyes to superior gaze (left or right according to eye involved). Rarely is he aware of diplopia and carries his head in a normal position.

BIBLIOGRAPHY. Swan K: The syndrome of congenital epiblepharon and inferior oblique insufficiency. Am J Ophthalmol 39:130–136, 1955
Duke-Elder S: System of Ophthalmology, vol 3, p 2. St Louis, CV Mosby, 1963

SWANSON

Synonyms. Anhidrosis—pain insensitivity; dysautonomia familial II; pain insensitivity—anhidrosis; sensory—autonomic neuropathy IV; HSAN-IV; see Biemond.

Symptoms. Both sexes. From birth. Unexplained episodes of fever; self-mutilating behavior, congenital insensibility to pain; mild mental retardation; low IQ (70).

Signs. Thermal and traumatic injuries when child begins to crawl. Analgesia (loss of superficial and deep sensitivity); hyporeflexia; pupillary abnormalities from partial to complete Horner syndrome (see); vasomotor instability; anhidrosis; aplasia of dental enamel; blond hair; blue eyes.

Etiology. Developmental defect. Suggested abnormality in differentiation of neural crest; autosomal recessive trait. See also Christ-Siemens-Touraine.

Pathology. No uniform findings. Absence of small myelinated and unmyelinated fibers. Sweat glands present in the skin but not innervated. Meningeal thickening and cystic changes.

Diagnostic Procedures. Lack of sweating also after intense physical or pharmacologic stimulation. Spontaneous lacrimation, but lack of response to Mecholyl or neostigmine. *Urine.* Abnormal vanillylmandelic and homovanyllinic acid assays.

Therapy. Careful handling of child. Padding of area susceptible to trauma.

Prognosis. Poor. Infection, traumatic lesion, self-mutilation.

BIBLIOGRAPHY. Swanson AG: Congenital insensitivity to pain with anhidrosis. A unique syndrome in two male siblings. Arch Neurol 8:299–306, 1963
Brown JW, Podosin R: A syndrome of the neural crest Arch Neurol 15:294–301, 1966
Axelrod FB, Pearson J, Tapperby J, et al: Congenital sensor neuropathy with skeletal dysplasia. J. Pediatr 102:727–730, 1983
Adams RD, Victor M: Principles of Neurology, 5th ed, p 1148. New York, McGraw-Hill, 1993

SWEAT RETENTION

Synonyms. Anhidrosis; hypohidrosis; thermogenic anhidrosis. See Ross.

Symptoms. Occurs when patient exposed to high temperature and high humidity. Malaise; weakness; flushing; pruritus; headache; nausea.

Signs. Tachycardia; tachypnea; fever.

Etiology. Idiopathic or all causes that prevent sweating (inability to produce or to deliver to skin surface): congenitally absent or deficient sweat glands; dermatitis; ectodermal dysplasia scars; neurogenic factors; miliaria; endocrine and metabolic conditions. Usually inherited as X-linked trait (see Christ-Siemens-Tourine); autosomal recessive inheritance reported as well.

Diagnostic Procedures. Colorimetric test. Absence of sweating.

Therapy. Removal to cooler, dryer place with breeze. Treatment, when feasible, of determining causes.

Prognosis. Severe hyperthermia may develop, sometimes with fatal consequences.

BIBLIOGRAPHY. Wolkin J, Goodman JI, Kelley WE: Failure of sweat mechanism in desert. JAMA 124:478–482, 1944
Mahloudji M, Livingston KE: Familial and congenital simple anhidrosis. Am J Dis Child 113:477–479, 1967
Crump IA, Danks DM: Hypohidrotic ectodermal dysplasia: A study of sweatpore in the X-linked forms and in a family with probable autosomal recessive inheritance. J Pediatr 78:466–473, 1971
MacKie RM: Melanocytic naevi and malignant melanoma. In Champion RH, Burton JL, Ebling FJG (eds): Rook/Wilkinson/Ebling Textbook of Dermatology, 5th ed, p 1757. Oxford, Blackwell Scientific, 1992

SWEDISH TYPE PORPHYRIA

Synonyms. Waldenström's I; intermittent acute porphyria; IAP; porphyria hepatica I; porphyria intermittens acuta; pyrroloporphyria.

Symptoms. Both sexes affected. Female to male ratio, 3:2; usual onset in young adulthood. Abdominal symptoms. Intermittent, recurrent attack of pain (colicky type) (85–95%); localized or generalized constipation (48–84%). Vomiting, occasionally severe (43–88%). Muscle weakness (42–68%). Attacks may last days or months. During attack, slight fever may be present (9–37%). Weight loss, emaciation, electrolyte imbalance with dehydration may result. Neurologic symptomatology. Highly variable; polyneuritis including cranial nerves; autonomic system abnormalities; cerebral function derangement with motor, sensorial (9–38%) and psychotic manifestations (40–58%). Convulsions (10–20%). Absence of photosensitivity and of increased mechanical fragility of skin.

Signs. Abdomen usually soft; no rebound tenderness; stomach distended. Neurologic findings highly variable. Blood hypertension (36–54%). During attack, sinus tachycardia (28–80%)

Etiology. Autosomal dominant inheritance. Deficiency of porphobilinogen (PBG) deaminase with which concomitant factors (steroid hormones, drugs, nutrition) determine clinical syndrome. Women probably have more frequent episodes because of menstrual cycles.

Pathology. High concentration of PBG in liver.

Diagnostic Procedures. *Blood.* During attack, leukocytosis may be present. Electrolyte imbalance (when severe vomiting); hyponatremia. *Urine.* Excretion of high amount of PBG and d-aminolevulinic acid (ALA) (rough correlation of their amounts with attacks); in intermittent periods values may approach normality). *X-ray.* Of GI. Areas of distention proximal to areas of spasm.

Therapy. Avoid dangerous drugs (especially barbiturates). Symptomatic: narcotic analgesics for pain relief. High carbohydrate intake ameliorates symptoms; hematin IV.

Prognosis. Attacks may last for various lengths of time; occasionally fatal. Usually followed by periods of latency lasting weeks or years. Death rate highest in third decade. Some of these patients undergo repeated abdominal operations before the diagnosis is made.

BIBLIOGRAPHY. Günther H: Die Haematoporphyrie. Dtsch Arch Klin Med 105:89–146, 1911
Waldenström J: Studien über Porphyrie. Acta Med Scand (Suppl) 82:1–254, 1937
Lee GR: Porphyria. In Lee GR, Bithel TC, Foerster J, et al (eds): Wintrobe's Clinical Hematology, 9th ed, pp 1282–1287. Philadelphia, Lea & Febiger, 1993

SWEET

Synonym. Acute febrile neutrophilic dermatosis.

Symptoms and Signs. Occurs in women. Onset in middle age. Infection precedes onset. High persistent fever; eruption of painful plaques on skin of limbs, face, and neck. Later, pustules.

Etiology. Unknown. Possibly, hypersensitivity to infective agent.

Pathology. Skin. Focal infiltration of neutrophils and lymphocytes; moderate leukocytolysis. Moderate vascular endothelial swelling and vasodilatation.

Diagnostic Procedures. *Blood.* Culture; moderate leukocytosis.

Therapy. Antibiotics ineffective. Steroids effective as long as administered.

Prognosis. Condition lasts 2 weeks or more. Repeated relapses (usually preceded by infections).

BIBLIOGRAPHY. Sweet RD: An acute febrile neutrophilic dermatosis. Br J Dermatol 76:349–356, 1964
Spector JI, Zimbler H, Levine R, et al: Sweet's syndrome, association with acute leukemia. JAMA 244:1131–1132, 1980
Ryan TJ: Cutaneous vasculitis. In Champion RH, Burton JL, Ebling FJG (eds): Rook/Wilkinson/Ebling Textbook of Dermatology, 5th ed, pp 1928–1929. Oxford, Blackwell Scientific, 1992

SWYER

Synonyms. Gonadal dysgenesis (46, XY); pure gonadal dysgenesis 46, XY. See Golberg-Maxwell and Turner.

Symptoms and Signs. Complete form: female phenotype; failure of puberty and fertility. No stigma of Turner syndrome (see). Tall stature; eunuchoid proportion. Primary amenorrhea. Incomplete forms: genital ambiguity with bilateral dysgenetic testes and muellerian derivatives.

Etiology. Failure of fetal testes to develop and thus the fetus develops on female phenotype. Clinically and genetical heterogeneity. Sporadic and familial (X-linked recessive or sex-limited dominant autosomal inheritance).

Pathology. Streak gonads at the site where ovaries may be expected containing androgen-secreting hilus cells; small uterus and fallopian tubes.

Diagnostic Procedures. *Chromosome study,* 46, XY karyotype. *Echography.* Demonstration of presence of uterus. *Blood.* At time of anticipated puberty, evidence of absent gonadal activity in presence of increased gonadotropins. Sex steroids levels remaining very low; gonadotropins increasing progressively with age.

Therapy. As in Turner (see). Prophylactic gonadectomy and estrogen substitution at puberty.

Prognosis. With treatment, good response and good psychological adjustment. High incidence of neoplasia (germinomas; gonadoblastomas).

BIBLIOGRAPHY. Swyer GIM: Male pseudohermaphroditism: A hitherto undescribed form. Br Med J 2:709–712, 1955
Frasier SD, Bashore RA, Mosier HD: Gonadoblastoma associated with pure gonadal dysgenesis in monozygous twins. J Pediatr 64:740–745, 1964
Forest MG: Diagnosis and treatment of disorders of sexual development. In De Groot LJ (ed): Endocrinology, 3rd ed, pp 1902–1903. Philadelphia, WB Saunders, 1995

SWYER-JAMES

Synonyms. Mac Leod; unilateral pulmonary emphysema; lung, unilateral, hyperlucent; pulmonary artery functional hypoplasia.

Symptoms. Onset in childhood and adolescence. Recurrent pulmonary infections.

Signs. Unilateral diminished pulmonary expansion, faint breath sounds, and fine rales.

Etiology. Acquired condition, secondary to necrotizing bronchitis, probably viral in origin, with onset in early infancy, damaging peripheral bronchial passages with consequent emphysema and bronchiolectasis and functional insufficiency of pulmonary artery and its branches. Agenesis and congenital hypoplasia of pulmonary artery are usually accompanied by major symptomatology owing to cardiovascular and pulmonary anomaly, which allows the differentiation of the two conditions.

Pathology. Obliteration of peripheral capillaries of affected lung. Bronchiolectasis; some alveolar emphysematous zones are collapsed. Chronic inflammatory changes.

Diagnostic Procedures. *X-ray.* Of chest. Must be done in inspiration and forced expiration. Hyperlucency of affected lung or lobe; decreased peripheral vascular marking with small hilar shadow. *CT scan. MRI.* Reinforce the findings of radiography. *Fluoroscopy.* Heart and mediastinum shift toward affected lung in inspiration and away in expiration. *Bronchoscopy.* No obstruction of major bronchi. *Bronchography.* Decreased or absent filling at periphery. Unusual bronchial pattern; small bronchioles terminating in clubs or pools. *Angiography.* In the affected side, decreased filling of pulmonary artery. *Isotopic V/Q study* shows hypoperfusion.

Therapy. Antibiotic for acute or chronic pulmonary infections. When syndrome does not react to treatment and interferes with work and well-being of patient because of persistence of definite syndrome, surgery is indicated.

Prognosis. Variable according to intensity of symptoms and response to treatment.

BIBLIOGRAPHY. Swyer PR, James GCW: Case of unilateral pulmonary emphysema. Thorax 8:133–136, 1953
McLeod WM: Abnormal translucency of one lung. Thorax 9:147, 1954
Avital A, Shulman DL, Baryishay E, et al: Differential lung function in an infant with the Swyer-James syndrome. Thorax 44:298–302, 1989
Weatherall DJ, Ledingham JGG, Warrell DA: Oxford Textbook of Medicine, p 2778. Oxford, Oxford Med Pub, 1996

SYDENHAM

Synonyms. Saint Vitus dance; chorea acute; chorea minor; rheumatic chorea.

Symptoms. Occurs in children 5–13; more frequently in females. Involuntary, purposeless, irregular, short-lasting movements (choreiform) initially in one limb. Anxiety; irritability; weakness; face movements that simulate smirking expressions. Voice changes may also be observed; dysarthria may be severe. Movements cease during sleep. Emotional instability.

Signs. Hypotonic musculature; flaccidity; passive motion that allows unusual and otherwise uncomfortable positions. Tendon reflexes variable; no sensory changes; psychological changes; possibly fever.

Etiology. Unknown. Association with rheumatic fever, tonsillitis, less frequently typhus, malaria, or other infections, or completely independent. Phenothiazine drugs, haloperidol may cause chorea.

Pathology. Diffuse cerebral edema; congestion of corpus striatum. Three orders of changes: inflammatory, degenerative, and vascular. But no precise localization of lesions.

Diagnostic Procedures. *CSF.* Mildly increased pressure; mild pleocytosis; increased glucose. *Blood.* Sedimentation rate; antistreptolysin titer; C-reactive protein.

Therapy. Rest; quiet; protection from harmful movements. Phenobarbital; paraldehyde; phenothiazine; haloperidol. Salicylates or other specific therapy if rheumatic fever present.

Prognosis. Variable; mild form recovers in weeks; exacerbation may prolong form for years. Death may result from exhaustion or associated cardiac complication. Relapses after months or years in 33% of cases.

BIBLIOGRAPHY. Sydenham T: Schedula monitoria de novae febris ingressu Londini, Kettilby, 1636
Begbie J: Remarks on rheumatism and chorea; their relation and treatment. Month J Med Sci 7:740–754, 1847
Adams RD, Victor M: Principles of Neurology, 5th ed, p 67. New York, McGraw-Hill, 1993
Weatherall DJ, Ledingham JGG, Warrell DA: Oxford Textbook of Medicine, p 4012. Oxford, Oxford Med Pub, 1996

SYLVESTER (P.E.)

Synonym. Friedreich ataxia—optic atrophy—sensorineural deafness.

Symptoms and Signs. Both sexes. From childhood. Neural deafness, optic atrophy, ataxia; muscle wasting of shoulder girdle and arms; mental dullness.

Etiology. Unknown. Autosomal dominant inheritance.

Pathology. Degeneration of optic nerves, posterior columns, spinocerebellar and corticospinal tracts.

Prognosis. Variable progressivity.

BIBLIOGRAPHY. Sylvester PE: Some unusual findings in a family with Friedreich's ataxia. Arch Dis Child 33:217–221, 1958
Adams RD, Victor M: Principles of Neurology, 5th ed, p 1002. New York, McGraw-Hill, 1993

SYNBLEPHARON

Symptoms and Signs. Partial or complete adherence of the eyelid to the eyeball. Inability to close eyelids effectively. Diplopia.

Etiology. Defect owing to inflammation, injury, or burns. Congenital type, usually of recessive inheritance, possibly dominant. Frequently associated with ankyblepharon, microphthalmos, ankyloblepharon filiforme adnatum or with cleft palate. This manifestation is present in various congenital syndromes.

Pathology. Affects lower lid more frequently. Bands of fibrous tissue between globe and lid.

Therapy. Prevention by daily probing. Mucous membrane grafts.

Prognosis. Frequent recurrence. Disfigurement, lagophthalmus.

BIBLIOGRAPHY. Torczynski E: Developmental anomalies of the eye. In Garner A, Klintworth GK (eds): Pathobiology of Ocular Disease: A Dynamic Approach, 2nd ed, pp 1330–1331. New York, Marcel Dekker, 1994

SYNCOPAL MIGRAINE

Symptoms and Signs. More frequent in adolescent females, frequently associated with menstrual cycle. Premonitory aura of migraine is followed by consciousness loss. Slow onset. At awaking severe headache (occipital area).

Etiology. Unknown. Postulated brain stem ischemia or prolonged localized basilar artery spasm. Hyperresponsiveness of dopamine receptors is an alternative explanation.

Therapy. See Migraine.

Prognosis. That of migraine.

BIBLIOGRAPHY. Bickerstaff ER: Impairment of consciousness in migraine. Lancet 2:1057–1070, 1961
Sicuteri F, Boccuzzi M, Fanciullacci M, et al: A new nonvascular interpretation of syncopal migraine. Adv Neurol 33:199–210, 1982
Lewis RP, Budoulas H, Schaal SF, et al: Diagnosis and management of syncope. In Schlant RC, Alexander RW: Hurst's The Heart, 8th ed, p 935. New York, McGraw-Hill, 1994

SYPHILID, TUBEROSERPIGINOUS

Synonym. Lewis.

Symptoms and Signs. Both sexes affected. Skin lesions similar to those of lupus vulgaris affecting eyelids, nose, and ears and, possibly, also extremities and trunk. Lower eyelids more frequently affected. Conjunctival lesions; corneal ulcers.

Etiology. Syphilis.

Therapy. Specific.

Prognosis. Lesions could be arrested by treatment.

BIBLIOGRAPHY. Schreck E: Veraenderungen des Sehorgans bei Haut-und-Geschlechtskrankheiten. In: Gottron HA, Schoenfeld V (eds). Dermatologie und Venerologie (IV) Stuttgart, Thieme, 1960
Korting GW: The Skin and Eye, p 26. Philadelphia, WB Saunders, 1973

SYRINGOMYELIA

Synonym. Morvan I; including segmental sensory dissociation–brachial amyotrophy.

Symptoms. Both sexes equally affected. Insidious onset in third to fourth decade. (1) Cervical lesions (most frequent); unilateral numbness of finger; localized analgesia (loss of pain and temperature; preservation of touch and deep sensibilities). At onset, in one arm and upper part of chest; then involving both sides. Later, weakness and atrophy of hands (claw deformity) and loss of deep reflexes. Stiffness of neck; deep boring spontaneous pain. (2) Lumbar lesion, unilateral and then bilateral. Same symptoms as in the preceding in lower extremities and pelvic girdle. (3) Medulla oblongata lesions (syringobulbia); same symptoms as in the preceding in the face.

Signs. Insensitivity to pain and temperature in areas affected. Burns, scars, and injuries. Trophic changes, ulcerations, Charcot joints may be seen. Muscular atrophy and fasciculation. Spasticity; ataxia; neurogenic bladder. Horner syndrome frequently seen.

Etiology. Possibly neoplasm; disorderly proliferation of ependyma; anomalies of blood supply. Probably congenital in origin. Both autosomal dominant and recessive traits have been reported. Mechanism postulated: prevention of normal flow of CSF by a congenital failure of opening of outlet of IV ventricle, resulting in pulse-wave of pressure transmitted into the cord through central canal and causing its dilatation (syrinx) and diverticulum.

Pathology. At onset, proliferation of glial cells in the region of central canal; then cavity formation spreading longitudinally. Gliosis is not limited to central gray matter, but tends to send projection ventrally and dorsally. Cervical cord most frequent site of origin. Four types have been classified. *Type I.* Syringomyelia with obstruction of foamen magnum and dilatation of central canal (a) with Chiari Type I malformation; or (b) with other type of obstruction of foramen. *Type II.* Without obstruction of foramen (idiopathic). *Type III.* With other diseases of spinal cord (tumors, trauma, arachnoiditis, pachymengitis, etc.). *Type IV.* Pure hydromyelia with or without hydrocephalus.

Diagnostic Procedures. *CSF.* Increase of total protein (50% of cases) does not differentiate from tumors. *CT scan. MRI.*

Therapy. Deep roentgen radiation (has been discontinued). Surgery, results according to etiology.

Prognosis. Slowly progressing for years.

BIBLIOGRAPHY. Olliver d'Angier 1827. Quoted by Ballantine

Morvan AM: De la parésie analgésique a panaris des extrémitiés supérieures ou paréso-analgésie des extrémités supérieures. Gaz Hebd Med Paris 20:580–583; 624–626, 1883

Ballantine HT, Ojemann RG, Drew JH: Syringohydromyelia. In Krayenbuehl H, Maspes PE, Sweet WH (eds): Progress in neurological surgery, vol 4, pp 227–245. New York, Karger, 1971

Brown LK, Stacy C, Schick A, Miller A: Obstructive sleep apnea in syringo-myelia-syringobulbia. NY State J Med 88:152–154, 1988

Adams RD, Victor M: Principles of Neurology, 5th ed, pp 1110–1113. New York, McGraw-Hill, 1993

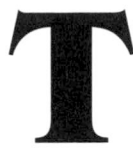

TACHYPNEA, TRANSIENT NEWBORN

Synonym. Respiratory distress type II.

Symptoms and Signs. Usually full-term infants. Elevated respiratory rate on first day of life; some retraction and grunting; slight cyanosis; no rales or rhonchi. Respiratory rate remains elevated for 2–5 days.

Etiology. Unknown. It may represent a delay in resorption of fluid from lungs.

Pathology. Postulated reduction of compliance of the lung from delay of resorption of alveolar fluid and distention of periarterial space.

Diagnostic Procedures. *ECG.* Normal. *X-ray.* Of chest. Suggestive of vascular engorgement or passive vascular congestion (poorly defined margins). Lack of reticulogranular pattern. Slight cardiomegaly (mean ratio 0.60). *Blood.* pH and PCO$_2$; standard bicarbonate within normal limits.

Therapy. Symptomatic; oxygen.

Prognosis. Recovery with disappearance of radiologic findings between first and fifth days.

BIBLIOGRAPHY. Avery ME, Gatewood OB, Brumley G: Transient tachypnea of newborn: Possible delayed resorption of fluid at birth. Am J Dis Child 111:380–385, 1966
Rawlings JS, Smith FR: Transient tachypnea of the newborn: An analysis of neonatal and obstetric risk factors. Am J Dis Child 138:869–871, 1984
Shohat M, Levy G, Levy I, et al: Transient tachypnea of the newborn and asthma. Arch Dis Child 64:277–279, 1989

TAFFY CANDY

Synonyms. Mitral regurgitation; chordal elongation; primary chordal dysplasia; secondary chordal dysplasia. See also Papillary muscle.

Symptoms and Signs. Gradual or sudden, severe mitral regurgitation symptomatology.

Etiology. Inappropriate elongation of anterior leaflet chordae. In course of rheumatic fever, myocardial infarction; without underlying abnormalities.

Pathology. Chordae of anterior leaflet elongated and thinned out, especially in the middle; all the features of mitral regurgitation.

Diagnostic Procedures. *ECG. Angiocardiography. X-ray.* Of chest. *Two-dimensional echocardiography with color flow imaging and spectral Doppler interrogation. Cardiac catheterization. Radionuclide studies.*

Therapy. Medical or surgical.

Prognosis. Fair with treatment. May evolve into chordal rupture.

BIBLIOGRAPHY. Cobbs BW Jr: In Hurst JW, Logue RB (eds): The Heart, 1st ed, p 88. New York, McGraw-Hill, 1966
Gaasch WH, O'Rourke RA, Cohn LH, et al: Mitral valve disease. In Schlant RC, Alexander RW: Hurst's The Heart, 8th ed, pp 1493, 1495. New York, McGraw-Hill, 1994

TAIJIN KYOFU SHO

Symptoms and Signs. In Japan. Distinctive phobia: intense fear that proper body or its parts or functions are offensive to people.

Etiology. Psychotic disorder, culture bound. Locally included in diagnostic system for mental disorders.

BIBLIOGRAPHY. Lin K-M: Cultural influences on the diagnosis of psychotic and organic disorders. In Mezzich JE, Kleinman A, Fabrega H, et al: Culture and Psychiatric Diagnosis. Washington, American Psychiatry Press, 1995
Kaplan HI, Sadock BJ: Comprehensive Textbook of Psychiatry, 6th ed, p 1053. Baltimore, Williams & Wilkins, 1995

TAKAHARA

Synonyms. Acatalasia; acatalasemia.

Symptoms. Common in Japanese and Koreans; reported in Caucasians as well. Asymptomatic (50%). Exeptionally affected after puberty. Chronic, severe infection of mouth; gangrenous lesions, including alveolar destruction.

Etiology. Deficiency of enzyme catalase in tissues and cells, including blood, erythrocytes. Autosomal recessive inheritance with heterozygotes with intermediate levels of red-cell catalase activity.

Pathology. Gangrenous lesion of mouth owing to lack of resistance to normal flora; no other serious pathology.

Diagnostic Procedures. Addition of hydrogen peroxide to whole acatalasic blood produces methemoglobin, black-brown color (normal blood remains pink).

Therapy. Antibiotics; local surgical excision, tooth extraction. Whole blood transfusion to raise catalase level in period of need. Crystalline catalase suspension for topical treatment.

Prognosis. Lesions respond in part to antibiotic treatment and measures to prevent infections. After healing, lesions may produce scarring that may impair mouth opening.

BIBLIOGRAPHY. Takahara S: Progressive oral gangrene probably due to lack of catalase in the blood. Lancet 2:1101–1104, 1952
Matsunaga T, Seger R, Hoger P, et al: Congenital acatalasemia: A study of neutrophil functions after provocation with hydrogen peroxide. Pediatr Res 19:1187–1190, 1985
Eaton JWMAM: Acatalasemia. In Scriver CR, Beaudet AL, Sly WS, et al: The Metabolic and Molecular Bases of Inherited Disease, 7th ed, pp 2375–2376. New York, McGraw-Hill, 1995

TAKAYASU

Synonyms. Martorell II; Martorell-Fabre; Raeder-Arbitz; Ash-Upmark; aortic arch arteritis; brachiocephalic arteritis; reversed coarctation, pulseless; young female aortic arch arteritis.

Symptoms. Prevalent in young women. Symptoms may be intermittent. Usually, unilateral transient amblyopia or persistent blindness. Aphasia; transient hemiparesis; headache; vertigo; syncope, convulsions. Weakness and pain in the muscles of mastication; occasionally, weakness, numbness, or pain exertion of upper limb.

Signs. Atrophy and pigmentation on skin of face; ulceration of nose and palate. Cataracts. In fundus: anastomosis about the disk; atrophy of iris, optic nerve, atrophy or pigmentation of retina. Weakness of pulse in the arm; decrease of blood pressure on the arm; tendency to hypertension of the legs. Bruit on upper chest and neck. Marked pulmonary hypertension can occur, in the absence of symptoms referrable to systemic vasculitis.

Etiology. Unknown. Idiopathic arteritis; possibly autoimmune condition.

Pathology. Arteritis confined to first few centimeters of innominate, common carotid, and subclavian arteries, adjacent thoracic aorta. The pulmonary vessels can be the principal vessels involved. Microscopically, all layers of arteries are involved; round cell (and occasionally giant cell) infiltration. Elastica disrupted; medial atrophy and fibrosis.

Diagnostic Procedures. *Blood.* Normal red cell and white cell number; sedimentation rate increased; hypergammaglobulinemia. *X-ray.* Notching of upper ribs; occasionally, calcification of ascending arch and descending aorta. *Aortography. Endomyocardial biopsy.*

Therapy. Chronic anticoagulation and corticosteroid (result equivocal). Surgery with excision and graft replacement of part of artery involved; bypass for multiple occlusions.

Prognosis. Poor; survival varies 1–15 years from onset of symptoms.

BIBLIOGRAPHY. Takayasu M: A case with peculiar changes of the central retinal vessels. Acta Soc Ophthalmol (Jpn) 12:554, 1908
Haas A, Stiehm R: Takayasu's arteritis presenting as pulmonary hypertension. Am J Dis Child 140:372–374, 1986
Hall S, Buchbinder R: Takayasu's arteritis. Rheum Dis Clin No Am 16:411–422, 1990
Weatherall DJ, Ledingham JGG, Warrell DA (eds): Oxford Textbook of Medicine, 3rd ed, pp 2377–2380. Oxford, Oxford Med Pub, 1996

TALMA

Synonyms. Acquired myotonia. Myotonia, percussion.

Symptoms and Signs. Onset in adult life. Prolonged contraction of some muscles after electric or mechanical stimulation, with delayed relaxation. Strong voluntary contraction also followed by delayed relaxation.

Etiology. Unknown. It follows or is associated with acute infections, intoxications, and traumas.

Therapy. Symptomatic. Quinine; procaine.

Prognosis. Variable. Usually, regression of the myotonic phenomenon.

BIBLIOGRAPHY. Talma S: Over myotonia acquisita. Med Tschr Geneesk 28:321–328, 1892
Weatherall DJ, Ledingham JGG, Warrell DA (eds): Oxford Textbook of Medicine, 3rd ed, pp 4151–4153. Oxford, Oxford Med Pub, 1996

TANGIER*

Synonyms. Alpha-lipoprotein deficiency; analphalipoproteinemia; familial HDL deficiency; high-density lipoprotein deficiency.

Symptoms. Both sexes affected. Age of detection from childhood to fourth or fifth decade. Usually asymptomatic. In some cases, intermittent diarrhea; recurrent mild sensory symptoms, at distal part of extremities (pain and temperature); bilateral motor weakness, usually proximal, occasionally also distal; in one case observed also dissociated loss of pain and temperature (syringo-like syndrome).

Signs. Enlargement of tonsils with typical orange color. If tonsils removed, remaining follicles show the same color. Muscle wasting. Occasionally, splenomegaly and moderate lymphadenopathy, and, still less frequently, moderate hepatomegaly, corneal infiltration (in adult). Premature coronary heart condition in some patients. Abnormal rectal mucosa.

Etiology. May be a mutation in a gene that regulates synthesis of Apo-Gln-I characterized by almost complete absence of plasma high-density lipoproteins and cholesterol ester storage in many tissues. Lipoprotein instability causes cholesterol deposit in reticuloendothelial macrophages. Autosomal recessive inheritance with different penetrability.

Pathology. Storage of large amount of cholesterol esters in reticuloendothelial tissues. Tonsil, pharyngeal, and rectal mucosae show typical orange color. Spleen, liver, and lymph nodes may be enlarged with the presence of foam cells. Muscle biopsy shows neurogenic myopathy changes.

Diagnostic Procedures. *Blood.* Plasma cholesterol below 120 mg/100 ml; phospholipids reduced; triglycerides normal or elevated. Lipoproteins study shows practically an absence of high-density lipoprotein. Hyperuricemia (only in adults). *Biopsy.* Of lymph node and bone marrow. Presence of foam cells. *Electromyography.*

Therapy. No treatment presently indicated.

Prognosis. Benign course. To date has not affected longevity. Possibility of increased incidence of vascular pathology considered.

BIBLIOGRAPHY. Fredrickson DS, Altrocchi PH, Avioli LV, et al: Tangier disease. Ann Intern Med 55:1016–1031, 1961
Makrides SC, Ruiz-Opazo N, Hayden M, et al: Sequence and expression of Tangier Apo A-I-gene. Eur J Biochem 173:465–471, 1988
Winder AF: Disorders of lipid and lipoprotein metabolism. In Garner A, Klintworth GK (eds): Pathobiology of Ocular Disease: A Dynamic Approach, 2nd ed, pp 1106–1107. New York, Marcel Dekker, 1994
Assmann von Eckardstein A, Brewer HB Jr: Familial high density lipoprotein deficiency: Tangier disease. In Scriver CR, Beaudet AL, Sly WS, et al: The Metabolic and Molecular Bases of Inherited Disease, 7th ed, pp 2053–2072. New York, McGraw-Hill, 1995

TAPETAL-LIKE REFLEX

Synonym. Retinitis pigmentosa-3; RP 3; retinitis pigmentosa, X-linked. See Flecked retina.

Symptoms and Signs. In females (heterozygous) no visual defect. Ring scotoma; retina and choroid: bright yellow greenish spots in posterior polar region. Retinitis pigmentosa may be associated.

Etiology. Unknown. Sex-linked heterozygous transmission.

Pathology. Degenerative changes in Bruch membrane (?).

Therapy. None.

Prognosis. Benign lesion.

BIBLIOGRAPHY. Niccol W: A family with bilateral developmental defects of the macula. Trans Ophthalmol Soc UK 58:763, 1938
Ciccarelli EC: A new syndrome of tapetal-like fundic reflexes with ring scotomata: Report of two cases. Arch Ophthalmol 67:316–320, 1962
Dahl N, Sundvall M, Pettersson U, et al: Genetic mapping of loci for X-linked retinitis pigmentosa. Clin Genet 40:435–440, 1991
Bird AC, Jay B, Hussain AA, et al: Retinal photoreceptor disorders. In Garner A, Sarks S, Sarks JP: Degenerative and related disorders of the retina and choroid. In Garner A, Klintworth GK (eds): Pathobiology of Ocular Disease: A Dynamic Approach, 2nd ed, p 1210. New York, Marcel Dekker, 1994

TAPIA

Synonym. Nucleus ambigous—hypoglossal; vagohypoglossal.

Symptoms. Dysarthria and dysphagia.

Signs. Ipsilateral paralysis of tongue, soft palate, vocal cord; hemiatrophy of tongue.

Etiology. Trauma; aneurysm of carotid artery, malignancy determining

---

*Named after the Chesapeake Bay island where first cases were identified.

paralysis of the hypoglossal (XII) nerve and partial paralysis of the vagus (X) nerve. Occasional involvement of the XI.

Pathology. Extracranial lesion of hypoglossal (XII) and vagus (X) (partial) nerves. Fracture of skull; luxation of atlas; aneurysm or malignancy.

Diagnostic Procedures. *X-ray. CT scan. MRI.* Of skull. *Angiography.*

Therapy. Symptomatic.

Prognosis. Depends on etiology.

BIBLIOGRAPHY. Tapia AG: Un caso de paralisis del lado derecho de la laringe y de la lengua; con paralisis del esterno-cleido-mastoidea y trapecio del mismo lado; acompanado de hemiplejia total temporal del lado izquierdo del cuerpo. Siglo Méd Madrid 52:211–213, 1905

Tapia AG: Un nouveau syndrome; quelques cas d'hémiplégie du larynx et de la langue avec ou sans paralysie du sternocléido-mastoïdien et du trapèze. Arch Int Laryngol 22:780–785, 1906

Schmidt D, Tiel K: In Schmidt D, Malin JP (eds): Erkrankungen der Hirnnerven 2 Aufl. Stuttgart, 1991

TARLOV CYST

Synonyms. Perineural cysts, spinal nerve roots.

Symptoms and Signs. In adults. From asymptomatic or cause of sciatica, or equine cauda syndrome (see). Cysts on the sacral or coccygeal posterior nerve roots in the region of passage through dura mater; the larger cyst compress the corresponding anterior and posterior roots.

Etiology. Unknown. Inflammatory? Traumatic? Degeneration?

Pathology. Cysts containing clear fluid that do not communicate with subarchnoid space. Cysts arising between perinerium and endoneurium usually dorsally and extending around circumference of nerve root and ganglion that may be destroyed.

Diagnostic Procedures. *CT scan. MRI.*

Therapy. Excision.

Prognosis. Rapid recovery from treatment if carried out in time.

BIBLIOGRAPHY. Tarlov IM: Perineurial cysts of the spinal nerve roots. Arch Neurol Psychiat (Chicago) 40:1067–1074, 1938

Wilkins RH, Odom GL: Spinal extradural cysts. In Vinken PJ, Bruyn GW: Handbook of Clinical Neurology, vol 22, pp 146–152. Amsterdam, North-Holland, 1975

TARSAL TUNNEL

Synonym. Jogger foot.

Symptoms. Intermittent burning pain, paresthesias, cyanosis, coldness, and numbness of foot following prolonged standing or walking; sometimes progressing in intensity during the day; occasionally, pain at night. Usually more pronounced in toes and sole. Removal of shoe, massage, and sometimes walking relieve pain. Radiation of pain to calf occasionally experienced.

Signs. Presence of area of hypoesthesia and diminished two-point discrimination. Tinel sign or formication sign positive (percussion over or just below the point of original nerve section gives rise to tingling sensation in the periphery). Atrophy of abductor hallucis (in advanced state) or occasionally hypertrophy of abductor hallucis. In some patients, fat ankle and foot.

Etiology and Pathology. Post-traumatic fibrosis; presence of accessory of hypertrophic abductor hallucis muscle; tenosynovitis or spontaneous entrapment resulting in chronic compression from fascial bands of posterior tibial nerve beneath flexor retinaculum and deep fascia along medial border of foot.

Diagnostic Procedures. *Electromyography.* Nerve conduction studies.

Local injection with cortisone, tourniquet test. To produce temporary passive congestion and an ischemic element.

Therapy. Local steroid injection; weight reduction; surgical decompression of nerve.

Prognosis. Good with treatment.

BIBLIOGRAPHY. Pollock LJ, Davis L: Peripheral Nerve Injuries, pp 32; 484–493. New York, Hoeber, 1933

Keck C: The tarsal tunnel syndrome. J Bone Joint Surg (Am) 44:180–182, 1962

Ricciardi-Pollini PT, Moneta MR, Falez F: The tarsal tunnel syndrome: A report of eight cases. Foot Ankle 6:146–149, 1985

Klippel JH, Dieppe PA: Rheumatology, pp 3.4.11, 5.19.9–5.19.10. St Louis, CV Mosby, 1994

TARUI

Synonyms. Glycogen storage defect (type VII); glycogenosis (type VII); muscle phosphofructokinase deficiency. PFKM deficiency.

Symptoms and Signs. Both sexes affected. Identical to McArdle syndrome (see). Easy fatigability. Muscle stiffness on vigourous exercise. Occasionally, myoglobinuria. No neurological anomalies.

Etiology. Autosomal recessive inheritance.

Diagnostic Procedures. *Blood.* Reticulocytosis; reduced red cell life span; reduction of red cell phosphofructokinase activity. In some cases hemolysis. Ischemic exercise does not cause rise in venous lactate. *Biopsy.* Of muscle. Increase of glucose 6-phosphate and fructose 6-phosphate and decrease of fructose, 1, 6-diphosphate. Phosphofructokinase activity equal to 1–3% of normal. Glycogen storage. *Urine.* Occasionally myoglobinuria.

Therapy. No specific treatment. Avoidance of strenuous exercise to avoid acute attacks and oral ingestion of fructose to relieve symptoms.

Prognosis. Good.

BIBLIOGRAPHY. Tarui S, Okuno G, Ikura Y, et al: Phosphofructokinase deficiency in skeletal muscle: A new type of glycogenosis. Biochem Biophys Res Com 19:517–523, 1965

Danon MJ, Servidei S, Di Mauro S, et al: Late onset muscle phosphofructokinase deficiency. Neurology 38:956–960, 1988

Haller RG, Lewis SF: Glucose-induced exertional fatigue in muscle phosphofructokinase deficiency. N Engl J Med 324:364–369, 1991

Chen YT, Burchell A: Glycogen storage diseases. In Scriver CR, Beaudet AL, Sly WS, et al: The Metabolic and Molecular Bases of Inherited Disease, 7th ed, pp 954–955. New York, McGraw-Hill, 1995

TAUSSIG-BING

Synonyms. Double outlet right ventricle III; pulmonic stenosis absence; right ventricle origin of both great arteries; supracrystal septal defect.

Symptoms and Signs. Onset at birth. Cyanosis; dyspnea on exertion; underdevelopment; cardiomegaly; systolic murmur in left third intercostal space; loud second pulmonic sound.

Etiology. Congenital vascular malformation.

Pathology. Ventricular septal defect anterosuperior to the crista supraventricularis, close to the pulmonary valve, without pulmonary stenosis. Aorta completely transposed arising from right ventricle, levoposition of large pulmonary artery that overrides left ventricle without arising completely from it. High ventricular septal defect; right ventricular hypertrophy.

Diagnostic Procedures. *ECG. X-ray.* Of chest. *Angiocardiography. Cardiac catheterization. Two-dimensional echocardiography with color flow imaging and spectral Doppler interrogation. Blood.* Moderate polycythemia.

Therapy. Medical treatment and surgical correction.

Prognosis. Permanent and progressive cyanosis. Clubbing of fingers becomes evident after survival for a few years. Patient may live to second to fourth decade.

BIBLIOGRAPHY. Taussig HB, Bing RJ: Complete transposition of aorta and levoposition of pulmonary artery. Am Heart J 37:551–559, 1949
What Is the Taussig-Bing Malformation? (editorial). Circulation 38:445–449, 1968
Pacifico AD, Kirklin JK, Colvin EV, et al: Intraventricular tunnel repair for Taussing-Bing heart and related cardiac anomalies. Circulation 74(Suppl 1):53–60, 1986
Nugent EW, Plauth WH, Edwards JE, et al: The pathology, pathophysiology recognition and treatment of congenital heart disease. In Schlant RC, Alexander RW: Hurst's The Heart, 8th ed, pp 1811–1813. New York, McGraw-Hill, 1994
Perloff JK: The Clinical Recognition of Congenital Heart Disease, 4th ed, pp 499–505. Philadelphia, WB Saunders, 1994

TAY

Synonyms. Ichthyosis—trichothyodystrophy; trichothyodystrophy, congenital ichthyosis; IBIDS.

Symptoms. Both sexes. From birth. Nonbullous ichthyosiform erythroderma, growth and mental retardation, progerioid lack of subcutaneous fat; short brittle hair; dysplastic nails; photosensitivity; congenital cataracts; spasticity; ataxia; decreased fertility.

Etiology. Unknown. Autosomal recessive inheritance.

Pathology. Ichthyosis (see). Typical sulfur deficiency in the hair.

Therapy. Symptomatic.

Prognosis. Poor.

BIBLIOGRAPHY. Tay CH: Ichthyosisform erythroderma, hair shaft abnormalities and mental and growth retardation: A new recessive disorder. Arch Dermatol 104:4–13, 1971
Happle R, Grobe H, et al: The Tay syndrome (congenital ichthyosis with trichothyodystrophy). Eur J Pediatr 141:147–152, 1984
Blomquist HK, Back O, Fagerlund M, et al: Tay or IBIDS syndrome: A case with growth and mental retardation, congenital ichthyosis and brittle hair. Acta Pediat Scand 80:1241–1245, 1991

TAYBI

Synonyms. Otopalatodigital; OPD.

Symptoms. Both sexes affected. Females show variable degrees of expression. Moderate deafness (conductive); mild mental deficiency; limited elbow extension.

Signs. Small stature; frontal and occipital prominence; hypertelorism; small nose and mouth; partial anodontia; cleft soft palate; short trunk. Short broad phalanges of thumbs and toes; short nails.

Etiology. Mapping of OpDI gene to XQ28. X-linked semidominant inheritance.

Diagnostic Procedures. *X-ray. CT scan. MRI.* Thick cranial bones; absence of frontal and sphenoidal sinuses; failure of neural arch fusion. Accessory ossification center at base of second metatarsal; short metacarpals third, fourth, fifth.

Prognosis. Death in first weeks or months of life

BIBLIOGRAPHY. Taybi H: Generalized skeletal dysplasia with multiple anomalies. Am J Roentgenol Rad Ther Nucl Med 88:450–457, 1962
Gorlin RJ, Poznanski AK, Heudon I: The oto-palato-digital (O.P.D.) syndrome in females. Oral Surg 35:218–224, 1973
Biancalana V, Le Marec B, Odent S, et al: Oto-palato-digital syndrome

type. In Further Evidence for Assignment of the Locus to X Q 28. Hum Genet 88:228–230, 1991

TAYBI-LINDER

Synonyms. Dwarfism; skeletal dysplasia; brain abnormalities.

Symptoms and Signs. Both sexes. Low birth weight, dwarfism, microcephaly, bulging eyes, spade-like hands. Convulsion, cyanotic attacks.

Etiology. Autosomal recessive inheritance.

Pathology. Brain abnormalities: large, midline parasagittal hemispheral defect and absent corpus callosum, common ventricular cavity. Alteration of cerebral cortex, absence of lamina pattern, heterotopic gray matter scattered in the subcortical white matter. Various skeletal abnormalities: spine, iliac wings and limbs. Cartilage cells irregularly aligned at the zones of provisional calcification.

Prognosis. Death within first year.

BIBLIOGRAPHY. Taybi H, Linder D: Congenital familial dwarfism with cephaloskeletal dysplasia. Radiology 89:275–281, 1967
Kaufman RL: Dwarfism skeletal dysplasia and brain abnormalities. In Vinken PJ, Bruyn GW: Handbook of Clinical Neurology, vol 43, pp 385–386. Amsterdam, North-Holland, 1982
Lavollay B, Faure C, Filipe G, et al: Nanisme familial congenital avec dysplasie cephalo-skeletique (syndrome de Taybi-Linden). Arch Fran Pediatr 41:57–60, 1984

TAYLOR

Synonyms. Congestion fibrosis; dysmenorrhea, congestive; pelvic congestion; pelvic sympathetic.

Symptoms. Affects women of childbearing age. Onset of symptoms especially in premenstrual period. Menometrorrhagia; ill-defined pelvic pain; emotional lability.

Signs. Cervix: soft, bluish; excess of cervical mucus. Uterus; symmetric enlargement; pain on uterus examination. Congested painful breasts; frequently varicosities of legs.

Etiology. Diagnosis of exclusion once chronic inflammatory disease ruled out. Possibly a "stress disease," psychogenic in origin, manifested in women who (1) had insecure family life in childhood, (2) are unable to function adequately as women, (3) reveal signs of immaturity and dependency. May be a result of pregnancy and its excessive hormonal effects on the vessels of reproductive organs.

Pathology. Circulatory engorgement of pelvic viscera; slight boggy hypertrophy of uterus; telangiectasia and lymphectasia involving also the cervix. Varicosity of veins of broad ligaments; ovaries enlarged, soft, edematous.

Therapy. Reassurance and symptomatic treatment. Understanding that it may be treated by psychotherapy. Hysterectomy if severe pain and incapacitation.

Prognosis. Responding to treatment.

BIBLIOGRAPHY. Taylor HC Jr: Vascular congestion and hyperemia. Their effect on structure and function in the female reproductive system. Am J Obstet 57:211–230, 637–653, 654–668, 1949
Stearus HC, Sneeden VD: Observations on the clinical and pathologic aspects of the pelvic condition syndrome. Am J Obstet Gynec 94:718–732, 1966

TAY-SACHS

Synonyms. Amaurotic familial infantile idiocy; cerebromacular degeneration; ganglioside infantile lipoidosis; GM-2 gangliosidosis (type I). Hexosaminidase A deficiency.

Symptoms. Affects Jewish population 100 times more frequently than other ethnic groups. The sexes are equally affected. Onset between birth and 10 months (average 6 months) in apparently normal infants. Insidious progression of feeding difficulties, weakness, growth retardation, restlessness, to motor deterioration. Abnormal movements; convulsions; hyperacusis; visual difficulty. Variants with onset in juvenile and adult age usually have a chronic course.

Signs. Doll-like facies. Fine hair. Macrocephaly (after 16 months of life). Extremities spastic, hyperreflexic initially, then flaccid and paralyzed. Blindness. Fundus shows typical cherry-red spot in the macula.

Etiology. Autosomal recessive inheritance. Severe deficiency of hexosaminidase A. Mutations in the HEXA and HEXB genes result in many allelic conditions sharing main features but with different clinical history.

Pathology. Brain. Atrophic with ventricular dilatation (initially); marked atrophy and smaller ventricles (later). Consistency firm or leathery. Ballooning of ganglion cells. Astrocyte and microglia hypertrophic (foamy or fat granule cells). Myelin degeneration. Visceral organs. No evidence of pathologic changes, except for (occasionally) lipid inclusion.

Diagnostic Procedures. *Blood. Serum and leukocytes.* Assay of hexosaminidase (absence of hexosaminidase A). *Fibroblast culture.* Assay of hexosaminidase. *X-ray.* No significant changes. *Urine.* Absence of mucopolysaccharide.

Therapy. No specific therapy. Symptomatic and general intensive case.

Prognosis. Invariably fatal by the age of 3 or 4 years.

BIBLIOGRAPHY. Tay W: Symmetrical changes in the region of the yellow spot in each eye of an infant. Trans Ophthalmol Soc UK 1:55–57, 1881
Sachs B: On arrested cerebral development, with special reference to its cortical pathology. J Nerv Ment Dis 14:541–553, 1887
Neufeld EF: Natural history and inherited disorders of a lysosomal enzyme beta-hexosaminidase. J Biol Chem 264:10927–10930, 1989
Barnes D, Misra VP, Young EP, et al: An adult onset hexosaminidase: A deficiency syndrome with sensory neuropathy and internuclear ophthalmoplegia. J Neurol Neurosurg Psychiatr 54:1112–1113, 1991
Gravel RA, Clarke JTR, Kaback MM: The G m2 gangliosidoses. In Scriver CR, Beaudet AL, Sly WS, et al: The Metabolic and Molecular Bases of Inherited Disease, 7th ed, pp 2848–2849. New York, McGraw-Hill, 1995

TELFER

Synonym. Piebald—neurologic defect.

Symptoms and Signs. Both sexes. Piebald trait. Leukoderma of dorsal and ventral areas (involving in particular pubic hair, a white forelock, and variable patterns of forehead, trunk, arms, and legs). Cerebellar ataxia; mental (IQ 56–86) and physical development impaired; deafness (variable, sometime only in one ear, ranging from mild high frequency to profound). Fundus and irises normal.

Etiology. Autosomal dominant inheritance.

BIBLIOGRAPHY. Telfer MA, Sugar M, Jaeger EA, et al: Dominant piebald trait (white forelock and leukoderma) with neurological impairment. Am J Hum Genet 23:383–389, 1971
Finucane B, Scott CI Jr, Kurtz MB: Concurrence of dominant piebald trait and fragile X syndrome. Am J Hum Genet 48:815, 1991

TEMTAMY

Synonyms. Brachydactyly type A4; brachymesophalangy II and V.

Symptoms and Signs. Brachymesophalangy of second and fifth digits. Absence of middle phalanges of lateral four toes. Mild radial clino-

dactyly of fifth and fourth fingers. Feet: absence of middle phalanges of lateral four toes.

Etiology. Autosomal dominant inheritance.

BIBLIOGRAPHY. Jeanselme B, Joannon NI: Brachydactylie symmetrique familiale. Rev Anthrop 33:1–23, 1923
Temtamy SA, McKusick VA: The Genetics of Hand Malformation. New York, Alan R. Liss, 1978

TENNIS ELBOW

Synonyms. Golfer elbow; tennis elbow; epicondylitis; radiohumeral bursitis.

Symptoms. Pain in the elbow, at first, intermittent, then persistent. Radiating to forearm, occasionally to the hand. Stabs of pain cause weakness of hand and object dropping. Limited functions.

Signs. Tenderness on pressure over radiohumeral area of elbow; pain with resisted extension; no pain with flexion.

Pathology. Inflammatory signs in aponeurosis, bursa, periosteum. Fibrosis; tear of common extensor tendon in median epicondyle area.

Etiology. Strain of arm extensors, frequently associated with tennis (backhand).

Therapy. Massage; physical therapy; anti-inflammatory agents, or in severe cases, injection of hydrocortisone into tendon distal to epicondyle. Or surgery: section of orbicular ligament of radius and division of common extensor.

Prognosis. Tennis elbow with medical treatment, recovery in 12 months; golfer elbow, faster recovery.

BIBLIOGRAPHY. Wright PE: Shoulder and elbow injuries. In Crenshaw AH (ed): Campbell's Operative Orthopedics, 7th ed, p 2515. St Louis, CV Mosby, 1987
Weatherall DJ, Ledingham JGG, Warrell DA (eds): Oxford Textbook of Medicine, 3rd ed, p 2995. Oxford, Oxford Med Pub, 1996

TENNIS LEG

Synonym. Calf muscle rupture.

Symptoms. During strong exercise (tennis) audible snap in the leg, sudden intense pain in the calf that may extend to popliteal space, enhanced by passive dorsiflexion of ankle.

Signs. Marked tenderness on the calf; local discoloration.

Etiology. Sudden muscular contraction with rupture of one calf muscle during violent exercise.

Therapy. Strapping to immobilize ankle in plantar flexion; after weeks, massage and gradual exercises.

Prognosis. Several weeks before all symptoms subside.

BIBLIOGRAPHY. Weatherall DJ, Ledingham JGG, Warrell DA (eds): Oxford Textbook of Medicine, 3rd ed, p 2996. Oxford, Oxford Med Pub, 1996

TENSION-FATIGUE

Symptoms and Signs. Male to female ratio, approximately 1:3. Long-standing fluctuant or intermittent symptoms: vocal fatigue, reduction of voice quality, painful speaking, tension headache, and other musculoskeletal tension symptoms.

Etiology. Chronic stress and physical fatigue.

Diagnostic Procedures. *Laryngoscopy; frequency (pitch) analysis; waveform analysis; spectrography; laryngeal airway resistance.*

Therapy. Rest.

Prognosis. High percentage of good response to treatment.

BIBLIOGRAPHY. Koufman JA, Blalock PD: Functional voice disorders. Otolaryngol Clin N Am 24:1059–1073, 1991

TERRIEN

Synonyms. Marginal degeneration of Terrien; gutter dystrophy; peripheral furrow keratitis; senile marginal atrophy; Fuch marginal degeneration.

Symptoms and Signs. Onset at all ages (the youngest case described was age 9). Two-thirds were more than 40 years old. Acute onset of severe ocular pain, usually associated with conjunctival hyperemia, lacrimation, and photophobia. The attacks last 2 days to a week; the durations are consistent for each individual patient. The attack usually recurs, and can affect one eye or both.

Etiology. Unknown. The condition is believed to be degenerative in origin, with secondary inflammatory symptoms.

Pathology. Peripheral, fine, yellow punctate stromal opacities frequently associated with mild superficial corneal vascularization. Progressive thinning leads to peripheral gutter formation.

Diagnostic Procedure. *Slit-lamp examination.*

Therapy. None. Topical corticosteroids have not relieved the symptoms or halted the attacks.

Prognosis. Recurrent episodes can interfere with the patient's normal life. Vision can gradually deteriorate because of increasing corneal astigmatism.

BIBLIOGRAPHY. Duke-Elder S: Textbook of Ophthalmology, vol 8, p 909. London, Kingston, 1965
Austin P, Brown SI: Inflammatory Terrien's marginal corneal disease. Am J Ophthalmol 92:189–192, 1981
Robin JB, Schanzlin DJ, Verity SM: Peripheral corneal disorders. Surv Ophthalmol 31:1–36, 1986
Pouliquen Y, Renard G, Savoldelli M: Keratoconus associated with Terrien's marginal degeneration: A clinical and ultrastructural study. Acta Ophthalmol Suppl (Copenh.) 192:174–181, 1989

TERRIEN-VIEL

Synonyms. Posner-Schlossman; unilateral recurrent glaucoma; glaucomatocyclitic crisis.

Symptoms. Both sexes affected. Occurs in subjects presenting allergic diathesis. Periodic slight blurring of vision, and colored halos, without visual field losses. Occasionally, eye pain during episodes.

Signs. Possibly, heterochromia. Features of (usually) unilateral benign glaucoma: high intraocular pressure; enlarged pupil, anisocoria; trace of aqueous flare; chamber angle open; possible presence of keratitic precipitates.

Etiology. Unknown. Allergy, hypothalamic disturbances with neurosympathetic functional impairment considered.

Diagnostic Procedures. *Ophthalmoscopy. Tonometry. Gonioscopy. Allergy test.*

Therapy. Diuretics; topical treatment with antiinflammatory agents and antibiotics.

Prognosis. Crises last from few hours to few weeks.

BIBLIOGRAPHY. Terrien F, Viel P: De certaines glaucomes soi-disant primitifs. Bull Soc Fr Ophthalmol 42:349–368, 1929
Posner A, Schlossman A: Syndrome of unilateral recurrent attacks of glaucoma with cyclic symptoms. Arch Ophthalmol 39:517–535, 1948
Joseph J, Grierson I: Anterior segment changes in glaucoma. In Garner A, Klintworth GK (eds): Pathobiology of Ocular Disease: A Dynamic Approach, 2nd ed, p 450. New York, Marcel Dekker, 1994

TERRY

Synonyms. Prematurity retinopathy; retrolental fibroplasia.

Symptoms. Occurs in premature underweight infants who are exposed to atmosphere with increased oxygen content. Visual disturbances, up to blindness.

Signs. Pupillary light reflexes absent. Ophthalmoscopic examination shows bilateral opaque retrolental membrane. Vessels are dilated, tortuous, later obliterated. Ciliary body drawn anteriorly; ciliary process around dilated pupil; shallow anterior chamber.

Etiology. Immaturity and periods of retinal hyperoxia are considered to be major factors in the development of the syndrome. The syndrome can develop (in rare instances) in the premature or the full-term healthy infant who has received little or no oxygen therapy.

Pathology. Hemorrhages; retinal edema; proliferation of vascular retinal tissue and successive organization and substitution with fibrous tissue and contraction. Retinal detachment.

Therapy. Prevention by control of amount of oxygen given (the least concentration and for short periods). The biologic antioxidant tocopherol (vitamin E) is being studied as a means of protecting infants who are at risk for the syndrome (premature); preliminary studies suggest that use of tocopherol can be successful.

Prognosis. Blindness may result from this lesion. Before etiology was discovered 5 out of 25 premature infants developed this condition. Unfortunately this complication has not yet completely disappeared.

BIBLIOGRAPHY. Terry TL: Extreme prematurity and fibroblastic overgrowth of persistent vascular sheath behind each crystalline lens: Preliminary report. Am J Ophthalmol 25:203–204, 1942
Merritt JC, Sprague DH, Merritt WE, et al: Retrolental fibroplasia: A multifactional disease. Anesth Analg 60:109–111, 1981
Bachynski BN, Kincaid MC, Nussbaum J, Green WR: A hemorrhagic form of zone I retinopathy of prematurity. J Pediatr Ophthalmol Strabismus 26:56–60, 1989
Garner A: Vascular diseases. In Garner A, Sarks S, Sarks JP: Degenerative and related disorders of the retina and choroid. In Garner A, Klintworth GK (eds): Pathobiology of Ocular Disease: A Dynamic Approach, 2nd ed, pp 1684–1689. New York, Marcel Dekker, 1994

TERSON

Synonym. Subarachnoid hemorrhage; ocular hemorrhage.

Symptoms. Onset at all ages. Both sexes affected. Sudden loss of consciousness; reduced vision.

Signs. Weakness of extraocular muscles and, occasionally, uncoordinated gaze; anisocoria; intraocular hemorrhages; papilledema.

Etiology. Syndrome may be spontaneous, follow trauma or rupture of brain aneurysm. Subarachnoid hemorrhages are associated in 5% of cases with intraocular hemorrhages, in 6% of cases with papilledema.

Pathology. Subarachnoid hemorrhage; preretinal, peripapillary hemorrhages; papilledema; secondary hemorrhage in the optic nerve.

Diagnostic Procedures. *Cerebrospinal fluid.* Presence of red cells. *CT scan. Angiography.*

Therapy. Control of cerebral edema: osmotic diuretics, corticosteroids. Surgery for clipping of brain aneurysm; intensive care.

Prognosis. The association subarachnoid–intraocular hemorrhages: unfavorable prognosis. Death rate double that in single subarachnoid hemorrhage.

BIBLIOGRAPHY. Paton L: Ocular symptoms in subarachnoid hemorrhage. Trans Ophthalmol Soc UK 44:110–126, 1924

Tureen LL: Lesions of the fundus associated with brain hemorrhage. Arch Neurol Psychiatr 42:664–678, 1939

Castren GA: Pathogenesis and treatment of Terson's syndrome. Acta Ophthalmol 41:430–434, 1963

Fahmy JA: Vitreous hemorrhage in subarachnoid hemorrhage. Terson's syndrome. Report of a case with macular degeneration as a complication. Acta Ophthalmol 50:137–143, 1972

Albert DM, Jakobiec FA: Principles and Practice of Ophthalmology, pp 1030, 3420. Philadelphia, WB Saunders, 1994

TESTOTOXICOSIS, FAMILIAL

Synonyms. Precocious puberty, male limited; gonadotropin, independent sexual precocity.

Symptoms and Signs. Male. Sexual development at about 3 year of age, accelerated growth and development of secondary sexual characteristics. Spontaneous erections. Severe acne; aggressive behavior. Final: short stature (150–160 cm), normal size penis, small, soft testis, normal reproduction.

Etiology. Unknown. Sporadic and autosomal dominant inheritance (sisters normal), however, X-linked mutation cannot be excluded.

Pathology. Testis biopsy: Leydig cells: nuclear and cytoplasmic characteristics of fully differentiated normal cells. Adrenals normal.

Diagnostic Procedures. *Blood.* Testosterone level in the child at puberal to adult range; gonadotropins are in the normal range. Absence of suppressive effects of potent gonadotropin-releasing hormone analogs. *X-ray.* Of skeleton. Bone age superior.

Therapy. A combination of two androgen and estrogen synthesis blockading agents (spironolactone, testolactone) given for at least 6 months restores both normal growth rate and bone maturation and control acne, and mentioned symptoms. Ketaconazole (testosterone synthesis inibitor).

Prognosis. Good. Short stature if not treated; normal reproduction.

BIBLIOGRAPHY. Schedewie HK, Reiter EO, Beitins IZ, et al: Testicular Leydig cell hyperplasia as cause of familial sexual precocity. J Clin Endocrinol Metabol 52:271–278, 1981

Gondos B, Egli CA, Rosenthal SM, et al: Testicular changes in gonadotropin-independent familial male sexual precocity: Familial testotoxicosis. Arch Pathol Lab Med 109:990–995, 1985

Manasco PK, Girton ME, Diggs RL, et al: A novel testis-stimulating factor in familial male precocious puberty. N Engl J Med 324:227–231, 1991

Weatherall DJ, Ledingham JGG, Warrell DA (eds): Oxford Textbook of Medicine, 3rd ed, p 1702. Oxford, Oxford Med Pub, 1996

THALAMIC MEDIAL

Symptoms and Signs. Vegetative troubles (body temperature, cardiovascular, gastrointestinal, and respiratory) mental changes (mood changes, hallucinations, deficits of memory, confusion up to dementia).

Etiology and Pathology. Vascular, degenerative, or neoplastic origin.

BIBLIOGRAPHY. Martin JJ: Thalamic syndromes. In Vinken PJ, Bruyn GW: Handbook of Clinical Neurology, vol 2, pp 485–486. Amsterdam, North-Holland, 1969

THALASSEMIA SYNDROMES

Various classifications of these syndromes exist.

CLINICAL CLASSIFICATIONS

1. THALASSEMIA MINIMA

Synonym. Microcythemia minima.

Symptoms. Asymptomatic with barely detectable erythrocyte anomaly. See Silvestroni-Bianco.

2. β-THALASSEMIA MINOR

Synonym. Heterozygous β-thalassemia. See Rietti-Greppi-Micheli, also Jaksch-Hayem-Luzet.

Symptoms. Wide spectrum of symptoms and signs, all related to chronic moderate anemia; hemolysis and splenomegaly. Chronic ulcers in the legs may be observed.

Etiology. Heterozygous beta chain defects.

Pathology. Increased red cell production, medullary and occasionally extramedullary; secondary bone changes. Generalized hemochromatosis; splenomegaly.

Diagnostic Procedures. *Blood.* Hypochromic microcytic, moderate anemia; anisopoikilocytosis; schistocytosis; target cells; reticulocytosis; moderate hyperbilirubinemia; increased low osmotic resistance. *Bone marrow.* Erythroid hyperplasia. *X-ray.* Of skeleton. Osteoporosis. Hemoglobin electrophoresis. Increased A2 fraction, occasionally increased hemoglobin F.

Therapy. Symptomatic.

Prognosis. Variable, from normal life span to symptoms associated with chronic anemia.

3. THALASSEMIA INTERMEDIA

Symptoms. Intermediate between thalassemia minor and Cooley syndrome.

4. COOLEY SYNDROME

Synonyms. Beta-thalassemia (type I); erythroblastic anemia; thalassemia major; Mediterranean; homozygous β-thalassemia.

Symptoms and Signs. Both sexes affected. Clinical onset insidious at 3–6 months of age. Severe weakness; pallor; mongoloid facies; large head; oxycephaly; enlargement of abdomen; splenomegaly; hepatomegaly; stunted growth; jaundice; recurrent febrile episodes; cardiac dilatation; hemorrhagic manifestation.

Etiology. Homozygous beta chain defects. True homozygosity for one or another thalassemia gene or double heterozygosity for any two different β-thalassemia genes.

Pathology. Marked medullary and extramedullary erythropoiesis; hepatosplenomegaly; hematochromatosis. Bone changes secondary to the erythropoietic proliferation.

Diagnostic Procedures. *Blood.* Severe anemia. Marked anisopoikilocytosis, poor in pigment; target cells; marked distortion and deformation of cells; nucleated red cells with various degrees of immaturity. Marked reticulocytosis; osmotic fragility usually markedly decreased. Usually, leukocytosis with some immature forms; hyperbilirubinemia; serum iron high; iron-binding capacity markedly decreased or absent. *Urine.* Increased urobilinogen and urobilin; increased aminoaciduria. *Stool.* High coproporphyrin. *X-ray.* Of skeleton. Marked thickening of diploë of skull with perpendicular striations between thinned tables. Long bones, decreased density of medulla and thinning of cortex, mosaic pattern.

Therapy. Symptomatic; blood transfusion. Splenectomy moderately beneficial in some cases. Corticosteroids in some cases. Desferrioxamine plus vitamin C.

Prognosis. Very severe. Ultimately fatal in few months to years.

Biochemical Classification. Various classifications of these syndromes exist. We report one of the last classifications. For individual syndromes see clinical and hematologic classification under specific titles.

5. ALPHA-THALASSEMIA SYNDROMES

1. Heterozygous α-thalassemia 2 or "silent carrier" state (no symptoms)
2. Heterozygous α-thalassemia 1 or α-thalassemia trait (no symptoms)
3. HbH disease: double heterozygosity for α-thalassemia 1 + α-thalassemia 2 (see)
4. Hydrops fetalis with Hb Bart's: homozygous α-thalassemia 1
5. Hb Constant spring syndromes (see)
6. $\alpha + \beta$ thalassemia

6. BETA-THALASSEMIA SYNDROMES

1. Heterozygous β-thalassemia, β-thalassemia trait, or β-thalassemia minor (see).
    a. With elevated HbA$_2$ + elevated HbF
    b. With normal HbA$_2$ + elevated HbF: delta-thalassemia (δ-thalassemia) or F-thalassemia
    1. GγAγ($\delta\beta$) thalassemia
    2. Gγ(A$\gamma\delta\beta$) thalassemia
    c. With normal HbA$_2$ and HbF
    1. "Silent carrier" including Hb Knossos
    2. Concomitant $\delta + \beta$ thalassemia, in cis or trans
    3. $\gamma\delta\beta$-thalassemia
    4. Other: atypical $\delta\beta$-thalassemia; concomitant iron deficiency
    d. Hb Lepore trait
2. Homozygous β-thalassemia, Cooley anemia or β-thalassemia major (see Cooley)
    a. True homozygosity for one or another β-thalassemia gene
    b. Double heterozygosity for any two different β-thalassemia genes
3. β-thalassemia intermedia (see)

7. RARE FORMS OF THALASSEMIA

1. γ-thalassemia
2. δ-thalassemia
3. $\gamma\delta\beta$-thalassemia

8. INTERACTING THALASSEMIA

1. α-thalassemia + α-chain variant
    a. HbQ/α-thalassemia (like HbH disease)
    b. HbG/α-thalassemia (mild anemia)
2. α-thalassemia + β-chain variant
    a. Sickle/β-thalassemia (see sickle)
    b. HbC/β-thalassemia (mild anemia)
    c. HbE/β-thalassemia (like homozygous thalassemia)

9. HEREDITARY PERSISTENCE OF FETAL HEMOGLOBIN

1. Pancellular (no symptoms)
    a. G$\gamma^A\gamma$($\delta\beta$) HPFH
    b. Hb Kenya (G γ HPFH)
    c. Black G $\gamma\beta$-HPFH with high HbF
    d. Greek A γ-HPFH
    e. Chinese A γ-HPFH
2. Heterocellular (no symptoms)
    a. Swiss type G $\gamma^A\gamma$ HPFH
    b. British type Aγ-HPFH
    c. Other: Seattle type G$\gamma^A\gamma$-HPFH; Atlanta type-Black G$\gamma\beta$ + HPFH with low HbF; Saudi high HbF determinant

BIBLIOGRAPHY. Cooley TB, Lee P: Series of cases of splenomegaly in children with anemia and peculiar bone change. Trans Am Pediatr Soc 37:29, 1925

Marks PA: Thalassemia syndromes. Biochemical, genetic and clinical aspects. N Engl J Med 275:1363–1369, 1966

Bunn HF, Forget BG: Hemoglobin: Molecular Genetic and Clinical Aspects, pp 333–335. Philadelphia, WB Saunders, 1986

Lukens JN: The thalassemias and related disorders: Quantitative disorders of hemoglobin synthesis. In Lee GR, Bithel TC, Foerster J, et al (eds): Wintrobe's Clinical Hematology, 9th ed. Philadelphia, Lea & Febiger, 1993

THANATOPHORIC DWARFISM

Synonyms. Osteochondrodysplasia, lethal.

Symptoms and Signs. Male to female ratio, 2:1. Onset in fetal life. Feeble fetal activity and polyhydramnios. At birth, reduced length (40 cm average), shortened limbs. Head enlarged; small face; enlarged fontanelles; high forehead; frontal bossing; bulging eyes; saddle nose. Abdomen protuberant. Thorax narrow; short ribs. Absence of primitive reflexes. Marked hypotonia. Respiratory distress and cardiac failure.

Etiology. Unknown. Sporadic. Genetics still confused. Various possibilities of inheritance. Possibly various conditions reported under this heading. One variety associated with cloverleaf skull (possibly autosomal dominant) and one called Glasgow variant (possibly autosomal recessive) have been reported. Other variants include Torrance type, St Diego type, Luton (or Middlesex) type.

Pathology. Nodular masses epiphyseal cartilage; slanting of bony trabeculae of growth plates; fibrous band interposed between epiphyses and metaphyses. In brain, microgyria, absent corpus callosum, temporal lobe, and cerebellum disorganized. Extramedullary hematopoiesis.

Diagnostic Procedures. *X-ray.* Of spine. Short flattened vertebrae ("H configuration"); wide intervertebral disk of pelvis; squarish; reduced height; small sciatic notch; medial spurs. Of limbs. Marked bowing of femora.

Prognosis. Death usually within first 3 days of life.

BIBLIOGRAPHY. Maroteaux P, Laury M, Robert JM: Le nanisme thanatophore. Presse Med 75:2519–2522, 1967

Isaacson G, Blakemore KJ, Chervenak FA: Thanatophoric dysplasia with cloverleaf skull. Am J Dis Child 137:896–898, 1983

Andersen PE Jr: Prevalence of lethal osteochondrodysplasia in Denmark. Am J Med Genet 32:484–489, 1989

THANOS

Synonyms. Craniosynostosis; hyperostoses; epibulbar dermoids; linear verrocous epidermal nevus. See Proteus.

Symptoms and Signs. Both sexes. From fourth to seventh month. Craniosynostosis, facial asymmetry. Hypertelorism, epibulbar dermoids, nose broad strabismus, myopia, progressive visual impairment up to blindness. Mental deficiency. Linear verrocous epidermal nevi. Kyphoscoliosis. Limbs normal.

Etiology. Unknown. Sporadic. Not yet fully delineated syndrome.

Diagnostic Procedures. Progressive hyperstoses of skull. Hyperostoses in sites of minor bony traumas.

BIBLIOGRAPHY. Thanos C: Craniosynostosis, boni exostoses, epibulbar dermoids, epidermal nevus and slow development. Syndrome Ident 5:19–21, 1977

THIBIERGE-WEISSENBACH

This eponym is used to describe different diseases included in a spectrum that goes from progressive systemic sclerosis with calcinosis to the CRST syndrome (see).

BIBLIOGRAPHY. Thibierge G, Weissenbach RJ: Concrétions calcaires soucutanées et sclérodermie. Ann Dermatol Syph 2:129–155, 1911

Dellipiani AW, George M: Syndrome of sclerodactyly, calcinosis. Raynaud's phenomenon, and telangiectasia. Br Med J 4:334–345, 1967

Le Roy EC, Black C, Fleischmajer R, et al: Sclerodrema (systemic sclerosis) classification subsets and pathogenesis. J Rheumatol 15:202–295, 1988

THIEFFRY AND SORRELL-DEJERINE

Synonyms. Thieffry-Kohler; osteolysis hereditary; ostheolysis idiopathic multicentric; hyperhydroxyprolinemia—osteolysis; osteolysis hereditary—carpal bones—nephropathy.

Symptoms and Signs. Both sexes affected. Marfanoid appearance; frontal bossing; micrognathia; scoliosis; pes cavus; overlapping toes; plantar cysts. During childhood, onset of a progressive painless osteolysis beginning in the carpal and tarsal bones and spreading distally and proximally to other bones. Occasionally, osteolysis may be asymmetric. Hypertension and signs of renal failure.

Etiology. Sporadic and autosomal dominant cases reported. Still confused clinical entity (possibly a cluster of different disorders)

Diagnostic Procedures. *Blood.* Elevated hydroxyproline and alkaline phosphatase levels. *Urine.* Hydroxyproline.

BIBLIOGRAPHY. Thieffry S, Sorrell-Dejerine J: Forme spéciale d'ostéolysis essentielle héréditaire et familiale a stabilization spontanée, survenant dans l'énfance. Presse Méd 66:1858–1861, 1958

Kohler E, Babbitt D, Huizenga B, et al: Hereditary osteolysis. Radiology 108:99–105, 1973

Fryns JP: Osteolyse essentielle a debut carpien et tarsien. J Genet Hum 30(Suppl 5):423–428, 1982

Pai GS, MacPherson RI: Idiopathic multicentric osteolysis: Report of two cases and a review of the literature. Am J Med Genet 29:929–936, 1988

Shinohara O, Kubota C, Kimura M, et al: Essential osteolysis associated with nephropathy corneal opacity and pulmonary stenosis. Am J Med Genet 41:482–486, 1991

THIEMANN

Synonyms. Thiemann-Fleischer; phalangeal avascular necrosis; digital osteoarthropathy; metaphyseal dysplasia; epiphyseal tarda; MEDT IIIa. See also Multiple epiphyseal dysplasia syndromes and acroosteolysis.

Symptoms. Both sexes affected. Onset in infancy and up to 18 years of age. In finger joints, pain with limitation of movements.

Signs. Fusiform enlargement of proximal interphalangeal joints, especially of medial finger, less frequently of other digits. Later, possible digital shortening.

Etiology. Unknown. In some cases autosomal dominant inheritance proved; in others cases the recessive type suspected.

Pathology. Avascular osteolysis in epiphyseal-diaphyseal zone of digits.

Diagnostic Procedures. *X-ray.* Of hands and feet. Destruction of cartilages; lacunae of bone reabsorption; hazy outline; shortening of phalangeal epiphyses.

Therapy. Symptomatic.

Prognosis. Severe deformities. Spontaneous arrest after closure of epiphyses. Eventual regeneration of cartilage.

BIBLIOGRAPHY. Thiemann H: Juvenile Epiphysenstoerungen, idiopathische Erkrankung der Epiphysenknoepel der Fingerphalangen.

Fortschr Roengtenol 14:79–87, 1909–1910

Gewanter H, Baum J: Thiemann's disease. J Rheum 12:150–153, 1985

THIES-SCHWARZ

Synonym. Eruptive milia; milia eruptive.

Symptoms. Onset in adult life. Development of nodules without apparent reason.

Signs. Milia-like nodules on face and upper trunk, 1–5 mm, symmetric; some show a central black comedo.

Etiology. Unknown. Sporadic (original T–S). Possible autosomal dominant inheritance also reported.

Pathology. Deformed follicles joined by epitheliomal strands with dermis and epidermis. Occasionally, horn cysts. The affected follicles are enclosed in a sheath of connective tissue.

Diagnostic Procedure. *Biopsy.* Of skin.

Therapy. Comedo may be removed but will reform. Dermabrasion.

Prognosis. Some cases develop a trichoepithelioma-like tumor.

BIBLIOGRAPHY. Thies W, Schwarz E: Multiple eruptive milia. An organoid follicle hamartoma. Arch Klin Exp Dermatol 214:21–34, 1961

MacKie RM: Tumors of the skin appendages. In Burton JL, Cunlife WJ: Subcutaneous fat. In Champion RH, Burton JL, Ebling FJG (eds): Rook/Wilkinson/Ebling Textbook of Dermatology, 5th ed, p 1509. Oxford, Blackwell Scientific, 1992

THIRST DEFICIENCY SYNDROMES

Synonyms. Adipsic hypernatremia; hypodipsic hypernatremia; hypernatremia adipsic. Includes hypernatremia essential.

Symptoms and Signs. Patients never experience thirst, and if left to themselves do not drink. From minor forms where rarely develop life-threatening hyponatremia to forms where wide swings from hypernatremia to hyponatremia occur and a life-threatening situation may arise.

Etiology and Pathology. From a variety of pathological processes involving putative thirst receptors in the anterior circumventricular organs of hypothalamus or their neural connections: primary and secondary neoplastic conditions; vascular; granulomatous; or miscellaneous (trauma, cysts, hydrocephalus, etc.).

Diagnostic Procedures. *Vasopressin assay* and *blood* and *urine* sodium levels: variable disorders may be identified from normal osmoregulated AVP secretion with total absence of osmoregulated thirst; to variable reduction of AVP secretion in response to osmotic stimuli up to complete lack of response.

Therapy. Treatment of underlying cause if possible; adequate fluid intake.

Prognosis. Variable according to nature and degree of derangements.

BIBLIOGRAPHY. Baylis PH: Vasopressin and its neurophysin. In DeGroot LJ (ed): Endocrinology, 3rd ed, p 417. Philadelphia, WB Saunders, 1995

THOMAS

Symptoms and Signs. Occurs in subjects who underwent partial thyroidectomy. Association of clinical manifestations of hypothyroidism and Marie-Bamberg (see).

BIBLIOGRAPHY. Thomas HMJ: Acropachy. Secondary superiosteal new bone formation. Arch Intern Med 51:571–588, 1933

THOMPSON (A.H.)

Synonyms. Congenital optic atrophy. Eponym used to indicate a congenital type (autosomal dominant inheritance) of atrophy of optic nerve characterized by nystagmus and blindness.

BIBLIOGRAPHY. Thompson AH, Cashell GTW: A pedigree congenital optic atrophy entrancing sixteen affected cases in six generations. Proc R Soc Med 28:1415–1426, 1935

THOMSEN

Synonyms. Myotonia congenital dominant; myotonia dystrophica; DMC.

Symptoms. Prevalent in males; onset at birth or shortly after, or at puberty with sudden onset. Muscular hypertrophy, common, tendency to athletic habitus. After a period of rest, difficulty in relaxing muscles. Frequently limited to extremities only. Difficulty in initiating walking, then normal ambulation. Difficulty in releasing grip. Masticatory, laryngeal, and ocular muscles may also be affected. Emotions and cold enhance symptoms; warmth decreases them. Five varieties have been described: first, the Thomsen classic; the others with partial symptomatology to end in the fifth with isolated myotonia on percussion of the tongue.

Signs. Firm and solid muscle.

Etiology. Autosomal dominant inheritance. Gene defect probably of chloride channel gene: Chromosome 7 is imputated. Five varieties of dominant myotonia have been proposed with variable clinical expression.

Pathology. In muscles, increase of myofibril number and sarcoplasm. Sarcolemmal nuclei and also the connective interstitial tissue increased. Later stages, atrophic changes appear.

Diagnostic Procedures. *Biopsy.* Of muscle. *Electromyography.*

Therapy. Symptomatic; quinine; procainamide. Cortisone and chlorothiazide (to cause K+ depletion). Apparent benefit from antazoline and trimeprazine.

Prognosis. Cataracts, muscular wasting may develop, and other features of myotonic dystrophy, now considered identical disease.

BIBLIOGRAPHY. Thomsen J: Tonische Krämpfe in willkürlich beweglichen Muskeln in Folge von ererbter psychischer Disposition (Ataxia muscularis [?]). Arch Psychiatr Nervenkr 76:706–718, 1875–1876
Becker RE: Myotonia congenita and syndromes associated with myotonia. VIII, Top Hum Genet, Stuttgart, George Thieme, 1977
Hughes EF, Wilson J: Response to treatment with antistamines in a family with myotonia congenita. Lancet 337:28–30, 1991
Koch MC, Steinmeyer K, Lorenz C, et al: The skeletal muscle chloride channel in dominant and recessive human myotonia. Science 257:797–800, 1992
Weatherall DJ, Ledingham JGG, Warrell DA (eds): Oxford Textbook of Medicine, 3rd ed, p 4152. Oxford, Oxford Med Pub, 1996

THOMSEN (O.)

Synonyms. Polydactyly (preaxial IV). Polysyndactyly; preaxial polysyndactyly; syndactyly. See Greig syndrome.

Symptoms and Signs. Preaxial polydactyly of hands or feet more severe of variable grade.

Etiology. Autosomal dominant with variable expression.

Diagnostic Procedures. *X-ray.* Of hand. Dysplastic distal phalanges with a central hole (specific finding of this form).

BIBLIOGRAPHY. Thomsen O: Einige Eigentumlichkeiten der Erblichen Poly und Syndaktylie bei menschen. Acta Med Scand 65:609, 1927
Baraitner M, Winter RM, Brett EM: Greig cephalopolysyndactyly: Report of 13 individuals in three families. Clin Genet 24:257–265, 1983
Reynolds JF, Sommer A, Kelly TE: Preaxial polydactyly type 4: Variability in a large kindred. Clin Genet 25:267–272, 1984

THOMSON (M.S.)

Synonym. Atrophic heredofamilial dermatosis.

Symptoms and Signs. Skin changes identical to those observed in Rothmund (see). Cataracts were not reported in any of the cases described by Thomson.

Etiology. Unknown. Autosomal recessive trait. Likely represents a forme fruste of Rothmund.

BIBLIOGRAPHY. Thomson MS: A hitherto undescribed familial disease. Br J Dermatol 35:455–462, 1923
Silver HK: Rothmund-Thomson syndrome: An oculocutaneous disorder. Am J Dis Child 111:182–190, 1966
Gorlin RJ, Cohen MM Jr, Levin LS: Syndromes of Head and Neck, 3rd ed, p 488. New York, Oxford Univ Press, 1990

THORACIC OUTLET

Synonyms. Shoulder girdle compression; neurovascular shoulder compression. This eponym includes various syndromes previously described as separate entities that all share the same physiopathology and characteristics:

1. Naffziger or Adson; cervical rib-without cervical rib; Coote-Hanauld; Haven; Nonne II; scalenus anticus
2. Cervical rib or first thoracic rib, Rust
3. Falconer-Weddell. Costoclavicular; military posture
4. Wright; hyperabduction; subcoracoid-pectoralis minor
5. Low ligaments simulating cervical ribs

Symptoms. Usually in adult life after trauma to the shoulder (cervical rib), stretching of arm (cervical rib, Wright-Falconer-Weddell), pregnancy, military service (Falconer-Weddell described cases in soldiers carrying military packs) or not in relation to particular posture (Naffziger). More frequent in females (cervical rib), usually unilateral. Exercise increases pain, rest reduces it. Pain from neck to hand, usually on the ulnar side, or pain over deltoid extending to the arm, greatest at the elbow. Paresthesia, weakness of affected arm, occasionally hyperesthesia in painful areas, vasomotor alterations.

Signs. Edema, venous congestion of arm, pulse decreased particularly in fourth to fifth finger (Falconer-Weddell), Adson maneuver induces symptoms. Reflexes reduced or absent on affected arm. Tender point at scalenus anticus (Naffziger), supraclavicular bruit if axillary artery aneurysm, bony mass palpable in supraclavicular fossa (cervical rib).

Etiology. Compression of neurovascular bundle at thoracic outlet (first rib, clavicle, scalenus muscle) owing to various causes: cervical rib, muscular malformation (scalenus anticus, Naffziger), ligaments simulating scalenus anticus (Law's) forced hyperabduction with weight load (Falconer-Weddell, Wright). Some cases with familial incidence reported.

Pathology. Atrophy of muscles, neuritis, possible occurrence of aneurysm of axillary artery, or thrombosis of vein.

Diagnostic Procedures. *Adson test.* (Costoclavicular and hyperabduction maneuvers) Positive. *X-ray.* Shows supernumerary rib. *Electromyography. Arteriography.*

Therapy. In case of hyperabduction simple correction of posture is sufficient. In other cases surgery with resection of first thoracic rib, which is usually done by subaxillary approach (Roos technique).

Prognosis. Good with therapy.

BIBLIOGRAPHY. Hunauld FJ: Communication to the Royal Academy of Sciences in 1740. Amsterdam, 1744
Willshire: Supernumerary first rib. Lancet 2:633, 1860
Naffziger HC: The scalenus syndrome. Surg Gynecol Obstet 64:119–120, 1937
Murphy T: Brachial neuritis caused by pressure of first rib. Aust Med J 15:582–585, 1910
Law AA: Adventitious ligaments simulating cervical ribs. Ann Surg 72:497, 1920
Adson AW, Caffey IR: Cervical rib: A new method of approach for relief of symptoms by division of the scalenus anticus. Ann Surg 85:839–857, 1927
Haven H: Neurocirculatory scalenus anticus syndrome in the presence of developmental defect of the first rib. Yale J Biol Med 11:443–458, 1938–1939
Falconer MA, Weddell G: Costoclavicular compression of subclavian artery and vein: Relation to scalenus anticus syndrome. Lancet 2:539–543, 1943
Wright IS: The neurovascular syndrome produced by hyperabduction of the arms. Am Heart J 29:1–19, 1945
Thoracic outlet. In Vastamaeki M: Current Trends in Hand Surgery, pp 315–340. Netherlands, Excerpta Medica, 1995

THORN

Synonyms. Pseudo-Addison; renal tubular salt-wasting; salt-losing nephritis; aldosterone secretion, compensatory increase.

Symptoms. Prevalent in males. Onset at all ages; most often in young adulthood. Polyuria and nicturia present in 50% of cases before diagnosis. Thirty percent of patients had history of gastritis and prolonged intake of large amount of alkali. Salt-craving only in a few cases. During acute episodes: nausea; vomiting; anorexia; weakness; muscle cramps; fainting; mental confusion.

Signs. Increased skin pigmentation (bronzing); dehydration; blood pressure usually normal.

Etiology. Not a separate disease entity but a syndrome observed in chronic renal diseases. When salt intake falls below level of urinary salt loss.

Pathology. *Kidney.* Chronic pyelonephritis. *Adrenal.* Enlargement. *Parathyroid.* Hyperplasia. Occasional calcification of vessels and nephrolithiasis.

Diagnostic Procedures. *Urine.* Specific gravity fixed; albuminuria and altered tests of renal function. High urinary aldosterone; 17-ketosteroids normal or elevated. Lack of response to administration of desoxycorticosterone acetate (DOCA). *Blood.* Moderate to severe azotemia; acidosis; low serum sodium; serum potassium frequently elevated; occasional depression.

Therapy. A mixture of NaCl and NaHCO₃ in equal parts, 1–2 g two to three times daily with meals. Monitoring of serum sodium levels: with the progression of the disease, sodium restriction may become necessary.

Prognosis. Varies according to degree of renal impairment. With treatment, prompt relief of symptoms and survival of 20 more years in relative comfort. If no treatment, death may ensue following attack. With progression of renal pathology, loss of salt decreases and patient develops edema, hypotension, cardiac failure.

BIBLIOGRAPHY. Thorn GW, Koepf GF, Clinton M Jr: Renal failure simulating adrenocortical insufficiency. N Engl J Med 231:76–85, 1944
Hughes JM: Salt-losing nephritis: A case report and a review. Arch Intern Med 114:190–195, 1964
Ehrlich EN, Friedman AL, Shenker Y: Hormonal regulation of electro-
lyte and water metabolism. In De Groot LJ (ed): Endocrinology, 3rd ed, pp 1702–1703. Philadelphia, WB Saunders, 1995

THROMBOCYTOPATHIA, HEREDITARY

AUTOSOMAL DOMINANT

Includes: Thrombopathic thrombocytopenia; isolated thrombocytopenia; the association Thrombocytopenia, deafness, renal disease (see Alport, Epstein, Fechtner, etc.); Montreal platelet (giant platelets, see); pseudo von Willebrand disease; bis-albuminemia; gray platelet (see); Garcia (see); in various generalized disorders: i.e., May-Hegglin (see).

AUTOSOMAL RECESSIVE

Includes: Bernard-Soulier (see); hereditary thrombotic thrombocytopenic purpura; and as a feature of other disorders (Chediak-Steinbrink-Higashi, see); Fanconi (see) and variants; and various errors of metabolism.

X-LINKED RECESSIVE

Includes: Wiscott-Aldrich (see) and variants (see Vestermark-Vestermark); isolated thrombocytopenia; thrombocytopenia-increased IgA-renal disease; thrombocytopenia-platelets dysfunction-unbalanced globin chain synthesis (hemolysis).

BIBLIOGRAPHY. Bernheim J, Dechavanne M, Bryon PA, et al: Thrombocytopenia, macrothrombocytopathia, nephritis and deafness. Am J Med 61:145–150, 1976
Milton JC, Frojmovic MM: Shape-changing agents produce abnormally large platelets in a hereditary "giant platelet" syndrome (MPS). J Lab Clin Med 93:154–161, 1979
Aranda E, Dorandes S: Garcia's disease: Cyclic thrombocytopenic purpura in a child and abnormal platelet counts in his family. Scand J Haematol 18:39–46, 1977
High KA, Roberts HR: Molecular Basis of Thrombosis and Hemostasis. New York, Marcel Dekker, 1995

THROMBOCYTOPENIA, HYPERSPLENIC PRIMARY

Synonym. Primary hypersplenism; hypersplenism, primary.

Symptoms and Signs. Both sexes affected. Onset at all ages. Variable degree of hemorrhagic manifestations; splenomegaly.

Etiology. Unknown. Selective dysfunction of spleen with trapping and destruction of platelets (?). Often associated with other features of hypersplenism, anemia, neutropenia (see Doan-Wright). With time frequently the presence of an underlying disease may became evident: cirrhosis sarcidosis Hodgkin; felty, Gaucher, etc.

Therapy. Splenectomy.

Prognosis. Return to normal platelet value after splenectomy.

BIBLIOGRAPHY. Cooney DP, Smith BA: The pathophysiology of hypersplenic thrombocytopenia. Arch Intern Med 121:332–337, 1968
Bowdler AJ: Splenomegaly and hypersplenism. Clin Haematol 12:467–488, 1983
Bithell TC: Miscellaneous forms of thrombocytopenia. In Lee GR, Bithel TC, Foerster J, et al (eds): Wintrobe's Clinical Hematology, 9th ed, pp 1367–1368. Philadelphia, Lea & Febiger, 1993

THURMAN-HILLIER

Synonyms. Levoisomerism LV-RA communication; left ventricular to right atrial communication; right atrial from left ventricular communication.

Symptoms and Signs. Both sexes equally affected. Present at birth. Holosystolic murmur located over sternum or right sternal edge; apical or tricuspid midsystolic murmur occasionally present. On palpation, right ventricular impulse extremely prominent. Frequently present polysplenia

Etiology. Congenital cardiac defect.

Pathology. Communication between left ventricle and right atrium in the region of membranous septum inferior to the crista supraventricularis, in some cases below level of tricuspid annulus (Thurman) and in others above the insertion of septal leaflets of tricuspid valve.

Diagnostic Procedures. *ECG.* Peaked P-waves in right atrial enlargement. Possibly, atrial arrhythmias. Similar pattern with normal septal defect. *X-ray.* Bronchial tomogaphy. *CT scan.* Prominent pulmonary trunk; small aorta; large left ventricle; right ventricle and atrium extremely enlarged (ball-like shape in frontal position). *Echocardiography.* Two-dimensional echocardigraphy with Doppler color flow mapping.

Therapy. Medical management for intercurrent respiratory infections; prevention of bacterial endocarditis and failure. Surgery if indicated.

Prognosis. Fair.

BIBLIOGRAPHY. Thurman J: Aneurysms of the heart; with cases. Med Chir Trans Lond 21:187–265, 1838
Hillier T: Congenital malformation of the heart. Perforation of the septum ventriculorum, establishing a communication between the left ventricle and the right auricle. Trans Pathol Soc Lond 10:110, 1858–1859
Perloff JK: The Clinical Recognition of Congenital Heart Disease, 4th ed, pp 21–52. Philadelphia, WB Saunders, 1994

THURSTON

Synonyms. Oral–facial digital type V.

Symptoms and Signs. Both sexes. From birth. Median cleft of vermilion of upper lip. Post axial polydactyly (6 or 7) of hands and feet.

Etiology. Unknown.

BIBLIOGRAPHY. Thurston EO: A case of median hare-lip associated with other malformations. Lancet 996–997, 1909
Gopalakrishna A, Thatte RL: Median cleft lip associated with bimanual hexadactyly and bilateral accessory toes: Another case. Br J Plast Surg 35:354–355, 1982

THYGESON

Synonyms. Keratitis superficialis punctata; punctata superficial keratitis.

Symptoms and Signs. Small bilateral punctiform lesions spread on superficial layers of cornea; 20 or more in number, most common centrally in the papillary area. Corneal sensitivity may be reduced.

Etiology. Unknown. Viral origin suspected.

Pathology. Mild epithelial edema, infiltration with polymorphonucleates and later with lymphocytes.

Therapy. Topical instillation of steroids.

Prognosis. Recurrence every 3–4 years.

BIBLIOGRAPHY. Thygeson P: Superficial punctate keratitis. JAMA 144:1544–1549, 1950
Lemp MA, Chambers RW, Lundy J: Viral isolate in superficial punctate keratitis. Arch Ophthalmol 91:8–10, 1974
Easty DL, Williams C: Viral and rickettsial disease. In Garner A, Klint-

worth GK (eds): Pathobiology of Ocular Disease: A Dynamic Approach, 2nd ed, p 234. New York, Marcel Dekker, 1994

THYROTOXIC STORM, APATHETIC

Synonyms. Lahey II; Lahey apathetic form; apathetic hyperthyroidism; includes Zondek comatose form.

Symptoms and Signs. Occurs in hyperthyroidal patients. Extreme weakness and wasting; emotional apathy; otherwise generally oligosymptomatic except for normal or slight elevation of temperature and presence of other minor symptoms of hypothyroidism, that became evident only if searched for. Absence of delirium and agitation typical of thyrotoxic storm (see Waldenström II).

Etiology. See Waldenström II.

Therapy. Propanolol or similar. Adrenergic blocker agents useful.

BIBLIOGRAPHY. Lahey EH: The crisis of exophthalmic goiter. N Engl J Med 199:255–257, 1928
Toft AD (ed): Hyperthyroidism (Symposium). Clin Endocrinol Metab 14:(whole issue), 1985
McKenzie JM, Zakarija M: Hyperthyroidism. In De Groot LJ (ed): Endocrinology, 3rd ed, p 687. Philadelphia, WB Saunders, 1995

TIBIAL COMPARTMENT, ANTERIOR

Synonyms. March; March gangrene; tibial compartment anterior; pretibial.

Symptoms. Pain of muscles of anterior tibial region; sensory loss in foot and leg. Pretibial exercise pain in chronic states.

Signs. Redness, swelling, tenderness in anterior tibial region.

Etiology. Injury of muscle or overstraining causes compression of tibial arteries and lymphatics. Anterior tibial nerve lesion (?); spasm, or thrombosis or embolism of anterior tibial artery (?); accumulation of fluid in the anterior tibial compartment.

Pathology. Biopsy of muscle shows various degrees of necrosis. In chronic stage, possible tendonitis.

Therapy. Bed rest; analgesic; fasciotomy in refractory cases.

Prognosis. If fasciotomy performed in time, good recovery; if excessively delayed, irreversible changes and persistent neuromyopathy.

BIBLIOGRAPHY. Bhild CG: Noninfective gangrene following fractures of lower leg. Ann Surg 116:721–728, 1942
Dawson DM, Hallett M, Millender LH: Entrapment Neuropathies, 2nd ed. Boston, Little, Brown, 1990
Weatherall DJ, Ledingham JGG, Warrell DA (eds): Oxford Textbook of Medicine, 3rd ed, p 4159. Oxford, Oxford Med Pub, 1996

TIDAL PLATELET DYSGENESIS

Synonyms. Platelet tidal dysgenesis.

Symptoms and Signs. Hemorragic manifestations, alternated every 20–30 days with hypocoagulation phenomena.

Etiology. Unknown.

Diagnostic Procedures. *Blood.* Thrombocytopenia alternating with thrombocytosis. *Bone marrow.* Same sequence manifested by megakariocystic hypoplasia alternating with hyperplasia.

Therapy. None effective.

BIBLIOGRAPHY. Bernard J, Caen J: Purpura thrombopenique et megacaryocytopenic cycliques mensuels. Nouv Rev Fr Hemat 2:378, 1962

Engstrom K: Periodic thrombocytopenia or tidal platelet dysgenesis in a man. Scand J Haematol 3:290, 1966

Bithell TC: Miscellaneous forms of thrombocytopenia. In Lee GR, Bithel TC, Foerster J, et al (eds): Wintrobe's Clinical Hematology, 9th ed, p 1366. Philadelphia, Lea & Febiger, 1993

TIÈCHE-JADASSOHN

Synonyms. Jadassohn-Tièche; blue nevus; melanofibroma; chromatophoroma.

Symptoms. Both sexes affected. Female to male ratio, 2.5:1. Onset in infancy or adolescence.

Signs. On the face, forearms, hands, or thighs (less frequently on other areas), appearance of a solitary nevus, dark blue, round or oval, with sharp border, smooth and slightly raised.

Etiology. Unknown.

Pathology. Mixture of melanocytes, fibrous and collagen fibers, and dendritic, bipolar, and fusiform cells.

Therapy. Excision and plastic surgery (for cosmetic reasons).

Prognosis. Benign.

BIBLIOGRAPHY. Tièche M: Uber Melanome ("chromatophorome") der Haut. "Blaue Naevi." Virchows Arch 186:212–228, 1906

Jadassohn J: Dermatologie, p 429. Wien, 1938

MacKie, RM: Melanocytic naevi and malignant melanoma. In Champion RH, Burton JL, Ebling FJG (eds): Rook/Wilkinson/Ebling Textbook of Dermatology, 5th ed, pp 1538–1539. Oxford, Blackwell Scientific, 1992

TIETZE

Synonyms. Costal chondritis; chondropathia tuberosa; chondrocostal junction. See SAPHO.

Symptoms. Pain in one or more costal cartilages, enhanced by motion, coughing, sneezing; radiation to neck, shoulder, and arm.

Signs. Swelling of upper costal cartilage; tenderness and slight hyperemia of skin overlying fusiform swelling. Second rib most frequently affected.

Etiology. Unknown.

Pathology. Nonsuppurative inflammation of rib cartilage; perichondritis.

Diagnostic Procedures. *ECG.* To rule out cardiac conditions. *X-ray.* Of chest.

Therapy. Steroid infiltration when pain is severe.

Prognosis. Benign condition, lasting weeks or months; relapses possible.

BIBLIOGRAPHY. Tietze A: Ueber eine eigenartige Häufung von Fällen mit Dystrophie der Rippenknorpel. Berl Klin Wochenschr 58:829–831, 1921

Kayser HL: Tietze's syndrome: A review of literature. Am J Med 21:982–989, 1956

O'Rourke RA: Chest pain. In Schlant RC, Alexander RW: Hurst's The Heart, 8th ed, p 465. New York, McGraw-Hill, 1994

TILING-WERNICKE

Obsolete.

Synonyms. Old eponym used to denote ophthalmoplegia.

BIBLIOGRAPHY. Thurel R: Les syndromes pseudobulbaires. Thesis Paris, 1929

Bruyn GW, Gathier JC: The operculum syndrome. In Vinken PJ, Bruyn GW: Handbook of Clinical Neurology, vol 2, p 777. Amsterdam, North-Holland, 1969

TIXIER

Obsolete.

Synonyms. Childhood hemolytic anemia; Hutinel-Tixier. Acute fulminating hemolytic crisis in debilitated newborns.

BIBLIOGRAPHY. Hutinel VH: La pseudo-chlorose des nourrissons. Med Mod Paris 19:193, 1908

Tixier L: Les anémies infantiles. Pediatrie Prat (Lille) 10:526–535, 1912; 11:512–517, 1913

Tixier L: Les anémies. Paris, Flammarion, 1923

TODD POSTEPILEPTIC PARALYSIS

Synonym. Ictal and periictal mental. Includes post-epileptic furor; post-epileptic paranoid hallucinatory. A sequela of Jacksonian attacks, manifested by temporary weakness or paralysis of arm or leg, lasting a few hours or days.

BIBLIOGRAPHY. Todd RB: Clinical Lectures on Paralysis, 2nd ed. London, Churchill, 1856

Adams RD, Victor M: Principles of Neurology, 5th ed, p 285. New York, McGraw-Hill, 1993

Weatherall DJ, Ledingham JGG, Warrell DA (eds): Oxford Textbook of Medicine, 3rd ed, pp 4237–4238. Oxford, Oxford Med Pub, 1996

TODESERWARTUNG

Synonym. Death expectancy. See Survivor syndrome.

Symptoms. Occurs in residents of old-age homes. Hypochondriasis, hysteria, dependency, and impulsivity; varieties of somatic complaints purely functional or elaboration of existing deficit. Attitude of not getting involved with other residents; lack of communication between residents; loss of self-esteem; assumption of role of passive child and exploitation of the advantages deriving from it.

Etiology. Attitude assumed to repress thoughts of death and withdrawal from reality.

Therapy. Find ways to substitute meaningful social interaction and feeling of self-esteem and utility.

BIBLIOGRAPHY. Berman MI: The Todeserwartung syndrome. Geriatrics 21:187–192, 1966

McCann IL, Pearlman LA: Psychological trauma and the adult survivor: Theory, therapy and transformation. New York, Brunner-Mazel, 1990

TOGLIA

Synonym. Dysostosis Toglia.

Symptoms and Signs. *Skull.* Open suture. *Facies.* "Oldish"; deep-set eyes; flat nose; prognathism. *Limbs.* Spade-like hands and short fingers.

Etiology. Unknown. Familial occurrence. Single report. Unclassifiable.

BIBLIOGRAPHY. Toglia JU: Hereditary dysostosis. Tex J Med 62:23–41, 1966

Aita JA: Congenital Facial Anomalies with Neurological Defects. Springfield, IL, Charles C Thomas, 1969

TOLOSA-HUNT

Synonyms. Ophthalmoplegia dolorosa; painful ophthalmoplegia. See orbital apex.

Symptoms. Both sexes affected. Onset most frequent in fifth decade. Unilateral, steadily progressive retro-orbital pain. May also be of recurrent type (remission for months or years) of scintillating scotoma. Blurred vision up to complete blindness.

Signs. Paresis of oculomotor (III), trochlear (IV), abducens (VI), and first branch of trigeminal (V) nerves (may follow or be concomitant with manifestation of pain). Decrease of corneal sensitivity; decreased pupillary reaction or fixity. Absence of systemic signs.

Etiology. Various causes that result in inflammatory lesions of cavernous sinus.

Pathology. According to etiology. Inflammatory changes of cavernous sinus; no other structure involved.

Therapy. According to etiology. Corticosteroids for granulomatous lesions.

Prognosis. May last days or weeks. Spontaneous or therapeutic remission (residual neurologic defects possible). Recurrence in months or years.

BIBLIOGRAPHY. Tolosa E: Periarteritic lesions of carotid siphon with clinical features of carotid infraclinoidal aneurysm. J Neurol Neurosurg Psychiatr 17:300–302, 1954
Hunt WE, Meacher JN, Le Fever HE, et al: Painful ophthalmoplegia: Its relation to indolent inflammation of the cavernous sinus. Neurology 11:56–62, 1961
Spector R, Fiandaca M: The "sinister" Tolosa-Hunt syndrome. Neurology 36:198–203, 1986
Garner A, Klintworth GK: Tumors of the orbit, optic nerve and lacrimal sac. In Garner A, Klintworth GK (eds): Pathobiology of Ocular Disease: A Dynamic Approach, 2nd ed, p 1581. New York, Marcel Dekker, 1994

TOOTH-NAIL

Synonyms. Witkop tooth—nail; nails—teeth; hypodontia; nail dysgenesis.

Symptoms and Signs. Hypocalcified enamel hypoplasia to coniform crowns; onycholysis; nails spoon-shaped and slow growing; subungueal hyperkeratosis; fine slow growing hair.

Etiology. Autosomal dominant inheritance. Heterogeneity cannot be excluded.

BIBLIOGRAPHY. Weech AA: Hereditary ectodermal dysplasia (congenital ectodermal defect). Am J Dis Child 37:766–790, 1929
Witkop CJ Jr: Genetic diseases of the oral cavity. In Tiecke RW (ed): Oral Pathology. New York, McGraw-Hill, 1965
Ellis J, Dawber RPR: Ectodermal dysplasia: A family study. Clin Exp Dermatol 5:295–304, 1980

TORG

Synonyms. Osteolysis, hereditary, multicentric.

Symptoms and Signs. From birth. Fusiform enlargement of digits and contraction in flexion of knee, hip, and elbows.

Etiology. Autosomal recessive inheritance.

Diagnostic Procedures. X-ray. Osteoporosis, cortex thin, enlarged; tubular and long bones; collapse and resorption of carpal and tarsal bones.

BIBLIOGRAPHY. Torg JS, Di George AM, Kirpatick JA Jr, et al: Hereditary

multicentic osteolysis with recessive transmission: A new syndrome. J Pediatr 75:243–252, 1969

TORIELLO

Synonym. Brachial arch, X-linked.

Symptoms and Signs. Male; microcephaly, downslanting palpebral fissures, high palate, low-set ears, bilateral deafness, moderately webbed neck, short stature, mental retardation. Occasional cryptorchidism and subvalvular pulmonic stenosis.

Etiology. Autosomal X-linked inheritance.

Pathology. See Signs. Defects of brachial arch.

BIBLIOGRAPHY. Toriello HV, Higgins JV, Abrahamson J, et al: X-linked syndrome of brachial arch and other defects. Am J Med Genet 21:137–142, 1985

TORN ANTERIOR CRUCIATE LIGAMENT

Synonyms. Anterior cruciate ligament tear; knee anterior cruciate ligament tear; cruciate ligaments tear.

Symptoms and Signs. Usually occurs during athletic competition, following a deceleration twisting of the knee: "pop" from deep within the joint, preventing further activity and followed within hour by intense effusion.

Etiology. Trauma causing an isolated tear of the anterior cruciate ligament.

Diagnostic Procedures. Surgical exposure. Through enlarged anterior medial incision.

Therapy. Surgical repair.

Prognosis. If undiagnosed beyond 10 days lesion is rarely amenable to repair.

BIBLIOGRAPHY. Feagin JA: Jr: The syndrome of torn anterior cruciate ligament. Orthop Clin North Am 10:81–90, 1979
Insall JN, Windsor RE, Scott WN, et al (eds): Surgery of the Knee. New York, Churchill Livingstone, 1993

TORNWALDT

Synonyms. Nasopharyngitis chronica, pharyngeal bursitis.

Symptoms. Occipital headache; sensation of mucus accumulation back of the nose; expectoration.

Signs. Nasopharynx covered by mucopurulent material.

Etiology. Chronic inflammation of infected pharyngeal bursa or median recess extending to fauces and pharynx.

Pathology. Nasopharyngeal mucosa congested, with signs of chronic inflammation. Abscess of pharyngeal tonsils.

Diagnostic Procedures. Culture and antibiotic sensitivity of agents involved.

Therapy. Antibiotics; surgery occasionally indicated.

Prognosis. Prompt recovery with adequate treatment.

BIBLIOGRAPHY. Tornwaldt GL: Ueber die Bedeutung der Bursa pharyngea für die Erkennung und Behandlung gewisser Nasenrachenraum Krankheiten. Wiesbaden, Bergmann, 1885
James AE, MacMillan AS, MacMillan AS Jr, et al: Tornwaldt's cyst. Br J Radiol 41:902–904, 1968

Sabiston DC: Textbook of Surgery, 14th ed, pp 1619–1620. Philadelphia, WB Saunders, 1991

TORRE-MUIR

Synonyms. Muir-Torre; sebaceous tumors; keratoacanthomas; visceral malignancy.

Symptoms and Signs. Both sexes. Multiple sebaceous tumors (occasionally solitary, usually relatively indolent): adenoma, carcinoma, and epithelioma often in the same patient; different skin lesions including keratoacantoma. Internal malignancies affect gastrointestinal system, especially colon, only occasionally the urogenital tract. Malignancies may be multiple and arise in different locations.

Etiology. Autosomal dominant inheritance. It belongs to the cancer family syndrome.

Pathology. See Symptoms.

Therapy. Symptomatic: surgery, radiation, etc. Manifestations exacerbated by immunosuppression.

Prognosis. Low incidence of metastases. Survival often good.

BIBLIOGRAPHY. Muir GG, Bell AY, Barlow KA: Multiple primary carcinomata of the colon, duodenum and larynx associated with keratoacanthomata of the face. Br J Surg 54:191–195, 1967
Torre D: Multiple sebaceous tumors. Arch Dermat 98:549–551, 1968
Rothenberg J, Lambert WC, Vail JT, et al: The Muir-Torre (Torre's) syndrome: The significance of a solitary sebaceous tumor. J Am Acad Dermat 23:638–640, 1990
Weatherall DJ, Ledingham JGG, Warrell DA (eds): Oxford Textbook of Medicine, 3rd ed, p 3795. Oxford, Oxford Med Pub, 1996

TORTICOLLIS

Synonyms. Caput obstinatum; crooked neck; stiff neck; twisted neck. See also Spasmodic torticollis.

CONGENITAL

Symptoms and Signs. Onset in first months of life. Inclination of head and rotation of occiput. Palpation of exostosis on clavicle at point of insertion of sternocleidomastoid muscle; eyebrow of affected side slopes downward; face broadened and vertically shortened; cranial vault deformed.

Etiology. Many causes are responsible for this condition: (1) intrauterine theory; (2) birth trauma theory; (3) infections theory; (4) neurogenic theory; or as sequela of chronic encephalitis; (5) ischemic theory; (6) combinations of the preceding. Autosomal dominant and recessive inheritance described.

Pathology. *In early phase.* Vacuolization and degeneration of muscle fibers of lower half of sternocleidomastoid muscle. *Later.* Connective tissue replacement with normal muscle fiber left.

Therapy. Psychotherapy does not help. Supporting padded collar of some help. Tenotomy or in severe cases section of intraspinal portion of spinal accessory nerves and upper three or four anterior roots of spinal cord gives good results.

Prognosis. Good response to early treatment. Ten percent show involvement of other muscles of body; may become static or spontaneously regress.

ACQUIRED

Symptoms and Signs. Painful contraction of sternocleidomastoid muscle, with inclination and deviation of head.

Etiology. Infection, neoplastic, traumatic, psychogenic, paralytic factors.

Pathology, Therapy, and Prognosis. According to etiology.

BIBLIOGRAPHY. Taylor F: Induration of sternomastoid muscle. Trans Pathol Soc Lond 26:224–227, 1875
Lidge RT, Bechtol RC, Lambert CN: Congenital muscular torticollis; etiology and pathology. J Bone Joint Surg 39:1165–1182, 1957
Thompson F, McManus S, Colville J: Familial congenital muscular torticollis case report and review of literature. Clin Orthop Rel Res 202:193–196, 1986
Weatherall DJ, Ledingham JGG, Warrell DA (eds): Oxford Textbook of Medicine, 3rd ed, p 4018. Oxford, Oxford Med Pub, 1996

TOURAINE I

Eponym used to indicate the association of retinal angioid streaks and cardiovascular lesions. Today recognized as manifestation (or subsyndrome) of Groenblod-Strandberg-Touraine (see).

BIBLIOGRAPHY. Touraine MA: L'élastorrhexie systématisée. Bull Soc Fr Dermatol 47:255–273, 1940

TOURAINE III

Synonym. Purpura telangiectasica arciformis.

Symptoms and Signs. Variant of Majocchi (see). Fewer, larger arciform lesions.

BIBLIOGRAPHY. Touraine A: Le purpura annulaire télangiectasique de Majocchi et ses parentes (less capillarites ectasiantés). Presse Med 57:934–936, 1949

TOURAINE-SOLENTE-GOLÉ

Synonyms. Audry II; Brugsch (same condition plus acromicria); Friedreich-Erb-Arnold; Roy; Roy-Jutras; Hehlinger; acropachyderma; megalia cutis et osseum; primary hypertrophic osteoarthropathy; osteodermopathic; pachydermoperiostitis. See Cutis verticis gyrata syndrome.

Symptoms and Signs. Prevalent (almost exclusively) in males. Onset after puberty, up to third decade. Skin of forehead, face, scalp, hands, and feet becomes thick and furrowed. Hyperhidrosis of hands and feet; increased sebaceous secretion. Hands and feet become enormous; nails are watch crystal-like. Arms and legs appear cylindrical. Effusions of ankles, knees, and occasionally other joints. General health, mental status not affected.

Etiology. Unknown. Primary form autosomal dominant (?) inheritance with variable expressivity; sex influenced. Hypertrophic osteoarthropathy (secondary form) is a form closely related or identical (see Marie-Bamberg).

Pathology. *Bones.* Peripheral periostitis with diffuse irregular periosteal ossification (usually leg bones); in severe forms all bones may be involved (except cranium). *Skin.* Hypertrophy of connective tissue and epidermis.

Diagnostic Procedures. *X-ray.* Of skeleton and chest. *Biopsy.* Of skin. *Blood.* Low sodium. *Urine.* Normal sodium excretion.

Therapy. Symptomatic.

Prognosis. Progressing for 5–10 years, and then remaining stabilized for rest of life. Reduced activity capacity. Life expectancy normal.

BIBLIOGRAPHY. Friedreich M: Hyperostose des gesammten Skeletoes. Virchows Arch (Pathol Anat) 43:83–87, 1868
Audry C: Pachydermia occipitale vorticelée (cutis verticis gyrata). Ann Dermatol Syph 10:257–258, 1909

Labbe M, Renault P: Hypertrophic osteodermopathy. Bull Mem Soc Med Hop Paris 1:1065–1067, 1926

Touraine A, Solente G, Golé L: Un syndrome ostéodermopathique: La pachyderme plicaturée avec pachypériostose des extrémités. Presse Med 42:1820–1824, 1935

Brugsch HG: Acropachyderma with pachyperiostitis: Report of case. Arch Intern Med 68:687–700, 1941

Harper J: Genetics and genodermatoses. In Champion RH, Burton JL, Ebling FJG (eds): Rook/Wilkinson/Ebling Textbook of Dermatology, 5th ed, pp 362–363. Oxford, Blackwell Scientific, 1992

TOURNIQUET PARALYSIS

Synonym. Pressure paralysis.

Symptoms. Paralysis with hypotonia or atonia but no atrophy distal to application of tourniquet. No paresthesia after tourniquet is removed; real hyperalgesia.

Signs. Sensory examination shows loss of touch, light pressure sensations, vibration, and position sense while cold and warm sensations, pain, and pilomotor reflexes are preserved. Color and temperature of skin normal.

Etiology. Compression of nerves.

Pathology. Absence of neuroma at the point of injury.

Diagnostic Procedures. *Electric stimulation of nerves.* Block of conduction: in motor nerve lack of stimulation above and good response below the injury. Sensory fibers tingling sensation when stimulation is above the lesion and no tingling when stimulation is below lesion.

Therapy. None.

Prognosis. Good. Return to function in short time. When paralysis complete, impairment of motor and sensory function can last 3 months or longer.

BIBLIOGRAPHY. Duchenne de Boulogne GBA: De l'électrisation localisée et son Application à la Pathologie et à la Thérapeutique, 2nd ed. Paris, Bailière, 1861

Moldaver J: Tourniquet paralysis syndrome. Arch Surg 58:136–144, 1954

TOWNES-BROCKS

Synonyms. Anus imperforate—hand, foot, ear anomalies; deafness sensorineural—imperforate anus—hypoplastic thumbs. See VATER.

Symptoms and Signs. Both sexes. From birth. Anus imperforate; anomalies of hands (triphalangeal thumb and others) and feet (absent bones, supernumerary thumbs, fusion of metatarsal bones). Sensorineural deafness (mild), satyr ears. Possibly associated hypoplastic kidney, radial dysplasia.

Etiology. Autosomal dominant inheritance.

Pathology, Diagnostic Procedures, Therapy, and Prognosis. See Anus, imperforate; orthopedic and ORL consultation.

BIBLIOGRAPHY. Townes PL, Brocks E: Hereditary syndrome of imperforate anus with hand, foot and ear anomalies. J Pediatr 81:321–326, 1972

Aylsworth AS: The Townes-Brock syndrome: A member of the anus-hand-ear family of syndromes. Am J Hum Genet 37:A43, 1985

Konig R, Schick U, Fuchs S: Townes-Brocks syndrome. Eur J Pediatr 150:100–103, 1990

TOXIC MEGACOLON

Synonym. Megacolon toxic.

Symptoms and Signs. Systemic toxicity, fever, tachycardia, abdominal distention.

Etiology. Complication of idiopathic, ulcerative colitis, Crohn disease; observed also in intestinal infections (amebiasis, typhoid, cholera, etc.). Other contributing causes antibiotics; cathartics; opiates; anticholinergics.

Pathology. Mucosal denudation and inflammatory changes of submucosal strata.

Diagnostic Procedures. *Blood.* Leukocytosis. Frequently hypokalemia. *X-rays.* Dilatation of colon.

Therapy. Colon decompression (intestinal tube). Fluid and electrolytes balance. Cortical steroid (attention to K^+ depletion). Broad-spectrum antibiotics. Intensive therapy and eventually surgery.

Prognosis. Severe.

BIBLIOGRAPHY. Grant CSA, Dozois RR: Toxic megacolon: Ultimate fate of patients after successful medical managements. Am J Surg 147:106–110, 1984

Greenstein AJ: Surgical management and ultimate outcome. In Haubrich WS, Schaffner F, Berk JE (eds): Bockus Gastroenterology, 5th ed, vol 2, pp 1530–1531. Philadelphia, WB Saunders, 1995

TRANSIENT THYROTOXICOSIS

Synonym. Levi; silent thyroidiotis; includes postpartum thyroiditis. See Flajani.

Symptoms and Signs. Those of typical thyrotoxicosis (see Flajani) without tenderness of thyroid; significant ocular signs; or pretibial myxedema, that spontaneously regress within weeks or months (occasionally passing through a phase of hypothyroidism and of single or repeated relapses).

Etiology. Unknown. Could be considered a form of painless thyroiditis (?).

Pathology. *Biopsy.* Fibrosis (minimal) and lymphocyte infiltration, not typical for Hashimoto (see) or De Quervain (see) absence of granulomatous reaction.

Diagnostic Procedures. Antithyroglobulin and antimicrosomal antibodies: Presence not uncommon l.

BIBLIOGRAPHY. Taft AD (ed): Hyperthyroidism (Symposium). Clin Endocrinol Metab 14(2): (whole issue), 1985

McKenzie JM, Zakarija M: Hyperthyroidism. In De Groot LJ (ed): Endocrinology, 3rd ed, pp 677–678. Philadelphia, WB Saunders, 1995

TRANSPLANT LUNG

Symptoms and Signs. Occurs in patients after homotransplantation; onset follows a rejection crisis or decrease in dose of corticosteroids. Fever; at onset absence of malaise or fatigue. Symptoms and signs of diffuse bilateral pulmonary infiltrates, mostly at bases and hilus.

Etiology. Unknown. Immune mechanism (virus, fungi, infection [?]).

Pathology. Thickened alveolar membranes; features of infection (fungal, bacterial). Frequently observed, presence of cytomegalic inclusions.

Diagnostic Procedures. *X-ray.* Diffuse bilateral pulmonary infiltrates. *Pulmonary function tests.* Abnormalities consistent with alveolar-capillary block, demonstrable before clinical and x-ray findings. *Blood. Sputum.* To demonstrate virus or fungus.

Therapy. (1) Increase dose of corticosteroid or other immunosuppressing agents; (2) reduce hypoxia; (3) specific antibiotic treatment.

Prognosis. With prompt and adequate treatment, possibility of recovery high.

BIBLIOGRAPHY. Rifkind D, Starzl TE, Marchioro TL, et al: Transplantation pneumonia. JAMA 189:808–812, 1964

Slapak M, Lee HM, Hume DM: Transplant lung: A new syndrome. Br Med J 1:80–84, 1968

Fraser RS, Paré JAP, Fraser RG, Paré PD: Synopsis of Disease of the Chest, 2nd ed. Philadelphia, WB Saunders, 1994

TRANSSEXUALISM

Synonyms. Paranoia metamorphosis sexualis; psychopathia transsexualis; psychosexual inversion; "Scythes maladie des."

Symptoms. Prevalent in males (3–7 times). Intense desire for sexual transformation with procedures to accomplish a complete identification of the male with the female sex or vice versa, by surgical and hormonal means. Cooperation of the physician is sought to reach such transformation: castration, penectomy, and plastic construction of an artificial vagina or mastectomy and hysterectomy, and hormone administration.

Etiology. No organic or genetic etiology (as general rule). Some patients show some sexual underdevelopment. Psychological and sociological factors in early parent-child relationship play an important role in etiology, plus some unknown biologic factor (possibly). It may, in some cases, be considered a paranoid state.

Diagnostic Procedures. *Chromosome and hormone studies. Psychological evaluation.*

Therapy. Psychotherapy. In some cases, decision to operate and treat this patient to accomplish his aim is prompted by uncontrollable suicide or self-mutilation tendency.

Prognosis. Variable. Some individuals, once measures are taken, become deluded that metamorphosis has been accomplished, and that they really belong to different sex. Integrate if new role is not challenged. Many keep insisting on new operations to further transformation, such as ovary or uterus transplantation to become pregnant.

BIBLIOGRAPHY. Friedreich J: Versuch Einer Leterargeschichte der Pathologic und Therapie der psychischen Krankheiten. Wurzburg, 1830

Pauly IB: Male psychosexual inversion: Transsexualism. A review of 100 cases. Arch Gen Psychiatr 13:172–181, 1965

The physician's guide to sexual counseling (special issue). Med Aspects Hum Sex 20:(whole issue), 1986

Kaplan HI, Sadock BJ: Comprehensive Textbook of Psychiatry, 6th ed, pp 651, 1330, 1348. Baltimore, Williams & Wilkins, 1995

TRAUMATIC MYOSITIS OSSIFICANS

Synonyms. Calcified hematoma; myositis ossificans traumatica; myositis ossificans circumscripta; ossifying hematoma.

Symptoms. Both sexes affected. Onset at all ages. More frequent in young active persons with athletic habits or occupations requiring exertion and physical contact that may injure muscles. A particular type (myositis ossificans circumscripta) is determined by repeated minor traumas. From asymptomatic to painful mass and motion limitation becoming evident 1–4 weeks after traumatic event. Minor traumas type is responsible for minor motor limitation and discomfort.

Signs. Palpable mass at site of injury. Most frequent sites are quadriceps femoris, brachialis anticus.

Etiology. Unknown. Trauma of periosteum and displacement of osteoblasts into muscle: activation of osteoblasts, present metaplastic change.

Pathology. Hematoma followed by aseptic inflammation, proliferation of connective tissue, and formation of cartilage and bone island containing residual muscle fibers.

Therapy. Rest. Symptomatic. Surgery. Diphosphonate 5 mg/kg/day

orally for no more than 6 months to prevent and reduce swellings. Prednisone also can be tried.

Prognosis. Spontaneous regression possible

BIBLIOGRAPHY. Fay OJ: Traumatic periosteal bone and callus formation: The so-called traumatic ossifying myositis. Surg Gynecol Obstet 19:174–190, 1914

Weatherall DJ, Ledingham JGG, Warrell DA (eds): Oxford Textbook of Medicine, 3rd ed, p 3093. Oxford, Oxford Med Pub, 1996

TRAVELER DIARRHEA

Synonyms. Pharaoh curse.

Symptoms and Signs. Worldwide. It varies according to populations and regions visited. Warm, developing regions higher risk. Both sexes, more frequent in younger people who do not comply with the traditional recommendation, "boil it, cook it, peel it, or forget it." Bacterial pathogens (escherichia coli, shigella, salmonella, campylobacter, aeromonas, plesiomonas, etc.) viral agents, parasites, preformed toxins, or other dietary factors. Onset within first week of travel. Occurrence of three or more loose stool each day usually accompanied by abdominal cramping, fever, vomiting.

Etiology. Bacterial pathogens (escherichia coli, shigella, salmonella, campylobacter, aeromonas, plesiomonas, etc.) preformed toxins, or other dietary factors.

Diagnostic Procedures. *Stool.* Examination for infective agents. Only when needed.

Therapy. Antimicrobial prophylaxis (limited to time of administration). High fluid intake, antimicrobial agent specific or broad spectrum and loperamidum chloridrate 2 mg after each bowel movement.

Prognosis. Short duration, in 20% of cases 24 hours or less and in 60% 2–7 days.

BIBLIOGRAPHY. Okhuysen PC, Ericsson CD: Traveler's diarrhea: Prevention and treatment. Med Clin N Am 76:1357–1373, 1992

TREACHER-COLLINS

Synonyms. Collins. Treacher-Collins-Franceschetti; mandibulofacial. See Franceschetti, Pierre Robin, and Nager-Reynier.

Symptoms and Signs. Prevalent in Caucasians, but occurs in all major ethnic groups. Notching of lower eyelids with antimongoloid obliquity of palpebral fissures; flattening of malar bones. When associated with mandible defects, external ears defect, and deafness, it is more exactly called Franceschetti syndrome (see); when associated with micrognathia, glossoptosis, and cleft palate, Pierre Robin syndrome.

Etiology. See First arch syndrome(s). Autosomal dominant inheritance proposed. Changes observed are strikingly similar to those of vitamin A toxicity.

Pathology. Absence or hypoplasia of zygomatic arch.

Diagnostic Procedures. *Chromosomal studies.* Normal pattern. *X-ray. Ultrasonography.*

Therapy. Symptomatic.

Prognosis. In syndrome with only the classic signs, good.

BIBLIOGRAPHY. Berry GA: Note on congenital defect (coloboma) of lower lid. Lond Ophthalmol Hosp Rep 12:255–277, 1889

Collins E: Case with symmetrical congenital notches in outer part of each lower lid, and defective development of malar bones. Trans Ophthalmol Soc UK 20:190–192, 1900

Sulik KK, Johnston MC, Smiley SJ, et al: Mantidulofacial dysostosis

(Treacher Collins syndrome): A new proposal for its pathogenesis. Am J Med Genet 27:359–372, 1987

Jabs EW, Li X, Coss CA, et al: Mapping the Treacher Collins syndrome locus to 5q31.3–q33.3. Genomics 11:193–198, 1991

TREFT

Synonym. Optical atrophy—deafness—ophthalmoplegia—myopathy.

Symptoms and Signs. Visual loss by age 11, deafness by age 14. Myopathic changes, difficulty of balance. Ptosis of lids, ophthalmoplegia.

Etiology. Unknown. Autosomal dominant.

BIBLIOGRAPHY. Treft RL: Unique hereditary syndrome found, involves vision and hearing loss. Ophthalmol Times, July 12–13, 1983

TREVOR

Synonym. Trevor-Fairbank; Mouchet-Belot; dysplasia epiphysealis-hemimelia; hemimelic epiphyseal dysplasia; tarsomegaly; tarsoepiphyseal aclasis.

Symptoms and Signs. Occasionally manifested at birth, usual presentation 2–14 years. Male to female ratio, 3:1. With or without pain. Asymmetric excessive growth of one or several epiphyses of carpal and tarsal (more frequent) bones and less frequently than other ones. There may be painful flatfoot. Upper limbs rarely involved. Occasionally associated, chondromas and osteochondromas.

Etiology. Unknown. Sporadic cases and one family with possible autosomal dominant inheritance.

Pathology. Exostosis arising from epiphysis, apophysis, or round bones with cartilaginous cap.

Prognosis. Evolution stops after epiphyseal plate fusion.

BIBLIOGRAPHY. Mouchet A, Belot J: La tarsomegalie. J Radiol 10:289–293, 1926

Fairbank TJ: Dysplasia epiphysealis hemimelica (tarso-epiphyseal aclasis). J Bone Joint Surg 38:237, 1956

Trevor D: Tarsoepiphysealis aclasis: A congenital error of epiphyseal development. J Bone Joint Surg 32B:204–213, 1950

Sherlock DA, Benson MKD: Dysplasia epiphysealis hemimelica of the hip. Acta Orthop Scand 57:173–175, 1986

Rimoin DL, Lachman RS: Genetic disorders of the osseous skeleton. In Beithon P (ed): McKusick's Heritable Disorders of Connective Tissue, 5th ed, p 667. St Louis, CV Mosby, 1993

TRICEPS SURAE

Symptoms and Signs. This disorder may be simple or may represent a combination of several functional and anatomic disturbances of ambulation. Spasticity or actual shortening of gastrocnemius and soleus.

Etiology. Involvement of gastrocnemius and soleus, which form the triceps surae, in cerebral palsy patient with spasticity or with marked tension; associated with athetosis. It may also occur as compensatory in response to disturbance of other antigravity muscles, or be evidence of overflow mechanism initiated in other part of the body or extremities.

Therapy. Surgical correction: to decrease spasticity; eliminate clonus; restore functional or anatomic length; restore knee extension; correct pes planus or equinus; decrease overflow to or from the muscles by neurectomies; tendon lengthening, or transplant.

Prognosis. Surgery in well-evaluated patient may offer great advantages over conservative therapy.

BIBLIOGRAPHY. Baker LD: Triceps surae syndrome in cerebral palsy. Operation to aid its relief. Arch Surg 68:216–221, 1954

TRICHODENTO-OSSEOUS

Synonyms. Amelogenesis imperfecta—osteosclerosis; taurodontism—curly hair—osteosclerosis; TDO.

Synonyms. Both sexes affected. Present from birth. Asymptomatic.

Signs. *Hair.* Kinky, strikingly curly. *Nails.* Brittle; desquamating. *Head.* Frontal bossing, dolichocephaly; square jaw; small, spaced teeth, with deficient enamel and periapical abscesses. Teeth are lost in second or third decade.

Etiology. Autosomal dominant inheritance.

Diagnostic Procedures. *X-ray.* Of skeleton. Moderate increase of bone density; increased pulp chamber of teeth. Occasionally, partial craniosynostosis. *Blood.* Serum acid phosphatase increased.

Therapy. Care of teeth.

Prognosis. Good except for eventual teeth loss.

BIBLIOGRAPHY. Robinson GC, Miller JR, Worth HM: Hereditary enamel hypoplasia: Its association with characteristic hair structure. Pediatrics 37:489–502, 1966

Lichtenstein J, Warson R, Jorgenson R, et al: The tricho-dento-osseous (T.D.O.) syndrome. Am J Hum Genet 24:569–582, 1972

Shapiro SD, Quattromani FL, Jorgenson RJ, et al: Tricho-dento-osseous syndrome: Heterogeneity or clinical variability. Am J Med Genet 16:225–236, 1983

TRICHORHINOPHALANGEAL

Synonym. Giedion. See also Langer-Giedion.

Symptoms and Signs. Both sexes affected. Present from birth. Repeated respiratory infections. *Head.* Sparse hair (especially in frontotemporal zone), fine and brittle; eyebrows broad and medially narrowing; cilia scant; ears large; nose bulbous and flabby; philtrum prominent; upper lip thin; mild micrognathia; occasionally, oral malformations. *Skeleton.* Variable growth retardation; in middle childhood, fingers deform (swelling at proximal interphalangeal joints, clinobradydactyly). Thumbs and great toes short. Nails thin.

Etiology. Unknown. Both autosomal dominant and recessive inheritance reported; chromosome rearrangement also described.

Diagnostic Procedures. *Blood.* Hypoglycemia. *X-ray.* Typical cone-shaped epiphyses of fingers and toes. Scoliosis and lordosis in some cases. Bone age usually retarded.

Therapy. Symptomatic. Orthopedic and surgical correcting measures.

Prognosis. Hand deformation tends to arrest itself at puberty. Mental retardation, occasionally cerebrovascular accident.

BIBLIOGRAPHY. Klingmüller G: Ueber eigentümliche Kostitutionsanomalien der 2 Schwestern und ihre Beziehungen zu neneun entwicklungspathologischen Befunden. Hautarzt 7:105–113, 1956

Giedion A: Das Tricho-rhino-phalangeal syndrome. Helv Paediatr Acta 2:475–482, 1966

Sanchez JM, Labarta JD, De Negrotti TC, et al: Complex translocation in a boy with trichorhinophalangeal syndrome. J Med Genet 22:314–318, 1985

TRICUSPID ATRESIA

Symptoms. Both sexes affected. Male predominance. Extremely variable according to associated defects or lack of them. Retarded growth and development; from birth progressive cyanosis, after crying or feeding, hypoxic spells, dyspnea, lethargy, consciousness loss.

Signs. Underdevelopment; edema; clubbing. Pulse normal. On palpation, left ventricular impulse without right ventricular impulse. First and second heart sounds usually single. Absence of pulmonic ejection sound. Murmur absent or variable according to coexisting malformations. Prominent third sound (increased pulmonary blood flow and left failure).

Etiology. Congenital malformation.

Pathology. Atresic tricuspid valve; hypoplasia of right ventricle; interatrial communication; large left ventricle. Variable presence or absence of pulmonary blood flow; and origin and spatial relation of great arteries.

Diagnostic Procedures. *ECG.* Sinus rhythm; P-waves abnormal; PR interval normal or short, seldom prolonged; QRS axis left deviation. *X-ray.* Reduction of pulmonary vessels; aorta enlarged. *Heart.* Size normal (initially); absence of right ventricle; hypertrophy of left ventricle; apex elevated above diaphragm; various differences according to associated malformations. *Two-dimensional echocardiography with color flow imaging and spectral Doppler interrogation.* Hypoplastic right side of heart, no record of tricuspid valve. *Cardiac catheterization.*

Therapy. Surgery for palliation; repeated if symptoms return (see Prognosis).

Prognosis. Longevity according to adequacy of interatrial communication and pulmonary arteries flow. From death in first few months (60–75%) to (seldom) longer survival. Return of symptoms 5–10 years after intervention indicates need for second operation.

BIBLIOGRAPHY. Holmes WF: Case of malformation of the heart. Trans Med Chir Soc Edinb 1:252–259, 1824
Rashkind WJ: Tricuspid atresia: A historical review. Ped Cardiol 2:85, 1982
Perloff JK: The Clinical Recognition of Congenital Heart Disease, 4th ed, pp 614–634. Philadelphia, WB Saunders, 1994
Van Mierop LHS, Kutsche LM: Embryology of the heart. In Schlant RC, Alexander RW: Hurst's The Heart, 8th ed. New York, McGraw-Hill, 1994

TRICUSPID REGURGITATION–PROTEIN-LOSING ENTEROPATHY

Synonym. See Protein-losing gastroenteropathy.

Symptoms and Signs. Occurs in patients with tricuspid regurgitation secondary to rheumatic heart. Development of protein-losing enteropathy; edema.

Etiology. Suggested that elevated systemic venous pressure leads to congestion of bowel lymphatics and loss of lymph in gastrointestinal tract.

Diagnostic Procedures. *Blood.* Hypoproteinemia; lymphocytopenia. *Skin.* Anergy; inability to reject skin graft and other immunologic deficiencies. *X-ray.* Of chest. *ECG. Cardiac catheterization. Echocardiography.*

Therapy. Correction of venous hypertension.

Prognosis. Poor.

BIBLIOGRAPHY. Strober W, Cohen LS, Waldmann TA, et al: Tricuspid regurgitation: A newly recognized cause of protein-losing enteropathy, lymphocytopenia and immunologic deficiency. Am J Med 44:842–850, 1968
Golberg RL, Calleja GA: Protein-losing gastroenteropathy. In Haubrich WS, Schaffner F, Berk JE (eds): Bockus Gastroenterology, 5th ed, vol 2, p 1073. Philadelphia, WB Saunders, 1995

TRIGGER FINGER AND THUMBS

Symptoms. In children younger than 2 years or adults usually after age 45. Local tenderness (not prominent complaint) on the thumbs or one or more fingers (middle and ring more frequently).

Signs. Nodule or fusiform swelling on the flexor tendon that moves with tendon, causing a relative stenosis of the sheath (triggering) and snapping.

Etiology. Congenital, collagen diseases, rheumatoid arthritis.

Therapy. Congenital form usually resolves within first 2 years. In adult, sectioning of the proximal annulus.

BIBLIOGRAPHY. Fahey JJ, Bellinger JA: Trigger in adult and children. J Bone Joint Surg 36A:1200–1212, 1954

TRIGGER POINT

Used to designate any of the syndromes where a local area of tenderness exists, and the stimulation of such areas elicits the pain or symptoms of a referred area thus simulating many different conditions.

Therapy. Injection of procaine into trigger area leads to relief of pain in most instances.

TRIHYDROXYCOPROSTANIC ACIDEMIA

Synonym. Cholestasis intrahepatic; trihydroxycoprostanic acid. See Zelweger; Refsum; Adrenoleukodystrophy.

Symptoms and Signs. Neonatal jaundice.

Etiology. Autosomal recessive. Impaired transformation of trihydroxycoprostanic acid to cholic acid.

Diagnostic Procedures. *Bile.* Absence of primary bile acid, cholic acid, and presence of trihydroxycoprostanic acid.

BIBLIOGRAPHY. Eyssen H, Parmentier G, Campermolle F, et al: Trihydroxycoprostanic acid in the duodenal fluid of two children with intrahepatic bile duct anomalies. Biochim Biophys Acta 273:212–221, 1972
Setchell KDR, Street JM: Inborn errors of bile acid synthesis. Semin Liver Dis 7:85, 1987

TRILAMINAR MUSCLE FIBER MYOPATHY

Synonyms. Myopathy, trilaminar muscle fibers.

Symptoms and Signs. In infants. Marked rigidity, reduced spontaneous movements; hard muscles on palpation; sometime tremor, hypotonic muscles.

Pathology. Muscle: Trilaminar fibers with outer zone resembling sarcoplasmic masses, a middle zone of myofibrils and an inner zone of glycogen.

Diagnostic Procedures. *Muscle biopsy. EMG. Blood. CK.* Normal.

Therapy. None.

Prognosis. Death at an early age.

BIBLIOGRAPHY. Ringee SP, Neville Heduster MC, et al: A new congenital neuromuscolar disease with trilaminar muscle fibers. Neurology 28:282–289, 1978
Goebel HH, Lenard HG: Congenital myopathies. In Rowland LP, Di Mauro S (eds): Handbook of Clinical Neurology 18: The Myopathies, p 331. Amsterdam, Elsevier, 1992

TRIOSEPHOSPHATE ISOMERASE DEFICIENCY

Synonyms. Enzymopathic hemolytic anemia (TPI); TPI deficiency; anemia, hemolytic, enzymopathic.

Symptoms and Signs. Both sexes affected. Onset in infancy. Chronic hemolysis or hemolytic crisis. In homozygous, atypical progressive neurologic syndrome after first year of life (paraparesis, weakness, and hypotonia); splenomegaly; recurrent infections; possible sudden death.

Etiology. Deficiency of triosephosphate isomerase in red cells and leukocytes. Autosomal recessive inheritance.

Pathology. Not specific.

Diagnostic Procedures. *Blood.* Red cell and leukocyte deficiency of TPI. Slight macrocytosis; some red cells with fingerlike projection (acanthocytes). Hyperbilirubinemia. Autohemolysis almost completely corrected by glucose or ATP. A spot test that allows visual assessment of TPI activity useful for provisional diagnosis.

Therapy. Symptomatic. Occasional blood transfusions. Splenectomy of no benefit.

Prognosis. Poor. Unexplained death.

BIBLIOGRAPHY. Schneider AS, Valentine WN, Hattori M, et al: Hereditary hemolytic anemia with triosephosphate isomerase deficiency. N Engl J Med 272:229–235, 1965

Clay SA, Shore NA, Landing BH: Triosephosphate isomerase deficiency: A case report with neuropathological findings. Am J Dis Child 136:800–802, 1982

Rosa R, Prehu MO, Calvin MC, et al: Hereditary triosephosphate isomerase deficiency. Seven new homozygous cases. Hum Genet 71:235–240, 1985

Lukens JN: Hereditary hemolytic anemias associated with abnormalities of erythrocyte anaerobic glycolysis and nucleotide metabolism. In Lee GR, Bithell TC, Foerster J, et al (eds): Wintrobe's Clinical Hematology, 9th ed, p 997. Philadelphia, Lea & Febiger, 1993

TRIPLE X

Synonyms. Jacob (P.A.); superfemale; XXX.

Symptoms and Signs. Incidence 1:800 live female births. Low birth weight. Often asymptomatic and not associated with characteristic phenotype; but increased incidence of clinodactyly of fourth finger and epicanthal folds, ofter very tall; long legged. Occasionally, mental retardation (delayed language development and pitch problems); sometimes, menstrual irregularities, early menopause; microcephaly; hypertelorism; strabismus; abnormal dentition.

Etiology. Presence of an extra X chromosome, owing to nondisjunction. Frequently associated with autosomal trisomies. Single trisomy X may not be considered a characteristic syndrome.

Pathology. Presence of double chromatin bodies.

Therapy. Early diagnosis and language therapy, in adolescence therapy to prevent excessive tallness.

Prognosis. Majority of individuals exist unrecognized. Many have proved fertile, and some conceived children may be phenotypically and cytogenetically normal, or present aneuploidy.

BIBLIOGRAPHY. Jacobs PA, Baikie AG, Court-Brown WM, et al: Evidence for the existence of the human "superfemale." Lancet 2:423–425, 1959

Kohn G, Winter JSD, Mellman WJ: Trisomy X in three children. J Pediatr 72:248–252, 1968

Gorlin RJ, Cohen MM Jr, Levin LS: Syndromes of Head and Neck, p 63. New York, Oxford, 1990

TROCHANTERIC

Symptoms and Signs. Deep aching pain in the region of great trochanter, usually radiated to the thigh. Occasionally, radiation to the hip, and dorsolateral aspect of foot. In other instances, radiation to lower part of back, lower portion of abdomen, and medial portion of buttock.

Etiology. Trauma.

Diagnostic Procedures. *X-ray. Blood.* To assess lesions and evaluate any coexisting disease.

Therapy. Ultrasound therapy may aggravate the syndrome; infiltrations (procaine-hydrocortisone) usually relieve the symptoms.

Prognosis. According to etiology.

BIBLIOGRAPHY. Hays MB: Trochanteric syndrome. J Bone Joint Surg 45:657, 1963

TROELL-JUNET

Synonym. Acromegaly; goiter; skull hyperostosis; diabetes.

Symptoms and Signs. Reported only in females. Those of acromegaly, toxic goiter (usually nodular type), and Morgagni (see); diabetes mellitus also frequently associated.

Etiology. See multiple endocrine adenomatosis.

Pathology. Pituitary adenoma (eosinophilic, and in one case chromophobic). Nodular type of goiter. Acromegalic and Morgagni syndrome changes.

Diagnostic Procedures. *X-rays. Hormonal studies.* See Acromegaly.

Therapy. Removal of pituitary adenoma and symptomatic.

Prognosis. Poor.

BIBLIOGRAPHY. Troell A: "Syndroma morgagni" hos patienter med samtidig akromegali och tyreotoxikos. Seven Lak Tidn 35:763–771, 1938

Junet RM: Histopathologic du squelette acromegalique et ses modifications sous l'influence de l'hyperthroidisme. Geneva, Thèse No. 1681, 1938

Moore S: Troell-Junet syndrome. Acta Radiol 39:485–493, 1953

TROPICAL EOSINOPHILIA

Synonyms. Frimodt-Moller; Weingarten; Meyers-Kouvenaar; tropical eosinophilic lung; eosinophilia tropicale. See Eosinophilic lung, secondary.

Symptoms. Occurs in Near and Far East, primarily in Indians. May appear in persons of other races coming back from the Orient. Chronic productive cough, malaise, and wheezing, with spontaneous remissions and relapses.

Signs. In chest, bilateral rales localized to middle and basilar areas.

Etiology. An atypical host response to various filariae including Wuchereria bancrofti and Brugia malayi.

Pathology. Eosinophilic bronchopneumonia; histiocytic infiltration often associated with fibrosis; mixed cell exudate with eosinophils, lymphocytes; marked fibrosis.

Diagnostic Procedures. *Blood.* Eosinophilia. High titers of filarial antibodies: IgE levels more than 1000 U ml. *Sputum.* Eosinophils. *X-ray.* Of lung. Symmetric middle and basilar zone infiltrations.

Therapy. Diethylcarbamazine, preceded by antihistamines; corticosteroids. Ivermectin in repeated courses.

Prognosis. Chronic course; rapid improvement with treatment; some patients develop chronic pulmonary insufficiency and failure from development of pulmonary fibrosis. Not as benign as previously considered.

BIBLIOGRAPHY. Frimodt-Moller C, Barton RM: Pseudo-tuberculous condition associated with eosinophilia. Indian Med Gaz 75:607–613, 1940

Weingarten RJ: Tropical eosinophilia. Lancet 1:103–105, 1943

Udwadia FE: Tropical eosinophilia: A correlation of clinical, histopathologic and lung function studies. Dis Chest 52:531–538, 1967

Athens JW: Variation of leukocytes in disease. In Lee GR, Bithell TC,

Foerster J, et al (eds): Wintrobe's Clinical Hematology, 9th ed, p 1575. Philadelphia, Lea & Febiger, 1993

Weatherall DJ, Ledingham JGG, Warrell DA (eds): Oxford Textbook of Medicine, 3rd ed, p 2806. Oxford, Oxford Med Pub, 1996

TROPICAL SPASTIC PARAPARESIS

Synonyms. Cassava; ataxic neuropathy of Nigeria. See Lathyrism.

Symptoms and Signs. Relatively common in tropical climates. Sporadic or epidemic acute onset. Painful paresthesias followed by weakness of the legs, dysarthria; visual complaints or slowly progressing spastic weakness of legs.

Etiology. Variable agents considered: insufficiently detoxified Cassava (cyanide intoxication), Lathyrism infections (see), etc.

BIBLIOGRAPHY. Osuntokun BO, Bademosi O: Disease of peripheral nerves as seen in the Nigerian African. Afr J Med Sci 10:33–38, 1981

Adams RD, Victor M: Principles of Neurology, 5th ed, p 862. New York, McGraw-Hill, 1993

Weatherall DJ, Ledingham JGG, Warrell DA (eds): Oxford Textbook of Medicine, 3rd ed, pp 490, 3995. Oxford, Oxford Med Pub, 1996

TROPICAL SPLENOMEGALY

Synonyms. African macroglobulinemia; Bengal splenomegaly; cryptogenic splenomegaly; idiopathic splenomegaly; big spleen.

Symptoms. Found in tropical and subtropical regions with endemic malaria. Predominant in females. Asthenia; fatigue.

Signs. Marked splenomegaly.

Etiology. Unknown. Malaria considered a direct or indirect agent, but no conclusion reached. Abnormal immune response.

Pathology. In spleen different findings in different regions. In New Guinea, more sinus dilatation and less lymphatic proliferation than in cases in Africa. Reticuloendothelial biopsy shows lack of malarial pigment.

Diagnostic Procedures. *Blood.* Anemia a constant feature; search for malaria parasites negative, or few parasites. In Nigeria, peripheral blood and bone marrow lymphocytosis. In Uganda and New Guinea, absence of lymphocytosis. Increased concentration of IgM immunoglobulin in serum.

Therapy. Proguanil (also if malarial parasites are absent), lifelong treatment. Splenectomy not indicated because of risk of bacterial infections and fatal attacks of malaria, although in selected cases has been beneficial.

Prognosis. With proguanil, slow and progressive decrease in size of spleen and improvement of general health (over months). With cessation of treatment, full relapse in 3 months.

BIBLIOGRAPHY. Conferences and Meeting: Tropical splenomegaly syndrome. Br Med J 4:614, 1967

Athens JW: Disorders primarily involving the spleen. In Lee GR, Bithel TC, Foerster J, et al (eds): Wintrobe's Clinical Hematology, 9th ed, p 1710. Philadelphia, Lea & Febiger, 1993

Weatherall DJ, Ledingham JGG, Warrell DA (eds): Oxford Textbook of Medicine, 3rd ed, pp 857–858, 3591. Oxford, Oxford Med Pub, 1996

TROTTER

Synonyms. Morgagni sinus; peritubal.

Symptoms. Predominant in males. Onset from adolescence to old age. Deafness (first or early symptom), middle ear type; severe neurologic pain in the ear, side of head, lower jaw, side of tongue (third branch of trigeminal nerve); anesthesia of lower jaw (later symptoms) in the region of the mental foramen; defective mobility of soft palate, trismus (later stage).

Signs. (1) Fullness without ulceration in the lateral wall of nasopharynx (firm thickening) that eventually extends to adjacent muscles. (2) Asymmetry of soft palate (observed when it is relaxed). (3) Eustachian catheterization may produce bleeding, temporary relief of deafness. (4) Unilateral or bilateral cervical and retropharyngeal glands (frequently, first sign).

Etiology. Lateral nasopharyngeal lesion of neoplastic nature. Also occurring as development of the Jacod syndrome (for extension of an intracranial lesion) or of the pterygopalatine fossa syndrome. The Trotter syndrome may precede or follow the pterigopalatine syndrome, or occur in combination.

Pathology. Neoplastic lesion not invading the mucous membrane, spreading into sinus of Morgagni, and involving adjacent muscles. Cervical lymph nodes, liver, and skeleton metastasis.

Diagnostic Procedures. *X-ray.* Of skull. Involvement of foramen ovale. *Biopsy.*

Therapy. Deep X-ray therapy; surgery to reach lesion for radium implantation.

Prognosis. Very poor. Treatment only palliative.

BIBLIOGRAPHY. Trotter W: On certain clinically obscure malignant tumours of the nasopharyngeal wall. Br Med J 2:1057–1059, 1911

Asherson N: Trotter's syndrome and associated lesions. J Laryngol Otol 65:349–366, 1951

Bingas B: Tumors of the base of skull. In Vinken PJ, Bruyn GW (eds): Handbook of Clinical Neurology, vol 17, pp 136–233. Amsterdam, North-Holland, 1994

TROUSSEAU

Synonyms. Carcinogenic thrombophlebitis; thrombophlebitis migrans; recurrent thrombophlebitis.

Symptoms. Repeated episodes of pain extending over a period of months or years. Extremities most frequently affected areas.

Signs. Red, tender, raised, short cord-like nodules under the skin, usually disappearing with little or no residual damage before next lesions appear.

Etiology. Unknown. Frequent association with carcinoma (especially of the pancreas, lung, breast, colon, stomach). Possibly, release of thromboplastin-like substance from neoplasia.

Pathology. Segmental thrombosis of veins; infiltration of media and of adventitia; clot firmly attached.

Diagnostic Procedures. Search for hidden malignancy.

Therapy. No specific treatment necessary.

Prognosis. The thrombi disappear spontaneously. Low incidence of pulmonary thrombosis. In idiopathic form, disappearance of condition without treatment. If sign of malignancy, according to nature and degree of development of this lesion.

BIBLIOGRAPHY. Trousseau A: Lectures delivered in 1862

Thompson AV: Thrombosis of visceral veins in visceral cancer. Clin J 67:137–140, 1938

Sibrack LA, Gouterman IH: Cutaneous manifestations of pancreatic disease. Cutis 21:763–768, 1978

Rio B: Manifestations dématologiques des tumeurs malignes nonhematopoiétiques. Encyl Med Chir. Paris France Sang 13036 F 207, 1986

Malamani GD, Agata G, Grandi A, et al: Trombocitosi secondarie e reattive. Significato clinico-epidemiologico a proposito di 385 casi di osservazione personale. Rec Prog Med 79:15–18, 1988

Levine MN: Cancer patients. In Goldhaber SZ (ed): Prevention of Venous Thromboembolism. New York, Marcel Dekker, 1992

TROYER*

Synonyms. Spasting paraparesis (childhood); distal muscle wasting. See Struempell.

Symptoms and Signs. Amish group in Ohio. Onset in early childhood, dysarthria, distal muscle wasting, delayed and difficulties in walking becaming more severe up to inability to walk by 3–4 decades, occasionally drooling and cerebellar signs.

Etiology. Autosomal recessive inheritance.

Pathology. Thenar, hypotenar, and dorsal interosseous more affected muscles.

Prognosis. See Symptoms.

BIBLIOGRAPHY. Cross HE, McKusick VA: The Troyer syndrome: a recessive form of spastic paraplegia with distal muscle wasting. Arch Neurol 16:473–485, 1967

Neuhanser G, Wiffler C, Opits JM: Familial spastic paraplegia with distal muscle wasting in the Old Order Amish: atypical Troyer syndrome or new syndrome. Clin Genet 9:315–323, 1976

TRYPSINOGEN DEFICIENCY

Synonyms. Trypsin-1 included.

Symptoms and Signs. Present from birth. Severe growth failure; edema; pallor; hypochromotrichia. In an affected female associated imperforate anus

Etiology. Chromosomal defect location 7q32–qter. Autosomal recessive inheritance.

Diagnostic Procedures. *Blood.* Anemia; moderate reticulocytosis; severe neutropenia; severe hypoproteinemia; all protein fractions low. *Sweat.* Chloride test. Negative. *Urine.* Normal. *Duodenal aspirate.* Complete lack of trypsinogen.

Therapy. Protein hydrolysate.

Prognosis. Optimal response to treatment. Growth progresses regularly and all clinical and hematologic features disappear.

BIBLIOGRAPHY. Townes PL: Trypsinogen deficiency disease. J Pediatr 66:275–285, 1965

Townes PL, Bryson MF, Miller G: Further observations on trypsinogen deficiency disease: Report of a second case. J Pediatr 71:220–224, 1967

Emi M, Nakamura Y, Okawa M, et al: Cloning, characterization and nucleotide sequences of two cDNAs encoding human pancreatic trypsinogens Gene 41:305–310, 1986

Adibi SA: Protein digestion and absorption of its products. In Haubrich WS, Schaffner F, Berk JE (eds): Bockus Gastroenterology, 5th ed, vol 2, p 966. Philadelphia, WB Saunders, 1995

TUBERAL ARTERIES

Synonyms. See other thalamic syndromes.

Symptoms and Signs. Similar to other thalamic syndromes with fewer strictly thalamic symptoms. (See other thalamic syndromes.)

BIBLIOGRAPHY. Martin JJ: Thalamic syndromes. In Vinken PJ, Bruyn GW:

Handbook of Clinical Neurology, vol 2, p 486. Amsterdam, North-Holland, 1969

TUBULAR AGGREGATE MYOPATHY

Synonyms. Myopathy tubular aggregate.

Symptoms and Signs. Onset in childhood or adult life. Aspecific clinical features typical for congenital myopathies: cramps and myalgia on exertion.

Etiology. Autosomal dominant inheritance. It could be owing to an alteration of calcium permeability of muscle.

Pathology. Tubular aggregate: non specific inclusions chiefly in type II fibers; that react positively with WADH and negatively with MAG preparations, located in subsarcolemmal regions. The aggregates originate from sarcoplasmic reticulum.

Diagnostic Procedures. *Muscular biopsy.* EMG.

Therapy. Symptomatic.

Prognosis. Stable condition.

BIBLIOGRAPHY. De Groot JG, Arts WF: Familial myopathy with tubular aggregates. J Neurol 227:35–41, 1982

Pierobon-Bermioli S, Armani M, Ringel SP, et al: Familial neuromuscular diseases with tubular aggregates. Muscle Nerve 8:291–298, 1985

Goebel HH, Lenard HG: Congenital myopathies. In Rowland LP, Di Mauro S (eds): Handbook of Clinical Neurology, vol 18: Myopathies, p 331. Amsterdam, Elsevier, 1992

TUBULAR INSUFFICIENCY, ACUTE

Synonyms. Tubular necrosis acute, ATN; acute renal failure, ARF; kidney acute tubular necrosis; renal tubular acute insufficiency.

Symptoms. Oliguria of variable degree (50–75 ml/day to 1000 ml/day or more) and according to severity of syndrome; anorexia; nausea; vomiting; dry mouth.

Signs. Facies drawn; postural hypotension in 25% of cases; cardiac arrhythmias; seizures; lethargy up to coma.

Etiology. Assumption of nephrotoxins: antibiotics; various drugs; organic solvents; radiographic contrast materials; metals. Ischemia; hypovolemia; shock; hemolytic crisis or crush syndrome (see Bywaters).

Pathology. In acute phase, large edematous kidney. Histologically uniform pattern with diffuse lesions of various degrees of severity up to necrosis, but intact basement membrane or "Patchy pattern" with proximal and distal tubular cell involvement associated with disruption of basement membrane. Glomeruli usually normal in appearance.

Diagnostic Procedures. *Urine.* Specific gravity lower than 1.020; osmolality 280–320 mOsm/kg water; sodium in excess of 20 mEq/liter. Renal failure index greater than 2 or 3. Fractional excretion Na (FENA). Proteinuria, red cells, hemoglobin, casts according to etiology. *Blood.* Metabolic acidosis; increase in blood urea nitrogen (BUN) and creatinine, potassium phosphate; decrease in sodium, calcium, and carbon dioxide. *Electrocardiography.* Signs of hyperkalemia. In atypical cases consider renal biopsy and arteriography of renal and splanchnic vessels.

Therapy. Prophylaxis. Avoidance of use of (or prolonged therapy with) nephrotoxic agents; cure water balance when using radiographic contrast materials in particular pathologic conditions; rapid correction of hypovolemic conditions. Diuretics: mannitol, furosemide, and follow up with glucose-saline infusions; if they fail, establishment of fluid administration according to minimal balance and to provide caloric support (if gastrointestinal tract not usable). Dialysis. Antihypertensive agents. In diuretic phase follow water and electrolyte loss, and provide for caloric and plastic needs. Early diagnosis and treatment of infections.

---

*Family name of majority of patients.

Prognosis. According to determining causes. Post-traumatic 50–70% mortality; medical 25–30%. Nonoliguric cases 26%; oliguric cases 50%. Diffuse pattern: better prognosis than for patchy pattern. Recovery may be complete, or near normal renal function.

BIBLIOGRAPHY. Eliahou HE, Bata A: The diagnosis of acute renal failure Nephron 2:287–295, 1965
Brenner BN, Lazurus JM (eds): Acute Renal Failure. Philadelphia, WB Saunders, 1983
Meeks ACG, Sinus DG: Treatment of renal failure in neonates. Arch Dis Child 63:1372–1376, 1988
Elihou HE: Oliguria and anuria. In Massry SG, Glassock RJ: Textbook of Nephrology, 3rd ed, pp 543–546. Baltimore, Williams & Wilkins, 1995

TUBULOINTERSTITIAL IMMUNE COMPLEX

Synonyms. Antitubular basement membrane.

Symptoms and Signs. The characterizing element (see Pathology) generally is not an isolated finding.

Etiology. Seen in association with systemic lupus erythematoides, Sjoegren; mixed cryoglobulinemia, cutaneous vasculitis

Pathology. Immune complex and complement deposition along the tubulo basement membrane.

BIBLIOGRAPHY. Leheman DH, Wilson CB, Dixon FJ: Extraglomerular immunoglobulin deposits in human nephritis. Am J Med 58:765–786, 1975
Neilson EG: Pathogenesis and therapy of interstitial nephritis. Kidney Int 35:1257–1270, 1989

TUBULOINTERSTITIAL NEPHROPATHY

Synonyms. Interstitial nephritis; Tin; see also karyomegalic interstitial nephritis.

Symptoms and Signs. *Acute Form.* Rapid deterioration of renal function. *Chronic Form.* Frequently initially asymptomatic, then according to deterioration of renal function.

Etiology. *Acute.* Antibiotics; multiple myeloma; lymphoproliferative disorders; immunopathies; analgesics; metabolic disorders; infections sickle hemoglobinopathy; idiopathic. *Chronic.* Heavy metals immunopathies; myeloma; hypercalcemia, amyloidosis; granulomatous diseases; hemoglobinopathies; metabolic infections diabetes; transplanted kidney, idiopathic

Pathology. *Kidney.* Edema and inflammatory cells infiltration (mononuclear rather then polymorphic) of interstitium; absence of interstitial fibrosis and sparing of glomeruli and vessels, variable degree of tubular injury without atrophy; interest of basement membrane and basilar surface of cells; relative sparing of luminal side of cells.

Diagnostic Procedures. *Blood. Urine.* Variable patterns according to degree of involvement and progression of renal function. *Biopsy.* Diagnostic, see Pathology.

Therapy. That of associate condition and symptomatic for kidney failure. Trials with steroids.

Prognosis. Usually progression to end-stage kidney disease.

BIBLIOGRAPHY. Neilson EG: Pathogenesis and therapy of interstitial nephritis. Kidney Int 35:1257–1270, 1989

TUBULOINTERSTITIAL NEPHROPATHY, UVEITIS

Synonyms. T.I.N.U.; reno-ocular.

Symptoms and Signs. Those of tubulointerstitial nephropathy (see) with associated uveitis.

Etiology. Unknown

Therapy and Prognosis. Good response to brief course of steroid therapy.

BIBLIOGRAPHY. Eknoyan G: Tubulointerstitial nephropathies. In Massry SG, Glassock RJ: Textbook of Nephrology, 3rd ed, pp 752–760, 1040. Baltimore, Williams & Wilkins, 1995

TUCKER

Synonyms. Paget-like amyotrophic sclerosis. Pagetoid neuroskeletal.

Symptoms and Signs. Both sexes equal distribution. Onset insidious after 30 years of age. Weakness and then atrophy of muscles of legs and proximal part of arms. Progression to total motor incapacitation: tetraparesis and dementia. Respiratory insufficiency.

Etiology. Unknown. Possibly autosomal dominant inheritance

Pathology. *Bone.* Thickening and spotty sclerosis.

Diagnostic Procedures. *Blood.* Increased alkaline phosphatases. *X-ray.* Skeleton (see Pathology). *Nerve conduction studies.* Normal. *Electromyogram.* Muscle denervation. *Muscle biopsy.* Atrophy from muscle denervation.

Therapy. None.

Prognosis. Death at about age 60.

BIBLIOGRAPHY. Tucker WS Jr, Hubbard WH, Stricker JD, et al: A new familial disorder of combined lower motor neuron degeneration and skeletal disorganization. Trans Assoc Am Phys 95:126–134, 1982
Adams RD, Victor M: Principles of Neurology, 5th ed, p 994. New York, McGraw-Hill, 1993

TUFFLI-LAXOVA

Synonym. Ectodermal dysplasia adrenal cyst.

Symptoms and Signs. One case (male) reported: aplasia cutis verticis, hypohidrosis, nipple hypoplasia; onychodysplasia, delayed teeth eruption. Large adrenal cyst. Mother presented analogous features.

Etiology. Autosomal dominant inheritance.

BIBLIOGRAPHY. Tuffli GA, Laxova R: New autosomal dominant form of ectodermal dysplasia. Am J Med Genet 14:381–384, 1983

TUNBRIDGE-PALEY

Synonym. Optic atrophy—deafness—diabetes.

Symptoms and Signs. Onset in childhood. Primary optic atrophy and perceptive hearing loss in patients with juvenile diabetes mellitus.

Etiology. Unknown. Familiar. Frequent association with Friedreich, Refsum, Laurence-Moon-Biedel syndromes, dementia, and epilepsy.

Pathology. Optic atrophy, retinal pigmentation.

Therapy. None.

Prognosis. Poor.

BIBLIOGRAPHY. Tunbridge RE, Paley RG: Primary optic atrophy in diabetes mellitus. Diabetes 5:295–296, 1956
Ikkos DG: Association of juvenile diabetes mellitus, primary optic atrophy, and perceptive hearing loss in 3 sibs, with additional diabetes insipidus in one case. Acta Endocrinol 65:95–102, 1970

TUOMAALA-HAAPANEN

Synonym. Brachymetapody—anodontiasis—albinoidism.

Symptoms and Signs. Finnish family. Both sexes. *Facies.* Oxycephaly; alopecia; antimongoloid lid fissures; hypoplastic tarsus; nystagmus; strabismus; cataract; fovea hypoplasia; myopia; wide nose bridge; micrognatia; anodontia. *Limbs.* Short digits. *Skin.* Depigmentation.

Etiology. Unknown. Familial occurrence reported.

BIBLIOGRAPHY. Tuomaala P, Haapanen E: Three siblings with similar anomalies of the eyes, bones and skin. Acta Opthalmol 46:365–371, 1968

TURCOT

Synonyms. Turcot-Després-St. Pierre; colon polyposis—brain tumor—glioma polyposis. See Gardner.

Symptoms and Signs. Those of colon polyposis (see intestinal polyposis, familial) and central nervous system tumor. Skin. Café au lait spots.

Etiology. Autosomal recessive condition; only two cases (in brother and sister born from consanguineous marriage) reported.

Pathology. Polypoid adenomatosis of colon; medulloblastoma of spinal cord in one case; glioblastoma of frontal lobe in the other one. Various types of brain tumors reported.

Diagnostic Procedures. *X-rays. Intestine. Endoscopic examination. Cerebral CT scan. MRI.*

Prognosis. Poor.

BIBLIOGRAPHY. Turcot J, Després MP, St. Pierre F: Malignant tumors of central nervous system associated with familial polyposis of colon: Report of two cases. Dis Colon Rectum 2:465–468, 1959
McKusick VA: Genetic factors in intestinal polyposis. JAMA 182:271–277, 1962
Chowdhary VM, Boehme DH, Al-Jishi M: Turcot syndrome (glyoma-polyposis): Case report. J Neurosurg 63:804–807, 1985
Kropilak M, Jagelman DG, Fazio VW, et al: Brain tumors in familial adenomatous polyposis. Dis Colon Rectum 32:778–782, 1989
Weatherall DJ, Ledingham JGG, Warrell DA (eds): Oxford Textbook of Medicine, 3rd ed, p 1990. Oxford, Oxford Med Pub, 1996

TÜRK

See Duane.

Symptoms and Signs. Limitation of abduction of affected eye beyond midline; retraction of bulb on abduction.

Etiology. Birth injury (?). Considered incomplete Duane syndrome.

Pathology. Fibrous degeneration of external rectus muscle.

Therapy. Surgery to correct strabismus.

BIBLIOGRAPHY. Türk S: Ueber Retractionsbewegungen der Augen. Dtsch Med Wochenschr 22:199–201, 1896

TURNER

Synonyms. Bonnevie-Ullrich; Morgagni-Turner-Albright; Seresewski-Turner; Ulrich-Turner; ovarian dwarfism; genital dwarfism; gonadal dysgenesis (XO); monosomy X; pterygolymphangiectasia; XO.

Symptoms. Frequency 1/2500 live females. Wide spectum of clinical presentations. Female phenotype. Onset in childhood. Retardation of linear growth; primary amenorrhea; lack of development of secondary sex characteristic.

Signs. Short stature (105–130 cm). Lack of axillary hair and very scanty or absent pubic hair. Breasts underdeveloped. Lymphedema. Congenital abnormalities of various nature associated: webbed neck; cubitus valgus; ptosis; strabismus; nystagmus; cardiac abnormalities: coarctation of aorta (70%), or other cardiovascular lesions almost constantly affecting left heart. Lymphedema of extremities (30–40%). Occasionally, anomalies of bone development such as protuberance of sternum, high palate, underdeveloped mandible.

Etiology. Genetic abnormality owing to sex chromatin abnormalities. Karyotype generally XO (80%): lack of one of the sex chromosomes. In 20%, sex chromatin positive for various chromosomal abnormalities: XX (one chromosome abnormal); mosaicism XO (XX and even XO (XX) XXX). Familiar case rare.

Pathology. Absent, or rudimentary, gonads. Usually, absence of proliferation of epithelial layer. In some cases, germinal element of cortical (ovary) or medullary (testicular) origin may be found. The gonadal dysgenesis syndrome and its variants represent a continuum that ranges from typical pattern (see preceding) to normal male or female.

Diagnostic Procedures. *Sex chromatin study.* Chromosome determination. *Culposcopy. Blood. Urine.* Gonadodotropins, particularly FSH, elevated during infancy and after 10 years of age. GH levels lower from 8 years of age on; thyroid and adrenal hormones normal level.

Therapy. GH alone or in combination with oxandrolone or ethinylestradiol (or both) (no definitive conclusion on benefits on final growth from these treatments). Estrogen replacement either by continuous method or cyclic fashion. Therapy should be started as early as age 14 or 15 and should be continued as long as menstrual period continues. Malformation somatic or heart: surgical corrections.

Prognosis. Use of estrogen prevents premature aging and decreases incidence of cardiovascular and coronary artery diseases.

BIBLIOGRAPHY. Morgagni GB: Epistola Anatomica Medica, XLVII: Article 20, 1768
Ulrich O: Über typische Kombinationsbilder multiple Abartungen. Z Kinderheilkd 49:271–276, 1930
Turner HH: A syndrome of infantilism, congenital webbed neck and cubitus valgue. Endocrinology 23:566–574, 1938
Carothers AD, Frackiewicz A, De Mey R, et al: A collaborative study of the aetiology of Turner syndrome. Ann Hum Genet 43:355–368, 1980
Forest MG: Diagnosis and treatment of disorders of sexual development. In De Groot LJ: Endocrinology, 3rd ed, pp 1908–1910. Philadelphia, WB Saunders, 1995

TURNER-KIESER

Synonyms. Chatelain; Fong; Oesterreicher-Turner; Touraine II; arthro–osteo–onychodysplasia; iliac horns; HOOD (hereditary osteo-onycho–dysplasia); nail patella; osteo–onychodysostosis.

Symptoms. Usually not discovered until second or third decade; males and females equally affected. Usually asymptomatic or (in a few cases) weakness, difficulty in climbing stairs, dislocation of patella.

Signs. *Nails.* Large spectrum of symmetric abnormalities from anonychia to minimal longitudinal ridging, hypoplasia, thinness affecting all of patients. *Elbow.* Inability to extend fully, pronate, or supinate. Flexion usually normal; prominence of medial epicondyle (90%). *Knees.* Patellae usually smaller than normal or absent. Frequent dislocation; prominence of medial femoral condyles and decrease in the size of lateral femoral condyles (90%). *Pelvis.* Palpable iliac horns arising from central area of external iliac fossa, bilateral, symmetric (70%). *Eyes.* Anomalies of iris pigmentation (darker around inner margin; lighter at the periphery, 45%). Other abnormalities occasionally observed: anomalies of scapula; lumbar lordosis; clinodactyly; early arthritic joint changes.

Etiology. Unknown. Genetic defect, autosomal dominant (single gene?), variable expression with possible linkage with loci for determination of ABO blood group.

Pathology. Information fragmentary. In knee, absence of anterior cruciate ligament, osteoarthritic changes. In kidney, glomerulonephritis in different phases.

Diagnostic Procedures. *Urine.* Proteinuria (in about 40%); increased mucoproteins. *X-ray. Of elbow.* Prominence of medial epicondyle of humerus; dysplasia with or without luxation. *Of knee.* Hypoplasia of lateral femoral condyle and hypoplasia or absence of patella. *Of pelvis.* Iliac horns (pathognomonic).

Therapy. Symptomatic.

Prognosis. Very good.

BIBLIOGRAPHY. Little EM: Congenital absence or delayed development of patella. Lancet 2:781–784, 1897

Oesterreicher W: Nagel-und Skelettananomalien. Wien Klin Wochenschr 42:632, 1929

Turner JW: Hereditary arthrodysplasia associated with hereditary dystrophy of nails. JAMA 100:882–884, 1933

Kieser W: Die Sog. Flughaut beim ihre Bezieehung Zum Status dysraphicus und ihre Erbichkleit. Z Menschl Vererb 2:594–619, 1939

Fong EE "Iliac horns" (symmetrical bilateral cental, posterior ilac processes). Case Report Radiol 47:517–518, 1946

Taguchi T, Takebayashi S, Nishimura M, et al: Nephropathy of nail patella syndrome. Ultrastruct Pathol 12:175–183, 1988

TURPIN

Synonym. Bronchiectasis—megaesophagus—osteopathy.

Symptoms and Signs. Present from neonatal period. Repeated respiratory infections with chronic respiratory insuffiency, cough, and purulent sputum. Coughing on swallowing liquids.

Etiology. Congenital malformation.

Pathology. Association of bronchiectasis, megaesophagus, and osteopathy (vertebral and costal malformations). Frequently, tracheobronchial fistula.

Diagnostic Procedures. *X-ray.* Of lung, gastrointestinal tract, and skeleton. See Pathology.

Therapy. Surgery when indicated and feasible. Antibiotics.

Prognosis. Poor.

BIBLIOGRAPHY. Turpin R et al: Image claire, cervicale, traduction radiographique d'un mégaoesophagus groupment dysmorphique particulier. J Fr Med Chir Thor 3:436–439, 1949

TWIN-TO-TWIN TRANSFUSION

Synonyms. Neonatal arteriovenous transfusion; intrauterine parabiotic; see Pena-Shokier; TTS.

Symptoms and Signs. Incidence 3–5:1000 pregnancies. One of the twins (recipient) is bigger, polycythemic, hypervolemic. He shows increased cardiac size with myocardial hyperplasia and arterial hypertension, both systemic and pulmonary. The other twin (donor) is pale, with hypovolemia, undersized visceral organs. Disparity of body growth between the two twins. The recipient twin is usually associated with polyhydramnios. Two cases of the syndrome have been described in which the donor twin exhibited blueberry muffin-like macules and papules associated with cutaneous erythropoiesis (that is considered to be owing to persistence or reactivation of fetal dermal erythropoiesis secondary to prolonged, severe intrauterine anemia).

Etiology. Results from transfusion of blood from one fetus to the other; occurs only in monozygous twins. Various pathogenetic theories: donor pumps blood into recipient through third circulation; loss of proteins from donors into recipient changes osmotic pressure and cause fluid transfer over the placenta; increased atriopeptin in recipient; increased atriopeptin and decreased antidiuretic hormone in recipient; compression of donor placental vessels; compression of donor velamentous inserted cord; uteroplacental insufficiency affecting donor; growth stimuli of donor promotes growth of recipient.

Pathology. See Symptoms and Signs. The transfusion occurs via anastomotic channels between the two circulations. These channels are artery-to-artery, artery-to-vein, vein-to-vein.

Diagnostic Procedures. Examination of placenta on delivery. Suspicion if (1) hydramnios with twin pregnancy is noticed and (2) disparity of growth between two twins is observed. *Echography. Placentography.* With radioactive isotopes. *Skin biopsy.* Of blueberry muffin lesion.

Therapy. Blood transfusion to donor (undersized) twin. Removal of blood from recipient twin. Placental vascular laser surgery may improve perinatal outcome for monozygotic twins even further.

Prognosis. Increased perinatal mortality. Up to 70%; perinatal morbidity is also significantly high.

BIBLIOGRAPHY. Schotz F: Die Gefassverbindunger der Placenta kreislaufe eineuger Zwillinge, ihre Entwickelung und ihre Flogen. Arc Gur Gynaekol 30:335–381, 1887

Herlitz G: Zur Kenntnis der anaemischen und polyzytmischen Zustnde bei Neugeboren sowie des Icterus gravis neonatorum. Acta Paediatr 29:211–241, 1941

Lopriore E, Vandenbussche FPHA, Tiersma ESM, et al: Twin-to-twin transfusion syndrome: New perspectives. J Med Ped 127:675–680, 1995

TYLOSIS–ESOPHAGUS CARCINOMA

Synonym. Keratosis palmo; plantaris; esophagus carcinoma.

Symptoms and Signs. Both sexes affected. Onset between third and sixth decades. Keratosis of palms and soles; development of symptoms and signs of carcinoma of the esophagus.

Etiology. Unknown. Autosomal dominant inheritance.

Pathology. Hyperkeratosis of palms and soles. Squamous cell carcinoma of esophagus (usually lower third).

Diagnostic Procedures. *Esophagoscopy. X-ray. Biopsy.*

Therapy. Surgery if feasible.

Prognosis. Poor.

BIBLIOGRAPHY. Howel-Evans W, McConnell RB, Clarke CA, et al: Carcinoma of the esophagus with keratosis palmaris et plantaris (tylosis): A study of two families. Q J Med 27:413–429, 1958

Shine I, Allison PR: Carcinoma of the esophagus with tylosis (keratosis palmaris et plantaris). Lancet 1:951–953, 1966

Yesudian P, Premalatha S, Thambiah AS: Genetic tylosis with malignancy: A study of a South Indian pedigree. Br J Dermatol 102:597–600, 1980

Weatherall DJ, Ledingham JGG, Warrell DA (eds): Oxford Textbook of Medicine, 3rd ed, pp 202, 1981, 3723. Oxford, Oxford Med Pub, 1996

TYLOSIS–OPTIC ATROPHY

Symptoms and Signs. Prevalent in females. Thickening of skin of palms and soles (tylosis), occasionally of the ears as well. Development of optical atrophy late in life.

Etiology. Unknown. Possibly, sex-linked dominant inheritance.

BIBLIOGRAPHY. Dimsdale H: Hereditary optic atrophy in family with keratodermia palmaris et plantaris (tylosis). Proc R Soc Med 42:796, 1949

TYPHLITIS

Synonyms. Cecitis; necrotizing colitis; neutropenic enterocolitis; ileocecal neutropenic enterocolitis, acute.

Symptoms and Signs. In neutropenic patients. In leukemia, during induction therapy, remission, or relapse; in chemotherapy; in aplastic anemia; immunosupression after organ transplantation; in cyclic neutropenia. Fever, abdominal pain, distension, lower intestinal bleeding. Presence of tender palpable mass in the right side of abdomen.

Etiology. Neutropenia, spontaneous or induced by chemotherapy and cortisone, decrease host resistance to bacteria causing inflammation and infarction of cecum from selected intestinal flora.

Pathology. Edematous dusky cecum, cloudy peritoneal fluid; mucosal ulceration and necrosis of affected section of bowel.

Diagnostic Procedures. *Plain abdominal film.* Fluid-filled cecum, dilatation of small bowel. In some cases pneumatosis intestinalis. *Ultrasonography.* Fluid-filled cecum. *Barium enema.* Atonic, spastic, distorted cecum.

Therapy. *Medical.* Bowel rest, nasogastric suction, total parenteral nutrition, antibiotics, antifungines, transfusion. *Surgical.* Right hemicolectomy with anastomosis or ileostomy. In relapsing cases prophylactic hemicolectomy is advised.

Prognosis. A function of recovery of an adequate neutrophil level.

BIBLIOGRAPHY. Wagner ML, Rosenberg HS, Fernback DJ, et al: Typhlitis: A complication of leukemia in childhood. AJR 109:341–350, 1970
Katz JA, Wagner ML, Gresik MV, et al: Typhlitis: An 18 year experience and postmortem review. Cancer 65:1041–1047, 1990
Kuster GGR: The appendix. In Haubrich WS, Schaffner F, Berk JE (eds): Bockus Gastroenterology, 5th ed, pp 1804–1805. Philadelphia, WB Saunders, 1995

TYROSINEMIA, NEONATAL

Symptoms and Signs. Occurs usually in premature infants. Apparently asymptomatic and harmless.

Etiology. Temporarily delayed development of enzymes necessary to metabolize tyrosine. Combination of pHp–pD immaturity, elevated dietary phenylalanine, and tyrosine intake and ascorbate deficiency. The importance of this syndrome is in relation to differential diagnosis with the hereditary tyrosinemia-tyrosiluria syndromes.

Pathology. None.

Diagnostic Procedures. *Plasma. Urine.* High tyrosine level.

Therapy. Vitamin C and dietary proteins restriction.

Prognosis. Good. Adverse effect on development not eliminated in all cases. Metabolic defect disappears with treatment or spontaneously.

BIBLIOGRAPHY. Avery ME, Clow CL, Menkes JH, et al: Transient tyrosinemia of the newborn: Dietary and clinical aspects. Pediatrics 39:378–384, 1967
Mitchell GA, Lambert M, Tanguay RM: Hypertyrosinemia. In Scriver CR, Beaudet AL, Sly WS, et al: The Metabolic and Molecular Bases of Inherited Disease, 7th ed, p 1077. New York, McGraw-Hill, 1995

TYROSINEMIA–TYROSILURIA, HEREDITARY SYNDROMES

TYROSINEMIA TYPE I OR TYROSINOSIS

Synonyms. Tyrosiluria; hepatorenal tyrosinemia; fumaryl acetoacetase deficiency.

Symptoms. Prevalence in French Canadian population of Quebec. Both sexes affected. Normal at birth; onset at 2–8 weeks of age. Initial presentation following infection or catabolic stress: fever, lethargy, irritability, drowsiness, anorexia, vomiting, diarrhea, epistaxia, hematemesis, acute episode of peripheral neuropathy (painful crises). Chronic form cirrhosis and high risk of hepatic hepatocellular carcinoma (37% in patient older than 2 years, overestimated [?]).

Signs. Peculiar (cabbage) urine odor; jaundice; hematuria; melena; ecchymosis; abdominal distention; hepatosplenomegaly; paralytic crises; edema; autonomic signs (hypertension tachycardia, ileus). From mild tubular dysfunction to overt renal failure. Occasionally hypertrophic cardiomyopathy.

Etiology. Deficiency of fumaril acetoacetate (FAA) hydrolase.

Pathology. Generalized edema and hemorrhages. *Liver.* Degenerative changes; vacuolization. *Kidney.* Interstitial edema; marked renal tubular dilatation. *Pancreas.* Islet cell hyperplasia.

Diagnostic Procedures. *Blood.* Anemia; high reticulocytes; leukocytosis; thrombocytopenia; prothrombin deficiency; partial thromboplastin generation prolonged. Bilirubin high; alkaline phosphatase high; esterified cholesterol low; sulfobromophthalein abnormal; total protein low; glucose low. Tyrosine increased; other amino acids in normal range. *Urine.* High excretion of tyrosine and methionine.

Therapy. Diet with low tyrosine and phenylalanine. High doses of vitamin C. Liver transplantation. Promising new therapeutical agent: 2-(2-nitro-4-trifluoromethylbenzoyl)-1-3-cycloexanedione (NTBC).

Prognosis. Poor. Death in months frequently from respiratory insufficiency. If patients survive, they develop Baber syndrome.

BABER SYNDROME

Symptoms and Signs. Occurs in patients initially presenting the chronic form or survivors of the acute form. Same as the preceding, but with reduced intensity. Failure to thrive and dwarfism. Rickets.

Etiology. Considered a variant in the evolution of the preceding, or hepatic dysfunction of unknown origin.

Pathology. *Liver.* Firmer than normal; nodular cirrhosis; various degree of fibrosis; inflammatory (lymphomono) infiltration; bile stasis. *Kidney.* Edema; marked tubular dilatation; foci of calcium deposits. *Pancreas.* Hyperplasia of Langerhans islets (50%).

Diagnostic Procedures. As preceding. Most cases develop Fanconi syndrome (see), hypophosphatemic rickets, and disturbance of water and electrolyte metabolism.

Therapy. As preceding. Rickets resistant to vitamin D.

Prognosis. Unknown if patients may survive into adulthood.

TYROSINEMIA TYPE II

See Richner-Hannart.

TYROSINEMIA TYPE III

Synonyms. 4-Hydroxyphenylpyruvate dioxygenase; hydroxyphenylpyruvate dioxygenase deficiency, pHPPD deficiency.

Symptoms and Signs. Two cases, a boy and a girl, neither hepatorenal or cutaneous symptoms. *The boy.* Convulsions; cerebral atrophy; decreased myelinization of nerve (bioptic finding) *The girl.* Normal up to 17 months of age then temporary ataxia (few days); mild ataxia recurred following thyrosine load; then normal development and persistent hyperthyrosinemia.

Etiology. pHPPD deficiency. Mode of inheritance possibly autosomal recessive.

BIBLIOGRAPHY. Medes G: A new error of tyrosine metabolism: Tyrosinosis. Biochem J 26:917–940, 1932

Baber MD: A case of congenital cirrhosis of the liver with renal tubular defects akin to those in the Fanconi syndrome. Arch Dis Child 31:335–339, 1956

Conference on Hereditary Tyrosinemia, Hosp for Sick Children, Toronto, Ontario. Can Med Assoc J 97:1045–1101, 1967

Tanguay RM, Valet JP, Lescault A, et al: Different molecular basis for fumarylacetoacetate hydrolase deficiency in two clinical forms of hereditary tyrosinemia (type I). Am J Hum Genet 47:308–316, 1990

Mitchell GA, Lambert M, Tanguay RM: Hypertyrosinemia. In Scriver CR, Beaudet AL, Sly WS, et al: The Metabolic and Molecular Bases of Inherited Disease, 7th ed, pp 1077–1106. New York, McGraw-Hill, 1995

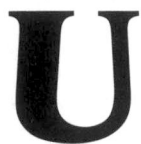

U

U.G.H.

Synonym. Uveitis—glaucoma—hyphema.

Symptoms and Signs. Uveitis; glaucoma; hyphema.

Etiology. Defective anterior chamber lens, or caused by toxics incorporated into plastic of the lens, or warped intraocular lens.

BIBLIOGRAPHY. Pallin SL: Condition mimicking UGH syndrome said unrelated to presence of IOL. Ophthal Times, Aug 1983, p 50
Scroggs MW, Klintworth GK: Drugs and toxins. In Garner A, Klintworth GK (eds): Pathobiology of Ocular Disease: A Dynamic Approach, 2nd ed, p 1175. New York, Marcel Dekker, 1994

UHL

Synonym. Parchment heart.

Symptoms. Age of clinical presentation 1–57 years. Dyspnea; fatigue; chest pain, and syncope on exertion.

Signs. Generally acyanotic; widely split and soft second heart sound; right ventricular third sound nonspecific systolic murmur.

Etiology. Congenital malformation.

Pathology. Normal tricuspid valve; atrophy of right ventricular wall; chamber dilatation. Fibrosis of right ventricular wall with irregular islands of myocardial tissue. Right ventricular thrombi found at death.

Diagnostic Procedures. Prominent α wave in jugular venous pulse. *X-ray.* Of chest. Cardiomegaly. *Angiography.* Excludes Ebstein anomaly and shows large noncontractile right ventricle. *ECG. Two-dimensional echocardiography with color flow imaging and spectral Doppler interrogation. Cardiac catheterization.*

Therapy. Medical management. Surgery not generally recommended; only of palliative type; attempts to be carefully evaluated.

Prognosis. Poor.

BIBLIOGRAPHY. Osler W: The Principles and Practice of Medicine, 7th ed, p 820. New York, Appleton-Century-Crofts, 1905
Segall HN: Parchment heart (Osler). Am Heart J 40:948, 1950
Uhl HMS: A previously undescribed congenital malformation of the heart: Almost total absence of the myocardium of right ventricle. Bull Johns Hopkins Hosp 91:197–205, 1952
Perloff JK: The Clinical Recognition of Congenital Heart Disease, 4th ed, pp 267–268. Philadelphia, WB Saunders, 1994
Weatherall DJ, Ledingham JGG, Warrell DA (eds): Oxford Textbook of Medicine, 3rd ed, p 2414. Oxford, Oxford Med Pub, 1996

UHTHOFF

Synonyms. See Multiple sclerosis.

Symptoms and Signs. In patients with multiple sclerosis, reduction of visual activity accentuated by vigorous exercise (or by a hot bath).

BIBLIOGRAPHY. Van Diemen HA, Van Dongen MH, Dammers SW, et al: Increased visual impairment after excercise (Hithoff's phenomenon) in multiple sclerosis: Therapeutic possibilities. Eur Neurol 32:231–234, 1992

Guthrie TC, Nelson DA: Influence of temperature changes on multiple sclerosis: Critical review of mechanism and research potential. J Neur Sci 129:1–8, 1995

ULCERATIVE COLITIS, IDIOPATHIC

Synonyms. Colitis gravis; thromboulcerative colitis.

Symptoms. Both sexes affected with equal incidence. Onset at all ages, more frequently at 20–40 years of age. Occasionally, insidious onset with simple appearance of bloody mucus on outside of stool. Usually, abrupt onset with diarrhea (day and night), soft, mushy, or loose with mixed blood. Tenesmus; abdominal pain of various degrees relieved by defecation. Gastric symptoms and anorexia may occur. Anxiety manifestation usually precipitating and accompanying attacks. Weight loss frequent; fever occasional. Frequently, rheumatoid arthritis manifestations; less frequently, erythema multiforme, pyoderma gangrenosum. In children, infantilism may be found. Three clinical patterns may be recognized: (1) Relapsing, remitting type. (a) Mild; without fever; self-limited; each attack lasting 1–3 months; (b) Severe; fever; blood loss; toxemia. (2) Chronic, continuous type. Duration, 6 months or longer mild or severe. (3) Acute, fulminating type (rare, 5%); fever; hemorrhages; perforation or obstruction.

Signs. During attacks, pallor, weakness, weight loss, tenderness over colon. Rectal examination painful; nutritional deficiency.

Etiology. Multifactorial origins. Suspected: immune mechanisms; microbial aspects; psychogenic relationship; genetic aspects.

Pathology. Ulceration of colon with island of normal mucosa (pseudopolyps); microscopic: microabscesses in crypts of mucosal glands; aspecific inflammatory reaction around ulcers; metadysplastic mucosal regeneration and fibrotic changes.

Diagnostic Procedures. *Sigmoidoscopy.* Reveals typical lesions. *Blood.* Microcytic anemia; hypoproteinemia; electrolytes alteration. *X-ray.* Colon shortened; hose appearance; loss of haustral marking. *Stool.* Negative culture.

Therapy. According to clinical type: diet; salicylazosulfapyridine; mesalamine, olsalazine, if no response after 2–4 weeks corticosteroids; sedatives; azathioprine, cyclosporine. Severe disease methylprednisolone 50 mg a day and eventually proctocolectomy with successive reconstruction through pouches. In fulminating type: blood replacement, electrolyte balance, parental alimentation.

Prognosis. Spontaneous remission and relapses characterize course of the condition. In chronic continuous type, development of carcinoma after 5 years frequent. Death from complications, circulatory collapse, hemorrhage, hypokalemia, liver cirrhosis, perforation, marasmus.

BIBLIOGRAPHY. Wilks W, Moxon W: Lectures on Pathological Anatomy. London, Churchill, 1875
Sales DJ, Kirsner JB: The prognosis of inflammatory bowel disease (review). Arch Int Med 143:294–299, 1983
Podolsky DK: Inflammatory bowel disease (two parts). N Engl J Med 325:928–1008, 1991
Ulcerative colitis. In Haubrich WS, Schaffner F, Berk JE (eds): Bockus Gastroenterology, 5th ed, vol 2, pp 1326–1363. Philadelphia, WB Saunders, 1995

ULLMANN

Obsolete.

Synonyms. Angiomatosis systemica; systemis hamartosis. See Sturge Webber, von Hippel-Lindau, Rendu-Osler.

Symptoms and Signs. Angiomatosis of nervous system extending to the visceral field.

Etiology. Diagnosis that attempts to comprise all cases of angiomatosis affecting the nervous system, skin and viscera and that do not fall into the major nosologically defined angiomatoses that may also present this diffuse involvement. Do we need this syndrome?

BIBLIOGRAPHY. Ullmann K: Ueber das Wesen der Angiomatosis Mschr Ohrenheik 65:1147–1165, 1931
Kissel P, Dureux JB: Ullmann syndrome: Systemic angiomatosis. In Vinken PJ, Bruyn GW (eds): Handbook of Clinical Neurology, vol 22, pp 446–454. Amsterdam, North-Holland, 1972

ULLRICH-BONNEVIE

Synonyms. Bonnevie-Ullrich; pterygolymphangiectasia. See Turner and Noonan. Obsolete.

Symptoms. Present from birth. Pterygium colli; lymphedema of the hands and feet; various congenital disorders of bones, muscle, and viscera; dwarfism.

Etiology. To be identified with Turner (see) and/or Noonan (see).

BIBLIOGRAPHY. Ullrich O: Ueber typiche kombinationsbilder Multipler Abartungen. Z Kinderheilkd 49:271–276, 1930
Bonnevie K: Embryological analysis of gene manifestation in Little and Bagg's abnormal mouse tribe. J Exp Zool 67:443–520, 1934

ULLRICH-FEICHTEIGER

Synonyms. Bortholin; anophthalmia—cleft lip and palate—polydactyly; dyscraniopylophalangy. See also Fraser. Obsolete.

Symptoms and Signs. Anophthalmia or microphthalmia; cleft lip or palate (or both); polydactyly.

Etiology. Unknown. Sporadic occurrence. (Some cases reported are likely D1 trisomy.)

BIBLIOGRAPHY. Ullrich O: Der Status Bonnevie-Ullrich in Rahmenanderer "Dyscranio-Dysphalangien." Ergebn Inn Med Kinderheilkd NF2:412–420, 1951
Warburg M: Anophthalmos complicated by mental retardation and cleft palate. Acta Ophthalmol 38:394–404, 1960
Weatherall DJ, Ledingham JGG, Warrell DA (eds): Oxford Textbook of Medicine, 3rd ed, p 4147. Oxford, Oxford Med Pub, 1996

ULNAR-FIBULAR DIMELIA, PECULIAR FACIES, TIBIA-RADIUS ABSENCE

Synonyms. Mirror hand.

Symptoms and Signs. Both sexes (A man and his daughter). From birth. Hand and foot syndactyly and polydactyly. Bilateral clefts enlarging margins of nares. Duplication of fibula and ulna bilaterally and missing radius and tibia.

Etiology. Autosomal dominant inheritance.

Therapy. Correction of digital webs in hand and feet and removal of supernumerary toes.

BIBLIOGRAPHY. Guilo Obsequente (IV century), quoted by Burman M: An historical perspective of double hands and double feet. The survey of the cases reported in the 16th and 17th centuries. Bull Hosp Joint Dis 29:241–254, 1968
Sandrow RE, Sullivan PD, Steel HH: Hereditary ulnar and fibular dimelia with peculiar facies. J Bone Joint Surgery 52:367–370, 1970

ULNAR NERVE COMPRESSION (WRIST AND HAND) SYNDROMES

Synonyms. Guyon canal; ulnar tunnel; ulnar-carpal canal. See also Entrapment and Gessler. Frequently affects gold polishers, oyster openers, cutlery workers, motorcyclists, bowlers (bowler thumb). According to the site of compression, three different syndromes result.

TYPE I

Symptoms and Signs. Gradual onset. Motor weakness of all hand muscles innervated by ulnar nerve, with sensory deficit of palmar surfaces of hypothenar eminence and index and little fingers, on dorsum of medial side of the hand.

Etiology. Pressure on the ulnar nerve just proximal to or within the ulnar tunnel.

Pathology. Any of the following lesions may cause the compression and relative syndromes: ganglion (28.7%); occupational neuritis (23.5%); laceration (10.3%); arteritis, thromboangiitis (8.1%); fracture of metacarpal (2.9%); other bone fractures; aberrant muscles; bursitis.

Diagnostic Procedures. *X-ray.* Of hand and wrist, cervical spine, shoulder, and elbow if indicated. Electromyography and nerve conduction studies. *Blood.* For evidence of generalized disorders: diabetes mellitus, rheumatoid arthritis; scleroderma.

Therapy. Conservative therapy: immobilization; cortisone injection; change of occupation. If unsuccessful, surgical decompression and exploration of nerve and its branches.

Prognosis. Good with adequate treatment.

TYPE II

Symptoms and Signs. Motor weakness of muscles innervated by deep branch of ulnar nerve; normal sensation in the hand.

Etiology. Pressure on the deep branch of ulnar nerve at the exit from the ulnar tunnel or at the hook of hamate at origin of abductor and flexor digiti minimi brevis manus and in opponens digiti minimi muscles.

Pathology. See Type I.

Diagnostic Procedures. See Type I.

Therapy. See Type I.

Prognosis. See Type I.

TYPE III

Symptoms and Signs. Sensory deficits in the volar surface of hypothenar eminence and in the ring and little fingers; absence of muscle weakness or atrophy. On dorsum, normal sensation.

Etiology. Pressure on the superficial branch of the ulnar nerve in the ulnar tunnel or at hook of hamate or in palmaris brevis. Arteritis of ulnar artery and direct trauma along the ulnar border of the hand are among the causes of compression of this particular type of the syndrome.

Pathology. See Type I.

Diagnostic Procedures. See Type I.

Therapy. See Type I. If arteritis is responsible for the syndrome, resection of affected segment of the artery.

Prognosis. See Type I.

BIBLIOGRAPHY. Guyon F: Note sur une disposition anatomique propre à la face antérieure de la région du poignet et non encore décrite par le docteur. Boll Soc Anat Paris 6:184–186, 1861

Hunt JR: Thenar and hypothenar types of neural atrophy of the hand. Am J Med Sci 141:224–241, 1911

Shea JD, McClain EJ: Ulnar nerve compression syndromes at and below the wrist. J Bone Joint Surg 51:1095–1103, 1969

Vastamaeki M: Current Trends in Hand Surgery. Netherlands, Excerpta Medica, 1995

Weatherall DJ, Ledingham JGG, Warrell DA (eds): Oxford Textbook of Medicine, 3rd ed, pp 4096–4097. Oxford, Oxford Med Pub, 1996

UMBER

Synonyms. Sament-Schwartz; nonketotic hyperosmolar coma; hyperglycemic dehydration.

Symptoms and Signs. Most frequent in middle-aged patients with no previous history of diabetes; in most cases iatrogenic precipitating causes (e.g., drugs, fluid restrictions applied to the treatment of variable associated illness). Dehydration; weakness (leading symptoms); polyuria and polydipsia (may persist for weeks before becoming appreciated and correctly interpreted). Consciousness alterations from drowsiness to frank coma; focal neurologic findings (transitory). Shock, infections frequently associated.

Etiology. Persistent osmotic diuresis leading to dehydration; sodium and potassium deficits and severe hyperglycemia in absence of marked hyperketonemia.

Pathology. In brain, findings still debated: edema; localized brain infections; subdural hemorrhages. Increased frequency of pancreatitis; pulmonary embolus; and thromboembolic phenomena.

Diagnostic Procedures. *Blood.* Hyperosmolarity; hyperglycemia; absence of marked elevation of ketone bodies; high blood urea nitrogen; creatinine ratio exceeds 30.

Therapy. Rapid partial correction of dehydration and shock prevention or treatment; Potassium balance. Specific treatment for basic illness. Insulin in graduated doses (20–25 IU) intramuscularly or intravenously in albumin to produce a more sustained, gradual fall of plasma glucose over a period of hours.

Prognosis. Very variable according to reported series. Mortality approximately 40–50%.

BIBLIOGRAPHY. Umber F: Stoffwechsel krankheiten. II. Diabetes mellitus. Med Wochenschr (Munich) 71:1324–1326, 1924

Sament S, Schwartz MB: Severe diabetic stupor without ketosis. S Afr Med J 31:893–894, 1957

Forster DW, McGarry JD: Diabetes mellitus acute complications, ketoacidosis, hyperosmolar coma lactic acidosis. In De Groot LJ (ed): Endocrinology, 3rd ed, pp 1516–1518. Philadelphia, WB Saunders, 1995

UNDERWOOD

Synonyms. Sclerema adiposum; sclerema neonatorum; preagonal induration.

Symptoms. Both sexes affected. Onset during first week of life (in premature or debilitated children) or later associated with severe disorders. Prodromata represented by respiratory or gastrointestinal manifestations.

Signs. Small, weak infant. Cyanosis; progressive hardening of skin of buttocks, thighs, and calves, then of rest of body, with the exception of genitalia, palms, and soles. Skin assumes a mottled white color. Body temperature progressively decreases.

Etiology. Unknown. Exposure to cold is frequently the precipitating factor of shock, circulatory failure, and temperature fall.

Pathology. Hardening of subcutaneous fat; scanty histologic changes. Swollen trabeculae.

Diagnostic Procedures. Identification of basic pathology.

Therapy. Incubator. Antibiotics (for treatment of underlying condition). Corticosteroids (of doubtful utility). Repeated exchange transfusions may reduce mortality.

Prognosis. Extremely severe. The 80% mortality may be reduced to 50% with adequate treatment. The outcome, however, is bound to the basic pathology.

BIBLIOGRAPHY. Underwood M: A Treatise on the Diseases of Children. London, Matthews, 1784

Atherton DJ: The neonate. In Champion RH, Burton JL, Ebling FJG (eds): Rook/Wilkinson/Ebling Textbook of Dermatology, 5th ed, pp 411–412. Oxford, Blackwell Scientific, 1992

UNNA (P.G.)

Synonyms. Seborrheic dermatitis; seborrheic eczema, pityrosporal dermatitis.

Symptoms. Pruritus most frequently affecting scalp, external ear, and retroauricular area, or less frequently, generalized with localizations between scapulae and over sternal region and groin.

Signs. Scales of scalp (dandruff) and seborrheic dermatitis of areas indicated; exfoliative dermatitis with or without secondary eczematization may superimpose.

Etiology. As causative agent or cofactor has been indicated: the yeast pityrosporum ovale. Cases with autosomal dominant inheritance reported.

Pathology. Hyperkeratosis; parakeratosis; intracellular and extracellular edema; slight or moderate acanthosis. Frequently, perifolliculitis; cutis infiltrates with polymorphs, lymphocytes (occasionally, plasma cells); presence of clumps of cocci in epidermis and stratum corneum. Elastic and connective tissues not affected.

Diagnostic Procedures. *Biopsy.* Of skin (area not scrubbed too vigorously, so that scales are not removed). *Blood.* Normal.

Therapy. Regular washing and frequent use of a detergent (including selenium sulfide, zinc pyrithione and tar) shampoo. Corticosteroids alone or with antibiotics. Ketonazole (temporary action). Salicylic acid to reduce scaling. Effective also benzoyl peroxide and lithium succinate (5%) ointment and isotretinoin.

Prognosis. No effective treatment except in those cases where the condition is manifestation of a reversible systemic process.

BIBLIOGRAPHY. Unna PG: Das sebborhoische Ekzem Mschr Pract Derm 6:829–846, 1887

Burton JL: Eczema, lichenification, prurigo and erytroderma. In Champion RH, Burton JL, Ebling FJG (eds): Rook/Wilkinson/Ebling Textbook of Dermatology, 5th ed, pp 545–551. Oxford, Blackwell Scientific, 1992

UNRULY HAIR

Synonyms. Pili trianguli et canaliculi. See Wooly hair; Span-glass hair; Uncombable hair.

Symptoms and Signs. Both sexes equal incidence. Difficulty in combing hair in infancy up to about 5 years of age.

Etiology. Hair malformation inherited as autosomal dominant.

Diagnostic Procedures. *Electron microscopy:* Hair triangular cross-section and longitudinal groove.

Prognosis. Hair gradually becoming normal.

BIBLIOGRAPHY. Strond JD, Mehregan AH: Spun glass hair: A clinico-pathologic study of an unusual hair defect. In Brown S (ed): The First Human Hair Symposium, pp 103–107. New York, Medcom Press, 1973

Herbert AA, Charrow J, Esterly NB, et al: Uncombable hair (pili tri-anguli et canaliculi) evidence of a dominant inheritance with complete penetrance based on scanning electron microscopy. Am J Med Genet 28:185–193, 1987

UNVERRICHT

Synonyms. Lundborg-Unverricht; familial myoclonia; myoclonus epilepsy progessive; baltic myoclonus epilepsy. See Janz; M.E.R.R.F.; Lafora.

Symptoms and Signs. Irregular, fast contraction of groups of muscles bilaterally symmetrical but asynchronous, mostly in proximal muscles of limbs. Seizures starting 6–13 years of age, first mild then progressively more violent with myoclonus, precipitated by slight stimulus following after 1–5 years. Emotional lability. Loss of mental power; amaurosis ataxia. Terminal stage: parkinsonism and muscle innervated by bulbar centers affected.

Etiology. Unknown. Sporadic in some cases hereditary condition autosomal recessive or less frequently X-linked inheritance.

Pathology. Numerous intracellular bodies found in extrapyramidal center. Degenerative changes in Purkinje cells and neurons in the medial part of thalamus. Absence of Lafora bodies.

Diagnostic Procedures. *EEG.* Wave and spike formation 3/sec in all cortical leads, associated with jerks. *Blood.* Decrease of mucoprotein content reported in a patient and siblings.

Therapy. Phenobarbital; L-5 hydroxytryptophan; clonazepam valproate, drug of choice; antibiotics for frequent episodes of pneumonia.

Prognosis. Incapacitation by the age of 20 years in severe cases. Death in young adulthood (10–20 years after onset). Frequent suicides.

BIBLIOGRAPHY. Unverricht H: Die Myoclonie. Berlin, Franz Dewticke, 1891

Wienker TF, Von Reutern GM, Ropers HH: Progressive myoclonus epilepsy: A variant with probable X-linked inheritance. Hum Genet 49:83–89, 1979

Marseille Consensus Group: Classification of progressive myoclonus epilepsies and related disorders. Ann Neurol 28:113–116, 1990

Kyllerman M, Sommerfelt K, Hedatrom A, et al: Clinical and neuro-physiological development of Unverricht-Lundborg disease in four Swedish siblings. Epilepsia 32:900–909, 1991

Weatherall DJ, Ledingham JGG, Warrell DA (eds): Oxford Textbook of Medicine, 3rd ed, pp 3988, 4014. Oxford, Oxford Med Pub, 1996

UPBEAT NYSTAGMUS-VERTIGO

Synonyms. Vertigo—upbeat nystagmus. See also Downbeat nystagmus vertigo.

Symptoms and Signs. Both sexes. Rare in children. Upbeat nystagmus in the primary position of gaze not suppressed by fixation, modulated by static head tilt. Associated oscillopsia and postural imbalance.

Etiology. Tone imbalance of the vertical semicircular canal reflexes modulated by otolithes, brainstem tumors, infarction, hematoma, multiple sclerosis, encephalitis, abscess, Wernicke's, drug intoxication. Described congenital form.

Pathology. Pontomesencephalic junction lesion or pontomedullary junction.

Diagnostic Procedures. *EEG. CT scan. MRI imaging. Electronystagmography.*

Therapy. Physical exercise. Baclofen (?).

Prognosis. According to etiology.

BIBLIOGRAPHY. Stengel E: Zur Frage der Heredolokalisation bei spontanem Vertikalnystagmus. Zeitschr Ges Neurol Psychiatr 153:417–424, 1935

Forsythe WI: Congenital hereditary vertical nystagmus. J Neurol Neurosurg Psychiatr 18:196–198, 1955

Brandt T: Vertigo: Its multisensory syndromes, pp 109–116. London, Springer-Verlag, 1991

UPINGTON*

Synonyms. Perthes-like hip; enchondromata; ecchondromata. See Ollier, Maffucci.

Symptoms and Signs. Those of Perthes (see) enchondromata and ecchondromata.

Etiology. Possibly autosomal dominant inheritance.

BIBLIOGRAPHY. Schweitzer G, Jones B, Timme H: Upington disease: a familial dyschondroplasia. S Afr Med J 45:994–1000, 1971

URBACH-WIETHE

Synonyms. Rössle-Urbach-Wiethe; hyalinosis cutis et mucosae; lipoid proteinosis; proteinosis-lipoidosis.

Symptoms. Both sexes affected. Onset in infancy. Inability to cry. Itching of the eyes. Hoarseness.

Signs. Generalized papules; plaques and ulcers of skin and mucosae. Predilection for lips, mouth, pharynx, vocal cords, eyelids, neck, hands, fingers, knees, elbows, and scrotum. Apparently no visceral symptoms or signs. Possibly, macrocheilia, macroglossia.

Etiology. Lysosomal storage disease. Autosomal recessive inheritance (most likely). Association with diabetes mellitus.

Pathology. Early lesions: hyaline thickening of capillary walls. Intermediate lesions: eosinophilic hyalinosis bands around capillaries in dermis and hyaline wrapping around sweat glands. Late lesions: substitution of dermal collagen and elastic tissue by hyaline material, with atrophy of glands. Lipid deposits in hyalinized areas. Epithelium overlying lesions usually becomes hyperplastic and hyperkeratotic.

Diagnostic Procedures. *Blood.* Phospholipids increased. *Urine.* Increased excretion of amino acids (tyrosine). *X-ray.* Possibly, calcification of sella turcica. *Biopsy.* Of skin. See Pathology.

Therapy. Insulin indicated also in absence of hyperglycemia. Surgical removal of growths on vocal cord.

Prognosis. Relatively benign, progressive course.

BIBLIOGRAPHY. Urbach E, Wiethe C: Lipoidosis cutis et mucosae. Virchows Arch (Pathol Anat) 273:285–319, 1929

Haneke E, Hornstein OP, Meisel-Stosiek M, et al: Hyalinosis cutis et mucosae in siblings. Hum Genet 68:342–345, 1984

Stine OC, Smith KD: The estimation of selection coefficients in Afrikaners: Huntigton disease, porphyria variegata and lipoid proteinosis. Am J Med Genet 46:425–458, 1990

Winder AF: Disorders of lipid and lipoprotein metabolism. In Garner A,

---

*District of Cape Province (South Africa).

Klintworth GK (eds): Pathobiology of Ocular Disease: A Dynamic Approach, 2nd ed, p 1111. New York, Marcel Dekker, 1994

UREA ENZYMOPATHIES

Synonym. Hyperammonemia.

1. N-acetylglutamate synthetase deficiency (AGA deficiency). One case described. Mental retardation; ataxia.
2. Carbamoyl phosphate synthetase deficiency (CPSD).
3. Ornithine carbamoyl transferase deficiency (OCTD) see Russell III.
4. Citrullinemia (ASASD) (see).
5. Argininosuccinate lyase deficiency (argininosuccinic aciduria) (ASALD) (see).
6. Arginase deficiency (see).
7. Hyperornithinemia syndromes (see Simell-Takki); hyperornithinemia-hyperammonemia-homocitrullinuria).
8. Lysinuric protein intolerance (hyperdibasic aciduria). Perheentupa-Visakorpi (see).
9. Hyperlysinemia periodic (see); persistent hyperlysinemia that is not associated with hyperammonemia.
10. Rett (see).

Hyperammonemia may be present also in other disorders of amino acid metabolism.

BIBLIOGRAPHY. Brusilow SW, Horwich AL: Urea cycle enzymes. In Scriver CR, Beaudet AL, Sly WS, et al: The Metabolic and Molecular Bases of Inherited Disease, 7th ed, pp 1187–1232. New York, McGraw-Hill, 1995

UREMIC CARDIAC

Synonym. Cardiouremica.

Symptoms and Signs. Occurs in patients with chronic uremia, treated with a selected low-protein diet. Pronounced cardiomegaly; gallop rhythm; severe hypotension; pericarditis with or without pericardial effusion; arrhythmias; marked sensitivity to cardiac glycosides.

Etiology. Considered a progression of the uremia or secondary to dietetic factors, prolonged anemia, or prolonged hypertension.

Diagnostic Procedures. *Blood. Urine.* All features of chronic uremia. Low hematocrit (which remains low after recovery from syndrome). *X-ray.* Of chest. Cardiomegaly. *ECG.* Venous pressure.

Therapy. Hemodialysis or kidney homotransplantation.

Prognosis. Recovery. Abnormal findings disappear or markedly improve as soon as treatment with hemodialysis or peritoneal dialysis is started.

BIBLIOGRAPHY. Bailey GL, Hampers CL, Merrill JP: Annual Meeting of American Society Artificial Internal Organs. JAMA 200:8–30, 1967
Kikeri D, Mitch WE: The heart and kidney disease. In Schlant RC, Alexander RW: Hurst's The Heart, 8th ed, p 1964. New York, McGraw-Hill, 1994

UREMIC-NEUROMYOPATHIC

Synonyms. Uremic myopathy; uremic polyneuropathy; tetanic uremic neuromyopathy. Still not well defined or universally accepted symptom complexes that develop in patients with chronic uremia. Four different syndromes may be recognized.

UREMIC POLYNEUROPATHY

Symptoms. Occurs in young males with chronic uremia. Initially, painful burning sensation of feet; followed by progression to lower extremities, paresthesias, painful cramps, and weakness. Same symptoms but much milder in upper extremities. Distal segment more affected than proximal. Trunk and face spared.

Signs. Feet sensitive to light touch and pressure. Atrophy of leg muscles. Sensory loss of feet and legs, less pronounced on arms and hands. Tendon reflexes abolished.

Etiology. Unknown. Possibly, metabolic defect resulting in polyneural alteration (specific nature not determined).

Pathology. Disappearance of a proportion of large medullated fibers, maximal degree on feet. Less pronounced lesions on proximal part of nerves. Anterior horn cells of spinal cord; chromatolysis limited to lumbosacral and cervical enlargements. No evidence of regeneration. Atrophic muscles (denervation atrophic type).

Diagnostic Procedures. *Blood.* All findings of chronic uremia. *Electromyography. Biopsy* of muscle and peripheral nerve.

Therapy. Dialysis; renal transplantation.

Prognosis. Progressive form; treatment results in slow improvement of nerve function.

UREMIC MYOPATHY

Symptoms. Occurs in older subjects than previous syndrome; not prevalent in males. Asthenia and weakness of muscles of both pelvic and scapular region. Alteration of subjective sensitivity.

Signs. Atrophy of scapular and pelvic girdle muscles. Tendon reflex normal; idiomuscular reflexes abolished.

Etiology. Unknown. Muscular atrophy secondary to metabolic defect (specific nature not determined).

Pathology. Muscular tissue fiber atrophy; degenerative changes, occasional disintegration, and necrosis of muscle fibers; moderate hyperplasia of sarcolemma. Lack of inflammatory changes. Fibroadipose involution.

Diagnostic Procedures. *Blood.* All features of chronic uremia. *Biopsy.* Of muscle. See Pathology. *Electromyography.*

Therapy. Symptoms do not respond to dialysis.

Prognosis. Poor.

UREMIC NEUROMYOPATHY

Combination of symptoms, signs, and pathologic findings of the two previously described syndromes.

TETANIC NEUROMYOPATHY

Synonym. Uremic twitch, convulsive.

Symptoms and Signs. Severe, painful, and unrelenting tonic contraction of muscles. Myoclonus and convulsions may also be present.

Signs. Rigid extension of the legs; plantar flexion, internal rotation of the feet. Abdomen rigid and painful. Injection of calcium and magnesium does not affect symptomatology (in one patient myospasm so intense as to tear abdominal rectus muscle: blue discoloration simulating Cullen sign).

Etiology. Unknown. Neuromyopathy owing to chronic renal failure.

Pathology. Chronic uremia.

Diagnostic Procedures. *Blood.* High blood urea nitrogen; calcium, magnesium normal. *Urine.* Findings of chronic renal failure.

Prognosis. Syndrome preceding death by hours or months.

BIBLIOGRAPHY. Merklen P, Gounelle H: Uremie musculaire. Medicine 12:225–229, 1931
Tenckhoff HA, Boen FST, Jebsen RH et al: Polyneuropathy in chronic renal insufficiency. JAMA 192:1121–1124, 1965

Serratrice G, Toga M, Roux H, et al: Neuropathies, myopathies et neuromyopathies chez des urémiques chroniques. Presse Med 75:1835–1838, 1967

Biasioli S, D'Andree G, Feriani S, et al: Uremic encephalopathy: An update. Clin Nephrol 25:57–63, 1986

Adams RD, Victor M: Principles of Neurology, 5th ed, pp 887–889, 1144–1145. New York, McGraw-Hill, 1993

UROGENITAL TRACT AND EAR MALFORMATIONS

Synonym. Renal, genital, middle ear (Winter).

1. Urogenital tract and external ear (Potter syndrome [see]).
2. Urogenital tract and middle ear (Winter). Combination of renal hypoplasia, internal genital, and middle ear malformations, possibly caused by autosomal recessive gene inheritance.

BIBLIOGRAPHY. Longenecker CG, Ryan RF, Vincent RW: Malformations of the ear as a clue to urogenital anomalies: Report of six additional cases. Plast Reconstr Surg 35:303–309, 1965

Winter JSD, Millman WJ: A familial syndrome of renal, genital, and middle ear anomalies. J Pediatr 72:88–93, 1968

Turner GA: Second family with renal, vaginal, and middle ear anomalies. J Pediatr 76:641, 1970

Warkany J: Congenital Malformations, p 1037. Chicago, Year Book Med Pub, 1971

USHER

Synonyms. Von Graefe; Graefe-Sjögren; deafness-retinitis pigmentosa; retinitis pigmentosa-deafness; includes Lindenov-Hallgren, Hallgren. See also Graefe-Sjögren.

Symptoms. Time of onset unknown. Family history of poor night vision, blue-green color blindness, or total blindness. During childhood, progressive hearing loss (evident at age 4–6) and secondary lack of speech development. Usually, a few years later (average age 9) progressive poor night vision, degeneration of peripheral visual fields, tunnel vision, blindness. Mental deficiency and psychosis (25%). In the family described by Hallgren cataract at 40 years of age

Signs. Physical examination normal (see Diagnostic Procedures).

Etiology. Anatomic and metabolic conditions causing deafness and retinitis are unknown. Autosomal recessive inheritance and X-linked. Four types have been subclassified (Davenport):

Type I. Profound congenital deafness; onset of retinitis by age 10.

Type II. Moderate to severe progressive congenital deafness; onset of retinitis in the teens.

Type III. Retinitis at puberty with progressive hearing loss.

Type IV. A possible X-linked form.

Another classification (Fishman) has two types: The first with earlier and more severe: night blindness, vision loss, hearing loss; unintelligible speech, vestibular reflexes, and ataxia. The second with less severe and delayed manifestations.

Pathology. In eyes, rod degeneration preceding the typical pigment deposits on the retina. No adequate microscopic studies of cochlear lesions.

Diagnostic Procedures. *Audiography.* Pure tone threshold losses of variable severity. Intracochlear defect. *Electroretinography.* Early signs of retinal degeneration detected by abnormal dark-adapted electroretinogram.

Therapy. Early diagnosis of hearing loss allows prevention of lack of speech development and improves secondary retarded speech.

Prognosis. Hearing loss is usually not rapidly progressing. Eye lesions may progress to total blindness.

BIBLIOGRAPHY. Von Graefe AF: Exceptionelles Verhalten des Gesichtsfeldes bei Pigmententartung der Nethaut Graefe. Arch Klin Exper Ophthal 4:250–253, 1858

Usher CH: On the inheritance of retinitis pigmentosa with notes of cases. Roy Lond Ophthalmol Hosp Rep 19:130–236, 1914

Lindenov H: The Etiology of Deaf-Mutism with Special Reference to Heredity. Copenhagen, E Munksgaard, 1945

Hallgren B: Retinitis pigmentosa combined with congenital deafness: with vestibulo-cerebellar ataxia and mental abnormality in a proportion of cases. Acta Psychiatr Neurol Scand 34:9–101, 1951

Tamayo ML, Bernal JE, Tamayo GE, et al: Usher syndrome: Results of a screening program in Columbia. Clin Genet 40:304–311, 1991

UVEAL EFFUSION

Symptoms and Signs. Described in mild form of Hunter (see). Visual impairment. Serious detachment of peripheral choroid and ciliary body, detachment of retina.

Etiology. See Hunter. Scleral thickening from glycosaminoglycan deposition causing obstruction of vortex vein and preventing transport of extravascular proteins out of eye.

Pathology. Chronic exudative detachment of uvea and retina, increased colloid osmotic pressure.

BIBLIOGRAPHY. Vine AK: Uveal effusion in Hunter's syndrome: Evidence that abnormal sclera is responsible for uveal effusion syndrome. Retina 6:57–60, 1986

UYEMURA

Synonyms. Fundus albipunctatus—hemeralopia—xerosis; night blindness I; nyctalopia—xerosis—fundus albipunctatus.

Symptoms. Occurs more often in males. Onset in childhood or young adulthood. Night blindness (transitory); conjunctival xerosis.

Signs. Fundus oculi grayish-white appearance and densely covered by yellowish-white spots.

Etiology. Deficiency of vitamin A. To be differentiated from retinitis punctata albescens, fundus albipunctatus, and Oguchi. Unclear genetic role.

Therapy. Vitamin A.

Prognosis. Quick recovery with treatment.

BIBLIOGRAPHY. Uyemura M: Ueber eine merkwürdige Augenhintergrundveräderung bei zwei Fällen von idiopathischer Hemeralopie. Klin Monatsbl Augenheilkd 81:471–473, 1928

Fuchs A: White spots of the fundus combined with night blindness and xerosis (Uyemura's syndrome). Am J Ophthalmol 48:101–103, 1959

Krill AE, Martin D: Photopic-abnormalities in congenital stationary nightblindness. Invest Ophthalmol 10:625–636, 1971

Krill AE: Hereditary Retinal and Choroidal Diseases. Hagerstown, MD, Harper & Row, 1977

Bird AC, Jay B, Hussain AA, et al: Retinal photoreceptor disorders. In Garner A, Klintworth GK (eds): Pathobiology of Ocular Disease: A Dynamic Approach, 2nd ed, p 1225. New York, Marcel Dekker, 1994

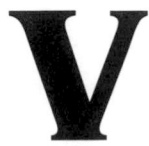

VAANDRAGER-PENA

Synonyms. Spondylometaphyseal dysplasia type C-IV; metaphyseal chondrodysplasia; spondylometaphyseal dysostosis type C-IV; Pena.

Symptoms and Signs. Present from birth. Metaphyseal dysostosis primarily involving vertebrae and pelvis (coxa vara) and resulting in dwarfism.

Etiology. Probably, autosomal recessive inheritance.

BIBLIOGRAPHY. Vaandrager GJ: Metafysaire dystosis? Nederl T Geneesk 104:547–552, 1960

Pena J: Dysostosis metafisaria. Una revision, con aportacion de una observation familiar. Una forma nueva de la enfermaded? Radiologia (Madrid) 47:3–22, 1965

Kozlowski K, Sikorska B: Dysplasia metaphysaria Typ Vaandrager-Pena. Z Kinderheilkd 108:165–170, 1970

VAGAL BODY TUMOR

Symptoms. Relatively equal sex distribution. Average age at onset 37 years. Frequently asymptomatic. Duration of symptoms and signs before diagnosis variable, up to 3 years. Sudden hoarseness; dull pain on side of the neck; syncope; difficulty in swallowing; disturbed balance.

Signs. Mass in high anterolateral side of neck (more frequently the right side). Peritonsillar structures displaced medially (50%); hemiatrophy of tongue (rare); Horner syndrome (rare).

Etiology. Unknown. Tumor of vagal body.

Pathology. Nodular, ovoid, encapsulated mass, 2–6 cm in diameter, below base of skull, near foramen jugulare, contiguous with vagus (X) nerve. Infiltration of jugular foramen occasionally observed. Microscopically, chemodectoma cluster of "balls" of polyhedral cells, thin vascular fibrus septa. Metastasis rare.

Therapy. Surgical excision; X-ray treatment.

Prognosis. May be cured by surgical excision. This tumor seems to have more of a tendency to metastasize than glomus jugular tumor and carotid body tumor.

BIBLIOGRAPHY. White EG: Die Structur des Glomus caroticum, seine Pathologie und Physiologie und seine Beziehung zum Nerven-system. Beitr Pathol Anat 96:177–227, 1935

Oberman HA, Holtz F, Sheffer LA, et al: Chemodectomas (nonchromaffin paragangliomas) of the head and neck: A clinicopathologic study. Cancer 21:838–851, 1968

Arts HA, Fagan PA: Vagal body tumors. Otolaryngol Acad Neck Surg 105:78–85, 1991

VAHLQUIST-GASSER

Synonyms. Gasser I; infantile granulocytopenia, benign; granulocytopenia, chronic infantile; neutropenia, chronic, benign, of infancy–childhood.

Symptoms. Negative family history. Onset at infancy or early childhood. Male to female ratio, 1:1.5. Trivial infections; paronychia; gingivitis; ulcerations; furunculosis; respiratory tract infection. Child appears healthy in intervals between infections.

Signs. None or moderate lymphadenopathy in connection with infections. Moderate splenomegaly in some cases.

Etiology. Unknown. Disturbance of leukocytogenesis; no familial tendency.

Pathology. Cytologic examination of pus reveals the presence of neutrophils.

Diagnostic Procedures. *Blood.* Moderate leukopenia or normal total leukocyte count; absolute and relative neutropenia; eosinophils normal or increased; no anemia or thrombocytopenia. Leukocyte response to epinephrine variable, occasionally normal. Protein electrophoretic pattern: no consistent changes. *Bone marrow.* Cellularity normal or slightly increased. Variable lymphocytosis. Erythroid series normal; myeloid-erythroid ratio normal. Myeloid series normal, except for almost total absence of mature neutrophils. Megakaryocytic series normal. Histoid series normal. Response to local stimulus (window technique) absence of neutrophils. Leukoagglutinine test positive in 78% of cases and immunofluorescent test for antibodies, 88.5%; circulating immune complexes frequently present.

Therapy. Antibiotics; no response to steroids or splenectomy. Urinary CSF produces transient increases in neutrophils.

Prognosis. Good. Infections controlled by antibiotics. Spontaneous recovery frequent at 1–4 years of age.

BIBLIOGRAPHY. Hotz A: Zur Differentialdiagnose-Agranulocytose-Leukamie. Z Kinderheilkd 65:529–540, 1949

Vahlquist B, Anjou N: Granulocytopénie chronique bénigne. Acta Haematol (Basel) 8:199–208, 1952

Gasser C, Vrtilek MR: Essentielle chronische Granulocytopenie in Kindersalter. Schweiz Med Wochenschr 52:1122–1123, 1952

Athens JW: Neutropenia. In Lee GR, Bithel TC, Foerster J, et al (eds): Wintrobe's Clinical Hematology, 9th ed, p 1601. Philadelphia, Lea & Febiger, 1993

VAIL

Synonym. Vidian neuralgia. See Horton II.

Symptoms. Prevalent in adult females. Usually unilateral, often nocturnal, severe pain in nose, face, eyes, ears, head, neck, and shoulders. Nasal sinusitis symptoms frequent.

Etiology and Pathology. Irritation or inflammation of vidian nerve, secondary to infection of sphenoidal sinus. Relationship of this syndrome with Sluder not clear.

Diagnostic Procedures. Cocainization of sphenopalatine ganglion.

Therapy. Therapy of sinus disease; procaine alcohol injection of sphenopalatine ganglion.

Prognosis. Good result with injection.

BIBLIOGRAPHY. Vail HH: Vidian neuralgia, with special reference to eye and orbital pain in suppuration of petrous apex. Ann Otol Rhinol Laryngol 41:837–856, 1932

Bell WE: Orofacial Pains Classification: Diagnosis Management. Chicago, Year Book Med Publ, 1985

Olen J (chairman): Classification and diagnostic criteria for headache disorders: Cranial neuralgia and facial pain. Cephalalgia 8:(Suppl 7), 1988

Cady RK, Fox AW: Treating the Headeache Patient. New York, Marcel Dekker, 1994

Weatherall DJ, Ledingham JGG, Warrell DA (eds): Oxford Textbook of Medicine, 3rd ed, p 2610. Oxford, Oxford Med Pub, 1996

VALENTIN

Synonyms. Glenoid hypoplasia; scapular—neck dysplasia.

Symptoms and Signs. In children. Usually asymptomatic. Shoulder pain, and limited motion; recurrent dislocation. Premature development of osteoarthritis.

Etiology. Unknown. Sporadic. Reported cases of autosomal dominance.

Diagnostic Procedures. *X-rays.* Hypoplasia of scapular neck; widened glenohumeral space; altered articular surface; hypoplasia of humeral head and neck.

BIBLIOGRAPHY. Valentin B: Die Kongenital Schulterluxation. Z Orthop Chir 55:229, 1931

Zozlowski K, Scougall S: Congenital bilateral glenoid hypoplasia: A report of four cases. Br Radiol 60:705–706, 1987

VALSUANI

Synonyms. Wills-Metha; pernicious anemia gravidica; gravidic pernicious anemia; pregnancy, pernicious anemia.

Symptoms and Signs. Those of Addison-Biermer (see) appearing during pregnancy and receding after its termination.

Etiology. Deficiency of folic acid.

Pathology. See Addison-Biermer.

Therapy. Folic acid plus iron. Diagnosis and proper treatment of infections.

Prognosis. Prompt remission with treatment.

BIBLIOGRAPHY. Valsuani E: Cachessia puerperale raccolta nella clinica ginecologica dell'ospedale Maggiore di Milano, Bernardoni, 1870

Wills L, Metha MM: Studies in "pernicious anemia" of pregnancy. I. Preliminary report. Indian J Med Res 17:777–792, 1930

Wintrobe MM, Lukens JN, Lee GR: The approach to the patient with anemia. In Lee GR, Bithell TC, Foerster J, et al (eds): Wintrobe's Clinical Hematology, 9th ed, p 733. Philadelphia, Lea & Febiger, 1993

VAN ALLEN

Obsolete.

Synonyms. Amyloid IV; amyloidosis, Iowa type; formerly amyloidosis, neuropathy-nephropathy. See amyloidosis.

Symptoms and Signs. Occurs in patients of English-Scottish-Irish descent. Both sexes involved. Age at onset 26–44 years (average 35). Neuropathy dominates at onset, involving all four extremities. Severe peptic ulcer disease; frequently, hearing loss and blurred vision (cataracts but no vitreous opacities). Commonly, impotence and sphincter disturbances. Seldom, foot ulcers or cardiomegaly. Later evidence of nephropathy.

Etiology. Autosomal dominant inheritance suggested.

Pathology. Widespread amyloidosis.

Diagnostic Procedures. *Blood.* Normal; later, evidence of nephropathy. *Biopsy.*

Therapy. Symptomatic. Dialysis. No effective treatment of systemic amyloidosis.

Prognosis. Average survival 12 years. Usual cause of death, development of generalized amyloidosis.

BIBLIOGRAPHY. Van Allen MW, Frolich JA, Davis JR: Inherited predisposition to generalized amyloidosis. Neurology 19:10–25, 1969

Benson MD: Amyloidosis. In Scriver CR, Beaudet AL, Sly WS, et al: The Metabolic and Molecular Bases of Inherited Disease, 7th ed, pp 4159–4191. New York, McGraw-Hill, 1995

VAN BOGAERT-HOZAY

Synonyms. Hozay; acro-osteolysis; facial abnormalities. See Hajdu-Cheney; Nelaton.

Symptoms and Signs. Both sexes affected. Onset at 3 years of age. *Facies.* Asymmetric; nose flat and wide with broad bridge; pronounced zygomatic arcs; hypertelorism; hypoplasia of cilia and eyebrows; eyelid ptosis; alternating squint; astigmatism and myopia; arched palate. *Extremities.* Short; sudden arrest of growth; acrocyanosis; short, thick phalangeal joints. From normal to mild mental retardation.

Etiology. Unknown. Possible autosomal recessive inheritance.

BIBLIOGRAPHY. Van Bogaert L: Essai de classement et d'interprétation de quelques acro-ostéolyses mutilantes et non mutilantes actuelment connues. Acta Neurol Psych Belg 53:90–115, 1953

Hozay J: Sur une dystrophie familiale particulière. Inibition précoce de la croissance et osteolyse non mutilante acrales avec dysmorphie faciale. Rev Neurol (Paris) 89:245–258, 1953

Durner W: Das van Bogaert-Hozay syndrom. Eine Falldemonstration. Klin Monatsbl Augenheilkd 162:658–660, 1973

Kircher D: In memoriam Ludo van Bogaert (1897–1989). Neuropathol Exp Neurol 49:185–187, 1990

VAN BOGAERT-SCHERER-EPSTEIN

Synonyms. Thiébaut; cerebrotendinous cholesterolosis; spinal cholesterolosis; CTX.

Symptoms and Signs. Both sexes affected. Onset at different ages. Onset in childhood with dementia; evolving in adolescence with progressive ataxia, spasticity, and cataracts, and finally in adulthood with tendinous xanthoma, severe spastic ataxic syndrome, bulbar paralysis, and distal muscle wasting. Hepatosplenomegaly. Palmar and plantar xanthomas.

Etiology. Autosomal recessive inheritance. Defect in bile acid synthesis with incapacity to form cholic and chenodeoxycholic acids. Enterohepatic recirculation is thus defective, the liver synthetizes increased quantities of cholesterol and cholestanol, which are deposited in tissues.

Pathology. *Tendon.* Granulomatous lesions with deposits of cholesterol. *Brain.* Atrophy with granulomatous lesions in the white matter; demyelinization; cystic spaces with foamy cells, crystals of cholesterol. Cerebellum and brain stem similar lesions. *Eyes.* Cataract. Xanthomas also in lungs.

Diagnostic Procedures. *Blood.* Cholesterol triglyceride and phospholipid normal in most cases, elevated in others, especially at later stages. Cholestanol levels range from 1.3–15 mg/dl (3–20 times higher than normal value in plasma). *Biopsy.* Measurement of cholestanol levels in xantomatous tissue.

Therapy. Good results with chenodeoxycholic acid. Cholestyramine absolutely not indicated.

Prognosis. See Symptoms and Signs. Patient may reach fifth or sixth decade. Arrest of disease with therapy.

BIBLIOGRAPHY. Van Bogaert L, Scherer HJ, Epstein E: Une forme cerebralé de cholestérinose généralisée. Paris, Masson, 1937

Thiébaut F: Paraplégies spasmodiques et xanthomes tendineux associés. Des rapports de ce syndrome avec le cholestérinose cérébrospinal. Rev Neurol (Paris) 74:313–315, 1942

Salen G, Shefer S, Berginer VM: Familial diseases with storage of sterol other than cholesterol: Cerebrotendinous xanthomatosis and sitosterolemia with xanthomatosis. In Schettler G, Habenicht AJR: Principles and Treatment of Lipoprotein Disorders. Ijmuiden, Netherlands, Springer, 1994

VAN BUCHEM

Synonyms. Buchem; endosteohyperostosis; hyperostosis corticalis generalisata; leontiasis ossea generalisata; hyperphosphatasemia tarda. See craniodyaphyseal dysplasia and Worth.

Symptoms. More frequent in males. Onset in puberty; onset of clinical manifestation from 20–50 years of age. Usually asymptomatic for a long period except in cases where mental retardation is associated. In due course patients may present paralysis of facial nerve, optic atrophy, and perceptive deafness.

Signs. Prognathism absent; wide chin; occasionally, mild exophthalmos.

Etiology. Unknown. Autosomal recessive inheritance.

Pathology. Cranium, jaw, clavicles, and ribs. Thickened compact aspect and absence of diplöe. Long bones. Thickening of cortical zone and periosteal irregularities.

Diagnostic Procedures. *Blood.* Normal or minor anemia. *Urine.* Normal. *Ophthalmoscopy.* Papillary edema. *X-ray.* See Pathology.

Therapy. When signs of compression become manifest, decompression of nerves.

Prognosis. Does not limit physical activity. Its progression involves facial (VII) nerve paralysis, optic (II), and acoustic (VIII) nerve damage.

BIBLIOGRAPHY. Garland LH: Generalized leontiasis ossea. Am J Roentgen 55:37–43, 1946

Halliday J: A rare case of bone dystrophy. Br J Surg 37:52–63, 1949

Van Buchem FSP, Hadders HN, Ubbens R: Uncommon familial systemic disease of skeleton: Hyperostosis cortical generalisata familiaris. Acta Radiol 44:109–120, 1955

Fryns JP, van den Berghe H: Facial paralysis at the age of two months as a first clinical sign of van Buchem disease (endosteal hyperostosis). Eur J Pediatr 147:99–100, 1988

Weatherall DJ, Ledingham JGG, Warrell DA (eds): Oxford Textbook of Medicine, 3rd ed, p 3090. Oxford, Oxford Med Pub, 1996

VAN DER BOSH

Symptoms and Signs. From birth. Mental deficiency; choroideremia; acrokeratosis verruciformis; anhidrosis; skeletal deformities.

Etiology. Possibly X-linked recessive inheritance.

BIBLIOGRAPHY. Van der Bosh J: A new syndrome in three generations of a Dutch family. Ophthalmologica 137:422–423, 1959

VANISHING BILE DUCT

Symptoms and Signs. Those of obliterative colangitis and ductopenia. Within 3 months from liver transplantation.

Etiology. Immune response leading to destruction of small bile ducts stimulated by VBDS, HLA mismatch, and cytomegalovirus infection.

Pathology. Obliterative cholangitis.

Diagnostic Procedures. Assay for CMV DNA.

Therapy. Prophylactic measures by acyclovir and ganciclovir, and better immunosupression with triple-drug regimens.

Prognosis. Rejection of transplanted liver.

BIBLIOGRAPHY. Ludwig J, Wiesner RH, Batts KP, et al: The acute vanishing bile duct syndrome (acute irreversible rejection) after orthotopic liver transplantation. Hepatology 7:476–483, 1987

Arnold JC, Portmann BC, O'Grady JC, et al: Cytomegalovirus infection persists in the liver graft in vanishing bile duct syndrome. Hepatology 16:494–496, 1992

Weatherall DJ, Ledingham JGG, Warrell DA (eds): Oxford Textbook of Medicine, 3rd ed, pp 2059, 2079, 2114, 2129. Oxford, Oxford Med Pub, 1996

VANISHING LUNG SYNDROMES

Eponym used to indicate a radiologic sign common to many diseases: Decrease of roentgenographic density. See also Swyer-James, Wilson-Mikity, and Burke. This may be owing to the following physiopathologic conditions:

1. Increased air. Unchanged blood and tissue (local, owing to bronchial obstruction or general asthma, bronchiolitis).
2. Increased air. Decreased blood and tissue (owing to diffuse obstructive emphysema, or bullae and cysts).
3. Normal amount of air. Decreased blood and tissue (local: lobar emphysema, embolism without infarction; general: decreased blood flow).
4. Reduction of all three components.
5. Pulmonary artery agenesis.

BIBLIOGRAPHY. Burke RN: Vanishing lung: A case report of bullous emphysema. Radiology 28:367–371, 1937

Fraser RS, Paré JAP, Fraser RG, Paré PD: Synopsis of Diseases of the Chest, 2nd ed. Philadelphia, WB Saunders, 1994

VANISHING TESTIS

Synonyms. Anorchism; castrate; functional castrate; testicular agenesis; embryonic testicular regression.

Symptoms. In childhood, normal development including external genitalia (at birth penis and scrotum may be small); no development of secondary sex characteristics at pubertal age and acquisition of typical eunuchoid phenotype.

Etiology. Unknown. Destruction of testis between seventh and fourteenth week of intrauterine life (infection [?], torsion [?], vascular accident [?]) in 46, XY phenotypic male; X-linked inheritance in some cases.

Pathology. Condition is unilateral in 97% of cases. Muellerian structures are absent, Wolffian are normal, vas deferens are rudimentary, and epididymis is absent; prepuberal testis hyalinization.

Diagnostic Procedures. *Blood.* Highest gonadotropin level of all testicular disorders and extremely low testosterone. Administration of human chorionic gonadotropin (HCG) fails to enhance testosterone production. *MRI. Laparoscopy. Surgical exploration.*

Therapy. Long-acting testosterone, starting in the early teenage years and continuing for life.

Prognosis. Correction of all development defects with adequate treatment.

BIBLIOGRAPHY. Koopman J: Congenital anorchia: Case. Geeneesk Gids 8:309–330, 1930

Josso N, Briard ML: Embryonic testicular regression syndrome. J Pediatr 97:200–204, 1980

Abeyaratue MR, Aherne WA, Scott JES: The vanishing testis. Lancet II:822–826, 1969

Winters SJ: Clinical disorders of the testis. In De Groot LJ (ed): Endocrinology, 3rd ed, p 2391. Philadelphia, WB Saunders, 1995

VAN LOHUIZEN

Synonyms. Phlebectasia congenita-livedo reticularis (past terminology); reticulate vascular nevus; cutis maculata teleangiectatica congenita. See Cutis marmorata.

Symptoms and Signs. Present from birth. Progeriod general aspect. Localized or generalized network of dilated veins in the skin, associated with spider nevi and small ulcers.

Etiology. Unknown. Usually sporadic. Autosomal recessive occurrence also reported.

Pathology. In many cases no abnormalities (functional disorder) in other ill-defined capillary dilatation in the dermis and often in the subcutis.

Therapy. None, especially during early years. In case of persistent lesions argon or dye laser may be tried.

Prognosis. Spontaneous improvement. Seldom, lesions may persist and develop varicose veins and hypertrophy of extremities involved.

BIBLIOGRAPHY. Van Lohuizen CHJ: Ueber eine seltene angeborene Hautanomalie (cutis Marmorata Telangiectatica Congenita). Acta Derm Venereol 3:202–211, 1922

Del Giudice SM, Nydorf ED: Cutis marmorata teleangiectatica with multiple congenital anomalies. Arch Derm 122:1060–1061, 1986

Atherton DJ: Naevi and other developmental defects. In Champion RH, Burton JL, Ebling FJG (eds): Rook/Wilkinson/Ebling Textbook of Dermatology, 5th ed, pp 496–498. Oxford, Blackwell Scientific, 1992

VAN NECK

Synonyms. Odelberg; ischiopubic osteochondropathy; osteitis pubis.

Symptoms. Onset few weeks after prostate or bladder intervention, herniorrhaphy in children, or childbirth. Pain in pubic symphysis area, radiating down the inner side of thighs. Cough and strains may enhance the pain. Analgesis gait; low fever.

Signs. Point tenderness. Spasm of abdominal and hip muscles.

Etiology. Osteomyelitis of pubic bones secondary to adjacent areas trauma. Various factors implied in the pathogenesis (neurovascular, endocrine, infective).

Pathology. Erosion of bone, with sclerosing and periosteal reaction.

Diagnostic Procedures. *X-ray.* Normal initially; signs of osteolysis perisymphyseal within 2–4 weeks.

Therapy. Anti-inflammatory drugs; immobilization; surgery.

Prognosis. Possible spontaneous remission; however, symptoms may last many months.

BIBLIOGRAPHY. Odelberg A: Some cases of destruction of the ischium of doubtful etiology. Arch Chir Scand 56:273–284, 1923

Van Neck M: Ostéocondritis du pubis. Arch Fr Belg Chir 27:238–240, 1924

Richardson EG: Miscellaneous nontraumatic disorders. In Crenshaw AH (ed): Campbell's Operative Orthopedics, 7th ed, pp 1060–1062. St Louis, CV Mosby, 1987

VAQUEZ-OSLER

Synonyms. Osler II; erythremia; erythrocytosis megalosplenica; myelopathic polycythemia; cryptogenic polycythemia; polycythemia rubra; polycythemia vera; splenomegalic polycythemia.

Symptoms. Slightly more prevalent in males. Onset middle or late life, reported occasionally in childhood (see Erythrocytosis in childhood). Insidious onset. Headache (48%); weakness (47%); dizziness (43%); transitory syncope; visual disturbances (31%); ringing in the ears; exertional dyspnea (26%); intense itching, especially after bath (43%); sensitivity to cold; epistaxis and gum bleeding; pain in the limbs (26%); paresthesia (29%). Sense of weight or swelling in the abdomen and occasional pain in left quadrant (24%).

Signs. Color of face "rubber"; change in color also on distal extremities of limbs, with cyanotic hue. Ecchymoses of various sizes; purpura (8%). Eyes congested; conjunctiva and mucosae deep red; in eye grounds; engorgement of vessels. Clubbing of fingers and toes (rare). Hepatomegaly (40–50%). See Mosse and Budd-Chiari. Splenomegaly (90%), hard and smooth.

Etiology. Unknown. Belongs to the group of myeloproliferative syndromes (see).

Pathology. Plethoric engorgement of all organs; enlarged thrombosed veins; diffuse hemorrhages in skin, membranes, serosa, meninges, and various organs. *Spleen.* Enlarged; infarct; thrombosis; cysts; atrophic follicles; hypertrophic pulp; foci of extramedullary hematopoiesis. *Liver.* Enlarged and hyperemic; occasionally, extramedullar hematopoiesis. *Stomach and duodenum.* Frequently, ulcers are found.

Diagnostic Procedures. *Blood.* Red cells 7–10 million; hemoglobin increased to 18–24 g/100 ml; leukocytes over 10,000 with shift to the left. Leukocyte alkaline phosphatase values above normal; platelets increased as high as 3–6 million; blood viscosity markedly increased; sedimentation rate greatly delayed. Total blood volume typically increased. Uric acid normal or elevated. *Bone marrow.* Hypercellular; hyperplasia of all series. *Urine.* Normal or seldom proteinuria.

Therapy. Phlebotomies; hydroxyurea (apparently least toxic agent for chronic treatment, however, still under evaluation); radioactive phosphorus (32P); busulfan and chlorambucil (*Caution:* They may be leukemogenic); antihistamines (for prutitus); treatment of eventual hyperuricemia.

Prognosis. The disease has a progressive, rather prolonged course. Untreated cases 50% mortality within 18 months from first symptoms; with treatment median survival approximately 12 years. Hemorrhages, cardiovascular insufficiency among leading cases of death. Transformation (or evolution) into myeloid leukemia or erythroleukemia rather frequent.

BIBLIOGRAPHY. Vaquez H: Sur une forme spéciale de cyanose s'accompagnant d'hyperglobulie excessive et persistente. C R Bull Med Paris 44:384–388, 1892

Osler W: Chronic cyanosis with polycythemia and enlarged spleen: A new clinical entity. Am J Med Sci 126:187–201, 1903

Athens JW: Polycytemia vera. In Lee GR, Bithell TC, Foerster J, et al (eds): Wintrobe's Clinical Hematology, 9th ed, pp 1999–2017. Philadelphia, Lea & Febiger, 1993

VARADI

Synonyms. Oro–facial–digital type VI; polydactyly—cleft lip/palate, lingual lump—cerebral anomalies: See Mohr; Joubert-Bolthauser, and Hooft-Jongbloet.

Symptoms and Signs. In endogamic Gypsies. Episodes of tachypnea or hypopnea. *Facies.* Hypertelorism, epicanthal folds, broad nasal tip, cleft lip. Rotary nystagmus, oculomotor apraxia, esotropia, angulated ears. Occasionally microphthalmia. Intraoral frenulae, lingual limps palate cleft or high arched. *Limbs.* Hands postaxial polydactyly, less frequently clinodactyly and syndacyly. *Feet.* Bilateral preaxial polydactyly. *Internal anomalies.* Heat, kidney, gonads. Cerebellar defects: motor incoordination delayed or absent speech. Severe mental retardation.

Etiology. Autosomal recessive inheritance.

Pathology. See Signs. Typical: cerebellar defects (including agenesis of vermis or hypoplasia or Dandy-Walker malformation).

Diagnostic Procedures. *Fetal sonography.* (See Signs.) MRI. Hypoplasia of cerebellar vermis.

Therapy. Symptomatic.

Prognosis. Death at an early age.

BIBLIOGRAPHY. Gustavson K-H, Kreuger A, Petersson PO: Syndrome characterized by lingual malformation, polydactyly, tachnypea and psychomotor retardation (Mohr syndrome). Clin Genet 2:261–266, 1971

Varadi V, Szabo L, Papp Z: Syndrome of polydactyly; cleft lip/palate or lingual lump and psychomotor retardation in endogamic gypsies. J Med Genet 17:119–122, 1980

Munke M, McDonald DM, Cronister A, et al: Oral facial-digital syndrome type VI (Varadi syndrome): Further clinical delineation. Am J Med Genet 35:360–369, 1990

VARIOT-PIRONNEAU

Obsolete.

Symptoms and Signs. Similar to Hutchinson-Gilford syndrome (see).

Etiology. Adrenal or pluriglandular deficiency. Familiar occurrence. See multiendocrine deficiency syndromes.

BIBLIOGRAPHY. Variot, Pironneau: Nanisme avec dystrophie osseuse et cutanée speciales: Soupçon d'agénésie des capsules surrénales. Bull Soc Pédiatr Paris 12:307–314, 1910

Valenzano L, Valenzano G: Osservazioni su due casi di: "Sindrome di Rummo e Ferrarini." Boll Ist Dermatol S Gallicano 6:55–72, 1970

VASA PREVIA

Synonym. Placenta vasa previa.

Symptoms. Occurs during the third trimester of pregnancy. Usually rupture of the amniotic sac and slight to moderate vaginal bleeding.

Signs. Irregularities in the fetal heart tones; bradycardia during uterine contractions; vaginal bleeding.

Etiology. Velamentous insertion of the umbilical vessels torn with rupture of the amniotic sac, or rupture because of pressure of the presenting part.

Pathology. Placenta pale; velamentous insertion of the umbilical vessels; rupture in one or more of the umbilical vessels.

Diagnostic Procedures. *Vaginal blood.* Tested for fetal hemoglobin, which is alkaline resistant (adult hemoglobin is not).

Therapy. Once diagnosed, rapid delivery, either vaginally or abdominally.

Prognosis. Maternal: excellent. Fetal: poor, associated with increased mortality.

BIBLIOGRAPHY. Torrey WE Jr: Vasa previa. Am J Obstet Gynecol 63:146–152, 1952

Naftolin F, Mishell DR Jr: "Vasa previa:" Report of 3 cases. Obstet Gynecol 26:561–565, 1965

Dougall A, Baird CH: Vasa praevia-report of three cases and review of literature. Br J Obstet Gynaecol 94:712–715, 1987

VASOVAGAL

Synonyms. Gowers; Nothnagel II; vasodepressor syncope. See orthostatic syncope; Da Costa and Weisenburg.

Symptoms. Most common form of syncope. Onset at any age. *Precipitating factors.* Emotion; fatigue; minor trauma with pain; lack of food or sleep; indigestion; close environment; the sight of blood; or no factor. Patient before syncope is standing, occasionally sitting, never lying down. *Warning symptoms.* Sudden weakness; sweating; dizziness; epigastric discomfort; paresthesia; palpitation; sialorrhea. Syncope may be prevented by lying down when warning symptoms appear. *Syncope.* Loss of consciousness for a few seconds or minutes; occasionally, tonic and clonic movements. After regaining consciousness usually no residue; occasionally nervousness, dizziness, headache. Some patients may experience all symptoms and signs without, however, reaching the complete loss of consciousness.

Signs. Pallor; cold skin; sweating; moderate cyanosis; weak pulse. Bradycardia (sometimes preceded by tachycardia); hypotension.

Etiology. Sudden reflex; loss of peripheral resistance creating a temporary cerebral anoxia.

Diagnostic Procedures. Rule out epilepsy and heart conditions.

Therapy. None. Sympathomimetic drugs only in severe cases.

Prognosis. Good. Attack appears at irregular intervals or according to precipitating factors. During attack patient may injure himself.

BIBLIOGRAPHY. Foster M: Textbook of Physiology, pp 297, 345. London, Macmillan, 1888

Lewis RP, Budoulas H, Schaal SF, et al: Diagnosis and management of syncope. In Schlant RC, Alexander RW: Hurst's The Heart, 8th ed. New York, McGraw-Hill, 1994

Weatherall DJ, Ledingham JGG, Warrell DA (eds): Oxford Textbook of Medicine, 3rd ed, p 2267. Oxford, Oxford Med Pub, 1996

VASQUEZ-HURST-SOTOS

Symptoms and Signs. Evidence of hypogenitalism, gynecomastia, obesity, short stature, skeletal defects (scoliosis, etc.), mental retardation.

Etiology. X-linked inheritance.

BIBLIOGRAPHY. Vasquez SB, Hurst DI, Sotos JF: X-linked hypogonadism, gynecomastia, mental retardation, short stature and obesity: A new syndrome. Pediatrics 83:280–284, 1979

V.A.T.E.R.

Synonyms. Vertebral defects; anal atresia–TE fistula–radial–renal dysplasia; including V.A.T.E.R.S. (and S for single umbilical artery). See Goldenhar.

Symptoms. Both sexes affected. Present from birth. Failure to thrive; slow development, normal intelligence.

Signs. Association of three or more of the following defects: Vertebral anomalies (70%). Ventricular septal defects (53%). Anal atresia (80%). Tracheoesophageal fistula (esophageal atresia) (70%). Radial dysplasia (69%). Renal anomalies (53%). Single umbilical artery (39%). Other abnormalities: inguinal hernias; small intestinal malformations; choanal atresia; cleft lip and/or palate.

Etiology. Unknown. Sporadic occurrence.

Therapy. Symptomatic, medical and surgical.

Prognosis. Variable. If surviving, normal brain function.

BIBLIOGRAPHY. Say B, Gerald PS: A new polydactyly, imperforate anus, vertebral anomalies syndrome. Lancet II:688, 1968

Quan L, Smith DW: The VATER association Vertebral defects, anal atresia, T-E fistula, with esophageal atresia: Radial and Renal dysplasia: A spectrum of associated defects. J Pediatr 82:104–107, 1973

Weaver DD, Mapstone CL, Yu Pao-lo: The VATER association: Analysis of 46 patients. Am J Dis Child 140:225–229, 1986
Jones KL: Smith's Recognizable Patterns of Human Malformation. Philadelphia, WB Saunders, 1988

VENA CAVA, INFERIOR, OBSTRUCTION

Symptoms. According to site and rapidity of obstruction. Vomiting; diarrhea.

Signs. Edema in legs; enlargement of superficial veins of legs, abdomen, chest; occasionally, ascites.

Etiology and Pathology. Congenital; aneurysm; thrombosis; intra-abdominal malignancy; infection; trauma; cirrhosis. Retroperitoneal fibrosis; primary or metastatic (renal cell carcinoma) tumors.

Diagnostic Procedures. *Urine.* Albuminuria. *Blood.* Hyperbilirubinuria, and other liver function tests altered; increased blood urea nitrogen.

Therapy. Surgery difficult. According to etiology. Symptomatic.

Prognosis. Depends on etiology and site of obstruction. Rapid obstruction above renal artery, usually fatal.

BIBLIOGRAPHY. Pleasants J: Obstruction of the inferior vena cava with a report of eighteen cases. Johns Hopkins Hosp 16:363–558, 1911
Joyce JW: The diagnosis and management of diseases of the peripheral arteries and veins. In Schlant RC, Alexander RW: Hurst's The Heart, 8th ed. New York, McGraw-Hill, 1994
Joyce JW: The diagnosis and management of diseases of the peripheral arteries and veins. In Schlant RC, Alexander RW: Hurst's The Heart, 8th ed, p 2193. New York, McGraw-Hill, 1994

VENA CAVA, SUPERIOR, OBSTRUCTION

Synonym. Superior mediastinal.

Symptoms. Predominant in males. Observed at all ages, maximum frequency at 40–50 years of age. *Neck and face.* Venous distention and edema. Dyspnea; orthopnea; dysphagia; hoarseness; epistaxis; headache; vertigo; tinnitus; somnolence; syncope.

Signs. Edema and cyanosis of face, neck, shoulder, and arms; suffused conjunctivae. Varicose veins over shoulder, upper thorax. No edema of lower parts of the body or marked preference of edema for upper part so that a clear line of demarcation may be noticed (short cape edema). Edema and cyanosis of mucous membrane of mouth, pharynx, larynx, hydrothorax; occasionally hydropericardium.

Etiology and Pathology. Any cause compressing or infiltrating superior vena cava and obstructing its circulation. Mediastinal neoplasms and aneurysm of aorta, carcinoma of lung or adjacent structures, thyroid adenoma, and idiopathic causes. Ormond syndrome (see).

Diagnostic Procedures. *X-ray.* Of chest. *CT scan. MRI. Angiography. ECG.*

Therapy. Surgery with decompression whenever feasible. Roentgen therapy.

Prognosis. Depends on etiology and degree of damage.

BIBLIOGRAPHY. Corvisart: Essai sur les Maladies et les Lesions Organiques du Coeur, p 350. Paris, 1806
McArt BA, Ramsey FB, Tosik WA, et al: Surgical reversal of superior vena cava syndrome; report of a case caused by intrathoracic goiter and associated with roentgenographic hilar vascular shadow simulating neoplasm of chest. Arch Surg 69:4–11, 1954
Lokich JJ, Goodman R: Superior vena cava syndrome: Clinical management. JAMA 231:58–61, 1975
Parish JM, Marschke RF Jr, Dines DE, et al: Etiologic considerations in superior vena cava syndrome. Mayo Clin Proc 56:407–413, 1981

Joyce JW: The diagnosis and management of diseases of the peripheral arteries and veins. In Schlant RC, Alexander RW: Hurst's The Heart, 8th ed, p 2193. New York, McGraw-Hill, 1994

VENTRICULAR SEPTAL ANEURYSM

Symptoms and Signs. Both sexes affected. Usually asymptomatic; however, defect may cause complication: conduction disturbances; systemic embolism; aortic or tricuspid regurgitation; obstruction or right ventricular outflow; perforation causing a shunt; subacute bacterial endocarditis.

Etiology. Congenital malformation.

Pathology. Membranous septum continuous with aorta lies above muscular septum; the formed aneurysm protrudes into right ventricle or atrium or both.

Diagnostic Procedures. *ECG. Two-dimensional echocardiography with color flow imaging and spectral Doppler interrogation. Cardiac catheterization. X-ray.* Variable findings.

Therapy. If needed, surgical correction.

Prognosis. Extremely variable. Occasionally, autopsy finding in old persons.

BIBLIOGRAPHY. Laennec RTH.:Traite de l'Auscultation Mediate et des Maladies de Poumons et du Coeur. Ed 2, Paris, JS Chaude, 1826
Freedom RM, White RD, Pieroni DR, et al: The natural history of the so-called aneurysm of the membraneous ventricular septum in childhood. Circulation 49:375–384, 1974
Hoeffel JC, Henry M, Flizet M, et al: Radiologic patterns of aneurysm of the membranous septum. Am Heart J 91:450–456, 1976
Perloff JK: The Clinical Recognition of Congenital Heart Disease, 4th ed, pp 400–401. Philadelphia, WB Saunders, 1994

VENTRUTO

Synonyms. Strabismus-craniosynostosis.

Symptoms and Signs. Both sexes. At birth. Strabismus. Craniosynostosis. Hands and feet: not symmetric anomalies. Synphalangism. Carpal-tarsal fusion. Brachydactyly, absent or hypoplastic nails. Dysplastic hip joints.

Etiology. Autosomal dominant inheritance.

BIBLIOGRAPHY. Ventruto V, Di Girolamo R, Festa B, et al: Family study of inherited syndrome with multiple congenital deformities: symphalangism, carpal and tarsal fusion, brachydactyly, craniosynostosis, strabismus, hip osteochondritis. J Med Genet 13:394–398, 1976
Cohen MM Jr: Craniosynostosis: Diagnosis evaluation and management. New York, Raven Press, 1986

VERALLO-HASERICK

Synonym. Lymphomatoid pityriasis lichenoides.

Symptoms and Signs. Those of Mucha-Habermann (see) with papules, and purpura, plaques, and edema.

Etiology. Unknown.

Pathology. Histology of skin shows colonization with atypical lymphocytes (high nucleus: cytoplasm ratio) and abnormal mitosis.

Therapy. Topical steroids; photochemotherapy (UVB or PUVA).

Prognosis. Chronic course; small number of patients proceed to full Alibert-Bazin (see).

BIBLIOGRAPHY. Verallo VM, Haserick JR: Mucha-Habermann's disease simulating lymphoma cutis: Report of two cases. Arch Derm 94:295–299, 1966

MacKie RM: Lymphomas and leukemias. In Champion RH, Burton JL, Ebling FJG (eds): Rook/Wilkinson/Ebling Textbook of Dermatology, 5th ed, p 2133. Oxford, Blackwell Scientific, 1992

VERBOV

Synonym. Anonychia; flexural pigmentation.

Symptoms and Signs. Both sexes. *Extremities.* Nails of fingers and toes absent; palmar and plantar skin dry, thin, and peeling. *Hair.* Coarse and sparse. *Teeth.* Early caries. *Groin. Axillae.* Mottled hyper-hypopigmentation.

Etiology. Autosomal dominant inheritance.

BIBLIOGRAPHY. Verbov J: Anonychia with bizarre flexural pigmentation: An autosomal dominant dermatosis. Br J Derm 92:469–474, 1975

VERBRYCKE

Synonym. Cholecystohepatic flexure adhesion.

Symptoms. In upright position, dull pain in epigastrium or upper right quadrant; nausea.

Signs. Tenderness and some protective splinting of muscles on right upper quadrant (nonconstant).

Etiology and Pathology. Adherence between gallbladder and hepatic flexure of colon.

Diagnostic Procedures. *Cholecystography.* Normal function of gallbladder. *Barium enema.* Simultaneous examinations of colon and gallbladder reveal the lesion.

Therapy. Cholecystectomy.

Prognosis. Excellent with surgery.

BIBLIOGRAPHY. Verbrycke JR Jr: Adhesions of cholecystohepatic flexure, new syndrome with specific test. JAMA 114:314–316, 1940
Matolo NM (ed): Symposium on biliary disease. Surg Clin N Am 61:765 (whole issue), 1981

VERGER-DEJERINE

Synonyms. Déjerine-Mouzon; Head-Holmes; distorted spacial perception; visual disorientation; cortical sensory; anterior parietal lobe; parietal lobe, anterior. See Riddoch.

Symptoms. Inability to localize stationary or moving object in the three planes of space because of lack of ability to estimate distance and improper judgment of size and length of objects. Visual acuity good; stereoscopic vision seldom lost. In some cases, associated, loss of sense of limb position and movement of body, without participation of primary modalities of sensation and sensory and visual inattention, difficulty in maintaining fixation when object moves; visual agnosia. Possibly body neglect.

Signs. Failure to accommodate and to converge on close object; absence of blinking reflex.

Etiology and Pathology. Bilateral cerebral lesions, posterior part of parietal lobe or surface of occipital lobe. Trauma, hemorrhage.

Diagnostic Procedures. *CT scan. MRI. EEG. Evoked potentials.*

Therapy and Prognosis. According to nature and extent of lesions. Generally poor.

BIBLIOGRAPHY. Verger H: Sur la valeur semeiologique de la stereo-agnosie. Rev Neurol 2:1201–1205, 1902
Head H, Holmes G: Sensory disturbances from cerebral lesions. Brain 34:102, 1911
Déjerine J, Mouzon J: Un nouveau type de syndrome sensitif corticale observè dans un cas de monoplégic corticale dissociée. Rev Neurol 28:1265, 1914–1915
Holmes G: Disturbances of visual orientation. Br J Ophthalmol 2:449–468, 1918
Riddoch G: Visual disorientation in homonymous half fields. Brain 58:376–382, 1935
Adams RD, Victor M: Principles of Neurology, 5th ed, p 145. New York, McGraw-Hill, 1993

VERMA-NAUMOFF

Synonym. Naumoff chondrodystrophy, polydactyly III; short rib polydactyly III; SRP-3; polydactyly, neonatal chondrodystrophy III. See Saldino-Noonan.

Symptoms and Signs. At birth. Fifty percent males. Similar to, but milder manifestations, than Saldino Noonan (see), except for less severe changes in the ilia and long bones. Polydactyly frequently not present; fibulas normal or hypoplastic.

Etiology. Autosomal recessive inheritance.

Pathology. See Saldino-Noonan, plus PAS positive chondrocytic cytoplasmic inclusions (that are not present in Saldino-Noonan).

Diagnostic Procedures. *X-rays. Echography.* Midgestational for prenatal diagnosis. Features less evident if compared with type I (see).

Prognosis. Lethal form.

BIBLIOGRAPHY. Verma IC, Bhargava S, Agarwal S: An autosomal recessive form of lethal chondrodystrophy with severe thoracic narrowing, rhyzoacromelic type of micromelia, polydactyly and genital anomalies. Birth Defects 11:167–174, 1975
Naumoff P, Young LW, Mazer J, et al: Short rib-polydactyly syndrome type 3. Radiology 122:443–447, 1977
Bernstein R, Isdale J, Pinto M, et al: Short rib-polydactyly syndrome: A single or heterogeneous entity? A re-evaluation prompted by four new cases. J Med Genet 22:46–53, 1985
Rimoin DL, Lachman RS: Genetic disorders of the osseous skeleton. In Beithon P (ed): McKusick's Heritable Disorders of Connective Tissue, 5th ed, p 590. St Louis, CV Mosby, 1993

VERMIS AGENESIS

Synonyms. Dandy-Walker (see); Eisenring-Robb-Andermann; Rossi (V).

Symptoms and Signs. The simple agenesis of vermis is not responsible for the clinical manifestations. Patients with vermis agenesis may have intelligence, development, and life span within normal limits. The clinical manifestations are owing to the associated defects. Psychomotor retardation, hypotonia, incoordination, headache, convulsions, and other signs related to obstruction of ventricular system (when present) such as hydrocephalus, midline central nervous system malformations; cranioschisis, myelomeningocele. A better defined syndrome associated with agenesis of vermis has been reported (see Joubert).

Etiology. Unknown. Both agenesis of vermis and associated malformations may be owing in some cases to primitive maldevelopment (familial and sporadic), in others to internal hydrocephalus that has led to the abnormalities during fetal life. Autosomal recessive inheritance to be considered.

Pathology. Two types of defects: complete or partial agenesis. Other midline malformations often encountered, but not necessarily associated (see Symptoms and Signs).

Diagnostic Procedures. *X-ray. CT brain scan. MRI.*

Therapy. Symptomatic or neurosurgical.

Prognosis. Extremely variable according to degree of associated lesions: from death few days after birth to normal life span. The agenesis of vermis per se is not responsible for neurologic or psychic development disorders.

BIBLIOGRAPHY. Rossi V: Un caso di mancanza del lobo mediano del cervelletto con presenza della fossetta occipitale media. Sperimentale 45:518–528, 1891
Joubert M, Eisenring JJ, Robb JP, et al: Familial agenesis of the cerebellar vermis. Neurology 19:813–825, 1969

VERNET

Synonyms. Foramen lacerum posterior; jugular foramen.

Symptoms. Hoarseness; taste alterations; dysphagia for solid food; nasal regurgitation of fluids.

Signs. Paralysis of palate, pharynx, and larynx. Posterior wall of pharynx deviates to unaffected side when tongue is protruded. Tachycardia; paralysis and atrophy of sternocleidomastoid and upper portion of trapezius muscles.

Etiology and Pathology. Trauma; aneurysm; neoplasia involving glossopharyngeal (IX), vagus (X), spinal accessory (XI) nerves in the region of the jugular foramen.

Diagnostic Procedures. *X-rays.* Of skull and esophagus. *Angiography. Brain isotope scan. CT scan. MRI.*

Therapy. Surgery when indicated to remove pressure.

Prognosis. Depends on etiology.

BIBLIOGRAPHY. Vernet M: Les paralysies laryngées associés (thesis), p 233. Lyon, 1916
Vernet M: The classification of syndromes of associated laryngeal paralysis. Med Rev NY:449–458, 1918
Wilson H, Johnson DH: Jugular foramen syndrome as a complication of metastatic cancer of the prostate. So Med J 77:92–93, 1984
Weatherall DJ, Ledingham JGG, Warrell DA (eds): Oxford Textbook of Medicine, 3rd ed, p 3880. Oxford, Oxford Med Pub, 1996

VERTIGO, BENIGN PAROXYSMAL, IN CHILDHOOD

Synonyms. BVP, Basser; vertigo benign, paroxysmal.

Symptoms and Signs. In children 1–4 years. Both sexes. Sudden transient attacks (seconds to minutes) of incapacitating vertigo, postural imbalance, gait of ataxia associated with nystagmus, pallor, nausea, vomiting, no headache or impairment of consciousness. Child is frightened, unable to move, and clutches on to a person or object. Torticollis may be feature of syndrome.

Etiology. In two thirds of cases family history of hemicrania. Hemicrania equivalent, transient vertebro basilar constriction with ischemia of vestibular nuclei.

Diagnostic Procedures. *CT scan. MRI. EEG. Caloric testing:* Normal.

Therapy. Usually none because attacks are self-limited.

Prognosis. Attacks of varying frequency (10/year), sometimes in clusters that cease spontaneously for months or years.

BIBLIOGRAPHY. Basser LS: Benign paroxymal vertigo of childhood. Brain 87:141, 1964

Brand T: Vertigo: Its Multisensory Syndromes, pp 177–179. London, Springer-Verlag, 1912

VERTIGO, BENIGN RECURRENT

Synonyms. BRV; Slater; migraine vertigo.

Symptoms and Signs. Both sexes. Onset 5–55 years. Prevalent in females, personal of family history of migraine precipitated by menstruation, alcohol, lack of sleep, stress. Incapaciting vertigo, postural imbalance, and gait ataxia, spontaneous nystagmus, nausea, vomiting, no headache or impairment of consciousness.

Etiology. Migraine equivalent. Transient vertebrobasilar constriction with ischemia of vestibular nuclei.

Diagnostic Procedures. *CT scan. ECG. MRI. Caloric testing.*

Therapy. Migraine therapy (see). Ergotamine not useful.

Prognosis. Attack of varying frequency, benign course.

BIBLIOGRAPHY. Slater R: Benign recurrent vertigo. J Neurol Neurosurg Psychiat 42:363–367, 1979
Brand T: Vertigo: Its Syndromes, pp 179–180. London, Springer-Verlag, 1991
Herdman SJ, Tusa RJ, Zee DS: Single treatment approaches to benign paroxysmal positional vertigo. Arch Otorinolaryng Head Neck Surg 119:450–454, 1993

VERTIGO, POSITIONAL NYSTAGMUS, HYPEROSMOLAR

Synonyms. Hyperosmolar vertigo, positional nystagmus; including Positional alcohol nystagmus (PAN).

Symptoms and Signs. Same as Barany but lasting longer (hours) and not induced by head tilting.

Etiology. Gravity differential between cupola and endolymph causing either a positional (alcohol, glycerol, heavy water [D_2O], macroglobulinemia) or a positioning vertigo–nystagmus (cupololithiasis).

Diagnostic Procedures. According to pre-existing pathology.

Therapy. That of basic condition.

Prognosis. According to etiology. Lasting from 1 hour (glycerol) to 12 hours (alcohol).

BIBLIOGRAPHY. Brandt T: Vertigo: Its Multisensory Syndromes, pp 153–158. London, Springer-Verlag, 1991

VESICA PUDICA

Synonym. Shy bladder.

Symptoms and Signs. Inability to initiate urinary flow (or a long delay) when other person is watching or waiting in line in public toilets; or when the micturition has to be performed in unusual places (train, airplane, or in the open country).

Etiology. Psychoneurologic reflex. Of interest only because it may help some people once they hear about its existence in other people.

VESICOURETERAL REFLUX

Synonyms. Innes Williams; megaureter-megacystis; primary ureteral reflux; VUR.

Symptoms. Repeated urinary tract infections in children, temporarily cured by antibiotics.

Signs. Dilated, refluxing ureters and a large, thin-walled bladder.

Etiology. Primary ureteral reflux. The ureteral reflux may be caused by lack of development of trigonal muscles, or other mechanisms. The so-called megacystis with thin-walled bladder is secondary and caused by the distensibility of the bladder walls of children. Multifactorial or mendelian (autosomal dominant) trait reported.

Diagnostic Procedures. *Urine.* Culture. Excretory urography. Normal or scarred dilated calices and irregular ureters. Cystourethrography. Large, thin-walled bladder extending outside bony pelvis; ureters and pelvis ballooned out; normal voiding of urethra and emptying of bladder.

Therapy. Assessment of degree of reflux. *Grade 1* (lower ureteral filling) and *Grade 2* (ureteral and pelvicaliceal without pelvic dilatation). Antibiotics (1-year trial); if failure, surgery. *Grade 3* (grade 2 plus pelvic dilatation). Antibacterial agents or surgery debated. *Grade 4.* Direct surgery followed by antibiotics. Tunnel reimplantation of ureters, anchoring the bladder wall near the neck, without revising the bladder neck (Politano-Leadbetter technique).

Prognosis. Good with adequate and timely treatment.

BIBLIOGRAPHY. Kretschmer HL, Greer JR: Insufficiency at the ureterovesical junction. Surg Gynecol Obstet 21:228–231, 1915

Paquin AJ Jr, Marshal VF, McGovern JH: The megacystis syndrome. J Urol 83:634–646, 1960

Harrow BR: The myth of the megacystis syndrome. J Urol 98:205, 1967

Forland M: Urinary tract infections. In Massry SG, Glassock RJ: Textbook of Nephrology, 3rd ed, pp 774–775. Baltimore, Williams & Wilkins, 1995

Weatherall DJ, Ledingham JGG, Warrell DA (eds): Oxford Textbook of Medicine, 3rd ed, pp 3214–3220. Oxford, Oxford Med Pub, 1996

VESSEL

Synonyms. Cushing symphalangism; symphalangism, proximal.

Symptoms and Signs. Symphalangism. Fusion of carpal and tarsal bones. Conductive deafness frequent association. Strabismus.

Etiology. Unknown. Autosomal dominant inheritance.

Therapy. Surgical approach to correct symphalangism unsuccessful.

BIBLIOGRAPHY. Cushing H: Hereditary ankylosis of proximal phalanges joints (symphalangism). Genetics 1:90–106, 1916

Vessel ES: Symphalangism, strabismus and hearing loss in mother and daughter. N Engl J Med 263:839–842, 1960

Cremer C, Theunissen E, Kuijpers W: Proximal symphalangy and stages ankylosis. Arch Otolaryngol 111:765–767, 1985

VESTERMARK-VESTERMARK

Synonyms. Wiskott-Aldrich variant; Canales-Mauer; sex-linked thrombocytopenia. See Thrombocytopenias, X-linked.

Symptoms and Signs. Appears almost only in males. Only one female reported (lyonization). Onset in childhood. Purpura; epistaxis; easy bruising; pallor; absence of eczema.

Etiology. Sex-linked inheritance. Raised question of its distinctness from Wiskott-Aldrich.

Diagnostic Procedures. *Blood.* Hypochromic anemia; thrombocytopenia; leukoctyes normal or decreased. Evidence of immunologic defect. *Bone marrow.* Normal or moderate erythroid hyperplasia.

Therapy. Moderate response to corticosteroids. Occasional benefit from splenectomy.

Prognosis. Greatest severity in childhood, then chronic course.

BIBLIOGRAPHY. Vestermark B, Vestermark S: Familial sex-linked thrombocytopenia. Arch Pediatr 53:369–370, 1964

Ata M, Fisher OD, Holman CA: Inherited thrombocytopenia. Lancet 1:119–123, 1965

Canales L, Mauer AM: Sex-linked hereditary thrombocytopenia as a variant of Wiskott-Aldrich syndrome. N Engl J Med 277:899–901, 1967

Cohn J, Hange M, Andersen V, et al: Sex-linked hereditary thrombocytopenia with immunologic defect. Hum Hered 25:309–317, 1975

Donner M, Schwartz M, Carlson KU, et al: Hereditary X-linked thrombocytopenia maps to the same chromosomal region as the Wiskott-Aldrich syndrome. Blood 72:1849–1853, 1988

VESTIBULAR AREFLEXIA, FAMILIAL

Synonyms. Verhagen; familial vestibular areflexia.

Symptoms and Signs. Onset about 40 years, progressive hearing loss, tinnitus, head movement dependent. Oscillopsia and instability in the dark (vestibular areflexia).

Etiology. Autosomal dominant inheritance.

BIBLIOGRAPHY. Verhagen WIM, Huygen PLM, Horstink NWIM: Familial congenital vestibular areflexia. J Neurol Neurosurg Psychiatr 50:933–935, 1987

Verhagen WIM, Huygen PLM: Familial progressive vestibulocochlear dysfunction. Arch Neurol 48:262, 1991

VESTIBULAR EPILEPSY

Synonyms. Epilepsy vestibular. See Sensory seizures syndromes.

Symptoms. Both sexes. Onset at various ages. Sudden rotational or linear vertigo with contraversive to lesion body or head and eye rotation lasting seconds or minutes. Occasionally tinnitus, controlateral paresthesia, contraversive nystagmus. Nausea usually moderate or absent.

Etiology. Congenital lesions, tumors, hemorrhage, ischemia, trauma, infections, and intoxications (cysplatinum). Epileptic discharges of vestibular cortex.

Pathology. Lesion involving intraparietal sulcus, superior temporal gyrus, or caudal part of postcentral gyrus.

Diagnostic Procedures. *EEG.* Abnormal pattern and lateral temporal epileptic foci. *CT scan. MRI.*

Therapy. Anticonvulsants: carbamazepine, phenytoine, valproate. Surgery for focal epilepsy.

Prognosis. According to etiology.

BIBLIOGRAPHY. Bumke O, Foerster O (eds): Handbuch der Neurologie, vol 6. Berlin, Springer, 1936

Brandt T: Vertigo: Its Multisensory Syndromes, pp 91–97. London, Springer Verlag, 1991

VESTIBULAR NEURITIS

Synonyms. Dix-Hallpike; Pedersen; neurolabyrinthitis; epidemic vertigo; vestibular neuronitis.

Symptoms. Occurs in young adulthood or from third to fifth decades. Onset abrupt, associated with upper respiratory infections. Vertigo (without concomitant auditory dysfunction); nausea and vomiting. Head movements enhance the symptoms. Tinnitus rare.

Signs. Fever, gait, and stance disturbed. Fall toward lesioned ear; horizontal rotatory spontaneous nystagmus (fast phase away from lesioned ear). Absent response to caloric stimulation on one side, nystagmus with quick component to the opposite side. Normal hearing; occasionally response positive on both sides.

Etiology. Viral neuritis of vestibular nerve, but limited usually to the superior division (horizontalsemicircular canal paresis) and sparing the inferior part. Labyrinthine or vestibular nerve ischemia considered also among the etiologic hypothesis.

Pathology. From rare autopsies. Lesions of nerve fibers to horizontal and anterior semicircular canal.

Diagnostic Procedures. *Cochlear function.* Normal. *Hearing.* Normal. *Caloric response.* Reduced bilaterally.

Therapy. During first 1–3 days of nausea and vomiting, vestibular sedatives: dramamine 50–100 mg every 6 hours, or scopolamine 0.6 mg. After physical exercise (modified Cawthorne-Cocksey) to rest or central compensation.

Prognosis. Transient and benign condition. Gradual recovery in 1–6 weeks.

BIBLIOGRAPHY. Ruttin Zur Differentialdiagnose der Labyrinth-und Hoernerverkrankungen. Z Ohrenheilk 57:327–331, 1909
Pedersen E: Epidemic vertigo: Clinical picture, epidemiology and relation to encephalitis. Brain 82:566–580, 1959
Dix MR, Hallpike CS: The pathology, symptomatology and diagnosis of certain common disorders of vestibular system. Proc R Soc Med 45:341–347, 1962
Brandt T: Vertigo: Its Multisensorial Syndromes, p 29. London, Springer-Verlag, 1991
Weatherall DJ, Ledingham JGG, Warrell DA (eds): Oxford Textbook of Medicine, 3rd ed, p 3876. Oxford, Oxford Med Pub, 1996

VESTIBULAR PARALYSIS, BILATERAL

Symptoms and Signs. Patients stagger and walk zigzag, more so after dark; cannot swim and become disoriented in the water; have no sense of depth with the eyes closed but no difficulty with eyes open. Loss of hearing is often associated.

Etiology and Pathology. Infective process bilaterally affecting the vestibular system in any site between the semicircular canals and the vestibular nuclei in the brain. Usually, vasculitic type of lesions (e.g., scrub typhus, scarlet fever, syphilis). Neoplasms.

Diagnostic Procedures. *Rotation and caloric stimulation.* Does not elicit vertigo, unsteadiness, nausea; nystagmus because of inability to maintain ocular fixation. *Galvanic stimulation.* Elicits nystagmus and unsteadiness in semicircular canal lesions but not in central lesions (ganglion, nerves, nuclei). *Audiometry.* Hearing lost in central lesions, not in semicircular canal lesions. *Search for specific agent of infection.* Culture, complement fixation, antibodies.

Therapy. Specific for infection or neoplasm.

Prognosis. Lesions may be persistent.

BIBLIOGRAPHY. James W: The sense of dizziness in deaf-mutes. Am J Otol 4:239–254, 1882
Chusid J, DeGutierrez-Mahoney CG: Syndrome of bilateral vestibular paralysis. J Nerv Ment Dis 103:172–180, 1946
Brandt T: Vertigo: Its Multisensorial Syndromes. London, Springer-Verlag, 1991

VIBRATORY ANGIOEDEMA

Synonym. Angioedema, vibratory.

Symptoms and Signs. Stimulation of frictional or vibratory type triggers severe local reaction followed by generalized erythema and cephalea.

Etiology. Autosomal dominant inheritance.

Diagnostic Procedures. *Venous blood.* From area submitted to stimulation, increase of amine levels.

BIBLIOGRAPHY. Patterson R, Mellies CJ, Blankenship ML, et al: Vibratory angioedema: A hereditary type of physical hypersensitivity. J Allergy Clin Immun 50:174–182, 1972
Lawlor F, Black AK, Breathnach AS, et al: Vibratory angioedema: Lesion induction, clinical features, laboratory and ultrastructural findings and response to therapy. Br J Dermatol 120:93–96, 1989
Weatherall DJ, Ledingham JGG, Warrell DA (eds): Oxford Textbook of Medicine, 3rd ed, pp 1225–1227. Oxford, Oxford Med Pub, 1996

VIDAL

Synonyms. Toyama, Brocq I; pityriasis circinata; pityriasis rotunda; pseudoichthyosis acquired.

Symptoms. Common in Far East populations, less in South Africans, Bantus, Egyptians, and West Indians; onset at 7–76 years of age. Pregnancy or infection may precipitate onset.

Signs. Appearance of solitary or multiple round patches of dry scaling, without inflammatory changes, on the buttocks, thighs, abdomen, back, arms.

Etiology. Unknown. Genetic factors postulated.

Pathology. Mild hyperkeratitic changes in areas affected.

Therapy. None. Keratin stripping: temporary effect.

Prognosis. Life-long lesions.

BIBLIOGRAPHY. Vidal E: Du lichen (Lichen, prurigo, strophulus) Ann Dermatol Syph (Paris) 7:133–154, 1866
Toyama I: Isshu no Kasshoku enkei rakushosei hifubyo ni tsnite. Jpn Derm 6:91–105, 1906
Arndt KA, Pane BS, Stern RS, et al: Treatment of pityriasis rosea with UV radiation. Arch Dermatol 9:381–382, 1983
Highet AS, Kurtz J: Viral infections. In Champion RH, Burton JL, Ebling FJG (eds): Rook/Wilkinson/Ebling Textbook of Dermatology, 5th ed, p 950. Oxford, Blackwell Scientific, 1992

VILANOVA-AGUADÉ

Synonyms. Nodular migratory panniculitis; sclerodermiform panniculitis; erythema nodosum migrans. See Bazin and Whitfield syndromes.

Symptoms. Seldom in males; previous history of acute tonsillitis frequent. Trauma often preceding first lesion. Nodule or plaque (singly or in crops) on one leg (usually ankle region) expanding or joining to form a large erythematous plaque of hard successive eruptions. Consistent for weeks or months; always limited to legs.

Etiology. Unknown. Variant of erythema nodosum (see). Alpha 1 proteinase inhibitor deficiency in same cases.

Pathology. *Early.* Epithelial proliferation occluding capillaries and small vessels. Infiltration with lymphocytes, monohisticytes, and fibroblasts. *Later.* Only giant cells. Skin and subcutaneous restitutio ad integrum as lesion regresses.

Therapy. Treatment of focal infections if identified. Potassium iodide 360–900 mg/day for 4 weeks (watch for side effects). Dapsone?

Prognosis. Spontaneous remission after variable time. Recurrences also after long periods.

BIBLIOGRAPHY. Vilanova X, Piñol Aguadé JP: Hypodermite nodulaire subaiguë migratrice. Ann Derm Syph 83:369–404, 1956
Vilanova X, Piñol Aguadé JP: Subacute nodular migratory panniculitis. Br J Derm 71:45–50, 1959

Ryan TJ: Cutaneous vasculitis. In Champion RH, Burton JL, Ebling FJG (eds): Rook/Wilkinson/Ebling Textbook of Dermatology, 5th ed, pp 1938–1939. Oxford, Blackwell Scientific, 1992

VILLARET

Synonyms. Parotid posterior space; retroparotid space. See Collet-Sicard.

Symptoms and Signs. Ipsilateral paralysis of soft palate, pharynx, and vocal cords (see Collet-Sicard), associated with Horner syndrome.

Etiology and Pathology. Trauma, infections, neoplasm involving last four cranial nerves (ninth through 12th) and cervical sympathetic chain.

Diagnostic Procedures. *X-ray.* Of skull. *Angiography. CT brain scan. MRI. Culture.* If infection.

Therapy. Surgical, according to etiology, to relieve nerve involved.

Prognosis. Depends on etiology.

BIBLIOGRAPHY. Villaret M: Le syndrome nerveux de l'espace rétro-parotidien postérieur. Rev Neurol (Paris) 23:188–190, 1916
Adams RD, Victor M: Principles of Neurology, 5th ed, p 591. New York, McGraw-Hill, 1993

VILLARET-DESOILLES

Synonyms. Peters-Hoevels; maxillofacial dysostosis; dysostosis maxillofacial dysplasia.

Symptoms and Signs. Bilateral hypoplasia of malar bones; antimongoloid obliquity of lids without colobomas; open bite; excessive development of lower jaw.

Etiology. Unknown. Autosomal dominant inheritance.

BIBLIOGRAPHY. Villaret R, Desoilles H: L'hypoplasie primitive familiale du maxillaire supérieur. Ann Med 32:378–381, 1932
Peters A, Hoevels O: Die dysostosis maxillofacialis, eine erbliche, typische Fehlbildung des I. Visceralbogens. Z menschl Vererb Konstitutionslehre 35:434–444, 1960
Melnick M, Eastman JR: Autosomal dominant maxillofacial dysostosis. Birth Defects Orig Art Series XIII (3B):39–44, 1977

VINCENT

Synonyms. Plaut; fusospirochetal gingivitis.

Symptoms and Signs. In young adults and smokers. Sudden onset. Pain; bleeding of gums; typical foul breath; regional lymphoadenitis; hypertermia; intense malaise. At the level of interdental spaces in particular punched-out ulcers sometimes diffusing to oropharyngeal mucosa with marked erythema (Vincent angina).

Etiology. Mixed bacterial, Gram-negative (fusobacterial, veillonella, bacteriodes, leptotrichia) responsible for the lesions by endotoxin activity; plus predisposing factors (poor oral hygiene, defective restoration and pericoronitis, lowered general resistance).

Pathology. Gingival acute inflammatory reaction leading to polynuclear and fibrinous infiltration and necrosis with thrombosis of small vessels.

Diagnostic Procedures. *Culture.* Of swabs.

Therapy. Metronidazole; phenoxymethyl penicillin. Topical hydrogen peroxide and other oxidizing agents useful. Forceful rinsing with saline.

Prognosis. Without proper treatment, acute phase may spontaneously regress but frequently leaves recurrent ulcerative gingivitis; halitosis, recession, gingival bleeding.

BIBLIOGRAPHY. Plaut HC: Studien zur bacteriellen Diagnostick der Diphtherie und der anginen. Deut Med Wschr 20:920–923, 1894
Vincent JH: Sur l'étiologie et sur les lésions anatomo-pathologiques de pouriture d'hopital. Ann Inst Pasteur 10:488–510, 1896
Lehner T: The mouth and the salivary glands. In Weatherall DJ, Ledingham JGG, Warrell DA (eds): Oxford Textbook of Medicine, 3rd ed, pp 1852–1853. Oxford, Oxford Med Pub, 1996

VISCEROSPINAL SYNDROMES

This term designates confusing intra-abdominal symptoms that are manifestations of a radiculitis or myositis (see Trigger point). Symptoms of appendicitis, gallbladder disease, ureteral colic, and cardiovascular diseases may be found. Treatment of nerve irritation, once the trigger point is identified, leads to the disappearance of all symptoms.

BIBLIOGRAPHY. Ussher NT: Spinal curvatures-visceral disturbances in relation thereto. Calif West Med 38:423–428, 1933
Ussher NT: The viscerospinal syndrome: A new concept of visceromotor and sensory changes in relation to deranged spinal structures. Ann Intern Med 13:2057–2090, 1940
Strong EK, Davila JC: The cluneal nerve syndrome: A distinct type of low back pain. Indust Med S 26:417–429, 1957
Haubrich WS: Abdominal pain. In Haubrich WS, Schaffner F, Berk JE (eds): Bockus Gastroenterology, 5th ed, vol 2, p 28. Philadelphia, WB Saunders, 1995

VISSER

Synonyms. Aldosterone deficiency I; 18-hydroxylase deficiency; salt-wasting; hypoaldosteronism, primary; corticosterone methyloxidase, type I deficiency; CMO I deficiency; see adrenal hyperplasia syndromes.

Symptoms and Signs. Rare. From birth. Dehydration; intermittent fever; seldom, vomiting; failure to gain weight. Alterations of sexual characteristics are not present.

Etiology. Autosomal recessive inheritance. Deficiency of 18-hydroxylase; which converts corticosterone to aldosterone, hence no aldosterone production.

Pathology. At autopsy. Adrenals grossly normal. Histology. Glomerulosa with tubular empty areas.

Diagnostic Procedures. *Blood.* Hypernatremia; hypokalemia. *Urine.* 17-ketosteroids; 17-ketogenic steroids and hydroxycorticosteroids: normal total excretion; aldosterone absent.

Therapy. Desoxycorticosterone acetate.

Prognosis. Good results with therapy.

BIBLIOGRAPHY. Visser HKA, Cost WS: A new hereditary defect in the biosynthesis of aldosterone: urinary C21-corticosteroid pattern in three related patients with salt losing syndrome suggesting an 18-oxidation defect. Acta Endocrinol 47:589–612, 1964
White PC, New MI, Dupond B: Congenital adrenal hyperplasia. N Engl J Med 316:1580–1586, 1987
Melby JC, Azar ST: Hypoaldosteronism and mineralocorticoid resistance. In De Groot LJ (ed): Endocrinology, 3rd ed, pp 1804–1805. Philadelphia, WB Saunders, 1995

VISUAL VERTIGO

Synonyms. Ocular vertigo, visual ataxia, height vertigo, fisiological visual vertigo, distance vertigo.

Symptoms and Signs. In all subjects with appropriate stimulation consisting of: distortion of tilt of three-dimensional visual environment (tilted rooms, distorting mirrors), height (critical distance between eye and visual surroundings), moving visual fields, angular motion, etc. Vertigo and nystagmus receding after suppression of stimuli.

Etiology. Physiological mechanism owing to critical distance between eye and visual surroundings.

BIBLIOGRAPHY. Darwin E: Zoonomia or the laws of organic life. Vol I of Johnson J: Vertigo, pp 227–239. London, 1794
Bandt T: Vertigo: Its Multisensory Syndromes, pp 233–275. London, Springer-Verlag, 1991

VITROCORNEAL TOUCH

Synonyms. Cataract extraction; postcataract extraction; vitreous touch; intermittent touch postinsertion or iatrogenic endothelial damage; pseudophathic bullous kerathopathy.

Symptoms. Onset usually 2–3 weeks after cataract extraction or after intraocular lens implantation. Severe visual loss and irregular astigmatism because of irregularity of corneal surface.

Signs. Central cornea shows area of diminished transparency and edema; iris bombé; bullous keratopathy.

Etiology. Collection of fluid between corneal epithelial cells or inhibition of epithelial cells usually initially involving the basal layer and then leading to intracellular edema. The hydrophic swelling may lead to necrosis of affected cells and formation of intraepithelial microcysts. The bulla is created when cleavage plane forms between corneal epithelium and underlying Bowan membrane.

Pathology. In late stages bullous canthi is replaced by organized fibrous tissue.

Therapy. Penetrating keratoplastic. Corneal transplantation.

Prognosis. Good results with corneal transplantation.

BIBLIOGRAPHY. Leahey BD: Bullous keratitis vitreous from contact. Arch Ophthalmol 46:22–28, 1951
Gostin SB: Vitrocorneal touch syndrome. So Med J 65:741–766, 1972
Drews RC: Intermittent touch syndrome. Arch Ophthalmol 100:1440–1441, 1982
Klintworth GK, Garner A: The causes types and morphology of cataracts. In Garner A, Klintworth GK (eds): Pathobiology of Ocular Disease: A Dynamic Approach, 2nd ed, p 519. New York, Marcel Dekker, 1994

VOCAL CORD NODULES

Symptoms and Signs. Female predominance. Most frequent functional voice disorder in children, frequently associated with vocal abuse, singing out of range high-stress occupations. Longstanding fluctuant voice dysfunction with changes in voice quality.

Etiology. Vocal abuse.

Diagnostic Procedures. *Laryngoscopy. Frequency (pitch) analysis. Waveform analysis. Spectrography. Laryngeal airway resistance.*

Therapy. Voice rest and therapy; refrain from smoking.

Prognosis. High percentage of good response to treatment.

BIBLIOGRAPHY. Koufman JA, Blalock PD: Functional voice disorders. Otolaryngol Clin N Am 24:1059–1073, 1991

VOCAL PROCESS ULCER/GRANULOMA

Symptoms and Signs. Onset acute (days to weeks); occasionally intermittent for months, painful speaking, vocal fatigue, changes in voice quality.

Etiology. Associated with chronic throat clearing; endotracheal injury (i.e., intubation); vocal abuse; gastroesophageal reflux; poor breath support (use of long uninterrupted sentences).

Pathology. Unilateral or bilateral vocal process ulceration or granuloma.

Diagnostic Procedures. *Laryngoscopy. Frequency (pitch) analysis. Waveform analysis. Spectrography. Laryngeal airway resistance.*

Therapy. Voice rest and therapy; refrain from smoking; anti-inflammatory agents.

Prognosis. High percentage of good response to treatment.

BIBLIOGRAPHY. Koufman JA, Blalock PD: Functional voice disorders. Otolaryngol Clin N Am 24:1059–1073, 1991

VOERNER I

Synonyms. Vörner; haloderma; knuckle pads-keratosis palmoplantaris; hyperkeratosis, localized epidermolytic; palmoplantar keratoderm-epidermolytic variant; keratoderma, epidermolytic palmoplantar. See other keratoderma syndromes.

Symptoms and Signs. Both sexes. From early infancy: Those of keratosis palmoplantar. Frequently associated with knuckle-pad-like lesions.

Etiology. Familial occurrence (autosomal dominance and possibly recessive inheritance) reported.

Pathology. Differentiating characteristic is the presence of histologic and kinetic findings of epidermolysis.

Diagnostic Procedures. *Blood.* Reported increase of IgE in one family.

Therapy. See other keratolytic syndromes.

BIBLIOGRAPHY. Voerner H: Zur kenntnis des Keratomas hereditarium palmare et plantare. Arch Dermatol Syph 56:3–31, 1901
Schwann J: Keratosis palmaris et plantaris cum surditate congenita et leukonychia totally unguium. Dermatologica 126:335–353, 1963
Nogita T, Nakagawa H, Ishibashi Y: Hereditary epidermolytic palmoplantar keratoderma with knuckle pad-like lesions over finger joints. Br J Dermatol 125:496, 1991

VOERNER II

Synonyms. Nevus anemicus; nevus avasculosus.

Symptoms. Both sexes affected. Onset at birth or in early childhood. Asymptomatic.

Signs. On face, chest, or back of neck, irregularly shaped area of pale skin, occasionally multiple areas. Diascopic pressure cancels difference with surrounding skin. Cold-heat application does not produce erythema, in contrast to surrounding skin.

Etiology. Developmental (functional) anomaly. Consistent with autosomal dominant inheritance. Impaired blood supply.

Pathology. Normal histology.

Diagnostic Procedures. *Diascopy. Iontophoresis.* With acetylcholine. No dilatation, epinephrine does not increase pallor of the affected area.

Therapy. None. Cosmetic cream.

Prognosis. Lesion persisting for life.

BIBLIOGRAPHY. Piorkowski FO: Nevus Anemicus (Voerner). Arch Derm Syph 54:374–377, 1944
Butterworth T, Walter JD: Observation on pharmacologic responses of Voerner's nevus anemicus. Arch Derm Syph 66:333–339, 1952
Cardoso H, Vignale R, Abren de Sastre H: Familial naevus anemicus. Am J Hum Genet 27:24A, 1975

Atherton DJ: Naevi and other developmental defects. In Champion RH, Burton JL, Ebling FJG (eds): Rook/Wilkinson/Ebling Textbook of Dermatology, 5th ed, pp 494–495. Oxford, Blackwell Scientific, 1992

VOGT (A.) I

Synonym. Nuclear diffuse cataract; aculeiform cataract, including: frosted cataract; coralliform cataract (Nettleship); fusiform cataract; pisciform cataract; spirochetiform cataract, dilacerated cataract; spear cataract.

Symptoms. Variable degree of visual impairment.

Signs. Frost-like, whitish threads in superficial layers of embryonic nucleus that may be diffusely gray (congenital diffuse nuclear cataract of Vogt) or white (total nuclear cataract) or extending between anterior and posterior pole (fusiform cataract) or other varieties: pisciform cataract; spirochetiform, floriform, spear, dilacerated.

Etiology. Unknown. Autosomal dominant inheritance; recessive also suspected.

Pathology. Fine granular deposits (breaks) in Bawman layer.

Therapy. Corneal transplantation.

BIBLIOGRAPHY. Nettleship E: Seven new pedigrees of hereditary cataract. Trans Ophthal Soc UK 29:188–211, 1909

Vogt A: Weitere Ergebmisse der Spaltlampen Mikroscopie des vorden Bulbusatschnittes (Cornea, Vorderkrammer, Iris, vorder Glaskorper, Conjunctive, Lidrendev). Albrecht Von Graefes Arch Ophthalmol 106:63–103, 1921

Gifford SR, Puntenney I: Coralliform cataract and a new form of congenital cataract with crystals in the lens. Arch Ophthalmol 17:885–892, 1937

Jordan M: Stammbaumuntersuchungen bei Cataracta stellata coralliformis. Klin Monatsbl Augenheilkd 126:467–469, 1955

Klintworth GK, Garner A: The causes, types and morphology of cataracts. In Garner A, Klintworth GK (eds): Pathobiology of Ocular Disease: A Dynamic Approach, 2nd ed, p 493. New York, Marcel Dekker, 1994

VOGT (A.) II

Synonym. Cornea guttata. See Vogt I.

Symptoms and Signs. Both sexes affected with equal incidence. Onset after 40 years of age (70%). Variable visual impairment. Cornea with numerous central fine, wart-like excrescences on Descemet membrane, which spreads progressively toward periphery.

Etiology. Autosomal dominant inheritance (?).

Pathology. Endothelium of cornea hexagonal aspect disturbed; cells irregular in shape and size; golden brown pigmentation; pigment deposition on corneal posterior surface.

BIBLIOGRAPHY. Vogt A: Weitere Ergebnisse der Spaltlampen mikroscopie des vorden Bulbusabschnittes. III. Augeborene und Fruherworbene linsenveranderung. Albrecht von Graefes Arch Ophthalmol 107:196–240, 1922

Klintworth GK, Garner A: The causes types and morphology of cataracts. In Garner A, Klintworth GK (eds): Pathobiology of Ocular Disease: A Dynamic Approach, 2nd ed, p 493. New York, Marcel Dekker, 1994

VOGT (A.) III

Synonyms. Cornea farinata; floury cornea. See Vogt I.

Symptoms and Signs. Both sexes affected. Onset in old age. Variable visual impairment. In the cornea, fine, floury, dusty layer in a restricted area of posterior stroma, anterior to Descemet membrane.

Etiology. Unknown. Type of heredity not established.

BIBLIOGRAPHY. Vogt A: Neure Ergebnisse der Spaltlampen mikroscopie. Schweiz Med Wochenschr 53:989–995, 1923

Klintworth GK, Garner A: The causes types and morphology of cataracts. In Garner A, Klintworth GK (eds): Pathobiology of Ocular Disease: A Dynamic Approach, 2nd ed. New York, Marcel Dekker, 1994

VOGT (A.) IV

Synonyms. Crocodile shagreen; mosaic corneal degeneration.

Symptoms and Signs. Both sexes affected. Onset at 15–72 years of age. Variable visual impairment. Unilateral or bilateral cornea flat, gray, polygonal opacities at Bowman membrane level (axial mosaic). A deep crocodile shagreen or a tear in Bowman layer may be associated.

Etiology. Autosomal dominant inheritance if associated with megalocornea; X-lined inheritance; or acquired form from trauma.

Pathology. Calcific band keropathy, small basophilic granules in Bowman layer, in post-traumatic cases evident break of Bowman layer.

Prognosis. May have a progressive course

BIBLIOGRAPHY. Vogt A: Lehrbuch und Atlas der Spaltlampen Mikroscopie des Lebenden Augens. Berlin, Springer, 1930

Krochmer JH, Dubord PJ, Rodriguez MM, et al: Corneal posterior crocodile shagreen and polymorphic amyloid degeneration: A histopathologic study. Arch Ophthal 101:54–59, 1983

Klintworth GK: Degenerations depositions and miscellaneous reaction of the ocular anterior segment. In Garner A, Klintworth GK (eds): Pathobiology of Ocular Disease: A Dynamic Approach, 2nd ed, p 757. New York, Marcel Dekker, 1994

VOGT-KOYANAGI-HARADA

Synonyms. Alopecia; poliosis; uveitis; vitiligo; deafness; cutaneous—uveo—oto; VKH. See Harada.

Symptoms and Signs. Onset at 20–50 years. No sex or race preference. *Prodromal phase (meningeal).* Nausea; emesis; fever; headache; drowsiness; vertigo. Various other neurologic signs may appear during this phase, or later; Kernig, Brudzinski signs; acute brain syndrome; paresis of cranial nerves (usually unilateral); hemiparesis; aphasia. *Ophthalmic phase.* One or two weeks later, eye irritation; photophobia; and rapid vision loss. Signs of granular inflammation of iris, ciliary body, and retina. According to degree of inflammation, edema; secondary glaucoma; and partial or total detachment of retina may develop. *Convalescent phase.* During the course of several weeks, intermittent symptoms and progression after the subsidence of acute stage, the following additional manifestations appear: poliosis; leukoderma; alopecia; skin pigmentation, sensitive, easily sunburned, paresthetic; canities; dysacusia; tinnitus. Acute neurologic signs and ocular symptoms and signs remit, whereas neurologic and ophthalmic damage may persist unchanged or improved (see Prognosis).

Etiology. Unknown. Viral inflammation theory. Allergic sensitivity of pigmented structures.

Pathology. Central nervous system. During acute stage diffuse adhesive inflammatory arachnoiditis in the brain and spinal cord. *Eyes.* Typical acute bilateral uveitis; retinal detachment. After convalescent stage, from complete remission and reattachment of retina, to permanent detachment, cataracts, scarring, and retraction of entire globe. *Skin.* Irregular spot of depigmentation (neurotrophic type); hair depigmentation frequently following distribution of cutaneous nerves.

Diagnostic Procedures. Acute phase. *Cerebrospinal fluid.* Pleocytosis and increase of protein and pressure. *EEG.* Changes. *Blood.* Normal; serology negative. *Urine.* Normal. *X-rays.* Negative. *Skin tests.* For tuberculosis, coccidioidomycosis, and blastomycosis: negative.

Therapy. Large doses of steroids.

Prognosis. Through the different phases, the natural course of the disease is of about 1 year with possible relapse during this period and no further progression or relapses later. From complete remission to serious sequelae: blindness; total or partial deafness; personality changes and psychosis; persistent aphasia. Neurologic deficit and endocrine complications from involvement of pituitary gland. Steroids may shorten the course and prevent most of the complications.

BIBLIOGRAPHY. Vogt A: Fruhzeitiges ergrauen der Zilien und bemerkungen über den sogenannten plotzlichen Eintritt dieser Veranderung. Klin Augenheilkd 44:228–242, 1906
Harada E: Beitrage zur klinischen Kernitis von nichteitriger Choroiditis. Nippon Ganka Gakkai Zasshi 30:356–361, 1926
Koyanagi Y: Dysakusis, Alopecia und Poliosis bei schwerer Uveitis nichttraumitischen Ursprunges. Klin Monatsbl Augenheilkd 82:194–211, 1929
Forster CS: Ocular manifestations of immune disease. Garner A, Klintworth GK (eds): Pathobiology of Ocular Disease: A Dynamic Approach, 2nd ed, pp 174–176. New York, Marcel Dekker, 1994
Weatherall DJ, Ledingham JGG, Warrell DA (eds): Oxford Textbook of Medicine, 3rd ed, p 4074. Oxford, Oxford Med Pub, 1996

VOGT-VOGT

Synonym. Status dysmyelinatus.

Symptoms and Signs. Onset in first year of life. Athetoid movements replaced successively by rigidity leading to a condition of helplessness with limbs in weird postures and spasms.

Etiology. Unknown.

Pathology. Shrinkage of caudate nucleus, globus pallidus, subthalamic nucleus. Myelin sheaths in affected areas are absent.

Therapy. Symptomatic.

Prognosis. Death in second decade.

BIBLIOGRAPHY. Vogt C, Vogt O: Zum Lehre der Erkrankungen des striäten systems. J Psychol Neurol 18:627–846, 1920
Adams RD, Victor M: Principles of Neurology, 5th ed, p 837. New York, McGraw-Hill, 1993

VOHWINKEL

Synonyms. Nockermann; mutilating keratoderma; keratoderma mutilating hereditarium; deafness-keratopachydermia-ainhum.

Symptoms. Both sexes affected. Onset early infancy. Hyperhidrosis; keratosis pilaris; hourglass nail; development of tylosis and fissure with ainhum-like constriction (see Ainhum) and with spontaneous amputation of fingers. Absence of leukonychia. Deafness. Symptoms and signs of hypogonadism. Years after onset of tylosis, development of symptoms and signs of syringomyelia.

Etiology. Unknown. Autosomal dominant inheritance.

Therapy. Etretinate.

BIBLIOGRAPHY. Vohwinkel KH: Keratoma hereditarium mutilans. Arch Derm Syph 158:354–364, 1929
Tatz K: Pityriasis rubra pilaris with ainhum and syringomyelia. Br J Derm 58:123–126, 1946
Nockermann PF: Erbliche Hornhautverdickung mit Schnuerfurchen an Fingern und Zehen und Innenohrschwerhoerigkeit. Med Welt 37:1894–1900, 1961

Aksu F, Mietens C: Keratopachydermie mit Schnuerfurchen an Fingern und Zehen und Innenohrschwerhoerigkeit. Paediatr Prax 23:303–310, 1980
Rivers JK, Duke EE, Justus DW: Etretinate management of keratoma hereditaria mutilans in four family members. J Am Acad Dermatol 13:43–49, 1985
Griffiths WAD, Leigh IM, Marks R: Disorders of keratinization. In Champion RH, Burton JL, Ebling FJG (eds): Rook/Wilkinson/Ebling Textbook of Dermatology, 5th ed, pp 1374–1375. Oxford, Blackwell Scientific, 1992

VOICE FUNCTIONAL DISORDERS

Psychophonoasthenia (see)

Habituated hoarseness (see)

Inappropriate falsetto (see)

Vocal abuse
a. Tension-fatigue (see)
b. Bogart-Bacall (see)
c. Vocal cord nodules (see)
d. Reinke edema (see)
e. Vocal process; Ulcer/Granuloma (see)

Postoperative dysphonia (see Habituated hoarseness)

Relapsing aphonia (see Psychophonoasthenia)

See also Spasmodic dysphonia

BIBLIOGRAPHY. Koufman JA, Blalock PD: Functional voice disorders. Otolaryngol Clin N AM 24:1059–1073, 1991

VOLKMANN I

Eponym used to indicate tibiotarsal dislocation causing a congenital deformity of the foot.

BIBLIOGRAPHY. Volkmann R: Ein Fall von hereditaerer kongenitaler Luxation beider Sprunggelekne. Dtsch Z Chir 2:538–542, 1873

VOLKMANN II

Synonyms. Ischemic contracture; myositis fibrosa; post-traumatic muscle contraction. See compartment syndromes.

Symptoms. Burning pain, weakness, or paralysis or paresthesia in hand and forearm.

Signs. Hand cyanosis; swelling; coldness. Fingers in fixed contracted flexion. Radial pulse absent or weak. Atrophic changes of skin of forearm and hand.

Etiology. Spastic or organic occlusion of artery or vein of arm. Fracture; extrinsic compression (splint-tourniquet).

Pathology. Muscle fibers degenerated and necrotic; fibrotic changes. Ischemic degeneration of nerve fibers.

Diagnostic Procedures. *X-rays. Arteriography.*

Therapy. Removal of obstruction. Splitting the deep fascia in front of the elbow within 36 hours after injury.

Prognosis. Good if immediately treated. If unrecognized, it results in chronic, permanent deformity with atrophy of forearm and hand, abduction of thumb and flexion of fingers.

BIBLIOGRAPHY. Volkmann R: Die ischaemischen Muskellahmungen und Kontracturen. Zentralbl Chir 8:801–803, 1881

Sabiston DC: Textbook of Surgery, 14th ed, pp 1619–1620. Philadelphia, WB Saunders, 1991

Adams RD, Victor M: Principles of Neurology, 5th ed, p 1190. New York, McGraw-Hill, 1993

VOLTOLINI

Synonym. Labyrinthitis acute; vertigo—meningitis. See Menière and vestibular neuritis.

Symptoms. Occurs in young children. Onset after infectious diseases. Intense otalgia; vertigo; bilateral deafness; delirium; loss of consciousness; signs of meningeal irritation.

Etiology. Infection.

Diagnostic Procedures. Lack of labyrinth excitability.

Therapy. Antibiotics.

Prognosis. Severe. Progressive, leading to permanent deafness.

BIBLIOGRAPHY. Voltolini FER: Die acute Entzuendung des hauetigen Labyrinthes, gewoehlich irrthuemlich fuer Meningitis gehalten. Mschr Ohrenh 1:9–14, 1867

Brandt T: Vertigo: Its Multisensory Syndromes. London, Springer-Verlag, 1991

VON BEKHTEREV-STRÜMPELL

Synonyms. Marie-Strümpell; ankylosing spondylitis; juvenile spondylitis; rheumatoid spondylitis; rhizomelic spondylitis; spondylitis ossificans ligamentosa II; spondylosis deformans.

Symptoms. Prevalent in males, onset insidious in second or third decade. Lumbar pain with radiation, limited flexibility of spine; pain in the chest (pleuritic type); generalized arthralgia. Back stiff after a period of inactivity.

Signs. Loss of normal lumbar lordosis; reduced mobility of spine. Other articulations eventually become involved. Kyphosis, scoliosis, forward displaced head and total rigidity of spine eventually develop.

Etiology. Unknown. Autosomal hereditary transmission reported in some cases.

Pathology. Minimal chronic inflammatory changes, fibrosis, and eventually calcification of capsules and intervertebral ligaments. Ankylosis and periarticular osteoporosis.

Diagnostic Procedures. *X-ray. CT scan. MRI.* Bamboo spine; extensive spondylosis. *Blood.* Rheumatoid arthritis (R.A.) test.

Therapy. Corticosteroids (very good response in approximately 80% of cases); analgesics; roentgen therapy; physical therapy.

Prognosis. Chronic course evolving to complete spinal rigidity in 10–15 years (bamboo spine) with temporary remission and exacerbation. Rapid progressive course in some cases. Pulmonary diseases frequently develop.

BIBLIOGRAPHY. Connor B, Marie P: Les rheumatismes deformants. Trib Med 27:27–30, 1895 Phil Trans 19:21, 1695

Bekhterev VM: Oderevenelast' pozvonochikas iskrivleniemego, kak osobia forma zabolevaniia. Vrach St Petersburg 13:899–903, 1892

Strümpell A: Bemerkung über die chronische Ankylosirende Entzündung der Wirbelsäule un der Hüftgelenke. Dtsch Z Nervkr 11:338–342, 1897

Weatherall DJ, Ledingham JGG, Warrell DA (eds): Oxford Textbook of Medicine, 3rd ed, pp 2965–2968. Oxford, Oxford Med Pub, 1996

VON BERGMANN

Synonyms. Bergmann diaphragmatic hernia; gastrocardiac; hiatus hernia; paraesophageal hernia; sliding diaphragmatic hernia. See Winkelstein.

Symptoms. Occurs in old age in males and in middle age in females. Frequently manifested when lying down or after meals. Symptoms of variable nature and intensity: increase of intra-abdominal pressure; epigastric or midthoracic pain; radiation to left costal margin or shoulder and arm; sudden weight loss; chronic inflammation of esophagus. Symptoms may mimic coronary, colic, duodenal pains. Symptoms today referred to gastroesophageal reflux (see Winkelstein).

Signs. On chest auscultation, gurgling sounds, emphysema. Sliding hernia prevalent in males. Paraesophageal hernia in females.

Etiology. Cases with autosomal recessive or X-linked inheritance. Variable chromosomal alterations observed in some cases: mosaic isochrome 12p trisomy 1,8, etc.

Pathology. Paraesophageal hernia with or without herniation of cardias into thoracic cavity.

Diagnostic Procedures. *X-ray.* Of digestive tract. *Blood.* Usually, hypochromic anemia.

Therapy. According to grade and symptomatology. Diet: do not overload the stomach, do not eat close to bed time; use of nonabsorbable antacids, acid-suppressing agents. Surgery.

Prognosis. Good with surgical correction.

BIBLIOGRAPHY. von Bergmann G: Das "Epiphrenale syndrom" seine Beziehung zur Angina pektoris und zum Cardiospasmus. Dtsch Med Wochenschr 58:605–609, 1932

Cunha F: Recurrent "hiatus hernia" syndrome of von Bergmann. Am J Dig Dis Nutrition 1:170–172, 1934

Norio R, Kaariainen H, Rapola J, et al: Familial congenital diaphragmatic defects: Aspects and etiology, prenatal diagnosis and treatment. Am J Med Genet 17:471–483, 1984

Haubrich WS: Diaphragmatic hernias. In Haubrich WS, Schaffner F, Berk JE (eds): Bockus Gastroenterology, 5th ed, pp 439–444. Philadelphia, WB Saunders, 1995

VON ECONOMO

Synonyms. Economo; Economo-Cruchet; encephalitis lethargica; sleeping sickness (African); Nona.

Symptoms. Occurs in epidemic form. Both sexes affected. Onset at all ages. Febrile onset. Headache; dizziness; fatigue; irritability; choreiform movements. Later, parkinsonism (see). Oculogyric crisis; disorder of behavior.

Signs. Variable in different patients and course of the disease according to neurologic lesions and degree of recovery. Motor, sensorial lesions, and alterations.

Etiology. Trypanosomiasis (in African sleeping sickness).

Pathology. *Brain.* Hyperemia; petechiae in basal ganglia of midbrain; pons; destruction of nerve fibers; lymphocytic infiltration.

Diagnostic Procedures. *Cerebrospinal fluid.* Increase in pressure, proteins, and cells. *Viral cultures.*

Therapy. Symptomatic. L-Dopa and other antiparkinsonian agents.

Prognosis. Variable course and sequelae.

BIBLIOGRAPHY. von Economo C: Encephalitis lethargica. Wien Klin Wochenschr 30:581–585, 1917

Adams RD, Victor M: Principles of Neurology, 5th ed, pp 654–655. New York, McGraw-Hill, 1993

VON EULENBERG

Synonyms. Eulenberg; normokalemic periodic paralysis (type B); paramyotonia congenita; PC; see Gamstrop.

Symptoms. Both sexes equally affected. Onset in first decade. Between attacks, asymptomatic. Precipitating factors: sleep; rest after exertion; alcohol; cold and dampness; mental stress. Attack: flaccid paralysis of all muscles except facial expression, mastication, deglutition, speech, and respiration. In some cases, jaw muscle may be affected. Limited muscle groups may be affected.

Signs. Hyporeflexia of affected muscles.

Etiology. Unknown. Simple autosomal dominant inheritance. Paramyotonia (or cold-sensitive myotonia), according to majority of myologists, represents the end of a spectrum extending to periodic paralysis (see Gamstrop), since many cases show both conditions. In addition it does not appear justifiable to separate normokalemic from hyperkalemic paralysis since, in these two syndromes, serum potassium levels do not (always) correlate with muscle weakness PC and HPP (hyperkalemic periodic paralysis) are allelic disorders of the skeletal muscle sodium channel.

Pathology. Subsarcolemmal vacuolization observed. No degenerative changes.

Diagnostic Procedures. Administration of potassium chloride precipitates attack. *Blood.* Serum potassium normal during and between attacks. Occasionally hypocalcemia during attacks. *Electromyography.*

Therapy. If mild, no treatment required. In severe attacks calcium gluconate may restore power; if unsuccessful, glucose plus insulin and chlorothiazide must be tried. Continuous use of diuretics (chlorothiazide) prevents attacks; if myotonic symptoms prevail: antiarrhytmic agents phenytoine, quinine, procainamide, mexiletine and others; however, patients spontaneously, often discontinue drugs because of their severe collateral effects versus their beneficial effects.

Prognosis. Chronic recurrent condition. Some patients develop polymyopathy with persistent weakness.

BIBLIOGRAPHY. Von Eulenberg A: Ueber eine familiare, durch 6 Generationen Verfolgbare. Form Kongenitaler Paramyotonic. Neurol Zentralbl 5:265–272, 1886

Poskauzer DC, Kerr DNS: A third type of periodic paralysis with normokalemia and favorable response to sodium chloride. Am J Med 31:328–342, 1961

Danowski TS, Fisher ER, Vidalon C, et al: Clinical and ultrastructural observations in a kindred with normo-hyperkalemic periodic paralysis. J Med Genet 132:20–28, 1975

Barchi RL: The nondystrophic myotonic syndromes. In Rowland LP, Di Mauro S (eds): Handbook of Clinical Neurology, vol 18: Myopathies, p 261. Amsterdam, Elsevier, 1992

VON GIERKE IA

Synonyms. Cori type I glycogenosis; Gierke; von Creveld-von Gierke; glycogen storage disease Ia; glucose 6-phosphate deficiency; glycogen storage (type I); glycogenosis (type I); hepatorenal glycogenosis; hepatonephromegalia glycogenica.

Symptoms. Both sexes affected. Clinical onset during first year of life. Convulsion (hypoglycemic); failure to thrive. Bleeding tendency. Epistaxis; oozing after surgery. Occasionally, steatorrhea.

Signs. Retarded growth without disproportion, lumbar lordosis; adiposity; skin yellowish xanthomas over joints and buttocks. Large abdomen; marked hepatomegaly; no spleen enlargement. Kidney enlarged. Bilateral, symmetric, yellow paramacular lesions of eye fundus. Gout-related signs. Chronic pancreatitis as complication of hyperlipemia.

Etiology. Genetic heterogeneity. Type I in particular demonstrates

pleiotropism with simulation of primary gout and xanthomatosis. Deficiency of glucose 6-phosphatase. Autosomal recessive inheritance.

Pathology. Accumulation of glycogen in various tissues. Liver becomes markedly enlarged and kidneys are particularly involved. Liver and renal adenomata.

Diagnostic Procedures. *Blood.* Mild anemia; marked hypoglycemia; hyperlactacidemia; marked hypertriglyceridemia; hypercholesterolemia; increase of fatty acids; acetonemia; hyperuricemia; low serum phosphate; normal alkaline phosphatases. *Urine.* Acetonuria; glucosuria; occasionally, aminoaciduria. *Biopsy.* Of liver. Absence of enzymatic activity.

Therapy. Correction of hypoglycemia (multiple feedings day and night). Uncooked starch. Allopurinol. Prevention of acidosis and infections. L-Thyroxine-glucagon. Good results with portal diversions, portocaval shunting, and liver transplantation.

Prognosis. Poor. If treated and death is prevented for 4 years, disease becomes less severe. Liver adenomas may progress to hepatoma or liver carcinoma.

BIBLIOGRAPHY. von Gierke E: Hepato-Nephromegalia glykogenica (Glykogenspeicherkrankeit der Leber und Nieren). Beitr Pathol Anat 82:497–513, 1929

Chen YT, Scheinman JI, Park HK, et al: Amelioration of proximal renal tubular dysfunction in type I glycogen storage disease with dietary therapy. N Engl J Med 323:590–593, 1990

Kikuchi M, Hasegawa K, Handa I, et al: Chronic pancreatitis in a child with glycogen storage disease type I. Eur J Pediatr 150:852–53, 1991

Chen YT, Burchell A: Glycogen storage diseases. In Scriver CR, Beaudet AL, Sly WS, et al: The Metabolic and Molecular Bases of Inherited Disease, 7th ed, pp 944–949. New York, McGraw-Hill, 1995

VON GIERKE IB

Synonyms. Glycogen storage disease type IB; glucose-6-phosphate transport defect.

Symptoms and Signs. Both sexes. From birth. Protuberant abdomen and diarrhea, growth failure, hepatomegaly. Second decade: yellowish red spots on legs and hypertension, repeated infections, hemorrhages.

Etiology. Autosomal recessive inheritance. Functional defect in transport system of glucose that is not liberated from glucose-6-phosphate.

Pathology. Liver adenomas; eruptive xanthomas; hypersplenism with sequestration of iron (persistent feature).

Diagnostic Procedures. *Blood.* Hyperlipemia; hypochromic anemia, platelet dysfunction, leucocytopenia, deficient chemiotaxis; In vitro enzyme assay: glucose-6-phosphatase activity is present but striking limitation of glucose transport across cell membrane of polymorphonucleates. *CT scan. Scintography. MRI.* Adenomas in liver.

Therapy. Portocaval anastomosis; granulocyte colony stimulating factor to treat neutropenia.

Prognosis. Improvement with treatment.

BIBLIOGRAPHY. Senior B, Loridan L: Functional differentiation of glycogenoses of the liver the use of glycerol. N Engl J Med 279:965–970, 1968

Schroten H, Roesler J, Breidenbach T, et al: Granulocytes and granulocyte macrophage colony stimulating factors for treatment of neutropenia in glycogen storage disease type IB. J Pediat 119:748–754, 1991

Chen YT, Burchell A: Glycogen storage diseases. In Scriver CR, Beaudet AL, Sly WS, et al: The Metabolic and Molecular Bases of Inherited Disease, 7th ed, pp 944–949. New York, McGraw-Hill, 1995

VON GIERKE IC

Synonyms. Glycogen storage disease Ic.

Symptoms and Signs. Classic clinical features of von Gierke I.

Etiology. Autosomal recessive inheritance. Defect in translocase specific for G6P.

Pathology. See von Gierke I.

VON GIERKE ID

Synonyms. Glycogen storage disease Id.

Symptoms and Signs. Only one case described. Classic clinical features of von Gierke I.

Etiology. Defect in microsomal glucose transport from deficiency of GLUT 7 (hepatic microsomal glucose transport protein).

BIBLIOGRAPHY. Nordlie RC, Sukalski KA, Munoz JM, et al: Type I C, a novel glycogenosis: Underlying mechanism. J Biol Chem 258:9739–2944, 1983
Burchell A: Molecolar pathology of glucose-6-phosphatase. FASEB J 4:2978–2988, 1990
Chen YT, Burchell A: Glycogen storage diseases. In Scriver CR, Beaudet AL, Sly WS, et al: The Metabolic and Molecular Bases of Inherited Disease, 7th ed, pp 944–949. New York, McGraw-Hill, 1995

VON HERRENSCHWAND

Synonyms. Herrenschwand; Passow; sympathetic heterochromia. See also Fuch III.

Symptoms and Signs. Hemifacial decreased sweating; enophthalmos; ptosis; heterochromia (unilateral iris): myosis.

Etiology. Represents the combination of heterochromia and Horner. May be caused by sympathetic palsy (traumatic, surgical, or owing to secondary infections), or transmitted as irregular autosomal dominant trait. Associated also with other syndromes: Waarderburg; Marfan, etc.

Pathology. See Horner.

Diagnostic Procedures. Differential diagnosis with Fuch III: typical architecture and trabeculae of deeper iris layers remain well outlined.

Therapy. Once the cause is found the same as in Horner.

Prognosis. According to etiology.

BIBLIOGRAPHY. von Herrenschwand F: Ueber verschiedene Arten von Heterochromia iridis. Klin Monatsbl Augenheilkd 60:467–494, 1918
Gladstone RM: Development of significance of heterochromia of the iris. Arch Neurol 21:184–192, 1969

VON HIPPEL-LINDAU*

Synonyms. VLH; Hippel; Hippel-Czermak; Lindau-von Hippel; retinocerebello angiomatosis; angiomatosis retinae; cerebello retina angiomatosis; hemoangioblastomatosis cerebello retinae.

Symptoms. Onset 4–68 years (mean, 26.3). Headache; dizziness; unilateral ataxia; mental changes; blindness; or others related to variable localization (see Signs).

Signs. In eyes (75%), tortuous aneurysms of retinal vessels, exudates on fundus, subretinal yellowish spot. Signs of presence of: pheochromocytoma (see) in 19%, renal carcinoma in 23%, hemangioblastoma in spinalcord (14%), in cerebellum or brain stem (54%); abdominal cysts (kidney, pancreas, liver, speen, etc., 50%).

Etiology. Unknown. Autosomal dominant inheritance. The VHL gene is in the region 3p25–p26, near the tip of the short arm of chromosome 3.

Pathology. In 50% of patients, involvement of only one organ. *Brain.* Cystic, hemorrhagic lesion in lateral lobes of cerebellum with mural nodules; vascular epithelialized channels; foamy fat cells. *Retina.* Subretinal hemorrhages; aneurysm with dilatation and tortuosity of vessels; destruction of nerve elements. Frequently associated, simple renal cyst or renal carcinoma, pancreatic cysts, and solid or cystic tumors of epididymis; pheochromocytoma.

Diagnostic Procedures. *Spinal tap.* Increased in pressure. *Angiography. Brain isotope scan. CT scan. MRI (or MIBG). Sonography of abdominal region. Blood. Polycythemia. Urine.* Increase of catecholamines. *Ophthalmoscopy.* Papilledema and see signs. Genetic studies focused on the short arm of chromosome 3.

Therapy. Photocoagulation; (laser) cryotherapy of retinal lesions. Neurosurgery; aspiration of cyst and removal of nodules; according to eventual manifestations from presence of renal, pheochromocytoma, pancreatic, and epididymal cyst. Gene therapy is currently tried.

Prognosis. According to time of onset, type and extent of lesions and timing and adequacy of therapeutical interventions. Mean age of death, 41 years.

BIBLIOGRAPHY. von Hippel E: Vorstellung eines Patienten mit einem sehr ungewöhnlichen Aderhautleiden. Bericht 24 Versammlung Ophthalmol Ges. 269, 1895
Lindau A: Studien über Kleinhincysten. Acta Pathol Microbiol Scand (Suppl):1–128, 1926
Maher ER, Yates JRW, Harries R, et al: Clinical features and natural history of van Hippel-Lindau disease. Quart J Med 77:1151–1163, 1990
Editorial: Von Hippel-Lindau disease. The Lancet 337:1065, 1991
Neumann HP, Eggert HR, Scheremet R, et al: Lesions of the central nervous system in von Hippel-Lindau Syndrome. J Neurol Neurosurg Psychiatr 55:898–901, 1993
Weatherall DJ, Ledingham JGG, Warrell DA (eds): Oxford Textbook of Medicine, 3rd ed, pp 3987–3988. Oxford, Oxford Med Pub, 1996

VON MIKULICZ

Synonyms. Mikulicz-Sjögren; Mikulicz-Radecki; dacryosialoadenopathy.

Symptoms. Dryness of mouth and absent or decreased lacrimation; vision blurring.

Signs. Symmetric, painless, hard tumefactions of lacrimal and salivary glands, gradually progressing.

Etiology. Lymphoid leukemia; lymphomas; sarcoidosis; tuberculosis; syphilis; idiopathic; associated with thiouracil treatment; familial possible.

Pathology. Atrophy of acinar parenchyma and replacement with lymphoid cells.

Diagnostic Procedures. *Blood.* For diagnosis of leukemia. *Bone marrow. X-ray.* Of chest. *Sputum.* Smear and culture. *Mantoux skin test. Serology. Sialography. Ultrasonography.*

Therapy. According to etiology: roentgen; chemotherapy; corticoids; antibiotics.

Prognosis. That of primary condition. Remissions and relapses or cure of the syndrome may be observed according to the response to the specific treatment.

BIBLIOGRAPHY. von Mikulicz J: Ueber eine eigenartige symmetrische Erkrankung der Tränen und Mundspeicheldrüsen. Beitr Chir Fortschr Gewidmet, Stuttgart, Theodor Billroth, pp 610–630, 1892
von Mikulicz J: Concerning a peculiar symmetrical disease of the lacrimal and salivary glands. Med Classics 2:165–186, 1937
Penfold CN: Mikulicz syndrome. J Oral Maxillofac Surg 43:900–905, 1985

---

*For information and family assistance: VHL Family Alliance 171 Clinton Road Brookline, MA 02146 (617) 232-5946; (800) 767-4VHL; Fax (617) 734-8233

Weatherall DJ, Ledingham JGG, Warrell DA (eds): Oxford Textbook of Medicine, 3rd ed, pp 1861, 4182. Oxford, Oxford Med Pub, 1996

VON RECKLINGHAUSEN I

Synonyms. Recklinghausen phakomatosis; neurofibromatosis, NF1.

Symptoms. Onset in childhood. Becomes more active at puberty, during pregnancy, and at menopause. Asymptomatic or pain when tumor produces pressure on adjacent structures. Occasionally, mental retardation, cretinism, and growth abnormalities; delay in sexual development; spontaneous fractures; hemifacial hypertrophy.

Signs. Café au lait skin pigmentation. Multiple tumors of different consistencies along the course of cutaneous nerves; kyphoscoliosis; acromegaly. Occasionally (not rarely), proptosis, ptosis, ocular muscle palsy, unilateral hydrophthalmos, optic atrophy.

Etiology. Unknown. Congenital autosomal dominant inheritance. High spontaneous mutation 30–50% of cases new mutations. Gene for NF1 resides on chromosome 17q11.2. In some families or in isolated cases, reported male linkage and recessive inheritance.

Prognosis. Benign tumor (fibroma mollusca) arising from covering cells of peripheral nervous system; tumor of meninges, optic (II) nerve, and central nervous system frequent. Osteodysgenesis; subperiosteal tumors. Possible association with gliomatous tumors of brain or spinal cord.

Diagnostic Procedures. *Biopsy. EEG. CT scan. MRI. X-ray.*

Therapy. Removal of tumors that produce symptoms.

Prognosis. Tumor benign and usually does not regrow after removal. Prognosis depends on ocular and central nervous system involvement. Malignant change (5–10%) mostly in males.

BIBLIOGRAPHY. von Recklinghausen FD: Ueber die multiplen Fibrome der Haut und ihre Beziehung zu den multiplen Neuromen. Festschr. Feier Funfundzwanzigjahrigen Best Pathol Inst Berlin. Berlin, A. Hirschwald, 1882

Riccardi VM, Eichner JE: Neurofibromatosis: Phenotype, Natural History and Pathogenesis. Baltimore, Johns Hopkins Univ Press, 1986

Gutmann DH, Collins FS: Von Recklinghousen neurofibromatosis. In Scriver CR, Beaudet AL, Sly WS, et al: The Metabolic and Molecular Bases of Inherited Disease, 7th ed, pp 677–696. New York, McGraw-Hill, 1995

VON ROKITANSKY

Synonyms. Rokitansky II. Corrected great arteries transposition.

Symptoms. Male predominance. Pure defect (rare). Asymptomatic.

Signs. Second sound accentuated at left of sternum.

Etiology. Congenital heart defect.

Pathology. Mirror images of atrioventricular valves (resembling normal contralateral valves); aorta arises from a morphologic right ventricle and pulmonary trunk arises from a morphologic left ventricle. Common associated condition (80%): ventricular septal defect.

Diagnostic Procedures. *ECG.* Left ventricular hypertrophy; prolonged P-R interval; in lead I, high P-waves; II or III heart block. *Angiocardiography.* Pulmonary main artery medial to aorta; right ventricle smooth outline. *Cardiac catheterization. Two-dimensional echocardiography with color flow imaging and spectral Doppler interrogation.*

Therapy. Surgical approach and correction of associated defects are dictated by anatomic reversal of ventricles and conduction system.

Prognosis. Normal survival (in pure form); some patients may, however, develop "spontaneous" heart failure.

BIBLIOGRAPHY. Von Rokitansky KF: Die Defecte der Scheidewande des Hertzens. Vienna, W Braumiller, 1875

Perloff JK: The Clinical Recognition of Congenital Heart Disease, 4th ed, pp 67–90. Philadelphia, WB Saunders, 1994

VON ROKITANSKY-CUSHING

Synonyms. Rokitansky-Cushing; Cushing ulcer; neurogenic gastrointestinal bleeding. Eponym used to indicate the gastrointestinal hemorrhagic complication arising after head injury or neurosurgery. See Curling ulcer.

BIBLIOGRAPHY. Von Rokitansky CV: Handbuch der pathologischen Anatomie kien Braumueller-Seidel, vol 8, 1842

Cushing H: Peptic ulcers and the interbrain. Surg Gynecol Obstet 55:1–34, 1932

VON SALLMAN-PATON-WITKOP

Synonyms. Sallman. Witkop-von Sallman intraepithelial benign hereditary dyskeratosis, HBID; dyskeratosis hereditary, benign intraepithelial.

Symptoms. Both sexes affected. Onset in infancy or childhood, progressing to adolescence. Photophobia; lacrimation, especially in the summer months.

Signs. Eye, oral, and labial mucosae smooth; opalescent plaques; thicker lesions folded (see Cannon). Eyes small; pingueculae or foamy gelatinous plaques over conjunctiva.

Etiology. Unknown. Autosomal dominant inheritance.

Pathology. Acanthosis; vacuolated cells; eosinophilic cells; parakeratosis and hyperkeratosis.

Diagnostic Procedures. *Biopsy.* Conjunctival cell smears. Presence of waxy eosinophilic cells and "cell within cell" pattern.

Therapy. Symptomatic.

Prognosis. Lesions progress to adolescence, then remain stable. Benign condition.

BIBLIOGRAPHY. Witkop CJ Jr, Shankle CH, Graham JB, et al: Hereditary benign intraepithelial dyskeratosis. Arch Pathol 70:696–711, 1960

Von Sallman L, Paton D: Hereditary benign intraepithelial dyskeratosis. Arch Ophthalmol 63:421–429, 1960

McLean IW, et al: Hereditary benign intraepithelial dyskeratosis. Ophthal 88:164–168, 1981

Schields CL, Schilds JA, Eagle RC Jr: Hereditary benign intraepithelial dyskeratosis. Arch Ophthal 105:422–423, 1987

VON WILLEBRAND

Synonyms. Angiohemophilia; vascular hemophilia; Minot-von Willebrand; pseudohemophilia; constitutional thrombopathy.

Symptoms. Frequency per million, 5–10. Both sexes equally affected. Onset usually in early childhood. Manifestation of bleeding among affected individuals extremely variable in intensity. Bleeding tendency; easy bruising; epistaxis; bleeding from gums and female genitalia; occasionally, also from urinary and gastrointestinal tracts. Hemathrosis rare. Inconstant, prolonged bleeding from trauma or surgery.

Etiology. Acquired form is exceptional; associated with various hematologic, immunologic, or neoplastic process. Autosomal dominant transmission with variable penetrance and expressivity; 70–90% autosomal dominant, the rest autosomal recessive. Certain families have both kinds of transmission, indicating a double heterozygosity. Reduction of von Willebrand factor (vWF) or anomalies; reduction of factor VIII. According to the deficits, various forms have been described:

Type I. Frequency 70–80%. Reduction of vWFAg, vWFRCo, and factor VIII (this may be normal in some cases). Aggregation ristocetin absent; multimer distribution normal but slightly reduced. Autosomal dominant or double heterozygotes. Treatment: DDAVP.

Type IIA and Type IB. Frequency Type A 10–12%, type B 3–5%; vWFAg decreased; vWFRCo in type A highly decreased (+++), in type II (++) factor VIII normal or decreased; aggregation ristocetin in type A absent, in type B increased; multimer distribution in type A abnormal with absence of high molecular forms, in type IIb absence of multimer with high molecular weight. Autosomal dominant or recessive inheritance. Treatment: vWF concentrate.

Type II N. Frequency not determined; vWFAg and vWFRCo normal; factor VIII decreased (++); aggregation ristocetin absent. Treatment: vWF concentrate. Autosomal recessive inheritance.

Type III. Frequency 1–3%: vWFAg, vWFRCo, and aggregation ristocetin absent; factor VIII highly decreased (+++); multimers absent. Autosomal recessive inheritance. Treatment: vWF concentrate.

Diagnostic Procedures. In full expression, morphologic and functional alteration of platelets and deficiency of factor VIII; however, any combination of these abnormalities may be observed. See types. Usually the following pattern is observed: tourniquet test usually normal; bleeding time may be prolonged; partial thromboplastin time (PPT), and clotting time pathologic; prothrombin consumption impaired; thromboplastin generation test (TGT) plasma defect; thrombin and prothrombin time normal; vWF decreased or normal; ristocetin platelet aggregation absent except in type IIB. Electrophoretic study of multimeres (on gel of agarose with a dissociant agent and revelation by specific marked antibodies).

Therapy. Whole blood, plasma, or plasma fraction containing factor VIII. New synthesis of factor VIII seems to follow transfusion. Fresh frozen plasma, cryoprecipitate; DDAVP (only in mild cases). In women sex hormones to ameliorate menometrorrhagias.

Prognosis. Severity of bleeding tendency decreases with age and during pregnancy.

BIBLIOGRAPHY. Minot GR: Familial hemorrhagic condition associated with prolongation of bleeding time. Am J Med Sci 175:301–306, 1928
von Willebrand EA: Hereditary pseudohemofilia; description; previously observed cases. Finska Lak Sallsk Handl 68:87–112, 1926
von Willebrand EA: Ueber hereditaere Pseudohaemophilie. Acta Med Scand 76:521–550, 1931
von Willebrand EA, Jürgen R: Ueber eine neue vererbbares Bluterkrenkheit; Die konstitutionelle Thrombopathie. Dtsch Arch Klin Med 175:453–483, 1933
Fressinaud E, Meyer D, Maladie de Willebrand ED: Thecniques Encycl. Méd Chir (Paris-France) Hématologie 13–021–A-50 1994 9p
Rick ME: Diagnosis and management of von Willebrand's syndrome. Med Clin N Am 78:609–623, 1994

VOODOO DEATH

Synonyms. Curse death; wish dying; rootwork.

Symptoms. Occurs in African and West Indian societies, particularly in Haiti. Short, ritual-induced hysterical states; convulsions; twilight states; excitement. Voodoo death in people who, believing they are under magic spells, die.

Etiology. Unknown. Explanation for voodoo death: state of hopeless resignation that through sympathetic or parasympathetic imbalance reduces resistance to shock (?). Possibility of poisoning, organic illness, or refusal of food or water must be considered.

BIBLIOGRAPHY. Richter CP: On the phenomenon of sudden death in animals and men. Psychosomat Med 19:191–198, 1967
Kaplan HI, Sadock BJ: Comprehensive Textbook of Psychiatry, 6th ed, p 1057. Baltimore, Williams & Wilkins, 1995

VOORHOEVE

Synonym. Osteopathia striata.

Symptoms and Signs. Asymptomatic. Radiologic syndrome.

Etiology. Unknown. Condition differs from osteoporosis, Engelmann, Ribbing, and other bone affections since only cancellous bone is involved. Occurs as a feature in Goltz, in Pierre Robin (see), and in two specific syndromes; osteopathia striata-cranial stenosis (see) and osteopathia striata-pigmentary dermopathy (see).

Diagnostic Procedures. *X-ray.* Multiple condensations of cancellous bone tissue, beginning at the epiphyseal line and extending into diaphysis. Any long bones may be involved; in the ilium "sunburst" aspect around acetabulum. Normal ^{99m}Tc pyrophosphate uptake.

BIBLIOGRAPHY. Voorhoeve N: L'image radiologique non encore décrite d'un anomalie du squelette. Les rapports avec la dyschondroplasie et l'osteopathia condensans disseminata. Acta Radiol (Stockh) 3:407–427, 1924
Bernard C, Hoeffel JC, Merle M, et al: A propos d'un cas d'osteopathie striée. Sem Hop Paris 60:573–576, 1984

VULPIAN-BERNHARDT

Synonyms. Muscular atrophy progessive, spino-muscular atrophy. See Kugelberg-Welander; Aran-Duchenne; Becker.

Symptoms and Signs. Disease of adult life, weakness, fasciculation (50%), and with time atrophy of neck and shoulder muscles progressing to the involvement first of arms, hands, and trunk, and seldom of legs; leading to lordosis, winged scapulas. Absence of sensory disturbances and mental retardation.

Etiology. Sporadic occasionally autosomal dominant inheritance. It belongs to a confused group of motor neuron diseases that includes several syndromes with scapulohumeral muscular atrophy. Claimed characteristics of this syndrome seem the pattern of progression.

Pathology. Degenerative process of anterior horn cells muscular atrophy affecting primarily the shoulder girdle region.

Diagnostic Procedures. *Blood.* Serum enzymes increase particularly creatinine kinase. *Electromyogram.*

Therapy. Symptomatic, orthopedic, physiotherapeutic.

Prognosis. Variable. Usually very slow progression with stasis or even temporary remission. Ability to walk may be lost ten years after onset of disease or even later. Condition compatible with normal life span.

BIBLIOGRAPHY. Vulpian A: Maladies du système nerveux, vol 2. Paris, Octave Doin, 1886
Bernardt M: Ueber eine hereditaere Form der progressiven spinalen mit Bulbaerpralyse complicierten Muskleatrophie. Virchows Arch Pathol Anat 115:197–216, 1889
Kugelberg E: Chronic proximal (pseudomyopathic) spinal muscular atrophy Kugelberger-Wdelander syndrome. In Vinken PJ, Bruyn GW: Handbook of Clinical Neurology, vol 22, pp 75–76. Amsterdam, North-Holland, 1975

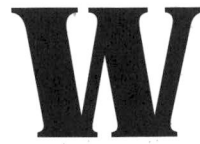

W*

Synonym. Pallister (W).

Symptoms. Mental retardation; seizures.

Signs. *Facies.* Frontal bossing; hypertelorism; antimongoloid palpebral fissures; broad, flat nose bridge; notch of upper lip and submucous cleft of hard palate; absence of upper incisors. *Limbs.* Subluxation of elbow; camptodactyly; pes cavus.

Etiology. Unknown. X-linked trait.

BIBLIOGRAPHY. Pallister PD, Hermann J, Springer JW, et al: The W syndrome. Birth Defects Orig Art Ser X (7):51–60, 1974
Martin AO, Perrin JC, Muir WA, et al: An autosomal dominant midline cleft syndrome resembling familial holoprosencephaly. Clin Genet 12:65–72, 1977

WAARDENBURG I AND II

Synonyms. Klein-Waardenburg; Mende; Van der Hoeve-Halberstam-Gualdi; embryonic fixation; interoculoiridodermatoauditory dysplasia; ptosis-epicanthus. Including Fisch-Renwick. See Albinism syndromes and Meesmann (possibly identical condition).

Symptoms. No sex preference. Reported in all ethnic groups. Complete form rare; various combinations of various characteristics (forme fruste; or incomplete found in different members of affected families). Evident at birth. Deafness (in 20% of cases).

Signs. The syndrome has been divided into type WS1 with dystopia canthorum and type WS2 without dystopia and with higher frequency of deafness; there is also a WS III (see Klein-Waardenburg), and a pseudo-Waardenburg with unilateral congenital ptosis and without dystopia canthorum. Other signs: high nose bridge (78%); hypertrichosis of the eyebrows tending to join at midline (45%); hypopigmentation and hypoplasia of iris stroma in one or both eyes (25%); median white forelock of varying size, from a few hairs to obvious large forelock (17%). (This sign may be evident at birth and disappear during first year of life, or begin after puberty.) Some patients may also present white patches of the skin or areas of increased pigmentation.

Etiology. Unknown. Congenital familial ectodermal dysplasia; autosomal dominant transmission.

Pathology. Not many reports; examination of auditory pathway in one case with deafness revealed absence of Corti organ and atrophy of spiral ganglion and nerve.

Diagnostic Procedures. *Chromosome studies.* Normal. No biochemical (blood, urine) abnormalities.

Therapy. Eye surgery for cosmetic reasons and epiphora.

Prognosis. Good quoad vitam.

BIBLIOGRAPHY. Van der Breggen FA: Een familiare oogafwijking en een aangeboren symmetrische misvorming van handen en voeten. Ned Tijdschr Geneeskd 59:1874–1876, 1915
Van der Hoeve J: Abnorme Länge der Tränenrohrchen mit Ankyloblepharon. Klin Monatsbl Augenheilkd 56:232; 238, 1916

Klein D: Albinisme partial (leucism) avec surdimutité, blépharophimosis ey dysplasie myo-ostéo-articulaire. Helv Paediatr Acta 5:38–58, 1950
Waardenburg PJ: A new syndrome combining developmental anomalies of the eyelids, eyebrows and nose root with pigmentary defects of the iris and head and with congenital deafness. Am J Hum Genet 3:195–253, 1951
Nork TM, Shihab ZM, Young RSL, and Price J: Pigment distribution in Waardenburg's syndrome: a new hypothesis. Graefe's Arch Clin Exp Ophthalmol 224:487–492, 1986
da Silva EO: Waardenburg I syndrome: A clinical and genetic study of two large Brasilian kindreds and literature review. Am J Med Genet 40:65–74, 1991
King RA, Hearing VJ, Creel DJ, et al: Albinism. In Scriver CR, Beaudet AL, Sly WS, et al: The Metabolic and Molecular Bases of Inherited Disease, 7th ed, pp 4379–4380. New York, McGraw-Hill, 1995
Zoghbi H, Ballabio A: Waardenburg syndrome. In Scriver CR, Beaudet AL, Sly WS, et al: The Metabolic and Molecular Bases of Inherited Disease, 7th ed, pp 4575–4580. New York, McGraw-Hill, 1995

WAARDENBURG-JONKERS

Synonyms. Corneal dystrophy; Waardenburg-Jonkers.

Symptoms. Both sexes affected. Present from first year of life. Eye irritation episodes; progressive vision reduction, and reduction of corneal sensibility.

Signs. Cornea stroma shows multiple opacities similar to snowflakes or hailstones that increase with age in number to involve the epithelium.

Etiology. Autosomal dominant inheritance.

Therapy. Corneal transplantation.

Prognosis. Progressive vision loss.

BIBLIOGRAPHY. Waardenburg PJ, Jonkers GA: A specific type of dominant progressive dystrophy of the cornea developing after birth. Acta Ophthalmol (Copenh). 39:919–923, 1961

WAARDENBURG-SHAH

Synonym. Waardenburg variant; Shah-Waardenburg; Hirshsprung-pigmentary anomaly.

Symptoms and Signs. Both sexes. From birth. White forelock and eyebrows and eyelashes. Signs of intestinal obstruction. Isochromia irides (approximately 50%). Absence of dystopia canthorum, broad nose, or white patches or deafness.

Etiology. Autosomal recessive inheritance suggested as well as dominant.

Pathology. Microcolon; proximal ileum dilatation and collapse of distal ileum and colon.

Diagnostic Procedures. *X-ray. Barium enema.*

Therapy. Ileostomy.

Prognosis. Poor. Frequent failure of the ileostomy to function.

BIBLIOGRAPHY. Shah KN, Dalal SJ, Desai MP, et al: White forelock, pigmentary disorder of irides and long segment Hirschsprung disease:

Possible variant of Waardenburg syndrome. J Pediatr 99:423–435, 1981

Badner JA, Chakravarti A: Waardenburg syndrome and Hirschsprung disease: Evidence for pleiotropic effects of a single dominant gene. Am J Med Genet 35:100–104, 1990

Zoghbi H, Ballabio A: Waardenburg syndrome. In Scriver CR, Beaudet AL, Sly WS, et al: The Metabolic and Molecular Bases of Inherited Disease, 7th ed, p 4576. New York, McGraw-Hill, 1995

WADIA-SWAMI

Synonym. Cerebellar degeneration, slow eye movement; spinocerebellar degeneration, slow eye movements. See Jervis.

Symptoms and Signs. Described in India and the United States. Manifestations of spinocerebellar degeneration plus abnormal eye movements: absent scanning and slow tracking. Progressive mental deterioration.

Etiology. Unknown. Cerebellar degeneration and possibly also paramedian pontine reticular formation. Autosomal dominant inheritance, a possible recessive form also described.

Prognosis. Rapidly progressing course; death within 10 years from onset.

BIBLIOGRAPHY. Wadia NH, Swami RK: A new form of heredo-familial spinocerebellar degeneration with slow eye movements (nine families). Brain 94:359–374, 1971

Starkman S, Kaul S, Fried J, et al: Unusual abnormal eye movements in a family with hereditary spino-cerebellar degeneration. Neurology 22:402, 1972

Whyte MP, Dekaban AS: Familial cerebellar degeneration with slow eye movements, mental deterioration and incidental nevus of Ota (oculodermal melanocytosis). Dev Med Child Neurol 18:373–380, 1976

WAGENER-KEITH

Obsolete eponym used to indicate the symptom complex: headache, monoplegia, or hemiplegia; seizures; variable degree of visual impairment; asthenia, dyspnea, and peripheral edemas associated with blood hypertension.

BIBLIOGRAPHY. Wagener HP, Keith NM: Cases of marked hypertension, adequate renal function and neuroretinitis. Arch Intern Med 34:374–387, 1924

WAGNER-STICKLER

Synonyms. Cervenka; David-Stickler; Stickler; arthroophthalmopathy, hereditary; clefting; hyaloid-retina degeneration, palatoschisis. Possibly part of a spectrum including Marshall; Weissenbacher-Zweymuller, Pierre Robin, Kniest, SED congenita.

Symptoms. Both sexes affected. Onset variable according to presence or development of findings. Loss of visual acuity. In second decade, myopia, scotomas.

Signs. *Facies.* Anomalies; hypoplastic maxilla; saddle nose; palatoschisis. Epicanthus. *Eyes.* Nystagmus; abnormal anterior chamber angle; iris atrophy; vitreous degeneration with streaks in posterior hyaloid membrane; cataract; keratopathy. *Extremities.* Joint hyperextensibility (finger, elbow, knee); tapering fingers; genu valga; hip deformities; talipes equinovarus.

Etiology. Irregular dominant inheritance with variable expression.

Diagnostic Procedures. *X-ray.* Of skeleton. See Signs. *Ophthalmos-*

copy. Various types of retinal degeneration (after 19 years of age); choroidal sclerosis, pseudoedema, and pale optic disk.

Therapy. Symptomatic.

Prognosis. Poor. Frequently, death before full syndrome becomes manifest.

BIBLIOGRAPHY. Wagner H: Ein bisher unberkauntes Erbleiden des Auges (Degeneratio hyaloideo-retinalis hereditaria), beobachtet in Kanton Zuerich. Klin Monatsbl Augenheilkd 100:840–857, 1938

Daniel R, Kanski JJ, Claaspool MG: Hyalo-retinopathy in the clefting syndrome. Br J Ophthalmol 58:96–102, 1974

Libergarb RM, Hirose T, Holmes LB: The Wagner-Stickler syndrome: A study of 22 families. J Pediatr 99:394–399, 1981

Fitch N: Update on the Marshall-Smith-Weaver controversy. Am JMed Genet 20:559–562, 1985

Gorlin RJ, Cohen MM, Levin LS: Syndromes of Head and Neck, 3rd ed, pp 288–289. New York, Oxford Univ Press, 1990

WAGNER-UNVERRICHT

Synonyms. Dermatomyositis; dermatomucomyositis; DM; neuromyositis; polymyositis gregarina.

Symptoms. Prevalent in females (2:1). Onset in infancy rare, in childhood usually before 10 years; in adult, predominant in fourth to sixth decades. Variable symptoms according to prevalent skin or muscular involvement. Malaise; fever; weakness. Erythematous rash (heliotrope rash with blue purple discoloration); edema of eyelids and periorbital. Erythema usually involves face, forearms, upper back. Hands present scaly reddish plaques, especially periungually and over back of joints (Gottron rash). Cuticles irregular, thickened, and distorted, areas of fingers rough and craked with "dirty" horizontal lines resembling mechanic hands; visible capillary loops under nail. When acute phase fades, telangiectatic erythema and pigmentation or depigmentation remains. Subcutaneous calcifications may be extensive and protrude through skin (ulcers and infections). Other types of skin lesions occasionally seen: bullous urticaria, erythema nodosum, or multiform type, hypertrichosis. Muscle weakness, especially shoulder and pelvic girdles; difficulty in swallowing; respiratory difficulty; tachycardia (in 30% of cases). Amyopathic or sine myositis forms may be present.

Etiology. Possibly, autoimmune mechanism; association with neoplastic disease (15–20% of adult cases). Complement deposition in capillaries that leads to necrosis and reduction of number and then muscle fiber destruction.

Pathology. In skin lesion, lymphocytic infiltration, perivascular or in clusters (histiocytes, plasma cells, and eosinophils may be present). Later, homogenization and sclerosis of collagen leading to atrophic changes. Calcification occasionally seen. Muscle involvement frequently localized (seen on biopsy of affected muscles): paleness; flabbiness; fibrosis; calcification according to stage. Vacuolar degeneration of fibers; lymphocytic infiltration. In blood vessels, eosinophilic thickening and thrombosis. Endomysial inflammation predominantly perivascular, perifascicular atrophy (diagnostic for DM even in absence of inflammation).

Diagnostic Procedures. *Biopsy.* Of skin and muscle. *Blood.* SGOT; SGPT; and LDH negative. *X-ray.* Skin and muscle calcification; search for malignancy. *ECG. Electromyography.*

Therapy. If malignancy, surgery, or chemotherapy. Rest in acute phase. Corticosteroids (high doses, then maintenance). Physical therapy to prevent contracture.

Prognosis. In fulminating cases (20%), death during first year. In children 5–16 years survival (75%). Removal of cancer may cure dermatomyositis. In chronic forms, survival variable from 2 to several years. Death from respiratory infections, malnutrition, cardiac failure.

BIBLIOGRAPHY. Wagner E: Fall einer seltener Muskelkrankheit. Arch Theilk 4:282–283, 1863
Unverricht H: Ueber eine eigentnemliche Form von akuter Muskelentzuendung mit einem der Trichinose aehnelnden. Krankheitsbilde Munch Med Wchnschr 4:488–492, 1887
Dalakas MC: Inflammatory myopathies. In Rowland LP, Di Mauro S (eds): Handbook of Clinical Neurology, vol 18: Myopathies, p 369. Amsterdam, Elsevier, 1992

WAISMAN

Synonyms. Parkinsonism early onset, mental retardation; basal ganglia, mental retardation BGMR.

Symptoms. Those of Parkinson seizures (see). Early onset.

Signs. Megalocephaly, frontal bossing.

Etiology. Unknown. X-linked recessive inheritance.

Diagnostic Procedures. See Parkinson's. *X-rays. CT scan. MR imaging.* No basal ganglia calcification. *Karyotype.* Normal.

Therapy. See Parkinson.

Prognosis. Good general health. Normal longevity.

BIBLIOGRAPHY. Lexona R, Brown ES, Hogan K, et al: An X-Linked recessive basal ganglia disorder with mental retardation. Am J Med Genet 21:681–689, 1985
Gregg RG, Metrenberg AB, Hogan K, et al: Waisman syndrome, a human X-linked recessive basal ganglia disorder with mental retardation: Localized to Xq27.3–qter. Genomics 9:701–706, 1991
Ellenberg JH, Koller WC, Langston JW: Etiology of Parkinson Disease. New York, Marcel Dekker, 1995

WALDENSTRÖM II

Synonym. Macroglobulinemia, primary.

Symptoms. More common in males; onset in sixth and seventh decades. Lassitude; weakness (44%); weight loss (23%); hemorrhagic manifestations (37%); frequent infections; visual troubles (8%) (often first chief complaint); hemorrhagic manifestation (44%); Raynaud phenomenon (3%); neurologic symptoms (11%).

Signs. Pallor; microlymphadenopathy (30%); hepatosplenomegaly (38%); fundus oculi, purpura (15%).

Etiology. Unknown. Primary plasma cell dyscrasia. Genetic predisposition and role of various inflammatory and nonreticular neoplasms discussed. To be differentiated from a stable gammaglobulin production abnormality; gammopathy, benign monoclonal. A genetic basis (autosomal dominant) reported in some families.

Pathology. Hemorrhagic lesions. In bone marrow, presence of small atypical lymphomonocytoid cells, increase of mast cells.

Diagnostic Procedures. *Blood.* Anemia; leukopenia; thrombocytopenia. Rouleau formation; Sia test and formol-gel test positive. High sedimentation rate; in some varieties (macrocryogel globulins) low sedimentation rate. Increased serum viscosity and presence of cold agglutinin. *Electrophoresis.* Demonstration of homogeneous typical protein fraction in globulin zone (more frequently in gamma zone). Ultracentrifugation of protein, demonstration of macroglobulin. IgM sedimentation 19S and other fractions more rapidly sediment. *Bone marrow.* Frequently dry tap. Infiltration by abnormal lymphoid cells; demonstration by immunofluorescence of monoclonal IgM on their cytoplasm and surface. *Urine.* Bence-Jones protein in some cases.

Therapy. If marked hypervicosity in emergency: plasmapheresis Chlorambucil; cyclophosphamide, penicillamine; corticosteroids. In secondary form, specific treatment; fludarabine and cladribine worth a trial.

Prognosis. Linked to response to treatment; progressive condition with death in months or few years.

BIBLIOGRAPHY. Waldenström J: Incipient myelomatosis or "essential" hyperglobulinemia with fibrinogenopenia: A new syndrome? Acta Med Scand 117:216–247, 1944
Renier G, Ifrah Chevalier A, et al: Four brothers with Waldenstrom's macroglobulinemia. Cancer 64:1554–1559, 1989
Kantarjian HM, Alexanian R, Koller CA: Fludarabine therapy in macroglobulinemic lymphoma. Blood 75:1928–1931, 1990
Foerster J: Waldenström's macroglobulinemia. In Lee GR, Bithell TC, Foerster J, et al (eds): Wintrobe's Clinical Hematology, 9th ed, pp 2250–2259. Philadelphia, Lea & Febiger, 1993

WALDENSTRÖM III

Synonyms. Acute thyrotoxic encephalopathy; thyroid storm.

Symptoms. Occurs in patients affected by Flajani syndrome (see). Onset usually in advanced age. The crisis is precipitated by various medical (including the rare radioiodine-induced thyroid storm), surgical, or metabolic factors. Severe vomiting; diarrhea; rapid weight loss; fever that is slightly elevated at onset and that rapidly rises to extreme values; severe dyspnea. This variety of thyrotoxic storm is characterized by a prevalent neurologic component represented by dysphagia, dysphonia, labioglossopharyngeal paralysis, oculomotor paralysis; choreiform movements, and transitory palsies among the variable involvement of a number of other organ systems: cardiac, gastrointestinal, hepatic renal, etc.

Signs. Those of Flajani (see).

Etiology. Excessive production of thyroid hormones and particular sensitivity of central nervous system and peripheral nervous system.

Diagnostic Procedures. See Flajani syndrome.

Therapy. It is a major medical emergency and needs intensive treatment and continuous monitoring of vital functions. Methymazole (15 mg every 6 hours) orally or parenterally. Propylthiuracil (150–250 mg every 6 hours) 1 hour after the administration of one of the previously mentioned drugs. Sedation; oxygen; digitalization; rehydration; cooling by physical means (mattress); antibiotics; if hypoadrenalism suspected, hydrocortisone (100–200 mg) or equivalent must be given before initiating the specific (previously mentioned) treatment. Other useful drugs are reserpine or guanethidine (every 8 hours), propanolol (every 6 hours).

Prognosis. Severe. May be improved by the previously mentioned treatment, which brings the crisis under control.

BIBLIOGRAPHY. Waldenström J: Acute thyrotoxic encephalo or myopathy: Its cause and treatment. Acta Med Scand 121:251–294, 1945
Mackin JF, Canary JJ, Pittman CS: Thyroid storm and its management. N Engl J Med 29:1396–1398, 1974
Toft AD (ed): Hyperthyroidism (Symposium). Clin Endocrinol Metab (whole issue), 1985
McKenzie JM, Zakarija M: Hyperthyroidism. In De Groot LJ (ed): Endocrinology, 3rd ed, pp 704–705. Philadelphia, WB Saunders, 1995

WALDENSTRÖM-UVEOPAROTITIS

Synonym. Waldenström uveoparotitis. See also Heerfordt.

Symptoms and Signs. Variety of Heerfordt (see), with addition of hallucinatory manifestations, lethargy, peripheral polyneuritis, areflexia of patella, and Achilles tendon. Presence of Babinski sign.

Etiology. See Heerfordt.

BIBLIOGRAPHY. Waldenström J: Some observations on uveoparotitis and allied conditions with special references to the symptoms from the nervous system. Acta Med Scand 91:53–68, 1937

WALKER-WARBURG

Synonyms. Pagon I; Chemke; cerebrocular dysgenesis; COD; lissencephaly type II; hydrocephalus—agyria—retinal dysplasia; HARD; HARD + Y—Warburg.

Symptoms. Both sexes. At birth. Blindness. (Usually retinal detachment that develops at third trimester of gestation.)

Signs. Hydrocephalus. In some cases encephalocele; retinal detachment; eye anomalies (microphthamlia, angle anomalies, iris hypoplasia, cornal opacity, cataracts, retinal detachment, etc.); hypertelorism; micrognathia.

Etiology. Autosomal recessive inheritance.

Pathology. *Brain.* Agyria, thick cortex, absent cortical layers; hypoplasia or absence of olfactory and optic pathways.

Diagnostic Procedures. *Ultrasonography* for prenatal diagnosis.

Therapy. Symptomatic.

Prognosis. Death within 3 months (65%) to 1 year (100%).

BIBLIOGRAPHY. Walker AE: Lissencephaly. Arch Neurol Psychol 48:13–29, 1942
Warburg M: The heterogeneity of microphthalmia in the mentally retarded. Birth Defects 7:136–154, 1971
Chemke J, Czernobilsky B, Mundel G, et al: A familial syndrome of central nervus system and ocular malformations. Clin Genet 7:1–7, 1975
Pagon RA, Chandler JW, Collie WR, et al: Hydrocephalus, agyria, retinal dysplasia, encephalocele (HARD+ E) syndrome: An autosomal recessive condition. Birth Defects 14:232–241, 1978
Warburg M: Hydrocephaly. Am J Ophthalmol 85:88–95, 1978
Dobyns WB, Agon RA, Armstong D, et al: Diagnostic criteria for Walker-Warburg syndrome (Warburg's syndrome Hard +/–E syndrome). J Med Genet 32:195–210, 1989

WALLENBERG

Synonyms. Vieseaux-Wallenberg; cerebellar artery, postinferior; cerebellar peduncle; dorsolateral medullary; lateral bulbar; lateral medullary.

Symptoms. Occurs usually in patients over 40 years of age. Sudden or gradual onset. Vertigo; vomiting; hiccup; dysphagia; diplopia, ipsilateral course; ataxia; pain or analgesia; loss of temperature sensitivity ipsilateral side of the face; contralateral hypoesthesia for pain and temperature of extremities and trunk. Seldom, contralateral hemiparesis.

Signs. Ipsilateral enophthalmos; ptosis; coarse nystagmus; loss of corneal reflex; miosis; lack of coordination; ipsilateral hypotonia; ipsilateral paralysis soft palate, pharynx, vocal cord.

Etiology. Thrombosis of posterior, inferior, cerebellar, or vertebral artery or both. Arteriosclerotic vascular disease, syphilis, and other types of occlusive disease.

Pathology. Infarction of lateral medulla, inferior part of cerebellum, spinal tract, nucleus ambiguous, restiform body, vestibular nucleus.

Diagnostic Procedures. *Spinal tap. EEG. Angiography. CT scan. MRI.*

Therapy. Anticoagulant.

Prognosis. Symptoms may disappear abruptly; complete recovery usually in months. Facial neuralgia, crossed neuralgia of extremities and trunk persist for a longer time.

BIBLIOGRAPHY. Wallenberg A: Acute bulbäraffection (Embolie der Art. Cerebellar post, inf. sinstr. ?). Arch Psychiatr 27:504–540, 1895
Lemarquis P, Bartolomei F: A propos d'un nouveau cas de syndrome de Wallenberg après manipulations du rachis cervical. Sem Hop Paris 67:1486–1488, 1991
Weatherall DJ, Ledingham JGG, Warrell DA (eds): Oxford Textbook of Medicine, 3rd ed, p 3858. Oxford, Oxford Med Pub, 1996

WALTER-BOHMANN

Old eponym used to indicate symptoms complex occurring after cholecystectomy or cholecystoduodenostomy: pallor; cold sweat; hypothermia; tachycardia and polypnea (see Postcholecystectomy).

BIBLIOGRAPHY. Akel S: Kolesistektomiden soura goeruelen bir Walter-Bohmann syndrom V. Tuerk tip Cem Mec 21:255–256, 1956

WALTON

Synonyms. Benign congenital hypotonia; congenital benign muscular hypoplasia; muscular benign hypoplasia. See Floppy infant syndromes.

Symptoms. Onset in neonatal period. Extreme muscular weakness. Same symptoms as in Werdnig-Hoffmann (see), but late in developing, however, patients obtain a good range of spontaneous movements. Arms affected to a lesser degree than legs.

Signs. Reflexes may be depressed or normal; no fasciculations. Muscles extremely flabby.

Etiology. Unknown. Delay of development of neuromuscular apparatus.

Pathology. Biopsy of muscle. Smallness of all muscle fibers; increase of connective tissue or fat, or degenerative changes.

Diagnostic Procedures. Difficult to differentiate at early stage from Werdnig-Hoffmann, except by muscle biopsy.

Therapy. Symptomatic.

Prognosis. Good. Seldom persists beyond first decade. Progressive improvement. Some contortionists may have had this syndrome in infancy.

BIBLIOGRAPHY. Sobel J: Essential or primary hypotonia in young children. Med J Rec 124:225–230, 1926
Walton J: Amyotonie congenita. Lancet I:1023–1028, 1956
Zellweger H, Afifi A, McCormick WF, et al: Benign congenital muscular dystrophy: a special form of congenital hypotonia. Clin Pediatr 6:544–553, 1967
Adams RD, Victor M: Principles of Neurology, 5th ed, pp 1247, 1249. New York, McGraw-Hill, 1993

WANDERING PACEMAKER

Synonyms. Atrioventricular nodal rhythm; shifting pacemaker.

Symptoms. Frequently asymptomatic. Occasionally, palpitation, choking from sensation of fullness in neck.

Signs. Bradycardia. Undue variations of first heart sound; irregularity may induce suspicion of presence of atrial fibrillation.

Etiology. Suppression of successive pacemakers and successive takeover by following centers. Usually, shifting back and forth between sinus and A-V nodes. In normal heart, caused by fluctuating vagal tone.

Diagnostic Procedures. *ECG.* Changes in size, shape of P-waves; P-Q intervals shortened to less than 0.10 second; rate alterations.

Therapy. None. Decrease of vagal tone.

Prognosis. Transitory phenomenon of no clinical importance.

BIBLIOGRAPHY. Meyerburg RJ, Kessler KM, Castellanos A: Recognition, clinical assessment and management of arrhytmias and conduction disturbances. In Schlant RC, Alexander RW: Hurst's The Heart, 8th ed, p 729. New York, McGraw-Hill, 1994

WARDROP

Synonym. Onychia maligna.

Symptoms and Signs. Fetid ulceration of fingertips with eventual loss of nails.

Etiology. Primary or secondary infective process of nail beds.

BIBLIOGRAPHY. Wardrop H: An account of some diseases of the toes and fingers, with observation on their treatment. Med Chir Trans 5:129–143, 1814
Barak R, Dawber RPR (eds): Diseases of the Nail and Their Management. Oxford, Blackwell Scientific, 1994

W.A.R.G.

Synonyms. Wilms tumor—aniridia—mental retardation—gonadoblastoma. See Drash.

Symptoms and Signs. Aniridia, mental retardation, and Wilms tumor (see) that may became detectable several months or years after birth and only occasionally, bilateral gonadoblastoma and sexual anomalies

Etiology. Congenital condition. Microdilation of 11p13 chromosome.

Diagnostic Procedures. *Chromosomal studies. Echography.*

Therapy. Symptomatic. Surgery.

Prognosis. Poor.

BIBLIOGRAPHY. Riccardi VM, Sujansky E, Smith AC, et al: Chromosomal imbalance in the aniridia-Wilms association: 11 interstitial deletion. Pediatrics 61:604–610, 1978
Turleau C, de Grouchy J, Dufier JL, et al: Aniridia, male pseudohermaphroditism, gonadoblastoma, mental retardation and del 11p13. Hum Genet 57:300–306, 1981

WARTENBERG

Synonyms. Cheiralgia parestetica; chiralgia parestetica. See also acroparesthesia.

Symptoms and Signs. Paresthesia, dysesthesia, or hyperesthesia (burning pain) in the distal third of forearm; local cutaneous discoloration.

Etiology and Pathology. Injury (blunt trauma) or compression (entrapment) of radial nerve (from repeated rotation of arm) as the nerve emerges from beneath the brachioradialis tendon.

Diagnostic Procedures. Diagnostic nerve blocking.

Therapy. Splinting; rest; antiinflammatory; surgical decompression.

Prognosis. Good with conservative or surgical treatment.

BIBLIOGRAPHY. Wartenberg R: Brachialgia statica paresthetica (nocturnal arm dysesthesias). J Nerv Ment Dis 99:877–887, 1944
Zemel N: Neurovascular disorders. In Jobe FW: Operative Techniques in Upper Extremity Sport Injuries. St Louis, CV Mosby, 1996

WATERHOUSE-FRIEDERICHSEN

Synonyms. Marchand-Waterhouse-Friederichsen; adrenal apoplexy; adrenal hemorrhage; meningococcal adrenal; purpura meningococcemia. See Addisonian syndromes.

Symptoms. Occurs usually in infants or children, occasionally in adults. Increased irritability; headache; nausea; vomiting; abdominal pain; diarrhea. Fever initially moderate, then high.

Signs. Pallor; clammy skin; cyanosis; petechial rash; neck stiffness; convulsion; dyspnea; tachycardia; hypotension; coma; dehydration; oliguria.

Etiology. In large majority of cases, meningococcemia. Seen also with other infections (diphtheria; pneumococcus; staphylococcus; smallpox).

Pathology. That of acute infection; necrosis and hemorrhage of adrenal cortex; large skin hemorrhage.

Diagnostic Procedures. *Blood.* Culture; serology; low sodium and chlorides; high potassium. *CT scan. MRI.*

Therapy. Treatment of sepsis; control of shock; adrenal hormone therapy.

Prognosis. Death in 24–48 hours if treatment not given rapidly. Permanent adrenal insufficiency not recorded in patients who survive.

BIBLIOGRAPHY. Marchard F: Ueber eine eigentümliche Erkrangkung des Sympathicus, der Nebennieren der peripherischen Nerven (ohne Bronzehaut). Virchows Arch (Pathol) 81:477–502, 1880
Waterhouse R: A case of suprarenal apoplexy. Lancet I:577–578, 1911
Friederichsen C: Nebeunieren-apoplexie bei Kleinen Kinderh. Jahrb Kinderheilkd 87:109–125, 1918
Loriaux DL, McDonald WJ: Adrenal insufficiency. In De Groot LJ (ed): Endocrinology, 3rd ed, pp 1731–1740. Philadelphia, WB Saunders, 1995
Weatherall DJ, Ledingham JGG, Warrell DA (eds): Oxford Textbook of Medicine, 3rd ed, pp 536, 1510, 1653, 3658, 4052. Oxford, Oxford Med Pub, 1996

WATER INTOXICATION

Synonyms. Dilution; overhydration. See Hyponatremia and Schwartz-Bartter syndromes.

Symptoms. *Chronic type.* Slow accumulation of water; weakness; sleepiness; apathy; anorexia; nausea; vomiting; sialorrhea; lacrimation; watery diarrhea; perspiration not excessive; progression to behavioral changes, seizures, and coma. *Acute type.* Decreased attention; strange behavior; confusion; aphasia; incoordination; apathy alternated with violent behavior; marked muscle weakness.

Signs. Skin warm, moist; pitting edema. Muscle twitching; tendon hyporeflexia; Babinski sign (later). Hemiplegia may develop. Signs of pulmonary edema, especially if heart condition pre-exists.

Etiology. Administration of water in excess of kidney excretion capacity. Psychogenic water drinker. Usually iatrogenic excessive water administration, especially in patients with excessive antidiuretic hormone (ADH) secretion, in postoperative stage with low renal blood flow, or with Addisonian syndromes (see), acute renal insufficiency, congestive heart failure. May occur from large enema in hyponatremic patients, and in infants with megacolon.

Diagnostic Procedures. *Blood.* Hemoglobin, hematocrit decreased; macrocytosis with decrease of mean hemoglobin concentration. Sodium low; potassium low, normal or high in severe form. Blood urea nitrogen normal, or low (except if previously increased). Bicarbonates low. *Urine.* Volume variable; specific gravity low; sodium and chloride, low or normal.

Therapy. *Acute treatment.* Initiate and maintain rapid diuresis with IV furosemide; replace the sodium and potassium lost in urine (3% saline seldom required). *Chronic treatment.* Restrict water; discontinue hypotonic solutions; administer demeclocycline, furosemide.

Prognosis. Guarded. Varies in accordance with the etiology and the general fitness of the patient.

BIBLIOGRAPHY. Goldberger E: A Primer of Water, Electrolyte, and Acid-base Syndromes, 3rd ed. Philadelphia, Lea & Febiger, 1965

Berl T: Psychosis and water balance. N Engl J Med 318(7):441–442, 1988

Weatherall DJ, Ledingham JGG, Warrell DA (eds): Oxford Textbook of Medicine, 3rd ed, p 4125. Oxford, Oxford Med Pub, 1996

WATSON

Synonyms. Noonan neurofibromatosis; neurofibromatosis–Noonan; pulmonic stenosis—café au lait spots; café au lait spots—pulmonic stenosis; von Recklinghausen and Noonan. See LEOPARD.

Symptoms and Signs. Both sexes. Cafe-au-lait spots; signs of pulmonic stenosis reduced intelligence; short stature; for another group reported neurofibromatosis signs, short stature, ptosis midface hypoplasia, webbed neck, and weakness.

Etiology. Autosomal dominant inheritance postulated. (The two groups as described were considered by some authors as distinct syndromes; successive reports found shared features between the two groups, thus presently they are considered as a unique entity or the coincidence of two relatively frequent conditions.)

Therapy. Cardiac surgery.

Prognosis. According to different degrees of the manifestations.

BIBLIOGRAPHY. Watson GH: Pulmonary stenosis, cafe-au-lait spots, and dull intelligence. Arch Dis Child 42:303–307, 1967

Partington MW, Burggraf GW, Fay JE, et al: Pulmonary stenosis, cafe-au-lait spots and dull intelligence: The Watson syndrome revised. Proc Greenwood Genet Ctr 4:105, 1985

Allanson JE, Upadhyaya M, Watson GH, et al: Watson syndrome: Is it a subtype of type I neurofibromatosis? J Med Genet 28:752–756, 1991

WATSON-ALAGILLE

Synonyms. Alagille; arteriohepatic dysplasia, AHD; cholestasis, peripheral pulmonary stenosis; hepatofacial, neurocardiac, vertebral; hepatic ductal hypoplasia, multiple malformations.

Symptoms. Uncommon. Both sexes affected. Neonatal jaundice; pruritus, retarded physical, mental, and sexual development.

Signs. Broad forehead, pointed mandibula, bulbous nose, posterior embryotoxon, retinal pigmentary changes. Heart murmurs and other signs of pulmonar valve stenosis and peripheral arterial stenosis. Absence of deep tendon reflexes. Finger foreshortening.

Etiology. Autosomal dominant inheritance. It appears to be a possible variant of von Recklingausen I.

Pathology. Liver cholestasis and inflammation; paucity of intrahepatic bile ducts. Pulmonary valve and peripheral pulmonary arterial stenosis.

Diagnostic Procedures. *ECG. X-rays.* Cardiovascular defects; vertebral defects; limb deformities; other variable skeletal defects. *Ultrasonography.* Liver diffuse hepatic increase in echogenicity, loss of normal structures. *Hepatobiliary scintigraphy.* Changes similar to those of biliary atresia. *Blood.* Transaminase (SGPT) chronic elevation. *Liver biopsy.*

Therapy. Cardiosurgery and/or liver transplantation may be considered according to conditions. Medical treatment of cholestasis.

Prognosis. Patients reach adult age.

BIBLIOGRAPHY. Watson GH, Miller V: Arteriohepatic dysplasia: Familial pulmonary arterial stenosis with neonatal liver disease. Arch Dis Child 48:459–466, 1973

Alagille D, Odievre M, Gautier M, et al: Hepatic ductular hypoplasia associated with characteristic facies, vertebral malformations, retard-

ed physical, mental and sexual development and cardiac murmur. J Pediatr 86:63–71, 1975

Alagille D, Estrada A, Hadchduel M, et al: Syndromic paucity of intralobular bile ducts (Alagille syndrome or arteriohepatic dysplasia). Review of 80 cases. J Pediatr 110(2):195–200, 1987

Weatherall DJ, Ledingham JGG, Warrell DA (eds): Oxford Textbook of Medicine, 3rd ed, pp 2014, 2015. Oxford, Oxford Med Pub, 1996

WEARY

Synonyms. Sclerosing poikiloderma, hereditary; poikiloderma sclerosing, hereditary. See keratosis syndromes.

Symptoms and Signs. Described in a large Negro family. Onset early childhood. Generalized poikiloderma. Sclerosing palms and soles linear hyperkeratotic and sclerotic bands in the limbs flexures.

Etiology. Autosomal dominant inheritance.

BIBLIOGRAPHY. Weary PE, Hsu YT, Richardson D: Hereditary sclerosing poikiloderma: Report of two families with an unusual and distinctive genodermatosis. Arch Dermatol 100:413–422, 1969

WEATHERALL

Synonyms. ATR-X; alpha thalassemia, mental retardation; hemoglobin H disease, mental retardation; HbH with multiple congenital anomalies. See ATR16.

Symptoms and Signs. Rare. In North European families. From birth, mental retardation (IQ 50–70) and multiple congenital anomalies.

Etiology. X-linked inheritance. ATR-X locus localized to an interval of approximately 11cM between the loci DXS106 and DXYS1X (Xq12–q21.31).

Diagnostic Procedures. *Hemoglobin electrophoresis.*

Therapy. Symptomatic.

Prognosis. Poor.

BIBLIOGRAPHY. Borochowitz D, Levin SE, Krawitz S, et al: Hemoglobin-H disease in association with multiple congenital abnormalities. Clin Ped 9:432–435, 1970

Weatherall DJ, Higgs DR, Bunch C, et al: Hemoglobin H disease and mental retardation: A new syndrome or a remarkable coincidence? N Engl J Med 305:607–612, 1981

Gibbons RJ, Suyhers GK, Wilkie AOM, et al: X-linked-thalassemia/mental retardation (ATR-X) syndrome: Localization to Xq12–q21.31 by X inactivation and linkage analysis. Am J Hum Genet 51:1136–1149, 1992

WEAVER

Synonyms. Weaver-Smith.

Symptoms and Signs. Males are affected three times as frequently as females. Females may have a milder form of the syndrome. Large birth size and accelerated growth; mild hypertonia; hoarse cry. Loose skin; thin hair. *Head.* Wide frontal area; flat occiput; hypertelorism; large ears; long philtrum; micrognathia; hoarse voice. *Extremities.* Elbow and knee reduced extension; broad distal femur and ulna; broad thumbs; camptodactyly; thin nails. Umbilical hernia. Neoplasia may develop.

Etiology. Sporadic. A mesenchymal defect resulting in early mineralization of the ossification centers has been suggested. Neurologic deficits may be caused by instability of cervical spine.

Diagnostic Procedures. *X-rays. CT scan. MRI. Polytomography dynamic:* accelerated bone maturation, and splaying of distal part of long bones (femur; ulna). The cervical spine must be evaluated with plain flexion and extension views of the lateral aspect of cervical region to assess the question of instability.

Prognosis. Accelerated physical growth continuing in infancy; however, overgrowth seems to be a variable in both onset and duration.

Therapy. Stabilization of the unstable cervical spine, either by immobilization or surgery.

BIBLIOGRAPHY. Weaver DD, Graham CB, Thomas IT, et al: A new overgrowth syndrome with accelerated skeletal maturation, unusual facies, and camptodactyly. J Pediatr 84:547–552, 1974
Ardinger HH, Hanson JW, Harrod MJ, et al: Further delineation of Weaver syndome. J Pediatr 108:228–235, 1986
Muhonen MG, Menez AH: Weaver syndrome and instability of upper cervical spine. J Pediatr 116:596–599, 1990

WEAVER-LIKE

See Weaver (may be a separate entitity) and Marshal-Smith.

BIBLIOGRAPHY. Stoll C, Talon P, Mengus L, et al: A Weaver-like syndrome with endocrinological abnormalities in a boy and mother. Clin Genet 8:225–259, 1985

WEBER-CHRISTIAN

Synonyms. Pfeifer-Weber-Christian; nodular nonsuppurative panniculitis; spondylopanniculitis.

Symptoms. Occurs in every age group. No sex dominance. Prodromal symptoms; malaise; low fever; oropharyngeal infections; mild arthralgia or arthritis.

Signs. Subcutaneous nodules of various diameters (1–12 cm) in all parts of body, more frequently on the thighs. Hands, face, and feet usually spared. Usually tender; seldom painful. Redness of overlying skin; after acute phase, pigmentation and then atrophy of skin. Nodules (seldom) rupture with extrusion of yellow fatty fluid. Splenomegaly; anterior uveitis, and acute exudative central choroiditis in some cases. Relapses frequent.

Etiology. The syndrome is probably the result of an inborn error in the regulation of the inflammatory response leading to uncontrolled fever, leukocytosis, and local inflammatory reactions directed mainly, but not exclusively, against fat but also, for instance, against vessels; in fact distinction between panniculitis and various vasculitis is blurred. Among the various causes of panniculitis one must consider pancreatic enzyme p; 1-antitrypsin deficiency; immunologic disorders; cellular proliferative diseases; cold; facticial; steroids; etc.

Pathology. *Early lesion.* Fat-laden macrophages. *Larger lesion.* Small central area of fat necrosis with halo of lymphocytes, polymorphonuclear and macrophages. *Old lesions.* Decrease of necrotic material and fibrotic changes. Blood vessels in the nodules usually normal; occasionally moderate vasculitic changes or thrombosis or both. Liver usually shows fatty changes and necrosis. Macrophages may be found in many organs (lymph nodes, spleen, pancreas, lung).

Diagnostic Procedures. *Blood.* During acute phase, moderate to marked leukopenia with moderate relative lymphocytosis and moderate anemia. Leukocytosis in involution phase. Biopsy of subcutaneous node. *X-ray.* Occasionally, calcification of nodules has been reported.

Therapy. Symptomatic. Corticosteroids: methylprednisolone dosages of up to 2 mg/kg four times a day during acute episodes of fever, pain, and pulmonary symtoms; during remissions, 0.25–0.5 mg/kg/day. Attempts to further reduce the dosage or to use alternate-day therapy have often resulted in recurrence of panniculitis.

Prognosis. Febrile period (acute) of different lengths (weeks); then spontaneous regression. Frequent relapses in months or years. Myocar-

dosis, coronary occlusion, granulomatous pneumonitis, ileus, liver cirrhosis, myelofibrotic pancytopenia, glaucoma, and retroperitoneal fibrosis may develop as complications of this syndrome.

BIBLIOGRAPHY. Pfeifer V: Ueber einen Fall von herdweiser Atrophie des subkutanen Fettgewebes. Dtsch Arch Klin Med 50:438–449, 1892
Weber FP: A case of relapsing nonsuppurative nodular panniculitis showing phagocytosis of subcutaneous fat-cells by macrophages. Br J Derm 37:301–311, 1925
Christian HA: Relapsing, febrile, nodular nonsuppurative panniculitis. Arch Intern Med 42:338–351, 1928
Sorensen R, Abramowsky C, Stern RC: Ten-year course of early-onset Weber-Christian syndrome with recurrent pneumonia: a suggestion for pathogenesis. Pediatrics 78:115–120, 1986
Burton JL, Cunlife WJ: Subcutaneous fat. In Champion RH, Burton JL, Ebling FJG (eds): Rook/Wilkinson/Ebling Textbook of Dermatology, 5th ed, pp 2140–2142. Oxford, Blackwell Scientific, 1992

WEBER-COCKAYNE

Synonyms. Cockayne-Touraine; acanthosis bullosa; epidermolysis bullosa localized; hand-feet epidermolysis bullosa; includes Kallin (name of patient). See also Fox, Goldscheider, and Herlitz syndromes.

Symptoms and Signs. Both sexes affected. Onset in infancy, especially in warm season. Occasionally delayed to early adult life (wearing heavy boots). After minor trauma formation of bullae on palms and soles. Sharp pain when bullae rupture. Hyperhidrosis. If associated anadontia, hair and nail disorders: Kallin syndrome.

Etiology. Autosomal dominant inheritance. In Kallin possibly recessive inheritance.

Pathology. Subepidermal bullae with clear fluid; scarce or absent signs of inflammation. Elastic tissue broken or frayed.

Diagnostic Procedures. *Biopsy.* Of skin. See Pathology.

Therapy. Protection from trauma, especially during warm season.

Prognosis. Chronic condition.

BIBLIOGRAPHY. Elliot GT: Two cases of epidermolysis bullosa. J Cutan Genitourin Dis 13:10–18, 1895
Weber FP: Recurrent bullous eruption of the feet in a child. Proc R Soc Med 19:72, 1926
Cockayne EA: Recurrent bullous eruption of the feet. Br J Derm 50:358–362, 1938
Haldane JBS, Poole RA: A new pedigree of recurrent bullous eruption on the feet: Four generations of foot blister. J Hered 33:17–18, 1985
Pye RJ: Bullous eruptions. In Champion RH, Burton JL, Ebling FJG (eds): Rook/Wilkinson/Ebling Textbook of Dermatology, 5th ed, pp 1626–1627. Oxford, Blackwell Scientific, 1992

WEBER-GUBLER

Synonyms. Weber (H); alternating oculomotor; cerebellar peduncle; superior alternating hemiplegia; Leyden oculomotor alternating paralysis; ventral medial midbrain.

Symptoms and Signs. Ipsilateral oculomotor (III) nerve paresis; contralateral spastic paresis of lower face, tongue, and extremities. External strabismus; fixed dilated pupil; ptosis.

Etiology. Vascular occlusion of paramedian area of midbrain; parasellar aneurysm tumor.

Pathology. Hemorrhage; thrombosis of ventral part of midbrain with involvement of nucleus or oculomotor (III) nerve.

Diagnostic Procedures. *Spinal tap. Angiography. CT brain scan. MRI.*

Therapy. According to etiology.

Prognosis. Variable, usually poor.

BIBLIOGRAPHY. Weber H: A contribution to the pathology of the crura cerebri. Med Chir Tr (Lond) 46:121–139, 1863
Adams RD, Victor M: Principles of Neurology, 5th ed, p 1173. New York, McGraw-Hill, 1993

W.E.B.I.N.O.

Synonym. Wall-eyed bilateral internuclear ophthalmoplegia.

Symptoms and Signs. Distinctive disordered ocular motility of bilaterally impaired adduction and dissociated nystagmus of the abducting eye on horizontal gaze in either direction.

Etiology. The condition has been observed in demyelinating diseases, arteriosclerotic cerebrovascular disease, trauma, Arnold-Chiari malformation, syphilis, periarteritis nodosa, glioma, and cryptococcal meningitis, and lymphoma after intrathecal chemotherapy and cranial irradiation.

Diagnostic Procedures, Therapy, Prognosis. Those of the underlying disorder.

BIBLIOGRAPHY. Daroff RB, Hoyt WF: Supranuclear disorders of ocular control systems in man. In Bach YR, Rita P, Collins CC (eds): The Control of Eye Movements, p 223. New York, Academic Press, 1971
Lepore FE, Nissenblatt MJ: Bilateral internuclear ophthalmoplegia after intrathecal chemotherapy and cranial irradiation. Am J Ophthalmol 92:851–853, 1981
Klintworth GK: Ocular involvement in disorders of the nervous system. In Garner A, Klintworth GK (eds): Pathobiology of Ocular Disease: A Dynamic Approach, 2nd ed, pp 1713, 1714, 1733. New York, Marcel Dekker, 1994

WEGENER

Synonyms. Klinger; arteritis—pulmonary—nephropathy; granulomas—arteritis—glomerulonephritis; granulomatosis pathergic; necrotizing respiratory granulomatosis.

Symptoms. Occurs in individuals of both sexes. Onset at all ages. At onset persistent rhinitis; malaise; fever; cough; severe weight loss; hemoptysis; seizures, hypertension. ELK system (E = ear-nose-throat, L = lung, K = kidney) may be affected in toto or separately; involvement of the kidney alone is not considered diagnostic.

Signs. Ulceration of midline structure of face. Upper respiratory tract (E): serohematic discharge, perforation of nasal septum, ulcerated mucosae, otitis. *Eyes.* Proptosis, necrotizing scleritis, perforation of globe, central artery occlusion, uveitis, dacriocystitis. *Lung (L).* Usually no signs or respiratory failure, cough, dyspnea; hemoptysis. *Kidney (K)* (85% incidence). Slowly progressive kidney dysfunction or advanced renal failure. *Skin.* Papulonecrotic lesions of extremities purpura, and telangiectasia (late stage), urticaria, pyoderma gangrenosum. *Nervous system.* Mononeuritis multiplex owing to nerve ischemia, multiple crania nerves palsies, amaurosis fugax, cerebral infarction, transverse myelitis. *Joints.* Symmetic polyarthritis.

Etiology. Unknown. Possibly, an autoimmune disease. It is considered the generalized form of the lethal midline granuloma (see).

Pathology. In skin; necrotic granulomatous lesions, necrotizing vasculitis (artery and veins). Hyaline and fibrinoid thrombi in all organs, but always predominantly involving upper respiratory tract, lungs, and kidneys (focal necrotizing glomerulonephritis).

Diagnostic Procedures. *Biopsy. X-ray.* Of chest: multiple nodules with or without cavitation, rarely diffuse alveolar filling. Interstitial pattern uncommon. *Urine.* Albuminuria; casts; hematuria. *Blood.* Anemia, high blood urea nitrogen, and creatinemia; transient eosinophilia; hyperglobulinemia, rheumatoid factor positivity. Sputum cytology. *Kidney biopsy.* See Pathology. Anticytoplasmic autoantibody is diagnostic for Wegener.

Therapy. Relative effectiveness of steroids, nitrogen mustard, azathioprine, chlorambucil, cyclophosphamide. Antibiotics for secondary infections. Trimetoprim/sulfamethoxazole in monotherapy.

Prognosis. Progressive. Spontaneous remissions of 2 or 3 months that temporarily interrupt progressive fatal course are occasionally observed. Mortality 28% at 5 years; major cause kidney failure.

BIBLIOGRAPHY. Klinger H: Grenzformen der Periarteritis nodosa. Frank Zt Pathol 42:455–480, 1931
Wegener F: Ueber generalisierte septische gefosser Krankungen. Verhandl Dtsch Pathol Ges 29:202–210, 1936
Lê Thi Huong Du, Wechsler B, Cabane J, et al: Granulomatose de Wegener. Aspects cliniques, problèmes nosologiques. Revue de la Littérature à propos de 30 observations. Ann Med Intern 139:169–182, 1988
Weatherall DJ, Ledingham JGG, Warrell DA (eds): Oxford Textbook of Medicine, 3rd ed, pp 2801–2802, 3011–3012. Oxford, Oxford Med Pub, 1996

WÊGIERKO

Obsolete.

Synonym. Third diabetic coma. See Umber.

Symptoms. Eponym used to indicate a cluster of neurologic symptoms: vomiting; anorexia; insomnia; restlessness; hallucination; depression; coma, which occurs in diabetic patients without hyperketonemia or hyperglycemia. A hypothalamic lesion suspected by the author, but no autopsy findings are reported. The author also reported a mortality of 100% in his cases.

BIBLIOGRAPHY. Wêgierko H: Typowy Zespòl objawów klinicznych u chorych na cukrzyce, zakończozony s'mierciâ w špiaczce bez zakwaszenia Ketonowegâ ("trzecia špiâczka"). Pol Typ Lek 11:2020–2033, 1956

WEIL II

Synonyms. Fielder II; Landouzy-Mathieu-Weil; Landouzy II; Mathieu; Vasilev; spirochetal jaundice; icterohemorrhagic leptospirosis; spirochetosis.

Symptoms and Signs. Prevalent in male, teenage, and young to middle-age adults. Onset during hot months, in people directly or indirectly exposed to excretions of any of a wide variety of domestic and wild animals. Biphasic illness; acute infection manifestation at onset: headache; fever; muscle aching. Distinct features appear on third to sixth day and slowly progress: jaundice; generalized hemorrhages (epistaxis; hemoptysis, GI gastrointestinal bleeding); and a combination of hepatic and renal manifestations (with one of the two predominating). Hepatic tenderness and enlargement; renal involvement (see Diagnostic Procedures).

Etiology. Usually owing to *Leptospira* icterohaemorrhagiae, occasionally other leptospirae. Direct toxic damage owing to leptospiral antigens.

Pathology. Hemorrhages and bile staining of skeletal muscles, kidney, liver, adrenals, stomach, spleen, lung, and brain. Focal microscopic, vacuolization of sarcoplasm with neutrophilic infiltrations. In kidney, hemoglobin, myoglobin casts, interstitial neutrophilic infiltration of cortex and medulla; glomeruli usually spared. Other tissue changes not diagnostic.

Diagnostic Procedures. *Blood.* From leukopenia to marked leukocytosis (neutrophilia 70%); anemia; demonstration of hemolysis. Seldom, thrombocytopenia. Hyperbilirubinemia; azotemia. Cultural and serologic studies for identification of Leptospira. Dark-field examination. *Urine.* Proteinuria; red cell casts; urobilinuria.

Therapy. Penicillin; streptomycin; tetracyclines (given within first 4 days). Doxycycline (as prophylactic agent 200 mg per os once a week). Fluid and electrolytes balance.

Prognosis. Average mortality 10%. Severity of form correlates with duration of disease: in anicteric patients, no deaths reported; with jaundice, 15–40% mortality.

BIBLIOGRAPHY. Landouzy LTJ: Typhus hépatique. Gaz Hôp Paris 56:913–914, 1883

Weil A: Ueber eine eigenthümliche, mit Milztumor, Icterus und Nephritis einhergehende, acute Infektionskrankheit. Dtsch Arch Klin Med 39:209–232, 1886

Sperber SJ, Schleupner CJ: Leptospirosis: A forgotten cause of aseptic meningitis and multisystem febrile illness. South Med J 82:1285–1288, 1989

Weatherall DJ, Ledingham JGG, Warrell DA (eds): Oxford Textbook of Medicine, 3rd ed, pp 700–701. Oxford, Oxford Med Pub, 1996

WEILL-MARCHESANI

Synonyms. Marchesani; Marfan inverted; brachymorphia—spherophakia; mesodermal hypoplastic dystrophy. M-W; spherophakia—brachymorphia. Includes GEMSS (glaucoma—lens ectopia—microspherophakia—stiffness of joints—shortness).

Symptoms. Onset of ocular symptoms in first decade, myopia with or without glaucoma; blindness in one-third of cases. Inability to flex or extent the fingers completely, or to make a fist. Possibly, defective hearing.

Signs. In eyes: spherophakia, microphakia, subluxated lenses (50%). Short stature (average 148 cm), short extremities, and brachydactyly. In some cases, cardiac murmur. Teeth malformed; maxillary hypoplasia.

Etiology. Unknown. Considered a result of a basic embryologic mesodermal defect. Marchesani considers this syndrome to be the opposite of Marfan and represents the hyperplastic (brachydactyly) variant of the latter. Inherited condition of homozygous recessive genotype; dominant inheritance also suggested. Full form or partial form may be manifested. GEMSS autosomal dominant inheritance.

Diagnostic Procedures. *X-ray.* Of hand. Symmetric shortening and widening of metacarpals and phalanges and retardation of carpal ossification. Feet and toes may share in the process of delayed ossification. *Ophthalmoscopy.* See Signs. Retinal pigment degeneration; optic atrophy.

Therapy. Ophthalmologic procedures to correct myopia and pressure. Medical and surgical (removal of lens to prevent glaucoma).

Prognosis. The patients are short and proportioned. Eye pathology sometimes corrected, sometimes proceeding to blindness.

BIBLIOGRAPHY. Weill G: Ectopie des cristallins et malformations génèrales. Ann Ocul (Paris) 169:21–44, 1932

Marchesani O: Brachydaktylie und angeborene Kugellinse als Systemar-Krankung. Klin Monatsbl Augenheilkd 103:392–406, 1939

Hailk GM Sr, Terrell WL, Hailk GM Jr: The Weill-Marchesani syndrome: Report of two cases and a review. LA State Med Soc 142:25–32, 1990

Kunz M, Paulus W, Sollberg S, et al: Sclerosis of the skin in the GEMSS syndrome: An overproduction of normal collagen. Arch Dermatol 131:1170–1174, 1995

WEINBERG

Synonyms. Dysplasia tarda of lower limb; MEDT (type IIa); lower limbs dysplasia.

Symptoms and Signs. Present from birth. Epiphyseal dysplasia of lower limbs. Occasionally, minor abnormality of vertebrae.

Etiology. Autosomal dominant inheritance. It represents one of the various forms of spondiloepiphyseal dysplasia tarda (see).

BIBLIOGRAPHY. Weinberg H, Frankerl M, Mekin J, et al: Familial epiphyseal dysplasia of lower limbs. J Bone Joint Surg (Br) 42:313–332, 1960

Beighton P: McKusick's Heritable Disorders of Connective Tissue, 5th ed, pp 622–625. St Louis, CV Mosby, 1993

WEINBERG-HIMELFARB

Synonyms. Endocardial dysplasia; endocardial fibroelastosis, EFE; subendocardial sclerosis; primary endocardial fibroelastosis.

Symptoms. Both sexes equally affected. Onset in infancy or early childhood, seldom at older age. Dyspnea; cough; irritability; anorexia; vomiting; weakness; chest pain; failure to thrive.

Signs. Diaphoresis; tachypnea; tachycardia; pulmonary rales; hepatomegaly; acyanosis; absence of cardiac murmurs.

Etiology. Two forms described. Primary or idiopathic with no other heart disease; secondary with left-sided congenital heart condition (aorta coarctation, stenosis, mitral stenosis, or atresia). It has been discussed as a separate entity. Three types of inheritance reported autosomal dominant and recessive, and X-linked. But majotity of cases are sporadic.

Pathology. Diffuse opaque thickening of endocardium. Typical endocardial scarring. Proliferation of collagenous and elastic tissue. Left ventricle exclusively or predominantly involved. Two types described: dilated heart type; nondilated type (rare). In first type, possibly, association with mitral insufficiency with chordae tendinae short and thick; seldom, aortic valve insufficiency.

Diagnostic Procedures. *ECG.* Sinus rhythm; left ventricular hypertrophy. *X-ray.* Cardiomegaly (dilated type); hilar and intrapulmonary vessels show venous congestion. *Angiography. Fluoroscopy.* Pulsation on cardiac margin; weak wavy contraction. *Two-dimensional echocardiography with color flow imaging and spectral Doppler interrogation.* Markedly dilated left ventricle, a thin free wall and greatly decreased contractility. *Biopsy.*

Therapy. Symptomatic. L-Carnitine, steroids, digitalis, diuretics. Antibiotics for pulmonary complications. Heart transplantation.

Prognosis. Death usually before completion of second year of life. Survival after 5 years of age unusual. Particularly poor if condition becomes manifest in first month of life.

BIBLIOGRAPHY. Weinberg T, Himelfarb AJ: Endocardial fibroelastosis (so-called fetal endocarditis). Bull Johns Hopkins Hosp 72:299–306, 1943

Perloff JK: The Clinical Recognition of Congenital Heart Disease, 4th ed, pp 189–197. Philadelphia, WB Saunders, 1994

Towbin JA, Roberts R: Cardiovascular diseases due to genetic abnormalities. In Schlant RC, Alexander RW: Hurst's The Heart, 8th ed, p 1741. New York, McGraw-Hill, 1994

WEISENBURG

Synonym. Glossopharyngeal neuralgia. See Reichert.

Symptoms. Unilateral lancinating, paroxysmal pain usually starting in the tonsillar region, lateral pharynx, or base of tongue, radiating deeply into the ear. Irritated by eating, talking, or movement of pharynx or tongue with occasionally increased salivation. Rarely recurrent episodes of syncope. Sinus bradycardia, hypotension.

Signs. Induction of the symptoms by stimulating one of the trigger points.

Etiology and Pathology. Irritation of entire glossopharyngeal (IX) nerve. Neoplasia; inflammation.

Therapy. Intracranial section of glossopharyngeal (IX) nerve. Carbamazepine. To control syncopal episodes: atropine or, if uncontrollable, a pacemaker.

Prognosis. Cured by treatment. Sectioning of the glossopharyngeal (IX) nerve results in unilateral anesthesia of soft palate and pharyngeal wall, and anesthesia and loss of taste of posterior third of the tongue.

BIBLIOGRAPHY. Weisenburg TH: Cerebellopontine tumor diagnosed for six years as a tic douloureux. The symptoms of irritation of ninth and twelfth cranial nerves. JAMA 54:1600–1604, 1910
St John JN: Glossopharyngeal neuralgia associated with syncope and seizures. Neurosurgery 10:380–383, 1982
Adams RD, Victor M: Principles of Neurology, 5th ed, p 1178. New York, McGraw-Hill, 1993

WEISMANN-NETTER

Synonyms. Weismann-Netter-Stuhl; tibioperoneal diaphyseal pachyperiostosis; toxopachyostéose diaphysaire tibio-péronière.

Symptoms and Signs. Equal distribution both sexes. Dwarfism; mental retardation; bowing of legs, minor alterations of the arms.

Etiology. Familial incidence (autosomal dominant) reported.

Diagnostic Procedures. *X-ray.* Selective thickening of affected bones. Diaphyseal bowing may be present in other long bones; squaring of iliac bones. Dural calcification.

BIBLIOGRAPHY. Weismann-Netter R, Stuhl I: D'une osteopathie congénitale éventuellement familiale surtout définie par l'incurvation antéro-postérieure et l'épaississement des deux os de la jambe (toxopachyostéose diaphysaire tibiopéronière). Presse Med 62:1618–1622, 1954
Amendola MA, Brower, AC, Tisnado J: Weismann-Netter-Stuhl syndrome: toxopachyperiostéose diaphysaire tibio-péronière. Am J Roentgen 135:1211–1215, 1980
Robinow M, Johnson GF: The Weismann-Netter syndrome. Am J Med Genet 29:573–579, 1988

WEISS

Synonym. Storage pool platelet deficiency, SPD.

Symptoms and Signs. Mild or moderate hemorrhagic tendency.

Etiology. Autosomal dominant inheritance. Hereditary condition frequently associated with other platelet anomalies: Hermanski-Pudlak (see); Chediak-Higashi (see); Wiskott-Aldrich (see).

Diagnostic Procedures. *Blood.* Decrease of adenosine diphosphate in the dense granules of platelets. It may either affect the delta or the alpha granules or the two types.

Prognosis. Fair.

BIBLIOGRAPHY. Weiss HJ, Chervenick PA, Zalusky R, et al: A familial defect in platelet function associated with impaired release of adenosine diphosphate. N Engl J Med 281:1264–1270, 1969
Weiss HJ, Lages BA: Platelet malondialdehyde production and aggregation responses induced by arachidonate, prostaglandin-G2, collagen and epinephrine in 12 patients with storage pool deficiency. Blood 58:27–33, 1981
Herve P, Drouet L, Dosquet C, et al: Primary pulmonary hypertension in a patient with a familial platelet storage pool disease role of serotonine. Am J Med 89:117–120, 1990
Holmsen HN, Weiss HJ: Hereditary defect in the platelet release reaction caused by a deficiency in the storage pool of platelet adenine nucleotides. Br J Haemat 19:643–649, 1991

WEISS-BAKER

Synonym. See Carotid sinus.

Symptoms. With patient in any position, loss of consciousness.

Signs. No change in pulse rate or arterial pressure. Attacks may be preceded or accompanied by focal neurological signs.

Etiology. See Carotid sinus.

BIBLIOGRAPHY. Weiss S, Baker JP: The carotid sinus reflex in health and disease: Its role in the causation of fainting and convulsions. Medicine 12:297–354, 1933
Lewis RP, Budoulas H, Schaal SF, et al: Diagnosis and management of syncope. In Schlant RC, Alexander RW: Hurst's The Heart, 8th ed, pp 932–933. New York, McGraw-Hill, 1994

WEISSENBACHER-ZWEYMULLER

Synonym. W-Z. Possibly part of a spectrum including Marshall, Wagner-Stickler, Pierre Robin, Kniest, SED congenita.

Symptoms and Signs. Rare. At birth. Micrognathia; rhizhomelic chondrodysplasia (dumbbell-shaped femora and humeri). Successively myopia conductive hearing loss.

Etiology. Disease of connective tissue resulting in delayed maturation. Autosomal dominant inheritance. Considered neonatal expression of Wagner syndrome (see) or part of the continuum: Stickler-Marshall-OSMED-Micrognatic dwarfism.

Diagnostic Procedure. *X-rays.* Long bones: dumbbell widening of metaphyses; ischial, pubic bones: bulbous deformities; vertebrae: coronal clefts.

Prognosis. Regression of bone changes and successive almost normal growth.

BIBLIOGRAPHY. Weissenbacher G, Zweymuller E: Gleichzeitiges Vorkommen eines Syndromes von Pierre Robin und einer fetalen Chondrodysplasie. Monatsschr Kinderh 112:315–317, 1964
Kelly TE, Wells HH, Tuck KB: The Weissenbacher-Zweymuller syndrome: Possible neonatal expression of the Stickler's syndrome. Am J Med Genet 11:113–119, 1982
Galil A, Carmi R, Goldstein E, et al: Weissenbacher-Zweymuller syndrome: Long term follow-up of growth and psychomotor development. Dev Med Child Neurol 33:1104–1109, 1991

WELLS

Synonyms. Eosinophilia—granulomatous dermatitis; granulomatous dermatitis; cellulitis eosinophilic.

Symptoms and Signs. Both sexes affected. Variable age (29–70). *First stage.* Localized redness and edema of skin (sparing the face) that in 2 or 3 days spreads, with central involution and, possibly, blistering (occasionally hemorrhagic). *Second stage.* Formation of dermal mass, overlying skin slate colored, with violet edge. *Third stage.* Evolution toward a pale solid, morphea-like mass and, finally, regression.

Etiology. Unknown. Related to allergic vasculitis, Schulman, and other hypereosinophilic syndromes.

Pathology. Three stages: *First.* Dermal edema; intradermal leukocytes (eosinophils prevalent) masses. *Second.* Granulomatous dermatitis; eosinophil infiltrates around fibrinoid flame masses, surrounded by a palisade of histiocytes and giant cells. *Third.* Histiocyte necrobiosis and persistence of flame figures. No evidence of vasculitis at any stage, but evidence of eosinophilic infiltration in fascia and muscles as well.

Diagnostic Procedures. *Blood. Bone marrow.* Increase in eosinophils. *Biopsy.* Of skin. See Pathology.

Therapy. Corticosteroids.

Prognosis. Duration 1 year with variability of severity.

BIBLIOGRAPHY. Wells GC: Recurring granulomatous dermatitis with eosinophilia. Trans St Johns Hosp Dermatol Soc 37:46–56, 1971

Spigel GT, Ninikelmann RK: Wells' syndrome: Recurrent granulomatous dermatitis, with eosinophilia. Arch Derm 119:611–613, 1979

Contant G: Blètry O Pathologie de l'eosinophile aspect cliniques prognostic and therapeutiques. Enciclopedie Med Sang 13–009–A10, p 2. 1994

WERDNIG-HOFFMANN

Synonyms. Hoffmann (J.) I; spinal muscular atrophy infantile, SMAI; muscular atrophy, infantile; PHYI. See Kugelberg-Welander. See Floppy infant syndromes.

Symptoms. Present at birth or onset in newborn in half of cases. In other half, onset within first year of life. Symmetric paralysis of trunk and limbs, so that head cannot be turned, and infant cannot turn over. Loss of sucking ability.

Signs. Tendon reflexes depressed or absent; muscular wasting; fasciculation of tongue and other muscles. Respiratory embarrassment.

Etiology. Unknown. Autosomal recessive inheritance; possibly, dominant with incomplete expression.

Pathology. In central nervous system, paucity of cells on anterior horn, no glial or inflammatory reaction, demyelinized anterior root and peripheral nerves. Muscle thin with atrophic fibers.

Diagnostic Procedures. *Biopsy.* Of muscle. *Electromyography.*

Therapy. Symptomatic.

Prognosis. Death between third month and end of fourth year.

BIBLIOGRAPHY. Werdnig G: Zwei frühinfantile hereditäre Fälle von progressive Muskelatrophie unter dem Bilde der Dystrophie aber auf neurotischer Grundlage. Arch Psychiatr Nervenkr 22:437–480, 1891

Hoffmann J: Ueber chronische spinale Muskelatrophie im Kindersalter, auf familiarer Basis. Dtsch Z Nervenkr 3:427–470, 1893

Hausmanowa-Petrusewics I, Zaremba J, et al: Chronic proximal spinal muscular atrophy of childhood and adolescence: Problems of classification and genetic counselling. J Med Genet 22:350–353, 1985

Daniels RJ, Thomas NH, MacKinnon RN, et al: Linkage analysis of spinal muscular atrophy. Genomics 12:335–339, 1992

Weatherall DJ, Ledingham JGG, Warrell DA (eds): Oxford Textbook of Medicine, 3rd ed, p 3988. Oxford, Oxford Med Pub, 1996

WERLHOF

Synonyms. Idiopathic thrombocytopenic purpura; ITP; purpura hemorrhagica.

ACUTE IDIOPATHIC THROMBOCYTOPENIA

Symptoms. Both sexes equally affected. Prevalent in children (85% under 8 years of age). Usually, infection 1 or 2 weeks prior to onset. Sudden skin and mucosa purpura.

Signs. Purpura; ecchymosis; no palpable spleen.

Etiology. Idiopathic; following infection (in children) or drug administration or exposure to chemicals (in adult).

Pathology. Generalized hemorrhagic manifestation.

Diagnostic Procedures. *Blood.* Anemia (occasionally secondary to blood loss), normal leukocytes; thrombocytopenia; shortened platelet survival time; demonstration of antiplatelet factors. *Bone marrow.* Normal number of megakaryocytes.

Therapy. Transfusion if needed; corticosteroid or adrenocorticotropic hormone (ACTH); intravenous IgG.

Prognosis. Self-limited course of 1 week or a few months in 90% of cases; 10% of cases become chronic.

CHRONIC IDIOPATHIC THROMBOCYTOPENIC PURPURA

Symptoms. Prevalent in females (3:1); onset usually in adult life, except the cases with acute onset (see the preceding). The onset is usually insidious. Increased bruisability; prolonged menses; mild bleeding manifestations.

Signs. Spleen normal or slightly enlarged.

Etiology. Unknown. Possibly, autoimmune disorder.

Diagnostic Procedures. *Blood.* Moderate anemia may be present, leukocytes normal. Moderate thrombocytopenia (40,000–80,000); platelet survival shortened. Demonstration of serum antiplatelet factors.

Therapy. Corticosteroids; ACTH; splenectomy; intravenous IgG.

Prognosis. Chronic condition. Complete cure probably never occurs spontaneously. Clinical remission and relapses (occasionally, at time of menses or with infection, vaccination, or other stressing situations), with or without variation of platelet number; however, platelet numbers never reach normal values, and they always show a shortened life span. Cure by splenectomy in almost 70% of cases. Mortality from this condition 6.8% in one large series.

RECURRENT IDIOPATHIC THROMBOCYTOPENIC PURPURA

Symptoms. As in the preceding, recurrent episodes with complete clinical and hematologic remissions (return to normal of platelet number and to normal life span).

BIBLIOGRAPHY. Werlhof PG: Disquisitio Medica et Philologica ed Variolis et Anthracibus. Brunswick, 1735

Frank E: Die essentielle Thrombopenie. Berl Klin Wochenschr 52:454–458, 1915

Imbert CL, Shaison G: Interet des immunoglobines dans le traitment du purpura thrombopenique idiopathique. Encycl Med Chir Sang 13019 A 10:7, 1987

WERMER

Synonyms. Endocrine adenoma-peptic ulcer complex; MEA; MEN I; multiple endocrine adenomatosis I; multiple endocrine neoplasias I; pluriglandular adenomatosis I. See Zollinger-Ellison.

Symptoms and Signs. Both sexes affected with same frequency. Onset at all ages, after first decade. Protean symptomatology related to the various endocrine glands involvement: parathyroid, pancreas (Zollinger-Ellison, insulinoma, glucagonoma, Vipoma, Poma, somastatinoma), pituitary or other possibly associated tumors. Thyroid, carcinoid, adrenocortical, lipoma. Hyperfunction of any single gland for some time, usually at onset. Peptic ulcer symptoms most common initial feature. Hypoglycemic crisis; headache; visual field defects; amenorrhea; diarrhea; weight loss.

Etiology. Genetic basis. Two types of oncogenes dominant and recessive have been described. MEN 1 gene localized to chromosome 11q13.

Pathology. Adenomas or hyperplasia of multiple glands: parathyroid (88%); pancreas (81%); pituitary (65%); adrenals (19%). Lesions of nonendocrine organs found in the same patients are also manifestations of the syndrome (e.g., gastrointestinal tract pathology).

Diagnostic Procedures. *Blood. Urine. X-ray.* Of skull and gastrointestinal tract. According to clinical manifestation.

Therapy. Surgery when feasible and medical treatment of specific hormonal and secondary metabolic alterations.

Prognosis. Cause of death frequently related to syndrome manifestations such as hypoglycemic coma or to complications of surgery.

BIBLIOGRAPHY. Erdheim J: Zur normalen und pathologischen Histologie

der Glandula thyroidea, parathyroidea und Hypophysis. Beitz Pathol Anat Allg Pathol 33:158–236, 1903
Wermer P: Genetic aspects of adenomatosis of endocrine glands. Am J Med 16:363–371, 1954
Schimke RN: Genetic aspects of multiple endocrine neoplasia. Am Rev Intern Med 35:25–31, 1984
Thakker RV: Multiple endocrine neoplasia. In De Groot LJ (ed): Endocrinology, 3rd ed, pp 2815–2831. Philadelphia, WB Saunders, 1995

WERNER (C.W.O.)

Synonym. Progeria of adult. See also Rothmund-Thompson.

Symptoms. Fully developed during second and third decades of life, tendency to occur in brother and sister. Normal birth; early physical and mental development. In adolescence, growth failure, hypogonadism, lack of sexual desire, and appearance of typical signs

Signs. Short stature; sexual underdevelopment; canities (hair becoming gray); premature baldness; development of atrophic dermatitis (see Pathology) of lower legs, feet, upper arms, hands, and partially on the face. Nose beaked; eyes prominent; extremities slender (atrophy of subcutaneous fat and muscles); development of bilateral cataracts and finally signs of arteriosclerosis, completing the picture of presenility. This syndrome may also occur in forme fruste with only some of the signs present.

Etiology. Unknown. Autosomal recessive inheritance.

Pathology. Skin: circumscribed areas of hyperkeratosis and atrophy; skin becoming tightly pulled over bony prominence; hair follicle and sweat glands scarce and not well developed; no proliferative or necrotizing arteritis; elastic fiber of corium loose but unaltered. Generalized arteriosclerotic changes; hypertrophic arthritis; osteoporosis; tissue calcification.

Diagnostic Procedures. *Biopsy.* Of skin. *X-ray.* Hormone excretion studies. *Blood.* Sugar (frequently diabetes mellitus develops). Increased number of both anti-double-stranded and anti-single-stranded DNA antibodies in the IgG class.

Therapy. Surgery for cataract; skin grafting for ulcer; none specific.

Prognosis. Average life span of 47 years.

BIBLIOGRAPHY. Werner CWO: Ueber Katarakt in Verbindung mit Sclerodermie Inaug Disser Kiel, 1904
Thannhauser SJ: Werner's syndrome (progeria of adult) and Rothmund's syndrome; two types of closely related heredofamilial atrophic dermatoses with juvenile cataracts and endocrine features: Critical study with five new cases. Ann Intern Med 23:559–626, 1945
Bauer EA, Uitto J, Tan EM, et al: Werner's syndrome: Evidence for preferential regional expression of a generalized mesenchymal cell defect. Arch Derm 124:90–101, 1988
Goto M, Rubenstein M, Weber J, et al: Genetic linkage of Werner syndrome to five markers on chromosome 8. Nature 355:735–738, 1992

WERNER (P.)

Synonym. Mesomelic dwarfism Werner. See ulna-fibula hypoplasia and Nievergelt.

Symptoms and Signs. Both sexes affected. Present from birth. Polydactyly (hands and feet); absent thumbs; short legs (absent or rudimentary tibia); reduced knee movements.

Etiology. Autosomal dominant inheritance with variable expressivity. Lethal autosomal recessive form.

Diagnostic Procedures. *X-ray.* Absence or short tibias; altered growth of arm bones. Spine and head normal. Thick humerus, hypoplastic platella.

Therapy. *Surgical.* Amputation of extra finger. Pollicization. Feet bracing; prosthesis.

Prognosis. According to degree of lesions. Corrective measures may improve mobility and height of patient.

BIBLIOGRAPHY. Werner P: Ueber einen seltenen Fall von Zwergwuchs. Arch Gynaekol 104:278–300, 1919
Kozlowski K, Eklof O: Werner mesomelic dysplasia. J Belge Radiol 70:337–339, 1987
Rimoin DL, Lachman RS: Genetic disorders of the osseous skeleton. In Beithon P (ed): McKusick's Heritable Disorders of Connective Tissue, 5th ed, p 636. St Louis, CV Mosby, 1993

WERNICKE APHASIA

Synonyms. Bastian; Pick-Wernicke; aphasia receptive; sensory aphasia; temporoparietal.

Symptoms and Signs. Lack of comprehension of spoken language, alexia, and agraphia. Voluble speech; paraphasia.

Etiology and Pathology. Lesion on posterior temporoparietal lobe of dominant hemisphere. Vascular, infective, traumatic, neoplastic etiology.

Diagnostic Procedures. *X-ray. Angiography. Brain isotope scan.*

Therapy. According to etiology.

Prognosis. Depends on etiology. When vascular lesion, progressive improvement frequently is noticed.

BIBLIOGRAPHY. Wernicke K: Der Aphasische Symptomekomplex. Breslau, M Chohn und Weigert, 1874
Adams RD, Victor M: Principles of Neurology, 5th ed, pp 413–414, 418–419. New York, McGraw-Hill, 1993
Weatherall DJ, Ledingham JGG, Warrell DA (eds): Oxford Textbook of Medicine, 3rd ed, pp 3850, 3851, 3968. Oxford, Oxford Med Pub, 1996

WERNICKE (C.) II

Synonym. Neurosis cramps.

Symptoms. In state of fear or anxiety, painful muscular cramps in various parts of the body.

Etiology. Psychogenic mechanism the precipitating factor.

BIBLIOGRAPHY. Wernicke C: Ein Fall von Crampus-Neurose. Klin Wochenschr 41:1121–1124, 1904

WERNICKE-KORSAKOFF

Synonyms. Gayet-Wernicke; Wernicke I; Meynert; Korsakoff (pure encephalopathy); cerebral beriberi; encephalopathia hemorrhagica superioris; polyencephalitis transketolase defect; alcohol-induced encephalopathy; anamnestic confabulatory (Korsakov); association of Wernicke encephalopathy and Korsakoff anamnestic (see) syndromes.

Symptoms. More frequent in Europeans. Anorexia; insomnia; anxiety; confusion; drowsiness; vomiting; progressive dementia.

Signs. Nystagmus; partial to complete ophthalmoplegia (most commonly, external recti); paralysis of conjugate gaze; ptosis; impairment of pupil reactions; ataxia; prostration; coma. Peripheral neuritis frequently associated. Severe form (Gayet also defined).

Etiology. Inborn error of metabolism of transketolase that makes cells more susceptible to thiamine deficiencies. This defect presumably is autosomal recessive. Frequently observed in alcoholic, nutritionally deficient patients and chronic hemodialysis patients.

Pathology. *Brain.* Generalized production of new blood vessels (granulation tissue-like); proliferation of vascular endothelium; thickening of blood walls; dilatation of vessels; small hemorrhages; fibroblasts into scars; destruction of nervous tissue and invasion by neuroglia. Hemorrhage and scar widespread in corpora mammilari.

Diagnostic Procedures. *Blood.* Hypochromic anemia (usually); elevated pyruvic acid. *Isoenzyme studies. Spinal tap. EEG.*

Therapy. Thiamine. Propranolol has been tried with some success.

Prognosis. Early treatment with thiamine reverses condition rapidly and completely. The Korsakov may persist after vitamin replacement and abstinence with persisting ante- and retrograde amnesia, confabulation and with a poor prognosis. If untreated, coma and death.

BIBLIOGRAPHY. Gayet M: Affection encéphalique (Encéphalique diffuse probable). Localisée aux étages supérieurs des pédoncules (cerébraux et aux couches optiques, ainsi qu'au plancher du quatrième ventricule et aux parosis latérales du troisème). Observation recueille. Arch Physiol Norm Pathol, Paris, 2:341–351, 1875

Wernicke C: Lehrbuch der Gehirnkrankeiten fur Aerzte und Studirende. Kassel, T Fisher, 1881

Korsakoff SS: Ob alkogol' nour paraliche. Vest Psikhiat (Moskva) 4:1887

Dreyfus PM: Thoughts on the physiopathology of Wernicke disease. Ann NY Acad Sci 215:367–369, 1973

Mukherjee AB, Svoronos S, Ghazanfari A, et al: Transketolase abnormality in cultured fibroblasts from familial chronic alcoholic men and their male offspring. J Clin Invest 79:1039–1043, 1987

Weatherall DJ, Ledingham JGG, Warrell DA (eds): Oxford Textbook of Medicine, 3rd ed, pp 4126–4127. Oxford, Oxford Med Pub, 1996

WEST

Synonyms. Generalized flexion epilepsy; infantile spasm; jack-knife convulsion; massive myoclonia; salaam spasms.

Symptoms. Onset during first year of life. Convulsion in infancy, characterized by fast recurrence, nodding of the head, with or without bending of entire body. Occasionally, opisthotonos with or without rapid movements of arms (less frequently legs) reminiscent of Moro reflex. Mental retardation; visual problems.

Etiology. Many causes suggested. Brain damage from trauma, anoxia, or degenerative, metabolic factors and infective agents. Possibly X-linked inheritance.

Pathology. According to etiology.

Diagnostic Procedures. *EEG.* Hypsarrhythmia. *Blood. CSF. Cultures. Metabolic studies.*

Therapy. Anticonvulsive therapy: diphenylhydantoin; phenobarbital; trimethadione. Cortical steroids. ACTH initiated early.

Prognosis. Poor for mental development.

BIBLIOGRAPHY. West WJ: On a peculiar form of infantile convulsions. Lancet I:724–725, 1840–41

Feldman RA, Schwartz JF: Possible association between cytomegalovirus infection and infantile spasms. Lancet I:180–181, 1968

Doose H: Epilepsien im Kindes-und Jugendalter. Desin Hamburg, 1988

Adams RD, Victor M: Principles of Neurology, 5th ed, pp 276, 282. New York, McGraw-Hill, 1993

WEST INDIES ATAXIC–SPASTIC

Synonyms. Jamaican paraplegic ataxic–spastic. Tropical spastic paraparesis. See Leber II. See Grierson-Gopalan.

ATAXIC GROUP

Described originally in the West Indies; observed also in besieged population during wars in Europe, the Middle and Far East, and Africa. Presently considered part of an enlarged Frierson-Gopalan syndrome (see).

Symptoms. Either sex. Insidious onset. Bilateral symptoms; deafness; decrease in vision; central or paracentral scotoma (never complete blindness). Other symptoms precede leg symptoms by years. Weakness; unsteadiness of gait; numbness and burning of lower legs and feet.

Signs. Ataxia, mild spasticity, Babinski sign; symmetric, confined to or exclusive of lower extremities. Wasting of leg muscles and foot drop (in long-lasting cases). Fundus oculi: various degrees of bilateral optic atrophy, marked temporal pallor.

Etiology. Unknown. No vitamin deficiency or consistent spirochetal infections demonstrated.

Pathology. Unknown.

Diagnostic Procedures. *CSF.* Normal. *Gastric analysis.* Achlorhydria or hypochlorhydria. *Blood.* Occasionally hypochromic anemia. *X-ray.* Normal. *Serology.* For syphilis; positive only in some cases.

Prognosis. Relatively benign condition. All symptoms and signs progress steadily for months, then become stationary.

SPASTIC GROUP

Symptoms. Occurs in early middle age, in both sexes. Sudden onset. First symptoms unilateral. Mild nerve deafness (infrequent); weakness; pain and numbness of legs; lumbar backache; occasionally, severe paraplegia developing in a few days. Later, bladder dysfunction.

Signs. Leg spasticity; Babinski sign, loss of abdominal reflexes (not constant); mild spasticity of upper limbs. Jaw jerk reflex exaggerated. Eye pupils may be slightly irregular and reaction is sluggish to light and accommodation.

Etiology. Unknown. Possible role of syphilis and yaws considered, but features of this syndrome are atypical. Toxins, vitamin deficiencies also may play a role.

Pathology. Inflammatory changes of variable degree; destruction of myelin; particularly in pyramidal, spinocerebellar; dorsomedial tracts, and thickening of blood vessels.

Diagnostic Procedures. *CSF.* Moderate increase (in 40%) in lymphocytes or proteins, or both; abnormal colloidal gold reactions. *Blood.* Hypergammaglobulinemia. *Gastric analysis.* Hypochlorhydria or achlorhydria. *X-ray.* Negative. *Serology.* For syphilis. Positive only in some cases. Negative in spinal fluid.

Therapy. Symptomatic; physical therapy.

Prognosis. Progression of symptoms for weeks or months, occasionally for years. Variable degree of impairment. Bladder dysfunction in most cases. (Described also, a group with both ataxic and spastic features.)

BIBLIOGRAPHY. Montgomery RD, Cruickshank EK, Robertson WB, et al: Clinical and pathological observations on Jamaican neuropathy: A report on 206 cases. Brain 87:425–462, 1964

Adams JH, Blackwood W, Wilson J: Further clinical and pathological observations on Leber optic atrophy. Brain 89:15–26, 1966

Adams RD, Victor M: Principles of Neurology, 5th ed, pp 773, 882. New York, McGraw-Hill, 1993

WESTPHAL-BERNHARD

Obsolete.

Synonyms. Papilitis stenosans, benign.

BIBLIOGRAPHY. Westphal K: Muskelfunktion Nervensystem und Pathologie der Gallenwege 3. Die Motilitaetsneurose der Gallenwege und ihre Beziehungen zu deren Pathologie, zur Stauung, Entzuendung, Steinbildung usw. Z klin Med 96:95, 1923

WESTPHAL-LEYDEN

Obsolete.

Synonyms. Westphal ataxia; Leyden ataxia; Goekay-Tuekel ataxia acute; chorea—akinetic—rigidity variety. See Choreiform.

Symptoms and Signs. Both sexes affected. Onset in childhood. Vomiting; vertigo; proximal muscle rigidity; convulsive seizures; mental abnormalities. Choreic movements (rare).

Etiology. Unknown. Nosologic confused condition. Possibly autosomal dominant inheritance.

Diagnostic Procedures. *EEG. Angiography. CT brain scan. MRI.*

Therapy. Haloperidol; chlorpromazine.

Prognosis. Death within 10 years. Final stage indistinguishable from Huntington chorea (see).

BIBLIOGRAPHY. Westphal C: Eigenthümliche mit Einschlafen verbundene Anfälle. Arch Psychiatr 7:631–635, 1877
Leyden E: Ueber akute Ataxia. Z Klin Med 18:576–587, 1890

WESTPHAL-PILTZ

Synonyms. Piltz-Westphal; neurotonic pupillary reaction.

Symptoms and Signs. Pupillary contraction occurring after vigorous closing of eyes. Delayed reaction to light, followed by slow dilatation of pupil.

Etiology. Unknown. See Pupillotonic syndrome.

BIBLIOGRAPHY. Westphal A: Ueber ein bischer nicht beschriebene Pupillenphänomen. Neurol Centralbl (Leipz) 18:161–164, 1899
Piltz J: Das vagotonische Pupillenphänomen, von Somogyi. (Wiener Klin Wschr 1913 NR 33). Neurol Centralbl (Leipz) 33:1124, 1914

WEYERS II

Synonyms. Miller; Neger-De Reyner; Treacher Collins; Curry-Hall; acrodysostosis; Weyers acrodysplasia; Weyers dysostosis acrofacialis. See Meyer-Schwicherath.

Symptoms and Signs. Both sexes affected. Present from birth. Postaxial hands and feet hexadactyly and fusion of fifth and sixth metatarsals and metacarpals. Cleft of mandibular symphysis; anomalies of lower incisors and oral vestibule.

Etiology. Autosomal dominant inheritance.

BIBLIOGRAPHY. Weyers H: Ueber eine korrelierte Missbildung der Kiefer und Extremitaetenakren. (Dysostosis acro-facialis) Fortsch Roentgen 77:562–567, 1952
Curry CJR, Hall BD: Polydactyly, conical teeth, nail dysplasia, and short limbs: A new dominant autosomal malformation syndrome. Birth Defects 15:253–263, 1979
Roubicek M, Spranger J: Weyers' acrodental dysostosis in a family. Clin Genet 26:587–590, 1984

W.H.I.M.

Synonyms. Whart—Hypogammaglubulinemia—Infection—Mielok athesis; Wetzler.

Symptoms and Signs. Both sexes. Repeated sinopulmonary bacterial infections; cervical and vulvar chronic papillovirus infections; hands verrucae vulgaris.

Etiology. Unknown. Possibly autosomal dominant inheritance.

Diagnostic Procedures. *Blood.* Hypogammaglobulinemia; neutropenia. Neutrophyls show cytosplasmic vacuoles and hypersegmentation with dense lobules. *Bone marrow.* Hypercellularity, shift to the right of granulopoiesis (myelokathesis = retention of myeloid cells at bone marrow level): normal erythropoiesis, megakaryocytes, and lymphocytes.

Therapy. Antibiotics, antiviral agents, gamma globulin.

Prognosis. Repeated severe infections; eventually septicemia causes death.

BIBLIOGRAPHY. Mentzer WC, Johnston RB Jr, Baeher RL, et al: An unusual form of chronic neutropenia in a father and daughter with hypogammaglobulinemia. Br J Haemat 36:313–322, 1977
Wetzler M, Talpaz M, Kleinerman ES, et al: A new familial immunodeficiency disorder characterized by severe neutropenia: A defective marrow release mechanism and hypogammaglobulinemia. Am J Med 89:663–672, 1990

WHIPPLE

Synonyms. Lipophagic intestinal granulomatosis; intestinal lipodystrophy. See Malabsorption syndromes.

Symptoms. Predominant in males. Onset usually between fourth and seventh decades. Migratory arthralgia; diffuse abdominal discomfort; intermittent diarrhea with frothy, bulky, foul-smelling stool. Cough; dyspnea; weakness; weight loss; intermittent fever. Occasionally: sensory and motor changes, and other severe neurologic manifestations (observed usually in patients not treated or treated later after onset, seldom occurring as first manifestation); cardiac impairment in approximately 50% of cases.

Signs. Grayish pigmentation of skin; occasionally, purpura; edema; emaciation. Abdomen: generalized tenderness; doughy consistency. Lymphadenopathy; ascites; polyserositis.

Etiology. Unknown. Host susceptibility factors and not yet identified or confirmed organism.

Pathology. Thickening of intestinal wall; white patches; bluish discoloration of serosa. Enlarged mesenteric lymph nodes. Mucosa: velvety; clubbed villi. Presence of macrophage containing periodic acid-Schiff (PAS)-positive material in jejunal lamina propria and in various organs: heart; adrenals; lymph nodes, subcutaneous fat. With high magnification many bacilli may be seen.

Diagnostic Procedures. *Stool.* Rich in fat and fatty acid. *Blood.* Hypochromic anemia; increased sedimentation rate; hypoproteinemia; hypocholesterolemia; glucose tolerance test normal or flat. *Gastric analysis.* Decreased free acid. *Biopsy.* Of lymph node and jejunae mucosa (see Pathology). *X-ray. CT scan. MRI.* Deficiency in small intestine and brain.

Therapy. Antibiotics (continued indefinitely, intermittently). Corticosteroids give temporary remission.

Prognosis. Dramatic response to treatment with disappearance of symptoms and signs. Weight gain; increased well-being.

BIBLIOGRAPHY. Whipple, GH: A hitherto undescribed disease characterized anatomically by deposits of fat and fatty acids in the intestinal and mesenteric lymphatic tissues. Bull Johns Hopkins Hosp 18:382–391, 1907
Allchin and Heeb quoted by Morgan AD: The first recorded case of Whipple disease. Gut 2:370–372, 1961
Fleming JL, Wiesner RH, Shorter RG: Whipple's disease: Clinical, bio-

chemical and histopathologic features and assessment of treatment in 29 patients. Mayo Clin Proc 63:539–551, 1988

Shifrin HD: Whipple's disease. In Haubrich WS, Schaffner F, JE Berk (eds): Bockus Gastroenterology, 5th ed, vol 2, pp 1183–1194. Philadelphia, WB Saunders, 1995

WHITE LIVER

Synonyms. Fatty metamorphosis viscerae; steatosis of liver; visceral steatosis. See Wolman.

Symptoms and Signs. Both sexes. Onset congenital. Progressive muscle hypotonia; lethargy; coma; hemorrhagic condition; jaundice.

Etiology. Possibly lack of one of the mechanisms of excretion of triglycerides formed in hepatocytes. Autosomal recessive inheritance.

Pathology. Heart, liver, kidney fatty infiltration (fatty acids 15 times normal amount) and increase of triglycerides.

Diagnostic Procedures. *Blood.* Milky serum with chylomicrons and high pre-beta and high quantity of high-density lipoproteins; hypoglycemia; hypocalcemia.

Therapy. Symptomatic.

Prognosis. Death in first days after birth or within a few weeks.

BIBLIOGRAPHY. Peremans J, Degraef PJ, Strubbe G, et al: Familial metabolic disorder with fatty metamorphosis of the viscera. J Pediatr 69:1108–1112, 1966

Chesney RW, Sveum RJ, Lacey M, et al: A three month old infant with seizures, hypoglycemia, and apnea. Am J Med Genet 16:373–388, 1983

Schaffner F: Nonalcoholic fatty liver. In Haubrich WS, Schaffner F, Berk JE (eds): Bockus Gasroenterology, 5th ed, p 2246. Philadelphia, WB Saunders, 1995

WHITE MATTER

Synonyms. Hemiplegia, bilateral cerebral blindness deafness decerebration.

Symptoms and Signs. Includes most of leukodystrophies, familial (see individual syndromes).

BIBLIOGRAPHY. Adams RD, Victor M: Principles of Neurology, 5th ed, p 840. New York, McGraw-Hill, 1993

WHITFIELD

Synonym. Erythema induratum; Whitfield. See Bazin, Vilanova-Aguadé.

Symptoms. Predominent in women. Onset in middle age. Aching of legs after prolonged standing; generalized malaise; minor systemic complaints.

Signs. Edema of ankles; crops of painful tender nodules erupting after exposure to cold, minor traumas, general infections. No erythrocyanosis; no ulceration.

Etiology. Allergic mechanism possible; association with tuberculosis (in that case Bazin, see) venous stasis may play some role. See also Vilanova-Aguadé.

Pathology. Vasculitis of different degrees. Pattern clouded by venous involvement with edema and fibrosis and thrombosis of small vessels with areas of tuberculoid granulomata; caseation rare.

Therapy. Elevation of legs; rest; elastic stockings. Elimination infective foci.

Prognosis. Chronic recurrences with precipitating factors.

BIBLIOGRAPHY. Whitfield A: On the nature of the disease known as erythema induratum scrofulosorum. Am J Med Sci 122:828–834, 1901

Savin JA: Mycobacterial infections. In Champion RH, Burton JL, Ebling FJG (eds): Rook/Wilkinson/Ebling Textbook of Dermatology, 5th ed, p 1053. Oxford, Blackwell Scientific, 1992

WHITMORE

Synonyms. Stanton; melioidosis (means "similar to distemper in asses"); pneumoenteritis; pseudocholera.

Symptoms. Endemic in Southeast Asia; rare in the Western Europe. Occasionally seen in drugs users. Men more frequently affected than women. Onset 2 or more days after exposure. From asymptomatic to acute, subacute, and chronic. Chills; cough; bloody sputum; abdominal pain; diarrhea; prostration.

Signs. Acute (most frequent). Signs of pneumonia; empyema; lung abscess; splenomegaly; jaundice; hyperthermia. Subacute. Lymphadenitis; signs of osteomyelitis; numerous abscesses (pulmonary, cutaneous, liver, spleen); occasionally, pyelonephritis. Latent. For years recrudescent; may become activated after long periods of latency by intercurrent trauma, burns, surgery.

Etiology. Pseudomonas pseudomallei (Whitmore bacillus).

Pathology. Lesions prevalent in the lung; extensive abscesses: outer border hemorrhagic; medial zone neutrophilic leukocytes; inner core formed by necrotic debris with multinucleated histiocytes (giant cells), marked karyorrhexis. Similar abscesses (but less frequently) in any other viscera or organs (e.g., subcutaneous, brain, eye, heart, liver, spleen, lymph node).

Diagnostic Procedures. *Pus culture.* Presence of specific agents. *Isotope scan.* Of affected organ. *Blood.* Bacteriemia; leukocytosis (up to 20,000); complement fixation; hemoagglutination.

Therapy. Choice of antibiotics for acute form based on sensitivity studies; tetracycline, chloramphenicol, kanamycin, sulfadiazine for at least 30 days. TMS-SMX (trimethoprim/sulfamethoxalole 1/5). Surgical drainage.

Prognosis. Variable. Without treatment, mortality from apparent infection 95%; with treatment, in septicemic form mortality 50%.

BIBLIOGRAPHY. Whitmore A: An account of glander-like disease occurring in Rangoon. J Hygiene 13:1–34, 1913

The choice of antimicrobial drugs. Med Lett Drugs Ther 34:49, 1992

WIDAL-RAVAUT

Obsolete.

Synonyms. Abrami; Hayem-Widal; hemolytic anemia. The syndromes indicated by these eponyms are now recognizable as Coombs test-positive immunohemolytic anemia. As a group, all syndromes present variable degrees of hemolytic anemia, different times of onset but usually evident in infancy and childhood, absence of spherocytosis or increased osmotic fragility, as a rule not benefiting, or only mildly benefiting, from splenectomy. Dacie described two types. *Dacie type I hemolytic syndrome.* Oval macrocytosis; normal autohemolysis, with addition of glucose decreased autohemolysis to a lesser extent than in normal cells. *Dacie type II hemolytic syndrome.* Round macrocytosis, autohemolysis, and potassium loss greater than normal, and unaffected by addition of glucose.

BIBLIOGRAPHY. Hayem G: Sur une variéte particulière d'ictère chronique. Ictère infectieux chronique splénomégalique. Press Méd 6:121, 1898

Widal F, Ravaut P: Ictère chronique acholurique congénital chez un homme de vingt-neuf ans. Bull Mem Soc Med Hôp Paris 19:984–991, 1902

Dacie JV, Mollison PL, Richardson N, et al: Atypical congenital haemolytic anaemia. Q J Med 22:79–98, 1953

Engelfriet CP, Vań Tveer MB, Maas NEL, et al: Autoimmune haemolytic anaemias. In Clinical Immunology and Allergy, vol 1, p 251. London, Baillière Tindall, 1987

WIEACKER

Synonyms. Wieacker-Wolff; WWS.

Symptoms and Signs. In males. At birth: contractures of feet, slowly progressive muscle athophy (prevalently distal) dyspraxia of eyes, face and tongue muscles; mild mental retardation.

Etiology. X-linked phenotype (carrier females).

BIBLIOGRAPHY. Wieacker P, Wolff G, Wienker TF, et al: A new X-linked syndrome with muscle atrophy, congenital contractures, and oculomotor apraxia. Am J Med Genet 20:597–606, 1985
Wieacker P, Wolff G, Wienker TF: Close linkage of the Wieacker-Wolff syndrome to DNA segment DXYS1 in proximal Xq. Am J Med Genet 28:245–253, 1987

WIEDEMANN

Synonyms. Lenz; thalidomide phocomelia; fetal thalidomide.

Symptoms and Signs. Occurs in newborns of mothers who consumed thalidomide during gestation period (most critical period 37th–50th day after last menstrual period). No sex preference. Varying degrees of limb deformities, from amelia to minor thumb anomalies. Deformities prevalent in upper extremities; involvement bilateral but generally asymmetric. Other associated anomalies include cranial malformation, hydrocephalus, meningomyelocele, colobomas, macrophthalmia or anophthalmia, saddle nose, cleft palate, webbed neck, capillary hemangioma of the face, cardiovascular anomalies, and malformation of gastrointestinal and genitourinary tracts. Usually normal intelligence. Sometimes may cause clinical pattern similar to CHARGE syndrome (see).

Etiology. Ingestion of thalidomide during gestational period.

Pathology. See Signs.

Diagnostic Procedures. *X-ray. Chromosome studies.* Pattern normal.

Therapy. Orthopedic and surgical procedures.

Prognosis. Depends on degree and type of the lesions.

BIBLIOGRAPHY. Weidenbach A: Total Phocomelie. Zentralbl Gynaekol 81:2048–2052, 1956
Wiedemann HR: Hinweis auf eine derzeitige Häufung hypo-und aplastischer. Fehlbildungen der Gliedmassen Med Welt 2:1863–1866, 1961
Stephens TD: Proposed mechanisms of action in thalidomide embriopathy. Teratology 38:229–239, 1988
Schardein JL: Chemically Induced Birth Defects, 2nd ed. New York, Marcel Dekker, 1993

WIEDEMANN-RAUTENSTRAUCH

Synonyms. Progeroid neonatal, pseudohydrocephalic progeroid; neonatal progeroid.

Symptoms and Signs. Both sexes, from birth. *Facies.* Aged, small, frontal, and bitemporal bossing (pseudohydrocephalic). Fontanelles tends to close late, hair sparse, scalp vein prominent, nose small, ears low set, mouth small, chin prominent. *Body.* At birth small and successive slow growth, scarce fat, prominence of vessels and muscles; abdomen prominent. *Hand and feet.* Large; fingers: long. Deficient psychic

and motor development. Nystagmus; reduced vision, hypotonia, trunkal ataxia, dysmetria, intentional tremor. Recurrent respiratory infection.

Etiology. Autosomal recessive inheritance.

Pathology. Brain: extensive demyelination occasional tigroid pattern, macrophages with accumulation of neutral fat and myelin (sudonophilic leukodystrophy).

Therapy. Symptomatic.

Prognosis. Death prior to 5 years of age.

BIBLIOGRAPHY. Rautenstrauch T, Snigula F, Krieg T, et al: Progeria: A cell culture study and clinical report of familial incidence. Eur J Pediatr 124:101–111, 1977
Wiedemann HR: An identified neonatal progerioid syndrome. Follow-up report. Eur J Pediatr 130:65–70, 1979
Toriello HV:Wiedemann-Rautenstrauch syndrome. J Med Genet 27:256–257, 1990

WIHTIGO

Synonyms. Windigo.

Symptoms and Signs. Confined with some Indian tribes of North America. Belief that one person can be transformed into a giant monster, who eats human flesh. Frequently fear of the transformation arises when loss of appetite or nausea owing to any pathological reason is present.

Etiology. Psychotic disorder culture bound.

BIBLIOGRAPHY. Lin K-M: Cultural influences on the diagnosis of psychotic and organic disorders. In Mezzich JE, Kleinman A, Fabrega H, et al: Culture and Psychiatric Diagnosis. Washington, American Psychiatry Press, 1995

WILDERVANCK

Synonyms. Acoustic cervico—oculo; cervico—oculo—acoustic. See also Klippel-Feil and Mondini dysplasia and Duane.

Symptoms. Prevalent in females. Present from birth. Deafness or deaf-mutism (Mondini dysplasia). Epileptic attacks. Mental retardation.

Signs. Torticollis and short, webbed neck. Orbit: bulbar retraction. Nystagmus; paresis of abducens (VI) nerve. Heterochromia iridis. Cleft palate. Dextrocardia.

Etiology. Unknown. Hereditary polygenic with limitation to females.

BIBLIOGRAPHY. Wildervanck LS: Klippel-Feil syndrome associated with abducens paralysis, bulbar retraction and deaf-mutism. Ned Tijdschr Geneeskd 96:2751–3122, 1952
Wildervanck LS: Een Cervico-oculo-acoustic Nerve Syndroom Ned Tijdschr Geneeskd 104:2600–2605, 1960
Cremers CWRJ, Hoogland GA, Kuypers W: Hearing loss in the cervico-oculo-acoustic (Wildervanck) syndrome. Arch Otolaryngol 110:54–57, 1984

WILLAN-PLUMBE

Synonyms. Alphos; lepra alphos; lepra Willan; psora; psoriasis.

Symptoms. Both sexes equally affected. Onset at any age. Very rare before age of 3 years; peak at puberty and following childbirth. Typical lesions appear occasionally after infective diseases or trauma, or in any part of the skin (face usually spared). Skin lesions: uniform, thick, typically intense red, scaling. Lesions may present different morphology: guttate; nummular; rupioid; exfoliative; pustular. Some features are present according to site of involvement. Nail involvement: pitting; discoloration; subungual keratosis; onycholysis. Nail involvement frequently associated with arthritis. Two clinical syndromes recognized. (1) Stable erythrodermic psoriasis. Exfoliative phase appearing suddenly or as an evolution of chronic form; involving all skin; sparing only limited areas. Itching mild or absent. Local treatment well tolerated. (2) Unstable erythrodermic psoriasis. Sudden or following infection, treatment, or complicating arthropathic form. Entire skin surface involved; fever; severe malaise; severe itching. Intolerance to treatment.

Etiology. Unknown. Autosomal dominant trait.

Pathology. Upper dermis: micropustules; acanthosis; absent or reduced granular layer; hyperparakeratosis; polymorph invasion; parakeratotic scaling.

Diagnostic Procedures. *Biopsy. Blood.* Hypocalcemia or hyperuremia (or both) in some cases.

Therapy. Methotrexate; triacetyl azauridine; corticosteroids (danger of rebound). Local treatment: ultraviolet light; tar baths; coal-tar ointment; dithranol paste; salicylic acid ointment; local corticosteroids. (In acute form: bland application; in chronic form: stronger application.)

Prognosis. Unpredictable. Spontaneous or therapeutic remission. Frequent relapses. Stable form has best prognosis. Unstable form may be fatal or convert to stable form.

BIBLIOGRAPHY. Willan R: Description and Treatment of Cutaneous Diseases, pp 132–188. London, 1796–1808

Plumbe S: A Practical Treatise of the Skin. London, Underwood, 1824

Propping P, Hohenschutz C, Voigtlander V: Increased birth weight in psoriasis–another expression of a "thrifty genotype"? Hum Genet 71:92, 1985

Happle R: Somatic recombination may explain linear psoriasis. J Med Genet 28:337, 1991

Weatherall DJ, Ledingham JGG, Warrell DA (eds): Oxford Textbook of Medicine, 3rd ed, pp 667–679. Oxford, Oxford Med Pub, 1996

WILLIAMS-BEUREN

Synonyms. Beuren; supravalvular aortic stenosis, SAS; elfin face; hypercalcemia-supravalvular aortic stenosis; hypercalcemic face. See Hypercalcemia, infantile.

Symptoms. Affects both sexes. Onset at birth or early infancy. Feeding problem, anorexia; vomiting; slow weight gain; retarded physical and mental development. Various degrees of hypotonia; easy fatigability; occasionally, chest pain and syncope. Reduction of exercise tolerance.

Signs. Height and weight below third percentile. Facial abnormalities: elfin face (broad forehead, heavy cheeks, pointed chin). Bilateral corneal opacities. Tooth enamel hypoplasia; malocclusion; cavities. Unequal blood pressure between two arms. In heart; harsh ejection systolic murmur, with thrill maximum at second intercostal space. Absent aortic systolic click; occasionally, aortic diastolic murmur.

Etiology. Unknown. Primary disturbance begins in utero. Possibly autosomal dominant inheritance. Increased intestinal calcium absorption, and possibly, abnormality of vitamin D metabolism.

Pathology. See Signs. Supravalvular aortic stenosis associated with some degree of generalized hypoplasia of entire aorta or normal aorta caliber. Coexistence of multiple peripheral pulmonary stenosis. Hypoplasia of several organs. In kidney, calcium deposition, arterial hyperplasia.

Diagnostic Procedures. *Blood.* Hypercalcemia (frequently present in this condition, values even above 16 mg/dl recorded) or normal calcium and phosphorus. Hypercholesterolemia (occasional). Hypercalcemia and hypercholesterolemia usually disappear during second or third decade of life. *X-ray.* Metaphyseal osteosclerosis and craniostenosis. *Angiocardiography. Cardiac catheterization. ECG. Urine.* Endogenous creatine clearance decreased. *Chromosome study.* Normal pattern. *Echocardiography.*

Therapy. Vascular surgery; low calcium and vitamin D diet. Glucocorticoids in the doses used for vitamin D intoxication, adjusted for body weight, reverse hypercalcemia

Prognosis. Depends on degree of malformations and surgical correction.

BIBLIOGRAPHY. Langdon-Down JLH: Observations on an Ethnic Classification of Idiots. Clinical Lectures and Report. London, 1866

Fanconi G, Girardet, P, Sclesinger B, et al: Chroniche Hypercalcaemia, Kombiniert mit Osteosklerose, Hyperazotaemia, Minderwunhs und Kongenitalen Missbildungen. Helv Paediatr Acta 7:314–341, 1952

Williams JCP, Barratt-Bayes BG, Lowe JB: Supravalvular aortic stenosis. Circulation 24:1311–1318, 1961

Beuren AJ, Apitz J, Harmianz B: Supravalvular aortic stenosis in association with mental retardation and certain facial appearance. Circulation 26:1235–1240, 1962

Jones KL: Williams syndrome: An historical perspective of its evolution, natural history and etiology. Am J Med Genet Suppl 6:89–96, 1990

Weatherall DJ, Ledingham JGG, Warrell DA (eds): Oxford Textbook of Medicine, 3rd ed, pp 3095, 4111. Oxford, Oxford Med Pub, 1996

WILLIAMS-CAMPBELL

Synonyms. Bronchial cartilage absence, bronchiectasis; bronchomalacia.

Symptoms and Signs. Onset in early childhood. Pneumonia as complication of exanthematous disease of infancy, followed by pulmonary infections with cough and purulent sputum.

Etiology. Absence of bronchial annular cartilage causing development of bronchiectasis. Familial occurrence reported (autosomal recessive type).

Diagnostic Procedures. *X-ray. Pulmonary function studies.*

Therapy. Antibiotics. Fluidification of secretions.

Prognosis. Poor

BIBLIOGRAPHY. Williams H, Campbell P: Generalized bronchiectasis associated with deficiency of cartilage in the bronchial tree. Arch Dis Child 35:182–191, 1960

Mitchell RE, Bury RG: Congenital bronchiectasis due to deficiency of bronchial cartilage (Williams-Campbell syndrome): A case report. J Pediatr 87:230–234, 1975

Davis PB, Hubbard VS, McCoy R, et al: Familial bronchiectasis. J Pediatr 102:177–185, 1983

Fraser RS, Paré JAP, Fraser RG, Paré PD: Synopsis of Disease of the Chest, 2nd ed. Philadelphia, WB Saunders, 1994

WILLIGE-HUNT

Synonyms. Hunt corpus striatum juvenile parkinsonism; Hunt (JR) II; pallidopyramidal paralysis agitans; parkinson juvenile. See Parkinson and Hunt (J.R.) II; striatonigral degeneration.

Symptoms and Signs. Both sexes affected. Onset at 10–30 years of age or earlier. Tremor; bradykinesia; dysarthria; rigidity; fixed facies. Symptoms less intense than in Parkinson. Tendency to faint. Mental function intact; no reflex changes. Orthostatic hypotension (frequent association with Shy-Drager syndrome, see).

Etiology. Autosomal dominant and recessive inheritance. Sporadic or multifactorial inheritance.

Pathology. Decrease of large cells and increase of glial cells in the globus pallidus; same findings, but less evident, in other basal ganglia.

Diagnostic Procedures. See Parkinson.

Therapy. Except in few early cases levodopa may have no effect or make the symptoms more intense (lack of dopamine receptors [?]).

Prognosis. Slower progression of symptoms than in Parkinson. Long survival; possibly normal life expectancy.

BIBLIOGRAPHY. Willige H: Ueber Paralysis agitans im Hugendlichen Alter Z Ges Neurol Psychiatr 4:520, 1911

Hunt JR: Progressive atrophy of the globus pallidus (primary of the pallidal system). A system disease of the paralysis agitans type, characterized by atrophy of the motor cells of the corpus striatum. A contribution to the functions of the corpus striatum. Brain 40:58–148, 587, 1917

Ellenberg JH, Koller WC, Langston JW: Etiology of Parkinson Disease, New York, Marcel Dekker, 1995

WILLVONSEDER

Synonyms. Menkes variant (see).

Symptoms and Signs. All males. Onset before puberty mild intellectual loss; followed by dysarthria, clumsiness of all extremities, with lurching, ataxic gait. No abnormal reflexes but hyper-reflexia. Then tremor of head, trunk, and upper extremities. Splenomegaly under stress.

Etiology. Possibly X-linked. Autosomal recessive not excluded.

Pathology. Not available.

Prognosis. Slow progression.

BIBLIOGRAPHY. Willvonseder R, Goldstein NP, McCall JT, et al: A hereditary disorder with dementia, spastic dysarthria, vertical eye movement paresis, gait disturbance, splenomegaly, and abnormal copper metabolism. Neurology 23:1039–1049, 1973

WILMS

Synonyms. Embryonal kidney adenomyosarcoma; Birch-Hirschfeld; embryonal kidney carcinosarcoma; embryonal mixed tumor; embryonal kidney; nephroblastoma. See Brusa-Torricelli.

Symptoms. Both sexes affected. Onset before 5 years of age in 75% of cases, reported also in adults. Initially, asymptomatic; later, moderate local pain, or acute abdominal pain, nausea, vomiting, apathy, fever.

Signs. Pallor; weight loss; abdominal distention; blood hypertension (75–95%); palpable mass in kidney lodge; peripheral edema; ascites; varicocele; hematuria.

Etiology. Unknown. Neoplasia arising from embryonic metanefric blastema. Usually sporadic, but cases of autosomic dominant transmission have been reported. Mutations of 11p13 have been retained responsible for tumor.

Pathology. Neoplastic kidney invasion of great variety of cells like abortive renal element of mesodermal and epithelial type; occasionally bilateral.

Diagnostic Procedures. *Urine.* Albuminuria; increased lactic dehydrogenase (LDH). *Biopsy.* Of kidneys. See Pathology. *Renal function tests.* Altered. *X-ray.* Mass related to kidney; variously deformed kidney structures.

Therapy. Surgical excision. Chemotherapy. Roentgen therapy.

Prognosis. Very poor. Rapid diffusion of neoplasia; diffuse metastasis to all organs. In firm nonmetastatic tumor treated within first year, the prognosis is better, with possibility of cure in 60% of cases, and in children younger than 1 year of age close to 90%.

BIBLIOGRAPHY. Birsh-Hirschfeld FV: Sarkomatoese Druesengeschwueste der Niere im Kindersalter (Embryonales Adenosarcom). Deitr Pathol Anat 24:343–362, 1898

Wilms M: Die Mischgeschwueste. I. Die Mischgeschwuelste der Niere. Leipzig, 1899

D'Angio GJ, Beckwith JB, Breslow NE, et al: Wilms' tumor: An update. Cancer 45(7 Suppl):1791–1798, 1980

Haber DA, Housman DE: Wilms tumor. In Scriver CR, Beaudet AL, Sly WS, et al: The Metabolic and Molecular Bases of Inherited Disease, 7th ed, pp 665–676. New York, McGraw-Hill, 1995

WILSON-MIKITY

Synonyms. Cystic pulmonary emphysema; interstitial prematurity fibrosis; lung cystic emphysema; neonatal cystic pulmonary emphysema; bubbly lung; chronic neonatal pulmonary disease, pulmonary dysmaturity; bronchopulmonary dysplasia.

Symptoms. Seen most commonly in premature infants usually of less than 32 weeks gestation and birth weight below 1500 g, onset occurring between birth and end of first month of life (average at eighth day). The syndrome is characterized by insidious onset of dyspnea, tachypnea, retractions, and cyanosis.

Signs. Cyanosis; auscultation of lung clear or rales, rhonchi, or wheezing; tachypnea; rib recession.

Etiology. Premature birth with immaturity of the lung; oxygen injury (increased generation of oxygen radicals); positive pressure ventilation with barotrauma; pulmonary edema, possible role of infection by ureoplasma ureolyticum.

Pathology. Lung histology: inequality of terminal air space size; variation of alveolar walls (increase of reticulum and elastic fibers and increased cellularity). Occasionally, unusual prominent bands of muscle in the wall of terminal bronchioles. Absence of clear-cut increase of pulmonary fibrosis.

Diagnostic Procedures. *X-ray.* Of chest. This essentially is a radiologic diagnosis. Three stages of the condition may be recognized: (1) Acute. Bilateral diffuse reticulonodular pattern with small, round, radiolucent foci; generalized hyperaeration. (2) Intermediate (in weeks or months). Coarse streaking from hilus into upper lobe; focal lucent areas disappear; generalized hyperaeration persists. (3) Clearing. Complete disappearance of findings between fourth and 11th months of age. Pulmonary function tests. Dynamic lung: "compliance" significantly reduced; static lung: "Compliance" within normal limit. *Sputum. Culture. Biopsy.* Of lung (only with severe symptoms).

Therapy. Treatment consists of supportive measures: oxygen for cyanosis, digitalization and diuretics for cardiac failure, acid-base correction, and assisted ventilation when indicated. New therapies: exogenous surfactant (derived from calf and pig lungs from human amniotic fluid, or artificially produced); exogenous superoxide dismutase; nutritional factors; high frequency positive pressure ventilation, high frequency jet ventilation, high frequency oscillation.

Prognosis. A few patients may die during acute stage; majority slowly recover completely. Radiologic findings disappear as well within 4–11 months. Chronic respiratory problems may last for whole life span.

BIBLIOGRAPHY. Wilson MC, Mikity VG: A new form of respiratory disease in premature infants. Am J Dis Child 99:489–499, 1960

Nortthway WH: Bronchopulmonary dysplasia then and now. Arch Dis Child 65:1076–1080, 1990

Fraser RS, Paré JAP, Fraser RG, Paré PD: Synopsis of Disease of the Chest, 2nd ed. Philadelphia, WB Saunders, 1994

WILSON (S.A.K.)

Synonyms. Kinnier Wilson; Westphal-Strümpell; lenticular progressive degeneration; pseudosclerosis hepatolenticular degeneration.

Symptoms. Slight prevalence in males. Onset in childhood to early adulthood. Occasionally acute onset with fulminant hepatic failure (jaundice, vomiting), hemolytic crisis, arthritis, renal colics with emission of stones, renal tubular acidosis. Females more often present with hepatic failure, males more often with neurological symptoms. In group of Eastern Europe extraction, later onset. Tremor beginning on extremity and successively extending to head and body. Weakness; drooling; dysarthria; mental changes. Later stage: anarthria, dysphagia.

Signs. *Eyes.* Pigmentation of periphery of cornea (Kayser-Fleischer ring). *Skin.* Discoloration; occasionally, jaundice; spider angiomas. Hepatosplenomegaly. *Bone or joint changes and muscular wasting.* From mild to severe incoordination; choreic movements; dystonic spasm convulsions; plastic rigidity of extremities.

Etiology. Autosomal recessive inheritance. Gene concerned near 13q14 linked to esterase D locus. Specific defect is not known but the two chief disturbances are (1) reduction of rate of incorporation of copper in ceruloplasmin and (2) reduced biliary excretion of copper. The accumulated metal deposits in hepatocytes and successively in central nervous system.

Pathology. *Brain.* Basal ganglia brown pigmentation and cavitation. Increased number of glial cells throughout brain. *Liver.* Coarse nodular cirrhosis, postnecrotic type with active regeneration. Esophageal varices; ascites. Copper content increased in brain, liver (100 mg/g of tissue), kidney, and cornea.

Diagnostic Procedures. *Blood.* Hemolytic anemia; hypocupremia; hypoceruloplasminemia (less than 20 mg/dl of serum). *Liver function test.* Cirrhosis pattern. *Urine.* Hypercupriuria (variable); hyperaminoaciduria; hematuria. *Biopsy.* Of liver. *X-ray.* Osteoporosis.

Therapy. Dietary restriction of copper. Dimercaprol intramuscularly and (better) penicillamine (orally 1 g/day over 10 years of age and adult; 0.5–0.75 under this age). Continue treatment in spite of lack of apparent clinical improvement; triethylene tetramine dihydrochloride is another nontoxic, good, potential drug. Zinc sulfate can be a low toxic and well tolerated alternative for D-penicillamine. Liver transplant successfully carried out.

Prognosis. Progressive; fatal. Benefit of treatment directly correlated to time treatment was initiated. Good results with transplantation and penicillamine reported.

BIBLIOGRAPHY. Westphal C: Ueber eine dem Bilde der cerebrospinalen graven Degeneration ähnliche Erkrankung des centralen Nervensystems ohne anatomischen Befund, nebst einigen Bemerkungen öcüber paradoxe Contraction. Arch Psychiatr Berl 14:87–134, 1883

Wilson SAK: Progressive lenticular degeneration: a familial nervous disease associated with cirrhosis of the liver. Brain 34:295–509, 1911–1912

Danks DM: Disorders of copper metabolism. In Scriver CR, Beaudet AL, Sly WS, et al: The Metabolic and Molecular Bases of Inherited Disease, 7th ed, pp 2217–2223. New York, McGraw-Hill, 1995

WINCHESTER

Symptoms and Signs. Both sexes. From birth. Visual impairment from peripheral corneal opacities. Short stature; severe joints contractures, abnormal (coarse) facies.

Etiology. Autosomal recessive inheritance. Mucoplysaccharide storage disorder. Non-lysosomal connective tissue disease.

Pathology. Joint changes simulating rheumatoid arthritis; generalized osteoporosis; dissolution of carpal and tarsal bones.

Diagnostic Procedures. *X-ray.* See pathology. *Urine.* Normal mucopolysaccharides. *Skin fibroblast cultures.* Metachromatic changes and increase of uronic acid.

BIBLIOGRAPHY. Winchester P, Grossman H, Lim WN, et al: A new acid mucoplysaccharidosis with skeletal deformities simulating rheumatoid arthritis. AM J Roentgen 106:121–128, 1969

Winter RM: Winchester's syndrome. J Med Genet 26:772–775, 1989

WINCKEL

Obsolete.

Synonyms. Charrin-Winckel; cyanosis afebrilis icterica perniciosa cum hemoglobinuria; neonatal hemoglobinuria.

Symptoms and Signs. Occurs in newborns. Recurrent crises of jaundice, cyanosis, hemorrhagic manifestation, and hemoglobinuria.

Etiology. Unknown.

BIBLIOGRAPHY. Charrin S: Maladie bronzée hematique des enfants nouveau-nés (tubulhematie renale de M. Parrot) (thesis). Paris, 1873

Winckel F: Ueber eine bisher miet bescheriebene endemisch aufgetretene Erkrankung Neugeborener. Dtsch Med Wochenschr 5:303–307, 415–418; 431–436; 447–450, 1879

Rook A, Wilkinson DS, Ebling FJG, et al: Textbook of Dermatology, 4th ed, pp 2134–2135. Oxford, Blackwell Scientific, 1986

WINDIGO

Symptoms and Signs. Reported but never actually observed by anthropologists or psychologists, in Northern Algonkian peoples of Canada; compulsive desire to eat human flesh.

BIBLIOGRAPHY. Kalan HI, Sadock BJ: Comprehensive Textbook of Psychiatry, p 258. Baltimore, Williams & Wilkins, 1985

WINDSHIELD WIPER

Synonyms. Movement of intraocular lens.

Symptoms and Signs. Defects of vision after IOL implantation after cataract extraction.

Etiology. Small diameter of IOL allows movement.

Pathology. Ruptured zonules; lateral tilt and decentration of intraocular lens.

Diagnostic Procedures. Ophthalmoscopy: typical aspect of loop of lens eroding ciliary body.

Therapy. Replacement with wider IOL.

BIBLIOGRAPHY. Simcoe CW: Simcoe posterior chamber lens: Therapy, techniques and results. Am Intraocular Implant Soc J 7:154–157, 1981

Apple DJ, Rabb MF: Ocular Pathology, 4th ed, p 147. St Louis, Mosby Year Book, 1991

WINKELSTEIN

Synonyms. Gastroesophageal reflux; GERD; peptic esophagitis.

Symptoms and Signs. Both sexes. All ages. More frequent in middle old age. Heartburn (sine qua non for diagnosis) exacerbated by eating, bending, and lying down; postural regurgitation; dysphagia. Chest pain. Otorynologic symptoms: excess salivation, hoarseness, postnasal drip, persistent coughing, globus (see) throat clearing; sore throat, choking spells; laryngospasm. Pulmonary symptoms: asthma; secondary pulmonary diseases gastric content microaspiration; bronchocostriction; bradichardia.

Etiology. Hiatal hernia causing intrathoracic displacement of lower esophageal stricture (LES) (theory considered from 1940–1960). Reduced LES determining low basal LES pressure or inappropriate LES adaptive responses (theory considered in the decade 1970) and from

1980 to present, inappropriate relaxation of LES. Variable conditions may be associated with this disease: Chalasia of infancy; pregnancy; scleroderma (see), Zollinger-Ellison (see); Heller esophagogastric myotomy; ablation of pylorus with alkaline reflux.

Pathology. Epithelial basal cell hyperplasia, and proximity of papillae to epithelial surface, inflammatory changes (not costant); Barrett esophagus (see) may be associated.

Diagnostic Procedures. *Endoscopy. Biopsy. Upper gastrointestinal X-ray; scintigraphy; esophageal manometry; acid perfusion of esophagus; ambulatory esophageal monitoring.*

Therapy. Changes in eating habits (small meals, no hot food, coffee, chocolate, peppermint, ethanol, fat) no lying down after meals, and sleep with head elevated. Control of gastric acidity by antacid, mucosal cytoprotection (sucralfate), and systemic agents (blockers of H2-receptor blocking, proton pump, or selective muscarinic). Prokinetic agents (bethanechol, metoclopramide, domperidone, cisapride) and finally in refractory cases surgery (partial fundoplication).

Prognosis. Variable response to medical approach from excellent to poor; good to surgical.

BIBLIOGRAPHY. Winkelstein A: Peptic esophagitis: A new clinical entity. JAMA 104:906, 1935
Ogorek CO: Gastroesophageal reflux disease. In Haubrich WS, Schaffner F, Berk JE (eds): Bockus Gastroenterology, 5th ed, pp 445–467. Philadelphia, WB Saunders, 1995

WINKLER

Synonym. Chondrodermatitis helicis.

Symptoms. Ten times more frequent in men. Onset after 40 years of age. Severe pain in the ear initiated by pressure, interfering with sleep (in women less intense). In men (90%) the helix in the right ear more frequently involved.

Signs. Single and occasionally multiple globular nodules of 1 cm or larger and raised 0.5 cm hyperemia of surrounding skin. Skin usually scaly or crusty. In women both ears equally affected and localization is usually in the antihelix and tragus.

Etiology. Predisposing factors: anatomical development defects of vascular supply; age. Causative factors: trauma; cold.

Pathology. Acantholysis and hyperkeratosis of epidermis with parakeratosis in center of nodule. Edema; homogenization; fibrinoid necrosis; vascular granulation of dermis. Perichondral tissue: fibrinoid degeneration and, according to involvement, various degrees of degeneration and reactive changes.

Therapy. Surgical excision or for early lesion intralesional steroids.

Prognosis. Recurrences possible (avoid pressure or trauma to the helix).

BIBLIOGRAPHY. Winkler M: Knoetchenfoermige Erkrankung am Helix. (Chondrodermatitis nodularis chronica helicis). Arch Derm Syph 121:278–285, 1915–16
Wilkinson JD: The external ear. In Champion RH, Burton JL, Ebling FJG (eds): Rook/Wilkinson/Ebling Textbook of Dermatology, 5th ed, pp 2674–2675. Oxford, Blackwell Scientific, 1992

WISKOTT-ALDRICH

Synonyms. Aldrich; Aldrich-Huntley; Aldrich-Dees; eczema; infections; thrombocytopenia triad. SeeThrombocytopenia, X-linked syndromes.

Symptoms. Occurs in infancy and childhood, only in males. Eczema; easy bruisability; hemorrhage; recurrent infections, especially otitis media; bloody diarrhea.

Signs. Petechiae and hematomas; eczema; otitis media; periosteal hemorrhages.

Etiology. Unknown. Sex-linked recessive condition. Primary inability to process certain polysaccharide antigens as required for normal induction of an immunoresponse (Cooper et al.).

Pathology. Manifestation of a broad spectrum of infective diseases: viral; bacterial; fungal; pneumocystis carinii. Hemorrhagic manifestation affecting all organs. If surviving, widespread malignancies of lymphoreticular type develop at later age.

Diagnostic Procedures. *Blood.* Anemia; thrombocytopenia; lymphopenia; hypogammaglobulinemia (IgM and isoagglutinins levels low; IgA and IgE elevated); impaired delayed hypersensitivity. *Bone marrow.* Normal megakaryocytes; decreased platelet production; microplatelets; thrombi in lymph node vessels.

Therapy. Bleeding treated by transfusion of fresh platelets irradiated. Splenectomy useful. Gammaglobulin contraindicated. Bone marrow transplantation has been performed with success. The transplantation was preceded by high-dose immunosuppression with cyclophosphamide.

Prognosis. A patient treated with bone marrow transplantation is still alive and in good health after 15 years.

BIBLIOGRAPHY. Wiskott A: Familiarer Angeborener Morbus Werlhoffi. Monatsschr Kinderheilkd 68:212–216, 1937
Aldrich RA, Steinberg AG, Campbell DC: Pedigree demonstrating a sex-linked recessive condition characterized by draining ears, eczematoid dermatitis and bloody diarrhea. Pediatrics 13:133–139, 1954
Meuwissen H, Bortin M, Bach F, et al: Long term survival after bone marrow transplantation: A 15-year follow-up report of a patient with Wiskott-Aldrich syndrome. J Pediatr 105:365–369, 1984
Atherton DJ: The neonate. In Champion RH, Burton JL, Ebling FJG (eds): Rook/Wilkinson/Ebling Textbook of Dermatology, 5th ed, pp 427–429. Oxford, Blackwell Scientific, 1992

WISSLER-FANCONI

Obsolete.

Synonyms. Subsepsis hyperergia; subsepsis allergica.

Symptoms. Most frequent in children and young adults. Intermittent fever; recurring exanthemas of various types; transient rheumatoid arthralgia and occasionally pleuritic pain.

Signs. Slight transient jaundice; nonpalpable or slightly enlarged spleen; no lymph node enlargement; occasionally, pleuritic and pneumonic signs.

Etiology. Unknown. Supposed allergic reaction to moderate bacteremia. Possibly, allied to rheumatic fever and rheumatoid arthritis. Diagnosis reached by exclusion of other known fever-producing diseases.

Diagnostic Procedures. *Blood.* High sedimentation rate; anemia; leukocytosis (neutrophilia; normal number of eosinophils); blood and throat cultures negative; antistreptolysin titer frequently elevated; lupus erythematosus (L.E.) test negative. Transient signs of myocardial involvement (electrocardiographic) or liver or kidney involvement.

Therapy. Lack of response to antibiotics (except for an initial temporary moderate decrease of temperature). Steroids in moderate or high dose not always effective; antihistamines helpful to alleviate symptoms.

Prognosis. Spontaneous recovery and recurrences. Possibility that this syndrome represents a prodromal stage of rheumatoid arthritis that will eventually develop its full-blown pattern. See Cheshire cat syndrome.

BIBLIOGRAPHY. Wissler H: Ueber eine Besondere Form sepsisahnlicher Krankheiten (subsepsis hyperergica). Monatsschr Kinderheilkd 94:1–15, 1943
Fanconi G: Über einen Fall von Subsepsis allergica Wissler. Helv Paediatr Acta 1:532–537, 1946

Bottiger LE, Landegren J: Wissler's syndrome. Acta Med Scand 174:415–420, 1963

Bywaters FGL: Still's disease in the adult. Ann Rheum Dis 30:121–133, 1971

WITCHCRAFT

Synonyms. Urticaria artefacta contact.

Symptoms and Signs. Epidemia of urticaria-like lesions developing after hairdo by the daughter of the owner (only in one peculiar hairdresser shop).

Etiology. Application of benzyl ester of nicotinic acid to the customer's head skin that causes edema and prurigo, although not affecting the inside of hands of the "witch." The reason for such behavior was a retaliatory reaction to the father's annoyance for her pregnancy.

Prognosis. Short lasting.

BIBLIOGRAPHY. Bandman HJ, Wahl B: Contact urticaria artefacta (witchcraft syndrome). Contac Derm 8:145–146, 1982

WITCH MILK

Symptoms and Signs. Galactorrhea in the newborn. Both sexes.

Etiology. Unknown. Former theories about an association between this disorder and hypothyroidism with other endocrinopathies are not accepted today. It is attributed to the high level of estradiol and progesterone produced by the mother during fetal life.

Pathology. Breast nodules significantly larger than those of children without galactorrhea.

Therapy. None. Pressing the infant breast can be dangerous (inflammation and breast abscesses).

Prognosis. Good. Galactorrhea may persist for 2 months.

BIBLIOGRAPHY. Forbes TR: Witch's milk and witches' marks. Yale J Biol Med 22:219–225, 1950
Madlon-kay DJ: Witch's milk. Galactorrhea in the new-born. Am J Dis Child 140:252–253, 1986
Santen EJ: Gynecomastia. In De Groot LJ (ed): Endocrinology, 3rd ed, p 2474. Philadelphia, WB Saunders, 1995

WITHDRAWAL EMERGENT

Synonym. Neuroleptic withdrawal dyskinetic; tardive dyskinesia. See Neuroleptic malignant.

Symptoms and Signs. In children and adolescents after discontinuation or reduction of neuroleptics. Choreoathetoid and myoclonic movements of the trunk, extremities, and orofacial region.

Etiology. Neuroleptic removal. Dopamine receptor hypersensitivity.

Therapy. Adjustment of medication dosage. Benadryl administration may be useful.

Prognosis. Good after weeks; spontaneous regression of signs.

BIBLIOGRAPHY. Gualtieri CT, Quade D, Hicks RE, et al: Tardive dyskinesia and other clinical consequences of neuroleptic treatment in children and adolescents. Am J Psychiatr 141a:20–23, 1984
Adams RD, Victor M: Principles of Neurology, 5th ed, p 935. New York, McGraw-Hill, 1993

WITKOP

Synonyms. Mucoepithelial dysplasia.

Symptoms and Signs. Both sexes. In infancy severe tearing and photophobia, nystagmus, eventually corneal vascularization, development of pannus, cataracts (at 4–6 years of age) leading to blindness before puberty. Mucosae: oral, vaginal, nasal, urethral, anal: fiery red and eroded (end of first year). Skin (except hands and feet) presents follicular keratosis. Scanty hair. Easy burning on sun exposure. Chronic rinorrhea, diarrea, bladder infections, recurrent respiratory infections. Spontaneous pneumothorax.

Etiology. Autosomal dominant inheritance.

Pathology. Mucosae: deficiency of keratinization and dyskeratosis, numerous basal and parabasal cells, nuclear atypia and vacuoalization of cytoplasm.

Therapy. Antibiotics. Antimycotic agents. Symptomatic.

Prognosis. Death for cor pulmonale and fibrocystic type of lung disease in third to fourth decade.

BIBLIOGRAPHY. Okamoto GA, Hall JG, Ochs H, et al: New syndrome of chronic mucocutaneous candidiasis. Birth Defects Orig Art Ser 13 (3B):117–125, 1977
Witkop CJ Jr: Clinical, histologic, cytologic and ultrastructural characteristics of the oral lesions from hereditary mucoepithelial dysplasia: Disease of gut junction and desmosomal formation. Oral Surg 46:645–657, 1978
Urban MD, Schosser R, Spohn W, et al: New clinical aspects of hereditary mucoepithelial dysplasia. Am J Med Genet 39:338–341, 1991

WITTMAAK-EKBOM

Synonyms. Ekbom; anxietas tibialis; asthenia crurum paresthetica; leg jitter; restless legs; acromelalgia, painful legs, moving toes.

Symptoms. Recurrent, unpleasant, peculiar creeping or crawling sensation in the legs, occasionally in the thighs or feet, felt deep inside the muscle or bones, which prevents the patient from keeping the involved extremities still. Bilateral and symmetric involvement or preponderant on one side; seldom affecting the arms and hands in "tono minor." Seldom true pain. Worst in the evening and at night or when the patient rests for some time. Sometimes lasting only a short period, sometimes hours. Sensation is relieved by movement, but reappears a short time after patient returns to bed. Important cause of severe insomnia.

Signs. None or cold feet and lower legs.

Etiology. Unknown. Psychic factor of some importance (symptoms appearing especially during boring programs, movies, television, theater). Iron-deficiency anemia a possible etiologic factor. Hereditary (dominant transmission) implicated. In pregnancy present in 10% of cases; disappears after delivery.

Diagnostic Procedures. *Blood.* Moderate anemia; serum iron low in some cases.

Therapy. If anemia and iron deficiency, correction of condition will relieve symptoms. Most patients will not need treatment; reassurance of the benign nature of the syndrome may suffice. For those who require drug therapy, a trial with one of the following drugs can be suggested: levodopa, benserazide, carbidopa, clonazepam, carbamazepine, and for resistant cases, chlorpromazine.

Prognosis. In some cases, spontaneous remission. Some cured by treatment of anemia. In pregnancy, symptoms disappear after delivery. Patient with aching pain is resistant to all kinds of treatment.

BIBLIOGRAPHY. Willis T: The London Practice of Physick, p 404. London, Bassett Crooke, 1685
Wittmaak T: Pathologie und Therapie der Sensibilitat-Neurosen, p 459. Leipzig, Schafer, 1861
Ekbom KA: Asthenia crurum paraesthetica ("irritable legs"): A new syndrome consisting of weakness, sensation of cold and nocturnal paresthesia in legs, responding to certain extent to treatment with

priscol and doryl. Note on paresthesis in general. Acta Med Scand 118:197–209, 1944

Gibb WRG, Lees AJ: The restless legs syndrome. Postgrad Med J 62:329–333, 1986

Clough C: Restless legs syndrome. Br Med J 294:262–263, 1987

Weatherall DJ, Ledingham JGG, Warrell DA (eds): Oxford Textbook of Medicine, 3rd ed, p 4159. Oxford, Oxford Med Pub, 1996

WOLCOTT-RALLISON

Synonyms. Epiphyseal dysplasia, early diabetes mellitus; diabetes mellitus, epiphyseal dysplasia.

Symptoms. Very rare. Both sexes. Symptoms become evident during first weeks of life, seizures. From second year: joint pains, walking difficulties.

Signs. Normal facies. Tooth discoloration; skin abnormalities; hepatosplenomegaly; multiple bone fractures, dwarfism; small stature.

Etiology. Autosomal recessive inheritance; abnormality in collagen synthesis.

Pathology. *Bone.* Nonspecific changes; scarse chondrocytes; resorption zone z poorly vasculized, thick collagen fibers. *Liver and spleen.* Fat infiltration.

Diagnostic Procedures. *X-rays.* Spondyloepiphyseal dysplasia. *Blood.* Insulin dependent diabetes. Features of renal failure.

Therapy. Slow-acting insulin. Symptomatic.

Prognosis. That of juvenile diabetes. Dwarfism.

BIBLIOGRAPHY. Wolcott CD, Rallison ML: Infancy onset diabetes mellitus and multiple epiphyseal dysplasia. J Pediatr 80:292–297, 1972

Stoss H, Pesch HJ, Poptiz B, et al: Wolcott-Rallison syndrome: diabetes mellitus-spondyloepiphyseal dysplasia. Eur J Pediatr 138:120–129, 1982

Rimoin DL, Lachman RS: Genetic disorders of the osseous skeleton. In Beithon P (ed): McKusick's Heritable Disorders of Connective Tissue, 5th ed, p 616. St Louis, CV Mosby, 1993

WOLFF-PARKINSON-WHITE

Synonyms. WPW; anomalous atrioventricular excitation; false bundle-branch block; pre-excitation.

Symptoms and Signs. Most patients asymptomatic. Onset at young age. Episodes of paroxysmal tachycardia in 10% of cases.

Etiology. Congenital variation in the heart conduction system; bypassing of the delay at A-V node and early excitation of a portion of ventricles.

Pathology. None.

Diagnostic Procedures. ECG. WPW pattern: short P-R interval with prolonged QRS complex. *Vectorcardiography. Echocardiography.*

Therapy. Response to drugs usually unpredictable. Most paroxysms resolve spontaneously. Digitalis, although contraindicated by many authors, found useful. Digitalis plus quinidine best results; propranolol (considered by others as drug of choice). Counter-shock if paroxysm is persistent; procainamide or lidocaine considered useful. As last resort, surgical division of accessory path.

Prognosis. Usually benign condition, but severe condition in some cases. Patients who develop tachyarrhythmia present atrial flutter (4%); atrial fibrillation (16%); atrial tachycardia (70%); and unidentified supraventricular tachycardia (10%).

BIBLIOGRAPHY. Wolff L, Parkinson J, White PD: Bundle branch block with short P-R interval in healthy young people prone to paroxysmal tachycardia. Am Heart J 5:685–704, 1930

Lamb LE: Wolff-Parkinson-White syndrome. Postgrad Med 43:173–176, 1968

Myerburg RJ, Kessler KM, Castellanos A: Recognition clinical assessment and management of conduction disturbances. In Schlant RC, Alexander RW: Hurst's The Heart, 8th ed, pp 717–720. New York, McGraw-Hill, 1994

WOLF-HIRSCHORN

Synonyms. Chromosome 4 p (partial deletion); partial monosomy 4;46; 4B.

Symptoms. Present from birth. Slow growth; repeated respiratory infections; seizures (minor or grand mal, characteristic); severe mental deficiency; hypotonia. Absence of cat cry (characteristic).

Signs. *Head.* Microcephaly; doliochocephaly; hypertelorism; lids antimongoloid slant; broad nasal root; beaked nose; strabismus; iris coloboma; speckled irides; cleft lip or palate (characteristic); fish-like mouth; micrognathia; ear malformations. *Extremities.* Simian creases; altered dermal ridges. Talipes equinovarus. *Genitals.* Hypospadias; cryptorchidism. Cardiac malformations.

Etiology. Partial deletion of chromosome 4 of B group.

Diagnostic Procedures. Chromosome studies. See Etiology.

Therapy. Symptomatic.

Prognosis. Short life expectancy (one-third die before 3 years of age). Survivors show slow growth and repeated infections.

BIBLIOGRAPHY. Sidbury JB, Schmickel RD, Gray M: Findings in a patient with apparent deletion of short arms on one of the B group chromosomes. J Pediatr 65:1098, 1964

Wolf U, Porsch R, Baitsch H, et al: Deletion on short arms of a B-chromosome without "cri du chat" syndrome. Lancet I:769, 1965

Hirschhorn K, Cooper HL, Firchein IL: Deletion of short arms of chromosome 4–5 in a child defects of mid-line fusion. Humangenetik 1:479–482, 1965

Centerwall WR, Thompson WP, Allen IE, et al: Translocation 4p-Syndrome: A general review. Am J Dis Child 129:366–370, 1975

Quarrell OWJ, Snell RG, Curtis MA, et al: Paternal origin of the chromosomal deletion resulting in Wolf-Hirschhorn syndrome. J Med Genet 28:256–259, 1991

WOLFRAM

Synonyms. Marquardt-Loriaux; Turnbridge-Paley; diabetes insipidus—diabetes mellitus—optic atrophy—deafness; DIDMOAD.

Symptoms and Signs. Both sexes affected. Present from childhood. Bilateral optic atrophy; extensive visual loss, with small paracentral islands of remaining function; diabetes mellitus; diabetes insipidus, later, development of neurosensory deafness; in some cases, neurogenic bladder and autonomic dysfunction; blood hypertension.

Etiology. Hereditary condition. Retrograde or anterograde transsynaptic degeneration (?). Autosomal recessive inheritance suggested. Possible linkage with brachydactyly type E (see).

Diagnostic Procedures. *Blood.* Hyperglycemia, anemia. *Urine.* Hyperalaninuria. *Electroretinography.* Primary lesion of central optic pathway, with relative sparing of the external retinal layers located more in the cone than in the rod system. *EEG.* Abnormal pattern (?).

Therapy. Symptomatic. Controlled trials with cyclosporin A and azathioprine, pancreas transplant. Megaloblastic anemia responsive to thiamine.

Prognosis. Very poor quoad functionem and quoad vitam.

BIBLIOGRAPHY. Von Graefe A: Ueber die mit Diabetes vorkommenden. Stoerungen Arch Ophthalmol 18:4:230–234, 1858

Gregg JB: Primary optic atrophy in juvenile diabetes. Am J Ophthalmol 18:856–858, 1935

Wolfram DJ, Wagener HP: Diabetes mellitus and simple optic atrophy among siblings: Report of four cases. Mayo Clinic Proc 13:715–718, 1938

Salih MAM, Tuvemo T: Diabetes insipidus, diabetes mellitus optic atrophy and deafness (DIDMOAD syndrome): A clinical study in two Sudanese families. Acta Paediat Scand 80:567–572, 1991

Muir A, Schatz D, Maclaren NK: Polyglandular failure syndromes. In De Groot LJ (ed): Endocrinology, 3rd ed, p 3020. Philadelphia, WB Saunders, 1995

WOLFSON

Symptoms and Signs. Irritative roots pain, high sedimentation rate, increased alkaline phosphatase.

Etiology. Metastatic malignancy to the spine.

BIBLIOGRAPHY. Wolfson SA, Reznick S, Gunther L: Early diagnosis of malignant metastases to the spine: A clinical syndrome. JAMA 116:1044–1048, 1941

WOLMAN

Synonyms. Adrenal calcification; familial xanthomatosis; acid lipase deficiency (fatal form); xanthomatoses; calcified adrenals. Includes Wolman—hypolipoproteinemia—acathocytosis. See also Cholesterol ester hydrolase deficiency.

Symptoms. Relative high incidence in Israel in Jews of Iraqi or Iranian origin. Recently less severe cases who have reached adult life have been reported. Both sexes affected. Onset in first weeks of life. Forceful vomiting; abdominal distention; watery diarrhea; failure to thrive. Occasionally low fever. Initially mentally bright and alert; by ninth or tenth week, reduction of activity.

Signs. Hepatomegaly; progressive pallor, from sixth week. Optic fundus normal; occasionally, tendon hyperreflexia, clonus, positive Babinski.

Etiology. Autosomal recessive inheritance. Deficient activity of acid cholesteryl ester hydrolase (or acid lipase) causing accumulation of cholesterol esters and triglycerides in tissues. In one report hypolipoproteinemia and acanthocytosis have been added to the classic features of the syndrome, thus suggesting the possibility of an additional distinct entity (Eto Y).

Pathology. *Adrenal glands.* Normal configuration; enlarged, bright yellow, firm, containing calcified tissue. Zona glomerulosa and fasciculata well-preserved; cells swollen; vacuolated. Zona inner fasciculata and reticularis replaced by large cells with vacuolated foamy cytoplasm, with necrosis, lipid infiltration, and calcifications. *Medulla.* Narrow but normal. *Liver.* Hepatomegaly; yellow; architecture variably distorted; cells large and vacuolated. *Spleen, lymph nodes, thymus.* Large foamy cells. Other organs and tissues. Variable degree of cell vacuolization.

Diagnostic Procedures. *Blood.* Total lipids, cholesterol, and triglycerides normal or low. Anemia. Lymphocyte vacuolization. Tissue extracts. Qualitative and quantitative cholesterol and triglyceride alterations. *Fibroblast culture.* Severe deficiency of acid ester hydrolase activity. *X-ray. CT scan. MRI.* Adrenal calcification.

Therapy. Lovostatine appears of scarce or no effect.

Prognosis. Death in first few months of life.

BIBLIOGRAPHY. Alexander WS: Nieman-Pick disease. Report of a case

showing calcification in the adrenal glands. NZ Med J 45:43–45, 1946

Abramov A, Schorr S, Wolman M: Generalized xanthomatosis with calcified adrenals. Am J Dis Child 91:282–286, 1956

Wolman M, Sterk VV, Gatt S, et al: Primary family xanthomatosis with involvement and calcification of the adrenals: Report of two more cases in siblings of a previously described infant. Pediatrics 28:742–757, 1961

Eto Y, Kitagawa T: Wolman's disease with hypolipoproteinemia and acanthocytosis: Clinical and biochemical observations. J Pediatr 77:862–867, 1970

Assman G, Seedorf U: Acid lipase deficiency: Wolman disease and cholesterol ester storage disease. In Scriver CR, Beaudet AL, Sly WS, et al: The Metabolic and Molecular Bases of Inherited Disease, 7th ed, pp 2563–2587. New York, McGraw-Hill, 1995

WOMEN WHO FALL

Symptoms. Occurs only in females. Usually begins in late childhood and persists in adulthood. Stumbling and falling without any apparent reason.

Signs. None.

Etiology. Psychiatric disturbance. Precipitating factors are emergence into consciousness of aggressive or erotic impulses. To be differentiated from myoclonic syndrome and epileptic syndromes.

Diagnostic Procedures. *Psychoanalysis. EEG.*

Therapy. Psychiatric treatment.

Prognosis. When properly recognized and treated, good result. Correction of the basic personality derangement more difficult.

BIBLIOGRAPHY. Leuba J: Women who fall. Int J Psychoanalysis 31:6–7, 1950

WOODS-PENDLETON

Symptoms and Signs. Reported in 1921 in China. Both sexes, all ages. Abrupt onset, no fever, repeated failure of muscles of equilibrium, followed by dysarthria, in some cases vertigo, hearing troubles, lethargy, in all cases involuntary movements superimposed on attempted voluntary movements, sudden loss of normal postural and muscle tone, torsion spasms, athetoid, etc. Hemiparesis in two cases.

Etiology. Unknown. Possibly toxic degeneration of pallidum.

Pathology. Autopsy in one case revealed symmetrical focal necrosis of caudal half and dorsal two thirds of pallidum. Big clear cells (Alzheimer II type) observed in all brain.

Prognosis. Course may be abortive, of brief duration with complete recovery or progressive and fatal in short or long term (2 years).

BIBLIOGRAPHY. Woods AH, Pendleton L: Fourteen simultaneous cases of an acute degeneration stiatal disease. Necropsy of one case revealing gross necrosis of globus pallidus (symmetrical) and substantia nigra. Arch Neurol Psychiatr (Chicago) 13:549–568, 1925

WOODS-SCHAUMBURG

Synonyms. Nigro–spino–dental degeneration; nuclear ophthalmoplegia. See Azorean neurologic.

Symptoms and Signs. Onset in adolescence or early adulthood. Ataxia, hyper-reflexia ophthalmoplegia, marked extrapyramidal rigidity, severe distal motor weakness. Prominent bulbar signs.

Etiology. Unknown.

Pathology. Spino-cerebellar tract and pons degeneration; olivary complex normal cerebellum: normal granules and Purkinje cells. Dentate nucleus, substantia nigra, and anterior horn cells and nuclei of cranial nerves; marked loss of cells.

Therapy. Anti cholinergic and dopaminergic medication for rigidity control.

Prognosis. Slowly progressive.

BIBLIOGRAPHY. Woods BT, Schaumburg HH: Nigro-spino-dentatal degeneration with nuclear ophthalmoplegia: A unique and partially treatable clinico-pathological entity. J Neurol Sci 17:149–166, 1972

Boller F, Segarra JM: Spino-pontine degeneration. In Vinken PJ, Bruyn GW (eds): Handbook of Clinical Neurology, vol 21, p 401. Amsterdam, North-Holland, 1975

WOOLLY HAIR

Symptoms and Signs. Hair, short, curled, woolly in Caucasian subjects.

Etiology. Dominant and recessive forms.

BIBLIOGRAPHY. Mohr OL: Woolly hair: A dominant mutant character in man. J Hered 23:467–473, 1985

Mortimer PS: Unruly hair. Br J Derm 113:467–473, 1985

Taylor AEM: Hereditary woolly hair with ocular involvement. Br J Dermatol 123:523–525, 1990

WORINGER-KOLOPP

Synonyms. Epidermotropic lymphoblastoma; pagetoid reticulosis. See also Alibert-Bazin.

Symptoms and Signs. Rare. Asymptomatic. Affects young adults. Isolated plaque on distal part of legs, slowly expanding.

Etiology. Unknown. Particular form of T-cell lymphoma (may be a variant of Alibert-Bazin).

Pathology. Acanthotic epidermis colonized by two populations of cells: small lymphocytes with surface membrane markers of suppressor cells or T-helper subsets (T4 + T8 +); second type larger and paler cells (related to histocytes, Langerhans cells or Merkel cells [?]). These cells show strong staining for lysozyme.

Diagnostic Procedures. *Biopsy.* Of skin.

Therapy. Surgical excision and low-dose radiotherapy.

Prognosis. Very slow local extension.

BIBLIOGRAPHY. Woringer F, Kolopp P: Lesion erythemato-squameuse polycyclique de l'avantbras evoluant depuis 6 ans chez un garconnet de 13 ans histologiquement infiltrant intraepidermique d'apparence tumorale. Ann Derm Syph 10:945, 1939

Denean JG, Wood GS, Becksverd J, et al: Woringer-Kolopp disease (pagetoid verticulosis): Four cases with histopathologic, ultrastructural and immunohistologic observations. Arch Derm 120:1045, 1984

MacKie RM: Lymphomas and leukemias. In Champion RH, Burton JL, Ebling FJG (eds): Rook/Wilkinson/Ebling Textbook of Dermatology, 5th ed, p 2130. Oxford, Blackwell Scientific, 1992

WORTH

Synonyms. Endosteal hyperostosis Worth; hyperostosis corticalis generalisata, benign-torus palatinus osteosclerosis, autosomal dominant; hyperostosis corticalis generalisata congenita. See van Buchem.

Symptoms. Both sexes. Usually asymptomatic. Onset in late childhood. Benign. Cough, seldom headaches and involvement of cranial (facial, optic, auditory) nerves.

Signs. *Face.* Prominent forehead, progressive enlargement of mandible; increase of gonial angle; widening of nasal root. Absence of exophthalmos, hypertelorism, nasal obstruction, increase of head circumference.

Etiology. Autosomal dominant.

Diagnostic Procedures. Thickened, but normal, mature lamellar bone.

Diagnostic Procedures. *Blood.* Increased alkaline phosphatase. *X-rays. CT scan. MRI.* Endo-osteal sclerosis of calvarium loss of diploe, osterosclerosis, and hyperosteosis of the mandible; endosteal sclerosis of long bones and pelvis.

Therapy. Symptomatic, Craniotomy.

Prognosis. Benign evolution in the majority of cases.

BIBLIOGRAPHY. Worth HM, Wollin DG: Hyperostosis corticalis generalisata congenita. J Canad Assoc Radiol 17:67–74, 1966

Perez-Vicente JA, Rodriguez De Castro E, Lafuente J, et al: Autosomal dominant endosteal hyperostosis: Report of a Spanish family with neurological involvement. Clin Genet 31:161–169, 1987

WRINKLY SKIN

WSS. See also Ehler-Danlos.

Symptoms. Onset from birth. Muscle hypotonia. Severe myalgia and decreasing visual acuity. Delayed growth.

Signs. Normal face. Body skin, including palms and soles, is markedly wrinkled and shows a decreased elasticity. Venous pattern over chest. Dwarfism; kyphosis; scapular winging. Mental retardation and microcephaly also reported as parts of the syndrome.

Etiology. Autosomal recessive inheritance.

Pathology. Absence of abnormality of elastic fibers and collagen of skin.

Therapy. Symptomatic.

Prognosis. Dwarfism. Mental retardation.

BIBLIOGRAPHY. McKusick VA: Heritable Disorders of Connective Tissue, 4th ed. St Louis, CV Mosby, 1972

Gazit E, Goodman RM, Bat-Miriam Katznelson M, et al: The wrinkly skin syndrome: A new heritable disorder of connective tissue. Clin Genet 4:186–192, 1973

Hurvitz SA, Baumgarten A, Goodman RM: The wrinkly skin syndrome: A report of case and review of the literature. Clin Genet 38:307–313, 1990

W-T*

Synonyms. Anemia hypoplastic, congenital anomalies, leukemia; pancytopenia, congenital anomalies. See Fanconi.

Symptoms and Signs. Both sexes. From birth. Variable congenital malformations: clinodactyly, elbow and hands anomalies. Severe anemia and/or pancytopenia that may initiate at various ages from infancy to adulthood, and that sometimes evolves into leukemia: monocytic, lymphocytic.

Etiology. Unknown. Autosomal dominant inheritance.

Diagnostic Procedures. *Bone marrow.* Refractory anemia, pancytopenic leukemia infiltration. *X-rays.* Variable bone and joint anomalies, especially upper limbs.

Therapy. Anemia refractory to all type of treatments.

---

*Initials of surnames of first two families described.

Prognosis. Leukemia cause of death at various ages.

BIBLIOGRAPHY. McDonald R, Goldschidt B: Pancytopenia with congenital defects (Fanconi anemia). Arch Dis Child 35:367–372, 1960
Gonzales CH, Durkin-Stamm MV, Geimer NK, et al: The W-T syndrome: A new autosomal dominant pleitropic trait of radial-ulnar hypoplasia with high risk of bone marrow failure and/or leukemia. Birth Defects Orig Art Ser XIII (3B):31–38, 1977
Smith ACM, Hays T, Harvey LA, et al: WT syndrome: A third family. Am J Hum Genet 41:A84, 1987

WUNDERLICH

Synonyms. Perirenal hematoma; perirenal apoplexy.

Symptoms and Signs. Both sexes affected. Onset at all ages. Usually secondary to direct trauma, causing contusion or compression of kidney, acting on the lumbar region or on the hypochondrium. Hematuria. Abdominal mass. Contraction makes the physical demonstration of the perirenal hematoma difficult, but in severe cases, inspection and palpation confirm the presence of the mass, which usually progressively enlarges to reach even the iliac fossa. In the following days wide lumbar zone discoloration; occasionally, the hematoma may emerge in the inguinoscrotal region. Shock is frequent.

Etiology. Trauma direct or (seldom) indirect or other lesions causing a perirenal hematoma.

Pathology. Simple ecchymosis: subcapsular hemorrhage, with parenchymal ecchymosis and capsula intact. Interstitial fracture: capsula intact and parenchymal lesions.

Diagnostic Procedures. *Blood.* Central venous pressure decreased. Anemia. Blood pressure. Hypotension. *Urine.* Hematuria. *CT scan.*

Therapy. Treatment and stabilization of patient; if persistent, hematuria and shock progressing in spite of treatment, surgical intervention.

Prognosis. Variable according to degree, speed of progression, and treatment.

BIBLIOGRAPHY. Wunderlich CA: Grundriss der speziellen Pathologie und Therapie. Stuttgart, Ebner Seubert, 1858
Baetan PN Jr, McAninich JW, Federlem P, et al: Computerized tomographic staging of renal trauma: 85 consecutive cases. J Urol 136:563–570, 1986

WYBURN-MASON

Synonym. Cerebroretinal arteriovenous aneurysm. See Bonnet-Dechance-Blanc, Klippel-Trenaunay-Weber, Sturge-Weber, and von Hippel-Lindau.

Symptoms. More frequently in males. Present from birth. Onset of symptons in third decade, gradual or sudden. Loss of vision in one eye; severe headache; vomiting; sudden proptosis. When hemorrhage of midbrain, neck rigidity, meningitis symptoms, loss of consciousness, tinnitus, deafness, aphasia, cerebellar signs may be present. In some patients, mental retardation, psychotic symptoms.

Signs. Multiple cutaneous facial nevi, vascular, occasionally pigmented, usually ipsilateral to affected eye and in area of distribution of trigeminal (V) nerve. Eye: papilledema; nystagmus; ptosis; fundus shows arteriovenous aneurysm between veins and arteries. Signs of increased intracranial pressure or brain hemorrhage according to location. Other congenital anomalies may be associated.

Etiology. Unknown. Possible autosomal dominant inheritance.

Pathology. Arteriovenous aneurysm of one or both sides of midbrain. Arteriovenous aneurysm or other types of congenital anomalies of retina. Vascular (pigmented or not) facial nevi.

Diagnostic Procedures. *X-ray.* Of skull. *Angiography. CT brain scan. MRI.*

Therapy. Symptomatic. Surgery occasionally indicated.

Prognosis. When hemorrhages occur in mid-brain, poor.

BIBLIOGRAPHY. Wyburn-Mason R: Arteriovenous aneurysm of midbrain and retina, facial naevi and mental changes. Brain 66:163–203, 1943
Burke EC, Winkelmann RK, Strickland MK: Disseminated hemangiomatosis: the newborn with central nervous system involvement. Am J Dis Child 108:418–424, 1964
Atherton DJ: Naevi and other developmental defects. In Champion RH, Burton JL, Ebling FJG (eds): Rook/Wilkinson/Ebling Textbook of Dermatology, 5th ed, p 493. Oxford, Blackwell Scientific, 1992

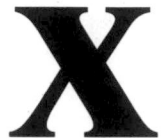

XANTHINURIA

Two types.

CLASSICAL XANTHINURIA

Synonym. Xanthine oxydase deficiency type I and II.

Symptoms and Signs. Rare. Prevalent in males. Some cases can be completely asymptomatic (20%). From birth to eighth decade; 50% children of ten years of age or less. Excretion of renal calculi. In 10%: myopathy, arthropathy, duodenal ulcers.

Etiology. Autosomal recessive inheritance. Isolated deficiency of xanthine oxydase (type I deficiency) or dual deficiency of xanthine dehydrogenase and related enzyme aldehyde oxydase (type II deficiency). Iatrogenic forms may be a result of treatment with xanthine dehydrogenase inhibitor allopurinol or aggressive treatment of malignancies, associated with massive uric acid production.

Diagnostic Procedures. *Blood.* Hypouricemia. *Urine.* Hypouricosuria; increased excretion of oxypurines (xanthine, hypoxanthine).

Pathology. Calculi. Xanthine.

Therapy. Alkali; light liquid intake.

Prognosis. From asymptomatic to renal failure owing to stone formation.

MOLIBDENUM, COFACTOR DEFICIENCY

Symptoms and Signs. Few cases described. Those of the classical form plus neurologic signs (intractable seizures from neonatal period).

Etiology. Autosomal recessive inheritance deficiency of all three enzymes: xanthine dehydrogenase, sulfite oxidase, and aldehyde oxidase, owing to congenital absence of a common molybdenum-containing cofactor essential for all three. Acquired (prolonged parenteral therapy with consequent molybdenum deficiency).

Therapy. Administration of molybdenum.

Prognosis. Poor in congenital cases.

BIBLIOGRAPHY. Dent CE, Philpot GR: Xanthinuria, an inborn error (or deviation) of metabolism. Lancet I:182–185, 1954

Fildes RD: Hereditary xanthinuria with severe urolythiasis occurring in infancy as renal tubular acidosis and hypercalciuria. J Pediat 115:277–280, 1989

Simmonds HA, Reiter S, Nishino T: Hereditary xanthinuria. In Scriver CR, Beaudet AL, Sly WS, et al: The Metabolic and Molecular Bases of Inherited Disease, 7th ed, pp 1781–1797. New York, McGraw-Hill, 1995

XANTHURENIC ACIDURIA

Synonym. Kynureninase deficiency. See Hunt (A.D.), Rundles-Falls, and Hartnup.

Symptoms and Signs. Both sexes affected. Present from infancy. Mental retardation; variable symptoms; mild stomatitis or cheilosis; high occurrence of urticaria, anemia, bronchial asthma, and diabetes in the families of affected probands.

Etiology. Autosomal recessive inheritance. Defect of kynureninase (a vitamin B_6 dependent enzyme) in tryptophan metabolism.

Diagnostic Procedures. *Urine.* Excessive excretion of xanthurenic acid, kynurenic acid, 3-hydroxy-kynurenine and kynurenine following tryptophan loading. Urinary abnormalities temporarily abolished by large dose of pyridoxine.

Therapy. Pyridoxine. Responsive and unresponsive forms are known.

Prognosis. Mental retardation. May reach adulthood.

BIBLIOGRAPHY. Knapp A: Ueber eine neue hereditäre, von Vitamin-B_6 abhängige Störung im Tryptophan-Stoffwechsel. Clin Chim Acta 5:6–13, 1960

Tada K, Yokoyama Y, Nakagawa H, et al: Vitamin B_6 dependent xanthurenic aciduria. Tohoku J Exp Med 93:115–124, 1967

Levy HL, Hartnup disorder: In Scriver CR, Beaudet AL, Sly WS, et al: The Metabolic and Molecular Bases of Inherited Disease, 7th ed, p 3633. New York, McGraw-Hill, 1995

XEROCYTOSIS

Synonym. Desiccosis. See Black Heel and Purpura traumatica.

Symptoms and Signs. Both sexes. After activities, based on impact of hands and feet on unyielding surface (marching, jogging, karate, free-style swimming): fatigue, pallor, jaundice, darkened urine.

Etiology. Membrane protein of red cell abnormality with increased permeability to cations and higher loss of K than Na. Autosomal dominant trait proposed.

Diagnostic Procedures. *Blood.* Increased mechanical fragility of red cells. Free hemoglobin in plasma; hyperbilirubinuria. *Urine.* Hematuria after exercise.

BIBLIOGRAPHY. Glader BE, Fortier N, Albala MM, et al: Congenital hemolytic anemia associated with dehydrated erythrocytes and increased potassium loss. N Engl J Med 191:491–496, 1974

Nolan GR: Hereditary xerocytosis: A case history and review of the literature. Pathology 16:151–154, 1984

XIPHOID PROCESS

Synonyms. Hypersensitive xiphoid; xiphoidadenia; xiphoidalgia.

Symptoms. Deep, slightly nauseating, dull pain in differing intensity from mild to agonizing in anterior chest; occasionally radiating to epigastrium, back, shoulders, arm, or precordium. Occurs also during night and interferes with sleep. Onset not instantaneous, lasting from minutes to days; recurrences for weeks or months, rarely for years. Precipitating causes: bending; stooping; lifting; head turning; eating large meal; walking.

Signs. Palpation of xiphoid process reproduces typical pain and associated manifestations (sine qua non sign for the diagnosis).

Etiology. Unknown. Xiphoidalgia may be present without association with other diseases or in concomitance with coronary artery, gallbladder, gastrointestinal diseases.

Pathology. Unknown. In cases in which the process was removed, perichondritis and periostitis have been described.

Diagnostic Procedures. All studies to rule out concomitant conditions. *ECG*. *X-ray*. Of gastrointestinal tract, cholecystography. According to other symptoms and signs of these diseases.

Therapy. Procaine infiltration of xiphoid area; ethyl chloride spray. If underlying disease, specific treatment. Psychological reassurance on benign nature of the process. Surgery in refractory cases.

Prognosis. Responds optimally to treatment (especially procaine infiltration). Untreated, lasts for months. Recurrences are common.

BIBLIOGRAPHY. Junghanns H: Der Schwertfortsatzschemerz (Xyphoideodinie). Zentralbl Chir 67:628–629, 1940
Lipkin M, Fulton LA, Wolfson EA: The syndrome of the hypersensitive xiphoid. N Engl J Med 253:591–597, 1955

X-LINKED HYPOGAMMAGLOBULINEMIA, GROWTH HORMONE DEFICIENCY

Synonyms. Hypogammaglobulinemia—X-linked-growth hormone deficiency.

Symptoms and Signs. From early infancy recurrent sinopulmonary infections, short stature, delayed puberty, and retarded bone growth.

Etiology. Congenital defect that apparently maps to the same region of the X chromosome as XLA.

Diagnostic Procedures. *Blood*. Reduction of all immunoglobulins; circulating B-cells are rare; failure to respond to immunologic stimulation with antibodies production; cellular immunity normal, growth hormone level reduced.

Therapy. Immunoglobulins and growth hormone administration.

BIBLIOGRAPHY. Fleisher TA, White RM, Broder S, et al: X-linked hypogammaglobulinemia and isolated growth hormone deficiency. N Engl J Med 302:1429–1434, 1980
Barrett DJ, Butler JL, Cooper MD: Antibody deficiency diseases. In Scriver CR, Beaudet AL, Sly WS, et al: The Metabolic and Molecular Bases of Inherited Disease, pp 3885–3887. New York, McGraw-Hill, 1995

XX, MALE

Synonyms. 46, XX.

Symptoms and Signs. Incidence 1 in 200,000 newborn males. Male phenotype, small testes and phallus, feminine distribution of pubic hair. Mentally from normal to feeble-minded. Reduced libido. Resembles Klinefelter (see) but smaller stature. Recognized in adult life because of hypogonadism, gynecomastia or infertility.

Etiology. Double XX (to be distinguished from XX true hermaphrodite). In 80% of XX, males with normal male genitalia one to the X chromosomes carries the testes-determining factor (TDF) designated also SRY (sex determining region of the Y).

Pathology. *Testes*. See Klinefelter. Absence of spermatogonia, hyalinization and partial or total obliteration of tubules containing only Sertoli cells and occasionally hyperplasia of the Leydig cells. No evidence of mullerian or ovarian duct tissue.

Diagnostic Procedures. *Blood*. High levels of FSH and LH and low testosterone. Chromosomal study: 46, XX.

Therapy. Emotional support. Testosterone supplementation. Treat eventual cryptorchidism.

Prognosis. Infertility. Good quoad vitam.

BIBLIOGRAPHY. De la Chapelle A: Nature and origin of males with XX sex chromosomes. Am J Hum Genet 24:71–105, 1972
Fetchner PY, Marcantonio SM, Jaswaney V, et al: The role of sex determining region Y gene in the etiology of 46, XX maleness. J Clin Endocrin Metab 76:690–695, 1993

XXXXY

Synonyms. Fraccaro.

Symptoms and Signs. Males affected. Present from birth. Variable pattern of features. Most common elements in over 50% of cases: at birth, low weight and stature; muscle hypotonia; joint laxity; mental retardation (average IQ 34). Characteristic facies. *Head*. Hypertelorism; upward slanted eyelids; inner epicanthic folds; strabismus; depressed nasal bridge; wide nose tip; prognathism; ear deformations. Short neck. *Extremities*. Short limited elbow pronation; clinodactyly; coxa vara and genu varum; pes planus. Abnormal dermal ridge count. *Genitalia*. Cryptorchidism, small testis. Possibly numerous other abnormalities. Congenital heart disease (20%).

Etiology. XXXXY aneuploidy.

Diagnostic Procedures. *Chromosome studies*. Three X-chromatin masses in all nuclei of buccal smear of subject with 49 chromosomes. *X-ray*. Retarded bone maturation; sclerotic cranial sutures; thick sternum; radioulnar synostosis; and other signs indicated in the preceding.

Therapy. Testosterone.

Prognosis. Dwarfism. Sterility. Lack of development of secondary sexual characteristics.

BIBLIOGRAPHY. Fraccaro M, Kaijser K, Lindsten J: A child with 49 chromosomes. Lancet II:724–726, 1960
Penrose LS: Finger-print pattern and sex chromosomes. Lancet I:298–300, 1967
Christensen MF, Therkelsen AJ: A case of the XXXXY chromosome anomaly with maternal X chromosomes and diabetic glucose tolerance. Acta Paediatr Scand 59:706–710, 1970
Thompson MW, McInnes RR, Willard HF: Genetics in Medicine, 5th ed. Philadelphia, WB Saunders, 1991

XYY

Synonym. YY; Klinefelter variant.

Symptoms. Onset in early childhood. Behavioral problems (tantrum; aggressivity); psychic dullness; weakness and poor coordination; later, psychosexual derangements.

Signs. At birth, occasionally increased length; in childhood, accelerated growth (at 5–6 years). Chest and shoulder, poor development. In adolescence, nodulocystic acne. Facial asymmetry; long ears; large teeth; long fingers.

Etiology. Chromosomal abnormality: XYY.

Diagnostic Procedures. *X-ray*. Of skeleton. Increased length; relatively reduced breadth; occasionally, synostosis. *EEG*. Occasionally, altered. *ECG*. Occasionally, prolonged P-R.

Therapy. Institutionalization for delinquency frequently required.

BIBLIOGRAPHY. Sanderberg AA, Koepf GF, Ishihara T, et al: XYY Human male. Lancet II:488–489, 1961
Harrison MJG, Tennent TG: Neurological anomalies in XYY males. Br J Psychiatry 120:447–448, 1972
Baghdassarian A, Bayard F, Digamber S, et al: Testicular function in XYY men. Johns Hopkins Med J 136:15–29, 1979
Thompson MW, McInnes RR, Willard HF: Genetics in Medicine, 5th ed. Philadelphia, WB Saunders, 1991

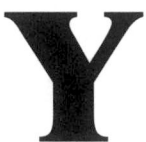

Y

YELLOW NAIL

Synonyms. Samman; bronchiectasis, lymphedema, yellow nails.

Symptoms and Signs. Onset at all ages. Usually becoming apparent late in life. Slow-growing nails of fingers and toes, usually remaining smooth. Cross-ridging and hump may be present, becoming progressively curved from side to side, with insufficient cuticles. Color change to pale yellow or slightly green with darker border; proximal part remains of normal color. Onycholysis of one or more fingernails may occur. Edema of the ankle usually becoming evident (occasionally years) after nail changes have been noticed. Facial edema or Nonne-Milroy-Meige syndrome in both legs may be observed. Thoracic signs related to presence of bronchiectasis and recurrent pleural effusion at later stage.

Etiology. Unknown. Associated occasionally with malignancy, nephrotic syndrome; hypothyroidism; immunodeficiency and D-penicillamine treatment.

Pathology. Hypoplasia or atresia of lymphatics. Dense fibrous tissue replaces subungueal stroma with ectatic vessels.

Diagnostic Procedures. Lymphangiography. Shows abnormalities.

Therapy. Symptomatic. Recurrent infections from bronchiectasis and pleural effusion may indicate surgical treatment.

Prognosis. According to associations. Nail lesions may disappear independently from treatment.

BIBLIOGRAPHY. Heller J: In Jadassohn: Handbuch der Haut-und Geschlechtskrankheiten XIII. Berlin, Springer, 1927
Samman PD, White WF: The "yellow nail" syndrome. Br J Derm 76:153–157, 1964
DeCoste SD, Imber MJ, Baden HP: Yellow nail syndrome. J Am Acad Dematol 22:608–611, 1990

YESUDIAN

Synonym. Ichthyosis, split hair, aminoaciduria. See Netherton and Tay.

Symptoms and Signs. Both sexes. From birth. Ichthyosis (lamellar) and split hairs. Mental retardation.

Etiology. Unknown. Autosomal recessive inheritance.

Diagnostic Procedures. *Blood. Urine.* Increase of arginine, alanine, lysine, serine, absence of proline and hydroxyproline.

BIBLIOGRAPHY. Yesudian P, Srinivas K: Ichthyosis with unusual hair shaft abnormalities in siblings. Br J Derm 96:199–203, 1977

YOUNG

Synonyms. Barry-Perkins-Young; azoospermia, obstructive; sinopulmonary infections; sinusitis, infertility.

Symptoms and Signs. History of bronchitis and chronic sinusitis from childhood; infertility (fertility block occasionally developed after puberty, since in some cases patient may have had children in the past).

Etiology. Autosomal recessive inheritance postulated.

Pathology. Sinusitis; bronchiectasis. Testis. Failure of the vasa efferentia to join together in the epidymis, inspissated material in the head of epididymis, lipid inclusion in the epithelial cells.

Diagnostic Procedures. *X-ray.* Of chest. *Bronchography. Sperm analysis.*

Therapy. Microsurgery of efferents may restore fertility.

BIBLIOGRAPHY. Young D: Surgical treatment of male infertility. J Reprod Fertil 23:541–542, 1970
Handelsman DJ, Conway AJ, Boylan LM, et al: Young's syndrome: Obstructive azoospermia in chronic sinopulmonary infections. N Engl J Med 310:3–9, 1984
Kahn MA, Noaah MS, Bashi SA, et al: Young's syndrome. Eur J Respir Dis 70:62–64, 1987
Hendry WF, Levison DA, Parkinson MC, et al: Testicular obstruction clinicopathological studies. Ann R Coll Surg Engl 72:396–407, 1990
Fraser RS, Paré JAP, Fraser RG, Paré PD: Synopsis of Diseases of the Chest, 2nd ed. Philadelphia, WB Saunders, 1994

YOUNG-PAXSON

Synonyms. Paxson; obstetric-gynecological crush.

Symptoms and Signs. Occurs following obstetric conditions: retroplacental hemorrhage; trauma of labor; rupture of uterus; observed also in twisted ovarian cyst with bloody extravasation. Tissue injury; shock, at times absent or minimal; urinary suppression progressing to anuria; hypertension; symptoms and signs of uremia.

Etiology. Extensive trauma and prolonged tissue ischemia (same as in Bywater).

Pathology. In kidney, pigmentary casts occluding tubules with degeneration of tubular epithelium.

Diagnostic Procedures. *Blood.* Hyperkalemia; hyperazotemia (peak at fifth to ninth day following injury). *Urine.* Hematuria; pigmentary and granular casts. *ECG.* Signs of hyperkalemia.

Therapy. Fluid balance and liquid diet with minimum protein and potassium, calcium intravenously, cation exchange enemas (to remove potassium). If transfusion indicated, removal of plasma to avoid administration of potassium; if acidosis, small amount of sodium bicarbonate. Hemodialysis often indicated. When diuresis starts, liberal amount of fluid and careful control of electrolyte balance.

Prognosis. Guarded. Less severe than in the past because of medical management and prevention of complications: infection, lung edema, cardiac insufficiency.

BIBLIOGRAPHY. Young J: Renal failure after utero-placental damage. Br Med J 2:715–718, 1942
Paxson NF, Golub LJ, Hunter RM: The crush syndrome in obstetrics and gynecology. JAMA 131:500–504, 1946

YUNIS-VARON

Synonym. Cleidocranial dysplasia; micrognathia; absent thumbs and distal aphalangia.

Symptoms and Signs. Very rare (seven cases from two families). From birth. *Head.* Macrocrania (diastasis of sutures); micrognathia; retracted and poorly delineated lips. *Limbs.* Absent thumbs and distal phalanges of fingers; hypoplasia of proximal phalanx of big toe. Absent clavicles; pelvic dysplasia; bilateral hip dislocation.

Etiology. Unknown. Autosomal recessive inheritance.

Diagnostic Procedures. *X-rays.* Micrognathia, hypoplasia facial bones, separated sutures, hypoplasia (up to agenesis) of clavicle, iliac bones, thumbs, other phalanges of hands and feet; cardiomegaly.

BIBLIOGRAPHY. Yunis E, Varon H: Cleidocranial dysostosis, severe micrognathism: Bilateral absence of thumbs and first metatarsal bone and distal aphalangia: A new genetic syndrome. Ann J Child 134:649–653, 1980

Partington MW: Cardiomyopathy added to the Yanis-Veron syndrome. Proc Greenwood Genet Ctr 7:224–225, 1988

Garrett C, Berry AC, Simpson RH, et al: Yunis-Varon syndrome with severe osteodysplasty. J Med Genet 27:114–121, 1990

Z

ZACKAY

BIBLIOGRAPHY. Zackai EH, Sly WS, McAlister WH: Microcephaly, mild mental retardation, short stature, and skeletal anomalies in siblings. Am Dis Child 124:111–115, 1972

ZAHN

Synonyms. Pseudoinfarct of liver. See also Liver peliosis. Eponym used to indicate a pseudoinfarct resulting from the occlusion of small branches of portal vein formed by dilatation of sinusoids and atrophy of neighboring lobules and hepatocytes, without necrotic component. They are seen after splenectomy. Usually asymptomatic.

BIBLIOGRAPHY. Zahn FW: Ueber die Folgen des Verschusses der Lungenarterien und Fortaderäste durch Embolie. Verh Ges Dtsch Natur Aerzt 2 (2 part):9–11, 1898

ZAHORSKY II

Synonyms. Mikulicz aphthae; von Mikulicz aphthae; angina herpetica, aphthosis; canker sores; herpes angina; MiRAS (minor recurrent stomatitis).

Symptoms. Both sexes equally affected before puberty; after, more prevalent in females. Onset from late childhood to third decade, increased incidence, then decreased. Small red macules in oral mucosa, seldom genital location, which rapidly break, leaving shallow painful ulcers.

Etiology. Unknown. Genetic basis, stress, trauma, food allergy etc. Various viruses and bacteria have been recurrently implicated.

Pathology. Early lymphocytic infiltration around lobules and ducts of salivary glands; no primary vascular changes.

Therapy. Topical tetracycline suspension and steroid applied every 2–3 hours; levamisole; metronidazole; chlorhexidine gel; topical tetracycline.

Prognosis. Extremely variable; lesions last 7–10 days; no scar. Recurrence more or less periodic.

BIBLIOGRAPHY. Zahorsky J: Herpangina. Arch Pediatr NY 41:181–184, 1924
Graykowski EA, Barile MF, Lee WB, et al: Recurrent aphthous stomatitis. Clinical, therapeutic, histopathologic, and hypersensitivity aspects. JAMA 196:637–644, 1966
Scully C: The oral cavity. In Champion RH, Burton JL, Ebling FJG (eds): Rook/Wilkinson/Ebling Textbook of Dermatology, 5th ed, pp 2710–2711. Oxford, Blackwell Scientific, 1992

ZAMBONI

Synonyms. Diesel fumes inhalation; pulmonary edema in ice hockey player; nitrogen dioxide in ice skating.

Symptoms and Signs. In ice skaters after 1.5 hours of skating, shortness of breath and cough with clear frothy sputum, tachycardia, tachypnea.

Etiology. Inhalation of oxides of nitrogen (produced by a Zamboni machine that is used to resurface the ice of rink).

Pathology. Noncardiogenic pulmonary edema.

Diagnostic Procedures. *X-ray.* Of chest. Bilateral perihilar infiltrates.

Therapy. Symptomatic.

Prognosis. Complete clearing of the findings in 2–3 days.

BIBLIOGRAPHY. Roger RB, Morgan WKC: Diesel fumes potential health effects, fact and fiction. J Occup Health Safety Aust NZ 6:525–531, 1990
Soparcar Mayers I, Edouard L, et al: Toxic effects from nitrogen dioxide in ice-skating. Can Med Ass J 148:1181–1182, 1993
Morgan WKC: "Zamboni" disease. Arch Int Med 155:2479–2480, 1995

ZANGE-KINDLER

Synonym. Cisternal block. Eponym used to indicate a block of spinal fluid circulation at the level of the cisterna magna, caused by any space-occupying lesion of posterior cranial fossa with the classic symptoms of increased intracranial tension: nausea; vomiting; cephalalgia; choked disks; stupor and mental clouding.

BIBLIOGRAPHY. Zange J: Ueber Subarchnoidealblock, insbesondere den der Cisterna cerebellomedullaris ("Zisternenblock") (Entstehungsbedingungen des letzteren, klinische Feststel lung und liquor-diagnostische Bedeutung, namentlich bei entzuendlichen Erkrankungen im Schaedel). Munch Med Wchnschr 73:1150–1152, 1926
Kindler W: Vorteile und Gefahren des diagnostischen Zinternenstiches. Wien Klin Wchnschr 41:632–634, 1928
Vick NA: Grinker's Neurology, 7th ed. Springfield, IL, Charles C Thomas, 1976

ZANOLI-VECCHI

Synonyms. Convulsive post-spinal-operative; postoperative spinal hemorrhage. See Spinal cord injury—progressive confusional. Spinal shock.

Symptoms and Signs. Occurs after surgical intervention on the spine. Convulsion; loss of consciousness; apnea.

Etiology. Spinal hemorrhage and siphoning of blood into cerebral ventricles.

Therapy. Diazepam for the control of convulsions; intensive care; tracheal intubation and respiratory assistance. Treatment of circulatory shock with fluids, atropine, and dopamine.

BIBLIOGRAPHY. Zanoli R, Vecchi B: Syndrome convulsiva postoperatoria da emorachide. Gaz Sanit 27:421–423, 1956

ZAPPERT

Synonyms. Cerebellar acute ataxia in children; hypertonic-dyskinetic infantile cerebral ataxia.

Symptoms and Signs. Onset at age 1–12 years. Symptoms developing in healthy children or following infections (e.g., measles, chickenpox, scarlet fever). Ataxia of station and gait; intentional tremor; slurred speech; vomiting, convulsion; unconsciousness; delirium; nystagmus.

Etiology. Unknown. Hypoxia and hypoglycemia (?). Hyperthermia most frequent cause; hypothermia usually better tolerated.

Pathology. Unknown. Loss of some of Purkinje cells, swelling pyknosis, if survive longer complete degeneration of Purkinje cells and gliosis and degeneration of the dental nuclei.

Diagnostic Procedures. *CSF.* Normal or pleocytosis and increased protein. *CT brain scan. MRI.* Diffuse atrophy of various degrees. *EEG.* Normal or diffuse activity.

Therapy. Symptomatic.

Prognosis. Variable, from death to recovery usually in 3–6 weeks, rarely exceeding 3 months. In some cases, residual mental deficiency.

BIBLIOGRAPHY. Zappert J: Ueber den acuten zerebralen Tremor im frühen Kindesalter. Monatsschur Kinderh 8:133–149, 1909

Goldwyn A, Waldman AM: Acute cerebellar ataxia in children: A report of three cases. J Pediatr 42:75–79, 1953

Adams RD, Victor M: Principles of Neurology, 5th ed, pp 829–830. New York, McGraw-Hill, 1993

ZAR

Synonyms. Spirit possession.

Symptoms and Signs. In Asia and North Africa, and Middle East. Dissociative episodes including singing, weeping, laughing, shouting, hitting the head against wall; apathy, anorexia, refuse to work, or openly establishing relationship with a possessing spirit.

Etiology. Psychotic disorder culture bound. Not considered pathological behavior locally.

BIBLIOGRAPHY. Lin K-M: Cultural influences on the diagnosis of psychotic and organic disorders: In Mezzich JE, Kleinman A, Fabrega H, et al: Culture and Psychiatric Diagnosis. Washington, American Psychiatry Press, 1995

Kaplan HI, Sadock BJ: Comprehensive Textbook of Psychiatry, 6th ed. Baltimore, Williams & Wilkins, 1995

ZEEK

Synonym. Hypersensitivity angiitis. See Kussmaul-Maier.

Symptoms and Signs. Male to female ratio, 1.3:1. Respiratory disease in previous year (56%); drug reaction in previous year (38%); middle ear infection (31%); hypertension (25%). Except for the variation in frequency previously mentioned, all symptoms and signs overlap with Kussmaul-Maier syndrome (see).

Etiology. Hypersensitivity arteritis. See Kussmaul-Maier. The Zeek variety of polyarteritis has been differentiated on the basis of anatomopathologic findings (see) and the frequent pulmonary involvement.

Pathology. The main features differentiating Zeek from Kussmaul-Maier syndrome are the lack of involvement of large muscular arteries and no predilection for sites of bifurcation. Presence of vasculitis of pulmonary arteries; frequent splenic hilar vasculitis and splenic follicular arteriolitis; interstitial inflammation; focal necrosis; extravascular granulomas.

Diagnostic Procedures. Same as Kussmaul-Maier. *Blood.* More prominent eosinophilia.

Therapy. See Kussmaul-Maier.

Prognosis. Slightly better than in Kussmaul-Maier.

BIBLIOGRAPHY. Zeek PM, Smith CC, Weeter JC: Studies on periarteritis

nodosa; differentiation between vascular lesions of periarteritis nodosa and of hypersensitivity. Am J Pathol 24:889–917, 1948

Moskowitz RW, Baggenstoss AH, Slocumb CH: Histopathologic classification of periarteritis nodosa: A study of 56 cases confirmed at necropsy. Proc Staff Meet Mayo Clin 38:345–357, 1963

Winkelmann RK, Ditto WB: Cutaneous and visceral syndromes of necrotizing or "allergic" angiitis: A study of 38 cases. Medicine 43:59–89, 1964

Ryan TJ: Cutaneous vasculitis. In Rook/Wilkinson/Ebling Textbook of Dermatology, pp 1920–1921. London, Blackwell Scientific, 1992

ZELLWEGER

Synonyms. Cerebrohepatorenal; hepatocerebrorenal; renohepatocerebral; CHR. See Adrenoleukodystrophy, autosomal neonatal.

Symptoms. Onset in fetal life; prevalent in females. Feeble fetal activity. After birth (breech presentation prevalent), marked generalized hypotonia (poor or absent Moro reflex). Respiratory problems. Failure to thrive; vomiting; mental retardation; variable seizures.

Signs. Several combinations of the following features: low birth weight; jaundice; short stature; moderate muscle hypotonicity or (rarely) hypertonicity. Typical face: high forehead, upslanting palpebral fissures, hypoplastic supraorbital ridges, epicanthal folds. Eye abnormalities: cataracts, glaucoma corneal clouding, Brushfield spots, pigmentary retinopathy, optic nerve dysplasia, hypertelorism. Broad nose; upturned nares; micrognathia; arched palate; posterior palatal cleft; abnormal ears; hypospadias; cryptorchidism. Hands with horizontal upper palmar creases; short fingers and toes; camptodactyly; syndactyly. Limited extension of knee; equinovarism. Hepatomegaly. Occasionally, heart signs consistent with septal defect or patent ductus arteriosus.

Etiology. Autosomal recessive inheritance. Absence of perioxisomes in the liver and reduction in all other organs, that determine: defective synthesis of plasmalogens, increased tissue levels of VLCFA (very long chain fatty acids) and medium and long chain, dicarboxylic aciduria (modest), age-related tissue accumulation of phytanic acid, accumulation of bile acid metabolites (THCA) and (DHCA), and accumulation of pipecolic acid.

Pathology. *Brain.* Small; macrogyria and polymicrogyria; sudanophilic leukodystrophy. Neuropathologic studies have revealed disturbed neuronal migration resulting in a malformed cerebral cortical plate. *Liver.* Variable unspecific findings; in some cases, cirrhosis; intrahepatic biliary dysgenesis. Absence of perioxisomes. *Kidneys.* Cortical cysts. Extramedullary hematopoiesis. Tissue iron increased. Congenital heart disease may be associated. *Eye.* Multiple abnormalities of optic nerve. *Adrenals.* Pattern similar to adrenoleucodystrophy (see). *Cartilage.* Calcific stippling of patella.

Diagnostic Procedures. *Blood.* Hyperbilirubinemia; hypoprothrombinemia; hypoproteinemia; elevated serum iron and iron-binding capacity. Hyperpipecolic acid. Screening for the presence of coprostanic acids and the C29 dicarboxylic bile acid in serum or urine is a reliable method for detection of syndrome and confirmation of diagnosis. *Electromyography.* Normal. *Chromosome studies.* Normal. *Nerve conduction velocity.* Normal. *X-ray.* See Signs; pattern of chrondrodystrophia calcificans characterized by multiple punctate calcifications in the epiphyses. *Isotope scan* (of kidney) and pyelography.

Therapy. Symptomatic.

Prognosis. Almost never achieve psychomotor development. Death within few weeks or months of life, often owing to hemorrhages.

BIBLIOGRAPHY. Bowen P, Lee CSN, Zellweger H, et al: A familial syndrome of multiple congenital defects. Bull Johns Hopkins Hosp 114:402–414, 1964

Wanfers RJA, van Roermund CWT, Schutgens RBH, et al: The inborn errors of peroxisomal beta-oxidation: A review. J Inherit Metab Dis 13:4–36, 1990

Shimozawa N, Tsukamoto T, Suzuki Y, et al: A human gene responsible for Zellweger syndrome that affects peroxisome assembly. Science 255:1132–1134, 1992

Garner A: Metabolic disorders involving metals. In Garner A, Klintworth GK (eds): Pathobiology of Ocular Disease: A Dynamic Approach, 2nd ed, pp 1141–1142. New York, Marcel Dekker, 1994

Weatherall DJ, Ledingham JGG, Warrell DA (eds): Oxford Textbook of Medicine, 3rd ed, pp 1442–1443. Oxford, Oxford Med Pub, 1996

ZENKER

Synonyms. Hypopharyngeal diverticulum; included Killian-Jamieson diverticulum (lateral protrusion of pharyngeal mucosa).

Symptoms and Signs. In sixth to seventh decade, often asymptomatic. Food ingested several hours previously may be regurgitated without dysphagia. Annoying bubbling sensation in the back of throat. Excessive salivation, drooling, choking on food or saliva. Hoarseness. Special maneuvers may empty the diverticulum.

Etiology. Protrusion of pharyngeal mucosa between fibers of inferior constrictor muscle of the pharynx and transverse fibers of cricopharyngeal muscle.

Pathology. Pharyngeal mucosa diverticulum of different sizes containing food.

Diagnostic Procedures. *X-ray.* With Valsalva manouver. *Endoscopy.* Very dangerous. *Manometry. Ultrasonography. CT scan.*

Therapy. Dietary advice: easily swallowable foods. Surgery when diverticulum becomes troublesome (crycopharyngeal myotomy).

Prognosis. Good with therapy.

BIBLIOGRAPHY. Ludlow A: A case of obstructed deglutition from a preternatural dilatation and bag formed in the pharynx: Medical observations and inquiries by a Society of Physicians in London, 2nd ed, p 85, 1769

Van Overbeek JJM: The Hypopharyngeal Diverticulum. Amsterdam, Van Goruum Assen, 1977

Lindgren S, Ekberg O: Crycopharyngeal myotomy in the treatment of dysphagia. Clin Otol Laryngol 15:221–227, 1990

Haubrich WS, Schaffner F, Berk JE (eds): Bockus Gastroenterology, 5th ed, pp 524–527. Philadelphia, WB Saunders, 1995

ZIEGLER

Synonyms. Cachectic endocarditis; nonbacterial thrombotic endocarditis; NBTE; indeterminate endocarditis; marantic endocarditis.

Symptoms. Both sexes affected. Age range 18–90 years. Usually occurs in patients with prolonged disease or cachexia, but observed also in early stage of many other diseases. Symptoms owing to peripheral arterial embolization. Fever may be present.

Signs. Usually systolic murmur (33%).

Etiology. Unknown. Associated with malignancy or other acute or chronic disease, even psychosis. Attempted correlation also with disseminated intravascular coagulation.

Pathology. Five types of lesions described: small single node along edge of closure of valve; large nonverrucous node on valve; small multiverrucous friable lesions on valve edge; (embolizing); fibrous tab, result of collagen degeneration on valve edge (nidus for thrombus).

BIBLIOGRAPHY. Lebman E: Characterization of various forms of endocarditis. JAMA 80:813, 1923

Gross L, Friedberg C: Nonbacterial thrombotic endocarditis. AMA Arch Intern Med 58:620–640, 1936

Durack DT: Infective and non infective endocarditis. In Schlant RC, Alexander RW: Hurst's The Heart, 8th ed, p 1688. New York, McGraw-Hill, 1994

ZIEHEN-OPPENHEIM

Synonyms. Schwalbe-Ziehen-Oppenheimer; dystonia lenticularis; dystonia musculorum deformans; torsion dystonia; torsion spasm; see Paraspasm, bilateral and Spasmodic torticollis, which may be considered localized forms of this syndrome. Includes Dystonia idiopathic (see OXPHOS syndromes).

Symptoms. Onset 5–15 years of age, frequently in Semitic peoples. Usually unilateral; gradual onset. Foot becomes flexed, inverted, or adducted; abnormal movements spread to entire leg and then spread to other one, and finally to whole musculature, particularly of trunk and neck. During sleep the patient relaxes; while awake, continuously turns and twists.

Signs. Reflexes difficult to elicit or exaggerated. Babinski sign absent.

Etiology. Unknown or symptomatic of infections or vascular, toxic, neoplastic lesions of extrapyramidal system. The autosomal dominant variety (not ethnic background) onset at later age and slower and more benign course. Hereditary autosomal recessive and autosomal dominant. (This variety correlated with elevation of serum dopamine-beta-hydroxylase.)

Pathology. Degenerative changes of putamen, caudate nuclei, and other extrapyramidal centers. In symptomatic lesion, according to etiology.

Diagnostic Procedures. Establishment of idiopathic or secondary type. *CSF. Blood. X-ray.* Of skull. *Arteriography. CT scan. MRI.*

Therapy. Disappointing. Early in the course beneficial: L-dopa and belladonna groups of drugs; bromocriptine. Diazepam; chlorpromazine; haloperidol; carbomazepine. Various neurosurgical procedures: root sections; spinal cord operations; thalamus lesions. Attempts to utilize biofeedback mechanisms.

Prognosis. Progressing to confinement in bed.

BIBLIOGRAPHY. Schwalbe MW: Eine eigentuemliche tonische Krampffor mit histerischen Symptomen. Berlin, G Schade, 1908

Ziehen GT:Ein Fall von toniher Torsionsneurose Demonstrationen im Psychiatrischen Verein zu Berlin. Zentralbl Nervenkr 30:109–110, 1911

Oppenheim H: Ueber eine eigenartige Krampfkrankheit des kindlichen und jugendlichen Alters. (Dysbasia lordotica progressiva, Dystonia musculorum deformans). Zentralbl Nervenkr 30:1090–1109, 1911

Thomalla C: Ein Fall von Torsionsspasmus mit Sektionsbefund und seine Beziehungen zur Athétose doppel Wilsoncheni Krankheit und Pseudosklerose. Z Ges Neurol Psychiatr 41:311–343, 1918

Fletcher NA: The genetics of idiopathic torsion dystonia. J Med Genet 27:409–412, 1990

Adams RD, Victor M: Principles of Neurology, 5th ed, pp 984–985. New York, McGraw-Hill, 1993

ZIEVE

Synonyms. Alcoholic hyperlipemia; hemolytic anemia-hyperlipemic alcoholic; hepatopancreatic alcoholic; transitory alcoholic hyperlipemia.

Symptoms. Prevalent in middle-aged male patients. History of recent alcohol intake; onset insidious; weakness; fatigability; anorexia; nausea; vomiting and pain (dull cramps) in upper part of abdomen; varying in intensity, changing location. More frequent on right side than left. The acute pain lasts from minutes to hours and never subsides completely.

Signs. Moderate hepatomegaly; occasionally, mild splenomegaly. Weight loss; jaundice.

Etiology. Alcoholic intake with specific liver and pancreas damage. It has not been shown that all the features of the syndrome are causally interrelated.

Pathology. *Liver.* Minimal to moderate cirrhotic findings, and fatty infiltration. *Pancreas.* Cellular and obstructive type of pancreatitis.

Diagnostic Procedures. *Blood.* Anemia hemolytic type (shorter survival time; increased reticulocytes; increased bilirubin). Hyperlipemia: milky, cloudy plasma; hypercholesterolemia; hyperphospholipemia; increase of neutral fat and fatty acids; hyperuricemia; amylase normal; white blood cells usually increased. Platelets usually increased. *Bone marrow.* Marked normoblastic hyperplasia; presence of large phagocytic histiocytes with lipid granules. *Biopsy.* Of liver.

Therapy. Abstinence from alcohol; adequate diet.

Prognosis. Spontaneous remission of hemolytic anemia, hyperlipemia, jaundice, and pains with abstinence from alcohol occurs within 4–6 weeks.

BIBLIOGRAPHY. Zieve L: Jaundice, hyperlipemia and hemolytic anemia: a heretofore unrecognized syndrome associated with alcoholic fatty liver and cirrhosis. Ann Intern Med 48:471–496, 1958

Balcerzak SP, Westerman MP, Heinle EW: Mechanism of anemia in Zieve's syndrome. Am J Med Sci 255:277–287, 1968

Criqui MH, Cowan LD, Tyroler HA, et al: Lipoproteins as mediators for the effect of alcohol consumption and cigarette smoking on cardiovascular mortality. Am Epiodemiol 126–129, 1987

Weatherall DJ, Ledingham JGG, Warrell DA (eds): Oxford Textbook of Medicine, 3rd ed, p 2082. Oxford, Oxford Med Pub, 1996

ZINSSER-COLE-ENGMAN

Synonyms. Cole; Cole-Rauschkalb-Toomey; Engman; dyskeratosis congenita. See Fanconi anemia.

Symptoms. Almost exclusively in males. Onset at 5–13 years. Dysonychia with shedding, complete destruction; repeated suppurative paronychia. Later development of reticulate grayish pigmentation, mostly on neck and thighs but also involving entire trunk. Atrophy and telangiectases. Face red, atrophic; maculated skin. Macules on back of hands and feet. Palmar and sole keratosis; hyperhidrosis; bullae. Mucosal lesions: oral; small erosions evolving to leukoplakia; on conjunctiva similar lesions; excessive lacrimation. Defect of teeth. Hypotrichia-cicatricial alopecia. Physical and mental development may be retarded. In the majority of cases testicular atrophy.

Etiology. Unknown. Sex-linked recessive inheritance.

Pathology. Skin changes not specific; parakeratosis; hyperkeratosis; acanthosis. Gastrointestinal tract mucosa may show same lesions as the oral.

Diagnostic Procedures. *Blood.* (In some cases) anemia or pancytopenia; Fanconi type (see Fanconi).

Therapy. Etretinate. Bone marrow transplantation for pancytopenia.

Prognosis. Malignant transformation in areas of leukoplakia, occasionally also from atrophic zone. Death from carcinoma at 30–50 years of age. In *forme fruste* (only dysonychia and pigmentation), normal life expectancy.

BIBLIOGRAPHY. Zinsser F: Atrophia cutis reticularis cum pigmentatione, dystrophia unguium et leukoplakia oris (poikilodermia atrophicans vascularis Jacobi). Ikonogr Derm (Kyoto), fas 5 219–223, 1906

Engman MF: A unique case of reticular pigmentation of the skin with atrophy. Arch Derm Syph Suppl 13:685–687 1926

Cole HN, Rauschkolb JE, Toomey J: Dyskeratosis congenita with pigmentation, dystrophia unguis and leukokeratosis oris. Arch Derm Syph 21:71–95, 1930

Garb J: Dyskeratosis congenita with hypoplastic anemia: A stem cell defect. Am J Hemat 20:85–87, 1985

Davidson HR, Connor JM: Dyskeratosis congenita. J Med Genet 25:843–846, 1988

Harper J: Genetics and genodermatoses. In Champion RH, Burton JL, Ebling FJG (eds): Rook/Wilkinson/Ebling Textbook of Dermatology, 5th ed, pp 354–357. Oxford, Blackwell Scientific, 1992

ZIPRKOWSKI-ADAM

Synonyms. Deafness-Albinism recessive; albinism-deafness recessive.

Symptoms and Signs. Congenital deafness. Total albinism.

Etiology. Autosomal recessive inheritance.

BIBLIOGRAPHY. Ziprkowski L, Adam A: Recessive total albinism and congenital deaf mutism. Arch Dermatol 89:151–155, 1964

ZIPRKOWSKI-MARGOLIS

Synonyms. Margolis; Woolf (considered different form from some Authors); Reed; albinism-deaf-mutism (sex-linked); albinism-deafness, sex-linked; ADFN; ALDS.

Symptoms and Signs. Only males. Those of oculocutaneous albinism; piebaldism is possible. Sensorineural deafness from birth.

Etiology. Sex-linked inheritance. Locus has been mapped to Xq probably in the region Xq13-q26.

BIBLIOGRAPHY. Ziprkowski LA, Krakowski A, Adam A, et al: Partial albinism and deaf mutism due to a recessive sex-linked gene. Arch Derm 86:530–539, 1962

Margolis E: A new hereditary syndrome: Sex-linked deaf-mutism associated with total albinism. Acta Genet (Basel) 12:12–19, 1962

Woolf CM, Dolowitz DA, Aldous HE: Congenital deafness associated with piebaldism. Arch Otolaryngol 82:244–250, 1965

Reed WB, Stone VM, Boder E, et al: Pigmentary disorders in association with congenital deafness. Arch Derm 95:176–186, 1967

Shiloh Y, Litvak G, Ziv Y, et al: Genetic mapping of X-linked albinism—deafness syndrome (ADFN) to Xq26.3-q27.1. Am J Hum Genet 47:20–27, 1990

ZOLLINGER-ELLISON

Synonyms. Z-E; Strøm-Zollinger-Ellison; gastrinoma; multiple partial adenomatosis; multiple partial endocrine adenomatosis; pancreatic ulcerogenic tumor; polyglandular adenomatosis. See Wermer.

Symptoms. Males affected slightly more frequently than females. Peak of onset third to fifth decades (10% in first two decades of life). Peptic ulcer pain (in 90% of cases), severe, refractory to usual medical or surgical measures (short of total gastrectomy); hematemesis or melena (45%); vomiting (25%); diarrhea (36%); abdominal pain (50%). Pancreatic tumor seldom produces local symptoms.

Signs. Dehydration (60%).

Etiology. Islet cell adenoma of pancreas secreting a gastrin-like material. Usually malignant, metastasizing tumor; in 10% of cases syndrome determined by simple diffuse islet cell hyperplasia; autosomal dominant inheritance.

Pathology. Malignant or benign tumor of islet cells of pancreas (difficult to differentiate microscopically) but distinguished by the presence of invasion and metastasis, or simple diffuse hyperplasia of islet cells. In many patients primary tumor located in stomach or duodenum, classified as nonbeta cell tumor. Stomach: hypersecretion; multiple stomach and duodenal or proximal jejunal ulcers.

Diagnostic Procedures. *Gastric aspiration.* Massive hypersecretion of acid gastric juice. *Stool.* Diarrhea with steatorrhea frequently observed. Relieved by gastric aspiration. *X-ray. CT scan. MRI.* Multiple ulcers or abnormally located ulcers; marked hypertrophy of gastric folds; duodenal ileus; small bowel pattern; rapid barium transit through small bowel and to localize the tumor and metastasis. *CT brain scan* (positive 20% of cases), cerebral angiography (positive 20% of cases). Percutaneous transhepatic portal-venous sampling with gastrin measured in blood samples (not considered any longer useful).

Therapy. Medical. H2-receptor blockers, cimetidine or ranitidine, acid inhibition of parietal cells (measures highly effective 90% of cases). Surgery not routinely recommended (as in the recent past), but (except in case with precise localization) limited to surgical exploration. Total gastrectomy recommended for patients who do not respond to medical treatment.

Prognosis. According to size, localization, and metastasis of tumor, association with other tumors (MEN-I, see). Removal of tumors: cure of hypersecretion and ulcers.

BIBLIOGRAPHY. Strøm R: A case of peptic ulcer and insulinoma. Acta Chir Scand 104:252–260, 1952–1953

Zollinger RM, Ellison EH: Primary peptic ulcerations of the jejunum associated with islet cell tumors of the pancreas. Ann Surg 142:709–728, 1955

Ellison EH, Wilson SD: The Zollinger-Ellison syndrome updated. Surg Clin N Am 47:1115–1124, 1967

Zollinger RM, Ellison EL, O'Dorisio TM, et al: Thirty years experience with gastrinoma. World J Surg 8:552–560, 1984

Wilding JPH, Ghatei MA, Bloom SR: Hormones of the gastrointestinal tract. In De Groot LJ (ed): Endocrinology, 3rd ed, pp 2884–2885. Philadelphia, WB Saunders, 1995

ZONDEK-BROMBERG-ROZIN

Synonym. Pituitary (anterior) hyperhormonotrophic.

Symptoms. Occurs in female patients 20–30 years old; not seen in nulliparae. Prolonged, abundant uterine bleeding; anemia; galactorrhea; thyroidotoxic manifestation (tachycardia, perspiration, diarrhea); nervous symptoms; weight loss; secondary sterility.

Signs. Pallor; emaciation; enlargement of thyroid with signs of thyrotoxicosis (exophthalmos). *Breast.* Areolar hyperpigmentation with flaccid breast. *Uterus.* Enlargement; palpable cystic ovaries.

Etiology and Pathology. Overproduction of estrogenic, thyrotropic, lactotrophic hormones owing to hyperplasia of the hypophysis or to hypothalamic pathology (?).

Diagnostic Procedures. *Blood.* Anemia; hypoglycemia with occasionally flat curve in glucose tolerance test. *Urine.* Increased urinary estrogens and no increase in gonadotropin (FSH); hyperestrogenic. *Vaginal smear. Hysterosalpingography.* Normal. *Milk.* Does not coagulate on boiling. *Basal metabolic rate.* Increased. *X-ray of skull.* Normal with no alteration of sella.

Therapy. X-ray or ablation of hypophysis seems to be indicated for the treatment of this rare syndrome.

BIBLIOGRAPHY. Zondek B, Bromberg YM, Rozin S: Anterior pituitary hyperhormonotrophic syndrome (excessive uterine bleeding, galactorrhea, hyperthyroidism). J Obstet Gynaecol B Emp 58:525–537, 1951

Dowling JT, Richards JB, Freinkel N, et al: Nonpuerperal galactorrhea. Arch Intern Med 107:885–893, 1961

Christy MP, Warren MP: Disease syndromes of the hypothalamus and anterior pituitary. In De Groot LJ, Cahill FG Jr, Odell WD, et al (eds): Endocrinology, p 237. New York, Grune & Stratton, 1979

ZOON

Synonyms. Plasma cell balanitis; pseudo-erythroplasmic balanitis.

Symptoms and Signs. Occurs in middle-aged and old men. Indolent plaques on glans and prepuce with shiny, moist skin, stippling of skin, "cayenne pepper" on the surface.

Etiology. Unknown. Possibly, aspecific chronic balanitis.

Pathology. Plasma cell infiltration and deposit of hemosiderin.

Therapy. Topical cortisone ointment; gentamycin ointment. Circumcision permanent cure.

Prognosis. Chronic benign condition that temporarily disappears with application of steroids.

BIBLIOGRAPHY. Zoon JJ: Balantis circumscripta chronica met plasmacellen-infiltrant. Ned Tijdsch Geneesk 94:1529–1530, 1950

Ive FA: The umbilical perianal and genital regions. In Champion RH, Burton JL, Ebling FJG (eds): Rook/Wilkinson/Ebling Textbook of Dermatology, 5th ed, pp 2812–2813. Oxford, Blackwell Scientific, 1992

Weatherall DJ, Ledingham JGG, Warrell DA (eds): Oxford Textbook of Medicine, 3rd ed, p 3768. Oxford, Oxford Med Pub, 1996

ZUELZER-OGDEN

Obsolete. The term refers to megaloblastic anemia with a superimposed infection and deficiency of vitamin C, observed in children.

BIBLIOGRAPHY. Zuelzer WW, Ogden FN: Megaloblastic anemia in infancy. Am J Dis Child 71:211–243, 1946

ZUNICH

Synonyms. Neuroectodermal Zunich; ichthyosiform dermatosis Zunich.

Symptoms. Both sexes. Early onset. Ichthyosiform migratory dermatosis; visual impairment, deafness (conductive type). Seizures, mental retardation.

Signs. Bilateral ocular coloboma. Cleft palate. Heart congenital malformation (Fallot great vessel transposition).

Etiology. Autosomal recessive inheritance.

BIBLIOGRAPHY. Zunich J, Kaye CI: New syndrome of congenital ichthyosis with neurologic abnormalities. Am J Med Genet 15:331–333, 1983

Zunich J, Esterly NB, Kaye CI: Autosomal recessive transmission of neuroectodermal syndrome. Arch Dermatol 124:1188–1189, 1988

Index

A

B

C

D

E

F

G

H

J

L

M

N

P

Q

R

S

W